COMMUNITY NURSING DEFINITIONS

Community-Oriented Nursing Practice is a philosophy of nursing service delivery that involves the generalist or specialist public health and community health nurse providing "health care" through community diagnosis and investigation of major health and environmental problems, health surveillance, and monitoring and evaluation of community and population health status for the purposes of preventing disease and disability and promoting, protecting, and maintaining "health" in order to create conditions in which people can be healthy.

Public Health Nursing Practice is the synthesis of nursing theory and public health theory applied to promoting and preserving health of populations. The focus of practice is the community as a whole and the effect of the community's health status (resources) on the health of individuals, families, and groups. Care is provided within the context of preventing disease and disability and promoting and protecting the health of the community as a whole. Public Health Nursing is population focused, which means that the population is the center of interest for the public health nurse. *Community Health Nurse* is a term that is used interchangeably with *Public Health Nurse.*

Community-Based Nursing Practice is a setting-specific practice whereby care is provided for "sick" individuals and families where they live, work, and go to school. The emphasis of practice is acute and chronic care and the provision of comprehensive, coordinated, and continuous services. Nurses who deliver community-based care are generalists or specialists in maternal-infant, pediatric, adult, or psychiatric-mental health nursing.

SELECT EXAMPLES OF SIMILARITIES AND DIFFERENCES BETWEEN COMMUNITY-ORIENTED AND COMMUNITY-BASED NURSING

	COMMUNITY-ORIENTED NURSING		COMMUNITY-BASED NURSING
	PUBLIC HEALTH NURSING—POPULATION FOCUSED/POPULATION CENTERED		
Philosophy	PRIMARY focus is on "health care" of communities and populations	SECONDARY focus is on "health care" of individuals, families, and groups in community to unserved clients by health care system	Focus is on "illness care" of individuals and families across the life span
Goal	Prevent disease; preserve, protect, promote, or maintain health	Prevent disease; preserve, protect, promote, or maintain health	Manage acute or chronic conditions
Service context	Community and population health care "the greatest good for the greatest number"	Personal health care to unserved clients	Family-centered illness care
Community type	Varied: local, state, nation, world community	Varied, usually local community	Human ecological
Client characteristics	• Nation • State • Community • Populations at risk • Aggregates • Healthy • Culturally diverse • Autonomous • Able to define problem • Client primary decision maker	Individuals/families at risk—if unserved by health care system • Usually healthy • Culturally diverse • Autonomous • Able to define own problem • Client primary decision maker	• Individuals • Families • Usually ill • Culturally diverse • Autonomous • Client able to define own problem • Client involved in decision making
Practice setting	• Community • Organization • Government • Community agencies	• May be organization • May be government • Community agencies • Home • Work • School • Playground	• Community agencies • Home • Work • School
Interaction patterns	• Governmental • Organizational • Groups • May be one-to-one	• One-to-one • Groups • May be organizational	• One-to-one
Type of service	• Indirect • May be direct care of populations	• Direct care of at-risk persons • Indirect (program management)	• Direct illness care
Emphasis on levels of prevention	• Primary	• Primary • Secondary—screening • Tertiary—maintenance and rehabilitation	• Secondary • Tertiary • Maybe primary

	COMMUNITY-ORIENTED NURSING		COMMUNITY-BASED NURSING
	PUBLIC HEALTH NURSING—POPULATION FOCUSED/POPULATION CENTERED		
Roles	**Client and delivery oriented: community/population**	**Client and delivery oriented: individual, family, group**	**Client and delivery oriented: individual, family**
	• Educator	Individual/family oriented—as needed	• Caregiver
	• Consultant	• Caregiver	• Educator
	• Advocate	• Social engineer	• Counselor
	• Planner	• Educator	• Advocate
	• Collaborator	• Counselor	• Care manager
	• Data collector/evaluator	• Advocate	
	• Health status monitor	• Case manager	
	• Social engineer		
	• Community developer/partner		
	• Facilitator		
	• Community care agent		
	• Assessor		
	• Policy developer/maker		
	• Assuror of health care		
	• Enforcer of laws/compliance		
	• Disaster responder		
	Population oriented	**Group Oriented**	**Group Oriented**
	• Program manager, aggregates	• Leader, personal health management	• Leader, disease management
	• Health initiator	• Change agent, screening	• Change agent, managed care services
	• Program evaluator	• Community advocate	
	• Counselor	• Case finder	
	• Change agent-population health	• Community care agent	
	• Educator	• Assessment	
	• Population advocate	• Policy developer	
		• Assurance	
		• Enforcer of laws/compliance	
Priority of nurses' activities	• Community development	• For individual and family clients—as needed	• Care management, direct care
	• Community assessment/monitoring	• Case finding	• Patient education
	• Health policy/politics	• Client education	• Individual and family advocacy
	• Community education	• Community education	• Interdisciplinary practice
	• Interdisciplinary practice	• Interdisciplinary practice	• Continuity of care provider
	• Program management	• Case management, direct care	
	• Community/population advocacy	• Program planning, implementation	
		• Individual and family advocacy	

The terms *public health nurse* and *community health nurse* have been used interchangeably for at least 30 years. They continue to be used interchangeably by providers and those educated as community health nurses. However, the two terms are being merged into the term *public health nurse*. The two columns of this chart represent the scope of contributions made to health care delivery by the community-oriented nurse. A distinction may be made between the public health nurse's roles and functions, as can be seen here and compared with the newest nurse role/function of the community-based nurse.

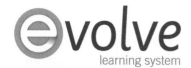
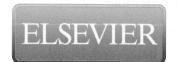
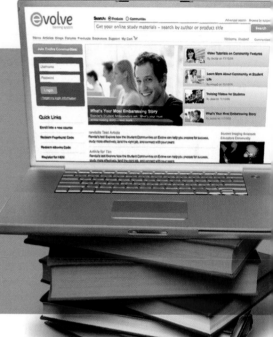

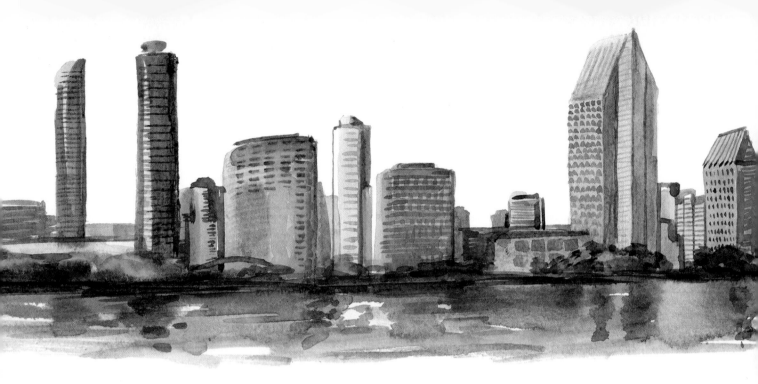

Public Health Nursing

Population-Centered
Health Care in the Community

8th
EDITION

Revised Reprint

Marcia Stanhope, RN, DSN, FAAN
Endowed Professor and Good Samaritan Chair Holder
Community Health Nursing
University of Kentucky
Lexington, Kentucky

Jeanette Lancaster, RN, PhD, FAAN
Medical Center Professor
School of Nursing
University of Virginia
Charlottesville, Virginia

ELSEVIER

Elsevier
3251 Riverport Lane
Maryland Heights, Missouri 63043

Notice

Knowledge and best practice in this field are constantly changing. As new research and experience broaden our knowledge, changes in practice, treatment and drug therapy may become necessary or appropriate. Readers are advised to check the most current information provided (i) on procedures featured or (ii) by the manufacturer of each product to be administered, to verify the recommended dose or formula, the method and duration of administration, and contraindications. It is the responsibility of the practitioner, relying on their own experience and knowledge of the patient, to make diagnoses, to determine dosages and the best treatment for each individual patient, and to take all appropriate safety precautions. To the fullest extent of the law, neither the Publisher nor the Authors assume any liability for any injury and/or damage to persons or property arising out of or related to any use of the material contained in this book.

The Publisher

Previous editions copyrighted 1984, 1988, 1992, 1996, 2000, 2004, 2008.
ISBN: **9780323241731**

Library of Congress Cataloging-in-Publication Data

Public health nursing : population-centered health care in the community / [edited by] Marcia Stanhope, Jeanette Lancaster. -- 8th ed.
        p. ; cm.
    Includes bibliographical references.
    ISBN 978-0-323-08001-9 (hardback : alk. paper) 1. Community health nursing. I. Stanhope, Marcia.
II. Lancaster, Jeanette.
    [DNLM: 1. Community Health Nursing. 2. Public Health Nursing. WY 106]
    RT98.C6562 2012
    610.73'43—dc23   2011021948

Content Strategist: Nancy O'Brien
Content Development Specialist: Jennifer Shropshire
Content Coordinator: Kelly Albright
Publishing Services Manager: Jeff Patterson
Project Manager: Jeanne Genz
Design Direction: Kim Denando

Printed in the United States of America

Last digit is the print number: 9 8 7 6 5 4 3

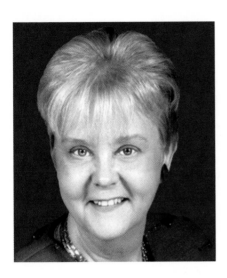

Marcia Stanhope, RN, DSN, FAAN

Marcia Stanhope is currently Professor at the University of Kentucky College of Nursing, Lexington, Kentucky. She was appointed to the Good Samaritan Endowed Chair in Community Health Nursing 8 years ago. She has practiced community and home health nursing, has served as an administrator and consultant in home health, and has been involved in the development of a number of nurse-managed centers. She has taught community health, public health, epidemiology, primary care nursing, and administration courses. Dr. Stanhope is the former Associate Dean and formerly directed the Division of Community Health Nursing and Administration at the University of Kentucky. She has been responsible for both undergraduate and graduate courses in population-centered, community-oriented nursing. She has also taught at the University of Virginia and the University of Alabama, Birmingham. Her presentations and publications have been in the areas of home health, community health and community-focused nursing practice, nurse-managed centers, and primary care nursing. Dr. Stanhope holds a diploma in nursing from the Good Samaritan Hospital, Lexington, Kentucky, and a bachelor of science in nursing from the University of Kentucky. She has a master's degree in public health nursing from Emory University in Atlanta and a doctorate of science in nursing from the University of Alabama, Birmingham. Dr. Stanhope is the co-author of four other Elsevier publications: *Handbook of Community-Based and Home Health Nursing Practice, Public and Community Health Nurse's Consultant, Case Studies in Community Health Nursing Practice: A Problem-Based Learning Approach,* and *Foundations of Community Health Nursing: Community-Oriented Practice.*

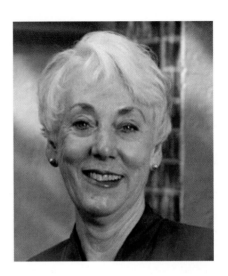

Jeanette Lancaster, RN, PhD, FAAN

Jeanette Lancaster is currently the Medical Center Professor of Nursing at the University of Virginia School of Nursing in Charlottesville, Virginia. She served as dean of the School of Nursing at the University of Virginia from 1989 until 2008. From 2008 to 2009 she served as a visiting professor at the University of Hong Kong where she taught courses in public health nursing and worked with faculty to develop their scholarship programs. She has practiced psychiatric nursing and taught both psychiatric and community health nursing. She formerly directed the master's program in community health at the University of Alabama, Birmingham, and served as dean of the School of Nursing at Wright State University in Dayton, Ohio. Her publications and presentations have been largely in the areas of community and public health nursing leadership and change and the significance of nurses to effective primary health care. Dr. Lancaster is a graduate of the University of Tennessee Health Science Center Memphis. She holds a master's degree in psychiatric nursing from Case Western Reserve University and a doctorate in public health from the University of Oklahoma. Dr. Lancaster is the author of another Elsevier publication, *Nursing Issues in Leading and Managing Change* and the co-author of *Foundations of Community Health Nursing: Community-Oriented Practice.*

It seems amazing that the work on the first edition of this text began in 1980. This eighth edition marks over three decades of colleagueship between the two of us and with some of the contributors. Other contributors have joined the project in editions beyond the first one, and we are grateful to each of you. We could not have developed a text as important as this one has been without your contributions.

Jeanette Lancaster and Marcia Stanhope

Swann Arp Adams, PhD
Assistant Professor, College of Nursing
Department of Epidemiology and
    Biostatistics, Arnold School of Public
    Health
University of South Carolina
Columbia, South Carolina
Chapter 12: Epidemiology

Debra Gay Anderson, PhD, PHCNS-BC
Associate Professor
College of Nursing
University of Kentucky
Lexington, Kentucky
Chapter 28: Family Health Risks

Dyan A. Aretakis, RN, MSN, FNP-BC
Project Director
Teen Health Center
University of Virginia Health System
Charlottesville, Virginia
Chapter 35: Teen Pregnancy

Linda K. Birenbaum, PhD, RN
Public Health Program Supervisor
Washington County Health & Human
    Services
Hillsboro, Oregon
*Chapter 27: Family Development and Family
    Nursing Assessment*

Jean C. Bokinskie, PhD, RN
Assistant Professor, Nursing Department
Concordia College
Moorhead, Minnesota
*Chapter 45: The Nurse in the Faith
    Community*

Nisha Botchwey, MCRP, PhD
Associate Professor of Urban and
    Environmental Planning and Public
    Health Sciences
University of Virginia
Charlottesville, Virginia
*Chapter 17: Promoting Healthy Communities
    Using Multilevel Participatory Strategies*

Kathryn H. Bowles, PhD, RN, FAAN
Associate Professor
New Courtland Center for Transitions and
    Health
University of Pennsylvania
Philadelphia, Pennsylvania
*Chapter 41: The Nurse in Home Health and
    Hospice*

**Angeline Bushy, PhD, RN, PHCNS-BC,
    FAAN**
Professor & Bert Fish Chair
College of Nursing
University of Central Florida
Daytona Beach, Florida
*Chapter 19: Population-Centered Nursing in
    Rural and Urban Environments*

Jacquelyn C. Campbell, PhD, RN, FAAN
Anna D. Wolf Chair
The Johns Hopkins University School of
    Nursing
National Director
Robert Wood Johnson Foundation Nurse
    Faculty Scholars
Baltimore, Maryland
Chapter 38: Violence and Human Abuse

Ann H. Cary, PhD, MPH, RN, A-CCC
Professor and Director—School of Nursing
Robert Wood Johnson Foundation
    Executive Nurse Fellow
Loyola University
New Orleans, Louisiana
Chapter 22: Case Management

Cynthia E. Degazon, PhD, RN
Professor Emerita
Hunter College of the City University of
    New York
New York, New York
*Chapter 7: Cultural Diversity in the
    Community*

Janna Dieckmann, PhD, RN
Clinical Associate Professor
School of Nursing
University of North Carolina at Chapel Hill
Chapel Hill, North Carolina
*Chapter 2: History of Public Health and
    Public and Community Health Nursing*

Diane Downing, PhD, RN
Adjunct Faculty
School of Nursing and Health Studies
Georgetown University
Washington, District of Columbia
*Chapter 46: Public Health Nursing at Local,
    State, and National Levels*

Amanda Fallin, MSN, RN
Instructor
University of Kentucky
Lexington, Kentucky
Chapter 28: Family Health Risks

James J. Fletcher, PhD
Professor Emeritus of Philosophy
Department of Philosophy
George Mason University
Fairfax, Virginia
*Chapter 6: Application of Ethics in the
    Community*

Monty Gross, PhD, RN, CNE
Associate Professor of Nursing
James Madison University
Harrisonburg, Virginia
*Chapter 30: Major Health Issues and Chronic
    Disease Management of Adults Across the
    Life Span*

Patty J. Hale, PhD, RN, FNP, FAAN
Professor & Graduate Program Director
Department of Nursing
James Madison University
Harrisonburg, Virginia
*Chapter 14: Communicable and Infectious
    Disease Risks*

Susan B. Hassmiller, PhD, RN, FAAN
Senior Advisor for Nursing
Robert Wood Johnson Foundation
Princeton, New Jersey
*Chapter 23: Public Health Nursing and the
    Disaster Management Cycle*

**DeAnne K. Hilfinger Messias, PhD, RN,
    FAAN**
Professor
College of Nursing and Women's and
    Gender Studies
University of South Carolina
Columbia, South Carolina
Chapter 12: Epidemiology

Linda J. Hulton, PhD, RN
Professor of Nursing
James Madison University
Harrisonburg, Virginia
*Chapter 30: Major Health Issues and Chronic
    Disease Management of Adults Across the
    Life Span*

**Anita Hunter, PhD, APRN – CPNP,
    FAAN**
Professor & Chair, Department of Nursing
Dominican University of California
San Rafael, California
Chapter 4: Perspectives in Global Health Care

Bonnie Jerome-D'Emilia, PhD, RN, MPH
Assistant Professor of Nursing
Director of RN-BSN Program
Camden College of Arts and Sciences
Department of Nursing
Rutgers, The State University of New Jersey
Camden, New Jersey
*Chapter 3: Public Health and Primary
   Health Care Systems and Healthcare
   Transformation*

Joanna Rowe Kaakinen, PhD, RN
Professor, School of Nursing
University of Portland
Portland, Oregon
*Chapter 27: Family Development and Family
   Nursing Assessment*

Katherine K. Kinsey, PhD, RN, FAAN
Administrator
Philadelphia Nurse-Family Partnership
Mabel Morris Early Head Start
First Steps Autism Spectrum Disorder (ASD)
   Program
National Nursing Centers Consortium
Philadelphia, Pennsylvania
*Chapter 21: The Nursing Center: A Model for
   Nursing Practice in the Community*

**Pamela A. Kulbok, DNSc, RN,
   PHCNS-BC, FAAN**
Professor of Nursing and Chair
Department of Family, Community, and
   Mental Health Systems
Coordinator of Public Health Leadership
University of Virginia
Charlottesville, Virginia
*Chapter 17: Promoting Healthy Communities
   Using Multilevel Participatory Strategies*

Kären M. Landenburger, PhD, RN
Professor of Nursing
Director, Education
University of Washington Tacoma
Tacoma, Washington
Chapter 38: Violence and Human Abuse

Susan C. Long-Marin, DVM, MPH
Epidemiology Manager
Mecklenburg County Health Department
Charlotte, North Carolina
*Chapter 13: Infectious Disease Prevention and
   Control*

Karen S. Martin, RN, MSN, FAAN
Health Care Consultant
Martin Associates
Omaha, Nebraska
*Chapter 41: The Nurse in Home Health and
   Hospice*

Mary Lynn Mathre, RN, MSN, CARN
Substance Abuse Consultant
President and Co-founder of Patients Out
   of Time
Howardsville, Virginia
*Chapter 37: Alcohol, Tobacco and Other Drug
   Problems*

Robert E. McKeown, PhD, FACE
Professor and Chair
Department of Epidemiology & Biostatistics
Arnold School of Public Health
Director, Health Sciences Research Core
University of South Carolina
Columbia, South Carolina
Chapter 12: Epidemiology

Mary Ellen T. Miller, PhD, RN
Assistant Professor
DeSales University
Center Valley, Pennsylvania
and
Co-Chair Wellness Centers Committee
National Nursing Center Consortium
Philadelphia, Pennsylvania
*Chapter 21: The Nursing Center: A Model for
   Nursing Practice in the Community*

Marie Napolitano, PhD, RN, FNP
Director—Doctorate of Nursing Practice
   Program
School of Nursing
University of Portland
Portland, Oregon
Chapter 34: Migrant Health Issues

**Linda Olson Keller, DNP, CPH,
   APHN-BC, RN, FAAN**
Clinical Associate Professor
University of Minnesota School of Nursing
Minneapolis, Minnesota
*Chapter 9: Population-Based Public Health
   Nursing Practice: The Intervention Wheel*

Susan B. Patton, DNSc, PNP, BC
Associate Professor
College of Nursing
University of Tennessee Health Science
   Center
Memphis, Tennessee
Chapter 44: The Nurse in Forensics

Bonnie Rogers, DrPH, COHN-S, LNCC
Director, NC Occupational Safety and Health
   and Education and Research Center
Director, Occupational Health Nursing
   Program
School of Public Health
University of North Carolina
Chapel Hill, North Carolina
*Chapter 43: The Nurse in Occupational
   Health*

Molly A. Rose, PhD, RN
Professor
Thomas Jefferson University
Jefferson School of Nursing
Philadelphia, Pennsylvania
*Chapter 39: The Advanced Practice Nurse in
   the Community*

Cynthia Rubenstein, PhD, RN, CPNP-PC
Department of Nursing
James Madison University
Harrisonburg, Virginia
Chapter 29: Child and Adolescent Health

Barbara Sattler, DrPH, RN, FAAN
Professor and Director
Environmental Health Education Center
University of Maryland School of Nursing
Baltimore, Maryland
Chapter 10: Environmental Health

Juliann G. Sebastian, PhD, RN, FAAN
Dean and Professor
College of Nursing
University of Missouri—St. Louis
St. Louis, Missouri
*Chapter 32: Vulnerability and Vulnerable
   Populations: An Overview*
*Chapter 40: The Nurse Leader in the
   Community*

George F. Shuster III, RN, DNSc
Associate Professor
College of Nursing
University of New Mexico
Albuquerque, New Mexico
*Chapter 18: Community as Client: Assessment
   and Analysis*

Mary Cipriano Silva, PhD, RN, FAAN
Professor Emerita
School of Nursing
George Mason University
Fairfax, Virginia
*Chapter 6: Application of Ethics in the
   Community*

Kellie Smith, MSN, RN
Instructor
Jefferson School of Nursing
Thomas Jefferson University
Philadelphia, Pennsylvania
*Chapter 39: The Advanced Practice Nurse in
   the Community*

Jeanne Merkle Sorrell, PhD, RN, FAAN
Professor Emerita
School of Nursing
George Mason University
Fairfax, Virginia
*Chapter 6: Application of Ethics in the
   Community*

Sharon A.R. Stanley, PhD, RN, RS
Chief Nurse and Director
Disaster Health & Mental Health Services
American Red Cross
Washington, District of Columbia
Chapter 23: Public Health Nursing and the Disaster Management Cycle

Sharon Strang, DNP, APRN, FNP-BC
Assistant Professor of Nursing
Department of Nursing
James Madison University
Harrisonburg, Virginia
Chapter 30: Major Health Issues and Chronic Disease Management of Adults Across the Life Span

Sue Strohschein, MS, RN/PHN, APRN, BC
Culture of Excellence Project Coordinator
University of Minnesota School of Nursing
Minneapolis, Minnesota
Chapter 9: Population-Based Public Health Nursing Practice: The Intervention Wheel

Francisco S. Sy, MD, DrPH
Director
Division of Extramural Activities & Scientific Programs
National Center on Minority Health & Health Disparities
National Institutes of Health
Bethesda, Maryland
Chapter 13: Infectious Disease Prevention and Control

Anita Thompson-Heisterman, MSN, PMHCNS, BC, PMHNP, BC
Assistant Professor
School of Nursing
and
University of Virginia
Nurse Practitioner
Department of Neurology
University of Virginia
Charlottesville, Virginia
Chapter 36: Mental Health Issues

Lisa Pedersen Turner, MSN, RN
College of Nursing
University of Kentucky
Lexington, Kentucky
Chapter 42: The Nurse in the Schools

Lynn Wasserbauer, PhD, FNP, RN
Nurse Practitioner
Strong Memorial Hospital
University of Rochester Medical Center
Rochester, New York
Chapter 31: Special Needs Populations

Carolyn Antonides Williams, PhD, RN, FAAN
Professor, Dean Emeritus
College of Nursing
University of Kentucky
Lexington, Kentucky
Chapter 1: Population-Focused Practice: The Foundation of Specialization in Public Health Nursing

Elke Jones Zschaebitz, MSN, FNP
Formerly, Instructor
School of Nursing
University of Virginia
Charlottesville, Virginia
Chapter 11: Genomics

ANCILLARY AUTHORS

Elizabeth E. Friberg, DNP, RN
Assistant Professor
University of Virginia School of Nursing
Charlottesville, Virginia
Instructor's Manual
Student Quiz

Lisa Pedersen Turner, MSN, RN
College of Nursing
University of Kentucky
Lexington, Kentucky
PowerPoint Lecture Slides
Case Studies

Anna K. Wehling Weepie, DNP, RN, CNE
Associate Professor
Allen College
Waterloo, Iowa
Testbank
Community Assessment Applied

REVIEWERS

Judith Alexander, PhD, RN, PHCNS, NEA-BC
Associate Professor
College of Nursing
University of South Carolina
Columbia, South Carolina

Carol S. Brown, PhD, APRN, BC
President
Community Health and Environment, LLC
Mankato, Minnesota

Jacquelyn Burchum, DNSc, FNP-BC, CNE
Associate Professor
College of Nursing
University of Tennessee Health Science
    Center
Memphis, Tennessee

Christine Eisenhauer, MSN, APRN-CNS
Assistant Professor
Division of Nursing
Mount Mary College
Yankton, South Dakota

Elizabeth Furlong, PhD, RN, JD
Associate Professor
School of Nursing
and
Faculty Associate
Center for Health Policy and Ethics
Creighton University
Omaha, Nebraska

Georgia A. Moore, PhD, MSNed, RN
Nursing Education Consultant
Department of Nursing
Nursing Education and Technology
    Consultants
Louisville, Kentucky

Teresa O'Neill, PhD, APRN, MN, RNC
Professor
Department of Nursing and Allied Health
Our Lady of Holy Cross College
New Orleans, Louisiana

ACKNOWLEDGMENTS

Once again, for the eighth edition of this text, we would like to thank our families, friends, and colleagues for their support and encouragement in this project. We particularly would like to thank our colleagues at the University of Kentucky College of Nursing and the University of Virginia School of Nursing for their support and assistance. Special thanks go to Nancy O'Brien, Carlie Bliss, Jennifer Shropshire, and Kevin Clear at Elsevier and to Lisa Turner at the University of Kentucky, who have been steadfast and compassionate in their work with us on this edition.

A Special Thanks

To the seventh edition contributors who have chosen to pass the torch to other contributors for the eighth edition. Your expertise, thoughtful development of chapter content, and devotion to education of the next generation of PHNs is much appreciated. You will be missed.

Brenda Afzal, Edie Devers Barbero, Christine DiMartile Bolla, Marjorie Buchanan, Sudruk Chitthathairatt, Marcia Cowen, Kathleen Fletcher, Doris Glick, Jean Goeppinger, Cynthia Gustafson, Diane Hatton, Kathleen Huttlinger, Lisa Kaiser, Susan Kennel, Shirley Cloutier Laffrey, Sharon Lock, Carol Lynn Maxwell-Thompson, Lillian Mood, Lisa Onega, Mary Riner, Jennifer Schaller-Ayers, Heather Ward, and Judith Lupo Wold.

We would like to express our gratitude to two contributors who are deceased and who contributed a great deal to the success of previous editions of the book.

Linda Kay Birenbaum, who passed away in 2010, co-authored the chapter "Family Development and Family Nursing Assessment" in the sixth and seventh editions. Dr. Birenbaum was well known for her research expertise and grant writing that helped advance the science of nursing by increasing our understanding of families and children in pediatric oncology nursing, particularly in assessing children's bereavement when a sibling dies from cancer. She taught nursing research and community health nursing at both the University of Portland and Oregon Health Sciences University. Her friends describe her as a colleague who had a great laugh and could find humor in most situations. She was devoted to her family, friends, cancer research, and her cats.

Janet Ihlenfeld authored the chapter "The Nurse in the Schools" in the sixth and seventh editions. She spent many years teaching at the Department of Nursing at D'Youville College in Buffalo, New York. Her practice focused on child health and community health nursing. She was considered an expert in helping nursing students learn about both of these content areas by supervising them in well-child settings including daycare centers and high schools.

We are grateful to have had the opportunity to work with both of these nursing educators and authors. They will each be missed.

Marcia Stanhope
Jeanette Lancaster

Since the last edition of this text, many changes have occurred in society as well as in health care. The rapid and often startling changes in society are influencing the amount and ways in which health care is delivered. Many of the industrial nations around the world are engaged in health care reform, and a major driver for reform is the enormous cost of providing health care to citizens. The human, financial, infrastructure, and other costs associated with war, natural and human-made diseases, and civil uprising continue to affect many nations, including the United States.

The world, as many people know, has changed dramatically in the past few decades because of such disruptions as the two Gulf Wars and the continuing wars in Iraq and Afghanistan, the bombing of the World Trade Center, several massive hurricanes (most notably Hurricane Katrina), the oil spill in the Gulf of Mexico, and the floods, earthquakes, tornados, and other storms that cost lives, homes, and livelihoods.

In the past, limited funds have been available for disaster preparedness. In recent years the money needed to ensure greater safety from disasters has increased. The need to provide the necessary help and support to deal with possible and real health disruptions has strengthened the role of public health professionals. If there is a bright spot to the concerns about terrorism, war, and limited financial resources, it is that far more people understand the importance and value of public health to individuals, families, communities, and nations.

In the Association of State and Territorial Directors of Nursing's document, "Why does every state need public health nursing leadership in their state health?" many of the current public health nursing needs are cited (ASTDN, 2008). They contend that effective public health nursing practice relies on effective senior level nursing leadership. They highlight these critical roles for public health nurses:

- Emergency and disaster planning and response to hurricanes, floods, fires, and tornados
- Infectious disease monitoring and prevention, tracking outbreaks
- Community health education and school nursing
- Health fairs and preventive health screenings
- Chronic disease management in populations
- Monitoring and preventing environmental health issues such as food safety and lead poisoning
- Valuable resources for advisory boards, coalitions, and community health programs (p 1)

Chapters in this text include all of the critical roles listed above as well as guidance in how to deal with other major issues including the quality of care, the cost of care, and access to care. The growing shortage of nurses and other health care providers will only increase the concerns about these issues. One of the ways in which quality of care could be improved would include new uses of technology to manage an information revolution. Great improvements in quality would require a restructuring of how care is delivered, a shift in how funds are spent, changing the workplace, and using more effective ways to manage chronic illness. There will be costs associated with these quality improvements.

The United States continues to have a problem of increasing health care costs. At present these costs are consuming about $2.5 trillion, or 17% of the Gross Domestic Product. The costs of health care have risen by $1 trillion in 4 years (CMS, 2010). These enormous costs are imposing heavy burdens on employer's and consumers. Despite these costs, the number of uninsured continues to grow and is estimated to be around 49.4 million (U.S. Census Bureau, 2010). This number of uninsured is larger than the population of either Canada or Australia. Despite spending more money per person in the United States for illness care than any other country, Americans are not the healthiest of all people. The infant mortality and life expectancy rates—indexes of health care—while improving, are not close to what they should be given the amount spent on health care. Some of the most important factors leading to the high health care costs are diagnostic and treatment technologies, drugs, an aging population, more chronic illness, shortages in health care workers, and medical-legal costs. Lifestyle continues to play a big role in morbidity and mortality. It is embarrassing that overall, citizens in the United States are the most obese citizens in any industrialized nation. In addition, half of all deaths are still caused by tobacco, alcohol, and illegal drug use; diet and activity patterns; microbial agents; toxic agents; firearms; sexual behavior; and motor vehicle accidents.

In the last two decades the greatest improvements in population health have come from public health achievements such as immunizations leading to eliminating and controlling infectious diseases; motor vehicle safety; safer workplaces; lifestyle improvements reducing the risk of heart disease and strokes; safer and healthier foods through improved sanitation; clean water and food fortification programs; better hygiene and nutrition to improve the health of mothers and babies; family planning; fluoride in drinking water; and recognition of tobacco as a health hazard. Continued changes in the public health system are essential if death, illness, and disability resulting from preventable problems are to continue to decline.

The need to focus attention on health promotion, lifestyle factors, and disease prevention led to the development of a major public policy about health for the nation. This policy was designed by a large number of people representing a wide range of groups interested in health. The policy, first introduced in 1979, was updated in 1990 and in 2000; it is reflected in the most recent document updated in 2010, titled *Healthy People 2020*. These four

National Health Expenditures Fact Sheet, CMS, 2011. Retrieved June 20, 2011 from http://www.cms.gov.nationalhealthExpendata/25–NHE–factsheet.asp.

National Center for Health Statistics: Health: United States, 2009 with special feature on technology, Hyattsville, Md, 2010. U.S. Government Printing Office.

U.S. Census Bureau: U.S. population check, 2010. Available at http://www.census.gov/main/www/popclock.html. Accessed August 13, 2010.

documents have identified a set of national health promotion and disease prevention objectives for each of four decades. Examples of these objectives are highlighted in chapters throughout the text.

The most effective disease prevention and health promotion strategies designed to achieve the goals and objectives of *Healthy People 2020* are developed through partnerships between government, businesses, voluntary organizations, consumers, communities, and health care providers. According to *Healthy People 2020*, the partners who join a newly established consortium will work to achieve these goals and objectives of *Healthy People 2020*.

Healthy People 2020 emphasizes the concept of social determinants of health—that is, the notion that health is impacted by many social, economic, and environmental factors that extend far beyond individual biology of disease. This means that improving health requires a broad approach to including the concept of health in all policies and creating environments where the healthy choice is the easy choice. To develop healthy communities, individuals, families, communities, and populations must commit to these approaches. Also, society, through the development of health policy, must support better health care, the design of improved health education, and new ways of financing strategies to alter health status.

The regrettable fact is that few health indicators have been substantially improved since *Healthy People 2010* was released in 2000. *Healthy People 2020* retains many of the original objectives and adds new ones. What does this mean for nurses who work in public health? Because people do not always know how to improve their health status, the challenge of nursing is to create change. Nursing takes place in a variety of public and private settings and includes disease prevention, health promotion, health protection, surveillance, education, maintenance, restoration, coordination, management, and evaluation of care of individuals, families, and populations, including communities.

To meet the demands of a constantly changing health care system, nurses must have vision in designing new and changing current roles and identifying their practice areas. To do so effectively, the nurse must understand concepts and theories of public health, the changing health care system, the actual and potential roles and responsibilities of nurses and other health care providers, the importance of health promotion and disease orientation, and the necessity to involve consumers in the planning, implementing, and evaluating of health care efforts.

Since its initial publication 30 years ago, this text has been widely accepted and is popular among nursing students and nursing faculty in baccalaureate, BSN-completion, and graduate programs. The text was written to provide nursing students and practicing nurses with a comprehensive source book that provides a foundation for designing population-centered nursing strategies for individuals, families, aggregates, populations, and communities. The unifying theme for the book is the integrating of health promotion and disease prevention concepts into the many roles of nurses. The prevention focus emphasizes traditional public health practice with increased attention to the effects of the internal and external environment on health of communities. The focus on interventions for the individual and family emphasizes the aspects of population-centered practice

with attention to the effects of all of the determinants of health, including lifestyle, on personal health.

CONCEPTUAL APPROACH TO THIS TEXT

The term *community-oriented* has been used to reflect the orientation of nurses to the community and the public's health. In 1998, the Quad Council of Public Health Nursing comprised of members from the American Nurses Association Congress on Nursing Practice; the American Public Health Association Public Health Nursing section; the Association of Community Health Nursing Educators; and the Association of State and Territorial Directors of Public Health Nursing developed a statement on the *Scope of Public Health Nursing Practice*. Through this statement, the leaders in public and community health nursing attempted to clarify the differences between public health nursing and the newest term introduced into nursing's vocabulary during health care reform of the 1990s, *community-based nursing*. The Quad Council recognized that the terms *public health nursing* and *community health nursing* have been used interchangeably since the 1980s to describe population-focused, community-oriented nursing, and community-focused practice. They decided to make a clearer distinction between community-oriented and community-based nursing practice. In 2007, the definitions were further refined and nurses once referred to as public health nurses and community health nurses are now referred to only as public health nurses in the revised standards of practice.

In this textbook, two different levels of care in the community are acknowledged: community-oriented care and community-based care. Two role functions for nursing practice in the community are suggested: public health nursing (community health nursing), and community-based nursing. This text focuses only on public health nursing (community health nursing), using the term *community-oriented nursing*, which encompasses a focus on populations within the community context or *population-centered nursing practice*.

For the fifth edition of this text, with consultation from C. A. Williams (author) and June Thompson (Mosby editor), Marcia Stanhope developed a conceptual model for community-oriented nursing practice. This model was influenced by a review of the history of community-oriented nursing from the 1800s to today. Marcia Stanhope studied Betty Neuman's model intensively while in school, which influenced this model.

The model itself is presented as a caricature of reality—or an abstract, with a description of the characteristics and the philosophy upon which community-oriented nursing is built.

The *model* is shown as a flying balloon (see inside front cover of this book). The balloon represents community-oriented nursing and is filled with the knowledge, skills, and abilities needed in this practice to carry the world (the basket of the balloon) or the clients of the world who benefit from this practice. The *subconcepts* of public health nursing with the community and populations as the center of care are the *boundaries* of the practice. The public health foundation pillars of assurance, assessment, and policy development hold up the world of communities, where people live, work, play, go to school, and worship. The ribbons flying from the balloon indicate the interventions used by nurses.

These ribbons (interventions) serve to provide lift and direction, tying the services together for the clients that are served. The intervention names and the services are listed on the inside cover of this book. The *propositions* (statements of relationship) for this model are found in the definitions of practice, public health functions, clients served, specific settings, interventions, and services. Many *assumptions* have served as the basis for the development of this model. Community-oriented nursing is a specialty within the nursing discipline. The practice has evolved over time, becoming more complex. The practice of nursing in public health is based on a philosophy of care rather than being setting specific. It is different from community-based nursing care delivery. The development of community-oriented nursing has been influenced by public health practice, preventive medicine, community medicine, and shifts in the health care delivery system. Community-oriented nursing requires nurses to have specific competencies to be effective providers of care.

The definition of community-oriented nursing appears on the inside front cover of this book. This practice includes both public health and community health nurses. Community-based nurses differ from community-oriented nurses in many ways. These differences are described in the table on the inside back cover of this book. The differences are described as they relate to philosophy of care, goals, service, community, clients served, practice settings, ways of interacting with clients, type of services offered to clients, prevention levels used, goals, and priority of nurses' activities.

The four concepts of nursing, person (client), environment, and health are described for this model. These concepts appear in many works about nursing and in almost every educational curriculum for undergraduate students. Each of the four concepts may be defined differently in these works because of the beliefs of the persons writing the definitions.

In this text *nursing* is defined as community-oriented with a focus on providing "health care" through community diagnosis and investigation of major health and environmental problems. Health surveillance, monitoring, and evaluating community and population status are done to prevent disease and disability, and to promote, protect, preserve, restore, and maintain health. This in turn creates conditions in which clients can be healthy. The person, or client, is the world, nation, state, community, population, aggregate, family, or individual.

The boundaries of the client *environment* may be limited only by the world, nation, state, locality, home, school, work, playground, religion, or individual self. *Health,* in this model, involves a continuum of health rather than wellness, with the best health state possible as the goal. The best possible level of health is achieved through measures of prevention as practiced by the nurse.

The nurse engages in autonomous practice with the client, who is the primary decision maker about health issues. The nurse practices in a variety of environments, including, but not limited to, governments, organizations, homes, schools, churches, neighborhoods, industry, and community boards. The nurse interacts with diverse cultures, partners, other providers in teams, multiple clients, and one-to-one or aggregate relationships. Clients at risk for the development of health problems are a major focus of nursing services. Primary prevention–level strategies are the key to reducing risk of health problems. Secondary prevention is done to maintain, promote, or protect health whereas tertiary prevention strategies are used to preserve, protect, or maintain health.

The community-oriented nurse has many roles related to community clients and roles that relate specifically to practice with populations (or population-centered) (see inside back cover). Community-oriented nurses engage in activities specific to community development, assessment, monitoring, health policy, politics, health education, interdisciplinary practice, program management, community/population advocacy, case finding, and delivery of personal health services when these services are otherwise unavailable in the health care system. This conceptual model is the framework for this text.

ORGANIZATION

The text is divided into seven sections:

- **Part One, Perspectives in Health Care and Population-Centered Nursing,** describes the historical and current status of the health care delivery system and public health nursing practice, both domestically and internationally.

- **Part Two, Influences on Health Care Delivery and Population Centered Nursing,** addresses the economics, ethics, policy and cultural issues that affect public health, nurses, and clients.

- **Part Three, Conceptual and Scientific Frameworks Applied to Population-Centered Nursing Practice,** provides conceptual models and scientific bases for public health nursing practice. Selected models from nursing and related sciences are also discussed.

- **Part Four, Issues and Approaches in Population-Centered Nursing,** examines the management of health care, quality and safety, and populations in select community environments and groups, as well as issues related to managing cases, programs, and disasters.

- **Part Five, Health Promotion with Target Populations Across the Life Span,** discusses risk factors and population-level health problems for families and individuals throughout the life span.

- **Part Six, Vulnerability: Issues for the Twenty-First Century,** covers specific health care needs and issues of populations at risk.

- **Part Seven, Nurse Roles and Functions in the Community,** examines diversity in the role of public health nurses and describes the rapidly changing roles, functions, and practice settings.

NEW TO THIS EDITION

New content has been included in the eighth edition of *Public Health Nursing: Population-Centered Health Care in the Community* to ensure that the text remains a complete and comprehensive resource:

- **NEW!** Chapter 4, Perspectives in Global Health Care, has been expanded to present a much broader and in-depth global health perspective that is consistent with health trends and nursing practice.

- **NEW!** Chapter 11, Genomics in Public Health Nursing, discusses the growing field of genetics/genomics and includes information that public health nurses need in order to include this science into their practice.
- **NEW!** Chapter 30, Major Health Issues and Chronic Disease Management of Adults Across the Life Span, focuses on health problems and issues related to populations across the lifespan.
- **NEW!** Chapter 44, The Nurse in Forensics, expands the content that has been included in previous editions of the chapter related to violence and human abuse and applies this specialized area to the work of public health nurses.
- **NEW!** Boxes titled "Linking Content to Practice" have been included in most chapters that connect many of the key statements and practice guides in nursing and public health to the practice of public health nursing.
- **NEW!** Chapter boxes pertaining to the work of *Healthy People* have all been updated to include objectives from *Healthy People 2020* that apply to the content of the chapters.
- **NEW!** In select chapters, content is applied to Quality and Safety Education for Nurses (QSEN).

PEDAGOGY

Other key features of this edition are detailed below.

Each chapter is organized for easy use by students and faculty.

ADDITIONAL RESOURCES

Additional Resources listed at the beginning of each chapter direct students to chapter-related tools and resources contained in the book's Appendixes or on its Evolve website.

OBJECTIVES

Objectives open each chapter to guide student learning and alert faculty to what students should gain from the content.

KEY TERMS

Key Terms are identified at the beginning of the chapter and defined either within the chapter or in the glossary to assist students in understanding unfamiliar terminology.

CHAPTER OUTLINE

Finally, the Chapter Outline alerts students to the structure and content of the chapter.

DID YOU KNOW? Boxes

Provide students with interesting facts that lend insight into the chapter content.

WHAT DO YOU THINK? Boxes

Stimulate student debate and classroom discussion.

HOW TO Boxes

Provide specific, application-oriented information.

NURSING TIP Boxes

Emphasize special clinical considerations for nursing practice.

EVIDENCE-BASED PRACTICE

Evidence-Based Practice boxes in each chapter illustrate the use and application of the latest research findings in public health, community health, and community-oriented nursing.

THE CUTTING EDGE Boxes

Highlight significant issues and new approaches in community-oriented nursing practice.

PRACTICE APPLICATION

At the end of each chapter a case situation helps students understand how to apply chapter content in the practice setting. Questions at the end of each case promote critical thinking while students analyze the case.

KEY POINTS

Key Points provide a summary listing of the most important points made in the chapter.

CLINICAL DECISION-MAKING ACTIVITIES

Clinical Decision-Making Activities promote student learning by suggesting a variety of activities that encourage both independent and collaborative effort.

The back of the book contains the following resources:
- The **Appendixes** provide additional content resources, key information, and clinical tools and references.

EVOLVE STUDENT LEARNING RESOURCES

Additional resources designed to supplement the student learning process are available on this book's website at http://evolve.elsevier.com/Stanhope, including:
- **Community Assessment Applied:** A student resource providing tools and exercises to practice community assessment
- **Case Studies** with questions and answers
- **Student Quiz** questions with answers
- **WebLinks** for direct access to websites keyed to specific chapter content
- **Answers to Practice Application** provide suggested solutions to the Practice Application questions at the end of each chapter.
- **Glossary** with complete definitions of all key terms and other important community and public health nursing concepts
- **Resource Tools** to accompany select chapters

INSTRUCTOR RESOURCES

Several supplemental ancillaries are available to assist instructors in the teaching process:
- **Instructor's Manual**, with Annotated Lecture Outlines, Chapter Key Points, Clinical Decision-Making, Critical Analysis Questions with Answers
- **Computerized Test Bank** with 1200 NCLEX®-style questions and answers
- **PowerPoint Lecture Slides** for each chapter
- **Image Collection** with illustrations from the text
- **Answers to Practice Application** questions
- **Glossary of Key Terms**

CONTENTS

PART 3 Conceptual and Scientific Frameworks Applied to Population-Centered Nursing Practice

PART 5   Health Promotion with Target Populations Across the Life Span

Appendixes

Perspectives in Health Care and Population-Centered Nursing

Since the late 1800s, public health nurses have been leaders in making improvements in the quality of health care for individuals, families, and aggregates, including populations and communities. As nurses around the world collaborate with one another, it is clear that, from one country to another, population-centered nursing has more similarities than differences.

Important changes in health care have been taking place since the early 1990s, and there is every reason to think that the changes that will occur as a result of the health care reform work in the United States will be significant. Although considerable controversy surrounds the implementation of the Patient Protection and Affordable Care Act of 2010, it seems clear that change will occur.

The areas in health care that have posed the greatest problems for patients over the years have been access, quality, and cost. These problems are still present. Too many people have either no insurance or inadequate insurance, access to quality care is unevenly distributed across the country, and the cost of health care continues to grow for consumers, employers, insurers, and state and federal governments.

Some of the key areas of emphasis in the current efforts to reform health care include preventing disease, coordinating care, and shifting care from the hospital to the home or community facilities where possible. In the coming years, a large growth in the number of nurses employed in home health care and in nursing care facilities is expected. An area targeted for growth is that of the federal community health centers. The health care legislation signed into law in May 2010 authorized $11 billion for community health centers. Nurses comprise the largest category of employees in those centers. It is also expected that more new graduates will go directly into community health work rather than working for a few years in the hospital before making that transition. This trend supports the recommendations that nurses need to be prepared at the baccalaureate level regardless of their first program in nursing.

Over the years, funding for public health has decreased while the needs for population based services have increased. The key question is whether health care reform will support what is needed to provide population-based care in America's communities. There is much discussion about the new emphasis on prevention, community-oriented care, continuity, and the important role that nurses will play in health care. With anticipation that many of these projections will become a reality and that nurses will become increasingly key practitioners in promoting the health of the people, they must understand the history of public health nursing and the current status of the public health system.

There are some early indicators that health care reform will increase support for prevention. The government website http://www.healthcare.gov/learn/index/html provides easy-to-understand information about health care changes. Two sections on the website may be of particular interest to students in public health nursing: "Health Finder" and "Let's Move."

Part One presents information about significant factors affecting health in the United States. Changing the level and quality of services and the priorities for funding requires that nurses be involved, informed, courageous, and committed to the task. The chapters in Part One are designed to provide essential information so that nurses can make a difference in health care by understanding their own roles and their functions in population-centered practice and by understanding how the public health system differs from the primary care system. With terrorism, wars, and natural disasters, the importance of public health and the nurses who work within those systems is escalating.

Explanations are offered about exactly what it is that makes population-centered nursing unique. Often this form of nursing is confused with community-based nursing practice. There is a core of knowledge known as "public health" that forms the foundation for population-centered community and public health nursing. This core has historically included epidemiology, biostatistics, environmental health, health services administration, and social and behavioral sciences. In recent years, new areas of focus within public health have included informatics, genomics, communication, cultural competence, community-based participatory research, evidence-based practice, policy and law, global health, ethics, and forensics. This book covers both the traditional and the newer content either in a full chapter or as a section in one or more chapters.

CHAPTER 1

Population-Focused Practice: The Foundation of Specialization in Public Health Nursing

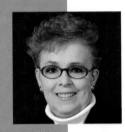

Carolyn A. Williams, RN, PhD, FAAN

Dr. Carolyn A. Williams is Dean Emeritus and Professor at the College of Nursing at the University of Kentucky, Lexington, Kentucky. Dr. Williams began her career as a public health nurse. She has held many leadership roles, including President of the American Academy of Nursing; membership on the first U.S. Preventive Services Task Force, Department of Health and Human Services; and President of the American Association of Colleges of Nursing. She received the Distinguished Alumna Award from Texas Woman's University in 1983. In 2001 she was the recipient of the Mary Tolle Wright Founder's Award for Excellence in Leadership from Sigma Theta Tau International, and in 2007 she received the Bernadette Arminger Award from the American Association of Colleges of Nursing.

ADDITIONAL RESOURCES

evolve WEBSITE

http://evolve.elsevier.com/Stanhope
- *Healthy People 2020*
- WebLinks—Of special note, see the link for this site:
  - Guide to Community Preventive Services
- Quiz
- Case Studies
- Glossary
- Answers to Practice Application

- Resource Tools
  - Resource Tool 5.A: Schedule of Clinical Preventive Services
  - Resource Tool 45.A: Core Competencies and Skill Levels for Public Health Nursing

APPENDIXES
- Appendix F.1: Instrumental Activities of Daily Living (IADL) Scale
- Appendix G.1: Examples of Public Health Nursing Roles and Implementing Public Health Functions
- Appendix H: Focus on Quality and Safety Education for Nurses

OBJECTIVES

After reading this chapter, the student should be able to do the following:
1. State the mission and core functions of public health and the essential public health services.
2. Describe specialization in public health nursing and community health nursing and the practice goals of each.
3. Contrast clinical community health nursing practice with population-focused practice.
4. Describe what is meant by population-focused practice.
5. Name barriers to acceptance of population-focused practice.
6. State key opportunities for population-focused practice.
7. Recognize quality performance standards program in public health.

KEY TERMS

aggregate, p. 12
assessment, p. 7
assurance, p. 7
capitation, p. 18
community-based nursing, p. 16
Community Health Improvement Process (CHIP), p. 8

community health nurses, p. 15
cottage industry, p. 18
integrated systems, p. 18
managed care, p. 4
policy development, p. 7
population, p. 12
population-focused practice, p. 11

public health, p. 7
public health core functions, p. 7
public health nursing, p. 9
Quad Council, p. 9
subpopulations, p. 12
—*See Glossary for definitions*

The second decade of the twenty-first century finds the United States entering an era when more public attention is being given to efforts to protect and improve the health of the American people and the environment. The continuing increase in the cost of medical care also has the attention of the public and policy makers. Despite what many see as a failure to make fundamental changes in the delivery and financing of health care, significant change has occurred. Federal and state initiatives, private market forces, the development of new scientific knowledge and new technologies, and the expectations of the public are bringing about changes in the health care system. With the national legislation that passed in 2010—the Patient Protection and Affordable Care Act (www.healthcare.gov/law/introduction/index.html)—which in part was designed to increase access to care, concerns have been raised about the availability of adequate numbers of professional personnel to provide services, particularly in primary care and strained health care facilities. Despite some of the insurance reforms in the legislation, many citizens and businesses remain concerned about their ability to maintain affordable insurance coverage; at the national level serious concern exists regarding the growing cost of health care as a part of federal expenditures (Orszag, 2007; 2010). Other health system concerns focus on the quality and safety of services, warnings about bioterrorism, and global public health threats such as infectious diseases and contaminated foods. Because of all of these factors, the role of public health in protecting and promoting health, as well as preventing disease and disability, is extremely important.

Whereas the majority of national attention and debate surrounding national health legislation has been focused primarily on insurance issues related to medical care, there are indications of a renewed interest in public health and in population-focused thinking about health and health care in the United States. For example, the Patient Protection and Affordable Care Act contains a number of provisions that address health promotion and prevention of disease and disability. These include (1) establishing the National Prevention, Health Promotion and Public Health Council to coordinate federal prevention, wellness, and public health activities and to develop a national strategy to improve the nation's health, and (2) creating a Prevention and Public Health

Fund to expand and sustain funding for prevention and public health programs, and (3) improving prevention by covering only proven preventive services and eliminating state cost sharing for preventive services, including immunizations recommended by the U.S. Preventive Services Task Force. Also grants and technical assistance will be available to employers who establish wellness programs (PPACAHCEARA, healthcare.gov, 2010).

Although populations have historically been the focus of public health practice, populations are also the focus of the "business" of managed care; therefore public health practitioners and managed care executives are both population oriented. Increasingly, managed care executives and program managers are using the basic sciences and analytic tools of the field of public health. They focus particularly on epidemiology and statistics to develop databases and approaches to making decisions at the level of a defined population or subpopulation. Thus a population-focused approach to planning, delivering, and evaluating nursing care has never been more important.

Where is public health nursing in all of the changes swirling around in the world of health and health care? This is a crucial time for public health nursing, a time of opportunity and challenge. The issue of growing costs together with the changing demography of the U. S. population, particularly the aging of the population, is expected to put increased demands on resources available for health care. In addition, the threats of bioterrorism, highlighted by the events of September 11, 2001, and the anthrax scares, will divert health care funds and resources from other health care programs to be spent for public safety. Also important to the public health community is the emergence of modern-day epidemics (such as the mosquito-borne West Nile virus, and the H1N1 influenza virus) and globally induced infectious diseases such as avian influenza and other causes of mortality, many of which affect the very young. Most of the causes of these epidemics are preventable. What has all of this to do with nursing?

Understanding the importance of community-oriented, population-focused nursing practice and developing the knowledge and skills to practice it will be critical to attaining a leadership role in health care regardless of the practice setting. The following discussion explains why those who practice population-focused nursing in the context of community-based programs directed to populations will be in a very strong position to affect the health of populations and the decisions about how scarce resources will be used.

PUBLIC HEALTH PRACTICE: THE FOUNDATION FOR HEALTHY POPULATIONS AND COMMUNITIES

During the last 20 years, considerable attention has been focused on proposals to reform the American health care system. These proposals focused primarily on containing cost in medical care financing and on strategies for providing health insurance coverage to a higher proportion of the population. In the national health legislation that passed in 2010, The Patient Protection and Affordable Care Act, the majority of the provisions and the vast majority of the discussion of the bill focused on those issues (PPACAHCEARA, 2010).

Because physician services and hospital care combined account for over half of the health care expenditures in the United States, it is understandable that changes in how such services would be paid for would receive much attention (kaiseredu.org, 2010). However, many times the most benefit from the least cost is sought in the wrong place. As stated in the Public Health Services Steering Committee Report on the Core Functions of Public Health (1998), reform of the medical insurance system was thought to be necessary, but it was not adequate to improve the health of Americans.

Historically, gains in the health of populations have come largely from public health changes. Safety and adequacy of food supplies, the provision of safe water, sewage disposal, public safety from biological threats, and personal behavioral changes, including reproductive behavior, are a few examples of public health's influence. The dramatic increase in life expectancy for Americans during the 1900s, from less than 50 years in 1900 to 77.9 years in 2007, is credited primarily to improvements in sanitation, the control of infectious diseases through immunizations, and other public health activities (USDHHS, 2010a). Population-based preventive programs launched in the 1970s were also largely responsible for the more recent changes in tobacco use, blood pressure control, dietary patterns (except obesity), automobile safety restraint, and injury control measures that have fostered declines in adult death rates. There has been more than a 50% decline in stroke and coronary heart disease deaths. Overall death rates for children have declined by about 40% (USDHHS, 2010).

Another way of looking at the benefits of public health practice is to look at how early deaths can be prevented. The U.S. Public Health Service estimates that medical treatment can prevent only about 10% of all early deaths in the United States. However, population-focused public health approaches have the potential to help prevent approximately 70% of early deaths in America through measures targeted to the factors that contribute to those deaths. Many of these contributing factors are behavioral, such as tobacco use, diet, and sedentary lifestyle. Other factors that affect health are the environment, social conditions, education, culture, economics, working conditions, and housing (*Healthy People 2020*, USDHHS, 2010b).

> **DID YOU KNOW?**   *The concept of using a population (or aggregate) approach in the practice of public health nursing began to be seriously discussed in the 1970s.*

Public health practice is of great value. The Centers for Medicare and Medicaid Services (CMS) (2010) estimated that in 2008 only 3% (up from 1.5% in 1960) of all national health expenditures support population-focused public health functions, yet the impact is enormous. Unfortunately, the public is largely unaware of the contributions of public health practice. Federal and private monies were sparse in their support of public health, so public health agencies began to provide personal care services for persons who could not receive care elsewhere. The health departments benefited by getting Medicaid and Medicare funds. The result was a shift of resources and energy away from public health's traditional and unique population-focused perspective to include a primary care focus (USDHHS, 2002).

Because of the importance of influencing a population's health and providing a strong foundation for the health care system, the U.S. Public Health Service and other groups strongly advocated a renewed emphasis on the population-focused essential public health functions and services, which have been most effective in improving the health of the entire population. As part of this effort, a statement on public health in the United States was developed by a working group made up of representatives of federal agencies and organizations concerned about public health. The list of essential services presented in Figure 1-1 represents the obligations of the public health system to implement the core functions of assessment, assurance, and policy development. The How To box further explains these essential services and lists the ways public health nurses implement them (U.S. Public Health Service, 1994/update 2008).

> **HOW TO** **Participate, as a Public Health Nurse, in the Essential Services of Public Health**
>
> 1. *Monitor health status to identify community health problems.*
>   - *Participate in community assessment.*
>   - *Identify subpopulations at risk for disease or disability.*
>   - *Collect information on interventions to special populations.*
>   - *Define and evaluate effective strategies and programs.*
>   - *Identify potential environmental hazards.*
> 2. *Diagnose and investigate health problems and hazards in the community.*
>   - *Understand and identify determinants of health and disease.*
>   - *Apply knowledge about environmental influences of health.*
>   - *Recognize multiple causes or factors of health and illness.*
>   - *Participate in case identification and treatment of persons with communicable disease.*
> 3. *Inform, educate, and empower people about health issues.*
>   - *Develop health and educational plans for individuals and families in multiple settings.*
>   - *Develop and implement community-based health education.*
>   - *Provide regular reports on health status of special populations within clinic settings, community settings, and groups.*
>   - *Advocate for and with underserved and disadvantaged populations.*

PUBLIC HEALTH IN AMERICA

Vision:
Healthy people in healthy communities

Mission:
Promote physical and mental health and
prevent disease, injury, and disability

Public health
- Prevents epidemics and the spread of disease
- Protects against environmental hazards
- Prevents injuries
- Promotes and encourages healthy behaviors
- Responds to disasters and assists communities in recovery
- Ensures the quality and accessibility of health services

Essential public health services by core function
Assessment
1. Monitor health status to identify community health problems
2. Diagnose and investigate health problems and health hazards in the community

Policy Development
3. Inform, educate, and empower people about health issues
4. Mobilize community partnerships to identify and solve health problems
5. Develop policies and plans that support individual and community health efforts

Assurance
6. Enforce laws and regulations that protect health and ensure safety
7. Link people to needed personal health services and assure the provision of health care when otherwise unavailable
8. Assure a competent public health and personal health care workforce
9. Evaluate effectiveness, accessibility, and quality of personal and population-based health services

Serving All Functions
10. Research for new insights and innovative solutions to health problems

FIGURE 1-1 Public health in America. (From U.S. Public Health Service: *The core functions project,* Washington, DC, 1994/update 2000, Office of Disease Prevention and Health Promotion. Update 2008.)

- Ensure health planning, which includes primary prevention and early intervention strategies.
- Identify healthy population behaviors and maintain successful intervention strategies through reinforcement and continued funding.
4. Mobilize community partnerships to identify and solve health problems.
   - Interact regularly with many providers and services within each community.
   - Convene groups and providers who share common concerns and interests in special populations.
   - Provide leadership to prioritize community problems and development of interventions.
   - Explain the significance of health issues to the public and participate in developing plans of action.

5. Develop policies and plans that support individual and community health efforts.
   - Participate in community and family decision-making processes.
   - Provide information and advocacy for consideration of the interests of special groups in program development.
   - Develop programs and services to meet the needs of high-risk populations as well as broader community members.
   - Participate in disaster planning and mobilization of community resources in emergencies.
   - Advocate for appropriate funding for services.
6. Enforce laws and regulations that protect health and ensure safety.
   - Regulate and support safe care and treatment for dependent populations such as children and frail older adults.
   - Implement ordinances and laws that protect the environment.

- Establish procedures and processes that ensure competent implementation of treatment schedules for diseases of public health importance.
- Participate in development of local regulations that protect communities and the environment from potential hazards and pollution.

7. Link people to needed personal health services and ensure the provision of health care that is otherwise unavailable.
   - Provide clinical preventive services to certain high-risk populations.
   - Establish programs and services to meet special needs.
   - Recommend clinical care and other services to clients and their families in clinics, homes, and the community.
   - Provide referrals through community links to needed care.
   - Participate in community provider coalitions and meetings to educate others and to identify service centers for community populations.
   - Provide clinical surveillance and identification of communicable disease.

8. Ensure a competent public health and personal health care workforce.
   - Participate in continuing education and preparation to ensure competence.
   - Define and support proper delegation to unlicensed assistive personnel in community settings.
   - Establish standards for performance.
   - Maintain client record systems and community documents.
   - Establish and maintain procedures and protocols for client care.
   - Participate in quality assurance activities such as record audits, agency evaluation, and clinical guidelines.

9. Evaluate effectiveness, accessibility, and quality of personal and population-based health services.
   - Collect data and information related to community interventions.
   - Identify unserved and underserved populations within the community.
   - Review and analyze data on health status of the community.
   - Participate with the community in assessment of services and outcomes of care.
   - Identify and define enhanced services required to manage health status of complex populations and special risk groups.

10. Research for new insights and innovative solutions to health problems.
    - Implement nontraditional interventions and approaches to effect change in special populations.
    - Participate in the collecting of information and data to improve the surveillance and understanding of special problems.
    - Develop collegial relationships with academic institutions to explore new interventions.
    - Participate in early identification of factors that are detrimental to the community's health.
    - Formulate and use investigative tools to identify and impact care delivery and program planning.

From the Association of State and Territorial Directors of Nursing: Public health nursing: a partner for healthy populations, Washington, DC, 2000, ASTDN.

Definitions in Public Health

In 1988 the Institute of Medicine published a report on the future of public health, which is now seen as a classic and influential document. In the report, public health was defined as "what we, as a society, do collectively to assure the conditions in which people can be healthy" (IOM, 1988, p. 1). The committee stated that the mission of public health was "to generate organized community effort to address the public interest in health by applying scientific and technical knowledge to prevent disease and promote health" (IOM, 1988, p. 1; Williams, 1995).

It was clearly noted that the mission could be accomplished by many groups, public and private, and by individuals. However, the government has a special function "to see to it that vital elements are in place and that the mission is adequately addressed" (IOM, 1988, p. 7). To clarify the government's role in fulfilling the mission, the report stated that assessment, policy development, and assurance are the public health core functions at all levels of government.

- Assessment refers to systematically collecting data on the population, monitoring the population's health status, and making information available about the health of the community.
- Policy development refers to the need to provide leadership in developing policies that support the health of the population, including the use of the scientific knowledge base in making decisions about policy.
- Assurance refers to the role of public health in ensuring that essential community-oriented health services are available, which may include providing essential personal health services for those who would otherwise not receive them. Assurance also refers to making sure that a competent public health and personal health care workforce is available. More recently, Fielding (2009) made the case that assurance also should mean that public health officials should be involved in developing and monitoring the quality of services provided.

Public Health Core Functions

The Core Functions Project (U.S. Public Health Service, 1994/2008) developed a useful illustration, the Health Services Pyramid (Figure 1-2), which shows that population-based public health programs support the goals of providing a foundation for clinical preventive services. These services focus on disease prevention; on health promotion and protection; and on primary, secondary, and tertiary health care services. All levels of services shown in the pyramid are important to the health of the population and thus must be part of a health care system with health as a goal. It has been said that "the greater the effectiveness of services in the lower tiers, the greater is the capability of higher tiers to contribute efficiently to health improvement" (U.S. Public Health Service, 1994/2008). Because of the importance of the basic public health programs, members of the Core Functions Project argued that all levels of health care, including population-based public health care, must be funded or the goal of health of populations may never be reached.

Several new efforts to enable public health practitioners to be more effective in implementing the core functions of assessment, policy development, and assurance have been undertaken at the national level. In 1997 the Institute of Medicine published *Improving Health in the Community: A Role for Performance*

Monitoring (IOM, 1997). This monograph was the product of an interdisciplinary committee, co-chaired by a public health nursing specialist and a physician, whose purpose was to determine how a performance monitoring system could be developed and used to improve community health.

The major outcome of the committee's work was the Community Health Improvement Process (CHIP), a method for improving the health of the population on a community-wide basis. The method brings together key elements of the public health and personal health care systems in one framework. A second outcome of the project was the development of a set of 25 indicators that could be used in the community assessment process (see Chapter 18) to develop a community health profile (e.g., measures of health status, functional status, quality of life, health risk factors, and health resource use) (Box 1-1). A third product of the committee's work was a set of indicators for specific public health problems that could be used by public health specialists as they carry out their assurance function and monitor the performance of public health and other agencies.

In 2000 the Centers for Disease Control and Prevention (CDC) established a Task Force on Community Preventive Services (CDC, 2000). The Task Force worked to collect evidence on the effectiveness of a variety of community interventions to prevent morbidity and mortality. The effort has resulted in a versatile set of resources that can be used by public health specialists and others interested in a community-level approach to health improvement and disease prevention. Information is available on 16 topics, which include health problems/issues such as obesity, vaccines, asthma, cancer, diabetes, and concerns such as violence, tobacco, nutrition, and worksite initiatives (CDC, 2005). The materials, which include systematic reviews of research, can be used to help make choices about policies and programs that have been shown to be effective (CDC, 2010). The material can be found at the project's website, www.thecommunityguide.org/index.html. Collaborative efforts such as the Task Force on Community Preventive Services are important because they provide tools for public

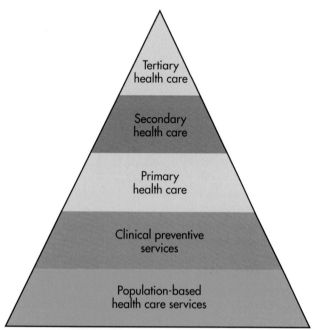

FIGURE 1-2 Health Services Pyramid.

BOX 1-1   INDICATORS USED TO DEVELOP A COMMUNITY HEALTH PROFILE

Sociodemographic Characteristics
- Distribution of the population by age and race/ethnicity
- Number and proportion of persons in groups such as migrants, homeless, or the non–English speaking, for whom access to community services and resources may be a concern
- Number and proportion of persons aged 25 and older with less than a high school education
- Ratio of the number of students graduating from high school to the number of students who entered ninth grade 3 years previously
- Median household income
- Proportion of children less than 15 years of age living in families at or below the poverty level
- Unemployment rate
- Number and proportion of single-parent families
- Number and proportion of persons without health insurance

Health Status
- Infant death rate by race/ethnicity
- Numbers of deaths or age-adjusted death rates for motor vehicle crashes, work-related injuries, suicide, homicide, lung cancer, breast cancer, cardiovascular diseases, and all causes, by age, race, and sex as appropriate
- Reported incidence of AIDS, measles, tuberculosis, and primary and secondary syphilis, by age, race, and sex as appropriate
- Births to adolescents (ages 10 to 17) as a proportion of total live births
- Number and rate of confirmed abuse and neglect cases among children

Health Risk Factors
- Proportion of 2-year-old children who have received all age-appropriate vaccines, as recommended by the Advisory Committee on Immunization Practices
- Proportion of adults aged 65 and older who have ever been immunized for pneumococcal pneumonia; proportion who have been immunized in the past 12 months for influenza
- Proportion of the population who smoke, by age, race, and sex as appropriate
- Proportion of the population aged 18 and older who are obese
- Number and type of U.S. Environmental Protection Agency air quality standards not met
- Proportion of assessed rivers, lakes, and estuaries that support beneficial uses (e.g., approved fishing and swimming)

Health Care Resource Consumption
- Per capita health care spending for Medicare beneficiaries—the Medicare-adjusted average per capita cost (AAPCC)

Functional Status
- Proportion of adults reporting that their general health is good to excellent
- Average number of days (in the past 30 days) for which adults report that their physical or mental health was not good

Quality of Life
- Proportion of adults satisfied with the health care system in the community
- Proportion of persons satisfied with the quality of life in the community

health practitioners, many of whom are public health nursing specialists, to enable them to be more effective in dealing with the core functions.

Core Competencies of Public Health Professionals

To improve the public health workforce's abilities to implement the core functions of public health and to ensure that the workforce has the necessary skills to provide the 10 essential services listed in Figure 1-1, a coalition of representatives from 17 national public health organizations has been working since 1992 on collaborative activities to "assure a well-trained, competent workforce and a strong, evidence-based public health infrastructure." (USPHS, 1994/2008). In the spring of 2010 this Council, funded by the CDC and DHHS, adopted an updated set of Core Competencies ("a set of skills desirable for the broad practice of public health") (Council on Linkages, 2010) for all public health professionals, including nurses. The 72 Core Competencies are divided into eight categories (Box 1-2). In addition, each competency is presented at three levels (tiers), which reflect the different stages of a career. Specifically, Tier 1 applies to entry level public health professionals without management responsibilities. Tier 2 competencies are expected in those with management and/or supervisory responsibilities, and Tier 3 is expected of senior managers and/or leaders in public health organizations. It is recommended that these categories of competencies be used by educators for curriculum review and development and by agency administrators for workforce needs assessment, competency development, performance evaluation, hiring, and refining of the personnel system job requirements. A detailed listing of these competencies can be found at www.phf.org/link/index.htm.

Using an earlier version of the Council on Linkage's Core Competencies as a starting point, a group of public health nursing organizations called the Quad Council developed levels of skills to be attained by public health nurses for each of the competencies. Skill levels are specified for the generalist/staff nurse and the specialist in public health nursing (Quad Council, 2003/2009). See Resource Tool 45.A on the Evolve website for the Public Health Nursing Core Competencies.

National Public Health Performance Standards Program

In the same time period, the Institute of Medicine released a report, "Who Will Keep the Public Healthy?" (2003b) that identified eight content areas in which public health workers should be educated—informatics, genomics (Box 1-3), cultural competence, community-based participatory research, policy, law, global health, and ethics—in order to be able to address the emerging public health issues and advances in science and policy.

Another broad initiative within the field of public health is the National Public Health Performance Standards Program, a high-level partnership initiative started in 1998 and led by the Office of Chief of Public Health Practice, CDC. The collaborative partners are the American Public Health Association, Association of State and Territorial Health Officials, National Association of County and City Health Officials, National Association of Local Boards of Health, National

---

BOX 1-2   CATEGORIES OF PUBLIC HEALTH WORKFORCE COMPETENCIES

- Analytic/assessment
- Policy development/program planning
- Communication
- Cultural competency
- Community dimensions of practice
- Basic public health sciences
- Financial planning and management
- Leadership and systems thinking

Compiled from Centers for Disease Control and Prevention: *Genomics and disease prevention: Frequently asked questions,* 2010. Accessed 1/11/11 from http://www.cdc.gov/genomics/faq.htm; Centers for Disease Control and Prevention: *Genomics and disease prevention. Genomic competencies for the public health workforce,* 2009. Accessed 1/11/10 from http://www.cdc.gov/genomics/training/competencies/intro.htm.

Network of Public Health Institutes, and the Public Health Foundation. The overall goal of the program is "to improve the practice of public health, the performance of public health systems, and the infrastructure supporting public health actions" (CDC, Governance—Public Health Performance Assessment, 2005). The performance standards, collectively developed by the participating organizations, set the bar for the level of performance that is necessary to deliver essential public health services. Four principles guided the development of the standards. First, they were developed around the ten Essential Public Health Services (see previous How To box). Second, the standards focus on the overall public health system rather than on single organizations. Third, the standards describe an optimal level of performance. Finally, they are intended to support a process of quality improvement.

States and local communities seeking to assess their performance can access the Assessment Instruments developed by the program and other resources such as training workshops, on-site training, and technical assistance to work with them in conducting assessments (CDC, 2010).

THE CUTTING EDGE   *The Council on Linkages (2001, updated 2010) developed a set of competencies for all public health professionals. The Quad Council developed skill levels for each of the 34 competencies needed by public health nurses.*

From Council on Linkages Between Academia and Public Health Practice: Core competencies for public health professional, Washington, DC, 2001, updated 2010 Public Health Foundation/Health Resources and Services Administration; Quad Council of Public Health Nursing Organizations: Scope and standards of public health nursing practice, Washington, DC, 1999, revised 2005, American Nurses Association, 2007.

PUBLIC HEALTH NURSING AS A FIELD OF PRACTICE: AN AREA OF SPECIALIZATION

Most of the proceeding discussion has been about the broad field of public health. Now the attention turns to public health nursing. What is public health nursing? Is it really a specialty,

BOX 1-3   GENOMICS IN PUBLIC HEALTH

The work of the Human Genome Project, which was completed in 2003 and identified all of the genes in human DNA, has provided information about the role of genes in health and disease that is now essential for all public health workers. Genetic and genomic science is leading to new understanding of the health and human illness continuum. All nurses need to use genetic and genomic information and technology when providing care. Why is genomics important? The Centers for Disease Control and Prevention (CDC) defines genetics as "the study of inheritance, or the way traits are passed down from one generation to another" (CDC, 2006) or the study of individual genes and their impact on relatively rare single gene disorders (Guttmacher and Collins, 2002). Genomics is a newer term that "describes the study of all the genes in a person, as well as interactions of those genes with each other and with that person's environment" (CDC, 2006b). Genomics would include the influence of psychosocial and cultural factors (Guttmacher and Collins, 2002). Because of the crucial importance of the study of the broader concept—genomics—to public health, the CDC has identified competencies, or the applied skills and knowledge, that members of the public health workforce need to effectively practice public health. Overall, a public health worker should be able to perform the following:

- Demonstrate basic knowledge of the role that genomics plays in the development of disease.
- Identify the limits of his/her genomic expertise.
- Make appropriate referrals to those with more genomic expertise.

All public health professionals should be able to perform the following:

- Apply the basic public health sciences (including behavioral and social sciences, biostatistics, epidemiology, informatics, environmental health) to genomic issues and studies and genetic testing, using the genomic vocabulary to attain the goal of disease prevention.

- Identify ethical and medical limitations to genetic testing, including uses that do not benefit the individual.
- Maintain up-to-date knowledge on the development of genetic advances and technologies relevant to his/her specialty or field of expertise and learn the uses of genomics as a tool for achieving public health goals related to his/her field or area of practice.
- Identify the role of cultural, social, behavioral, environmental, and genetic factors in development of disease, disease prevention, and health-promoting behaviors, as well as their impact on medical service organizations and delivery of services to maximize wellness and prevent disease.
- Participate in strategic policy planning and development related to genetic testing or genomic programs.
- Collaborate with existing and emerging health agencies and organizations; academic, research, private, and commercial enterprises (including genomic-related businesses); and agencies, organizations, and community partnerships to identify and solve genomic-related problems.
- Participate in the evaluation of program effectiveness, accessibility, cost benefit, cost-effectiveness, and quality of personal and population-based genomic services in public health.
- Develop protocols to ensure informed consent and human subject protection in research.

In addition, the CDC lists genomic competencies for the following groups: (1) public health leaders/administrators, (2) public health professionals in clinical services evaluating individuals and families, (3) individuals in epidemiology and data management, (4) individuals in population-based health education, (5) individuals in laboratory sciences, and (6) public health professionals in environmental health. Many of the following chapters will have boxes that list the competencies pertaining to the content of the chapter.

Compiled from Centers for Disease Control and Prevention: *Genomics and disease prevention: Frequently asked questions,* 2010. Accessed 1/11/11 from http://www.cdc.gov/genomics/faq.htm; Centers for Disease Control and Prevention: *Genomics and disease prevention. Genomic competencies for the public health workforce,* 2009. Accessed 1/11/11 from http://www.cdc.gov/genomics/training/competencies/intro.htm; and Guttmacher A, Collins F: Genomic medicine: a primer, *N Engl J Med* 347:1512-1520, 2002.

and if so, why? Public health nursing is a specialty because it has a distinct focus and scope of practice, and it requires a special knowledge base. The following characterizations distinguish public health nursing as a specialty:

- *It is population-focused.* Primary emphasis is on populations whose members are free-living in the community as opposed to those who are institutionalized.
- *It is community-oriented.* There is concern for the connection between the health status of the population and the environment in which the population lives (physical, biological, sociocultural). There is an imperative to work with members of the community to carry out core public health functions.
- *There is a health and preventive focus.* The primary emphasis is on strategies for health promotion, health maintenance, and disease prevention, particularly primary and secondary prevention.
- *Interventions are made at the community or population level.* Political processes are used as a major intervention strategy to affect public policy and achieve goals.
- *There is concern for the health of all members of the population/community, particularly vulnerable subpopulations.*

NURSING TIP   *The primary features of public health nursing as a specialty are population focus, community orientation, health promotion and disease prevention emphasis, and population-level concern and interventions, which frequently are at the level of public policy, such as anti-smoking laws, the requirement of immunizations for entry to school, and seat belt legislation.*

In 1981 the public health nursing section of the American Public Health Association (APHA) developed *The Definition and Role of Public Health Nursing in the Delivery of Health Care* to describe the field of specialization (APHA, 1981). This statement was reaffirmed in 1996 (APHA, 1996). In 1999 the American Nurses Association, with input from three other nursing organizations—the Public Health Nursing Section of the APHA, the Association of State and Territorial Directors of Public Health Nursing, and the Association of Community Health Nurse Educators—published the *Scope and Standards of Public Health Nursing Practice* (Quad Council, 1999). In this document, the 1996 definition was supported. The scope and standards have been revised and continue to support the above definition. Public health nursing is defined as the practice of promoting and protecting the health of populations using knowledge from nursing, social, and public health sciences (APHA, 1996). Public health nursing is further described as **population-focused practice** that emphasizes the promotion of health, the prevention of disease and disability, and the creation of conditions in which all people can be healthy (Quad Council, 1999, rev 2005). Public health nursing practice takes place through assessment, policy development, and assurance activities of nurses working in partnerships with many others within communities, individuals, families, various community organizations, and groups of concerned citizens, community officials, and other community leaders.

Educational Preparation for Public Health Nursing

Targeted and specialized education for public health nursing practice has a long history. In the late 1950s and early 1960s, before the integration of public health concepts into the curriculum of baccalaureate nursing programs, special baccalaureate curricula were established in several schools of public health to prepare nurses to become public health nurses. Today it is generally assumed that a graduate of any baccalaureate nursing program has the necessary basic preparation to function as a beginning staff public health nurse.

Since the late 1960s, public health nursing leaders have agreed that a specialty in public health nursing requires a master's degree. Today, a master's degree in nursing is necessary to be eligible to sit for a certification examination. In the future, the Doctor of Nursing Practice (DNP), which the American Association of Colleges of Nursing has proposed as the expected level of education for specialization in an area of nursing practice (AACN, 2004, 2006), will probably be required to sit for certification. The educational expectations for public health nursing were highlighted at the 1984 Consensus Conference on the Essentials of Public Health Nursing Practice and Education sponsored by the U.S. Department of Health and Human Services (USDHHS) Division of Nursing. The participants agreed "that the term 'public health nurse' should be used to describe a person who has received specific educational preparation and supervised clinical practice in public health nursing" (Consensus Conference, 1985, p. 4). At the basic or entry level, a public health nurse is one who "holds a baccalaureate degree in nursing that includes this educational preparation; this nurse may or may not practice in an official health agency but has the initial qualifications to do so" (Consensus Conference, 1985, p. 4). Specialists in public health nursing are defined as those who are prepared at the graduate level, with either a master's or a doctoral degree, "with a focus in the public health sciences" (Consensus Conference, 1985, p. 4) (Box 1-4). The consensus statement specifically pointed out that the public health nursing specialist "should be able to work with population groups and to assess and intervene successfully at the aggregate level" (Consensus Conference, 1985, p. 11).

The Association of Community Health Nursing Educators reaffirmed the results of the 1984 Consensus Conference (ACHNE, 2003). The educational requirements are reaffirmed by ACHNE (2009) and in the revised *Scope and Standards of Public Health Nursing Practice* and include both clinical specialists and nurse practitioners who engage in population-focused care as advanced practice registered nurses in public health (Quad Council, 1999, rev 2005). The latest iteration of the *Scope and Standards of Practice for Public Health Nursing* was published by the American Nurses Association in 2007 (ANA, 2007).

BOX 1-4   AREAS CONSIDERED ESSENTIAL FOR THE PREPARATION OF SPECIALISTS IN PUBLIC HEALTH NURSING

- Epidemiology
- Biostatistics
- Nursing theory
- Management theory
- Change theory
- Economics
- Politics
- Public health administration
- Community assessment
- Program planning and evaluation
- Interventions at the aggregate level
- Research
- History of public health
- Issues in public health

From Consensus Conference on the Essentials of Public Health Nursing Practice and Education, Rockville, MD, 1985, U.S. Department of Health and Human Services, Bureau of Health Professions, Division of Nursing.

LEVELS OF PREVENTION

Examples in Public Health

Primary Prevention
The public health nurse develops a health education program for a population of school-age children that teaches them about the effects of smoking on health.

Secondary Prevention
The public health nurse provides toxin screenings for migrant workers who may be exposed to pesticides.

Tertiary Prevention
The public health nurse provides a diabetes clinic for a defined population of adults in a low-income housing unit of the community.

Population-Focused Practice Versus Practice Focused on Individuals

The key factor that distinguishes public health nursing from other areas of nursing practice is the focus on populations, a focus historically consistent with public health philosophy. Box 1-5 lists principles upon which public health nursing is built. Although public health nursing is based on clinical nursing practice, it also incorporates the population perspective of public health. It may be helpful here to define the term *population*.

BOX 1-5   EIGHT PRINCIPLES OF PUBLIC HEALTH NURSING

1. The client or "unit of care" is the population.
2. The primary obligation is to achieve the greatest good for the greatest number of people or the population as a whole.
3. The processes used by public health nurses include working with the client(s) as an equal partner.
4. Primary prevention is the priority in selecting appropriate activities.
5. Selecting strategies that create healthy environmental, social, and economic conditions in which populations may thrive is the focus.
6. There is an obligation to actively reach out to all who might benefit from a specific activity or service.
7. Optimal use of available resources to assure the best overall improvement in the health of the population is a key element of the practice.
8. Collaboration with a variety of other professions, organizations, and entities is the most effective way to promote and protect the health of the people.

From Quad Council of Public Health Nursing Organizations: *Scope and standards of public health nursing practice*, Washington, DC, 1999, revised 2005, 2007 with the American Nurses Association.

A population, or aggregate, is a collection of individuals who have one or more personal or environmental characteristics in common. Members of a community who can be defined in terms of geography (e.g., a county, a group of counties, or a state) or in terms of a special interest or circumstance (e.g., children attending a particular school) can be seen as constituting a population. Often there are subpopulations within the larger population, such as—for example, high-risk infants under the age of 1 year, unmarried pregnant adolescents, or individuals exposed to a particular event such as a chemical spill. In population-focused practice, problems are defined (by assessments or diagnoses), and solutions (interventions), such as policy development or providing a particular preventive service, are implemented for or with a defined population or subpopulation (examples are provided in the Levels of Prevention box). In other nursing specialties, the diagnoses, interventions, and treatments are carried out at the individual client level.

Professional education in nursing, medicine, and other clinical disciplines focuses primarily on developing competence in decision making at the individual client level by assessing health status, making management decisions (ideally *with* the client), and evaluating the effects of care. Figure 1-3 illustrates three levels at which problems can be identified. For example, community-based nurse clinicians, or nurse practitioners, focus on individuals they see in either a home or a clinic setting. The focus is on an individual person or an individual family in a subpopulation (the *C* arrows in Figure 1-3). The provider's emphasis is on defining and resolving a problem for the individual; the client is an individual.

In Figure 1-3 the individual clients are grouped into three separate subpopulations, each of which has a common characteristic (the *B* arrows). Public health nursing specialists often define problems at the population or aggregate level as opposed to an individual level. Population-level decision making is different from decision making in clinical care. For example, in a

clinical, direct care situation, the nurse may determine that a client is hypertensive and explore options for intervening. However, at the population level, the public health nursing specialist might explore the answers to the following set of questions:

1. What is the prevalence of hypertension among various age, race, and sex groups?
2. Which subpopulations have the highest rates of untreated hypertension?
3. What programs could reduce the problem of untreated hypertension and thereby lower the risk of further cardiovascular morbidity and mortality for the population as a whole?

Public health nursing specialists are usually concerned with more than one subpopulation and frequently with the health of the entire community (in Figure 1-3, arrow *A*: the entire box containing all of the subgroups within the community). In reality, of course, there are many more subgroups than those in Figure 1-3. Professionals concerned with the health of a whole community must consider the total population, which is made up of multiple and often overlapping subpopulations. For example, the population of adolescents at risk for unplanned pregnancies would overlap with the female population 15 to 24 years of age. A population that would overlap with infants under 1 year of age would be children from 0 to 6 years of age. In addition, a population focus requires considering those who may need particular services but have not entered the health care system (e.g., children without immunizations or clients with untreated hypertension).

Public Health Nursing Specialists and Core Public Health Functions: Selected Examples

The core public health function of assessment includes activities that involve collecting, analyzing, and disseminating information on both the health status and the health-related aspects of a community or a specific population. Questions such as whether the health services of the community are available to the population and are adequate to address needs are considered. Assessment also includes an ongoing effort to monitor the health status of the community or population and the services provided. Excellent examples of assessment at the national level are the efforts of the USDHHS to organize the goal setting, data collecting and analysis, and monitoring necessary to develop the series of publications describing the health status and health-related aspects of the U.S. population. These efforts began with *Healthy People* in 1980 and continued with *Promoting Health, Preventing Disease: 1990 Health Objectives for the Nation, Healthy People 2000, Healthy People 2010,* and are now moving forward into the future with *Healthy People 2020* (USDHHS, 1979, 1991, 2000, 2010). (*Healthy People 2020* retrieved at http://www.healthy people.gov/hp2020/objectives/topicareas.aspx.)

Many states and other jurisdictions have developed publications describing the health status of a defined community, a set of communities, or populations. Unfortunately, it is difficult to find published descriptions of health assessments on particular communities unless they demonstrate new methods or reveal unusual findings about a community. Such working documents and data sets should be available in specific settings, such as a county or state health department, and should be used by public health practitioners to develop services.

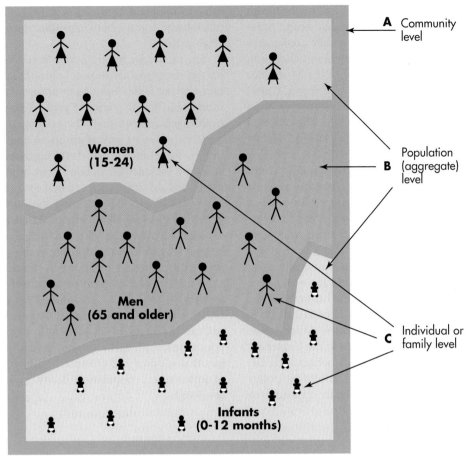

FIGURE 1-3 Levels of health care practice.

In 2004, Turnock (2009) described a survey conducted to determine the extent to which local health departments were performing the core public health functions. The questions asked about *assessment* included (1) whether there was a needs assessment process in place that described the health status of the community and community needs, (2) whether there had been a survey of behavioral risk factors within the last 3 years, and (3) whether an analysis had been done of "the determinants and contributing factors of priority health needs, adequacy of existing health resources, and the population groups most affected." The results were disappointing and suggested that in 1993 less than 40% of the population in the United States were served by a health department which was effectively addressing the core function of public health. In this study, compliance with the performance measures was highest for practices related to the assurance function and lowest for practices related to policy development (Turnock, 2009). It should be part of the public health nurse specialist's role within a local health department to participate in and provide leadership for assessing community needs, the health status of populations within the community, and environmental and behavioral risks; looking at trends in the health determinants; identifying priority health needs; and determining the adequacy of existing resources within the community (see the Evidence-Based Practice box), and engaging in policy-development efforts.

EVIDENCE-BASED PRACTICE

This research used a participatory approach to explore environmental health (EH) concerns among Lac Courte Oreilles (LCO) Ojibwa Indians in Sawyer County, Wisconsin. The project focused on health promotion and community participation. Community participation was accomplished through a steering committee that consisted of the primary author and LCO college faculty and community members. The assessment method used was a self-administered survey mailed to LCO members in Sawyer County.

Concern for environmental issues was high in this tribal community, and what they would mean to future generations. Concern was higher among older members and tribal members living on rather than off the reservation. Local issues of concern included environmental issues such as motorized water vehicles, effects from global warming, effects of aging septic systems on waterways, unsafe driving, and contaminated lakes/streams. Health concerns included diabetes, cancer, stress, obesity, and use of drugs and alcohol. The LCO community can use survey results to inform further data needs and program development.

Nurse Use

The community was most interested in developing a program on drug and alcohol use. The community participation in the assessment would promote a greater possibility that a drug and alcohol program would be successful.

Severtson C, et al: A participatory assessment of environmental health concerns in an Ojibwa community, *Public Health Nurs* 19:47-58, 2002.

Policy development is both a core function of public health and a core intervention strategy used by public health nursing specialists. Policy development in the public arena seeks to build constituencies that can help bring about change in public policy. In an interesting case study of her experience as director of public health for the state of Oregon, Christine Gebbie (1999), a nurse, describes her experiences in developing a constituency for public health. This enabled her to mobilize efforts to develop statewide goals for *Healthy People 2000* as well as to update Oregon's disease reporting laws. Gebbie's experiences as a state director of public health illustrate how a public health nursing specialist can provide leadership at a very broad level. Gebbie left Oregon to go to Washington, DC, to serve in the federal government as President Clinton's key official in the national effort to control acquired immunodeficiency syndrome (AIDS). Clearly, Gebbie is an example of an individual who has provided leadership in policy development at both state and national levels. Another public health nursing specialist who has and continues to provide strong policy leadership is Ellen Hahn, DNS, Director of the Kentucky Center for Smoke-Free Policy (www.mc.uky.edu/tobaccopolicy/), which is based at the University of Kentucky's College of Nursing. Through her research Dr. Hahn has developed evidence to support important policy changes (anti-smoking ordinances) to reduce exposure to tobacco smoke in Kentucky, a state that has a long tradition of a tobacco culture, both in production of tobacco and in use (Hahn, 2008).

The third core public health function, *assurance,* focuses on the responsibility of public health agencies to make certain that activities have been appropriately carried out to meet public health goals and plans. This may result in public health agencies requiring others to engage in activities to meet goals, encouraging private groups to undertake certain activities, or sometimes actually offering services directly. Assurance also includes the development of partnerships between public and private agencies to make sure that needed services are available and that assessing the quality of the activities is carried out (see the Evidence-Based Practice box, p 15). A recent report suggested that much more attention should be paid by public health officials to the quality of direct care services provided by clinicians in their communities (Fielding, 2009). It is important to point out that when personal services to individuals are offered by public health agencies to ensure that they can get care they might not receive without the intervention of the official agency, the goal is to "promote knowledge, attitudes, beliefs, practices and behaviors that support and enhance health with the ultimate goal of improving… population health" (Quad Council, 1999, rev 2005).

♥ HEALTHY PEOPLE 2020

In 1979 the surgeon general issued a report that began a 30-year focus on promoting health and preventing disease for all Americans. The report, entitled *Healthy People,* used morbidity rates to track the health of individuals through the five major life cycles of infancy, childhood, adolescence, adulthood, and older age.

In 1989 *Healthy People 2000* became a national effort of representatives from government agencies, academia, and health organizations. Their goal was to present a strategy for improving the health of the American people. Their objectives are being used by public and community health organizations to assess current health trends, health programs, and disease prevention programs.

Throughout the 1990s, all states used *Healthy People 2000* objectives to identify emerging public health issues. The success of the program on a national level was accomplished through state and local efforts. Early in the 1990s, surveys from public health departments indicated that 8% of the national objectives had been met, and progress on an additional 40% of the objectives was noted. In the mid-course review published in 1995, it was noted that significant progress had been made toward meeting 50% of the objectives.

In light of the progress made in the past decade, the committee for *Healthy People 2010* proposed the following two goals:
- To increase years of healthy life
- To eliminate health disparities among different populations

The hope was to reach these goals by such measures as promoting healthy behaviors, increasing access to quality health care, and strengthening community prevention.

The major premise of *Healthy People 2010* was that the health of the individual cannot be entirely separate from the health of the larger community. Therefore the vision for *Healthy People 2010* was "Healthy People in Healthy Communities."

The vision for *Healthy People 2020* is: A society in which all people live long, healthy lives.

The overarching goals for 2020 are:
- To eliminate preventable disease, disability injury, and premature death
- To achieve health equity, eliminate disparities, and improve the health of all groups
- To create social and physical environments that promote good health for all
- To promote healthy development and healthy behaviors across every stage of life

In contrast to previous years, *Healthy People 2020* has a web-accessible database which will be searchable, multilevel, and interactive to be more useful.

The first draft of the objectives for 2020 is now available on the website: www.healthypeople.gov/hp2020/advisory/phase1/default.htm.

Compiled from U.S. Department of Health and Human Services: *Healthy People 2000: national health promotion and disease prevention objectives,* DHHS Publication No. 91-50212, Washington, DC, 1991, U.S. Government Printing Office; U.S. Department of Health and Human Services: *Healthy People 2010: understanding and improving health,* ed 2, Washington, DC, 2000, U.S. Government Printing Office; and U.S. Department of Health, Education, and Welfare: *Phase 1 Report: Recommendations for the Framework and Format of Healthy People 2020,* www.healthypeople.gov/hp2020/advisory/phase1/default.htm; *Healthy People: the surgeon general's report on health promotion and disease prevention,* DHEW Publication No. 79-55071, Washington, DC, 1979, U.S. Government Printing Office.

EVIDENCE-BASED PRACTICE

The purpose of this study was to evaluate whether an 8-week support and education program could be beneficial for parents at high risk for parenting problems and at potential for child abuse. The participants were parents of infants and toddlers, and the project was aimed at alleviating parental stress and improving parent-child interaction among parents who attended an inner-city clinic. Participants were 199 parents of children 1 through 36 months of age. Serious life stress including poverty, low social support, personal histories of childhood maltreatment, and substance abuse defined the parents at risk. Program effects were evaluated in terms of improvement in self-reported parenting stress and observed parent-child interaction. Positive effects were documented for the group as a whole and within each of three subgroups: two community samples and a group of mothers and children in a residential drug treatment program. Program attendance and the amount of gain in observed parenting skills were the factors related to a positive outcome.

Nurse Use

This program was offered in partnership with academic researchers and the public clinic. The nurses in this agency can ensure better outcomes in parenting by providing a long-term program for high-risk parents.

From Huebner C: Evaluation of a clinic-based parent education program to reduce the risk of infant and toddler maltreatment, *Public Health Nurs* 19:377-389, 2002.

PUBLIC HEALTH NURSING AND COMMUNITY HEALTH NURSING VERSUS COMMUNITY-BASED NURSING

The concept of public health should include all populations within the community, both free-living and those living in institutions. Furthermore, the public health specialist should consider the match between the health needs of the population and the health care resources in the community, including those services offered in a variety of settings. Although all direct care providers may contribute to the community's health in the broadest sense, not all are primarily concerned with the population focus—the big picture. All nurses in a given community, including those working in hospitals, physicians' offices, and health clinics, may contribute positively to the health of the community. However, the special contributions of public health nursing specialists include looking at the community or population as a whole; raising questions about its overall health status and associated factors, including environmental factors (physical, biological, and sociocultural); and *working with the community* to improve the population's health status.

Figure 1-4 is a useful illustration of the arenas of practice. Because most community health nurses and many staff public health nurses, historically and at present, focus on providing direct personal care services—including health education—to persons or family units outside of institutional settings (either in the client's home or in a clinic environment), such practice falls into the upper right quadrant (section *B*) of Figure 1-4. However, specialization in public health nursing is population-focused and focuses on clients living in the community and is represented by the box in the upper left quadrant (section *A*) (see the Nursing Tip on p 10).

There are three reasons, in addition to the population focus, that the most important practice arena for public health nursing is represented by section *A* of Figure 1-4, the population of free-living clients:

1. Preventive strategies can have the greatest impact on free-living populations, which usually represent the majority of a community.
2. The major interface between health status and the environment (physical, biological, sociocultural) occurs in the free-living population.
3. For philosophical, historical, and economic reasons, prevention-oriented population-focused practice is most likely to flourish in organizational structures that serve free-living populations (e.g., health departments, health maintenance organizations, health centers, schools, and workplaces).

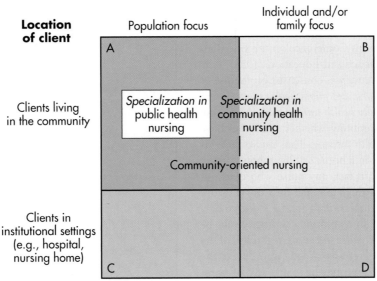

FIGURE 1-4 Arenas for health care practice.

What roles in the health care system do public health nursing specialists (those in section *A* of Figure 1-4) have? Options include director of nursing for a health department, director of the health department, state commissioner for health, director of maternal and child health services for a state or local health department, director of wellness for a business organization, and director of preventive services for an integrated health system. Nurses can occupy all of these roles, but, with the exception of director of nursing for a health department, they are in the minority. Unfortunately, nurses who occupy these roles are often seen as "administrators" and not as public health nursing specialists. However, those who work in such roles have the opportunity to make decisions that affect the health of population groups and the type and quality of health services provided for various populations.

Where does the staff public health nurse or community health nurse fit on the diagram? That depends on the focus of the nurse's practice. In many settings, most of the staff nurse's time is spent in community-based direct care activities, where the focus is on dealing with individual clients and individual families, in which the practice falls into section *B* of Figure 1-4. Although a staff public health nurse or a community health nurse may not be a public health nurse specialist, this nurse may spend some time carrying out core public health functions with a population focus, and thus that part of the role would be represented in section *A* of Figure 1-4. In summary, the field of public health nursing can be seen as primarily encompassing two groups of nurses:

- Public health nursing specialists, whose practice is community-oriented and uses population-focused strategies for carrying out the core public health functions (section *A*)
- Staff public health nurses or community health nurses, who are community-based, who may be clinically oriented to the individual client, and who combine some population-focused strategies and direct care clinical strategies in programs serving specified populations (section *B*)

Figure 1-4 also shows that specialization in public health nursing, as it has been defined in this chapter, can be viewed as a specialized field of practice with certain characteristics within the broad arena of community health nursing and community-based nursing. This view is consistent with recommendations developed at the Consensus Conference on the Essentials of Public Health Nursing Practice and Education (1985). One of the outcomes of the conference was consensus on the use of the terms *community health nurse* and *public health nurse*. It was agreed that the term *community health nurse* could apply to all nurses who practice in the community, whether or not they have had preparation in public health nursing. Thus nurses providing secondary or tertiary care in a home setting, school nurses, and nurses in clinic settings (in fact, any nurse who does not practice in an institutional setting) may fall into the category of *community health nurse*. Nurses with a master's degree or a doctoral degree who practice in community settings could be referred to as *community health nurse specialists*, regardless of the area of nursing in which the degree was earned. According to the conference statement: "The degree may be in any area of nursing, such as maternal/child health, psychiatric/mental health,

or medical-surgical nursing or some subspecialty of any clinical area" (Consensus Conference, 1985, p. 4). The definitions of the three areas of practice have changed, however, over time.

In 1998 the Quad Council began to develop a statement on the scope of public health nursing practice (Quad Council, 1999). The council attempted to clarify the differences between the term *public health nursing* and the term introduced into nursing's vocabulary during health care reform of the 1990s: *community-based nursing*. The authors recognized that the terms *public health nursing* and *community health nursing* had been used interchangeably since the 1980s to describe population-focused, community-oriented nursing practice and community-based practice. However, the Council decided to make a clearer distinction between community-oriented and community-based nursing practice. In contrast, **community-based nursing** care was described as the provision or assurance of personal illness care to individuals and families in the community, whereas community-oriented nursing was the provision of disease prevention and health promotion to populations and communities. It was suggested that there be two terms for the two levels of care in the community: *community-oriented care* and *community-based care*. Three role functions were suggested for nursing practice: public health nursing and community health nursing (both of which are considered community-oriented) and community-based nursing (see the list of definitions presented in Box 1-6).

BOX 1-6   DEFINITIONS OF THE FOUR KEY NURSING AREAS IN THE COMMUNITY

- *Community-oriented nursing practice* is a philosophy of nursing service delivery that involves the generalist or specialist public health and community health nurse. The nurse provides health care through community diagnosis and investigation of major health and environmental problems, health surveillance, and monitoring and evaluation of community and population health status for the purposes of preventing disease and disability and promoting, protecting, and maintaining health to create conditions in which people can be healthy.
- *Public health nursing practice* is the synthesis of nursing theory and public health theory applied to promoting and preserving the health of populations. The focus of public health nursing practice is the community as a whole and the effect of the community's health status (including health care resources) on the health of individuals, families, and groups. Care is provided within the context of preventing disease and disability and promoting and protecting the health of the community as a whole.
- *Community health nursing practice* is the synthesis of nursing theory and public health theory applied to promoting, preserving, and maintaining the health of populations through the delivery of personal health care services to individuals, families, and groups. The focus of community health nursing practice is the health of individuals, families, and groups and the effect of their health status on the health of the community as a whole.
- *Community-based nursing practice* is a setting-specific practice whereby care is provided for clients and families where they live, work, and attend school. The emphasis of community-based nursing practice is acute and chronic care and the provision of comprehensive, coordinated, and continuous services. Nurses who deliver community-based care are generalists or specialists in maternal/infant, pediatric, adult, or psychiatric/mental health nursing.

In Figure 1-4, the words *specialization in community health nursing* span boxes *A* and *B*. This suggests that there is a need and a place for a nursing specialty in community health; the nurse in this specialty is more than a clinical specialist with a master's degree who practices in a community-based setting, as was suggested by the Consensus Conference more than 25 years ago. Although in 1984 these nurses were referred to as community health nurses, today they are referred to as nurses in community-based practice. Those who provide community-oriented service to specific subpopulations in the community and who provide some clinical services to those populations may be seen as nurse specialists in community health. Although such practitioners may be community-based, they are also community-oriented as public health specialists but are usually focused on only one or two special subpopulations. Preparing for this specialty includes a master's or doctoral degree with emphasis in a direct care clinical area, such as school health or occupational health, and ideally some education in the public health sciences. Examples of roles such specialists might have in direct clinical care areas include case manager, supervisor in a home health agency, school nurse, occupational health nurse, parish nurse, and a nurse practitioner who also manages a nursing clinic.

| **WHAT DO YOU THINK?** *Are public health nursing, community health nursing, and community-based nursing practice all the same?* |

Sections *C* and *D* of Figure 1-4 represent institutionalized populations. Nurses who provide direct care to these clients in hospital settings fall into section *D*, and those who have administrative responsibility for nursing services in institutional settings fall into section *C*. See Box 1-6 for detailed definitions of the four key nursing areas in the community that are depicted in Figure 1-4.

ROLES IN PUBLIC HEALTH NURSING

In community-oriented nursing circles, there has been a tendency to talk about public health and community health nursing from the point of view of a role rather than the functions related to the role. This can be limiting. In discussing such nursing roles, there is a preoccupation with the direct care provider orientation. Even in discussions about how a practice can become more population focused, the focus is frequently on how an individual practitioner, such as an agency staff nurse, can adopt a population-focused practice philosophy. Rarely is attention given to how nurse administrators in public health (one role for public health nursing specialists) might reorient their practice toward a population focus, which is particularly important and easier for an administrator to do than for the staff nurse. This is because many agencies' nursing administrators, supervisors, or others (sometimes program directors who are not nurses) make the key decisions about how staff nurses will spend their time and what types of clients will be seen and under what circumstances. Public health nursing administrators who are prepared to practice in a population-focused manner will be more effective than those who are not prepared to do so.

Although their opportunities to make decisions at the population level are limited, staff nurses benefit from having a clear understanding of population-focused practice for three reasons:

- First, it gives them professional satisfaction to see how their individual client care contributes to health at the population level.
- Second, it helps them appreciate the practice of others who are population-focused specialists.
- Third, it gives them a better foundation from which to provide clinical input into decision making at the program or agency level and thus to improve the effectiveness and efficiency of the population-focused practice.

A curriculum was proposed by representatives of key public health nursing organizations and other individuals that would prepare the staff public health nurse or generalist to function as a community-oriented practitioner (Association of State and Territorial Directors of Nursing, 2000). Box 1-7 lists the areas of study (which can be found in this book) that are essential to prepare the public health nurse generalist at the baccalaureate level.

Unfortunately, nursing roles as presently defined are often too limited to include population-focused practice, but it is important not to think too narrowly. Furthermore, roles that entail population-focused decision making may not be defined as nursing roles (e.g., directors of health departments, state or regional programs, and units of health planning and evaluation; directors of programs such as preventive services within a managed care organization). If population-focused public health nursing is to be taken seriously, and if strategies for assessment, policy development, and assurance are to be implemented at the population level, more consideration must be given to organized systems for assessing population needs and managing care. Clearly, public health nurse specialists must move into positions where they can influence policy formation.

BOX 1-7 AREAS OF STUDY TO PREPARE THE PUBLIC HEALTH STAFF NURSE
• Epidemiology
• Skills to effect organizational change
• Measurement of health status and organizational change
• How people connect to organizations
• Environmental health
• Policy
• Negotiation, collaboration, communication
• Advocacy
• Data analysis, statistics
• Health economics
• Interdisciplinary teams
• Program evaluation
• Coalition building
• Population-based principles, interventions
• Politics of health
• How to build on differences, diversity
• Quality-improvement approach

This means, however, that some nurses will have to assume positions that are not traditionally considered nursing.

Redefining nursing roles so that population-focused decision making fits into the present structure of nursing services may not be difficult in some circumstances at the present time, but future needs will require that nurses be prepared to make such decisions (IOM, 2010). At this point, it may be more useful to concentrate on identifying the skills and knowledge needed to make decisions in population-focused practice (see Appendix G.1), to define where in the health care system such decisions are made, and then to equip nurses with the knowledge, skills, and political understanding necessary for success in such positions. Although some of these positions are in nursing settings (e.g., administrator of the nursing service and top-level staff nurse supervisors), others are outside of the traditional nursing roles (e.g., director of a health department).

CHALLENGES FOR THE FUTURE

Barriers to Specializing in Public Health Nursing

One of the most serious barriers to the development of specialists in public health nursing is the mindset of many nurses that the only role for a nurse is at the bedside or at the client's side (i.e., the direct care role). Indeed, the heart of nursing is the direct care provided in personal contacts with clients. On the other hand, two things should be clear. First, whether a nurse is able to provide direct care services to a particular client depends on decisions made by individuals within and outside of the care system. Second, nurses need to be involved in those fundamental decisions. Perhaps the one-on-one focus of nursing and the historical expectations of the "proper" role of women have influenced nurses to view less positively other ways of contributing, such as administration, consultation, and research. Fortunately, things are changing. Within and outside of nursing, women have taken on every role imaginable. Further, the number of male nurses is steadily growing; nursing can no longer be viewed as a profession practiced by women exclusively. These two developments have opened doors to new roles that may not have been considered appropriate for nurses in the past.

A second barrier to population-focused public health nursing practice consists of the structures within which nurses work and the process of role socialization within those structures. For example, the absence of a particular role in a nursing unit may suggest that the role is undesirable or inaccessible to nurses. In another example, nurses interested in using political strategy to make changes in health-related policy—an activity clearly within the domain of public health nursing—may run into obstacles if their goals differ from those of other groups. Such groups may subtly but effectively lead nurses to conclude that their involvement takes their attention away from the client and it is not in their own or in the client's best interest.

A third barrier is that few nurses receive graduate-level preparation in the concepts and strategies of the disciplines basic to public health (e.g., epidemiology, biostatistics, community development, service administration, and policy formation). As mentioned previously, master's level programs for public health nursing do not give the in-depth attention to population

assessment and management skills that other parts of the curriculum, particularly the direct care aspects, receive. In 1995 Josten et al noted that with few exceptions, graduate programs in public health and community health nursing have not aggressively developed the population-focused skills that are needed. A web review of master's programs in public health nursing in April 2006 indicated the number of programs with a population focus was declining. For individuals who want to specialize in public health nursing, these skills are as essential as direct care skills, and they should be given more attention in graduate programs that prepare nurses for careers in public health. Fortunately, the curricular expectations for academic programs leading to the Doctor of Nursing Practice (DNP) include serious attention to preparing nurses to develop a population perspective as well as the analytical, policy, and leadership skills necessary to be successful as a specialist in public health nursing (AACN, 2006).

Developing Population-Focused Nurse Leaders

The massive organizational changes occurring in the health delivery system present a unique opportunity to establish new roles for nurse leaders who are prepared to think in population terms. In a book that is now viewed as a classic, Starr (1982) described the trend toward the use of private capital in financing health care, particularly institution-based care and other health-related businesses. The movement can be thought of as the "industrialization" of health care, which currently is operated very much like a cottage industry, or a small business. Health care reform is seeking to change this focus.

The implications and consequences of this movement are enormous. First, the goal was to provide investors a return on their investment. Other aspects included more attention to the delivery of primary and community-based care in a variety of settings; less emphasis on specialty care; the development of partnerships, alliances, and other linkages across settings in an effort to build integrated systems, which would provide a broad range of services for the population served; and an increasing adoption of capitation, a payment arrangement in which insurers agree to pay providers a fixed sum for each person per month or per year, independent of the costs actually incurred. With the spread of capitation, health professionals have become more interested in the concept of populations, sometimes referred to by financial officers and others as *covered lives* (i.e., individuals with insurance that pays on a capitated basis). For public health specialists, it is a new experience to see individuals involved in the business aspects of health care, and frequently employed by hospitals, thinking in population terms and taking a population approach to decision making.

This new focus on populations, coupled with the integration of acute, chronic, and primary care that is occurring in some health care systems, is likely to create new roles for individuals, including nurses, who will span inpatient and community-based settings and focus on providing a wide range of services to the population served by the system. Such a role might be director of client care services for a health care system, who would have administrative responsibility for a large program area. There will also be a demand for individuals who can design programs of preventive and clinical services to be offered to targeted subpopulations and those who can implement the services. Who will decide what services will be given to which subpopulation and by which providers? How will nurses be prepared for leadership in the emerging and future structures for health care delivery and health maintenance?

Physician leaders are recognizing that physicians need to be prepared to use population-focused methods, such as epidemiology and biostatistics, to make evidence-based decisions in the development of programs and protocols. The attention being given to preparing nurses for administrative decision making seems to be declining. This may be a result of (1) the recent lack of federal support for preparing nurse administrators, and (2) the growing popularity of nurse practitioner programs. However, it is time that nurse leaders give more attention to preparing nurses for leadership in the area of population-focused practice. Perhaps it is time to combine the specialty in public health nursing and nursing administration. As suggested some time ago by Williams (1985), some DNP programs are combining much of the preparation for specialization in public health nursing and administration into a systems-oriented curriculum with differentiation in the application to practice. This makes sense because regardless of how the population is defined, there will be a growing need for nurses with population-level assessment, management, and evaluation skills to assume leadership roles (IOM, 2010).

The primary focus of the health care system of the future will be on community-oriented strategies for health promotion and disease prevention, and on community-based strategies for primary and secondary care. Directing more attention to developing the specialty of public health nursing as a way to provide nursing leadership may be a good response to the health care system changes. Preparing nurses for population-focused decision making will require greater attention to developing programs at the doctoral level that have a stronger foundation in the public health sciences, while providing better preparation of baccalaureate-level nurses for community-oriented as well as community-based practice.

Some observers of public health have anticipated that if access to health care for all Americans becomes a reality, public health practitioners can turn over the delivery of personal primary care services to other providers such as health maintenance organizations and integrated health plans, and return to the core public health functions. However, assurance (making sure that basic services are available to all) is a core function of public health. Thus even under the condition of improved access to care, there will still be a need to monitor subpopulations in the community to ensure that necessary care is available and that its quality is at an acceptable level. When these conditions are not met, public health practitioners will have to find a solution.

Shifting Public Policy Toward Creating Conditions for a Healthy Population

A major challenge for the future is the need for public health nursing specialists to be more aggressive in their practice of the core public health function of policy development, one of the major ways public health specialists intervene, with the focus on actively engaging in influencing public decisions that will create conditions for a healthy population. This is necessary at the local, state, and national levels and encompasses a wide range of concerns from the availability of adequate nutrition to the maintenance of a healthy and safe environment in schools, to the reduction of secondhand smoke, to assuring access to needed health services. Policy development is not a solitary activity; it involves working with many groups and coalitions. Also, policy development is not just the responsibility of public health specialists; it is important that all professional nurses become more serious and adept in the process of policy development.

In the just released report, *The Future of Nursing: Leading Change, Advancing Health* (IOM, 2010) a key message is that "Nurses should be full partners, with physicians and other health professionals, in redesigning health care in the United States" (pp 1-11). In discussing this message, the report states that "to be effective in re-conceptualized roles, nurses must see policy as something they can shape rather than something that happens to them" (pp 1-11). In other words, nurses need to be key actors. However, the report also makes clear that nurses need to be prepared for leadership in that area.

The history of public health nursing shows that a common attribute of leaders is to move forward to deal with unresolved problems in a positive, proactive way. This is the legacy of Lillian Wald at the Henry Street Settlement, and many others who have met a need by being innovative. Within the context of the core public health function of policy-making, public health nursing clearly has an opportunity to affect public decisions that will help create conditions for a healthy population and influence the provision of needed services to populations in the community, particularly those that are most vulnerable. As a specialty, public health nursing can have a positive impact on the health status of populations, but to do so "it will be necessary to have broad vision; to prepare nurses for leadership roles in policy making and in the design, development, management, monitoring, and evaluation of population-focused health care systems and to develop strategies to support nurses in these roles" (Williams, 1992, p 268).

LINKING CONTENT TO PRACTICE

In this chapter emphasis is placed on defining and explaining public health nursing practice with populations. The three essential functions of public health and public health nursing are assessment, policy development, and assurance. The Council on Linkages: Core Competencies for Public Health Professionals revised June 11, 2009 describes the skills of public health professionals, including nurses. In assessment function, one skill is assessment of the health status of populations and their related determinants of health and illness. For policy development, one of the skills is development of a plan to implement policy and programs. For the assurance function, one skill that public health nurses will need is to incorporate ethical standards of practice as the basis of all interactions with organizations, communities, and individuals. These skills can also be linked to the ten essential services of public health nursing found on pp 5-7. Assessment of health status is a skill needed for implementing essential service 1, the monitoring of health status to identify community problems. Development of a plan for policy and program implementation is a skill needed for essential service 5 to support individual and community health efforts. Incorporating ethical standards is done in essential service 3 when informing, educating, and empowering people about health issues.

CHAPTER REVIEW

PRACTICE APPLICATION

Population-focused nursing practice is different from clinical nursing care delivered in the community. If one accepts that the specialist in public health nursing is population-focused and has a unique body of knowledge, it is useful to debate where and how public health nursing specialists practice. How does their practice compare with that of the nurse specialist in community health nursing or community-based nursing?

A. In your public health class, debate with classmates which nurses in the following categories practice population-focused nursing:
   1. School nurse
   2. Staff nurse in home care
   3. Director of nursing for a home care agency
   4. Nurse practitioner in a health maintenance organization
   5. Vice president of nursing in a hospital
   6. Staff nurse in a public health clinic or community health center
   7. Director of nursing in a health department
   • Provide reasons for your choices.

B. Choose three categories in the preceding list, and interview at least one nurse in each of the categories. Determine the scope of practice for each nurse. Are these nurses carrying out population-focused practice? Could they? How?

Answers can be found on the Evolve site.

KEY POINTS

• Public health is what we, as a society, do collectively to ensure the conditions in which people can be healthy.

• Assessment, policy development, and assurance are the core public health functions; they are implemented at all levels of government.

• *Assessment* refers to systematically collecting data on the population, monitoring of the population's health status, and making available information about the health of the community.

• *Policy development* refers to the need to provide leadership in developing policies that support the health of the population; it involves using scientific knowledge in making decisions about policy.

• *Assurance* refers to the role of public health in making sure that essential community-wide health services are available, which may include providing essential personal health services for those who would otherwise not receive them. Assurance also refers to ensuring that a competent public health and personal health care workforce is available.

• Its setting is frequently viewed as the feature that distinguishes public health nursing from other specialties. A more useful approach is to use the following characteristics: a focus on populations that are free-living in the community, an emphasis on prevention, a concern for the interface between the health status of the population and the living environment (physical, biological, sociocultural), and the use of political processes to affect public policy as a major intervention strategy for achieving goals.

• According to the 1985 Consensus Conference sponsored by the Nursing Division of the U.S. Department of Health and Human Services, *specialists in public health nursing* are defined as those who are prepared at the graduate level, either master's or doctoral, "with a focus in the public health sciences" (Consensus Conference, 1985). This is still true today.

• Population-focused practice is the focus of specialists in public health nursing. This focus on populations and the emphasis on health protection, health promotion, and disease prevention are the fundamental factors that distinguish public health nursing from other nursing specialties.

• A *population* is defined as a collection of individuals who share one or more personal or environmental characteristics. The term *population* may be used interchangeably with the term *aggregate*.

CLINICAL DECISION-MAKING ACTIVITIES

1. Define the following for your personal understanding, and suggest ways to check whether your understanding is correct:
   A. Essential functions of public health
   B. Specialist in public health nursing
   C. Nurse specialist in the community

2. State your opinion about the similarities and/or differences between a clinical nursing role and the population-focused role of the public health nursing specialist. What are some of the complex issues in distinguishing between these roles?

3. Review the model of public health nursing practice of the APHA as described in this chapter. Can you elaborate on the differences between the staff nurse and the specialist nurse?

4. With three or four classmates, identify some nurses in your community who are in an administrative role and discuss with them the following:
   A. The way they define the populations they are serving
   B. Strategies they use to monitor the population's health status
   C. Strategies they use to ensure that the populations are receiving needed services
   D. Initiatives they are taking to address problems

5. Do additional questions need to be asked to determine their views on population-focused practice and the responsibilities of the staff nurse? Elaborate.

REFERENCES

American Association of Colleges of Nursing: *AACN position statement on the practice doctorate in nursing*, Washington, DC, 2004, AACN.

American Association of Colleges of Nursing: *The essentials of doctoral education for advanced nursing practice*, Washington, DC, 2006, AACN.

American Public Health Association: *The definition and role of public health nursing in the delivery of health care: a statement of the public health nursing section*, Washington, DC, 1981, APHA.

American Public Health Association: *The definition and role of public health nursing: a statement of the APHA public health nursing section, March 1996 update*, Washington, DC, 1996, APHA.

American Nurses Association: *Public Health Nursing: scope and standards of practice*, Washington, DC, 2007, ANA.

Association of Community Health Nursing Educators: *Essentials of baccalaureate nursing education for entry level community/public health nursing*, Wheat-Ridge, CO, 2009, ACHNE.

Association of Community Health Nursing Educators: *Essentials of Master's level nursing education for advanced community/public health nursing practice*, Lathrop, NY, 2003, ACHNE.

Association of State and Territorial Directors of Nursing: *Public health nursing: a partner for healthy populations*, Washington, DC, 2000, ASTDN.

Centers for Disease Control and Prevention: *Genomics and disease prevention: Frequently asked questions*, 2010. Accessed 1/11/11 from http://www.cdc.gov/genomics/faq.htm.

Centers for Disease Control and Prevention: *Genomics and disease prevention: Genomic competencies for the public health workforce*, 2009. Accessed 3/28/06 from http://www.cdc.gov/genomics/training/competnecies/intro.htm.

Centers for Disease Control and Prevention: *Governance: Public health performance assessment, national public health performance standards program*. Accessed 10/7/10 from www.phf.org/nphpsp/.

Centers for Disease Control and Prevention: *Guide to community preventive services 2000*, 2000. Retrieved 12/1/10 from http://www.cdc.gov/.

Centers for Disease Control and Prevention: *Guide to community preventive services 2005*, 2005. Retrieved 12/1/10 from http://www.thecommunityguide.org/library/book/default.htm.

Centers for Disease Control and Prevention: *Guide to community preventive services*, 2010. Retrieved 10/7/10 from www.thecommunityguide.org/index.html.

Centers for Medicare and Medicaid Services, Office of the Actuary, National Health Statistics Group: *National health care expenditures data*, Washington, DC, January, 2010, CMS. Accessed 10/6/10 from www.kaiseredu.org/issue-modules/us-health-care-costs/background-brief.

Consensus Conference on the Essentials of Public Health Nursing Practice and Education, Rockville, MD, 1985, U.S. Department of Health and Human Services, Bureau of Health Professions, Division of Nursing.

Council on Linkages Between Academia and Public Health Practice: *Core competencies for public health professionals*, Washington, DC, 2010, Public Health Foundation/Health Resources and Services Administration.

Fielding J: Commentary: public health and health care quality assurance—strange bedfellows? *The Milbank Quarterly* 87:581–584, 2009.

Gebbie K: Building a constituency for public health, *J Public Health Manag Pract* 3:1, 1999.

Guttmacher A, Collins F: Genomic medicine: a primer, *New Engl J Med* 347:1512–1520, 2002.

Hahn EJ, Rayens MK, Butler KM, Zhang M, Durbin E, Steinke D: Smoke-free laws and adult smoking prevalence, *Preventive Medicine* 47:206–209, 2008.

Huebner C: Evaluation of a clinic-based parent education program to reduce the risk of infant and toddler maltreatment, *Public Health Nurs* 19:377–389, 2002.

Institute of Medicine: *The future of public health*, Washington, DC, 1988, National Academy Press.

Institute of Medicine: *Improving health in the community: a role for performance monitoring*, Washington, DC, 1997, National Academy Press.

Institute of Medicine: *The future of nursing: leading change, advancing health*, Washington, DC, 2010, National Academy Press.

Institute of Medicine: *Who will keep the public healthy?* Washington, DC, 2003, National Academy Press.

Josten L, et al: Public health nursing education: back to the future for public health sciences, *Fam Community Health* 18:36, 1995.

Kaiseredu.org. 2010: Health policy explained. Retrieved December 1, 2010.

Kentucky Center for Smoke-Free Policy. Retrieved October 7, 2010 from www.mc.uky.edu/tobaccopolicy/

National Public Health Performance Standards Program. Retrieved October 6, 2010 from www.phf.org/nphpsp/.

Orszag PR: *Health care and the budget: issues and challenges for reform. Statement before the Committee on the Budget, United States Senate*, Washington, DC, June 21, 2007, Congressional Budget Office.

Orszag PR, Emanuel EJ: Health care reform and cost control, *N Engl J Med* 363:601–603, 2010.

Patient Protection and Affordable Care Act & Health Care and Education Affordability Reconciliation Act, 2010. Retrieved December 1, 2010 from www. healthcare.gov.

Public Health Services Steering Committee: Public health in America, 1998. Retrieved 4/1/03 from http://www.health.gov/phfunctions/public.htm.

Quad Council of Public Health Nursing Organizations: *Scope and standards of public health nursing practice*, Washington, DC, 1999, American Nurses Association, revised 2005.

Quad Council of Public Health Nursing Organizations: *Competencies for Public Health Nursing Practice*, Washington, DC, 2003, ASTDN, revised 2009.

Severtson C, et al: A participatory assessment of environmental health concerns in an Ojibwa community, *Public Health Nurs* 19:47–58, 2002.

Starr P: *The social transformation of American medicine*, New York, 1982, Basic Books.

Turnock B: *Public health: what is it and how does it work?* ed 4, Boston, 2009, Jones and Bartlett.

U.S. Department of Health, Education, and Welfare: *Healthy People: the Surgeon General's report on health promotion and disease prevention*, DHEW Publication No. 79-55071, Washington, DC, 1979, U.S. Government Printing Office.

U.S. Department of Health and Human Services: *Healthy People 2000: national health promotion and disease prevention objectives*, DHHS Publication No. 91-50212, Washington, DC, 1991, U.S. Government Printing Office.

U.S. Department of Health and Human Services: *Healthy People 2010: understanding and improving health*, ed 2, Washington, DC, 2000, U.S. Government Printing Office.

U.S. Department of Health and Human Services: *Health US: 2000*, Washington, DC, 2002, National Center for Statistics.

U.S. Department of Health and Human Services: *National Center for Statistics*, Washington, DC, 2010a. Retrieved December 1, 2010 from http://www.cbsnews.com/stories/2005/12/08/health/printable1109413.shtml.

U.S. Department of Health and Human Services: *Healthy People 2020: the road ahead*, 2010b. Retrieved October 8, 2010 from www.healthypeople.gov/hp2020/default.asp.

U.S. Preventive Services Task Force: *Guide to clinical preventive services*, ed 3, Baltimore, 2000, Williams & Wilkins.

U.S. Public Health Service: *The core functions project*, Washington, DC, 1994/update 2008, Office of Disease Prevention and Health Promotion.

Williams CA: Population-focused community health nursing and nursing administration: a new synthesis. In McCloskey JC, Grace HK, editors: *Current issues in nursing*, ed 2, Boston, 1985, Blackwell Scientific.

Williams CA: Public health nursing: does it have a future? In Aiken LH, Fagin CM, editors: *Charting nursing's future: agenda for the 1990s*, Philadelphia, 1992, Lippincott.

Williams CA: Beyond the Institute of Medicine report: a critical analysis and public health forecast, *Fam Community Health* 18:12, 1995.

CHAPTER 2

History of Public Health and Public and Community Health Nursing

Janna Dieckmann, PhD, RN

Janna Dieckmann began her nursing practice in 1974 as a public health nurse with the Visiting Nurse Association of Cleveland, Ohio, and also practiced many years with the Visiting Nurse Association of Philadelphia. Today she is a clinical associate professor at The University of North Carolina at Chapel Hill, where she teaches public health nursing, health promotion, and health policy. She uses written and oral historical materials to research the history of public health nursing and care of the chronically ill, and to comment on contemporary health policy.

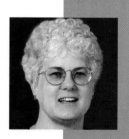

ADDITIONAL RESOURCES

ℯvolve WEBSITE
http://evolve.elsevier.com/Stanhope
- *Healthy People 2020*
- WebLinks
- Quiz
- Case Studies

- Glossary
- Answers to Practice Application

APPENDIX
- Appendix H: Focus on Quality and Safety Education for Nurses

OBJECTIVES

After reading this chapter, the student should be able to do the following:

1. Interpret the focus and roles of public health nurses through a historical approach.
2. Trace the ongoing interaction between the practice of public health and that of nursing.
3. Discuss the dynamic relationship between changes in social, political, and economic contexts and nursing practice in the community.
4. Outline the professional and practice impact of individual leadership on population-centered

nursing, especially the leadership of Florence Nightingale and Lillian Wald.
5. Identify structures for delivery of nursing care in the community such as settlement houses, visiting nurse associations, official health organizations, and schools.
6. Recognize major organizations that contributed to the growth and development of population-centered nursing.

KEY TERMS

American Nurses Association, p. 36
American Public Health Association, p. 29
American Red Cross, p. 28
district nursing, p. 25
district nursing association, p. 26
Florence Nightingale, p. 25
Frontier Nursing Service, p. 30

Lillian Wald, p. 27
Mary Breckinridge, p. 30
Metropolitan Life Insurance Company, p. 30
National League for Nursing, p. 36
National Organization for Public Health Nursing, p. 29
official (health) agencies, p. 32

settlement houses, p. 27
Sheppard-Towner Act, p. 30
Social Security Act of 1935, p. 32
Town and Country Nursing Service, p. 28
visiting nurse, p. 26
William Rathbone, p. 26
—*See Glossary for definitions*

Nurses use historical approaches to examine both the profession's present and its future. In doing so, several different questions are asked: First, who is the population-centered nurse? In the past, population-centered nurses have been called public health nurses, district nurses, and visiting nurses; sometimes they have even been called school nurses, occupational health nurses, and home health nurses. Second, how does the past contribute to who the population-centered nurse is today? Next, what are the places and times in which these nurses have worked and continue to work? When a conscious process of critique and insight is used to look into past actions of the specialty, what can be discovered? Must contemporary nurses agree with or endorse past actions of the profession? And last, how might knowledge of population-centered nursing history serve not only as a source of inspiration, but also as a creative stimulus to solve the new and enduring problems of the current period? This chapter serves as an introduction to these questions through tracing the development of population-centered nursing and the evolution of this approach to nursing practice.

CHANGE AND CONTINUITY

For more than 125 years, public health nurses in the United States have worked to develop strategies to respond effectively to prevailing public health problems. The history of population-centered nursing reflects changes in the specific focus of the profession while emphasizing continuity in approach and style. Nurses have worked in communities to improve the health status of individuals, families, and populations, especially those who belong to vulnerable groups. Part of the appeal of this nursing specialty has been its autonomy of practice and independence in problem solving and decision making, conducted in the context of a multidisciplinary practice. Many varied and challenging public health nursing roles originated in the late 1800s when public health efforts focused on environmental conditions such as sanitation, control of communicable diseases, education for health, prevention of disease and disability, and care of aged and sick persons in their homes.

Although the manifestations of these threats to health have changed over time, the foundational principles and goals of public health nursing have remained the same. Many communicable diseases, such as diphtheria, cholera, and typhoid fever, have been largely controlled in the United States, but others continue to affect many lives, including human immunodeficiency virus (HIV), tuberculosis, and hepatitis. Emerging communicable diseases, such as H1N1 influenza, underscore the truth that health concerns are international. Even though environmental pollution in residential areas has been reduced, communities are now threatened by overcrowded garbage dumps and pollutants affecting the air, water, and soil. Natural disasters continue to challenge public health systems, and bioterrorism and other human-made disasters threaten to overwhelm existing resources. Research has identified means to avoid or postpone chronic disease, and nurses implement strategies to modify individual and community risk factors and behaviors. Finally, with the growing population percentage of older adults in the United States and their preference to remain at home, additional nursing services are required to sustain the frail, the disabled, and the chronically ill in the community.

Contemporary nursing roles in the United States developed from several sources and are a product of various ongoing social, economic, and political forces. This chapter describes the societal circumstances that influenced nurses to establish community-based and population-centered practices. For the purposes of this chapter, the term *nurse* will be used to refer to nurses who rely heavily on public health science to complement their focus on nursing science and practice. The nation's need for community and public health nurses, the practice of population-centered nursing, and the organizations influencing public health nursing in the United States from the nineteenth century to the present are discussed.

PUBLIC HEALTH DURING AMERICA'S COLONIAL PERIOD AND THE NEW REPUBLIC

Concern for the health and care of individuals in the community has characterized human existence. All people and all cultures have been concerned with the events surrounding birth, death, and illness. Human beings have sought to prevent, understand, and control disease. Their ability to preserve health and treat illness has depended on the contemporary level of science, use and availability of technologies, and degree of social organization.

In the early years of America's settlement, as in Europe, the care of the sick was usually informal and was provided by household members, almost always women. The female head of the household was responsible for caring for all household members, which meant more than nursing them in sickness and during childbirth. She was also responsible for growing or gathering healing herbs for use throughout the year. For the increasing numbers of urban residents in the early 1800s, this traditional system became insufficient.

American ideas of social welfare and the care of the sick were strongly influenced by the traditions of British settlers in the New World. Just as American law is based on English common law, colonial Americans established systems of care for the sick, poor, aged, mentally ill, and dependents based on England's Elizabethan Poor Law of 1601. In the United States, as in England, local poor laws guaranteed medical care for poor, blind, and "lame" individuals, even those without family. Early county or township government was responsible for the care of all dependent residents but provided almshouse charity carefully, economically, and only for local residents. Travelers and wanderers from elsewhere were returned to their native counties for care. The few hospitals that existed were found only in the larger cities. In 1751, Pennsylvania Hospital was founded in Philadelphia, the first hospital in what would become the United States.

Early colonial public health efforts included the collection of vital statistics, improvements to sanitation systems, and control of any communicable diseases introduced through seaports. Colonists lacked a continuing and organized mechanism for ensuring that public health efforts would be supported and enforced. Epidemics intermittently taxed the limited local organization for health during the seventeenth, eighteenth, and nineteenth centuries (Rosen, 1958).

After the American Revolution, the threat of disease, especially yellow fever, brought public support for establishing government-sponsored, or official, boards of health. New York City, with a population of 75,000 by 1800, had established basic public health services, which included monitoring water quality, constructing sewers and a waterfront wall, draining marshes, planting trees and vegetables, and burying the dead (Rosen, 1958).

Increased urbanization and beginning industrialization in the new United States contributed to increased incidence of disease, including epidemics of smallpox, yellow fever, cholera, typhoid, and typhus. Tuberculosis and malaria remained endemic at a high incidence rate, and infant mortality was about 200 per 1000 live births (Pickett and Hanlon, 1990). American hospitals in the early 1800s were generally unsanitary and staffed by poorly trained workers; institutions were a place of last resort. Physicians received a limited education through proprietary schools or simple apprenticeship. Medical care was difficult to secure, although public dispensaries (similar to outpatient clinics) and private charitable efforts attempted to address gaps in the availability of sickness services, especially for the urban poor and working classes. Environmental conditions

in urban neighborhoods, including inadequate housing and sanitation, were additional risks to health. Table 2-1 presents milestones of public health efforts that occurred during the seventeenth, eighteenth, and nineteenth centuries.

The federal government's early efforts for public health aimed to secure America's maritime trade and major coastal cities by providing health care for merchant seamen and by protecting seacoast cities from epidemics. The Public Health Service, still the most important federal public health agency in the twenty-first century, was established in 1798 as the Marine Hospital Service. The first Marine Hospital opened in Norfolk, Virginia, in 1800. Additional legislation to establish quarantine regulations for seamen and immigrants was passed in 1878.

During the early 1800s, experiments in providing nursing care at home focused on moral improvement and less on illness intervention. The Ladies' Benevolent Society of Charleston, South Carolina, provided charitable assistance to the poor and sick beginning in 1813. In Philadelphia, lay nurses after a brief training program cared for postpartum women and newborns in their homes. In Cincinnati, Ohio, the Roman Catholic Sisters of Charity began a visiting nurse service in 1854 (Rodabaugh and Rodabaugh, 1951). Although these early programs provided services at the local level, they were not adopted elsewhere, and their influence on later public health nursing is unclear.

During the mid-nineteenth century, national interest increased in addressing public health problems and improving urban living conditions. New responsibilities for urban boards of health reflected changing ideas of public health, as the boards

TABLE 2-1	MILESTONES IN THE HISTORY OF PUBLIC HEALTH AND COMMUNITY HEALTH NURSING: 1600-1865
YEAR	**MILESTONE**
1601	Elizabethan Poor Law written
1751	Pennsylvania House founded in Philadelphia
1789	Baltimore Health Department established
1798	Marine Hospital Service established; later became Public Health Service
1812	Sisters of Mercy established in Dublin, Ireland, where nuns visited the poor
1813	Ladies' Benevolent Society of Charleston, South Carolina, founded
1836	Lutheran deaconesses provide home visits in Kaiserwerth, Germany
1851	Florence Nightingale visits Kaiserwerth for 3 months of nurse training
1855	Quarantine Board established in New Orleans; beginning of tuberculosis campaign in the United States
1859	District nursing established in Liverpool, England, by William Rathbone
1860	Florence Nightingale Training School for Nurses established at St. Thomas Hospital in London, England
1864	Red Cross established in the United States

began to address communicable diseases and environmental hazards. Soon after it was founded in 1847, the American Medical Association (AMA) formed a hygiene committee to conduct sanitary surveys and to develop a system to collect vital statistics. The Shattuck Report, published in 1850 by the Massachusetts Sanitary Commission, called for major innovations: the establishment of a state health department and local health boards in every town; sanitary surveys and collection of vital statistics; environmental sanitation; food, drug, and communicable disease control; well-child care; health education; tobacco and alcohol control; town planning; and the teaching of preventive medicine in medical schools (Kalisch and Kalisch, 1995). However, these recommendations were not implemented in Massachusetts until 1869, and in other states much later.

In some areas, charitable organizations addressed the gap between known communicable disease epidemics and the lack of local government resources. For example, the Howard Association of New Orleans, Louisiana, responded to periodic yellow fever epidemics between 1837 and 1878 by providing physicians, lay nurses, and medicine. The Association established infirmaries and used sophisticated outreach strategies to locate cases (Hanggi-Myers, 1995).

NIGHTINGALE AND THE ORIGINS OF TRAINED NURSING

The origins of professional nursing are found in the work of Florence Nightingale in nineteenth-century Europe. With tremendous advances in transportation, communication, and other forms of technology, the Industrial Revolution led to deep social upheaval. Even with the advancement of science, medicine, and technology in the two previous centuries, nineteenth-century public health measures continued to be very basic. Organization and management of cities improved slowly, and many areas lacked systems of sewage disposal and depended on private enterprise for water supply. Previous caregiving structures, which relied on the assistance of family, neighbors, and friends, became inadequate in the early nineteenth century because of human migration, urbanization, and changing demand. During this period, a few groups of Roman Catholic and Protestant women provided nursing care for the sick, poor, and neglected in institutions and sometimes in the home. For example, Mary Aikenhead, also known by her religious name Sister Mary Augustine, organized the Irish Sisters of Charity in Dublin (Ireland) in 1815. These sisters visited the poor at home and established hospitals and schools (Kalisch and Kalisch, 1995).

In nineteenth-century England, the Elizabethan Poor Law continued to guarantee medical care for all. This minimal care, provided most often in almshouses supported by local government, sought as much to regulate where the poor could live as to provide care during illness. Many women who performed nursing functions in almshouses and early hospitals in Great Britain were poorly educated, untrained, and often undependable. As the practice of medicine became more complex in the mid-1800s, hospital work required skilled caregivers. Physicians and hospital administrators sought to advance the practice of nursing. Early experiments yielded some improvement in care, but Florence Nightingale's efforts were revolutionary.

Florence Nightingale's vision of trained nurses and her model of nursing education influenced the development of professional nursing and, indirectly, public health nursing in the United States. In 1850 and 1851, Nightingale had carefully studied nursing "system and method" by visiting Pastor Theodor Fliedner at his School for Deaconesses in Kaiserwerth, Germany. Pastor Fliedner also built on the work of others, including Mennonite deaconesses in Holland who were engaged in parish work for the poor and the sick, and Elizabeth Fry, the English prison reformer. Thus mid-nineteenth century efforts to reform the practice of nursing drew on a variety of interacting innovations across Europe.

The Kaiserwerth Lutheran deaconesses incorporated care of the sick in the hospital with client care in their homes, and their system of district nursing spread to other German cities. American requests for the deaconesses to respond to epidemics of typhus and cholera in Pittsburgh provided only temporary assistance since local women were uninterested in the work. The early efforts of the Lutheran deaconesses in the United States ultimately focused on developing systems of institutional care (Nutting and Dock, 1935).

Nightingale soon found a way to implement her ideas about nursing. During the Crimean War (1854–1856) between the alliance of England and France against Russia, the British military established hospitals for sick and wounded soldiers at Scutari (in modern Turkey). The care of the sick and wounded soldiers was severely deficient, with cramped quarters, poor sanitation, lice and rats, insufficient food, and inadequate medical supplies (Kalisch and Kalisch, 1995; Palmer, 1983). When the British public demanded improved conditions, Nightingale sought and received an appointment to address the chaos. Because of her wealth, social and political connections, and knowledge of hospitals, the British government sent her to Asia Minor with 40 ladies, 117 hired nurses, and 15 paid servants.

In Scutari, Nightingale progressively improved soldiers' health outcomes using a population-based approach that strengthened environmental conditions and nursing care. Using simple epidemiological measures, she documented a decreased mortality rate from 415 per 1000 at the beginning of the war to 11.5 per 1000 at the end (Cohen, 1984; Palmer, 1983). Paralleling Nightingale's efforts in Scutari, public health nurses typically identify health care needs that affect the entire population, mobilize resources, and organize themselves and the community to meet these needs.

Nightingale's fame was established even before she returned to England in 1856 after the Crimean War. She then organized hospital nursing practice and established hospital-based nursing education to replace the untrained lay nurses with Nightingale nurses. Nightingale also emphasized public health nursing: "The health of the unity is the health of the community. Unless you have the health of the unity, there is no community health" (Nightingale, 1894, p. 455). She differentiated "sick nursing" from "health nursing." The latter emphasized that nurses should strive to promote health and prevent illness. Nightingale (1946, p. v) wrote that nurses' task is to "put the constitution in such a state as that it will have no disease, or that it can recover from disease." Proper nutrition, rest, sanitation, and hygiene were necessary for health. Nurses continue to focus on the vital role of health promotion, disease prevention, and environment in their practice with individuals, families, and communities.

Nightingale's contemporary and friend, British philanthropist **William Rathbone,** founded the first **district nursing association** in Liverpool, England. Rathbone's wife had received outstanding nursing care from a Nightingale-trained nurse during her terminal illness at home. He wanted to offer similar care to relieve the suffering of poor persons unable to afford private nurses. With Rathbone's advocacy and economic support between 1859 and 1862, the Liverpool Relief Society divided the city into nursing districts and assigned a committee of "friendly visitors" to each district to provide health care to needy people (Kalisch and Kalisch, 1995). Building on the Liverpool experience, Rathbone and Nightingale recommended steps to provide nursing in the home, and district nursing was organized throughout England. Florence Sarah Lees Craven shaped the profession through her book *A Guide to District Nursing,* which recommended, for example, that nursing care during the illness of one family member provided the nurse with influence to improve the health status of the whole family (Craven, 1889).

AMERICA NEEDS TRAINED NURSES

As urbanization increased during America's Industrial Revolution, the number of jobs for women rapidly increased. Educated women became elementary school teachers, secretaries, or saleswomen. Less-educated women worked in factories of all kinds. The idea of becoming a trained nurse increased in popularity as Nightingale's successes became known across the United States. During the 1870s, the first nursing schools based on the Nightingale model opened in the United States.

Trained nurse graduates of the early schools for nurses in the United States usually worked in private duty nursing or held the few positions as hospital administrators or instructors. Private duty nurses might live with families of clients receiving care, to be available 24 hours a day. Although the trained nurse's role in improving American hospitals was very clear, the cost of private duty nursing care for the sick at home was prohibitive for all but the wealthy.

The care of the sick poor at home was made economical by having home-visiting nurses attend several families in a day rather than attend only one client as the private duty nurse did. In 1877 the Women's Board of the New York City Mission hired Frances Root, a graduate of Bellevue Hospital's first nursing class, to visit sick poor persons to provide nursing care and religious instruction (Bullough and Bullough, 1964). In 1878 the Ethical Culture Society of New York hired four nurses to work in dispensaries, a type of community-based clinic. In the next few years, visiting nurse associations (VNAs) were established in Buffalo, New York (1885), Philadelphia (1886), and Boston (1886). Wealthy people interested in charitable activities funded both settlement houses and VNAs. Upper-class women, freed of some of the social restrictions that had previously limited their public life, became interested in the charitable work of creating, supporting, and supervising the new

visiting nurses. Public health nursing in the United States began with organizing to meet urban health care needs, especially for the disadvantaged.

The public was interested in limiting disease among all classes of people not only for religious reasons as a form of charity, but also because the middle and upper classes feared the impact of communicable diseases believed to originate in the large communities of new European immigrants. In New York City in the 1890s, about 2.3 million people lived in 90,000 tenement houses. Deplorable environmental conditions for immigrants in urban tenement houses and sweatshops were common across the northeastern United States and upper Midwest. "Slum dwellers were ravaged by epidemics of typhus, scarlet fever, smallpox, and typhoid fever, and many of them died or developed tuberculosis" (Kalisch and Kalisch, 1995, p. 172). From the beginning, nursing practice in the community included teaching and prevention (Figure 2-1). Nursing interventions, improved sanitation, economic improvements, and better nutrition were credited with reducing the incidence of acute communicable disease by 1910.

New scientific explanations of communicable disease suggested that preventive education would reduce illness. The **visiting nurse** became the key to communicating the prevention campaign, through home visits and well-baby clinics. Visiting nurses worked with physicians, gave selected treatments, and kept temperature and pulse records. Visiting nurses emphasized education of family members in the care of the sick and in personal and environmental prevention measures, such as hygiene and good nutrition (Figure 2-2). Many early visiting nurse agencies employed only one nurse, who was supervised by members of the agency board, usually composed of wealthy or socially prominent ladies who were not nurses. These ladies were critically important to the success of visiting nursing through their efforts to open new agencies, financially support existing agencies, and render the services socially acceptable. The work of both visiting nurses and their lady supporters reflected changing societal roles for women as it became more acceptable for women to be active in public arenas than it had been earlier in the nineteenth century.

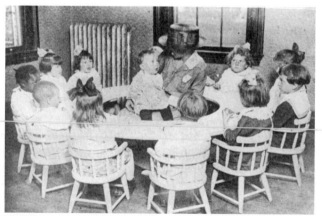

FIGURE 2-1 A Red Cross nurse tells a health story to children. (From Pickett SE: *The American National Red Cross: its origin, purpose, and service,* 1924, American Red Cross. Courtesy of the American Red Cross. All rights reserved in all countries.)

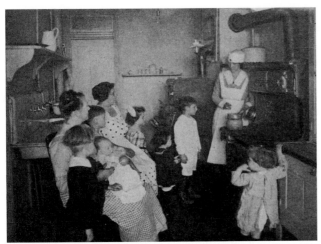

FIGURE 2-2 A Red Cross nutrition worker in the home. (From Pickett SE: *The American National Red Cross: its origin, purpose, and service,* 1924, American Red Cross. Courtesy of the American Red Cross. All rights reserved in all countries.)

For example, in 1886 two Boston women approached the Women's Education Association to seek local support for district nursing. To increase the likelihood of financial support, they used the term *instructive district nursing* to emphasize the relationship of nursing to health education. The Boston Dispensary provided support in the form of free outpatient medical care. In 1886 the first district nurse was hired, and in 1888 the Instructive District Nursing Association became incorporated as an independent voluntary agency. Sick poor persons, who paid no fees, were cared for under the direction of a trained physician (Brainard, 1922).

Other nurses established settlement houses—neighborhood centers that became hubs for health care, education, and social welfare programs. For example, in 1893 Lillian Wald and Mary Brewster, both trained nurses, began visiting the poor on New York's Lower East Side. The nurses' settlement they established became the Henry Street Settlement and later the Visiting Nurse Service of New York City. By 1905 the public health nurses had provided almost 48,000 visits to more than 5000 clients (Kalisch and Kalisch, 1995). Lillian Wald emerged as the established leader of public health nursing during its early decades (Box 2-1; Figure 2-3). Other settlement houses influenced the growth of community nursing including the Richmond (Virginia) Nurses' Settlement, which became the Instructive Visiting Nurse Association; the Nurses' Settlement in Orange, New Jersey; and the College Settlement in Los Angeles, California.

NURSING TIP   *Learning about the organizational history of a practice agency, such as a visiting nurse association, may provide important perspectives on current agency values, decision-making structures, service areas, and clinical priorities.*

Jessie Sleet (Scales), a Canadian graduate of Provident Hospital School of Nursing (Chicago), became the first African-American public health nurse when she was hired by the New York Charity Organization Society in 1900. Although it was hard for her to find an agency willing to hire her as a district nurse,

BOX 2-1   LILLIAN WALD: FIRST PUBLIC HEALTH NURSE IN THE UNITED STATES

Beyond New York City, Lillian Wald took steps to increase access to public health nursing services through innovation. She persuaded the American Red Cross to sponsor rural health nursing services across the country, which stimulated local governments to sponsor public health nursing through county health departments. Beginning in 1909, Wald worked with Dr. Lee Frankel of the Metropolitan Life Insurance Company (MetLife) to implement the first insurance payment for nursing services. She argued that keeping working people and their families healthier would increase their productivity. MetLife found that nursing care for communicable diseases, injuries, and mothers and children reduced mortality and saved money for this life insurance company. MetLife nursing services continued for 44 years, yielding accomplishments in (1) providing home nursing services on a fee-for-service basis, (2) establishing an effective cost-accounting system for visiting nurses, and (3) reducing mortality from infectious diseases.

Convinced that environmental conditions as well as social conditions were the causes of ill health and poverty, Wald became actively involved in using epidemiological methods to campaign for health-promoting social policies. She advocated for creation of the U.S. Children's Bureau as a basis for improving the health and education of children nationally. She fought for better tenement living conditions in New York City, city recreation centers, parks, pure food laws, graded classes for mentally handicapped children, and assistance to immigrants. She firmly believed in women's suffrage and considered its acceptance in 1917 in New York State to be a great victory. Wald supported efforts to improve race relations and championed solutions to racial injustice. She wrote *The House on Henry Street* (1915) and *Windows on Henry Street* (1934) to describe this public health nursing work.

Backer BA: Lillian Wald: connecting caring with action, *Nurs Health Care* 14:122, 1993; Cristy TE: Lillian D. Wald: portrait of a leader. In Kelly LY: *Pages from nursing history,* New York, 1984, American Journal of Nursing Co., pp 84-88; Dock LL: The history of public health nursing, *Public Health Nurs* 14:522, 1922; Dolan J: *History of nursing,* ed 14, Philadelphia, 1978, Saunders; Duffus RL: *Lillian Wald: neighbor and crusader,* New York, 1938, Macmillan; Frachel RR: A new profession: the evolution of public health nursing, *Public Health Nurs* 5:86, 1988; Wald LD: *The house on Henry Street,* New York, 1915, Holt; Wald LD: *Windows on Henry Street,* Boston, 1934, Little, Brown; Williams B: *Lillian Wald: angel of Henry Street,* New York, 1948, Julian Messner; Zerwekh JV: Public health nursing legacy: historical practical wisdom, *Nurs Health Care* 13:84, 1992.

she persevered and was able to provide exceptional care for her clients until she married in 1909. At the Charity Organization Society in 1904 to 1905, she studied health conditions related to tuberculosis among African-American people in Manhattan using interviews with families and neighbors, house-to-house canvases, direct observation, and speeches at neighborhood churches. Sleet reported her research to the Society board, recommending improved employment opportunities for African-Americans and better prevention strategies to reduce the excess burden of tuberculosis morbidity and mortality among the African-American population (Buhler-Wilkerson, 2001; Hine, 1989; Mosley, 1994; Thoms, 1929).

In 1909 Yssabella Waters published her survey titled *Visiting Nursing in the United States,* which documented the concentration of visiting nurse services in the northeastern quadrant of the nation. In 1901 New York City alone had 58 different

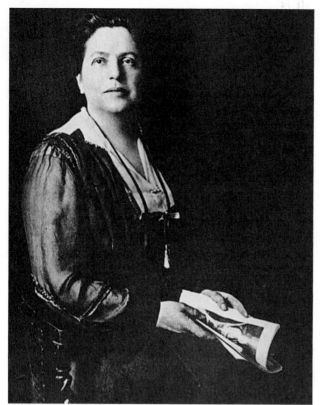

FIGURE 2-3 Lillian Wald. (Courtesy of the Visiting Nurse Service of New York.)

organizations with 372 trained nurses providing care in the community. However, nationally, 68% of visiting nurses were employed in single-nurse agencies. In addition to VNAs and settlement houses, a variety of other organizations sponsored visiting nurse work, including boards of education, boards of health, mission boards, clubs, churches, social service agencies, and tuberculosis associations. With tuberculosis then responsible for at least 10% of all mortality, visiting nurses contributed to its control through gaining "the personal cooperation of patients and their families" to modify the environment and individual behavior (Buhler-Wilkerson, 1987, p. 45). Most visiting nurse agencies depended financially on the philanthropy and social networks of metropolitan areas. As today, fund-raising and service delivery in less densely populated and rural areas was challenging.

WHAT DO YOU THINK?   *Lillian Wald demonstrated an exceptional ability to develop approaches and programs to solve the health care and social problems of her times. How would you apply this creativity to today's health care challenges? If Lillian Wald were looking over your shoulder, what would she recommend?*

The **American Red Cross**, through its Rural Nursing Service (later the **Town and Country Nursing Service**), provided a framework to initiate home nursing care in areas outside larger cities. Wald secured initial donations to support this agency, which provided care of the sick and instruction in sanitation and hygiene in rural homes. The agency also improved living conditions in villages and isolated farms. The Town and Country nurse dealt with diseases such as tuberculosis, pneumonia, and typhoid fever with a resourcefulness born of necessity. The rural nurse might use hot bricks, salt, or sandbags to substitute for hot water bottles; chairs as back-rests for the bedbound; and boards padded with quilts as stretchers (Kalisch and Kalisch, 1995). In the 2 years after World War I, the 100 existing Red Cross Town and Country Nursing Services expanded to 1800, and eventually to almost 3000 programs in small towns and rural areas. This service demonstrated the importance and feasibility of public health nursing across the country at local and county levels. Once firmly established by the Red Cross, ongoing responsibilities for these new agencies were passed on to local voluntary agencies or local government.

Occupational health nursing began as industrial nursing and was a true outgrowth of early home visiting efforts. In 1895 Ada Mayo Stewart began work with employees and families of the Vermont Marble Company in Proctor, Vermont. As a free service for the employees, Stewart provided obstetric care, sickness care (e.g., for typhoid cases), and some post-surgical care in workers' homes. Unlike contemporary occupational health nurses, Stewart provided very few services for work-related injuries. A graduate of the Waltham (Massachusetts) Training School, Stewart continued to wear the Waltham nursing student uniform, and added a plain coat and hat. Although her employer provided a horse and buggy, she often made home visits on a bicycle. Before 1900 a few nurses were hired in industry, such as in department stores in Philadelphia and Brooklyn. Between 1914 and 1943, industrial nursing grew from 60 to 11,220 nurses, reflecting increased governmental and employee concerns for health and safety at work (AAIN, 1976; Kalisch and Kalisch, 1995).

SCHOOL NURSING IN AMERICA

In New York City in 1902, more than 20% of children might be absent from school on a single day. The children suffered from the common conditions of pediculosis, ringworm, scabies, inflamed eyes, discharging ears, and infected wounds. Physicians began to make limited inspections of school students in 1897, and they focused on excluding infectious children from school rather than on providing or obtaining medical treatment to enable children to return to school. Familiar with this community-wide problem from her work with the Henry Street Nurses' Settlement, Wald sought to place nurses in the schools and gained consent from the city's health commissioner and the Board of Education for a 1-month demonstration project.

Lina Rogers, a Henry Street Settlement resident, became the first school nurse. She worked with the children in New York City schools and made home visits to instruct parents and to follow up on children excluded or otherwise absent from school. The school nurses found that "many children were absent for lack of shoes or clothing, because of malnourishment, or because they were serving their families as babysitters" (Hawkins, Hayes, and Corliss, 1994, p. 417). The school nurse experiment made such a significant and positive impact that it became permanent, with 12 more nurses appointed 1 month later. School nursing was soon implemented in Los Angeles, Philadelphia, Baltimore, Boston, Chicago, and San Francisco.

THE PROFESSION COMES OF AGE

Established by the Cleveland Visiting Nurse Association in 1909, the *Visiting Nurse Quarterly* initiated a professional communication medium for clinical and organizational concerns. In 1911 a joint committee of existing nurse organizations convened, under the leadership of Wald and Mary Gardner, to standardize nursing services outside the hospital. Recommending formation of a new organization to address public health nursing concerns, 800 agencies involved in public health nursing activities were invited to send delegates to an organizational meeting in Chicago in June 1912. After a heated debate on its name and purpose, the delegates established the National Organization for Public Health Nursing (NOPHN) and chose Wald as its first president (Dock, 1922). Unlike other professional nursing organizations, the NOPHN membership included both nurses and their lay supporters. The NOPHN sought "to improve the educational and services standards of the public health nurse, and promote public understanding of and respect for her work" (Rosen, 1958, p. 381). With greater administrative resources than any of the other national nursing organizations existing at that time, the NOPHN was soon the dominant force in public health nursing (Roberts, 1955).

The NOPHN sought to standardize public health nursing education. Visiting nurse agencies found that graduates of the hospital schools were unprepared for home visiting. It became apparent that the basic curriculum of many schools of nursing was insufficient. Because diploma schools of nursing emphasized hospital care of clients, public health nurses would require additional education to provide services to the sick at home and to design population-focused programs. In 1914, in affiliation with the Henry Street Settlement, Mary Adelaide Nutting began the first post-training-school course in public health nursing at Teachers College in New York City (Deloughery, 1977). The American Red Cross provided scholarships for graduates of nursing schools to attend the public health nursing course. Its success encouraged development of other programs, using curricula that might seem familiar to today's nurses. During the 1920s and 1930s, many newly hired public health nurses had to verify completion or promptly enroll in a certificate program in public health nursing. Others took leave for a year to travel to an urban center to obtain this further education. Correspondence courses (distance education) were even acceptable in some areas, for example, for public health nurses in upstate New York.

Public health nurses were also active in the American Public Health Association (APHA), which was established in 1872 to facilitate interprofessional efforts and promote the "practical application of public hygiene" (Scutchfield and Keck, 1997, p. 12). The APHA targeted reform efforts toward contemporary public health issues, including sewage and garbage disposal, occupational injuries, and sexually transmitted diseases. In 1923 the Public Health Nursing Section was formed within the APHA to provide nurses with a forum to discuss their concerns and strategies within the larger context of the major public health organization. The Section continues to serve as a focus of leadership and policy development for public health nursing.

PUBLIC HEALTH NURSING IN OFFICIAL HEALTH AGENCIES AND IN WORLD WAR I

Public health nursing in voluntary agencies and through the Red Cross grew more quickly than public health nursing sponsored by state, local, and national government. In the late 1800s, local health departments were formed in urban areas to target environmental hazards associated with crowded living conditions and dirty streets, and to regulate public baths, slaughterhouses, and pigsties (Pickett and Hanlon, 1990). By 1900, 38 states had established state health departments, following the lead of Massachusetts in 1869; however, these early state boards of health had limited impact. Only three states—Massachusetts, Rhode Island, and Florida—annually spent more than 2 cents per capita for public health services (Scutchfield and Keck, 1997).

The federal role in public health gradually expanded. In 1912 the federal government redefined the role of the U.S. Public Health Service, empowering it to "investigate the causes and spread of diseases and the pollution and sanitation of navigable streams and lakes" (Scutchfield and Keck, 1997, p. 15). The NOPHN loaned a nurse to the U.S. Public Health Service during World War I to establish a public health nursing program for military outposts. This led to the first federal government sponsorship of nurses (Shyrock, 1959; Wilner, Walkey, and O'Neill, 1978).

During the 1910s, public health organizations began to target infectious and parasitic diseases in rural areas. The Rockefeller Sanitary Commission, a philanthropic organization active in hookworm control in the southeastern United States, concluded that concurrent efforts for all phases of public health were necessary to successfully address any individual public health problem (Pickett and Hanlon, 1990). For example, in 1911 efforts to control typhoid fever in Yakima County, Washington, and to improve health status in Guilford County, North Carolina, led to establishment of local health units to serve local populations. Public health nurses were the primary staff members of local health departments. These nurses assumed a leadership role on health care issues through collaboration with local residents, nurses, and other health care providers.

The experience of Orange County, California, during the 1920s and 1930s illustrates the role of the public health nurse in these new local health departments. Following the efforts of a private physician, social welfare agencies, and a Red Cross nurse, the county board created the public health nurse's position, which began in 1922. Presented with a shining new Model T car sporting the bright orange seal of the county, the nurse focused on the serious communicable disease problems of diphtheria and scarlet fever. Typhoid became epidemic when a drainage pipe overflowed into a well, infecting those who drank the water and those who drank raw milk from an infected dairy. Almost 3000 residents were immunized against typhoid. Weekly well-baby conferences provided an opportunity for mothers to learn about care of their infants, and the infants were weighed and given communicable disease immunizations. Children with orthopedic disorders and other disabilities were identified and referred for medical care in Los Angeles. At the end of a successful first year of public health nursing work, the Rockefeller Foundation and the California Health Department recognized the favorable outcomes and provided funding for more public health professionals.

The personnel needs of World War I in Europe depleted the ranks of public health nurses, even as the NOPHN identified a need for second and third lines of defense within the United States. Jane Delano of the Red Cross (which was sending 100 nurses a day to the war) agreed that despite the sacrifice, the greatest patriotic duty of public health nurses was to stay at home. In 1918 the worldwide influenza pandemic swept the United States from the Atlantic coast to the Pacific coast within 3 weeks and was met by a coalition of the NOPHN and the Red Cross. Houses, churches, and social halls were turned into hospitals for the immense numbers of sick and dying. Some of the nurse volunteers died of influenza as well (Shyrock, 1959; Wilner, Walkey, and O'Neill, 1978).

PAYING THE BILL FOR PUBLIC HEALTH NURSES

Inadequate funding was the major obstacle to extending nursing services in the community. Most early VNAs sought charitable contributions from wealthy and middle-class supporters. Even poor families were encouraged to pay a small fee for nursing services, reflecting social welfare concerns against promoting economic dependency by providing charity. In 1909, as a result of Wald's collaboration with Dr. Lee Frankel, the Metropolitan Life Insurance Company began a cooperative program with visiting nurse organizations that expanded availability of public health nursing services. The nurses assessed illness, taught health practices, and collected data from policyholders. By 1912, 589 Metropolitan Life nursing centers provided care through existing agencies or through visiting nurses hired directly by the company. In 1918 Metropolitan Life calculated an average decline of 7% in the mortality rate of policyholders and almost a 20% decline in the mortality rate of policyholders' children under age 3. The insurance company attributed this improvement and their reduced costs to the work of visiting nurses. Voluntary health insurance was still decades in the future; public and professional efforts to secure compulsory health insurance seemed promising in 1916 but had evaporated by the end of World War I.

Nursing efforts to influence public policy bridged World War I and included advocacy for the Children's Bureau and the Sheppard-Towner Program. Responding to lengthy advocacy by Wald and other nurse leaders, the Children's Bureau was established in 1912 to address national problems of maternal and child welfare. Children's Bureau experts conducted extensive scientific research on the effects of income, housing, employment, and other factors on infant and maternal mortality. Their research led to federal child labor laws and the 1919 White House Conference on Child Health.

Problems of maternal and child morbidity and mortality spurred the passage of the Maternity and Infancy Act (often called the Sheppard-Towner Act) in 1921. This act provided federal matching funds to establish maternal and child health divisions in state health departments. Education during home visits by public health nurses stressed promoting the health of mother and child as well as seeking prompt medical care during pregnancy. Although credited with saving many lives, the Sheppard-Towner Program ended in 1929 in response to charges by the AMA and others that the legislation gave too much power to the federal government and too closely resembled socialized medicine (Pickett and Hanlon, 1990).

Some nursing innovations were the result of individual commitment and private financial support. In 1925 Mary Breckinridge established the Frontier Nursing Service (FNS) to emulate systems of care used in the Highlands and islands of Scotland (Box 2-2; Figure 2-4). The unique pioneering spirit of the FNS influenced development of public health programs geared toward improving the health care of the rural and often inaccessible populations in the Appalachian region of southeastern Kentucky (Browne, 1966; Tirpak, 1975). Breckinridge introduced the first nurse-midwives into the United States when she deployed FNS nurses trained in nursing, public health, and midwifery. Their efforts led to reduced pregnancy complications and maternal mortality, and to one-third fewer stillbirths and infant deaths in an area of 700 square miles (Kalisch and Kalisch, 1995). Today the FNS continues to provide comprehensive health and nursing services to the people of that area and sponsors the Frontier School of Midwifery and Family Nursing.

AFRICAN-AMERICAN NURSES IN PUBLIC HEALTH NURSING

African-American nurses seeking to work in public health nursing faced many challenges. Nursing education was absolutely segregated in the South until at least the 1960s, and elsewhere was also generally segregated or rationed until mid-century. Even public health nursing certificate and graduate education programs were segregated in the South; study outside the South for southern nurses was difficult to afford and study leaves from the workplace were rarely granted. The situation improved somewhat in 1936, when collaboration between the United States Public Health Service and the Medical College of Virginia (Richmond) established a certificate program in public health nursing for African-American nurses for which the federal government paid nurses' tuition. Discrimination continued during nurses' employment: African-American nurses in the American South were paid significantly lower salaries than their white counterparts for the same work. In 1925 just 435 African-American public health nurses were employed in the United States, and in 1930 only 6 African-American nurses held supervisory positions in public health nursing organizations (Buhler-Wilkerson, 2001; Hine, 1989; Thoms, 1929).

BOX 2-2   MARY BRECKINRIDGE AND THE FRONTIER NURSING SERVICE

Born in 1881 into the fifth generation of a Kentucky family, Mary Breckinridge devoted her life to the Frontier Nursing Service (FNS) and to promoting the health care of disadvantaged women and children. Educated by tutors and in private schools, Breckinridge considered becoming a nurse only after her first husband died. In 1907 she entered St. Luke's Hospital School of Nursing in New York City. She later married for a second time, but her daughter died at birth and her son died at age 4 in 1918. In post–World War I France, Breckinridge administered maternal/child and public health programs, including a "goat crusade" in which Americans donated goats to provide milk for hungry European infants. In Great Britain, she became one of the first Americans to receive a nurse-midwifery certificate. At this time, nurse- midwifery training was not available in the United States. Breckinridge returned to the United States to take the 1-year public health nursing course at Teacher's College of Columbia University in New York.

Passionate about helping the children of rural America and prepared to begin her life's work, Breckinridge returned to Kentucky early in 1925. She had determined that Kentucky's mountain region was an excellent place to demonstrate the value of public health nursing to improving the health of disadvantaged families living in remote areas. She thought that if it were possible to establish a nursing center in rural Kentucky, the program could be duplicated anywhere. Breckinridge used her family inheritance to start the Frontier Nursing Service. Establishing the first FNS health center in a five-room cabin in Hyden, Kentucky, required not only nursing skills, but also construction of the cabin, other buildings, and later the FNS hospital. Each step was difficult, including securing a water supply, electric power, and sewage disposal, and stabilizing a mountain terrain prone to landslides. Despite these obstacles, six outpost nursing centers were built between 1927 and 1930. When the FNS hospital in Hyden was completed in 1928, physicians began providing service. Financial support for FNS nursing and medical care ranged from client families' labor exchange and farm product donation to fund-raising through annual family dues, philanthropy, and direct fund-raising by Breckinridge herself.

Serving nearly 10,000 people distributed over 700 square miles, the FNS provided nursing and midwifery services 24 hours a day and established medical, surgical, and dental clinics. Reduced death rates were especially remarkable considering the environmental conditions these rural Kentuckians faced. Many area homes lacked heat, electricity, and running water. During the 1930s, nurses lived in one of the six outposts. Transportation was difficult, as nurses, midwives, and couriers climbed mountains by foot and rode horses great distances. Like her staff, Breckinridge traveled through the remote mountains of Kentucky on her horse, Babette, providing food, supplies, and health care to mountain families. Breckinridge documented her experiences in the book *Wide Neighborhoods, a Story of the Frontier Nursing Service.*

Over the years, hundreds of nurses have worked with the FNS. Since Breckinridge died in 1965, FNS has continued to grow and provide needed services to people in the mountains of Kentucky. FNS remains a vital means to providing health services to rural families and as a creative model for nursing service delivery through its home health agency, outpost clinics, primary care centers, the Frontier School of Midwifery and Family Nursing, and the Mary Breckinridge Hospital.

Breckinridge M: *Wide neighborhoods, a story of the Frontier Nursing Service,* New York, 1952, Harper; Browne H: A tribute to Mary Breckinridge, *Nurs Outlook* 14:54, 1966; Buhler-Wilkerson K: *No place like home: a history of nursing and home care in the United States,* Baltimore, 2001, Johns Hopkins Press; Frontier Nurse Service homepage: http://www.frontiernursing.org/History/History.shtm; Goan, MB: *Mary Breckinridge: the Frontier Nursing Service and rural health in Appalachia.* Chapel Hill, NC, 2008, University of North Carolina Press; Holloway JB: Frontier Nursing Service 1925-1975, *J Ky Med Assoc* 13:491, 1975; Tirpak H: The Frontier Nursing Service: fifty years in the mountains, *Nurs Outlook* 33:308, 1975.

African-American public health nurses had a significant impact on the communities they served (Figure 2-5). The National Health Circle for Colored People was organized in 1919 to promote public health work in African-American communities in the South. One strategy adopted was providing scholarships to assist African-American nurses to pursue university-level public health nursing education. Bessie M. Hawes, the first recipient of the scholarship, completed the program at Columbia University (New York) and was then sent by the Circle to Palatka, Florida. In this small, isolated lumber town, Hawes' first project was to recruit school-girls to promote health by dressing as nurses and marching in a parade while singing community songs. She conducted mass meetings, led mother's clubs, provided school health education, and visited the homes of the sick. Eventually she gained the community's trust, overcame opposition, and built a health center for nursing care and treatment (Thoms, 1929).

BETWEEN THE TWO WORLD WARS: ECONOMIC DEPRESSION AND THE RISE OF HOSPITALS

The economic crisis during the Depression of the 1930s deeply influenced the development of nursing. Not only were agencies and communities unprepared to address the increased needs and numbers of the impoverished, but decreased funding for nursing services reduced the number of employed nurses in hospitals and in community agencies. Federal funding led to a wide variety of programs administered at the state level, including new public health nursing programs. The NOPHN's tenacious effort to ensure inclusion of public health nursing in federal relief programs secured success after a flurry of last-minute telegrams and lobbying efforts.

The Federal Emergency Relief Administration (FERA) supported nurse employment through increased grants-in-aid for state programs of home medical care. FERA often purchased nursing care from existing visiting nurse agencies, thus supporting more nurses and preventing agency closures. The FERA program focus varied among states; the state FERA program in New York emphasized bedside nursing care, whereas in North Carolina, the state FERA prioritized maternal and child health, and school nursing services. Some Depression-era federal programs built new services; public health nursing programs of the Works Progress Administration (WPA) were sometimes later incorporated into state health departments. In West Virginia, as elsewhere, the Relief Nursing Service had a dual purpose—to assist unemployed nurses and to provide nursing care for families on relief. Fundamental services included: "(1) providing bedside care and health supervision for the family in the home; (2) arranging for medical and hospital care for emergency and obstetric cases; (3) supervising the health of children in emergency relief nursery schools; and (4) caring for patients with tuberculosis" (Kalisch and Kalisch, 1995, p. 306).

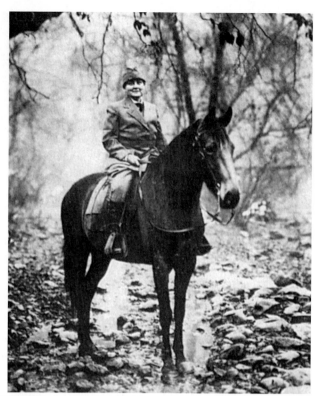

FIGURE 2-4 Mary Breckinridge, founder of the Frontier Nursing Service. (Courtesy of the Frontier Nursing Service of Wendover, Kentucky.)

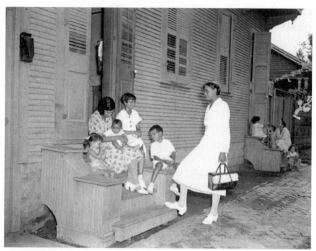

FIGURE 2-5 African-American nurse visiting a family on the door-step of their home. (Courtesy of the New Orleans Public Library WPA Photograph Collection.)

In another Depression-era program, more than 10,000 nurses were employed by the Civil Works Administration (CWA) programs and assigned to official health agencies. "While this facilitated rapid program expansion by recipient agencies and gave the nurses a taste of public health, the nurses' lack of field experience created major problems of training and supervision for the regular staff" (Roberts and Heinrich, 1985, p. 1162).

A 1932 survey of public health agencies found that only 7% of nurses employed in public health were adequately prepared (Roberts and Heinrich, 1985). Basic nursing education focused heavily on the care of individuals, and students received limited information on groups and the community as a unit of service. Thus in the 1930s and early 1940s, new graduates continued to be inadequately prepared to work in public health and required considerable remedial orientation and education from the hiring agencies (NOPHN, 1944).

Public health nurses continued to weigh the relative value of preventive care compared with bedside care of the sick. They also questioned whether nursing interventions should be directed toward groups and communities or toward individuals and their families. Although each nursing agency was unique and services varied from region to region, voluntary VNAs tended to emphasize care of the sick, whereas official public health agencies provided more preventive services. Not surprisingly, the conflicting visions and splintering of services between "visiting" and "public health" nurses further impeded development of comprehensive population-centered nursing services (Roberts and Heinrich, 1985). In addition, some households received services from several community nurses representing several agencies (e.g., visits for a postpartum woman and new baby, for a child sick with scarlet fever, and for an older adult sick in bed). Nurses believed this confused families and duplicated scarce nursing resources. One solution was the "combination service"—the merger of sick care services and preventive services into one comprehensive agency, most often administered through local health departments. On the other hand, compared with nursing in VNAs, nurses in official agencies may have had less control over their practice roles because physicians and politicians often determined services and personnel assignments in public health departments.

INCREASING FEDERAL ACTION FOR THE PUBLIC'S HEALTH

Expansion of the federal government during the 1930s affected the structure of community health resources. Credited as "the beginning of a new era in public nursing" (Roberts and Heinrich, 1985, p. 1162), Pearl McIver in 1933 became the first nurse employed by the U.S. Public Health Service. In providing consultation services to state health departments, McIver was convinced that the strengths and ability of each state's director of public health nursing would determine the scope and quality of local health services. Together with Naomi Deutsch, director of nursing for the federal Children's Bureau, and with the support of nursing organizations, McIver and her staff of nurse consultants influenced the direction of public health nursing. Between 1931 and 1938, greater than 40% of the increase in public health nurse employment was in local health agencies. Even so, nationally more than one third of all counties still lacked local public health nursing services.

The Social Security Act of 1935 was designed to prevent reoccurrence of the problems of the Depression. Title VI of this act provided funding for expanded opportunities for health protection and promotion through education and employment of public health nurses. More than 1000 nurses completed educational programs in public health in 1936. Title VI also provided $8 million to assist states, counties, and medical districts in the establishment and maintenance of adequate health services, as well as $2 million for research and investigation of disease (Buhler-Wilkerson, 1985, 1989; Kalisch and Kalisch, 1995).

A categorical approach to federal funding for public health services reflected the U.S. Congress's preference for funding specific diseases or specific groups, rather than providing dollar allocations to local agencies. In categorical funding, resources are directed toward specific priorities rather than toward a comprehensive community health program. When funding is directed by established national preferences, it becomes more difficult to respond to local and emerging problems. Even so, local health departments shaped their programs according to the pattern of available funds (e.g., maternal and child health services and crippled children [1935], venereal disease control [1938], tuberculosis [1944], mental health [1947], industrial hygiene [1947], and dental health [1947]) (Scutchfield and Keck, 1997). Categorical funding continues to be a preferred federal approach to address health policy objectives.

EVIDENCE-BASED PRACTICE

No Place Like Home: A History of Nursing and Home Care in the United States (2001) is a book-length analysis of the development of nursing care for those at home. Buhler-Wilkerson traces how the care of the sick moved from a domestic function to a charitable or public responsibility provided through visiting nurse associations and official health agencies. The central dilemma she raises is, "why, despite its potential as a preferred, rational, and possibly cost-effective alternative to institutional care, home care remains a marginalized experiment in caregiving" (p. xi).

Buhler-Wilkerson follows the origins of home care from its beginnings in Charleston, South Carolina, to its expansion into northern cities at the end of the nineteenth century. She interprets the founding of public health nursing by Lillian Wald "as a new paradigm for community-based nursing practice within the context of social reform" (p. xii), and she particularly analyzes the effects of ethnicity, race, and social class. She traces the difficulties of organizing and financing care of the sick in the home, including the work of private duty nurses and the role of health insurance in shaping home services. The concluding section of the book highlights contemporary themes of "chronic illness, hospital dominance, financial viability, and struggles to survive" (p. xii) and projects the future of home care.

Buhler-Wilkerson brings to bear the stories of clients' needs and nurses' work against the financial challenges that have characterized home care. While focusing on one element, this book raises important questions for nurses' work across elements of community/public health nursing. Clearly identified need does not by itself open the doors to adequate financing for nursing care of the sick, for public health nursing, or for population care for health promotion.

Nurse Use

This book points out the complex issues involved in trying to provide the most effective care to clients. The needs of clients and their families may not entirely correlate with what is financially available. A lesson for each of us to learn is the following: identified need does not always influence the availability of funds to provide the desired care.

From Buhler-Wilkerson K: *No place like home: a history of nursing and home care in the United States,* Baltimore, 2001, Johns Hopkins Press.

WORLD WAR II: EXTENSION AND RETRENCHMENT IN PUBLIC HEALTH NURSING

The U.S. involvement in World War II in 1941 accelerated the need for nurses, both for the war effort and at home. The Nursing Council on National Defense was a coalition of the national nursing organizations that planned and coordinated activities for the war effort. National interest prioritized the health of military personnel and workers in essential industries. Many nurses joined the Army and Navy Nurse Corps. Through the influence and leadership of U.S. Representative Frances Payne Bolton of Ohio, substantial funding was provided by the Bolton Act of 1943 to establish the Cadet Nurses Corps, leading to increased enrollment in schools of nursing at undergraduate and graduate levels. Under management by the U.S. Public Health Service, the Nursing Council for National Defense received $1 million to expand facilities for nursing education. Training for Nurses for National Defense, the GI Bill, the Nurse Training Act of 1943, and Public Health and Professional Nurse Traineeships provided additional educational funds that expanded both the total number of nurses and the number of nurses with preparation in public health nursing (McNeil, 1967).

As more and more nurses and physicians left civilian hospitals to meet the needs of the war, responsibility for client care was shifted to families, non-nursing personnel, and volunteers. "By the end of 1942, over 500,000 women had completed the American Red Cross home nursing course, and nearly 17,000 nurse's aides had been certified" (Roberts and Heinrich, 1985, p. 1165). By the end of 1946, more than 215,000 volunteer nurse's aides had received certificates.

In some cases, public health nursing expanded its scope of practice during World War II. For example, nurses increased their presence in rural areas, and many official agencies began to provide bedside nursing care (Buhler-Wilkerson, 1985; Kalisch and Kalisch, 1995). The federal Emergency Maternity and Infant Care Act of 1943 (EMIC) provided funding for medical, hospital, and nursing care for the wives and babies of servicemen. Health services seeking EMIC funds were required to meet the high standards of the U.S. Children's Bureau, thus increasing quality of care for all. In other situations, nursing roles were constrained by wartime and postwar nursing shortages. For example, the Visiting Nurse Society of Philadelphia ceased home birth services, drastically reduced industrial nursing services, and deferred care for the long-term chronically ill client.

Reflecting the complex social changes that occurred during the war years, immediately after the war local health departments faced sudden increases in client demand for care of emotional problems, accidents, alcoholism, and other responsibilities new to the domain of official health agencies. Changes in medical technology offered new possibilities for screening and treatment of infectious and communicable diseases, such as antibiotics to treat rheumatic fever and venereal diseases, and photofluorography for mass case finding of pulmonary tuberculosis. Local health departments expanded, both to address underserved areas and to expand types of services, and they often fared better economically than the voluntary agencies.

TABLE 2-2   MILESTONES IN HISTORY OF COMMUNITY HEALTH AND PUBLIC HEALTH NURSING: 1866-1945

YEAR	MILESTONE
1866	New York Metropolitan Board of Health established
1872	American Public Health Association established
1873	New York Training School opens at Bellevue Hospital, New York City, as first Nightingale-model nursing school in the United States
1877	Women's Board of the New York Mission hires Frances Root to visit the sick poor
1885	Visiting Nurse Association established in Buffalo
1886	Visiting nurse agencies established in Philadelphia and Boston
1893	Lillian Wald and Mary Brewster organized a visiting nursing service for the poor of New York, which later became the famous Henry Street Settlement
	Society of Superintendents of Training Schools of Nurses in the United States and Canada was established (in 1912 became known as the National League for Nursing)
1895	Associated Alumnae of Training Schools for Nurses established (in 1911 became the American Nurses Association)
1902	School nursing started in New York (Lina Rogers)
1903	First nurse practice acts
1909	Metropolitan Life Insurance Company provides first insurance reimbursement for nursing care
1910	Public health nursing program instituted at Teachers College, Columbia University, in New York
1912	National Organization for Public Health Nursing formed with Lillian Wald as first president
1914	First course in public health nursing offered by Adelaide Nutting for graduates of diploma programs to secure Teacher's College (New York) degree
1918	Vassar Camp School for Nurses organized
	U.S. Public Health Service (PHS) establishes division of public health nursing to work in the war effort; worldwide influenza epidemic begins
1919	*Public Health Nursing* textbook written by Mary S. Gardner
1921	Maternity and Infancy Act (Sheppard-Towner Act) passed
1925	Frontier Nursing Service using nurse-midwives established
1933	Pearl McIver becomes first nurse employed by PHS
1935	Passage of Social Security Act
1941	Beginning of World War II
1943	Passage of Bolton-Bailey Act for nursing education and Cadet Nurse Program established
	Division of Nursing begun at PHS
	Lucille Petry appointed chief of Cadet Nurse Corps
1944	First basic program in nursing accredited as including sufficient public health content

Job opportunities for public health nurses grew because they continued to constitute a large proportion of health department personnel. Between 1950 and 1955, the proportion of U.S. counties with full-time local health services increased from 56% to 72% (Roberts and Heinrich, 1985). With more than 20,000 nurses employed in health departments, VNAs, industry, and schools, public health nurses at the middle of the twentieth century continued to have a crucial role in translating the advances of science and medicine into saving lives and improving health.

In 1946 representatives of agencies interested in community health met to improve coordination of various types of community nursing and to prevent overlap of services. The resulting guidelines proposed that a population of 50,000 be required to support a public health program and that there should be 1 nurse for every 2200 people. Nursing functions should include health teaching, disease control, and care of the sick. Communities were encouraged to adopt one of the following organizational patterns (Desirable organization, 1946):

- Administration of all community health nurse services by the local health department

- Provision of preventive health care by health departments, and provision of home visiting for the sick by a cooperating voluntary agency
- A combination service jointly administered and financed by official and voluntary agencies with all services provided by one group of nurses

Table 2-2 highlights significant milestones in public health nursing from the mid-1800s to the mid-1900s.

THE RISE OF CHRONIC ILLNESS

Between 1900 and 1955, the national crude mortality rate decreased by 47%. Many more Americans survived childhood and early adulthood to live into middle and older ages. Although in 1900 the leading causes of mortality were pneumonia, tuberculosis, and diarrhea/enteritis, by mid-century the leading causes had become heart disease, cancer, and cerebrovascular disease. Nurses helped to reduce communicable disease mortality through immunization campaigns, nutrition education, and provision of better hygiene and sanitation. Additional factors included improved medications, better housing, and innovative emergency and critical care services. Studies such as the National Health Survey of 1935-1936 had documented the national transition from communicable to chronic disease as the primary cause of significant illness and death. However, public policy and nursing services were diverted from addressing the emerging problem, first by the 1930s Depression and then by World War II.

As the aged population grew from 4.1% of the total in 1900 to 9.2% in 1950, so did the prevalence of chronic illness. Faced with a client population characterized by extended life spans and increased longevity after chronic illness diagnosis, nurses addressed new challenges related to chronic illness care, long-term illness and disability, and chronic disease prevention. In official health agencies, categorical programs focusing on a single chronic disease emphasized narrowly defined services, which might be poorly coordinated with other community programs. Screening for chronic illness was a popular method of both detecting undiagnosed disease and providing individual and community education.

Some VNAs adopted coordinated home care programs to provide complex, long-term care to the chronically ill, often after long-term hospitalization. These home care programs established a multidisciplinary approach to complex client care. For example, beginning in 1949, the Visiting Nurse Society of Philadelphia provided care to clients with stroke, arthritis, cancer, and fractures using a wide range of services, including physical and occupational therapy, nutrition consultation, social services, laboratory and radiographic procedures, and transportation services. During the 1950s, often in response to family demands and the shortage of nurses, many visiting nurse agencies began experimenting with auxiliary nursing personnel, variously called housekeepers, homemakers, or home health aides. These innovative programs provided a substantial basis for an approach to bedside nursing care that would be reimbursable by commercial health insurance (such as Blue Cross) and later by Medicare and Medicaid.

> **THE CUTTING EDGE** *Nurse historians are increasingly using oral history methodology to uncover and preserve the history of public health nurses on audiotapes and in written transcripts.*

The increased prevalence of chronic illness also encouraged a resurgence in combination agencies—the joint operation of official (city or county) health departments and voluntary visiting nurse agencies using a unified staff. Nurses wanted services to be provided in a coordinated, cost-effective manner respectful to the families served as well as to avoid duplication of care. Where nursing services were specialized, one household might simultaneously receive care from three different agencies for postpartum and newborn care, tuberculosis follow-up, and stroke rehabilitation. In cities with combination agencies, a minimum number of nurses provided improved services, ensuring continuity of care at a cheaper price. No longer would an agency "pick up and drop a baby," but instead would follow the child through infancy, preschool, school, and into adulthood as part

of one public health nursing program using one client record. The "ideal program" of the combination agency proved difficult to fund and administer, however, and many of the combination services implemented between 1930 and 1965 later retrenched into their former divided, public and private structures.

During the 1950s, public health nursing practice, like nursing in general, increased its focus on the psychological elements of client, family, and community care. To be more effective as helping persons, nurses sought improved understanding of their own behavior, as well as the behavior of their clients and their co-workers. The nurse's responsibility for health and human needs expanded to include stress and anxiety reduction associated with situational or developmental stressors, such as birth, adolescence, and parenting. Public health nurses sought a comprehensive approach to mental health that avoided dividing persons into physical components and emotional components (Abramovitz, 1961).

DECLINING FINANCIAL SUPPORT FOR PRACTICE AND PROFESSIONAL ORGANIZATIONS

During the 1930s and 1940s hospitals became the preferred place for illness care and childbirth. Improved technology and the concentration of physicians' work in the acute care hospital were influential, but the development of health insurance plans such as Blue Cross provided a means for the middle class to seek care outside the traditional arena of the home. Federal health policy after World War II supported the growth of institutional care in hospitals and nursing homes instead of community-based alternatives.

Financing for voluntary nursing agencies was greatly reduced in the early 1950s when both the Metropolitan and John Hancock Life Insurance Companies stopped funding visiting nurse services for their policyholders. The life insurance companies had found nursing services financially beneficial when communicable disease rates were high in the 1910s and 1920s, but reductions in communicable disease rates, improved infant and maternal health, and increased prevalence of expensive chronic illnesses reduced sponsor interest in financing home visiting. The American Red Cross also discontinued its programs of direct nursing service by the mid-1950s.

The NOPHN had long sought additional approaches for funding public health nursing. Beginning in the 1930s, the NOPHN collaborated with the American Nurses Association (ANA) through the Joint Committee on Prepayment. Both organizations had identified the growth potential of early health insurance innovations. Voluntary nursing agencies developed a variety of initiatives to secure health insurance reimbursement for nursing services, including demonstration projects and educational campaigns directed toward nurses, physicians, and insurers. Blue Cross and other hospital insurance programs gradually adopted a formula that exchanged unused days of hospitalization coverage for post-discharge nursing care at home. Unlike organized medicine and hospital associations, nursing organizations contributed substantially to securing federal medical insurance for the aged, which was implemented as the Medicare program in 1966. The support of the ANA, so integral to the passage of Medicare legislation, was recognized by President Lyndon Baines Johnson at the 1965 ceremony to sign the bill.

Despite the success and importance of the NOPHN, by the late 1940s its membership had declined and financial support was weak. At the same time, the nursing profession as a whole sought to reorganize its national organizations to improve unity, administration, and financial stability. Three existing organizations—the NOPHN, the National League for Nursing Education, and the Association of Collegiate Schools of Nursing—were dissolved in 1952. Their functions were distributed primarily to the new National League for Nursing. The American Nurses Association, which merged with the National Association of Colored Graduate Nurses, continued as the second national nursing organization. Occupational health nursing and nurse-midwifery organizations declined to join the consolidation, and both nursing specialties have continued to set their own course. Despite the optimism of the national reorganization and its success in some areas, the subsequent loss of independent public health nursing leadership and focus resulted in a weakened specialty.

> **DID YOU KNOW?** *Nurses, including public and community health nurses, interested in the history of nursing can join the American Association for the History of Nursing (AAHN), which holds annual research meetings. Look for the AAHN on the internet at www.aahn.org.*

PROFESSIONAL NURSING EDUCATION FOR PUBLIC HEALTH NURSING

The National League for Nursing enthusiastically adopted the recommendations of Esther Lucile Brown's 1948 study of nursing education, reported as *Nursing for the Future*. Her recommendation to establish basic nursing preparation in colleges and universities was consistent with the NOPHN's goal of including public health nursing concepts in all basic baccalaureate programs. The NOPHN believed that this would remedy the preparation problems found among many nurses new to the practice and would thus upgrade the public health nursing profession. Unfortunately, the implementation of the plan fell short, and training programs in public health nursing for college and university faculty were very brief. The population focus of public health nursing toward groups and the larger community was compromised and became less distinct in the hands of educators who themselves lacked education and practice in public health nursing.

During the 1950s, public health nursing educators carefully considered steps to enhance undergraduate and graduate education. Education for public health nurses was actually divided between schools of nursing and schools of public health. Although both claimed legitimacy, collegiate education for nurses gradually moved completely into schools of nursing. The Haven Hill (1951) and Gull Lake (1956) Conferences clarified roles and definitions, built expectations for graduate education, and set standards for undergraduate field

experiences. As public health nursing education drew closer to university schools of nursing, it adopted and applied broad principles characteristic of general nursing education. For example, rather than have the education director of the placement agency teach nursing students as done previously, collegiate programs themselves hired faculty who provided direct student supervision at community placements (NOPHN, 1951; Robeson and McNeil, 1957). Ruth Freeman was an innovative thinker and important nursing leader in this period, whose influential public health nursing books were widely read (Box 2-3).

NEW RESOURCES AND NEW COMMUNITIES: THE 1960s AND NURSING

Beginning in earnest in the late 1940s but on the basis of advocacy begun in the late 1910s, policymakers and social welfare representatives sought to establish national health insurance. In 1965 Congress amended the Social Security Act to include health insurance benefits for older adults (Medicare) and increased care for the poor (Medicaid). Unfortunately, the revised Social Security Act did not include coverage for preventive services, and home health care was reimbursed only when ordered by the physician. Nevertheless, this latter coverage prompted the rapid proliferation of home health care agencies with for-profit agencies seeing new opportunities. Many local and state health departments rapidly changed their policies to allow the agencies to provide reimbursable home care as bedside nursing. This often resulted in reduced health promotion and disease prevention activities. From 1960 to 1968, the number of official agencies providing home care services grew from 250 to 1328, and the number of for-profit agencies continued to grow (Kalisch and Kalisch, 1995).

COMMUNITY ORGANIZATION AND PROFESSIONAL CHANGE

Social changes during the 1960s and 1970s influenced both nursing and public health. "The emerging civil rights movement shifted the paradigm from a charitable obligation to a political commitment to achieving equality and compensation for racial injustices of the past" (Scutchfield and Keck, 1997, p 328). New programs addressed economic and racial differences in health care services and delivery. Funding was increased for maternal and child health, mental health, mental retardation, and community health training. Beginning in 1964, the federal Economic Opportunity Act provided funds for neighborhood health centers, Head Start, and other community action programs. Neighborhood health centers increased community access for health care, especially for maternal and child care. The work of Nancy Milio in Detroit, Michigan, is an example of this commitment to action with the community. Milio built a dynamic decision-making process that included neighborhood residents, politicians, the Visiting Nurse Association and its board, civil rights activists, and church leaders. The Mom and Tots Center emerged as a neighborhood-centered service to provide maternal and child

BOX 2-3   RUTH FREEMAN: PUBLIC HEALTH EDUCATOR, ADMINISTRATOR, CONSULTANT, AUTHOR, AND LEADER OF NATIONAL HEALTH ORGANIZATIONS

Public health nursing by the 1940s had emerged from its pioneer experiences and began to develop into a professional discipline capable of functioning in an increasingly complex health care system. To meet the challenges of providing health services to diverse communities, nursing needed leaders who possessed the necessary intellectual and political capabilities to keep the profession in the forefront of the national public health care movement. Ruth Freeman was one of these leaders.

Born in Methune, Massachusetts, on December 5, 1906, Freeman was the oldest of three children in a middle-class family. Encouraged by an aunt to become a nurse, Freeman entered the nursing program at Mount Sinai Hospital in New York City in 1923. As a student, she discovered not only that nursing was about caring for people, but also that it was intellectually challenging and offered many professional opportunities. After graduating in 1927, Freeman accepted a staff position at the Henry Street Visiting Nurse Service. This position profoundly influenced her career and her view of the power of nursing to help people deal with their illnesses and social problems. Recalling these formative years, Freeman noted that the families taught her an important nursing lesson: "that dying wasn't a calamity, that 'making do' was not demeaning, and helping was not controlling" (Safier, 1977, p. 68). Her Henry Street mentors, including Lillian Wald, reinforced her developing philosophy that the family was the principal decision-maker in their health activities, and that patience and optimism were essential characteristics of an effective nurse (Safier, 1977).

Recognized by faculty in her Columbia University baccalaureate program for her ability to lead, Freeman began her teaching career at the New York University Department of Nursing in 1937. She moved to the University of Minnesota School of Public Health to teach and to learn how health care was provided in rural communities. Freeman's insistence that she remain actively engaged in public health work allowed her opportunities to integrate the newly emerging social and biological knowledge into the direct care of clients. Her ability to use this information to alleviate health problems in the community enriched her students' education, and through her many articles and national presentations, she greatly influenced the practice of public health nurses and physicians in the nation.

Freeman's reputation as an innovative thinker and effective administrator led to the positions director of nursing at the American Red Cross and consultant to the National Security Board in Washington, DC (1946–1950). This experience solidified her belief in the interprofessional nature of community health services and the need for professional nurses to serve as administrators of health agencies and organizations. To ensure her own academic competency, she earned an MA degree from Columbia University in 1939 and an EdD from New York University in 1951 (Kaufman, 1988).

A new position at the Johns Hopkins University School of Hygiene and Public Health (1950–1971) led Freeman to becoming a professor of public health administration and coordinator of the nursing program. During her tenure at Hopkins, her talents as teacher, author, consultant, and organizational leader flourished. Author of over 50 publications, several of her books, including *Public Health Nursing Practice, Administration in Public Health Services* (with E. M. Holmes), and *Community Health Practice*, became widely used texts in nursing programs. Her ability to provide insightful leadership led to her election and appointment to numerous national posts, including president of the National League of Nursing (1955–1959), president of the National Health Council (1959–1960), and many of the major committees of the American Public Health Association. Freeman also served as a member of the 1958 White House Conference on Children and Youth and as a consultant to the World Health Organization and the Pan American Health Organization (Bullough, Church, and Stern, 1988).

The numerous national and international awards bestowed on her acknowledged Freeman's unique contributions to the professionalization of nursing and the improvement of public health services. These included the prestigious Pearl McIver Award from the American Nurses Association, the Bronfman Prize awarded by the American Public Health Association, and the Florence Nightingale Medal given by the International Red Cross. She was named, in 1981, an honorary member of the American Academy of Nursing, and in 1984, 2 years after her death, she was awarded American nursing's highest honor, election to the American Nurses Association's Nursing Hall of Fame (Bullough et al, 1988; Kaufman, 1988; Safier, 1977).

Contributed by Barbara Brodie, PhD, RN, FAAN, Director Emeritus of the Center for Nursing Historical Inquiry, University of Virginia, Charlottesville. Bullough V, Church OM, Stern A: *American nursing: a biographic dictionary*, New York, 1988, Garland; Kaufman M, editor: *Dictionary of American nursing biography*, New York, 1988, Greenwood Press; Safier G: *Contemporary American leaders in nursing: an oral history*, New York, 1977, McGraw-Hill.

health services and a day-care center. Milio (1971) recorded this story in her book, *9226 Kercheval: The Storefront That Did Not Burn.*

HOW TO   Conduct an Oral History Interview

1. Identify an issue or event of interest.
2. Research the issue or event using written materials.
3. Locate a potential oral history interviewee or narrator.
4. Obtain the agreement of the narrator to be interviewed. Arrange an interview appointment.
5. Research the narrator's background and the time period of interest.
6. Write an outline of questions for the narrator. Open-ended questions are especially helpful.
7. Meet with the narrator. Bring a tape recorder and extra tapes to the interview.
8. Interview the narrator. Ask one brief question at a time. Give the narrator time to consider your question and answer it.
9. Ask clarifying questions. Ask for examples. Give encouragement. Allow the narrator to tell his or her story without interruption.
10. After the interview, transcribe the interview tape and prepare a written transcript.
11. Carefully compare the written transcript to the narrator's recorded interview. It may be appropriate to have the narrator review and edit the written transcript.
12. If you have made written arrangements with the narrator, place the oral history tape and transcripts in an appropriate archives or library (highly recommended).

Oral history is a type of nursing research. Please consider that oral history interviews may require formal consent by the interviewee or narrator before the interview, as well as prior approval of the research from an institutional review board.

An example of oral history is found at: Gates MF, Schim SS, Ostrand L: Uniting the past and the future in public health nursing: the Michigan oral history project, Public Health Nurs *11*:3, 1994.

New personnel also added to the flexibility of the public health nurse to address the needs of communities. Beginning in 1965 at the University of Colorado, the nurse practitioner movement opened a new era for nursing involvement in primary care that affected the delivery of services in community health clinics. Initially, the nurse practitioner was often a public health nurse with additional skills in the diagnosis and treatment of common illnesses. Although some nurse practitioners chose to practice in other clinical areas, those who continued in public health settings made sustained contributions to improving access and providing primary care to people in rural areas, inner cities, and other medically underserved areas (Roberts and Heinrich, 1985). As evidence of the effectiveness of their services grew, nurse practitioners became increasingly accepted as cost-effective providers of a variety of primary care services.

PUBLIC HEALTH NURSING FROM THE 1970s TO THE PRESENT

During the 1970s, nursing was viewed as a powerful force for improving the health care of communities. Nurses made significant contributions to the hospice movement, the development of birthing centers, day care for older adult and disabled persons, drug abuse programs, and rehabilitation services in long-term care. Federal evaluation of the effectiveness of care was emphasized (Roberts and Heinrich, 1985).

By the 1980s, concern grew about the high costs of health care in the United States. Programs for health promotion and disease prevention received less priority as funding was shifted to meet the escalating costs of acute hospital care, medical procedures, and institutional long-term care. The use of ambulatory services including health maintenance organizations was encouraged, and the use of nurse practitioners increased. Home health care weathered several threats to adequate reimbursement and, by the end of the decade, had secured favorable legal decisions that increased its impact on the care of the sick at home. Individuals and families assumed more responsibility for their own health because health education, always a part of nursing, became increasingly popular. Advocacy groups representing both consumers and professionals urged the passage of laws to prohibit unhealthy practices in public such as smoking and driving under the influence of alcohol. Sophisticated media campaigns contributed to changing health behaviors and improving health status. As federal and state funds grew scarce, fewer nurses were employed by official public health agencies. Committed and determined to improve the health care of Americans, nurses continued to press for greater involvement in official and voluntary agencies (Kalisch and Kalisch, 1995; Roberts and Heinrich, 1985).

The National Center for Nursing Research (NCNR), established in 1985 within the federal National Institutes of Health near Washington, DC, had a major impact on promoting the work of nurses. Through research, nurses analyze the scope and quality of care provided by examining the outcomes and cost-effectiveness of nursing interventions. With the concerted efforts of many nurses, NCNR gained official institute status within the National Institutes of Health in 1993, becoming the National Institute of Nursing Research (NINR).

> **WHAT DO YOU THINK?**   *The emphasis on public health in nursing has been varied and has changed over time. Given this chapter's review of the important issues that nursing can address, what priorities would you set for the work of contemporary public health nurses?*

By the late 1980s, public health as a whole had declined significantly in its effectiveness in accomplishing its mission and in shaping the public's health. Significant reductions in local and national political support, financing, and outcomes were vividly described in a landmark report by the Institute of Medicine, *The Future of Public Health* (IOM, 1988). The IOM study group found America's public health system in disarray and concluded that, although there was widespread agreement about what the mission of public health should be, there was little consensus on how to translate that mission into action. Not surprisingly, the IOM reported that the mix and level of public health services varied extensively across the United States (Williams, 1995).

The Future of Public Health (IOM, 1988) determined that "contemporary public health is defined less by what public health professionals know how to do than by what the political system in a given area decides is appropriate or feasible" (p. 4). Nurses working in health departments saw underfunding reduce the breadth and depth of their role. When local public health departments provided insufficient care, voluntary agencies such as VNAs stepped in to assist vulnerable groups. However, without adequate funding for care of the poor, VNAs faced hard economic choices, and some closed their doors.

As described later in the chapter in the history of *Healthy People*, the *Healthy People* initiative has influenced goals and priority setting in both public health and nursing. In 1979 *Healthy People* proposed a national strategy to improve significantly the health of Americans by preventing or delaying the onset of major chronic illnesses, injuries, and infectious diseases. The initiative's specific goals and objectives provide a framework for periodic evaluation, leading to a new set of detailed objectives every decade. Implementation of these strategies has influenced the work of nurses through their employment in health agencies and through participation in state or local *Healthy People* coalitions. The most recent initiative, the development of *Healthy People 2020* objectives, has built on the work of *Healthy People 2010*. Some objectives in *Healthy People 2010* have been met; others are being retained in *Healthy People 2020*, and new ones have been added. *Healthy People 2020* objectives are included in each chapter.

The health care debate in the 1990s focused on cost, quality, and access to direct care services. Despite considerable interest in health care reform and securing universal health insurance coverage, the core economic debate—who will pay for what—emphasized reform of medical care rather than comprehensive changes in health promotion, disease prevention, and health care. In 1993, the American Health Security Act received insufficient Congressional support. Reflecting the weakness of public health, the aims of public health were never clearly considered in the proposed program. Proposals to reform existing services failed to apply the lesson learned from the *Healthy People* initiative—that health promotion and disease prevention appear to yield reductions in costs and illness/injury incidence while increasing years of healthy life.

TABLE 2-3 MILESTONES IN THE HISTORY OF COMMUNITY HEALTH AND PUBLIC HEALTH NURSING: 1946 TO 2010

YEAR	MILESTONE
1946	Nurses classified as professionals by U.S. Civil Service Commission
	Hill-Burton Act approved, providing funds for hospital construction in underserved areas and requiring these hospitals to provide care to poor people
	Passage of National Mental Health Act
1950	25,091 nurses employed in public health
1951	National organizations recommend that college-based nursing education programs include public health content
1952	National Organization for Public Health Nursing merges into the new National League for Nursing
	Metropolitan Life Insurance Nursing Program closes
1964	Passage of Economic Opportunity Act
	Public health nurse defined by the American Nurses Association (ANA) as a graduate of a BSN program
	Congress amended Social Security Act to include Medicare and Medicaid
1965	ANA position paper recommended that nursing education take place in institutions of higher learning
1977	Passage of Rural Health Clinic Services Act, which provided indirect reimbursement for nurse practitioners in rural health clinics
1978	Association of Graduate Faculty in Community Health Nursing/Public Health Nursing (later renamed as Association of Community Health Nursing Educators)
1979	Publication of *Healthy People: The Surgeon General's Report on Health Promotion and Disease Prevention*
1980	Medicaid amendment to the Social Security Act to provide direct reimbursement for nurse practitioners in rural health clinics
	ANA and APHA developed statements on the role and conceptual foundations of community and public health nursing, respectively
1983	Beginning of Medicare prospective payment system
1985	National Center for Nursing Research established in the National Institutes of Health (NIH)
1988	Institute of Medicine publishes *The Future of Public Health*
1990	Association of Community Health Nursing Educators publishes *Essentials of Baccalaureate Nursing Education*
1991	Over 60 nursing organizations joined forces to support health care reform and publish a document entitled *Nursing's Agenda for Health Care Reform*
1993	American Health Security Act of 1993 published as a blueprint for national health care reform; the national effort, however, failed, leaving states and the private sector to design their own programs
1994	NCNR becomes the National Institute for Nursing Research, as part of the National Institutes of Health
1996	Public health nursing section of American Public Health Association, *The Definition and Role of Public Health Nursing*, updated
1998	*The Public Health Workforce: An Agenda for the 21st Century* published by the U.S. Public Health Service to look at the current workforce in public, health, and educational needs, and the use of distance learning strategies to prepare future public health workers
1999	The Public Health Nursing Quad Council through the American Nurses Association works on new scope and standards of a public health nursing document, which differentiates between community-oriented and community-based nursing practice
2001	Significant interest in public health ensues from concerns about biological and other forms of terrorism in the wake of the intentional destruction of buildings in New York City and Washington, DC, on September 11
2002	Office of Homeland Security established to provide leadership to protect against intentional threats to the health of the public
2003	The Quad Council of Public Health Nursing Organizations finalizes *Public Health Nursing Competencies*
2003–2005	Multiple natural disasters including earthquakes, tsunamis, and hurricanes demonstrated the weak infrastructure for managing disasters in the United States and other countries and emphasized the need for strong public health programs that included disaster management
2007	An entirely new *Public Health Nursing Scope and Standards of Practice* is released through the ANA, reflecting the efforts of the Quad Council of Public Health Nursing Organizations
2010	The *Patient Protection and Affordable Care Act* is signed by President Barack Obama

In 1991 the ANA, the American Association of Colleges of Nursing, the National League for Nursing, and more than 60 other specialty nursing organizations joined to support health care reform. The coalition of nursing organizations emphasized key health care issues of access, quality, and cost, and proposed a range of interventions designed to build a healthy nation through improved primary care and public health efforts. Professional nursing's continued support for improved health care access and reduced cost was rewarded in 2010 with the passage of the federal Patient Protection and Affordable Care Act. Public health nursing must continue to advocate for extension of public health services to prevent illness, promote health, and protect the public (Table 2-3).

During the 1990s and 2000s, the Quad Council of Public Health Nursing Organizations supported the efforts of its organizational members and public health organizations to establish mechanisms to improve quality of care and to advance the public health nursing profession in the twenty-first century. For example, the certification of public health nurses with graduate degrees was reinforced through collaborative agreements with the American Nurses Credentialing Center (ANCC). The Association of Community Health Nursing Educators developed important position papers on graduate education for advanced practice public health nursing (2007) and on faculty qualifications for community/public health nursing educators (2009). The Association of State and Territorial Directors of Nursing asserted the importance of public health nurses within public health systems through the publication of *Every State Health Department Needs a Public Health Nurse Leader* (2008).

Since 1990, new and continuing challenges have triggered growth and change in nursing. Where existing organizations have been unable to meet community and neighborhood needs, nurse-managed health centers provide a diversity of nursing services, including health promotion and disease/injury prevention. New populations in communities continue to challenge schools of nursing, health departments, rural health clinics, and migrant health services to provide the range of services to meet specific needs, including the needs of new immigrants. Transfer of official health services to private control has sometimes reduced professional flexibility and service delivery. Many nurses leave public health nursing to work in acute care where the salaries are often higher. This is even more prominent in times of a nursing shortage. The Association of Community Health Nurse Educators calls for increased graduate programs to educate public health nurse leaders, educators, and researchers. Natural disasters (such as floods, hurricanes, and tornados) and human-made disasters (including explosions, building collapses, and airplane crashes) require innovative and time-consuming responses. Preparation for future disasters and potential bioterrorism demands the presence of well-prepared nurses. Some states hear new calls to deploy school nurses in every school; a new recognition of the link between school success and health is making the school nurse essential. Many of these stories are detailed in the chapters that follow.

> **DID YOU KNOW?** *Many colleges and universities offer courses on the history of nursing, the history of medicine, and the history of health care.*

 HEALTHY PEOPLE 2020

History of the Development of *Healthy People*

In 1979 the groundbreaking *Healthy People: The Surgeon General's Report on Health Promotion and Disease Prevention* asserted that "the health of the American people has never been better" (p. 3). But this was only the prologue to deep criticism of the status of American health care delivery. Between 1960 and 1978, health care spending increased 700%—without striking improvements in mortality or morbidity. During the 1950s and 1960s, evidence accumulated about chronic disease risk factors, particularly cigarette smoking, alcohol and drug use, occupational risks, and injuries. But these new research findings were not systematically applied to health planning and to improving population health.

In 1974 the Government of Canada published A New Perspective on the Health of Canadians (Lalonde, 1974), which found death and disease to have four contributing factors: inadequacies in the existing health care system, behavioral factors, environmental hazards, and human biological factors. Applying the Canadian approach, in 1976 U.S. experts analyzed the 10 leading causes of U.S. mortality and found that 50% of American deaths were the result of unhealthy behaviors, and only 10% were the result of inadequacies in health care. Rather than just spending more to improve hospital care, clearly prevention was the key to saving lives, improving the quality of life, and saving health care dollars.

A multidisciplinary group of analysts conducted a comprehensive review of prevention activities. They verified that the health of Americans could be significantly improved through "actions individuals can take for themselves" and through actions that public and private decision makers could take to "promote a safer and healthier environment" (p. 9). Like Canada's *New Perspectives*, *Healthy People* (1979) identified priorities and measurable goals. *Healthy People* grouped 15 key priorities into three categories: key preventive services that could be delivered to individuals by health providers, such as timely prenatal care; measures that could be used by governmental and other agencies, as well as industry, to protect people from harm, such as reduced exposure to toxic agents; and activities that individuals and communities could use to promote healthy lifestyles, such as improved nutrition.

In the late 1980s, success in addressing these priorities and goals was evaluated, new scientific findings were analyzed, and new goals and objectives were set for the period from 1990 to 2000 through *Healthy People 2000: National Health Promotion and Disease Prevention Objectives* (U.S. Public Health Service, 1991). This process was repeated 10 years later to develop goals and objectives for the period 2000 to 2010, and for 2010 to 2020. Recognizing the continuing challenge to using emerging scientific research to encourage modification of health behaviors and practices, *Healthy People 2020* addresses health equity, elimination of disparities, and improved health for all groups across the life span through disease prevention, improved social and physical environments, and healthy development and health behaviors.

Like the nurse in the early twentieth century who spread the gospel of public health to reduce communicable diseases, today's population-centered nurse uses *Healthy People* to reduce chronic and infectious diseases and injuries through health education, environmental modification, and policy development.

Lalonde M: *A new perspective on the health of Canadians*, Ottawa, Canada, 1974, Information Canada; U.S. Department of Health and Human Services: *Healthy People 2010: understanding and improving health*, ed 2, Washington, DC, 2000, U.S. Government Printing Office; U.S. Department of Health and Human Services: *Healthy People 2020: the road ahead*. Available at: http://www.healthypeople.gov/hp2020/. Accessed December 2, 2010; U.S. Department of Health, Education, and Welfare: *Healthy People: the surgeon general's report on health promotion and disease prevention*, DHEW Publication No. 79-55071, Washington, DC, 1979, U.S. Government Printing Office; U.S. Public Health Service: *Healthy People 2000: national health promotion and disease prevention objectives*, Washington, DC, 1991, U.S. Government Printing Office.

PUBLIC HEALTH NURSING TODAY

Today, nurses look to their history for inspiration, explanation, and prediction. Information and advocacy are used to promote a comprehensive approach to address the multiple needs of the diverse populations served. Nurses will seek to learn from the past and to avoid known pitfalls, even as they seek successful strategies to meet the complex needs of today's vulnerable populations. As plans for the future are made, as the public health challenges that remain unmet are acknowledged, it is the vision of what nursing can accomplish that sustains these nurses. As seen in the box below, nurses continue to rely on both nursing and public health standards and competency guides to help chart their practice.

The ANA's *Scope and Standards of Public Health Nursing Practice*, the Council on Linkages' *Domains and Core Competencies*, and the Quad Council's *Public Health Nursing Competencies* each include the processes of assessment, analysis, and planning. Each also incorporates the importance of communication, cultural competency, policy, and public health skills in their recommendations for effective public health nurse practice. Specific to this chapter, the Council on Linkages (2009) features a core competency under the domain of public health sciences skills: "Identifies prominent events in the history of the public health profession." Moreover, the Quad Council (2009) builds on this competency with an application to nursing under Domain #6, that a public health nurse "Identifies and understands the historic development and foundation of the fields of public health and public health nursing."

LINKING CONTENT TO PRACTICE

Public Health Nursing, a major journal in the field of public health nursing, publishes articles that very broadly reflect contemporary research, practice, education, and public policy for population-based nurses. Begun in 1984, *Public Health Nursing (PHN)* was published quarterly through 1993, and has been a bimonthly journal since 1994. Sarah E. Abrams (the Historical Editor) and Judith C. Hays are the journal's current editors (2010).

More than any other journal, *PHN* has assumed responsibility for preserving the history of public health nursing and for publishing new historical research on the field. The contemporary *Public Health Nursing* shares its name with the official journal of the National Organization for Public Health Nursing in the period 1931 to 1952 (earlier names were used for the official journal from 1913 to 1931, which built on the *Visiting Nurse Quarterly*, published 1909 to 1913).

The contemporary *Public Health Nursing* presents a wide variety of articles, including both new historical research and reprints of classic journal articles that deserve to be read and re-applied by modern public health nurses. One historical article reprinted in *PHN* addressed a nurse's 1931 work on county drought relief that underscores continuing professional themes of case-finding, collaboration, and partnership (Wharton, 1999). Another historical reprint recalled the important 1984 dialogue between two public health nurse leaders, Virginia A. Henderson and Sherry L. Shamansky, with an added contextual introduction from Dr. Abrams (Abrams, 2007). Original historical research presented in *PHN* is extremely varied, from public health nursing education, to public health nurse practice in Alaska's Yukon, to excerpts from the oral histories of public health nurses.

Contemporary nurses find inspiration and possibilities for modern innovations in reading the history of public health nursing in the pages of *PHN*.

Abrams SE: Nursing the community, a look back at the 1984 dialogue between Virginia A. Henderson and Sherry L. Shamansky, *PHN* 24:382, 2007; reprinted from *PHN* 1:193, 1984; Wharton AL: County drought relief: a public health nurse's problem. *PHN* 16(4):307-308, 1999; reprinted from *PHN* 23, 1931.

CHAPTER REVIEW

PRACTICE APPLICATION

Mary Lipsky has worked for the county health department in a major urban area for almost 2 years. Her nursing responsibilities include a variety of services, including consultations at a senior center, maternal/newborn home visits, and well-child clinics. As she leaves work each evening and returns to her own home, she keeps thinking about her clients. Why was it so difficult today to qualify a new mother and her baby to receive WIC (women, infants, and children) nutrition services? Why must she limit the number of children screened for high lead levels, when last year the health department screened twice as many children? Several children last month seemed asymptomatic, but the laboratory found lead levels that were high enough to cause damage. One of the mothers Ms. Lipsky is acquainted with is having a difficult time emotionally. Why is it so difficult to find a behavioral health provider for her? And the health department still cannot find a new staff dentist! And families on welfare cannot find a private dentist to care for their children.

A. Why might it be difficult to solve these problems at the individual level, on a case-by-case basis?

B. What information would you need to build an understanding of the policy background for each of these various populations? Answers can be found on the Evolve site.

KEY POINTS

- A historical approach can be used to increase understanding of public health nursing in the past, as well as its current dilemmas and future challenges.
- The history of public health nursing can be characterized by change in specific focus of the specialty but continuity in approach and style of the practice.
- Public health nursing, referred to in this text as population-centered nursing, is a product of various social, economic, and political forces; it incorporates public health science in addition to nursing science and practice.
- Federal responsibility for health care was limited until the 1930s when the economic challenges of the Depression permitted reexamination of local responsibility for care.
- Florence Nightingale designed and implemented the first program of trained nursing, and her contemporary, William Rathbone, founded the first district nursing association in England.

KEY POINTS—cont'd

- Urbanization, industrialization, and immigration in the United States increased the need for trained nurses, especially in public health nursing.
- Increasing acceptance of public roles for women permitted public health nursing employment for nurses, as well as public leadership roles for their wealthy supporters.
- The first trained nurse in the United States, who was salaried as a visiting nurse, was Frances Root; she was hired in 1887 by the Women's Board of the New York City Mission to provide care to sick persons at home.
- The first visiting nurses' associations were founded in 1885 and 1886 in Buffalo, Philadelphia, and Boston.
- Lillian Wald established the Henry Street Settlement, which became the Visiting Nurse Service of New York City, in 1893. She played a key role in innovations that shaped public health nursing in its first decades, including school nursing, insurance payment for nursing, national organization for public health nurses, and the United States Children's Bureau.
- Founded in 1902 with the vision and support of Lillian Wald, school nursing sought to keep children in school so that they could learn.
- The Metropolitan Life Insurance Company established the first insurance-based program in 1909 to support community health nursing services.
- The National Organization for Public Health Nursing (founded in 1912) provided essential leadership and coordination of diverse public health nursing efforts; the organization merged into the National League for Nursing in 1952.
- Official health agencies slowly grew in numbers between 1900 and 1940, accompanied by a steady increase in public health nursing positions.
- The innovative Sheppard-Towner Act of 1921 expanded community health nursing roles for maternal and child health during the 1920s.
- Mary Breckinridge established the Frontier Nursing Service in 1925, which influenced provision of rural health care.
- African-American nurses seeking to work in public health nursing faced many challenges, but ultimately had significant impact on the communities they served.

- Tension between the nursing role of caring for the sick and the role of providing preventive care, and the related tension between intervening for individuals and intervening for groups have characterized the specialty since at least the 1910s.
- As the Social Security Act attempted to remedy some of the setbacks of the Depression, it established a context in which public health nursing services expanded.
- The challenges of World War II sometimes resulted in extension of nursing care and sometimes in retrenchment and decreased public health nursing services.
- By mid-twentieth century, the reduced prevalence of communicable diseases and the increased prevalence of chronic illness, accompanied by large increases in the population more than 65 years of age, led to examination of the goals and organization of public health nursing services.
- Between the 1930s and 1965, organized nursing and community health nursing agencies sought to establish health insurance reimbursement for nursing care at home.
- Implementation of Medicare and Medicaid programs in 1966 established new possibilities for supporting community-based nursing care but encouraged agencies to focus on services provided after acute care rather than on prevention.
- Efforts to reform health care organization, pushed by increased health care costs during the last 40 years, have focused on reforming acute medical care rather than on designing a comprehensive preventive approach.
- The 1988 Institute of Medicine report documented the reduced political support, financing, and impact that increasingly limited public health services at national, state, and local levels.
- In the late 1990s, federal policy changes dangerously reduced financial support for home health care services, threatening the long-term survival of visiting nurse agencies.
- *Healthy People 2000, Healthy People 2010,* and recent disasters and acts of terrorism have brought renewed emphasis on prevention to nursing.

CLINICAL DECISION-MAKING ACTIVITIES

1. Interview nurses at your clinical placement about the changes they have seen during their years in a population-centered nursing practice. How do these changes relate to the changing needs of the community or the population?

2. Identify the visible record of nursing agencies in your community. Note the buildings, plaques, and display cases, for example, that are records of the past provision of nursing care in community settings. What forces have influenced these agencies over time? Which factors do they wish to make known publicly, and which factors are less apparent?

3. Secure a copy of your clinical agency's recent annual report. How is the history of the agency presented? How does this agency's history fit in with the points made in this chapter? What are your conclusions about how this agency's past influences its present?

4. Interview older relatives for their memories of public health nursing care received by them, their families, and their friends. When they were younger, how was the public health nurse perceived in their community? What interventions were used by the public health nurse? How was the public health nurse dressed? How has the position of the public health or community health nurse changed?

5. Of what element or aspect of the history of public health nursing would you like to learn more? At your nursing library, review a period of 10 years of one journal from the past to identify trends in how this element or aspect was addressed. What conclusions do you reach?

6. The work and impact of several nursing leaders is reviewed or noted in this chapter. Of these leaders, which one strikes you as most interesting? Why? Locate and read further articles or books about this leader. What personal strengths do you note that supported this nurse's leadership?

REFERENCES

Abramovitz AB, editor: *Emotional factors in public health nursing: a casebook,* Madison, WI, 1961, University of Wisconsin Press.

American Association of Industrial Nurses: *The nurse in industry: a history of the American Association of Industrial Nurses, Inc.,* New York, 1976, AAIN.

Association of State and Territorial Directors of Nursing: *Every state health department needs a public health nurse leader,* 2008. Available at: http://www.astdn.org/. Accessed December 2, 2010.

Backer BA: Lillian Wald: connecting caring with action, *Nurs Health Care* 14:122, 1993.

Brainard A: *Evolution of public health nursing,* Philadelphia, 1922, Saunders.

Breckinridge M: *Wide neighborhoods, a story of the Frontier Nursing Service,* New York, 1952, Harper.

Browne H: A tribute to Mary Breckinridge, *Nurs Outlook* 14:54, 1966.

Buhler-Wilkerson K: Public health nursing: in sickness or in health? *Am J Public Health* 75:1155, 1985.

Buhler-Wilkerson K: Left carrying the bag: experiments in visiting nursing, 1877-1909, *Nurs Res* 36:42–45, 1987.

Buhler-Wilkerson K: *False dawn: the rise and decline of public health nursing, 1900-1930,* New York, 1989, Garland.

Buhler-Wilkerson K: *No place like home: a history of nursing and home care in the United States,* Baltimore, 2001, Johns Hopkins Press.

Bullough V, Bullough B: *The emergence of modern nursing,* New York, 1964, Macmillan.

Bullough V, Church OM, Stern A: *American nursing: a biographic dictionary,* New York, 1988, Garland.

Cohen IB: Florence Nightingale, *Sci Am* 250:128, 1984.

Council on Linkages Between Academic and Public Health Practice: *Core competencies for public health professionals.* Washington DC, 2010, Public Health Foundation/Health Resources and Services Administration.

Craven FSL: *A guide to district nursing,* New York, 1984, Garland (originally published in London, 1889, Macmillan).

Cristy TE: Lillian D. Wald: portrait of a leader. In Kelly LY, editor: *Pages from nursing history,* New York, 1984, American Journal of Nursing Co, pp 84–88.

Deloughery GL: *History and trends of professional nursing,* ed 8, St Louis, 1977, Mosby.

Desirable organization for public health nursing for family service, *Public Health Nurs* 38:387, 1946.

Dock LL: The history of public health nursing, *Public Health Nurs* 14:522, 1922.

Dolan J: *History of nursing,* ed 14, Philadelphia, 1978, Saunders.

Duffus RL: *Lillian Wald: neighbor and crusader,* New York, 1938, Macmillan.

Goan MB: *Mary Breckinridge: the Frontier Nursing Service and rural health in Appalachia,* Chapel Hill, NC, 2008, University of North Carolina Press.

Hanggi-Myers L: The Howard Association of New Orleans: precursor to district nursing, *Public Health Nurs* 12:78, 1995.

Hawkins JW, Hayes ER, Corliss CP: School nursing in America: 1902-1994: a return to public health nursing, *Public Health Nurs* 11:416, 1994.

Hine DC: *Black women in white: racial conflict and cooperation in the nursing profession, 1890-1950,* Bloomington, 1989, Indiana University Press.

Holloway JB: Frontier Nursing Service 1925-1975, *J Ky Med Assoc* 13:491, 1975.

Institute of Medicine: *The future of public health,* Washington, DC, 1988, National Academy of Science.

Kalisch PA, Kalisch BJ: *The advance of American nursing,* ed 3, Philadelphia, 1995, Lippincott.

Kaufman M, editor: *Dictionary of American nursing biography,* New York, 1988, Greenwood Press.

Lalonde M: *A new perspective on the health of Canadians,* Ottawa, Canada, 1974, Information Canada.

McNeil EE: *Transition in public health nursing,* Feb 27, 1967, John Sundwall Lecture, University of Michigan.

Milio N: *9226 Kercheval: the storefront that did not burn,* Ann Arbor, MI, 1971, University of Michigan Press.

Mosley MOP: Jessie Sleet Scales: first black public health nurse, *ABNF J* 5:45, 1994.

National Organization for Public Health Nursing: Approval of Skidmore College of Nursing as preparing students for public health nursing, *Public Health Nurs* 36:371, 1944.

National Organization for Public Health Nursing: *Proceedings of work conference: Collegiate Council on Public Health Nursing Education,* New York, 1951, NOPHN.

Nightingale F: *Notes on nursing: what it is, and what it is not,* Philadelphia, 1946, Lippincott.

Nightingale F: Sick nursing and health nursing. In Billings JS, Hurd HM, editors: *Hospitals, dispensaries, and nursing,* New York, 1984, Garland (originally published in Baltimore, 1894, Johns Hopkins Press).

Nutting MA, Dock LL: *A history of nursing,* New York, 1935, Putnam.

Palmer IS: *Florence Nightingale and the first organized delivery of nursing services,* Washington, DC, 1983, American Association of Colleges of Nursing.

Pickett G, Hanlon JJ: *Public health: administration and practice,* St Louis, 1990, Mosby.

Pickett SE: *The American National Red Cross: its origin, purpose, and service,* ed 2, New York, 1924, Century.

Quad Council of Public Health Nursing Organizations: *Competencies for Public Health Nursing Practice,* Washington DC, 2003, ASTDN, revised 2009.

Roberts DE, Heinrich J: Public health nursing comes of age, *Am J Public Health* 75:1162–1165, 1985.

Roberts M: *American nursing: history and interpretation,* New York, 1955, Macmillan.

Robeson KA, McNeil EE: *Report of conference on field instruction in public health nursing,* New York, 1957, National League for Nursing.

Rodabaugh JH, Rodabaugh MJ: *Nursing in Ohio: a history,* Columbus, OH, 1951, Ohio State Nurses' Association.

Rosen G: *A history of public health,* New York, 1958, MD Publications.

Safier G: *Contemporary American leaders in nursing: an oral history,* New York, 1977, McGraw-Hill.

Scutchfield FD, Keck CW: *Principles of public health practice,* Albany, NY, 1997, Delmar.

Shyrock H: *The history of nursing,* Philadelphia, 1959, Saunders.

Thoms AB: *Pathfinders: a history of the progress of colored graduate nurses,* New York, 1929, Kay Printing House.

Tirpak H: The Frontier Nursing Service: fifty years in the mountains, *Nurs Outlook* 33:308, 1975.

U.S. Department of Health and Human Services: *Healthy People 2010: understanding and improving health,* ed 2, Washington, DC, 2000, U.S. Government Printing Office.

U.S. Department of Health, Education, and Welfare: *Healthy People: the Surgeon General's report on health promotion and disease prevention,* DHEW Publication No. 79-55071, Washington, DC, 1979, U.S. Government Printing Office.

Wald LD: *The house on Henry Street,* New York, 1915, Holt.

Wald LD: *Windows on Henry Street,* Boston, 1934, Little, Brown.

Waters Y: *Visiting nursing in the United States,* New York, 1909, Charities Publication Committee.

Williams B: *Lillian Wald: angel of Henry Street,* New York, 1948, Julian Messner.

Williams CA: Beyond the Institute of Medicine report: a critical analysis and public health forecast, *Fam Community Health* 18:12, 1995.

Wilner DM, Walkey RP, O'Neill EJ: *Introduction to public health,* ed 7, New York, 1978, Macmillan.

Zerwekh JV: Public health nursing legacy: historical practical wisdom, *Nurs Health Care* 13:84, 1992.

CHAPTER 3

Public Health and Primary Health Care Systems and Health Care Transformation

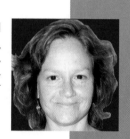

Bonnie Jerome-D'Emilia, PhD, MPH, RN

Dr. Bonnie Jerome-D'Emilia is an Assistant Professor of Nursing at Rutgers, The State University of New Jersey, in Camden, New Jersey. Dr. Jerome-D'Emilia is the director of the RN to BSN program at the University and teaches community health, leadership, management, and health policy courses. She taught previously at the University of Virginia School of Nursing, where she coordinated the Health Systems Management Master's program and distance learning. Her research and publications focus on diffusion of innovation in health care and specifically in the treatment of breast cancer in the United States.

ADDITIONAL RESOURCES

ⓔvolve WEBSITE
http://evolve.elsevier.com/Stanhope
- *Healthy People 2020*
- WebLinks
- Quiz

- Case Studies
- Glossary
- Answers to Practice Application
- Resource Tool
  - Resource Tool 3.A: Declaration of Alma Ata

OBJECTIVES

After reading this chapter, the student should be able to do the following:

1. Describe the trends that are influencing the evolution of the health care system in the early decades of the twenty-first century.
2. Define public health and primary health care and explain the nursing roles in each.
3. Evaluate the effectiveness of the United States primary health care system to meet the established goals of Alma Ata as the basis for primary health care.
4. Describe the current public health system in the United States.
5. Compare and contrast the responsibilities of the federal, state, and local public health systems.

KEY TERMS

Affordable Health Care for America Act, p. 60
American Recovery and Reinvestment Act of 2009, p. 48
disease prevention, p. 54
disparities, p. 45
electronic health record, p. 51

globalization, p. 52
health care reform, p. 45
Healthy People 2020, p. 54
Institute of Medicine, p. 45
managed care, p. 54
medically underserved areas, p. 56
primary health care, p. 53

public health, p. 45
public health system, p. 56
sentinel events, p. 50
World Health Organization, p. 52
—*See Glossary for definitions*

It has been said about health care that the only constant is change. Yet if we look back at predictions made in the final years of the twentieth century, the changes that have come to pass are not those that were expected. We thought in 2000 that although our health care system was expensive, and that access and quality were not optimal, the infrastructure was such that we could meet the challenges of the major killers of the time—cardiovascular disease and cancer. However, we had not yet considered the report published by the Institute of Medicine that found that between 44,000 and 98,000 people die each year as a result of preventable medical errors (IOM, 2000). In addition, we had not yet lived through the nightmare of September 11, 2001, when we learned that terrorism could strike on American soil, or August 29, 2005, when category 3 Hurricane Katrina generated flooding in New Orleans that resulted in the worst natural disaster in U.S. history. We had not yet witnessed the release of a global pandemic warning, which followed the occurrence of the H1N1 flu in Mexico, where 854 cases of the flu and 59 deaths were observed between March 18 and April 23, 2009 (WHO, 2010a). Subsequent transmission across large geographical areas spread laboratory confirmed flu cases to 212 countries, resulting in some 15,292 deaths by February 2010 (WHO, 2010b). Nor had we experienced the release of vast reserves of oil in the Gulf of Mexico in April 2010, affecting the lives of people, animals, and the water and land themselves.

We had not yet begun to fund the Global Health Initiative, in which the U.S. government would eventually invest $63 billion over 6 years to assist partner countries to improve the provision of care in the following areas: HIV/AIDS, malaria, tuberculosis, maternal and child health, nutrition, family planning and reproductive health, and neglected tropical diseases. This initiative, which emphasizes a "women and girl approach" in the provision of health care (in recognition of the central role of women in the health of their families and communities) also recognizes that the United States cannot fund these programs indefinitely, and so self sustainability must be integrated into the partner countries' health systems (Office of U.S. Global AIDS Coordinator, 2010). Most significantly, we had not foreseen that the Presidential election of 2008 would usher in a major battle in health care reform that may change the face of health care in the

United States for decades to come. Perhaps we need to reconsider the magnitude of the changes that have bombarded the health care system in the first decade of the twenty-first century, and state instead that the only constant is revolutionary change.

This chapter discusses a health care system in flux and evolving to meet domestic and global challenges. The health care system in the United States, the trends that affect this system, and the impact of these trends on public health are described. The primary health care and public health systems in the United States are described and differentiated, and the changing priorities of these systems to meet the nation's needs are identified. Nurses play a pivotal role in meeting these needs, and so the role of the nurse in the health system is presented. Box 3-1 lists selected definitions that will help explain concepts introduced in this chapter.

CURRENT HEALTH CARE SYSTEM IN THE UNITED STATES

While technology, disasters (both man-made and natural), and global health crises influence how we think about our health care system, the ongoing indicators of cost, access, and quality continue to cause disparities in the U.S. health care system. Further debate on these issues will drive improvements that will lead nurses into new roles, tasks, and challenges in the decade ahead.

Cost

Beginning in 2008, a historic weakening of the national and global economy—the "Great Recession"—lead to the loss of 7 million jobs in the United States (Economic Report, 2010). Even as the Gross Domestic Product (GDP), an indicator of the economic health of a country, declined in 2009, health care spending continued to grow and reached $2.5 trillion in the same year (Truffer et al, 2010). In the years between 2010 and 2019, national health spending is expected to grow at an average annual rate of 6.1%, reaching $4.5 trillion by 2019, for a share of approximately 19.3% of the GDP. This translates into a projected increase in per capita spending from $8046 in 2009 to $13,387 in 2019 (Centers for Medicare and Medicaid Services, 2009a).

BOX 3-1   DEFINITIONS OF SELECTED TERMS

- *Disease prevention:* Activities that have as their goal the protection of people from becoming ill because of actual or potential health threats.
- *Disparities:* Racial or ethnic differences in the quality of health care, not based on access or clinical needs, preferences, or appropriateness of an intervention.
- *Electronic health record:* A computer-based client health record.
- *Globalization:* A trend toward an increased flow of goods, services, money, and disease across national borders.
- *Health:* A state of complete physical, mental, and social well-being; not merely the absence of disease or infirmity (WHO, 1948).
- *Health promotion:* Activities that have as their goal the development of human attitudes and behaviors that maintain or enhance well-being.
- *Institute of Medicine:* A part of the National Academy of Sciences, and an organization whose purpose is to provide national advice on issues relating to biomedical science, medicine, and health.
- *Primary care:* The provision of integrated, accessible health care services by clinicians who are accountable for addressing a large majority of personal health care needs, developing a sustained partnership with clients, and practicing in the context of family and community.
- *Primary health care:* A combination of primary care and public health care made universally accessible to individuals and families in a community, with their full participation, and provided at a cost that the community and country can afford (WHO, 1978).
- *Public health:* Organized community and multidisciplinary efforts, based on epidemiology, aimed at preventing disease and promoting health (Terris, 1988).

Terris M: Epidemiology and leadership in public health in the Americas, *J Public Health Pol* 9(2):250-260, 1988.
World Health Organization: *Primary health care,* Geneva, 1978, WHO.

TABLE 3-1   ACTUAL AND PROJECTED NATIONAL HEALTH EXPENDITURES, 2004-2019

YEAR	2004	2009	2014	2019
Percent GDP	15.6	17.3	17.4	19.3
Per capita spending (dollars)	6327	8046	10,048	13,387

From Centers for Medicare and Medicaid Services: National health projections 2009-2019, forecast summary and selected tables, table 1, 2009. Available at http://www.cms.hhs.gov/NationalHealthExpendData/downloads/proj2009.pdf. Retrieved December 3, 2010.
GDP, Gross Domestic Product.

Table 3-1 shows the increases in spending from actual expenditures in 2004 to projections for 2019, a 19% increase in GDP and a 52% increase in per capita spending for this time period. These projections reflect the effects of the recession (beginning in 2008) which included a shift toward more public spending to offset the decline of employer-sponsored insurance. For example, as jobs are lost, employer-sponsored insurance is lost as well, so the numbers of Medicaid recipients rose 6.5% and Medicaid spending increased 9.9% (Truffer et al, 2010). In addition to this increase in public spending, private spending declined, which reflects both the increasing number of uninsured among the newly unemployed as well as the decline of disposable income that could be used to pay for out-of-pocket health care expenses. Although the economy strengthened in 2010, jobs did not correspondingly increase, and this slow return to pre-recession employment kept private spending down. By 2012, it is expected that public payment for health care services (programs such as Medicare, Medicaid and the Children's Health Insurance Plan) will account for over half the health care purchased in the United States (Truffer et al, 2010).

Figure 3-1 illustrates how health care dollars were spent in the year 2008. The largest share of health care expenditures goes to pay for hospital care, with physician services being the next largest item. It is obvious when looking at this chart that the amount of money that has gone to pay for public health services is much lower than the other categories of expenditures. Other significant drivers of the increasingly high cost of health care include:

- Prescription drugs and technology: Prescription drug expenses, although only 10% of health care expenditures in 2008, have been growing rapidly and will continue to do so. Development of new drugs and technologically advanced treatments entail high costs in research and development and lead to an increased demand among consumers (Kaiser Family Foundation, 2009a).
- Chronic disease: At the beginning of the twentieth century, infectious diseases such as pneumonia, flu, and tuberculosis were the major causes of death, and a man who was born in 1900 could expect to die before age 50 (Arias, 2007). At the end of the twentieth century, heart disease and cancer had eclipsed infectious disease as the major causes of death, resulting in the increased costs of prolonged care including nursing home and home health care, as well as costs of medication and treatment.

Following the "Great Recession," the economic rebound will likely coincide with the burgeoning Medicare enrollment of the aging Baby Boomer population. These new Medicare enrollees will increase Medicare expenditures for the foreseeable future. Medicaid recipients can be expected to decline as jobs are added to the economy, and the percentage of workers covered by employer-sponsored insurance should rise to reflect that growth. Costs will rise as private insurers pass the increased costs of health care onto employers as increased premiums. Employers then pass these premium increases onto their workers, along with higher co-pay and deductible expenses. Although workers' salaries have not kept pace, employer-sponsored insurance premiums have grown 119% since 1999 (Kaiser Family Foundation, 2009a), and the inability of workers to pay this increased cost has lead to a rise in the percentage of working families who are uninsured.

Access

As costs continue to rise for the provision of health care services, the number of people who can afford to pay for even the most basic care has declined. The U.S. Census Bureau reported that the number of uninsured rose to 46.3 million in 2008 from

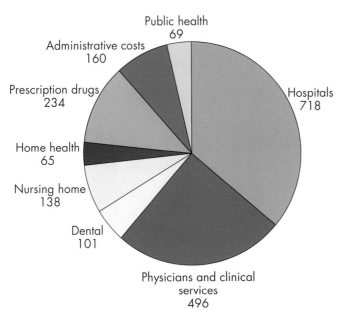

BOX 3-2 GOVERNMENT-FINANCED REIMBURSEMENT PROGRAMS

Medicare
- Federal government pays
- 45 million beneficiaries in 2008
- People age 65 or older
- Some people under age 65 with disabilities
- People with end-stage renal disease requiring dialysis or a kidney transplant

Medicaid
- Federal and state share expenses
- 43.5 million enrollees in 2008
- State administered; state programs vary
- Low-income families with children who meet eligibility requirements
- Disabled who meet eligibility requirements
- Poor elderly "dual eligibles"

Children's Health Insurance Program (CHIP)
- Created by Balanced Budget Act of 1997
- 7 million enrollees in 2008
- Federal and state share expenses although federal share is capped each year
- State administered; state programs vary
- Coverage of children to age 19 if not already insured
- For low-income uninsured children above Medicaid eligibility limits

FIGURE 3-1 Where the money went in 2008: health care spending in billions of dollars. (Data extracted from Centers for Medicare and Medicaid Services: National health expenditures aggregate, per capita amounts, percent distribution, and average annual percent growth, by source of funds: selected calendar years 1960-2008, Table 2, 2009. Available at http://www.cms.hhs.gov/NationalHealth ExpendData/downloads/tables.pdf. Accessed December 3, 2010.)

45.7 million in 2007, although the percentage of uninsured in the U.S. population remained unchanged at 15.4% of the non-elderly population (DeNavas-Walt, Proctor, and Smith, 2009). In addition, there was a shift to public funding as the number of people insured through private health insurance (including employer-sponsored insurance) decreased by 1 million and the number of people receiving government-provided insurance increased by 4.4 million recipients (DeNavas-Walt, Proctor, and Smith, 2009).

Although 61% of the non-elderly population continues to obtain health insurance through their employer as a benefit, employment does not guarantee insurance (Rowland, Hoffman, and McGinn-Shapiro, 2009). As costs for insurance premiums rise, employers either shift more of these costs to their employees or decline to offer employment-based health coverage at all. This becomes clear when we consider that 9 in 10 (91%) of the middle-class uninsured come from families with at least one full-time worker in jobs that do not offer health insurance or where coverage is unaffordable (Rowland, Hoffman, and McGinn-Shapiro, 2009).

Government programs such as Medicare, Medicaid, and the Children's Health Insurance Program (CHIP), all described in Box 3-2, play a significant role in meeting the needs of the uninsured. However, as workers lose jobs and employer-sponsored insurance and turn to publically funded programs, states face substantial budget shortfalls, prompting some immediate cuts in the health programs that rely on state funding (Medicaid and CHIP). The continuing growth in the number of uninsured reminds us that there is a significant gap in coverage.

In 2008, 10.8% of white, non-Hispanic Americans were uninsured, compared with 19.1% of African-Americans, 17.6% of Asians, and 30.7% of Latinos (U.S. Census Bureau, 2009). The risk of being uninsured is particularly high for immigrants who are not citizens: 44.7% of non-citizens were uninsured in 2008 (U.S. Census Bureau, 2009). There is a strong relationship between health insurance coverage and access to health care services. Insurance status determines the amount and kind of health care people are able to afford, as well as where they can receive care. The uninsured receive less preventive care, are diagnosed at more advanced disease states, and once diagnosed tend to receive less therapeutic care in terms of surgery and treatment options. A recent study found that as many as 27,000 deaths were the result of a lack of insurance in 2006 (Dorn, 2008).

Even those individuals and families with insurance coverage may find themselves medically underserved. The medically underserved includes those whose insurance does not pay adequately for medical care needed, whose coverage includes high cost sharing and strict limits on covered services, as well as those who live in areas lacking in health care providers. A study in 2007 found that 56 million people in the United States lacked adequate access to primary health care because of shortages of primary health care providers in their communities (National Association of Community Health Centers, 2009). Those who are poor, minority group members, and non-English speakers have the greatest barriers to access.

The uninsured or underinsured have a safety net. There are now more than 6600 federally funded community health centers throughout the United States. The community health

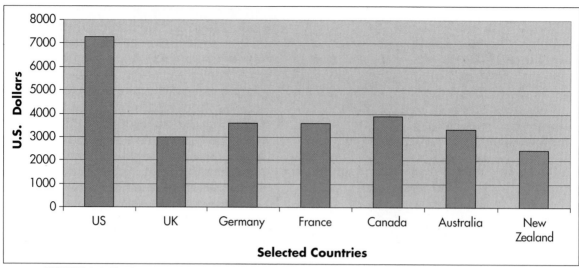

FIGURE 3-2 Total expenses per capita in U.S. dollars, 2007. (Data extracted from OECD Health Data 2009. Available at http://www.oecd.org/document/16/0,3343,en_2649_34631_2085200_1_1_1_1,00.html. Accessed December 3, 2010.)

center is the backbone of the safety net system. These centers are public and non-profit and receive funding from the federal government. Characteristics of these centers (USDHHS, n.d.a) include the following:

- They must be located in or serve a high need or medically underserved community, which can be rural or urban.
- They must provide comprehensive primary care services and supportive services such as translation and transportation services.
- Their services must be available to all residents of their service areas. Fees are adjusted based on the clients' ability to pay.
- They must be governed by a community board that is composed of a majority of health center clients to represent the population served.

Federally funded community health centers offer a broad range of health and social services, provided by nurse practitioners, physician assistants, physicians, social workers, and dentists. Among the 18 million who received care in these clinics in 2007, one out of every five clients were low-income, uninsured individuals; one in four were low income and members of minority populations; and one in seven were rural residents (National Association of Community Health Centers, 2009).

The **American Recovery and Reinvestment Act of 2009** (ARRA), an economic stimulus package designed to offset some of the losses related to the recession, provided $2 billion in additional funding for the nation's community health centers, including a substantial amount of money to cover the increased demand for services that is likely to occur in a time of rising unemployment. Nineteen states also increased funding for community health centers, although 13 states decreased funding in 2009 because of budgetary shortfalls.

Per capita health spending in the United States continues to exceed spending in the other industrialized countries. Canada, with medical practice styles fairly similar to those in the United States, spent only $5452 per person in 2009, 32% less than the United States (Canadian Institute for Health Information,

2010). In addition, although the United States spends more on health care than any other country (Figure 3-2), when compared with Australia, Canada, Germany, New Zealand, and the United Kingdom, the United States ranks last among these countries in infant mortality and life expectancy (Figure 3-3) (Davis et al, 2007). In 2006, in an international ranking of 191 national health care systems, the United States ranked 43rd for adult female mortality, 42nd for adult male mortality, and 36th for life expectancy (Doe, 2009). These rankings were based on the extent to which the money spent on public health and medical care in these 191 countries improved health, reduced disparities, protected families from impoverishment resulting from medical expenses, and provided services that respect the dignity of clients (Murray and Frenk, 2010).

As the nation's economy stagnated, it became obvious that the high cost of public funding for health care would only serve to increase the ballooning national deficit. Yet the inequities in access would likely increase unless disparities caused by lack of insurance were addressed as well. The 2008 election ushered in a renewed interest in health reform. Not since President Clinton's failed effort to pass the Health Security Act in 1993 has an administration attempted a major health reform initiative. The most recent reform efforts were incremental changes or additions to the present system, such as the Children's Health Insurance Program, passed by President Clinton, and Medicare Part D, the prescription drug coverage addition to the Medicare program, passed during President George W. Bush's time in office.

President Obama placed the goal of major and systemic health care reform on the top of his agenda and, soon after taking office, instructed the Democratic majorities in the House of Representatives and the Senate to draft a proposal. Debate ensued with much concern over the financial implications of various reform efforts such as the public option, individual mandates, and the health insurance exchange (defined in Box 3-3). Although partisan politics threatened to derail the President's efforts to pass a major health reform bill in 2010, public concern over health care's rising costs and lack of access

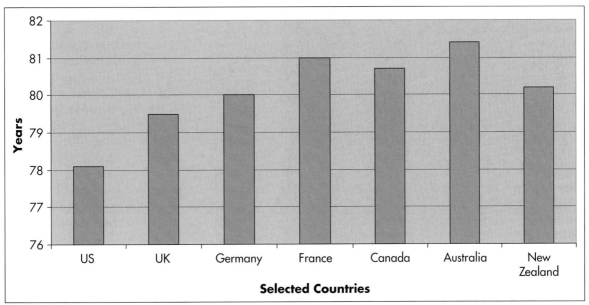

FIGURE 3-3 Life expectancy of the total population for births in 2007. (Data extracted from OECD Health Data 2009. Available at http://www.oecd.org/document/16/0,3343,en_2649_34631_2085200_1_1_1_1, 00.html. Accessed December 3, 2010.)

BOX 3-3   DEFINITIONS OF SELECTED HEALTH CARE REFORM OPTIONS

- *Public option:* A government-run health insurance plan, like Medicare, that would compete with private insurers in a Health Insurance Exchange.
- *Individual mandate:* Those who do not have insurance and refuse to subscribe to health insurance will be required to pay a tax penalty.
- *Insurance mandate:* Eliminates preexisting disease clauses, discrimination based on age or gender, lifetime limits on coverage, and rescissions in which insurance companies suddenly withdraw coverage when the individual becomes very sick. Allows young adults to remain on parent's insurance until age 26.
- *Health insurance exchange:* A virtual marketplace in which the uninsured can go to comparison shop for a health plan.

---

remained high. Indeed, rising health care costs were often cited as the most pressing economic problem in the nation (Teixeira, n.d.). Although the final health care reform bill was more realistically called health insurance reform, its passage by the 111th Congress in March of 2010 was historic; its full enactment, which will take place through 2018, will usher in an era of expanded access to health care in the United States.

WHAT DO YOU THINK? *Enrollment in the Medicaid program increased by 3.29 million from June 2008 to June 2009, a 7.5% increase for a total of almost 60 million Americans. Increased enrollment of children accounted for 60% of this growth. An additional 3.3% of the growth in enrollment was an increase in elderly and disabled beneficiaries, who, although they comprise only one quarter of Medicaid enrollees, account for more than two thirds (68% in 2006) of program spending. Although the elderly and individuals with disabilities are a minority of the Medicaid population, they are responsible for the majority of program costs because of their intensive use of services, including long-term care (Kaiser Family Foundation, 2009).*

Quality

Quality of care leaped to the forefront of concern about health care following the 1999 release of the Institute of Medicine (IOM) report, *To Err Is Human: Building a Safer Health System* (IOM, 2000). In this groundbreaking report, as many as 98,000 deaths a year were attributed to preventable medical errors. Some of the untoward events categorized in this report included adverse drug events and improper transfusions, surgical injuries and wrong-site surgeries, suicides, restraint-related injuries or death, falls, burns, pressure ulcers, and mistaken client identities. Beyond the cost in human lives, preventable medical errors result in total costs of between $17 billion and $29 billion per year in hospitals nationwide (IOM, 2000). Significant to nurses, the IOM estimated that the number of lives lost to preventable medication errors alone represented more than 7000 deaths annually, with a cost of about $2 billion nationwide. Although the IOM report made it clear that the majority of medical errors today were not produced by provider negligence, lack of education, or lack of training, questions were raised about the nurse's role and workload and its effect on client safety. In a follow-up report, *Keeping Patients Safe: Transforming the Work Environment of Nurses,* the IOM (2003) stated that nurses' long work hours pose one of the most serious threats to client safety, since fatigue slows reaction time, saps energy, and diminishes attention to detail. The group called for state regulators to pass laws barring nurses from working more than 12 hours a day and 60 hours a week—even if by choice (IOM, 2003).

The IOM recommended financial and regulatory incentives to lead to a safer health care system. These recommendations called for the need to stop blaming and punishing individuals for errors and to begin identifying and correcting systems failures by designing safety into the process of care. The Joint Commission (TJC) responded to the report and has developed National Patient Safety Goals specific for each of its accreditation and certification programs (Bleich, 2005). TJC encourages hospitals to report sentinel events, defined as an unexpected occurrence involving death, severe physical or psychological injury, or the risk of injury or death (Liang, 2000; The Joint Commission, 2009). In 2006, TJC began making unannounced hospital inspections.

This culture of safety has made providers and consumers more conscious of safety, but medical errors and untoward events continue to occur. As a means to improve consumer awareness of hospital quality, the Centers for Medicare and Medicaid Services (CMS) began publishing a database of hospital quality measures, Hospital Compare, in 2005. Hospital Compare, a consumer-oriented website that provides information on how well hospitals provide recommended care in such areas as heart attack, heart failure, and pneumonia is available through the CMS website (www.cms.gov). In a further effort, the CMS, in 2008, announced that it will no longer reimburse hospitals for care provided for "preventable complications" such as hospital-acquired infections.

DID YOU KNOW? *The process by which medical errors are identified and addressed in many facilities uses an approach called root cause analysis. As part of an overall process for identifying prevention strategies by looking at changes that need to be made, root cause analysis asks those most familiar with the problem to scrutinize a problem situation until there is no further room for questions. The goal of the root cause analysis is to generate specific prevention strategies, but it is also designed to engender a culture of safety in the organization that uses it. The Joint Commission requires that hospitals submit a root cause analysis within 45 days of a sentinel event that has been voluntarily reported or discovered during a survey (The Joint Commission, 2009).*

TRENDS AFFECTING THE HEALTH CARE SYSTEM

Because of the rising national concern with cost, access, and quality of care, it is expected that significant change will occur within the next decade or two. Several trends may shape future changes in the structure of the health care system. These trends include demographics of the population at large and the health care workforce, technology in treatment and in information management, and the recognition that global influences can shape our future.

Demographics

Seventy-seven million babies were born between the years of 1946 and 1963, giving rise to the Baby Boomer generation (Center for Health Communication, 2004). The oldest members of this group turn 65 in 2011, and on average they are expected to live to the age of 83, with many surviving until 90. This generational bubble overwhelmed schools and challenged social norms in childhood and adolescence. Can we expect them to do less as they enter late middle and early old age? Life expectancy has been higher for this group (see Figure 3-3), with much of this increase expected to be attributable to longevity at older age.

In 2007, the number of Medicare beneficiaries reached 44 million, or 15% of the U.S. population, but by 2030 that same population is projected to grow to 79 million (Umans and Nonnemaker, 2009). The cost of Medicare and its share of the GDP is expected to rise astronomically, causing many to think there will be a Medicare shortfall in the middle of this century. The vastly increased numbers of elderly and their greater percentage of the population mean that there will be fewer workers paying taxes into the Medicare system at the same time that the elderly will be consuming more health resources.

A second and equally important demographic trend is the rise in the nation's foreign-born population: 38.1 million in 2007, or 12.6% of the total U.S. population (U.S. Census Bureau, 2008). Within the foreign-born population, 31% were born in Mexico and an estimated 35 million (12.3%) speak Spanish at home. Following Mexico, the next largest source of immigrants was Asia, and these two geographic areas accounted for 80% of the nation's foreign-born population in 2007 (Frey et al, 2010).

Twenty-first–century America already looks demographically different than twentieth-century America. The 2000 census showed that America was more ethnically, racially, culturally, and linguistically diverse than ever before. In 2003 the Census Bureau announced that Hispanics now outnumber African-Americans in the United States. States with the largest percentage of foreign-born populations are California, New York, and New Jersey, yet the states with the fastest-growing immigrant populations in 2008 were South Carolina, Georgia, Nevada and Tennessee (Migration Policy Institute, 2010). The Hispanic population is growing most rapidly in the Southeast, the Asian population centers are in the Sun Belt and high-tech areas of the United States, and the African-American population is growing rapidly in the large Southern cities of Atlanta, Houston, and Washington DC (Frey et al, 2010).

The Changing Health Care Workforce

To care for a population that is aging—yet living longer—and is rapidly becoming diverse requires a strong and flourishing health care workforce, yet the workforce faces challenges today.

- In 2000, the national supply of registered nurses working fulltime was estimated at 1.89 million while the demand was estimated at 2 million, a shortage of 110,000 (6%). By 2020, the shortage is projected to grow to an estimated 340,000.
- In a July 2002 report by the Health Resources and Services Administration, 30 states were found to have shortages of registered nurses in the year 2000. The shortage is projected to intensify over the next two decades, with 44 states and the District of Columbia expected to have RN shortages by the year 2020 (Kaiser Family Foundation, 2008).
- According to projections from the U.S. Bureau of Labor Statistics published in 2004, more than 1 million new and replacement nurses will be needed by 2012. The U.S. Department of Labor has identified registered nursing as the top occupation in terms of job growth through the year 2012 (U.S. Department of Labor, 2008).
- According to an American Association of Colleges of Nursing's report, preliminery data showed that U.S. nursing schools turned away 52,115 qualified applicants to baccalaureate and

graduate nursing programs in 2009 because of a lack of faculty, although other factors such as limitations in clinical sites, classroom space, and clinical preceptors as well as budget constraints were also to blame (AACN, 2005).

In addition to the widespread nursing shortage, chronic, severe workforce shortages among the allied health professions currently exist throughout the United States. According to the U.S. Department of Labor, allied health professionals represent 60% of the American health care workforce, and a shortage of some 1.6 million to 2.5 million allied health workers is predicted by 2020 (Medical News Today, 2006).

Missing Persons: The Lack of Diversity in the Health Care Workforce

Minorities are underrepresented in the physician and nurse workforce relative to their proportion of the total population, but they are overrepresented in lower-paying health professions such as nurse aides and home health aides. The Pew Commission (Grumbach et al, 2003), a national and interprofessional group of health care leaders, suggests that increasing minority representation in the health workforce not only is a commitment to diversity, but also will improve the health care delivery system. The two main arguments that diversity improves health care delivery are: (1) minority health professionals can be expected to practice in underserved areas at a greater rate, and (2) health professionals who share the same culture and language with the clients they serve can provide more effective care (USDHHS, n.d.c; AACN, 2009a).

Technology

Since 2004, when President Bush called for the nationwide adoption of electronic medical records, there has been increased focus on the widespread adoption of innovative technology in health care. This focus has been felt from nursing education, with the increasing number of online nursing programs, to the bedside where personal digital assistants (PDAs) have replaced the pharmacology textbook and bedside computer charting has replaced the paper chart.

The development and refinement of new technologies such as telehealth has opened up new clinical opportunities for nurses, particularly in the management of chronic conditions, home care, rehabilitation, and long-term care. However, along with new opportunities come new challenges and pitfalls. Telehealth, defined as the use of electronic communication networks to transmit client-related information, has been used by the Department of Veterans Affairs to decrease hospitalizations by 20% by improving at-home monitoring of chronically ill clients (Merrill, 2009). And the EmotaMe, an "emotional networking" system unveiled for testing in March 2010, uses concepts from computer games, social networking, and videoconferencing to allow health care providers and family members to monitor and provide emotional, social, and physical support to at-home elderly (Milliard, 2010). Yet while telehealth is seen as a cost-effective way to diagnose and treat rural and isolated clients and to educate rural doctors and nurses, concerns linger about privacy, security, and reimbursement for services provided at a distance and perhaps across state lines.

NURSING TIP   *Maintaining a client's privacy and confidentiality is more than good nursing practice: it is the law. Palm Pilots, PDAs, and Blackberries are rapidly becoming necessities in nursing practice. However, the Internet does not typically provide a secure medium for transferring confidential information unless both parties are using encryption technologies. Be sure to check with your facility's health information services department or privacy office for advice and assistance before you use your PDA or e-mail device in the provision of client care.*

In the hospital, technology has allowed providers to perform feats of health care that would have been unimaginable just a decade ago. With ultrasound, video-assisted and laser surgery, filmless radiology, robotic pharmacy dispensing, wireless monitoring, and virtual intensive care units, hospitals can provide state-of-the-art care to the sickest of clients. Advanced technology is also being introduced into the health care system as a method of ensuring client safety and improving the quality of care in ways that were addressed by the IOM report on medical errors. The electronic health record (EHR) has been called the most important innovation for client safety, and has been endorsed by Health and Human Services (HHS) Secretary Leavitt (under President Bush) as the means to create a system in which information is digital, privacy protected, and interchangeable (Leavitt, 2010).

An innovative use of the electronic health record to meet the needs of the public health workforce is the ability to embed reminders or guidelines within the EHR. The Practice Partner Research Network's Colorectal Cancer Screening in Primary Care study looked at the inclusion of reminders for colon cancer screening within a large national group of physicians sharing an EHR system. In this study, evidence-based guidelines were incorporated into progress note templates along with links to previous screening results, and a Health Maintenance section of the EHR was updated with age- and gender-appropriate screening targets. Although screening literature documents the need to overcome barriers that keep clients from following up on screening, such as lack of knowledge and insurance, having a health care provider encourage the need for screening is often the most important factor in fostering client compliance (Shokar, Nguyen-Oghalai, and Wu, 2009). The use of office policies, reminder systems, and communication strategies are crucial tools to enable doctors and nurses to encourage their clients to meet screening goals, and in this study, embedded tools within the EHR resulted in rates of up to 78% in the highest provider practices (Nemeth, Nietert, and Ornstein, 2009).

Publically funded community health centers lag behind private sector health care in adopting and implementing the EHR. In a study by the National Association of Community Health Centers, only 8% of health centers have incorporated the use of electronic records compared with 18% of private physician practices. The overwhelming majority of the community centers cited financial need as the factor that prevented adoption (Smith, 2007). The American Recovery and Reinvestment Act of 2009 included funding to allow community centers to afford the transition to electronic records.

Hamilton Community Health Network (Health Care for the Homeless)—a 25-physician, six-center network serving the population of Flint, Michigan, where one in four residents are poor and uninsured—received a $2 million grant to improve facilities and introduce an EHR system (Business Wire, 2009).

Some of the benefits of the EHR for public health (Bower et al, 2005) include the following:

- 24-hour availability of records with downloaded laboratory results and up-to-date assessments
- Coordination of referrals and facilitation of interprofessional care in chronic disease management
- Incorporation of protocol reminders for prevention, screening, and management of chronic disease
- Improvement of quality measurement and monitoring
- Increased client safety and decline in medication errors

Public health systems share the same reason for limited use of EHRs as community centers, which is a lack of funds to support this work.

In the aftermath of Hurricane Katrina, it became clear that an electronic recording system of health care data including medication lists and diagnoses would have alleviated some of the chaos experienced by many of the displaced residents of New Orleans. Forced to evacuate with little but the clothes on their backs and a personal memento or two, many were not able to recall their precise medical history details. Recent efforts to develop networks for storing client data over time and through the continuum of care have been introduced. Two such methods are the personal health record (PHR) and the health information exchanges (HIE).

The PHR is an electronically maintained record of an individual's health information, managed by the individual with information from health care providers. Data that would be included in the PHR includes demographics, general medical information, allergies, hospitalizations, operations, medications, immunizations, and clinical tests. Although the PHR may be the ultimate resource for the knowledgeable, proactive health care consumer, many barriers such as a lack of standardized information and the inability to share information among providers has hindered the adoption of the PHR. Another significant barrier to the implementation of the PHR is the digital divide that prevents those with limited access to technology and low literacy levels from participating (Hinman and Davidson, 2009).

The HIE is a regional network of integrated data-sharing incorporating client information from local hospitals as well as clinics or provider practices within one database. As of 2007, 32 fully operational HIEs existed in the United States. HIEs are expected to have a major role in the National Health Information Network. An HHS program has been proposed that would link health care information systems across the nation together to allow clients, physicians, hospitals, public health agencies, and other authorized users to share clinical information. However, without considerable federal funding and the development of standardized systems of information gathering and sharing, this effort will take many years to come to fruition (Hinman and Davidson, 2009).

HOW TO   **Prevent Medication Errors for Clients in the Community**

Instruct your clients that when they obtain their medicine from the pharmacy, they should ask, "Is this the medicine that my doctor prescribed?" The Food and Drug Administration receives 300 notices each month of drug errors and classifies the type of error that was made. The most common types of errors involved administering an improper dose (41%), giving the wrong drug (16%), and using the wrong route of administration (16%) (U.S. Food and Drug Administration, 2009). Rather than simply trusting the pharmacy to provide the correct medication, consumers should know what drugs they are taking and how they should be taken, make sure they understand the administration instructions, keep a list of all medications they take (including over-the-counter supplements), and verify medication if unsure of what they have been given.

Global Influences

Globalization is a process of change and development across national boundaries and oceans, involving economics, trade, politics, technology, and social welfare. The recent outbreaks of SARS (in 2003) and H1N1 flu (in 2009), as well as a resurgence of polio in Africa and Asia and the prevalence of HIV/AIDS in Africa, have encouraged a global view of health and wellness, since diseases can no longer be contained to one area of the world. With immigration, trade, and air travel, no country on earth, no matter how technologically sophisticated, is completely safe from infectious disease.

Emerging infectious diseases have produced new demands for disease surveillance, and information technology has met the demand for immediate and widespread response. Outbreak reports must be assessed for accuracy and rapidly transmitted so that control efforts can be initiated and scientific evidence can be collected. However, with rapid transmission of information, the quality of information may be questionable, resulting in unnecessary public anxiety and confusion. Rumors that later prove to be unsubstantiated may lead to inappropriate responses, causing disruption in trade and economic loss.

As the pace of globalization has increased in the recent past, interest has grown in the development of collective action plans to meet global health needs. The World Health Organization (WHO), comprised of 192 member countries, provides leadership on global health, shapes worldwide research and policy agendas, and monitors trends and responses to disease threats on a global level. In May 2005 the WHO introduced a new set of International Health Regulations to manage public health emergencies of international concern. The new rules have been proposed to prevent, protect against, control, and provide a public health response to the international spread of disease. Under the revised regulations, countries have much broader obligations in preventive measures as well as detection and response to public health emergencies of international concern. In recent years the worldwide outbreak of the H1N1 flu and the massive earthquake in Haiti have challenged the capacity of developing and developed nations to respond to public health emergencies. Following the 7.0 Richter Scale earthquake in the impoverished nation of Haiti, the WHO lead an effort to conduct a public health risk assessment that will provide technical guidance to Haitian health professionals and those from the United Nations and non-governmental organizations on the major public health threats faced by the population (WHO, 2010c).

ORGANIZATION OF THE HEALTH CARE SYSTEM

A large and growing number and range of facilities and providers comprise the health care system. Facilities include physicians' and dentists' offices, hospitals, nursing homes, mental health facilities, ambulatory care centers, free-standing clinics, and public health and home health agencies. Providers include nurses, advanced practice nurses, physicians and physician assistants, and dentists and dental hygienists, as well as a large array of allied health professionals with specialized knowledge and circumscribed roles. Although the setting and the provider may vary from setting to setting, there is a clear division between two components of our system: the private system and the public health system. The main difference between private health care and the public health care system in the United States is who funds and determines the structure of the provision of care. For example, in private health care, a physician or nurse practitioner can decide to open a practice anywhere, and as long as they are licensed in that state and follow the laws of that state in their practice, they are free to pursue their livelihood. Clients will be expected to pay for services through insurance; through government programs such as Medicare, Medicaid or CHIP; or out-of-pocket (if uninsured). In the public health care system, the government, either at the federal or state level, has funded the setting of the care (center or clinic); providers who see clients at that setting are paid a salary by the government for all services rendered. Most people in the United States receive their care through contact with the private health care system, but the public system is an increasingly important safety net for the uninsured or underinsured needing care; as the health care reform effort continues, the public system may begin to play a larger role. The provision of primary health care via the public health care system will be the main focus for the rest of this chapter.

THE CUTTING EDGE *House Resolution 4601, introduced into the House of Representatives in February 2010, is a bill to amend the Public Health Service Act to establish the Office of the National Nurse. The National Nurse, who will be the Chief Nurse of the U.S. Public Health Service, will provide guidance for community prevention efforts. The office of the National Nurse will raise the visibility of nursing and help the public become aware of the role of nurses in public health.*

Primary Health Care System

The two concepts *primary care* and *primary health care* may sound similar, but the services provided are different. Primary care, as defined here, is a component of the private health care system. It is the care provided by a physician, physician assistant, or nurse practitioner, trained in family practice, pediatrics,

---

BOX 3-4 LEVELS OF CARE

- *Primary care:* Basic care; first contact with a health provider and health system; includes preventive, curative, and rehabilitative care
- *Secondary care:* Provided by a specialist health care provider usually after referral from a primary care provider
- *Tertiary care:* Requires specialized skills, technology, and support services available at only larger or more technically advanced teaching hospitals
- *Quaternary care:* Requires highly specialized skills, technology, and support services, usually an academic medical center; one hospital may provide the majority of such services within a geographic area

---

or internal medicine. This is care provided to the individual at the first level of contact with the health care system (e.g., if a mother brings her baby to a pediatrician for a well baby visit). Box 3-4 presents the four levels of health care defined by contact with the health care system. Primary health care (PHC), the focus of the public health system in the United States, is defined as a broad range of services, including, but not limited to, basic health services, family planning, clean water supply, sanitation, immunization, and nutrition education. It consists of programs designed to be affordable for the recipients of the care and the governments that provide them (United Nations, 2009).

In primary health care the emphasis is on prevention, and the means of providing the care are based on practical, scientifically sound, culturally appropriate, and socially acceptable methods. This care is provided at the community level and is accessible and acceptable to the community and inviting of community participation (United Nations, 2009; WHO, 2005).

Primary Health Care Workforce

The primary health care workforce consists of a multidisciplinary team of health care providers. Team members include primary care generalists and public health physicians, nurses, dentists, pharmacists, optometrists, nutritionists, community outreach workers, mental health counselors, translators, and other allied health professionals. Community members are also considered important to the team.

Primary Health Care Initiative

The primary health care movement officially began in 1977 when the 30th WHO Health Assembly adopted a resolution accepting the goal of attaining a level of health that permitted all citizens of the world to live socially and economically productive lives. At the international conference in 1978 in Alma Ata, Russia, it was determined that this goal was to be met through PHC. This resolution, the *Declaration of Alma Ata,* became known by the slogan "Health for All (HFA) by the Year 2000" (WHO, 2005), which captured the official health target for all the member nations of the WHO. In 1998, the program was adapted to meet the needs of the new century and deemed "Health for All in the 21st Century." Health is defined by WHO (WHO, 1946) as a state of complete physical, mental, and social well-being and not merely the absence of disease or infirmity, thus providing for the broad scope of primary health care.

In 1981 the WHO established global indicators for monitoring and evaluating the achievement of HFA, including health policy, social and economic development, provision of health care, and health status. These indicators are addressed in yearly reports; WHO provides an expert assessment of global health, relevant to all countries, yet focused on a specific goal or agenda. The purpose of these reports is to provide an international audience with the information they need to make policy and funding decisions. The report of World Health Day 2005 presents statistics on infant and maternal mortality and stresses the importance of access to care for every woman and child from pregnancy through childhood (WHO, 2010d). All countries that are members of the United Nations may become members of WHO by accepting its Constitution, but one cannot expect all member countries to interpret the yearly reports with the same sense of urgency. Although the original definition of PHC, with its emphasis on social and economic opportunity, may be represented differently by member nations, it is important to remember the Alma Ata declaration as the basis for PHC, and to understand the global evolvement of this strategy over the past three decades. For this reason, the complete declaration is presented in Resource Tool 3.A.

The United States, as a WHO member nation, has endorsed primary health care as a strategy for achieving the goal of health for all in the twenty-first century. However, the PHC emphasis on broad strategies, community participation, self-reliance, and a multidisciplinary health care delivery team is not the primary method of delivery for health care in the United States. Although objectives are developed at the federal level and programs are initiated to meet those objectives, much of the health care in this country is delivered in the cure-oriented private sector. Still, it is relevant for us to consider the federal guidelines developed to promote the primary health care of Americans.

The national health plan for the United States identifies **disease prevention** and health promotion as the areas of most concern in the nation. Each decade since the 1980s has been measured and tracked according to health objectives set at the beginning of the decade. The U.S. Public Health Service of the DHHS publishes the objectives after gathering data from health professionals and organizations throughout the country.

Healthy People 2020, which was officially launched in December 2010 is comprised of a large number of objectives related to 38 topic areas. These objectives are designed to serve as a road map for improving the health of all people in the United States during the second decade of the twenty-first century. These objectives are described by four main goals (USDHHS, 2009):

- Elimination of preventable disease, disability, injury and premature death
- Achievement of health equity
- Elimination of health disparities
- Creation of social and physical environments that will promote good health and healthy development and behavior at every stage of life

These goals provide the framework with which measurable health indicators can be tracked. The emphasis on the social and physical environment moves *Healthy People 2020* from the traditional disease-specific focus to a more holistic view of health consistent with a public health frame of reference (Krisberg, 2008). This in turn will encourage public health nurses to broaden their scope to all aspects of their clients' lives that may need assessment and intervention, including where they live, the condition of their home, and how the appropriateness of their environment may change as the client ages. The Healthy People 2020 box presents indicators of *Healthy People 2020* related to access to care.

 HEALTHY PEOPLE 2020

Selected objectives that pertain to public health and primary health care are listed here:

- AHS-1: Increase the proportion of persons with health insurance.
- AHS-2: Increase the proportion of insured persons with coverage for clinical preventive services.
- AHS-3: Increase the proportion of persons with a usual primary care provider.
- AHS-6: Reduce the proportion of individuals who are unable to obtain or delay in obtaining necessary medical care, dental care, or prescription medicines.
- AHS-7: (Developmental) Increase the proportion of persons who receive appropriate evidence-based clinical preventive services.

From U. S. Department of Health and Human Services. *Healthy People 2020.* Available at http://www.healthypeople.gov/2020topicsobjectives 2020/default.aspx. Accessed December 27, 2010.

Primary Care

Primary care, the first level of the private health care system, is delivered in a variety of community settings, such as physicians' offices, urgent care centers, community health centers, and nurse-managed centers. Depending on the geographic location, these settings may be more or less accessible. The main tool by which Americans access the primary care system is through insurance programs, either private (primarily employment-based) or governmental (e.g., Medicare, Medicaid, CHIP). Those with private insurance may have an option of using a fee-for-service system in which they have relatively free choice of provider and their insurance pays all or at least a significant percentage of the provider's charges. However, the majority of the insured are covered through a managed care model in which the insurer has control of provider, services covered, and the fees paid.

Managed care, defined as a system in which care is delivered by a specified network of providers who agree to comply with the care approaches established through a case management process, was a strategy chosen by the federal government as a means to control the rising costs of traditional fee-for-service health care. The Managed Care Act of 1973, which required employers to offer a managed care option as an alternative to regular insurance plans, ushered in an era of cost control by integrating the means of insuring care with the delivery of care. The crucial factors of a managed care organization (MCO) are a specified network of providers and the use of a gatekeeper to control access to providers and services. Early MCOs, such as the group and staff model health maintenance organizations (HMOs), were a form of health care in which an insurer collected premiums and paid a negotiated fee to a group of doctors

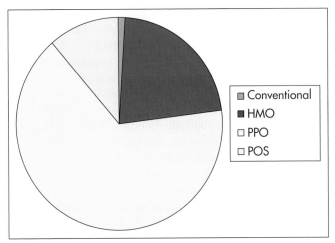

FIGURE 3-4 Distribution of health plan enrollment for covered workers, 2009. (Data extracted from Kaiser Family Foundation: 2009: Kaiser/HRET survey of employer-sponsored health benefits, 1999-2009. Available at http://facts.kff.org/chart.aspx?ch=1052. Accessed December 3, 2010.)

to provide care, or as in the staff model, the HMO employed the doctors directly. Kaiser Permanente is an example of such an HMO (Green and Rowell, 2008). Less restrictive models—such as the preferred provider organization (PPO) in which a group of health care providers agree to provide services at discounted rates to an enrolled population, or the point of service (POS) model in which an insurer allows enrollees to use providers outside of a specified network for an additional fee—are now quite commonly integrated into most insurance plans. Figure 3-4 illustrates the breakdown of enrollment by plan type in 2009.

The government has tried to reap the benefits of cost savings by introducing the managed care model into Medicare and Medicaid with varying levels of success. Part C, the Medicare Advantage program, incorporates private insurance plans into the Medicare program including HMO and PPO managed care models and private fee-for-service plans. These plans receive payments from Medicare to provide Medicare benefits, including hospital, physician, and often, prescription drug benefits. Of the nation's 45 million Medicare enrollees in 2008, 10.2 million are enrolled in a Medicare Advantage managed care option (Kaiser Family Foundation, 2009b).

Medicaid has made large-scale use of the managed care model within its various state programs. Medicaid managed care enrollment grew rapidly in the 1990s, with the percentage of beneficiaries enrolled in managed care plans increasing from 9% in 1990 to 59% of the Medicaid population in 2003. By 2009 all states enrolled a proportion of their Medicaid population in MCOs, and in 2009 70% of Medicaid beneficiaries were enrolled in MCOs (Kaiser Family Foundation, 2010). CHIP programs tend to be managed similarly to state Medicaid programs, thus resulting in the use of MCOs for these children as well.

The cost savings expected with the development of the MCO model were short-lived. Initially it was assumed that the elimination of unnecessary services and the restriction of excess utilization through the use of a gatekeeper would save money and

satisfy clients. The enticement of low out-of-pocket expenses and minimal paperwork was not sufficient to satisfy clients who had been used to free access to the providers of their choice and unlimited service with little awareness of the expense— the defining features of the fee-for-service model. Consumer groups began to question restrictions on care, such as 1-day hospital stays for childbirth and denials of bone marrow transplantation for breast cancer clients. Hospitals presented legal challenges to the limited networks of participating facilities that MCOs chose to form. Providers withdrew from plans if reimbursement was too low. All of these factors and more lead to the less restrictive models of MCOs now in use, such as PPOs and POS plans.

Primary Care Workforce

Primary care developed in the 1960s as a need to reexamine the role of the general practitioner. The Millis Commission (Millis, 1966) expressed concern that a knowledge explosion, development of new technologies, and an increasing number of new specialties were threatening the role of the general practitioner. The specialty of family practice and the arrival of nurse practitioners (NPs) and physician assistants (PAs) emerged in response to the need to provide primary care.

Currently, primary care providers include generalists who possess skills in health promotion and disease prevention, assessment and evaluation of symptoms and physical signs, management of common acute and chronic medical conditions, and identification and appropriate referral for other needed health care services. The health care personnel trained as primary care generalists include family physicians, general internists, general pediatricians, NPs, clinical nurse specialists (CNSs), PAs, and certified nurse-midwives (CNMs). Some physicians with special training in preventive medicine, public health, or obstetrics/gynecology also deliver primary care.

NPs, CNSs, and CNMs—considered advanced practice nursing specialties—are vital members of the primary care and primary health care teams. NPs receive advanced training, either at the master's or doctoral levels, and many pursue certification by examination in a specialty area, such as pediatrics, adult, gerontology, obstetrics/gynecology, or family. Training emphasizes clinical medical skills (history, physical, and diagnosis) and pharmacology, in addition to the traditional psychosocial- and prevention-focused skills that are normally thought of as nursing. According to the ANA, nearly 60% to 80% of primary and preventive care traditionally done by physicians can be done by an NP for less money. The cost-effectiveness of the advanced practice nurse reflects a variety of factors related to the employment setting, liability insurance, and the cost of education. In 2008 there were approximately 158,348 nurse practitioners in the United States (USDHHS, 2010a). NPs have been given the authority to prescribe medication by state law in all 50 states, although legislation varies by state (Byrne, 2009). Some work as independent practitioners and can be reimbursed by Medicare or Medicaid for services rendered.

There were 18,492 nurse midwives in the United States in 2008 (USDHHS, 2010b). In 2005 there were 306,377 vaginal births attended by CNMs in the United States, or 10.7% of all live births for that year (Declercq, 2009). CNM practitioners receive an average of 1.5 years of specialized education beyond nursing school, and all but 4 of the 43 accredited programs in the United States are at the master's level. CNMs are required to pass a national certification examination before practice. CNMs provide well-woman gynecological and low-risk obstetrical care including prenatal, labor and delivery, and postpartum care. CNMs have prescriptive authority in some form in all 50 states. Medicaid reimbursement is mandatory in every state, and 31 states mandate private insurance reimbursement for midwifery services (Brigham and Women's Hospital, 2010).

CNSs currently number 59,242, a drop of 22.4% from 2004 (USDHHS, 2010b). With advanced nursing degrees, typically at the master's level, CNSs are experts in a specialized area of clinical practice such as mental health, gerontology, cardiac or cancer care, and public health or neonatal health. CNSs provide primary care, but often work in consultation, research, education, and administration. Some work independently or in private practice and can be reimbursed by Medicare and Medicaid.

A new category of advanced practice nurse is the DNP, or Doctorate in Nursing Practice. In 2004, the member schools of the American Association of Colleges of Nursing (AACN) voted to endorse the policy that all advanced practice nurses must be educated at the doctoral level by 2015 (AACN, 2009b). By 2008 there were 92 DNP programs in the United States with another 102 programs in various stages of development. There were 3415 students enrolled in these programs and 361 students graduated with the DNP degree in that year (AACN, 2009b). The DNP role is a clinical role, and it can be expected that nurses educated at that level will soon be moving into all areas of public health in which an advanced degree in nursing is required.

Public Health System

The public health system is mandated through laws that are developed at the national, state, or local level. Examples of public health laws instituted to protect the health of the community include a law mandating immunizations for all children entering kindergarten and a law requiring constant monitoring of the local water supply. The public health system is organized into many levels in the federal, state, and local systems. At the local level, health departments provide care that is mandated by state and federal regulations.

The Federal System

The HHS is the agency most heavily involved with the health and welfare concerns of U.S. citizens. The organizational chart of HHS (Figure 3-5) shows the office of the secretary and the divisions that report to the secretary. HHS is charged with regulating health care and overseeing the health status of Americans. Newer areas of interest to public health are the Office of Public Health Preparedness, the Center for Faith-Based and Neighborhood Partnerships and the Office of Global Affairs. The Office of Public Health Preparedness was added to assist the nation and states to prepare for bioterrorism after September 11, 2001. The Center for Faith-Based and Neighborhood Partnerships

is considered the HHS's liaison to grassroots level community support. Goals of the Center put forth by President Obama in 2009 (USDHHS, n.d.b) include the following:

- Strengthen the role of community organizations in the economic recovery and poverty reduction.
- Reduce unintended pregnancies and support maternal and child health.
- Promote responsible fatherhood and healthy families.
- Foster interfaith dialogue and collaboration with leaders and scholars around the world, and at home.

The Office of Global Health Affairs represents the HHS to other countries and international organizations and works with other countries in various health programs (USDHHS, 2010c).

The U.S. Public Health Service (PHS) is a major component of the HHS. The PHS consists of eight agencies: Agency for Healthcare Research and Quality; Agency for Toxic Substances and Diseases Registry; Centers for Disease Control and Prevention; Food and Drug Administration; Health Resources and Services Administration; Indian Health Service; National Institutes of Health; and Substance Abuse and Mental Health Services Administration.

The Health Resources and Services Administration (HRSA) consists of four bureaus: Bureau of Primary Health Care, Maternal and Child Health Bureau, Bureau of Health Resources Development, and Bureau of Health Professions. The HRSA directs grant programs that improve the nation's health by expanding access to primary care for low-income and uninsured people, focusing on mothers and their children, people with HIV/AIDS, and residents of rural areas (USDHHS, n.d.c).

The HRSA also serves as a national focus for efforts to assure the delivery of health care to residents of **medically underserved areas** and to persons with special health care needs. Through HRSA's Consolidated Health Center Program, 6000 health center delivery sites in every state, Puerto Rico, the U.S. Virgin Islands, and the Pacific Basin are funded and offer primary care services including screenings, diagnostic and laboratory tests, immunizations, and gynecological care. Many sites offer oral health, mental health, substance abuse services, and pharmacy services (USDHHS, 2008). To improve access to health care in health manpower shortage areas, the Bureau assists states and communities in the placement of physicians, dentists, and other health professionals through the National Health Service Corps (NHSC). An adequate supply of health care providers for placement in underserved areas is ensured through the NHSC scholarship program and the NHSC loan repayment programs. Nurses are represented throughout the ranks of HHS and particularly HRSA in many senior and policy-making positions, as well as staffing the centers that provide care to the underserved throughout the nation.

A component of HRSA, the Bureau of Health Professions, includes separate divisions for nursing, medicine, dentistry, public health, and allied health professions. The federal government looks to the Division of Nursing to provide the competence and expertise for administering nurse education legislation, interpreting trends and needs of the nursing component of the nation's health care delivery system, and maintaining a liaison with the nursing community and with

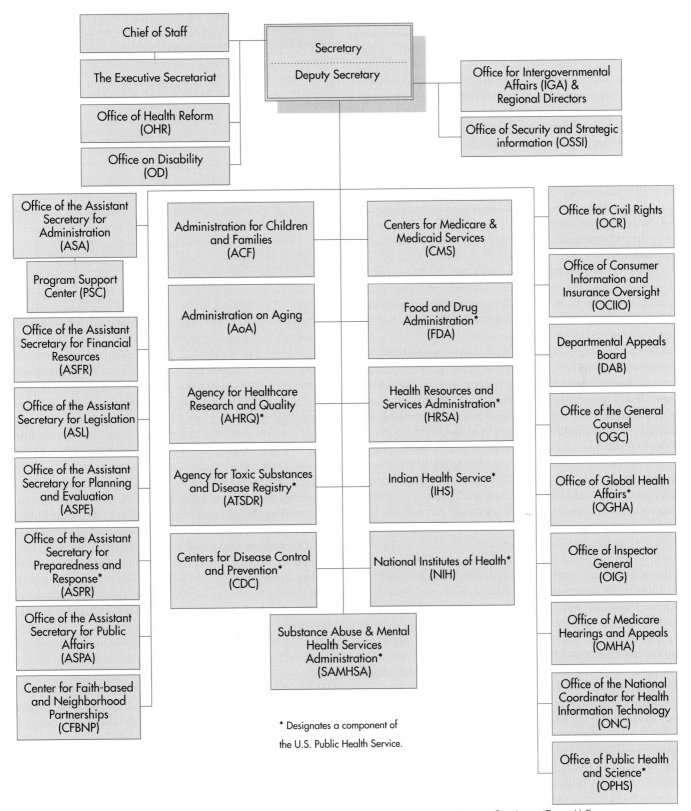

FIGURE 3-5 Organizational chart of the U.S. Department of Health and Human Services. (From U.S. Department of Health and Human Services: U.S. Department of Health and Human Services Organizational Chart, n.d. Available at http://www.hhs.gov/about/orgchart/#text. Accessed December 3, 2010.)

international, state, regional, and local health interests. As the federal focus for nursing education and practice, the Division of Nursing identifies current and future nursing issues.

The National Institutes of Health (NIH) is the world's premier medical research organization, supporting 325,000 scientists and researchers at more than 3000 institutions nationwide, investigating diseases including cancer, Alzheimer's disease, diabetes, arthritis, heart ailments, and AIDS (USDHHS, 2010d). Twenty-seven separate health institutes and centers are included in the NIH structure, including the National Institute for Nursing Research (NINR), which is the focal point of the nation's nursing research activities. The NINR promotes the growth and quality of research in nursing and client care, provides important leadership, expands the pool of experienced nurse researchers, and serves as a point of interaction with other bases of health care research.

The Agency for Healthcare Research and Quality (AHRQ) supports research on health care systems, health care quality and cost issues, access to health care, and effectiveness of medical treatments. It provides evidence-based information on health care outcomes and quality of care.

The Food and Drug Administration (FDA) ensures the safety of foods and cosmetics, and the safety and efficacy of pharmaceuticals, biological products, and medical devices. Besides the approval and monitoring of products, the FDA promotes food safety and tracks food-borne illnesses, and is also responsible for the safety of the nation's blood and plasma supply. In 2009 the FDA was given oversight over tobacco products with the implementation of the Family Smoking Prevention and Tobacco Control Act. Under this Act, the FDA has been tasked with setting performance standards, reviewing premarket applications for new tobacco products, determining requirements for new warning labels, and establishing and enforcing advertising and promotion restrictions (USDHHS, 2010e).

The main job of the Centers for Disease Control and Prevention (CDC) is to protect lives and improve health through health promotion, prevention of disease, and emergency preparedness (CDC, 2010). The CDC provides a system of health surveillance to monitor and prevent disease outbreaks (including bioterrorism), implement disease prevention strategies, and maintain national health statistics, as well as providing for immunization services, workplace safety, and environmental disease prevention. The CDC also guards against international disease transmission, with personnel stationed in more than 25 foreign countries. The CDC has started the new decade with a focus on supporting state and local health departments, improving global health, implementing measures to decrease leading causes of death, strengthening surveillance and epidemiology, and reforming health policies (CDC, 2010).

Other HHS agencies outside of the PHS include the Centers for Medicare and Medicaid Services (CMS), which administers Medicare and Medicaid; the Administration for Children and Families, which oversees 60 programs that promote the economic and social well-being of children, families, and communities, including the state–federal welfare program, Temporary Assistance for Needy Families, and Head Start; and the Administration on Aging, which supports a nationwide aging network,

---

BOX 3-5 TYPICAL PROGRAMS IN A STATE HEALTH DEPARTMENT

Epidemiology, Environmental and Occupational Health
Communicable Disease Service
Consumer, Environmental and Occupational Health Services
Cancer Epidemiology Services
Health Infrastructure Preparedness and Emergency Response
HIV/AIDS Services
Family Health Services
Public Health and Environmental Laboratories
Senior Services and Health Systems
Health Facilities Evaluation and Licensing
Senior Benefits Utilization and Management
Budget and Finance
Hospital Finance and Charity Care
Information Technology
Vital Statistics and Registration

---

providing services to the elderly, especially to enable them to remain independent, and providing policy leadership on issues concerning the aging. The U.S. Public Health Service Commissioned Corps is a uniformed service of more than 6000 health professionals who serve in many HHS and other federal agencies. The Surgeon General is head of the Commissioned Corps.

An important agency and a relatively recent addition to the federal government, the Department of Homeland Security (DHS), was created in 2002. The mission of the DHS is to prevent and deter terrorist attacks and protect against and respond to threats and hazards to the nation. The goals for the department include awareness, prevention, protection, response, and recovery. The DHS works with first responders throughout the United States and, through the development of programs such as the Community Emergency Response Team (CERT), trains people to be better prepared to respond to emergency situations in their communities. Nurses working in state and local public health departments as well as those employed in hospitals and other health facilities may be called upon to respond to acts of terrorism or natural disaster in their careers, and the DHS, along with the FDA and CDC, is developing programs to ready nurses and other health care providers for an uncertain future.

The State System

When the United States faced a pandemic flu outbreak in 2009, the federal government and the public health community quickly prepared to meet the challenge of educating the public and health professionals about the H1N1 flu and making vaccinations available. In addition to standing ready for disaster prevention or response, state health departments have other equally important functions, such as health care financing and administration for programs such as Medicaid, providing mental health and professional education, establishing health codes, licensing facilities and personnel, and regulating the insurance industry. State systems also have an important role in direct assistance to local health departments, including ongoing assessment of health needs. Box 3-5 provides a list of typical state health department programs, and the Levels of Prevention

BOX 3-6   EXAMPLES OF PROGRAMS PROVIDED BY LOCAL HEALTH DEPARTMENTS

AIDS community care
Animal shelter
Blood pressure
Cancer
Cancer and chronic illness prevention
Cholesterol screening
Communicable disease prevention and control
Dental services
Division of Public Health
Flu shots, adult
Health insurance
Lyme disease information
Mental health
Mosquito control
Nursing home services
Prescription savings program
Public health
Rabies clinics
SARS (severe acute respiratory syndrome)
Senior health
Sexually transmitted disease
Substance abuse services
Tick-borne diseases
Transportation
Tuberculosis
West Nile virus
Workplace health information

Note: Not all health departments will offer this comprehensive array of services. Visit your local health department to determine what is available in your area.

 ## LEVELS OF PREVENTION

Public Health Care System

Primary Prevention
Teach parents about the need for appropriate immunization for their children.

Secondary Prevention
Implement a family-planning program to prevent unintended pregnancies for teen girls who attend the primary health care clinic.

Tertiary Prevention
Provide a self-management asthma program for children with chronic asthma to reduce their need for hospitalization.

box provides a list of interventions for levels of preventive care typically found in the public health system.

Nurses serve in many capacities in state health departments as consultants, direct service providers, researchers, teachers, and supervisors, as well as participating in program development, planning, and evaluation of health programs. Many health departments have a division or department of nursing.

Every state has a board of examiners of nurses. The board may be found either in the department of licensing boards of the health department or in an administrative agency of the governor's office. Created by legislation known as a State Nurse Practice Act, the examiners' board is made up of nurses and consumers. A few states have other providers or administrators as members. The functions of this board are described in the practice act of each state and generally include licensing and examination of registered nurses and licensed practical nurses; approval of schools of nursing in the state; revocation, suspension, or denial of licenses; and writing of regulations about nursing practice and education.

The Local System

The local health department has direct responsibility to the citizens in its community or jurisdiction. Services and programs offered by local health departments vary depending on the state and local health codes that must be followed, the needs of the community, and available funding and other resources. For example, one health department might be more involved with public health education programs and environmental issues, whereas another health department might emphasize direct client care. Local health departments vary in providing sick care or even primary care. A list of health department programs, taken from an urban-suburban county health department in a mid-Atlantic state, is shown in Box 3-6.

Public health nursing is defined as the practice of protecting and promoting the health of populations using knowledge from nursing, social, and public health sciences (APHA, 1996). In the United States, nurses make up the largest portion of the public health workforce, primarily at the local level, and this area of nursing has been hard hit by the nation-wide nursing shortage (ANA, 2007). More often than at other levels of government,

LINKING CONTENT TO PRACTICE

As discussed in Chapter 1, the objectives of *Healthy People 2020* have direct application to the system of health care, including the public health system. In addition, two other key initiatives are highlighted here to emphasize the congruence with the goals of public health and those of health care in general. Specifically, The Council on Linkages of the Public Health Foundation has defined a set of Core Competencies that public health workers should possess. These competencies are not specific for nurses, but can be adopted by all public health providers. The goal of developing cross disciplinary competencies is to facilitate collaboration among public health nurses and other public health professionals to improve the nation's health (Quad Council, 2003). In 2009 the Council revised the original set of Core Competencies to include:

- Use of community input when developing policies
- Health disparities
- Health equity
- Social determinants of health
- Ethics
- Continuous Quality Improvement (CQI)
- Listing the basic public health sciences
- Ability to assess health literacy of population served
- Personal development opportunities for all public health workers

These Competencies are expected to be useful in the development of educational programs for students interested in pursuing public health careers as well as in practice in public health programs (Public Health Foundation, n.d.).

public health nurses at the local level provide direct services. Some of these deliver special or selected services, such as follow-up of contacts in cases of tuberculosis or venereal disease, or providing child immunization clinics. Others provide more general care, delivering services to families in certain geographic areas. This method of delivery of nursing services involves broader needs and a wider variety of nursing interventions. The local level often provides an opportunity for nurses to take on significant leadership roles, with many nurses serving as directors or managers.

Since the tragedy of September 11, 2001, state and local health departments have increasingly focused on emergency preparedness and response. In case of an event, state and local health departments in the affected area will be expected to collect data and accurately report the situation, to respond appropriately to any type of emergency, and to ensure the safety of the residents of the immediate area, while protecting those just outside the danger zone. This level of knowledge—to enable public health agencies to anticipate, prepare for, recognize, and respond to terrorist threats or natural disasters such as hurricanes or floods—has required a level of interstate and federal–local planning and cooperation that is unprecedented for these agencies. Whether participating in disaster drills or preparing a local high school for use as a shelter, nurses will play a major role in meeting the challenge of an uncertain future.

TRANSFORMATION OF THE HEALTH CARE SYSTEM: WHAT DOES THE FUTURE HOLD?

This chapter describes the functioning of the current health care system. The U.S. health care system has a number of flaws. On some dimensions, American medicine is the best in the world. The American health care system has new technologies and provides amazing new procedures and treatments that offer hope to many who would have faced certain death in the past. Yet, quality of care varies across the nation, and unequal access with resultant health disparities, along with continually rising costs, leads to dissatisfaction for consumers, providers, and policy makers.

Much research has been, and will continue to be, done on these problems, and much money has been spent trying to alleviate concerns and provide reassurance that the U.S. health care system remains the best in the world. Grand schemes for change that come with high price tags will probably not be the most effective means of transformation. Evidence-based practice had been thought to hold the most promise to fix what is broken in the health care system. What are the essentials of evidence-based practice that can meet our needs? Evidence-based medicine has been defined as the careful and conscious use of current best evidence in making decisions about the care of individual clients (Sackett, Rosenberg, and Gray, 1996). However, this description does not lend itself to the management of public health. What we have today are decades of evidence as to what does *not* work. Piecemeal improvements have not been successful. Incremental, patchwork changes such as CHIP or the Medicare Prescription Drug Act meet the needs of one population while squeezing funding and benefits from another, leaving other aspects of the safety net weakened. To solve the health care crisis requires the institution of a rational health care system, a system that balances equity, cost, and quality. The fact that 47 million are uninsured (Johnson, 2008), that wide disparities exist in access, and that a large proportion of deaths each year are attributable to preventable causes (errors as well as tobacco and alcohol abuse) indicates that the American system is currently not serving the best interests of the American population.

The United States is the only industrialized nation in the world that does not guarantee health care to all of its citizens. In addition, although many agree that health care is a basic human right, it is unclear how to make that belief a reality. The discrepancy between these two ideas is based on the U.S. concept of the health care marketplace. Unlike other industrialized countries, the United States has allowed and encouraged the growth of the private health care delivery system as the main source of health care. Despite the large amount of money spent on Medicare and Medicaid, until the United States adopts the concept of a single payer (i.e., the federal government) as the source for all health care financing and removes the responsibility from employers and insurance companies to fill this need, we cannot expect to have a system in which at least a basic level of primary care is accessible, free, and of acceptable quality for all U.S. citizens and residents.

During the Presidential election of 2008, the subject of health care reform was hotly debated. Candidate Barack Obama proposed a major overhaul of the system with the result that the 45 million Americans who were then uninsured would be covered by affordable insurance similar to the plan that federal employees enjoy. He vowed to end insurance restrictions based on preexisting illness, pledged to increase emphasis on preventive care, and offered that employers and the federal government will be paying for much of the proposed changes (Organizing for America, 2007).

President Obama made the reform of the nation's health care system the major priority of his agenda in his first year in office. He then instructed the Congress, with large Democratic majorities in both houses, to develop the policies that would result in the largest health care reform effort since the passage of Medicare and Medicaid in 1965. Many options were debated by the House of Representatives and the Senate, and much political turmoil ensued as the Republicans in Congress promised to derail the process. Some policies such as the individual mandate, the public option and the health insurance exchange were debated exhaustively (see Box 3-3 for descriptions of the policy options in health care reform). A crucial vote was held in Congress on March 21 at which 216 Congressmen (all Democrats) voted to support The Affordable Health Care for America Act and 212 Congressmen (including 34 Democrats) voted to defeat the legislation. Although President Obama went on to sign the Act into law on March 23, because the House of Representatives had approved some minor changes to the law, it was returned to the Senate for a final vote through the procedure of reconciliation, and was passed into law on March 25, 2010.

The Affordable Health Care for America Act will require most Americans to have health insurance coverage; allow 16 million people to join Medicaid; and subsidize private coverage for low- and middle-income people. The Congressional Budget Office determined the law would cost about $938 billion over 10 years, but would reduce the federal deficit by $138 billion over that same period of time (Stolberg, 2010).

Organized nursing, through the agency of the ANA, expressed support of President Obama's proposed health care reform as the year-long battle to pass this legislation ensued. In the following statement from the ANA health care reform toolkit, it is apparent that nurses have much to gain from a less fragmented, more rational system (ANA, 2009):

> *As the largest single group of clinical health care professionals within the health system, licensed registered nurses are educated and practice within a holistic framework that views the individual, family and community as an interconnected system that can keep us well and help us heal. Registered nurses are fundamental to the critical shift needed in health services delivery, with the goal of transforming the current 'sick care' system into a true 'health care' system."*
>
> *(ANA, 2009)*

An important piece of the health care reform legislation promises federal government support for nursing workforce development programs. These programs recruit new nurses into the profession, promote career advancement within nursing, and improve client care delivery. These programs are also used to direct RNs into areas with the greatest need, including departments of public health, community health centers, and hospitals that treat large numbers of poor and uninsured. Other provisions of the legislation propose increased funding for the National Health Service Corps, federal support for Nurse Managed Health Centers, increased opportunities for scholarship and loan repayment for nursing students in undergraduate and graduate education, and establishment of a National Public Health Corps modeled on the National Health Service Corps, to address public health workforce shortages.

The many provisions included in the 2010 health care reform legislation will promote a culture change in the thinking about health care, education and training of health care providers, and financing of our health care system. A change of this magnitude, affecting so many aspects of citizens' lives, is not easily made. As with other changes proposed for our health care system, such as managed care, the end product of change is not always of the quality that had been expected. However, it is likely that the health care system of the United States will evolve in the twenty-first century. Whether President Obama's reform agenda is passed in its entirety or major provisions are left for future political decision making, whether change is transformative or evolutionary, nurses will be poised to respond and play an active role in whatever configuration the system assumes.

EVIDENCE-BASED PRACTICE

It is often said that the states are the laboratories of democracy. One state, Massachusetts, began an experiment in health reform in 2006. Within 2 years after health reform legislation became effective, only 2.6% of Massachusetts residents were uninsured, the lowest percentage ever recorded in any state (Dorn, Hill, and Hogan, 2009).

Although other states have experimented with various programs to decrease the number of uninsured, the Massachusetts plan has had the most success. The health reform plan rests upon an individual mandate that requires everyone who can afford insurance to purchase coverage. Those unable to afford insurance receive subsidies that allow low-income individuals and families to purchase coverage. A new state-run program, Commonwealth Care (CommCare), provides benefits to adults who are not eligible for Medicaid but whose incomes fall below 300% of the federal poverty level.

To understand how the state was so successful in this effort toward universal coverage, a group of evaluators met with 15 key informants representing hospitals, community health centers, insurance companies, Medicaid, and CommCare. Several factors, it was found, have contributed to the historic level of coverage seen in the state. Rather than requiring consumers to complete separate applications for programs such as Medicaid, CHIP, or CommCare, a single application system provides entry to all the state programs. If an uninsured client was admitted to a hospital or visited a community health center, his eligibility was automatically evaluated and, if eligible, the client would be automatically converted to CommCare coverage, even without completing an application. A "Virtual Gateway" has been developed through which staff of community-based organizations have been trained to complete online applications on behalf of consumers, and to provide education and counseling about insurance options to underserved communities. By holding back reimbursement to providers who do not help consumers sign up for one of the available insurance options, hospitals and health centers are motivated to dedicate staff to provide education and counseling to the formerly uninsured. The result is that at least half of the new enrollees in Medicaid and CommCare have been enrolled without filling out any forms on their own. In addition to these efforts, shortly after the reform legislation was enacted, the state financed a massive public education effort to inform consumers about their new options.

Nurse Use

As health reform begins on the national level, nurses can play a crucial role in driving down the number of uninsured. Even if programs such as Massachusetts' integrated application system are not enacted on a larger scale, nurses should educate themselves so that they can encourage clients to apply and take advantage of all available coverage options. Taking an active role in consumer educational programs is a natural extension of a nurse's role as a client advocate. Nurses can promote legislation to simplify enrollment processes and encourage the development of shared databases for community health care providers, thus preventing consumers from falling through the cracks in our fragmented health care system.

Dorn S, Hill I, and Hogan S: The secrets of Massachusetts' success: why 97 percent of state residents have health coverage: state health access reform evaluation, 2009 Robert Wood Johnson Foundation. Available at http://www.urban.org/uploadedpdf/411987_massachusetts_success_brief.pdf. Accessed December 3, 2010.

CHAPTER REVIEW

■ PRACTICE APPLICATION

Rachel Green is a BSN student in her first community clinical rotation at a local health department clinic. Assisting Mary Toms (the pediatric nurse practitioner) with well-child visits, Ms. Green meets Karen Sloan and her 6-month-old daughter, Ann. Ms. Sloan has recently found a job at the local Target store, and although she will earn enough money to pay her bills and child care expenses, Ms. Sloan is concerned about her daughter's health care. "I will receive insurance for myself if I work full time and my mother can watch Ann," she explains. "But if I work I can't get Medicaid and will have to come to the department of health or go to the emergency department if my daughter gets sick."

Ms. Sloan does not want to share this information with Ms. Toms, since she is afraid it will hurt her feelings, but instead asks Ms. Green if she should take the new job. What should Ms. Green do?

A. Encourage Ms. Sloan to give up the job at Target and stay home with her daughter. The literature shows that a child of 6 months will be negatively affected by a change in caregiver.
B. Encourage Ms. Sloan to continue using the department of health for Ann's care, because she does not want Ms. Toms to think she is turning away her clients.
C. Wait until Ms. Toms enters the room and then tell her that Ms. Sloan does not want to continue bringing her daughter to the center, since reporting observations is more important than earning Ms. Sloan's trust.
D. Tell Ms. Sloan about the CHIP program and give her an application. Advise Ms. Toms of Ms. Sloan's concerns after the appointment.

Answers can be found on the Evolve site.

■ KEY POINTS

- In the years between 2010 and 2019, national health spending is expected to grow at an average annual rate of 6.1%, reaching $4.5 trillion by 2019.
- By 2012 it is expected that programs such as Medicare, Medicaid and the Children's Health Insurance Plan will account for over half the health care purchased in the United States.
- The U.S. Census Bureau reported that the number of uninsured rose to 46.3 million in 2008, from 45.7 million in 2007.
- The uninsured receive less preventive care, are diagnosed at more advanced disease states, and, once diagnosed, tend to receive less therapeutic care in terms of surgery and treatment options. A recent study found that as many as 27,000 deaths in 2006 were the result of a lack of insurance (Dorn, 2008).
- A study in 2007 found that 56 million people in the United States lacked adequate access to primary health care because of shortages of primary health care providers in their communities. Those who are poor, minority group members, and non-English speakers have the greatest barriers to access.
- Among the 18 million who received care in community health centers in 2007, one out of every five clients were low-income, uninsured individuals, one in four were low income and members of minority populations, and one in seven were rural residents (NACHC, 2009).
- Globalization is a process of change and development across national boundaries and oceans, involving economics, trade, politics, technology, and social welfare.

- Primary health care, the focus of the public health system in the United States, is defined as a broad range of services, including, but not limited to, basic health services, family planning, clean water supply, sanitation, immunization, and nutrition education.
- The United States, as a WHO member nation, has endorsed primary health care as a strategy for achieving the goal of health for all in the twenty-first century.
- The emphasis on the social and physical environment moves *Healthy People 2020* from the traditional disease-specific focus to a more holistic view of health consistent with a public health frame of reference.
- The U.S. Department of Health and Human Services (HHS) is the agency most heavily involved with the health and welfare concerns of U.S. citizens.
- Public health nursing is defined as the practice of protecting and promoting the health of populations using knowledge from nursing, social, and public health sciences.
- The United States is the only industrialized nation in the world that does not guarantee health care to all of its citizens.
- The passage of health care reform by the 111th Congress in March of 2010 was historic, and its full enactment, which will take place through 2018, will usher in an era of expanded access to health care in the United States.

CLINICAL DECISION-MAKING ACTIVITIES

1. Visit your local health department and obtain a list of their services. Do these services fit with the guidelines developed by *Healthy People 2020*? How would you measure the facility's success or failure in meeting the indicators of *Healthy People 2020*?

2. Ask a provider in the health department what he or she thinks is the most pressing need in that geographic area. Do you agree that the services provided by this agency address the most important problems in the local community? What services would you add?

3. Interview a nurse practitioner and a primary care physician about their scope of practice. Compare and contrast their roles and how they function. Is there a place in the primary care system for these two types of providers?

4. Some disabled people choose not to work for fear that they will lose their Medicaid benefits, and that private insurance will not cover their needs. Are they justified in remaining unemployed given the circumstances? If you could fix the system so that the disabled could return to work, what changes would need to be made?

5. Many people immigrate legally and illegally to the United States every year. As a nurse, you may come in contact with clients who have become ill in their native countries but are seeking care in the United States, or clients who are in the United States illegally and become sick or injured. Under the new health care reform law, undocumented immigrants are not eligible for insurance benefits. What are your thoughts on the decision to exclude these residents from the expanded insurance options?

REFERENCES

American Association of Colleges of Nursing: *New data show that enrollment in baccalaureate nursing programs expands for the 10th consecutive year*, 2010. Available at http://www.aacn.nche.edu/media/newsreleases/2010/baccgrowth.html. Accessed February 15, 2011.

American Association of Colleges of Nursing: *Fact sheet: enhancing diversity in the nursing workforce*, 2009a. Available at http://www.aacn.nche.edu/Media/pdf/diversityFS.pdf. Accessed December 3, 2010.

American Association of Colleges of Nursing: *Fact Sheet: The Doctor of Nursing Practice (DNP)*, 2009b. Available at http://www.aacn.nche.edu/media/FactSheets/dnp.htm. Accessed December 3, 2010.

American Nurses Association: Quad Council of Public Health Nursing Organizations: *The public health nursing shortage: a threat to the public's health*, 2007. Available at http://www.astdn.org/downloadablefiles/Final Nursing Shortage Paper.pdf. Accessed December 3, 2010.

American Nurses Association: *Health care reform: Key provisions related to nursing: House (H.R. 3962) and Senate (H.R. 3590)*, 2009. Available at http://www.rnaction.org/site/DocServer/Key_Provisions_Related_to_Nursing-House_and_Senate.pdf?docID=981. Accessed December 3, 2010.

American Public Health Association: *Public Health Nursing Section: 1996: Definition and role of public health nursing*, Washington, DC, 1996, American Public Health Association.

Arias E: *National vital statistics reports: United States life tables, 2004*, 56(9), 2007. Available at http://www.cdc.gov/nchs/data/nvsr/nvsr56/nvsr56_09.pdf. Accessed December 3, 2010.

Bleich S: *Medical errors: five years after the IOM report: Commonwealth Fund Issue Brief*, 2005. Available at http://www.commonwealthfund.org/usr_doc/830_Bleich_errors.pdf. Accessed December 3, 2010.

Bower A, Girosi F, Meili R, et al: Can electronic medical record systems transform health care? Potential health benefits, savings, and costs, *Health Affairs* 24(5):1103–1117, 2005.

Brigham and Women's Hospital: *Basic facts about certified nurse-midwives*, 2010. Retrieved from http://www.brighamandwomens.org/Departments_and_Services/obgyn/Services/midwifery/Patient/facts.aspx.

Business Wire: *Federal grant allows community health center to adopt GE Healthcare's electronic medical record*, 2009. Available at http://www.thefreelibrary.com/Federal+Grant+Allows+Community+Health+Center+to+Adopt+GE+Healthcare%27s.-a0209237608. Accessed December 3, 2010.

Byrne W: *U.S. Nurse Practitioner prescribing law: a state-by-state summary*, 2009. Available at http://www.medscape.com/viewarticle/440315#NY. Accessed March, 2010.

Canadian Institute for Health Information: *National health expenditure trends, 1975 to 2009*, 2010. Available at http://secure.cihi.ca/cihiweb/dispPage.jsp?cw_page=PG_2490_E&cw_topic=2490&cw_rel=AR_31_E#full. Accessed March 2010.

Centers for Disease Control and Prevention: *Vision, mission, core values, and pledge*, 2010. Available at http://www.cdc.gov/about/organization/mission.htm. Accessed December 3, 2010.

Center for Health Communication, Harvard School of Public Health: *Reinventing aging: baby boomers and civic engagement*, Boston, MA, 2004, Harvard School of Public Health. Available at http://www.hsph.harvard.edu/chc/reinventingaging/Report.pdf. Accessed December 3, 2010.

Centers for Medicare and Medicaid Services: *National health expenditure data*, 2009a. Available at http://www.cms.gov/NationalHealthExpendData/. Accessed December 3, 2010.

Centers for Medicare and Medicaid Services: *National health expenditures aggregate, per capita amounts, percent distribution, and average annual percent growth, by source of funds: Selected calendar years 1960-2008, Table 2*, 2009c. Available at http://www.cms.hhs.gov/NationalHealthExpendData/downloads/tables.pdf. Accessed December 3, 2010.

Council on Linkages Between Academic and Public Health Practice: *Core competencies for public health professionals*, Washington, DC, 2010, Public Health Foundation/Health Resources and Services Administration.

Davis K, Schoen C, Schoenbaum S, et al: *Mirror, mirror on the wall: An international update on the comparative performance of American health care: The Commonwealth Fund*, 2007. Available at http://www.commonwealthfund.org/Content/Publications/Fund-Reports/2007/May/Mirror–Mirror-on-the-Wall–An-International-Update-on-the-Comparative-Performance-of-American-Healt.aspx. Accessed December 3, 2010.

Declercq E: Births attended by certified nurse-midwives in the United States in 2005, *J Midwifery Womens Health* 54(1):95–96, 2009. Available at http://www.midwife.org/siteFiles/legislative/DeClerq_article_Jan_Feb_2009.pdf. Accessed December 3, 2010.

DeNavas-Walt C, Proctor BD, Smith JC: *Income, poverty and health insurance coverage in the United States: Current population reports*, 2009. Available at http://www.census.gov/prod/2009pubs/p60-236.pdf. Accessed December 3, 2010.

Doe J: *WHO Statistical information system (WHOSIS)*, Geneva, 2009, World Health Organization.

Dorn S: *Uninsured and dying because of it: Updating the Institute of Medicine analysis on the impact of uninsurance on mortality*, Urban Institute, 2008. Available at http://www.urban.org/UploadedPDF/411588_uninsured_dying.pdf. Accessed December 3, 2010.

Dorn S, Hill I, Hogan S: *The secrets of Massachusetts' success: why 97 percent of state residents have health coverage: state health access reform evaluation*, 2009, Robert Wood Johnson Foundation. Available at http://www.urban.org/uploadedpdf/411987_massachusetts_success_brief.pdf. Accessed December 3, 2010.

Economic Report of the President U.S. Government Printing Office, 2010. Available at http://www.whitehouse.gov/sites/default/files/microsites/economic-report-president.pdf. Accessed December 3, 2010.

Frey WH, Berube A, Singer A, Wilson JH: *Getting current: Recent demographic trends in metropolitan America,* Brookings Institution, 2010. Available at http://www.brookings.edu/reports/2009/03_metro_demographic_trends.aspx. Accessed December 3, 2010.

Green MA, Rowell JC: *Understanding health insurance: a guide to billing and reimbursement,* ed 9, Clifton Park, NJ, 2008, Delmar Cengage Learning.

Grumbach K, Coffman J, Muñoz C, et al: *Strategies for improving diversity in the health professions,* 2003, Center for California Health Workforce Studies, University of California, San Francisco Education Policy Center, University of California, Davis. Available at http://www.calendow.org/uploadedFiles/strategies_for_improving_the_diversity.pdf. Accessed December 3, 2010.

Hinman AR, Davidson AJ: Linking children's health information systems: clinical care, public health, emergency medical systems, and schools, *Pediatrics* 123:S67–S73, 2009.

Institute of Medicine: *To err is human: building a safer health system,* 2000. Available at http://www.nap.edu/openbook.php?isbn=0309068371. Accessed December 5, 2010.

Institute of Medicine: *Keeping patients safe: Transforming the work environment of nurses,* Washington, DC, 2003, National Academy Press. Available at http://www.nap.edu/openbook.php?isbn=0309090679. Accessed December 5, 2010.

Johnson TD: Census Bureau: number of U.S. uninsured rises to 47 million Americans are uninsured: almost 5 percent increase since 2005, *Nations Health* 37(8), 2008. Available at http://www.medscape.com/viewarticle/567737. Accessed March 2010.

Kaiser Family Foundation: *Addressing the nursing shortage: background brief,* 2008. Available at http://www.kaiseredu.org/topics_im.asp?imID=1&parentID=61&id=138. Accessed December 3, 2010.

Kaiser Family Foundation: *Kaiser/HRET survey of employer-sponsored health benefits, 1999-2009,* 2009a. Available at http://facts.kff.org/chart.aspx?ch=1052. Accessed March 2010.

Kaiser Family Foundation: *Medicare: a primer,* 2009b. Available at http://kff.org/medicare/upload/7615-02.pdf. Accessed December 3, 2010.

Kaiser Family Foundation: *Kaiser Commission on Medicaid and the Uninsured: Medicaid and managed care: key data, trends, and issues,* 2010. Available at http://kff.org/medicaid/upload/8046.pdf. Accessed December 3, 2010.

Krisberg K: *Healthy People 2020* Tackling social determinants of health: input sought from health work force, *Nation's Health* 38(10), 2008. Available at http://www.medscape.com/viewarticle/587569. Accessed March 2010.

Leavitt MO: In: *U.S. Department of Health and Human Services: Personalized health care: pioneers, partnerships, progress,* 2010. Available at http://www.hhs.gov/myhealthcare/news/phc-report.pdf. Accessed February 15, 2011.

Liang BA: Risks of reporting sentinel events, *Health Affairs* 19(5):112, 2000. Available at http://content.healthaffairs.org/cgi/reprint/19/5/112.pdf. Accessed December 3, 2010.

Medical News Today: *Allied health professions week highlights: workforce shortage crisis,* 2006. Available at http://www.medicalnewstoday.com/articles/56473.php. Accessed December 3, 2010.

Merrill M: *Healthcare IT News: Telehealth boon expected for chronic care patients,* 2009. Available at http://www.healthcareitnews.com/news/telehealth-boon-expected-chronic-care-patients. Accessed December 3, 2010.

Migration Policy Institute: *2008 American community survey and census data on the foreign born by state,* 2010. Available at http://www.migrationinformation.org/datahub/acs census.cfm. Accessed December 3, 2010.

Milliard M: *Healthcare IT News: New 'emotional networking' product aims to complement telehealth,* 2010. Available at http://www.healthcareitnews.com/news/new-emotional-networking-product-aims-complement-telehealth. Accessed December 3, 2010.

Millis JS: *The graduate education of physicians: report of the citizens' commission on graduate medical education,* Chicago, 1966, American Medical Association.

Murray CJL, Frenk J: Ranking 37th—Measuring the performance of the U.S. health care system, *N Engl J Med* 362(2), 2010. Available at http://healthcarereform.nejm.org/?p=2610&query=home. Accessed December 3, 2010.

National Association of Community Health Centers: *Primary care access: an essential building block of health reform,* 2009. Available at http://www.nachc.com/client/documents/pressreleases/PrimaryCareAccessRPT.pdf. Accessed December 3, 2010.

Nemeth LS, Nietert PJ, Ornstein SM: High performance in screening for colorectal cancer: a Practice Partner Research Network (PPRNet) case study, *J Am Board Family Med* 22:141–146, 2009.

Office of U.S. Global AIDS Coordinator: *Implementation of the Global Health Initiative: Consultation Document,* 2010. Accessed at http://www.pepfar.gov/documents/organization/136504.pdf. Accessed December 3, 2010.

Organizing for America: *Cutting costs and covering America: a 21st century health care system,* 2007. Available at http://www.barackobama.com/2007/05/29/cutting_costs_and_covering_ame.php. Accessed December 3, 2010.

Public Health Foundation: *Core competencies for public health professionals,* n.d. Available at http://www.phf.org/resourcestools/Pages/Core_Public_Health_Competencies.aspx. Accessed March 2010.

Quad Council of Public Health Nursing Organizations: *Competencies for Public Health Nursing Practice,* Washington, DC, 2003, ASTDN, revised 2009.

Rowland D, Hoffman C, McGinn-Shapiro M: *Focus on health reform: Health care and the middle class: More costs and less coverage*: KaiserFamily Foundation, 2009. Available at http://kff.org/healthreform/upload/7951.pdf. Retrieved December 3, 2010.

Sackett DL, Rosenberg WM, Gray JA, et al: Evidence-based medicine: what it is and what it isn't, *Br Med J* 312:71–72, 1996.

Shokar NK, Nguyen-Oghalai T, Wu ZH: Factors associated with a physician's recommendation for colorectal cancer screening in a diverse population, *Family Med* 41(6):427–433, 2009. Available at https://www.stfm.org/fmhub/fm2009/June/Navkiran427.pdf. Accessed December 3, 2010.

Smith D: *Bringing affordable EMR capabilities to community health centers: HealthLeaders News,* 2007. Available at http://www.healthleadersmedia.com/content/TEC-88521/Bringing-Affordable-EMR-Capabilities-to-Community-Health-Centers.html. Accessed December 3, 2010.

Stolberg SG: Obama signs health care overhaul bill, with a flourish, *New York Times,* March 23, 2010. Available at http://www.nytimes.com/2010/03/24/health/policy/24health.html?nl=us&emc=politicsemailema1. Accessed December 3, 2010.

Teixeira R: *What the public really wants in health care:* The Century Foundation: Center for American Progress, n.d. Available at http://tcf.org/publications/healthcare/wtprw.healthcare.pdf. Accessed December 3, 2010.

Terris M: Epidemiology and leadership in public health in the Americas, *J Public Health Pol* 9(2):250–260, 1988.The Joint Commission. Sentinel event alert. 1998. Available at www.jointcommission.org/assets/1/18/SEA_5.Pdf. Accessed February 15, 2011.

The Joint Commission: Facts about the National Patient Safety Goals 2009. Available at http://www.jointcommission.org/assets/1/18/National_Patient_Safety_Goals_12_09.pdf. Accessed December 3, 2010.

Truffer CJ, Keehan S, Smith S, et al: Health spending projections through 2019: The recession's impact continues, *Health Affairs* 29(3), 2010. Available at http://content.healthaffairs.org/cgi/reprint/hlthaff.2009.1074v1. Retrieved December 3, 2010.

Umans B, Nonnemaker KL: The Medicare beneficiary population, *AARP Public Policy Institute,* 2009. Available at http://assets.aarp.org/rgcenter/health/fs149_medicare.pdf. Accessed December 3, 2010.

United Nations: *Department of Economic and Social Affairs: Division for Sustainable Development: Agenda 21: Section I: Social and Economic Dimensions: Chapter 6: Protecting and Promoting Human Health,* 2009. Available at http://www.un.org/esa/dsd/agenda21/res_agenda21_06.shtml. Accessed December 3, 2010.

U.S. Census Bureau: *U.S. Census Bureau News: One-in-five speak Spanish in four states new Census Bureau data show how America lives,* 2008. Available at http://www.census.gov/newsroom/releases/archives/american_community_survey_acs/cb08-cn67.html. Accessed December 3, 2010.

U.S. Census Bureau: *US Census Bureau News: Income, poverty and health insurance coverage in the United States: 2008,* 2009. Available at http://www.census.gov/newsroom/releases/archives/income_wealth/cb10-144.html. Accessed December 3, 2010.

U.S. Department of Health and Human Services: Health Resources and Services Administration: n.d.a. The Health Center Program: what is a health center? Available at http://bphc.hrsa.gov/about/. Accessed December 3, 2010.

U.S. Department of Health and Human Services: About faith-based and community initiatives, n.d.b. Available at http://www.hhs.gov/fbci/about/index.html. Accessed December 3, 2010.

U.S. Department of Health and Human Services: Health Resources and Services Administration: Bureau of Health Professions: changing demographics and the implications for physicians, nurses, and other health workers, n.d.c. Available at http://bhpr.hrsa.gov/healthworkforce/reports/changedemo/default.htm. Accessed December 3, 2010.

U.S. Department of Health and Human Services: US Department of Health and Human Services Organizational Chart, n.d.d. Available at http://www.hhs.gov/about/orgchart/#text. Accessed December 3, 2010.

U.S. Department of Health and Human Services: *2008: Health Resources and Services Administration: Bureau of Primary Health Care: Health Centers: America's primary care safety net reflections on success, 2002-2007.* Rockville, MD , 2008. Available at http://bhpr.hrsa.gov/interdisciplinary/acicbl/reports/second/1.htm. Accessed December 5, 2010.

U.S. Department of Health and Human Services: *Healthy People 2020.* Available at http://www.healthypeople.gov/2020topics objectives2020/default.aspx. Accessed January 1, 2011.

U.S. Department of Health and Human Services: Health Resources Services Administration: *National sample survey of Registered Nurses, 2008: Initial findings,* 2010a. Available at http://www.acnpweb.org/i4a/pages/index.cfm?pageid=3353. Accessed December 3, 2010.

U.S. Department of Health and Human Services Health Resources and Services Administration: *Initial findings from the 2008 national sample survey of Registered Nurses,* 2010b. Available at http://bhpr.hrsa.gov/healthworkforce/rnsurvey/initialfindings2008.pdf. Accessed December 3, 2010.

U.S. Department of Health and Human Services: *About the Office of Global Health Affairs,* 2010c. Available at http://www.globalhealth.gov/office/index.html. Accessed December 3, 2010.

U.S. Department of Health and Human Services: *National Institutes of Health: About NIH,* 2010d. Available at http://www.nih.gov/about/#mission. Accessed December 3, 2010.

U.S. Department of Health and Human Services: *U.S. Food and Drug Administration: About the Center for Tobacco Products,* 2010e. Available at http://www.fda.gov/AboutFDA/CentersOffices/AbouttheCenterforTobaccoProducts/default.htm. Accessed December 3, 2010.

U.S. Department of Labor: Bureau of Labor Statistics: *Economic News Release, Table 6, the 30 occupations with the largest employment growth,* 2008. Available at http://www.bls.gov/news.release/ecopro.t06.htm. Accessed December 3, 2010.

U.S. Food and Drug Administration: *Strategies to reduce medication errors: working to improve medication safety,* 2009. Available at http://www.fda.gov/Drugs/ResourcesForYou/Consumers/ucm143553.htm. Accessed December 3, 2010.

World Health Organization: Preamble to the Constitution of the World Health Organization as adopted by the International Health Conference, New York, 19-22 June 1946; signed on 22 July 1946 by the representatives of 61 states (Official Records of the World Health Organization, no. 2, p. 100) and entered into force on April 7, 1948. Available at http://www.who.int/about/definition/en/. Accessed December 3, 2010.

World Health Organization: *Primary health care,* Geneva, 1978, WHO.

World Health Organization: Declaration of Alma Ata, WHO Regional Office for Europe, 2005. Available at http://www.euro.who.int/AboutWHO/Policy/20010827_1. Accessed December 3, 2010.

World Health Organization: *Global alert and response: influenza-like illness in the United States and Mexico,* 2010a. Available at http://www.who.int/csr/don/2009_04_24/en/index.html. Accessed December 3, 2010.

World Health Organization: *Global Alert and Response: Pandemic (H1N1) 2009—update 87,* 2010b. Available at http://www.who.int/csr/don/2010_02_12/en/index.html. Accessed December 3, 2010.

World Health Organization: *Public health risk assessment and interventions: earthquake: Haiti,* 2010c. Available at http://www.who.int/diseasecontrol_emergencies/publications/haiti_earthquake_20100118.pdf. Accessed December 3, 2010.

World Health Organization: *World Health Day 2005: Make every mother and child count, WHO Regional Office for Europe,* 2010d. Available at http://www.who.int/world-health-day/previous/2005/en/. Accessed December 3, 2010.

CHAPTER 4

Perspectives in Global Health Care

Anita Hunter, PhD, APRN–CPNP, FAAN*

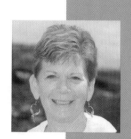

Dr. Anita Hunter has been a pediatric nurse practitioner since 1975, working with the vulnerable populations of children and families living in poor urban and rural communities. Her work with culturally diverse populations expanded to the international arena in 1994 when she began taking students and faculty on clinical immersion experiences. These immersion medical missions have extended into Northern Ireland, Ghana, Mexico, the Dominican Republic, and Uganda; each evolving into sustainable health initiatives within each country. In conjunction with her prior academic role as Director of MSN Programs and the International Nursing Office at the University of San Diego, Dr. Hunter also serves as the Medical Director for the Holy Innocents Children's Hospital Uganda NGO (non-governmental organization) that oversees the development and management of the Holy Innocents Children's Hospital in Uganda. Dr. Hunter is the Chairperson, Department of Nursing at Dominican University of California.

ADDITIONAL RESOURCES

evolve WEBSITE
http://evolve.elsevier.com/Stanhope
- *Healthy People 2020*
- WebLinks
- Quiz
- Case Studies

- Glossary
- Answers to Practice Application
- Resource Tool
  - Resource Tool 4.A: Millennium Development Goals Report 2010

OBJECTIVES

After reading this chapter, the student should be able to do the following:

1. Identify the major aims and goals for global health that have been presented by the *Millennium Global Developmental Goals* (2009).
2. Identify the health priorities of Health for All in the 21st Century (HFA21).
3. Analyze the role of nursing in global health.
4. Explain the role and focus of a population-based approach for global health.
5. Discuss the many causes of global health problems.
6. Identify some solutions for at least one of these global health problems.
7. Describe how global health is related to economic, industrial, environmental, and technological development.
8. Compare and contrast the health care system in a developed country with one in a lesser-developed country.
9. Define burden of disease.
10. Explain how countries can prepare for natural and manmade disasters and the role of nurses in these efforts.
11. Describe at least five organizations that are involved in global health.

*Dr. Hunter greatly acknowledges the original authors of this chapter: Kathleen Huttlinger, PhD, FNP and Jennifer M. Schaller-Ayers, PhD, RN, BC, as well as the manuscript review and consultation of a review committee from the U.S. Army Center for Health Promotion and Preventive Medicine. The mention of the U.S. Army, Army organizations, and/or Army personnel in this chapter is not to be interpreted or construed, in any manner, to be official U.S. Army endorsement of same or to represent or express the official opinion of the U.S. Army.

KEY TERMS

OUTLINE

This chapter presents an overview of the major public health problems of the world, along with a description of the role and involvement of nurses in global and community health care settings. It describes health care delivery from a global and population health perspective, illustrates how health systems operate in different countries, presents examples of organizations that address global health, and explains how economic development relates to health care throughout the world.

OVERVIEW AND HISTORICAL PERSPECTIVE OF GLOBAL HEALTH

Why is it important for nurses to understand and attend to global health issues? Why be concerned about population health at the global level? What is a nurse's responsibility to global health? Such questions have been asked of this author over the last 15 years while working in the global arena. Her response is framed by the following: philosophically, we should be global citizens, caring about and for the greater than 80% of the world that is impoverished, starving, and dying from preventable conditions. What once were the unique health challenges of people in less-developed countries, such as loss of human rights, lack of access to food, housing, safety, and health care, are now common problems of people all over the world. Global warming, destruction of natural resources, increasing global violence, the declining global economy, and the depletion of food supplies

all contribute to the current global health crisis. Preventable conditions like malaria, malnutrition, communicable diseases, chronic health problems, and conditions related to environmental pollution are taxing the health care systems of many nations. Immigrants from developing nations often bring these conditions with them. Understanding global health and factors that contribute to the immigrant's health problems better prepares the nurse to develop interventions that are culturally congruent, culturally responsive, and culturally acceptable to the people for whom interventions are planned.

Nursing has been actively engaged in global health (Lewis, 2005) since the turn of the twentieth century, as nurses served in each of the World Wars, Korea, Vietnam, and the wars of the twenty-first century, striving to save the lives of combatants and non-combatants. Dealing with the collateral damage of war, nurses became committed to help intervene before wars began with the intent that addressing the factors that contributed to war might change the outcome and prevent it. In 1977 attendees at the annual meeting of the World Health Assembly stated that all citizens of the world should enjoy a level of health that would permit them to lead a socially and economically productive life. This goal was to have been achieved by the year 2000; however, man-made and natural disasters, political corruption, lack of infrastructures in lesser-developed nations, and unforeseen obstacles have inhibited this goal from being achieved. The goals of Health for All by the Year 2000 (HFA2000) were extended into the next century with the document Health for

All in the 21st Century (HFA21). These goals have continued to be promoted by numerous health-related conferences held around the world, including the International Council of Nurses (ICN). Therefore, nurses must be globally astute and involved in helping to ensure that these goals are obtained by the people of the world.

In 1978 concern for the health of the world's people was voiced at the International Conference on Primary Health Care that was held in Alma Ata, Kazakhstan, in what was then Soviet Central Asia. The conference, sponsored by the World Health Organization (WHO) and the United Nations Children's Fund (UNICEF), had representatives from 143 countries and 67 organizations. They adopted a resolution that proclaimed that the major key to attaining HFA2000 was the worldwide implementation of primary health care (Lucas, 1998). These global partners continue to evolve the *Healthy People* doctrine. The third iteration of *Healthy People entitled Healthy People 2020* was released in December 2010.

♥ HEALTHY PEOPLE 2020

Selected Objectives that Apply to Global Health Care

- EH-1: Increase the proportion of persons served by community water systems who receive a supply of drinking water that meets the regulations of the Safe Drinking Water Act.
- EH-5: Reduce waterborne disease outbreaks arising from water intended for drinking among persons served by community water systems.
- FP-1: Increase the proportion of pregnancies that are intended.
- GH-1: Reduce the number of cases of malaria reported in the United States.
- HIV-1: Reduce the number of new HIV diagnoses among adolescents and adults.
- MICH-3: Reduce the rate of child deaths.

From U.S. Department of Health and Human Services: *Healthy People. 2020 topics and objectives.* Available at http://www.healthypeople.gov/2020/topicsobjectives2020/default.aspx. Accessed January 1, 2011.

Since the Alma Ata conference, there has been growing interest in global health and how best to attain it. People around the world want to know and understand the issues and concerns that affect health on a global scale. This is important since many countries have not yet experienced the technological advancement in their health care systems that have been realized by more developmentally advanced countries. Many terms are used to describe nations that have achieved a high level of industrial and technological advancement (along with a stable market economy) and those that have not. For the purposes of this chapter, the term developed country refers to those countries with a stable economy and a wide range of industrial and technological development (e.g., the United States, Canada, Japan, the United Kingdom, Sweden, France, and Australia). A country that is not yet stable with respect to its economy and technological development is referred to as a lesser-developed country (e.g., Bangladesh, Zaire, Haiti, Guatemala, most countries in sub-Saharan Africa, and the island nation of Indonesia). Both developed and lesser-developed countries are found in all parts of the world and in all geographic and climatic zones.

Health problems exist throughout the world, but the lesser-developed countries often have more exotic sounding health care problems such as Buruli ulcers, leishmaniasis, schistosomiasis, brucellosis, typhus, yellow fever, and malaria (WHO, 2000a). Ongoing health problems needing control in lesser-developed countries include measles, mumps, rubella, and polio; the current health concerns of the more-developed countries are problems such as hepatitis, infectious diseases, and new viral strains such as the hantavirus, SARS, H1N1, and avian flu. Chronic health problems such as hypertension, diabetes, cardiovascular disease, obesity, cancer, the resurgence of human immunodeficiency virus/acquired immunodeficiency syndrome (HIV/AIDS) among adolescents and young adults, drug-resistant tuberculosis (TB); and the larger social, yet health-related, issues such as terrorism, warfare, violence, and substance abuse are now global issues (ICN, 2003). World travelers both serve as hosts to various types of disease agents and may expose themselves to diseases and environmental health hazards that are unknown or rare in their home country. Two examples of diseases from recent years that were once fairly isolated and rare but are now widespread throughout the world are AIDS and drug-resistant TB (IOM, 2009, 2010; WHO, 2004a) (Figure 4-1).

In addition to direct health problems, increasing populations, migration within countries, political corruption, lack of natural resources, and natural disasters affect the health and well-being of populations. Dr. Paul Farmer (2005) talks about the war on the poor; how many migrate to the city to find employment where limited employment opportunities exist. Such migration leads to the development of shanty towns often built on the outskirts of cities, on unstable ground, and in areas vulnerable to natural disasters such as hurricanes, tsunamis, and earthquakes such as those in Haiti, Chile, and Indonesia. These environments are unsanitary, unsafe, and a breeding ground for TB, dysentery, malnutrition, abuse of women and children, and mosquito and other insect or animal-borne diseases.

Nations plagued by civil war and political corruption are faced with chronic poverty, unstable leadership, and lack of economic development. The effects of war and conflict also have devastating effects on a country and the health of its population. The wars in Afghanistan, Iraq, and the West Bank of Palestine, to name a few, have had devastating mental and physical health consequences, leaving each country and its people with few health care services or other resources to sustain life. A recent research study about the long-term effects of children exposed to war (Asia, 2009) supports the negative health consequences of such exposure. For example, changes in biomarkers can lead to future chronic health conditions like cardiovascular disease, autoimmune conditions, cancer, and mental health problems. Serious nutritional problems and outbreaks of influenza have been reported. The increased incidence of violence against women and children, the hazards of unexploded weapons and land mines, and the occurrence of earthquakes and other natural disasters increase the health risks (USAID, 2005; WHO, 2002a,b).

WHAT DO YOU THINK?   *Many people believe that the wars in Iraq and Afghanistan have created a public health crisis. What do you think is the public health crisis, and what could nurses do to ameliorate one contributing factor to the crisis?*

As countries promote the objectives of HFA21, they realize that they need to improve their economies and infrastructures. They often seek funds and technological expertise from the wealthier and more-developed countries (UN, 2009; World Bank, 2005). According to the WHO, HFA21 is not a single, finite goal but a strategic process that can lead to progressive improvement in the health of people (WHO, 2002c). In essence,

it is a call for social justice and solidarity. Unfortunately, the lesser-developed nations lack the infrastructure necessary to achieve health promotion and living conditions, as many of these countries continue to deteriorate for the poor, and environments that breed infections are the norm (Figure 4-2).

The United Nations' (UNs') **Millennium Development Goals** (MDGs) were first agreed upon by world leaders at the Millennium Summit in 2000 (see Resource Tool 3.A on the book's Evolve site). The MDGs were developed to relieve poor health conditions around the world and to establish positive steps to improve living conditions (UN, 2005). By the year 2005, all member nations pledged to meet the goals described

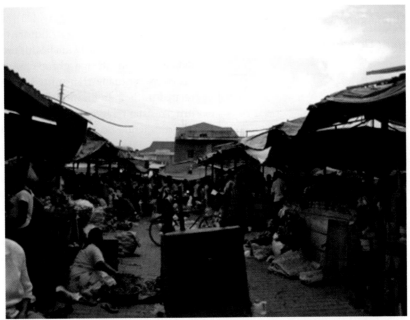

FIGURE 4-1 Open market in Uganda, where preventable diseases are rampant. (Courtesy A. Hunter.)

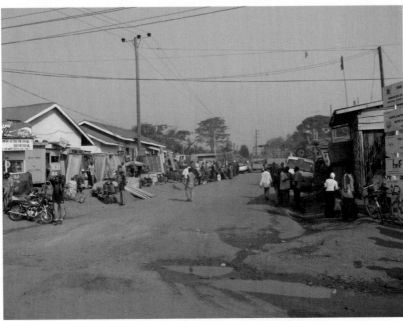

FIGURE 4-2 The streets of a typical town in Uganda. (Courtesy A. Hunter.)

in Box 4-1. These goals have continued to evolve as natural disasters and internal strife continue to affect the poor and the vulnerable. The Millennium Report (UN Millennium Development Report, 2009) describes the developed nations' responsibility to the betterment of those in lesser-developed nations. The revised goals highlight the global responsibility to eradicate poverty and hunger; achieve universal primary education for all children; promote gender equality and empower women; reduce child mortality; improve maternal health; combat HIV/AIDS, malaria, and other diseases; ensure environmental sustainability; and develop a global partnership for development. The U.S. has supported this mandate in its Global Health Initiatives (n.d.) as has the ICN. As economic agreements between countries remove financial and political barriers, growth and development are stimulated. Simultaneously, as global health problems that once seemed distant are brought closer to people around the globe, political and economic barriers between countries fall.

Despite efforts by individual governments and international organizations to improve the general economy and welfare of all countries, many health problems continue to exist, especially among poorer people. Many countries lack both political commitment to health care and recognition of basic human rights. They may fail to achieve equity in access to primary health care, demonstrate inappropriate use and allocation of resources for high-cost technology, and maintain a low status of women. Currently, the lesser-developed countries experience high infant and child death rates (Figure 4-3), with diarrheal and respiratory diseases as major contributory factors (WHO, 2010).

Other major worldwide health problems include nutritional deficiencies in all age groups, women's health and fertility problems, sexually transmitted diseases (STDs), and illnesses related to the human immunodeficiency virus (HIV), malaria, drug-resistant TB, neonatal tetanus, leprosy, occupational and environmental health hazards, and abuses of tobacco, alcohol, and drugs. Because of these continuing problems, the Director General of the WHO has made a commitment to renew all of the policies and actions of HFA21. The WHO continues to develop new and holistic health policies that are based on the concepts of equity and solidarity with an emphasis on the individual's, family's, and community's responsibility for health. Strategies for achieving the continuing goals of HFA21 include building

---

BOX 4-1   MILLENNIUM GOALS

Goal Number Millennium Development Goals (MDGs)

MDG 1: Eradicate extreme poverty and hunger
MDG 2: Achieve universal primary education
MDG 3: Promote gender equality and empower women
MDG 4: Reduce child mortality
MDG 5: Improve maternal health
MDG 6: Combat HIV/AIDS, malaria, and other diseases
MDG 7: Ensure environmental sustainability
MDG 8: Develop a global partnership for development

From United Nations: *UN millennium development goals (MDGs)*, 2005. Available at http://www.un.org/milleniumgoals/. Accessed December 5, 2010.

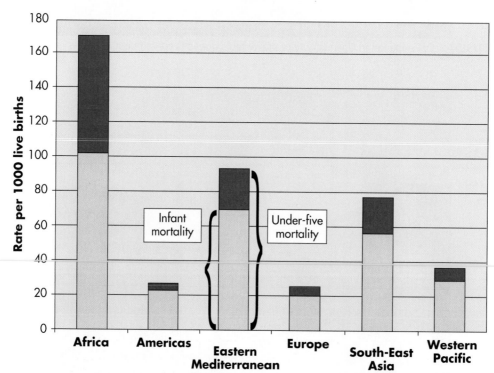

FIGURE 4-3 Under-five and infant mortality rates, by WHO region, 2003. (From World Health Organization: Health status statistics: mortality. Available at http://www.who.int/healthinfo/statistics/indneonatal mortality/en/. Accessed December 5, 2010.)

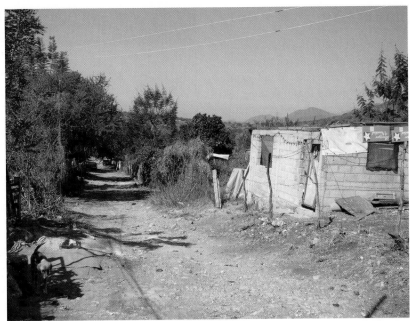

FIGURE 4-4 A community living in a dump in Miacatlan, Mexico. (Courtesy A. Hunter.)

on past accomplishments and the identification of global priorities and targets for the first 20 years of the new century (WHO, 2002).

Nurses need to be informed about global health. Many of the world's health problems directly affect the health of individuals who live in the United States. For example, the 103rd U.S. Congress passed the North American Free Trade Agreement (NAFTA), which opened trade borders between the United States, Canada, and Mexico in 1994 and allowed an increased movement of products and people. Along the United States–Mexico border, an influx of undocumented immigrants in recent years has raised concerns for the health of people who live in this area. For example, many immigrants have settled on unincorporated land, known as *colonias,* outside the major metropolitan areas in California, Arizona, New Mexico, and Texas. These colonies may have no developed roads, transportation, water, or electrical services (Figures 4-4 and 4-5).

Conditions in these settlements have led to an increase in disease conditions such as amebiasis and respiratory and diarrheal diseases. Environmental health hazards in the *colonias* are associated with poverty, poor sanitation, and overcrowded conditions (Brown, 2005). On a more positive note, NAFTA has provided an impetus and framework for the government of Mexico to modernize their medical system so that they can compete and respond to the demands of more global competition. Although some improvements have been made, there is still an overriding concern that environmental and health regulations in Mexico have not kept up with the pace of increased border trade (Malkin, 2009). The Mexican National Academy of Medicine continues to make health and environmental recommendations to the government, which illustrates the beneficial interactions that are occurring between Mexico, Canada, and the United States as part of this trade agreement. Nurses play a significant role in obtaining health for the indigent and

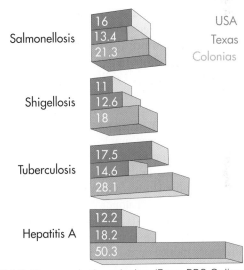

FIGURE 4-5 Diseases in the colonias. (From PBS Online, *The Forgotten Americans.* Available at http://www.pbs.org/klru/forgotten americans/focus/health.htm. Accessed December 5, 2010.)

undocumented persons who live along the border regions in Texas, New Mexico, Arizona, and California. Nurses supported by private foundations and by local and state public health departments often provide the only reliable health care in these areas.

Interestingly, Canadian worker groups were concerned that NAFTA would eventually lead to worsened working conditions as manufacturing plants move to the lower-wage and largely non-unionized southern United States and Mexico (Fuller, 2002); however, reports indicate that trade, standard of living, and employment opportunities have risen (Foreign Affairs and International Trade Canada International, 2009; Cahoon and Myles, 2004).

THE ROLE OF POPULATION HEALTH

Population health refers to the health outcomes of a group of individuals, including the distribution of such outcomes within the group, and includes health outcomes, patterns of health determinants, and policies and interventions that link these two (Kindig and Stoddard, 2010). It is an approach and perspective that focuses on the broad range of factors and conditions that have a strong influence on the health of populations (environment, genetics, ethnicity, pollution, and physical and mental stressors affecting a community). Using epidemiological trends, population health emphasizes health for groups at the population level rather than at the individual level and focuses on reducing inequities, improving health in these groups to reduce morbidity and mortality, and assessing emerging diseases and other health risks to a community (IOM, 2002). A population can be defined by a geographic boundary, by the common characteristics shared by a group of people such as ethnicity or religion, or by the epidemiological and social conditions of a community (Fox, 2001).

The factors and conditions that are important considerations in population health are called **determinants.** Population health determinants may include income and social factors, social support networks, education, employment, working and living conditions, physical environments, social environments, biology and genetic endowment, personal health practices, coping skills, healthy child development, health services, sex, and culture (Galea, 2008; Ibrahim et al, 2001). The determinants do not work independently of each other but form a complex system of interactions.

Canada is a leader in promoting the population health approach. Canada has been implementing programs using this framework since the mid-1990s and builds on a tradition of public health and health promotion. Box 4-2 presents the development of the Healthy Cities movement in Toronto. A Canadian document, the Lalonde Report (1974), proposed that changes in lifestyles or social and physical environments lead to more improvements in health than would be achieved by spending more money on existing health care delivery systems. The Canadian initiative was aimed at efforts and investments directed at root causes to increase potential benefits for health outcomes (Public Health Agency of Canada, 2005). A key was the identification and definition of health issues and of the investment decisions within a population that were guided by evidence about what keeps people healthy. Therefore a population health approach directs investments that have the greatest potential to influence the health of that population in a positive manner. Canada has since implemented a broad range of projects across the country and is a model that many U.S. communities have begun to adopt. The 2002 IOM report emphasized the need to assess the determinants affecting population health and initiate interventions to correct them because America's health status did not match the country's substantive investment in health (IOM, 2002).

International communities have also integrated the health determinants into public policies. At the 2009 Nairobi Global Conference on Health Promotion, over 600 participants

---

From Flynn B, Ivanov L: Health promotion through healthy communities and cities. In *Community & Public Health Nursing*, ed 6, St Louis, 2004, Mosby, pp 396-411.

> **BOX 4-2 EXAMPLES OF THE HEALTHY CITIES MOVEMENT**
>
> Toronto, Ontario was one of the first cities in North America to become involved in the Healthy Cities movement. Toronto began with a strategic planning committee to develop an overall strategy for health promotion. The committee conducted vision workshops in the community and a comprehensive environmental scan to help identify health needs in Toronto. The outcome was a final report outlining major issues, and it included a strategic mission, priorities, and recommendations for action. The Toronto Healthy City was involved in a number of projects. One of them, the Healthiest Babies Possible project, was an intensive antenatal education and nutritional supplement program for pregnant women who were identified by health and social agencies as being at high risk. The program included intensive contact and follow-up of women, along with food supplements. It has been successful in decreasing the incidence of low–birth-weight infants.
>
> Another example is Chengdu, China. Chengdu is located on the upper parts of the Yangtze River and is surrounded on four sides by the Fu and Nan Rivers and was one of the most polluted cities in southwestern China. The pollution created severe environmental problems as a result of industrial waste, raw sewage, and the intensive use of fresh water. The proliferation of slum and squatter settlements exacerbated the social, economic, and environmental problems of the city. The Fu and Nan Rivers Comprehensive Revitalization Plan was started in 1993 as a Healthy Community and City initiative to deal with the growing environmental problems. The principles of participatory planning and partnership were used to raise awareness of the problem among the general public and to mobilize major stakeholders to invest in a sustainable future for Chengdu and its inhabitants. The plan resulted in providing 30,000 households living in the slum and squatter settlements with decent and affordable housing, and with projects to deal with sewage and industrial waste. In addition, the plan was able to improve parks and gardens, turning Chengdu into a clean and green city with the natural flow of its rivers.

representing 100 countries adopted a Call to Action on addressing population health and finding ways to promote health at the global level. Health and development today face unprecedented threats by the financial crisis, global warming and climate change, and security threats. Since 1986, with the development of the first Global Conference, until 2009, a large body of evidence and experience has accumulated about the importance of health promotion as an integrative, cost-effective strategy, and as an essential component of health systems primed to respond adequately to emerging concerns (WHO, 2010).

As nurses work with immigrants from global arenas or become active participants in health care around the world, understanding such concepts as population health and the determinants of health for a population becomes more important than the most advanced acute care skills. These skills, though important, are intended to help an individual; population health skills sets can help the world.

PRIMARY HEALTH CARE

The role of **primary health care** is historically based on the worldwide conference that was held at Alma Ata (Tejada de Rivers, 2003). WHO and UNICEF still actively promote primary health care and maintain that the training of health workers needs to be based on current primary health care practices. They advocate for community members to be involved in all aspects of the planning and implementation of health services that are delivered to their respective communities.

The early recommendations in 1978 by WHO/UNICEF believed that a unified approach to creating primary care services globally was important. These aims continue to be reinforced and modified and were recently updated to incorporate MDGs (WHO, 2003a; Kekki, 2005). Such services included the following:

- An organized approach to health education that involves professional health care providers and trained community representatives
- Aggressive attention to environmental sanitation, especially food and water sources
- Involvement and training of community and village health workers in all plans and intervention programs
- Development of maternal and child health programs that include immunization and family planning
- Initiation of preventive programs that are specifically aimed at local endemic problems such as malaria and schistosomiasis in tropical regions
- Accessibility and affordability of services for the treatment of common diseases and injuries
- Availability of chemotherapeutic agents for the treatment of acute, chronic, and communicable diseases
- Development of nutrition programs
- Promotion and acceptance of traditional medicine

Global leaders have recognized the need to get nations committed to the health care agenda (the UNs' MDGs, 2009). Maeseneer et al (2008) presented 12 characteristics that define primary health care: it is general in scope, accessible, integrated (including health promotion, disease prevention, cure and care, rehabilitation and palliation), continuous, dependent on teamwork, holistic, personal (focusing on the person rather than the disease), family and community oriented, coordinated, confidential (respecting the client's privacy), and playing an advocacy role. An important effort is needed at the level of recruitment, education, and retention of primary health care workers, including primary care nurses, family physicians, and mid-level care workers. Professional organizations, clinical agencies, universities, and other institutions for higher education should continue to demonstrate their "social accountability" by training appropriate providers.

Mexico is an example of a country that has made a particular effort to implement primary health care services. Mexico has initiated a module program that is administered through the ministry of health. The program is characterized by village-based health posts, each of which is operated by a community volunteer and a health committee. The volunteer and committee are supervised by a nurse who operates from a regional health center. It is believed that this module system can address community needs and will ultimately lead to better use of services and resources (Nigenda, Ruiz, and Montes, 2001).

NURSING AND GLOBAL HEALTH

Nurses play a leadership role in health care throughout the world (Hancock, 2005). Those with public health experience provide knowledge and skill in countries where nursing is not an organized profession, and they give guidance to the nurses as well as to the auxiliary personnel who are part of the primary health care team (ICN, 2001a). In many areas in the developed world, nurses provide direct client care and help meet the education and health promotion needs of the community. They are viewed as strong advocates for primary health care, through social commitment to equality of health care and support of the concepts that are contained in the Alma Ata declaration (ICN, 2003).

Unfortunately, in the lesser-developed countries, the role of the nurse is defined poorly, if at all, and care often depends on and is directed by physicians (Buchan and Dal Poz, 2002). This author has seen health care systems in Africa, Mexico, and the Dominican Republic in which nursing is not valued and the ability of nurses to contribute to improving an individual's health, much less a community's health, is minimal. Much work is needed to raise the bar in the education of nurses in these countries so they have the skills necessary to make a difference; however, overcoming some of the cultural and gender-role barriers makes this process laborious (Figure 4-6).

Nurses have led in care delivery in such areas as the devastating tsunami in south Asia (ICN, 2005), and more recently after the earthquakes in Haiti and Chile in 2010. Other health interventions have been the interprofessional work of nursing and science to build and open the dedicated children's hospital in Uganda (Bolender and Hunter, 2010), the nurse-developed Ghana Health Mission (Hunter and McKenry, 2005), a quality improvement program in the Congo (DuMortier and Arpagaus, 2005), an emergency service program in Mongolia (Cherian et al, 2004), and a community-based TB program in Swaziland (Escott and Walley, 2005).

On a different continent, the role of nursing in China and Taiwan is noteworthy. Nursing in China is undergoing a dramatic change, largely because of an evolving political and economic environment. In the past, nursing was viewed as a trade, and the acquisition of nursing skills and knowledge took place in the equivalent of a middle school or junior high in the United States. Increasing pressure on the health care system in China is providing an impetus for education at the university level. The Chinese government has sent many nurses to the United States, Europe, and Australia to receive university-level education in nursing at the undergraduate and graduate levels in hopes that these individuals will return to China to provide the nursing and nursing education needed there (Anders and Harrigan, 2002). The author, in conjunction with a colleague (Dr. Mary Jo Clark), has consulted in Taiwan, helping them establish their nurse practitioner programs and to implement their doctoral programs in nursing. Part of that consultation involved the use of standardized clients as a component for certification and license to practice as a nurse practitioner. The United States is just beginning to entertain this idea.

In some countries, such as Chile, the physician-to-population ratio is higher than the nurse-to-population ratio. In these cases,

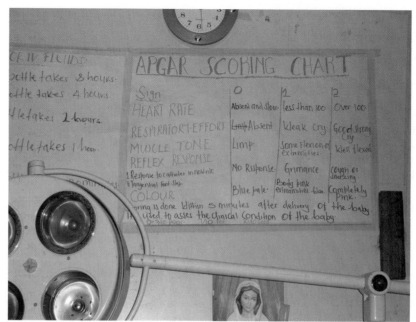

FIGURE 4-6 Uganda hospital information for nurses in labor and delivery. (Courtesy A. Hunter.)

physicians influence nursing practice and place economic and political pressure on local, regional, and national governments to control the services that nurses provide. In Chile, nurses have set up successful and cost-effective clinics to deliver quality primary care services, but they are constantly being threatened by physicians who want to remove the nurses and replace them with the more costly services of physicians (WHO, 2000a). Box 4-3 describes nursing and health care efforts in Zambia.

MAJOR GLOBAL HEALTH ORGANIZATIONS

Many international organizations have an ongoing interest in global health. Despite the presence of these well-meaning organizations, it is estimated that the lesser-developed countries still bear most of the cost for their own health care and that contributions from major international organizations actually provide for less than 5% of needed costs. Recent reports indicate that the majority of funds raised by international organizations are used for food relief, worker training, and disaster relief (IMVA, 2002). However, when considering the total effort, the poorer countries, such as those in sub-Saharan Africa, still receive the greatest amount of financial support from the more developed countries, often accounting for more than 20% of the poorer country's health care expenditures (IMVA, 2002; World Bank, 2005).

International health organizations are classified as multilateral organizations, bilateral organizations, or **non-governmental organizations (NGOs)** or **private voluntary organizations (PVOs)** (including philanthropic organizations). **Multilateral organizations** are those that receive funding from multiple government and non-government sources. The major organizations are part of the United Nations (UN), and they include the World Health Organization (WHO), the United Nations Children's Fund (UNICEF), the Pan American Health Organization (PAHO), and the World Bank. A **bilateral organization** is a single government agency that provides aid to lesser-developed countries, such as the U.S. Agency for International Development (USAID). NGOs or PVOs, including the philanthropic organizations, are represented by such agencies as Oxfam, Project Hope, the International Red Cross, various professional and trade organizations, Catholic Relief Services (CRS), church-sponsored health care missionaries, and many other private groups.

Specifically, the World Health Organization (WHO) is a separate, autonomous organization that, by special agreement, works with the UN through its Economic and Social Council. The idea for this worldwide health organization developed from the First International Sanitary Conference in 1902, a precursor to the WHO (Campana, 2005). The WHO was created in 1946 as an outgrowth of the League of Nations and the UN charter that provided for the formation of a special health agency to address the wide scope and nature of the world's health problems. The WHO, headed by a director general and five assistant generals, has three major divisions: (1) the World Health Assembly approves the budget and makes decisions about health policies, (2) the executive board serves as the liaison between the assembly and the secretariat, and (3) the secretariat carries out the day-to-day activities of the WHO. The principal work of the WHO is to direct and coordinate international health activities and to provide technical medical assistance to countries in need. More than 1000 health-related projects are ongoing within the WHO at any one time. Requests for assistance may be made directly to the WHO by a country for a project, or the project may be part of a larger collaborative endeavor involving many countries. Examples of current collaborative, multinational projects include comprehensive family planning programs in Indonesia, Malaysia, and Thailand; applied research on communicable disease and immunization in several

BOX 4-3   COMMUNITY HEALTH NURSING IN ZAMBIA

The Ministry of Health, Churches Health Association, the private Medical Practitioners, and the Traditional Healer Services provide health care in Zambia. By 1995 there were 86 hospitals and 1345 health centers in the country. About 60% of the bed capacity is provided by the government hospitals and health centers, 26% by mission hospitals, and 13% by the Zambia consolidated Copper Mines. At the time of independence, the population of Zambia was sparsely distributed, especially in the rural area, and there were inadequate health facilities. Health facilities were concentrated along the line of rail, and the provision of care was poor. This prompted the government to review the health care provision system after independence in 1964. The government then declared that health care services would be free for all, with the main health care services being curative rather than preventive. This policy was detrimental to Zambia, whose population was increasing.

In 1991 the government of the republic of Zambia, under the leadership of the Movement for Multiparty Democracy, introduced the concept of National Health Reforms whose vision is to provide equitable access to high-quality, cost-effective health care intervention as close to the family as possible. Health reforms stress the need for families and communities to be self-reliant and to participate in their own health care provision and development. The major component of the health policy reform is the restructured primary health care (PHC) program. This has been defined as the essential health care made universally accessible to individuals and families by means acceptable to them through their full participation and at a cost that the community and country can afford. The principles of PHC include community participation and intersectoral collaboration. Families are considered as a unit of service, as most health care provision starts with the family setting. The Zambian government is committed to the fundamental and humane principle in the development of the health care system to provide Zambians with the equity of access to cost-effective quality health care as close to the family as possible.

The National Health Reforms decentralized power to districts, and home-based care (HBC) was introduced. HBC was adopted and implemented in all districts as a way of cost sharing between the government, families, and community. HBC led to reduced congestion in hospitals, and government resources were not overstrained as families also took part in supplying the needed resources, time, and personnel (caregiver) when the clients were cared for at home.

Nurses provide about 75% of the health force in Zambia. The community health nursing component is one of the major components of the nursing curriculum at all levels of training. Basically, every general nurse is taught to operate as a community health nurse. However, to be registered as a public health nurse by the General Nursing Council of Zambia, one must undergo the following levels of training. The individual undergoes 3 years of training as a registered nurse followed by 1 year of training as a midwife. In the past they would then undergo 2 years of training at the University of Zambia to obtain a diploma in public health nursing. This was phased out when the bachelor of science in nursing degree was initiated. Currently, the individual pursues the bachelor of science in nursing degree and majors in community health nursing in the final year.

The main role of the community health nurse includes competence and skill in the care of individuals, families, and communities in the following ways:

1. Critically explore and analyze current developments in community health as they relate to different populations at different levels of care.
2. Apply health promotion models and theories to community health nursing practice.
3. Design, implement, and manage community-based projects, programs, and services.
4. Integrate community-based agents into the health care system.
5. Use epidemiology concepts in the management of communicable and noncommunicable diseases.

Courtesy Prudencia Mweemba, University of Zambia, School of Medicine, Department of Post Basic Nursing, Lusaka, Zambia, 2006.

East African nations; and projects that investigate the viability of administering AIDS vaccines to pregnant women in South Africa and Namibia. For further information about the WHO, visit http://www.who.int/en/online.

> **DID YOU KNOW?** *Mercy Corps International initiated the Kosovo Women's Health Promotion Project (2001), in which nurse-midwives actively participate in promoting midwifery care for positive reproductive outcomes. Kosovo is one of the countries where women's health care has suffered from the ravages of war.*

From Heymann M: Reproductive health promotion in Kosovo, J Midwifery Womens Health 46:74-81, 2001.

Another multilateral agency is the **United Nations Children's Fund (UNICEF)** (http://www.unicef.org). Formed shortly after World War II (WWII) to assist children in the war-ravaged countries of Europe, it is a subsidiary agency to the UN Economic and Social Council. After WWII, many social agencies realized that the world's children needed medical and other kinds of support. With financial assistance from the newly formed UN General Assembly, post-WWII programs were developed to control yaws, leprosy, and TB in children. Since then, UNICEF has worked closely with the WHO as an advocate for the health needs of women and children under the age of 5. In particular, there have been multinational programs aimed at the provision of safe drinking water, sanitation, education, and maternal and child health.

The **Pan American Health Organization (PAHO)** is one of the oldest continuously functioning multilateral agencies, founded in 1902, and predates the WHO. Presently, PAHO serves as a regional field office for the WHO in Latin America, with a focused effort to improve the health and living standards of the Latin American countries. PAHO distributes epidemiological information, provides technical assistance over a wide range of health and environmental issues, supports health care fellowships, and promotes health and environmentally related research, along with professional education. Focusing primarily on reaching people through their communities, PAHO works with a variety of governmental and non-governmental entities to address the health issues of the people of the Americas. At present, a primary concern of PAHO is the prevention and control of AIDS and other sexually transmitted diseases amongst the most vulnerable: mothers and children, workers, the poor, older adults, refugees, and displaced persons. With the earthquakes in Haiti and Chile, and the drought and starvation in Guatemala, PAHO's attentions are being directed toward crisis intervention (http://new.paho.org/hq). Other focused efforts include the provision of public information, the control and eradication of tropical diseases, and the development of health system infrastructures in the poorer Latin American countries. PAHO collaborates with individual countries and actively promotes multinational efforts as well. Recently PAHO has examined the effects of health care reform on nurses and midwifery in the Latin American countries and found that the reform changed the work environments, the scope of practice, and the relationship of nurses with other health care workers and providers. The role of PAHO in the development of healthy communities is discussed in Chapter 20.

The World Bank (http://www.worldbank.org) is another multilateral agency that is related to the UN. Although the major aim of the World Bank is to lend money to the lesser-developed countries so that they might use it to improve the health status of their people, it has collaborated with the field offices of the WHO for various health-related projects such as the control and eradication of the tropical disease onchocerciasis in West Africa, as well as programs aimed at providing safe drinking water and affordable housing, developing sanitation systems, and encouraging family planning and childhood immunizations. The World Bank also sponsors programs to protect the environment, as reflected by the $30 million project in Brazil to protect the Amazon ecosystem and reduce the effects on the ozone layer; to support people in lesser-developed countries to pursue careers in health care; and to improve internal infrastructures, including communication systems, roads, and electricity, all of which ultimately affect health care delivery.

Bilateral agencies operate within a single country and focus on providing direct aid to lesser-developed countries. The U.S. Agency for International Development (USAID) (http://www.usaid.gov) is the largest of these and supports long-term and equitable economic growth and advances U.S. foreign policy objectives by supporting economic growth, agriculture, and trade; global health; and democracy, conflict prevention, and humanitarian assistance. It provides assistance in five regions of the world: Sub-Saharan Africa, Asia, Latin America and the Caribbean, Europe and Eurasia, and the Middle East. All bilateral organizations are influenced by political and historical agendas that determine which countries receive aid. Incentives for engaging in formal arrangements may include economic enhancements for the benefit of both countries, national defense of one or both countries, or the enhancement and protection of private investments made by individuals in these nations. Something similar is present in other developed nations around the globe. For example, the Japanese government currently has an active collaborative arrangement with Indonesia to study ways to control the spread of yellow fever and malaria. France gives most of its aid to its former colonies.

Non-governmental organizations (NGOs) or private voluntary organizations (PVOs), as well as philanthropic organizations, provide almost 20% of all external aid to lesser-developed countries. NGOs and PVOs are represented by many different kinds of religious and secular groups. Representatives of these independent citizen organizations are increasingly active in policy-making at the United Nations. These organizations are often the most effective voices for the concerns of ordinary people in the international arena. NGOs include the most outspoken advocates of human rights, the environment, social programs, women's rights and more (Global Policy Forum, 2010). The author is the Medical Director for the Holy Innocents Children's Hospital Uganda NGO (www.holyinnocentsuganda.org) founded in San Diego, CA in 2007. Its mission was to build the first dedicated children's hospital in Uganda in order to address the unnecessary loss of lives of children from preventable conditions, especially malaria. In its first year of operation, the hospital with its 53 beds and an outpatient department has cared for over 16,000 children and become the regional "NICU" and a pediatric "tertiary" setting.

The International Red Cross (http://www.icrc.org) is one of the best-known NGOs. Although the Red Cross is most often associated with disaster relief and emergency aid, it lays the groundwork for health intervention as a result of a country's emergency. It is a volunteer organization that consists of approximately 160 individual Red Cross societies around the world, and it prides itself on its neutrality and impartiality with respect to politics and history. Therefore, it seeks permission from the country in which the disaster occurs before services are rendered.

Another NGO that provides health services and aid to countries experiencing warfare or disaster is Medicins San Frontieres (MSF) (http://www.msf.org), also home of Doctors without Borders. It is an international, independent, medical humanitarian organization that delivers emergency aid to people affected by armed conflicts, epidemics, health care exclusion, and natural or man-made disasters. Unlike the Red Cross, MSF does not seek government approval to enter a country and provide aid and it often speaks out against observed human rights abuses in the country it serves. MSF was the recipient of the Nobel Peace Prize in 1999 and the Conrad Hilton Prize in 1998.

The professional and trade organizations are PVOs that are found mostly in the more developed and industrialized countries. One of the most famous of the professional and technical organizations is the Institut Pasteur, which began in the 1880s. Its laboratories have facilitated the development of sera and vaccines for countries in need, have disseminated current health information, and have trained and provided fellowships for medical training and study in France.

Religious organizations, reflecting several denominations and religious interests, support many health care programs, including hospitals in rural and urban areas, refugee centers, orphanages, and leprosy treatment centers. For example, the Maryknoll Missionaries, sponsored by the Roman Catholic Church, carry out health service projects around the world. The missionaries comprise a large group of religious as well as lay people trained and educated in a variety of educational and health care professions. The Catholic Relief Services (CRS) (http://crs.org) is the official international humanitarian agency of the Catholic community in the United States. CRS alleviates suffering and provides assistance to people in need who are affected by war, starvation, famine, drought, and natural disasters, in more than 100 countries, without regard to race, religion, or nationality. Many Protestant and evangelical groups throughout the world function both as separate entities and as part of the Church World Service, which works jointly with secular organizations to improve health care, community development, and other needed projects. Other private and voluntary groups that assist with the worldwide health effort include CARE (http://www.care.org), Oxfam (www.oxfam.org.uk), and Third World First. Several of these organizations receive additional funding from developed countries including the United States, the United Kingdom, Sweden, Canada, and countries in Western Europe.

Philanthropic organizations receive funding from private endowment funds. A few of the more active philanthropic organizations that are involved in world health care include the W. K. Kellogg Foundation, the Milbank Memorial Fund, the Pathfinder Fund, the Hewlett Foundation, the Ford Foundation, the Rockefeller Foundation, the Carnegie Foundation, and the Gates Foundation. The purpose and programmatic goals of each organization differ widely with respect to funding, and their purposes often change as their governing boards change. Some of the worldwide health care activities that have been sponsored in the past include projects in public and preventive health; vital statistics; medical, nursing, and dental education; family planning programs; economic planning and development; and the formation of laboratories to investigate communicable diseases.

Many private and commercial organizations such as Nestle and the Johnson & Johnson Company provide financial and technical backing for investment, employment, and access to market economies and to health care. Although these organizations have been present throughout the world for more than 30 years, they have come under criticism for the promotion and marketing of infant formulas, pharmaceuticals, and medical supplies, especially to lesser-developed countries. The intense marketing that is done in these countries is known as *commodification,* turning health care into a business with clients as consumers and health care professionals from altruistic healers to business technicians (Lown, 2007; White, Henderson, and Petersen, 2002). There is global controversy as to the legitimacy of commodification. For example, the health commodification of pharmaceuticals in southern India is a concern because the companies give little consideration to the cultural and social structure of the country, thus interfering with the long-standing traditional Indian medical system. In southern India, good health and prosperity are related to certain social parameters bestowed to families and communities as a result of their conformity to the socio-moral order that was established by their ancestors, gods, and patron spirits (Segal, Demos, and Kronenfeld, 2003). The taking of pharmaceutical agents thus disrupts the social and cultural order of things that have been traditionally addressed by cultural practices. Similar controversies in other countries have involved infant formulas and oral rehydration therapies.

> **DID YOU KNOW?** *Information about volunteering for many NGOs and PVOs can be obtained from the Internet web pages included in the text. Nurses have developed global initiatives, participate in global health projects, and lead global health organizations such as Doctors without Borders. Becoming a global citizen is the responsibility of all.*

EVIDENCE-BASED PRACTICE

This research study examined the relationships among demographic characteristics, acculturation, psychological resilience, and symptoms of depression in midlife women from the former Soviet Union who immigrated to the United States. This cross-sectional study of 200 women revealed that the Russian immigrant women scored higher on the depression scales than those women native to the United States. Older women scored particularly high, but those younger women who learned English and held at least part-time jobs had lower scores.

Nurse Use

This study indicates that interventions that encourage the use of English may help decrease symptoms of depression in midlife immigrant Russian women.

How could you as a nurse encourage immigrant women to learn English and become more acculturated to their new life in the United States in order to decrease the potential for depression and isolationism? One suggestion could be the development of a support group comprised of newly immigrated with established immigrant women who can advise and mentor the new immigrant. What might be others?

Miller A, Chandler PJ: Acculturation, resilience, and depression in midlife women from the former Soviet Union, *Nurs Res* 51:26-32, 2002.

GLOBAL HEALTH AND GLOBAL DEVELOPMENT

Global health is not just a global public health agenda; it does not begin and end with the individual; it must consider all factors within a country that affect health, such as environment, education, national and local policies, health care and access to health care, economics (importing and exporting of goods, industry, technology), war, and public safety. This paradigm shift is called *global health diplomacy,* which refers to multilevel and multifactor negotiation processes involving environment, health, emerging diseases, and human safety. It is now recognized that to solve global health problems, one must build capacity for global health diplomacy by training public health professionals and diplomats respectively to prevent the imbalances that emerge between foreign policy and public health experts and the imbalances that exist in negotiating power and capacity between developed and developing nations (Kickbusch, Silberschmidt, and Buss, 2007). The cutting edge of global health diplomacy raises certain cautions regarding health's role in trade and foreign policies. Unfortunately, securing health's fullest participation in foreign policy does not ensure health for all, but it supports the principle that foreign policy achievements by any country in promoting and protecting health will be of value to all (Drager and Fidler, 2007).

Nurses cannot think in isolation about health for the global population; they must think more broadly to achieve their goals through a multidiscipline and multilevel approach involving such dimensions as economic, industrial, and technological development. An example of this global health diplomacy approach, developed by the author and her colleagues, is the Uganda Project. What began as a simple request to help a community in Uganda save the lives of children dying unnecessarily from preventable diseases has turned into a sustainable community development project. Serving as consultants to an NGO, led by the school of nursing at the University of San Diego, and working collaboratively with the departments of environmental science and business, students and faculty have provided volunteer service and consultation to the people of Mbarara, Uganda on the building, implementation, and sustainability of a children's hospital in their community. Such consultation involved addressing the training of health care professionals on pediatric care and lay health educators to help improve the health of the community; assessing and intervening on water quality issues affecting public health; and assessing and making recommendations for business ventures that could help support the fiscal sustainability of the hospital and improve the economics of the community. Future projects will include faculty and students from the school of peace studies to help the community learn how to deal with conflict and social justice issues and the school of education to help support the teacher training that might better serve the education of the children (Bolender and Hunter, 2010).

Access to services and the removal of financial barriers alone do not account for use of health services. In fact, the introduction of health care technology from developed countries to lesser-developed countries has led to less-than-satisfactory results. For example, during the 1980s in an eastern Mediterranean country, two thirds of the high-output x-ray machines were not in use because of a lack of qualified and trained individuals to carry out routine maintenance and repairs (World Bank, 2005). In another example, a hospital in a Latin American country was given a high-technology neonatal intensive care unit by a wealthier and more technologically advanced country. However, 70% of the infants died after discharge because there were no follow-up nutritional and prevention services, and many of them experienced malnutrition and complications from dehydration on return to their home communities. Countries devastated by war have lost their total infrastructures for food, trade, social justice, health, water, and public security as evident today in Afghanistan, the West Bank, Gaza, Darfur, and other war-torn countries. When implementing services for lesser-developed nations, it is essential to conduct needs assessments to learn what a community has, what a community wants, and what it can sustain. Quite simply, the aforementioned projects, although well-intended, failed because the most basic needs were not met, nor was recognition given to what resources and services the country could sustain.

On the basis of these examples, improvement in the overall health status of a population contributes to the economic growth of a country in several ways (World Bank, 2005; WHO, 2009):

- Reduction in production loss caused by workers who are absent from work because of illness
- Increase in the use of natural resources that, because of the presence of disease entities, might have been inaccessible
- Increase in the number of children who can attend school and eventually participate in their country's economic growth
- Monetary resources, formerly spent on treating disease and illness, now available for the economic development of the country

However, adequate health care coverage for individuals who live in lesser-developed countries is lacking because their governments reallocate financial resources from internal health needs and education to invest in the country's market economy, or to develop technology, or to pay off the interest on their national debt. Many countries also divert resources to develop the underlying infrastructure that they believe is needed for technological and industrial improvement. Unfortunately, when governments experience an economic crisis, household expenditures are adversely affected. Most often, the provision of health services in lesser-developed countries depends on the importation of drugs, vaccines, and other health care products (World Bank, 2005), which in turn depends on a network of foreign exchange that is influenced by economic and political factors. Because the economics of international development are complex, it is often difficult to convince governments to direct their resources away from perceived needs such as military and technology and, instead, place resources in health and educational programs. Ideally, the role of the more-developed countries is to assist lesser-developed countries to identify internal needs and to support cost-efficient measures and share their technology and industrial expertise (Peters and Fisher, 2004). It is important that nurses who work in international communities acknowledge the importance of the concept of global health diplomacy: culture, political, economic, technological, public health, social justice, foreign policy, and public safety. Provision of health services alone will not ease a country's health care plight (Figure 4-7).

HEALTH CARE SYSTEMS

The countries of the world present many different kinds of health care systems, but most consist of five fundamental elements (Basch, 1990): (1) usership, or who can use the system, (2) benefits, or what kind of coverage a citizen might expect, (3) providers who deliver health care, (4) facilities, or where the provision of health care takes place, and (5) power, or who controls access and usability of the system. Understanding some of these principles is highlighted when one compares the health care systems in the Netherlands, Japan, Canada, and Mexico. A recent report by Ray Suarez (2009) for PBS compared the health care system across five international arenas (Table 4-1).

The Netherlands

In the Netherlands, under a health policy reform movement in 2006, residents are required to purchase health insurance, which is provided by private health insurers (for-profit or non-profit) that compete for business. Everyone must be insured and the insurers are required to accept every resident in their coverage area, regardless of preexisting conditions. The government provides larger subsidies to insurers for participants who are sicker, are elderly, or have preexisting conditions. Tax credits are given to low-income clients to help them purchase insurance. People under age 18 are insured at no cost. There is a separate universal national social insurance program for long-term care, known as the AWBZ, or Exceptional Medical Expenses Act. Insurers offer a choice of policies at a range of costs. In some of the plans,

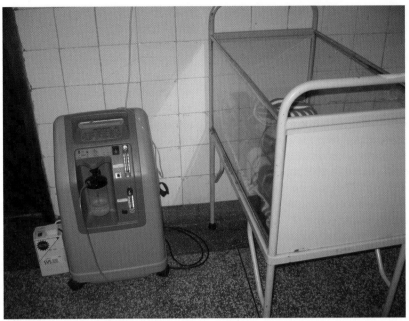

FIGURE 4-7 "NICU unit" in a local Ugandan community hospital: one oxygen concentrator and one suction machine. (Courtesy A. Hunter.)

TABLE 4-1	COMPARING INTERNATIONAL HEALTH CARE SYSTEMS				
	HEALTH SPENDING PER CAPITA	HEALTH COSTS COVERED BY GOVERNMENT	PERCENT GDP SPENT ON HEALTH CARE	INFANT DEATHS PER 1000	AVERAGE LIFE EXPECTANCY
Japan	$2581	81.3%	8.1%	3	83
Netherlands	$3481	80.0%	9.4%	4	80
Canada	$3673	70.4%	10.0%	5	81
United States	$6719	45.8%	15.3%	7	78
Mexico	$778	44.2%	6.6%	29	74

From World Health Organization, 2006. Available at http://www.pbs.org/newshour/globalhealth/july-dec09/insurance_1006.html. Accessed December 5, 2010.
GDP, Gross domestic product.

the insurer negotiates and contracts with the health provider, whereas more costly plans allow clients to choose their health provider and be reimbursed by the insurer. The insured also pay a flat-rate premium to their insurer for a policy. Everyone with the same policy pays the same premium, and lower-income residents receive a healthcare allowance from the government to help make payments.

Japan

In Japan, the first nation in Asia to create a comprehensive social insurance program, all citizens are required to have health insurance, either through an employer-based health insurance program or through the national health care program. Public assistance is available for those who cannot afford the premiums. The insurers are all not-for-profit and do not compete since they all cover the same services and drugs for the same price. The Japanese health ministry fixes health service prices and negotiates rates every 2 years with the health care industry. Clients have access to all health institutions and freely choose their provider. Covered services under Japan's system include

inpatient and outpatient care, home care, dental, prescriptions, long-term care, home nursing for the elderly and prosthetics, and a cash benefit for childbirth. Costs that are not covered include routine physical examinations, some dental services, and over-the-counter drugs.

Canada

Canada has a universal health care system that is publicly funded and administered and delivers care primarily through private providers. Private insurance exists but is prohibited by the government to cover the same benefits as the public plan called Medicare; however, private insurance can be purchased to cover any gaps in the coverage. Clients pay no co-pays or deductibles. Despite broad coverage, the Medicare system has been criticized for long waiting times on specialty coverage. Care is given either at public or private hospitals and facilities, and clients can choose their doctor. Each of the provincial and territorial governments is responsible for administering the single-payer system for universal hospital and medical services in the region. All medically necessary hospital and physician services are covered under the Medicare plan whereas dental care, outpatient prescription drugs, and rehabilitation services are not. Federal and provincial income taxes, as well as payroll taxes and sales tax, fund the program in Canada.

Mexico

Mexico has a fractionalized system with a variety of public programs. There is no universal coverage, but a social security–administered system does cover those who are employed. The private insurance market is mostly used by wealthy residents. The Seguro Popular program, created in 2003, has been set up to help cover more of the uninsured population. Poor families can participate in Seguro Popular for free, and people who do not participate in the insurance program can still access services through the ministry of health, although sometimes with some difficulty. The different public set-ups and private insurers all use different systems of medical facilities and providers, with a wide range of quality reported in those services. The social security system provides broad coverage for medical services, including primary care, acute care, ambulatory and hospital care, pregnancy and childbirth, as well as prescription medications. The Seguro Popular system provides access to an established set of essential medical services and the needed drugs for those conditions, as well as 17 high-cost interventions such as breast cancer treatment. The services are provided through government, usually state-run, facilities. Out-of-pocket payments by clients represent over half of financing for the Mexican health care system, whereas the public schemes are financed through general taxes and payment from the employer and employee, determined by salary. The Seguro Popular is also funded by taxes, contributions from the state and federal government, and payments by the families, as a percentage of income. Participants in Seguro Popular pay nothing at the time of delivery of the service.

There are positives and negatives to consider about alternative health care systems as experts strive to "fix the broken health care system" in the United States. One begins to realize how broken the system is when the United States is shown to have the highest health spending per capita of all nations, the highest percentage of GDP spent on health care, one of the lowest percentages of health care costs covered by the government, yet clearly not some of the best health indicators as reflected by the higher infant death rates compared with Japan, the Netherlands, and Canada.

The United Kingdom

It is also useful to examine the United Kingdom, with a tax-supported health system that is owned and operated by the government. Services are available to all citizens without cost or for a small fee. Administration of health services is conducted through a system of health authorities (Trusts). Each Trust plans and provides services for 250,000 to 1 million people. The services offered by each Trust are comprehensive, in that health care is available to all who want it and covers all aspects of general medicine, disability and rehabilitation, and surgery. Although physicians are the primary providers in this system, nurses and allied health professionals are also recognized and

used. Services are made available through hospitals, private physicians and allied health professional clinics, health outreach programs such as hospice, boroughs, and environmental health services. Physicians are paid by the number of clients they serve and not by individual visits.

Although the British system has come under criticism in past years, individual citizens still maintain a high level of support for government funding and control of their health services (Schoen, Davie, and DesRoches, 2000; Hutton, 2003). Clients, especially the elderly and new mothers, receive assistance from the district nurses (public health nurses). One of the hallmarks of the British system is a reduction in infant mortality, from 14.3 deaths per 1000 births in 1975 to 5.4 in 2002. Overall life expectancy in Great Britain also improved during the same period (77.2 years in 2000). This has been done while holding down gross spending on health care. A 2009 report by Sutherland found that the UK has seen a significant fall in mortality rates from the major killers: cancer, coronary heart disease, and stroke. It has the longest life expectancy of men and women, and client ratings of quality care are high all across the UK. Of concern is the rising health expenditure over the past 10 years (Sutherland, 2009).

THE CUTTING EDGE *In Southern Australia, a group of nutritionists developed and implemented a specialized nutrition program for the Umoona aboriginal community in Coober Pedy. This project focused on the fact that a great portion of ill health was attributed to diet-related illnesses. Working with aboriginal health workers, the nutritionists fashioned an intervention program that could be delivered by the health workers that was culturally appropriate, easily understood, and relevant to the aboriginal population.*

Zeunert S, Cerro N, Boesch L, et al: Nutrition project in a remote Australian Aboriginal community, Nutrition 12:102-106, 2002.

China

China has made tremendous strides since 1949 in providing access to health care for its citizens. At present, China is a large developing country with many human resources (Yun, Jie, and Anli, 2010). Nursing comprises a large segment of the health care workforce, yet there are too few nurses to meet the needs of the population. China, like the United States, is engaged in health care reform. China also has more physicians than nurses which is different than in most other areas of the world. Nurse density in China is higher in urban than in rural areas, and this poses a problem in a large country in which much of the territory is rural in nature. Like many other countries, China has made public health advances by controlling contagious diseases such as cholera, typhoid, and scarlet fever, and a reduction in infant mortality (Kennedy, 1999). These accomplishments in public health were credited to a political system that was and is largely socialistic and features a health care system that is described in socialistic terms as collective. The Chinese collective system emphasized the common good for all people, not individuals or special groups. This system was financed through cooperative insurance plans. The collective health care system was owned and controlled by the state and used barefoot doctors. The barefoot doctors were medical practitioners trained at the community level and who could provide a minimal level of health care throughout the country. Barefoot doctors combined Western medicine with traditional techniques such as acupuncture and herbal remedies. The government stressed an improvement in the quality of water supplies and disease prevention and implemented massive public health campaigns against sanitation problems, such as flies, mosquitoes, and the snails that spread schistosomiasis. Box 4-2 describes a Healthy Cities initiative that took place in Chengdu, China.

Today, health care in China is managed by the Ministry of Public Health, which sets national health policy. The current Chinese government continues to make health care a priority and has set goals to provide medical care to all of its citizens. The Chinese Government published the Healthcare Reform Plan in 2009. In developing this plan the government took into account recommendations from the WHO and the World Bank. Among the aims of the plan are to develop a system of health insurance to help people pay for catastrophic illness, to increase and improve the education for nurses in order to intervene in the growing nursing shortage, and to develop urban health centers. At present, a small percentage of Chinese nurses work in public health, and some authors attribute this to the low pay in these settings. Hospitals and clinics are typically located in urban areas, which means that the large rural population must travel a great distance for care, and even then, the care may be substandard and the wait time to receive care may be long. It is estimated that approximately 200 million people in China lack health insurance (Mikelonis and Fan, 2009). When the State Council published its health reform plan in April of 2009, a 3-year goal of "covering 90% of the Chinese population by 2011 and achieving universal health care by 2020" was established. The goal is to provide basic health care as a public service. This will require a significant investment of government funds to achieve the goal. The reform consists of 4 key pillars:

- Public health service
- Medical treatment
- Medical insurance
- Medical supply (Mikelonis and Fan, 2009, p 2)

In 2008, Premier Wen Jiabao signed the "Nursing Act" which aims to intervene in some of the problems facing nursing in China (Yun, Jie, and Anli, 2010). One of the goals of this act is to expand the scope of community nursing, and this goal is consistent with the first of the four pillars of the reform plan.

The nursing education system in China has developed rapidly. All college based nursing education was terminated during the period of the Cultural Revolution and only began again in the mid 1980s. At present the nursing education system includes associate degree, baccalaureate, master's degree and doctoral programs (Yun, Jie, and Anli, 2010).

Interestingly, the image of nursing has improved based on the effectiveness of nurses during recent public health crises and events that claimed international attention. Specifically, nurses played important and effective roles in caring for people during the disasters caused by the Severe Acute Respiratory Syndrome (SARS in 2003) and the Sichuan earthquake in 2008. More recently, nurses were well recognized in China for their considerable work during the 2008 Olympic Games in Beijing (Yun, Kie, and Anli, 2010).

MAJOR GLOBAL HEALTH PROBLEMS AND THE BURDEN OF DISEASE

Despite the gains that have been made in improving the health of so many around the globe, the increasing population, decreasing food and water sources, and increasing poverty related to a global economic crisis all contribute to a critical demise in health. The amount of debt incurred by lesser-developed countries has increased steadily over the last 20 years, and money that was once used for health care has been used to pay off growing debt. Communicable diseases that are often preventable are still common throughout the world and are more common in lesser-developed countries. Also, both developed and lesser-developed countries are seeking ways to cope with the aging of their populations—a population that presents governments with the burden of providing care for those who become ill with more expensive non-communicable and chronic forms of diseases and disabilities. Illnesses such as AIDS continue to raise concerns, especially in child-bearing women, adolescents, and young adults. Long-standing diseases such as TB, dysentery, and mosquito-borne diseases, especially malaria, still persist and have become drug resistant, adding to a growing burden of overextended health care delivery systems.

Mortality statistics do not adequately describe the outlook of health in the world. The WHO (2002) and the World Bank (2005) have developed an indicator called the global burden of disease (GBD). The GBD combines losses from premature death and losses of healthy life that result from disability. Premature death is defined as the difference between the actual age at death and life expectancy at that age in a low-mortality population. People who have debilitating injuries or diseases must be cared for in some way, most often by family members, and thus they no longer can contribute to the family's or a community's economic growth. The GBD represents units of disability-adjusted life-years (DALYs) (World Bank, 2005) (Box 4-4).

Since the 1990s the WHO has been assessing the trends for disabilities related to psychiatric disorders (WHO, 2002). Psychiatric and neurological conditions account for 28% of all years lived with disability, but only 1.4% of all deaths and 1.1% of years of life lost. Thus, psychiatric disorders, although traditionally not regarded as a major epidemiological problem, are shown by consideration of disability years to have a huge impact on population. In 2000, 1.28 billion DALYs were lost worldwide, which equates to 39 million deaths of newborn children or to 80 million deaths of people who reach age 50. Approximately 13.7 million children under age 5 died during the same year in lesser-developed countries. If these children could face the same risks as those in developed nations, the deaths would decrease by 90% to 1.1 million. This example demonstrates the importance of having accessible and affordable disease prevention programs for children around the world (World Bank, 2005). Overall, premature deaths throughout the world during 2002 accounted for more than two thirds of all

BOX 4-4 CALCULATING DISABILITY-ADJUSTED LIFE-YEARS

There are five components of disability-adjusted life-years (DALYs):

1. *Duration of time lost because of a death at each age:* Measurement is based on the potential limit for life, which has been set at 82.5 years for women and 80 years for men.
2. *Disability weights:* The degree of incapacity associated with various health conditions. Values range from 0 (perfect health) to 1 (death). Four prescribed points between 0 and 1 represent a set of accepted disability classes.
3. *Age-weighting function,* $C \times e^{-\beta x}$, where $C = 0.16243$ (a constant), $\beta = 0.04$ (a constant), $e = 2.71$ (a constant), and $x = $ age; this function indicates the relative importance of a healthy life at different ages.
4. *Discounting function,* $e^{-r(x-a)}$, where $r = 0.03$ (the discount rate), $e = 2.71$ (a constant), $a = $ age at onset of disease, and $x = $ age; this function indicates the value of health gains today compared with the value of health gains in the future.
5. *Health is added across individuals:* 2 people each losing 10 DALYs are treated as showing the same loss as 1 person losing 20 years.

"In summary, the disability-adjusted life-year (DALY) is an indicator of the time lived with a disability and the time lost due to premature mortality. The duration of time lost due to premature mortality is calculated using standard expected years of life lost with model life-tables. The reduction in physical capacity due to morbidity is measured using disability weights. The value of time lived at different ages has been calculated using an exponential function which reflects the dependence of the young and older adults on the adults. Streams of time have been discounted at 3%. Accordingly the number of DALYs lost due to disability at age 'x' can be calculated using the following formula" (Murray and Lopez, 1996, p 15):

$$DALY(x) = (D)(Cxe^{-\beta x})(e^{-r(x-a)})$$

where $D = $ disability weight (ranging from 1 [death] to 0 [perfect health]).

DALYs lost (WHO, 2002) with debilitating injuries and diseases accounting for one third.

Communicable diseases still account for the greatest proportion of calculated DALYs worldwide for both males and females, followed by non-communicable diseases and injuries. Infections and parasitic diseases remain a threat to the health of the majority of the world and are diseases seen in the United States in newly arriving immigrants. Studies demonstrate the continuing need for intervention for infectious and other kinds of communicable diseases. Conditions that contribute to one fourth of the GBD throughout the world include diarrheal disease, respiratory tract infections, worm infestations, malaria, and childhood diseases such as measles and polio. Sub-Saharan Africa demonstrated a GBD of 43% DALYs lost, largely because of preventable diseases among children (WHO/UNAIDS, 2002). Other countries and areas with comparable DALYs are India (29%) and the Middle Eastern crescent (29%). In adults, sexually transmitted disease (STDs) and TB combine to account for 70% of the world's GBD (World Bank, 2002).

According to the U.S. Global Health Policy fact sheet published by the Kaiser Family Foundation (Kaiser Family Foundation, 2010), globally there were 33 million people living with HIV in 2007, up from 29.5 million in 2001, the result of continuing new infections, people living longer with HIV, and general population growth. HIV is a leading cause of death worldwide and the number one cause of death in Africa. An estimated 8 in 10 people infected with HIV do not know it. HIV has led to a resurgence of TB, particularly in Africa, and TB is a leading cause of death for people with HIV worldwide. Women represent half of all people living with HIV worldwide, and more than half (60%) in sub-Saharan Africa. Globally, there were 2.5 million children living with HIV in 2009, 370,000 new infections among children, and 260,000 AIDS deaths. There are approximately 16.6 million AIDS orphans today (children who have lost one or both parents to HIV), most of whom live in sub-Saharan Africa (89%). Uganda's emphasis on ameliorating HIV/AIDS is a model for all African nations; however, there are still too many Ugandan children under 5 years old who are AIDS orphans. Unfortunately, despite the efforts of advocates, donors, and affected countries, there needs to be greater attention on the long overdue effort to expand access to antiretroviral therapy, which is still available to less than 10% of those who urgently require it.

Determining the total amount of loss, even using the GBD, is difficult because it does not address the many consequences of disease and injury such as post-trauma and infectious physical disabilities. Nor can it measure the short- or long-term effects of familial and marital dysfunction, family violence, or war. The following further elaborates on selected communicable diseases that still contribute substantially to the worldwide disease burden (TB, AIDS, and malaria) and other health problems such as maternal and women's health, diarrheal disease in children, nutrition, natural and man-made disasters.

Communicable Diseases

Prevention of communicable diseases is through immunization and improving environmental conditions. One example of the long-term benefits of immunizing children against communicable diseases is the successful campaign against smallpox that the WHO conducted during the 1960s and 1970s. Smallpox has been virtually eliminated throughout the world, with only occasional and incidental reporting from laboratory accidents and inoculation complications. The systematic and planned smallpox program formed the basis for a series of worldwide efforts that are now being implemented to control and eradicate other infectious and communicable diseases.

In 1974 the WHO formed the Expanded Programme on Immunization, which sought to reduce morbidity and mortality from diphtheria, pertussis, tetanus, TB, measles, and poliomyelitis throughout the world (WHO, 2002a). In the 2009 State of the World Report on immunizations and vaccines by the WHO, UNICEF, and the World Bank, it was noted that in developing countries, more vaccines are available and more lives are being saved; however, almost 20% of children born each year do not receive their complete immunization schedule for their first year of life. Although free vaccination clinics are brought to the people, they are often not used because of lack of knowledge, fear propagated by the traditional healers, and suspicion of anything offered by the government. Reaching these vulnerable children—typically in poorly served remote rural areas, deprived urban settings, fragile states, and strife-torn regions—is essential in order to meet the Millennium Development Goals (MDGs, United Nation, 2009).

For the first time in documented history, the number of children dying every year has fallen below 10 million—the result of improved access to clean water and sanitation, increased immunization coverage, and the integrated delivery of essential health interventions. WHO has estimated that if all the vaccines now available against childhood diseases were widely adopted, and if countries could raise vaccine coverage to a global average of 90%, by 2015 an additional 2 million deaths a year could be prevented among children under age 5. This level of vaccination would reduce child deaths by two thirds and achieve one of the MDG goals. It would also greatly reduce the burden of illness and disability from vaccine-preventable diseases and contribute to improving child health and welfare, as well as reducing hospitalization costs (WHO, 2009).

As discussed in Chapter 10, environmental sanitation is as important as the immunization of children. Around the world, many of the major health risks relate to interactions between people and their environment. For example, community drinking water sources can be contaminated by agricultural run-offs containing toxic pesticides and fertilizers, but they can also be contaminated by naturally occurring elements in the earth such as arsenic and fluoride. It is not uncommon for hospitals and HIV testing centers to dump waste products into the local rivers that often supply the local household water. Worldwide, environmental factors play a role in more than 80% of adverse outcomes reported by the WHO, including infectious diseases, injuries, mental retardation, and cancer, to name a few. Globalization and industrialization in the developing world have increased daily exposure to pollution and a wide array of chemicals in air, water, and food. At the same time, fecal pollution of drinking water sources caused by a lack of basic sanitation still exist. The effects of environmental risk factors are magnified by conditions often prevalent in poorer, undeveloped countries such as poor nutrition, poverty, lack of education about risks, and conflicts. Children are particularly susceptible to environmental risks because their systems are still developing. It is estimated that about one quarter of global disease is caused by avoidable environmental exposures; for young children in the developing world, causes of environmentally related deaths are acute respiratory infections, related to poor air quality, and diarrhea, related to poor drinking water quality. Each year, about 3 million children under the age of 5 die of environment-related diseases. There are projects that train and give technical assistance, data collection and analysis, laboratory analyses, research, surveillance, and emergency responses to international communities (Harvey, 2008).

As of 2008, 40% of the world's population still lacked access to improved sanitation. Estimates by the Joint Monitoring Program of UNICEF and the WHO predict that at the current rate of progress, approximately 2 billion people will still lack access to a clean environment by 2015. In sub-Saharan Africa 50% of people lack this basic human right, and their need may not be met until 2072 if the current rate continues (McMichael et al, 2008). Meanwhile, diarrhea remains the second highest single cause of child mortality worldwide. Access to sanitation is vital to ensuring health, dignity, and sustainable social and economic development for the world's poorest citizens (Harvey, 2008).

> **DID YOU KNOW?** *Twenty-nine billion people lack access to adequate sanitation and safe water. In sub-Saharan Africa, Nicaragua, Paraguay, Brazil, and Peru, less than 50% of the population has access to sanitation either in or near their homes. Why is this an important health fact for nurses to know and what could nursing do to help intervene?*

Tuberculosis

In 2004, about 2 million people died as a result of tuberculosis, and 8 to 9 million fell ill (Ruxin et al, 2005). Someone in the world is newly infected with TB bacilli every second. It is a leading killer of people with HIV, and up to 80% of TB clients are HIV positive in countries with a high prevalence of HIV. Between 5% and 10% of people who are infected with TB bacilli (but who are not infected with HIV) become sick or infectious at some time during their life. People with HIV are much more likely to develop TB; as are those infected with malaria, especially children because of the physiological damage to the liver, spleen, and hematological systems. A child or adult with any one of the three diseases mentioned is more prone to the other two, and this triad is the new scourge of impoverished nations. The WHO estimates that more than one third of the infectious disease deaths are due to this deadly triad of AIDS, TB, and malaria (Ginsberg, Sizemore, and Fauci, 2001).

The spread of multidrug-resistant TB highlights the global threat of poor TB control and of the failure to treat all clients properly. TB represents the largest cause of death from a single infectious agent, affecting nearly 3 million people each year. This statistic represents 25% of preventable premature adult deaths in lesser-developed countries (WHO, 2004a; United Nations, 2009). The growth of the world's population, including an increase in the number of older adults and the adverse effects of HIV, contributes to the large projected estimates for TB (WHO, 2004a). One third of the world's population, or 1.7 billion people, harbor the TB pathogen *Mycobacterium tuberculosis.* Clinical manifestations of the disease include pulmonary TB, which is the most widespread form; TB meningitis, which is a leading cause of childhood mortality; and extra-pulmonary TB of a variety of other organs. The WHO (2004a) reports that 1.7 million deaths resulted from TB in 2004, and Africa had the greatest number of deaths where the presence of HIV contributed to the rapid growth of TB. Chemotherapy reduces the number of individuals who die from TB; however, many lesser-developed countries do not have organized treatment and prevention programs and therefore lose more people each year to TB than to either malaria or measles (WHO, 2004a). The Stop TB Partnership, engaging nearly 300 governments and agencies, has brought consensus on approaches to global control of this disease, galvanized support, and launched new support mechanisms, such as the Global TB Drug Facility, an initiative to increase access to high-quality TB drugs. The Working Group on Tuberculosis recommends seven priorities to meet the MDG targets for this disease for 2015 (Ruxin et al, 2005).

Although TB is known worldwide, concern is greatest in certain areas: Southeast Asia (3 million new cases), sub-Saharan Africa (1.6 million cases), and Eastern Europe, where there is a reoccurrence of TB and a quarter of a million cases (WHO, 2004a). This compares with a record low number of cases, 14,111, in the United States in 2004 (CDC, 2005). However, foreign-born residents accounted for nearly 54% of the U.S. cases (CDC, 2005). Globally, approximately 3 million deaths were attributable to TB in 2000, which exceeds the number of deaths from measles and malaria—even more if one includes the almost 20% of HIV-infected individuals who die with active TB (Ginzberg et al, 2001). Most of these deaths occur in sub-Saharan Africa (Bleed et al, 2000).

Two factors are a threat to TB control and eradication. The first is the HIV virus. The appearance of HIV has added to the difficulty of treatment programs in both developed and lesser-developed countries. More important, HIV-positive individuals with infectious TB have an increased likelihood of transmitting TB to their families and to the community, further increasing the prevalence of this condition.

The second is the growing multidrug resistance of the TB bacillus to isoniazid and rifampin, the two drugs used to treat it. Resistance to these drugs is already evident around the world, including in the Mexico–Texas border communities. The WHO and other organizations maintain that a high priority should be given to TB control and eradication programs around the world. They advocate a short-term chemotherapy regimen for smear-positive clients as being one of the most cost-effective health interventions available (Ruxin et al, 2005).

The Bacille Calmette-Guérin (BCG) vaccine, which has been available since the 1920s, was promoted as an effective vaccine to induce active immunity against TB, especially children living in TB-endemic or high-risk TB areas that are impoverished and crowded. Although the effectiveness of BCG is still questionable, research studies have demonstrated that it is effective in preventing the more lethal forms of TB, including meningitis and miliary disease in children (WHO, 2005c). These same studies have demonstrated that more than 80% of the infants in lesser-developed countries have been vaccinated, with less coverage in sub-Saharan Africa. However, more studies are needed worldwide to determine the effect that BCG can have on the more infectious types of TB. Present indications are that BCG does not reduce the transmission of infectious types of TB.

The standard chemotherapeutic agents used in many countries for TB are isoniazid, thioacetazone, and streptomycin, and they are effective at converting sputum-positive cases to noninfectivity. The drug and the combinations that are used vary from country to country. To be effective, however, treatment must be carried out on a consistent basis, and many lesser-developed countries have difficulty getting clients to purchase the medications and to adhere to any treatment regimen. In 1990 the WHO Global Tuberculosis Program (GTB) promoted the revision of national TB programs to focus on short-course chemotherapy (SCC), with directly observed treatment (DOT). DOT programs

have been successful in the United States and in several lesser-developed countries, including Malawi, Mozambique, Nicaragua, and Tanzania, producing a cure rate of approximately 80%. The SCC program involves aggressive administration of chemotherapeutic drugs combined with short-term hospitalization. The key to the program lies in a well-managed system with a regular supply of anti-TB drugs to the treatment centers, follow-up care, and rigorous reporting and analysis of client information (WHO, 2004a). Despite these efforts, little progress has been made, and little international support has been given to placing TB control programs as a priority worldwide.

Lasting control of AIDS, TB, and/or malaria will depend on strengthening the health, economic, political, education, and other infrastructures necessary to sustain life and promote the well-being of the people. It will require sustained investment in physical infrastructure, drug distribution systems, management at all levels, and, most importantly, human resources such as the training and appropriate use of community health workers to deliver some essential services and education. Unfortunately, the failure of developed countries to fulfill their pledges of more development aid, and the failure of developing countries themselves to invest in health, are overarching barriers to health systems development. HIV/AIDS, TB, and malaria are only three of the challenges facing poor people. Only stronger, integrated health systems can provide a platform to sustain a successful fight against these diseases while advancing the other health priorities of developing countries, including child and maternal health and chronic disease.

NURSING TIP   *When conducting a health assessment interview, always ask if the client has recently traveled out of the United States or to one of the border areas along the United States–Mexico perimeter. People who travel abroad may bring back diseases that are hard to diagnose. In addition, people often cross the border into Mexico to fill a prescription for medicine because it is often less expensive than in the United States. Unfortunately, many times the medications brought back have been relabeled and are out of date.*

Acquired Immunodeficiency Syndrome

As discussed in Chapter 14, AIDS remains a major cause of morbidity and mortality throughout the world (WHO/UNAIDS, 2002). About 33.2 million people are infected with HIV in the world; of these, approximately 22.5 million are in sub-Saharan Africa where the adult infection prevalence is about 6%. Approximately 14,000 new HIV infections occur daily and over 90% of these are in developing countries. Of this 14,000, 7% are in children under 15 years of age, 15% are in individuals of 15 to 25 years of age, and 40% are in women. Perinatal infection has resulted in a large number of children being born with HIV. Between 30% and 50% of mother-to-child transmissions of HIV result from breastfeeding, and about a quarter of babies born to HIV-infected mothers are themselves infected (Kaiser Family Foundation, 2009).

Of greatest importance is the increasing incidence of this disease in adolescents, young adults, and heterosexuals. The reasons vary from young people believing that the disease can be cured with drugs and thus they can be less cautious (Varga, 2003), to cultural practices whereby older men marry virgins to cure them of AIDS or to prevent them from getting AIDS.

Worldwide prevention programs are important because failing to control this virulent disease will result in damaging and costly consequences for all countries in the future. Ideally, the goal is primary prevention of HIV. When prevention efforts fail at this level, the next goal is secondary prevention, or early diagnosis and treatment. In 2001, the director general of WHO appealed to the world's health professionals to establish targets for action to control and eradicate the spread of HIV/AIDS (WHO, 2002a). Specifically, WHO along with UNICEF, UNAIDS, women's health groups, and other international organizations promoted the use of nevirapine to prevent mother-to-child transmission of HIV. The regimen calls for a single dose of nevirapine to be given to the mother at delivery and a single dose to the newborn within 72 hours. WHO is recommending that nevirapine be included in the minimum standard package of care for HIV-positive women and their children (WHO/UNAIDS, 2002; Subways, 2004). Tertiary prevention with HIV includes both care of the client and instructing, guiding, and teaching the family how to care for the person with HIV.

📋 LEVELS OF PREVENTION

Global Health Care

Primary Prevention
Teach people how to avoid or change risky behaviors that might lead to contracting human immunodeficiency virus (HIV).

Secondary Prevention
Initiate screening programs for HIV.

Tertiary Prevention
Manage symptoms of HIV, provide psychosocial support, and teach clients and significant others about care and other forms of symptom management.

Malaria

Malaria causes over 1 million deaths—most in children younger than 5 years—and 300 to 500 million episodes of acute illness each year. This disease affects more than 50% of the world's population and hits tropical Africa the hardest. This region bears more than 90% of the global malaria burden. Malaria is caused by the *Anopheles* mosquito and is the only mosquito-borne disease that can be prevented and cured by pharmacological management (Hunter et al, 2007). It is caused by parasitic transmission from the infected female mosquito to its host. There are four types of malaria with the most serious form being the *Plasmodium falciparum,* which causes microvascular sequestration and obstruction in the brain, kidney, and liver leading to cerebral malaria, anemia, kidney failure, hypoglycemia, disseminated intravascular coagulation (DIC), fluid-electrolyte imbalance, and death (Hunter et al, 2007). Symptoms vary and range from mild to severe physiological responses (mild fever and chills to temperatures of 106° F with prolonged chills, seizures, and dehydration).

Malaria control is increasingly recognized as playing a key role in poverty reduction in countries in which it is endemic (Ruxin et al, 2005). Malaria continues to be one of the most important tropical parasitic diseases, and it kills more people than any other communicable disease except TB.

A range of effective antimalarial interventions exist for the prevention, treatment, and control of malaria. These include the use of insecticide-treated bednets (ITNs); indoor residual spraying; intermittent presumptive treatment during pregnancy; early diagnosis and prompt treatment with effective antimalarials; management of the environment to control mosquitoes; health education; and epidemic forecasting, prevention, and response (Ruxin et al, 2005). Methods of vector control vary widely, from using the larvae-eating fish tilapia to the use of insecticidal sprays and oils. Needless to say, the latter poses a potential threat to the environment in tropical areas where a delicate ecosystem is already threatened by other potential hazards such as lumbering and mining.

Countries that do not have strict environmental laws continue to use dichlorodiphenyltrichloroethane (DDT) sprays to control mosquito populations despite the advent of DDT-resistant mosquitoes. The non-DDT insecticide sprays, such as malathion, generally cost more, presenting an extra financial burden to lesser-developed countries. Methods for control and eradication that are being considered by malaria-ridden countries are environmental management, reduction and control of the source, and elimination of the adult mosquito. There are significant global efforts being made to "blanket" endemic communities with insecticide-treated mosquito nets. A multitude of NGO projects are distributing ITNs to contribute to this initiative: Project Mosquito Nets in Kenya (www.projectmosquitonet.org); Nothing But Nets (www.nothingbutnets.net/); Global Giving for Africa (www.globalgiving.org/projects/mosquito-nets-for-africa-families); Angola Mosquito Net Project (http://angolamosquitonetproject.com); and Holy Innocents Children's Hospital Uganda (www.holyinnocentsuganda.org) are examples of organizations actively engaged in preventing malaria and saving lives. It has been demonstrated that the incidence of malaria would be reduced 50% to 60% if children could be protected against the bites of infected mosquitoes by sleeping under a treated net (Lengeler, 2004).

However, coverage levels are inadequate in endemic countries, especially in poor communities. The successful experiences in Ethiopia, Vietnam, Madagascar, South Africa, and Tanzania indicate that sustained reductions in malaria morbidity and mortality can be achieved when programs are implemented through well-coordinated efforts that span regional and national levels. The 2010 report from the Roll Back Malaria (RBM) Partnership (WHO, March 18, 2010) (www.rollbackmalaria.org) confirms that current investment in malaria control is saving lives and providing far-reaching benefits for countries. However, it warns that without sustained and predictable funding, the significant contribution of malaria control toward the achievement of the MDGs could be reversed.

Although chemotherapeutic agents can be used for both protection and treatment of the disease, they are expensive and often cause side effects. However, evidence suggests that the *Plasmodium* sporozoites are becoming resistant to both treatment and preventive chemotherapeutic agents, especially chloroquine and its derivatives. Alternative therapies and/or combinations of medications such as fanisdar, amodiaquine, artemisinin, artemether, and atovaquone-proguanil are somewhat effective in treating malaria. Recent reports indicate that drug manufacturers in these endemic countries are diluting the drugs so clients, especially children, are not receiving therapeutic levels of the medications. Many children suffer the effects of partially treated malaria, and once hospitalized, IV quinine is the drug of choice. Unfortunately, quinine has significant neurotoxic and cardiovascular side effects that need monitoring (Hunter et al, 2007). Efforts are underway to develop an antimalarial vaccine, but so far the results have been unsuccessful. There is one candidate vaccine, known as RTS, S/AS01, which started Pivotal Phase III evaluation in May 2009 and is designed not for travelers but for children living in malaria-endemic areas. As discussed in Chapter 13, persons who live or travel to *Anopheles*-infested areas should protect themselves with mosquito netting, clothing that protects vulnerable parts of the body, repellents for both their bodies and their clothes, and antimalarial medications such as malarone or doxycycline.

Diarrheal Disease

The normal intestinal tract regulates the absorption and secretion of electrolytes and water to meet the body's physiological needs. More than 98% of the 10 L per day of fluid entering the adult intestines are reabsorbed (Keusch et al, 2010). The remaining stool water, related primarily to the indigestible fiber content, determines the consistency of normal feces from dry, hard pellets to mushy, bulky stools, varying from person to person, day to day, and stool to stool. This variation complicates the definition of *diarrhea*. For adults diarrhea is present when three or more liquid stools are passed in 24 hours. The frequent passage of formed stool is not diarrhea. Although young nursing infants tend to have five or more bowel movements per day, stools that are liquid without any formation and/or are more than what is normal for the child constitute diarrhea (Keusch et al, 2006). Definitions are complicated by the observable presence of blood, mucus, or parasites and the age of the affected person (WHO, 2005b).

Diarrhea, one of the leading causes of illness and death in children less than 5 years of age throughout the world, is most prominent in the lesser-developed countries despite recent initiatives by the WHO to correct this problem. Each year there are 1.6 million diarrheal deaths related to unsafe water, sanitation, and hygiene (WHO, 2005b). The prevalence of diarrheal disease was so pervasive during the 1970s and 1980s that the World Health Assembly established a global program to reduce mortality and morbidity in infants and young children who suffered from all forms of the disease. This program continues today.

Causes of diarrhea are just as varied and diverse as its definitions and perceptions. Some of the causes include: (1) viruses such as the rotavirus and Norwalk-like agents, (2) bacteria, including *Campylobacter jejuni, Clostridium difficile, Escherichia coli, Salmonella,* and *Shigella,* (3) environmental toxins, (4) parasites such as *Giardia lamblia* and *Cryptosporidium,* and (5) worms. Nutritional deficiencies can also cause diarrhea and are most often a result of

infectious agents. Of these, the rotavirus has emerged as a major world concern, hospitalizing 55,000 American children and killing 1 million children in the world each year (WHO, 2005b). Three major diarrhea syndromes exist:

- Acute watery diarrhea, which results in varying degrees of dehydration and fluid losses that quickly exceed total plasma and interstitial fluid volumes and is incompatible with life unless fluid therapy can keep up with losses. Such dramatic dehydration is usually due to rotavirus, enterotoxigenic *E. coli,* or *Vibrio cholerae* (the cause of cholera), and it is most dangerous in the very young.
- Persistent diarrhea, which lasts 14 days or longer, manifested by malabsorption, nutrient losses, and wasting; typically associated with malnutrition, either preceding or resulting from the illness itself. Even though persistent diarrhea accounts for a small percentage of the total number of diarrhea episodes, it is associated with a disproportionately increased risk of death.
- Bloody diarrhea, which is a sign of the intestinal damage caused by inflammation. Bloody diarrhea, defined as diarrhea with visible or microscopic blood in the stool, is associated with intestinal damage and nutritional deterioration, often with secondary sepsis. Mild dehydration and fever may be present. Bloody diarrhea should not be confused with dysentery, since dysentery is a syndrome consisting of the frequent passage of characteristic, small-volume, bloody mucoid stools, abdominal cramps, and tenesmus (a severe pain that accompanies straining to pass stool). Agents that cause bloody diarrhea or dysentery can also provoke a form of diarrhea that clinically is not bloody diarrhea, although mucosal damage and inflammation are present microscopically. The release of host-derived cytokines alters host metabolism and leads to the breakdown of body stores of protein, carbohydrate, and fat and the loss of nitrogen and other nutrients. Those losses must be replenished during the expected prolonged convalescence. For these reasons, bloody diarrhea calls for management strategies that are markedly different than those for watery or persistent diarrhea. New bouts of infection that occur before complete restoration of nutrient stores can initiate a downward spiral of nutritional status terminating in fatal protein-energy malnutrition (Keusch et al, 2006).

Diarrheal diseases are rampant among the impoverished. Poverty is associated with poor housing, crowding, dirt floors, lack of access to sufficient clean water or to sanitary disposal of fecal waste, cohabitation with domestic animals and zoonotic transmission of pathogens, and a lack of refrigerated storage for food. Unfortunately, even when the cause of the diarrhea is cured, poverty can restrict the ability to provide age-appropriate, nutritionally balanced diets or to modify diets so as to mitigate and repair nutrient losses. The lack of adequate, available, and affordable medical care increases the problem. Children suffer from an apparently never-ending sequence of infections, rarely receive appropriate preventive care, and too often only seek health care when they are already severely ill.

Dehydration is an immediate result of diarrhea and leads to a loss of fluid and electrolytes. The loss of up to 10% of the body's electrolytes can lead to shock, acidosis, stupor, and failure of the body's major organs (e.g., kidney, heart). Persistent diarrhea often leads to loss of body protein, an increased time-limited inability to digest and absorb dairy products, and increased susceptibility to infection. Every country should have as a major aim the prevention and control of diarrheal disease, especially in infants and children. Many countries have developed diarrhea control programs that improve childhood nutrition. These programs instruct in breastfeeding and weaning practices and promote oral rehydration therapy and the use of supplementary feeding programs (WHO, 2005b). However, all these programs must be considered in conjunction with improving the social and economic conditions that contribute to safe environmental, sanitary, and general living conditions of populations around the world.

| HOW TO | **Stay Current About Global Health** |

One of the ways to stay current with the world's health problems and advances is by reading the newspaper daily. Examples of newspapers that cover international health on an ongoing basis include the Wall Street Journal, USA Today, the Washington Post, and the New York Times. The following websites are examples of sources that pertain to international or global health:

- *U.S. Department of Health and Human Services: http://www. globalhealth.gov/*
- *Global Health Council: http://www.globalhealth.org/*
- *Centers for Disease Control and Prevention: http://www.cdc.gov/ globalhealth/*
- *World Health Organization: http://www.who.int/en/*
- *Pan American Health Organization: http://new.paho.org/*
- *World Bank: http://www.worldbank.org/*
- *Institute of Medicine: http://www.iom.edu/*
- *Millennium Development Goals: http://www.undp.org/mdg/*

EVIDENCE-BASED PRACTICE

This binational study explored the migration patterns and health experiences of indigenous Mixtec and Zapotec women from the state of Oaxaca in southern Mexico. The researcher discovered a high degree of independent decision-making among the women about migration and the various patterns of health-seeking behaviors for themselves and their families. Nearly always, their first recourse for treating health and illness conditions was the use of herbal and home remedies. They also used local public health departments and community clinics for children's well-care and immunizations, for acute episodes that were not responsive to treatment at home, and for themselves. They look for health care staff in the United States who are considerate of them as persons, who demonstrate affection and warmth to their children, and who are thorough and competent. Although some immigrant women have learned English, and all expressed a desire to learn, many work in the fields, in factories, and as domestics. These women lack the ability to speak English as a second language, are fully responsible for families, and have very complicated lives that present barriers to learning English. Some women speak their indigenous language and learned Spanish in northern Mexico before coming to the United States. Spanish-speaking immigrants are very responsive to health care workers who speak some Spanish.

Nurse Use
Being culturally sensitive and responsive means that nurses need to understand and value the practices and beliefs of the people with whom they work. Given this research study, how could you as a nurse incorporate the health beliefs of an immigrant from Mexico? One example might be the development of health information that integrates both traditional and Western health modalities when Mexican women are caring for their sick child. What might be others?

McGuire S: *Migration patterns and health experiences of Mixtec and Zapotec women*, dissertation research, 2002, University of San Diego, San Diego, California.

Maternal and Women's Health

Maternal health is central to the health of women, as well as the well-being of their children and families, and the economic productivity of their countries. A woman's ability to survive pregnancy and childbirth is closely related to how effectively societies invest in and realize the potential of women not only as mothers, but as critical contributors to sustaining families and transforming nations. When investments in women—as mothers, as individuals, as family members, and as citizens—lag, the economic cost of maternal death and illness is enormous.

Progress and investment in maternal health has lagged far behind estimates of what is needed to achieve MDG 5, Improve Maternal Health. Progress in the last 20 years on key maternal health indicators varies by outcome and region, but it has been uneven, inequitable, and inadequate overall. The two regions of the world with the worst maternal health status—South Asia and sub-Saharan Africa—show minimal signs of improvement largely because of poverty, disempowerment of women, and overall poor health status of women in developing countries. Women's reproductive health, especially their ability to control their fertility and avoid HIV infection, is also closely associated with their health as mothers.

Maternal health has widespread effects on children and families. A mother's death has profound repercussions for newborn and child health and survival. It also has grave implications for the long-term well-being of children—particularly girls—through its impact on their education, growth, and care, as well as intergenerational effects. Maternal ill health and related newborn mortality affect economic productivity, with estimated global costs of over $15 billion per year. Yet the total cost of preventing most of these maternal and newborn deaths ranges from only an estimated $4.1 to $6.1 billion per year. Although maternal death and disability represent a high burden of disease in the developing world, interventions to improve maternal health are available and cost-effective (Gill, Pande, and Malhotra, 2007).

In Uganda, Reproductive Health Uganda (RHU), formerly the Family Planning Association of Uganda (FPAU), provides services in 29 of the country's districts, targeting young people and marginalized groups to improve reproductive health. They offer family planning, HIV/AIDS testing and counseling, diagnosis and treatment of sexually transmitted infections (STIs), advocacy against female genital mutilation (FGM), post-abortion care to their high-risk constituency of internally displaced persons (IDPs), people at high risk of HIV/AIDS, young women in conflict-affected areas, sex workers, hawkers, saloonists, bicycle taxis, maids—any group subject to violence and disempowerment (www.rhu.or.ug). Despite FPAU's intent to improve the reproductive health of Ugandan women, there are barriers to the success of this initiative: continued cultural practice related to submissiveness of women and dependency on men for well-being of self and the children; bride wealth practices that give ownership to the man and permits beatings and other abuses of his wife; kinship patterns in which widowed women belong to the oldest brother; child care and all work related to the home and the children are performed by the women and girls; a woman's worth is still dependent on her ability to reproduce, even knowing that the more pregnancies a woman incurs, the less healthy the newborn and mother; and polygamy is practiced, allowing for transmission of STIs and HIV/AIDS (The Alan Guttmacher Institute, 2005).

WHO and UNICEF have continued their worldwide initiatives to reform the health care received by women and children in lesser-developed countries (USAID, 2005). However, studies on women's health indicate that most deaths to women around the world are related to pregnancy and childbirth. Every year, over half a million women die in pregnancy and childbirth around the world. This figure has altered little in the last 30 years. Equally distressing is the fact that worldwide, the ratio of maternal deaths to live births (the maternal mortality ratio) has remained essentially static during this period. Africa continues to have the highest maternal-child morbidity and mortality rate with 51% of all maternal deaths occurring in sub-Saharan Africa (Table 4-2). HIV currently accounts for 6.2% of maternal deaths in Africa and has reversed the progress made in maternal health in some countries (Gill et al, 2007; WHO, 2005b).

Throughout the world, women between 15 and 44 years of age account for approximately one third of the world's disease burden, and women between 45 and 59 for one fifth of the burden. This burden comprises diseases and conditions that are either exclusively or predominantly found in women, including maternal mortality and morbidity, cervical cancer, anemia, STIs, osteoarthritis, and breast cancer (World Bank, 2005). Although most of these conditions can be dealt with by cost-effective prevention and screening programs, many lesser-developed countries have ignored women's health issues other than those directly related to pregnancy and childbirth for two

major reasons: (1) women are not seen as valued members of society, and (2) most of the afflicted women are poor, malnourished, and cannot pay for health care services.

Sub-Saharan Africa accounts for the majority of the world's births. Although all countries profess they offer prenatal services and safe birthing services, most are unavailable, inaccessible, and unaffordable to women (USAID, 2005). An African woman's risk of dying from pregnancy-related causes is 1 in 20 (Gill et al, 2007; Raymond, Greenberg, and Leeder, 2005). Africa is followed by Bangladesh, Pakistan, and India. These three countries account for nearly half of the world's maternal deaths but only 29% of the world's births; they have more maternal deaths each week than Europe has in a year. Still, an accurate reporting of maternal deaths is difficult to obtain because many of the women who die are poor and live in remote areas, and their deaths are considered by many to be unimportant (Callister, 2005).

The primary causes of maternal mortality, particularly in lesser-developed countries, vary. They include hemorrhage, infection, convulsions, and coma caused by eclampsia and obstructed labor, and infections from unsanitary conditions and non-sterile and poorly performed abortions. Risk factors for maternal mortality include poor nutritional status, disease conditions, high parity, and age less than 20 and greater than 35 years. To date, little attention has been paid to the problem of maternal mortality, even though the reported incidences are high throughout the world. The WHO and the UN MDG 5 are addressing this problem by calling for government initiatives and actions to address maternal morbidity and mortality from obstetrical deaths as well as those that arise from indirect causes. MDG 5 aims to reduce the maternal mortality ratio by three quarters, improve the proportion of births attended by skilled health personnel, promote universal access to reproductive health, improve contraceptive rates, decrease adolescent birth rates, provide antenatal care coverage, and address the unmet need for family planning by 2015 (WHO, 2005). In some countries it is difficult to counsel women on family planning and spacing their children so as to promote maternal and fetal health when a woman's value depends on her ability to reproduce and over 50% of children die before they reach adolescence.

Even though programs in many countries have been initiated, safe motherhood initiatives are still needed throughout the world. These programs and initiatives need to include providing accessible family planning services and prenatal and postnatal health care services, ensuring access to safe abortion procedures, and improving the nutritional status of all women.

Nutrition and World Health

Many children around the world are underweight and have multiple micronutrient deficiencies such as iron, zinc, and vitamin A. Poor nutrition by itself or that associated with infectious disease accounts for a large portion of the world's disease burden (World Bank, 2005; Chan, 2008). Improved nutrition is related to stronger immune systems, decreased illness, better maternal and child health, longer life spans, and improved learning outcomes for children. Healthy protein balances are able to support major physiological stress with improved healing and ability to utilize protein-binding drugs; better nutrition

TABLE 4-2	LIFETIME RISK OF MATERNAL DEATHS IN SUB-SAHARAN AFRICA VERSUS INDUSTRIALIZED NATIONS
LIFETIME RISK OF MATERNAL DEATH	**1 IN __:**
Sub-Saharan Africa	22
Eastern/Southern Africa	29
West/Central Africa	17
Middle East/North Africa	140
South Asia	59
East Asia/Pacific	350
Latin America/Caribbean	280
CEE/CIS	1300
Industrialized countries	8000
Developing countries	76
Least developed countries	24
World	92

From Unicef/ChildInfo.org. Available at http://www.childinfo.org/images/maternal_mortality_progress_1.jpg. Accessed December 5, 2010.

is a prime entry point to ending poverty and a milestone to achieving better quality of life. Environmental and economic conditions related to poverty contribute to underconsumption of nutrients, especially those nutrients needed for protein building such as iodine, vitamin A, and iron. Worldwide, women and children suffer disproportionately from nutrition deficits, especially the micronutrients just mentioned (ICN, 2003).

For example, in war-torn Afghanistan, a critical shortage of fruits and vegetables led to an outbreak of scurvy that had devastating effects on the population, leaving them vulnerable to secondary diseases. In the same area, a vitamin A deficiency led to large numbers of people with night blindness (WHO, 2002b). Children in Haiti die daily from hunger; over 60% of the population is undernourished and children under the age of 5 suffer an even higher percentage. Over 800 million people (or one out of every five people in developing nations) are undernourished; and every few seconds, about every time one takes a breath, a child in the developing world dies of hunger and related diseases (Global Nutrition Alliance, 2010).

Poor nutrition also leads to stunting, or low height and weight for a given age. Stunting often results from eating foods that do not provide adequate energy or protein. Because protein foods are usually more expensive than non-protein food sources, many households reduce, or unconsciously eliminate, protein-rich foods to save money. Stunting is most prevalent in India (65%); Asia, not including India and China (50%); China (40%); and sub-Saharan Africa (40%) (World Bank, 2005). The author has cared for and watched many children with marasmus (total caloric deprivation) and Kwashiorkor (protein deficiency starvation) die who could have been saved if affordable protein and nutritious food were available. Usually this condition begins because an infant has been weaned away from breastfeeding after a year to make room for the next baby, and the food used in its place is mainly sugar and water or a starchy gruel. Kwashiorkor symptoms are apathy, muscular wasting, edema, and pigmentation loss in the skin and hair. Marasmus is a wasting away of the body tissues and symptoms are like kwashiorkor with fretfulness and an appearance of "skin and bones."

Iron deficiencies are also common in lesser-developed countries and severely affect women and children. When iron is low, fewer red blood cells are produced, and this reduces the capacity of the blood to transport oxygen. As a result, symptoms ranging from fatigue and inability to concentrate to impaired physical and cognitive development of children can occur. Iron deficiency anemia may also cause problems during pregnancy, particularly in developing countries where it can increase the risk of premature delivery, as well as the risk of maternal and fetal complications and death. Inadequate iron from food is the most common reason for iron deficiency anemia, especially among infants and children. Parasites, infections, stomach and digestive diseases, and blood loss during menstruation may also worsen anemia. A deficiency of iron in the diet can reduce appetite, physical productivity, the ability to learn, and growth.

Women are most susceptible to iron deficiency as a result of menstruation and childbearing. Women with iron deficiency can have an increased risk of hemorrhage during childbirth. A World Bank report (2005) indicates that 88% of all pregnant women in India are anemic, compared with 60% of the pregnant women in other parts of Asia. In developed, market-economy countries, only 15% of pregnant women experience iron deficiency anemia (WHO, 2002).

Other common dietary deficiencies include zinc, iodine, vitamin A, folic acid, and calcium. Zinc is important because it is an essential part of many enzymes and plays an important role in protein synthesis and cell division. The health consequences of zinc deficiency include poor immune system function, growth retardation, and delayed sexual maturity in children. Zinc deficiency is caused by low intake and/or low absorption of bioavailable zinc. Diets low in meat and fish increase the risk of zinc deficiency, because zinc is poorly bioavailable in cereals. Vitamin A is another essential nutrient in the human diet, contributing to the functioning of the retina, the growth of bone, and the immune response. Apart from preventable, irreversible blindness, vitamin A deficiency also causes reduced immune function, leading to an increased risk of severe infectious disease and anemia. It also increases the risk of death during pregnancy for both the mother and fetus and after birth for the newborn. An estimated 250 million preschool children in developing countries are affected by Vitamin A deficiency, although severe deficiency that causes blindness is declining (WHO, 2002).

The impact of malnutrition and dietary deficiencies is significant. Any malnourished condition in a population can increase susceptibility to illness. For example, the principal causes of death among malnourished persons are measles, diarrheal and respiratory disease, TB, pertussis, and malaria. The loss of life from these diseases can be measured as 231 DALYs worldwide, with one fourth of the 231 being directly attributable to malnourishment and dietary deficiencies. Individual governments and organizations such as the International Red Cross, WHO, and many international religious and private foundations have been active in promoting better nutrition. Worldwide initiatives directed at overcoming nutritional deficits include the following (World Bank, 2005): control of infectious diseases, nutritional education, control of intestinal parasites, micronutrient fortification of food, food supplementation, and food price subsidies.

Medecins Sans Fronteires (Doctors without Borders) was the first to use the life-saving supplement, invented in 2003 by a French scientist, called Plumpy'nut. Plumpy'nut requires no water preparation or refrigeration and has a 2-year shelf life, making it easy to deploy in difficult conditions to treat severe acute malnutrition. It is distributed under medical supervision, to humanitarian organizations for food aid distribution. The ingredients are: peanut paste; vegetable oil; powered milk; powdered sugar; vitamins A, B-complex, C, D, E, K; and minerals including calcium, phosphorus, potassium, magnesium, zinc, copper, iron, iodine, sodium, and selenium. These are combined in a foil pouch and each 92-g pack provides 500 kcal or 2.1 MJ.

Natural and Man-Made Disasters

As discussed in Chapter 23, earthquakes, floods, drought, and other natural hazards continue to cause tens of thousands of deaths, hundreds of thousands of injuries, and billions of dollars in economic losses each year around the world. EM-DAT, a global disaster database maintained by the Centre for Research on the Epidemiology of Disasters (CRED) in Brussels, records upwards of 600 disasters globally each year. Disaster frequency appears to be increasing (Vos, Rodriquez, Below, and Guha-Sapir, 2009). Disasters represent a major source of risk for the poor and wipe out development gains and accumulated wealth in developing countries.

Natural disasters such as earthquakes, tsunamis, and floods can often come at the least expected time. Others, such as hurricanes and cyclones, are increasing in severity and destruction. Droughts are increasing as the threat of global warming rises. Typically, the poor are the worst hit, for they have the least resources to cope and rebuild. Hurricane Katrina resulted in a 90,000 square mile disaster zone, equivalent to the area of Great Britain, and over 1800 died. The Indonesian tsunami of 2005 killed at least 230,000 people, and the livelihoods of millions were destroyed in over 10 countries affected by the tsunami. The earthquake in Haiti in 2010 destroyed a country and crushed the hopes of thousands of Haitians. Human activity is contributing to massive extinctions, from various animal species, to forests, and the ecosystems that support marine life. The costs associated with deteriorating or vanishing ecosystems is high. The World Resources Institute reports that there is a link between biodiversity and climate change, and rapid global warming can affect an ecosystem's chance to adapt naturally (World Resources Institute, 2010).

When poor countries face natural disasters, such as hurricanes, floods, earthquakes, and fires, the cost of rebuilding becomes even more of an issue when they are already burdened with debt. Often, poor countries suffer with many lost lives and/or livelihoods. Aid and disaster relief often does come in from international relief organizations, rich countries, and international institutions, but sometimes poor countries are still paying millions of dollars a week back in the form of debt repayment.

The aftermath of a natural disaster may be as devastating as the disaster itself. Inadequate shelter, unclean water, and lack of security are some of the most commonly reported problems, even a year after the event. The physical force of a disaster not only causes immediate injury and death, but each type of disaster can result in its own combination of physical injuries. In earthquakes, buildings and the objects inside them can fall, injuring those who live or work there. Floods can result in drowning, and wildfires can cause burns and illness from smoke inhalation.

In addition to the direct injury and death caused by the disaster's force, there can be other serious adverse effects on the well-being of those living in the area. The large numbers of people who are suddenly ill or injured can exceed the capacity of the local health care system to care for them. In addition to the burden of increased numbers of clients, the system itself can become a victim of the disaster. Hospitals may be damaged, roads blocked, and personnel unable to perform their duties. The loss of these resources occurs at a time when they are most critically needed. The disaster can also hamper the ability to provide routine, non-emergency health services. Many people may be unable to obtain care and medications for their ongoing health problems. The disruption of these routine services can result in an increase in illness and death in segments of the population that might not have been directly affected by the disaster.

The most serious consequences of natural disasters are related to mass population displacements, unsanitary conditions, lack of clean water, lack of nutritious foods, lack of safe housing, and the increased risk of diseases prevalent in crowded and unsanitary living conditions: typhoid fever, cholera, dysentery, TB, and infectious respiratory conditions (Waring and Brown, 2004).

Man-made disasters may be bioterrorism, chemical agents, pandemics and epidemics, radiation, and terrorism. A bioterrorism attack is the deliberate release of viruses, bacteria, or other germs (agents) used to cause illness or death in people, animals, or plants. These agents are typically found in nature, but it is possible that they could be changed to increase their ability to cause disease, to make them resistant to current medicines, or to increase their ability to be spread into the environment in order to threaten a government or intimidate or coerce a civilian population (Gostin et al, 2002). Bioterrorism is a significant public health threat that could produce widespread, devastating, and tragic consequences, and it would impose particularly heavy demands on international public health and health care systems. Nurses and other health personnel need to be aware and vigilant to the health consequences of terrorism and the potential use of biological agents to instill fear and to spread disease (ICN, 2001a, p 1).

A nation's capacity to respond to the threat of bioterrorism depends in part on the ability of health care professionals and public health officials to rapidly and effectively detect, diagnose, respond, and communicate during a bioterrorism event. The national health care community—including public health agencies, emergency medical services, hospitals, and health care providers—would bear the brunt of the consequences of a biological attack (Veneema, 2002). Attacks with biological agents are likely to be covert, rather than overt (CDC, 2000). Terrorists may prefer to use biological agents because of their difficulty to detect; they do not cause illness for several hours to several days (CDC, Bioterrorism Overview, n.d.).

A chemical emergency occurs when a hazardous chemical has been released and the release has the potential for harming people's health. Chemical releases can be unintentional, as in the case of an industrial accident, or intentional, as in the case of a terrorist attack. Sarin and ricin are the two most recent notorious chemicals used; however, mustard gas, cyanide, and tear gas have existed for decades.

Radiation poisoning occurs when an excess amount of radiation is released to harm people's health. These may be unintentional and intentional events. Intentional terrorist events are those designed to contaminate food and water with radioactive material; spread radioactive material into the environment by using conventional explosives (e.g., dynamite) called a dirty bomb or by using wind currents or natural traffic patterns; bomb or destroy a nuclear reactor; cause a truck or train carrying nuclear material to spill its load; or explode a nuclear weapon.

As discussed in Chapter 13, pandemics and epidemics may be intentional or unintentional (anthrax, cholera, ebola, lassa fever, plague, and smallpox, to name a few). A pandemic is an epidemic of infectious diseases that spread through human populations across a large region such as a continent or the globe (e.g., HIV/AIDS, smallpox, TB, H1N1, SARS). An epidemic is when new cases of a certain disease in a given human population exceed what is expected (cancer, heart disease, seasonal flu). The most recent pandemic (H1N1 [swine flu]) was an influenza virus that had never been identified as a cause of infections in people before. Genetic analyses of this virus have shown that it originated from animal influenza viruses and is unrelated to the human seasonal H1N1 viruses that have been in general circulation among people since 1977. The new virus also led to patterns of death and illness not normally seen in influenza infections. Most of the deaths caused by the pandemic influenza occurred among younger people, including those who were otherwise healthy. Pregnant women, younger children, and people of any age with certain chronic lung or other medical conditions appeared to be at higher risk of more complicated or severe illness. Many of the severe cases have been due to viral pneumonia, which is harder to treat than bacterial pneumonias usually associated with seasonal influenza. Many of these clients required intensive care that required 4 to 6 weeks of ICU services (WHO, 2010).

The word genocide was developed by a jurist named Raphael Lemkin in 1944. By combining the Greek word 'genos' (race) with the Latin word 'cide' (killing), genocide was defined by the United Nations in 1948 to mean any of the following acts committed with intent to destroy, in whole or in part, a national, ethnic, racial, or religious group, including: (a) killing members of the group, (b) causing serious bodily or mental harm to members of the group, (c) deliberately inflicting on the group conditions of life calculated to bring about its physical destruction in whole or in part, (d) imposing measures intended to prevent births within the group, and (e) forcibly transferring children of the group to another group (Albright and Cohen, 2008).

Genocide in the twentieth century includes such atrocities as the 1915-1918 Armenian elimination by Turkey when 2 million Armenians living in Turkey were removed from their historic homeland through forced deportations and massacres. The Ukrainian famine was designed by Stalin to destroy the Ukrainian people who were seeking independence from his rule. As a result, an estimated 7 million persons perished in a farming area known as the breadbasket of Europe, with the people deprived of the food they had grown with their own hands. The rape of Nanking occurred in 1937 when the Japanese Imperial Army marched into China's capital city of Nanking and proceeded to murder 300,000 out of 600,000 civilians and soldiers in the city. The 6 weeks of carnage represented the single worst atrocity during the World War II era in either the European or Pacific theaters of war. The Nazi Holocaust from 1938 to 1945 eliminated over 6 million people who did not fit into Hitler's ideal superior race, with most of the victims being Jewish. Khmer Rouge leader Pol Pot, from 1975 to 1979, wanted to form a Communist peasant farming society. His plan resulted in the deaths of 25% (2 million people) of the country's population from starvation, overwork, and executions. From 1992 to 1995 in the Republic of Bosnia-Herzegovina, the conflict between the three main ethnic groups (Serbs, Croats, and Muslims) resulted in a genocide committed by the Serbs against the Muslims in Bosnia. Over 200,000 people lost their lives. In Rwanda beginning April 6, 1994, and for the next 100 days, up to 800,000 Tutsis were killed by Hutu

militia using clubs and machetes, with as many as 10,000 killed each day. In the twenty-first century, the genocide in Darfur is still continuing. More than 400,000 civilians have been killed and 2.5 million people have been displaced from their homes. About the size of Texas, the Darfur region of Sudan is home to racially mixed Muslim tribes. In February 2003, frustrated by poverty and neglect, two Darfurian rebel groups launched an uprising against the Khartoum government. The government responded with a scorched-earth campaign, arming and bankrolling militias against the innocent civilians of Darfur.

Following genocide, there are biopsychological changes such as physical stress reactions (cardiovascular, neurological) and mental stress responses, especially post-traumatic stress disorders and depression. Many people flee and become refugees or internationally displaced people. These refugees flee to neighboring countries, placing social, political, and economic burdens on these countries. The author has been to the refugee camps in Uganda for refugees from Rwanda, the Congo, Kenya, and even northern Uganda whose people have been victims of the Liberation Rebel Army (LRA) as political turmoil continues to plague the civilians in East Africa. The victims of genocide often face discrimination in refugee camps or in their new country of permanent residence if they do not return home. Individuals who return to their home countries are often plagued with uncertainty regarding lost property and other belongings.

The biological and psychosocial effects of genocide are not exclusive to the child and adult victims, but affect the perpetrators as well. Marginalization and dehumanization place a mental toll on the victims that often result in negative cognitive, behavioral, affective, relational, and spiritual effects. Many perpetrators are forced into committing these acts, and achieving desensitization is necessary for a non-violent person to kill or to commit violent acts. This is evident in the boy soldiers of the LRA (some as young as 6 years old) who are forced to kill or be killed and become desensitized through the use of alcohol, drugs, and repeated exposure to death.

After genocidal conflicts have ceased, restoration of a country's infrastructure, as well as reconciliation, has to begin. The ramifications of genocide are widespread, and community leaders have to find the most effective ways of initiating the healing process. The U.N. has tried to develop strategies to prevent genocide from occurring and is encouraging initiatives that include appropriate comprehensive cultural competence in the delivery of services; supporting and organizing treatment and care that is fair and just to all members of specific societies, regardless of age, gender, race, cultural beliefs, religion, sexual orientation, affiliation, and civil status; encouraging international organizations to make mental and behavioral health a priority in conflict assistance throughout the various stages of genocide; and encouraging its member organizations to emphasize the importance of social work in regard to genocide in their respective countries (Albright and Cohen, 2008).

Surveillance Systems

Surveillance systems, discussed in Chapter 24, are used to track potential risks for intentional harm to the people of the world. Veneema (2002) discusses surveillance systems; however, these

BOX 4-5   WHAT CAN NURSING DO IN THE EVENT OF A DISASTER?

The International Council of Nursing (ICN) policy paper on disaster preparedness outlines actions, including risk assessment and multidisciplinary management strategies, as critical to the delivery of effective responses to the short-, medium-, and long-term health needs of a disaster-stricken population. These actions include the following:

HELP PEOPLE TO COPE WITH AFTERMATH OF TERRORISM

- Assist people to deal with feelings of fear, vulnerability, and grief.
- Use groups who have survived terrorist attacks as useful resources for victims.

ALLAY PUBLIC CONCERNS AND FEAR OF BIOTERRORISM

- Disseminate accurate information on the risks involved, preventive measures, use of antibiotics and/or vaccines, and reporting suspicious letters or packages to the police or other authorities.
- Address hoax messages, false alarms, and threats; any perceived threat to the public health must be investigated.

IDENTIFY THE FEELINGS THAT YOU AND OTHERS MAY BE EXPERIENCING

- In the aftermath of terror, even health care professionals can feel bias, hatred, vengeance, and violence toward ethnic or religious groups that are associated with terrorism. These feelings can compromise their ability to provide care for these groups. Yet as the ICN *Code of Ethics for Nurses* affirms, nurses are ethically bound to provide care to all people (ICN, 2000).
- Explain that feelings of fear, helplessness, and loss are normal reactions to a disruptive situation.

- Help people remember methods they may have used in the past to overcome fear and helplessness.
- Encourage people to talk to others about their fears.
- Encourage others to ask for help and provide resources and referrals.
- Remember that those in the helping professions (e.g., nurses, physicians, social workers) may find it difficult to seek help.
- Convene small groups in workplaces with counselors/mental health experts.

ASSIST VICTIMS TO THINK POSITIVELY AND TO MOVE TOWARD THE FUTURE

- Remind others that things will get better.
- Be realistic about the time it takes to feel better.
- Help people to recognize that the aim of terrorist attacks is to create fear and uncertainty.
- Encourage people to continue with the things they enjoy in their lives and to live their normal lives.

PREPARE NURSING PERSONNEL TO BE EFFECTIVE IN A CRISIS/EMERGENCY SITUATION (Incorporate disaster preparedness awareness in educational programs at all levels of nursing curriculum)

- Provide continuing education to ensure a sound knowledge base, skill development, and ethical framework for practice.
- Network with other professional disciplines and governmental and non-governmental agencies at local, regional, national, and international levels.

From ICN. Nursing Matters: Terrorism and bioterrorism: nursing preparedness. Available at http//www.icn.ch/publications/disaster-planning-and relief. Accessed December 27, 2010; International Council of Nurses (ICN): *Code of ethics for nurses,* Geneva, 2000, ICN.

systems are specifically designed to assess the risk for impending health crises. There are systems in place to assess the risks for other man-made and natural disasters to prevent the atrocities to mankind discussed previously. These systems may be on-the-ground specialists who acquire information about the political stability of nations, or they may be satellite systems that track weather, volcanic, and earthquake activities.

Veneema (2002) determined that to differentiate between an impending health care crisis and a hoax, it was imperative to understand the national and international systems of surveillance currently in place. How would a government find out that a deliberate outbreak had taken place? For the international system, the WHO monitors disease outbreaks through the Global Outbreak Alert and Response Network (WHO, 2004b; WHO Group of Consultants, 2001). This network, formally launched in April 2000, electronically links the expertise and skills of 72 existing networks from around the world, several of which were uniquely designed to diagnose unusual agents and handle dangerous pathogens. Its purpose is to keep the international community constantly alert to the threat of outbreaks and ready to respond. It has four primary tasks:

1. *Systematic disease intelligence and detection.* The first responsibility of the WHO network is to systematically gather global disease intelligence drawing from a wide range of resources, both formal and informal. Ministries of Health, WHO country offices, government and military centers, and academic institutions all file regular formal reports with the

Global Outbreak Alert and Response Network. An informal network scours world communications for rumors of unusual health events.

2. *Outbreak verification.* Preliminary intelligence reports from all sources, both formal and informal, are reviewed and converted into meaningful intelligence by the WHO Outbreak Alert and Response Team, which makes the final determination whether a reported event warrants cause for international concern.

3. *Immediate alert.* A large network of electronically connected WHO member nations, disease experts, health institutions, agencies, and laboratories is kept continually informed of rumored and confirmed outbreaks. The network also maintains and regularly updates an Outbreak Verification List, which provides a detailed status report on all currently verified outbreaks.

4. *Rapid response.* When the Outbreak Alert and Response Team determines that an international response is needed to contain an outbreak, it enlists the help of its partners in the global network. Specific assistance available includes targeted investigations, confirmation of diagnoses, handling of dangerous biohazards (biosafety level IV pathogens), client care management, containment, and logistical support in terms of staff and supplies.

In summary, if health care professionals and emergency responders are to be prepared to manage natural or manmade disasters, it is critical that there be cooperative efforts at the international, national, state, and local levels (Box 4-5). Such disaster response is not the domain of any one specialty; nurses, doctors, mental health experts, first responders, EMTs, volunteers, engineers, and many more need to be part of the team that helps people overcome the physical, emotional, social, and economic devastation. Nurses need to have political, historical, social, medical, nursing, and public health knowledge in order to be more effective in finding the resources their clients need to recover successfully.

🌐 LINKING CONTENT TO PRACTICE

The role and involvement of nurses in global health relies heavily on nursing standards of practice and core competencies of both nurses and other public health professionals. The role also varies from country to country. It is not surprising to learn that nursing plays a more active role in health care delivery in the more technologically advanced countries. The more developed countries have a defined role for nurses, whereas the role is less well defined, if it is defined at all, in lesser-developed countries. However, nurses need to remember that addressing the health of the people of the world is not restricted to meeting the physical health needs but, in order to be successful, must incorporate the concept of global health diplomacy. Physical, environmental, mental, political, fiscal, economic, safety, and educational "health" are intertwined in achieving the goals we all have for helping the people of the world obtain optimal well-being. Assessment of each of these areas is cited in standards of practice for nursing and public health professionals and is essential in the global nursing role. See the Quad Council on Nursing's competencies (2009), which incorporate those of the Council on Linkages core competencies for public health professionals (2009). Each set of competencies recommends analytic/assessment skills that are crucial to working in a global health arena. They also talk about the importance of cultural competence skills and communication skills that are relevant to the people with whom you are working.

During the last decade, some lesser-developed countries have implemented primary health care programs directed at prevention and management of important public health problems. With the increasing migration between and within countries because of war and famine, a greater need for nursing expertise to alleviate suffering of refugees and displaced persons has emerged. Starvation, disease, death, war, and migration underscore the need for support from the wealthier nations of the world.

More than 30 million refugees and internally displaced persons in lesser-developed countries currently depend on international relief assistance for survival. Death rates in these populations during the acute phase of displacement have been up to 60 times the expected rates. Displaced populations in Ethiopia and southern Sudan have suffered the highest death rates. In Afghanistan and in war-torn Iraq, infectious diseases accounted for one half of all admissions to the hospital—mostly malaria and typhoid fever. The greatest death rate has been in children 1 to 14 years old. The major causes of death have been measles, diarrheal diseases, acute respiratory tract infections, and malaria. In addition, poor sanitation in many hospitals and clinics and shortages of drugs and qualified health care workers produce huge gaps for needed health care services. Continued violence accounts for a population who is afraid to leave their homes to seek medical help.

Nurses from more developed countries are recruited to combat the major mortality in refugee camps: malnutrition, measles, diarrhea, pneumonia, and malaria. Nurses, collaborating with other experts, are following the principles of primary health care and are promoting adequate food intake, safe drinking water, shelter, environmental sanitation, and immunizations. These life-saving practices have been implemented in the following countries: Thailand (Myanmar refugees), Rwanda, Zaire, Angola, Afghanistan, the Sudan, Uganda, and the former Yugoslavia. Nurses are making a difference; however, nurses involved in this work must be culturally astute and responsive, be well educated about the world and well versed in the tasks required to achieve positive outcomes, able to critically reason, able to make decisions, able to identify who are appropriate team members, and be able to collaborate with the team. They ought not be afraid of taking risks, they should be action-oriented, and they need to be flexible and altruistic. Global health work is a labor of love, it is a giving of self to make a difference in the lives of others less fortunate, and it is the most rewarding work in which many nurses have ever been engaged.

Council on Linkages Between Academic and Public Health Practice: Core competencies for public health professionals, Washington, DC, 2010. Public Health Foundation/Health Resources and Services Administration.
Quad Council of Public Health Nursing Organizations. Competencies for Public Health Nursing Practice, Washington, DC, 2003, ASTDN, revised 2009.

CHAPTER REVIEW

▌ PRACTICE APPLICATION

You are sent to a country ravaged by war, in which many people are refugees. You are asked to work side by side with other nurses, both foreign and native to the country.

A. What would you do first to develop this group of nurses into a functioning team?

B. Which health and environmental problems would you attempt to handle early in your work?

C. Identify second-stage interventions and prevention once the initial crisis stage is relieved.

Answers can be found on the Evolve site.

▌ KEY POINTS

- Global health is a collective goal of nations and is promoted by the world's major health organizations.
- Global health cannot be achieved without using the constructs of global health diplomacy: addressing and finding solutions to physical, environmental, fiscal, economic, political, safety, educational, and trade issues.
- As the political and economic barriers between countries fall, the movement of people back and forth across international boundaries increases. This movement increases the spread of various diseases throughout the world.

KEY POINTS—cont'd

- Nurses play an active role in the identification of potential health risks at U.S. borders, with immigrant populations throughout the United States, and as participants in global health care delivery.
- Understanding a population approach is essential for understanding the health of specific populations.
- Universal access to health care for the world's populations relies on strong primary care.
- The major organizations involved in world health are: (1) multilateral, (2) bilateral and non-governmental or private voluntary, and (3) philanthropic.
- The health status of a country is related to its economic and technical growth. More technologically and economically advanced countries are referred to as *developed*, whereas those that are striving for greater economic and technological growth are termed *lesser developed*. Many lesser-developed countries shift financial resources from health and education to other internal needs, such as defense or economic development, and this shift does not help the poor.
- The global burden of disease (GBD) is a way to describe the world's health. The GBD combines losses from premature death and losses that result from disability. The GBD represents units of disability-adjusted life-years (DALYs).
- Critical global health problems still exist and include communicable diseases such as tuberculosis, measles, mumps, rubella, and polio; maternal and child health; diarrheal diseases; nutritional deficits; malaria; and AIDS.
- Natural and man-made disasters have become global health concerns.

CLINICAL DECISION-MAKING ACTIVITIES

1. In your class, divide into small groups and discuss how you might find out if there are immigrant communities in your area (you may need to contact your local health department, area social workers, or community social organizations and churches).
   A. Discuss how you can gain access to one of these immigrant groups.
   B. Upon gaining access, how would you go about determining what specific kinds of services the people need? What are their beliefs about health and health care? What customs regarding health were followed in their country of origin? How does the American health care system differ from the health care system in their country?
   C. As a nurse, what kinds of interventions can you implement with immigrant populations? What special skills or knowledge do you need to provide care to immigrant populations?
2. Write to one of the major international health organizations or visit their internet web page and obtain their mission and goal statements. What is the focus of their health-related activities? Does the organization that you identified have a specific role defined for nurses? How can a nurse who is interested become involved in their programs and activities?
3. Pick a country or area of the world outside the United States that interests you. Go to the library or use the internet to obtain information about the following:
   A. Status of health care in that country
   B. Major health concerns
   C. Global burden of disease (GBD)
   D. Whether this country is developed or lesser developed
   E. Which, if any, global health care organizations are involved with the delivery of health care in that country
4. Choose one or more of the following countries, and find out from your local or state health department the health risks that are involved in visiting that country: Indonesia, Zaire, Paraguay, Bangladesh, Kuwait, Kenya, Mexico, China, and Haiti.
5. Establish communication with nurses in a country of interest (via telecommunication [e.g., web, phone, blog]) to discuss the state of nursing in that country, their problems, and plans to overcome some of the barriers that obstruct them from achieving their professional goals.

REFERENCES

The Alan Guttmacher Institute: *Research Brief: Adolescents in Uganda: sexual and reproductive health*, 2005. Available at www.guttmacher.org/pubs/rib/2005/03/30/rib2-05.pdf. Accessed December 5, 2010.

Albright M, Cohen W: *Preventing genocide: a blueprint for U.S. policymakers*, 2008. Retrieved December 22, 2010 from http://media.usip.org/reports/genocide_taskforce_report.pdf.

Anders R, Harrigan R: Nursing education in China: opportunities for international collaboration, *Nurs Educ Perspect* 23:137, 2002.

Asia M: Effects of traumatic events exposure on neurohormonal diurnal patterns in Palestinian children, unpublished dissertation, 2009.

Audit Commission: *Educating and training the future health professional workforce for England*, 2005. Available at http://www.nao.org.uk/. Accessed December 5, 2010.

Basch PF: *Textbook of international health*, New York, 1990, Oxford University Press.

Bleed D, Dye C, Raviglione MC: Dynamics and control of the global tuberculosis epidemic, *Curr Opin Pulm Med* 6:174, 2000.

Bolender J, Hunter A: The Uganda project: a cross-disciplinary student-faculty research and service project to develop a sustainable community-development program, *College Undergraduate Research Journal*, 2010.

Brown GD: Protecting worker's health and safety in the globalizing economy through international trade treaties, *Int J Occup Environ Health* 11:207–209, 2005.

Buchan J, Dal Poz MR: Skill mix in the healthcare workforce: reviewing the evidence, *Bull World Health Organization* 80:575–580, 2002.

Cahoon M, Myles G: *Canada and NAFTA: a 10-year measure of success in Canadian-U.S. agricultural trade—North American Free Trade Agreement*, 2004. Available at http://findarticles.com/p/articles/mi_m3723/is_1_16/ai_114328141/. Accessed December 5, 2010.

Cairns M, Cisse B, Sokhna C, et al: Amodiaquine dosage and tolerability for intermittent preventive treatment to prevent malaria in children, *Antimicrob Agents Chemother* 54(3):1265–1274, 2010.

Callister LC: Global maternal mortality: contributing factors and strategies for change, *MCN, Am J Matern Child Nurs* 30:184–192, 2005.

Campana A: *Chronology and mandate of a specialized agency of the United Nations, Geneva Foundation for Medical Education and Research*, Geneva, 2005, WHO Foundation. Available at http://www.gfmer.ch/TMCAM/WHO_Minelli/A3.htm. Accessed December 5, 2010.

Centers for Disease Control and Prevention: Biological and chemical terrorism: strategic plan for preparedness and response, *MMWR Morbid Mortal Wkly Rep* 49(RR-4), 2000.

Centers for Disease Control and Prevention: *TB, data and statistics*, Atlanta, 2005, CDC.

Centers for Disease Control and Prevention: *Bioterrorism overview*, n.d. Available at http://www.bt.cdc.gov/bioterrorism/overview.asp. Accessed December 22, 2010.

Chan M: *The global nutrition challenge: getting a healthy start*, 2008. Retrieved December 2010 from http://www.who.int/dg/speeches/2008/20080618/en/index.html.

Cherian MN, Noel L, Buyanjargal Y, et al: Esssential emergency surgical procedures in resource-limited facilities: a WHO workshop in Mongolia, *World Hosp Health Serv* 40:24–29, 2004.

Commission on the Future of Health Care in Canada (CFHCC): *Home page*, 2005. Available at http://www.healthcarecommission.ca. Accessed December 5, 2010.

Council on Linkages Between Academic and Public Health Practice: *Core competencies for public health professionals*, Washington DC, 2010. Public Health Foundation/Health Resources and Services Administration .

Dobie M: *Why China's health needs fixing*, 2005a. Available at http://www.idrc.ca/books/reports/2001/04-02e.html. Accessed December 5, 2010.

Drager N, Fidler DP: Foreign policy, trade and health: at the cutting edge of global health diplomacy, *Bulletin WHO* 85(3):162, 2007.

DuMortier S, Arpagaus M: Quality improvement programme on the frontline: an international committee of the Red Cross experience in the Democratic Republic of Congo, *Int J Qual Healthcare*, 2005. (April 14, Epub ahead of print).

Dye C, Williams BG, Espinal MA, et al: Erasing the world's slow staining strategies to beat drug resistant tuberculosis, *Science* 15:75, 2002.

Escott S, Walley J: Listening to those on the frontline: lessons for community-based tuberculin programmes from a qualitative study in Swaziland, *Soc Sci Med*, 2005:(June 18, Epub ahead of print).

Farmer P: *Pathologies of power: health, human rights, and the new war on the poor*, Berkley, CA, 2005, University of California Press.

Fields RM, Margolin J: American Psychological Association, *Fact sheet on coping with terrorism*, 2001. Available at http://www.apa.org/. Accessed December 5, 2010.

Flynn B, Ivanov L: Health promotion through healthy communities and cities. In *Community & public health nursing*, ed 6, St Louis, 2004, Mosby, pp 396–411.

Foreign Affairs and International Trade Canada International: *The NAFTA's Impact Trade Results*, 2009. http://www.international.gc.ca/trade-agreements-accords-commerciaux/_agr-acc/nafta-alena/nafta5_section04.aspx?lang=eng:Accessed December 29, 2010.

Fox DM: The relevance of population health to academic medicine, *Acad Med* 76:6, 2001.

Fuller C: North America, Inc.: NAFTA chips away at Canadian healthcare, *Revolution* 3:11, 2002.

Galea S: Macrosocial determinants of population health, *Am J Epidemiol* 167(12):1518–1519, 2008.

Gill K, Pande R, Malhotra A: Women deliver for development, *Lancet* 13(370):1347–1357, 2007. Paper presentation at The Women Deliver Conference, October 2007.

Ginsberg AM, Sizemore C, Fauci AS: *Fighting the white plague, National Institute of Allergy and Infectious Diseases, National Institutes of Health.* Available at http://www3.niaid.nih.gov/news/newsreleases/2001/whiteplague.htm. Accessed December 5, 2010.

Global Health Initiatives, n.d. Available at http://www.pepfar.gov/ghi/136496.htm. Accessed December 5, 2010.

Global Issues: Social, political, economic and environmental issues that affect us all (2/14/2010) Available at http://www.globalissues.org/issue/587/health-issues. Accessed December 5, 2010.

Global Nutrition Alliance: http://www.globalnutritionalliance.org. Retrieved December, 2010.

Gostin I, Sapsin J, Teret S, et al: The Model State Emergency Health Powers Act: planning for and response to bioterrorism and naturally occurring infectious diseases, *JAMA* 288:622–628, 2002.

Hancock C: *Advancing the millennium development goals*, 2005. Available at http://www.icn.ch/. Accessed December 5, 2010.

Harvey P: Environmental sanitation crisis: more than just a health issue, *Env Health Insights* 2:77–81, 2008.

Health Canada: *Health care*, 2006. Available at http://www.hc-sc.gc.ca/ahc-ascli/index. Accessed November 9, 2006.

Heymann M: Reproductive health promotion in Kosovo, *J Midwifery Womens Health* 46(2):74–81, 2001.

Hunter A, Denman-Vitale S, Garzon L, et al: Global infections: recognition, management, and prevention, *Nurse Pract* 32(2):35–41, 2007.

Hunter A, McKenry L: An advanced practice international health initiative: The Ghana Health Mission, *Clin Excell Nurse Pract: Int J NPACE* 5(4):240–245, 2005.

Hutton J: PPPs review British health care system, *The Financial Post* , November 23, 2003.

Ibrahim MA, Savitz LA, Carey TS, et al: Population-based health principles in medical and public health practice, *J Public Health Manag Pract* 7:75, 2001.

Institute of Medicine (IOM): Committee on Summary Measures of Population Health, summarizing population health: directions for the development and application of population metrics, 1998.

Institute of Medicine (IOM): *The future of the public's health in the 21st century*, 2002.

Institute of Medicine (IOM): *Addressing the Threat of Drug-Resistant Tuberculosis: A Realistic Assessment of the Challenge.* Workshop Summary Released: August 26, 2009

Institute of Medicine (IOM): *Preparing for the Future of HIV/AIDS in Africa: A Shared Responsibility* Released November 29, 2010. Washington DC, National Academy Press.

International Council of Nurses: *Code of ethics for nurses*, Geneva, 2000, ICN.

International Council of Nurses: *ICN position statement on nurses and emergency preparedness*, Geneva, 2001a, ICN.

International Council of Nurses: *Tackling the UN millennium development goals (MDGs)*, Biennial report, Geneva, 2003, ICN. Available at http://www.globalissues.org/issue. Accessed December 5, 2010.

International Council of Nurses: *Disaster relief: donating to ICN member national nurses associations by the earthquake and tsunami in South Asia*, Publication 1–6, 2005.

International Medical Volunteer Association (IMVA): *The major international organizations*, Woodville, MA, 2002, IMVA.

Kaiser Family Foundation: *U.S. Global Health Policy. Fact sheet December, 2010.* http://www.kff.org/hivaids. Accessed December 28, 2010.

Kekki P: *Primary health care and the millennium development goals: issues for discussion*, Geneva, 2005, World Health Organization.

Kennedy B: *Serving the people: China's health care system may be headed for a crisis*, 1999. Available at http://asia.cnn.com/SPECIALS/1999/china.50/dispatches/09.23.health. Accessed December 5, 2010.

Keusch G, Fontaine O, Bhargava A, et al: Diarrheal diseases. In Jamison DT, Breman JG, Measham AR, et al: *Disease Control Priorities in Developing Countries*. Washington, DC, World Bank 2006. Available at http://www.ncbi.nlm.nih.gov/bookshelf/br.fcgi?book=dcp2&part=A2526. Accessed December 5, 2010.

Kickbusch I, Silberschmidt G, Buss P: Global health diplomacy: the need for new perspectives, strategic approaches and skills in global health, *Bulletin of the WHO* 85(3):161–244, 2007.

Kindig D, and Stoddard G: What is population health? Available at http://ajph.aphapublications.org/cgi/reprint/93/3/380.pdf. Accessed December 5, 2010.

Lalonde, M: A new perspective on the health of Canadians: health and welfare Canada, Ottawa, Ontario, 1974.

Lengeler C: Insecticide-treated bednets and curtains for preventing malaria, *The Cochrane Database of Systematic Reviews*, Issue 2, 2004.

Lewis S: *Health and human rights. A presentation made to the 23rd Quadrennial Congress, International Council of Nurses*, Tapei, May 23, 2005, Taiwan.

Lown B: The commodification of health care, *PNHP Newsletter*, 2007. Retrieved December 22, 2010 from http://www.pnhp.org/publications/the_commodification_of_health_care.php.

Lucas A: WHO at country level, *Lancet* 351:743, 1998.

Maeseneer JD, Shabir M, Yongyuth P, Kaufman A: Primary health care in a changing world, *Br J Gen Pract* 58(556):806–809, 2008.

Malkin E: Nafta's Promise, Unfulfilled, *The New York Times*, March 23, 2009. Available at http://www.nytimes.com/2009/03/24/business/worldbusiness/24peso.html. Accessed December 5, 2010.

Maurice J, Davey S: *State of the world's vaccines and immunization*, ed 3, Geneva Switzerland, 2009, WHO.

McMichael AJ, Friel S, Nyong A, et al: Global environmental change and health: impacts, inequalities, and the health sector, *BMJ* 336:191–194, 2008.

Miller A, Chandler PJ: Acculturation, resilience, and depression in midlife women from the former Soviet Union, *Nurs Res* 51:26–32, 2002.

Mikelonis G, Fan J: *Chinese health care reform: An overview*, September 28, 2009. Available at http://www.mercer.com/print/htm. Accessed December 27, 2010.

Mondy C, Cardenas D, Avila M: The role of an advanced practice public health nurse in bioterrorism preparedness, *Public Health Nurs* 20:422–431, 2003.

Murray C, Lopez A: *Global burden of disease: 1996*, pp 541-612, World Bank and Harvard School of Public Health publication, Cambridge, MA, 1996, Oxford University Press.

Nigenda G, Ruiz JA, Montes J: New trends in the regulation of medical practice in the context of health care reform: the Mexico case, *Rev Med Chil* 129:1343, 2001.

People and Ecosystems. World Resources Institute. Available at http://www.wri.org/ecosystems. Acessed July 10, 2010.

Peters A, Fisher P: The failures of economic development incentives, *J Am Planning Assoc* 70:27–37, 2004.

Public Health Agency of Canada: *Population health*, 2005. Available at http://www.phac_aspcia/ph_sp/phdd/determinants/2005. Accessed December 5, 2010.

Quad Council of Public Health Nursing Organizations. Competencies for Public Health Nursing Practice. Washington DC, 2003, ASTDN, revised 2009.

Qun Y: Bridging the health care gap: Amity's response to health care reforms in China, *Quart Bull Amity Found*, 2001. Available at http://www.amityfoundation.org/Amity/anl/Issue_56_1/gap.htm. Accessed December 5, 2010.

Raymond SU, Greenberg HM, Leeder SR: Beyond reproduction: women's health in today's developing world, *Int J Epidemiol* 34:1144–1148, 2005.

Ruxin J, Paluzzi JE, Wilson PA, et al: Emerging consensus in HIV/AIDS, malaria, tuberculosis, and access to essential medicines, *Lancet* 365:618–621, 2005.

Schoen C, Davie K, DesRoches C, et al: Equity in health care across five nations: summary findings from an international health policy survey, *Nurse Econ* 388:1–7, 2000.

Segal MT, Demos V, Kronenfeld JJ: *Gender perspectives on health and medicine: key themes*, New York, 2003, Elsevier.

Suarez R: Background report: comparing international health care systems, *Global Health Watch*, 2009. Available at http://www.pbs.org/newshour/globalhealth/july-dec09/insurance_1006.html. Accessed December 5, 2010.

Subways S: Africa: children's access to prophylaxis may improve after medical study, new WHO recommendations, *AIDS Treatment News* No. 407-408:8–9, 2004.

Sutherland K: *Quality in healthcare in England, Wales, Scotland, Northern Ireland: an intra-UK chartbook*. London, England: The Health Foundation. Available at http://www.health.org.uk/publications/research_reports/intrauk_chartbook.html. Accessed December 5, 2010.

Tejada de Rivers DA: Alma Ata revisited, *Magazine Pan American Health Organization* 8:345–350, 2003.

United Nations: *UN millennium development goals (MDGs)*, 2005. Available at http://www.un.org/milleniumgoals/. Accessed December 5, 2010.

United Nations: *UN Millennium Development Goals revised*, 2009. Available at http://www.un.org/milleniumgoals/. Accessed December 5, 2010.

USAID: *Frontlines: Afghan women visit clinics*, 2005. Available at http://www.usaid.gov/press/frontlines/fl_oct04/spotlight.html#2. Accessed December 5, 2010.

Varga C: Sexual and reproductive health among South African adolescents, *Stud Fam Plan* 34(3):160–172, 2003.

Veneema T: Chemical and biological terrorism: current updates for nurse educators, *Nurs Educ Perspect* 23:62–71, 2002.

Vos F, Rodriguez J, Below R, et al: *Annual disaster statistical review 2009*. Retrieved December 22, 2010 from Center for Research on Epidemiology of Disasters CRED: WHO Collaborating Center http://cred.be/sites/default/files/ADSR_2009.pdf.

Waring SC, Brown BJ: The threat of communicable diseases following natural disasters: A public health response, *Dis Manag Response* 3(2), 2004.

Weiner E: Preparing nurses internationally for emergency planning and response, *The Online Journal of Issues in Nursing* 11(3), 2006. Retrieved December 22, 2010 from: http://www.nursingworld.org/MainMenuCategories/ANAMarketplace/ANAPeriodicals/OJIN/TableofContents/Volume112006/No3Sept06/PreparingNurses.aspx

What is global environmental health? Available at http://www.cdc.gov/nceh/globalhealth/global.htm. Accessed March 10, 2010.

White K, Henderson S, Petersen A: *Consuming health: The commodification of health care*, London, 2002, Routledge.

World Bank: *World development report 2002: building institutions for markets*, New York, 2002, Oxford University Press.

World Bank: *A better investment climate for everyone: world development report*, Washington, DC, 2005, Oxford University Press.

World Health Organization: *World health report 2000*, Geneva, 2000a, WHO.

World Health Organization: *Global advisory group on nursing and midwifery*, Geneva, 2000b, WHO.

World Health Organization: *Health status statistics: mortality*. Available at http://www.who.int/healthinfo/statistics/indneonatalmortality/en/. Accessed December 5, 2010.

World Health Organization: *Reducing risks, promoting healthy life*, 2002, WHO.

World Health Organization: *Afghanistan health status update*, Geneva, 2002c, WHO.

World Health Organization: *WHO emergency and humanitarian action: Afghanistan*, Geneva, 2002b, WHO.

World Health Organization: *Health for all (press release)*, New York, 2002c, WHO.

World Health Organization: *Global meeting on future strategic directions for primary health care*, Geneva, 2003a, WHO.

World Health Organization: *Global tuberculosis control: surveillance, planning and financing*, Geneva, 2004a, WHO.

World Health Organization: *Health aspects of chemical and biological weapons: report of a WHO group of consultants*, ed 2, Geneva, 2004b, WHO.

World Health Organization: *Malaria*, Geneva, 2005a, WHO.

World Health Organization: *The international network to promote household water treatment and safe storage*, Geneva, 2005b, WHO.

World Health Organization: WHO estimates of the causes of death in children, *Lancet* 365(9465):1147–1152, 2005c.

World Health Organization Group of Consultants: *Updated report: health aspects of chemical and biological weapons*, Geneva, 2001, WHO.

World Health Organization/United Nations AIDS Program (WHO/UNAIDS): *WHO and UNAIDS continue to support use of nevirapine for prevention of mother-to-child HIV transmission (press statement)*, Geneva, March 22, 2002, WHO.

World Health Organization: *World health statistics*, 2009, WHO.

World Health Organization: *7th Global conference on health promotion*, 2010. Available at http://www.who.int/healthpromotion/conferences/7gchp/en/index.html. Accessed December 5, 2010.

World Health Organization: *Roll Back Malaria report confirms aid for malaria is working but predictable long-term funding is essential to achieve MDGs*, March 18, 2010, WHO.

World Health Organization, UNICEF, World Bank: *State of the World's Vaccines and immunizations*, ed 3, Geneva, WHO, 2009.

World Resources Institute. *What are the effects of climate change?* Retrieved December 22, 2010 from http://www.wri.org/publication/hot-climate-cool-commerce/what-are-effects-of-climate-change.

Yun H, Jie S, Anli J: Nursing shortage in China: state, causes, and strategy, *Nurs Outlook* 58(3):122–128, 2010.

Influences on Health Care Delivery and Population-Centered Nursing

As has been discussed in Part One, the U.S. health care system is criticized for its rapidly rising health care costs, unevenness in the level and quality of services provided from one area of the country to another as well as for people in different age and socioeconomic groups. There is also concern about the equality of access to health services. Since 2008, when the recession began in the United States, there have been an increasing number of people who live in poverty. The poverty rate in 2009 of 14.3% increased from 13.2% in 2008. In 2009 it was estimated that 43.6 million people in the United States were living in poverty. Some of the reasons for the poverty have to do with the decreased numbers of people who have full-time year-round jobs. Without the stability of a full-time, year-round job, many people are without adequate health insurance, and a sizable number of individuals and families have lost their homes because of foreclosures. There are many other Americans who have remained employed yet their salaries have not increased in the last 3 years. These flat salaries have not allowed the workers to keep pace with the increasing costs of consumer products and services.

Although the costs of health care have grown in recent years, local, state and federal funding for public health care has not grown. The vast majority of the money spent on health care in the United States is for acute care. Approximately 5% of the total health care budget is spent on the aspects of public health that could make a difference in the health of the citizens: health promotion and disease prevention. The allocation of funds may shift if significant health care reform does occur.

As mentioned, there are early indications that prevention, coordination, and community based care will be increasingly supported. As a result of the national debates—and some say "arguments" about health care reform—legal, economic, ethical, social, cultural, political, and health-policy issues have grown in importance. Now more than ever in the history of population-centered nursing, nurses must understand how these issues affect their practice and the outcomes of care. Nurses need to continue learning how their knowledge, skills, and voice can influence the decisions about health care. As health care, including public health care, changes, nurses as the largest public health provider workforce must be a force in redefining the renewed public health system. Understanding the issues that affect decisions about health care priorities is imperative. Knowledge is power.

The chapters in Part Two discuss important economic, ethical, cultural, and policy issues that affect nurses in general, and population-centered nurses specifically.

CHAPTER 5

Economics of Health Care Delivery

Marcia Stanhope, RN, DSN, FAAN

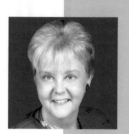

Dr. Marcia Stanhope is currently a professor at the University of Kentucky College of Nursing, Lexington, Kentucky. She has been appointed to the Good Samaritan Foundation Chair and Professorship in Community Health Nursing. She has practiced community and home health nursing and has served as an administrator and consultant in home health, and she has been involved in the development of two nurse-managed centers. She has taught community health, public health, epidemiology, primary care nursing, and administration courses. Dr. Stanhope formerly directed the Division of Community Health Nursing and Administration and was Associate Dean in the College of Nursing at the University of Kentucky. She has been responsible for both undergraduate and graduate courses in community-oriented nursing. She has also taught at the University of Virginia and the University of Alabama, Birmingham. Her presentations and publications have been in the areas of home health, community health and community-focused nursing practice, nurse managed centers, and primary care nursing.

ADDITIONAL RESOURCES

evolve WEBSITE
http://evolve.elsevier.com/Stanhope
- *Healthy People 2020*
- WebLinks
- Quiz
- Case Studies
- Glossary
- Answers to Practice Application
- Resource Tools

— Resource Tool 2.A: Select Major Historical Events Depicting Financial Involvement of Federal Government in Health Care Diversity

APPENDIX
Appendix G.4: The Health Insurance Portability and Accountability Act (HIPAA): What Does It Mean for Public Health Nurses?

OBJECTIVES

After reading this chapter, the student should be able to do the following:

1. Relate public health and economic principles to nursing and health care.
2. Describe the economic theories of microeconomics and macroeconomics.
3. Identify major factors influencing national health care spending.
4. Analyze the role of government and other third-party payers in health care financing.
5. Identify mechanisms for public health financing of services.
6. Discuss the implications of health care rationing from an economic perspective.
7. Evaluate levels of prevention as they relate to public health economics.

KEY TERMS

CHAPTER OUTLINE

Public Health and Economics
Principles of Economics
    Supply and Demand
    Efficiency and Effectiveness
    Macroeconomics
    Measures of Economic Growth
    Economic Analysis Tools
Factors Affecting Resource Allocation in Health Care
    The Uninsured
    The Poor
    Access to Care
    Rationing Health Care
    Healthy People 2020
Primary Prevention
The Context of the U.S. Health Care System
    First Phase
    Second Phase

    Third Phase
    Fourth Phase
    Challenges for the Twenty-First Century
Trends in Health Care Spending
Factors Influencing Health Care Costs
    Demographics Affecting Health Care
    Technology and Intensity
    Chronic Illness
Financing of Health Care
    Public Support
    Public Health
    Other Public Support
    Private Support
Health Care Payment Systems
    Paying Health Care Organizations
    Paying Health Care Practitioners

There is strong evidence to suggest that poverty can be directly related to poorer health outcomes. Poorer health outcomes lead to reduced educational outcomes for children, poor nutrition, low productivity in the adult workforce, and unstable economic growth in a population, community, or nation. However, improving health status and economic health is dependent on the "degree of equality" in policies that improve living standards for all members of a population including the poor. To move toward improving a population's health, there must be an "investment in public health" by all levels of government (Anderson et al, 2006).

Estimates indicate that public spending on health care makes a difference but needs the support of increased private health care spending to improve the overall health status of populations (Trust for America's Health, 2009). Several facts are known from the literature (Kaiser Family Foundation, 2009; Mantone, 2006; NCPP, 2007; RWJF, 2009; U.S. Census Bureau, 2010):

- Approximately 49.4 million (16%) of an estimated 308.4 million people in the United States are without health insurance. This number is expected to grow rapidly by 2015 (RWJF, 2009; U.S. Census Bureau, 2010).
- More than 8 in 10 (80%) of the uninsured are in working families (Kaiser Family Foundation, 2009).
- About 66% are from families with one or more full-time workers.
- 14% are from families with part-time workers.
- Only 19% of the uninsured are from families that have no connection to the workforce.
- Persons with money and/or health insurance are more likely to seek health care, but in 2009 the number without health insurance at some time in the year rose to 58% of the total population, including many middle income persons.
- The poor are not as healthy as persons with middle to higher incomes.
- The poor are more likely to receive health care through publicly funded agencies.
- Preventable hospitalizations can be reduced in vulnerable populations when public health and ambulatory clinics are available.
- An emphasis on individual health care will not guarantee improvement of a population or a community's health.

Approximately 97% of all health care dollars are spent for individual care whereas only 3% are spent on population level health care. The 3% includes monies spent by the government on public health as well as the preventive health care dollars spent by private sources. These numbers indicate that there is not a large investment in the public's health or population health in the United States (NCHS, 2010).

The United States spends more on health care than any other nation. The cost of health care has been rising more than the rate of inflation since the mid 1960s, yet the U.S. population does not enjoy better health as compared with nations that spend far less than the United States. The current health care system is at the point where it is not affordable (Turnock, 2008); Trust for America's Health, 2009). According to Trust for America's Health (2009), an estimated $10 per person invested in community-based prevention programs can lead to improved health status of the population and reduced health care costs. This return on investment represents medical cost savings only and does not include the significant gains that could be achieved in worker productivity, reduced absenteeism at work and school, and enhanced quality of life.

Nurses are challenged to implement changes in practice and participate in research, evidence-based practice, and policy activities designed to provide the best return on investment of health care dollars (i.e., to design models of care, at a reasonable price, that improve access or quality of care). Meeting this challenge requires a basic understanding of the economics of the U.S. health care system. Nurses should be aware of the effects of nursing practice on the delivery of cost-effective care.

PUBLIC HEALTH AND ECONOMICS

Economics is the science concerned with the use of resources, including the production, distribution, and consumption of goods and services. Health economics is concerned with how scarce resources affect the health care industry (McPake and Normand, 2008). Public health economics then focuses on the production, distribution, and consumption of goods and services as related to public health and where limited public resources might best be spent to save lives or best increase the quality of life (WordIQ.com, 2010). Economics provides the means to evaluate society's attainment of its wants and needs in relation to limited resources. In addition to the day-to-day decision-making about the use of resources, there is a focus on evaluating economics in health care (McPake and Normand, 2008). While in the past there has been limited focus on evaluating public health economics, it is becoming more obvious what evaluating public health and preventive care can do in terms of cost savings and, more importantly, quality of life (Trust for America's Health, 2009). This type of evaluation will help to present challenges to public policy makers (legislators). Public health financing often causes conflict because the views and priorities of individuals and groups in society may differ with those of the public health care industry. If money is spent on public health care, then money for other public needs, such as education, transportation, recreation, and defense, may be limited. When trying to argue that more money should be spent for population-level health care or prevention, data are becoming available that show the investment is a good one. Public health finance is a growing field of science and practice that involves the acquiring, managing, and using of monies to improve the health of populations through disease prevention and health promotion strategies. This field of study also focuses on evaluating the use of the money and the impact on the public health system (Honoré, 2008).

Although the public health system had been considered for many years as involving only government public health agencies such as health departments, today the public health system is known to be much broader and includes schools, industry, media, environmental protection agencies, voluntary organizations, civic groups, local police and fire departments, religious organizations, industry/business, and private sector health care systems, including the insurance industry. All can play a key role in improving population health (IOM, 2003; Trust for America's Health, 2009).

THE CUTTING EDGE *In 2010, a new health reform law, the Patient Protection and Affordable Care Act (PL 111-148) was passed by Congress and signed into law on March 23, 2010.*

The goal of public health finance is "to support population focused preventive health services" (Honoré, 2008). Four principles are suggested that explain how public health financing may occur.
- The source and use of monies are controlled solely by the government.
- The government controls the money, but the private sector controls how the money is used.
- The private sector controls the money, but the government controls how the money is used.
- The private sector controls the money and how it is used (Gillespie et al, 2004; Moulton et al, 2004).

When the government provides the funding and controls the use, the monies come from taxes, user fees (e.g., license fees and purchase of alcohol/cigarettes), and charges to consumers of the services. Services offered at the federal government level include the following:
- Policy making
- Public health protection
- Collecting and sharing information about U.S. health care and delivery systems
- Building capacity for population health
- Direct care services

Select examples of services offered at the state and local levels include the following:
- Maternal and child health
- Family planning
- Counseling
- Preventing communicable and infectious diseases
- Direct care services (see Chapter 46 for more examples)

When the government provides the money but the private sector decides how it is used, the money comes from business and individual tax savings related to private spending for illness prevention care. When a business provides disease prevention and health promotion services to its employees and sometimes families, such as immunizations, health screenings, and counseling, the business taxes owed to the government are reduced. This is considered a means by which the government provides money through tax savings to businesses to use for population health care.

When the private sector provides the money but the government decides how it is used, either voluntarily or involuntarily, the money is used for preventive care services for specific populations. A voluntary example is the private contributions made to reaching *Healthy People 2010* goals. An involuntary example is the Occupational Safety and Health Administration requiring industry to adhere to certain safety standards for use of machinery, air quality, ventilation, and eyewear protection to reduce disease and injury. This, for example, has the effect of reducing occupation-related injuries in the population as a whole.

When the private sector is responsible for both the money and its use of resources, the benefits incurred are many. For example, an industry may offer influenza vaccine clinics for

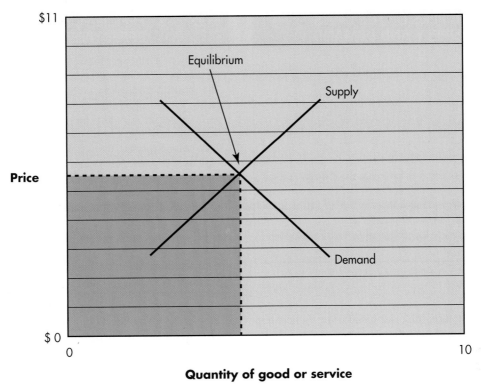

FIGURE 5-1 Supply-and-demand curve.

workers and families that may lead to "herd immunity" in the community (see Chapter 12 on epidemiology). A business or community may institute a "no-smoking" policy that reduces the risk of smoking-related illnesses to workers, family, and the consumers of the businesses' services. A voluntary philanthropic organization may give a local school money to provide preventive care and health education to the children of the school (Stanhope et al, 2008).

These are but a few examples of how public health services and the ensuring of a healthy population are not only government related. The partnerships between government and the private sector are necessary to improve the overall health status of populations.

PRINCIPLES OF ECONOMICS

Knowledge about health economics is particularly important to nurses because they are the ones who are often in a position to allocate resources to solve a problem or to design, plan, coordinate, and evaluate community-based health services and programs. Two branches of economics are important to understand for their application in health care: microeconomics and macroeconomics. **Microeconomic theory** deals with the behaviors of individuals and organizations and the effects of those behaviors on prices, costs, and the allocating and distributing of resources. Economic behaviors are based on: (1) individual or organization choices and the consumer's level of satisfaction with a particular good (product) or service, or use, and (2) the amount of money available to an individual or organization to spend on a particular good or service (its **budget limits**). Microeconomics applied to health care looks at the behaviors of

individuals and organizations that result from tradeoffs in the use of a service and budget limits.

The microeconomic example of the industry providing preventive services to its employees represents a behavior by the industry that provides for the use of a service and helps the industry's budget by reducing health care insurance premium costs. The terms of the Patient Protection and Affordable Health Care Act (2010) allow employers to provide incentive rewards to employees for participation in wellness programs. Providing the service also increases worker productivity and promotes a healthier workforce, thus enhancing economic growth (Hall, 2010).

Because of the unique characteristics of health care, some economists believe that health care is special. There are debates about whether health care markets can ensure that health care is delivered efficiently to consumers. Cost–benefit and cost-effectiveness analyses are techniques used to judge the effect of interventions and policies on a particular outcome, such as health status (Veney and Kaluzny, 2005).

Supply and Demand

Two basic principles of microeconomic theory are **supply** and **demand,** both of which are affected by price. A simple illustration of the relationship between supply and demand is provided in Figure 5-1. The upward-sloping supply curve represents the seller's side of the **market,** and the downward-sloping demand curve reflects the buyer's desire for a given product. As shown here, suppliers are willing to offer increasing amounts of a good or service in the market for an increasing price (Colander, 2008). The demand curve represents the amount of a good or service the consumer is willing to purchase at a certain price. This curve illustrates that when few quantities of a good or service are

BOX 5-1 PRINCIPLES OF THE LAWS OF SUPPLY AND DEMAND

The Law of Supply
- At higher prices, producers are willing to offer *more* products for sale than at lower prices.
- The supply increases as prices increase and decreases as prices decrease.
- Those already in business will try to increase productions as a way of increasing profits.

The Law of Demand
- People will buy more of a product at a lower price than at a higher price, if nothing changes.
- At a lower price, more people can afford to buy more goods and more of an item more frequently than they can at a higher price.
- At lower prices, people tend to buy some goods as a substitute for more-expensive goods.

From Curriculum Link, 2010. Available at www.curriculumlink.org. Accessed December 8, 2010.

BOX 5-2 EFFICIENCY VERSUS EFFECTIVENESS

To illustrate the differences between efficiency and effectiveness, consider the case of a nurse who is designing a community outreach program to educate high-risk, first-time mothers about the importance of childhood immunizations. The most *efficient* method to disseminate the information to a large number of mothers might be to have the child health team from the public health department hold an evening educational session, open to the public, at the health department. The most *effective* means of offering the program might be to link public health nurses with new mothers for one-on-one, in-home counseling, demonstration, and follow-up. The goals of the program could be stated as follows:
- To change the behavior of the mothers regarding providing immunizations for their children
- To increase community mothers' knowledge and awareness of infectious diseases
- To reduce the incidence of preventable infections in the community
- To decrease the number of hospital admissions

available in the marketplace, the price tends to be higher than when larger quantities are available. The point on the curve where the supply and demand curves cross is the equilibrium, or the point where producer and consumer desires meet. Supply and demand curves can shift up or down as a result of the following factors (McPate and Normand, 2008):
- Competition for a good or service
- An increase in the costs of materials used to make a product
- Technological advances
- A change in consumer preferences
- Shortages of goods or services

Box 5-1 provides a review of the laws of supply and demand.

Using the example of industry-offered health care, it is not likely that a small industry of fewer than 50 employees may be able to offer incentive based on-site illness prevention services. The demand may be great to keep employees healthy and on the job. The supply is limited by the cost and numbers of services available in the community. Therefore, the cost is likely to be higher for the small business than for the large industry that offers its own services.

Efficiency and Effectiveness

Two other terms are related to microeconomics: efficiency and effectiveness. Efficiency refers to producing maximal output, such as a good or service, using a given set of resources (or inputs), such as labor, time, and available money. Efficiency suggests that the inputs are combined and used in such a way that there is no better way to produce the service, or output, and that no other improvements can be made. The word *efficiency* often focuses on time, or speed in performing tasks, and the minimizing of waste, or unused input, during production. Although these notions are true, efficiency depends on tasks as well as processes of producing a good or service and the improvements made (Veney and Kaluzny, 2005).

Effectiveness, on the other hand, refers to the extent to which a health care service meets a stated goal or objective, or how well a program or service achieves what is intended. For example, the effectiveness of a mass immunization program is related to the level of "herd immunity" developed to reduce the problem that the program was addressing (see Chapter 12). Box 5-2 illustrates the differences between efficiency and effectiveness (Veney and Kaluzny, 2005).

Macroeconomics

Microeconomics focuses on the individual or an organization, whereas macroeconomic theory focuses on the "big picture"—the total, or aggregate, of all individuals and organizations (e.g., behaviors such as growth, expansion, or decline of an aggregate). In macroeconomics, the aggregate is usually a country or nation. Factors such as levels of income, employment, general price levels, and rate of economic growth are important. This aggregate approach reflects, for example, the contribution of all organizations and groups within health care, or all industry within the United States, including health care, on the nation's economic outlook.

> **DID YOU KNOW?** *When the media refer to "the economy," the phrase is typically used as a macroeconomic term to describe the wealth and financial performance of the nation as an aggregate. Health care contributes to the economy through goods and services produced and employment opportunities.*

The primary focuses of macroeconomics are the business cycle and economic growth. Business expands and contracts in cycles. These cycles are influenced by a number of factors, such as political changes (a new president is elected), policy changes (a new legislation is implemented, like the Patient Protection and Affordable Health Care Act of 2010), knowledge and technology advances (a new vaccine to treat H1N1 is placed on the market), or simply the belief by a recognized business leader that the cycle is or should be shifting (e.g., when the head of the Federal Reserve Board changes interest rates).

The human capital approach is a measure of macroeconomic theory (Goodwin et al, 2008). In this approach improving human qualities, such as health, are a focus for developing and spending money on goods and services because health is valued; it increases productivity, enhances the income-earning ability of people, and improves the economy. Therefore, there is a positive rate of return on the "investment in human capital." The individual, population, community, and nation all benefit. If the population is healthy, premature morbidity and mortality is reduced, chronic disease and disability are reduced, and economic losses to the nation are reduced.

Measures of Economic Growth

Economic growth reflects an increase in the output of a nation. Two common measures of economic growth are the **gross national product** (GNP) and the **gross domestic product** (GDP). GNP is the total market value of all goods and services produced in an economy during a period of time (e.g., quarterly or annually). GDP is the total market value of the output of labor and property located in the United States (USDHHS, 2004). GDP reflects only the national U.S. output, whereas GNP reflects national output plus income earned by U.S. businesses or citizens, whether within the United States or internationally. This discussion focuses on GDP, because U.S. health care spending reports are based on GDP (NCHS, 2010).

Nurses face microeconomic and macroeconomic issues every day. For example, they are influenced by microeconomics when referring clients for services, informing clients and others of the cost of services, assessing community need for a particular service, evaluating client access to services, and determining health provider and agency response to client needs. Nurses who work with aggregates of individuals and communities are faced with macroeconomic issues, such as health policies that make the development of new programs possible; local, state, and federal budgets that support certain programs; and the total effect that services will have on improving the health of the community and reducing the poverty level of the population. In short, knowledge about health economics can enhance a nurse's ability to understand and argue a position for meeting population health needs.

Economic Analysis Tools

The primary methods used to assess the economics of an intervention are **cost–benefit analysis** (CBA), **cost-effectiveness analysis** (CEA), and **cost-utility analysis** (CUA). CBA is considered the best of these methods. In simple form, CBA involves the listing of all costs and benefits that are expected to occur from an intervention during a prescribed time. Costs and benefits are adjusted for time and inflation. If the total benefits are greater than the total costs, the intervention has a *net positive value* (NPV). Future or continued funding is given to the intervention with the highest NPV. This technique provides a way to estimate overall program and social benefits in terms of net costs.

CBA requires that all costs and benefits be known and be able to be quantified in dollars; herein lies the major problem with its use. Although it is fairly easy to estimate the direct dollar costs of a health care program, it is often very difficult to quantify the non-dollar benefits and indirect costs. For example, benefits and costs could come in the form of increased income and expenses, which are fairly easy to measure. More difficult to measure are benefits such as improved community welfare resulting from a particular program, and the costs to the community that would result if the program did not exist. The value of *potential lives* lost because of lack of access to health care services is one example. The potential for a great number of lives lost from H1N1 resulted in the development of programs and monies invested with pharmaceutical companies in an attempt to reduce the risk of lives lost should the U.S. experience an epidemic from this disease risk. Although benefits could only be assumed from the cost investment, it was determined that the investment was essential (CDC, 2009).

CEA expresses the net direct and indirect costs and cost savings in terms of a defined health outcome. The total net costs are calculated and divided by the number of health outcomes. Although the data required for CEA are the same as for CBA, CEA does not require that a dollar value be put on the outcome (e.g., on an outcome such as quality of life). CEA is best used when comparing two or more strategies or interventions that have the same health outcome in the population. Both CEA and CBA are useful to nurses as they conduct community needs analyses and develop, propose, implement, and evaluate programs to meet community health needs. In both cases, the cost of a particular program or intervention is examined relative to the money spent and outcomes achieved.

An objective commonly used when CEA is performed in health care is improvement in **quality of adjusted life-years** (QALYs) for clients. QALYs are the sum of years of life multiplied by the quality of life in each of those years. The QALY assigns a value, ranging between 0 (death) and 1 (perfect health), to reflect quality of life during a given period of years (Hazen, 2007). In conducting a CEA, the cost of a program or an intervention is compared with real or expected improvements in clients' quality of life. The How To box lists the steps involved in conducting a CEA. The QALY is often used in malpractice suits to award money to clients who have been injured by health care.

HOW TO Do a Cost–Effectiveness Analysis (CEA)

In a CEA, the outcome of the service option is measured in a natural, non-monetary unit such as length of stay, years of life gained, therapeutic successes, or lives saved. Results are expressed as the net cost required to produce an outcome. The cost to outcome is expressed as a ratio of cost per unit of outcome, where the numerator is a monetary value corresponding to the net expenditure of resources and the denominator is the net improvement in health expressed in non-monetary terms. The steps for performing a CEA are as follows:

1. *Establish program or service goals and objectives.*
2. *Consider all possible alternatives to achieve the goal or objectives.*

DID YOU KNOW? *The value of money varies over time. Today's dollar is worth more than tomorrow's dollar. The causes include inflation and interest rates.*

3. *Measure net effects to reflect a change in health status or health outcome.*
4. *Analyze costs for each alternative (adjusting costs for time and inflation) and conduct final CEA on marginal costs rather than on total costs.*
5. *Use multivariate sensitivity analysis and modeling to assess the effect of random error on the cost-effectiveness ratio.*
6. *Combine CEA results with other types of information, not included in the CEA, to make the most appropriate therapeutic or policy decision.*

Depending on program or intervention goals, the most effective means of providing a service is not necessarily the least costly, particularly in the short run. This is particularly true in public health, when the cost-effectiveness of a preventive service may not be known until sometime in the future. For example, the total cost savings of a community no-smoking program might be difficult to project 10 years into the future. After 10 years, the number of lung cancer cases or deaths that have occurred can be compared with those in the 10 years before the program, and the cost-effectiveness of the no-smoking program can be shown. The Trust for America's Health (2008), along with a number of other agencies, is publishing reports that are beginning to show positive results and cost savings from prevention programs.

FACTORS AFFECTING RESOURCE ALLOCATION IN HEALTH CARE

The distribution of health care is affected largely by the way in which health care is financed in the United States. Third-party coverage, whether public or private, greatly affects the distribution of health care. Also, socioeconomic status affects health care consumption, since it determines the ability to purchase insurance or to pay directly out-of-pocket. The effects of barriers to health care access and the effects of health care rationing on the distribution of health care follow. Although the barriers are still issues, it remains to be determined how health care reform of 2010 will change the barriers to access and distribution.

The Uninsured

In 1996 68% of the total U.S. population had private health insurance. An additional 15% received insurance through public programs, and 17%, or 37 million, were uninsured. In 2006 the number of uninsured persons had increased to 46 million. The typical uninsured person is a member of the workforce or a dependent of this worker. Uninsured workers are likely to be in low-paying jobs, part-time or temporary jobs, or jobs at small businesses (Kaiser Family Foundation, 2009). These uninsured workers cannot afford to purchase health insurance, or their employers may not offer health insurance as a benefit. Others who are typically uninsured are young adults (especially young men), minorities, persons less than 65 years of age in good or fair health, and the poor or near poor. These individuals may be unable to afford insurance, may lack access to job-based coverage, or, because of their age or good health status, may

not perceive the need for insurance. Because of the eligibility requirements for Medicaid, the near poor are actually more likely to be uninsured than the poor.

Because of frustrations with the problems of lack of health insurance, The Patient Protection and Affordable Care Act was passed in 2010. This bill became law as a result of a promise to the American public by President Obama that health care reform would occur as part of his presidential agenda. Basically this law speaks to the following:

- Quality, affordable health care for all Americans
- A defined role of public programs
- Improving the quality and efficiency of health care
- Prevention of chronic disease and improving public health
- Health care workforce
- Transparency and program integrity
- Improving access to innovative medical therapies
- Community living assistance services and supports
- Revenue provisions

Prior to the passing of this act,

- Twenty-five states were considering making it mandatory for employers to provide insurance coverage
- Seven states were looking at approaches to universal coverage
- Six states were considering the development of universal health care plan commissions

However, only three states had passed comprehensive health care reform by 2008: Massachusetts, Maine, and Vermont. State fiscal capacity, structural deficits, and then a worsening economy and severe state budget shortfalls limited states' ability to further advance coverage initiatives. Although the experiences of pace-setting states will inform future federal action, the fiscal crisis makes it difficult for many states to achieve health care reform on their own.

As the health care reform debate progresses, the impact of federal reform on states will have differential effects. In general, states with more extensive poverty, higher budget shortfalls, lower eligibility levels for public programs, higher rates of uninsured, and more primary care shortages will be greatly affected (Kaiser Family Foundation, 2010a).

The Poor

Socioeconomic status is inversely related to mortality and morbidity for almost every disease. Poor Americans with an income below poverty level have a mortality rate nearly several times greater than that of middle-income Americans, even after accounting for age, sex, race, education, and risky health behaviors (e.g., smoking, drinking, overeating, and lack of exercise). Historically, the link between poor health and socioeconomic status resulted from poor housing, malnutrition, inadequate sanitation, and hazardous occupations. Today, explanations include the cumulative effects of a number of characteristics that explain the concept of poverty. These characteristics include low educational levels, unemployment or low occupational status (blue collar or unskilled laborer), low wages, being a child or an older person over the age of 65 years, or being a member of a minority group (NCHS, 2010).

Access to Care

Access to care is a public health issue *(Healthy People 2020)*. Medicaid is intended to improve access to health care for the poor. Although persons with Medicaid have improved access compared with the uninsured, Medicaid recipients are only about half as likely to obtain needed health services (e.g., medical-surgical care, dental care, prescription drugs, and eyeglasses) as the privately insured. Specifically, the poorest Americans have Medicaid insurance, yet they also have the worst health (Kaiser Family Foundation, 2009).

The primary reasons for delay, difficulty, or failure to access care include inability to afford health care and a variety of insurance-related reasons, including the insurer not approving, covering, or paying for care; the client having preexisting conditions; and physicians refusing to accept the insurance plan. Other barriers include lack of transportation, physical barriers, communication problems, child care needs, lack of time or information, or refusal of services by providers. In addition, lack of after-hours care, long office waits, and long travel distance are cited as access barriers. Community characteristics also contribute to individuals' ability to access care. For example, the limited prevalence of managed care and the limited number of safety net providers, as well as the wealth and size of the community, affect accessibility.

Because reimbursement for services provided to Medicaid recipients has been low, physicians are discouraged from serving this population. Thus, people on Medicaid frequently have no primary care provider and may rely on the emergency department for primary care services. Although physicians can respond to monetary incentives in client selection, emergency departments are required by law to evaluate every client regardless of ability to pay. Emergency department co-payments are modest and are frequently waived if the client is unable to pay. Thus, low out-of-pocket costs provide incentives for Medicaid clients and the uninsured to use emergency departments for primary care services.

With the Patient Protection and Affordable Health Care Act (PL 111-148), some of the issues and barriers that have previously existed may disappear. This depends on whether Congress decides to repeal all or part of PL 111-148 or change some of the mandates in the law. By 2014 Medicaid recipients may benefit from the law in its current structure as follows: (1) expansion of Medicaid to include all non-Medicare eligible persons under age 65 with incomes up to 133% of federal poverty level, (2) all Medicaid-eligible persons will be guaranteed a benchmark benefit package, and (3) states will be given the option to develop a basic health plan for uninsured individuals who do not qualify for the Medicaid program, at 133% to 200% of poverty level.

Poverty level income is adjusted annually for each state by the federal government to indicate how much money an individual or families may earn to qualify for subsidies such as food stamps, Medicaid, and Children's Health Insurance Program. In 2010 the federal poverty level for an individual was $10,830; for a family of four the poverty level was $22,050. If an individual was 133% of poverty level, then the individual earned no more than $14,403 (USDHHS, 2010).

LEVELS OF PREVENTION

Economic Prevention Strategies

Primary Prevention
Work with legislators and insurance companies to provide coverage for health promotion to reduce the risk of diseases.

Secondary Prevention
Encourage clients who are pregnant to participate in prenatal care and WIC to increase the number of healthy babies and reduce the costs related to preterm baby care.

Tertiary Prevention
Participate in home visits to mothers who are at risk for neglecting babies to reduce the costs related to abuse.

Rationing Health Care

Rationing health care in any form implies reduced access to care and potential decreases in acceptable quality of services offered. For example, a health provider's refusal to accept Medicare or Medicaid clients is a form of rationing. As with access to care, rationing health care is a public health issue. Where care is not provided, the public health system and nurses must ensure that essential clinical services are available. Managed care was thought to offer the possibility of more appropriate health care access and better-organized care to meet basic health care needs of the total population. A shift in the general approach to health care from a reactionary, acute-care orientation toward a proactive, primary prevention orientation is necessary to achieve not only a more cost-effective but also a more equitable health care system in the United States. PL 111-148, while providing coverage to more people, will not do away with rationing because the new law provides for a four-tiered plan (bronze, silver, gold, and platinum) by creating state-based American Health Benefit Exchanges. Persons at differing levels of poverty will have reductions in out-of-pocket expenses based on income up to 400% of poverty level and may receive tax credits and subsidies to assist with out-of-pocket expenses.

Healthy People 2020

Healthy People 2020 goals are examples of strategies to provide better access for all people. The Levels of Prevention box shows the levels of economic prevention strategies.

PRIMARY PREVENTION

Society's investment in the health care system has been based on the premise that more health services will result in better health, but non–health care factors also have an effect. Of the major factors that affect health—personal biology and behavior (or lifestyle), environmental factors and policies (including physical, social, health, cultural, and economic environments), social networks, living and working conditions, and the health care system—medical services are said to have the least effect. Behavior and lifestyle have been shown to have the greatest effect, with the environment and biology accounting for the greatest effect on the development of all illnesses (NCHS, 2009).

Despite the significant impact of behavior and environment on health, estimates indicate that 97% of health care dollars are spent on secondary and tertiary care. Such a reactionary, secondary-care system results in high-cost, high-technology, and disease-specific care and is consistent with the U.S. system's traditional emphasis on "sickness care." A more proactive investment in disease prevention and health promotion targeted at improving health behaviors, lifestyle, and the environment has the potential to improve health status of populations, thereby improving quality of life while reducing health care costs. The USDHHS has argued that a higher value should be placed on primary prevention. The goal of this approach is to preserve and maximize *human capital* by providing health promotion and social practices that result in less disease. An emphasis on primary prevention may reduce dollars spent and increase quality of life.

The return on investment in primary prevention through gains in human capital has not been acknowledged in the past, unfortunately. Consequently, large investments in primary prevention and public health care have not been made. Reasons given for this lack of emphasis on prevention in clinical practice and lack of financial investment in prevention include the following:

- Provider uncertainty about which clients should receive services and at what intervals
- Lack of information about preventive services
- Negative attitudes about the importance of preventive care
- Lack of time for delivery of preventive services
- Delayed or absent feedback regarding success of preventive measures
- Less reimbursement for these services than curative services
- Lack of organization to deliver preventive services
- Lack of use of services by the poor and elderly
- More out-of-pocket expenses for the poor and those who lack health insurance

A focus on prevention could mean reducing the need for and use of medical, dental, hospital, and health provider services. Under **fee-for-service** payment arrangements, this would mean that the health care system, the largest employer in the United States, would be reduced in size and would become less profitable. However, with the increasing costs of health care and consumer demand and the changes in financing mechanisms, there is a new trend toward financing more preventive care services.

Today, third-party payers are beginning to cover preventive services, recognizing that the growth of the health care system can no longer be supported. Under capitated health plans, health care providers stand to make money by keeping clients healthy and reducing health care use. Through combining client interests with financial interests of the health care industry, primary prevention and public health can be raised to the status and priority of acute care and chronic care. Despite difficulties, methods for determining prevention effectiveness, such as CEAs and CBAs, are becoming standard and used more widely. Two agendas for preventive services are published that promote the preventive agenda:

- The U.S. Preventive Services Task Force, Guide to Clinical Preventive Services (AHRQ, 2009) for clinicians in primary care that outlines the regular screening and risk factors to look for at various ages

HEALTHY PEOPLE 2020

Objectives Related to Access to Care

- AHS-1: Increase the proportion of persons with health insurance.
- AHS-2: (Developmental) Increase the proportion of insured persons with coverage for clinical preventive services.
- AHS-6: Reduce the proportion of individuals that experience difficulties or delays in obtaining necessary medical care, dental care, or prescription medicines.

- The Community Preventive Services Task Force (2006) that emphasizes population level interventions to promote primary prevention

Regardless of the method, prevention-effectiveness analyses (PEAs) are outcome oriented. This area of research seeks to link interventions with health outcomes and economic outcomes, and to reveal the tradeoffs between the two. In theory, support for increasing national investment in primary prevention is sound and long standing. Since the public health movement of the mid-nineteenth century, public health officials, epidemiologists, and nurses have been working to advance the agenda of primary prevention to the forefront of the health care industry. Today, these efforts continue across a number of disciplines and in both the public and the private sectors, and through the efforts for health care reform (PL 111-148, 2010).

THE CONTEXT OF THE U.S. HEALTH CARE SYSTEM

The U.S. health care system is a diverse collection of industries that are involved directly or indirectly in providing health care services. The major players in the industry are the health professionals who provide health care services, pharmacy and equipment suppliers, insurers (public/government and private), managed care plans (health maintenance organizations, preferred provider organizations), and other groups, such as educational institutions, consulting and research firms, professional associations, and trade unions. Today, the health care industry is large, and its characteristics and operations differ between rural and urban geographic areas.

In the twenty-first century, health policy and national politics reflect the importance of health care delivery in the general economy. Conflicts arise between competing special-interest groups who have different goals and objectives when it comes to the producing and consuming of health services. To some degree this is caused by federal and state policy changes about how health services are financed (public and private).

Figure 5-2 illustrates the four basic components that make up the framework of health services delivery: service needs and intensity, facilities, technology, and labor. **Intensity** is the extent of use of technologies, supplies, and health care services by or for the client. Intensity includes and is a partial measure of the use of technology (Kropf, 2005). **Medical technology** refers to the set of techniques, drugs, equipment, and procedures used by health care professionals in delivering medical care to individuals. It also includes information technology and the system within which such care is delivered (NCHS, 2010).

Health care systems have developed in four phases from the 1800s through 2000. These developmental stages correspond to different economic conditions. Developmentally, the four components of the health services delivery framework have changed over time, reflecting macro-level, or societal, changes in morbidity and mortality, national health policy, and economics (Figure 5-3).

First Phase

The first developmental stage (1800–1900) was characterized by epidemics of infectious diseases, such as cholera, typhoid, smallpox, influenza, malaria, and yellow fever. Health concerns

of the time related to social and public health issues, including contaminated food and water supplies, inadequate sewage disposal, and poor housing conditions (Lee and Estes, 2003). Family and friends provided most health care in the home. Hospitals were few in number and suffered from overcrowding, disease, and unsanitary conditions. Sick persons who were cared for in hospitals often died as a result of these conditions. Most people avoided being cared for in a hospital unless there was no alternative. In this first developmental phase, health care was paid for by individuals who could afford it, through bartering with physicians or through charity from individuals or organizations. The first county health departments were established in 1908.

Technology to aid in disease control was very basic and practical but in keeping with the knowledge of the time. The physician's "black bag" contained the few medicines and tools available for treatment. The economics of health care was influenced by the types of health care providers and the number of practitioners, and the labor force then was composed mostly of physicians and nurses who attained their skills through apprenticeships, or on-the-job training. Nurses in the United States were predominantly female, and education was linked to religious orders that expected service, dedication, and charity (Kovner, 2005). The focus of nursing was primarily to support physicians and assist clients with activities of daily living.

Second Phase

The second developmental stage (1900–1945) of U.S. health care delivery was focused on the control of acute infectious diseases. Environmental conditions influencing health began to improve, with major advances in water purity, sanitary sewage disposal, milk and water quality, and urban housing quality. The health problems of this era were no longer mass epidemics but individual acute infections or traumatic episodes (Lee and Estes, 2003).

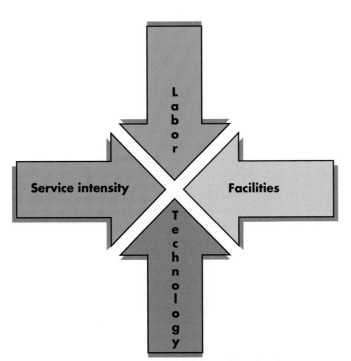

FIGURE 5-2 Components of health services development.

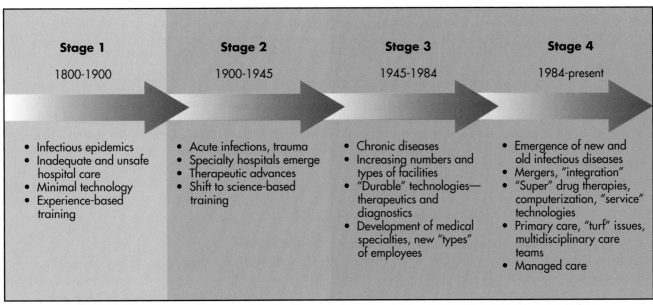

FIGURE 5-3 Developmental framework for health service needs and intensity, facilities, technology, and labor.

Hospitals and health departments experienced rapid growth during the late 1800s and early 1900s as technological advances in science were made (Kovner, 2005). In addition to private and charitable financing of health care, city, county, and state governments were beginning to contribute by providing services for poor persons, state mental institutions, and other specialty hospitals, such as tuberculosis hospitals. Public health departments were emphasizing case finding and quarantine. Although health care was paid for primarily by individuals, the Social Security Act of 1935 signaled the federal government's increasing interest in addressing social welfare problems.

Clinical medicine entered its golden age during this period. Major technological advances in surgery and childbirth and the identification of disease processes, such as the cause of pernicious anemia, increased the ability to diagnose and treat diseases. The first serological tests used as a tool for diagnosis and control of infectious diseases were developed in 1910 to detect syphilis and gonorrhea (Lee and Estes, 2003). The first virus isolation techniques were also developed to filter yellow fever virus, for example. The discovery and development of pharmacological agents, such as insulin in 1922 for control of diabetes, sulfa drugs in 1932 for treatment of infectious diseases, and antibiotics such as penicillin in the 1940s, eradicated certain infectious diseases, increased treatment options, and decreased morbidity and mortality (Lee and Estes, 2003).

Advances in technology and knowledge shifted physician education away from apprenticeships to scientifically based college education, which occurred as a result of the Flexner Report in 1910. It was the beginning of medical education as it is today. Nurses were trained primarily in hospital schools of nursing, with an emphasis on following and executing physicians' orders. Nurses in training were unmarried and under the age of 30. They provided the bulk of care in hospitals (Kovner, 2005). Public health nurses, who tracked infectious diseases and implemented quarantine procedures, worked more collegially with physicians (Kovner, 2005). In this period the university-based nursing programs were established to accommodate the expanding practice base of nursing. Client education became a nursing function early in the development of the health care delivery system.

Third Phase

The third developmental stage (1945–1984) included a shift away from acute infectious health problems of previous stages toward chronic health problems such as heart disease, cancer, and stroke. These illnesses resulted from increasing wealth and lifestyle changes in the United States. To meet society's needs, the number and types of facilities expanded to include, for example, hospital clinics and long-term care facilities. The Joint Commission on Accreditation of Hospitals, established in 1951 and later renamed The Joint Commission on Accreditation of Healthcare Organizations (and now called The Joint Commission [TJC]), focused on the safety and protection of the public and the delivery of quality care.

Changes in the overall health of American society also shifted the focus of technology, research, and development. Major technological advances included developments in the realms of chemotherapeutic agents; immunizations; anesthesia; electrolyte and cardiopulmonary physiology; diagnostic laboratories with complex modalities such as computerized tomography; organ and tissue transplants; radiation therapy; laser surgery; and specialty units for critical care, coronary care, and intensive care. The first "test tube baby" was born via in vitro fertilization, and other fertility advances soon emerged. Negative staining techniques for screening viruses via electronic microscope became available in the 1960s (Lee and Estes, 2003).

Health care providers constituted more than 5% of the total U.S. workforce during this period. The three largest health care employers were hospitals, convalescent institutions, and physicians' offices. Between 1970 and 1984 alone, the number of persons employed in the health care industry grew by 90%. The number of personnel employed in the community also increased. The expansion of care delivery into other sites, such as community-based clinics, increased not only the number but also the types of health care employees.

Technological advances brought about increased special training for physicians and nurses, and care was organized around these specialties. The ongoing shortage of nurses throughout the century was being seen in the 1970s and early 1980s. Nursing education expanded from hospital-based diploma and university-based baccalaureate education to include associate degree programs at the entry level. As the diploma schools of nursing began closing in the early- to mid-1980s, the number of baccalaureate and associate degree programs began to increase. Graduate nursing education expanded to include the nurse practitioner (NP) and clinical nurse specialist (CNS) to meet increasing demands for the education of nurses in a specialty such as public health. The first doctoral programs in nursing were instituted to build the scientific base for nursing and to increase the number of nurse faculty members.

The role of the commercial health insurance industry increased, and a strong link between employment and the providing of health care benefits emerged. Furthermore, the federal government's role expanded through landmark policy-making that would affect health care delivery well into the twenty-first century. Specifically, the passage of Titles XVIII and XIX of the Social Security Act in 1965 created the Medicare and Medicaid programs, respectively. The health care system appeared to have access to unlimited resources for growing and expanding.

Throughout the twentieth century, many public health advances were achieved. The life expectancy of U.S. citizens increased and has been related to public health activities. The most important achievements were in vaccinations, improved motor vehicle safety, safer workplaces, safer and healthier foods, healthier mothers and babies, family planning, fluoride in drinking water, and recognition of tobacco as a health hazard (CDC, 2001).

Fourth Phase

The fourth developmental stage (1984 to present) has been a period of limited resources, with an emphasis on containing costs, restricting growth in the health care industry, and reorganizing care delivery. For example, amendments were made to the Social Security Act in 1983 that created diagnostic-related groups and a prospective system of paying for health care provided to Medicare recipients. The 1997 Balanced Budget Act legislated additional federal changes in Medicare and Medicaid. Private-sector employer concerns about the rising costs of health care for employees and fear of profit losses spurred a major change in the delivery and financing of health care. Managed care systems were developed.

This period included drastic change in the settings and organization of health care delivery. Transforming health care organizations became commonplace, and buzz words of the period were reorganization, reengineering, restructuring, and downsizing. Organization mergers occurred at an increased rate to consolidate care, to save money, and to coordinate care across the continuum (i.e., from "cradle to grave"). Merger discussions focused on *horizontal integration*, which indicated the union of similar agencies (e.g., a merger of hospitals), and *vertical integration* between different types of organizations (e.g., an acute care hospital, long-term care institution, and a home health facility).

Initially these pressures brought about hospital closings and a shifting of care to other settings, such as ambulatory and community-based clinics and specialty diagnostic centers that offer technologies such as magnetic resonance imaging (MRI) and sonography. Rehabilitative, restorative, and palliative care, once delivered in the hospitals, was shifted to other settings, such as subacute care hospitals, specialty rehabilitation hospitals, long-term care institutions, and even individual homes. Although the basis of care delivery was no longer the traditional acute care hospital, the nature of the care delivered in hospitals changed remarkably, as evidenced by the following:

- Patients admitted to hospitals were more acutely ill.
- Length of stay for patients admitted to hospitals became shorter.
- Care delivery became more intense as a result of the first two items.

The widespread use of computers and the Internet enabled society to become increasingly sophisticated about health. The public's increasing knowledge about health care and awareness of health care advances influenced the demand for health care, such as diagnostic and therapeutic services for treatment. Furthermore, pharmaceutical companies and other technological suppliers actively marketed their products through television, printed advertisements, the Internet, and other sources, so clients rapidly became aware of the new technologies.

Health professionals were increasingly dependent on technology to care for clients. Distance, as a barrier to the diagnosis and treatment of disease, was overcome through the use of telehealth. The insurance industry became the principal buyer of technology for the client. They often made decisions about when and if a certain technology would be used for a client problem. Nurses became dependent on technologies to monitor client progress, make decisions about care, and deliver care in innovative ways.

The shift away from traditional hospital-based care to the community, together with the need to consider new models of care, brought about an increased emphasis on providing primary care, on developing care delivery teams, and on collaborating in practice and education. The substitution of one type of health personnel for another occurred to control care delivery costs. As examples, the NPs were replacing physicians as primary care providers, and unlicensed personnel were replacing staff nurses in hospitals and long-term care facilities. These replacements caused much debate, with territorial, or "turf," battles, for example, between physicians and nurses.

The increase in specialization by health professionals led to changes in certification, qualifications, education, and standards of care in health professions. These factors, in turn, caused an increase in the number and kinds of providers to meet the demands of the health care system. The Bureau of Labor Statistics (2006) predicted that health care employment would be among the top eight professional and related industries, with significant employment growth through 2014.

In the last part of the twentieth century, molecular tools were developed that provided a means of detecting and characterizing infectious disease pathogens and a new capacity to track the transmission of new threats, such as bioterrorism, and determine new ways to treat them.

Challenges for the Twenty-First Century

In the twenty-first century the emergence of new and the reemergence of old communicable and infectious diseases are occurring as well as larger food-borne disease outbreaks and acts of terrorism. In 2009, 70% of all deaths were related to chronic disease (CDC, 2010). One in every two Americans had a chronic disease. There is some concern that certain chronic diseases may be caused or intensified by infectious disease processes. Often there are complications that occur as a result of infectious disease, like HIV/AIDS and tuberculosis, which can result in chronic lung disease and certain types of cancer, because of the compromised immune system. Health behaviors and economics related to poverty are also continuing to build the path to acute and chronic health problems (e.g., the global obesity epidemic) (WHO, 2010). While some people choose to ignore behavioral factors related to obesity, such as physical activity and eating, those with insufficient income choose foods high in fat and sugar because those are the cheaper foods to obtain. The chronic disease burden is concentrated among the poor. Poor people are more vulnerable for several reasons, including increased exposure to risks and decreased access to health services. Chronic diseases can cause poverty in individuals and families and draw them into a downward spiral of worsening disease and poverty.

Investment in chronic disease prevention programs is going to be essential for many low- and middle-income countries struggling to reduce poverty. For the United States, this issue is addressed in the new health care reform program of 2010. Health promotion and protection, disease surveillance, emergency preparedness, new laboratory and epidemiologic methods, continued antimicrobial and vaccine development, and environmental health research are continuing challenges for this century. The role of technology has also intensified during this century. Technology is now defined as the application of science to develop solutions to health problems or issues such as the prevention or delay of onset of diseases or the promotion and monitoring of good health. Examples of technology include medical and surgical procedures (angioplasty, joint replacements, organ transplants), diagnostic tests (laboratory tests, biopsies, imaging), drugs (biologic agents, pharmaceuticals, vaccines), medical devices (implantable defibrillators, stents), prosthetics (artificial body parts), and new support systems (electronic medical records, e-prescribing, and telemedicine). The labor force is changing to include radiology oncologists, geneticists, and surgical subspecialists, as well as allied and support professions such as medical sonographers, radiation technologists, and laboratory technicians. These have all been created to support the use of specific types of technology.

The infrastructure necessary to support more complex technologies is also considered to be a part of health care technology. Use of electronic medical records and electronic prescribing are methods for coordinating the increasingly complex array of services provided, as well as allowing for electronic checks of quality to reduce medical errors for things like drug interactions. Because technologies have become a part of standard medical practice, there are concerns about whether they are consistently being used properly and about the quality of the information provided by tests, imaging, and other technological outputs (NCHS, 2010).

In addition to the labor force changes just described, physicians are increasingly moving away from solo practice to group practices, selling primary care practices to hospitals, working as hospital or corporation employees. The emerging role of hospital intensivists is growing, with hospitals employing physicians to be in-house and available to patients and to their community physicians to cover non-urgent, urgent, and emergent care while the patient is hospitalized. More nurse practitioners and physician assistants can be found working side by side with the physician in the community as a member of the office or clinic team.

Public health nurses are more involved with population-centered care, assessment of community needs, and the development or implementation of programs that meet the needs of certain populations. There is a move to provide more care to clients in the home, such as the programs to provide care to new mothers and babies who are defined as at-risk. Public health nurses play key roles in developing and implementing plans for bioterrorism and natural disasters in the community.

Nursing education is seeing a dramatic change in this century. There is a recommendation to move all advanced practice nursing to the level of the new doctoral program, begun in 2000, titled the Doctorate of Nursing Practice. This has the potential for closing specialists masters programs in nursing. This means the new BSN graduate, for example, can go into a doctoral program at graduation and become an advanced public health nurse or a nurse practitioner working in the community. The health care industry is one of the largest employers in the United States, and despite the economic downturn in 2008, has continued to grow. In addition, the largest number of employees in the industry are RNs (AACN, 2010; BLS, 2010).

Along with other changes in health care delivery and health insurance plans, PL 111-148 (2010) has proposed an emphasis on prevention and wellness by establishing the National Prevention, Health Promotion and Public Health Council to coordinate health promotion and public health activities as well as the creation of a prevention and public health fund to expand and sustain these activities. These activities are to assist in the development of a national strategy to improve health, reduce chronic disease rates, and address health disparities.

TRENDS IN HEALTH CARE SPENDING

Much has been written in the popular and scientific literature about the costs of U.S. health care and how society makes decisions about using available and scarce resources. Given that economics in general and health care economics in particular are concerned with resource use and decision-making, any discussion of the economics of health care must consider past and current health care spending. The trends shown here reflect public and private decisions about health care and health care delivery in the past. Past spending reflects past decision-making; likewise, past decisions reflect the values and beliefs held by society and policy makers that undergird policy making at any given point in time.

> **WHAT DO YOU THINK?** *Only 3% of all health care dollars are spent for the public's health. Is this a concern to you? Justify your answer.*

According to the Centers for Medicare and Medicaid Services (CMS) (formerly the Health Care Financing Administration), national health expenditures reached $2.5 trillion in 2009. This is compared to the $600 billion in health care dollars were spent in 1990 (CMS, 2010). The increase in health spending, from $2.34 trillion in 2008 to $2.47 trillion in 2009, was the largest one-year jump since 1960. CMS predicts total U.S. health spending in 2019 will be $4.5 trillion. Health spending has outpaced increases in the gross domestic product, accounting for 17.3% of the GDP by 2009. This means that over $17 of every $100 spent has been spent for health care. It also means that in 2009 approximately $8100 was spent on health care for every person in the U.S. population. The effect of this economic growth represents a large increase in contrast to the approximately 13% GDP spent between 1992 and 2001. The GDP was at 15.30% in 2003.

Figure 5-4 shows a breakdown of the distribution in health care expenses for 2007, and Table 5-1 shows the growth in U.S. health care expenditures between 1960 and 2019 (NCHS, 2010). Spending for health care increased from approximately $27 billion in 1960 to over $2 trillion in 2009. These numbers reflect per-person spending amounts of $143 in 1960 and over $8000 in 2009. In 2008 approximately $120 was spent per person for public health activities (Trust for America's Health, 2008).

The largest portions of health care expenses were for hospital care and physician services, respectively, in 2007 (NCHS, 2010). Only a small fraction of total health care dollars was spent on home health, public health, and research and construction

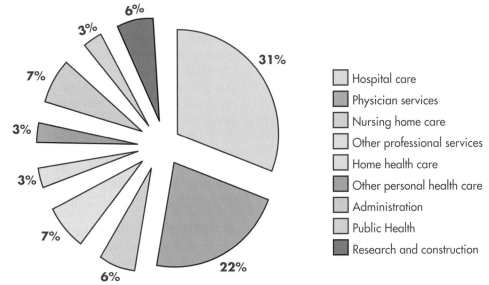

FIGURE 5-4 Distribution of U.S. health care expenditures, 2007. (From National Center for Health Statistics: *Health: United States, 2009, with special feature on medical technology,* Hyattsville, MD, 2010, U.S. Government Printing Office.)

TABLE 5-1	**HEALTH CARE EXPENDITURES: 1960-2019***		
CALENDAR YEAR	**TOTAL HEALTH EXPENDITURES (in billions of dollars)**	**TOTAL HEALTH EXPENDITURES PER CAPITA PER PERSON (in billions of dollars)**	**PERCENT OF GROSS DOMESTIC PRODUCT**
1960	26.7	143	5.1
1970	73.1	348	7.0
1980	245.8	1067	8.8
1990	696.0	2738	12.0
2000	1309.9	4560	13.3
2009	2472.2	8047	17.3
2010*	2569.6	8290	17.3
2019*	4482.7	13,387	19.3

From Centers for Medicare and Medicaid Services, Office of the Actuary: *National health care expenditures projections: 2004-2019,* January 2010. Available at http://www.cms.hhs.gov/NationalHealth ExpendData/downloads/proj2004.pdf. Accessed December 8, 2010. *Projected expenditures.

TABLE 5-2	**PROJECTED FEDERAL SPENDING FOR SOCIAL SECURITY, MEDICARE, MEDICAID AND CHIP IN 2010**	
SPENDING	**IN BILLIONS OF DOLLARS**	**FEDERAL (as percent of total dollars)**
Social Security	708	20.0
Medicare/Medicaid	753	21.0
CHIP	593	21.0
Subtotal	1461	42.0
Rest of government	2150	58.0
Total	3600	100.0

From Congressional Budget Office: *The budget and economic outlook,* Washington, DC, 2010, U.S. Government Printing Office. *CHIP,* Children's Health Insurance Program.

in 2007. The trends over time indicate that this is an ongoing pattern of spending.

FACTORS INFLUENCING HEALTH CARE COSTS

Health economists, providers, payers, and politicians have explored a variety of explanations for the rapid rate of increase in health expenses as compared with population growth. That individuals have, over time, consumed more health care is not an adequate explanation. The following factors are frequently cited as having caused the increases in total and per capita health care spending since 1960: inflation, changes in population demographics, and technology and intensity of services (NCHS, 2010).

Demographics Affecting Health Care

A major demographic change underway in the United States is the aging of the population. Population changes are also affected by illnesses such as acquired immunodeficiency syndrome and by chemical dependency epidemics. These changes have implications for providers' health services, and they affect the overall costs of health care. Because the majority of older adults and other special populations receive services through publicly funded programs, the growing health needs among these populations have great impact on costs, payments, and providers associated with Medicaid and Medicare programs (Table 5-2). As the population ages and the baby boom generation ages and retires, federal expenses for Social Security will increase (CBO, 2010). At 78 million strong, the oldest of the Boomers—born between 1946 and 1964—are already making unsustainable demands on federal entitlement programs like Medicare and Medicaid.

In its *Long-Term Outlook for Medicare, Medicaid and Total Health Care Spending,* the Congressional Budget Office (CBO) reports that spending for those programs will account for 3% each of GDP in 2009.

By 2035, in the absence of change, spending for Medicare alone (which is more likely to be impacted by aging Boomers) will have more than doubled to 8%, and by 2080 it will have grown to 15%.

The aging population is expected to affect health services more than any other demographic factor. In 1950 more than half of the U.S. population was under 30 years of age; in 1994 half of the population was 34 years of age or older. In 1990 individuals 65 and older comprised 12% of the population; in 2007 they comprised 12% of the population. By 2050 they are estimated to comprise up to 20% of the population. That is, 1 in 8 Americans were 65 and older in 1990; 1 in 5 are projected to be 65 and older in 2050. In addition, the number of individuals 85 and older is expected to double between 1990 and 2050 because the population is living longer, healthier lives.

Although many older adults are independent and active, they are likely to experience multiple chronic conditions that may become disabling. They are admitted to hospitals more often than the general population, and their average length of stay is more than 3 days longer than the overall average. They visit physicians more often and make up a larger percentage of nursing home residents than the general population.

Life expectancy and health status have been increasing in the United States. However, older adults continue to consume a large portion of financial resources. Health care providers are concerned about the growth in the older adult population because public funding sources, such as Medicare, have not been increasing their reimbursement rates sufficiently to cover inflation, and thus providers collect a smaller amount for visits by older adult clients each year.

The aging of the population also spurs concerns about funding their health care because of changes in the proportion of employed individuals to retired individuals. Persons in the workforce pay the majority of income taxes and all Social Security payroll taxes. The funding base for Medicare decreases as the population ages, as retirement rates increase, and as the numbers in the workforce decrease. As a result, some policy makers believe that Medicare and system reforms are needed to ensure adequate financing and delivery of health care services to an aging population (PL 111-148, 2010).

Health policy reform options being considered include increased age limits to become eligible for Medicare, **means testing** (i.e., determining a lack of financial resources) for Medicare eligibility, increased coverage for long-term care insurance, increased incentives for prevention, and less expensive and more efficient delivery arrangements and care settings (e.g., managed care arrangements). Meanwhile, the debate continues over how to best handle the future funding of the growing Medicare program. One example of a policy change to reduce the Medicare program burden is the new prescription plan (Medicare D) that was passed by Congress in 2005 and became effective in January 2006. This plan, while complicated, requires most Medicare recipients to provide a co-payment for prescription medications. Although controversial, the plan is thought to provide a positive impact for the elderly who could not afford to pay for their prescriptions, while reducing the cost burden for those who had to pay full price for prescriptions.

Technology and Intensity

The introduction of new technology enhances the delivery of care, but it also has the potential to increase the costs of care. As new and more complex technology is introduced into the system, the cost is typically high. However, clients often demand access to the technology, and providers want to use it. In an effort to keep health care costs down, however, payers have attempted to restrict the use of certain technologies. For example, the drug Viagra, developed for the treatment of impotence by Pfizer Pharmaceuticals, is a controversial technological advance that, as soon as it was available to the public, was in high demand and prescribed by providers. Initially, use was restricted by payers because of cost. It is now covered by some health insurance plans.

The adoption of new technology demands investment in personnel, equipment, and facilities. Furthermore, new technology adds to administrative costs, especially if the federal government provides financial coverage for the service or is involved in regulating the technology. Table 5-3 outlines federal policy that has impacted technology and the cost of health care over time.

Chronic Illness

Chronic illness is a new factor that is showing its impact on health care spending. Chronic disease accounted for 70% of deaths in 2007 (CDC, 2010). Using Medical Expenditure Panel Survey (MEPS) data, chronic medical conditions are identified by those costing the most, the number of bed days, work-loss days, and activity impairments. The most chronic medical condition was stroke.

FINANCING OF HEALTH CARE

Against the backdrop of today's chronic conditions, it must be appreciated that health care financing has evolved through the twentieth century from a system supported primarily by consumers to a system financed by third-party payers (public and private). Table 5-4 shows changes in the percentage of financing according to the source. From 1980 to 2010, the percentage of third-party public insurance payments increased slightly while the percent of out-of-pocket payments had declined. Combined state and federal governments paid the most in 2010.

TABLE 5-3 FEDERAL REGULATIONS CONTRIBUTING TO TECHNOLOGY/COST CONTROLS

YEAR	FEDERAL REGULATION
1906	Prescription drug regulation: Food, Drug, and Cosmetic Act, now the U.S. Food and Drug Administration (FDA)
1935	Social Security Act (PL 74-271): Provides grants-in-aid to states for maternal and child care, aid to crippled children, and aid to the blind and aged
1938	Food, Drug, and Cosmetic Act (PL 75-540): Establishes federal FDA protection for drug safety and protection for mis-branded goods, drugs, cosmetics
1946	Hill-Burton Act (PL 79-725): Enacts Hospital Survey and Construction Act providing national direct support for community hospitals; establishes rudimentary standards for construction and planning; establishes community service obligation
1954	Hill-Burton Act amended (PL 83-482): Expands scope of program for nursing homes, rehabilitation facilities, chronic disease hospitals, and diagnostic or treatment centers
1963	Community Mental Health and Mental Retardation Center Construction Act (PL 88-164)
1965	Medicare Title 18; Medicaid Title 19 (PL 89-97): Amendments to Social Security Act provide Medicare and Medicaid to support health care services for certain groups
1966	Comprehensive Health Planning Act (PL 89-749): For health services, personnel, and facilities in federal/state/local partnerships
1971	President Nixon introduces concept of HMOs as the cornerstone of his administration's national health insurance proposal
1972	Social Security Act Amendments (PL 92-603): Extend coverage to include new treatment technologies for end-stage renal disease; provide for professional standards review organizations to review appropriateness of hospital care for Medicare/Medicaid recipients
1973	HMO Act (PL 93-222): Provides assistance and expansion for HMOs
1975	National Health Planning and Resources Development Act (PL 93-641): Designates local health system areas and establishes a national certificate-of-need (CON) program to limit major health care expansion at local and state levels
1978	Medicare End-Stage Renal Disease Amendment: Provides payment for home dialysis and kidney transplantation; Health Services Research, Health Statistics, and Health Care Technology Act establishes national council on health care technology to develop standards for use
1981	Omnibus Budget Reconciliation Act of 1981 (PL 97-351): Consolidates 26 health programs into 4 block grants (preventatives, health services, primary care, and maternal and child health)
1982	Tax Equity and Fiscal Responsibilities Act (PL 97-248): Seeks to control costs by limiting hospital costs per discharge adjusted to hospital case mix
1983	Amended Social Security Act (PL 98-21): Establishes new Medicare hospital prospective payment system based on diagnosis-related groups (DRGs)
1986	1974 Health Planning and Resource Development Act (PL 93-641): Moves CON program to states
1989	Omnibus Reconciliation Act of 1989 (PL 101-239): Creates physician resource-based fee schedule to be implemented by 1992, with emphasis on high-tech specialties of surgery; creates Agency for Healthcare Policy and Research to research effectiveness of medical and nursing services, interventions, and technologies
1990	Ryan White Care Act (PL 101-381): Authorizes formula-based and competitive supplemental grants to cities and states for HIV-related outpatient medical services
1990	Safe Medical Devices Act (PL 101-629): Gives FDA authority to regulate medical devices and diagnostic products
1993	Omnibus Budget Reconciliation Act (OBRA 93) (PL 103-66): Cuts Medicare funding and ends ROE payments to skilled nursing facilities; provides support for immunizations for Medicaid children
1996	Health Insurance Portability and Accountability Act: Protects health insurance coverage for laid-off or displaced workers
1997	Balanced Budget Act of 1997: Creates a new program for states to offer health insurance to children in low-income and uninsured families
1998	Balanced Budget Act of 1997 (PL 105-33): Authorizes third-party reimbursement for Medicare Part B services for NPs and CNSs
2003	Medicaid Nursing Incentive Act (HR 2295): Expands direct reimbursement to all nurse practitioners and clinical nurse specialists and recognizes specialized services offered by advanced practice registered nurses such as primary care case management, pain management, and mental health services
2006	Medicare Part D: Provides a plan for prescription payments
2010	Patient Protection and Affordable Care Act passed and signed into law on March 23, 2010

EVIDENCE-BASED PRACTICE

Linking Improvements in Health-Related Quality of Life to Reductions in Medicaid Costs Among Students Who Use School-Based Health Centers

School-based health centers (SBHCs) have steadily increased in numbers across the United States over the last three decades. This shift in the delivery of health care for children is based on the assumption that access to health services in school increases access to health care and improves health status among children, especially for those children whose access to care is otherwise limited. Health status is often measured by health-related quality of life (HRQOL), which attempts to tap the current health perception of individuals.

The authors conducted a longitudinal study over 3 years to evaluate improvements in quality of life for 290 school children who used SBHCs and were linked to the Medicaid data base of Ohio. The study was conducted in Cincinnati, Ohio between 2000 and 2003 across two school districts. Of the 290 children, 71 had mental health diagnoses and 31 had asthma. The Pediatric Quality of Life Inventory was used to measure health-related quality of life. The authors were interested in whether changes in parent self-report and student self-report of the child's quality of life would predict changes in Medicaid costs. Each SBHC was open Monday through Friday and operated during the school year from September to May. A variety of health providers staffed the clinics, including nursing staff

The total score, physical, and psychosocial scores for both parent self-report ratings and student self-reports across time for the total sample as well as for each subsample were analyzed. For the total sample and children with asthma, parent ratings were higher than were student self-ratings across all measures and across each year. Moreover, both parents and students rated their physical health higher than their psychosocial health. In the mental health subsample, this pattern was present but less pronounced in years 1 and 2. In year 3, however, parent ratings were consistently lower than were their children's ratings across all measures of the Inventory.

Nurse Use

This cost-effectiveness analysis measured changes in costs in dollars associated with changes in HRQOL scores over the 3 years. This measure has been widely used for health care decision-making. This study is an example of the economic burden of chronic disease showing that regardless of cost savings, the children with chronic diseases will have higher costs than children who do not. Improvements in pediatric HRQOL translate into lower Medicaid costs, which supports the use of HRQOL as an outcome for evaluating SBHCs. This study also showed improvements in health care cost using SBHCs as a resource for school children accompanied by an improvement in quality of life.

Terrance J. Wade, PhD

Jeff Jianfei Guo, PhD

From American Public Health Association: AJPH First Look, *Am J Public Health* 100(9):1611-1616, September 2010. Published online ahead of print July 15, 2010.

TABLE 5-4   HEALTH SERVICES AND SUPPLIES, EXPENDITURES IN AGGREGATE DOLLARS BY SOURCE FOR SELECTED YEARS BETWEEN 1980 AND 2015

YEAR	TOTAL (BILLIONS)	OUT-OF-POCKET PAYMENTS	TOTAL THIRD-PARTY PAYMENTS	PRIVATE HEALTH INSURANCE	OTHER PRIVATE	PUBLIC: TOTAL
1980	Expense: $233.5	Expense: $58.3	Expense: $175.2	Expense: 468.2	Expense: $9.4	Expense: $97.6
	Percent: 100.00	Percent: 25	Percent: 75	Percent: 29.2	Percent: 4.0	Percent: 41.8
1990	Expense: $669.2	Expense: $137.8	Expense: $531.5	Expense: $232.6	Expense: $31.2	Expense: $267.6
	Percent: 100.0	Percent: 20.6	Percent: 79.4	Percent: 34.8	Percent: 4.7	Percent: 40.0
2000	Expense: $1264.5	Expense: $192.6	Expense: $1071.9	Expense: $454.8	Expense: $57.9	Expense: $559.2
	Percent: 100.0	Percent: 15.2	Percent: 84.8	Percent: 36.0	Percent: 4.6	Percent: 44.2
2010	Expense: $2570	Expense: $292	Expense: $2278	Expense: $829	Expense: $183	Expense: $1266
	Percent: 100.0	Percent: 11.4	Percent: 89	Percent: 32	Percent: 7	Percent: 49
2015	Expense: $3442	Expense: $372	Expense: $3070	Expense: $1076	Expense: $250	Expense: $1870
	Percent: 100.0	Percent: 11.0	Percent: 89	Percent: 31	Percent: 7	Percent: 51

From Centers for Medicare and Medicaid Services, Office of the Actuary: *National health care expenditures projections: 2004-2019,* August 2010.

Public Support

The U.S. federal government became involved in health care financing for population groups early in its history. In 1798 the federal government created the Marine Hospital Service to provide medical care for sick and disabled sailors, and to protect the nation's borders against the importing of disease through seaports. The Marine Hospital Service is considered the first national health insurance plan in the United States. The National Health Board was established in 1879 and was later renamed the United States Public Health Service (PHS). Within the PHS, the federal government developed a public health liaison with state and local health departments for the purpose of controlling communicable diseases and improving sanitation. Additional health programs were also developed to meet obligations to federal workers and their families within the PHS, the Department of Defense, and the Veterans Administration (VA) (see Chapters 3 and 8).

Medicare and Medicaid, two federal programs administered by the CMS, account for the majority of public health care spending. Table 5-5 compares these programs. The CMS is the federal regulatory agency within the U.S. Department of Health and Human Services (USDHHS) that is responsible for overseeing and monitoring Medicare and Medicaid spending. This agency routinely collects and reports actual health care use and

TABLE 5-5   COMPARISON OF MEDICARE AND MEDICAID PROGRAM FEATURES

FEATURE	MEDICARE	MEDICAID
Where to obtain information	Local Social Security Administration office	State welfare office
Recipients	Client is 65 years or older, is disabled, or has permanent kidney failure	Specified low-income and needy, children, aged, blind, and/or disabled; those eligible to receive federally assisted income
Type of program	Insurance	Insurance
Government affiliation	Federal	Joint federal/state
Availability	All states	All states
Financing of hospital insurance	Medicare Trust Fund, mandatory payroll deduction, recipient deductibles, trust fund interest	Federal and state governments
Financing of medical insurance	Recipient premium payments; general revenue, U.S. Treasury	Federal and state governments
Types of coverage	Inpatient and outpatient hospital services, skilled nursing facilities (SNFs), limited home health services	Inpatient and outpatient hospital services; prenatal care; vaccines for children; physician, dental, nurse practitioner, and nurse-midwife services; SNF services for persons 21 or older; family services; rural health clinic

From U.S. Department of Health and Human Services, Centers for Medicare and Medicaid Services: *Medicare and you,* Baltimore, MD, 2010, USDHHS.

spending and projects future spending trends. Through these programs, the federal government purchases health care services for population groups through independent health care systems, such as managed care organizations, private practice physicians, and hospitals.

Medicare

The Medicare program, established in Title XVIII of the Social Security Act of 1965, provides hospital insurance and medical insurance to persons aged 65 and older, to permanently disabled persons, and to persons with end-stage renal disease—altogether approximately 46 million people in 2009 (USDHHS, CMS, 2009). Medicare has two parts: Part A (hospital insurance) covers hospital care, home care, hospice care, and skilled nursing care (limited); Part B (non-institutional care insurance) covers "medically necessary" services like health care provider services, outpatient care, home health, and other medical services such as diagnostic services, and physiotherapy. In 1999 a program called Medicare Advantage was added to the program (Part C). This is an option that can be chosen for additional coverage. This option includes both Part A and B services. The Part C plans are coordinated care plans that include health maintenance organizations (HMOs), private fee-for-service plans, and medical savings accounts (MSAs). Part C provides for all health care coverage costs after a high deductible (NCHS, 2010).

Medicare Part A is primarily financed by a federal payroll tax that is paid by employers and employees. The proceeds from this tax go to the Hospital Insurance Trust Fund, which is managed by the CMS. If a person did not have federal payroll deductions, Part A can be obtained by paying a monthly premium. Part A coverage is available to all persons who are eligible to receive Medicare, with older adults comprising the majority of these individuals. There is concern about the future of the Medicare Trust Fund, since projected expenses may be more than the trust fund resources. Payments to hospitals for covered

services have been and continue to be higher than fund growth. Thus Medicare reimbursement policy has been changing in an attempt to control increasing hospital costs. Part A requires a deductible from recipients for the first 60 days of services with a reduced deductible for 61 to 90 days of service. The deductible has increased as daily hospital costs have increased. For skilled nursing facility (SNF) care, persons pay nothing for the first 20 days and a cost per day for days 21 through 100. After 100 days, persons must pay the total cost for care (CMS, 2009). The person pays zero for hospice care and home health.

The medical insurance package, Part B, is a supplemental (voluntary) program that is available to all Medicare-eligible persons for a monthly premium ($134 in 2010). The vast majority of Medicare-covered persons elect this coverage. Part B provides coverage for services other than hospital (physician care, outpatient hospital care, outpatient physical therapy, mental health, and home health care) that are not covered by Part A, such as laboratory services, ambulance transportation, prostheses, equipment, and some supplies. After a deductible, up to 80% of reasonable charges are paid for medical and other services. For mental health services, 55% of the costs are paid. Part B resembles the major medical insurance coverage of private insurance carriers. Figure 5-5 shows the total expenses of the Medicare program from 1970 to 2007.

Since the passing of the Medicare amendments to the Social Security Act in 1965, the cost of Medicare has increased dramatically. Hospital care continues to be the major factor contributing to Medicare costs. However, because of the shorter hospital stays, home health and nursing home costs have increased dramatically. As a result of rising health costs, Congress passed a law in 1983 that radically changed Medicare's method of payment for hospital services. In 1983 federal legislation (PL98-21) mandated an end to cost-plus reimbursement by Medicare and instituted a 3-year transition to a prospective payment system (PPS) for inpatient hospital services. The purpose of the new

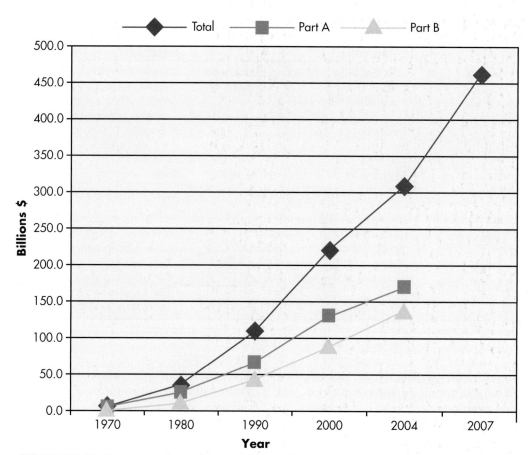

FIGURE 5-5 Medicare expenditures for selected years from 1970 to 2007. (From National Center for Health Statistics: *Health: United States, 2009, with special feature on medical technology*, Hyattsville, MD, 2010, U.S. Government Printing Office.)

hospital payment scheme was to shift the cost incentives away from the providing of more care and toward more efficient services. The basis for prospective reimbursement is the 468 diagnosis-related groups (DRGs). Also, the Balanced Budget Act of 1997 determined that payments to Medicare SNFs would be made on the basis of the PPS, effective July 1, 1998. The PPS payment rates cover SNF services, including routine, ancillary, and capital-related costs (HCFA, 1998). In 2001 CMS developed a PPS for DRGs for home health with Health Insurance Prospective Payment System (HIPPS) codes.

In 2006 the average amount spent for services for Medicare beneficiaries was approximately $8000 (Kaiser Family Foundation, 2010b). The average out-of-pocket spending is skewed to those beneficiaries who are older or have declining health. This is because of the limits in Medicare coverage, including certain preventive care, and the limited number of physicians and agencies who accept Medicare and Medicaid payment. Older adults who do not have supplemental insurance must cover the difference between the Medicare payment and the additional costs for services.

Medicaid

The Medicaid program, Title XIX of the Social Security Act of 1965, provides financial assistance to states and counties to pay for medical services for poor older adults, the blind, the disabled, and families with dependent children. The Medicaid program is jointly sponsored and financed with matching funds from the federal and state governments. In 2006 more than 57 million people were enrolled in Medicaid (NCHS, 2010). Medicaid expenditures from 1987 to 2007 are shown in Figure 5-6. Since the beginning of Medicaid, full payment has been provided for five types of services (NCHS, 2010):

- Inpatient and outpatient hospital care
- Laboratory and radiology services
- Physician services
- Skilled nursing care at home or in a nursing home for people more than 21 years of age
- Early periodic screening, diagnosis, and treatment (EPSDT) for those less than 21 years of age

The 1972 Social Security amendments added family planning to the list of full-pay services. States can choose to add prescriptions, dental services, eyeglasses, intermediate care facilities, and coverage for the medically indigent as program options. By law, the medically indigent are required to pay a monthly premium.

Any state participating in the Medicaid program is required to provide the six basic services to persons who are below state poverty income levels. Optional programs are provided at the discretion of each state. In 1989 changes in Medicaid required states to provide care for children less than 6 years of age and to pregnant women under 133% of the poverty level. For example, if the poverty level were $12,000, a pregnant woman could have a household income as high as $16,000 and still be eligible to

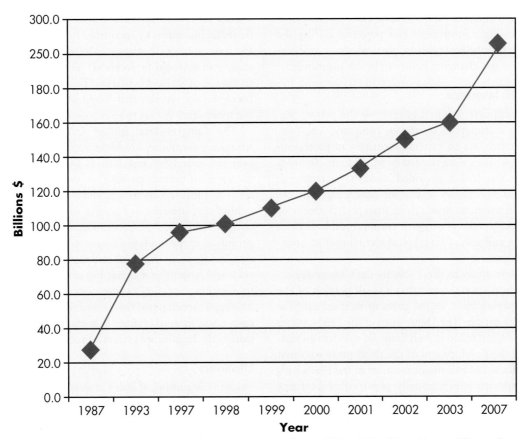

FIGURE 5-6 Medicaid expenditures for selected years from 1987 to 2007. (From National Center for Health Statistics: *Health: United States, 2009, with special feature on medical technology,* Hyattsville, MD, 2010, U.S. Government Printing Office.)

receive care under Medicaid. These changes also provided for pediatric and family nurse practitioner reimbursement. In the 1990s states were allowed to petition the federal government for a waiver. If the waiver was approved, the states could use their Medicaid monies for programs other than the six basic services. The first waiver to be approved was given to Oregon for their health care reform plan. Other states have received waivers to develop Medicaid managed care programs for special populations. The 2010 health care reform plan provides for new approaches to offering Medicaid services and incentives for states to offer Medicaid services rather than through the waiver option as described previously (PL 111-148, 2010).

The major expense categories for the Medicaid program have historically been skilled and intermediate nursing home care and inpatient hospital care. When combined, these two categories account today for 3% of all costs to the program (NCHS, 2010).

Public Health

Most public government agencies operate on an annual budget, and they plan for costs by estimating salaries, expenses, and costs of services for a year. Public health agencies, such as health departments and WIC programs (for women, infants, and children), receive primary funding from taxes, with additional money for select goods and services through private third-party payers. Selected public health programs receive

reimbursement for services as follows: through grants given by the federal government to states for prenatal and child health; through Medicare and Medicaid for home health, nursing homes, WIC programs, and EPSDT; and through collecting of fees on a sliding scale for select client services, such as immunizations.

In 2007 only 3% of all health care–related federal funds were expended for federal health programs such as WIC, versus 97% for other types of health and illness care (such as hospital and physician services). In addition to this 3% allotment, public health funds also come through states and territorial health agencies. State and local governments contributed 17.2% to public and general assistance, maternal and child health, public health activities, and other related services in 2007 (NCHS, 2010).

Other Public Support

The federal government finances health services for retired military persons and dependents through the TriCARE, the VA, and the Indian Health Service (IHS). These programs are very important in providing needed health care services to these populations (see Chapters 3 and 8).

Private Support

Private health care payer sources include insurance, employers, managed care, and individuals. Although insurance and consumers have been prominent health care payment sources for some time, the role of employers, managed care, and consumers became increasingly prominent and powerful during the first decade of the twenty-first century, particularly as concerns grew about the use and changing nature of health insurance.

Evolution of Health Insurance

Insurance for health care was first offered for the private sector in 1847 by a commercial insurance company. The purpose of the insurance was to provide security and protection when health care services were needed by individuals. The idea behind insurance was that it provided security, guaranteeing (within certain limits) monies to pay for health care services to offset potential financial losses from unexpected illness or injury related to accidents, catastrophic communicable diseases (such as smallpox and scarlet fever), and recurring (but unexpected) chronic illnesses.

A comprehensive study in the 1920s by the Committee on the Costs of Medical Care showed that a small portion of the population was paying most of the costs of medical care for the majority of the people. The Depression of the 1930s, rising medical costs, and the need to spread financial risk across communities spurred the development of the third-party payment system. The system began as a major industry in the 1930s with the Blue Cross system, which initially provided prepayment for hospital care. In 1939 Blue Shield created plans to provide physician payment. The Blue Cross plans began as tax-free, non-profit organizations established under special enabling legislation in various states.

In the 1940s and 1950s, hospital and medical–surgical coverage increased. Employee group coverage appeared, and profit-making commercial insurance underwriters began offering health insurance packages with competitive premiums. The commercial insurance companies could offer lower premium rates because of the methods used to set rates. Insurance and premium setting, in general, are based on the notion of risk pooling (i.e., insurance companies were willing to risk the unlikely event that all or even a large portion of individuals covered under a plan would need payment for health services at any given time). Blue Cross used a *community rate*, establishing a similar premium rate for all subscribers regardless of illness potential. In contrast, the commercial companies used an *experience rate*, in which the premium was based on an estimate of the illness *risk* or the number of claims to be made by the subscriber (Jacobs, 2002).

Premium competition, the offering of health insurance as a fringe benefit, and the use of health insurance as a negotiable collective bargaining item led to an increase in covered benefits, first-dollar coverage for medical care expenses, and increased employer-paid premiums. In turn, these factors pushed up insurance premium costs and health care costs and enabled insurance plans to cover high-cost segments of the population (the aged, poor, or disabled) because of the number of low-risk enrollees.

The health needs of high-risk populations led to the passage of Medicare and Medicaid legislation. These and other national health programs targeted health care coverage for specific population groups. Because these programs directed additional money into the health care system to subsidize care, there were financial incentives to encourage the providing of services (i.e., the more services that were ordered, the greater the amount of money that would be received). Other incentives were related to the use of services by clients (i.e., the more available the payment was for services that might otherwise have gone unused, the more services that were requested).

The Congressional Budget Office projected that private insurance premiums would on average increase about 5.1% per year between 1996 and 2007 (CBO, 2001). However, greater increases in premiums have occurred as a result of pressure from employers, consumers, and policy makers. Driving forces behind this pressure are quality of care, client dissatisfaction, clients' rights, and the concern that these areas are being compromised in the managed care system. Furthermore, the initial cost savings from managed care may have occurred already, and costs will have to be increased to simply maintain coverage, not to mention providing new services and technologies. Although managed care changed the structure of financing and delivery of care, it was soon recognized that managed care was not the solution to the health care system's problems (Lee and Estes, 2003).

Employers

Since the beginning of Blue Cross and Blue Shield, health insurance has been tied to employment and the business sector. This tie was strengthened during World War II to compensate, attract, and retain employees. Since that time, employers have played the major role in determining health insurance benefits. However, with the economic downturn in 2008, employers began to reduce their health insurance benefits or return the cost of insurance premiums to the employee.

> **DID YOU KNOW?** *If a client has health insurance, the payment to the provider is less than the payment made by the client who does not have health insurance.*

In 2005 approximately 70% of the population under 65 years of age had private health insurance, most of which was obtained through the workplace (NCHS, 2005). In 2009 the percentage had decreased to about 60% (Kaiser Family Foundation, 2009). In 2005 87% of employers paid 50% to 100% of the insurance premium (Kaiser Family Foundation, 2005). In 2009 employees paid a minimum of 26% to 36% of the health insurance premium with the employee's share of a family premium doubling in cost since 2000. For employees of small firms, the percentage of payment increased for all premiums (Kaiser Family Foundation, 2009). This substantial contribution to health care by the private business sector gave the employer a lot of health care buying power in making policy about what services insurance would cover. All but 600,000 of older Americans were covered by Medicare; low-income children can be covered by the Children's Health Insurance Program (CHIP) if enrolled by parents or guardians; and as previously described, some low-income adults were covered by Medicaid in 2008 (Kaiser Family Foundation, 2009). The new health reform law projects that an additional 32 million will be covered by 2016.

Before the growth of insurance (i.e., before 1930 and the beginning of Blue Cross), the health care consumer had more influence over health care costs because payment was out of pocket. Consumers made decisions about how they would spend their money, making certain tradeoffs—for example, about the type of health care they were willing to buy and how much they would pay. Entering the system was restricted in large part to those who could afford to pay for care, or to those few who could find care financed through charitable and philanthropic organizations. With the beginning of the insurance (or **third-party payer**) system, health care costs were set by payers, and they determined the type of care or service that would be offered and its price. This began to change somewhat in the 1980s with the increased use of managed care.

As the cost of health insurance has increased, some employers, in an effort to bypass the costs established by insurers, have found it less costly to self-insure. The employer does this by contracting directly with providers to obtain health care services for employees rather than going through health insurance companies. Some large businesses directly employ on-site providers for care delivery or offer on-site wellness programs. These programs within the private sector offer opportunities for nurses to provide wellness programs and health assessments to screen and monitor employees and their families. This move to self-insure resulted in savings to companies and reduced overall sick care costs (Hunt and Knickman, 2005).

In a truly competitive market, the consumer buys goods and services at will, knowing the costs and expected value of services bought and can choose the provider of those services. In the health system where a third party pays for the services, this transaction has less meaning. The third party makes decisions about the level and type of care that will be purchased for clients and determines how payment will be made. The service provider and client have no influence on how services will be reimbursed. However, the consumer may select the payer/plan and indeed may influence the system through political channels.

In 2007 individuals paid only approximately 14% of total health expenditures out-of-pocket (NCHS, 2010). However, these figures do not reflect the amount of money the consumer pays in taxes to finance government-supported programs such as Medicare and Medicaid, insurance premiums, and money paid for supplemental insurance to cover the gaps in a primary health insurance policy or Medicare.

The average monthly cost for private health insurance has increased greatly through the years. Premiums reflect a shift of the health care cost burden from employers to employees as the percentage of employer contributions to health care declines. The decrease in employer contribution to health insurance premiums parallels the economic downturn of 2008, the move away from traditional insurance plans, and the move toward managed care plans or self insurance plans by both small and large employers or toward dropping health insurance as a benefit. In 2008, 2 million people lost employer health insurance coverage (Kaiser Family Foundation, 2009).

From an economic point of view, the shift in responsibility for the cost of health insurance is not bad. In theory, this shift makes consumers more knowledgeable about (sensitive to) the price of health services. This means that they have more information for health care decision-making and may consider price in making the decision to access types of health care services. Satisfaction with the quality of service rests with the person buying the insurance and receiving health care. As with employers, employees may choose health insurance voluntarily. Therefore three factors—the shifting of responsibility for health insurance premiums to employees, the changing demographics of the workforce in general, and the loss of employment due to the economic downturn—have resulted in a decline in employee enrollment in health insurance plans. Employees are choosing to use their resources to meet basic needs and are assuming the risks of having an illness for which they may have to pay. A minor health problem can lead to major medical debt for someone without health insurance (Kaiser Family Foundation, 2009). The PL 111-148 includes a mandate for all citizens and legal residents to have qualifying health coverage. Employers will be required to offer coverage also, except for employers with less than 50 employees. These two requirements are to be in effect by 2014 unless repealed by Congress.

Given that access to health insurance is tied to employment, there was growing concern in the late 1980s and early 1990s about the employment layoffs and downsizing occurring in private business. Those who lost their jobs lost their ability to pay for health insurance and to qualify to purchase insurance privately. The Health Insurance Portability and Accountability Act of 1996 (HIPAA) was enacted to protect health insurance coverage for workers and families after a job change or loss (HCFA, 1999; Nichols et al, 1998). Although this has increased the number of people who have access to health insurance and health care, there are claims that individual premiums are high, that insurance companies have lost their ability to pool risks, and that HIPAA is just one more federal control mechanism undermining competitive market influences.

Managed Care Arrangements

Managed care is the term used for a variety of health care arrangements that integrate the financing and the delivery of health care. Managed care offers an array of services to purchasers, such as employers, Medicaid, or Medicare, for a set fee. These are called *risk-based plans*. This fee, in turn, is used to pay providers through preset arrangements for services delivered to individuals who are covered (NCHS, 2010). The concept of managed care is based on the notion that the use of costly care could be reduced if consumers had access to care and services that would prevent illness through consumer education and health maintenance. Therefore, managed care uses disease prevention, health promotion, wellness, and consumer education (Hunt and Knickman, 2005). In addition to the risk-based plan whereby the managed care organization accepts the set fee to cover all costs of care for the enrollee, there are cost-based plans. An example of such a managed care organization is the primary care case management (PCCM) organization often used by Medicaid programs. These PCCMs are comprised of a variety of health care providers contracted with states to locate, coordinate, and monitor covered primary care and other services on a per client case management fee payment. Whereas HMOs assume risks for the costs of care, the PCCMs do not (NCHS, 2010).

BOX 5-3   TYPES OF MANAGED CARE

1. Health Maintenance Organization (HMO)
An HMO is a provider arrangement whereby comprehensive care is provided to plan members for a fixed, "per member per month" fee. Common features include the following:
   a. Capitation
   b. Use of designated providers
   c. Point-of-service care, or receiving care from nondesignated plan providers
   d. One of the following models:
      (1) Staff model, whereby physicians are HMO employees
      (2) Group model, whereby a physician group practice contracts with the HMO to provide care
      (3) Individual practice association (IPA), whereby the HMO contracts with physicians in solo, small group practices, or physician networks to provide care
      (4) Mixed model, whereby the HMO uses a combination group/IPA arrangement
2. Preferred Provider Organization (PPO)
A PPO is a provider arrangement whereby predetermined rates are established for services to be delivered to members. Common features include the following:
   a. Hospital and physician providers
   b. Discounted rate setting
   c. Financial incentives to encourage plan members to select PPO providers
   d. Expedited claims' payment to providers

From Folland S, Goodman AC, Stano M: *The economics of health and health care,* New York, 1993, Macmillan; U.S. Department of Health and Human Services: *Health: United States, 1998,* DHHS Publication No. (PHS) 98-1232, Washington, DC, 1998, U.S. Government Printing Office.

Two common types of managed care are health maintenance organizations (HMOs) and preferred provider organizations (PPOs). Box 5-3 provides an overview of HMOs and PPOs. Although they seem relatively new to many clients of care, HMOs have actually been around since the 1940s. The Health Maintenance Organization Act was enacted in 1972, and since that time, the number of individuals receiving care through HMOs and other types of managed care organizations has increased considerably. Managed care is based, in part, on the principles of managed competition. Managed competition was introduced in health care in the late 1980s and early 1990s to address the increasing costs of health care and to introduce quality into the forefront of discussions. Managed competition simply means that clients make decisions and choose the health care services they want on the basis of the quality or reputation of the service. To make decisions, they use knowledge and information about health care problems, care, and providers, and they look at the costs of care. However, health care is a complex market and not one in which information about health care, health problems, and the costs of care are easy to get.

Medical Savings Accounts

Another insurance reform discussion at the political level concerns medical savings accounts (MSAs). MSAs are touted as a way of turning health care decision-making control over to the individuals receiving care. MSAs are tax-exempt accounts available to individuals who work for small companies, usually established through a bank or insurance company, that enable the individuals to save money for future medical needs and expenses (IRS, 2005). Money is contributed to an MSA by the employer, and the initial money put into an MSA does not come out of taxable income. Also, interest earned in MSAs is tax free, and unused MSA money can be held in the account from year to year until the money is used. MSAs, in theory, would allow individuals to make cost/quality tradeoffs and would require that individuals become knowledgeable about health care, become involved in health care decision-making, and take responsibility for the decisions made. Providers, in turn, must be willing to provide and disclose information to individuals and give up control of health care decision-making. The HIPAA and MSAs are examples of health insurance reform efforts, and these efforts will very likely remain in the forefront of political discussions for some time to come, especially with the health care reform discussions.

HEALTH CARE PAYMENT SYSTEMS

Several methods have been used by public and private sources to pay health care providers for health care services. These include retrospective and prospective reimbursement for paying health care organizations, and fee-for-service and capitation for paying health care practitioners (Hunt and Knickman, 2005).

Paying Health Care Organizations

Retrospective reimbursement is the traditional reimbursement method, whereby fees for the delivery of health care services in an organization are set after services are delivered (Hunt and Knickman, 2005). In this scenario, reimbursement is based on either organization costs or charges. The cost method reimburses organizations on the basis of cost per unit of service (e.g., home health visit, patient-day) for treatment and care. Costs include all or a percentage of added, allowable costs. Allowable costs are negotiated between the payer and provider and include items such as depreciation of building, equipment, and administrative costs (e.g., administrative salaries, utilities, and office supplies) (Hunt and Knickman, 2005). For example, the unit of service in home health is the visit, and the agreed-on price is a set amount of money that the home health agency will be paid for a home visit in the region of the United States in which the home care agency is located.

The *charge method* reimburses organizations on the basis of the price set by the organization for delivering a service (Hunt and Knickman, 2005). In this case, the organization determines a charge for providing a particular service, provides the service to a client, and submits a bill to the payer; the payer in turn provides payment for the bill. With this method, the charge may be greater than the actual cost to the agency to deliver the service. When the charge method is used, the client often has to pay the difference between what is paid and what is charged.

Prospective reimbursement, or payment, is a more recent method of paying an organization, whereby the third-party payer establishes the amount of money that will be paid for the delivery of a particular service before offering the services to the client (Hunt and Knickman, 2005). Since the establishment of prospective payment in Medicare in 1983, private insurance has followed by requiring pre-approvals before clients can receive certain services, such as hospital admission or mammograms more than once a year (Hunt and Knickman, 2005). Under this payment scheme, the third-party payer reimburses an organization on the basis of the payer's prediction of the cost to deliver a particular service; these predictions vary by case mix (i.e., different types of clients, with different types, levels, and intensities of health problems), the client's diagnosis, and geographic location. This process is used in the DRG system of the hospital (Hunt and Knickman, 2005).

Similarly, ambulatory care services received by Medicare recipients are classified into ambulatory payment classes (APCs), which reflect the type of ambulatory clinical services received and resources required (CMS, 2005a). Prospective payment to skilled nursing facilities is also adjusted for case mix and geographic variations (CMS, 2005b).

Positive and negative incentives are built into these reimbursement schemes. The retrospective method of payment encourages organizations to inflate prices in one area to offset agency losses in another. These losses can result from providing service to non-paying clients or from providing care to clients covered under plans that do not cover the total costs of delivering a service (Hunt and Knickman, 2005). The major disadvantage of this system is that little regard is given to the costs involved. This practice of charging a payer at a higher rate to cover losses in providing care is referred to as *cost-shifting*.

Prospective cost reimbursement encourages agencies to stay within budget limits and adds an incentive for providing less service to contain or reduce costs. If an organization provides care to a particular patient or group of patients and keeps the costs of delivering the service lower than the amount of reimbursement, the provider keeps the difference; however, if the provider's costs exceed the reimbursement, the provider must assume the risk and pay the difference. The major disadvantage of this method is that organizations tend to overemphasize controlling costs and sometimes compromise quality of care.

A growth in contracting, or competitive bidding, for health care services, intended to create incentives for providers to compete on price, has occurred as managed care has increased in health care markets. For example, contracting has been used by states to provide Medicaid services to eligible persons. Hospitals and other health care providers who do not have a contract with the state to provide services are not eligible to receive Medicaid payments for client care. Managed care organizations also use this approach to negotiate with health care organizations, such as hospitals, for coverage of services to be provided to covered enrollees, often called *covered lives*.

Paying Health Care Practitioners

The traditional method of paying health care practitioners is known as fee-for-service (Hunt and Knickman, 2005) and is like the retrospective method just described. The practitioner determines the costs of providing a service, delivers the service to a client, and submits a bill for the delivered service to a third-party payer; the payer then pays the bill. This method is based on usual, customary, and reasonable (UCR) charges for specific services in a given geographic region, determined by periodic regional evaluations of physician charges across specialties (Hunt and Knickman, 2005). Historically, Medicare, Medicaid, and private insurance companies have used this method of reimbursing physicians.

A major effort to regulate and control the costs of physician fees was introduced in 1990 in the Omnibus Reconciliation Act. After a study by the Physician Payment Review Commission established by Congress, the *resource-based relative value scale* (RBRVS) was established. The RBRVS method reimburses physicians for specific services provided and the amount of resources required to deliver the service. Resources are defined broadly and include not only the costs of providing the service, but also the training that is required to provide a particular service and the time required to perform certain procedures, including client diagnosis and treatment. The RBRVS method of reimbursement, adopted by Medicare in 1991, acknowledges the breadth and depth of knowledge required by primary care physicians in the community to provide services aimed at prevention, health promotion, teaching, and counseling.

Capitation is similar to prospective reimbursement for health care organizations. Specifically, third-party payers determine the amount that practitioners will be paid for a unit of care, such as a client visit, before the delivery of the service, thereby placing a limit on the amount of reimbursement received per patient (Hunt and Knickman, 2005). In contrast to a fee-for-service arrangement, where the practitioner determines both the services that will be provided to clients and the charges for those services, practitioners being paid through capitation are given the rate they will be paid for a client's care, regardless of specific services provided. Therefore, for example, physicians and nurse practitioners are aware in advance of the payment they will receive to perform a routine, uncomplicated physical examination or a more complex, detailed physical examination, diagnosis, and treatment (Hunt and Knickman, 2005).

In capitated arrangements, physicians and other practitioners are paid a set amount to provide care to a given client or group of clients for a set period of time and amount of money. This arrangement, typically used by managed care organizations, is one whereby the practitioner contracts with the managed care organization to provide health care services to plan members for a preset and negotiated fee. The agreed-upon fee is negotiated between the practitioner and the managed care organization before the delivery of services and is set at a discounted rate, and the practitioner and managed care organization come to a legal agreement, or contract, for the delivery and payment of services. The managed care organization pays the predetermined fee to the practitioner, often before the delivery of services, to provide care to plan members for a set period (Hunt and Knickman, 2005).

Reimbursement for Nursing Services

Historically, practitioners eligible to receive reimbursement for health care services included physicians only. However, nurses who function in certain capacities, such as NPs, CNSs, and midwives, also provide primary care to clients and receive reimbursement for their services. Being recognized as primary care providers and eligible to receive reimbursement has not been an easy achievement.

> **NURSING TIP**   *There are currently more than 250 nurse-managed clinics in the United States providing population-based preventive services, primary care, or specific wellness programs. Most are receiving financial support through Medicare, Medicaid, contracts, gifts, grants, and private donations.*

Hospital nursing care costs have traditionally been included as part of the overall patient room charge and reimbursed as such. Other agencies, such as home health care agencies, include nursing care costs with administrative costs, supplies, and equipment costs. Nursing organizations, such as the American Nurses Association, have long advocated that nursing care should become a separate budget item in all organizations so that cost studies can show the efficiency and effectiveness of the nursing profession.

Spurred by efforts to control the costs of medical care, effective January 1, 1998, NPs and CNSs were granted third-party reimbursement for Medicare Part B services only, under Public Law 105-33 (ANA, 1999). This new law set reimbursement for NPs and CNSs at 85% of physician rates for the same service, an extension of previous legislation that allowed the same reimbursement rate to NPs and CNSs practicing in rural areas (Buppert, 1999). This law was passed after years of work in this area, including research documenting NP and CNS contributions to health care delivery and client outcomes and after active lobbying efforts by professional nursing organizations. Reimbursement for these nurses has not changed to any extent since the 1990s.

In addition, data about the cost/benefit ratio, efficiency, and effectiveness of nursing care in general have been collected. Today, more than 250 nurse-managed clinics provide health care services to individuals in the United States who might not otherwise have access to health care, such as older adults, the homeless, and schoolchildren. All of these events have moved the discipline toward more autonomy in nursing practice and are serving as a means for evaluating and documenting nurses' contributions to health care delivery (Sebastian and Stanhope, 2005).

LINKING CONTENT TO PRACTICE

The balance of interest within society and health care will continue to shift toward a focus on quality, safety, and elimination of health disparities through public and private sector partnerships. Health care system concerns of the twenty-first century are expected to focus on examining the quality of health care relative to the costs of care delivered, reduction in disparities, access to care, and health care reform. These changes will result from continued efforts of both the public and private sectors to reform the U.S. health care system. The current era of health care delivery will be noted as a time of vast changes in all sectors of health care delivery.

Nurses must plan for future changes in health care financing by becoming aware of the costs of nursing services, identifying aspects of care where cost savings can be safely achieved, and developing knowledge on how nursing practice affects and is affected by the principles of economics. Nursing must continue to focus on improving the overall health of the nation, defining its contribution to the health of the nation, deriving the value of nursing care, and ensuring its economic viability within the health care marketplace. Nurses must effect changes in the health care system by providing leadership in developing new models of care delivery that provide effective, high-quality care and by assuming a greater role in evaluating client care and nurse performance. It is through their leadership that nurses will contribute to improved decision-making about allocating scarce health care resources, and promoting primary prevention as an answer to improve many of the current population level health outcomes.

CHAPTER REVIEW

PRACTICE APPLICATION

Connie, a nursing student, has identified a caseload of five families in a chronic disease program offered by the local public health department. She is interested in assessing the costs of care to her clients and to the agency. Connie approaches the public health nurse administrator and asks the following questions:

A. How is the agency reimbursed for chronic disease management?

B. Does the client have a responsibility for paying for services?

C. Are nursing care costs known?

D. Are services rationed to clients? On what basis?

E. What effect will the chronic disease management program have on the community population?

Answers can be found on the Evolve site.

KEY POINTS

- From 1800 to 2000, the U.S. health care delivery system experienced four developmental stages, with different emphases on health care economics. With the twenty-first century, the health care delivery system entered another developmental stage.
- Four basic components provide the framework for the development of delivery of health care services: service needs and intensity, facilities, technology, and labor (workforce).

- Three major factors have been associated with the growth of the health care delivery system: price inflation, changes in population demographics, and technology and service intensity.
- Chronic disease is becoming a major health factor affecting health care spending with one in two Americans experiencing at least one chronic disease.

KEY POINTS—cont'd

- Health care financing has evolved through the twentieth century from a system financed primarily by the consumer to a system financed primarily by third-party payers. In the twenty-first century, the consumer is being asked to pay more.
- To solve the problems of rising health care costs, a number of plans for future payment of health care are being considered; all include some form of rationing.
- Excessive and inefficient use of goods and services in health care delivery has been viewed as the major cause of rising health care costs.
- Economics is concerned with use of resources, including money, to fulfill society's needs and wants.
- Health economics is concerned with the problems of producing services and programs and distributing them to clients.
- The goal of public health economics is maximum benefits from services of public health providers, leading to health and wellness of the population.
- The goal of public health is providing the most good for the most people.
- Nurses need to understand basic economic principles to avoid contributing to rising health care costs.
- The GNP reflects the market value of goods and services produced by the United States.
- The GDP reflects the market value of the output of labor and property located in the United States.

- Microeconomic theory shows how supply and demand can be used in health care.
- Macroeconomic theory helps one look at national and community issues that affect health care.
- Social issues, economic issues, and communicable disease epidemics mark the problems of the twenty-first century.
- Medicare and Medicaid are two government-funded programs that help meet the needs of high-risk populations in the United States.
- A majority of the U.S. population has health insurance. The remaining uninsured segment represents millions of people, mostly the working poor, older adults, and children, and those who lost jobs in the economic downturn of 2008.
- Poverty has a detrimental effect on health.
- Health care rationing has always been a part of the U.S. health care system and will continue to be with the proposed new health care reform.
- Nurses are cost-effective providers and must be an integral part of health care delivery.
- *Healthy People 2020* is a document that has established U.S. health objectives.
- Human life is valued in health economics, as is money. An emphasis on changing lifestyles and preventive care will reduce the unnecessary years of life lost to early and preventable death.

CLINICAL DECISION-MAKING ACTIVITIES

1. Define the following terms in your own words: economics, health economics, public health economics, public health finance, gross national product, gross domestic product, consumer price index, and human capital. How do these terms relate to your work as a nurse?
2. Compare the advantages and disadvantages of applying economics to public health care issues. Be specific.
3. Compare and contrast efficiency and effectiveness of a public health program. What factors make these difficult to control?
4. Apply the concepts of supply and demand to an example from population health. Be precise in your answer.

5. Review Chapter 6. Debate in class the ethical implications of the goal of rationing. Focus your debate on the implications for nursing practice. What are some of the complexities of this question?
6. Invite a public health nurse administrator to meet with your class or clinical conference group. Ask how inflation, changes in population, and technology have changed the public health care delivery system and nursing practice. How could we check for ourselves to find the answers?

REFERENCES

Agency for Healthcare Research and Quality, Guide to Clinical Preventive Services, 2009, Rockville, MD, September 2009, AHRQ Publication No. 09–IP006.

American Association of Colleges of Nursing: *Nursing shortage fact sheet*, Washington, DC, May 2010, AACN.

American Nurses Association: *Medicare reimbursement for NPs and CNSs*, Silver Springs, MD, 1999, The Association.

Anderson E, de Renzio P, Levy S: *The role of public investment in poverty reduction: theories, evidence and methods*, London, 2006, Overseas Development Institute.

Buppert C: HEDIS for the primary care provider: getting an "A" on the managed care report card, *Nurse Pract* 24:84–94, 1999.

Bureau of Labor Statistics, U.S. Department of Labor: *Occupational outlook handbook, 2004-2005* edition, Washington, DC, 2006, Superintendent of Documents, U.S. Government Printing Office.

Bureau of Labor Statistics, U.S. Department of Labor: *Career guide to industries*, 2010-11 edition, Washington, DC, 2010, Superintendent of Documents, U.S. Government Printing Office.

Centers for Disease Control and Prevention: Ten great public health achievements—United States 1900-1999. In Lee P, Estes C, editors: *The nation's health*, Boston, 2001, Jones and Bartlett.

Centers for Disease Control and Prevention: *H1N1 outbreaks*, 2009. Available at http://www.cdc.gov. Accessed December 8, 2010.

Centers for Medicare and Medicaid Services: *Medicare hospital outpatient payment system*, 2005a. Available at http://www.cms.hhs.gov/apps/media/press/release.asp?Counter=376. Accessed December 8, 2010.

Centers for Medicare and Medicaid Services: *Medicare and you*, Baltimore, MD, September 2009, USDHHS.

Centers for Medicare and Medicaid Services: *Overview: case mix prospective payment for SNFs balanced budget*, 2005b. Available at http://www.cms.hhs.gov/SNFPPS/01_overview.asp. Accessed December 8, 2010.

Centers for Medicare and Medicaid Services: Office of the Actuary: *National health care expenditures projections*, U.S. Department of Health and Human Services, 2010. Available at http://www.cms.hhs.gov/MedicareEnRpts. Accessed December 8, 2010.

Colander D: *Microeconomics*, ed 7, London, 2008, McGraw-Hill.

Community Preventive Services Task Force: *Role of the task force*, 2006. Available at http://www.thecommunityguide.org/about/task-force-members.html, page last updated 05/09/06. Accessed December 8, 2010.

Congressional Budget Office: *The budget and economic outlook*, Washington, DC, August 2001, U.S. Government Printing Office.

Congressional Budget Office: *The budget and economic outlook*, Washington, DC, August 2010, U.S. Government Printing Office.

Gillespie KN, Kurz RS, McBride T, et al: Competencies for public health finance: an initial assessment and recommendations, *J Public Health Manag Pract* 10:458–466, 2004.

Goodwin N, Nelson JA, Ackerman F, Weisskopf T: *Microeconomics in Context*, M.E. Sharpe, New York, 2008, Armonk.

Hall B: *A new day: what the Patient Protection and Affordable Care Act means to the incentive industry Incentive*, June/July 2010. Available at www.incentivemag.com. Accessed December 8, 2010.

Hazen GB: Adding extrinsic goals to the quality-adjusted life year model, *Decision Analysis* 4(1):1–3, 2007.

Health Care Financing Administration: *Case mix prospective payment for SNF's Balanced Budget Act of 1997*, Washington, DC, 1998, USDHHS.

Health Care Financing Administration: *HIPAA: the Health Insurance Portability and Accountability Act of 1996*, Washington, DC, 1999, USDHHS.

Honoré PA: *DHA public health finance and quality: examining the connection*, Rockville, MD, 2008, U.S. Department of Health and Human Services.

Hunt KA, Knickman JR: Financing for health care. In *Health care delivery in the United States*, New York, 2005, Springer.

Institute of Medicine: *The future of the public's health in the 21st century*, Washington, DC, 2003, The National Academic Press.

Internal Revenue Service: *Publication 969: health savings accounts and other tax-favored health plans*, 2005. Available at http://www.irs.gov/publications/p969/ar02.html. Accessed December 8, 2010.

Jacobs P: *The economics of health and medical care*, ed 5, Gaithersburg, MD, 2002, Aspen.

Kaiser Family Foundation: *Fastfacts*, Menlo Park, CA, 2010a, Kaiser Family Foundation.

Kaiser Family Foundation: *Medicaid facts: Medicaid and uninsured*, Menlo Park, CA, 2010b, June 2010, Kaiser Family Foundation.

Kaiser Family Foundation: *Medicare chart book*, ed 3, Menlo Park, CA, 2005, Kaiser Family Foundation.

Kaiser Family Foundation: *The uninsured: a primer key facts about Americans without health insurance*, Menlo Park, CA, October 2009, Kaiser Family Foundation.

Kovner C: The health care workforce in the United States. In Kovner A, editor: *Health care delivery in the United States*, New York, 2005, Springer.

Kropf R: Technology assessment in health care. In *Health care delivery in the United States*, New York, 2005, Springer.

Lee P, Estes C: *The nation's health*, Boston, 2003, Jones and Bartlett.

Mantone J: Stating the case for coverage, *Modern Healthcare* 6-7:16, 2006.

McPake B, Normand C: *Health economics: an international perspective*, New York, 2008, Routledge.

Moulton AD, Halverson PK, Honoré PA, Berkowitz B: Public health finance: a conceptual framework, *J Public Health Manag Pract* 10:377–382, 2004.

National Center for Health Statistics: *Health: United States, 2005, with chartbook on trends in the health of Americans*, Hyattsville, MD, 2005, U.S. Government Printing Office.

National Center for Health Statistics: *Health: United States*, Hyattsville, MD, 2009, U.S. Government Printing Office.

National Center for Health Statistics: *Health: United States, 2009, with special feature on medical technology*, Hyattsville, MD, 2010, U.S. Government Printing Office.

National Commission on Prevention Priorities (NCPP) Preventive Care: *A National Profile on Use, Disparities, and Health Benefits*, August 2007, Partnership for Prevention.

Nichols LM, Blumberg LJ: A different kind of "new federalism"? The Health Insurance Portability and Accountability Act of 1996, *Health Aff* 17:25–42, 1998.

Patient Protection and Affordable Care Act (PL 111-148), March 2010, healthcare.org.

Robert Wood Johnson Foundation: *Cover The Uninsured*, 2009. Available at www.covertheuninsured.org. Accessed December 8, 2010.

Sebastian J, Stanhope M: Survey of academic primary care nurse managed centers, a joint project of the Michigan Consortium Group and the University of Kentucky College of Nursing, 2005.

Stanhope M, Turner L, Riley P: Vulnerable populations, *Nurs Clin North Am* 43(3):xiii–xiv, 2008.

Trust for America's Health: *Prevention for a healthier America: investments in disease prevention yield significant savings, stronger communities*, Washington, DC, February 2009.

Trust for America's Health: *Blueprint for a healthier American*, Washington, DC, October 2008.

Turnock BJ: *Public health: what it is and how it works*, Boston, 2008, Jones and Bartlett.

U.S. Census Bureau: U.S. population clock, 2010. Retrieved 8/13/10 from http://www.census.gov/main/www/popclock.html.

U.S. Department of Health and Human Services: HHS federal poverty guidelines, *Federal Register* 75(184):45625–45629, August 3, 2010.

U.S. Department of Health and Human Services, Centers for Medicare and Medicaid: *National trends, 1966-2009*. Available at http://www.cms.hhs.gov/medicareEnrpts.

U.S. Department of Health and Human Services: *Healthy People 2020: a roadmap to improve all American's Health*, Washington, DC, 2010, USDHHS, Public Health Service.

U.S. Department of Health and Human Services: *Healthy People 2010: understanding and improving health*, Washington, DC, 2000, Public Health Service.

U.S. Department of Health and Human Services (USDHHS), Centers for Disease Control and Prevention, National Center for Health Statistics: *NCHS definitions: gross domestic product (GDP)*, 2004. Available at http://www.cdc.gov/nchs/datawh/nchsdefs/gdp.htm. Accessed June 13, 2006.

Veney J, Kaluzny A: *Evaluation and decision making for health services*, Washington, DC, 2005, Beard Books.

World Health Organization: *World health statistics, 2010*, Geneva, 2010, WHO.

CHAPTER 6

Application of Ethics in the Community

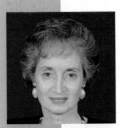

Mary Cipriano Silva, PhD, RN, FAAN

Mary Cipriano Silva is a professor emerita at George Mason University in Fairfax, Virginia. She is a nationally recognized and award-winning ethics scholar who has published extensively in health care ethics for over 35 years.

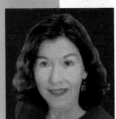

Jeanne Merkle Sorrell, PhD, RN, FAAN

Jeanne Merkle Sorrell is currently Senior Nurse Researcher at the Cleveland Clinic in Ohio, and professor emerita at George Mason University. Her current research focuses on ethical concerns of persons with Alzheimer's disease and their families and professional caregivers. She has incorporated her research findings into an award-winning educational video, *Quality Lives: Ethics in the Care of Persons with Alzheimer's,* and a play, *Six Characters in Search of an Answer,* which was selected for the 2007 Sigma Theta Tau International Nursing Media Award.

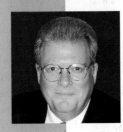

James J. Fletcher, PhD

James J. Fletcher is a professor emeritus of philosophy in the Department of Philosophy at George Mason University, where he specializes in bioethics. In addition to his research and teaching in bioethics, he is a member of the ethics committee and chair of the Human Research Review Committee of a community hospital. He sits on the Institutional Review Board of a local biotechnological company, serves as a member of Data and Safety Monitoring Boards for the National Institutes of Health, and is a member of a District Disciplinary Committee of the Virginia State Bar.

ADDITIONAL RESOURCES

Evolve WEBSITE

http://evolve.elsevier.com/Stanhope

- *Healthy People 2020*
- WebLinks—Of special note see the link for these sites:
  - International Council of Nurses Code of Ethics for Nurses
  - Online Journal of Issues in Nursing Ethics Column
  - American Nurses Association Center for Ethics and Human Rights
  - Bioethics Ethics Research at the Hastings Center
- Quiz
- Case Studies
- Glossary
- Answers to Practice Application

APPENDIX
- Appendix H: Focus on Quality and Safety Education for Nurses

OBJECTIVES

After reading this chapter, the student should be able to do the following:

1. Describe a brief history of the ethics of nursing practice.
2. Analyze ethical decision-making processes.
3. Compare and contrast ethical theories and principles, virtue ethics, the ethic of care, and feminist ethics.
4. Comprehend the ethics inherent in the core functions of public health nursing.
5. Analyze codes of ethics for nursing and for public health.
6. Apply the ethics of advocacy to nursing practice.

KEY TERMS

CHAPTER OUTLINE

Nurses who practice in the community focus on protecting, promoting, preserving, and maintaining health while preventing disease. These goals reflect the ethical principles of promoting good and preventing harm. In addition, nurses struggle with the rights of individuals and families versus the rights of local groups within a community. On the other hand, nurses struggle with the rights of a community or population versus the rights of individuals, families, and local groups within a community. These two types of struggle reflect the tensions between respect for autonomy, rights-based ethical theory, and community-based ethical theory.

Nurses also deal with consequence-based ethical theory, obligation-based ethical theory, and the ethical components of advocacy, justice, health policy, caring, women's moral experiences, and the moral character of health care practitioners. They are guided by codes of ethics and ethical decision-making frameworks. The purpose of this chapter, then, is to make explicit the preceding content as it relates to the ethics inherent in nursing.

HISTORY

The history of nursing is discussed in detail in Chapter 2. The focus here is a brief history of nursing and public health ethics and the relationship between them and nursing.

Modern nursing has a rich heritage of ethics and morality, beginning with Florence Nightingale (1820–1910). Her values and the moral significance she inculcated into the profession have endured. She saw nursing as a call to service and viewed the moral character of persons entering nursing as important. She also viewed nursing within a broad social context, where poor people mattered and where soldiers harmed in the Crimean War (1854–1856) did not have to endure unhealthy environments. Because of her commitment to poor individuals in communities, as well as her stances on primary prevention and population-based evidence that healthy environments save soldiers' lives, she is seen as nursing's first enduring moral leader who defined the community as her client.

In 1860, Nightingale established the first nursing program in London. It was hospital based, but the curriculum contained not only care of the sick, but also public health concepts with their inherent ethical tenets. Many of these programs were associated with religious institutions. Students, therefore, often received ethics courses with a slant toward a particular religion's values. Soon thereafter in the United States, the notion of hospital-based nursing programs took hold, but nursing practice in the community was not a part of the curricula.

In the 1960s, two seminal events occurred. First, the American Nurses Association (ANA) recommended that all nursing education should occur in institutions of higher education. As this process slowly took place, ethics, as a course per se, was removed from many schools of nursing, although ethical values remained. Second, because of major advances in science and technology that affected health care, the field of bioethics began to emerge and was reflected in nursing curricula. Today, the vast majority of nursing programs integrate bioethical content into their courses or have separate courses on this topic; some do both. Although some of these courses relate bioethics to community nursing, the emphasis has been primarily on acute care nursing.

DID YOU KNOW? *The term ethics comes from the Greek word ethos, meaning character, habit, or custom. In 1938 British-American anthropologist Gregory Bateson adapted the term ethos to refer to the distinguishing character or attitude of a specific people, culture, or group, as in, for example, the "American ethos."*

Nurses' codes of ethics are important in the history of public health nursing practice. The Nightingale Pledge is generally considered to be nursing's first code of ethics (ANA, 2001). After the Nightingale Pledge, a "suggested" code and a "tentative" code were published in the *American Journal of Nursing* but were not formally adopted. In 1950, however, the *Code for Professional Nurses* was formally adopted by the ANA House of Delegates. In 1956, 1960, 1968, 1976, and 1985, the code was amended or revised. In 2001, after 5 years of work, the *Code of Ethics for Nurses with Interpretive Statements* was adopted by the ANA House of Delegates (ANA, 2001).

Nurses should also be familiar with the first known international code of ethics, developed by the International Council of Nurses (ICN) in 1953 (ICN, 1953). Like the ANA code, the ICN code has undergone various revisions and adoptions. The most recent version of the *ICN Code of Ethics for Nurses* was adopted in 2006 (ICN, 2006).

In addition to codes of ethics, the nursing literature and nursing associations have consistently reflected a commitment to ethics, as well as an awareness of nursing's ethical obligations to society. From the 1980s to the present, the number of centers for nursing and health care ethics has increased steadily. The majority of these centers are located in academic settings; however, in 1991 the ANA founded its Center for Ethics and Human Rights. The historical contributions have affected the persistent ethicality of nursing. In 2008, the ANA published *Nursing and Health Care Ethics: A Legacy and a Vision*, which creatively assesses historical contributions of nursing scholars in ethics and explores a vision for the future scholarship of nursing ethics (Pinch and Haddad, 2008).

The bioethics movement of the late 1960s influenced not only nursing ethics, but also public health ethics. However, until recently, the relationship between public health and ethics was implicit rather than explicit (Callahan and Jennings, 2002; Petrini, 2010).

Finally, in 2000, public health professionals, individually and through their associations, initiated the writing of a code of ethics that was supported by the American Public Health Association (APHA). In 2001 the Public Health Code of Ethics was widely disseminated via the APHA website for critique (www.apha.org) and was adopted in 2002 (Olick, 2005). The code presents principles, rules, and ideals to guide public health practice but is not intended to provide a specific action plan for ethical decision making.

Before discussing ethics related to nursing practice in the community, some key ethical terms are defined in Box 6-1. Other ethical terms are defined within the context of the chapter.

BOX 6-1   KEY ETHICAL TERMS

Ethics is a branch of philosophy that includes both a body of knowledge about the moral life and a process of reflection for determining what persons ought to do or be, regarding this life.

Bioethics is a branch of ethics that applies the knowledge and processes of ethics to the examination of ethical problems in health care.

Moral distress is an uncomfortable state of self when one is unable to act ethically.

Morality is shared and generational societal norms about what constitutes right or wrong conduct.

Values are beliefs about the worth or importance of what is right or esteemed.

Ethical dilemma is a puzzling moral problem in which a person, group, or community can envision morally justified reasons for both taking and not taking a certain course of action.

Codes of ethics are moral standards that delineate a profession's values, goals, and obligations.

Utilitarianism is an ethical theory based on the weighing of morally significant outcomes or consequences regarding the overall maximizing of good and minimizing of harm for the greatest number of people.

Deontology is an ethical theory that bases moral obligation on duty and claims that actions are obligatory irrespective of the good or harmful consequences that they produce. Because humans are rational, they have absolute value. Therefore, persons should always be treated as ends in themselves and never as mere means.

Principlism is an approach to problem solving in bioethics that uses the principles of respect for autonomy, beneficence, nonmaleficence, and justice as the basis for organization and analysis.

Advocacy is the act of pleading for or supporting a course of action on behalf of a person, group, or community.

NURSING TIP *Our language often programs us to think in terms of opposites, such as right or wrong, so that we think we need to choose one or the other. Often, there are more than two sides to an ethical issue. When we try to understand the differing values of individuals and groups in a community, we find important points to consider on different sides of an ethical issue and focus not only on what we think is right, but also on what we should respect in each perspective of an ethical issue.*

ETHICAL DECISION MAKING

Ethical decision making is that component of ethics that focuses on the process of how ethical decisions are made. The process is the thinking that occurs when health care professionals must make decisions about ethical issues and ethical dilemmas. Ethical issues are moral challenges facing us or our profession. In nursing, one such challenge is how to prepare an adequate and competent workforce for the future. In contrast, ethical dilemmas are human dilemmas and puzzling moral problems in which a person, group, or community can envision morally justified reasons for both taking and not taking a certain course of action. One example of an ethical dilemma is how to allocate resources to two equally needy populations when the resources are sufficient to serve only one of the populations. Ethical theories, principles and decision-making frameworks help us think through these issues and dilemmas.

Ethical decision-making frameworks use problem-solving processes. They provide guides for making sound ethical decisions that can be morally justified. Many such frameworks exist in the health care literature, and some are presented in this chapter. A caveat, however, is in order. Weston (2006, p 22) notes that the first requirement of ethics is to *think* appreciatively and carefully about moral matters. We should not simply obey rules or authorities without thinking for ourselves; thinking for ourselves is both a moral responsibility and a hard-won right.

Keeping the preceding caveat in mind, the following generic ethical decision-making framework is presented:

1. Identify the ethical issues and dilemmas.
2. Place them within a meaningful context.
3. Obtain all relevant facts.
4. Reformulate ethical issues and dilemmas, if needed.
5. Consider appropriate *approaches* to actions or options (such as utilitarianism, deontology, principlism, virtue ethics, ethic of care, feminist ethics).
6. Make a decision and take action.
7. Evaluate the decision and the action.

The steps of a generic ethics framework are often non-linear, and, with the exception of step 5, they do not change substantially. The rationale for each of the seven steps is presented in Table 6-1. The six approaches to actions or options in the ethical decision-making framework (step 5) are outlined throughout the chapter in the "How To" boxes.

WHAT DO YOU THINK?   *Should a client be able to make a decision that meets his or her cultural or religious values if it contradicts the values of the health care providers or health care system?*

Two factors affect this ethical decision-making framework: (1) the growing multiculturalism of the American society, and (2) moral distress. First, nurses often deal with ethical issues and dilemmas related to the diverse and at times conflicting values that result from ethnicity. From a moral perspective, what should the nurse do when facing ethnicity conflicts?

Callahan (2000) offers useful insights into these conflicts. He describes four situations in which ethnic diversity can be judged in relationship to cultural standards:

1. Situations that place persons at direct risk of harm, whether psychological or physical
2. Situations in which ethnic cultural standards conflict with professional standards
3. Situations in which the greater community's values are jeopardized by specific ethnic values
4. Situations in which specific ethnic community customs are annoying but not problematic for the greater community

Callahan (2000, p 43) discusses how to judge diversity in the four situations. Regarding situation 1, he states that "we in America imposed some standards on ourselves for important moral reasons; and there is no good reason to exempt [ethnic] subgroups from those standards." Regarding situations 2 and 3, he suggests a thoughtful tolerance but also some degree of moral persuasion (not coercion) for ethnic groups to alter values so that they are more in keeping with what is normative in the American culture. However, Callahan notes that "in the absence of grievous harm, there is no clear moral mandate to interfere with those values" (p 43). Finally, regarding situation 4, he believes in moral tolerance of non-threatening ethnic traditions, since there is no moral mandate to do otherwise.

Second, since decision making is so central to the practice of nursing, and many decisions are not easy ones to make, spending more time on the experience of ethical or **moral distress** is useful. Moral or ethical distress occurs when a person is unable to act in a way that he or she thinks is right. You do not feel that you are able to act in a manner consistent with your own values, cultural expectations, and religious beliefs. When this conflict occurs, it can lead to a personal sense of failure in the kind of care you give and to subsequent performance issues and may lead to work and/or career dissatisfaction. However, there are ways to handle moral distress:

1. Identifying the type(s) of situations that lead to distress
2. Communicating that concern to your manager and examining ways to work toward addressing the stressor
3. Seeking support from colleagues

TABLE 6-1   RATIONALE FOR STEPS OF ETHICAL DECISION-MAKING FRAMEWORK

STEPS	RATIONALE
1. Identify the ethical issues and dilemmas.	Persons cannot make sound ethical decisions if they cannot identify ethical issues and dilemmas.
2. Place them within a meaningful context.	The historical, legal, sociological, cultural, psychological, economic, political, communal, environmental, and demographic contexts affect the way ethical issues and dilemmas are formulated and justified.
3. Obtain all relevant facts.	Facts affect the way ethical issues and dilemmas are formulated and justified.
4. Reformulate ethical issues and dilemmas if needed.	The initial ethical issues and dilemmas may need to be modified or changed on the basis of context and facts.
5. Consider appropriate approaches to actions or options.	The nature of the ethical issues and dilemmas determines the specific ethical approaches used.
6. Make decisions and take action.	Professional persons cannot avoid choice and action in applied ethics.
7. Evaluate decisions and action.	Evaluation determines whether or not the ethical decision-making framework used resulted in morally justified actions related to the ethical issues and dilemmas.

It is often useful to talk with colleagues. You may learn that they have similar concerns or that they have found ways to interrupt the stressful situation(s) (Carlock and Spader, 2007). Understanding both multiculturalism and moral distress enhances ethical decision making.

ETHICS

Definition, Theories, Principles

Ethics is concerned with a body of knowledge that addresses such questions as the following: How should I behave? What actions should I perform? What kind of person should I be? What are my obligations to myself and to fellow humans? There are general obligations that humans have as members of society. Among these general obligations are not to harm others, to respect others, to tell the truth, and to keep promises. Sometimes, however, a situation dictates that individuals tell a lie or break a promise because the consequences of telling the truth or keeping the promise may bring about more harm than good. For example, as a nurse you have promised a family that you will visit them at a certain time, but your schedule has gone awry because of unexpected circumstances. One of the other families you visit is in a state of crisis—their adolescent child is suicidal—and your nursing intervention is needed. Most nurses would agree that this is not a good time to keep the original promise. You are morally justified in breaking your promise because you fear that more harm than good would be done if it were kept.

HOW TO Apply the Utilitarian Ethics Decision Process

1. *Determine moral rules that are important to society and that are derived from the principle of utility.**
2. *Identify the communities or populations that are affected or most affected by the moral rules.*
3. *Analyze viable alternatives for each proposed action based on the moral rules.*
4. *Determine the consequences or outcomes of each viable alternative on the communities or populations most affected by the decision.*
5. *Select the actions on the basis of the rules that produce the greatest amount of good or the least amount of harm for the communities or populations that are affected by the actions.*
   (Remember that the utilitarian ethics decision process is one of the approaches in step 5 of the generic ethical decision-making framework.)

---

*Moral rules of action that produce the greatest good for the greatest number of communities or populations affected by or most affected by the rules.

This example illustrates several things about ethical thinking. First, ethical judgments are concerned with values. The goal of an ethical judgment is to choose that action or state of affairs that is good or right in the circumstances. Second, ethical judgments generally do not have the certainty of scientific judgments. For example, nurses diagnose a situation on the basis of the best available information and then choose the course of action that seems to provide the best ethical resolution to the issue. In some situations, the decision is based on outcomes or consequences. That approach to ethical decision making is called consequentialism. It maintains that the right action is the one that produces the greatest amount of good or the least amount of harm in a given situation. Utilitarianism is a well-known consequentialist theory that appeals exclusively to outcomes or consequences in determining which choice to make.

In other situations, nurses touch upon options open to fundamental beliefs. In such circumstances, these nurses may conclude that the action is right or wrong in itself, regardless of the amount of good that might come from it. This is the position known as deontology. It is based on the premise that persons should always be treated as ends in themselves and never as mere means to the ends of others.

HOW TO Apply the Deontological Ethics Decision Process

1. *Determine the moral rules (e.g., tell the truth) that serve as standards by which individuals can perform their moral obligations.*
2. *Examine personal motives for proposed actions to ensure that they are based on good intentions in accord with moral rules.*
3. *Determine whether the proposed actions can be generalized so that all persons in similar situations are treated similarly.*
4. *Select the action that treats persons as ends in themselves and never as mere means to the ends of others.*
   (Remember that the deontological ethics decision process is one of the approaches in step 5 of the generic ethical decision-making framework.)

Members of the health professions have specific obligations that exist because of the practices and goals of the profession. These health care obligations have been interpreted in terms of a set of principles in bioethics. The primary principles are respect for autonomy, nonmaleficence, beneficence, and distributive justice, as shown in Box 6-2. These principles have dominated

---

BOX 6-2 **ETHICAL PRINCIPLES**

Respect for autonomy: Based on human dignity and respect for individuals, autonomy requires that individuals be permitted to choose those actions and goals that fulfill their life plans unless those choices result in harm to another.

Nonmaleficence: Nonmaleficence requires that we do no harm. It is impossible to avoid harm entirely, but this principle requires that health care professionals act according to the standards of due care, always seeking to produce the least amount of harm possible.

Beneficence: This principle is complementary to nonmaleficence and requires that we do good. We are limited by time, place, and talents in the amount of good we can do. We have general obligations to perform those actions that maintain or enhance the dignity of other persons whenever those actions do not place an undue burden on health care providers.

Distributive justice: Distributive justice requires that there be a fair distribution of the benefits and burdens in society based on the needs and contributions of its members. This principle requires that, consistent with the dignity and worth of its members and within the limits imposed by its resources, a society must determine a minimal level of goods and services to be available to its members.

the development of the field of bioethics since its inception in the 1960s (Walker, 2009). This approach has been called **principlism,** and one of its best descriptions and fullest articulations is in the sixth edition of *Principles of Biomedical Ethics* by Beauchamp and Childress (2008). This approach to ethical decision making in health care arose in response to life-and-death decision making in acute care settings, where the question to be resolved tended to concern a single localized issue such as the withdrawing or withholding of treatment (Holstein, 2001). In these circumstances, preserving and respecting a client's autonomy became the dominant issue.

Despite its success as a basis for analysis in bioethics, principlism has come under attack (e.g., Callahan, 2000, 2003; Walker, 2009), and there are grounds for the criticism. First, the principles are said to be too abstract and narrow to serve as guides for action. Second, the principles themselves can conflict in a given situation, and there is no independent basis for resolving the conflict. Third, some persons claim that effective ethical problem solving must be rooted in concrete, individual experiences. Fourth, ethical judgments are alleged to depend more on the judgment of sensitive persons than on the application of abstract principles.

HOW TO Apply the Principlism Ethics Decision Process

1. *Determine the ethical principles (respect for autonomy, nonmaleficence, beneficence, justice) that are relevant to an ethical issue or dilemma.*
2. *Analyze the relevant principles within a meaningful context of accurate facts and other pertinent circumstances.*
3. *Act on the principle that provides, within the meaningful context, the strongest guide to action that can be morally justified by the tenets foundational to the principle.*

(Remember that the principlism ethics decision process is one of the approaches in step 5 of the general ethical decision-making framework.)

The dominance of the principle of respect for autonomy has been challenged by critics concerned about decision making in non–acute care settings, where the ethical decision is more likely to be about, for example, long-term care or access to health care for persons of diverse cultures (Callahan and Jennings, 2002; Walker, 2009). Thus, whereas autonomy may be stressed in acute care settings, an overemphasis on autonomy may inhibit ethical decisions in public health. In public health, beneficence and distributive justice are frequently a greater issue than autonomy. For this reason, it is useful to look at other models for ethical decision making, including models that expand the focus of nursing beyond the individual nurse-client relationship to the social environment and systems that impact health care (Bekemeier and Butterfield, 2005).

Utilitarianism and deontology were developed from the Enlightenment period's focus on universals, rationality, and isolated individuals. Each theory maintains that there is a universal first principle—the principle of utility for utilitarianism and the categorical imperative for deontology—that serves as a rational norm for our behavior and allows us to calculate the rightness or wrongness of each individual action. Both utilitarianism and deontology also follow the lead of classic liberalism in asserting that the individual is the special center of moral concern (Steinbock, Arras, and London, 2008). Giving priority to individual rights and needs means that these should not be sacrificed for the interests of society (Steinbock, Arras, and London, 2008). The focus on individual rights leads to complications in the interpretation of distributive or social justice.

Distributive or social justice refers to the allocation of benefits and burdens to members of society. *Benefits* refer to basic needs, including material and social goods, liberties, rights, and entitlements. Wealth, education, and public services are benefits. *Burdens* include such things as taxes, military service, and the location of incinerators and power plants. Justice requires that the distribution of benefits and burdens in a society be fair or equal. There is wide agreement that the distribution should be based on what one needs and deserves, but there is considerable disagreement as to what these terms mean. Three primary theories of distributive justice are defended today. They are the egalitarian, libertarian, and liberal democratic theories.

Egalitarianism is the view that everyone is entitled to equal rights and equal treatment in society. Ideally, each individual has an equal share of the goods of society, and it is the role of government to ensure that this happens. The government has the authority to redistribute wealth if necessary to ensure equal treatment. Thus, egalitarians are supportive of welfare rights—that is, the right to receive certain social goods necessary to satisfy basic needs, including adequate food, housing, education, and police and fire protection. The weaknesses of egalitarianism are both practical and theoretical. It would be practically impossible to ensure the equal distribution of goods and services in any moderately complex society. Assuming that such a distribution could be accomplished, it would require a coercive authority to maintain it (Coursin, 2009; Hellsten, 1998). Further, egalitarianism is unable to provide any incentive for each of us to do our best, since there is no promise of our merit being rewarded.

The *libertarian* view of justice holds that the right to private property is the most important right. Libertarians recognize only liberty rights—the right to be left alone to accomplish our goals. Hellsten (1998) notes, "The central feature of the libertarian view on distributive justice is that it is totally individualist. It rejects any idea that societies, states, or collectives of any form can be the bearers of rights or can owe duties" (p 822). Libertarians see a very limited role for government, namely, the protection of property rights of individual citizens through providing police and fire protection. While they also concede the need for jointly shared, publicly owned facilities such as roads, they reject the idea of welfare rights and view taxes to support the needs of others as coercive taking of their property. Given the libertarian rejection of the priority of the state, however, it is not clear where the right to property originates (Hellsten, 1998).

The *liberal democratic* theory is well represented by the work of John Rawls (2001). Rawls attempts to develop a theory that values both liberty and equality. He acknowledges that inequities are inevitable in society, but he tries to justify them by establishing a system in which everyone benefits, especially the least advantaged. This is an attempt to address the inequalities that result from birth, natural endowments, and historic circumstances. Imagining what he calls a "veil of ignorance" to keep us unaware of our actual advantages and disadvantages, Rawls would have us choose the basic principles of justice (p 15). Once impartiality is guaranteed, Rawls (2001, p 42) maintains that all rational people will choose a system of justice containing the following two basic principles:

Each person has the same indefeasible claim to a fully adequate scheme of equal basic liberties, which scheme is compatible with the same scheme of liberties for all; and social and economic inequalities are to satisfy two conditions: first, they are to be attached to offices and positions open to all under conditions of fair equality of opportunity; and second, they are to be to the greatest benefit of the least advantaged members of society (the difference principle).

As the veil of ignorance and the justice principles indicate, Rawls and other justice theorists all assume the Enlightenment concept of isolated, atomic selves in competition for scarce resources. The significance of justice, then, becomes the assurance of fairness to individuals. Violating the dictates of distributive justice is an offense to the dignity of the collective preferences of autonomous, rational moral agents. The interests of the community may be in conflict with the interests of individuals; yet, confined to the Enlightenment ideal, the needs of society are not directly addressed, nor is society given any priority.

This Enlightenment assumption has been challenged by a number of ethical theories loosely grouped together under the heading *communitarianism*. The dominant themes of **communitarianism** are that individual rights need to be balanced with social responsibilities; individuals do not live in isolation but are shaped by the values and culture of their communities (Wringle, 2006). Among the theories with a communitarian focus are virtue ethics, ethic of care, and feminist ethics.

Virtue Ethics

Virtue ethics is one of the oldest ethical theories; it belongs to a tradition dating back to the ancient Greek philosophers Plato and Aristotle. It is not concerned with actions, as utilitarianism and deontology are, but instead asks, What kind of person should I be? The goal of virtue ethics is to enable persons to flourish as human beings. According to Aristotle, **virtues** are acquired, excellent traits of character that dispose humans to act in accord with their natural good. During the seventeenth and eighteenth centuries, the Greek concept of the good as a principle of explanation went out of favor. Because virtue ethics was closely tied to the concept of the good, interest in virtues as an element of normative ethics also declined. Examples of virtues include benevolence, compassion, discernment, trustworthiness, integrity, and conscientiousness (Beauchamp and Childress, 2008).

There have been several attempts to revive virtue ethics (MacIntyre, 1984), including specific applications to the health care professions (Pellegrino, 1995). In a pluralistic society,

it may be difficult to reach agreement about what it means to flourish as a human being, thus fulfilling the goal of virtue ethics. Although it may not be possible to agree on a single end for human beings, many persons believe it is possible to agree on what is meant by the good for more restricted aspects of our lives.

The appeal to virtues results in a significantly different approach to moral decision making in health care (Olson, 2008). In contrast to moral justification via theories or principles, the emphasis is on practical reasoning applied to character development.

HOW TO Apply the Virtue Ethics Decision Process

1. *Identify communities that are relevant to the ethical dilemmas or issues.*
2. *Identify moral considerations that arise from a communal perspective and apply the consideration to specific communities.*
3. *Identify and apply virtues that facilitate a communal perspective.*
4. *Modify moral considerations as needed to apply to the specific ethical dilemmas or issues.*
5. *Seek ethical community support to enhance character development.*
6. *Evaluate and modify the individuals or community character traits that impede communal living.*
   (Remember that the virtue ethics decision process is one of the approaches in step 5 of the generic ethical decision-making framework.)

Modified from Volbrecht RM: Nursing ethics: communities in dialogue, Upper Saddle River, NJ, 2002, Prentice Hall, p 138.

Caring and the Ethic of Care

Caring in nursing, the ethic of care, and feminist ethics are all interrelated and, historically, all converged between the mid-1980s and early 1990s. Regarding caring in nursing, seminal work was done by nurse-scholars (e.g., Leininger, 1984; Watson, 2007), who wrote about caring as the essence of or the moral ideal of nursing. This conceptualization occurred as a response to the technological advances in health care science and to the desire of nurses to differentiate nursing practice from medical practice. The discussion of the centrality of caring to nursing is reflected in Eriksson's (2002) work on a caring science theory, which she sees as ethical in its essence. Proponents of caring support its premises; its detractors believe that nursing is not the only essentially caring profession and that caring, when placed within a broader societal context, represents the use of a disempowering concept to identify the essence of nursing. However, most nurses, including those who work in the community, would agree that there is a relationship between caring and ethics or morality.

HOW TO Apply the Care Ethics Decision Process

1. *Recognize that caring is a moral imperative.*
2. *Identify personally lived caring experiences as a basis for relating to self and others.*

3. Assume responsibility and obligation to promote and enhance caring in relationships.

(Remember that the care ethics decision process is one of the approaches in step 5 of the generic ethical decision-making framework.)

Carol Gilligan (1982) and Nel Noddings (1984) are often associated with the *ethic of care*. Gilligan (1982) speaks of a personal journey where, by listening and talking to people, she began to notice two distinct voices about morality and two ways of describing the interpersonal relationships between self and others. Contrary to what has been written about Gilligan and the two distinct voices (i.e., male and female) related to moral judgment, here is what she actually wrote: "The different voice I describe is characterized *not by gender* [italics added] but theme. Its association with women is an empirical observation, and it is primarily through women's voices that I trace its development. But this association is not absolute, and the contrasts between male and female voices are presented here to highlight a distinction between two modes of thought and to focus [on] a problem of interpretation rather than to represent a generalization about either sex" (Gilligan, 1982, p 2). Her 1982 book is based on three qualitative studies about conceptions of morality and self and about experiences of conflict and choice. From these studies she formulated her basic premises about responsibility, care, and relationships. These premises, in Gilligan's (1982) own voice, are as follows:

1. "Sensitivity to the needs of others and the assumption of responsibility for taking care lead women to attend to voices other than their own" (p 16).
2. "Women not only define themselves in a context of human relationships but also judge themselves in terms of their ability to care" (p 17).
3. "The truths of relationship, however, return in the rediscovery of connection, in the realization that self and other are interdependent and that life, however valuable in itself, can only be sustained by care in relationships" (p 127).

Noddings' (1984) personal journey started at a point different from that of Gilligan's. Noddings noticed that ethics was described in the literature primarily using principles and logic. The goal for Noddings' book, therefore, was to express a feminine view that could be accepted or rejected by women *or* men. The basic premises of Noddings (1984), in her own voice, are as follows:

1. "The essential elements of caring are located in the relation between the one caring and the cared-for" (p 9).
2. "Caring requires me to respond with an act of commitment: I commit myself either to overt action on behalf of the cared-for or I commit myself to thinking about what I might do" (p 81).
3. "We are not 'justified'—we are *obligated*—to do what is required to maintain and enhance caring" (p 95).
4. "Caring itself and the ethical ideal that strives to maintain and enhance it guide us in moral decisions and conduct" (p 105).

What both Gilligan and Noddings have in common has been called a **feminine ethic,** because they believe in the morality of responsibility in relationships that emphasize connection and caring. To them, caring is not a mere nicety but a moral imperative. Nevertheless, a long-term healthy debate has surrounded their premises.

HOW TO **Apply the Feminist Ethics Decision Process**

1. *Identify the social, cultural, legal, political, economic, environmental, and professional contexts that contribute to the identified problem (e.g., underrepresentation of women in clinical trials).*
2. *Evaluate how the preceding contexts contribute to the oppression of women.*
3. *Consider how women's lives are defined by their status in subordinate social groups.*
4. *Analyze how social practices marginalize women.*
5. *Plan ways to restructure those social practices that oppress women.*
6. *Implement the plan.*
7. *Evaluate the plan and restructure it as needed.*

(Remember that the feminist ethics decision process is one of the approaches in step 5 of the generic ethical decision-making framework.)

Modified from Volbrecht RM: Nursing ethics: communities in dialogue, Upper Saddle River, NJ, 2002, Prentice Hall, p 219.

Feminist Ethics

Although feminist ethics has begun to enter nursing, for many years, nurses appeared reluctant to embrace feminism and its ethics (Silva, 2008). Yet, according to Rogers (2006), the tenets of feminist ethics are highly relevant to public health. Rogers notes that a feminist perspective leads us to think critically about connections between gender, disadvantage, and health, as well as the distribution of power in public health processes. Because these issues have an impact on health, feminist perspectives and approaches are important for nursing practice.

But what is meant by *feminists* and *feminist ethics*? **Feminists** are women *and* men who hold a worldview advocating economic, social, and political equality for women that is equivalent to that of men. Consequently, feminists reject the devaluing of women and their experiences through systematic oppression based on gender. In analyzing the common good, feminists pay careful attention to power relations that constitute a community, rules that regulate it, and who pays and who benefits from membership in the community (Rogers, 2006). Feminists also can ascribe to the ethic of care.

Feminist ethics encompasses the tenets that women's thinking and moral experiences are important and should be taken into account in any fully developed moral theory, and that the oppression of women is morally wrong. Study of feminist ethics entails knowledge about and critique of classical ethical theories developed by men as well as ethical theories developed by women. Study of feminist ethics also entails knowledge about the social, cultural, political, legal, economic, environmental, and professional contexts that insidiously and overtly oppress women as individuals, or within a family, group, community, or society. Feminists and persons who ascribe to feminist ethics are not passive; they demand social justice and political action, preferably at the societal level and through legislation.

ETHICS AND THE CORE FUNCTIONS OF POPULATION-CENTERED NURSING PRACTICE

In Chapter 1, the three foundational pillars or core functions of public health nursing (i.e., assessment, policy development, and assurance) were identified and discussed. This discussion, however, did not include the basic assumption that public health nursing is an ethical endeavor, with moral leadership at its core. Now the links of these three core functions to ethics are described.

Assessment

To review, "assessment refers to systematically collecting data on the population, monitoring the population's health status, and making information available about the health of the community" (Williams and Stanhope, 2008, p 7). Underlying this core function are at least three ethical tenets. The first relates to competency related to knowledge development, analysis, and dissemination. An ethical question related to competency is, Are the persons assigned to develop community knowledge adequately prepared to collect data on groups and populations? This question is important because the research, measurement, and analysis techniques used to gather information about groups and populations usually differ from the techniques used to assess individuals. Wrong research techniques can lead to wrong assessments, which in turn may hurt rather than help the intended group or population. A startling example of this is the case of Henrietta Lacks, whose cancerous cervical cells were taken without her or her families' knowledge or permission and have now launched a medical revolution and a multimillion-dollar industry as the HeLa cells used in countless medical experiments (Skloot, 2010).

The second ethical tenet relates to virtue ethics or moral character. An ethical question related to moral character is, Do the persons selected to develop, assess, and disseminate community knowledge possess integrity? Beauchamp and Childress (2008) define *integrity* as the holistic integration of moral character. The importance of this virtue is self-evident: without integrity, the core function of assessment is endangered. Persons with compromised integrity are easy prey for potential or real scientific misconduct. An example of a failure of integrity for nurses would be bias in collecting or reporting based on racism or homophobic grounds.

The third ethical tenet relates to "do no harm." An ethical question related to "do no harm" is, Is disseminating appropriate information about groups and populations morally necessary and sufficient? The answer to "morally necessary" is yes, but to "morally sufficient," it is no. The fallacy with dissemination is that there is no built-in accountability that what is disseminated will be read or understood. If not read or understood, harm could come to groups and populations regarding their health status.

Policy Development

To review, "Policy development refers to the need to provide leadership in developing policies that support the health of the population, including the use of the scientific knowledge base in making decisions about policy" (Williams and Stanhope, 2008, p 7). Underlying this core function are at least three ethical tenets. First, an important goal of both policy and ethics is to achieve the public good (Silva, 2002). According to several recent accounts, the concept of "the public good" is rooted in citizenship (e.g., Denhardt and Denhardt, 2000; Rogers, 2006; Ruger, 2008). For example, Denhardt and Denhardt (2000) view citizenship, or what they call "democratic citizenship" (p 552), as a stance in which citizens play a more substantial role in policy development. For this to occur, however, citizens must be willing not only to be informed about policy, but also to do what is in the best interests of the community. The approach is basically one in which the voice of the community is the foundation upon which policy is developed, rather than the voice of community *and* public health administrators.

The second ethical tenet purports that service to others over self is a necessary condition of what is "good" or "right" policy (Silva, 2002). Denhardt and Denhardt (2000) offer three perspectives on this matter:

- *Serve rather than steer.* An increasingly important role of the public servant (e.g., nurses and administrators) is to help citizens articulate and meet their shared interests rather than to attempt to control or steer society in new directions (p 553).
- *Serve citizens, not customers.* The public interest results from a dialogue about shared values rather than the aggregation of individual self-interests. Therefore, public servants do not merely respond to the demands of "customers" but focus on building relationships of trust and collaboration with and among citizens (p 555).
- *Value citizenship and public service above entrepreneurship.* The public interest is better advanced by public servants and citizens committed to making meaningful contributions to society rather than by entrepreneurial managers acting as if public money were their own (p 556).

These three perspectives have service at their core, and service has always been one of the enduring values of nursing.

The third ethical tenet purports that what is ethical is also good policy (Silva, 2002). What is ethical should be the singular foundational pillar upon which nursing is based. Moral leadership is critical to policy development because it is the highest human standard and therefore should result in ethical health care policies.

Assurance

To review, "assurance refers to the role of public health in ensuring that essential community-oriented health services are available, which may include providing essential personal health services for those who would otherwise not receive them. Assurance also refers to making sure that a competent public health and personal health care workforce is available" (Williams and Stanhope, 2008, p 7). Underlying this core function are at least two ethical tenets.

The first purports that all persons should receive essential personal health services or, put in terms of justice, "to each person a fair share" or, reworded, "to all groups or populations a fair share." This is an egalitarian perspective of justice. This perspective does not mean that all persons in a society should share all of society's benefits equally, but that they should share at least those benefits that are essential. Few persons who see justice as fairness would disagree that basic health care for all is essential for social justice within a society.

The second ethical tenet purports that providers of public health services are competent and available. Although the *Public Health Code of Ethics* (PHLS, 2002) does not speak directly to workforce availability, it does speak directly to ensuring professional competency of public health employees. In addition to the *Public Health Code of Ethics*, the *Healthy People 2020* objectives (USDHHS, 2009) not only address competencies, but also note workforce needs; a new objective (HP 2020-6) calls for an increased number of health care professionals certified in geriatrics.

The *Healthy People 2020* objectives address the need for all public health workers not only to have knowledge of public health, but also to have additional competencies as needed to fulfill their job responsibilities. Specific areas of knowledge include information technology, biostatistics, environmental health, and cultural and linguistic competence. The objectives also address needs of future public health leaders, who must be educated to meet new challenges in health care. Emphasis is also given to the availability and provision of life-long learning opportunities for public health employees.

NURSING CODE OF ETHICS

As noted in the history section of this chapter, the *Code of Ethics for Nurses with Interpretive Statements* was adopted by the ANA House of Delegates in 2001. The three purposes of the 2001 code are the following:

- To be a succinct statement of the ethical obligations and duties of every individual who enters the nursing profession
- To be the profession's non-negotiable ethical standard
- To be an expression of nursing's own understanding of its commitment to society (p 5)

These purposes are reflected in the nine provisional statements of the code. The Code of Ethics for nurses and its interpretive statements apply to population-centered nurses, although the emphasis for each type of nursing sometimes varies. (For

the ANA Code of Ethics for Nurses, see http://www.nursingworld.org/MainMenuCategories/EthicsStandards/CodeofEthicsforNurses.aspx.)

THE CUTTING EDGE *The American Nurses Association has produced* Guide to the Code of Ethics for Nurses: Interpretation and Application, *which serves as a companion reader to the Code of Ethics for Nurses (Fowler, 2008). This reader contains specific applications to nursing practice for each of the Code's nine interpretive statements.*

Whereas provisions 1 through 3 focus on the recipients of nursing care, provisions 4 through 6 focus on the nurse. This focus addresses nurses' accountability, competency, and contributions to their employment conditions.

Provisions 7 through 9 focus on the bigger picture of both the nursing profession and national and global health concerns. Regarding the nursing profession, the emphasis is on professional standards, active involvement in nursing, and the integrity of the profession. All nurses have a responsibility to meet these obligations. Regarding national and global health concerns, the emphasis is on social justice and reform. According to the ANA code (2001), "The nurse has a responsibility to be aware not only of specific health needs of individual clients but also of broader health concerns such as world hunger, environmental pollution, lack of access to health care, violation of human rights, and inequitable distribution of nursing and health care resources" (p 23). The ANA code (2001) also stresses political action as the mechanism to effect social justice and reform regarding such issues as homelessness, violence, and stigmatization. The Levels of Prevention box presents actions related to ethics.

PUBLIC HEALTH CODE OF ETHICS

The *Public Health Code of Ethics* (PHLS, 2002) was noted in the history section of this chapter. This code consists of a preamble; 12 principles related to the ethical practice of public health (Box 6-3); 11 values and beliefs that focus on health, community, and action; and a commentary on each of the 12 principles. The preamble asserts the collective and societal nature of public health to keep people healthy. The 12 principles incorporate the ethical tenets of preventing harm; doing no harm; promoting good; respecting both individual and community rights; respecting autonomy, diversity, and confidentiality when possible; ensuring professional competency; manifesting trustworthiness; and promoting advocacy for disenfranchised persons within a

---

♥ HEALTHY PEOPLE 2020

There are two new objectives outlined in *Healthy People 2020* related to access to health services:

- AHS-1: Increasing the proportion of persons who receive appropriate evidence-based clinical preventive services

- AHS-4: Increasing the proportion of practicing primary care providers, including nurse practitioners
  Both of these areas related to access to care reflect important ethical considerations for nurses.

From U.S. Department of Health and Human Services: *Healthy People 2020.* Available at http://www.healthypeople.gov/2020/topicsobjectives 2020/default.aspx. Accessed January 1, 2011.

BOX 6-3 PRINCIPLES OF THE ETHICAL PRACTICE OF PUBLIC HEALTH (A SECTION OF THE *PUBLIC HEALTH CODE OF ETHICS*)

1. Public health should address principally the fundamental causes of disease and requirements for health, aiming to prevent adverse health outcomes.
2. Public health should achieve community health in a way that respects the rights of individuals in the community.
3. Public health policies, programs, and priorities should be developed and evaluated through processes that ensure an opportunity for input from community members.
4. Public health should advocate and work for the empowerment of disenfranchised community members, aiming to ensure that the basic resources and conditions necessary for health are accessible to all.
5. Public health should seek the information needed to implement effective policies and programs that protect and promote health.
6. Public health institutions should provide communities with the information they have that is needed for decisions on policies or programs and should obtain the community's consent for their implementation.

7. Public health institutions should act in a timely manner on the information they have, within the resources and the mandate given to them by the public.
8. Public health programs and policies should incorporate a variety of approaches that anticipate and respect diverse values, beliefs, and cultures in the community.
9. Public health programs and policies should be implemented in a manner that most enhances the physical and social environment.
10. Public health institutions should protect the confidentiality of information that can bring harm to an individual or community if made public. Exceptions must be justified on the basis of the high likelihood of significant harm to the individual or others.
11. Public health institutions should ensure the professional competencies of their employees.
12. Public health institutions and their employees should engage in collaborations and affiliations in ways that build the public's trust and the institution's effectiveness.

Reprinted with permission from the Public Health Leadership Society: *Public Health Code of Ethics,* American Public Health Association (APHA), 2002. Available at http://phls.org.CMSuploads/Principles-of-the-Ethical-Practice-of-PH-Version-2.2-68496.pdf. Members of the PHLS ethics work group who created the *Public Health Code of Ethics* include Elizabeth Bancroft (Centers for Disease Control and Prevention, Los Angeles County), Kitty Hsu Dana (APHA), Jack Dillenberg (Arizona School of Health Sciences), Joxel Garcia (Connecticut Department of Health), Kathleen Gensheimer (Maine Department of Health), V. James Guillory (University of Health Sciences, Kansas City, MO), Teresa Long (Department of Health, Columbus, OH), Ann Peterson (Virginia Department of Health), Michael Sage (Centers for Disease Control and Prevention), Liz Schwarte (Public Health Leadership Society), James Thomas (University of North Carolina), Kathy Vincent (Alabama Health Department), Carol Woltring (Center for Health Leadership Development and Practice, Oakland, CA). The ethics project was funded in part by the Centers for Disease Control and Prevention.

---

community. Examples of values and beliefs include a right to health care resources, the interdependency of humans living in the community, and the importance of knowledge as a basis for action.

When the *Code of Ethics for Nurses* and the *Public Health Code of Ethics* are assessed, some commonalities emerge. These codes provide general ethical principles and approaches that are both enduring and dynamic. They guide nurses and public health personnel in thinking about the underlying ethics of their profession. Although the two codes do not specify (nor should they specify) details for every ethical issue, other mechanisms such as standards of practice, ethical decision-making frameworks, and ethics committees help work out the details. Nevertheless, the preceding two codes address most approaches to ethical justification, including traditional and emerging ethical theories and principles, humanist and feminist ethics, virtue ethics, professional-individual and/or community relationships, and advocacy. Many websites provide further information on codes of ethics and other ethical concerns in public health; all can be accessed through the WebLinks section of this book's Evolve website. Some of them are noted in the Additional Resources feature at the beginning of the chapter.

ADVOCACY AND ETHICS

Advocacy is an important concept in nursing that embodies an ethical focus grounded in quality of life. The American Public Health Association (APHA) represents a powerful

LEVELS OF PREVENTION

Ethics

Primary Prevention
Use the *Code of Ethics for Nurses* to guide your nursing practice.

Secondary Prevention
If you are unable to behave in accordance with the *Code of Ethics for Nurses* (e.g., you speak in a way that does not communicate respect for a client), take steps to correct your behavior. You could explain to the client your error and apologize.

Tertiary Prevention
If you have treated a client or staff member in a way that is inconsistent with ethics practices, seek guidance on other choices you could have made.

voice for public health advocacy, focusing on finding ways to involve health care professionals in influencing policies related to protection of all Americans and their communities from preventable, serious health threats and helping to ensure access to health care and eliminating health disparities (APHA, n.d.). The APHA notes the critical need to shift from a nation focused on treating individual illness to one that also promotes population-based health services that encourage preventive and early intervention practices. Also, the field of genetics has increasingly become an important ethical focus in public health; two new *Healthy People 2020* objectives relate to genomics (G HP2020-1, G HP2020-2).

TABLE 6-2 CONTRAST OF SOCIAL JUSTICE AND MARKET JUSTICE AS AN ADVOCACY FRAMEWORK

MARKET JUSTICE VALUES	SOCIAL JUSTICE VALUES
Self-determination and self-discipline	Shared responsibility
Individual values and self-interest	Interconnection and cooperation among individuals in a community
Personal efforts key to desired benefits	Community shares responsibility for providing basic benefits
Limited responsibilities for good of the community	Important obligations for the collective good
Limited government intervention	Government involvement is necessary
Voluntary focus on individual moral behavior	Community well-being supersedes individual focus on well-being

Adapted from Dorfman L, Wallack L, Woodruff K: More than a message: framing public health advocacy to change corporate practices. *Health Educ Behav* 32:320-336, 2005.

Codes and Standards of Practice

Several codes and standards of practice address advocacy. Four are noted here. Advocacy is addressed in codes of ethics put forth by the ANA (2001) and the Public Health Leadership Society (PHLS) (2002), as well as in the ANA (2007) *Public Health Nursing: Scope & Standards of Practice* and the PHLS *Skills for the Ethical Practice of Public Health* (Thomas, 2004).

According to the ANA (2001) *Code of Ethics for Nurses,* "The nurse promotes, advocates for, and strives to protect the health, safety, and rights of the patient" (p 12). The focus of the interpretive statements regarding advocacy is the nurse's responsibility to take action when the client's best interests are jeopardized by questionable practice on the part of any member of the health team, the health care system, or others.

The *Public Health Code of Ethics* (PHLS, 2002) and the PHLS *Skills for the Ethical Practice of Public Health* (Thomas, 2004) state that public health should advocate for disenfranchised community members, aiming to ensure that the basic resources necessary for health are accessible to all. The PHLS's code addresses two important issues: that the voice of the community should be heard and that the marginalized or underserved in a community should receive "a decent minimum" (p 4) of health resources.

According to the ANA *Public Health Nursing: Scope & Standards of Practice* (2007), public health nurses have a moral mandate to establish ethical standards when advocating for health care policy. The preceding standards extend the prior two concepts of advocacy by moving advocacy into the policy arena, particularly health and social policy as applied to populations. When approaching advocacy from the viewpoint of social justice, it is important for nursing organizations to acknowledge neglect of social justice issues and for individual nurses to advocate that their organizations address socially unjust systems that impact health care for the vulnerable in our society (Bekemeier and Butterfield, 2005).

Conceptual Framework for Advocacy

One framework that can be used to define helpful behaviors for advocacy is to contrast social justice and market justice (Dorfman, Wallack, and Woodruff, 2005). As noted earlier in this chapter, it is important to recognize the potential conflict of individual versus society. With communitarianism, individual rights need to be balanced with social responsibilities. When using a framework that contrasts social justice and market justice, the biggest barrier to achieving social justice is the competing concept of market justice. Market justice is grounded in the assumption that the best way to meet the needs of individuals in a society is to avoid regulations. The focus is on individual, not shared, needs (Table 6-2). A focus on market justice, rather than social justice, influences public dialogue about public health needs. It is important that existing values and beliefs in the society be understood in order to frame the public health message appropriately in terms of social justice values that relate to changes that they seek. Health care professionals must develop media skills to compete effectively with adversaries in public debate and learn to frame their advocacy initiatives.

Practical Framework for Advocacy

Bateman (2000) takes a practical approach to advocacy. He places the advocate's core skills (i.e., interviewing, assertiveness and force, negotiation, self-management, legal knowledge and research, and litigation) within the context of six ethical principles for effective advocacy, as shown in Box 6-4. His focus is on the individual client, although the focus could also apply to groups and communities.

Regarding the first ethical principle, Bateman (2000) is sensitive to the ethical conflict between clients' best interests and the best interests of groups, communities, or societies but does not elaborate on this conflict. The second ethical principle, which puts the client in charge, works in tandem with the first principle. It goes like this: "This is what I think we can do. What do you want me to do?" (Bateman, 2000, p 51). Of course, the advocate can refuse the request if self or others may be harmed. By following the third ethical principle, the client is empowered to make knowledgeable decisions. The fourth ethical principle addresses standards of practice. The fifth ethical principle addresses fairness and respect for persons (population-centered nursing is more collaborative in nature than independent). The last ethical principle, confidentiality, ensures that information will be shared only on a need-to-know basis.

BOX 6-4 ETHICAL PRINCIPLES FOR EFFECTIVE ADVOCACY

1. Act in the client's* best interests.
2. Act in accordance with the client's wishes and instructions.
3. Keep the client properly informed.
4. Carry out instructions with diligence and competence.
5. Act impartially and offer frank, independent advice.
6. Maintain client confidentiality.

Modified from Bateman N: *Advocacy skills for health and social care professionals,* Philadelphia, 2000, Jessica Kingsley, p 63.
*Client may be a person, group, or community.

EVIDENCE-BASED PRACTICE

As health care becomes increasingly complex, practitioners may experience conflicting ethical concerns in meeting health care expectations of clients. Very little research has been done to explore the link between ethics-related work factors, job satisfaction, and intent to leave one's job. One study examined the extent to which ethics stress and adequacy of organizational resources affected nurses and social workers' job satisfaction and their intent to leave their current position. Ethics stress was defined as an occupational stress that reflects the emotional, physical, and psychosocial consequences of moral distress. The study surveyed 1215 randomly selected nurses and social workers in four regions of the United States. The questionnaire addressed six domains: description of the workplace ethical climate; availability and type of organizational resources to assist with ethical issues; type and frequency of ethical issues encountered; ethics stress; job satisfaction and intent to leave; and sociodemographic and practice characteristics.

Findings indicated that 32.5% of respondents felt powerless and 34.7% felt overwhelmed with ethical issues in the workplace. Respondents also reported frustration (52.8%) and fatigue (40%) when they could not resolve ethical issues. Ethics stress had a stronger relationship to job satisfaction than did the influence of staffing on decision to leave. Researchers concluded that a positive ethical climate and job satisfaction protected against respondents' intentions to leave their job; perceptions of adequate or extensive institutional support for dealing with ethical issues were also positive factors in intent to stay in the workplace. Unexpectedly, black nurses reported more ethics stress and were three times more likely than white nurses to want to leave their position.

Nurse Use

Although much of the research on job satisfaction and turnover has focused on the effect of staffing levels, data from this study suggest that a positive ethical climate, in which one is respected and seen as a valued member of the health care team, is one of the strongest influences in helping practitioners deal with ethics stress and decide not to leave their positions. Data from the study suggest that investing in institutional ethics support and resources for employees and establishing a positive ethical climate for practice could be important factors in enhancing job satisfaction and reducing turnover. In turn, at a reasonably low cost, this could have a positive effect on client care and quality outcomes. Future research should explore cultural variables and effects of ethics stress and turnover intentions in black nurses and other minority groups in the workplace.

From Ulrich C, O'Donnell P, Taylor C, et al: Ethical climate, ethics stress, and the job satisfaction of nurse and social workers in the United States, *Soc Sci Med* 65(8):1708–1719, 2007.

Advocacy and Bioterrorism

Before the terrorist attacks in the United States on September 11, 2001, the subject of terrorism was not a major focus in philosophical discussions (Terrorism, 2007). The September 11th attack, however, brought a frightening new awareness of the vulnerability of individuals and groups in our society and the need for advocacy. Although some countries have been forced to live with the knowledge of this type of vulnerability for years, today's reality of global terrorism means that nurses must thoughtfully reflect on and debate ethical issues that arise with the threat, action, and aftermath of terrorism. They also must carefully consider their own responsibilities in terms of moral obligation to respond and make themselves available in a crisis that threatens the well-being of a community.

WHAT DO YOU THINK? *A news photographer, Raymer (2009), suggests that it is important to think about ways in which terrorism issues are framed by the media. He notes that journalists tend to frame events in terms of compassion and suffering because they do not want to appear to be taking sides on an issue but that in telling the story in terms of individual experiences, the media may be evading their responsibility to make difficult judgments about the facts they discover. What do you think about the way in which the media frames events related to bioterrorism?*

As noted at the beginning of this chapter, population-centered nursing is concerned with protecting, promoting, preserving, and maintaining health while preventing disease. These goals that address the promotion of good and prevention of harm are intimately related to ethics and bioterrorism. It is often difficult to balance goals for the protection of the public and protection of the individual, as evidenced by an incident in which airport security personnel ordered a 4-year-old disabled child to remove his leg braces to go through a metal detector, even though his mother told the screeners that the child could not walk without the braces (Airport security, 2010). Silva and Ludwick (2003) provide a helpful framework for reflection on the need for advocacy related to bioterrorism in the principles of nonmaleficence, beneficence, and distributive justice. These principles can guide nurses as they learn to speak out against violence and terrorism, work with agencies in the community for short-term and long-term efforts to do good and avoid harm, and participate in policy debates that attempt to determine fair distribution of scarce resources to fight terrorism globally. The ANA Center for Ethics and Human Rights maintains a helpful list of resource information addressing biodefense at http://www.nursingworld.org/MainMenuCategories/ThePracticeofProfessionalNursing/EthicsStandards/CENR.aspx.

Advocacy and Health Care Reform

In the current focus on health care reform, it is critical that nurses advocate for reform that embodies ethical considerations that have been discussed in this chapter. Dr. Mary Wakefield, Administrator of the Health Resources and Services Administration (HRSA), noted that not only should nurses participate in implementing new directions for health care, but that it is important that they help to envision these new directions (Wakefield, 2008). Nurses can be an important voice in advocating for access to consistent, effective, efficient health care for all in our society. Wakefield notes that educating the public can be a unique challenge because clever sound bites and attack ads in the media can lure consumers into thinking that the status quo is the best option. Nurses are an important part of the health care industry and are respected by the public; they can make meaningful contributions toward health care reform through advocating for clients and families. The signing of the 2010 health care bill by President Obama, after many years of controversial attempts at health care reform, provides an excellent opportunity for nurses to advocate for tying health care for all to ethics and social justice.

 LINKING CONTENT TO PRACTICE

Throughout this chapter, there has been application of the content related to ethics in public health nursing and the many documents that influence the role of public health nurses. These include the ANA Scope and Standards of Public Health Nursing, the ANA Code of Ethics, the core functions of public health as outlined by the Institute of Medicine, and the Healthy People 2020 objectives. Ethics is also an integral part of the Core Competencies for Public Health Professionals. Skill 8 in the section on analytic/assessment skills says that a public health professional uses "ethical principles in the collection, maintenance, use, and dissemination of data and information" and skill 2 under leadership and systems thinking says a professional "incorporates ethical standards of practice as the basis of all interactions with organization, communities, and individuals."

Council on Linkages Between Academic and Public Health Practice: *Core competencies for public health professionals*, Washington, DC, 2010. Public Health Foundation/Health Resources and Services Administration.

CHAPTER REVIEW

PRACTICE APPLICATION

The retiring director of the division of primary care in a state health department had recently hired Ann Green, a 34-year-old nurse with a master's degree in public health, to be director of the division. Ms. Green's work involved the monitoring of millions of dollars of state and federal money as well as the supervising of the funded programs within her division.

Ms. Green received many requests for funding from a particular state agency that served a poor, large district. The poor people of the district primarily consisted of young families with children and homebound older adults with chronic illnesses. Over the past 3 years, the federal government had allocated considerable money to the state agency to subsidize pediatric primary care programs, but no formal evaluation of these programs had occurred.

The director of the state agency was a physician who had been in this position for over 20 years. He was good at obtaining funding for primary care needs in his district, but the statistics related to the pediatric primary care program seemed implausible—that is, few physical examinations were performed on the children, which had resulted in extra money in the budget. This unspent federal money was being used to supplement home health care services for the indigent homebound older adults in his district. The thinking of the physician was that he was doing good by providing some needed services to both indigent groups in his district. Ms. Green felt moral discomfort because she did not have either the money or the personnel to provide both services. What should she do?

A. What facts are the most relevant in this scenario?

B. What are the ethical issues?

C. How can Ms. Green resolve the issues?

(The preceding case and answers are adapted and paraphrased from a real practice application shared by J. L. Chapin on the inappropriate distribution of primary health care funds. [In Silva M, editor: *Ethical decision making in nursing administration*, Norwalk, CT, 1990, Appleton & Lange.])

Answers can be found on the Evolve site.

KEY POINTS

- Nursing has a rich heritage of ethics and morality, beginning with Florence Nightingale.
- During the late 1960s, the field of bioethics began to emerge and influence nursing.
- Ethical decision making is the component of ethics that focuses on the process of how ethical decisions are made.
- Many different ethical decision-making frameworks exist; however, underlying each of them is the problem-solving process.
- Ethical decision making applies to all approaches to ethics: utilitarianism, deontology, principlism, virtue ethics, the ethic of care, and feminist ethics.
- Cultural diversity makes ethical decision making more challenging.
- Moral distress can lead to a personal sense of failure in providing nursing care and may lead to work and/or career dissatisfaction.
- Classical ethical theories are utilitarianism and deontology.

- Principlism consists of respect for autonomy, nonmaleficence, beneficence, and justice.
- Other approaches to ethics include virtue ethics, the ethic of care, and feminist ethics.
- The core functions of public health nursing (i.e., assessment, policy development, and assurance) are all grounded in ethics.
- Healthy People 2020 objectives address workforce competencies, training in essential public health services, and continuing education.
- The 2001 *Code of Ethics for Nurses* contains nine statements that address the moral standards that delineate nursing's values, goals, and obligations.
- The 2002 *Public Health Code of Ethics* contains 12 statements that address the moral standards that delineate public health's values, goals, and obligations.
- Advocacy is the act of pleading for or supporting a course of action on behalf of a person, group, or community.

- The *Code of Ethics for Nurses,* the *Public Health Code of Ethics, Skills for the Ethical Practice of Public Health,* and *Public Health Nursing: Scope & Standards of Practice* all address advocacy.
- Public health advocacy is composed of both products and processes.
- The products of advocacy are decreased morbidity and mortality.

- The processes of public health advocacy include, but are not limited to, identifying problems, collecting data, developing and endorsing regulations and legislation, enforcing policies, and assessing the policy process.
- Advocacy related to bioterrorism and health care reform is important for community and public health nurses.
- Effective advocacy incorporates ethical principles and concepts.

CLINICAL DECISION-MAKING ACTIVITIES

1. Think about the differences in duties between a nurse working in a critical care facility and a nurse working in a community care or public health setting. How might these differences lead to differences in ethical problems and decision making?
2. Interview a long-retired nurse about the most important ethical issues that this nurse faced when practicing in the community. Next, interview a nurse actively practicing in the community about the most important ethical issues that this nurse is now facing. Compare and contrast the ethical issues in the two interviews and place each within a historical context.
3. In a local or national newspaper, read one or more articles that discuss health care public policy with which you agree or

disagree. Compose a letter to the editor analyzing why you agree or disagree with the policy but only after you take into account any of your own biases or vested interests.
4. Analyze the 2001 *Code of Ethics for Nurses* and the 2002 *Public Health Code of Ethics,* critiquing them for clarity and relevance. Give specific examples to support your assessment. Compare and contrast the two codes.
5. Investigate whether your college or university has a plan for emergency readiness. How are nurses involved in the plan? What ethical implications are evident in the plan?

REFERENCES

Airport security forces disabled boy, 4, to remove leg braces or else no Disney world, February 17, 2010. Available at http://www.ethicsoup.com/2010/02/airport-security-forces-disabled-boy-4-to-remove-leg-braces-or-else-no-disney-world.html. Accessed December 9, 2010.

American Nurses Association: *Code of ethics for nurses with interpretive statements,* Washington, DC, 2001, American Nurses Publishing.

American Nurses Association: *Public health nursing: scope & standards of practice,* Washington, DC, 2007, American Nurses Publishing.

American Public Health Association. *Advocacy and policy,* n.d. Available at http://www.apha.org/advocacy. Accessed December 9, 2010.

Bateman N: *Advocacy skills for health and social care professionals,* Philadelphia, 2000, Jessica Kingsley.

Beauchamp TL, Childress JF: *Principles of biomedical ethics,* ed 6, New York, 2008, Oxford University Press.

Bekemeier B, Butterfield P: Unreconciled inconsistencies: a critical review of the concept of social justice in 3 national nursing documents, *ANS* 28:152–162, 2005.

Callahan D: Universalism and particularism fighting to a draw, *Hastings Cent Rep* 30:37, 2000.

Callahan D: Principlism and communitarianism, *J Med Ethics* 29:287–291, 2003.

Callahan D, Jennings B: Ethics and public health: forging a strong relationship, *Am J Public Health* 92:169, 2002.

Carlock C, Spader C: Communication and understanding: best vs distress, *Nurs Spectr.* Available at http://news.nurse.com/apps/pbcs.dll/article?AID=2007710080311. Accessed December 9, 2010.

Council on Linkages Between Academic and Public Health Practice: *Core competencies for public health professionals,* Washington, DC, 2010. Public Health Foundation/Health Resources and Services Administration.

Coursin CC: Inequalities affecting access to healthcare: a philosophical reflection, *Int J Hum Caring* 13(1):7–15, 2009.

Denhardt RB, Denhardt JV: The new public service: serving rather than steering, *Public Admin Rev* 60:549–552, 2000.

Dorfman L, Wallack L, Woodruff K: More than a message: framing public health advocacy to change corporate practices, *Health Educ Behav* 32:320–336, 2005.

Eriksson K: Caring science in a new way, *Nurs Sci Quart* 15:61, 2002.

Fowler MDM, editor: *Guide to the Code of Ethics for Nurses. Interpretation and application,* Silver Spring, MD, 2008, American Nurses Association.

Gilligan C: *In a different voice: psychological theory and women's development,* Cambridge, MA, 1982, Harvard University Press.

Hellsten S: Theories of distributive justice. In Chadwick R, editor: *Encyclopedia of applied ethics,* vol 1, New York, 1998, Academic Press, pp 815–827.

Holstein MB: Bringing ethics home: a new look at ethics in the home and the community. In Holstein MB, Mitzen PB, editors: *Ethics in community based elder care,* New York, 2001, Springer.

International Council of Nurses: *ICN code of ethics for nurses,* Geneva, 1953, ICN.

International Council of Nurses: *ICN code of ethics for nurses,* Geneva, 2006, ICN.

Leininger M, editor: *Care: the essence of nursing and health,* Thorofare, NJ, 1984, Slack.

MacIntyre A: *After virtue,* Notre Dame, IN, 1984, University of Notre Dame Press.

Noddings N: *Caring: a feminine approach to ethics & moral education,* Berkeley, CA, 1984, University of California Press.

Olick RS: From the column editor: ethics in public health, *J Public Health Manag Pract* 11:258–259, 2005.

Olson LL: Provision Six. In Fowler MDM, editor: *Guide to the Code of Ethics for Nurses: interpretation and application,* Silver Spring, MD, 2008, American Nurses Association, pp 72–88.

Pellegrino ED: Toward a virtue-based normative ethics for the health professions, *Kennedy Inst Ethics J* 5:253, 1995.

Petrini C: Theoretical models and operational frameworks in public health ethics, *Int J Environ Res Public Health* 7:189–202, 2010.

Pinch WJE, Haddad AM, editors: *Nursing and health care ethics: a legacy and a vision,* Silver Spring, MD, 2008, American Nurses Association.

Public Health Leadership Society: *Public Health Code of Ethics,* American Public Health Association (APHA), 2002. Available at http://www.apha.org/NR/rdonlyres/1CED3CEA-287E-4185-9CBD-BD405FC60856/0/ethicsbrochure.pdf. Accessed December 9, 2010.

Quad Council of Public Health Nursing Organizations. *Competencies for Public Health Nursing Practice,* Washington, DC, 2003, ASTDN, revised 2009.

Rawls J, Kelly E, editors: *Justice as fairness: a restatement,* Cambridge, MA, 2001, Harvard University Press.

Raymer S: Framing the suffering: journalism is about being faithful to the facts, *News Photographer* 64(2):12–13, 2009.

Rogers WA: Feminism and public health ethics, *J Med Ethics* 32:351–354, 2006.

Ruger JP: Ethics in American health 2: an ethical framework for health system reform, *Am J Public Health* 98(10):1756–1763, 2008.

Silva MC: Ethical issues in health care, public policy, and politics. In Mason D, Leavitt J, Chaffee M, editors: *Policy and politics in nursing and health care,* ed 4, Philadelphia, 2002, Saunders.

Silva MC: Provision Eight. In Fowler MDM, editor: *Guide to the Code of Ethics for Nurses: interpretation and application*, Silver Spring, MD, 2008, American Nurses Association, pp 72–88.

Silva MC, Ludwick R: Ethics and terrorism: September 11, 2001 and its aftermath, *Online J Issues Nurs*, January 31, 2003. Available at http://www.nursingworld.org/Main MenuCategories/ANAMarketplace/ ANAPeriodicals/OJIN/Columns/ Ethics/EthicsandTerrorism.aspx. Accessed June 23, 2010.

Skloot R: *The immortal life of Henrietta Lacks*, New York, 2010, Crown Publishers.

Steinbock B, Arras J, London AJ, editors: *Ethical issues in modern medicine*, ed 7, Boston, 2008, McGraw-Hill.

Terrorism: *Stanford Encyclopedia of Philosophy*, October 22, 2007. Available at at http://plato.stanford. edu/entries/terrorism. Accessed December 9, 2010.

Thomas J: *Skills for the ethical practice of public health*, Public Health Leadership Society, 2004. Available at http://phls.org/CMSuploads/ Skills-for-the-Ethical-Practice-of-Public-Health-68547.pdf. Accessed December 9, 2010.

Ulrich C, O'Donnell P, Taylor C, et al: Ethical climate, ethics stress, and the job satisfaction of nurse and social workers in the United States, *Soc Sci Med* 65(8):1708–1719, 2007.

U.S. Department of Health and Human Services: *Healthy People 2020 Public Meetings. 2009 Draft Objectives*. Available at http://www. healthypeople.gov/hp2020/Objecti ves/files/Draft2009Objectives.pdf. Accessed December 9, 2010.

Volbrecht RM: *Nursing ethics: communities in dialogue*, Upper Saddle River, NJ, 2002, Prentice Hall.

Wakefield MK: Envisioning and implementing new directions for health care, *Nurs Econ* 26(1):49–51, 2008.

Walker T: What principlism misses, *J Med Ethics* 35:229–231, 2009.

Watson J: *Nursing: human science and human care,* revised edition, Norwalk, CT, 2007, Jones & Bartlett.

Weston A: *A practical companion to ethics*, ed 3, New York, 2006, Oxford University Press.

Williams CA, Stanhope M: Population-focused practice: the foundation of specialization in public health nursing. In Stanhope M, Lancaster J, editors: *Public health nursing: population-centered health care in the community*, ed 7, St Louis, 2008, Mosby.

Wringle C: *Philosophy and education*, *Moral Education* 14, part 2, 74–82, 2006.

CHAPTER 7

Cultural Diversity in the Community

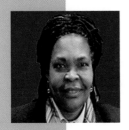

Cynthia E. Degazon, RN, PhD

Dr. Cynthia E. Degazon is professor emerita at Hunter College, City University of New York. She received a BS in nursing from Long Island University, and an MA in community health nursing and a PhD from New York University. For 18 years she has been preparing undergraduate and graduate nurses to provide culturally competent care to ethnically diverse populations. Dr. Degazon has given many national and international presentations, has authored several scholarly publications, and served on the editorial board of the Journal of Cultural Diversity.

ADDITIONAL RESOURCES

ᴇvolve WEBSITE
http://evolve.elsevier.com/Stanhope
- *Healthy People 2020*
- WebLinks
- Quiz
- Case Studies

- Glossary
- Answers to Practice Application

APPENDIX
- Appendix H: Focus on Quality and Safety Education for Nurses

OBJECTIVES

After reading this chapter, the student should be able to do the following:
1. Discuss the effect of culture on nursing practice.
2. Describe the process for developing cultural competency.
3. Describe major barriers to developing cultural competence.
4. Conduct a cultural assessment on a person from a culture different than the nurse's own culture.
5. Develop culturally competent nursing interventions to promote positive health outcomes for culturally diverse clients.
6. Analyze the role of the nurse as an advocate for providing culturally competent nursing care.

KEY TERMS

—*See Glossary for definitions*

Caring for culturally diverse groups has been a focus of nursing from its beginning. As early as 1893, under the leadership of Lillian Wald, nurses in New York City started public health nursing and provided home care to inner city people, particularly immigrants, who could neither read nor write the English language (Denker, 1994). Because nurses were not from the same cultural background as the immigrants, they had to deal with the cultural differences between themselves and the persons in their care. Today, the U.S. culture reflects a greater diversity of many cultures from all over the world. Thus, the need for nurses to provide culturally relevant care is greater than ever. Diversity in the U.S. across and within ethnic groups will most likely increase as descendants of immigrants are expected to account for most of the population growth in the coming decades (Pew Hispanic Center, 2008).

Data from the 2000 census showed a greater shift in population demographics than previously reported (U.S. Census Bureau, 2001). For example, in 1990 whites in 70 of the largest 100 U.S. cities represented more than 50% of the population; they are now a majority in only 52 of these cities. This pattern of a decreasing white population is attributed to a rapidly growing Hispanic population, a strong increase in Asians, and a modest increase in Americans of African descent. As a result, significant differences in beliefs about health and illness are becoming apparent among the various groups. Nurses who want to reflect their clients' beliefs of health and illness when intervening to promote and maintain wellness face many challenges.

Nurses need to understand the cultural views that affect perceptions of an illness, as well as the pathophysiology of the illness. According to the U.S. Department of Health and Human Services (2005), the nursing workforce is overwhelmingly white (81.8%): African-Americans account for 4.2%, Asian or Pacific Islanders 3.1%, Hispanics 1.7%, and Native Americans/Alaskan Natives 0.03%. The remaining 8.9% of nurses either categorized themselves as being of two or more races and non-Hispanic (1.4%) or did not respond to the question (7.5%). Given the minority population increase, and that clients prefer to be cared for by a nurse who is from the same ethnicity as themselves (Castro and Ruiz, 2009), the number of racially and ethnically diverse nurses who are available to provide care is insufficient. As a result, nurses must be prepared to meet all the needs of all their clients.

This chapter provides nurses with strategies to pursue a course of developing cultural competence as a means of providing culturally relevant nursing care for clients (individuals and aggregates, including families and communities) who are culturally different from the nurse's own culture. Emphasis is on clients from four culturally diverse groups: African-Americans, Asians, Native Americans/Alaskan Natives, and Hispanics. Although there is much cultural and ethnic diversity present within and among these groups, they are consistently identified in the literature as being more vulnerable, having less access to health care, receiving a poorer quality of health care, and having higher rates of chronic illnesses, and shorter life expectancies than white groups (CDC, 2009; Smedley, Stith, and Nelson, 2002; Agency for Healthcare Research & Quality, 2009a). However, evidence is beginning to show a narrowing of the gap between these groups for some of the access and quality measures.

IMMIGRANT HEALTH ISSUES

Immigration and the laws that pertain to it have been a subject of discussion and controversy for many years in the United States. The 1965 amendment of the Immigration and Nationality Act changed the quota system that discriminated against individuals from southern and eastern Europe (Center for Immigration Studies, 1995). The Refugee Act of 1980 provided a uniform procedure for refugees (based on the United Nations definition) to be admitted to the United States (U.S. Census Bureau, 2001). This included refugees from Cuba, Vietnam, Laos, Cambodia, and Russian Jewish refugees who may come to the U.S. for religious and political freedom as well as economic opportunities. The 1986 Immigration Reform and Control Act permitted illegal aliens already living in the United States an opportunity to apply for legal status if they met certain requirements. Table 7-1 summarizes the immigration patterns of selected immigrants by country of origin for the past 48 years.

TABLE 7-1 IMMIGRANTS BY COUNTRY OF LAST RESIDENCE: 1961 TO 2008 (NUMBERS IN THOUSANDS)

REGION/COUNTRY OF LAST RESIDENCE	1961-1970	1971-1980	1981-1990	1991-2000	2001-2006	2007	2008
All countries	3321.7	4493.3	7388.1	9095.4	6168.1	1052.4	1107.1
Africa	29.0	80.8	176.9	355.0	431.4	94.7	105.9
Asia	427.6	1588.2	2738.2	2795.7	2089.6	383.5	383.6
Europe	1123.5	800.3	761.6	1359.7	922.3	120.8	119.1
North America	1438.7	1685.9	3152.8	3947.1	2160.7	339.3	393.3
Oceania*	25.1	41.2	45.2	55.8	35.9	6.1	5.3
South America	257.9	295.7	461.8	539.7	510.8	106.5	98.6

From Office of Immigration Statistics, Office of Management, Department of Homeland Security: *2008 yearbook of immigration statistics,* Washington, DC, 2008, U.S. Government Printing Office.
*Australia, New Zealand, and the nearby islands.

Between 2001 and 2008, a smaller number of persons entered the United States than in the previous decade (Office of Immigration Statistics, 2008). It is estimated that the U.S. population consists of 33 million who are foreign-born, accounting for 12% of the total population (Congress of the United States, 2004). *Foreign-born* refers to all residents who were not U.S. citizens at birth, regardless of their current legal or citizen status.

More than two thirds of the foreign-born population lives in or around major metropolitan areas in six states: California, Texas, New York, Florida, Illinois, and New Jersey (Congress of the United States, 2004). They work in mainly service-producing and blue-collar sectors, but their employment in the information technology area is fast growing. The foreign-born are likely to be poorer (16.6%) than the U.S.-born population (11.5%), with the difference most pronounced for those under 18 years of age (foreign-born 28.5% vs. U.S. population 16.2%).

There are four categories of foreign-born. The first category is legal immigrants, also known as lawful permanent residents. This group constitutes about 85% of the immigrant population. They are not citizens but are legally allowed to live and work in the United States, usually because they fulfill labor demands or have family ties. Since 1997 legal immigrants have needed to live in the United States for 10 years to be eligible for all entitlements, such as Aid to Families of Dependent Children, food stamps, Medicaid, and unemployment insurance (National Immigration Forum, 2005). The second category of foreign-born consists of refugees and persons seeking asylum. These are people who seek protection in the United States because of fear of persecution (on the basis of race, religion, nationality, political view, or membership in a certain group) if they were to return to their homeland. Upon receiving such a status, refugees are immediately eligible to receive Temporary Assistance for Needy Families, Supplemental Security Income, and Medicaid. The third category of foreign-born is the nonimmigrants; these people are admitted to the United States for a limited duration and for a specified purpose. Non-immigrants include students, tourists, temporary workers, business executives, career diplomats and their spouses and children, artists, entertainers, and reporters. The fourth category of foreign-born is unauthorized immigrants, or undocumented or illegal aliens. These persons may have crossed a border into the United States illegally, or their legal permission to stay may have expired. They are eligible only for emergency medical services, immunizations, treatment for the symptoms of communicable diseases, and access to school lunches. A description of the immigrant populations and what benefits they are eligible to receive can be found in *A Description of Immigrant Population Health* (Congress of the United States, 2004).

Misperceptions abound about the economic value of allowing immigrants to enter, or to stay in, the United States. It is estimated that immigrants add about $10 billion to the economy annually, and that, in their lifetime in the United States, an immigrant family will pay $80,000 more in taxes than they consume in services (Mohanty et al, 2005). The dilemma for communities, however, is that the taxes are typically paid to the federal government, whereas the services the immigrants use are paid for by the states and localities. Although federal matching funds for Medicaid are not available to the states for immigrants, some states have found compelling public health reasons to use their own funds to cover even undocumented immigrant children, pregnant women with low incomes, disabled persons, and older adults (Okie, 2007).

People in the United States differ in their attitudes and support for policies that effect immigrants; there is also some misunderstanding about what determines an immigrant. National debate about immigration policy has intensified since the events of September 11, 2001. Since the attacks, a variety of immigration laws have been enacted (*Changes in Immigration Law,* 2008). Changes reflect tightened and more restrictive visa procedures as well as greater scrutiny given to all visas and entry documents. The complex issues involved with the foreign-born population and health care are beyond the scope of this discussion, but several issues will be discussed and suggestions made for nursing actions.

In addition to financial constraints on the provision of health care for immigrants, other factors need to be considered. Some of them are language barriers; differences in social, religious, and cultural backgrounds between the immigrant and the health care provider; and the use of traditional healing or folk health care practices that may be unfamiliar to their U.S. health care providers. Providers may lack knowledge about high-risk diseases in the specific immigrant groups for whom they care. For example, Southeast-Asians are often at risk for hepatitis B (with its attendant effects on the liver), tuberculosis, intestinal parasites, and visual, hearing, and dental problems. Most of these conditions are either preventable or treatable if managed correctly (Riedel, 1998).

DID YOU KNOW? *Definitions for immigrant differ, and immigrants may be legal or illegal. They come from all parts of the world and bring with them unique cultural, health care, and religious backgrounds.*

- *Access to health care may be limited because of immigrants' lack of benefits, resources, language ability, and transportation.*
- *Insured immigrants use less health care services than their U.S.-born counterparts.*
- *Nurses need to be astute in considering the cultural backgrounds of their immigrant clients and populations. Often, the family and community must be relied on to provide information, support, and other aid.*
- *Nurses need to know the major health problems and risk factors that are specific to immigrant populations, particularly the populations with whom they most often come in contact.*

Nurses need to understand the traditional healing practices that their clients use. Many of these treatments have proved effective and can be blended with traditional Western medicine. The key is to know what practices are being used so the blending can be knowledgeably done. Community members are excellent sources of this information, and nurses working with immigrant populations should use the community assessment, group work, and family techniques described in other chapters.

Often children and adolescents adjust to the new culture more easily than their elders. This can lead to family conflict and, at times, violence. Be alert for warning signs of family stress and tension. On the other hand, older family members can help translate their culture, beliefs, religious practices, support systems, and risk factors for the health care provider. They can also assist with decision making and provide support to enable the person or group seeking care to change behaviors and become more health promoting. Nurses need to understand the role of the family in immigrant populations and to treat individuals in the context of the families from which they come.

Similarly, the role of the community in the care of immigrants is important. Communities can help clients (and thus providers) with communication, crisis intervention, housing, emotional and other forms of support. Nurses need to carefully assess the community and learn what strengths, resources, and talents are available. As noted, cultural and religious beliefs influence behaviors, and community groups can explain their value and meaning to the nurse.

Horowitz (1998) has identified six steps that nurses can take to more effectively work with immigrant populations:

1. Know yourself: providers, like clients, are influenced by culture, values, and language.
2. Get to know the families and their health-seeking behaviors. You might try using a simple genogram, which places family members on a diagram. Ask who the family members are, where they live, and who is missing or dead. You might also ask them to talk about holiday celebrations: who comes, who is missing, and what do they do?
3. Get to know the communities that frequently interact with your clinical setting: read about them, take a course, get involved (e.g., volunteer to give talks), hold forums with free-flowing and two-way communication, and learn who the formal and informal resources are.
4. Get to know some of the traditional practices and remedies used by families and communities, so you can work with, not against, them.
5. Learn how a community deals with common illnesses or events.
6. Try to see things from the viewpoint of the client, family, and community.

CULTURE, RACE, AND ETHNICITY

The concepts of culture, race, and ethnicity play a strong role in understanding human behavior. In everyday living, these three terms are often used incorrectly. Nurses are expected to understand and appreciate the meaning of each term as they relate to providing culturally competent health care to clients of diverse cultures.

Culture

Culture is a set of beliefs, values, and assumptions about life that are widely held among a group of people and that are transmitted intergenerationally (Leininger, 2002a). Culture develops over time and is resistant to change. It takes many years for individuals to become familiar enough with a new value for it to become part of their culture. In response to the needs of its members and their environment, culture provides tested solutions to life's problems and, as a result, guides our thinking, discussions, and actions. Culture is important to nurses because it helps them to understand the beliefs and practices clients bring to the clinical setting, their responses to health and illness, and the type of health care they are expecting. Culture is applicable not only to minority groups, but also to groups of white Americans from European descent, such as the Irish, Italian, and Russian. Individuals learn about their culture during the processes of learning language and becoming socialized, usually as children. Parents and family, the most important sources for the transfer of traditions, teach both explicit and implicit behaviors of the culture. Explicit behaviors are straightforward and do not leave room for misinterpretation of what the person wants to communicate. Implicit behaviors are less exact and include the use of body language to communicate rather than persons saying verbally what is on their mind. An example of explicit versus implicit behavior is the choice of words in the following sign: "No smoking is permitted" versus "Thank you for not smoking." The former statement represents a culture that values directness, whereas the latter values indirectness.

Each culture has an organizational structure that distinguishes it from others and provides the structure for what members of the cultural group determine as appropriate or inappropriate behavior. The organizational elements of cultures have been described by Andrews and Boyle (2007), Giger

BOX 7-1 FACTORS INFLUENCING INDIVIDUAL DIFFERENCES WITHIN CULTURAL GROUPS

- Age
- Religion
- Dialect and language spoken
- Gender identity roles
- Socioeconomic background
- Geographic location in the country of origin
- Geographic location in the current country
- History of the subcultural group with which clients identify in their current country of residence
- History of the subcultural group with which clients identify in their country of origin
- Amount of interaction between older and younger generations
- Degree of assimilation in the current country of residence
- Immigration status*
- Conditions under which migration occurred*

Except where noted with an asterisk, from Orque M: Orque's ethnic/cultural system: a framework for ethnic nursing care. In Orque MS, Bloch B, Monrroy LSA, editors: *Ethnic nursing care: a multi-cultural approach,* St Louis, 1983, Mosby.

and Davidhizar (2008), Leininger (2002b), Purnell and Paulanka (2008), and Spector (2008). Such organizational elements include communication, family structure, child-rearing practices, religious practices, and physical space. In the case of communication, there are idiomatic expressions unique to each language. It is important that nurses know these organizational elements to provide appropriate care to persons of diverse cultures. This does not mean, however, that one should overlook or fail to incorporate the individuality of any person within any culture when developing a plan of care. Just as all cultures are not alike, all individuals within a culture are not alike. Sources of diversity include immigrant status, race, ethnicity, socioeconomic status, social class, sexual orientation, gender identity, and disability (Lipson and Dibble, 2005). Each individual should be viewed as a unique human being with differences that are respected. Box 7-1 summarizes factors that may influence individual differences within cultural groups.

Race

Race is primarily a social classification that relies on physical markers such as skin color to identify group membership (Brislin, 2000). Individuals may be of the same race but of different cultures. For example, African-Americans, who may have been born in Africa, the Caribbean, North America, or elsewhere, are a heterogeneous group, but they are often viewed as culturally and racially homogeneous. A frequent consequence of this is that the many cultural differences of these individuals from different countries are overlooked because of their similar racial characteristics (Degazon, 1994). This often blurs understanding of this culturally diverse group. One factor highlighting race's diminishing importance is the finding that the DNA composition for any two humans is 99.9% genetically identical and that the difference between them is only 1 in 1000. Another factor is the increasing number of interracial families that lead to

changes in physical appearances of individuals and make race less important in ethnic identity. In the United States, children of biracial parents are usually assigned the race of the mother. A social significance of race is that it allows for some groups to be separated, treated as superior, and given access to power and other valued resources, while others are treated as inferior and have limited access to power and resources (USDHHS, 2001).

Ethnicity

Ethnicity is the shared feeling of peoplehood among a group of individuals (Giger and Davidhizar, 2008). Ethnicity reflects membership in a cultural group and is based on individuals sharing similar cultural patterns (e.g., family structures, beliefs, and dietary habits). These patterns are developed in a socioeconomic context with historic and political underpinnings and are exceedingly resistant to change. Ethnicity represents the identifying characteristics of culture, such as race, religion, or national origin and affects beliefs, behaviors, and access to resources. It is influenced by education, income level, geographical location, and association with individuals from ethnic groups other than one's own. Therefore, there is a reciprocal relationship between the individual and society. Members of an ethnic group are likely to give up aspects of their identity and society when they adopt characteristics of another group's identity. However, when there is a strong ethnic identity, the individual maintains the values, beliefs, behaviors, practices, and ways of thinking of their group.

CULTURAL COMPETENCE

Many people are taught by and have knowledge of a dominant culture. As long as the person is operating within that culture, responses occur without thought to a variety of situations and do not require examination of the cultural context. However, in today's climate of multiculturalism, there is increasing emphasis from health care providers and organizations for nurses to provide culturally competent care. For example, a recent Mexican immigrant who speaks little English goes to a community health center because of a urinary tract infection. The nurse understands that she must use strategies that would allow her to effectively communicate with the client. She also understands that the client has the right to receive effective care that is based upon culturally informed nursing science, to judge whether she had received the care she wanted, and to follow up with appropriate action if she did not receive the expected care. Nurses must be culturally competent to modify nursing interventions that are specific to the needs of cultural and ethnic groups. Such actions have the potential to decrease racial and health disparities and foster effective health outcomes (Brondolo, Gallo, and Myers, 2009).

THE CUTTING EDGE *Standards for transcultural nursing have been developed to guide nurses in all areas of clinical practice in delivering culturally competent nursing care. The standards assist in demonstrating that nurses respect human rights and how culturally competent care can improve health outcomes, in focusing attention on transcultural nursing, in promoting the image of nursing within* *culturally diverse communities, and in advancing the practice of transcultural nursing. Specifically, nurses use the standards as a basis for describing, teaching, documenting, and evaluating culturally competent care.*

Cultural competence is a combination of culturally congruent behaviors, practice attitudes, and policies that allow nurses to use interpersonal communication, relationship skills, and behavioral flexibility to work effectively in cross-cultural situations. Cultural competence allows nurses to develop and form a sense of themselves and others within the context of their own culture (Campinha-Bacote, 2003; Leininger, 2002a). Nurses who strive to become culturally competent respect individuals from different cultures and value diversity. They function effectively when caring for clients from other cultures. Cultural competence reflects a higher level of knowledge than cultural sensitivity, which was once thought to be all that was needed for nurses to effectively care for their clients. In contrast, cultural sensitivity suggests that the nurse has basic knowledge of the client's culture but does not use the information to devise a plan of care that reflects the client's total cultural needs.

Culturally competent nursing care is guided by four principles (American Academy of Nursing Expert Panel, 1992):

1. Care is designed for the specific client.
2. Care is based on the uniqueness of the client's culture and includes cultural norms and values.
3. Care includes self-empowerment strategies to facilitate client decision making in health behavior.
4. Care is provided with sensitivity and is based on the cultural uniqueness of the client.

Nurses must work toward becoming culturally competent for a number of reasons. First, because the nurse's culture often differs from that of the client, the nurse may not be knowledgeable about the client's culture. Nurses come from a variety of cultural backgrounds and have their own cultural traditions. Each nurse has a unique set of cultural experiences that gives meaning and understanding to his or her behavior. Because the nursing profession is a subsystem of the U.S. health care system, nurses also bring biomedical beliefs and values to the practice environment that may differ from the client's beliefs and values. Because of these different beliefs and values, when the client and the nurse interact they may have different understandings about the meaning of the health issue and different ideas about what to do to promote and protect health. In these circumstances, cultural competence helps nurses use strategies that respect clients' values and expectations without diminishing the nurses' own values and expectations.

Second, care that is not culturally competent may further increase the gap in racial and health disparities between minority and majority populations. Failure to effectively respond to the health care needs and preferences of culturally and linguistically diverse individuals may: (1) increase barriers to equitable access to care, (2) inhibit effective communication between the client and the nurse, and (3) create obstacles in gathering assessment data, thus limiting the development and implementation of effective treatment plans. In the current climate of economic constraints, the health care industry is focused on cost-effectiveness, which means balancing cost and quality (Agency for Healthcare Research & Quality, 2009b).

Quality of care means that the client has access to health care and that the care is delivered by culturally competent nurses to support achieving positive health outcomes. Care that is not focused on the clients' values and ideas is likely to increase cost and diminish quality. For example, when clients are using both folk medicine and traditional Western medicine and nurses fail to assess and use this information in teaching, the clients may not get the full benefits of the treatment protocol. This suggests that positive outcomes, which are indicators of quality, may not be met. When quality is compromised, additional resources may be needed to achieve the health care outcomes. Increased use of resources means that cost is increased.

Third, the specific *Healthy People 2020* objectives for persons of different cultures need to be met (USDHHS, 2010). For this to be accomplished, the client's lifestyle and personal choices must be considered. For example, American health care professionals frequently view excessive drinking as a sign of disease and alcoholism as a mental illness. However, in the Native American/Alaskan Native culture, these signify a disharmony between the individual and the spirit world, and biomedical interventions alone may not be adequate to reduce alcoholism within this culture. Between 2001 and 2005, 11.7% of all deaths among Native Americans and Alaskan Natives were alcohol related. This was a rate two times higher than that in the general population and contributed to a loss of 6.4 more years of potential life compared with those in the general population (CDC, 2008). The national goal is to reduce this disparity. However, many Native Americans/Alaskan Natives view alcohol consumption as an acceptable way to participate in family celebrations and tribal ceremonies (Orlandi, 1992), and refusal to drink with family may be viewed as a sign of rejection. West (1993, p 234) suggested that nurses understand the possible ramifications of not having culturally competent staff available to care for the American Indian/Alaskan Native population. She stated, "If the government sends Indians to a health clinic where personnel do not understand the holistic health practices of Indians and where young white people serve as caregivers and authority figures, failure is likely to result." To have successful outcomes, nurses who develop population-based programs to reduce alcohol-related deaths must be willing to respect the cultural uniqueness of Native Americans and to explore individuals' life experiences to find the underlying causes of their behaviors. See the *Healthy People 2020* box that gives examples of health promotion objectives for selected minority groups who are at risk.

Developing Cultural Competence

Developing cultural competence is one of the core competencies for public health nurses (Quad Council, 2009). It is an ongoing life process that focuses on understanding every aspect of client care. It is challenging and at times painful as the nurse struggles to break with the old and adopt new ways of thinking and performing. Nurses develop cultural competence in different ways, but the key elements are experiences with clients from other cultures, an awareness of these experiences, and

HEALTHY PEOPLE 2020

***Goals and Objectives of** Healthy People 2020 Related to Cultural Issues*

Goal: Eliminate health disparities among different segments of the population as defined by gender, race or ethnicity, education, income, disability, living in rural areas, and sexual orientation.

Selected Objectives
- AHS-1: Increase the proportion of persons with health insurance.
- AHS-2: Increase the proportion of insured persons with clinical preventive services coverage.
- AHS-3: Increase the proportion of persons with a usual primary care provider.
- AHS-6: Increase the proportion of persons who have a specific source of ongoing care.
- AHS-7: Reduce the proportion of individuals who are unable to obtain or delay in obtaining necessary medical care, dental care, or prescription medicine.

From U.S. Department of Health and Human Services: *Healthy People 2020: understanding and improving health,* Washington, DC, 2010, U.S. Government Printing Office.

promotion of mutual respect for differences. In developing cultural competence, nurses may be guided by the two principles suggested by Leininger (2002a): (1) maintain a broad objective and open attitude toward individuals and their cultures, and (2) avoid seeing all individuals as alike. Because there are varying degrees of cultural competence, not all nurses may reach the same level of development.

Orlandi (1992) suggests that there are three stages in the development of cultural competence: culturally incompetent, culturally sensitive, and culturally competent (Table 7-2). Each stage has three dimensions—cognitive (thinking), affective (feeling), and psychomotor (doing)—that together have an overall effect on nursing care. (Stop now and describe your level of cultural competence with persons of a culture different from your own by staging each of these three dimensions.)

Campinha-Bacote (2003) offers a theoretical model to explain the process of developing cultural competence. The five constructs of the model are: (1) cultural awareness, (2) cultural knowledge, (3) cultural skill, (4) cultural encounter, and (5) cultural desire.

Cultural Awareness

Cultural awareness refers to the self-examination and in-depth exploration of one's own beliefs and values as they influence behavior (Campinha-Bacote, 2003). Culturally aware nurses are conscious of culture as an influencing factor on differences between themselves and others, and are receptive to learning about the cultural dimensions of the clients. They understand the basis for their own behavior and how it helps or hinders the delivery of competent care to persons from cultures other than their own (American Academy of Nursing Expert Panel, 1992). Culturally aware nurses recognize that health is expressed differently across cultures and that culture influences an individual's responses to health, illness, disease, and death. Culturally competent care can be delivered in a variety of modes consistent with the client's health values. For example, at a community outreach program, a nurse was teaching a racially mixed group the screening protocol for breast and cervical cancer detection. An African-American woman in the group refused to give the return demonstration for breast self-examination. When encouraged to do so, she said, "My breasts are much larger than those on the model. Besides, the models are not like me. They are all white." After hearing the client's comments, the nurse realized that she had made no reference in her talk to the influence of culture or race on screening for breast and cervical cancer.

The nurse then talked with the client, asked for her recommendations, and encouraged her to return the demonstration. The nurse coached the client through the self-examination process while pointing out that regardless of breast size, shape, and color, the technique is the same for feeling the tissue and squeezing the nipple to make certain that there is no discharge. Because this nurse was culturally aware, she neither became angry with herself or the client nor imposed her own values on the client. Rather, the client talked about her beliefs, attitudes, and feelings about screening for cancer that may have been influenced by her culture. The nurse understood that she had to tailor her teaching material to the needs of diverse client groups. Subsequently, she purchased a model of an African-American woman's breast to be used in future health education programs with African-American women.

If the nurse had not been culturally aware, she would have misunderstood the client's concerns and acted in a defensive manner. Such an interaction would have failed to identify client assets and barriers and appropriate intervention strategies. A confrontation might have ensued that would not have been

TABLE 7-2	THE CULTURAL COMPETENCE FRAMEWORK: STAGES OF COMPETENCE DEVELOPMENT		
	CULTURALLY INCOMPETENT	**CULTURALLY SENSITIVE**	**CULTURALLY COMPETENT**
Cognitive dimension	Oblivious	Aware	Knowledgeable
Affective dimension	Apathetic	Sympathetic	Committed to change
Psychomotor (skills)	Unskilled	Lacking some skills	Highly skilled
Overall effect	Destructive	Neutral	Constructive

From Orlandi MA: Defining cultural competence: an organizing framework. In Orlandi MA, editor: *Cultural competence for evaluators,* Washington, DC, 1992, U.S. Department of Health and Human Services.

BOX 7-2 EARLY CULTURAL AWARENESS

- Think about the first time you had contact with someone you realized was culturally different from you.
- Briefly describe the situation/event. How old were you? What were your feelings? What were your thoughts?
- What did your parents and other significant adults say about those who were culturally different from your family? What adjectives were used? What attitudes were conveyed?
- As you got older, what messages did you receive about minority groups from the larger community or culture?
- As an adult, how do you see others in the community talk about culturally different people? What adjectives are used? What attitudes are conveyed? How does this reinforce or contradict your earlier experience?
- What parts of this cultural baggage make it difficult to work with clients from different cultural groups?
- What parts of this cultural baggage facilitate your work with clients?

From Randall-David E: *Culturally competent HIV counseling and education,* McLean, VA, 1994, Maternal and Child Health Clearinghouse.

helpful to the client or the nurse. McKenna (2001) urges nurses to champion the cause for clients to have their cultural traditions respected when they seek health care from health care professionals. Box 7-2 identifies a number of questions that nurses may reflect on as they try to understand their own culture and the implications of their own cultural values. Table 7-3 offers a 10-point checklist on how to use cultural awareness and sensitivity to achieve effective client outcomes.

Cultural Knowledge

Cultural knowledge refers to the process of searching for and obtaining a sound educational understanding about culturally diverse groups (Campinha-Bacote, 2003). Emphasis is on learning about the clients' worldview from an emic (native) perspective. For example, cultural knowledge indicates that Middle Eastern women might not attend prenatal classes without encouragement and support from the nurse (Meleis, 2005). Attendance at prenatal classes is about the future of the baby while the mother's main focus may be on the present and what is happening in the immediate environment. An understanding of the client's culture decreases misinterpretation that the mother might undermine efforts to promote a healthy baby, and allows the nurse to select strategies to ensure the client's cooperation in providing the best care for the baby. In contrast, knowledge of Nigerian culture indicates that while women will start prenatal care as soon as pregnancy is confirmed, they view pregnancy and birth as natural events and may not continue to attend prenatal classes throughout the pre-natal phase (Ogbu, 2005). Although the behavior of the women from these two countries may be the same, the reason for their action is different. Leininger (2002a) points out that nurses who lack cultural knowledge may develop feelings of inadequacy and helplessness because they are often unable to effectively help their clients. When knowledge of the client's culture is missing or inadequate, it can contribute to negative situations such as clients' inadequate use of health resources. When nursing education fails to expose students to a variety of cultures, the students

TABLE 7-3 CULTURAL AWARENESS AND SENSITIVITY CHECKLIST

FOCUS	INSTRUCTIONS
1. Communication method	Identify the client's preferred method of communication. Make necessary arrangements if translators are needed.
2. Language barriers	Identify potential language barriers (verbal and nonverbal). List possible compensations.
3. Cultural identification	Identify the client's culture. Contact your organization's culturally specific support team (CSST) for assistance.
4. Comprehension	Double-check: Does the client and/or family comprehend the situation at hand?
5. Beliefs	Identify religious/spiritual beliefs. Make appropriate support contacts.
6. Trust	Double-check: Does the client and/or family appear to trust the caregivers? Remember to watch for both verbal and non-verbal cues. If not, seek advice from the CSST.
7. Recovery	Double-check: Does the client and/or family have misconceptions or unrealistic views about the caregivers, treatment, or recovery process? Make necessary adjustments.
8. Diet	Address culture-specific dietary considerations.
9. Assessments	Conduct assessments with cultural sensitivity in mind. Watch for inaccuracies.
10. Health care provider bias	Always remember, we all have biases and prejudices. Examine and recognize your own.

From Seibert PS, Stridh-Igo P, Zimmerman CG: A checklist to facilitate cultural awareness and sensitivity, *J Med Ethics* 28(3):143-146, 2002.

may have gaps in cultural knowledge on how to care for diverse groups. Although it is unrealistic to expect that nurses will have knowledge of all cultures, they should be aware of the impact of culture on behavior and know how to obtain cultural knowledge of cultural influences that affect groups with whom they most frequently interact (Figures 7-1 and 7-2). Clients provide a rich source of information about their own cultures.

DID YOU KNOW? *There are more than 325 federally recognized Native American/Alaskan Native tribes. Many of them share similar health beliefs and practices. For many, health is a reflection of living in harmony with nature, and illness occurs when there is disharmony. They believe that they should treat the earth and themselves with respect, and failure to do so creates an imbalance with nature and they are likely to become ill. Illness may be seen as a price they pay for past or future events. The diagnosis and treatment for such illnesses are provided by medicine men who perform various ceremonies to purify the individual. Nurses need to know that not all Native Americans and Alaskan Natives share these health beliefs and practices because differences occur as a result of education, employment, and assimilation with the dominant culture.*

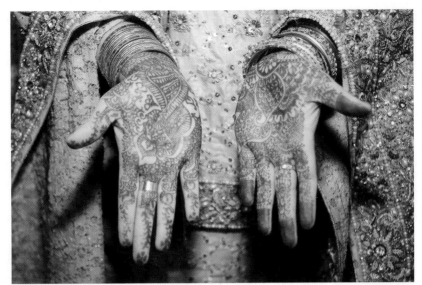

FIGURE 7-1 Henna on the hands of a Pakistani bride. Adorning hands and feet with Henna symbolizes good fortune for married women. There is the belief that when the Henna leaves a dark color, the bride will get plenty of love and care from her groom. Henna is a natural stain that remains on the skin for up to 4 weeks.

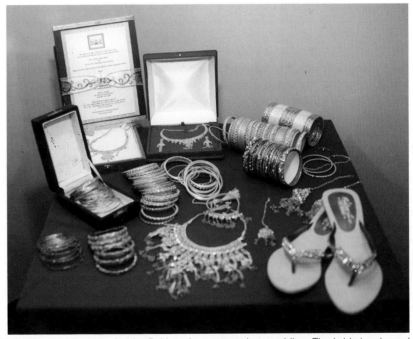

FIGURE 7-2 The jewelry worn by the Pakistani woman at her wedding. The bride is adorned with lots of gems because when she goes to her husband's home, she stands out as the most beautiful bride.

Cultural Skill

The third construct in developing cultural competence is cultural skill. **Cultural skill** refers to the ability of nurses to effectively integrate cultural awareness and cultural knowledge when conducting a cultural assessment and to use the findings to meet needs of culturally diverse clients (Campinha-Bacote, 2003). Culturally skillful nurses elicit from clients their perception of the health problem, discuss treatment protocol, negotiate acceptable options, select interventions that incorporate alternative treatment plans, and collaborate with all stakeholders. For example, culturally competent nurses use appropriate touch during conversation and modify the physical distance between themselves and others while meeting mutually agreed-upon goals.

Cultural Encounter

Cultural encounter is the fourth construct essential to becoming culturally competent. **Cultural encounter** refers to the process that permits nurses to seek opportunities to engage in cross-cultural interactions (Munoz and Luckmann, 2005). There

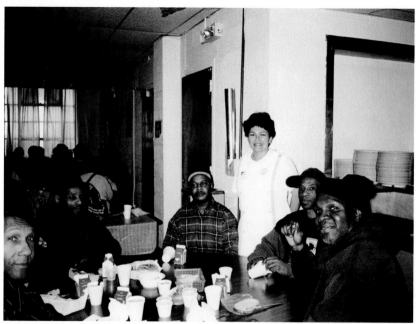

FIGURE 7-3 A Hispanic nursing student interacting with African-American men at a nutritional center. To interact in a culturally competent manner, the student needs to have an awareness of and knowledge about the differences between her culture and the men's culture and the skill to portray this in her behavior toward them.

are two types of cultural encounters: direct (face-to-face) and indirect. An example of a direct cultural encounter occurs when nurses learn directly from their Puerto Rican clients about spicy foods that they avoid during periods of breastfeeding. Indirect cultural encounters occur when nurses share these assessment findings with other nurses to help them develop their knowledge to effectively care for other Puerto Rican clients who are breastfeeding. The most important encounters are those in which nurses engage in effective communication, use appropriate language and literacy level, and learn about clients' life experiences and the significance of these experiences for health (Leininger, 2002a). In some communities, nurses may have few opportunities to work directly with persons of other cultures. Thus, when nurses come in contact with clients who are culturally different from the nurse, they should adapt general cultural concepts to the situation until they are able to learn directly from the clients about their culture (Figure 7-3). Developing cultural competence also comes from reading about, taking courses on, and discussing different cultures within multicultural settings.

Cultural Desire

Cultural desire is the fifth construct needed in the process of developing cultural competence. It refers to nurses' intrinsic motivation to want to engage in the previous four constructs necessary to provide culturally competent care (Campinha-Bacote, 2003). It is based on the humanistic value of caring for the individual. Nurses who have a desire to become culturally competent do so because they want to, rather than because they are directed to do so. They demonstrate a sense of energy and enthusiasm about the possibility of providing culturally competent nursing interventions. Unlike the other constructs, cultural desire cannot be directly taught in the classroom or in other educational or work settings. Nurses are more likely to demonstrate cultural desire when the environment at all levels of the organization reflects a philosophy that values cultural competence for all its clients.

Nurses should be aware that having cultural competence is not the same as being an expert on the culture of a group that is different from their own. A successful encounter may be judged on the basis of four aspects (Brislin, 2000):

1. The nurse feels successful about the relationship with the client.
2. The client feels that interactions are warm, cordial, respectful, and cooperative.
3. Tasks are done efficiently.
4. Nurse and client experience little or no stress.

Campinha-Bacote (2003) recommends that nurses should not be fearful of making mistakes, but should internalize and incorporate into their own world view selected beliefs, values, practices, lifeways, and problem-solving skills of other cultures from which they have the most frequent encounters. Box 7-3 provides several points to remember that could be helpful as they undertake the cultural competency journey.

Dimensions of Cultural Competence

Nurses integrate their professional knowledge with the client's knowledge and practices to maintain, protect, and restore the client's health. Leininger (2002a) suggests three modes of action, based on negotiation between the client and nurse, which guide the nurse to deliver culturally competent care: cultural preservation, cultural accommodation, and cultural repatterning. When these decisions and actions are used with

BOX 7-3 POINTS TO REMEMBER

- Culture is applicable to groups of whites, such as Italians or Irish, as well as to racial and ethnic minorities.
- During each interaction with clients, be sensitive to the cultural implications of the encounter.
- Ask questions to stimulate learning about how clients identify and express their cultural background.
- There is much diversity within groups and not all persons of the same racial or ethnic group may share the same culture. Assess both cultural group patterns as well as individual variations within a cultural group to avoid stereotyping.
- When misunderstandings arise, acknowledge the problem and take responsibility for your own error.
- Be knowledgeable about your own cultural heritage, biases, beliefs, values, and practices when providing care.
- Avoid making assumptions about non-verbal cues when interacting with clients from unfamiliar cultures.
- Use a variety of sources, including clients, to develop cultural knowledge.
- Developing cultural competence is an ongoing journey and an evolving process.

cultural brokering, the nurse is able to provide holistic care for culturally diverse clients (individual, family, or community).

Cultural Preservation

Cultural preservation refers to assistive, supportive, facilitative, or enabling nurse actions and decisions that help the clients of a particular culture to retain and preserve traditional values, so they can maintain, promote, and restore health. For example, acupuncture, an ancient Chinese practice of inserting needles in specific points on the skin through which life energy flows, is used to relieve pain or cure disease by restoring balance of yin and yang (Spector, 2008). This practice is being accepted by increasing numbers of Western practitioners as a legitimate treatment for many health problems. Thus, when Western practitioners integrate modalities, such as acupuncture, in the plan of care to maintain and protect the health of Asians who subscribe to the practice, they are providing care that is consistent with the clients' beliefs and values and helping to preserve their culture.

In another example, the nurse helps maintain cultural family values of Ms. Liu, a 73-year-old Chinese woman who was discharged from hospital to home care after surgery for cancer of the large intestine. During the home visit, the nurse discussed with the client and her husband about making a referral to have a home health aide assist with physical care and light housekeeping chores. The family was gracious but seemed hesitant to accept the referral. The nurse knew that the Chinese value the extended family network and family decision making. She asked the couple if they would like to discuss the situation with their daughters. Both the client and her husband seemed pleased with the idea, and the nurse promised to get back to them the next day. When the nurse returned for her visit, one of Ms. Liu's daughters was present and told the nurse that the family could manage without additional help. The three daughters had made a schedule to take turns caring for their parents.

The nurse accepted and supported the family's decision and told them that if they decided at a later time to accept the services of a home health aide, they should call the agency. The nurse then gave the family the telephone number of the agency, and scheduled the next follow-up visit with them.

Cultural Accommodation

Cultural accommodation refers to assistive, supportive, facilitative, or enabling nurse actions and decisions that help clients of a particular culture accept nursing strategies, or negotiate with nurses to achieve satisfying health care outcomes. Nurses may support and facilitate successful use of home burial of placenta alongside interventions from the biomedical health care system. For example, the delivery nurse was very helpful when Ms. Sanchez asked her not to discard a piece of the amniotic sac that was present on her grandbaby's face immediately after birth. Ms. Sanchez asked the nurse to give it to her instead. The grandmother believed that being born with a piece of the amniotic sac on the face was a visible sign that something special was going to happen in the person's life. The grandmother explained that after she dried the piece of the amniotic sac, she would keep it in a safe place. She would also spend extra time protecting the baby to prevent her from being harmed. Although the delivery room nurse was not knowledgeable about this practice, she was assistive and gave the grandmother the piece of the sac as she requested.

Cultural Repatterning

Cultural repatterning refers to assistive, supportive, facilitative, or enabling nurse actions and decisions that help people of a particular culture to change or modify a cultural practice for new or different health care patterns that are meaningful, satisfying, and beneficial. Successful repatterning is likely to occur when cultural values and beliefs are respected while at the same time there is a co-creation of interventions with the client to provide for a healthier health pattern than before the changes were developed. For example, a culturally competent school nurse who works with Mexican-Americans knows of the high incidence of obesity among women 20 years and older. Using this information, she developed a health education program for Mexican teenagers in the local high school. While respecting their cultural traditions, the nurse discussed weight management strategies with the teenagers. The nurse understood the teenagers' cultural issues pertaining to food and knew how to negotiate with them. She discouraged the use of fried foods (such as tortillas), sour cream, and regular cheese and encouraged and demonstrated the use of baked tortillas and salsa as dip and topping. In another example, a nurse discovered during her instructions on diabetes self-management that pregnant Haitian women were visiting an herbalist to obtain teas so they would not have to take insulin. The nurse asked for the names of the herbs in the teas that they were drinking and scheduled a conference with the pharmacist to discuss the specific ingredients in the herbs as well as ways that they might help clients meet their cultural needs. The nurse found out that one of the herbs contributed to high blood pressure, a problem that many of the women were experiencing. She negotiated with the women not to take the tea with the specific herb. The nurse understood the importance of supernatural causes of illness in the Haitian culture and sought cooperation from the herbalist. Another example of cultural repatterning occurs when nurses assist older Chinese clients to use low-sodium soy sauce, rather than soy sauce with high sodium, in their cooking as a means to more effectively manage their hypertension. Similarly, nurses should guide African-Americans to eat more broiled and less fried foods.

Culture Brokering

Culture brokering is advocating, mediating, negotiating, and intervening between the client's culture and the biomedical health care culture on behalf of clients. Nurses facilitate client access to health care as they are positioned to understand both cultures and resolve or lessen problems that result when individuals in either culture do not understand the other person's values. To illustrate, migrant workers tend to have high occupational mobility; many are poor and have limited formal education. They may seek health care only when they are ill and cannot work. Whenever a nurse from the mobile health care van interacts with them, the opportunity should be taken to teach about prevention, health maintenance, environmental sanitation, and nutrition, because it may be the only opportunity the nurse will ever have to care for that particular migrant worker. Nurses should also advocate for the rights of the migrant worker to receive quality health care. For example, the nurse may contact the migrant health services for follow-up or referral care for the migrant worker.

INHIBITORS TO DEVELOPING CULTURAL COMPETENCE

Nurses fail to provide culturally competent nursing care for a variety of reasons: they may have had minimal opportunity for learning about cross-cultural nursing; their supervisors may be encouraging them to increase productivity at the expense of quality; or they may be pressured by colleagues who are not knowledgeable about cultural concepts and are offended when others use the concepts. These and similar issues may result in nurse behaviors such as stereotyping, prejudice and racism, ethnocentrism, cultural imposition, cultural conflict, and culture shock.

Stereotyping

Stereotyping is ascribing certain beliefs and behaviors about a given racial and ethnic group to an individual without assessing for individual differences (Brislin, 2000). Stereotyping blocks the willingness of a person to be open and to learn about specific individuals or groups. When information is not immediately available, nurses may generalize about an individual's group behavioral pattern as a guide until they have had time to observe and assess the client's behavior. This can be a problem, and it may lead to a nurse's unwillingness to incorporate new and specific data about the client. New information may be distorted to fit with preconceived ideas. The generalizing that was a beginning point for understanding the individual becomes a

final point. The individual is thus stereotyped on the basis of the group's ascribed behavior (Galanti, 2008).

Stereotypes can be either positive or negative. For example, Asians are positively stereotyped as the "model" minority group, leading to an expectation that they will always behave in ways that reinforce the stereotypical notion. Other groups are stereotyped as "industrious and hard working." Nurses use negative stereotypes when they label an Native American/Alaskan Native who complains of abdominal pain as alcoholic because they suspect that there is a high incidence of alcoholism in the group and generalize from the group to the individual. Similarly, a nurse who believes that young African-American women are sexually permissive may label a woman in this group who is complaining of abdominal pain as having a sexually transmitted disease. Clients who perceive they are being stereotyped may respond with anger and hostility. This in turn perpetuates the stereotype and creates barriers to health-seeking behavior. To minimize the use of stereotypes, nurses should be aware of their biases and recognize the effect of socialization on individual differences. They should catch themselves before falling prey to stereotypical comments and correct others when they make such statements (Munoz and Luckmann, 2005).

Prejudice and Racism

Prejudice is the emotional manifestation of deeply held beliefs (stereotypes) about a group. These beliefs are directed toward a person who is a member of that group, and who is presumed to have the objectionable qualities ascribed to the group (Brislin, 2000). Prejudice usually refers to negative feelings. These feelings are often precursors for discriminatory acts based on prejudging, limited knowledge about, misinformation about, fear of, or limited contact with individuals from that group. Those who are prejudicial wish to deny the individuals, on the basis of factors such as race, skin color, ethnicity, or social standing, the opportunity to benefit fully from society's offerings of education, good jobs, and community activities.

Racism is a form of prejudice that occurs through the exercise of power by individuals and institutions against people who are judged to be inferior (e.g., in intelligence, morals, beauty, and self-worth) (Brislin, 2000). Individuals are denied certain opportunities (e.g., jobs, housing, education) typically enjoyed by the larger group because of some characteristic over which they have no control. When racism is acted upon, it results in perceived or actual harm to the individual. Three types of racism exist: individual, institutional, and cultural. Individual racism refers to discriminatory behavior or acts directed toward individuals or groups because of identified characteristics, such as skin color, hair texture, and facial features. Institutional racism refers to discriminatory behavior or acts by an institution, as expressed in policies, priority setting, and hiring and resource allocation practices that are directed toward individuals and groups and restrict their access to opportunities or resources. Institutional racism provides the structure for racism at the individual level to be accepted and condoned. Cultural racism refers to discriminatory behavior or acts directed by the dominant group toward another cultural group. The group is depicted in derogatory or stereotypical ways because of, for

BOX 7-4 TYPES OF PREJUDICE AND RACIST BEHAVIORS

Overt Intentional Prejudice/Racism

Two homeless women, one African-American and the other Irish, are clients at the neighborhood health care center. Both women are having financial difficulty. The African-American client's husband was laid off 4 years ago after his company closed. The Irish client is undergoing radiation treatment for metastatic cancer and has lost her job as a result of her prolonged illness. Both women are without health insurance. The nurse referred the Irish client to the social services department to enquire about available resources but did not refer the African-American woman. The nurse believed that minority clients have direct experience with some local and national government programs, know about available resources, and can negotiate the social system for themselves and family. In contrast, the nurse believed that because the Irish woman had a catastrophic illness and no prior experience negotiating government programs, she needed to advocate for her client. The nurse, not knowing the health-seeking behaviors of either client, stereotyped both women and intentionally used her informational power to help one client while denying assistance to the other client.

Overt Unintentional Prejudice/Racism

A nurse was assigned to make an initial home visit to two clients recently discharged from the hospital with a diagnosis of hypertension. The nurse performed physical assessments on both clients. He developed an extensive culturally relevant teaching plan with the Filipino client that included information on sodium restriction and its effect on kidney functioning, ways to integrate cultural foods into the diet, and support in lifestyle changes. With the Puerto Rican client, the nurse performed a routine physical assessment and did not discuss the client's culturally special dietary requirements. The nurse believed that the Puerto Rican client was not capable of understanding such complex information and was going to continue to seek help from her *cuarandera* (a folk practitioner) to manage the hypertension. At the end of his visit, the nurse said to this client, "Take care of yourself. See you next time." This nurse did not realize that he had stereotyped the client and that his actions were hurtful. He believed that he was providing quality care on the basis of the client's needs.

Covert Intentional Prejudice/Racism

A Native American nurse works in a home health agency that serves an ethnically diverse community. The nurse has observed that her assigned clients are always among the poorest and live in the unsafe areas of the community. Her non-minority nurse colleagues are not assigned to those sections of the community. In a recent staff meeting, she raised her observations with her nursing supervisors. On hearing her observations, the supervisors looked at the nurse in a skeptical manner and asked what she was talking about. This is covert racism because the nursing supervisors were aware of the informal policy that they assign minority nurses to clients in a particular area of the community. They had discussed the practice among themselves but would never admit to it. The supervisors thought that the best way for minority clients to be the recipients of culturally competent care was to assign a minority nurse to care for them.

Covert Unintentional Prejudice/Racism

A lesbian middle-class couple legally adopted a physically challenged child. Their insurance refuses to pay for the child's medical care. The nurse, who has been working for the agency for many years, is aware but failed to tell the parents that the baby can qualify for Medicaid through the handicapped insurance program, even though both parents work and their income is above the Medicaid guidelines' limit. This nurse was unaware that her dislike for the parents' sexual lifestyle influenced her thinking. She had in the past provided heterosexual couples with information on how to apply for Medicaid.

---

example, language or dress. All forms of racism can have individual, as well as community and population, effects.

The Tuskegee Syphilis Study is a well-known example of racism (Gamble, 1997). This study was conducted by the U.S. Public Health Service to observe the effects of syphilis on African-American men over a period of 40 years, beginning in 1932. When African-American men with syphilis were recruited for the study, they were told that they were being treated for "bad blood," and treatment for syphilis was withheld intentionally so that the study could be completed. As a result, hundreds of men lost their lives because of discriminatory policies that promoted substandard health care. The consequence of such racism has contributed to the belief among some African-Americans that research might be designed to harm them and that all care might be a part of a research study, especially government programs. Perceived racism can have physiological and psychological negative health outcomes to include high blood pressure, stroke, engaging in risky behaviors such as smoking and substance abuse, depression, and low self-esteem (Borrell et al, 2007; Richman et al, 2007; Smedley, Stith, and Nelson, 2002). Nurses too can exhibit prejudice and racism.

Prejudice and racism can be understood using a two-dimensional matrix: overt versus covert, and intentional versus unintentional. Locke and Hardaway (1992) depict four types of prejudice and racism that result from this matrix: overt intentional, covert intentional, overt unintentional, and covert unintentional. Overt intentional prejudice or racism means that the behavior is both apparent and purposeful. The nurse is aware of personal biases and beliefs and integrates them into a plan of action to negatively manage client problems. With overt unintentional, the behavior is apparent but not purposeful, and no harm is intended, although harm may result. Covert intentional means that the behavior is subtle and purposeful but the person tries to avoid being viewed as prejudicial or racist. Covert unintentional means that the person's behavior is neither apparent nor purposeful. The person is unaware of the behavior. Regardless of the type of prejudice or racism, the behavior is harmful to the client. Examples of each type of prejudice and racism are presented in Box 7-4.

Nurses may be recipients of prejudicial or racist acts (Fielo and Degazon, 1997), but they do not have to accept such behavior from clients. Rather, they should set limits, discuss the behavior with other colleagues, and avoid internalizing the behavior (Miles and Awong, 1997).

Ethnocentrism

Ethnocentrism, or cultural prejudice, is the belief that one's own cultural group determines the standards by which another group's behavior is judged. The implication is that one's own standards are better and superior than the other person's standards. Ethnocentric nurses favor their own professional values and find unacceptable that which is different from their culture. Their inability to accept different worldviews often leads them to devalue the experiences of others and judge them to be

EVIDENCE-BASED PRACTICE

A study was conducted to determine if the cultural competence of Nurse Practitioners was related to client satisfaction of Latinas (mainly Mexicans, 85.8%). The Nurse Practitioners (NPs) were female and Caucasians who had cultural competence training (93.3%) and had at least a master's degree (73.4%).

Findings show that the clients were highly unacculturated. Client satisfaction was positively associated with time clients spent with the NP, and with the NP's cultural skill, cultural competence, cultural encounter, cultural desire, cultural knowledge, American orientation, and ethnicity. These findings suggest that the more satisfied clients are more likely to have spent more time with the NP; to be more acculturated; to have NPs with greater cultural competence, cultural knowledge, cultural skill, cultural encounter, and cultural desire; and to be of Latina descent. An important indicator for client satisfaction was decreased waiting time to be seen by the NP.

Cultural competence was positively associated with NP ethnicity, cultural competence training, certification, interpersonal aspects of care, availability, and convenience of care. These findings suggest that NPs with greater cultural competence are more likely to be Latina, have received cultural competence training, possess certification, and have more acculturated clients. Other findings suggest that NPs with less cultural competence are less likely to speak Spanish and had received the RN degrees long ago and are older.

Nurse Use

Clients are often more satisfied with nursing care when they have an ethnic connection with the provider of that care. Nurses should obtain cultural competence certification and training since they make a difference in their practice and have the potential to contribute to effective client care outcomes.

Castro A, Ruiz E: The effects of nurse practitioner cultural competence on Latina patient satisfaction, *J Am Acad Nurs Pract* 21:278-286, 2009.

WHAT DO YOU THINK? *A 90-year-old South American woman refused to have an African-American nurse pre-pour her weekly medications in her home. The client requested that the community health agency replace the nurse with one who is white. What do you think the African-American nurse should have said to the client? Should the agency assign a nurse as requested, or should client services be terminated and the client transferred to another community health agency? What information would you seek to guide your decisions, and from where?*

---

inferior, and to treat those who are different from themselves with suspicion or hostility (Andrews and Boyle, 2007).

This behavior is in contrast to cultural blindness, in which there is an inability to recognize the differences between one's own cultural beliefs, values, and practices and those of another culture. The tendency is to believe that the recognition of racial, ethnic, religious, or gender differences is itself prejudicial and discriminatory. Hence, nurses who state that they treat all clients the same, regardless of cultural orientation, are demonstrating cultural blindness.

Cultural Imposition

The belief in one's own superiority, or ethnocentrism, may lead to cultural imposition. Cultural imposition is the act of imposing one's cultural beliefs, values, and practices on individuals from another culture. Nurses impose their values on clients when they forcefully promote biomedical traditions while ignoring the clients' value of non-Western treatments such as acupuncture, herbal therapy, or spiritualistic rituals. A goal for nurses is to develop an approach of cultural relativism, in which they recognize that clients have different approaches to health care, and that each culture should be judged on its own merit and not on the nurse's personal beliefs.

Cultural Conflict

Cultural conflict is a perceived threat that may arise from a misunderstanding of expectations when nurses are unable to respond appropriately to another individual's cultural practice because of unfamiliarity with the practice (Andrews and Boyle, 2007). Although cultural conflicts are unavoidable, the goal for nurses should be to manage conflicts so that they do not affect the delivery of culturally competent nursing care. Having knowledge of how conflict is managed in the particular culture may help to minimize the conflict. In any event, however, when resolving the conflict, it is important that all persons involved in the conflict have a way to "save face."

NURSING TIP *Respect all information that a client shares with you, even when the information is in conflict with your own value system.*

Culture Shock

Culture shock is the feeling of helplessness, discomfort, and disorientation experienced by an individual attempting to understand or effectively adapt to a cultural group whose beliefs and values are radically different from the individual's culture. When nurses experience culture shock, it may be a normal reaction to a client's beliefs and practices that are not allowed or approved in the nurse's own culture (Andrews and Boyle, 2007). Culture shock is brought on by anxiety that results from losing familiar signs and symbols of social interaction. As nurses change their practice environments and leave the safety of the hospital for community settings, they may experience heightened discomfort and feelings of powerlessness to confront differences between themselves and clients. This is especially true when nurses have little knowledge or exposure to the culture from which the client comes. For example, nurses who are unfamiliar with "cupping" may experience culture shock when Cambodians use this practice to relieve headaches, to reduce stress and sinus tension, or to delay the onset of colds. Being aware of the clients' own cultural beliefs and having knowledge of other cultures may help nurses to be more accepting of cultural differences.

CULTURAL NURSING ASSESSMENT

A cultural nursing assessment is "a systematic identification and documentation of the culture care beliefs, meanings, values, symbols, and practices of individuals or groups within a holistic perspective, which includes the worldview, life experiences, environmental context, ethnohistory, language, and diverse social structure influences" (Leininger, 2002b, pp 117-118). Cultural assessments should focus on those aspects relevant to the presenting problem, necessary intervention, and participatory education (Tripp-Reimer et al, 2001). Nurses use a component of data collection to help them identify and understand clients' beliefs about health and illness. By adopting a relativistic approach, nurses avoid judging or evaluating the clients in terms of their own culture.

A non-judgmental approach toward the client's culture is facilitated through having a skill set that includes understanding, eliciting, listening, explaining, acknowledging, recommending, and negotiating. It is vital that nurses listen to clients' perceptions of their problems and, in turn, that nurses explain to clients their own perceptions of the problems. Nurses and clients should acknowledge and discuss similarities and differences between the two perceptions to develop recommendations and suggestions for management of problems. A variety of tools are available to assist nurses in conducting cultural assessments (Andrews and Boyle, 2007; Leininger, 2002b; Tripp-Reimer, Brink, and Saunders, 1997). The focus of such tools varies, and selection is determined by the dimensions of the culture to be assessed.

During initial contacts with clients, nurses should perform a general cultural assessment to obtain an overview of the clients' characteristics (Tripp-Reimer, Brink, and Saunders, 1997). Nurses ask clients about their ethnic background, religious preference, family patterns, cultural values, language, education, and politics. Nurses also want to know about clients' perceptions of the health issue, causation, treatment, anticipated results, and the impact the issue might have on the client. Such basic data help nurses to understand the clients from their own point of view and to recognize their uniqueness, thus avoiding stereotyping. Data for an in-depth cultural assessment should be gathered over a period of time and not be restricted to the first encounter with the client. This gives both the client and the nurse time to get to know each other and, especially beneficial for the client, time to see the nurse in a helping relationship. An in-depth cultural assessment should be conducted in two phases: a data collection phase and an organization phase.

The data collection phase consists of three steps:

1. The nurse collects self-identifying data similar to those collected in the brief assessment.
2. The nurse raises a variety of questions that seek information on clients' perception of what brings them to the health care system, the illness, and previous and anticipated treatments.
3. After the nursing diagnosis is made, the nurse identifies cultural factors that may influence the effectiveness of nursing care actions.

In the organization phase, data related to the client's and family's views on optimal treatment choices are routinely examined, and areas of difference between the client's cultural needs and the goals of Western medicine are identified. Nurses may use Leininger's (2002a) three actions (discussed previously in this chapter) to guide them in selecting and discussing culturally appropriate interventions with clients.

The key to a successful cultural assessment lies in nurses being aware of their own culture. Randall-David (1989) developed a variety of principles that may be helpful as nurses conduct cultural assessments:

- Always be aware of the environment. Look around and listen to what is being said and understand non-verbal communications before taking action.
- Know about community social organizations such as schools, churches, hospitals, tribal councils, restaurants, taverns, and bars.
- Know the specific areas to focus on before beginning the cultural assessment.
- Select a strategy for gathering cultural data. Possible strategies include in-depth interviews, informal conversations, observations of the client's everyday activities or specific events, survey research, and a case method approach to study certain aspects of a client.
- Identify a confidante who will help "bridge the gap" between cultures.
- Know the appropriate questions to ask without offending the client.
- Interview other nurses or health care professionals who have worked with the specific individual, family, or community to get their input.
- Talk with formal and informal community leaders to gain a comprehensive understanding about significant aspects of community life.
- Be aware that all information has both subjective and objective aspects, and verify and cross-check the information that is collected before acting on it.
- Avoid the pitfalls that may occur when making premature generalizations.
- Be sincere, open, and honest with yourself and the client.

VARIATIONS AMONG CULTURAL GROUPS

Although all cultures are not the same, they do share basic organizational factors (Giger and Davidhizar, 2008). These factors—communication, space, social organization, time, environment control, and biological variations—should be explored in a cultural assessment because of their potential for highlighting differences between and among groups. Some of these factors and their variations are presented in Table 7-4. The Levels of Prevention box gives examples of cultural strategies for primary, secondary, and tertiary levels of prevention.

Communication

Effective communication is another one of the core competencies for public health professionals (Quad Council, 2009). Understanding variations in patterns of verbal and non-verbal communication as well as using vocabulary that a lay person would understand is an essential skill for nurses, since it helps to achieve therapeutic goals when working with individuals, families, and population systems. **Verbal communication** is the use of language in the form of words within a grammatical structure to express ideas and feelings and to describe objects. Variations in verbal communication among cultures are reflected in verbal styles, such as pronunciation, word meaning, voice quality, and humor. **Non-verbal communication** is the use of body

TABLE 7-4 CULTURAL VARIATIONS AMONG SELECTED GROUPS

	AFRICAN-AMERICANS	ASIANS	HISPANICS	NATIVE AMERICANS
Verbal communication	Asking personal questions of someone that you have met for the first time is seen as improper and intrusive	High level of respect for others, especially those in positions of authority	Expression of negative feelings is considered impolite	Speak in a low tone of voice and expect the listener to be attentive
Non-verbal communication	Direct eye contact in conversation is often considered rude	Direct eye contact among superiors may be considered disrespectful	Avoidance of eye contact is usually a sign of attentiveness and respect	Direct eye contact is often considered disrespectful
Touch	Touching one's hair by another is often considered offensive	It is not customary to shake hands with persons of the opposite sex	Touching is often observed between two persons in conversation	A light touch of the person's hand instead of a firm handshake is often used when greeting a person
Family organization	Usually have close extended family networks; women play key roles in health care decisions	Usually have close extended family ties; emphasis may be on family needs rather than individual needs	Usually have close extended family ties; all members of the family may be involved in health care decisions	Usually have close extended family; emphasis tends to be on family rather than on individual needs
Time perception	Often present oriented	Often present oriented	Often present oriented	Often past oriented
Perception	Harmony of mind, health, body, and spirit with nature	Balance between the "yin" and "yang" energy forces	Balance and harmony among mind, body, spirit, and nature	Harmony of mind, body, spirit, and emotions with nature
Alternative healers	"Granny," "root doctor," voodoo priest, spiritualist	Acupuncturist, acupressurist, herbalist	Curandero, espiritualista, yerbero	Medicine man, shaman
Self-care practices	Poultices, herbs, oils, roots	Hot and cold foods, herbs, teas, soups, cupping, burning, rubbing, pinching	Hot and cold foods, herbs	Herbs, corn meal, medicine bundle
Biological variations	Sickle cell anemia, mongolian spots, keloid formations, inverted "T" waves, lactose intolerance, skin color	Thalassemia, drug interactions, mongolian spots, lactose intolerance, skin color	Mongolian spots, lactose intolerance, skin color	Cleft uvula, lactose intolerance, skin color

LEVELS OF PREVENTION

Hypertension, Stroke, and Heart Disease Related to Cultural Differences

Primary Prevention
Provide health teaching about balanced diet and exercise. Based on the details of the individual's culture, the teaching should include members of the family and identification of culturally appropriate foods and the means to preparing them.

Secondary Prevention
Teach clients and/or family to monitor blood pressure. Teach about diet, keeping in mind the client's cultural preferences. Talk about health beliefs and cultural implications, such as the use of alternative therapies; make sure alternative therapies are compatible with any medications that may be prescribed.

Tertiary Prevention
If blood pressure cannot be controlled by diet and/or exercise, refer the client to a culturally appropriate medical practitioner for medication and supervision; advise the client to engage in a cardiac program that will oversee diet and exercise.

language or gestures to send information that cannot or may not be said verbally. Non-verbal styles include eye contact, gestures, touch, interjection during conversation, body posture, facial expression, and silence. For example, when gathering data from a Hispanic woman, the nurse should be aware that the style may be low-keyed and that the woman may avoid eye contact and be hesitant to respond to questions. This behavior should not be interpreted as lack of interest or inability to relate to others.

The need to understand cultural communication is underscored in the following example, when a nurse gave instructions to Asian clients about taking antituberculin drugs. The clients responded with a smile and a nod. The nurse interpreted this response to mean that the clients understood the instructions and that they had accepted the treatment protocol. A week later, when the clients returned for a follow-up visit, the nurse discovered that the medications had not been taken. The nurse knew that acceptance by, and avoidance of confrontation or disagreement with, those in authority are important behaviors in the Asian culture. Interventions were adjusted accordingly: the nurse repeated the medication instructions and gave the clients an opportunity to raise questions and concerns and to repeat the instructions that were given; the nurse also discussed the cultural meaning and treatment of tuberculosis. Other factors influencing communication relate to topics that are appropriate to be discussed, forms of address such as the use of first names or surnames, and whether it is permitted to wait until a person finishes speaking or to talk over each other (Hearnden, 2008).

🌐 LINKING CONTENT TO PRACTICE

As has been discussed throughout the chapter, cultural competent nursing care uses many of the standards, guidelines, and competencies from key nursing and public health documents. For example, the Council on Linkages (Council on Linkages, 2010) has a set of skills related to cultural competency and a set related to communication that are consistent with the information in this chapter. Likewise, the Quad Council further develops and applies the skills of the Council on Linkages related to both cultural competency and communication to public health nursing practice. As an example, the Council on Linkages states that a necessary skill in public health is to consider "the role of cultural, social, and behavioral factors in the accessibility, availability, acceptability and delivery of public health services." The Quad Council states that "public health nurses should consider the role of cultural, social, and behavioral factors in the accessibility, availability, acceptability and delivery of public health nursing services." Each of the competencies in the Council on Linkages core competencies is applied directly to public health nursing practice by the Quad Council (2009).

Using an Interpreter

When nurses do not speak or understand the client's language, they should make every effort to obtain assistance from an interpreter. **Interpreters** should be selected carefully, since all persons who speak the language may not be proficient in medical interpretation or in the cultural issues that are in play. Interpreters must also be able to understand what the clients are saying. Community members may be an excellent source since they understand not only the language, but also the cultural beliefs, expectations, and use of traditional health care practices. Interpreters may emphasize their personal preferences by influencing both nurses' and clients' decisions to select and participate in treatment modalities. Nurses can minimize this by learning basic words and sentences of the most commonly spoken languages in the community and observing client reactions when questions are posed. In addition, nurses should provide written material in the client's primary language, so that family members can reinforce information when at home with the client. Strategies that nurses may use to select and effectively use an interpreter are listed in the How To box.

HOW TO Select and Use an Interpreter

1. *When feasible, select an interpreter who has knowledge of health-related terminology.*
2. *Use family members with caution because of the client's need for privacy when discussing intimate matters. Family members may lack the ability to communicate effectively in both languages and may exhibit a bias that influences the client's decisions.*
3. *The sex of the interpreter may be of concern; in some cultures, women may prefer a female interpreter and men may prefer a male.*
4. *The age of the interpreter may also be of concern. For example, older clients may want a more mature interpreter. It is better to use adults rather than children as interpreters. Specifically, children tend to have limited understanding and language skills, and when used as interpreters, they may have difficulty interpreting the information. Children may also be uncomfortable with the content of the information being interpreted due to its personal or medical nature.*
5. *Differences in socioeconomic status, religious affiliation, and educational level between the client and the interpreter may lead to problems in translation of information.*
6. *Identify the client's origin of birth and language or dialect spoken before selecting the interpreter. For example, Chinese clients speak different dialects depending on the region in which they were born.*
7. *Avoid using an interpreter from the same community as the client to avoid a breach of confidentiality.*
8. *Clarify roles with the interpreter.*
9. *Introduce the interpreter to the client, and explain to the client what the interpreter will be doing.*
10. *Avoid using professional jargon, colloquialisms, abstractions, idiomatic expressions, slang, similes, and metaphors. Speak slowly and use words that are common in the client's culture.*
11. *Observe the client for non-verbal messages, such as facial expressions, gestures, and other forms of body language. If the client's responses do not fit with the question, the nurse should check to be sure that the interpreter understood the question.*
12. *Increase accuracy in transmission of information by asking the interpreter to translate the client's own words, and ask the client to repeat the information that was communicated.*
13. *At the end of the interview, review the material with the client to ensure that nothing has been missed or misunderstood.*

From Giger JN, Davidhizar R: Transcultural nursing: assessment and intervention, *ed 5, St Louis, 2008, Mosby; and Randall-David E:* Culturally competent HIV counseling and education, *McLean, VA, 1994, Maternal and Child Health Clearinghouse.*

DID YOU KNOW? *Health care institutions have a responsibility to effectively communicate with their clients. When an interpreter is not available to translate, the client may view this behavior as unacceptable and bring legal action against the agency.*

Space

Space is the physical distance between individuals during an interaction (Giger and Davidhizar, 2008). The amount of space varies among individuals and between cultures. When this space is violated, the nurse or the client may experience discomfort. There are four zones of interpersonal space—intimate space, personal distance, social distance, or public distance—that may be observed when they care for clients. Other cultural groups also have spatial preferences. To illustrate, Hispanics tend to be comfortable with less space because they like to touch persons with whom they are speaking. Filipinos may view touching strangers as inappropriate; therefore, nurses may stand farther away from Filipinos than from Hispanics. On the other hand, clients who are comfortable with closer distances may experience discomfort when nurses stand farther away, interpreting the behavior as rejecting. Nurses should take cues from clients to place themselves in the appropriate spatial zone and avoid misinterpretation of clients' behavior as they handle their spatial needs.

Social Organization

Social organization refers to the way in which a cultural group structures itself around the family to carry out role functions. In African-American culture, for example, family may include individuals who are unrelated or remotely related. Members of families depend on the extended family and kinship networks for emotional and financial support in times of crises. Mothers and grandmothers play important roles in African-American culture and may need to be included in health care decisions. The significance of family also varies across cultures. Members of Hispanic and Asian cultures tend to believe that the needs of the family come before those of the individual. In the Native American/Alaskan Native family, members honor and respect their elders and look to them for leadership, believing that wisdom comes with increasing age (West, 1993). When working with clients from these cultures, nurses should be aware that it can be counterproductive to exclude family involvement in decision making. At the same time, nurses should advocate for the individual, making sure that when families make decisions, the individual's needs are also being considered.

Time

Time, in the sense used here, refers to past, present, and future time as well as to the duration of and period between events. Some cultures assign greater or lesser value to events that occurred in the past, occur in the present, or will occur in the future. If members of a cultural group tend to be future oriented, they often will delay immediate gratification until future goals are accomplished. For example, some future oriented persons who value their potential longevity may moderate their dietary intake and engage in exercise activities to minimize future health risks. In contrast, other cultural groups may place greater value on present time and view it as being more important than future time. The future is unknown, but the present is known. When nurses discuss health promotion and disease prevention strategies with persons who have a present orientation, they should focus on the immediate benefits these clients would gain rather than emphasizing future outcomes. That is not to say that clients cannot or would not learn about preventing future problems, but nurses need to connect their teaching to the "here and now." It is important to listen carefully to what the clients say in order to gather information about their time orientation.

In cultures that focus on a past orientation (e.g., the Vietnamese culture), individuals may focus on wishes and memories of their ancestors and look to them to provide direction for current situations (Giger and Davidhizar, 2008). In a past-oriented culture, time is viewed as being more flexible than in a present-oriented culture. It has less of a fixed point, and individuals are not offended by being late or early for appointments. Nurses socialized in the Western culture may view time as money and

equate punctuality with correctness and being responsible. Working with clients who have a different time perception than the nurse can be problematic. Nurses should clarify the clients' perceptions to avoid misunderstandings. It is not feasible to expect that clients will change their behavior and adopt the nurse's schedule. Nurses should explain the importance of keeping appointments from the Western perspective. For example, the nurse can communicate a willingness to be flexible in scheduling appointments and explain to clients that the time will be set aside, specifically for them. Along with culture, socioeconomic status and religion may influence perception of time.

Environmental Control

Environmental control refers to the way in which individuals view their relationship with nature. Some cultural groups perceive individuals as having mastery over nature, being dominated by nature, or having a harmonious relationship with nature. Individuals who perceive mastery over nature (e.g., white Americans) believe that they can overcome the natural forces of nature. Such individuals would expect a cure for cancer through the use of medications, antibiotics, surgical interventions, radiation, and/or chemotherapy. They are willing to do whatever it takes to achieve health.

In contrast, those who view nature as dominant (e.g., African-Americans and Hispanics) believe that they have little or no control over what happens to them. They may not adhere to a cancer treatment protocol because of the belief that nothing will change the outcome and that their destiny has already been determined. These individuals are less likely to engage in illness prevention activities than those who have other worldviews.

Persons who view harmony with nature (e.g., Asians and Native Americans) may perceive that illness is disharmony with other forces and that medicine can only relieve the symptoms rather than cure the disease. They would look to find the treatment for the malignancy from the mind, body, and spirit connection, where healing comes from within. These groups are likely to look to naturalistic solutions, such as herbs, acupuncture, and hot and cold treatments, to resolve or cure a cancerous condition (Figure 7-4).

Biological Variations

Biological variations are the physical, biological, and physiological differences that exist between racial groups and distinguish one group from another. They occur in areas of growth and development, skin color, enzymatic differences, susceptibility to disease, and laboratory test findings (Andrews and Boyle, 2007; Giger and Davidhizar, 2008). For example, Western-born neonates are slightly heavier at birth than those born in non-Western cultures. Variations in growth and development may be influenced by environmental conditions such as nutrition, climate, and disease. Mongolian spots are bluish discolorations that may be present on the skin of African-American, Asian, Hispanic, and Native American/Alaskan Native babies. They may be mistaken for bruises. When nurses are exposed to situations involving biological variations of which they are unfamiliar, they may create embarrassing situations. Consider the following scenario: The school nurse observed a bluish discoloration on

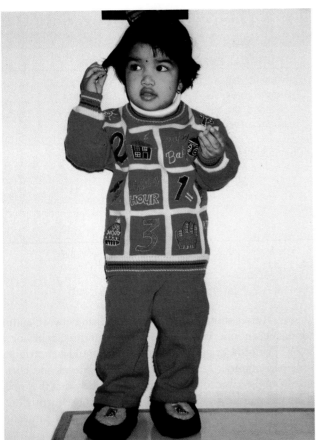

FIGURE 7-4 A child from Nepal living in the United States. The child has a black dot on her forehead to protect her from the "evil eye."

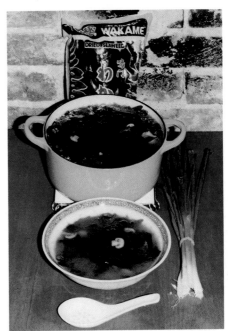

FIGURE 7-5 Mi-yuk kook (seaweed soup) is a Korean dish eaten by postpartum women to stop bleeding and to cleanse body fluids. It is also eaten every birthday.

BOX 7-5   ASSESSMENT OF DIETARY PRACTICES AND FOOD CONSUMPTION PATTERNS

- What is the social significance of food in the family?
- What foods are most frequently purchased for family consumption? Who makes the decision to buy the food?
- What foods, if any, are taboo (prohibited) for the family?
- Does religion play a significant role in food selection?
- Who prepares the food? How is it prepared?
- How much food is eaten? When is it eaten and with whom?
- Where does the client live and what types of restaurants does he or she frequent?
- Has the family adopted foods of other cultural groups?
- What are the family's favorite recipes?

---

the thigh of a Filipino child that she mistook for a bruise. The nurse reported her observation to the child protective agency in her state. When the child's mother arrived to pick her up at the end of the school day, she was accused of child abuse. The mother had to disprove the allegation before her child could be released into her care. Other common and obvious variations include eye shape, hair texture, adipose tissue deposits, shape of earlobes, thickness of lips, and body configuration.

Research findings suggest that sensitivity to codeine varies with ethnic background, and that Asian men experience significantly weaker effects from the drug than European men (Wu, 1997). Some Asian men are missing an enzyme called CYP2D6 that allows the body to metabolize codeine into morphine, which is responsible for the pain relief provided by codeine. When an individual is missing the enzyme, no amount of codeine will lessen the pain, and other pain-reducing medicines should be explored. A common enzyme deficiency is glucose-6-phosphate dehydrogenase (G6PD), which is responsible for lactose intolerance in many ethnic groups (Giger and Davidhizar, 2008).

CULTURE AND NUTRITION

Understanding the clients' nutritional practices is essential when completing a cultural assessment (Kaplan et al, 2004). Efforts to understand dietary patterns of clients should go beyond relying on membership in a defined group. Knowing clients' nutritional practices makes it possible to develop treatment regimens that would not conflict with their cultural food practices (Figure 7-5). Box 7-5 identifies several questions that nurses should ask when conducting a nutritional assessment.

In mutual goal setting with the client and nutritionist to change harmful dietary practices, the nurse might need to consult culturally oriented magazines. A number of popular magazines, such as *Essence, Ebony,* and *Latina,* have created new dishes from old family recipes using healthier ingredients. These dishes are tasty and resemble old traditions, yet they are not as harmful. Table 7-5 lists various dietary practices that are prevalent among some cultural groups in American society. Although the foods may differ culturally, excesses often lead to similar risk factors. Many of these practices may have their origin in religious as well as cultural traditions.

TABLE 7-5 **FOOD PREFERENCES AND ASSOCIATED RISK FACTORS IN SELECTED CULTURAL GROUPS**

CULTURAL GROUP	FOOD PREFERENCES	NUTRITIONAL EXCESS	RISK FACTORS
African-Americans	Fried foods, greens, bread, pork, rice, foods with high sodium and starch content	Cholesterol, fat, sodium, carbohydrates, calories	Obesity, coronary heart disease, diabetes
Asians	Soy sauce, rice, pickled dishes, raw fish, tea, balance between yin (cold) and yang (hot) concepts	Cholesterol, fat, sodium, carbohydrates, calories	Coronary heart disease, liver disease, cancer of the stomach, ulcers
Hispanics	Fried foods, beans and rice, chili, carbonated beverages, high-fat and high-sodium foods	Cholesterol, fat, sodium, carbohydrates, calories	Obesity, coronary heart disease, diabetes
Native Americans	Blue corn meal, fruits, game and fish	Carbohydrates, calories	Diabetes, malnutrition, tuberculosis, infant and maternal mortality

Data from Andrews MM, Boyle JS: *Transcultural concepts in nursing care,* ed 5, Philadelphia, 2007, JB Lippincott; Giger JN, Davidhizar R: *Transcultural nursing: assessment and intervention,* ed 5, St Louis, 2008, Mosby.

CULTURE AND SOCIOECONOMIC STATUS

The relationship between socioeconomic status and health disparities is reflected in life expectancy, infant death rates, low birth rates, and many other health measures (Kington and Smith, 1997; Sims, Sims, and Bruce, 2008). Minority groups may not have the same opportunities for education, occupation, income earning, and property ownership that the dominant group has. According to the U.S. Census Bureau (2001), in 1999 there were more white families than minorities below the poverty level. However, the proportion of poor families in a minority group is greater. For example, 7.3% of white families are living in poverty, whereas 21.9% of African-Americans and 20.9% of Hispanics are doing so. Consequently, minority families are disproportionately represented on the lower tiers on the socioeconomic ladder. Poor economic achievement is also a common characteristic found among populations at risk, such as those in poverty, the homeless, migrant workers, and refugees. Nurses should be able to distinguish between culture and socioeconomic issues and not misinterpret behavior as having a cultural origin, when in fact it should be attributed to socioeconomics. Data suggest that when nurses and clients come from the same social class, it is more likely that they operate from the same health belief model, and consequently there is less opportunity for misinterpretation and communication problems.

There is danger in believing that certain cultural behaviors, such as folk practices, are restricted to lower socioeconomic classes. Roberson (1987) found that health professionals, such as nurses and physicians, also used folk systems in conjunction with the biomedical system to promote their health and prevent disease. Therefore, nurses must conduct a cultural assessment for all individuals when they first come in contact with them. Nurses should have guidance in integrating cultural concepts with other aspects of client care to meet their clients' total health care needs.

CHAPTER REVIEW

PRACTICE APPLICATION

Mr. Nguyen, a 64-year-old man from rural Vietnam, entered the United States with his family 3 years ago through the refugee program. Mr. Nguyen was a farmer in his homeland, and since his arrival he has been unable to obtain a stable job that would allow him to adequately care for his family. His financial resources are limited and he has no insurance. He speaks enough English to interact directly with people outside his family and community. His oldest daughter, Shu Ping, is enrolled in a 2-year program to become a registered nurse.

The Nguyen family attends the neighborhood church with other Vietnamese families. Mr. Nguyen has been attending the clinic at the hospital but refuses to discuss with his family, even with Shu Ping, the reason for these visits. Shu Ping became increasingly concerned as she observed her father have insomnia, retarded motor activity, an inability to concentrate, and weight loss. However, Mr. Nguyen denied that he was not well. Shu Ping decided to discuss her concerns with a nurse, with whom she had developed an attachment, at the church. She invited the nurse to her home for lunch on a Saturday so she could meet her father and validate her impressions.

After several visits with the family, the nurse was able to establish a close enough relationship with Mr. Nguyen so that she could engage him in a discussion of his health. Because of her extensive work with other Vietnamese immigrants, the nurse was familiar with themes of loss and decided to focus her conversation with

Mr. Nguyen on his adjustment to the new community living, gains and losses as a result of immigration, and coping strategies. After several discussions with Mr. Nguyen, he confided in the nurse that he feared that he was dying because he had been diagnosed with cancer of the small intestine. He further revealed that he had not shared the diagnosis with the family because he did not want them to know of his "bad news." Mr. Nguyen had refused treatment because he knew that people never get better when they have cancer; they always die.

1. Which of the following actions best characterize the nurse's willingness to provide culturally competent care to Mr. Nguyen and his family?

   A. Discuss with the client his understanding of his diagnosis.

   B. Discuss with the client the prognosis for a person diagnosed with cancer of the small intestine in the United States.

   C. Discuss with the client the prognosis for a person diagnosed with cancer of the small intestine in Vietnam.

   D. Discuss the medical treatment and surgical intervention for cancer of the small intestine.

2. The way in which the nurse poses questions to Mr. Nguyen is very important and determines the kind of responses that the client gives to the nurse. What types of questions should the nurse pose to Mr. Nguyen to get the best responses from him?

3. Which resources should a community health agency have available to assist Mr. Nguyen with his health care concerns? Answers can be found on the Evolve site.

KEY POINTS

- The U.S. population is becoming increasingly diverse. Changes in immigration laws and policies have increased migration, contributed to changes in community demographics, and heightened the need to recognize the impact of culture on health care. There is a need for nurses, particularly population-centered nurses, to learn about the culture of the individuals to whom they give care.
- Culture is a learned set of behaviors that are widely shared among a group of people.
- Culture helps guide individuals in problem solving and decision making.
- Culturally competent nursing care is designed for a specific client, reflects the individual's beliefs and values, and is provided with sensitivity. Such nursing care helps to improve health outcomes and reduce health care costs.
- A culturally competent nurse uses cultural knowledge as well as specific skills, such as intracultural communication and cultural assessment, to select culturally appropriate interventions to care for the whole client.
- Nurses have four modes of action they may use to negotiate with clients and give culturally competent care: cultural preservation, cultural accommodation, cultural repatterning, and culture brokering.
- Barriers to providing culturally competent care are stereotyping, prejudice and racism, ethnocentrism, cultural imposition, cultural conflict, and culture shock.

- Nurses should perform a cultural assessment on every client with whom they interact. Cultural assessments help nurses understand clients' perspectives of health and illness and thereby guide them to providing culturally appropriate interventions. The needs of clients vary with their age, education, religion, and socioeconomic status.
- If nurses do not speak or understand the client's language, interpreters should be available to assist them in communicating with clients. In selecting an interpreter, nurses should not only consider the clients' cultural needs but also respect their right to privacy.
- Knowing the clients' dietary practices are an integral part of the assessment data. Efforts to understand dietary practices should go beyond relying on membership in a defined group and should include religious requirements.
- Members of minority groups are overrepresented on the lower tiers of the socioeconomic ladder. Poor economic achievement is also a common characteristic among populations at risk, such as those in poverty, the homeless, migrant workers, and refugees. Nurses should be able to distinguish between cultural and socioeconomic class issues and not interpret behavior as having a cultural origin when in fact it is based on socioeconomic class.

CLINICAL DECISION-MAKING ACTIVITIES

1. Select a culture that you would like to study. Go to an appropriate website and gather information about the cultural group. Identify the group's health-seeking behaviors. Discuss this information with at least one member of that cultural group. Compare and contrast information obtained from the two sources. How would you use this information in your clinical practice?

2. Recall the first time you encountered a client whose culture differed from yours. Discuss your assumptions about this client. What factors in your background led you to make these assumptions? How did your assumptions influence the care you gave the client and family members? Give specific examples.

3. Discuss how you would prepare for an interview with older clients about their cultural health beliefs and practices. Explore their use of Western and alternative health practices and determine the individual's decision-making process in seeking out

these health services. Who are the alternative health care specialists that practice in your community?

4. With the help of your local public health agency, explore the availability of culturally relevant policies and approaches for providing health care to major cultural groups in your community. On the basis of your findings, what gaps in services were evident? What input should the nurse give the agency personnel to augment services?

5. Which major ethnic and religious groups are represented in the community where you live? What resources are available to service their needs? What mechanisms are in place to facilitate access to these services by these groups?

6. On the basis of *Healthy People 2020* objectives, identify an at-risk aggregate in your community. What cultural content would you include when developing a health education program that promotes positive health behaviors for the group?

REFERENCES

Agency for Healthcare Research & Quality: *The National Healthcare Disparities Report, 2008*, Rockville, MD, 2009a, U.S. Department of Health and Human Services. Available at http://ftp.ahrq.gov/qual/nhdr08/nhdr08.pdf.Accessed December 10, 2010.

Agency for Healthcare Research & Quality: *The National Healthcare Quality Report, 2008*, Rockville, MD, 2009b, U.S. Department of Health and Human Services. Available at http://www.ahrq.gov/QUAL/nhqr08/nhqr08.pdf.Accessed December 10, 2010.

American Academy of Nursing Expert Panel on Culturally Competent Health Care: Culturally competent health care, *Nurs Outlook* 40:277–283, 1992.

Andrews MM, Boyle JS: *Transcultural concepts in nursing care*, ed 5, Philadelphia, 2007, Lippincott Williams & Wilkins.

Borrell LN, Jacobs DR, Williams DR, et al: Self-reported racial discrimination and substance use in the coronary artery risk development in adults study, *Am J of Epidemiol* 166:1068–1079, 2007.

Brislin R: *Understanding culture's influence on behavior*, ed 2, Fort Worth, TX, 2000, Harcourt Brace.

Brondolo E, Gallo LC, Myers HF: Race, racism and health: disparities, mechanisms, and interventions, *J Behav Med* 32:1–8, 2009.

Campinha-Bacote J: *The process of cultural competence in the delivery of healthcare services: a culturally competent model of care*, Cincinnati, OH, 2003, Transcultural CARE Associates.

Castro A, Ruiz E: The effects of nurse practitioner cultural competence on Latina clients satisfaction, *J Acad NP* 21:278–286, 2009.

Center for Immigration Studies: *Three decades of mass immigration*, Washington, DC, 1995, Center for Immigration Studies. Available at http://www.cis.org/articles/1995/back395.html Accessed December 9, 2010.

Centers for Disease Control and Prevention: Alcohol-attributable deaths and years of potential life lost among American Indians and Alaska Natives—United States, 2001-2005, *MMWR* 57:938–941, 2008.

Centers for Disease Control and Prevention: Differences in prevalence of obesity among black, white, and Hispanic adults—United States, 2006-2008, *Morb Mortal Wkly Rep* 58:740–744, 2009.

Changes in immigration law, 2008. Available at http://www.lawcom.com/immigration/chngs.shtml. Accessed December 9, 2010.

Congress of the United States: *A description of the immigrant population*, Washington, DC, 2004, U.S. Government Printing Office.

Council on Linkages Between Academic and Public Health Practice: *Core competencies for public health professional*, Washington, DC, 2010, Public Health Foundation/Health Resources and Services Administration.

Degazon CE: A contrast in ethnic identification, social support, and coping strategies among subgroups of African elders, *J Cult Div* 1:79–85, 1994.

Denker EP, editor: *Healing at home: visiting nurse service of New York, 1893-1993*, Dalton, MA, 1994, Studley Press.

Fielo S, Degazon CE: When cultures collide: decision making in a multicultural environment, *Nurs Health Care Perspect* 18:238–243, 1997.

Galanti GA: *Caring for patients from different cultures*, ed 4, Philadelphia, 2008, University of Pennsylvania Press.

Gamble VN: Under the shadow of Tuskegee: African Americans and health care, *Am J Public Health* 87:1773–1778, 1997.

Giger JN, Davidhizar R: *Transcultural nursing: assessment and intervention*, ed 5, St Louis, 2008, Mosby.

Hearnden M: Coping with differences in culture and communication in health care, *Nursing Standard* 23:49–57, 2008.

Horowitz C: The role of the family and the community in the clinical setting. In Loue S, editor: *Handbook of immigrant health*, New York, 1998, Plenum Press, pp 163–182.

Kaplan MS, Huguent N, Newman J, et al: The association between length of residence and obesity among Hispanic immigrants, *Am J Prevent Med* 27:323–326, 2004.

Kington RS, Smith JP: Socioeconomic status and racial ethnic differences in functional status associated with chronic diseases, *Am J Public Health* 8:805–810, 1997.

Leininger M: Essential transcultural nursing care concepts, principles, examples, and policy statements. In Leininger MM, McFarland M, editors: *Transcultural nursing: concepts, theories, research, and practices*, ed 3, New York, 2002a, McGraw-Hill, pp 45–69.

Leininger M: Part 1: The theory of culture care and the ethnonursing research method. In Leininger MM, McFarland M, editors: *Transcultural nursing: concepts, theories, research, and practices*, ed 3, New York, 2002b, McGraw-Hill, pp 71–98.

Lipson JG, Dibble SL, editors: *Providing culturally appropriate care in culture and clinical care*, San Francisco, 2005, UCSF Nursing Press, pp XII–XVII.

Locke DC, Hardaway YV: Moral perspectives in interracial settings. In Cochrane D, Manley-Casimir M, editors: *Moral education: practicalapproaches*, New York, 1992, Praeger.

McKenna M: A call for advocates for cultural awareness [editorial], *J Transcult Nurs* 12:5, 2001.

Meleis AI: Arabs. In Lipson JG, Dibble SL, editors: *Providing culturally appropriate care in culture and clinical care*, San Francisco, 2005, UCSF Nursing Press, pp 42–57.

Miles A, Awong L: When the patient is a racist, *Am J Nurs* 97(8):72, 1997.

Mohanty SA, Woolhandler S, Himmelstein DU, et al: Health care expenditures of immigrants in the United States: a nationally representative analysis, *Am J Public Health* 95:1431–1438, 2005.

Munoz CC, Luckmann J: *Transcultural communication in nursing*, ed 2, Clifton Park, NY, 2005, Thomson Delmar.

National Immigration Forum: *Immigration basics 2005*, Washington, DC, 2005, National Immigration Forum. Available at http://www.immigrationforum.org/images/uploads/ImmigrationBasics2005.pdf. Accessed May 17, 2010.

Office of Immigration Statistics, Office of Management, Department of Homeland Security: *2008 yearbook of immigration statistics*, Washington, DC, 2008, U.S. Government Printing Office.

Ogbu MA: Nigerians. In Lipson JG, Dibble SL, editors: *Providing culturally appropriate care in culture and clinical care*, San Francisco, 2005, UCSF Nursing Press, pp 243–259.

Okie S: Immigrants and health care—at the intersection of two broken systems, *N Engl J Med* 357(6):525–529, 2007.

Orlandi MA, editor: *Cultural competence for evaluators*, Washington, DC, 1992, U.S. Department of Health and Human Services.

Orque M: Orque's ethnic/cultural system: a framework for ethnic nursing care. In Orque MS, Bloch B, Monrroy LSA, editors: *Ethnic nursing care: a multi-cultural approach*, St Louis, 1983, Mosby.

Pew Hispanic Center: *Statistical portrait of Hispanics in the United States, 2006*, Washington, DC, 2008, Pew Hispanic Center.

Purnell LD, Paulanka BJ: *Transcultural health care*, ed 3, Philadelphia, 2008, FA Davis.

Quad Council of Public Health Nursing Organizations. *Competencies for Public Health Nursing Practice*, Washington, DC, 2003, ASTDN, revised 2009.

Randall-David E: *Strategies for working with culturally diverse communities and clients*, Bethesda, MD, 1989, Association of the Care of Children's Health.

Randall-David E: *Culturally competent HIV counseling and education*, McLean, VA, 1994, Maternal and Child Health Clearinghouse.

Richman LS, Pek J, Bennett GG, et al: Discrimination, dispositions, and cardiovascular responses to stress, *Health Psych* 26:675–683, 2007.

Riedel RL: Access to health care. In Loue S, editor: *Handbook of immigrant health*, New York, 1998, Plenum Press, pp 101–123.

Roberson MHB: Folk health beliefs of health professionals, *West J Nurs Res* 9:257–263, 1987.

Seibert PS, Stridh-Igo P, Zimmerman CG: A checklist to facilitate cultural awareness and sensitivity, *J Med Ethics* 28:143–146, 2002.

Sims M, Sims TL, Bruce MA: Race, ethnicity, concentrated poverty, and low birth weight disparities, *J Natl Black Nurses Assoc* 19:12–18, 2008.

Smedley BD, Stith AY, Nelson AR, editors: *Unequal treatment: confronting racial and ethnic disparities in health care*, Washington, DC, 2002, The National Academic Press.

Spector RE: *Cultural diversity in health and illness*, ed 7, Norwalk, CT, 2008, Appleton & Lange.

Tripp-Reimer T, Brink PJ, Saunders JM: Cultural assessment: content and process. In Spradley BW, Allender JA, editors: *Readings in community health*, ed 5, Philadelphia, 1997, Lippincott.

Tripp-Reimer T, Choi E, Kelley S: Cultural barriers to care: inverting the problem, *Diab Spect* 14:13–22, 2001.

U.S. Census Bureau: *Statistical abstract of the United States 2001*, Washington, DC, 2001, U.S. Government Printing Office.

U.S. Department of Health and Human Services: *Mental health: culture, race, and ethnicity. Supplement to Mental health: a report of the surgeon general*, Rockville, MD, 2001, U.S. Government Printing Office.

U.S. Department of Health and Human Services: *The Registered Nurse Population: findings from the 2004 national sample survey of registered nurses*, Washington, DC, 2005, U.S. Government Printing Office.

U.S. Department of Health and Human Services: *Healthy People 2020: understanding and improving health*, Washington, DC, 2010, U.S. Government Printing Office.

West EA: The cultural bridge model, *Nurs Outlook* 41:229–234, 1993.

Wu C: Drug sensitivity varies with ethnicity, *Sci News* 152:165, 1997.

CHAPTER 8

Public Health Policy

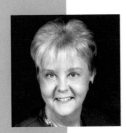

Marcia Stanhope, RN, DSN, FAAN

Dr. Marcia Stanhope is currently employed at the University of Kentucky College of Nursing, Lexington, Kentucky. She has been appointed to the Good Samaritan Foundation Chair and Professorship in Community Health Nursing. She has practiced community and home health nursing, has served as an administrator and consultant in home health, and has been involved in the development of two nurse-managed centers. At one time in her career, she held a public policy fellowship and worked in the office of a U.S. Senator. She has taught community health, public health, epidemiology, policy, primary care nursing, and administration courses. Dr. Stanhope formerly directed the Division of Community Health Nursing and Administration and served as Associate Dean of the College of Nursing at the University of Kentucky. She has been responsible for both undergraduate and graduate courses in population-centered nursing. She has also taught at the University of Virginia and the University of Alabama, Birmingham. Her presentations and publications have been in the areas of home health, community health and community-focused nursing practice, as well as primary care nursing.

ADDITIONAL RESOURCES

evolve WEBSITE
http://evolve.elsevier.com/Stanhope
- *Healthy People 2020*
- WebLinks

- Quiz
- Case Studies
- Glossary
- Answers to Practice Application

OBJECTIVES

After reading this chapter, the student should be able to do the following:

1. Discuss the structure of the U.S. government and health care roles.
2. Identify the functions of key governmental and quasi-governmental agencies that affect public health systems and nursing, both around the world and in the United States.
3. Differentiate between the primary bodies of law that affect nursing and health care.
4. Define key terms related to policy and politics.
5. State the relationships between nursing practice, health policy, and politics.
6. Develop and implement a plan to communicate with policy makers on a chosen public health issue.
7. Locate references related to nursing, public health, and health policy.

KEY TERMS

advanced practice nurse, p. 176
Agency for Healthcare Research and Quality, p. 170
American Association of Colleges of Nursing, p. 180
American Nurses Association, p. 169
block grants, p. 165
boards of nursing, p. 173
categorical funding, p. 172
categorical programs, p. 167

constitutional law, p. 173
devolution, p. 165
health policy, p. 164
judicial law, p. 173
law, p. 164
legislation, p. 173
legislative staff, p. 176
licensure, p. 174
National Institute of Nursing Research, p. 170
nurse practice act, p. 173
Occupational Safety and Health Administration, p. 169

Office of Homeland Security, p. 172
police power, p. 165
policy, p. 164
politics, p. 164
regulation, p. 173
U.S. Department of Health and Human Services, p. 164
World Health Organization, p. 168
—*See Glossary for definitions*

Nurses are an important part of the health care system and are greatly affected by governmental and legal systems. Nurses who select the community as their area of practice must be especially aware of the impact of government, law, and health policy on nursing, health, and the communities in which they practice. Insight into how government, law, and political action have changed over time is necessary to understand how the health care system has been shaped by these factors. Also, understanding how these factors have influenced the current and future roles for nurses and the public health system is critical for better health policy for the nation. Nurses have historically viewed themselves as advocates for the health of the population. It is this heritage that has moved the discipline into the policy and political arenas. To secure a more positive health care system, nurse professionals must develop a working knowledge of government, key governmental and quasi-governmental organizations and agencies, health care law, the policy process, and the political forces that are shaping the future of health care. This knowledge and the motivation to be an agent of change in the discipline and in the community are necessary ingredients for success as a population-centered nurse.

DEFINITIONS

To understand the relationship between health policy, politics, and laws, one must first understand the definitions of the terms. Policy is a settled course of action to be followed by a government or institution to obtain a desired end. Public policy is described as all governmental activities, direct or indirect, that influence the lives of all citizens (Birkland, 2005). Health policy, in contrast, is a set course of action to obtain a desired health outcome for an individual, family, group, community, or society. Policies are made not only by governments, but also by such institutions as a health department or other health care agency, a family, or a professional organization.

Politics plays a role in the development of such policies. Politics is found in families, professional and employing agencies,

and governments. Politics determines who gets what and when and how they get it (Birkland, 2005). Politics is the art of influencing others to accept a specific course of action. Therefore, political activities are used to arrive at a course of action (the policy). Law is a system of privileges and processes by which people solve problems based on a set of established rules; it is intended to minimize the use of force. Laws govern the relationships of individuals and organizations to other individuals and to government. Through political action, a policy may become a law, a regulation, a judicial ruling, a decision, or an order.

After a law is established, regulations further define the course of action (policy) to be taken by organizations or individuals in reaching an outcome. Government is the ultimate authority in society and is designated to enforce the policy whether it is related to health, education, economics, social welfare, or any other society issue. The following discussion explains the role of government in health policy.

GOVERNMENTAL ROLE IN U.S. HEALTH CARE

In the United States, the federal and most state and local governments are composed of three branches, each of which has separate and important functions. The *executive branch* is composed of the president (or state governor or local mayor) along with the staff and cabinet appointed by this executive, various administrative and regulatory departments, and agencies such as the U.S. Department of Health and Human Services (USDHHS). The *legislative branch* (i.e., Congress at the federal level) is made up of two bodies: the Senate and the House of Representatives, whose members are elected by the citizens of particular geographic areas.

> **DID YOU KNOW?** *There is a federal Division of Nursing, a section within the Health Resources and Services Agency (HRSA) of the USDHHS, that refines criteria for nursing education programs as funded by Congress and affirmed by the President.*

The *judicial branch* is composed of a system of federal, state, and local courts guided by the opinions of the Supreme Court. Each of these branches is established by the Constitution, and each plays an important role in the development and implementation of health law and public policy.

The executive branch suggests, administers, and regulates policy. The role of the legislative branch is to identify problems and to propose, debate, pass, and modify laws to address those problems. The judicial branch interprets laws and their meaning, as in its ongoing interpretation of states' rights to define access to reproductive health services to citizens of the states.

One of the first constitutional challenges to a federal law passed by Congress was in the area of health and welfare in 1937, after the 74th Congress had established unemployment compensation and old-age benefits for U.S. citizens (U.S. Law, 1937a). Although Congress had created other health programs previously, its legal basis for doing so had never been challenged. In *Stewart Machine Co. v. Davis* (U.S. Law, 1937b), the Supreme Court (judicial branch) reviewed this legislation and determined, through interpretation of the Constitution, that such federal governmental action was within the powers of Congress to promote the general welfare. It was obvious in 2008 and beyond that unemployment benefits are important to the economy and to individuals who lose jobs during a national economic crisis (BLS, 2010).

Most legal bases for the actions of Congress in health care are found in Article I, Section 8 of the U.S. Constitution, including the following:

1. Provide for the general welfare.
2. Regulate commerce among the states.
3. Raise funds to support the military.
4. Provide spending power.

Through a continuing number and variety of cases and controversies, these Section 8 provisions have been interpreted by the courts to appropriately include a wide variety of federal powers and activities. State power concerning health care is called **police power**. This power allows states to act to protect the health, safety, and welfare of their citizens. Such police power must be used fairly, and the state must show that it has a compelling interest in taking actions, especially actions that might infringe on individual rights. Examples of a state using its police powers include requiring immunization of children before being admitted to school and requiring case finding, reporting, treating, and follow-up care of persons with tuberculosis. These activities protect the health, safety, and welfare of state citizens.

Trends and Shifts in Governmental Roles

The government's role in health care at both the state and federal level began gradually. Wars, economic instability, and political differences between parties all shaped the government's role. The first major federal governmental action relating to health was the creation in 1798 of the Public Health Service (PHS). Then in 1890 federal laws were passed to promote the public health of merchant seaman and Native Americans. In 1934 Senator Wagner of New York initiated the first national health insurance bill. The Social Security Act of 1935 was passed to provide assistance to older adults and the unemployed, and it offered survivors' insurance for widows and children. It also provided for child welfare, health department grants, and maternal and child health projects. In 1948 Congress created the National Institutes of Health (NIH), and in 1965 it passed very important health legislation—creating Medicare and Medicaid to provide health care service payments for older adults, the disabled, and the categorically poor. These legislative acts by Congress created programs that were implemented by the executive branch. In March 2010, the most recent legislation passed and signed by President Obama to improve the health of the nation and access to care was the health reform law, the Patient Protection and Affordable Care Act (US LAW, PL 111-148). The legislation was designed to do the following:

- "Rein in the worst excesses and abuses of the insurance industry with some of the toughest consumer protections this country has ever known.
- Hold insurance companies accountable to keep premiums down and prevent denials of care and coverage, including for pre-existing conditions.
- Make health insurance affordable for middle class families and small businesses with one of the largest tax cuts for health care in history—reducing premiums and out-of-pocket costs.
- Provide the security of knowing that if a job is lost, changed, or a new business started, there will always be the ability to purchase quality, affordable care in a new competitive health insurance market that keeps costs down.
- Strengthen Medicare benefits with lower prescription drug costs for those in the 'donut hole,' chronic care, free preventive care, and nearly a decade more of solvency for Medicare.
- Improve the nation's fiscal health by reducing the federal deficit by more than $100 billion over the next decade, and more than $1 trillion in the decade after that." (Kaiser Family Foundation, 2010a)

The U.S. Department of Health and Human Services (USDHHS) (known first as the Department of Health, Education, and Welfare [DHEW]) was created in 1953. The Health Care Financing Administration (HCFA) was created in 1977 as the key agency within the USDHHS to provide direction for Medicare and Medicaid. In 2002 HCFA was renamed the Center for Medicare and Medicaid Services (CMS). During the 1980s, a major effort of the Reagan administration was to shift federal government activities, including federal programs for health care, to the states. The process of shifting the responsibility for planning, delivering, and financing programs from the federal level to the states is called **devolution**. Throughout the 1980s and 1990s, Congress has increasingly funded health programs by giving **block grants** to the states. Devolution processes including block granting should alert professional nurses that state and local policy has grown in importance to the health care arena. With the new health reform law, stimulus grants are being provided to state and local areas to improve health care access (HRSA, 2010).

The role of government in health care is shaped both by the needs and demands of its citizens and by the citizens' beliefs and values about personal responsibility and self-sufficiency. These beliefs and values often clash with society's sense of responsibility and need for equality for all citizens. A federal example of this ideological debate occurred in the 1990s over health care reform. The Democratic agenda called for a health care system that was universally accessible, with a focus on primary care and prevention. The Republican agenda supported more modest changes within the medical model of the delivery system. This agenda also supported reducing the federal government's role in health care delivery through cuts in Medicare and Medicaid benefits. The Democrats proposed the Health Security Act of 1993, which failed to gain Congress's approval. In an effort to make some incremental health care changes, both the Democrats and the Republicans in Congress passed two new laws. The Health Insurance Portability and Accountability Act (HIPAA) allows working persons to keep their employee group health insurance for up to 16 months after they leave a job (U.S. Law 107-105, 1996). The State Child Health Improvement Act (SCHIP) of 1997 provides insurance for children and families who cannot otherwise afford health insurance (U.S. Law, 1997).

With the new health care reform debates, numerous debates occurred in the House of Representatives and the Senate until there was agreement that the Senate version of the bill would be passed. On March 30, 2010 President Obama signed into law the Health Care and Education Reconciliation Act of 2010, which made some changes to the comprehensive health reform law and included House amendments to the new law (Kaiser, 2010a).

This discussion has focused primarily on trends in and shifts between different levels of government. An additional aspect of governmental action is the relationship between government and individuals. Freedom of individuals must be balanced with governmental powers. After the terrorist attacks on the United States in September (World Trade Center attack) and October (anthrax outbreak) of 2001, much government activity was being conducted in the name of protecting the safety of U.S. citizens.

WHAT DO YOU THINK? *Government has too much influence on the way health care services are delivered and on who receives care.*

It is interesting to note that before September 11, 2001, the congress and President, recognizing that the public health system infrastructure needed help, passed a law in 2000: "The Public Health Threats and Emergencies Act" (PL 106-505). This was the "first federal law to comprehensively address the public health system's preparedness for bioterrorism and other infectious disease outbreaks" (Frist, 2002, p 120). This legislation is said to have signaled the beginning of renewed interest in public health as the protector for entire communities. In June 2002 the Public Health Security and Bioterrorism Preparedness and Response Act was signed into law (PL 107-188) in December 2002, with $3 billion appropriated by Congress, to implement the following antibioterrorism activities:

- Improving public health capacity
- Upgrading of health professionals' ability to recognize and treat diseases caused by bioterrorism

- Speeding the development of new vaccines and other countermeasures
- Improving water and food supply protection
- Tracking and regulating the use of dangerous pathogens within the United States (Frist, 2002)

Yet it remains unclear just how much governmental intervention is necessary and effective and how much will be tolerated by citizens. For example, in 2010 approximately 49% of citizens were against the new health care reform acts, and the Republicans were seen as being obstructionists. A bill was also introduced into the House of Representatives to form a citizens' alliance for health care reform. From this example, it shows how unclear government actions are when looking at citizen reactions (The Citizens' Alliance, 2010).

Government Health Care Functions

Federal, state, and local governments carry out five health care functions, which fall into the general categories of direct services, financing, information, policy setting, and public protection.

Direct Services

Federal, state, and local governments provide direct health services to certain individuals and groups. For example, the federal government provides health care to members and dependents of the military, certain veterans, and federal prisoners. State and local governments employ nurses to deliver a variety of services to individuals and families, frequently on the basis of factors such as financial need or the need for a particular service, such as hypertension or tuberculosis screening, immunizations for children and older adults, and primary care for inmates in local jails or state prisons. The Evidence-Based Practice box presents a study that examined the use of a state health insurance program.

EVIDENCE-BASED PRACTICE

The purpose of this study was to examine the changes in access to care, use of services, and quality of care among children enrolled in Child Health Plus (CHPlus), a state health insurance program for low-income children that became a model for the State Child Health Insurance Program (SCHIP). A before-and-after design was used to evaluate the health care experience of children the year before and the year after enrollment in the state health insurance program. The study consisted of 2126 children from New York State, ranging from birth to 12.99 years of age. Results indicated that the state health insurance program for low-income children was associated with improved access, use, and quality of care. The development and implementation of SCHIP were an outcome of the soaring costs of health care and the fact that there are 11 million uninsured children in the United States. It was the largest public investment in child health in 30 years.

Nurse Use

This study supports the value of health policy and the need to evaluate the effectiveness of policy in accomplishing the purposes of the policy.

From U.S. Department of Health and Human Services: *Healthy People 2010: understanding and improving health,* ed 2, Washington, DC, 2000, U.S. Government Printing Office.

Financing

Governments pay for some health care services; the current percentage of the bill paid by the government is about 45.3%, and this is projected to increase to 47.6% by the year 2015. The government also pays for training some health personnel and for biomedical and health care research (NCHS, 2010). Support in these areas has greatly affected both consumers and health care providers. Federal governments finance the direct care of clients through the Medicare, Medicaid, Social Security, and SCHIP programs. State governments contribute to the costs of Medicaid and SCHIP programs. Many nurses have been educated with government funds through grants and loans, and schools of nursing, in the past, have been built and equipped using federal funds. Governments also have financially supported other health care providers, such as physicians, most significantly through the program of Graduate Medical Education funds. The federal government invests in research and new program demonstration projects, with NIH receiving a large portion of the monies. The National Institute of Nursing Research (NINR) is a part of the NIH and, as such, provides a substantial sum of money to the discipline of nursing for the purpose of developing the knowledge base of nursing and promoting nursing services in health care (NINR, 2010).

Information

All branches and levels of government collect, analyze, and disseminate data about health care and health status of the citizens. An example is the annual report *Health: United States, 2009*, compiled each year by the USDHHS (NCHS, 2010). Collecting vital statistics, including mortality and morbidity data, gathering of census data, and conducting health care status surveys are all government activities. Table 8-1 lists examples of available federal and international data sources on the health status of populations in the United States and around the world. These sources are available on the Internet and in the governmental documents' section of most large libraries. This information is especially important because it can help nurses understand the major health problems in the United States and those in their own states and local communities.

Policy Setting

Policy setting is a chief governmental function. Governments at all levels and within all branches make policy decisions about health care. These health policy decisions have broad implications for financial expenses, resource use, delivery system change, and innovation in the health care field. One law that has played a very important role in the development of public health policy, public health nursing, and social welfare policy in the United States is the Sheppard-Towner Act of 1921 (USDHHS, 2009; USDHHS, HRSA, 2010).

The Sheppard-Towner Act made nurses available to provide health services for women and children, including well-child and child-development services; provided adequate hospital services and facilities for women and children; and provided grants-in-aid for establishing maternal-child welfare programs. The act helped set precedents and patterns for the growth of modern-day public health policy. It defined the role of the federal government in creating standards to be followed by states in

TABLE 8-1	INTERNATIONAL AND NATIONAL SOURCES OF DATA ON THE HEALTH STATUS OF THE U.S. POPULATION	
ORGANIZATION	**DATA SOURCES**	
International		
United Nations	http://www.un.org/ *Demographic Yearbook*	
World Health Organization	http://www.who.int/en/ *World Health Statistics Annual*	
Federal		
Department of Health and Human Services	http://www.dhhs.gov National Vital Statistics System National Survey of Family Growth National Health Interview Survey National Health Examination Survey National Health and Nutrition Examination Survey National Master Facility Inventory National Hospital Discharge Survey National Nursing Home Survey National Ambulatory Medical Care Survey National Morbidity Reporting System U.S. Immunization Survey Surveys of Mental Health Facilities Estimates of National Health Expenditures AIDS Surveillance Nurse Supply Estimates	
Department of Commerce	http://www.commerce.gov U.S. Census of Population Current Population Survey Population Estimates and Projections	
Department of Labor	http://www.dol.gov Consumer Price Index Employment and Earnings	

conducting categorical programs, such as the Women, Infants, and Children (WIC) and Early Periodic Screening and Developmental Testing (EPSDT) programs. The act also defined the position of the consumer in influencing, formulating, and shaping public policy; the government's role in research; a system for collecting national health statistics; and the integrating of health and social services. This act established the importance of prenatal care, anticipatory guidance, client education, and nurse-client conferences, all of which are viewed today as essential nursing responsibilities.

Public Protection

The U.S. Constitution gives the federal government the authority to provide for the protection of the public's health. This function is carried out in numerous venues, such as by regulating air and water quality and protecting the borders from the influx of diseases by controlling food, drugs, and animal transportation, to name a few. The Supreme Court interprets and makes decisions related to public health, such as affirming a woman's rights to reproductive privacy (*Roe v. Wade*), requiring vaccinations, and setting conditions for states to receive public funds for highway construction/repair by requiring a minimum drinking age.

HEALTHY PEOPLE 2020: AN EXAMPLE OF NATIONAL HEALTH POLICY GUIDANCE

In 1979 the surgeon general issued a report that began a 30-year focus on promoting health and preventing disease for all Americans (DHEW, 1979). In 1989, *Healthy People 2000* became a national effort with many stakeholders representing the perspectives of government, state, and local agencies; advocacy groups; academia; and health organizations (USDHHS, 1991.

Throughout the 1990s states used *Healthy People 2000* objectives to identify emerging public health issues. The success of this national program was accomplished and measured through state and local efforts. The *Healthy People 2010* document focused on a vision of healthy people living in healthy communities. *Healthy People 2020* has four overarching goals, which can be found in the *Healthy People 2020* box; this box compares the goals of *Healthy People* documents from 2000 to 2020.

 HEALTHY PEOPLE 2020

A Comparison of the Goals of Healthy People 2000, Healthy People 2010, *and* Healthy People 2020

Healthy People 2000
Goals
- Increase the years of healthy life for Americans
- Reduce health disparities among Americans
- Achieve access to preventive services for all Americans

Healthy People 2010
Goals
- Increase quality and years of healthy life
- Eliminate health disparities

Healthy People 2020
Goals
- Attaining high quality, longer lives free of preventable disease, disability, injury, and premature death
- Achieving health equity, eliminating disparities, and improving the health of all groups
- Creating social and physical environments that promote good health for all
- Promoting quality of life, healthy development, and healthy behaviors across all life stages

From U.S. Department of Health and Human Services: Leading indicators. In *Healthy People 2000, 2010, & 2020,* Washington, DC, 1989, 1999, 2010, U.S. Government Printing Office.

ORGANIZATIONS AND AGENCIES THAT INFLUENCE HEALTH

International Organizations

In June 1945, following World War II, many national governments joined together to create the United Nations (UN). By charter, the aims and goals of the UN deal with human rights, world peace, international security, and the promotion of economic and social advancement of all the world's peoples. The UN, headquartered in New York City, is made up of six principal divisions, several subgroups, and many specialized agencies and autonomous organizations. With the approval and support of the UN Commission on the Status of Women, five world conferences on women have been held. At these conferences, the health of women and children and their rights to personal, educational, and economic security as well as initiatives to achieve these goals at the country level were debated and explored, and policies were formulated (United Nations, 1975, 1980, 1985, 1995, 2000).

One of the special autonomous organizations growing out of the UN is the World Health Organization (WHO). Established in 1946, WHO relates to the UN through the Economic and Social Council to achieve its goal to attain the highest possible level of health for all persons. "Health for All" is the creed of the WHO. Headquartered in Geneva, Switzerland, the WHO has six regional offices. The office for the Americas is located in Washington, DC, and is known as the Pan American Health Organization (PAHO). The WHO provides services worldwide to promote health, it cooperates with member countries in promoting their health efforts, and it coordinates the collaborating efforts between countries and the disseminating of biomedical research. Its services, which benefit all countries, include a day-to-day information service on the occurrence of internationally important diseases; the publishing of the international list of causes of disease, injury, and death; monitoring of adverse reactions to drugs; and establishing of world standards for antibiotics and vaccines. Assistance available to individual countries includes support for national programs to fight disease, to train health workers, and to strengthen the delivery of health services. The World Health Assembly (WHA) is the WHO's policy-making body, and it meets annually. The WHA's health policy work provides policy options for many countries of the world in their development of in-country initiatives and priorities; however, although WHA policy statements are important everywhere, they are guides and not law. The WHA's most recent policy statement on nursing and midwifery was released in 2003, and the current worldwide shortage of professional nurses is now on the WHO agenda and is being addressed by country (WHA, 2003; WHO, 2010).

The World Health Report, first published in 1995, is WHO's leading publication. Each year the report combines an expert assessment of global health, including statistics relating to all countries, with a focus on a specific subject. The main purpose of the report is to provide countries, donor agencies, international organizations, and others with the information they need to help them make policy and funding decisions. In the 2010 report, the WHO mapped out what countries can do to modify their financing systems so they can move more quickly toward this goal—universal coverage—and sustain the gains that have been achieved. The report builds on new research and lessons learned from country experience. It provides an action agenda for countries at all stages of development and proposes ways that the international community can better support efforts in low-income countries to achieve universal coverage and improve health outcomes (WHO, 2010).

The presence of nursing in international health is increasing. Besides offering direct health services in every country in the world, nurses serve as consultants, educators, and program planners and evaluators. Nurses focus their work on a variety of public health issues, including the health care workforce and education, environment, sanitation, infectious diseases, wellness promotion, maternal and child health, and primary care. Dr. Naeema Al-Gasseer of Bahrain has served as the scientist for nursing and midwifery at the WHO; Marla Salmon, dean of nursing at The University of Washington, chaired a Global Advisory Group on Nursing and Midwifery; and Linda Tarr Whelan served as the U.S. Ambassador to the UN Commission on the Status of Women. Virginia Trotter Betts, past president of the American Nurses Association (ANA), served as a U.S. delegate to both the WHA and the Fourth World Conference on Women in Beijing in 1995, where she participated on the negotiating team of the conference to develop a platform on the health of women across the life span. Many U.S. nurse leaders, such as Dr. Carolyn Williams, current author in this book, have been WHO consultants.

Federal Health Agencies

Laws passed by Congress may be assigned to any administrative agency within the executive branch of government for implementing, supervising, regulating, and enforcing. Congress decides which agency will monitor specific laws. For example, most health care legislation is delegated to the USDHHS. However, legislation concerning the environment would most likely be implemented and monitored by the Environmental Protection Agency (EPA), and that concerning occupational health by the Occupational Safety and Health Administration (OSHA) in the U.S. Department of Labor.

U.S. Department of Health and Human Services

The USDHHS is the agency most heavily involved with the health and welfare of U.S. citizens. It touches more lives than any other federal agency. The following agencies have been selected for their relevance to this chapter.

Health Resources and Services Administration. The Health Resources and Services Administration (HRSA) has been a long-standing contributor to the improved health status of Americans through the programs of services and health professions education that it funds. The HRSA contains the Bureau of Health Professions (BHPr), which includes the Division of Nursing as well as the Divisions of Medicine, Dentistry, and Allied Health Professions. The Division of Nursing is the key federal focus for nursing education and practice, and it provides national leadership to ensure an adequate supply and distribution of qualified nursing personnel to meet the health needs of the nation.

The Division of Nursing has the following strategic goals (USDHHS, 2010):

- Increase access to quality care through improved composition, distribution, and retention of the nursing workforce through financial assistance.

- Identify and use data, program performance measures, and outcomes to make informed decisions on nursing workforce issues.
- Increase cultural competence in the nursing workforce.
- Increase diversity in the nursing workforce

At the 122nd meeting of the Division of Nursing's National Advisory Council for Nursing Education and Practice (NACNEP), the participants discussed the role of public health nurses in participating in primary care in their communities. The speaker indicated several factors that need to be in place to support the public health nurse role:

- Baccalaureate standard for entry into practice
- Ongoing stable funding for health departments
- Competitive salaries commensurate with responsibilities
- Interventions grounded in and responsive to community needs
- Consideration of health determinants
- Experience in health promotion and prevention
- Long-term trusting relationships in the community (i.e., with clients)
- Established network of community partners
- Commitment to social justice and eliminating health disparities

Through the input of the NACNEP, the Division of Nursing sets policy for nursing nationally.

Centers for Disease Control and Prevention. The Centers for Disease Control and Prevention (CDC) serve as the national focus for developing and applying disease prevention and control, environmental health, and health promotion and education activities designed to improve the health of the people of the United States. The mission of the CDC is to promote health and quality of life by preventing and controlling disease, injury, and disability. The CDC seeks to accomplish its mission by working with partners throughout the nation and the world in the following ways:

- To monitor health
- To detect and investigate health problems
- To conduct research that will enhance prevention
- To develop and advocate sound public health policies
- To implement prevention strategies
- To promote healthy behaviors
- To foster safe and healthful environments
- To provide leadership and training

The mumps outbreak of Spring 2006 is an example of how the CDC fulfills its mission. The outbreak of mumps began in Iowa among college students. The CDC regularly collects data about mumps through the National Notifiable Disease Surveillance System on a weekly basis (CDC-MMWR Dispatch, 2006). Because of the recognized increase in mumps cases, states were asked to report aggregate numbers of cases twice a week along with mumps-related hospitalizations and complications. The CDC implemented an investigation to track the mumps cases and worked with state and local health departments to perform the following:

- Conduct mumps surveillance
- Assist with prevention and control activities
- Evaluate vaccine effectiveness

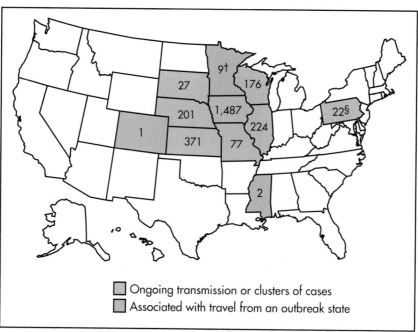

* N=2,597.
†Three cases related to the outbreak.
§Twelve cases related to the outbreak.

FIGURE 8-1 The number of reported mumps cases linked to multistate outbreak, by state—United States, January 1 to May 2, 2006. (From Centers for Disease Control and Prevention: *Epidemiology of mumps and multistate mumps outbreak, United States,* Atlanta, 2006, USDHHS.)

- Determine duration of immunity
- Evaluate risk factors for mumps

Before January 1, 2006, there had been about 300 cases per year between 2001 and 2003. In 5 months there were 2067 cases involving 10 states. Figure 8-1 presents a CDC map indicating cases per state (CDC, MMWR Dispatch, 2006).

National Institutes of Health. Founded in 1887, NIH today is one of the world's foremost biomedical research centers, and the federal focus point for biomedical research in the United States. The NIH is composed of 27 separate institutes and centers. The goal of NIH research is to acquire new knowledge to help prevent, detect, diagnose, and treat disease and disability, from the rarest genetic disorder to the common cold. The NIH mission is to uncover new knowledge that will lead to better health for everyone. The NIH works toward that mission by conducting research in its own laboratories; supporting the research of non-federal scientists in universities, medical schools, hospitals, and research institutions throughout the country and abroad; helping in the training of research investigators; and fostering communication of medical and health sciences' information (NIH, 2010a).

In late 1985 Congress overrode a presidential veto, allowing the creation of the National Center for Nursing Research within the NIH. In 1993 the Center became one of the divisions of the NIH and was renamed the **National Institute of Nursing Research** (NINR).

The research and research-related training activities previously supported by the Division of Nursing were transferred to the new Institute. The NINR is the focal point of the nation's nursing research activities. It promotes the growth and quality of research in nursing and client care, provides important leadership, expands the pool of experienced nurse researchers, and serves as a point of interaction with other bases of health care research. The mission of NINR is to promote and improve the health of individuals, families, communities, and populations. NINR supports and conducts clinical and basic research and research training on health and illness across the lifespan. The research focus encompasses health promotion and disease prevention, quality of life, health disparities, and end of life. NINR seeks to extend nursing science by integrating the biological and behavioral sciences, using new technologies to research questions, improving research methods, and developing the scientists of the future (NINR, 2010).

Agency for Healthcare Research and Quality. The Agency for Healthcare Research and Quality (AHRQ) is the lead federal agency charged with improving the quality, safety, efficiency, and effectiveness of health care for all Americans. As one of 12 agencies within the USDHSS, AHRQ supports health services research that will improve the quality of health care and promote evidence-based decision making. AHRQ is committed to improving care safety and quality by developing successful partnerships and generating the knowledge and tools required for long-term improvement. The goal of AHRQ research is to promote measurable improvements in health care in America. The outcomes are gauged in terms of improved quality of life and client outcomes, lives saved, and value gained for what we spend (AHRQ, 2009).

By examining what works and what does not work in health care, the AHRQ fulfills its missions of translating research findings into better client care and providing consumers, policy makers, and other health care leaders with information needed to make critical health care decisions. In 1999, Congress, through legislation, specifically directed AHRQ to focus on measuring and improving health care quality; promoting client safety and reducing medical errors; advancing the use of information technology for coordinating client care and conducting quality and outcomes research; and seeking to eliminate disparities in health care delivery for the priority populations of low-income groups, minorities, women, children, older adults, and individuals with special health care needs.

The AHRQ has published protocols for care of clients with a variety of health problems. These protocols have become the standards of health care delivery. The agency maintains a clinical practice guidelines clearinghouse for use by clinicians and others. In addition, the AHRQ has a project called "Put Prevention into Practice" to promote the use of standardized protocols for primary care delivery for clients across the age span (see Schedule of Clinical Preventive Services). These protocols can be used by nurses in planning disease prevention and health promotion activities for their clients.

Centers for Medicare and Medicaid Services. One of the most powerful agencies within the USDHHS is the CMS, which administers Medicare and Medicaid accounts and guided payment policy and delivery rules for services for 82 million people in 2007 (NCHS, 2010). In addition to providing health insurance, CMS also performs a number of quality-focused health care or health-related activities, including regulating of laboratory testing, developing coverage policies, and improving quality of care. CMS maintains oversight of the surveying and certifying of nursing homes and continuing care providers (including home health agencies, intermediate care facilities for the mentally retarded, and hospitals). It makes available to beneficiaries, providers, researchers, and state surveyors information about these activities and nursing home quality.

Federal Non-Health Agencies

Although the USDHHS has primary responsibility for federal health functions, several other departments of the executive branch carry out important health functions for the nation. Among these are the Defense, Labor, Agriculture, and Justice Departments.

Department of Defense

The Department of Defense delivers health care to members of the military, to their dependents and survivors, to National Guard and reserve members, and to retired members and their families. The assistant secretary of defense for health affairs administers a variety of health care plans for service personnel: TriCare Prime (a managed care arrangement) and an option for fee-for-service plans called TriCare Standard. In each branch of the uniformed services, nurses of high military rank are part of the administration of these health services (U.S. Department of Defense, 2010).

Department of Labor

The Department of Labor houses OSHA, which imposes workplace requirements on industries. These requirements shape the functions of nurses and the types of health services provided to workers in the workplace. A record-keeping system required by OSHA greatly affects health records in the workplace. Each state has an agency similar to OSHA that also monitors and inspects industries, as well as the health services delivered to them by nurses.

Needlestick injuries and other sharps-related injuries that result in occupational bloodborne pathogen exposure continue to be an important public health concern, especially to health care workers. In response to this serious situation, Congress passed the Needle Stick Safety and Prevention Act, which became law on November 6, 2000. To meet the requirements of this act, OSHA revised its Bloodborne Pathogen Standard to become effective on April 18, 2002. This act clarified the responsibility of employers to select safer needle devices as they become available and to involve employees in identifying and choosing the devices. The updated standard also required employers to maintain a log of injuries from contaminated sharps (Gerberding, 2003; OSHA, 2008).

Department of Agriculture

The Department of Agriculture houses the Food and Nutrition Service, which oversees a variety of food assistance activities. This service collaborates with state and local government welfare agencies to provide food stamps to needy persons to increase their food purchasing power. Other programs include school breakfast and lunch programs, WIC, and grants to states for nutrition education and training. Although these programs have been successful, the increasing use of the process of giving federal block grants to states (rather than implementing national programs) may threaten the effectiveness of these programs because of differences in how decisions are made at the state level on how to spend money on nutrition (USDA, 2010).

Department of Justice

Health services to federal prisoners are administered within the Department of Justice. The Federal Bureau of Prisons is responsible for the custody and care of approximately 210,000 federal offenders (Bureau of Federal Prisons, 2010). The Medical and Services Division of the Bureau of Prisons includes medical, psychiatric, dental, and health support services with community standards in a correctional environment. Health promotion is emphasized through counseling during examinations, education about effects of medications, infectious disease prevention and education, and chronic care clinics for conditions such as cardiovascular disease, diabetes, and hypertension. The Bureau also provides forensic services to the courts, including a range of evaluative mental health studies outlined in federal statutes. Health care for prisoners is highly regulated because of a series of court decisions on inmates' rights.

State and Local Health Departments

Depending on funding, public commitment and interest, and access to other resources, programs offered by state and local health departments vary greatly. Many state and local health officials report that employees in public health agencies lack skills in the core sciences of public health, and that this has hindered their effectiveness. The lack of specialized education and skill is a significant barrier to population-based preventive care and the delivery of quality health care to the public. Public health workforce specialists report that the number of retirees expected in this decade will result in a major shortage of public health workers, including nurses. More often than at other levels of government, nurses at the local level provide direct services. Some nurses deliver special or selected services, such as follow-up of contacts in cases of tuberculosis or venereal disease or providing child immunization clinics. Other nurses have a more generalized practice, delivering services to families in certain geographic areas (PHF, 2010; HRSA, 2005).

At the local and state levels, coordinating health efforts between health departments and other county or city departments is essential. Gaps in community coordination are showing up in glaring ways as states and communities scramble to address bioterrorism preparedness since September 11, 2001 and since such natural disasters as Hurricane Katrina.

IMPACT OF GOVERNMENT HEALTH FUNCTIONS AND STRUCTURES ON NURSING

The variety and range of functions of governmental agencies have had a major impact on the practice of nursing. Funding, in particular, has shaped roles and tasks of population-centered nurses. The designation of money for specific needs, or categorical funding, has led to special and more narrowly focused nursing roles. Examples are in emergency preparedness, school nursing, and family planning. Funds assigned to antibioterrorism cannot be used to support unrelated communicable disease programs or family planning.

The events of September 11, 2001, have had the public and the profession of nursing concerned about the ability of the present public health system and its workforce to deal with bioterrorism, especially outbreaks of deadly and serious communicable diseases. For example, smallpox vaccinations were stopped in 1972, but immunity lasts for only 10 years; although there have been no reported cases since the early 1970s, almost no one in the United States retains their immunity. Thus, the population is vulnerable to a smallpox outbreak, and smallpox could be used as a weapon of bioterrorism. Two laboratories in the world retain a small amount of the smallpox virus. Because of these potential threats, the U.S. government has begun to increase production of the vaccine (NIH, 2010b). Few public health professionals are knowledgeable of the symptoms, treatment, or mode of transmission of this disease. Most health professionals, including registered nurses (RNs), who currently work in the United States, have never seen a case of anthrax, smallpox, or plague—the three major biological weapons of concern in the world today. The USDHHS and the new federal Office of Homeland Security have provided funds to address this serious threat to the people of the United States. One of the first things being done is the rebuilding of the crumbling public health infrastructures of each state to provide surveillance, intervention, and communication in the face of future bioterrorism events and natural disasters. On December 19, 2006, President George W. Bush signed the Pandemic and All-Hazards Preparedness Act (PAHPA), which was intended to improve the organization, direction, and utility of preparedness efforts. PAHPA centralizes federal responsibilities, requires state-based accountability, proposes new national surveillance methods, addresses surge capacity, and facilitates the development of vaccines and other scarce resources (Hodge et al, 2007).

THE LAW AND HEALTH CARE

The United States is a nation of laws, which are subject to the U.S. Constitution. The law is a system of privileges and processes by which people solve problems on the basis of a set of established rules. It is intended to minimize the use of force. Laws govern the relationships of individuals and organizations to other individuals and to government. After a law is established, regulations further define the course of actions to be taken by the government, organizations, or individuals in reaching an agreed-on outcome. Government and its laws are the ultimate authority in society and are designed to enforce official policy whether it is related to health, education, economics, social welfare, or any other society issue. The number and types of laws influencing health care are ever increasing. Definitions of law (Catholic University of America, 2010) include the following:

- A rule established by authority, society, or custom
- The body of rules governing the affairs of people, communities, states, corporations, and nations
- A set of rules or customs governing a discrete field or activity (e.g., criminal law, contract law)

These definitions reflect the close relationship of law to the community and to society's customs and beliefs. The law has had a major impact on nursing practice. Although nursing emerged from individual voluntary activities, society passed laws to give formality to public health and, through legal mandates (i.e., laws), positions and functions for nurses in community settings were created. These functions in many instances carry the force of law. For example, if the nurse discovers a person with smallpox, the law directs the nurse and others in the public health community to take specific actions. In another example, in the mumps outbreak, a nurse and other health professionals are required to report mumps cases. This reporting requirement helps with locating and treating cases so cases can be treated or isolated as they occur to prevent further spreading of disease. Three types of laws in the United States have particular importance to the nurse: constitutional law, legislation and regulation, and judicial or common law.

DID YOU KNOW? *Persons with communicable diseases such as tuberculosis may be confined to a prison hospital if they are considered a threat to their community by failing to follow their treatment regimen.*

Constitutional Law

Constitutional law derives from federal and state constitutions. It provides overall guidance for selected practice situations. For example, on what basis can the state *require* quarantine or isolation of individuals with tuberculosis? The U.S. Constitution specifies the explicit and limited functions of the federal government. All other powers and functions are left to the individual states. The major constitutional power of the states relating to population-centered nursing practice is the state's right to intervene in a reasonable manner to protect the health, safety, and welfare of its citizens. The state has *police power* to act through its public health system, but it has limits. First, it must be a "reasonable" exercise of power. Second, if the power interferes or infringes on individual rights, the state must demonstrate that there is a "compelling state interest" in exercising its power. Isolating an individual or separating someone from a community because that person has a communicable disease has been deemed an appropriate exercise of state powers. The state can isolate an individual even though it infringes on individual rights (such as freedom and autonomy), under the following conditions (Watkins, 2006):

- There is a compelling state interest in preventing an epidemic.
- The isolation is necessary to protect the health, safety, and welfare of individuals in the community or the public as a whole.
- The isolation is done in a reasonable manner.

> **WHAT DO YOU THINK?** *The community's rights are more important than the individual's rights when there is a threat to the health of the public.*

The legal and medical communities along with AIDS (acquired immunodeficiency syndrome) activists rejected (and made the case) that the social quarantine of individuals with AIDS was unnecessary. Thus, individual freedom and autonomy of the individual come before "compelling state interest" unless science warrants another conclusion (Swendiman et al, 2010).

Legislation and Regulation

Legislation is law that comes from the legislative branches of federal, state, or local government. This is referred to as Statute Law because it becomes coded in the statutes of a government (Birkland, 2005). Much legislation has an effect on nursing. Regulations are specific statements of law related to defining or implanting individual pieces of legislation or statute law. For example, state legislatures enact laws (statutes) establishing boards of nursing and defining terms such as *registered nurse* and *nursing practice*. Every state has a board of nursing. The board may be found either in the department of licensing boards of the health department or in an administrative agency of the governor's office. Created by legislation known as a state nurse practice act, the board of nursing is made up of nurses and consumers. The functions of this board are described in the nurse practice act of each state and generally include licensing and examination of RNs and licensed practical nurses; licensing and/or certification of advanced practice nurses; approval of schools of nursing in the state; revocation, suspension, or denying of licenses; and writing of regulations about nursing practice and education. The state boards of nursing operationalize, implement, and enforce the statutory law by writing explicit statements *(rules)* on what it means to be an RN, and on the nurse's rights and responsibilities in delegating work to others and in meeting continuing education requirements.

All nurses employed in community settings are subject to legislation and regulations. For example, home health care nurses employed by private agencies must deliver care according to federal Medicare or state Medicaid legislation and regulations, so the agency can be reimbursed for those services. Private and public health care services rendered by nurses are subject to many governmental regulations for quality of care, standards of documentation, and confidentiality of client records and communications. All state health departments have a public health practice reference that governs the practice of nurses and others; and state public health laws that define the essential public health services that must be offered in the state as well as the optional services that may also be offered.

Judicial and Common Law

Both judicial law and common law have great impact on nursing. Judicial law is based on court or jury decisions. The opinions of the courts are referred to as *case law* (Birkland, 2005). The court uses other types of laws to make its decisions, including previous court decisions or cases. Precedent is one principle of common law. This means that judges are bound by previous decisions unless they are convinced that the older law is no longer relevant or valid. This process is called *distinguishing*, and it usually involves a demonstration of how the current situation in dispute differs from the previously decided situation. Other principles of common law such as justice, fairness, respect for individual's autonomy, and self-determination are part of a court's rationale and the basis upon which to make a decision.

LAWS SPECIFIC TO NURSING PRACTICE

Despite the broad nature and varied roles of nurses in practice, two legal arenas are most applicable to nurse practice situations. The first is the statutory authority for the profession and its scope of practice, and the second is professional negligence or malpractice.

Scope of Practice

The issue of scope of practice involves defining nursing, setting its credentials, and then distinguishing between the practices of nurses, physicians, and other health care providers. The issue is especially important to nurses in community settings, who have traditionally practiced with much autonomy.

Health care practitioners are subject to the laws of the state in which they practice, and they can practice only with a license. The states' nurse practice acts differ somewhat, but they are the most important statutory law affecting nurses. The nurse practice act of each state accomplishes at least four functions: defining the practice of professional nursing, identifying the scope of nursing practice, setting educational qualifications and other requirements for licensure, and determining the legal titles nurses may use to identify themselves. The usual and customary practice of nursing can be determined through a variety of sources, including the following:

- Content of nursing educational programs, both general and special
- Experience of other practicing nurses (peers)
- Statements and standards of nursing professional organizations
- Policies and procedures of agencies employing nurses
- Needs and interests of the community
- Updated literature, including research, books, texts, and journals

All of these sources can describe, determine, and refine the scope of practice of a professional nurse. Every nurse should know and follow closely any proposed changes in the practice acts of nursing, medicine, pharmacy, and other related professions. The nurse should always examine all legislation, rules, and regulations related to nursing practice. For example, a review of the Pharmacy Act will let the nurse know whether to question the right to dispense medications in a family planning clinic in a local health department. Defining the scope of practice forces one to clarify independent, interdependent, and dependent nursing functions.

Just as practice acts vary by state, so do the evolving issues and tensions of scopes of practice among the health professions. In past years, several state legislatures (working closely with the National Council of State Boards of Nursing) embarked on a legislative effort to develop the Interstate Nurse Licensure Compact. The compact allows mutual recognition of generalist nursing licensure across state lines in the compact states. By 2010, 24 states had adopted the compact (NCSBN, 2010).

Professional Negligence

Professional negligence, or *malpractice*, is defined as an act (or a failure to act) that leads to injury of a client. To recover money damages in a malpractice action, the client must prove all of the following:

1. That the nurse owed a duty to the client or was responsible for the client's care
2. That the duty to act the way a reasonable, prudent nurse would act in the same circumstances was not fulfilled
3. That the failure to act reasonably under the circumstances led to the alleged injuries
4. That the injuries provided the basis for a monetary claim from the nurse as compensation for the injury

Reported cases involving negligence and population-centered nurses are rare. However, the following is an example:

In *Williams v. Metro Home Health Care Agency et al* (U.S. Law, 2002), the client brought a malpractice action against Edward Schiro, RN, and his employer, a home health agency, alleging that the nurse's failure to visit and treat the client (a paraplegic) in a manner that followed physician orders caused the progression of a decubitus ulcer on his hip to the extent that surgical intervention was required. The physician orders called for three visits per week, and the client testified that the RN visited only once per week and had falsified the record as to the other visits.

The court determined that it was the nurse's duty to exercise the degree of skill used by other nurses in the community, along with his best judgment on client care to promote skin integrity. The failure of the nurse both to care for the client's decubiti and to instruct the client and his family concerning proper methods for self-care and assessment for decubitus ulcers contributed to the client's deteriorating skin integrity and condition.

> **DID YOU KNOW?** *In the eyes of the law, the "prudent nurse" used as the example, or standard, by which to judge the competency of a nurse's practice can be practicing anywhere in the United States and not just in the community in which the nurse works.*

An integral part of all negligence actions is the question of who should be sued. When a nurse is employed and functioning within the scope of employment, the employer is responsible for the nurse's negligent actions. This is referred to as the doctrine of *respondeat superior.* By directing a nurse to carry out a particular function, the employer becomes responsible for negligence, along with the individual nurse. Because employers are usually better able to pay for the injuries suffered by clients, they are sued more often than the nurses themselves, although an increasing number of judgments include the professional nurse by name as a co-defendant.

Thus, it is imperative that all nurses engaged in clinical practice carry their own professional liability insurance. Nurses may have personal immunity for particular practice areas, such as giving immunizations. In some states, the legislature has granted personal immunity to nurses employed by public agencies to cover all aspects of their practice under the legal theory of *sovereign immunity* (Cherry and Jacobs, 2005).

Nursing students need to be aware that the same laws and rules that govern the professional nurse govern them. Students are expected to meet the same standard of care as that met by any licensed nurse practicing under the same or similar circumstances. Students are expected to be able to perform all tasks and make clinical decisions on the basis of the knowledge they have gained or been offered, according to their progress in their educational programs and along with adequate educational supervision.

LEGAL ISSUES AFFECTING HEALTH CARE PRACTICES

Specific legal issues of nursing vary depending on the setting where care is delivered, the clinical arena, and the nurse's functional role. The law, including legislation and judicial opinions, significantly affects each of the following areas of nursing practice. Nurses responsible for setting and implementing program priorities need to identify and monitor laws related to each special area of practice.

School and Family Health

Nurses employed by health departments or boards of education may deliver school and family health nursing. School health legislation establishes a minimum of services that must be provided to children in public and private schools. For example, most states require that children be immunized against certain communicable diseases before entering school. Children must have had a physical examination by that time, and most states require at least one physical at a later time in their schooling. Legislation also specifies when and what type of health screening will be conducted in schools (e.g., vision and hearing testing). These requirements are found in statutory laws of states. Some states are now requiring a simple dental examination in schools for the purpose of referring children to a dental health professional if needed.

Statutes addressing child abuse and neglect make a large impact on nursing practice within schools and families. Most states require nurses to notify police and/or a social service agency of any situation in which they suspect a child is being abused or neglected. This is one instance in which the law mandates that a health professional breach client confidentiality to protect someone who may be in a helpless or vulnerable position. There is *civil immunity* for such reporting, and the nurse may be called as a witness in a court hearing of the case.

Occupational health is another special area of practice that has specific legal requirements as a result of state and federal statutes. Of special concern are the state workers' compensation statutes, which provide the legal foundation for claims of workers injured on the job. Access to records, confidentiality, and the use of standing orders are legal issues that have great practice significance to nurses employed in industries.

Home Care and Hospice

Home care and hospice services rendered by nurses are shaped through state statutes and have specific nursing requirements for licensure and certification. Compliance with these laws is directly linked to the method of payment for the services. For example, a service must be licensed and certified to obtain payment for services through Medicare. Federal regulations implementing Medicare/Medicaid have an enormous effect on much of nursing practice, including how nurses record details of their visits, record time spent in care activities, and document client care and the client's status and progress.

In addition, many states have passed laws requiring nurses to report elder abuse to the proper authorities, as is done with children and youth. Laws affecting home care and hospice services have focused on such issues as the right to death with dignity, rights of residents of long-term facilities and home health clients, definitions of death, and the use of living wills and advance directives. The legal and ethical dimensions of nursing practice are particularly important. Individual rights, such as the right to refuse treatment, and nursing responsibilities, such as the legal duty to render reasonable and prudent care, may appear to be in conflict in delivering home and hospice services. Much case discussion (sometimes including outside ethics consultation) may be needed to resolve such conflicts.

Correctional Health

Correctional health nursing practice is significantly shaped by federal and state laws and regulations and by recent Supreme Court decisions. The laws and decisions primarily relate to the type and amount of services that must be provided for incarcerated individuals. For example, physical examinations are required for all prisoners after they are sentenced. Regulations specify basic levels of care that must be provided for prisoners, and access to care during illness is a particular focus. Court decisions requiring adequate health services are based on constitutional law. If minimal services are not provided, it is a violation of a prisoner's right to freedom from cruel and unusual punishment. Such decisions provide a framework that strongly influences the setting of nursing priorities. For example, providing care to the sick would take priority over wellness or health education classes.

THE NURSE'S ROLE IN THE POLICY PROCESS

The number and types of laws influencing health care are increasing. Because of this, nurses need to be involved in the policy process and understand the importance of involvement of nursing to the clients they serve.

For nurses to effectively care for their client populations and their communities in the complex U.S. health care system, professional advocacy for logical health policy that considers equality is essential. Professional nurses working in the community know all too well about the health care problems they and their clients encounter daily, and it is through policy and political activism that both big-picture and long-term solutions can be developed.

Although the term *policy* may sound rather lofty, health policy is quite simply the process of turning health problems into workable action solutions. Health policy is developed on the three-legged stool of *access, cost,* and *quality.*

The policy process, which is very familiar to professional nurses, includes the following:

- Statement of a health care problem
- Statement of policy options to address the health problem
- Adoption of a particular policy option
- Implementation of the policy product (e.g., a service)
- Evaluation of the policy's intended and unintended consequences in solving the original health problem

Thus the policy process is very similar to the nursing process, but the focus is on the level of the larger society and the adoption strategies require political action. For most professional nurses, action in the policy arena comes most easily and naturally through participation in nursing organizations such as the ANA at the state level or the Association of Community Health Nursing Educators (ACHNE) or the Association of State and Territorial Directors of Nursing (ASTDN) at the national or state level, and in certain specialty organizations like the American Public Health Association (APHA).

NURSING TIP *The nurse's basic understanding of the political process should include knowing who the lawmakers are, how bills become laws (see Figure 8-2), the process of writing regulations (see Figure 8-3), and methods of influencing the process and shaping of health policy. With this knowledge, nurses can influence nursing practice.*

Legislative Action

It is often helpful to review the legislative and political processes that may have been a part of high school education. It becomes important material to remember as a professional career is embarked upon.

The people within geographic jurisdictions elect their legislative representatives and senators. An important part of the legislative process is the work of the legislative staff. These individuals do the legwork, research, paperwork, and other activities that move policy ideas into bills and then into law. In addition to the individual legislator's office, the congressional committee staffs are also important. They are usually experts in the content of the work of a committee, such as a health and welfare committee. Frequently, developing a working relationship with key legislative staffers can be as important to achieving a policy objective as the relationship with the policy maker (i.e., the legislator).

> **WHAT DO YOU THINK?** *As a former Speaker of the House of Representatives noted, "all politics is local." Therefore, should nurses focus their political activities only in the local community?*

The legislative process begins with ideas (policy options) that are developed into bills. After a bill is drafted, it is introduced to the legislature, given a number, read, and assigned to a committee. Hearings, testimony, lobbying, education, research, and informal discussions follow. If the bill is passed from the legislative committee, the entire House hears the bill, amends it as necessary, and votes on it. A majority vote moves the bill to the other House, where it is read and amended, and then a vote is taken. Figure 8-2 shows the necessary formal process of the legislative pathway.

Nurses can be involved in the legislative process at any point. Many professional nursing associations have legislative committees made up of volunteers, governmental relations staff professionals, and sometimes political action committees (PACs), all engaged in efforts to monitor, analyze, and shape health policy.

Common methods of influencing health policy outcomes include face-to-face encounters, personal letters, mailgrams, electronic mail, telephone calls, testimony, petitions, reports, position papers, fact sheets, letters to the editor, news releases, speeches, coalition building, demonstrations, and law suits. Depending on the issue, any of these can be effective. Although most business, including politics and the policy agendas, are dependent upon the Internet today for instant communication and quick response, all of these methods continue to be of great importance in influencing policy agendas. For example, if a face-to-face encounter is used with a legislator or a staffer, these persons can put a "face on the policy" agenda, and the reality that the policy affects real persons is an important consideration when the legislator or staff pushes the policy agenda forward. Guidelines on communication are provided in the How To box. Tips on communication and visiting legislators and their staffs, as well as general tips on political action, are presented in Boxes 8-1, 8-2, and 8-3. Political activities in which nurses can and should be involved include a wide variety of activities such as being informed voters (a must!), participating in a political party, registering others to vote, getting out the vote, fundraising for candidates, building networks or communication links for issues (e.g., a phone tree or Internet distribution list), and participating in organizations to ensure their effective involvement in health policy and politics.

HOW TO **Be an Effective Communicator**

- Use simple communications that will be readily understood.
- Choose language that clearly conveys information to individuals of diverse cultures, different ages, and different educational backgrounds.
- Oral or written communication needs to be targeted to the issue and free of terminology unique to medicine and nursing (i.e., jargon).
- State your expertise on the issue first.
- Briefly describe your education and experience.
- Identify the relevance of the issue beyond nursing.
- Provide information regarding the impact of the issue on the legislator's constituents.
- Present accurate, credible data.
- Do not oversell or give inaccurate information about the problem.
- Present information in an organized, thorough, concise form that is based on factual data (when available).
- Give examples.

The direct reimbursement of advanced practice nurses (APNs) in the Medicare program is one example of how nurses can use their influence. The inclusion of amendments to Medicare that authorized APN reimbursement regardless of specialty or client location in the Balanced Budget Act of 1997 required the sustained efforts of the ANA and other national nursing

---

BOX 8-1 **TIPS FOR VISITS WITH LEGISLATORS**

- Face-to-face visits are viewed as the most effective.
- Call ahead and ask how much time the staff or legislator is able to give you.
- When you arrive, ask if the appointment time is the same or if a scheduled vote on the House/Senate floor is going to need the legislator's attention.
- Engage in small talk at the beginning of the conversation only if the staff or legislator has time.
- Structure time so that the issue can be briefly presented. The visit will probably be 15 minutes or less.
- Allow an opportunity for the staff or Congress member to seek clarity or ask questions.
- Offer to provide additional information or find answers to questions asked.
- Do not assume that the legislator or the legislator's staff is well informed on the issue.
- Leave a one- or two-page fact sheet on the issue.
- Numbers count. If the views you express are shared by a local nurses' organization or by nurses employed at a health care facility, let the legislator know.
- Invite Congress members and their staffs to conferences or meetings of nurses' organizations, or to tour nursing facilities to meet others interested in the same policy issues.
- If appropriate, invite the media and let the legislator know.
- Follow up with a letter of thanks to both the legislator and the staffer.

Modified from Mason D et al: *Policy and politics in government*, ed 5, St Louis, 2007, Elsevier.

The Federal Level

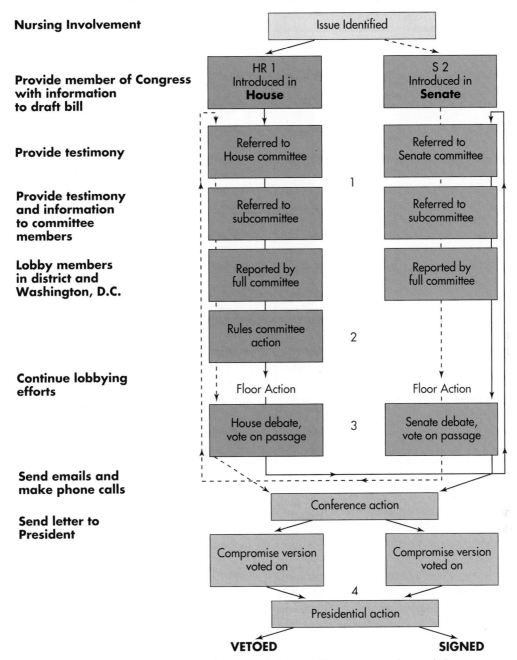

Nursing Involvement

Provide member of Congress with information to draft bill

Provide testimony

Provide testimony and information to committee members

Lobby members in district and Washington, D.C.

Continue lobbying efforts

Send emails and make phone calls

Send letter to President

Issue Identified

HR 1 Introduced in **House**

S 2 Introduced in **Senate**

Referred to House committee

Referred to Senate committee

Referred to subcommittee

Referred to subcommittee

Reported by full committee

Reported by full committee

Rules committee action

Floor Action

Floor Action

House debate, vote on passage

Senate debate, vote on passage

Conference action

Compromise version voted on

Compromise version voted on

Presidential action

VETOED   **SIGNED**

¹ A bill goes to full committee first, then to special subcommittees for hearings, debate, revisions, and approval. The same process occurs when it goes to full committee. It either dies in committee or proceeds to the next step.
² Only the House has a Rules Committee to set the "rule" for floor action and conditions for debate and amendments. In the Senate, the leadership schedules action.
³ The bill is debated, amended, and passed or defeated. If passed, it goes to the other chamber and follows the same path. If each chamber passes a similar bill, both versions go to conference.
⁴ The President may sign the bill into law, allow it to become law without his signature, or veto it and return it to Congress. To override the veto, both houses must approve the bill by a two-thirds majority vote.

FIGURE 8-2 How a bill becomes a law. (From Mason DJ, Keavitt JK, Chaffee MW: *Policy and politics in nursing and health care*, ed 5, St Louis, 2007, Elsevier.)

BOX 8-2   TIPS FOR WRITTEN COMMUNICATION WITH LEGISLATORS

- Communicate in writing to express opinions.
- Identify yourself as a nurse.
- Acknowledge the Congress member's work as positive or negative, but be courteous.
- Follow up on meetings or phone calls with a letter or e-mail.
- Share knowledge about a particular problem.
- Recommend policy solutions so the legislator or staff will know why you are writing.
- The letter should be typed, a maximum of two pages, and focused on one or two issues at most.
- The purpose of the letter should be stated at the beginning.
- Present clear and compelling rationales for your concern or position on an issue.
- If the purpose of the letter is to express disappointment regarding a stance on an issue or a vote that has been cast, the letter should be as positive as possible.
- Write letters thanking a Congress member for taking a particular position on an issue.
- A letter to the editor of the local newspaper or a nursing newsletter praising a legislator's position (with a copy forwarded to the legislator) is welcome publicity, especially during an election year.
- If you visited with the legislator or a staffer, review the major points covered in person and answer any questions that were raised during conversation.
- Have personal business cards and include them with letters.
- Address written correspondence as follows (the same general format applies to state and local officials):

U.S. Senator	U.S. Representative
Honorable Jane Doe	Honorable Jane Doe
United States Senate	House of Representatives
Washington, DC 20510	Washington, DC 20515
Dear Senator Doe:	Dear Representative Doe:

Modified from Mason D et al: *Policy and politics in government,* ed 5, St Louis, 2007, Elsevier.

BOX 8-3   TIPS FOR ACTION

- Become informed.
- Become acquainted with elected officials.
- Become involved in the state nurses' association.
- Build communication and leadership skills.
- Increase your knowledge about a range of professional issues.
- Expand and strengthen your professional network.
- Build relationships within the profession and with representatives of public and private sector organizations with an interest in health care.
- Be aware of what is taking place in health care beyond the environment and the practice in which you work.
- Communicate with legislators regularly and share expertise and perspective on issues related to health care and nursing.
- Offer your expertise to assist in developing new legislation, modifying existing legislation or regulations.
- Identify yourself as a nurse with associated education and expertise.
- Let people know that nurses are capable of functioning in many different roles and making substantial contributions.
- Be confident.
- Do not burn bridges.
- Be friendly.
- Lend a hand to other nurses. It benefits all of us.
- If you are new to the policy arena, find an experienced mentor to work with you.
- Volunteer, seek appointments, or participate in elections in campaigns.
- Explore opportunities for involvement through internships, fellowships, and volunteer work at all levels (local, state, and national).

Modified from Mason D, Keavitt JK, Chaffee MW: *Policy and politics in government,* ed 5, St Louis, 2007, Elsevier.

organizations over a long period (Nursing World, 2000). During that time, individual nurses provided testimony to Congress and to MEDPAC (the physicians' political action committee) on the importance of direct reimbursement to APNs. Many APNs worked closely and vigorously with their congressional representatives to lobby for this Medicare amendment. Even more wrote letters and provided position papers and fact sheets to help legislators understand the value of APNs. Although the process took more than 10 years to achieve fully, APN reimbursement in Medicare became a reality. Both the nursing profession and Medicare beneficiaries will benefit from the enhanced access of Medicare clients to APNs.

WHAT DO YOU THINK? *Which special interest group(s) has/have the most political influence in Washington, DC, today? Why?*

The ANA was likewise a strong supporter for the Patient Safety Act of 1997 (ANA, 1997). This law requires health care agencies to make public some information on nurse staff levels, staff mix, and outcomes, and it requires the USDHHS to review and approve all health care acquisitions and mergers. All

of these requirements are to determine any long-term effect on the health and safety of clients, communities, and staff.

On the state legislative level, all 50 states have passed title protection for APNs; this was achieved by individual nurses, state nurses associations, and various nursing specialty groups participating in the legislative process with the 50 state legislators. Title protection means that only certain nurses who meet state criteria can call themselves *advanced practice nurses*.

Regulatory Action

The regulatory process, although it may not be as visible a process as legislation, can also be used to shape laws and dramatically affect health policy. This process should be on the radar screen of professional nurses who wish to successfully participate in policy activity.

At each level of government, the executive branch can and, in most cases, must prepare regulations for implementing policy for new laws and new programs. These regulations are detailed, and they establish, fix, and control standards and criteria for carrying out certain laws. Figure 8-3 shows the steps in the typical process of writing regulations. When the legislature passes a law and delegates its oversight to an agency, it gives that agency the power to make regulations. Because regulations flow from legislation, they have the force of law.

The Process of Regulation

After a law is passed, the appropriate executive department begins the process of regulation by studying the topic or issue. Advisory groups or special task forces are sometimes formed to

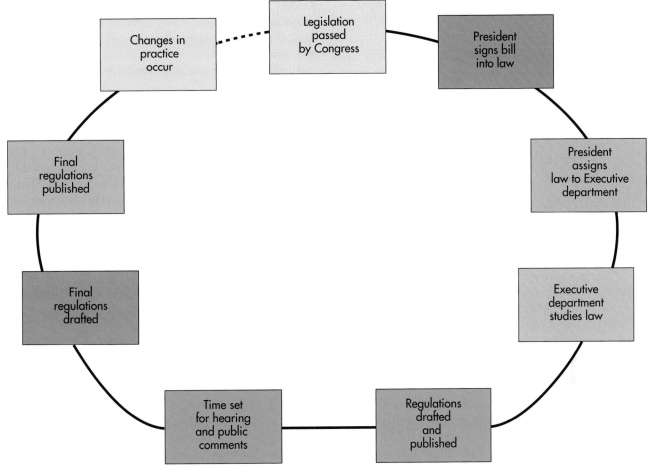

FIGURE 8-3 The process of writing regulations.

provide the content for the regulations. Nurses can influence these regulations by writing letters to the regulatory agency in charge or by speaking at open public hearings. Many letters are now accepted by Internet.

After rewriting, the proposed regulations are put into final draft form and printed in the legally required publication (e.g., at the federal level, the *Federal Register*). Similar registers exist in most states, where regulations from state executive departments, including state health departments, are published. Public comment is called for in written form or oral presentation within a given period.

Revisions made to proposed regulations are based on public comment and public hearing. Depending on the amount and content of the public reaction, final regulations are prepared or more study of the area and issues is conducted. Final published regulations carry the force of law. When regulations become effective, health care practice is changed to conform to the new regulations. Monitoring administrative regulations is essential for the professional nurse, who can influence regulations by attending the hearings, providing comments, testifying, and engaging in lobbying aimed at individuals involved in the writing of the regulations. Concrete written suggestions for revision submitted to these individuals are frequently persuasive and must be acknowledged by government in publishing the final rules. An excellent example of how nurses must continue to influence

health policy outcomes, even after positive legislation has passed, occurred after the passage of the Balanced Budget Act of 1997 (PL: 105-33 1997). The HCFA began to implement the BBA '97 through the publication of draft regulations seeking to define the how's of APN practice and Medicare reimbursement. The nursing community responded vigorously with negative opinions about the initial restrictive definitions and requirement. Their reactions were effective and reshaped the final regulations to recognize the state definitions for APN practice autonomy.

Final regulations, published in a *Code of Regulations* (both federal and state), usually lead to changes in practice. For example, Medicare regulations setting standards for nursing homes and home health are incorporated into these agencies' manuals. In the case of APN reimbursement, some Medicare fiscal intermediaries have had difficulty in recognizing APNs as appropriate providers, but professional nursing organization advocates have forcefully addressed these implementation barriers.

Nursing Advocacy

Advocacy begins with the art of influencing others (politics) to adopt a specific course of action (policy) to solve a societal problem. This is accomplished by building relationships with the appropriate policy makers—the individuals or groups that determine a specific course of action to be followed by a government or institution to achieve a desired end (policy outcome).

Relationships for effective advocacy can be built in a number of ways.

THE CUTTING EDGE *In January 2006, Medicare Part D—the prescription drug benefit policy—became effective. Public health professionals need to continue to assist many vulnerable persons to understand the value of enrolling in Part D, to educate them on how to use the benefits, and to ensure that the populations who are "dually" enrolled in both Medicare and Medicaid are registered. Coordinating efforts between civic, religious, and health care agencies to provide health education is a necessity.*

Kaiser Health News: Research Roundup: Lessons from Medicare Part D; Evaluating Medical Homes; Insuring Young Adults. Accessed January 22, 2011 from khn.org.

A letter or visit to the district, state, or national office of a legislator to discuss a particular policy or health care issue can be interesting, educational, and effective. Contributions of money, labor, expertise, or influence may also be welcomed by the policy makers involved in setting a course of action to obtain a desired health outcome for an individual, a family, a group, a community, or society (health policy). In addition, one may develop a grassroots network of community and professional friends with a mutual interest in health policy advocacy. The network may be able to promote health policy initiatives for the community. As one may know during the Obama presidential campaign, many advocacy networks were established via the Internet and monies were solicited using this process.

Many special-interest groups in health care have the potential, desire, and resources to influence the health policy process. A tremendous advantage that nursing has in advocating for issues and in influencing policy makers is the force of its numbers, since nursing is the largest of the health professions. However, nursing must organize its numbers in such a way that each nurse joins with others to speak with one voice. The greatest effect will be had when all nurses make similar demands for policy outcomes.

During 2002, the nursing profession spoke clearly, distinctly, and together on a serious problem for the health arena and for the profession: the nursing shortage. Health care facilities and employers were having ever-increasing difficulty finding experienced nurses to employ. In addition, the need for RNs was predicted to balloon in the next 20 years because of the aging of the U.S. population, technological advances, and economic factors. Demand for RNs was anticipated to increase by 22% by the year 2008. This increased demand for professional nurses, coupled with the expected retirement of a rapidly aging nursing workforce, placed a tremendous stress on the health care system. However, a workforce supply study published in 2009 estimated that by 2007 the number of nurses per capita (client) would begin to decline, and by 2020 supply would fall 20% short of demand. In December 2009, workforce analysts with the Bureau of Labor Statistics (BLS) projected that more than 581,500 new RN positions would be created through 2018, which would actually increase the size of the RN workforce by 22%. Employment of RNs is expected to grow much faster than the average when compared with all other professions. The workforce shortage resulted from a complex set of factors such as fewer young people entering the profession, declining nursing school enrollment, the aging of the current nurse workforce, and uncomfortable working conditions in which nurses felt pressured to "do more with less" (Bloom, 2002). On December 4, 2009, the BLS reported that the health care sector of the economy was continuing to grow, despite significant job losses in nearly all major industries. Hospitals, long-term care facilities, and other ambulatory care settings added 21,000 new jobs in November 2009, a month when 85,000 jobs were eliminated across the country. As the largest segment of the health care workforce, RNs likely will be recruited to fill many of these new positions. The BLS confirmed that 613,000 jobs have been added in the healthcare sector since the economic downturn began in 2008.

The American Association of Colleges of Nursing (AACN) remained concerned about the shortage of RNs and has worked with schools, policy makers, other organizations, and the media to bring attention to this health care crisis. AACN has worked to enact legislation, identify strategies, and form collaborations to address the nursing shortage (AACN, 2010).

Advocacy by expert and committed health professionals can bring about positive change for the profession, the community, and the clients that nurses serve. Keeping up to date on issues within government, professional organizations, law, and public policy is vitally important. Informed activism directed toward a professional role, image, and value for professional nurses, and toward a health care system in the United States that provides high-quality and affordable universal access to health care, should be a life-long commitment for all professional nurses.

LINKING CONTENT TO PRACTICE

An example follows of how the policy process works, involving a nursing organization and individual members. Whether you are a member of a group as described below, or working on your own to influence health policy, the steps described here apply.

Over a 15-month time frame, the American Nurses Association was involved in advocating for health care reform. During the Presidential campaign, candidates were educated about the nursing profession and ANA's *Agenda for Health System Reform*. ANA and its members participated in national media interviews and local media events. The message was that the association and its members believed that health care is a basic right. ANA collaborated with the nursing community to outline the profession's priorities as proposals were developed in Congress. Testimony was given before three key Congressional committees. ANA representatives met with White House and congressional health care reform staff, and took part in two presidential press conferences at the White House.

As reported by ANA, thousands of nurses joined ANA's health care reform team, sending letters to representatives of Congress, sharing their stories, and meeting with members of Congress. They also participated in rallies and events.

For more information on ANA's health care reform work, visit http://www.rnaction.org/toolkit.

CHAPTER REVIEW

PRACTICE APPLICATION

Larry was in his final rotation in the Bachelor of Science in nursing program at State University. He was anxious to complete his final nursing course, because upon graduation he would begin a position as a staff nurse specializing in school health at the local health department. His wife was expecting their first child, and she had been receiving prenatal care at the health department.

Larry was aware that a few years ago, the federal government had, by law, provided block grants to states for primary care, maternal-child health programs, and other health care needs of states. He had read the *Federal Register* and knew that the regulations for these grants had been written through USDHHS departments. He was aware that these regulations did not require states to fund specific programs.

Larry read in the local newspaper that the health department was closing its prenatal clinic at the end of the month. When his state had received its block grant, it decided to spend the money for programs other than prenatal care. Larry found that a 3-year study in his own state showed improved pregnancy outcomes as a result of prenatal care. The results were further improved when the care was delivered by population-centered nurses. After Larry's daughter was born, he read in the *Federal Register* that states could apply for federal stimulus funds and receive a grant for home visiting services to support mothers and new babies.

Larry was concerned that, as a student, he would have little influence on how such grant dollars would be spent. However, he decided to call his classmates together to plan a course of action.

What would such an action plan include?

Answers can be found on the Evolve site.

KEY POINTS

- The legal basis for most congressional action in health care can be found in Article I, Section 8, of the U.S. Constitution.
- The five major health care functions of the federal government are direct service, financing, information, policy setting, and public protection.
- The goal of the World Health Organization is the attainment by all people of the highest possible level of health.
- Many federal agencies are involved in government health care functions. The agency most directly involved with the health and welfare of Americans is the U.S. Department of Health and Human Services (USDHHS).
- Most state and local governments have activities that affect nursing practice.
- The variety and range of functions of governmental agencies have had a major impact on nursing. Funding, in particular, has shaped the role and tasks of nurses.
- The private sector (of which nurses are a part) can influence legislation in many ways, especially through the process of writing regulations.
- The number and types of laws influencing health care are increasing. Because of this, involvement in the political process is important to nurses.
- Professional negligence and the scope of practice are two legal aspects particularly relevant to nursing practice.
- Nurses must consider the legal implications of their own practice in each clinical encounter.
- The federal and most state governments are composed of three branches: the executive, the legislative, and the judicial.

- Each branch of government plays a significant role in health policy.
- The U.S. Public Health Service was created in 1798.
- The first national health insurance legislation was challenged in the Supreme Court in 1937.
- *Health: United States* (NCHS, 2010) is an important source of data about the nation's health care problems.
- In 1921 the Sheppard-Towner Act was passed, and it had an important influence on child health programs and population-centered nursing practice.
- The Division of Nursing, the National Institute of Nursing Research, and the Agency for Healthcare Policy and Research are governmental agencies important to nursing.
- Nurses, through state and local health departments, function as consultants, policy advocates, population level and direct care providers, researchers, teachers, supervisors, and program managers.
- The state governments are responsible for regulating nursing practice within the state.
- Federal and state social welfare programs have been developed to provide monetary benefits to the poor, older adults, the disabled, and the unemployed.
- Social welfare programs affect nursing practice. These programs improve the quality of life for special populations, thus making the nurse's job easier in assisting the client with health needs.
- The nurse's scope of practice is defined by legislation and by standards of practice within a specialty.

CLINICAL DECISION-MAKING ACTIVITIES

1. Conduct an interview with a local health officer. Ask for information from a 10-year period. Try to see trends in population size, health needs and corresponding roles, and activities of government that were implemented to meet these changes. What were some of the problems you identified?

2. Examine a current health department budget and compare it with a budget from previous years. Has there been any impact on health care because of changes in government spending (especially before and after the passing of the Patient Protection and Affordable Care Act)? Give an example.

CLINICAL DECISION-MAKING ACTIVITIES—cont'd

3. Locate your state register or other documents, such as newspapers, that publish proposed regulations. Select one set of proposed regulations and critique them. Submit your opinion in writing as public comment, or attend the hearing and testify on the regulations. Be sure to submit something in writing. Evaluate your participation by stating what you learned and whether the proposed regulations were changed in your favor.

4. Find and review your state nurse practice act and define your scope of practice. Give examples of your practice boundaries.

5. Contact your local public health agency to discuss the state's official powers in regulating epidemics, such as an H1N1 outbreak and anthrax exposures related to bioterrorism.

6. Explore the state's right to protect the health, safety, and welfare of its citizens.

7. Ask about the conflict between the state's rights and individual rights and how such issues are resolved.

8. Ask about the standards of care that apply to this issue and how it is decided which services offered to clients should be mandatory and which should be voluntary.

9. Explore how the role of public health differs in these epidemics compared with the past epidemics of smallpox and tuberculosis. Be specific.

REFERENCES

Agency for Healthcare Research and Quality: *At a glance,* AHRQ Pub No. 09-P0003, Bethesda, MD, May 2009, USDHHS.

American Association of Colleges of Nursing: *Fact sheet on the nursing shortage,* Washington, DC, May 2010, AACN.

American Nurses Association: Press release, *ANA applauds introduction of Patient Safety Act of 1997,* March 1997. Available at http://www.nursingworld.org. Accessed December 10, 2010.

Birkland T: *An introduction to the policy process,* ed 2, Armonk, NY, 2005, M.E. Sharpe.

Bloom B: Crossing the quality chasm: a new health system for the 21st century, *JAMA* 287:646–647, 2002.

Bureau of Federal Prisons: *Weekly population report.* Available at http://www.bop.gov. Accessed December 10, 2010.

Catholic University of America: *Definitions of law,* 2010. Available at http://www.faculty.cua.edu. Accessed August 2010.

CDC-MMWR Dispatch: *Update: multistate outbreak of mumps: United States, January 10,* May 2, 2006. Available at http://www.cdc.gov/mmwr/preview/mmwrhtml/mm55d518a1.htm. Accessed December 10, 2010.

Centers for Disease Control and Prevention: *Epidemiology of mumps and multistate mumps outbreak, United States,* Atlanta, 2006, USDHHS.

Cherry B, Jacobs S: *Contemporary nursing issues, trends and management,* St Louis, 2005, Elsevier.

The Citizens' Alliance for the Public Option. Available at HR676.org. Accessed December 10, 2010.

Department of Health, Education and Welfare: Improving health. In *Healthy People: the surgeon general's report on health promotion and disease prevention,* DHEW Publication No. 79-55-71, Washington, DC, 1979, U.S. Government Printing Office. Available at http://www.census.gov/statab/. Accessed July 2002.

Frist B: Public health and national security: the critical role of increased federal support, *Health Affairs* 21:117–130, 2002.

Gerberding J: Clinical practice: occupational exposure to HIV in health care settings, *N Engl J Med* 348:826–833, 2003.

Health Resources and Services Administration (HRSA): *City MatCH. City Lights: Reinventing MCH Practice: Rising to the Challenge, Committing to the Future, Maternal and Child Health Bureau,* Rockville, MD, 2009, USDHHS.

Health Resources and Services Administration: *Open opportunities,* Rockville, MD, 2010, USDHHS. Available at www.hrsa.gov. Accessed December 11, 2010.

Health Resources and Services Administration (HRSA): *Public health workforce study,* Rockville, MD, January 2005, USDHHS. Available at ftp://ftp.hrsa.gov/bhpr/nationalcenter/publichealth2005.pdf. Accessed December 10, 2010.

Hodge J, Gostin L, Vernick J: The Pandemic and All Hazards Preparedness Act: improving public health emergency response, *JAMA* 297:1708–1711, 2007.

Kaiser Family Foundation: *Fastfacts,* Menlo Park, CA, 2010b, Kaiser.

Kaiser Family Foundation: *Summary of New Health Reform Law,* PowerPoint "New Insurance Market rules, Menlo Park, CA, June 2010a, Kaiser. Accessed at www.healthreform.kff.org.

Mason DJ, Keavitt JK, Chaffee MW: *Policy and politics in nursing and health care,* ed 5, St Louis, 2007, Elsevier.

National Center for Health Statistics: *Health: United States, 2009, with special feature on medical technology,* Hyattsville, MD, 2010, U.S. Government Printing Office.

National Council of State Boards of Nursing: *Map of NLC states,* 2010. Available at https://www.ncsbn.org/158.htm. Accessed December 10, 2010.

National Institutes of Health: *Structure and goals,* Bethesda, MD, 2010a, USDHHS.

National Institutes of Health: *Smallpox vaccines,* Bethesda, MD, July 2, 2010b, USDHHS.

National Institute of Nursing Research: *National Institutes of Health: Funding opportunities,* Bethesda, MD, 2010, USDHHS.

Nursing World, Legislative Branch: *State government relations: advanced practice recognition with Medicaid reimbursement,* 2000. Available at http://www.nursingworld.org. Accessed December 10, 2010.

Occupational Health and Safety Administration: *Clarification of the use and selection of blood bourne pathogen safety devices,* Washington, DC, May 5, 2008, U.S. Department of Labor.

Public Health Foundation: *Improving public health infrastructure and performance through innovative solutions and measurable results,* Washington, DC, 2010, The Foundation.

Swendiman K, Elsea J: Federal and state quarantine and isolation authority: *CRS Report to Congress,* Washington, DC, August 2010, Legislative Attorneys American Law Division.

United Nations: *Report of the World Conference of the International Women's Year,* Mexico City, June 19 to July 2, Chapter I, Section A.2, Publication No. E.76.IV.1, New York, 1975, UN.

United Nations: *Report of the World Conference of the United Nations Decade for Women: Equality, Development and Peace,* Copenhagen, July 24-30, Chapter I, Section A, Publication No. E.80.IV.3, New York, 1980, UN.

United Nations: *Report of the World Conference to Review and Appraise Achievements of the United Nations Decade for Women: Equality, Development and Peace,* Nairobi, July 15-26, New York, 1985, UN.

United Nations: *Report of the Fourth World Conference on Women,* Beijing, September 4-15, Chapter I, Resolution 1, Annex I, Publication No. E.96.IV.13, New York, 1995, UN.

United Nations: *Women 2000: Gender Equality, Development and Peace for the 21st Century,* Beijing, 23rd session of the United Nations General Assembly, New York, 2000, UN.

U.S. Bureau of Labor Statistics (BLS): *Employment summary,* Washington, DC, December 4, 2009, U.S. Department of Labor.

U.S. Bureau of Labor Statistics (BLS): *The importance of unemployment benefits,* Washington, DC, August 2010, The U.S. Department of Labor.

U.S. Department of Agriculture: *Food and nutrition services: 40 years 1979-2009,* Washington, DC, 2010, USDA.

U.S. Department of Defense: *TRICARE Management Activity, The Military Health System,* 2010, Falls Church, VA. Available at www.tricare.com. Accessed December 10, 2010.

U.S. Department of Health and Human Services: Health Resources and Services Administration (HRSA): *America's children in brief: key national indicators of well-being,* Washington, DC, 2010, Maternal and Child Health Bureau.

U.S. Department of Health and Human Services: *Healthy People 2000: national health promotion and disease prevention objectives*, Washington, DC, 1991, U.S. Government Printing Office. Available at http://www.health.gov/healthypeople.

U.S. Department of Health and Human Services: *The division of nursing's national advisory committee on nursing education and practice*, Rockville, MD, 2010, Division of Nursing.

U.S. Department of Health and Human Services: Leading indicators. In *Healthy People 2010: understanding and improving health*, ed 2, Washington, DC, 2000, U.S. Government Printing Office.

U.S. Department of Health and Human Services: *Healthy People 2020*. Proposed *Healthy People 2020* Objectives, Washington, DC, 2009. Available at http://www.healthypeople.gov/hp2020/default.asp. Accessed December 10, 2010; page last updated November 3, 2009.

U.S. Law: 49 Stat 622, Title II, 1937a.

U.S. Law: 42 SC 301, *Stewart Machine Co. v. Davis*, 1937b.

U.S. Law: 105-33, Title XXL of the Social Security Act, BBA, 1997.

U.S. Law (Public Law 107-105): Health Insurance Portability and Accountability Act (HIPAA), 1996.

U.S. Law: 107-188: Public Health Security and Bioterrorism and Response Act, 2002.

U.S. Law (Public Law 111-148): Patient Protection and Affordable Care Act (PPACA), 2010.

U.S. Law (Title XXI of the Social Security Act, BBA '97): State Child Health Improvement Act (SCHIP), 1997.

U.S. Law (wl 1044712 La. App. 4 Cir.): *Williams v. Metro Home Health Care Agency et al*, 2002.

Watkins J: Bioterrorism: Cases: When public health agencies should have sweeping powers, *The Internet J Allied Health Sci Pract* 4(2):1–5, April 2006.

World Health Assembly: *Strengthening nursing and midwifery*, 56th session WHA, July 3, 2003. Available at http://www.who.org.

World Health Organization: *Health systems financing: the path to universal coverage*. The World Health Report, 2010. Available at http://www.who.org. Accessed December 10, 2010.

PART 3

Conceptual and Scientific Frameworks Applied to Population-Centered Nursing Practice

In 1988 the National Center for Nursing Research (NCNR) was established under the National Institutes of Health (NIH) to facilitate nursing research. In 1993 the U.S. Congress expanded the scope and functions of the NCNR and made it part of the NIH; it was renamed the National Institute of Nursing Research (NINR). The NINR is crucial to the profession's movement to build a stronger knowledge base for practice. Although no conceptual or theoretical model will meet the needs of all nurses, several nursing and public health models serve as frameworks for organizing educational programs and for making practice decisions.

In 1988 the Institute of Medicine report on the Future of Public Health identified the three primary or core functions of public health: (1) assessment through data collection and sharing of information, (2) policy development for family-, community-, and state-level health policies, and (3) assurance of available and necessary health services for clients. In 1993 the Public Health Nursing Directors of Washington State developed a model showing how nurses perform the three core functions with all clients: individuals, families, and communities. In 2000 the Council on Linkages initially developed a list of competencies required of public health workers to provide quality care. In 2003 the Quad Council of Public Health Nursing Organizations *then* applied the competencies to population-centered nursing practice. Both of these documents have been updated and continue to direct practice today. These competencies help nurses to recognize how they may implement the core functions of public health.

The scientific base provided by public health as a specialty remains the foundation for population-centered nursing. In 2003 two additional documents from the Institute of Medicine— *The Future of the Public's Health in the 21st Century* and *Who Will Keep the Public Healthy?*—further delineates the practice, education, and research needs for public health nursing. The chapters in Part Three support the tenants of these documents and provides information about how to use conceptual models, epidemiology, principles of education, and evidence to organize population-centered nursing practice to meet the core functions of public health. A new direction identified was emphasis on genomics. Each chapter provides both theory and practical application of the specific topic to the clinical area. This section provides readers with tools that can be used to influence population-centered nursing practice.

It has been estimated that the effect of the medical care system on the usual indexes for measuring health is about 10%. The remaining 90% is determined by factors over which health care providers have little or no direct control, such as lifestyle and social and physical environmental conditions. This text focuses on the processes and practices for promoting health, principally by the nurse, who is considered to be an ideal person to demonstrate and teach others how to promote health. To be effective, health promotion requires that people cease focusing on how to "fix" themselves and others only when they detect physical and emotional disequilibriums and that they instead assume personal responsibility for health promotion. Such a change in emphasis requires that health care providers incorporate health promotion techniques into their practice.

Concern currently exists that the environment's effects on health and social conditions are causing an increase in the rate of infectious diseases. Nurses are concerned with prevention, control, surveillance, case-finding, reporting, and maintenance strategies as they relate to communicable and infectious disease, to chronic disease processes, and to environment-related problems. Technological advances increasingly influence the environment and make it a potential threat to many aspects of health maintenance. Nurses must help others recognize how their actions as individuals, as well as in a composite group (aggregate) or community, are destroying vital parts of the environment. It has become increasingly important to base population-centered practice on the best available evidence found in the literature. Nationally, there is increased emphasis on developing more substantial evidence to improve health outcomes through population, community, and public health practices.

Population-Based Public Health Nursing Practice: The Intervention Wheel

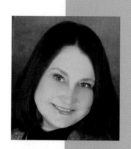

Linda Olson Keller, DNP, CPH, APHN-BC, RN, FAAN

Linda Olson Keller is a Clinical Associate Professor at the University of Minnesota School of Nursing. Her research focuses on evidence-based public health nursing practice and the infrastructure of the public health nursing workforce. She spent 20 years of her career in the Office of Public Health Practice at the Minnesota Department of Health. Dr. Olson Keller is certified in Public Health, board certified as an Advanced Public Health Nurse, and is a Fellow of the American Academy of Nursing. She is a frequent national speaker and consultant on public health leadership and practice.

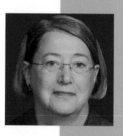

Sue Strohschein, MS, RN/PHN, APRN, BC

Sue Strohschein's public health nursing career spans more than 40 years and includes practice in both local and state health departments in Minnesota. She was a generalized public health nurse consultant for the Minnesota Department of Health for 25 years. Since 2008 she has been with the University of Minnesota School of Nursing as a senior research fellow.

ADDITIONAL RESOURCES

*e*volve **WEBSITE**
http://evolve.elsevier.com/Stanhope
- *Healthy People 2020*
- WebLinks

- Quiz
- Case Studies
- Glossary
- Answers to Practice Application

OBJECTIVES

After reading this chapter, the student should be able to do the following:

1. Identify the components of the Intervention Wheel.
2. Describe the assumptions underlying the Intervention Wheel.
3. Define the wedges and interventions of the Intervention Wheel.
4. Differentiate among three levels of practice (community, systems, and individual/family).
5. Apply the nursing process at three levels of practice.

KEY TERMS

◆ ◆ ◆

In these times of change, the public health system is constantly challenged to keep focused on the health of populations. The Intervention Wheel is a conceptual framework that has proved to be a useful model in defining population-based practice and explaining how it contributes to improving population health.

The Intervention Wheel provides a graphic illustration of population-based public health practice (Keller et al, 1998, 2004a,b). It was previously introduced as the Public Health Intervention Model and was known nationally as the "Minnesota Model"; it is now often simply referred to as the "Wheel." The Wheel depicts how public health improves population health through interventions with communities, the individuals and families that comprise communities, and the systems that impact the health of communities (Figure 9-1). The Wheel was derived from the practice of public health nurses (PHNs) and intended to support their work. It gives PHNs a means to describe the full scope and breadth of their practice.

This chapter applies the Intervention Wheel framework to public health nursing practice. However, it is important to note that other public health members of the interprofessional team such as nutritionists, health educators, planners, physicians, and epidemiologists also use these interventions.

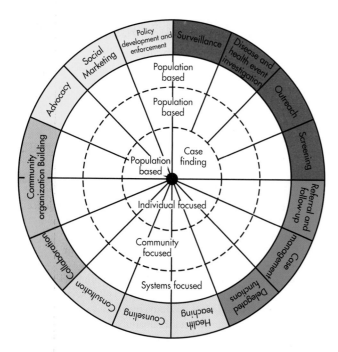

The Intervention Wheel is composed of three distinct elements of equal importance:

- First, the model is population based.

- Second, the model encompasses three levels of practice (community, systems, individual/family).

- Third, the model identifies and defines 17 public health interventions.

Each intervention and level of practice contributes to improving population health.

FIGURE 9-1 The Intervention Wheel components. (Used with permission from Keller LO, Strohschein S, Lia-Hoagberg B, Schaffer M: Population-based public health interventions: practice-based and evidence-supported, part I, *Public Health Nurs* 21:453-468, 2004.)

THE INTERVENTION WHEEL ORIGINS AND EVOLUTION

The original version of the Wheel resulted from a grounded theory process carried out by PHN consultants at the Minnesota Department of Health in the mid-1990s. This was a period of relentless change and considerable uncertainty for Minnesota's public health nursing community. Debates about health care reform and its impact on the role of local public health departments created confusion about the contributions of public health nursing to population-level health improvement. In response to the uncertainty, the consultant group presented a series of workshops across the state highlighting the core functions of public health nursing practice (see Chapter 1 for a description of these core functions). A workshop activity required participants to describe the actions they undertook to carry out their work. The consultant group analyzed 200 practice scenarios developed at the workshops that ranged from home care and school health to home visiting and correctional health. In the final analysis, 17 actions common to the work of PHNs regardless of their practice setting were identified. The analysis also demonstrated that most of these interventions were implemented at three levels: (1) with individuals, either singly or in groups, and with families, (2) with communities as a whole, and (3) with systems that impact the health of communities. A wheel-shaped graphic was developed to illustrate the set of interventions and the levels of practice (see Figure 9-1).

The interventions were subjected to an extensive review of supporting evidence in the literature through a grant from the federal Division of Nursing awarded to the Minnesota Department of Health in the 1990s. In 1999 the PHN consultant group at the Minnesota Department of Health designed and implemented a systematic process identifying more than 600 items from supporting evidence in the literature. These items were rated for their quality and relevancy by a group of graduate nursing students. The resulting subset of 221 items was further analyzed by two expert panels. One panel was composed of public health nursing educators and expert practitioners from five states (Iowa, Minnesota, North Dakota, South Dakota, and Wisconsin). The other panel was a similarly composed national panel. The result was a slightly modified set of 17 interventions. Figure 9-2 graphically illustrates the systematic critique. Each intervention was defined at multiple levels of practice; each was accompanied by a set of basic steps for applying the framework and recommendations for best practices.

Adoption of the model was rapid and worldwide. Since its first publication in 1998, the Intervention Wheel has been incorporated into the public/community health coursework of numerous undergraduate and graduate curricula. The Wheel serves as a model for practice in many state and local health departments and has been presented in Mexico, Norway, Poland, Hungary, Namibia, Kazakhstan, and Japan. It has served as an organizing framework for inquiry for topics ranging from doctoral dissertations (Sheridan, 2005) to the epidemiology of the lowly head louse (Monsen and Keller, 2002). The Wheel's strength comes from the common language it affords PHNs to discuss their work (Keller et al, 1998).

ASSUMPTIONS UNDERLYING THE INTERVENTION WHEEL

As with all conceptual frameworks and models, assumptions are made that help to explain the model or framework. The Intervention Wheel framework is based on 10 assumptions.

Assumption 1: Defining Public Health Nursing Practice

Public health nursing is defined as the practice of promoting and protecting the health of populations using knowledge from nursing, social, and public health sciences (APHA, 1996). The title "public health nurse" designates a registered nurse with educational preparation in both public health and nursing. The primary focus of public health nursing is to promote health and prevent disease for entire population groups. This is done by working with individuals, families, communities, and/or systems.

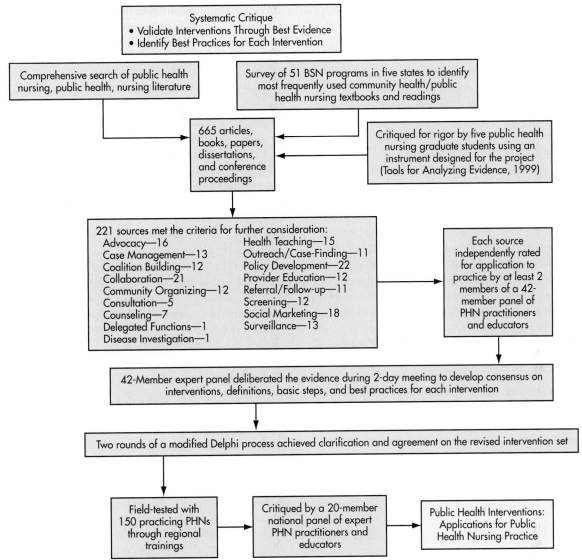

FIGURE 9-2 Development of a conceptual framework using an evidence-based process. (Used with permission from Keller LO, Strohschein S, Lia-Hoagberg B, et al: Population-based public health interventions: practice-based and evidence-supported, part I, *Public Health Nurs* 21:459, 2004.)

Assumption 2: Public Health Nursing Practice Focuses on Populations

The focus on populations as opposed to individuals is a key characteristic that differentiates public health nursing from other areas of nursing practice. A population is a collection of individuals who have one or more personal or environmental characteristics in common (Williams and Highriter, 1978). Populations may be understood as two categories. A population at risk is a population with a common identified risk factor or risk exposure that poses a threat to health. For example, all adults who are overweight and hypertensive constitute a population at risk for cardiovascular disease. All underimmunized or unimmunized children are a population at risk for contracting vaccine-preventable diseases. A population of interest is a population that is essentially healthy but that could improve factors that promote or protect health. For instance, healthy adolescents are a

population of interest that could benefit from social competency training. All first-time parents of newborns are a population of interest that could benefit from a public health nursing home visit. Populations are not limited to only individuals who seek services or individuals who are poor or otherwise vulnerable.

Assumption 3: Public Health Nursing Practice Considers the Determinants of Health

Health inequities are defined as health status inequalities that society deems to be avoidable or unnecessary (Kawachi, Subramanian, and Alemeida-Filho, 2002). Significant health disparities related to race, gender, age, and socioeconomic status exist within the United States. The *Health, United States, 2009* Chartbook (CDC, 2009) provides the following examples:

- In 2006, the U.S. rate of infant deaths per 1000 live births was 6.7. At least 29 other developed countries had lower infant mortality rates; the lowest was Hong Kong with 1.8 (Table 22, p 184).

- Between 2003 and 2005, the U.S. neonatal mortality rate per 1000 live births for all races was 4.6; across races and ethnicities the rates varied. For infants born to white women the rate was 3.7; for Black and African-American women, 9.2; for Hispanic or Latina women, 3.9; for American Indian or Alaskan Native, 4.3; for Asian or Pacific Islanders, 3.3 (Table 21, pp 182-183).

- In 2005 life expectancy at birth for men in the United States was 74.9 years; Hong Kong had greatest life expectancy with 77.8 years. For U.S. women, the life expectancy at birth in 2005 was 79.9; Japan ranked first with 85.5 (Table 23, p 187).

What are the factors driving these differences? Factors that influence health status across the life cycle are known as the determinants of health. They include: income, education, employment, social support, biology and genetics, physical environment, housing, transportation, and personal health practices.

Resolving health inequities and addressing the determinants of health are key distinguishing characteristics of public health nursing. In a recent interpretive qualitative study of PHNs' practice in Nova Scotia, researchers found that PHNs routinely implemented "ecosocial surveillance functions" that focused on monitoring changes in social determinants of health. The researchers observed that PHNs "…monitored both bottom-up changes in individual, family, and community determinants of health, and top-down vertical changes or policy directives in the larger system" (Meagher-Stewart et al, 2009, p 557).

DID YOU KNOW? *The practice of Lillian Wald, public health nursing's progenitor, offers plenty of examples of understanding determinants of health. Besides the services of PHNs, her Henry Street Settlement House offered numerous social programs, including drama and theater productions, vocational training for boys and girls, three kindergartens, summer camps for children, two large scholarship funds, study rooms staffed with people to help children with their homework, playgrounds for children, a neighborhood library, and classes in carpentry, sewing, art, diction, music, and dance. The photo below shows the settlement house's backyard playground.*

From Jewish Women's Archive: This day in history, March 10, 1893, Resource information for backyard of a Henry Street branch. Available at http://www.jwa.org/archive/jsp/gresInfo.jsp?resID=297. Accessed December 11, 2010.

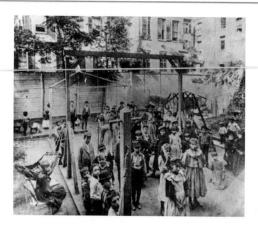

Assumption 4: Public Health Nursing Practice Is Guided by Priorities Identified Through an Assessment of Community Health

In the context of the Intervention Wheel, a community is defined as "a social network of interacting individuals, usually concentrated in a defined territory" (Johnston et al, 2000).

Assessing the health status of the populations that comprise the community requires ongoing collection and analysis of relevant quantitative and qualitative data. Community assessment includes a comprehensive assessment of the determinants of health. Data analysis identifies deviations from expected or acceptable rates of disease, injury, death, or disability as well as risk and protective factors. Community assessment generally results in a lengthy list of community problems and issues. However, communities rarely possess sufficient resources to address the entire list. This gap between needs and resources necessitates a systematic priority-setting process. Although data analysis provides direction for priority setting, the community's beliefs, attitudes, and opinions as well as the community's readiness for change must be assessed (Keller et al, 2002). PHNs, with their extensive knowledge about the communities in which they work, provide important information and insights during the priority-setting process.

DID YOU KNOW? *For a PHN employed by a unit of government, such as a city, county, or state public health department, a "community" is almost always a geopolitical unit. Core functions of governmental health departments are considered to be: assessment (identification of community problems); policy development (mobilization of necessary effort and resources); and assurance (making sure that vital conditions for keeping people healthy are in place) (Committee for the Study of the Future of Public Health, 1988). For these PHNs, accountability is to a board of elected officials and ultimately to the constituents who elect them. For PHNs employed by visiting nurse associations, and other non-governmental population-based entities, a service area is assigned by the agency. In these cases, accountability typically is to an appointed board of directors.*

Assumption 5: Public Health Nursing Practice Emphasizes Prevention

Prevention is "anticipatory action taken to prevent the occurrence of an event or to minimize its effect after it has occurred" (Turnock, 2009, p 516). Prevention is customarily described as a continuum moving from primary to tertiary prevention (Leavell and Clark, 1965; Novick and Mays, 2001; Turnock, 2009). The Levels of Prevention box provides definitions and examples of the levels of prevention.

A hallmark of public health nursing practice is a focus on health promotion and disease prevention, emphasizing primary prevention whenever possible. Although not every event is preventable, every event has a preventable component.

Assumption 6: Public Health Nurses Intervene at All Levels of Practice

To improve population health, the work of PHNs is often carried out sequentially and/or simultaneously at three levels of prevention (see Figure 9-2).

Community-level practice changes community norms, community attitudes, community awareness, community practices, and community behaviors. It is directed toward entire populations within the community or occasionally toward populations at risk or populations of interest. An example of community-level practice is a social marketing campaign to promote a community norm that serving alcohol to under-aged youth at high school graduation parties is unacceptable. This is a community-level primary prevention strategy.

Systems-level practice changes organizations, policies, laws, and power structures within communities. The focus is on the systems that impact health, not directly on individuals and communities. Conducting compliance checks to ensure that bars and liquor stores do not serve minors or sell to individuals who supply alcohol to minors is an example of a systems-level secondary prevention strategy practice.

📋 LEVELS OF PREVENTION

Examples of Interventions Applied to Definition of Prevention

Primary Prevention

Primary prevention promotes health and protects against threats to health. It keeps problems from occurring in the first place. It promotes resiliency and protective factors or reduces susceptibility and exposure to risk factors. Primary prevention is implemented before a problem develops. It targets essentially well populations. Immunizing against a vaccine-preventable disease is an example of reducing susceptibility; building developmental assets in young persons to promote health is an example of promoting resiliency and protective factors.

Secondary Prevention

Secondary prevention detects and treats problems in their early stages. It keeps problems from causing serious or long-term effects or from affecting others. It identifies risk or hazards and modifies, removes, or treats them before a problem becomes more serious. Secondary prevention is implemented after a problem has begun, but before signs and symptoms appear. It targets populations that have risk factors in common. Programs that screen populations for hypertension, obesity, hyperglycemia, hypercholesterolemia, and other chronic disease risk factors are examples of secondary prevention.

Tertiary Prevention

Tertiary prevention limits further negative effects from a problem. It keeps existing problems from getting worse. It alleviates the effects of disease and injury and restores individuals to their optimal level of functioning. Tertiary prevention is implemented after a disease or injury has occurred. It targets populations who have experienced disease or injury. Provision of directly observed therapy (DOT) to clients with active tuberculosis to ensure compliance with a medication regimen is an example of tertiary prevention.

From Keller LO, Strohschein S, Lia-Hoagberg B, Schaffer M: Population-based public health nursing interventions: a model from practice, *Public Health Nurs* 15:311-320, 1998.

Individual-level practice changes knowledge, attitudes, beliefs, practices, and behaviors of individuals. This practice level is directed at individuals, alone or as part of a family, class, or group. Even though families, classes, and groups are comprised of more than one individual, the focus is still on individual change. Teaching effective refusal skills to groups of adolescents is an example of individual secondary prevention strategy level of practice.

Assumption 7: Public Health Nursing Practice Uses the Nursing Process at All Levels of Practice

Although the components of the nursing process (assessment, diagnosis, planning, implementation, and evaluation) are integral to all nursing practice, PHNs must customize the process to the three levels of practice. Table 9-1 outlines the nursing process at the community, systems, and individual/family levels of practice.

Assumption 8: Public Health Nursing Practice Uses a Common Set of Interventions Regardless of Practice Setting

Interventions are "actions taken on behalf of communities, systems, individuals, and families to improve or protect health status" (ANA, 2010). The Intervention Wheel encompasses 17 interventions: surveillance, disease and other health investigation, outreach, screening, case finding, referral and follow-up, case management, delegated functions, health teaching, consultation, counseling, collaboration, coalition building, community organizing, advocacy, social marketing, and policy development and enforcement.

The interventions are grouped with related interventions; these wedges are color coordinated to make them more recognizable (Figure 9-3, A). For instance, the five interventions in the red wedge are frequently implemented in conjunction with one another. Surveillance is often paired with disease and health event investigation, even though either can be implemented independently. Screening frequently follows either surveillance or disease and health event investigation and is often preceded by outreach activities in order to maximize the number of those at risk who actually get screened. Most often, screening leads to case finding, but this intervention can also be carried out independently. The green wedge consists of referral and follow-up, case management, and delegated functions—three interventions that, in practice, are often implemented together (Figure 9-3, B). Similarly, health teaching, counseling, and consultation—the blue wedge—are more similar than they are different; health teaching and counseling are especially often paired (Figure 9-3, C). The interventions in the orange wedge—collaboration, coalition building, and community organizing—although distinct, are grouped together because they are all types of collective action and are most often carried out at systems or community levels of practice (Figure 9-3, D). Similarly, advocacy, social marketing, and policy development and enforcement—the yellow wedge—are often interrelated when implemented (Figure 9-3, E). In fact, advocacy is often viewed as a precursor to policy development; social marketing is seen by some as a method of carrying out advocacy.

TABLE 9-1   PUBLIC HEALTH NURSING PROCESS

PUBLIC HEALTH NURSING PROCESS	SYSTEMS LEVEL	COMMUNITY LEVEL	INDIVIDUAL/FAMILY LEVEL
Recruit additional partners.	Recruit additional partners (local, regional, state, national) from systems that are key to impacting and/or who have an interest in the health issue/problem.	Recruit community organizations, services, and citizens who are part of the community intervention that have an interest in this health issue/problem.	
Identify population of interest.	Identify those systems for which change is desired.	Identify the population of interest at risk for the problem.	Identify new and current clients in caseload who are at risk for the priority problem.
Establish relationship.	Begin/continue establishing relationship with system partners.	Begin/continue establishing relationship with community partners and population of interest.	Begin/continue establishing relationship with the family.
Assess priority.	Assess the impact and inter-relationships of the various systems on the development and extent of the health issue/problem.	Assess the health issue/problem (demographics, health determinants, past and current efforts). Identify the particular strengths, health risks, and health influences of the population of interest	Identify the particular strengths, health risks, social supports, and other factors influencing the health of the family and each family member.
Elicit perceptions.	Develop a common consensus among system partners of the health issue/problem and the desired changes.	Elicit the population of interest's perception of their strengths, problems, and health influences.	Elicit family's perception of their strengths, problems, and other factors influencing their health.
Set goals.	In conjunction with system partners, develop system goals to be achieved.	In conjunction with the population of interest, negotiate and come to agreement on community-focused goals.	In conjunction with the family, negotiate and come to agreement on meaningful, achievable, measurable goals.
Select health status indicators.	Based on systems goals, select meaningful, measurable health status indicators that will be used to measure success.	Based on the refined community goal/problem, select meaningful, measurable health status indicators that will be used to measure success.	Select meaningful, measurable health status indicators that will be used to measure success.
Select interventions.	Select system-level interventions considering evidence of effectiveness, political support, acceptability to community, cost-effectiveness, legality, ethics, greatest potential for successful outcome, non-duplicative, levels of prevention.	Select community-level interventions considering evidence of effectiveness, acceptability to community, cost-effectiveness, legality, ethics, non-duplicative, greatest potential for successful outcome.	Select interventions considering evidence of effectiveness, acceptability to family, cost-effectiveness, legality, ethics, greatest potential for successful outcome.
Select intermediate outcome indicators.	Determine measurable, meaningful intermediate outcome indicators.	Determine measurable and meaningful intermediate outcome indicators.	Determine measurable, meaningful intermediate outcome indicators.
Determine strategy frequency and intensity.	Using best practices, determine intensity, sequencing, frequency of interventions considering urgency, political will, resources.	Using best practices, determine intensity, sequencing, frequency of interventions.	Using best practices, determine intensity, sequencing, frequency of interventions.
Determine evaluation methods.	Determine evaluation methods for measuring process, intermediate, and outcome indicators.	Determine evaluation methods for measuring process, intermediate, and outcome indicators.	Determine evaluation methods for measuring process, intermediate, and outcome indicators.
Implement the interventions.	Implement the interventions.	Implement the interventions.	Implement the interventions.

TABLE 9-1   PUBLIC HEALTH NURSING PROCESS—cont'd

PUBLIC HEALTH NURSING PROCESS	SYSTEMS LEVEL	COMMUNITY LEVEL	INDIVIDUAL/FAMILY LEVEL
Regularly reassess interventions.	Regularly reassess the system's response to the interventions PHNs and modify plan as indicated.	Reassess the population of interest's response to the interventions on an ongoing basis and modify plan as indicated.	Reassess and modify plan at each contact as necessary.
Adjust interventions.	Adjust the frequency and intensity of the interventions according to the needs and resources of the community.	Adjust the frequency and intensity of the interventions accordingly.	Adjust the frequency and intensity of the interventions according to the needs and resources of the family.
Provide feedback.	Provide feedback to system's representatives.	Provide feedback to the population of interest and informal and formal organizational representatives.	Provide regular feedback to family on progress (or lack thereof) of client goals.
Collect evaluation.	Regularly and systematically collect evaluation information.	Regularly and systematically collect evaluation information.	Regularly and systematically collect evaluation information.
Compare results to plan.	Compare actual results with planned indicators.	Compare actual results with planned indicators.	Compare actual results with planned indicators.
Identify differences.	Identify and analyze differences in those systems that achieved outcomes compared with those that did not.	Identify and analyze differences in those in the population of interest who achieved outcomes compared with those who did not.	Identify and analyze differences in services received by families who achieved outcomes compared with those who did not.
Apply results to practice.	Apply results to identify needed systems changes. Depending on readiness of the system to accept the results, present results to decision makers and the general population.	Apply results to modify community interventions. Present results to community for policy considerations as appropriate.	Report results to supervisor and other service providers as appropriate. Apply results to personal practice and agency for policy considerations as appropriate.

The interventions on the right side of the Wheel (i.e., the red, green, and blue wedges) are most commonly used by PHNs who focus their work more on individuals, families, classes, and groups and to a lesser extent on work with systems and communities. The orange and yellow wedges, on the other hand, are more commonly used by PHNs who focus their work on effecting systems and communities. However, a PHN may use any or all of the interventions.

WHAT DO YOU THINK?   *No single PHN is expected to perform every intervention at all three levels of practice. From a management perspective, however, it is useful to ensure that a public health workforce has the capacity to implement all 17 interventions at all three practice levels. How could management ensure that a health agency has this capacity?*

Assumption 9: Public Health Nursing Practice Contributes to the Achievement of the 10 Essential Services

Implementing the interventions ultimately contributes to the achievement of the 10 essential public health services (see Chapter 1). The 10 essential public health services describe *what* the public health system does to protect and promote the health of the public. Interventions are the means through which public

health practitioners implement the 10 essential services. Interventions are the *how* of public health practice (Public Health Functions Steering Committee, 1995).

Assumption 10: Public Health Nursing Practice Is Grounded in a Set of Values and Beliefs

The Cornerstones of Public Health Nursing (Box 9-1) were developed as a companion document to the Intervention Wheel. The Wheel defines the "what and how" of public health nursing practice; the Cornerstones define the "why." The Cornerstones synthesize foundational values and beliefs from both public health and nursing. They inspire, guide, direct, and challenge public health nursing practice (Keller, Strohschein, and Schaffer, 2010).

USING THE INTERVENTION WHEEL IN PUBLIC HEALTH NURSING PRACTICE

The Wheel is a conceptual model. It was conceived as a common language or catalog of general actions used by PHNs across all practice settings. When those actions are placed within the context of a set of associated assumptions or relations among concepts, the Intervention Wheel serves as a conceptual model for public health nursing practice (Fawcett, 2005). It creates a structure for identifying and documenting

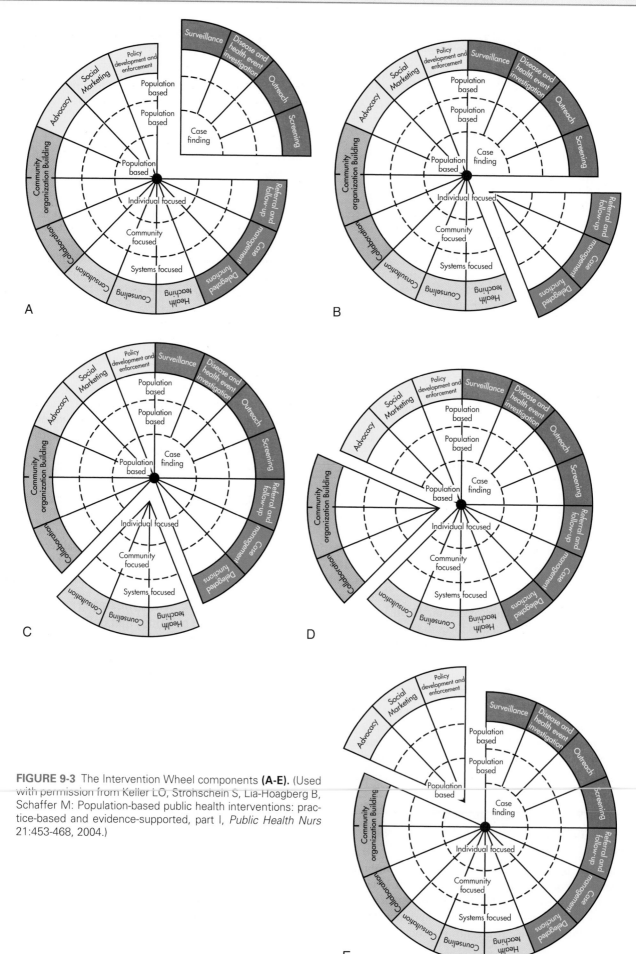

FIGURE 9-3 The Intervention Wheel components **(A-E).** (Used with permission from Keller LO, Strohschein S, Lia-Hoagberg B, Schaffer M: Population-based public health interventions: practice-based and evidence-supported, part I, *Public Health Nurs* 21:453-468, 2004.)

BOX 9-1 CORNERSTONES OF PUBLIC HEALTH NURSING

Public Health Nursing Practice:

- Focuses on the health of entire populations
- Reflects community priorities and needs
- Establishes caring relationships with the communities, families, individuals, and systems that comprise the populations PHNs serve
- Is grounded in social justice, compassion, sensitivity to diversity, and respect for the worth of all people, especially the vulnerable
- Encompasses the mental, physical, emotional, social, spiritual, and environmental aspects of health
- Promotes health through strategies driven by epidemiological evidence
- Collaborates with community resources to achieve those strategies, but can and will work alone if necessary
- Derives its authority for independent action from the Nurse Practice Act

CORNERSTONES FROM PUBLIC HEALTH	CORNERSTONES FROM NURSING
Population-based/focused	Relationship-based
Grounded in social justice	Grounded in an ethic of caring
Focus on greater good	Sensitivity to diversity
Focus on health promotion and disease prevention	Holistic focus
Does what others cannot or will not	Respect for the worth of all
Driven by the science of epidemiology	Independent practice
Organizes community resources	Long-term commitment to the community

interventions performed by PHNs and captures the nature of their work. The Intervention Wheel provides a framework, a way of thinking about public health nursing practice. The *Public Health Nursing: Scope and Standards of Practice* includes the Intervention Wheel as one of several public health nursing frameworks used in practice today (ANA, 2007).

COMPONENTS OF THE MODEL

As depicted in Figure 9-1, the model has three components: a population basis, three levels of practice, and 17 interventions.

Component 1: The Model Is Population Based

The upper portion of the Intervention Wheel clearly illustrates that all levels of practice (community, systems, and individual/family) are population based. Public health nursing practice is population focused. It identifies populations of interest or populations at risk through an assessment of community health status and an assignment of priorities.

DID YOU KNOW? *Are services to individuals and families population based?*

Services to individuals and families are population based only if they meet the following criteria: (1) Individuals receive services because they are members of an identified population, and (2) services to individuals clearly contribute to improving the overall health status of the identified population.

The population of Sherburne County (Minnesota) increased almost 175% in 25 years (Minnesota Departments of Education, Health, Human Services, and Public Safety, 2007). The numerous new housing developments characterized urban sprawl, which has been implicated in the current obesity epidemic in both children and adults (Dunton et al, 2009; Renalds, Smith, and Hale, 2010). The local health department staff was concerned about the prevalence of obesity in its population. Data from the Community Health Status Indicators' website showed that 24.1% of the population's adults were considered obese (USDHHS, 2010). A 2007 state student health survey documented that 25% of ninth-grade girls and 20% of ninth-grade boys in the county were overweight or obese. In this same age group, 76% of girls and 80% of boys reported they were active less than 30 minutes daily. It was clear that Sherburne County had an obesity problem (Minnesota Departments of Education, Health, Human Services, and Public Safety, 2007).

Reversing this trend required reducing barriers to exercise. Health department staff recognized the impact of urban sprawl on their built environment (Renalds, Smith, and Hale, 2010), or the "human-made space in which people live, work and recreate on a day-to-day basis" (Roof and Oleru, 2008). One of the first factors they considered was the walkability of their communities, or extent to which planned transportation networks and public spaces accommodate walking and other forms of physical exercise. Walkability includes: (1) continuous and well-maintained sidewalks, (2) easy access, path directness, and street network connectivity, (3) crossing safety, (4) absence of heavy and high-speed traffic, (5) pedestrian buffering from traffic, (6) land-use density and diversity, (7) street trees and landscaping, (8) visual interest and sense of place, and (9) security (Lo, 2009).

With these data, the public health staff engaged community members to determine the next steps to improve their community walkability. The department asked undergraduate nursing students who were in their public health nursing clinical program to design, implement, and evaluate a walkability project. The students walked over 100 miles and rated the walkability of three different Sherburne County communities. The students analyzed the results and presented recommendations for improvements to the city councils of the three communities. The findings were used by two of the three communities to secure funding for improvements to their community's walkability (Zoller, 2010).

DID YOU KNOW? *The mass production of the automobile in the 1920s killed the walkable city, which is why many older neighborhoods are deemed more pedestrian friendly and hospitable to walking. After the introduction of the automobile, and particularly after the 1950s, residential areas were built on discontinuous cul-de-sac designs rather than interconnected grids, block sizes grew, and activity centers such as parks and playgrounds were widely spaced. Streets and roadways were designed for the convenience of the motorist (Southworth, 2005), creating barriers for those wanting to walk or bicycle for transportation or physical fitness. Several methods are now available to measure a neighborhood's walkability.*

- *Walkability Checklist from Partnership for a Walkable America at: http://www.walkableamerica.org/*
- *Find your neighborhood's walkability score by zip code online at Walk Score: http://www.walkscore.com/*
- *Community Healthy Living Index at: http://www.ymca.net/communityhealthylivingindex/community_healthy_living_index.html*

Component 2: The Model Encompasses Three Levels of Practice

Public health nursing practice intervenes with communities, the individuals and families that comprise communities, and the systems that impact the health of communities. Interventions at each level of practice contribute to the overall goal of improving population health. The work of PHNs is accomplished at all levels. No one level of practice is more important than another; in fact, many public health priorities are addressed simultaneously at all three levels.

One public health priority that almost every PHN will encounter is the potential for the occurrence of vaccine-preventable disease because of delayed or missing immunizations. A recent task analysis of 60 PHNs from 29 states revealed that 93% of all PHNs participated in immunization activities (Keller, 2008). This held true regardless of the PHN's work setting (e.g., home, clinic, school, correctional facility, childcare center) or the population focus (e.g., maternal-child health, elderly chronic disease management, refugee health, disease prevention and control). Vaccine-preventable diseases, or diseases that may be prevented through recommended immunizations, include diphtheria, pertussis, tetanus, polio, mumps, measles, rubella, hepatitis A, hepatitis B, varicella, meningitis, *Haemophilus influenzae* type b (Hib), pneumococcal pneumonia, rotavirus, human papillomavirus (HPV), herpes zoster, and seasonal influenza (CDC, 2010b).

This section illustrates strategies for reducing the occurrence of vaccine-preventable diseases at all three levels of practice. These are only selected examples of strategies to improve immunization rates; it is not an inclusive list.

Community Level of Practice

The goal of community-level practice is to increase the knowledge and attitude of the entire community about the importance of immunization and the consequences of not being immunized. These strategies will lead to an increase in the percentage of people who obtain recommended immunizations for themselves and their children.

At the community level, PHNs work with health educators on public awareness campaigns. They perform outreach at schools, senior centers, county fairs, community festivals, and neighborhood laundromats.

PHNs conduct or coordinate audits of immunization records of all children in schools and childcare centers to identify children who are under-immunized. The PHNs refer them to their medical providers or administer the immunizations through health department clinics.

When a confirmed case of a vaccine-preventable disease occurs, PHNs work with epidemiologists to identify and locate everyone exposed to the index case. PHNs assess the immunization status of people who were exposed and ensure appropriate treatment.

In the event of an outbreak in the community, all PHNs have a role and ethical responsibility to take part in mass dispensing clinics. Mass dispensing clinics disperse immunizations or medications to specific populations at risk. For example, clinics may be held in response to an epidemic of mumps, a case of hepatitis A attributable to a foodborne exposure in a restaurant, or an influenza pandemic in the general population.

Systems Level of Practice

The goal of systems-level practice is to change the laws, policies, and practices that influence immunization rates, such as promoting population-based immunization registries and improving clinic and provider practices.

PHNs work with schools, clinics, health plans, and parents to develop population-based immunization registries. Registries, known officially by the Centers for Disease Control and Prevention (CDC) as "Immunization Information Systems," combine immunization information from different sources into a single electronic record. A registry provides official immunization records for schools, day-care centers, health departments, and clinics. Registries track immunizations and remind families when an immunization is due or has been missed.

PHNs conduct audits of records in clinics that participate in the federal vaccine program. PHNs ascertain if a clinic is following recommended immunization standards for vaccine handling and storage, documentation, and adherence to best practices. PHNs also provide feedback and guidance to clinicians and office staff for quality improvement.

PHNs also work with health care providers in the community to ensure that providers accurately report vaccine-preventable diseases as legally required by state statute.

Individual/Family Level of Practice

The goal of individual/family-level strategies is to identify individuals who are not appropriately immunized, identify the barriers to immunization, and ensure that the individual's immunizations are brought up to date.

At the individual level of practice, PHNs conduct health department immunization clinics. Unlike mass dispensing clinics, immunization clinics are generally available to anyone who needs an immunization and do not target a specific population. These clinics often provide an important service to individuals without access to affordable health care.

PHNs use the registry to identify children with delayed or missing immunizations. They contact families by phone or through a home visit. The PHNs assess for barriers and consult with the family to develop a plan to obtain immunizations either through a medical clinic or from a health department clinic. The PHN follows up at a later date to ensure that the child was actually immunized.

PHNs routinely assess the immunization status for clients in all public health programs, such as well-child clinics, family planning clinics, maternal-child health home visits, or case management of elderly and disabled populations, and they ensure that immunizations are up to date.

Component 3: The Model Identifies and Defines 17 Public Health Interventions

The Intervention Wheel encompasses 17 interventions: surveillance, disease and other health investigation, outreach, screening, case finding, referral and follow-up, case management, delegated functions, health teaching, consultation, counseling, collaboration, coalition building, community organizing, advocacy, social marketing, and policy development and enforcement.

All interventions, except case finding, coalition building, and community organizing, are applicable at all three levels of practice. Community organizing and coalition building cannot occur at the individual level. Case finding is the individual level of surveillance, disease and other health event investigation, outreach, and screening. Altogether, a PHN selects from among 43 different intervention-level actions.

Table 9-2 provides examples of the intervention at the three levels of practice for each of the 17 interventions.

- **Surveillance** describes and monitors health events through ongoing and systematic collection, analysis, and interpretation of health data for the purpose of planning, implementing, and evaluating public health interventions (adapted from *Mortality and Morbidity Weekly Review*, 2001).
- **Disease and other health event investigation** systematically gathers and analyzes data regarding threats to the health of populations, ascertains the source of the threat, identifies cases and others at risk, and determines control measures.
- **Outreach** locates populations of interest or populations at risk and provides information about the nature of the concern, what can be done about it, and how services can be obtained.

- **Screening** identifies individuals with unrecognized health risk factors or asymptomatic disease conditions in populations (Box 9-2).
- **Case finding** locates individuals and families with identified risk factors and connects them with resources.
- **Referral and follow-up** assists individuals, families, groups, organizations, and/or communities to identify and access necessary resources in order to prevent or resolve problems or concerns.
- **Case management** optimizes self-care capabilities of individuals and families and the capacity of systems and communities to coordinate and provide services.

DID YOU KNOW?   *Case management has long been a key service provided by PHNs. The origins of this intervention are attributed to PHNs who staffed the settlement houses prevalent around the turn of the century, such as Lillian Wald's Henry Street Settlement House in New York City. Wald and her colleagues provided direct patient care, as well as organized and mobilized family and community resources. Contemporary community-based case managers continue to address client needs and work to improve the quality of care provided to patients.*

From Scott J, Boyd M: Outcomes of community based nurse case management programs. In Cohen EL, Cesta TG, editors: Nursing case management: from essentials to advanced practice applications, *St Louis, 2005, Mosby, pp 129-140.*

- **Delegated functions** are direct care tasks a registered professional nurse carries out under the authority of a health care practitioner as allowed by law. Delegated functions also include any direct care tasks a registered professional nurse entrusts to other appropriate personnel to perform.
- **Health teaching** communicates facts, ideas, and skills that change knowledge, attitudes, values, beliefs, behaviors, and practices of individuals, families, systems, and/or communities (Box 9-3).

Text continued on p. 205.

BOX 9-2   SCREENING

A school nurse was approached by the school's health and physical education staff who expressed interest in implementing a BMI screening program for children in 4th through 8th grades. Their plan was to do height, weight, and BMI measurements during gym class and requested that the school nurse do the follow-up with the parents of children found to be overweight or obese and encourage that these children be seen by their family health care provider. Although aware that prevalence of obesity in that age group was growing, she was also aware that most local health care providers believed that "chunkiness" in the middle years was a natural occurrence for children. She was also aware that a cardinal rule of screening is that it is unethical to screen if effective treatment and other resources for follow-up do not exist.

In 2008 the U.S. Task Force on Community Preventive Services found insufficient evidence to recommend school-based programs to prevent or reduce obesity. In addition, the American Academy of Pediatrics expressed caution to schools when considering implementing such a program (AAP, 2009). Based on this knowledge, the school nurse suggested to the health and physical education staff that together they find other means of addressing the issue.

BOX 9-3   HEALTH TEACHING

Health teaching communicates facts, ideas, and skills that change knowledge, attitudes, values, beliefs, behaviors, practices, and skills of individuals, families, systems, and/or communities.

- Knowledge is familiarity, awareness, or understanding gained through experience or study.
- Attitude is a relatively constant feeling, predisposition, or set of beliefs directed toward an object, person, or situation, usually in judgment of something as good or bad, positive or negative.
- Value is a core guide to action.
- Belief is a statement or sense, declared or implied, intellectually and/or emotionally accepted as true by a person or group.
- Behavior is an action that has a specific frequency, duration, and purpose, whether conscious or unconscious.
- Practice is the act or process of doing something or the habitual or customary performance of an action.
- Skill is proficiency, facility, or dexterity that is acquired or developed through training or experience.

TABLE 9-2   EXAMPLES OF 17 INTERVENTIONS AT THREE LEVELS OF PRACTICE

INTERVENTIONS	SYSTEMS	COMMUNITY	INDIVIDUAL
Surveillance	PHNs participated in dead bird reporting (i.e., making "dead bird calls"). People were asked to report the sighting of dead birds to a health department as part of surveillance activities for the West Nile virus. PHNs collected dead birds found in atypical places, such as the middle of a backyard or on a hiking trail. Birds were tested until a positive was found in the county.	PHNs implemented a program that tracked the growth and development of all newborns in the county. Parents were mailed questionnaires at regular intervals that they completed and returned to the public health office. PHNs screened the questionnaires for potential problems or delays and contacted the families by phone or home visits to determine if further action was indicated.	Surveillance at the Individual Level is CASE FINDING (see Case Finding Intervention).
Disease and other health event investigation	During a flood, the PHNs spent part of the day doing "rounds" among the rows of people living in a large emergency shelter set up in a gymnasium. The PHNs were concerned about the stresses that this population experienced, so they assessed for withdrawal, depression, and inability to cope. The PHNs observed that the children were not coping well. They questioned parents and heard stories about night terrors and atypical behavior. In response, the PHNs requested child mental health counselors from the Emergency Response Team. They also worked with parents in the shelter to set up a "toddler corner" where children could play and act like children. Parents took turns staffing the corner.	A PHN worked with a Catholic church that served a parish with a rapidly growing Hispanic population to connect mothers and children with community resources. The priest mentioned that he was seeing an unusual number of stillbirths among his parishioners. His comment led the PHN into a series of questions and investigation. The PHN discovered that the church allowed its kitchen facilities to store foods brought from Mexico. Suspecting a possible foodborne contaminant, the PHN took samples to the health department lab for testing. A supply of queso blanco fresco obtained from the church's refrigerator was found to be contaminated with Listeria. After an outreach and education campaign within the parish and the community, the rate of stillbirths decreased.	Disease and other health event investigation at the Individual Level is CASE FINDING (see Case Finding Intervention).
Outreach	Prior to launching a universally offered home visiting program for newborns, focus group interviews revealed the best strategies to encourage participation were as follows: • Send letters or postcards announcing the program to pregnant women • Make hospital visits to moms after delivery • Include photos of visitors on business cards and brochures • Be recommended by trusted individuals, such as physicians, nurses, and other new mothers • Have program staff visit Lamaze and other childbirth education programs, and early childhood development classes	PHNs were part of a coalition that received a grant to do community education on depression to an elderly Hmong population. Many Hmong elders were isolated but did not view depression as a disease. The PHNs tailored an outreach event to the Hmong population during a community market. Even though the program targeted persons over 50, people were allowed to determine their own eligibility. That is, if they "felt old," they qualified. Second, since it was considered unlikely that the elders would come to the booth, the coalition members talked with elders in more casual settings, approaching elders sitting under shade trees or at their market booth. All the interviews were conducted in the Hmong language.	Outreach at the Individual Level is CASE FINDING (see Case Finding intervention).

		Screening at the Individual Level is CASE FINDING (see Case Finding Intervention).
Screening	Vision screening is a core PHN activity with the school-aged population. PHNs worked with a community group to determine why school children who failed vision screening and were referred did not receive the recommended follow-up. Issues included: the expense of eye-care services and glasses; lack of convenient appointment times with eye-care specialists; and whether parents valued eye care. The PHNs participated in a task force that facilitated an agreement among eye-care providers to schedule evening and weekend appointments, arranged support from the Lions International Service Club toward the purchase of eyewear, and communicated the need for follow-up to parents at parent–teacher conferences.	PHNs collaborated with a high school on a prevention program to address physical inactivity and unhealthy dietary behaviors. The PHNs conducted health screenings that gave each student a "snapshot" of his or her health (height, weight, BMI, blood pressure, total cholesterol, HDL). Students received a report of their nutritional and physical activity levels with information about how to begin building lifestyle changes. One hundred ninety-two students from five schools were screened and 71 were referred (37% referral rate). Upon completion of the educational components, students who were rescreened had a total cholesterol decrease of 219 points.
Case finding	Does not apply at this practice level	Does not apply at this practice level	A state's newborn blood screening program detected an infant with a possible case of congenital hypothyroidism. The information was sent to the infant's medical provider, who was expected to contact the family. The mother of the infant was a single Hispanic woman who did not speak English and did not respond to the clinic's numerous calls. The provider referred the situation to a PHN for assistance in locating the mother. After talking with contacts in the Hispanic community, the PHN located friends of the young mother who confirmed she had returned to Mexico with the infant. They did not know how to contact her but agreed to alert those within the Hispanic community of the seriousness of the baby's problem. About 2 months later the mother did return, sought the PHN's assistance, and received care for the baby.

Continued

TABLE 9-2 EXAMPLES OF 17 INTERVENTIONS AT THREE LEVELS OF PRACTICE—cont'd

INTERVENTIONS	SYSTEMS	COMMUNITY	INDIVIDUAL
Referral and follow-up	PHNs providing health services to inmates in a county jail noticed that individuals with mental health issues, chronic health concerns, chemical dependency issues, or homelessness frequently returned to jail. Few of these issues were typically addressed prior the inmates' release. The PHNs initiated RAPP (Release Advance Planning Program), a voluntary "discharge planning" process through which referrals and other arrangements with community resources could be made prior to the inmates returning to the community. Recidivism rates decreased by 57% by the third year of the program's operation.	PHNs often serve as community resource directories. PHNs are known by community members for their extensive knowledge of whom or where to call for a variety of problems or issues. For example, PHNs in a rural health department responded to calls ranging from rats to cockroaches to bedbugs, from septic tank failures to peeling paint, and from air quality to blue-green algae. The PHNs often followed up with community members to ensure that their issues were resolved.	A PHN received a referral on a mentally ill young man from a small town. He needed regular injections to prevent rehospitalization. When the PHN was unable to locate this client at home, she found him at his regular "hangout"—the local bar—where he only drank soda pop. While creatively maintaining confidentiality, the PHN worked with the bartender in this establishment to set up regular appointment times for the client.
Case management	Public health nurses representing 10 county health departments, medical clinics, a large health plan company, and the state health department worked together to provide coordinated prenatal care to improve birth outcomes. The group created an integrated prenatal care system that promoted early prenatal care, improved nutrition, and linked women to services in the communities.	PHNs provided case management for all frail elderly and disabled persons at risk for institutionalization but deemed eligible for community placement. Case management maintained this vulnerable population in their home or community and ensured that their needs were met within the allotted amount of money that would otherwise be spent on hospitalization or nursing home care.	A local physician reported a highly contagious active infectious tuberculosis (TB) case that was determined to be multi-drug resistant. The client did not speak English. The PHN coordinated his care with the physician, the state health department's TB unit, the CDC, and a home health agency. Neither the hospital outpatient department nor any home health agency would agree to treat this client in their facility or make home visits. (Continued under delegated functions below.)
Delegated functions	In a county of 120,000 residents, PHNs from the local health department led a coalition of hospitals, clinics, schools, and emergency managers in designing and implementing a community-wide mass immunization plan to administer influenza vaccine. The design included the establishment of administration protocols approved by the health department's medical advisor. The health department also served as the central distribution point for all vaccine available within the county.	PHNs administered immunizations at "drive-thru" flu clinics held in a county highway garage. Residents received their assessment and flu shots in their vehicles. This unique access increased the numbers of immunizations received by elderly and disabled residents, particularly those with limited mobility. The drive-thru clinic also reduced the exposure potential to infectious diseases that was inherent in regular clinic waiting rooms.	(See above case management.) In addition to doing daily direct observed therapy (DOT), the PHN was the only health care provider who would do weekly lab draws, daily IV therapy, and biweekly dressing changes for the first 7 months of treatment. Without PHN involvement, this client would have likely succumbed to TB. The client completed a full 18 months of therapy and recovered.

Health teaching	PHNs worked with the epidemiologist in their health department to develop "best practice" guidelines for pediculosis (lice) treatment from the perspectives of the scientific literature and the practice community. Recommendations included both suffocating and chemical agents. Clinics, schools, and pharmacists used the new guidelines. The public health department created an internal standardized pediculosis response procedure, and the county's social services department developed a new policy for school truancy issues related to pediculosis.	Several rural counties launched a program to help youth incorporate a healthy diet and exercise into their lives. A health fair was held in conjunction with parent–teacher conferences. Committees composed of youth and adults planned activities such as "Dance 'n' Dips," a dance followed by a dip at the city pool. Members of a church began offering evening exercise classes. A small town sponsored the "Run, Walk 'n Roll" that was open to runners, walkers, strollers, and wheelchairs. The "Toilet Paper" document, a monthly nutrition and health tip sheet designed to resemble toilet paper, was displayed in 152 bathrooms, next to the toilet paper dispensers. The tips were popular; PHNs reported that people came up to them on the street to discuss the tips. PHNs reported seeing changes in community attitudes.	A PHN works with pregnant and parenting teens at an alternative high school program that provides educational options for teens whose lives did not fit the traditional school day. The program included teens from a variety of cultures and backgrounds. The program had an onsite child care center; students were able to visit their child during the school day. The PHNs taught weekly prenatal classes in conjunction with life skills and child development classes. PHNs also worked with each student to look at family planning options. Their "Pregnancy Free Club" provided each student private time with a PHN to look at barriers that prevent the student from effectively using birth control. The program had a repeat adolescent pregnancy rate significantly lower than the national average, declining from a baseline of 25% to a mean of 4.7% over 9 years of the program.
Counseling	PHNs partnered with a community family center to promote prenatal attachment for families who were isolated, who had experienced previous pregnancy loss, or who had other attachment issues. The project promoted attachment to the baby through the use of doulas, guided videotaping, nutrition counseling, and relaxation through music and imagery.	In response to multiple deaths within an American Indian community, PHNs in a tribal health department worked with the community to design and implement a culturally appropriate grief and loss program. Interventions included drumming activities for youth, traditional healers, and peer counselors.	A PHN led monthly support groups for family members and volunteers providing in-home care to individuals with Alzheimer's disease. The PHN provided one-to-one caregiver coaching to those needing additional support.

Continued

TABLE 9-2 EXAMPLES OF 17 INTERVENTIONS AT THREE LEVELS OF PRACTICE—cont'd

INTERVENTIONS	SYSTEMS	COMMUNITY	INDIVIDUAL
Consultation	After hearing about the risk for serious infectious disease for children in day care, PHN day-care consultants from eight local health departments developed a curriculum on handwashing for children. They obtained a grant to develop a video in several languages and widely distributed the handwashing materials.	PHNs providing post-partum home visits to new mothers noted that women employed by a certain large company often gave up breastfeeding upon returning to work. Reasons included lack of private space to express milk and non-supportive supervisors. The PHNs approached the company's human resources director and presented a business case for breastfeeding. After several meetings the company agreed to revamp its policies on breastfeeding in the workplace and requested PHNs' assistance in providing training.	The older sister of an elderly bachelor farmer died. The sister had kept house and cooked for her brother for their entire adult lives. Upon her death, he was unable to live independently. Neighbors concerned for his well-being convinced him to talk with a PHN/social worker team to explore his preferences and determine the best options for a living situation that respected his need for self-determination. He eventually moved into an assisted living facility that met his needs.
Collaboration	PHNs changed the way they had traditionally related to the 26 medical clinics in their community. They visited each clinic quarterly to provide information about change in vaccine policy and improving the reporting of notifiable diseases as required by law. They also answered questions, promoted disease prevention programs, and resolved problems together, such as vaccine shortages. This relationship benefited the public health department and the medical clinics.	Everyone is a bully, is being bullied, or is a bystander. School nurses worked with a community action team to develop community assets—caring, encouraging environment for youth and valuing of youth by adults. Through strategies such as a mentoring program for at-risk elementary school students and a revitalized orientation program for ninth graders entering high school, the incidence of bullying behavior was reduced.	Over a period of years, a PHN was able to establish a trusting relationship with a Haitian client with HIV. Through her transactions with this client, the PHN came to understand her own values differently and honored the client's spiritual values and practices.
Coalition building	PHNs were part of a coalition that formed to address the exploding bedbug issue in the community. The coalition was a response to requests from local housing providers for assistance. Coalition members included PHNs along with property owners and managers, commercial pest management operators, university entomologists, and the local housing authority. They provided education about the eradication and prevention of bedbug infestations, cost implications and potential litigation issues to local apartment managers, fraternity house operators and housing officials.	A student health survey revealed a greater than expected number of overweight or obese children in a school district. A coalition of school nurses, educators, and health care providers concerned about childhood obesity developed a school-based program for elementary students. As a result of the work of this coalition, parents received a report card about their child's BMI. Parents also received educational materials that offered tips for healthy living and a directory of physical activity options. A follow-up evaluation revealed that parents who received a report card were more likely to have initiated dietary changes or a physical activity plan than parents who had not.	Coalition building is not implemented at the individual level of practice.

Community organizing	A local newspaper reported that a statewide student health survey revealed their school district had one of the highest teen alcohol-use rates in the state. Numerous letters to the editors questioned why the community was not doing anything about the problem and demanded community action. In response, a PHN from the public health department partnered with other community groups and organizations to develop a plan to address alcohol use in the community. The plan included enforcing existing laws, such as enforcing "not a drop" laws with minors and developing social media messages for adolescents that emphasized "Not everyone drinks...."	In response to a public safety meeting where 750 angry residents showed up to complain about what they saw as the deterioration of their community, a city health department dispersed a team of PHNs to develop "social capital." The PHNs facilitated the development of social connections, relationships, and trust in a community that had experienced an influx of mainly poor, minority renters. Their goal was to ensure that neighbors know and care about each other enough to run next door to borrow a cup of sugar or offer to help the elderly woman down the block. PHNs helped organize exercise classes, a farmer's market, community gardens, and neighborhood dinners, which were free with the only requirement that diners eat next to somebody they did not know.	Community organizing is not implemented at the individual level of practice.
Advocacy	A worker at a large meat packing plant that employed over 1000 people speaking 12 languages was diagnosed with active infectious tuberculosis (TB). Initially the plant managers were more concerned about losing production than being exposed. The PHNs worked with the managers to convince them that exposure to TB was a serious problem and that they could cooperate with public health without decreasing production. Although the managers would not mandate testing, they did allow PHNs to offer free Mantoux tests during work time on all three shifts to any employee who wanted to be tested. Over 700 employees were tested, with over 70 positives. Many of the employees with positive Mantoux tests lacked access to health care. The PHNs negotiated reduced clinic fees and secured community grant funds to pay for x-rays and prescribed treatment for infected persons who were uninsured and without resources. *(See individual advocacy example.)*	A visiting nurse agency (VNA) served many families with small children living at or below poverty level. Many were homeless, experiencing mental health issues, alcohol or drug abuse, or domestic violence. Club 100 was a voluntary organization of community women and men associated with the VNA. It is a program that reaches out into the community to ask people of means to help care for people who have very little. It paired men and women with VNA nurses and their at-risk family clientele. The volunteers of Club 100 were divided into teams that worked with a PHN. The PHN selected clients that would benefit from the program and presented the client's case to the team on a quarterly basis. The club provided "gifts" such as high chairs, strollers, diapers, books, toys, and tools to support family self-sufficiency and improved the lives of these men, women and children.	A PHN received a referral on a 9-month-old boy with a recent diagnosis of meningitis resulting from active TB. The child's parents were a young Hispanic couple who did not speak English. The child's mother was pregnant and stayed at home with her two small children. The family had no telephone and neither parent had a driver's license. The entire family reacted positively to the Mantoux tests that the PHN administered. At this point, the PHN arranged an appointment at the local clinic for the entire family, complete with transportation and interpreters. The father was found to have active infectious TB. He was ordered not to return to his job at the meat packing plant and consequently lost his health insurance. The PHN assisted the family in applying for medical assistance and other services for which they were eligible. *(The fact that a meat packing plant employee had infectious TB required this PHN to intervene at the systems level—see systems advocacy example.)*

Continued

TABLE 9-2 EXAMPLES OF 17 INTERVENTIONS AT THREE LEVELS OF PRACTICE—cont'd

INTERVENTIONS	SYSTEMS	COMMUNITY	INDIVIDUAL
Social marketing	A partnership of health departments, managed care organizations, pharmaceutical companies, health care insurers, and others sought to decrease unnecessary antimicrobial use and reduce the spread of antimicrobial resistance. "Moxie Cillin" and "Annie Biotic" were mascots that appeared on pamphlets, posters, stickers, and in person. They urged discontinuation of inappropriate requesting of antibiotics by parents and unnecessary prescribing of antibiotics by health care providers.	A PHN working in a small rural county was assigned to work on a Fetal Alcohol Syndrome prevention grant in partnership with the local hospital. The PHN coordinated the grant activities, which included mass media efforts such as billboards, radio spots read by local celebrities, and newspaper articles. Multiple posters were placed in every bar in the community, and local bartenders were engaged as partners in the effort to reduce alcohol use among pregnant women. After 2 years, the project documented an increase in community awareness, which is the first step in changing the community norm regarding alcohol use among pregnant women.	PHNs routinely conducted home safety checks with pregnant and parenting families to prevent childhood injuries. As incentives, they distributed safety kits that included items to child-proof a home, such as cupboard safety locks, outlet covers, door knob safety covers, and drawer latches. While having a PHN checking contents in cupboards and water temperatures may have felt intrusive to some families, the kits increased the number of families who were receptive to home safety checks.
Policy development and enforcement	Local health department PHNs and health educators partnered with law enforcement to establish ordinances prohibiting the sale of tobacco to underage youth. Part of the initiative included recruiting and training youth to conduct compliance checks, in which underage youth attempted to purchase cigarettes in retail stores. PHNs also created an electronic compliance tracking system that was eventually used by the entire state.	A PHN investigated a public health complaint about a fly problem originating from the manure pit of a farm that housed millions of chickens. Garbed in protective equipment, the intrepid PHN crawled under the chicken cages that dumped into the manure pits and found masses of maggots. After determining that the situation constituted a public health nuisance, the PHN successfully worked with the business owners to find a solution that involved the drying of manure to prevent the maggots from surviving.	A PHN received a referral regarding the safety of an 80-year-old woman living alone on a littered farm site. The woman lived with 18 cats in a house without heat that was ankle-deep with cans, clothes, and cat feces. The PHN initiated a vulnerable adult evaluation that resulted in a "not sufficiently vulnerable" finding under state statute. Through repeated contacts, the PHN was able to establish a trusting relationship; the women accepted a referral for care to a physician. However, she was not successful in changing the woman's living situation.

- **Counseling** establishes an interpersonal relationship with a community, system, family, or individual intended to increase or enhance their capacity for self-care and coping. Counseling engages the community, system, family, or individual at an emotional level.

| **NURSING TIP**   Differentiating Counseling from Psychotherapy |

Although PHNs do not provide psychotherapy, much of public health nursing deals with emotionally charged "client situations." These range from individuals attempting to cope with chronic pain, a couple grieving for the loss of their infant to SIDS, women involved with partners who batter them, or an elderly couple attempting to cope with the loss of all their possessions in a flood. Public health nursing also occurs at systems and community levels of practice. Examples of this are mediating a heated debate between providers competing for the same public contract to provide home health services or a PHN facilitating a community meeting on teen pregnancy prevention where the members are polarized around their beliefs. Although counseling as practiced by a PHN should have a therapeutic outcome (i.e., have a healing effect), it should not be confused with providing psychotherapy. Counseling is intended to clarify problems, relieve tension, facilitate problem solving, encourage friendship and companionship, enhance understanding, encourage insight, and relieve stress.

From Burnard P: Counseling skills for health professionals, *Cheltenham, England, 2005, Nelson Thomas Ltd.*

- **Consultation** seeks information and generates optional solutions to perceived problems or issues through interactive problem solving with a community, system, family, or individual. The community, system, family, or individual selects and acts on the option best meeting the circumstances.
- **Collaboration** commits two or more persons or organizations to achieve a common goal through enhancing the capacity of one or more of the members to promote and protect health (Freshman et al, 2010; Henneman et al, 1995).
- **Coalition building** promotes and develops alliances among organizations or constituencies for a common purpose. It builds linkages, solves problems, and/or enhances local leadership to address health concerns.
- **Community organizing** helps community groups to identify common problems or goals, mobilize resources, and develop and implement strategies for reaching the goals they collectively have set (Brown, 2007; Minkler, 1997).

| **DID YOU KNOW?**   *The Orange Wedge interventions are all* |

examples of collective action, or groups of people or organizations coming together for mutual gain or problem solving. Collective action is part of the American democratic tradition. Alexis de Tocqueville, writing in Democracy in America *in 1840, noted: "Americans are a peculiar people. If, in a local community, a citizen becomes aware of a human need that is not met, he thereupon discusses the situation with his neighbors. Suddenly a committee comes into existence. The committee thereupon begins to operate on behalf of the need, and a new common function is established. It is like watching a miracle."*

- **Advocacy** pleads someone's cause or acts on someone's behalf, with a focus on developing the capacity of the community, system, individual, or family to plead their own cause or act on their own behalf.
- **Social marketing** uses commercial marketing principles and technologies for programs designed to influence the knowledge, attitudes, values, beliefs, behaviors, and practices of the population of interest.

| **NURSING TIP**   Social Marketing |

In a 2009 article in the OJIN: Online Journal of Issues in Nursing, Berkowitz and Borchard declared a "call to action" for nursing to participate in the prevention of childhood obesity. They stress that both health promoting and health protecting strategies are needed, targeted at the individual, family, and community levels in multilevel coordinated programming. Skills in advocacy, collaborative leadership, and social marketing are highlighted as necessary for nursing success in these strategies. Regarding social marketing, the authors specify that the nurse "...must understand what the target audience is willing to give up or modify in terms of behavior in order to adopt (exchange) the new behavior (in place of) the old behavior." For example, a neighborhood group enlisted the support of their PHNs to develop a proposal requesting more sidewalks in a proposed housing project. The PHNs provided vital evidence that connected community "walkability" with community health.

- **Policy development** places health issues on decision-makers' agendas, acquires a plan of resolution, and determines needed resources. Policy development results in laws, rules, regulations, ordinances, and policies.
- **Policy enforcement** compels others to comply with the laws, rules, regulations, ordinances, and policies created in conjunction with policy development.

In addition to the definition and examples, each intervention has basic steps for implementation at each of the three levels (i.e., community, systems, and individual/family) as well as a listing of best practices for each intervention. The basic steps are intended as a guide for the novice public health nurse or the experienced public health nurse wishing to review his/her effectiveness. Box 9-4 describes the basic steps of the counseling intervention.

The best practices are provided as a resource for PHNs seeking excellence in implementing the interventions. They were constructed by a panel of expert public health nursing educators and practitioners after a thorough analysis of the literature. Many practices of public health nursing are either not researched or, if they are researched, not published. The process used to develop this model considered this limitation and met the challenge with the use of expert practitioners and educators. The best practices are a combination of research and other evidence from the literature and/or the collective wisdom of experts. Box 9-5 outlines an example of a set of best practices for the intervention of referral and follow-up, some supported by evidence and others supported by practice expertise.

BOX 9-4   BASIC STEPS FOR THE INTERVENTION OF COUNSELING*

Working alone or with others, PHNs . . .

1. Meet the "client"—the individual, family, system, or community.
2. Establish rapport by listening and attending to what the client is saying and how it is said.†
3. Explore the issues.
4. Gain the client's perception of the nature and cause of the identified problem or issue and what needs to change.‡
5. Identify priorities.
6. Gain the client's perspective on the urgency or importance of the issues; negotiate the order in which they will be addressed.
7. Establish the emotional context.
8. Explore, with the client, emotional responses to the problem or issue.
9. Identify alternative solutions.
10. Establish, with the client, different ways to achieve the desired outcomes and anticipate what would have to change in order for this to happen.
11. Agree on a contract.
12. Negotiate, with the client, a plan for the nature, frequency, timing, and end point of the interactions.
13. Support the individual, family, system, or community through the change.
14. Provide reinforcement and continuing motivation to complete the change process.
15. Bring closure at the point the PHN and client mutually agree that the desired outcomes are achieved.

*Complete version available at http://www.health.state.mn.us/divs/cfh/ophp/resources/docs/phinterventions_manual2001.pdf.
†Modified from Burnard P: *Counseling: a guide to practice in nursing*, Oxford, England, 1992, Butterworth-Heineman.
‡Understanding the client's cultural or ethnic context is important to perception. For further information, please see Sue DW, Sue D: *Counseling the culturally different: theory and practice*, ed 3, New York, 1999, Wiley.

BOX 9-5   BEST PRACTICES FOR THE INTERVENTION OF REFERRAL AND FOLLOW-UP

Best Practice
Successful implementation is increased when the . . .

• PHN respects the client's right to refuse a referral.
• PHN develops referrals that are timely, merited, practical, tailored to the client, client controlled, and coordinated.
• Client is an active participant in the process and the PHN involves family members as appropriate.
• PHN establishes a relationship based on trust, respect, caring, and listening.
• PHN allows for client dependency in the client–PHN relationship until the client's self-care capacity sufficiently develops.
• PHN develops comprehensive, seamless, client-sensitive resources that routinely monitor their own systems for barriers.

Evidence
• McGuire, Eigsti Gerber, Clemen-Stone, 1996 (expert opinion)
• Stanhope and Lancaster, 1984 (text)
• Will, 1977 (expert opinion)
• Wolff, 1962 (expert opinion)

Expert Panel Recommendation
• McGuire, Eigsti Gerber, Clemen-Stone, 1996 (expert opinion)
• Stanhope and Lancaster, 1984 (text)
• Will, 1977 (expert opinion)
• Wolff, 1962 (expert opinion)

McGuire S, Eigsti Gerber D, Clemen-Stone S: Meeting the diverse needs of clients in the community: effective use of the referral process, *Nursing Outlook* 44(5):218-222, 1996; Stanhope M, Lancaster J: *Community health nursing: process and practice for promoting health*, St Louis, 1984, Mosby, p 357; Will M: Referral: a process, not a form, *Nursing* 77:44-55, 1977; Wolff I: Referral—a process and a skill, *Nurs Outlook* 10(4):253-262, 1962.

ADOPTION OF THE INTERVENTION WHEEL IN PRACTICE, EDUCATION, AND MANAGEMENT

The speed at which the Intervention Wheel was adopted may be attributed to the balance between its practice base and its evidence-based support. The Intervention Wheel has led to numerous innovations in practice and education since it was first published in 1998 (Keller et al, 2004a). Further dissemination of the model has occurred through the hundreds of graduate and undergraduate schools of nursing that use the Intervention Wheel as a framework for teaching public health nursing.

The Intervention Wheel has been widely adopted as a framework for public health nursing practice:

• In 2007, the American Nurses Association officially recognized the Intervention Wheel as a framework in the Public Health Nursing Scope and Standards of Practice (ANA, 2007).
• The Los Angeles County Department of Health Services used the Intervention Wheel in their initiative to re-invigorate public health nursing practice—orientation, practice standards, documentation, recruitment, and retention—for their 500 public health nurse generalists and specialists (LACDHS, 2002; Avilla and Smith, 2003; Smith and Bazini-Barakat, 2003).
• The Massachusetts Association of Public Health Nurses used the Intervention Wheel as the framework for their state "Leadership Guide and Resource Manual" (Massachusetts Association of Public Health Nurses, 2009).
• PHNs in the Shiprock Service Unit of the Indian Health Service use the Wheel in their practice and adapted it to reflect the Navajo culture. The Navajo Intervention Wheel (Figure 9-4) is presented as a Navajo basket and uses the traditional colors of the Navajo nation.
• From 2001 to 2005, the Intervention Wheel served as the framework for a Division of Nursing grant that successfully brought together education and practice communities to collaboratively redesign the public health nursing student's clinical experience. Several of these collaboratives remain viable and active.
• PHN consultants at the Wisconsin Department of Health used the Intervention Wheel to differentiate levels of nursing practice in local health departments related to educational preparation and to outline the role of the associate degree and diploma nurse in public health. (Although the baccalaureate degree is the accepted standard for entry to public health nursing practice,

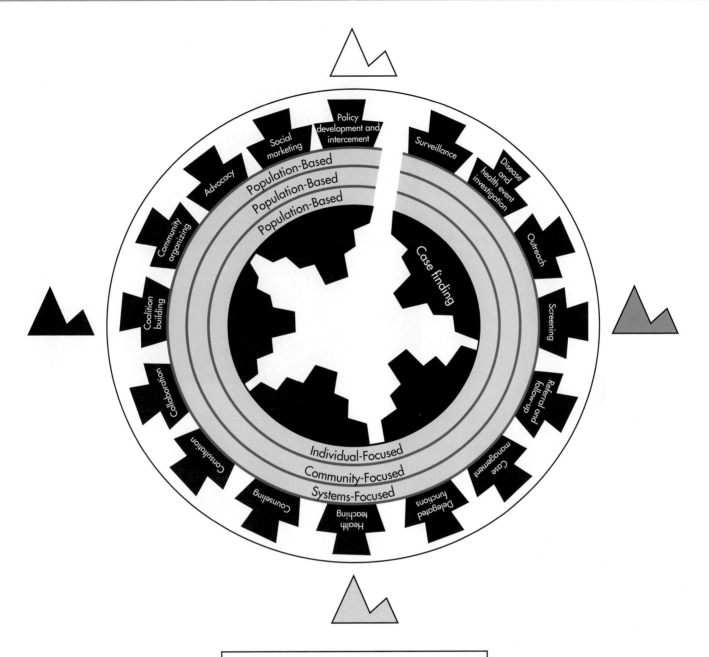

The Navajo basket represents mother earth (the tan area), the black design represents the four sacred mountains that surround the Navajo Nation, and the red area represents the rainbow, which symbolizes harmony. In Navajo philosophy, one should not enclose oneself without an opening. Therefore, the basket has an opening, or doorway, to receive all that is good/positive, and allow all the bad/negative to exit.

Neva Kayaani

FIGURE 9-4 Navajo Wheel. (Courtesy Shiprock Service Unit, Shiprock, NM, Indian Health Service.)

shortages of baccalaureate prepared nurses sometimes result in health departments employing associate degree and diploma nurses.)

- PHNs at the St. Paul-Ramsey County (MN) Department of Health used the Intervention Wheel to illustrate the activities of their refugee health program. Their display (Figure 9-5)

identified the most common interventions implemented with the refugee population and illustrated each intervention with a photograph.

The Wheel provides a meaningful frame of reference and common language for staff to communicate about the nature of their work and is used in orientation programs in several states.

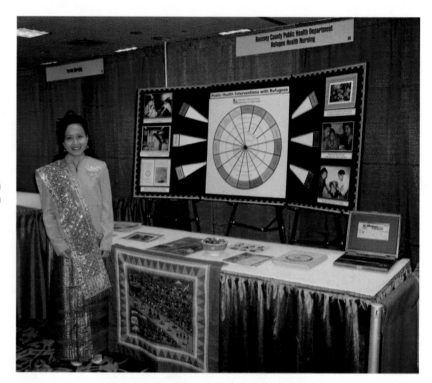

FIGURE 9-5 St. Paul-Ramsey County Public Health Family Health International Team. (Courtesy Sophia Emang, Public Health Nurse, St. Paul-Ramsey.)

- The Alaskan Public Health Nurse Leadership Academy uses the Intervention Wheel to familiarize new staff with population-based practice (http://www.hss.state.ak.us/dph/nursing/PFDs/Troshynski-Academy.pdf).
- Several universities have developed online applications of the Intervention Wheel, including the Virginia Commonwealth University (http://www.people.vcu.edu/~elmiles/interventions/) and the University of Minnesota School of Public Health (http://www.sph.umn.edu/ce/tools/wheel.asp).

The concepts of the model have also been used internationally. The Intervention Wheel was used in public health nursing projects in New Zealand and Ireland. The Institute of Primary Health & Ambulatory Care in the Townsville Health Service District, Queensland Health in Australia used the Intervention Wheel to develop a set of competencies (http://www.health.qld.gov.au/townsville/Clinicians/default.asp).

The significance of the contributions of the Intervention Wheel has been recognized by the nursing community. The authors of the Intervention Wheel received Sigma Theta Tau International and National Pinnacle Awards for Research Dissemination and a Creative Achievement Award from the American Public Health Association, Section of Public Health Nursing.

HEALTHY PEOPLE 2020

The objectives chosen to be highlighted in this chapter show how many of the interventions from the Wheel are applied in the *Healthy People 2020* document. It further indicates how appropriate these interventions are to improving the health of individuals, populations, and communities, thus improving the health of the nation.

APPLYING THE NURSING PROCESS IN PUBLIC HEALTH NURSING PRACTICE

PHNs use the nursing process at all levels of practice. PHNs must customize the components of the nursing process (assessment, diagnosis, planning, implementation, evaluation) to the three levels of practice. See Table 9-2 for an outline of the nursing process at the community, systems, and individual/family levels of practice.

APPLYING THE PROCESS AT THE INDIVIDUAL/FAMILY LEVEL

Community Assessment

During a health department's community assessment process, information on the health status of children was obtained from the following:

- Staff public health nurses who worked with families in clinics, schools, and homes
- Community partners who worked with families, including health care providers, mental health workers, social workers, and school personnel
- Preschool screening program data on the number of young children with developmental delays and problems for the past 5 years
- Data from the county social services department on the number of substantiated child maltreatment and neglect cases for the past 5 years

♥ HEALTHY PEOPLE 2020

Healthy People 2020 identifies action steps for 38 health priorities that the United States must take in order to achieve better population health by the year 2020. The 500 recommended objectives offer numerous opportunities for public health nurses to contribute though implementing interventions at any or all of the levels. Here are a few examples:

- AH-8: Adolescent Health Objective: *Increase the proportion of adolescents who have a wellness check-up in the past 12 months.* PHNs who provide well-child screening services in school settings or local health departments will need well-designed outreach interventions to convince teens that even healthy kids can benefit from check-ups. This will require consulting with parents and groups of teens themselves to identify what "benefits" would attract them and incorporating them into the outreach design. PHNs will also need to collaborate with other health care providers in the community to ensure that diagnostic and treatment services are available for teens who require additional services.
- DH-7: Disability and Secondary Conditions Objective: *Reduce the proportion of older adults with disabilities who use inappropriate medications.* The case management that PHNs provide to elderly or disabled populations in their communities includes an assessment of clients' medications to ensure compliance with the regimen prescribed by health care providers under delegated functions.
- ECBP-10: Education and Community-Based Programs Objective: *Increase the number of community-based organizations, providing population-based primary prevention services in the following areas: injury, violence, mental illness, tobacco use, substance abuse, unintended pregnancy, chronic disease programs, nutrition, and physical activity.* PHNs may convene coalitions to address an issue or serve as facilitators or participants of coalitions already organized. For instance, PHNs with expertise in substance use prevention might offer health teaching and consultation to a coalition organized to find ways to reduce substance use during pregnancy. It could also mean the establishment of a new screening and referral system among providers to identify early pregnant women and their partners struggling with drug or alcohol use and link with resources for treatment.

- EH-8.1: Environmental Health Objective: *Eliminate elevated blood lead levels in children.* PHNs providing services to families with young children assess (surveillance) the living conditions for lead. Housing constructed prior to 1978, the year lead-based paint for residential use was banned, is particularly suspect. Depending on the community's housing and lead-abatement codes, PHNs may provide health teaching and counseling to the families regarding the dangers of lead exposure to small children or provide advocacy on their behalf with housing authorities.
- MICH-18: Maternal Infant and Child Health Objective: *Decrease postpartum relapse of smoking among women who quit smoking during pregnancy.* A recent systematic review of the literature on effective strategies to prevent postpartum smoking relapse concluded that PHNs would more likely be effective in assisting new mothers to resist returning to smoking and exposing their child to second-hand smoke if they: (1) consistently used the U.S. Preventive Services Task Forces "5 A's" when counseling with smokers, (2) tailored health teaching regarding the dangers of second-hand smoke to the client's specific situation, (3) empowered the mother and family members to adopt a smoke-free home smoking policy, and (4) advocated for the importance of partners also quitting (Ashford et al, 2009).

From Ashford K, Hahn E, Hall L, et al: Postpartum smoking relapse and secondhand smoke, *Public Health Rep* 124:515-526, 2009.

THE CUTTING EDGE *The Intervention Wheel is being used to track health improvement in Milwaukee's Riverwest community, a community of about 7000 households. For this project interventions were integrated into the Automated Community Health Information System (ACHIS), a health information system that included the OMAHA system (Hildebrandt et al, 2003; Lundeen and Friedbacher, 1994). In this way, population interventions are linked to community health improvement and tracked over time. The "district nurses" electronically code their activities in the system, which generates data describing health improvement interventions on a continual basis for administrative and research purposes.*

Hildebrandt E, Baisch MJ, Lundeen SP, et al: Eleven years of primary health care delivery in an academic nursing center, J Prof Nursing 10(5):279-288, 2003; Lundeen SP, Friedbacher BE: The automated community health information system (ACHIS): a relational database application of the OMAHA System in a community nursing center. In SJ Grobe, ESP Pluyter-Wenting, editors: Nursing informatics: an international overview for nursing in a technological era, St Louis, 2003, Mosby, pp 393-397.

PHNs participated in the community meeting that prioritized the long list of issues identified in the community assessment. One of the top community priorities that emerged was the following: *Decreasing numbers of children at risk for delayed development, injury, and disease because of inadequate parenting by parents experiencing mental health problems.*

The community health plan developed a goal to decrease the number of children with delayed development, injury, and disease attributable to inadequate parenting. The local health department, with the support of community partners, decided they would address this priority through a home visiting strategy. Home visiting enhances a child's environment and increases the capacity of parents to behave appropriately. Although parental mental health problems are a major source of stress for children, this vulnerability can be tempered through support from others and a caring environment.

Home visiting to families is an example of practice at the individual level because the interventions are delivered to families with the goal of changing parental knowledge, attitudes, practices, and behaviors.

Public Health Nursing Process: Assessment of a Family

A PHN received a referral on Tyler, age 3. He was the only child of Ashley, a 19-year-old single mother with severe depression. Ashley lived in an old rented house in the small town where she grew up. She had a boyfriend who was not Tyler's biological father. Ashley survived on limited public assistance and occasional help from her mom.

The PHN assessed the resilience, assets, and protective factors as well as the problems, deficits, and health risks of this family. The PHN also tried to elicit Ashley's perception of her situation, which was difficult because of her depressed state. This step is important because often a client's perception of their problems or strengths may not align with the PHN's professional assessment.

All public health nursing practice is relationship based, regardless of level of practice. An established trust relationship increases the likelihood of a successful outcome. One of the PHN's main priorities was to establish a trusting relationship with Ashley. This was difficult because Ashley was seldom out of bed when the PHN arrived, but the PHN persisted and eventually developed the relationship.

Public Health Nursing Process: Diagnosis

- *Diagnosis:* Increased risk for delayed development, injury, and disease because of inadequate parenting by a primary parent experiencing depression
- *Population at risk:* Young children who are being parented by a primary parent who is experiencing mental health problems
- *Prevention level:* Secondary prevention, because the families have an identified risk

Public Health Nursing Process: Planning (Including Selection of Interventions)

Based on the assessment of this family, the PHN negotiated with Ashley to establish meaningful, measurable, achievable **intermediate goals.** In families experiencing mental illness (actually, in most families), behavior change occurs in very small steps. For this family, client goals included the following outcomes:

- Ashley will get out of bed at least 3 days in the week.
- Tyler will be dressed when the PHN arrives.
- Tyler will get to the bus on time 3 days in a row.
- The clutter will be cleaned off the steps.
- Ashley will call to make a doctor's appointment for Tyler's well-child check.
- Ashley will use "time outs" instead of spanking.
- Ashley will read a story to Tyler twice a week. (Intermediate indicators at the individual level of practice are changes in an individual's knowledge, attitudes, motivation, beliefs, values, skills, practices, and behavior that lead to desired changes in health status.)

The PHN also selected meaningful, measurable **outcome health status indicators** to measure the impact of the interventions on population health. Examples include no signs or reports of child maltreatment; child regularly attends preschool; child receives well-child examinations according to recommended schedule; child's immunizations are up to date; the family seeks medical care for acute illness as needed and does not seek medical care inappropriately; and child falls within normal limits on developmental tests.

The PHN selected the interventions, which included collaboration, case management, health teaching, delegated functions, and referral and follow-up. In selecting these interventions, the PHN considered evidence of effectiveness, political support, acceptability to the family, cost-effectiveness, legality, ethics, greatest potential for successful outcome, and level of prevention.

Public Health Nursing Process: Implementation

The PHN determined the sequence and frequency of her home visits based on her assessment of each family. Some families received home visits once a week, some twice a week, and others twice a month. The PHN visited this family weekly in the beginning and then spaced the home visits farther apart. She used the following interventions.

Collaboration

The PHN identified and involved as many alternative caregivers in Tyler's care as possible, including Tyler's biological father, aunt and uncle, and grandparents as well as Ashley's boyfriend.

Case Management

The PHN arranged childcare services and coordinated transportation for Tyler to spend significant portions of his day outside of the home.

Health Teaching

The PHN provided information on child growth and development, nutrition, immunizations, safety, medical and dental care, and discipline to Ashley and the alternative caregivers.

Delegated Functions (Public Health Nurse to Paraprofessional)

The PHN placed a family health aide in the home to provide role modeling for Ashley. As part of this intervention, the PHN monitored and supervised the aide.

Referral and Follow-up

Based on the assessment, the PHN referred Ashley to community resources and services that included early childhood services, legal aid, food stamps, mental health counselors, and transportation.

Public Health Nursing Process: Evaluation

The PHN reassessed and modified her plan at each home visit. She provided regular feedback to Ashley and the other caregivers on their progress. The PHN documented her results and compared them with the selected indicators. After 6 months of home visits, Ashley got out of bed most days of the week but rarely got dressed. Ashley was more successful in getting Tyler to the bus and to preschool. The family health aide helped Ashley clean the clutter off the steps. Ashley scheduled a doctor's appointment for Tyler's well-child visit but failed to get him to the appointment. Ashley was successful in learning to substitute "time outs" for spanking, with the help of the family aide. Tyler exhibited no signs of child maltreatment. He attended preschool regularly. Tyler was still behind on his immunizations because of the missed appointment. All of Tyler's developmental tests were within normal limits.

The PHN reported her results to her supervisor during their regular supervisory meetings. The PHN also talked with other PHNs who worked with similar families about common issues and best practices, and applied what she had learned to her practice.

APPLYING THE PUBLIC HEALTH NURSING PROCESS AT THE COMMUNITY LEVEL OF PRACTICE SCENARIO

Note: At the community level of practice, the community assessment, program planning, and evaluation process is the public health nursing process.

Community Assessment (Public Health Nursing Process: Assessment)

Childhood obesity is a rapidly growing community problem. An increasing number of children ages 2 to 11 are considered overweight, as defined by a body mass index (BMI) at or above the 95th percentile (based on CDC Growth Charts; Ogden 2010). The 2007-2008 National Health and Nutrition Examination Survey data estimated that 10% of boys and 10.7% of girls aged 2 to 5 were overweight in the United States. Among children aged 6 to 11 years, the percentages were 21.2% for boys and 18% for girls (Dakota County, 2010). Childhood obesity and hyperplasia of adipose cells are linked to obesity later in life.

A health department recognized the well-established association between overweight and obesity in childhood and the development of both continuing overweight/obesity as adults and a host of chronic diseases (CDC, 2010a). In response, the public health nursing director of a health department convened a childhood obesity prevention summit. Over 80 participants representing area health care providers, schools, child care, and governmental and community-based health organizations met for an entire day to discuss the problem and frame solutions.

Community Diagnosis (Public Health Nursing Process: Diagnosis)

The percentage of children aged 2 to 11 who are overweight or obese is unacceptable and threatens the future health status of the community.

- *Population of interest:* Children aged 2 to 11
- *Level of prevention:* Primary prevention

Community Action Plan: Public Health Nursing Process: Planning (Including Selection of Interventions)

At the conclusion of the summit, each organization represented committed to promoting healthy eating and physical activity habits for all residents, with an emphasis on parents of young children. The health department recognized that substantial portion of a child's caloric intake occurs at child care.

Based on its assessment of the community, the health department initiated a 24-week evidence-based program that promotes the consumption of fruits and vegetables by young children through intervention with licensed home childcare providers. "LANA the Iguana" (Learning About Nutrition Through Activities) encourages eating eight targeted fruits and vegetables: broccoli, sweet red pepper, cherry tomatoes, apricots, sugar snap peas, kiwi, sweet potatoes, and strawberries (Figure 9-6). These fruits and vegetables were featured in activities throughout the program related to menu changes, classroom activities, and family involvement.

Menu Changes

Home childcare providers increased opportunities for children to eat more fruits and vegetables by serving the targeted fruits and vegetables on the menu, alternating four for one week and

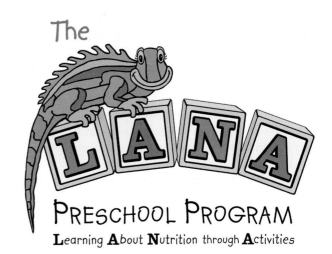

FIGURE 9-6 LANA the Iguana. (Used with permission from Minnesota Department of Health, Center for Health Promotion.)

four the next. Fruits and vegetables were served as the morning and afternoon snack every day.

Classroom Activities

Home childcare providers increased children's preference for and knowledge of fruits and vegetables by featuring one of the targeted fruits and vegetables each week throughout the program. During that week, the featured fruit or vegetable was the focus of tasting and cooking activities as well as the topic of stories and games.

Family Involvement

Home childcare providers gave families information about the program and activities to do at home. These included quick and easy kid-tested recipes and take-home fruit/vegetable tasting kits.

The PHNs selected their interventions, which included consultation, health teaching, social marketing, collaboration, and surveillance. In selecting these interventions, the PHNs considered evidence of effectiveness, acceptability to community, cost-effectiveness, legality, ethics, and greatest potential for successful outcome.

Community Implementation Plan (Public Health Nursing Process: Implementation)

1. *Social marketing:* LANA the Iguana was a social marketing program. It incorporated a range of age-appropriate social marketing techniques including iguana puppets and storybooks, recipe cards and activities. The PHNs promoted retention by providing home childcare providers with incentives, including two grocery store gift cards and plastic fruit/vegetable toys for the children. They worked with librarians to place LANA the Iguana kits (comprised of iguana puppets, activities, and storybooks) in the local library for parents to check out. PHNs also donned the LANA the Iguana costume to implement the curriculum directly to children as well as train the home childcare providers and parents.

2. *Health teaching:* The PHNs trained the home childcare providers on the LANA curriculum to ensure fidelity to the program.
3. *Consultation:* The public health nurses consulted with home childcare providers about the program on a regular and ongoing basis.
4. *Collaboration:* PHNs collaborated with health educators to develop and distribute LANA materials, including a curriculum guide, recipe books, storybooks, parent newsletters, and LANA the Iguana puppets. They also collaborated with public health nursing students to collect program evaluation data.
5. *Surveillance:* The PHNs collected data on the consumption of fruits and vegetables in the home childcare setting.

Community Evaluation (Public Health Nursing Process: Evaluation)

Follow-up surveys with the county's 75 licensed home childcare providers, who served about 500 children, found that 67% of children were more or much more likely to eat fruits and 78% were more likely to eat vegetables; 92% of children were more likely to try new foods; and 76% of providers offered fruits and vegetables more often at snack time (Dakota County, 2010). Establishing healthy eating habits among young children will lead to reduced levels of obesity.

APPLYING THE PUBLIC HEALTH NURSING PROCESS TO A SYSTEMS LEVEL OF PRACTICE SCENARIO

Health departments conduct assessments of community health status, a core function of public health, on an ongoing basis. The identification of some community problems emerges out of practice, rather than through a formal community assessment. This scenario is such an example.

Public Health Nursing Process: Assessment

For several years, PHNs had been very concerned about the poor living conditions in an apartment complex in which many of their clients lived. The walls were moldy, the carpet was unclean and deteriorated, and closet doors had fallen off their runners and struck children living in the apartment. The PHNs were suspect of the required cash payments that the manager required for repairs, extra security deposits, and increased rent after the birth of a baby.

Many of the tenants were undocumented Latinos and tried not to create problems. Most could not speak or read English well, and often signed lease agreements without taking note of damage or existing problems in the apartment and were therefore blamed for them. In addition, the manager blamed the tenants for the mold on the walls, implying that their cooking created too much humidity. Citing these "problems," the manager often gave bad references for the tenants, which made it difficult for them to move.

Over the years, the PHNs had diligently worked with their clients to correct these problems, but with little success. When the PHNs met with the manager to discuss the issues, he became

angry. As a result, the manager had the PHNs' cars towed whenever he saw them in the parking lot. The PHNs also had sought help from city officials, but the officials had no legal recourse to remedy the situation.

Finally, several events occurred that spurred the PHNs to action. One of the PHNs found a non-functioning smoke detector in an apartment during a home safety check. The family reported that the apartment manager had dismantled the smoke detector and left it that way. At the same time, another PHN was working with a family that was trying to move to a new, safer, cleaner apartment. The family had found a new apartment but could not move because the manager gave them a bad (although false) reference. The family no longer had a lease, but the manager said they could not move. The PHNs realized that there were many complex legal issues related to the living conditions of their clients.

Public Health Nursing Process: Diagnosis

- *Diagnosis:* Families at risk of illness and injury because of hazardous housing and abuse of legal rights
- *Population at risk:* Families living in hazardous housing in an apartment complex
- *Prevention level:* Secondary, because families are at risk for injury and illness

Public Health Nursing Process: Planning (Including Selection of Interventions)

At the systems level of practice, the goal is to change policies, laws, and structures. The PHNs' goals were to enforce the tenants' legal rights and improve the living conditions in the apartment complex. Their plan was to seek advice from a housing advocate service and connect their clients with legal counsel. Before they could pursue this plan, the PHNs consulted with their supervisor. Their supervisor supported their decision but also had to clear the plan with the health department director and the city manager.

The PHNs selected their interventions, which included consultation, referral and follow-up, advocacy, policy development, and surveillance. In selecting these interventions, the PHNs considered evidence of effectiveness, political support, acceptability to the family, cost-effectiveness, legality, ethics, greatest potential for a successful outcome, non-duplication, and level of prevention.

Public Health Nursing Process: Implementation

The PHNs worked with the tenants and the housing advocacy service to implement the following interventions.

Consultation

The PHNs consulted with attorneys at a housing advocate service.

Referral and Follow-up

The attorneys informed the PHNs that they needed to hear directly from the tenants in order to proceed. The PHNs set up a meeting time between the tenants and the attorneys from the housing advocate service.

Advocacy

The PHNs arranged for their public health interpreter to go door to door with an advocate from the housing service to invite tenants to the meeting. They also arranged for the interpreter to attend the meeting to interpret each family's concerns. The PHNs strongly encouraged all of the tenants to attend.

Policy Development

The public health nurses worked with the attorneys from the housing advocate service to develop the meeting agenda.

Surveillance

The PHNs continued to conduct ongoing monitoring of living conditions in the apartment complex.

LINKING TEXT CONTENT TO PRACTICE

The discussions of the application of the nursing process to a variety of clients on pages 208–213 and Tables 9-1 and 9-2 provide numerous examples of how the content in this chapter are applied in practice. Please review these for examples of how you may apply this model in your practice.

Public Health Nursing Process: Evaluation

Many of the tenants attended the meeting. As a result of the meeting, the attorney chose to have the rent paid to the court and put in escrow until a legal determination could be made. During this process the apartment owner became aware of these issues and dismissed the manager, who was discovered to have been acting fraudulently. A new manager was employed who worked to improve the living conditions of the apartments.

CHAPTER REVIEW

PRACTICE APPLICATION

Outreach locates populations of interest or populations at risk and provides information about the nature of the concern, what can be done about it, and how services can be obtained. Outreach activities may be directed at whole communities, at targeted populations within those communities, and/or at systems that impact the community's health. Outreach success is determined by the proportion of those considered at risk that receive the information and act on it.

The chance of a woman under the age of 30 developing breast cancer is 1 in 1985. From ages 30 to 39, a woman's chance of developing breast cancer is 1 in 229; from ages 40 to 49, it is 1 in 68; from ages 50 to 59, it is 1 in 37; from ages 60 to 69, it is 1 in 26; and from ages 70 to 79, it is 1 in 24 (Breast Cancer Action, 2007).

A health system decided to offer free mammograms in recognition of National Breast Cancer Month. They sponsored a mobile mammography van at a large shopping mall every Saturday in October. The van offered mammograms to everyone, regardless of age. The health system advertised the service by placing windshield flyers on all the cars in the shopping mall parking lot. The van provided 180 mammograms, mostly to women in their 30s who had health insurance that covered preventive services.
A. What is the population most at risk of breast cancer?
B. Did the mammograms in the parking lot reach this population?
C. What types of outreach would public health nurses conduct to reach the population at risk?
Answers can be found on the Evolve site.

KEY POINTS

- In these times of change, the public health system is constantly challenged to keep focused on the health of populations.
- The Intervention Wheel is a conceptual framework that has proved to be a useful model in defining population-based practice and explaining how it contributes to improving population health.
- The Wheel depicts how public health improves population health through interventions with communities, the individuals and families that comprise communities, and the systems that impact the health of communities.
- The Wheel serves as a model for practice in many state and local health departments.
- The Wheel is based on 10 assumptions.
- The Intervention Wheel encompasses 17 interventions.
- Other public health members of the interprofessional team such as nutritionists, health educators, planners, physicians, and epidemiologists also use these interventions.
- Implementing the interventions ultimately contributes to the achievement of the 10 essential public health services.
- The *Cornerstones of Public Health Nursing* was developed as a companion document to the Intervention Wheel.
- The original version of the Wheel resulted from a grounded theory process carried out by public health nurse consultants at the Minnesota Department of Health in the mid-1990s.

- The interventions were subjected to an extensive review of supporting evidence in the literature.
- The Wheel is a conceptual model. It was conceived as a common language or catalog of general actions used by public health nurses across all practice settings.
- The Intervention Wheel serves as a conceptual model for public health nursing practice and creates a structure for identifying and documenting interventions performed by public health nurses and captures the nature of their work.
- The Wheel has three main components: a population basis, three levels of practice, and 17 interventions.
- The Wheel has led to numerous innovations in practice and education since the original Intervention Wheel was first published in 1998.
- Public health nurses in the Shiprock Service Unit of the Indian Health Service adapted the Intervention Wheel to reflect the Navajo culture.
- Numerous graduate and undergraduate schools of nursing throughout the United States have adopted the Intervention Wheel as a framework for teaching public health nursing practice.

CLINICAL DECISION-MAKING ACTIVITIES

1. Describe the three components of the Intervention Wheel. How do the components relate to each other? Explain how you can apply them to your clinical practice.
2. Go to Chapter 1 and reread the definitions of the core functions of public health practice and look at the 10 essential services. How does the Wheel address the core functions? How does it relate to the 10 essential services?
3. Go to the Wheel website: www.health.state.mn.us/divs/cfh/ophp/resources/docs/wheel.pdf. Choose one of the 17 interventions to explore. Read about the recommended strategies to use when intervening with a client. Explain the level of practice and how you can apply the intervention. Give a concrete example.

REFERENCES

American Academy of Pediatrics: Active healthy living: prevention of childhood obesity through increased physical activity, *Pediatrics* 117(5):1834–1842, 2010. This policy is a revision of the policy posted on May 1, 2000.

American Nurses Association: *Public health nursings: scope and standards of practice*, Silver Spring, MD, 2007, ANA. Available at http://www.nursesbooks.org.

American Nurses Association Task Force: *Nursing social policy statement: the essence of the profession*, 2010 Edition, Washington, DC, 2010, American Nurses Publishing.

American Public Health Association, Public Health Nursing Section: *Definition and role of public health nursing*, Washington, DC, 1996, APHA.

Avilla M, Smith K: The reinvigoration of public health nursing: methods and innovations, *J Public Health Manag Pract* 9:16–24, 2003.

Barnard KE, Magyary D, Sumner G, et al: Prevention of parenting alteration for women with low social support, *Psychiatry* 51:248–253, 1988.

Berkowitz B, Borchard M: Advocating for the prevention of childhood obesity: a call to action for nursing, *OJIN: Online Journal of Issues in Nursing* 14(1-Manuscript 2), 2009. Available at http://www.nursingworld.org/MainMenuCategories/ANAMarketplace/ANAPeriodicals/OJIN/TableofContents/Vol142009/No1Jan09/Prevention-of-Childhood-Obesity.aspx. Accessed December 11, 2010.

Breast Cancer Action: *The facts and nothing but the facts*, 2007. Available at http://www.bcaction.org/Pages/GetInformed/Facts.html. Accessed December 11, 2010.

Brown MJ: *Building powerful community organizations: a personal guide to creating groups that can solve problems and change the world*, Arlington, MA, 2007, Long Haul Press.

Burnard P: *Counseling: a guide to practice in nursing*, Oxford, England, 1992, Butterworth-Heineman.

Centers for Disease Control and Prevention: *Health, United States, 2009*. Available at http://www.cdc.gov/nchs/data/hus/hus09.pdf#list figures. Accessed December 11, 2010.

Centers for Disease Control and Prevention: *Obesity: halting the epidemic by making health easier*, 2010a. Available at http://www.cdc.gov/chronicdisease/resources/publications/aag/pdf/2010/AAG_Obesity_2010_Web_508.pdf. Accessed December 11, 2010.

Centers for Disease Control and Prevention: *Vaccines and preventable diseases*, 2010b. Available at http://www.cdc.gov/vaccines/vpd-vac/default.htm. Accessed December 11, 2010.

Committee for the Study of the Future of Public Health: *The future of Public Health Institute of Medicine*, Washington, DC, 1988, National Academies Press.

Dakota County (MN) Public Health: Factsheet: tackling childhood obesity with Lana the Iguana. 2010. Available at http://www.co.dakota.mn.us

Dakota County (MN) Public Health: Research on the impact of LANA, 2006. Available at: http://www.co.dakota.mn.us/

Dunton G, Kaplan J, Wolch J, et al: Physical environmental correlates of childhood obesity: a systematic review, *Obesity Rev* 10:393–402, 2009.

Fawcett J: *Contemporary nursing knowledge: analysis and evaluation of nursing models and theories*, ed 2, Philadelphia, 2005, FA Davis, pp 4-25.

Freshman B, Rubino L, Chassiakos YR: *Collaboration across the disciplines in health care*, Sudbury, MA, 2010, Jones and Bartlett.

Henneman EA, Lee J, Cohn JI: Collaboration: a concept analysis, *J Adv Nurs* 21:103–109, 1995.

Jewish Women's Archive: *Resource information for Backyard of a Henry Street Branch*, 2010. Available at http://jwa.org/archive/jsp/gresInfo.jsp?resID=297. Accessed December 11, 2010.

Johnston RJ, Gregory D, Pratt G, Watts M, editors: *The dictionary of human geography*, ed 4, Oxford, England, 2000, Blackwell, pp 101–102.

Kawachi I, Subramanian SV, Almeida-Filho N: A glossary for health inequalities, *J Epidemiol Community Health* 56:647–652, 2002.

Keller LO: *Report on a public health nurse to population ratio*, Association of State and Territorial Directors of Nursing, 2008. Available at http://www.astdn.org/downloadablefiles/draft-PHN-to-Population-Ratio.pdf. Accessed December 11, 2010.

Keller LO, Strohschein S, Lia-Hoagberg B, Schaffer M: Assessment, program planning, and evaluation in population-based public health practice, *J Public Health Manag Pract* 8:30–43, 2002.

Keller LO, Strohschein S, Lia-Hoagberg B, Schaffer M: Population-based public health interventions: practice-based and evidence-supported, part I, *Public Health Nurs* 21:453–468, 2004a.

Keller LO, Strohschein S, Lia-Hoagberg B, Schaffer M: Population-based public health nursing interventions: a model from practice, *Public Health Nurs* 15:311–320, 1998.

Keller LO, Strohschein S, Schaffer M: Cornerstones of public health nursing, *Public Health Nurs*, 2010:(in press).

Keller LO, Strohschein S, Schaffer M, Lia-Hoagberg B: Population-based public health interventions: innovations in practice, teaching, and management, part II, *Public Health Nurs* 21:469–487, 2004b.

Leavell HR, Clark EG: *Preventive medicine for the doctor in his community*, ed 3, New York, 1965, McGraw-Hill.

Lo R: Walkability: what is it? *J Urbanism* 2(2):145–166, 2009.

Los Angeles County Department of Health Services: Public Health Nursing Administration. *Public health nursing administration model*, 2002. Available at http://lapublichealth.org/phn/whatphn.htm; narrative available at http://lapublichealth.org/phn/docs/Narrative2002.PDF. Accessed December 11, 2010.

Massachusetts Association of Public Health Nurses: Leadership guide and resource manual, 2009. Available at www.maphn.org. Accessed January 20, 2011.

McGuire S, Eigsti Gerber D, Clemen-Stone S: Meeting the diverse needs of clients in the community: effective use of the referral process, *Nurs Outlook* 44:218–222, 1996.

Meagher-Stewart D, Edwards N, Aston M, Young L: Population health surveillance practice public health nurses, *Public Health Nurs* 26(6):553–560, 2009.

Minkler M, editor: *Community organizing and community building for health*, New Brunswick, NJ, 1997, Rutgers University Press, p 30.

Minnesota Departments of Education, Health, Human Services, and Public Safety: *2007 Student Health Survey, Sherburne County*, 2007. Available at http://www.health.state.mn.us/divs/chs/mss/countytables/sherburne07.pdf. Accessed December 11, 2010.

Minnesota Department of Health, Division of Community Health Services: *Tools for analyzing evidence in support of public health nursing practice*, St. Paul, MN: Minnesota Department of Health.

Monsen K, Keller LO: A population-based approach to pediculosis management, *Public Health Nurs* 19:201–208, 2002.

Morbidity and Mortality Weekly Review: *Updated Guidelines for Evaluating Public Health Surveillance Systems* 50(RR13):1–35, 2001.

Novick LF, Mays GP: *Public health administration: principles for population-based management*, Gaithersburg, MD, 2001, Aspen, p 315.

Ogden CL, Carroll MD, Curtin LR, et al: Prevalence of high body mass index in U.S. children and adolescents, 2007-2008, *JAMA* 303(3):242–249, 2010.

Public Health Functions Steering Committee: *Public health in America*, 1995. Available at www.health.gov/phfunctions/public.htm. Accessed December 11, 2010.

Renalds A, Smith T, Hale P: A systematic review of built environment and health, *Fam Community Health* 33(1):68–78, 2010.

Roof K, Oleru N: Public health: Seattle and King County's push for the built environment, *J Env Health* 71(1):24–27, 2008.

Scott J, Boyd M: Outcomes of community based nurse case management programs. In Cohen EL, Cesta TG, editors: *Nursing case management: from essentials to advanced practice applications*, St Louis, 2005, Mosby, pp 129–140.

Sheridan NF: *Mapping a new future: primary health care nursing in New Zealand*, 2005. Available at http://researchspace.itss.auckland.ac.nz.

Smith K, Bazini-Barakat N: A public health nursing practice model: melding public health principles with the nursing process, *Public Health Nurs* 20:42–48, 2003.

Southworth M: Designing the walkable city, *J Urban Planning Dev* 131(4):246–257, 2005.

Stanhope M, Lancaster J: *Community health nursing: process and practice for promoting health*, St Louis, 1984, Mosby, p 357.

Sue DW, Sue D: *Counseling the culturally different: theory and practice*, New York, 1999, Wiley.

Turnock BJ: *Public health: what it is and how it works*, ed 4, Gaithersburg, MD, 2009, Aspen Publishers.

U.S. Department Health and Human Services: *Community health status indicators for Sherburne County (MN)*, 2007. Available at http://www.communityhealth.hhs.gov/RiskFactorsForPrematureDeath.aspx?GeogCD=27141&PeerStrat=45&state=Minnesota&county=Sherburne. Accessed December 11, 2010.

Walkability Checklist. (no date). Partnership for a Walkable America. Retrieved from: http://www.walkableamerica.org/checklist-walkability.pdf.

Williams CA, Highriter ME: Community health nursing: population focus and evaluation, *Public Health Rev* 7:197–221, 1978.

Zoller, Kara, personal communication, August 16, 2010.

CHAPTER 10

Environmental Health

Barbara Sattler, RN, DrPH, FAAN

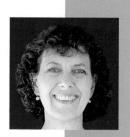

Dr. Barbara Sattler is a Professor and the Director of the Environmental Health Education Center at the University of Maryland School of Nursing, which hosts a graduate program for nurses in environmental health and a post-master's certificate in environmental health. She is the principal investigator and director of several grant-funded, environmental health–related projects. Over the years, Dr. Sattler's work has included lead poisoning prevention; healthy homes and schools; environmentally healthy and sustainable hospitals, safe drinking water; and community-based activities in areas of contaminated land. She has served on a number of federal advisory committees to the Environmental Protection Agency; on Institute of Medicine Committees, and on several state-level commissions, including the Governor's Commission on Environmental Justice. She is a founding member of the Alliance of Nurses for Healthy Environments. Her master's and doctorate degrees are in public health from Johns Hopkins University School of Public Health. She is a co-author of *Environmental Health and Nursing Practice* (Sattler and Lipscomb, 2002).

ADDITIONAL RESOURCES

evolve WEBSITE

http://evolve.elsevier.com/Stanhope
- *Healthy People 2020*
- WebLinks—Of special note see the link for these sites:
  - Envirotools
  - e-Commons.org Alliance of Nurses for Healthy Environments
  - National Library of Medicine online toxicology tutorial

- Quiz
- Case Studies
- Glossary
- Answers to Practice Application

APPENDIXES
- Appendix F.3: Comprehensive Occupational and Environmental Health History
- Appendix H: Focus on Quality and Safety Education for Nurses

OBJECTIVES

After reading this chapter, the student should be able to do the following:

1. Explain the relationship between the environment and human health and disease.
2. Understand the key disciplines that inform nurses' work in environmental health.
3. Apply the nursing process to the practice of environmental health.
4. Describe legislative and regulatory policies that have influenced the impact of the environment on health and disease patterns in communities.
5. Explain and compare the roles and skills for nurses practicing in the field of environmental health as well as those practicing in many other fields.
6. Incorporate environmental principles into practice.

KEY TERMS

agent, p. 222
bioaccumulated, p. 236
biomonitoring, p. 221
climate change, p. 223
compliance, p. 234
consumer confidence report, p. 227
environment, p. 222
environmental justice, p. 236
environmental standards, p. 234
epidemiological triangle, p. 222
epidemiology, p. 222
epigenetics, p. 221

geographic information systems (GISs), p. 222
global warming, p. 223
host, p. 222
indoor air quality, p. 226
Industrial Hygiene Hierarchy of Controls, p. 232
methylmercury, p. 236
monitoring, p. 234
non–point sources, p. 225
permit, p. 234
permitting, p. 234
persistent bioaccumulative toxins (PBTs), p. 236

persistent organic pollutants (POPs), p. 236
point sources, p. 225
precautionary principle, p. 230
right to know, p. 227
risk assessment, p. 228
risk communication, p. 233
risk management, p. 232
route of exposure, p. 233
toxicants, p. 229
toxicology, p. 221
—*See glossary for definitions*

OUTLINE

"Environmental health comprises those aspects of human health, including quality of life, that are determined by physical, chemical, biological, and social and psychological problems in the environment. It also refers to the theory and practice of assessing, correcting, controlling, and preventing those factors in the environment that can potentially affect adversely the health of present and future generations."

From *Protection of the Human Environment*, published by the World Health Organization
(2006, para. 1)

Our homes, schools, workplaces, and communities are the environments in which most of us can be found at any given time. Potential risks to health exist in each of these environments. As nurses, who are one of the most trusted conveyors of information to the public, it is our responsibility to understand as much as possible about these risks—how to assess them, how to eliminate/reduce them, how to communicate and educate about them, and how to advocate for policies that support healthy environments. In 2010, the American Nurses Association (ANA) established an environmental health standard, within the Scope and Standards of Professional Practice that define the profession of nursing (Box 10-1). This means that all nurses are now expected to have knowledge of and skills associated with environmental health.

There are many ways in which environmental health threats can occur. If you have children and regularly use insecticides in your home, you increase their risk of contracting leukemia. The more you use insecticides, the greater the risk of leukemia (Infante-Rivard et al, 1999; Turner et al, 2010). The greatest risk to the child occurs when the mother is exposed to insecticides indoors during pregnancy (Brown, 2004). Childhood leukemia is also associated with prenatal exposures by parents with occupational exposures to pesticides (Wigle et al, 2009). The use of professional pest control services at any time from 1 year before birth to 3 years after was associated with a significantly increased risk of childhood leukemia (Ma et al, 2002). Many playing fields where children compete in sports are regularly sprayed with pesticides.

BOX 10-1 AMERICAN NURSES ASSOCIATION'S PRINCIPLES OF ENVIRONMENTAL HEALTH FOR NURSING PRACTICE

1. Knowledge of environmental health concepts is essential to nursing practice.
2. The Precautionary Principle guides nurses in their practice to use products and practices that do not harm human health or the environment and to take preventive action in the face of uncertainty.
3. Nurses have a right to work in an environment that is safe and healthy.
4. Health environments are sustained through multidisciplinary collaboration.
5. Choices of materials, products, technology, and practices in the environment that impact nursing practice are based on the best evidence available.
6. Approaches to promoting a healthy environment respect the diverse values, beliefs, cultures, and circumstances of patients and their families.
7. Nurses participate in assessing the quality of the environment in which they practice and live.
8. Nurses, other health care workers, patients, and communities have the right to know relevant and timely information about the potentially harmful products, chemicals, pollutants, and hazards to which they are exposed.
9. Nurses participate in research of best practices that promote a safe and healthy environment.
10. Nurses must be supported in advocating for and implementing environmental health principles in nursing practice.

From American Nurses Association, *Principles of environmental health for nursing practice,* Silver Spring, MD, 2007.

In May 2010, the President's Cancer Panel proclaimed that the contribution that environmental carcinogens have made to the burden of cancer in the United States has been grossly underestimated. In addition to the main focus on chemical carcinogens, the panel noted the importance of radiation sources—ionizing and non-ionizing. In a letter to the President, they wrote: "The Panel urges you most strongly to use the power of your office to remove the carcinogens and other toxins from our food, water, and air that needlessly increase our health care costs, cripple our Nation's productivity and devastate American lives" (President's Cancer Panel, 2010).

With this call came a range of recommendations for reducing the risk of cancer, both through individual choices and through national policy (Box 10-2). The recommendations for individuals are found in Resource 10.A on the Evolve resources website. There is also a document online at http://deainfo.nci.nih.gov/advisory/pcp/pcp08-09rpt/PCPReport 08-09 508.pdf that has an excellent section on recommendations for policy and research.

An estimated 52 million homes in the United States contain some lead-based paint. Exposure to lead can cause premature births, learning disabilities in children, hypertension

---

BOX 10-2   GENETICS AND ENVIRONMENTAL HEALTH

The Institute of Medicine (Pope, Snyder, and Mood, 1995) defines environmental health as the freedom from illness or injury related to toxic agents and other environmental conditions that are potentially detrimental. With more than 80,000 chemicals currently in commerce and another 2000 novel chemicals being introduced annually (Congress of the United States, 1995; Rand, 2010), it has become increasingly difficult to ensure freedom from illness related to environmental exposures. Heavy metals, plasticizers, and pesticides are making their way into the human body through the air we breathe, water we drink, and food we consume. The publication *Third National Report on Human Exposure to Environmental Chemicals* (CDC, 2005) makes it abundantly clear that humans of all ages reflect the chemical world in which we live.

Connections between certain environmental exposures and adverse health outcomes have been strengthened by epidemiology and by laboratory and animal studies; examples include the relationships between smoking and risk of lung cancer (Alberg, Brock, and Samet, 2005), between thalidomide use and risk of birth defects (Goldman, 2001; Ema et al, 2010), and between arsenic exposure and risk of various cancers (Yoshida et al, 2004; Rahman et al, 2009). However, the relationship between other environmental exposures and overt disease is less well understood. Host factors such as age and genetics, chemical dose, and timing of exposures can modify the incidence of acute and chronic disease. Often, cause-and-effect relationships are not fully established, prompting the application of the precautionary principle (Wingspread Statement, 1998) and recognition that the absence of information does not necessarily mean the absence of harm.

Determining how genetic susceptibility contributes to disease risk from environmental exposures is a central theme of today's environmental health research (Hunter, 2005; Christiani et al, 2008). Scientists working on the Human Genome Project have provided a roadmap to the locations of the approximately 30,000 human genes (Collins, 2001). This information is critical for deciphering human variation and genomic changes that occur during the aging process. Scientists working on the Environmental Genome Project (2005) are focusing on small differences in human gene sequences that may explain disparate responses to environmental challenges. (See http://www.niehs.nih.gov/research/supported/programs.egp/a for information on the project). To date, approximately 400 environmentally responsive genes have been characterized as regulating cell division, cell signaling, cell structure, DNA repair, apoptosis, and metabolism. These efforts will help decipher connections between DNA sequence variation, environmental exposures, and disease susceptibility and should yield substantial public health benefits.

Risk assessment, risk reduction, and risk communication (the three "Rs") require a multidisciplinary approach with input from toxicologists, epidemiologists, earth scientists, and health professionals. Nurses play a key role in this process. Nurses frequently are the first to encounter clients with a history of hazardous exposures and are well positioned to initiate early interventions. A strong foundation in environmental health and genetics will promote a balanced approach for designing effective treatments and addressing larger policy issues. This chapter provides nurses with the skill set necessary for achieving these objectives, including tools for health assessment, summaries of current environmental laws, and a list of relevant websites, books, and publications to better understand environmental health and policies.

References

Alberg AJ, Brock MV, Samet JM: Epidemiology of lung cancer: looking to the future, *J Clin Oncol* 23:3175–3185, 2005.

Centers for Disease Control and Prevention: *Third national report on human exposure to environmental chemicals*, 2005. Available at http://www.cdc.gov/exposurereport/3rd/pdf/thirdreport_summary.pdf. Accessed December 15, 2010.

Christiani DC, Mahta AJ, Yu CL: Genetic susceptibility to occupational exposures, *Occup Environ Med* 65(6):430–436, 2008.

Collins RS: Contemplating the end of the beginning, *Genome Res* 11:641–643, 2001.

Congress of the United States, Office of Technology Assessment: *Screening and testing chemicals in commerce*, Publication No. OTA-BP-ENV-166, Washington, DC, 1995, Office of Technology Assessment. Available at http://www.wws.princeton.edu/ota/disk1/1995/9553_n.html. Accessed May 23, 2006.

Ema M, Ise R, Kato H, et al: Fetal malformations and early embryonic gene expression response in cynomolgus monkeys maternally exposed to thalidomide, *Reprod Toxicol* 29(1):49–56, 2010.

Environmental Genome Project, 2005. Available at http://www.niehs.nih.gov/envgenome/home.htm. Accessed December 15, 2010.

Goldman DA: Thalidomide use: past history and current implications for practice, *Oncol Nurs Forum* 28:471–479, 2001.

Hunter DJ: Gene-environment interactions in human disease, *Nat Rev Genet* 6:287–298, 2005.

Pope AM, Snyder MA, Mood LH, editors: *Nursing, health and environment*, Washington, DC, 1995, Institute of Medicine, National Academy Press, p 15.

Rahman MM, Ng JC, Naidu R: Chronic exposure of arsenic via drinking water and its adverse health impacts on humans, *Environ Geochem Health* 1:189–200, 2009.

Rand MD: Drosophotoxicology: the growing potential for *Drosophila* in neurotoxicology, *Neurotoxicol Teratol* 32(1):74–83, 2010.

Wingspread Statement on the Precautionary Principle: Racine, WI, January 1998, Conference, Wingspread Conference Center. Available at http://www.gdrc.org/u-gov/precaution-3.html. Accessed December 15, 2010.

Yoshida T, Yamauchi H, Sun GF: Chronic health effects in people exposed to arsenic via the drinking water: dose-response relationships in review, *Toxicol Appl Pharmacol* 198:243–252, 2004.

Developed by Anne R. Greenlee, PhD, Associate Professor, Oregon Health & Science University School of Nursing Center for Research on Occupational and Environmental Toxicology, La Grande, OR.

in adults, and many other health problems. Lead poisoning is a completely preventable disease (Figure 10-1). Of the top 20 environmental pollutants that were reported to the Environmental Protection Agency (EPA), nearly three fourths were known or suspected neurotoxics. In the United States alone, this accounted for more than a billion pounds of neurotoxicants being released into the air, water, and land (Goldman, 1998). Thirty million Americans drink water that exceeds one or more of the EPA's safe drinking water standards, and 50% of Americans live in an area that exceeds current national ambient air quality standards. When these standards are exceeded, there is an increased risk to the public for a wide range of health effects.

Although food labeling includes nutritional information, there is no requirement to label whether pesticides are used in the food production; whether non-therapeutic antibiotics were given to the livestock, poultry, or farmed fish; the presence of genetically engineered foods in a product; or whether recombinant bovine growth hormone was given to the dairy cows. Nurses have declared that the "right to know" about potentially hazardous exposures is one of the basic principles of environmental health (see Box 10-1). Nurses have a range of potential public health responsibilities in protecting the public from exposures and environmental health risks.

Nurses' environmental assessments begin with a set of questions: What exposures can you identify in your own home? Do you use pesticides? Does your home have lead-based paint? Is it chipping or peeling? Are any of your appliances or heat sources producing unhealthy levels of carbon monoxide? Have you checked your home for radon, the second largest cause of lung cancer in the United States? How about your workplace? Do you use latex gloves? Do you use medical equipment that contains mercury, such as mercury thermometers or sphygmomanometers, which can contribute to the environmental mercury load that has contaminated fish in lakes and streams in more than 40 states?

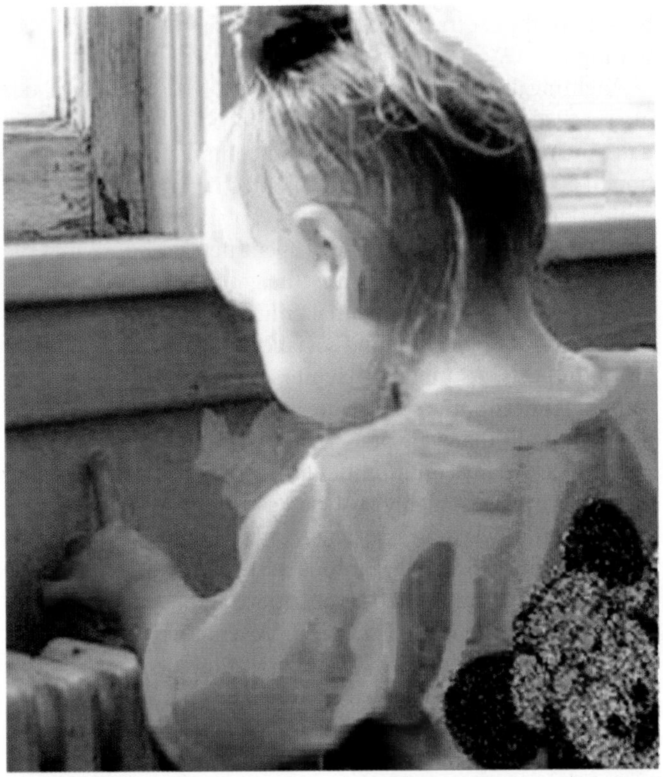

DID YOU KNOW? *There is a fish alert that warns pregnant women (or women who wish to become pregnant) to limit their fish consumption to one portion a week for certain fish, including tuna fish. Both the EPA and the Food and Drug Administration (FDA) have issued alerts because there are dangerously high amounts of mercury in certain fish that create risks for the unborn child's developing nervous system (see http://www.epa.gov/ost/fish or http://www.cfsan.fda.gov).*

Chemical, biological, and radiological exposures may contribute to health risks via the air we breathe (indoors and out), the water we drink, the food we eat, and/or the products we use. The mass media is alerting the *public* to health risks associated with foodborne illnesses, contaminated drinking water, indoor and outdoor air triggers to asthma (including mold),

FIGURE 10-1 Although much work has been done to reduce lead in paint, this remains a problem especially for children who pick at the paint and then eat it. Teach families to remove lead-based paint from their home. (From State of Hawaii Department of Public Health. Available at http://hawaii.gov/health/environmental/noise/asbestoslead/images2/child.jpg. Accessed December 15, 2010.)

LINKING CONTENT TO PRACTICE

Key documents that guide practice in both nursing and public health direct practitioners to be knowledgeable about and apply in their work principles related to environmental health. Specifically, the core competencies of the *Council on Linkages* has, with the domain of public health science skills, a competency that says practitioners will apply "the basic public health sciences (including, but not limited to, environmental health sciences, health services administration, and social and behavioral health sciences) to public health policies and programs." The Quad Council of Nursing further applies this competency specifically to public health nursing practice by adding that these skills are applied to public health nursing practice, policies, and programs. The most explicit set of principles are those developed by the ANA in their principles of environmental health for nursing practice.

The ANA (2007) lists 10 principles of environmental health. Although all 10 are essential, three are highlighted here. Nurses should know about environmental health concepts, participate in assessing the quality of the environment in which they practice, and live and use the Precautionary Principle (which is discussed later in the chapter) to guide their work. Another principle points out that healthy environments are sustained through multidisciplinary collaboration, which is a key concept discussed throughout the chapter.

From American Nurses Association: *ANA's principles of environmental health in nursing practice with implementation strategies*, Silver Spring, MD, 2007, author; Council on Linkages Between Academic and Public Health Practice: Core competencies for public health professionals: Washington, DC, 2010, Public Health Foundation/Health Resources and Services Administration; Quad Council of Public Health Nursing Organizations: Competencies for Public Health Nursing Practice, Washington, DC, 2003, ASTDN, revised 2009. Accessed December 15, 2010.

BOX 10-3 **GENERAL ENVIRONMENTAL HEALTH COMPETENCIES FOR NURSES**

Basic Knowledge and Concepts

All nurses should understand the scientific principles and underpinnings of the relationship between individuals or populations and the environment (including the work environment). This understanding includes the basic mechanism and pathways of exposure to environmental health hazards, basic prevention and control strategies, the interprofessional nature of effective interventions, and the role of research.

Assessment and Referral

All nurses should be able to successfully complete an environmental health history, recognize potential environmental hazards and sentinel illnesses, and make appropriate referrals for conditions with probable environmental causes. An essential component is the ability to access and provide information to clients and communities and to locate referral sources.

Advocacy, Ethics, and Risk Communication

All nurses should be able to demonstrate knowledge of the role of advocacy (case and class), ethics, and risk communication in client care and community intervention with respect to the potential adverse effects of the environment on health.

Legislation and Regulation

All nurses should understand the policy framework and major pieces of legislation and regulations related to environmental health.

From Pope AM, Snyder MA, Mood LH, editors: *Nursing, health, and environment,* Washington, DC, 1995, Institute of Medicine, National Academy Press.

♥ **HEALTHY PEOPLE 2020**

Examples of Objectives Related to Environmental Health

- EH-8.1: Eliminate elevated blood level levels in children.
- EH-9: Minimize the risks to human health and the environment posed by hazardous sites.
- EH-10: Reduce pesticide exposures that result in visits to the health care facility.
- EH-11: Reduce the amount of toxic pollutants released into the environment.
- EH-13: Reduce indoor allergen levels.
- EH-18: Decrease the number of U.S. homes that are found to have lead-based paint or related hazards.

From U.S. Department of Health and Human Services: *Healthy People 2020.* Available at http://www.healthypeople.gov/2020topicsobjectives 2020/default.aspx. Accessed January 1, 2011.

HISTORICAL CONTEXT

Historically, nurses and physicians have been taught little about the environment and environmental threats to health. In 1995 the IOM produced the report *Nursing, Health and Environment* (Pope, Snyder, and Mood, 1995), which recognized the environment as a significant determinant of health and acknowledged that this recognition is, in fact, deeply rooted in nursing's heritage. Pictures of and quotes from Florence Nightingale are used throughout the report, not only because she is a recognized symbol of nursing (i.e., the lady with the lamp), but also because of the central focus of environment in her practice and writings.

Nightingale is well-known for her work in the Crimea and is often called "the mother of biostatistics" for her skilled use of data, including her observations and compilation of information to compel action on conditions affecting population-based health. Early in the twentieth century, Lillian Wald, who coined the name "public health nurses," spent her life improving the environment of the Henry Street neighborhood and working her broad network of influential contacts to make changes in the physical environment and social conditions that had direct health impacts. As modern day nurses are rediscovering environmental health, they are reintegrating many of the observations and skills that were practiced by early nurse pioneers.

There are many communities like the ones that Lillian Wald served. Poverty is highly associated with health disparities. In addition, poverty is associated with living in sub-standard housing, living closer to hazardous waste sites, working in more hazardous jobs, having poorer nutrition, and having less access to quality health care (particularly preventative services). The term *environmental justice issue* refers to the disproportionate environmental exposures that poor people and people of color experience. Poor people and people of color often live in sub-standard housing and experience the risks from chipping and peeling paint, pests and use of pesticides, inadequate heating sources with attendant carbon monoxide exposure, and locations that are near industry, hazardous waste sites, and highways. These populations also often have poor access to fresh produce, work in the most hazardous jobs, and lack access to

---

and environmental threats from potential terrorists. If the general public knows this, then nurses must be a step ahead and be prepared to answer our clients' and communities' questions. Therefore, nurses must understand how to assess the health risks posed by the environment and develop educational and other preventive interventions to help individual clients and their families as well as communities understand and, when possible, decrease their risks. The Institute of Medicine (IOM) of the National Academy of Science recommends that all nurses have a basic understanding of environmental health principles and that these principles are integrated into all aspects of our practice, education, advocacy, policies, and research. In this chapter, we will explore the basic competencies recommended by the IOM. Box 10-3 presents the competencies recommended by the IOM report, *Nursing, Health and Environment* (Pope, Snyder, and Mood, 1995).

HEALTHY PEOPLE 2020 OBJECTIVES FOR ENVIRONMENTAL HEALTH

Environmental health is one of the priority areas of the *Healthy People 2020* objectives. The federal government has long recognized the importance of the relationship between environmental risks and the underlying factors contributing to diseases. Selected examples of the *Healthy People 2020* environmental health objectives are outlined in the *Healthy People 2020* box.

quality health care. These combined circumstances contribute to health disparities.

It is important to note how we began to understand the relationship between environmental chemical exposures and their potential for harm. There are several ways in which we have historically made such discoveries:

- When humans present with signs and symptoms that can be connected to a specific chemical exposure. This may occur with acute pesticide poisoning or carbon monoxide poisoning. It often occurs when workers are occupationally exposed. In such instances, the temporal and geographic relationships to the exposures and health effects help to identify health hazards *in the environment* (e.g., the diagnosis of mesothelioma from asbestos exposure).
- When large accidental releases of chemicals occur in a community that contaminate air, water, or food, resulting in health effects. Such events show us how toxic chemicals are to humans and animals. For example, in the Love Canal incident, outside of Buffalo, NY, a whole community was affected by hazardous chemicals that were dumped on the land where a housing development was built.
- In rare instances, when human environmental (and occupational) epidemiological studies have been performed. Through such studies, we have learned about the toxic effects of chemicals.

However, the most common way in which the relationships between chemical exposures and health risks are identified is when toxicologists study the effects of chemicals on animals and [we] then estimate what the effects might be on humans. This estimation process is called *extrapolation*. More than 100,000 man-made (synthetic) chemical compounds have been developed and introduced to our environment since World War II, and we are most often reliant on the data that are created in animal studies to warn us about their potential toxicity to humans. For many of these chemicals, no toxicity data are available (Sattler and Lipscomb, 2002). Surprisingly, there is no current requirement for original toxicological research to be completed when a product or process is being brought to market.

> **NURSING TIP** *When a woman is pregnant for the first time, this is an ideal time to help her assess and reduce or eliminate preventable environmental health risks in her home and workplace. A good environmental health history can help to uncover a number of exposures from the products she may use, the ways in which she addresses pests in her home and garden, or the way in which she may be setting up a new nursery room.*

We live in a radically different environment compared to a century ago. In addition to man-made pollutants contaminating our air, water, and food, many of the same pollutants are now also found in our bodies (including breast milk). In 2001, the Centers for Disease Control and Prevention began **biomonitoring**—the testing of human fluids and tissues for the presence of potentially toxic chemicals, as part of its National Health and Nutrition Exam Study. For instance, most Americans carry pesticides, solvents, heavy metals and other potentially toxic

chemicals in their bodies. In 2005 an Environmental Working Group tested the umbilical cord blood of newborn babies and found that they also contained a wide range of potentially harmful chemicals (EWG, 2005). Each of these potentially hazardous substances creates a health risk. Nurses need to understand the environmental exposures and the health effects that may be associated with chemicals.

ENVIRONMENTAL HEALTH SCIENCES

Toxicology

Toxicology is the basic science applied to understanding the health effects associated with chemical exposures. It is sometimes referred to as the "study of poisons." Its corollary in health care is pharmacology, which studies the human health effects, both desirable and undesirable, associated with drugs. In toxicology, only the negative effects of chemical exposures are studied. However, the key principles of pharmacology and toxicology are the same. Just as the dose of a drug makes the difference in its efficacy and its toxicity, the quantity of an air or water pollutant to which we may be exposed can determine whether or not we experience the risk of a health effect. In addition, the timing of the exposure—over the human life span—can make a difference. For example, during embryonic and fetal development, exposure to toxic chemicals can create immediate harm or create a critical pathway for future disease. Very young children, whose systems are still immature, are also more vulnerable to exposures. Just as is true of medications, the same dose that one would give an adult will have a much greater effect on a child and certainly on a fetus.

Both drugs and pollutants can enter the body from a variety of routes. Most drugs are given orally and absorbed by the gastrointestinal (GI) tract. Water- and food-associated pollutants, including pesticides and heavy metals, enter the body via the digestive tract. Some drugs are administered as inhalants, and some pollutants in the air (including indoor air) enter the body via the lungs. Some drugs are applied topically. In work settings, employees can receive dermal exposures from toxic chemicals when they immerse their unprotected hands in chemical solutions, especially solvents. Pollution can enter our body via the lungs (inhalation), GI tract (ingestion), skin, and even the mucous membranes (dermal absorption). Most chemicals cross the placental barrier and can affect the fetus, just as most chemicals cross the blood–brain barrier. In addition to direct damage to cells, tissues, organs and organ systems, there can be changes to the DNA from chemical exposures that can change gene expression which, in turn, can predict disease. This latter effect is the focus of a relatively new biological study: **epigenetics.** Scientists now understand that there are many variables that predict disease outcomes including environmental exposures.

In the same way that we consider age, weight, other drugs taken, and underlying health status of a client when we administer drugs, we must consider that these same factors may affect the way in which individual members of the community respond to environmental exposures. For example, children are much more vulnerable to virtually all pollutants. People who are immunosuppressed (people with HIV/AIDS or those on immunosuppressant drugs like steroids or anti-cancer medications) and have autoimmune diseases are especially at risk for food-borne and waterborne pathogens. This includes people who are HIV/AIDS positive, who have been prescribed chemotherapeutic drugs, or who are organ recipients. Because our communities are comprised of people of different ages and different health statuses, their vulnerabilities to the effects of pollution will also vary. When assessing a community's environmental health status, be sure to review the general health status of the community and to identify members who may have higher risk factors.

Chemicals are often grouped into categories or "families" so that it is often possible to understand the actions and risks associated with those groupings. Examples are metals and metallic compounds (e.g., arsenic, cadmium, chromium, lead, mercury), hydrocarbons (e.g., benzene, toluene, ketones, formaldehyde, trichloroethylene), irritant gases (e.g., ammonia, hydrochloric acid, sulfur dioxide, chlorine), chemical asphyxiants (e.g., carbon monoxide, hydrogen sulfide, cyanides), and pesticides (e.g., organophosphates, carbamates, chlorinated hydrocarbons). Although some common health risks exist within these families of chemicals, the possible health risks for each chemical should be evaluated individually when a potential human exposure exists. The best source of peer-reviewed information for this is the National Library of Medicine (NLM).

> **NURSING TIP**   *All nursing assessments, whether individual or community wide, must consider environmental exposures that may contribute to illness. With the identification of health risks, the development of a risk reduction plan should quickly follow.*

Epidemiology

Whereas toxicology is the science that studies the poisonous effects of chemicals, **epidemiology** is the science that helps us understand the strength of the association between exposures and health effects. Epidemiology is often used for occupationally related illnesses but has been used less often to study environmentally related diseases. It is difficult to characterize and/or distinguish from the many exposures that we all experience, and it can be challenging to find control groups when the environmental exposure of concern is in the air, water, or food.

Epidemiological studies have helped us to understand the association between learning disabilities and exposure to lead-based paint dust, asthma exacerbation and air pollution (Van den Hazel, Zuurbier, and Babisch, 2006), and GI disease and waterborne *Cryptosporidia* (Goldman, 2000). Environmental surveillance, such as childhood lead registries, provides data with which to track and analyze incidence and prevalence of health outcomes. The results of such analyses can help to target scarce public health resources. Scientists are now approaching epidemiology at the molecular level, looking at gene/environment interactions.

As described in Chapter 12, three major concepts—agent, host, and environment—form the classic **epidemiological triangle** (McKeown and Weinrich, 2000). (See Figure 12-2, *A* in Chapter 12.) This simple model belies the often complex relationships between **agent,** which may include chemical mixtures (i.e., more than one agent); **host,** which may refer to a community with people of multiple ages, genders, ethnicities, cultures, and disease

states; and **environment,** which may include dynamic factors such as air, water, soil, and food, as well as temperature, humidity, and wind. Limitations of environmental epidemiological data include reliance on occupational health studies to characterize certain toxic exposures. The occupational health studies were performed on healthy adult workers whose biological systems were different from those of neonates, pregnant women, children, people who are immunosuppressed, and the elderly. Nevertheless, nurses can review epidemiological studies regarding exposures of concern to their communities and use epidemiological techniques to assess environmental risks in communities.

Another research tool for environmental health studies is **geographic information systems (GIS),** a methodology that requires the coding of data so that it is related spatially to a place on Earth. By combining such geographically related data, maps can be created to note where the data may be related. For instance, by taking a data set that geographically notes where children under 10 years of age live and overlaying another data set that notes geographical areas designated by the age of housing stock, a public health nurse could see where there are the largest number of children who live in areas with older housing stock. With this information, the nurse could target a lead surveillance and educational program. Nurse researcher Mona Choi used GIS to study the relationship between air pollution and emergency visits for cardiovascular and pulmonary diagnosis. Community-based maps that are created using GIS technologies are helpful in educating community members and local policy makers. The maps can provide useful graphic depictions of public health problems.

Environmental health requires a combination of tried and tested nursing tools mixed with new tools, such as GIS, and the recognition that many disciplines may be involved in the identification and the resolution of environmental health issues.

EVIDENCE-BASED PRACTICE

A risk assessment was performed for population subgroups living on, and growing food on, urban sites. Soil collected in community gardens in urban areas was tested for the presence of heavy metals (e.g., lead, cadmium, copper, nickel, and zinc), which are known to be absorbed by garden vegetables. Risks from other exposure pathways were also estimated. A hazard index was created, and the results showed that food grown on 92% of the urban area presented minimal risk to the average person. However, more vulnerable subpopulations, including highly exposed infants and children, were at greater risk. This study indicates the importance of site-specific assessment in determining whether a site is suitable for use as an urban garden.

What advice should the public health nurse offer when neighbors are developing a community garden? Is there a government agency that will perform soil testing? What should be done if the soil has high heavy-metal contamination (Hough et al, 2004)?

Nurse Use

An alert has been issued by the federal government that the use of IV tubing that contains diethylhexyl phthalates (DEHP) can create a risk of testicular problems for neonatal boys. What "population-based" intervention can a hospital-based nurse develop to address this risk?

Hough RL, Breward N, Young SD, et al: Assessing potential risk of heavy metal exposure from consumption of home-produced vegetables by urban populations, *Environ Health Perspect* 112:215-225, 2004.

Nurse scientists Wade Hill and Patricia Butterfield developed a model for environmental risk interventions, which can be provided by public health nurses, that improves children's health by addressing home-related sources such as lead paint, contaminated drinking water, and environmental tobacco smoke, among others. These risks can cause health effects ranging from minor learning deficiencies to serious and life-threatening diseases such as cancer. Many of the environmental risks children encountered were prevented or reduced by taking practical and affordable steps (Hill and Butterfield, 2006).

Multidisciplinary Approaches

In addition to toxicology and epidemiology, there are a number of earth sciences to help us understand how pollutants travel in air, water, and soil. Geologists, meteorologists, physicists, and chemists all contribute information to help explain how and when humans may be exposed to hazardous chemicals, radiation (e.g., radon), and biological contaminants. Key public health professionals include food safety specialists, sanitarians, radiation specialists, and industrial hygienists.

The nature of environmental health demands a multidisciplinary approach to assess and decrease environmental health risks. For instance, in order to assess and address a lead-based paint poisoning case, we might include a housing inspector with expertise in lead-based paint or a sanitarian to assess the lead-associated health risks in the home; clinical specialists to manage the client's health needs; laboratories to assess the blood lead levels, as well as lead levels in the paint and house dust and drinking water; and then lead-based paint remediation specialists to reduce the lead-based paint risk in the home. We might also add a health educator and outreach worker to educate the family and encourage compliance with environmental health behaviors and clinical treatments. This approach could potentially involve the local health department, the state department of environmental protection, the housing department, a primary and tertiary care setting, and public or private sector labs. The nurse's responsibility is to understand the roles of each respective agency and organization, know the public health laws (particularly as they pertain to lead-based paint poisoning), and work with the community to coordinate services to meet their needs. The nurse also might set up a blood lead screening program through the local health department, educate local health providers to encourage them to systematically test children for lead poisoning, or work with advocacy organizations to improve the condition of local housing stock.

| **DID YOU KNOW?** *Although we have great scientific certainty about the toxicity of lead, and although lead-based residential paint has been banned in the United States since 1978, it is still manufactured and widely used throughout the developing world.*

GLOBAL WARMING/CLIMATE CHANGE

Global warming and the associated long-term warming trends over the last century have been well established, and climate change scientists are projecting substantial disruption in water supplies, agriculture, ecosystems, and coastal communities. There are two concurrent categories of roles for nurses: mitigation and response. There is still much we can do to mitigate the steep upward slope that we are now observing for temperatures, CO_2 levels, and sea water levels. Working at the individual, community, institutional (school, hospital, etc.), and governmental level, there is much work to be done to ensure energy-conserving policies and practices, rational transportation practices, and changes in our consumption patterns.

Regarding response preparation, public health nurses must lead the development of contingencies for long-term, high-heat weather conditions, as well as increased storm activities (that include more severe storm patterns) and the associated disaster preparedness. Nurses should also be prepared for threats to food security from shifting weather patterns that may not support food production as usual. Nurses should be prepared for population migration away from low-lying, coastal regions, creating a new type of refugee migration. The oil spill in the U.S. Gulf which was the largest in history has caused devastating damage to the Gulf of Mexico. It is expected that its effects on birds, fish, and other sea animals, as well as the environment, will last for many years to come. Since fish populations were affected, many fishermen have lost their jobs and the livelihood that they knew (Gulf Oil Spill, n.d.). This type of mobilization will be typical if the projections for global warming are not reversed.

ASSESSMENT

There are a number of ways to assess environmental health risks. For example, risks can be assessed by medium: air, water, soil, or food. In addition, exposures can be listed according to urban, rural, or suburban settings. Nurses may also divide the environment into functional locations such as home, school, workplace, and community. Each of these locations will have unique environmental exposures, as well as overlapping exposures. For instance, ethylene oxide, the toxic gas that is used in the sterilizing equipment in hospitals, is typically only found in a workplace. However, pesticides might be found in any of the four areas. When assessing environments, be sure to determine if an exposure is in the air, water, soil, and/or food and whether it is a chemical, biological, or radiological exposure.

Information Sources

The NLM has developed some of the most useful, comprehensive, and reliable sources of environmental health information. The NLM's website for ToxTown (http://toxtown.nlm.nih.gov/) is one of the best places to start when developing environmental assessment skills. Within ToxTown, there is a new Household Products page where nurses can research common products such as personal care products, cleaning products, pet care products, lawn care products, and others to see the potential health risks that may be associated with them. Also, chemicals can be researched by brand or chemical name or by Chemical Abstract System number. (The NLM website can be accessed through the WebLinks feature of this textbook's website or at www.nlm.nih.gov; at the website, search for the environmental assessment section.)

Another database that is specific to personal care products, which includes over 40,000 products that can be searched by brand name and specific product descriptors, is the *Safe Cosmetics* database (www.safecosmetics.org). This database provides information on how to protect your health such as by selecting products that have simpler ingredients and few synthetic chemicals and has a "skin deep" data base where readers can assess products for toxicity. For example, the site points out that even top selling brands of natural and organic products may have some toxic components. Specifically, they say that some top selling herbal shampoos contain 1,4-dioxane which is a synthetic chemical carcinogen. They also comment on the number of lipsticks that they found to contain lead. Note that in both the NLM and the Safe Cosmetic databases, the information is predicated on what the manufacturers place on the label as ingredients. If the manufacturer claims that a component is a "trade secret," it will not appear on the label. Rarely are the chemicals that make up a "fragrance" listed on the label; instead, it is likely to only read "fragrance" on the label. And finally, especially with pesticides, the label may merely say "inerts" without any further information regarding their chemical identify. Thus, it is sometimes impossible to make a true assessment about the health risks based on the information provided by the manufacturer.

As seen in Box 10-1, one of the ANA Environmental Health Principles is the tenet of the "Right to Know," which recommends the need for access to all information needed to make informed decisions and protect our health. There are still a number of ways in which full disclosure of chemical exposure is lacking in terms of air and water pollution, food contents, and product ingredients. Nurses can be advocates for increasing access to information through legislative and regulatory efforts both individually and through their professional organizations.

HOW TO Apply the Nursing Process to Environmental Health

If you suspect that a client's health problem is being influenced by environmental factors, follow the nursing process and note the environmental aspects of the problem in every step of the process:

1. *Assessment. Use your observational skills (e.g., windshield surveys); interview community members; ask your individual clients; and ask the families of your clients. Review Web-based data on existing exposures, such as air and water pollution monitoring data, drinking water testing, and contaminated soil.*
2. *Diagnosis. Relate the disease and the environmental factors in the diagnosis.*
3. *Goal setting. Include outcome measures that mitigate and eliminate the environmental factors.*
4. *Planning. Look at community policy and laws as methods to facilitate the care needs for the client; include environmental health personnel in planning.*
5. *Intervention. Coordinate medical, nursing, and public health actions to meet the client's needs. Ensure that the affected person or family is referred for appropriate clinical care.*
6. *Evaluation. Examine criteria that include the immediate and long-term responses of the client as well as the recidivism of the problem for the client.*

Public and private water utility companies are required to test drinking water in accordance with the EPA's drinking water standards. The results of this testing must be made available to consumers including an annual summary, called a Consumer Confidence Report. Nurses can check with their local drinking water supplier and request a copy of the Consumer Confidence Report, which is often found on the water suppliers' websites. This report will indicate the source of the drinking water and a review of any time the standards were exceeded in the previous year.

Environmental Exposure History

When working with individuals, it is important to include environmental health risks as part of a client's history. We are reminded to ask certain questions to assess exposures that may occur in all of the settings in which we spend time. A helpful mnemonic was developed to assist health professionals in remembering the areas of concern when taking an environmental history: "I PREPARE." The mnemonic (outlined in Box 10-4) can be used when interviewing an individual client or when assessing a family, or it can be adapted for use with a group of community members.

DID YOU KNOW?   *Radon, a naturally occurring element that is found in the earth's crust and can seep into basements and into ground water, is the second leading cause of lung cancer in the United States, second only to smoking.*

Environmental Health Assessment

Nurses have developed several exposure assessment tools, including forms for pregnant women, home and school assessments, community-wide assessments, and assessment tools for hospital-related exposures. The WebLinks on the Evolve site for this book include several examples of environmental assessment tools.

A windshield survey is a helpful first step in understanding the potential environmental health risks in a community. If the community is urban, the age and condition of the housing stock and potential trash problems (and the associated pest problems) can be determined easily by driving around the neighborhood. Note proximity to factories, dump sites, major transportation routes, and other sources of pollution. In rural communities, note if and when there are aerial and other types of pesticide and herbicide spraying, if people rely on wood-burning stoves, if there are industrial-type agricultural practices, and/or if there are contaminated waterways.

Some helpful tools supplement those used in a general community assessment when nurses focus on the environmental health risks in a community. The Right to Know section of this chapter (p 227) contains a description of the types of information that are available to the public about air and water pollutants, drinking water quality, and other environmental sources or exposures. In addition, Appendix F.3 presents an example of a community health assessment tool.

The term *nature-deficit disorder* was coined by author Richard Louv in his book *Last Child in the Woods* to describe what

BOX 10-4 THE "I PREPARE" MNEMONIC

- **I**nvestigate Potential Exposures
- **P**resent Work
- **R**esidence
- **E**nvironmental Concerns
- **P**ast Work
- **A**ctivities
- **R**eferrals and Resources
- **E**ducate

Do an Exposure History to

- Identify current or past exposures.
- Reduce or eliminate current exposures.
- Reduce adverse health effects.

Taking an Exposure History: Questions to Consider
I—Investigate Potential Exposures
Investigate potential exposures by asking:

- Have you ever felt sick after coming in contact with a chemical, such as a pesticide or other substances?
- Do you have any symptoms that improve when you are away from your home or work?

P—Present Work
At your present work:

- Are you exposed to solvents, dusts, fumes, radiation, pesticides, or other chemicals?
- Are you exposed to loud noise?
- Do you know where to find material safety data sheets for chemicals with which you work?
- Do you wear personal protective equipment?
- Are work clothes worn home?
- Do co-workers have similar health problems?

R—Residence

- When was your residence built?
- What type of heating do you have?
- Have you recently remodeled your home?

- What chemicals are stored on your property?
- Where is the source of your drinking water?

E—Environmental Concerns

- Are there environmental concerns in your neighborhood (i.e., air, water, soil)?
- What types of industries or farms are near your home?
- Do you live near a hazardous waste site or landfill?

P—Past Work

- What are your past work experiences?
- What job did you have for the longest period of time? Have you ever been in the military, worked on a farm, or done volunteer or seasonal work?

A—Activities

- What activities and hobbies do you and your family pursue?
- Do you burn, solder, or melt any products?
- Do you garden, fish, or hunt?
- Do you eat what you catch or grow?
- Do you use pesticides?
- Do you engage in any alternative healing or cultural practices?

R—Referrals and Resources
Use these key referrals and resources:

- Environmental Protection Agency (www.epa.gov)
- National Library of Medicine—Toxnet Programs (www.nlm.nih.gov)
- Agency for Toxic Substances and Disease Registry (www.atsdr.cdc.gov)
- Association of Occupational and Environmental Clinics (www.aoec.org)
- Occupational Safety and Health Administration (www.osha.gov)
- EnviRN website (www.enviRN.umaryland.edu)
- Local Health Department, Environmental Agency, Poison Control Center

E—Educate (A Checklist)

- Are materials available to educate the client?
- Are alternatives available to minimize the risk of exposure?
- Have prevention strategies been discussed?
- What is the plan for follow-up?

Prepared by Grace Paranzino, RN, MPH, for the Agency for Toxic Substances and Disease Registry. For more information, contact ATSDR at 1-888-42-ATSDR or visit ATSDR's website at http://www.atsdr.cdc.gov.

happens to young people who become disconnected from their natural world. Louv links this lack of nature to some of the most disturbing childhood trends, such as the rises in obesity, attention disorders, and depression (Louv, 2005). Policy makers, educators, and children's health advocates are considering their roles in addressing this issue.

Positive environmental factors such as green spaces (e.g., gardens and parks), streetscapes, bike paths, and water features within a community can positively contribute to a community's health. Recent attention has been paid to the importance of "walkable communities," access to nature, and other concerns included in the ideas about "Smart Growth" or "Sustainable Communities."

Air

Air pollution is a significant contributor to human health problems, and a sign that regulatory efforts are not completely effective. Nurses can have a role in addressing both the health problems and the policies affecting the exposures. Air pollution

BOX 10-5 CRITERIA AIR POLLUTANTS (NATIONAL AMBIENT AIR QUALITY STANDARDS)

- Ozone (ground level)
- Sulfur dioxide
- Nitrogen dioxide
- Particulate matter
- Carbon monoxide
- Lead

is divided into two major categories: point source and non–point source. **Point sources** are individual, identifiable sources such as smoke stacks. They are sometimes referred to as fixed sites. **Non–point sources** come from more diffuse exposures. For instance, the largest non–point source of air pollution is from mobile sources such as cars and trucks, which are the greatest single source of air pollution in the United States. The Clean Air Act regulates air pollution from point and non–point sources. Box 10-5 presents a listing of the air pollutants that comprise

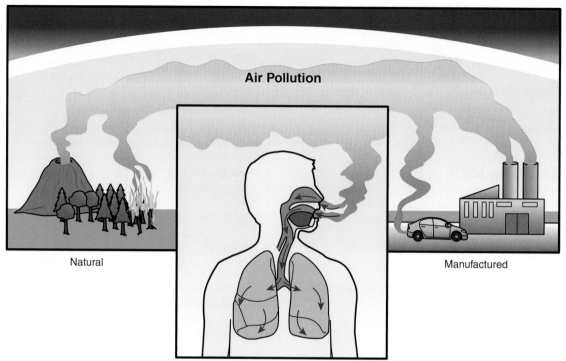

FIGURE 10-2 The air can become polluted both by natural sources as well as manufactured sources of pollution. These sources can have a cumulative effect on health. (Agency for Toxic Substances and Disease Registry: How Does Air Pollution Affect Me? Centers for Disease Control and Prevention, Atlanta, Georgia, retrieved March 2011 from http://www.atsdr.cdc.gov/general/theair/html.)

the "criteria pollutants"—a set of pollutants that the EPA uses to gauge the overall air quality. The burning of fossil fuel (e.g., diesel fuel, industrial boilers, and coal-fired power plants) and waste incineration are two other major contributors.

> **DID YOU KNOW?** *The mercury emitted from coal-fired power plants is the single largest source of mercury pollution in the United States—emitting 80,000 pounds a year into the air.*

Many people do not know that the mercury contained in a single fever thermometer is sufficient to contaminate a 25-acre lake and make fish unfit to eat. Although mercury thermometers have largely been replaced with mercury-free digital devices, the mercury persists in our fresh waterways and oceans from which we continue to get our fish. Health effects associated with air pollution include asthma and other respiratory diseases, cardiovascular diseases (including cardiac disorders and hypertension), cancer, immunological effects, reproductive health problems including birth defects, infant death, and neurological problems.

Indoor air quality (IAQ) is a growing public health concern in office buildings, schools, and homes and is reflected in the alarming rise in asthma incidence in the United States, particularly among children. The EPA and the American Lung Association both provide excellent materials on IAQ. The EPA has a free kit called *IAQ: Tools for Schools,* which includes a video and a number of helpful materials for people interested in improving the air quality in a school building. The major

culprits contributing to poor indoor air are carbon monoxide, dusts, molds, pests and pets, pesticides, cleaning and personal care products (particularly aerosols), lead, and of course environmental tobacco smoke.

Because environmental health implies a relationship between the environment and our health, we must assess both the environmental exposures and the human health status within a community. Health status is assessed by using local, state, and national health data or by collecting our own data, or a combination of the two. As we learn more about the exposures in our communities and their known or suspected health effects, we may target the health statistics we wish to review or collect (Figure 10-2).

> **DID YOU KNOW?** *You can learn about the major pollutants being released into your zip code area and other geographically related environmental information by accessing http://www.epa.gov/enviro/.*

Water

Water is necessary for all life forms. Human bodies consist of 70% water. Only 2.5% of the water on this planet is fresh water; the rest is salt water. Much of the freshwater is in the polar ice-caps, whereas groundwater makes up most of what remains, leaving only 0.01% in lakes, creeks, streams, rivers, and rainfalls. People's lives are inextricably tied to safe and adequate water. Water is necessary for the production of food. In the United States, all public water suppliers must test their water in accordance with the EPA's safe drinking water standards and they must summarize the results of their testing annually and make them available to their customers—those who pay water bills. Nurses can request this summary from the water suppliers that serve their communities. Private wells are not regulated and need not be tested except when they are first drilled. Nurses should encourage people with private wells to have them tested annually.

Pollution discharges into water bodies from industries and from wastewater treatment systems can contribute to the *degradation* of water quality. Water quality is also affected by non–point sources of pollution, such as storm water runoff from paved roads and parking lots, erosion from clear-cut tracts of land for timbering and mining, and runoff from chemicals added to soils such as pesticides and fertilizers.

> **DID YOU KNOW?** *One ton of virgin paper kills about 24 trees. Using recycled paper decreases unnecessary logging, and the associated environmental degradation caused by deforestation leads to the release of carbon, which contributes to greenhouse gases, and increased soil erosion, which compromises water quality. Eighty percent (80%) of the world's forests are gone.*

Land

Current and past land use can affect a community's health. Local governments dictate land use through zoning laws. For instance, zoning decisions can determine if a community will have a hazardous waste site built in its neighborhood or whether the land can only be used for residential purposes (housing). Historically, communities in which poor people and people of color live have been more likely to have undesirable and unhealthy industries. In many communities, prior use of the land has left a legacy of unhealthy contaminants. There are two designations for lands that may be contaminated: Superfund sites (highly contaminated sites, with associated health threats that are designated by the EPA) and Brownfield sites (land that has been used previously and may be perceived to pose health threats *and* which is now slated for redevelopment). Public health nurses can play an important role with both Superfund and Brownfield sites related to the health assessment.

> **THE CUTTING EDGE** *Antibiotics, codeine, 17β-estradiol (an estrogen replacement hormone), and acetaminophen (Tylenol) have been found in measurable quantities in U.S. streams and rivers.*

> **DID YOU KNOW?** *Of the thousands of personal care products on the market, including cosmetics, only 11% of them have been tested for potential health risks from the chemical ingredients.*

Food

Many health risks are associated with food and food production. In recent years, we have seen foodborne illnesses associated with *Salmonella* and *Escherichia coli* H:0157:H7 in chicken, eggs, and meats. Good food preparation practices, such as proper washing and using adequate cooking temperatures and time, can prevent foodborne illnesses associated with most pathogens. However, there are also environmental health risks posed by the presence of pesticide residues in our food; the use of recombinant bovine growth hormone (rBGH) that are given to many dairy cows; the administration of antibiotics to beef cattle, pigs, and chickens at non-therapeutic doses that are given to promote growth; and the use of genetically modified organisms (GMOs) for genetically engineered crops.

When assessing a community's environmental health risks, a nurse must consider air, water, soil, and food.

Right to Know

Several environmental statutes give the public the "right to know" about the hazardous chemicals in the environment. Under one of the "right to know" laws, health professionals and community members can easily access key information by zip code regarding major sources of pollution that are being emitted into the air or water in their community. The EPA has an "Envirofacts" section on its website that provides several sources of exposure data by zip code (http://www.epa.gov/enviro/).

When a water supplier provides drinking water to a community, the supplier, in contrast to individual wells, must test the water and report the results to its customers in the form of a consumer confidence report. Nurses should review the consumer confidence reports, sometimes referred to as "right to know" reports, to determine what pollutants have been found in the drinking water. If the drinking water poses an immediate health threat, the water provider must send emergency warnings out to the community via the local newspapers, radios, and television. A federal law, the Freedom of Information Act, allows citizens to request many different kinds of public documents, including information about environmental permits and inspections.

> **WHAT DO YOU THINK?** *Access to information on the existence of toxic substances leaching into the water table of a community should be withheld from the public until the government completes negotiations with the party responsible for the toxic substance.*

Employees have the "right to know" about the hazardous chemicals with which they work through the federal Hazard Communication Standard. This standard requires employers (including hospitals) to maintain a list of all of the hazardous chemicals that are used on site. Each of these chemicals should have an associated chemical information sheet known as a material safety data sheet (MSDS), which is written by the chemical manufacturer. These MSDSs are to be made available to any employee or his or her representative (e.g., a union) and should provide information about the chemicals that constitute the product, the health risks, and any special guidance on safe use or handling (e.g., requirements for protective gloves or respiratory tract protection). This standard is enforced by the Occupational Safety and Health Administration. For more extensive information on workplace health and safety, see http://www.osha.gov.

Risk Assessment

Currently, the EPA uses a process referred to as "risk assessment" when they develop health-based standards. The term **risk assessment** refers to a process to determine the probability of a health threat associated with an exposure. The following illustration of a chemical exposure demonstrates the four phases to a risk assessment:

1. Determining if a chemical is known to be associated with negative health effects (in animals or humans). For this, we rely on toxicological and/or epidemiological data. (Remember, the available toxicological data will probably be based on animal studies and these studies estimate the potential effects on humans, whereas the results of the epidemiological studies will be for human health effects.)

2. Determining whether the chemical has been released into the environment—into the air, water, soil, or food. This is accomplished by testing for the presence of the suspected chemical in the various media (air, water, soil, food). Environmental professionals such as sanitarians, food inspectors, air and water pollution scientists, environmental engineers, and others might be involved in this activity. When doing a risk assessment, it is important to note if there are multiple sources of the chemical in question. For example, is lead found in the drinking water, the ambient air, *and* in the paint within the houses of a given community?

3. Estimating how much and by which route of entry the chemical might enter the human body—inhalation, ingestion, dermally, or in utero exposure. This estimate can be based on a one-time exposure, a short-term exposure, or a projected lifetime exposure. (When federal standards are created for air, water, and other pollutants, they are based on an estimation of a lifetime exposure. However, in workplace settings the chemical exposure standards are based on an average exposure during a typical work shift or set for a maximum exposure at any given time.)

4. Characterizing the risk assessment process and taking into account all three of the previous steps. Is the chemical toxic? What is the source and amount of the exposure? What is the route and duration of the exposure for humans? The final synthesis attempts to predict the potential for harm based on the estimated exposure.

Both point and non–point sources of pollution must be considered. Remember, when a pollutant is a point source, it means that there is a single place from which the pollutant is released into the environment such as a smoke stack, a hazardous waste site, or an effluent pipe into a waterway. Non–point source implies a more diffuse source of pollution, such as traffic or fertilizer or pesticide runoff into waterways (whether from large-scale farming operations or from individual lawns and gardens). Another non–point source for both chemical and biological contamination is animal waste from wildlife or animal operations for food production (beef and dairy cows, hogs, and poultry). Manure can flow into nearby water bodies and result in coliform contamination and nutrient overload that can contribute to waterborne illnesses, as well as create conditions amenable to toxic algae growth, such as *Pfiesteria piscicida* (Burkholder et al, 2005).

All science is *subject to interpretation* and so is risk assessment. The reason that environmental laws are so often contentious is because there are economic interests at stake and not just public or ecological health concerns. In translating the risk assessment results for the purposes of policy development and recommendation for risk reduction activities, there are often several interpretations of each of the risk assessment steps that then result in differing recommendations for health-based standards. There are also areas of scientific uncertainty that contribute to variations in assessment of risk.

> **DID YOU KNOW?**   *New carpets release chemicals that can often be detected because of their odors. This is known as off-gassing, and these emissions can be harmful, especially for those who have allergies, asthma, or sensitivities to chemical products.*

Assessing Risks in Vulnerable Populations: Children's Environmental Health

Consider some of the current childhood health statistics for which environmental factors are associated: Asthma is at an all time high (Yang, 2005). More than 1 in 10 children and youth have a mental health problem, including hyperactivity disorder, anxiety, and depression (USPHS, 2000; Costello et al, 2003). Autism has increased 1000% since the mid-1980s (Previc, 2007). Developmental disorders and attention deficit hyperactivity disorder (ADHD) collectively are estimated to affect 17% of school-age children (AHRQ, 2002; Anney et al, 2006). Child and adolescent obesity has more than tripled since the 1960s (CDC, 2008). Several cancers have increased in children, including acute lymphocytic leukemia and cancers of the brain and nervous system (NCI, 2002). According to the American Cancer Society (ACS), about 5% of all cancers are strongly associated with heredity (ACS, 2010). The rest occur from environmental exposures and other damages that occur during our lifetimes.

Cancer is the second most common cause of death in children between 1 and 14 years, and nearly one-third of these cancers are leukemias. Over the past 25 years there has been great improvement in the 5-year survival rate of major childhood cancers. The 5 year survival rate for children for all cancer sites improved from 58% for those diagnosed between 1975 and 1977 and 81% for children diagnosed between 1999 and 2007 (Jemal et al, 2010). The list of possible causes of children's cancer includes the following: genetic abnormalities; ultraviolet and ionizing radiation; electromagnetic fields; viral infections; certain medications; food additives; tobacco; alcohol; and industrial and agricultural chemicals (Schmidt, 1998; Ross and Olshan, 2004; Bassil et al, 2007). Clearly, the environment is playing an important role.

> **WHAT DO YOU THINK?**   *When building a school, should the government require the same environmental assessment of the land as it would if a commercial enterprise, like a hotel, was being placed on the same site? (Currently, it requires less stringent environmental assessments.)*

Children are not just little adults. They are different in many ways, particularly with regard to their exposures and responses to the environment. As nurses, we know that infants and young children breathe more rapidly than adults, and this increase in respiratory rate translates to a proportionately greater exposure to air pollutants. While infants' lungs are developing, they are particularly susceptible to environmental toxicants. Although full function of the lungs is attained at approximately age 6, changes continue to occur in the lungs through adolescence (Dietert et al, 2000). Children are short and, as such, their breathing zones are lower than adults, causing them to have closer contact to the chemical and biological agents that accumulate on floors and carpeting. Children of color and poor children in America are disproportionately affected by a range of environmental health threats, including lead, air pollution, pesticides, incinerator emissions, and exposures from hazardous waste sites (Powell and Stewart, 2001; Faber and Krieg, 2002; Landrigan, Suk, and Amler, 1999; Silbergeld and Patrick, 2005; Suk and Davis, 2008).

> **DID YOU KNOW?** *Considerable electricity is wasted each day as a result of leaving the lights on; therefore saving 1 hour of wasted lighting daily will decrease the amount of carbon dioxide greenhouse gas emissions.*

In clinical settings, there is little that can be done to address a child's body burden of toxic chemicals; however, the nursing community as a profession has a weighty obligation to understand the science and risks associated with environmental pollutants and to engage in the political and economic decisions regulating the environment that have a profound effect on human health, especially the health of our children. This engagement occurs in policy-making arenas including legislative, regulatory, and international treaties. Nurses have increasingly become involved in the policy arena.

> **DID YOU KNOW?** *Children are more able to absorb calcium and other nutrients, an important mechanism for growing bodies. However, this increased process also enhances the uptake of potentially harmful chemicals such as lead and other heavy metals.*

Children's bodies also operate differently. Some of the protective mechanisms that are well developed in adults, like the blood–brain barrier, are immature in young children, thereby increasing their vulnerability to the effects of toxic chemicals. And finally, the kidneys of young children are less effective at filtering out undesirable toxic chemicals, and these chemicals then continue to circulate and accumulate.

Infants and young children drink more fluids per body weight than adults, thus increasing the dose of contaminants found in their drinking water, milk (hormones and antibiotics), and juices (particularly pesticides). If an adult were to drink a proportionate amount of water to an infant, the adult

---

BOX 10-6 PROVISIONS UNDER THE FOOD QUALITY PROTECTION ACT REGARDING PESTICIDE EXPOSURE TO CHILDREN FROM MULTIPLE SOURCES

New provisions under the Food Quality Protection Act of 1996 related to protection of infants and children:

- *Health-based standard:* A new standard of a reasonable certainty of "no harm" that prohibits taking into account economic considerations when children are at risk.
- *Additional margin of safety:* Requires that the EPA use an additional 10-fold margin of safety when there are adequate data to assess prenatal and postnatal development risks.
- *Account for children's diet:* Requires the use of age-appropriate estimates of dietary consumption in establishing allowable levels of pesticides on food to account for children's unique dietary patterns.
- *Account for all exposures:* In establishing acceptable levels of a pesticide on food, the EPA must account for exposures that may occur through other routes, such as drinking water and residential application of the pesticide.
- *Cumulative impact:* The EPA must consider the cumulative impact of all pesticides that may share a common mechanism of action.
- *Tolerance reassessments:* All existing pesticide food standards must be reassessed over a 10-year period to ensure that they meet the new standards to protect children.
- *Endocrine disruption testing:* The EPA must screen and test all pesticides and pesticide ingredients for estrogen effects and other endocrine disruptor activity.
- *Registration renewal:* Establishes a 15-year renewal process for all pesticides to ensure that they have up-to-date science evaluations over time.

From Environmental Protection Agency: *Food Quality Protection Act of 1996.* Available at http://www.epa.gov/pesticides/regulation/laws/fgpa/. Accessed December 15, 2010.

---

would have to drink about 50 glasses of water a day. Children also eat more per body weight, eat different proportions of food, and absorb food differently than adults (Bucubalis and Balisitreri, 1997; Tickner and Hoppin, 2000). How many adults could eat the same amount of raisins pound-for-pound as the average 2-year-old? Children consume much greater quantities of fruits and fruit juices than adults, once again adding exposure to doses of pesticide residues. The average 1-year-old drinks 21 times more apple juice, 11 times more grape juice, and nearly 5 times more orange juice per unit of body weight than the average adult (Rawn et al, 2004). The Food Quality Protection Act (FQPA) was passed to specifically address the consumption patterns and special vulnerabilities of children (Box 10-6).

Toxic chemicals can have different effects depending on the timing of exposure. During fetal development, there are periods of exquisite sensitivity to the effects of toxic chemicals. During such times, even extraordinarily small exposures can prevent or change a process that may permanently affect normal development. The brain undergoes rapid structural and functional changes during late pregnancy and in the neonatal period. Therefore, it is extremely important to *safeguard* women's environments when they are pregnant (Table 10-1).

TABLE 10-1	ENVIRONMENTAL AGENTS IMPLICATED IN ADVERSE REPRODUCTIVE OUTCOMES
EXPOSURE	**KNOWN/SUSPECTED EFFECT**
Anesthetic compounds	Infertility, spontaneous abortion, fetal malformations, low birth weight
Antineoplastics	Infertility, spontaneous abortion
Dibromochloropropane	Sperm abnormalities, infertility
Ionizing radiation	Infertility, microcephaly, chromosomal abnormalities, childhood malignancies
Lead	Infertility, spontaneous abortion, developmental disabilities
Manganese	Infertility
Organic mercury	Developmental disabilities, neurological abnormalities
Organic solvents	Congenital malformations, childhood malignancies
CBs, PBBs	Fetal mortality, low birth weight, congenital abnormalities, developmental disabilities

Data from Aldrich T, Griffith J: *Environmental epidemiology and risk assessment*, New York, 1993, Van Nostrand Reinhold.

> **DID YOU KNOW?**   *Developmental toxicants such as lead, mercury, and pesticides may directly interfere with any of the processes required for normal brain development.*

Alarmingly, 27 states have issued mercury contamination advisories for fish in *every* lake and river within their state's borders (EPA, 2009). According to the EPA, more than 1 million women in the United States of childbearing age eat sufficient amounts of mercury-contaminated fish to risk damaging brain development of their children. Nurses in all settings need to understand the implications that the fish advisories have for their clients and communities, and the contribution that the health sector has in creating this health risk, while at the same time counseling on the positive contribution of fish to a nutritionally balanced diet.

About 100,000 chemicals are used in the industrialized world. Almost all are man made; 15,000 of them are produced annually in quantities greater than 10,000 lb and 2800 of them are produced in quantities greater than 1 million lb per year (Goldman and Koduru, 2000). Of the 2800, only 7% have been tested for developmental effects and only 43% have been tested for any human health effects. As of December 1998, only 12 chemicals had complete tests for developmental neurotoxicity at the EPA (Schettler et al, 2000).

Companies are not required to divulge all the results of their private testing. A full battery of neurotoxicity tests is not required even for pesticides that may be sprayed in nurseries and labor and delivery areas, not to mention in homes. To make things even more complicated, risks from multiple chemical exposures are rarely considered when regulations are

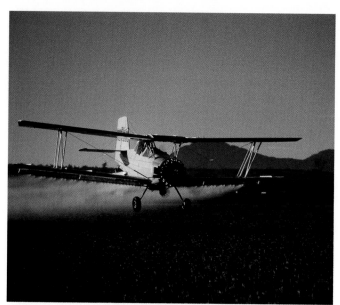

FIGURE 10-3 Agricultural aircraft is often used to apply fertilizers, pesticides, and fungicides to crops. (Copyright © 2011 Photos.com, a division of Getty Images. All rights reserved. Photo #87531230.)

drafted. Such an omission ignores the reality that both children and adults are exposed to many toxic chemicals, often concurrently. The only exception to this rule is in the case of regulations regarding pesticides that are used on food (Figure 10-3). This new exception was created by the 1996 FQPA, in which Congress acknowledged that children eat foods that may be contaminated by more than one pesticide residue. See Box 10-6 for the provisions under the FQPA.

PRECAUTIONARY PRINCIPLE

With thousands of chemical compounds now creating a chemical soup in air and water (in our bodies, in our breast milk), it is increasingly difficult to prove specific hypotheses regarding the relationship of exposure to a singular chemical and disease outcome in humans. It has been suggested that we adopt a "precautionary approach" when animal research and other indicators demonstrate a possible toxic relationship between a chemical and health effect. Box 10-7 presents the *Wingspread Statement on the Precautionary Principle*. This "precautionary approach" calls for action to reduce potentially toxic exposure to humans in light of data or other indicators, rather than delaying until more "conclusive" studies are performed. Nurses, who are trained in disease prevention, appreciate and should advocate for a precautionary approach when it may prevent injuries or illnesses. The ANA has adopted the precautionary principle as the basic tenet on which to guide its environmental advocacy work.

The bottom line is that life depends on the environment, and what humans do collectively can affect this vital resource for present and future generations. A central concept in Native American cultures is that humans are stewards, not proprietors, of the environment. Native Americans make the "Rule of Seven" central to all environmental decisions: What will be the effect on the seventh generation? A quote (Myths-Dreams-Symbols,

BOX 10-7 WINGSPREAD STATEMENT ON THE PRECAUTIONARY PRINCIPLE

In 1998 an international group of health and public health professionals, scientists, government officials, lawyers, grassroots activists, and labor activists met at a conference center called "Wingspread" in Wisconsin to define the "precautionary principle." The group issued the following consensus statement:

The release and use of toxic substances, the exploitation of resources, and physical alterations of the environment have had substantial unintended consequences affecting human health and the environment. Some of these concerns are high rates of learning deficiencies, asthma, cancer, birth defects and species extinctions, along with global climate change, stratospheric ozone depletion and worldwide contamination with toxic substances and nuclear materials.

We believe existing environmental regulations and other decisions, particularly those based on risk assessment, have failed to protect adequately human health and the environment the larger system of which humans are but a part.

We believe there is compelling evidence that damage to humans and the worldwide environment is of such magnitude and seriousness that new principles for conducting human activities are necessary.

While we realize that human activities may involve hazards, people must proceed more carefully than has been the case in recent history. Corporations, government entities, organizations, communities, scientists and other individuals must adopt a precautionary approach to all human endeavors.

Therefore, it is necessary to implement the Precautionary Principle: When an activity raises threats of harm to human health or the environment, precautionary measures should be taken even if some cause and effect relationships are not fully established scientifically. In this context the proponent of an activity, rather than the public, should bear the burden of proof.

The process of applying the Precautionary Principle must be open, informed and democratic and must include potentially affected parties. It must also involve an examination of the full range of alternatives, including no action.

From *Wingspread Statement on the Precautionary Principle*, Conference, Wingspread Conference Center, Racine, WI, January 1998. Available at http://www.gdrc.org/u-gov/precaution-3.html. Accessed December 15, 2010.

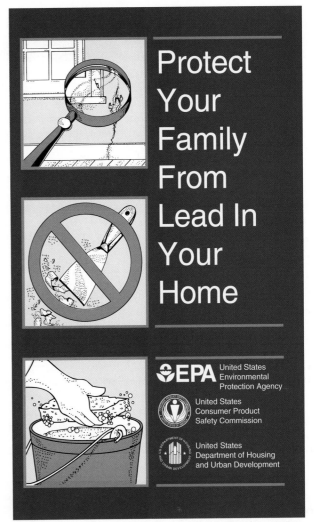

FIGURE 10-4 Lead can be found in many places in a home. Nurses should help families learn about these sources and take actions to remove the lead. (From U.S. Environmental Protection Agency. Available at http://www.epa.gov/lead/pubs/leadpdfe.pdf. Accessed December 29, 2010.)

2006) attributed to Chief Seattle, a nineteenth-century Native American, illustrates the need to think more holistically when we consider environmental impacts: "Whatever befalls the earth befalls the sons of the earth. Man did not weave the web of life; he is merely a strand in it. Whatever he does to the web, he does to himself."

Mary O'Brien, in her book *Making Better Environmental Decisions: An Alternative to Risk Assessments*, notes that we are repeatedly given a very short list of risk reduction choices, and that the public is not effectively engaged in the decision-making process. She suggests that a broader range of options would allow us to see the possibilities for further reducing (or even eliminating) risks and that the process should be much more democratic in nature. O'Brien suggests the best approach to making effective environmental decisions is to use information, emotion and a sense of relationship to others concurrently. By others she means other species, cultures and generations (O'Brien, 2000). Her method is consistent with a nursing approach. Using her approach will require that nurses more actively engage in assessing environmental health risks, developing risk reduction strategies, and supporting policies that embrace the precautionary principle.

REDUCING ENVIRONMENTAL HEALTH RISKS

Prevention is a core goal in every public health intervention. Preventing problems is less costly whether the cost is measured in resources consumed or in human effects. Education is a primary preventive strategy. As we explore the sources of environmental health risks in our communities, we can apply the basic principles of disease prevention when planning intervention strategies. For lead exposure, remediating a home with lead-based paint in order to make it lead safe applies the primary prevention strategy of removing the exposure (at least from that specific source of lead) (Figure 10-4). Good lead poisoning surveillance will not prevent lead exposure, but may help with early detection of rising blood lead levels. This surveillance is a secondary prevention strategy. Finally, when a symptomatic child is seen,

BOX 10-8 RISK REDUCTION: EVERYONE'S ROLE IN PROTECTING THE ENVIRONMENT

Everyone has a role in protecting the environment. The decisions and choices that we make as individuals and as a society can have a profound effect on the health of our environment. Our individual choices to drive versus use public transportation and our societal choice to invest in public transportation can significantly affect our air quality, which can quickly affect our collective health status.

In Atlanta, during the 1996 Olympics, residents of Atlanta and the surrounding area were encouraged to either work from home or take public transportation on the days that the Olympic games were engaged. This resulted in a significant drop in emergency department visits for asthma because there was less car-related pollution.

For car-related air pollution, there are many options for reducing pollution. We could:

- Take public transportation.
- Choose less polluting cars.
- Add an additional tax to polluting cars (thus creating an incentive for purchasing less polluting cars).
- Create a tax incentive to the car manufacturers for making less polluting cars (as well as the consumers who buy them).
- Encourage flexible work policies that allow people to work at home when possible.
- Build adequate sidewalks and paths in communities to encourage walking and biking.

Each of these is a risk management choice. Similar options could be described for water protection or the promotion of healthy indoor environments in buildings, such as schools.

BOX 10-9 INDUSTRIAL HYGIENE HIERARCHY OF CONTROLS*

- Substitute less hazardous or non-hazardous substances (e.g., using water-based vs solvent-based products).
- Isolate the hazardous chemicals from human exposure (e.g., use closed systems).
- Apply engineering controls (e.g., ventilation systems, including exhausts).
- Reduce the exposures through administrative controls (e.g., rotating employees).
- Use personal protective equipment (e.g., gloves, respirators, protective clothing).

From Levy B, Wegman D: *Occupational health: recognizing and preventing work-related disease and injury*, ed 4, Philadelphia, 2000, Lippincott Williams & Wilkins.
*In addition, education is a critical tool in the hierarchy of controls.

BOX 10-10 THE 3 Rs FOR REDUCING ENVIRONMENTAL POLLUTION

The 3 Rs adage of the environmentalist community—*reduce, reuse,* and *recycle*—helps us to consider ways to decrease our impact on the environment, and thereby decrease environmental health risks. These concepts can apply to our health care settings, as well as our homes. By recycling, we prevent the need to extract more resources from the earth in order to manufacture products. By recycling, we also prevent products from unnecessary landfilling or incineration. Choosing reusable products, versus single-use devices and products, similarly prevents the need for manufacturing more products and decreases the waste stream. Reducing our waste stream can also be accomplished generally by a reduction in consumption (buying less "stuff," as well as by reducing unnecessary packaging and other non-essential goods). The "Story of Stuff" (www.thestoryofstuff.org) provides an excellent overview of the "cradle to grave" travels of products and the full range of their human and ecological impacts.

it is important to have a health care system readily available in which specialists familiar with lead poisoning will provide swift medical interventions to reduce blood lead levels, thus reducing the risk of further harm. This is a tertiary prevention response. Box 10-8 presents examples of risk reduction strategies.

For workplace exposures, industrial hygienists have developed a "hierarchy of control" for avoiding or minimizing employee exposures to potentially hazardous chemicals. Industrial hygienists are public health professionals who specialize in workplace exposures to hazards—physical, chemical, and biological—that create the conditions for health risks (Box 10-9

presents the **Industrial Hygiene Hierarchy of Controls**). Once it is established that a human health threat exists, develop a plan of action—a way of eliminating or managing (reducing) the risk. **Risk management** should be informed by the risk assessment process and involves the selection and implementation of a strategy to eliminate or reduce risks. This can take many forms. Box 10-10 lists the 3 Rs for reducing environmental pollution. For example, in order to reduce the risk from exposure to ultraviolet rays, avoid being outside during peak sun hours, wear protective clothing, and/or wear sunscreen. To reduce exposure to dangerous heavy metals, special processes can be used at the water filtration plant that supplies the public water. Running the cold water tap for 1 or 2 minutes before collecting water for coffee or drinking each morning will reduce the presence of lead, which may have leached from old pipes overnight. Individuals, communities, and/or nations can work to reduce risks. In recent years, there have been global agreements to reduce persistent pollutants and decrease global warming.

Nursing interventions to reduce environmental health risks can also take many forms. Education is one example of a nursing intervention. By working with a wide array of community members, nurses can help a community understand the relationship between harmful environmental exposures and human health and guide the community toward risk reduction on the basis of both individual behavior changes as well as community-wide approaches.

Nurses work with individuals, families, and communities in all three levels of prevention. For example, in Planned Parenthood Clinics in the United States, as a form of primary prevention, clinicians ask clients about possible environmental health risks in their everyday lives and then direct them to safer products and healthier behaviors to decrease exposures from potentially toxic exposures. When pediatric clinics include lead screening as part of their protocols, they are apt to find children with elevated blood lead levels, which then allow them to act to decrease the child's environmental lead exposures. This intervention is secondary prevention. It does not actually prevent the exposure but calls for action based on evidence of exposure. If a child has a seriously high blood lead level, the child

LEVELS OF PREVENTION

Example Applied to Lead Exposure

Primary Prevention
Use only non-lead based paint.

Secondary Prevention
If lead is found in paint, remove this paint and replace with non-lead paint.

Tertiary Prevention
At the first sign of symptoms of lead exposure, take steps to reduce blood lead levels.

---

would be admitted to the hospital for chelation therapy, a process to decrease the body's burden of lead. This level of intervention is tertiary prevention. It neither prevents the exposure, nor focuses on decreasing the exposure, but rather focuses on decreasing the potential health sequela associated with elevated lead levels.

Risk Communication

Risk communication is both an area of practice and a skill that is a composite of two separate words: "risk" and "communication." *Risk* is a familiar term in nursing practice. It is recognized in counseling regarding risks of pregnancy, communicable disease (especially sexually transmitted disease), unintentional injury, and personal choices (e.g., smoking, alcohol consumption, and diet). Risk assessment in environmental health focuses on characterizing the hazard (the "source"), its physical and chemical properties, its toxicity, and the presence of or potential for the other elements in the exposure pathways—mode of transmission, **route of exposure,** receptor population, and dose. In their seminal work on risk communication, Sandman, Chess, and Hane (1991) noted that risk has traditionally been formulated as magnitude (the size, severity, extent of area, or population affected) multiplied by the probability (how likely exposure or damage is to occur) (Box 10-11). For example, an environmental risk assessment of a contaminated site would involve a calculation of the dose that might be received through all routes of exposure, the toxicity of the chemical, the size and vulnerability (age, health) of the population potentially exposed (resident, future resident, transient), and the likelihood of exposure. Sandman, Chess, and Hane also noted that the reaction to things that scare people and the things that kill people are often not related to the actual hazard. They have gone further to probe what is behind those differences and identified a list of 20 outrage factors to explain people's responses to risk (Box 10-12). They maintain that the outrage is just as predictable and open to intervention as the science of addressing the hazard.

"Communication" of risk involves understanding the outrage factors relevant to the risk being addressed so they can be incorporated in the message—the information—either to create action to ensure safety or prevent harm or to reduce unnecessary fear. An example of raising outrage to produce action can be seen in the shift from emphasis on smokers (voluntary) to victims of passive smoking (involuntary) to stimulate public

---

BOX 10-11 DEFINITIONS OF RISK

Risk has traditionally been defined by the following equation:

$$Risk = magnitude \times probability$$

There is a growing body of literature from practitioners and researchers who have studied the human reaction to risk—real and perceived. Sandman et al (1991) were the first to examine the "outrage" factor that can influence the way in which we perceive risk, particularly to environmental risks.

$$Risk = hazard + outrage$$

Addressing only the hazard is doing only half of the necessary work; addressing the response (outrage) is equally important.

From Sandman PM, Chess C, Hane BJ: *Improving dialogue with communities,* New Brunswick, NJ, 1991, Rutgers University.

BOX 10-12 OUTRAGE FACTORS: CHARACTERISTICS OF RISK THAT CONTRIBUTE TO THE PUBLIC'S FEELING OF OUTRAGE

SAFER = LESS OUTRAGE	LESS SAFE = MORE OUTRAGE
12 Principal Outrage Components	
Voluntary	Involuntary (coerced)
Natural	Industrial (artificial)
Familiar	Exotic
Not memorable	Memorable
Not dreaded	Dreaded
Chronic	Catastrophic
Knowable (detectable)	Unknowable (undetectable)
Individually controlled	Controlled by others
Fair	Unfair
Morally irrelevant	Morally relevant
Trustworthy sources	Untrustworthy sources
Responsive process	Unresponsive process
8 Secondary Outrage Components	
Affects average populations	Affects vulnerable populations
Immediate effects	Delayed effects
No risk to future generations	Substantial risk to future generations
Victims statistical	Victims identifiable
Preventable	Not preventable (only reducible)
Substantial benefits	Few benefits (foolish risk)
Little media attention	Substantial media attention
Little opportunity for collective action	Much opportunity for collective action

---

policy that limits or bans smoking in public places. When the emphasis on risk went from a voluntary choice of smokers to an involuntary exposure of non-smokers, the outrage level of the non-smoking public became high enough to result in legislation guaranteeing smoke-free public spaces (e.g., public buildings, airplanes, and restaurants).

On the other hand, outrage decreases when people receive information on the situation from a trusted source, and physicians and nurses are often cited in surveys as trusted sources of information on environmental risks (University of Newcastle upon Tyne, 2001-2002). The public trust is a compelling incentive to match professional knowledge and skills to a community's expectations. The outrage factor can also be a driving force in building credibility and trustworthiness in every person whose work involves interacting with the public.

Risk communication includes all the principles of good communication in general. It is a combination of the following:

- *The right information:* Accurate, relevant, in a language that audiences can understand. A good risk assessment is essential information for shaping the message.
- *To the right people:* Those affected and those who are worried but may not be affected. Information on the community is essential: geographic boundaries, who lives there (i.e., demographics), how they obtain information (e.g., flyers or newspapers, radio, television, word of mouth), where they congregate (e.g., school, church, community center), and who within the community can help plan the communication.
- *At the right time:* For timely action or to allay fear.

Ethics

Nurses need to understand ethics for making their own choices, in describing issues and options within groups, and in advocating for ethical choices. When the controversial points of an issue are about competing "goods"—such as jobs versus environmental protection or production versus conservation—the skillful nurse can change the discussion from "either/or" to "both" by opening new possibilities for both ethical and mutually satisfactory outcomes. Ethical issues likely to arise in environmental health decisions are as follows:

- Who has access to information and when?
- How complete and accurate is the available information?
- Who is included in decision making and when?
- What and whose values and priorities are given weight in decisions?
- How are short- and long-term consequences considered?

Governmental Environmental Protection

The government manages environmental exposures through the promulgation and enforcement of standards and regulations that may limit a polluter's ability to put hazardous chemicals into food, water, air, or soil. The government may also be involved in educating the public about risks and risk reduction. Many federal agencies are involved in environmental health regulation, such as the EPA, the FDA, and the Department of Agriculture. Every state has an equivalent state agency. At the city or county level, environmental health issues are most often managed by the local health department. However, environmental protection issues are typically directed by the state using both federal and state laws (Box 10-13).

Potentially harmful pollution that cannot be prevented must be controlled. The first step in the process of controlling pollution is permitting, a process by which the government places limits on the amount of pollution emitted into the air or water. A permit is a legally binding document.

Environmental standards may describe a permitted level of emissions, a maximum contaminant level (MCL), an action level for environmental clean-up, or a risk-based calculation; environmental standards are required to address health risks. It is the responsibility of potential polluters to operate within the standards. Compliance and enforcement are the next building blocks in controlling pollution. Compliance refers to the processes for ensuring that permit/standard requirements are met. Clean-up or remediation of environmental damage is another control step. Public information and involvement processes, such as citizen advisory panels or community forums, are integral to the development of standards, on-going monitoring, and remediation.

ADVOCACY

There are almost 3 million nurses in the United States today—approximately 1 in every 100 Americans is a registered nurse! Nurses can and should be a strong voice for a healthy environment. As informed citizens, nurses can take a variety of actions to protect the environmental health of families, clients, and communities. Nurses are perceived as trusted messengers and as reliable sources of environmental health information and as such, have a responsibility to be informed and take action in the best interest of public health. Often, legislators are called to vote on environmental legislation without a sound understanding of how the legislation may affect public health. Nurses can serve as a resource for state and federal legislators and their staff. Although every nurse may not be an expert in all aspects of environmental health, every nurse does have a basic education in human health and has a sufficient understanding of who may be most vulnerable to environmental insult. Nurses' thoughts about the potential impacts of new laws on the health of individuals and communities are valuable to legislators and other policy makers.

Grounded in science and using sound risk communication skills, nurses become the most credible sources of information at community gatherings, formal governmental hearings, and professional nursing forums. Nurses, as trusted communicators, must not be silent when they are informed about environmental health issues. Nurses work as advocates for environmental justice so that all members of the community have a right to live and work in an environment that is healthy and safe. They also volunteer to serve on state, local, or federal commissions, and they know about zoning and permit laws that regulate the impact of industry and land use on the community. Many nurse legislators began their careers by advocating for the rights of others. Nurses must read, listen, and ask questions. Then, as informed citizens, they will be leaders, fostering community action to address environmental health threats.

In 2008 the Alliance of Nurses for Healthy Environments was created to coalesce individual nurses and nursing organizations around issues associated with the environmental exposures and human health. This organization addresses the integration of environmental health into nursing education, practice (including greening the health care sector), research, and advocacy.

Environmental Justice and Environmental Health Disparities

Some diseases differentially affect different populations. Certain environmental health risks disproportionately affect poor people and people of color in the United States. If you are a

BOX 10-13 ENVIRONMENTAL LAWS

National Environmental Policy Act (NEPA)

The NEPA established the Environmental Protection Agency (EPA) and a national policy for the environment and provides for the establishment of a Council on Environmental Policy. All policies, regulations, and public laws shall be interpreted and administered in accordance with the policies set forth in this act.

Federal Insecticide, Fungicide, and Rodenticide Act (FIFRA)

FIFRA provides federal control of pesticide distribution, sale, and use. The EPA was given the authority to study the consequences of pesticide usage and requires users such as farmers and utility companies to register when using pesticides. Later amendments to the law required applicators to take certification examinations, registration of all pesticides used in the United States, and proper labeling of pesticides that, if in accordance with specifications, will cause no harm to the environment (summary from FIFRA, 1972).

Clean Water Act (CWA)

The CWA sets basic structure for regulating pollutants to U.S. waters. The law gave the EPA the authority to set effluent standards on an industry basis and continued the requirements to set water quality standards for all contaminants in surface water. The 1977 amendments focused on toxic pollutants. In 1987 the CWA was reauthorized, and again focused on toxic pollutants, authorized citizen suit provisions, and funded sewage treatment plants.

Clean Air Act

The Clean Air Act regulates air emissions from area, stationary, and mobile sources. The EPA was authorized to establish National Ambient Air Quality Standards (NAAQSs) to protect public health and the environment. The goal was to set and achieve the NAAQSs by 1975. The law was amended in 1977 when many areas of the country failed to meet the standards. The 1990 amendments to the Clean Air Act intended to meet unaddressed or insufficiently addressed problems such as acid rain, ground level ozone, stratospheric ozone depletion, and air toxics. Also in the 1990 reauthorization, a mandate for Chemical Risk Management Plans was included. This mandate requires industry to identify "worst case scenarios" regarding the hazardous chemicals that they transport, use, or discard (summary from Clean Air Act, 1970).

Occupational Safety and Health Act (OSHA)

The OSHA was passed to ensure worker and workplace safety. The goal was to make sure employers provide an employment place free of hazards to health and safety such as chemicals, excessive noise, mechanical dangers, heat or cold extremes, or unsanitary conditions. To establish standards for the workplace, the Act also created NIOSH (National Institute for Occupational Safety and Health) as the research institution for OSHA.

Safe Drinking Water Act (SDWA)

The SDWA was established to protect the quality of drinking water in the United States. The Act authorized the EPA to establish safe standards of purity and required all owners or operators of public water systems to comply with primary (health-related) standards.

Resource Conservation and Recovery Act (RCRA)

The RCRA gave the EPA the authority to control the generation, transportation, treatment, storage, and disposal of hazardous waste. The RCRA also proposed a framework to manage non-hazardous waste. The 1984 Federal Hazardous and Solid Waste Amendments to this Act required phasing out land disposal of hazardous waste. The 1986 amendments enabled the EPA to address problems from underground tanks storing petroleum and other hazardous substances.

Toxic Substances Control Act (TSCA)

The TSCA gives the EPA the ability to track the 75,000 industrial chemicals currently produced or imported into the United States. The EPA can require reporting or testing of chemicals that may pose environmental health risks and can ban the manufacture and import of those chemicals that pose an unreasonable risk. TSCA supplements the Clean Air Act and the Toxic Release Inventory.

Comprehensive Environmental Response, Compensation, and Liability Act (CERCLA or Superfund)

This law created a tax on the chemical and petroleum industries and provided broad federal authority to respond directly to releases or threatened releases of hazardous substances that may endanger public health or the environment.

Superfund Amendments and Reauthorization Act (SARA)

SARA amended the Comprehensive Environmental Response, Compensation, and Liability Act with several changes and additions. These changes included increased size of the trust fund; encouragement of greater citizen participation in decision making on how sites should be cleaned up; increased state involvement in every phase of the Superfund program; increased focus on human health problems related to hazardous waste sites; new enforcement authorities and settlement tools; emphasis of the importance of permanent remedies and innovative treatment technologies in cleanup of hazardous waste sites; and Superfund actions to consider standards in other federal and state regulations. (Under Superfund legislation, the Federal Agency for Toxic Substances and Disease Registry was established.)

Emergency Planning and Community Right to Know Act (EPCRA)

The EPCRA, also known as Title III of SARA, was enacted to help local communities protect public health safety and the environment from chemical hazards. Each state was required to appoint a State Emergency Response Commission that was required to divide their state into Emergency Planning Districts and establish a Local Emergency Planning Committee (LEPC) for each district.

National Environmental Education Act

The National Environmental Education Act created a new and better coordinated environmental education emphasis at the EPA. It created the National Environmental Education and Training Foundation.

Pollution Prevention Act (PPA)

The PPA focused industry, government, and public attention on reduction of the amount of pollution through cost-effective changes in production, operation, and use of raw materials. Pollution prevention also includes other practices that increase efficient use of energy, water, and other water resources, such as recycling, source reduction, and sustainable agriculture.

Food Quality Protection Act (FQPA)

The FQPA amended the Federal Insecticide, Fungicide, and Rodenticide Act and the Federal Food, Drug, and Cosmetic Act. The Act changed the way the EPA regulates pesticides. The requirements included a new safety standard of reasonable certainty of no harm to be applied to all pesticides used on foods.

Chemical Safety Information, Site Security, and Fuels Regulatory Act (Amendment to Section 112 of Clean Air Act)

This act removed from coverage by the Risk Management Plan (RMP) any flammable fuel when used as fuel or held for sale as fuel by a retail facility (flammable fuels used as a feedstock or held for sale as a fuel at a wholesale facility are still covered). The law also limits access to off-site consequence analyses, which are reported in RMPs by covered facilities.

poor person of color, you are more likely to live near a hazardous waste site or an incinerator, and more likely to have children who are lead poisoned. You are also more likely to have children with asthma, which has a strong association with environmental exposures. Campaigns to improve the unequal burden of environmental risks in communities of color and in poor communities are striving to achieve environmental justice or environmental equity (Mood, 2002; Butterfield and Postma, 2009).

In 1993 the Environmental Justice Act was passed, and in 1994 Executive Order 12898, "Federal Actions to Address Environmental Justice in Minority Populations," was signed. This Act and the subsequent actions created policies to more comprehensively reduce the incidence of environmental *injustice* by mandating that every federal agency act in a manner to address and prevent illnesses and injuries. Nursing interventions and involvement in environmental health policies can have a significant effect on the health disparities experienced by our most challenged communities.

Unique Environmental Health Threats from the Health Care Industry: New Opportunities for Advocacy

Many choices in the health care setting affect environmental health. Nurses often lead in reducing the use of mercury-containing products in hospitals. The use of mercury-containing thermometers and sphygmomanometers leads to a risk of breakage, which releases a highly toxic substance into the workplace. Further, when a hospital uses incineration to dispose of their waste, the mercury-containing products will create significant releases of mercury into the air, thus contaminating communities. This airborne mercury will be present in raindrops, and when it lands on water bodies (e.g., lakes, rivers, or oceans), it is converted by the microorganisms in the water to methylmercury, which is highly toxic to humans. The methylmercury is then bioaccumulated in the fish: as larger fish eat smaller fish, the body burden of methylmercury increases significantly.

Many synthetic chemicals that contaminate the environment are referred to as persistent bioaccumulative toxins (PBTs) or persistent organic pollutants (POPs). These are chemicals that do not break down in air, water, or soil, or in the plant, animal, and human bodies to which they may be passed. Ultimately, since humans are at the top of the food chain, these chemicals may come to reside in our bodies. For instance, lead, which should not be found in the human body, can be found in the long bones of almost any human in the world because of its ubiquitous use and presence in our environment.

Dioxin, another pollutant that contaminates our communities, is created, in part, by the health care industry. Dioxins are created when we manufacture or burn (incinerate) products that contain chlorine, such as bleached white paper or polyvinyl chloride (PVC) plastics. Once released into the environment, they are consumed by agricultural animals (e.g., beef and dairy cows, hogs, and poultry) and fish, where they are stored in fat cells as they work their way up the food chain. This phenomenon has resulted in dioxin deposition in breast tissue and been found in both cow and human milk. Virtually all women now have dioxin in their breast tissue. Dioxin, an endocrine-disrupting chemical and a strong carcinogen, is associated with several

neurodevelopmental problems including learning disabilities and is now in every human's body. The solution to this problem is to remove dioxins from the environment.

An international campaign called Health Care Without Harm is working to reduce and eliminate mercury and PVC plastic in the health care industry, as well as the elimination of incineration of medical waste. The ANA was a founder of the Health Care Without Harm campaign, and nurses have taken many leadership roles in the activities in the United States and around the world. The Health Care Without Harm website (http://www.noharm.org) and the ANA's website (http://www.nursingworld.org/rnnoharm/) provide outstanding information and resources about pollution prevention in the health care sector.

REFERRAL RESOURCES

There is no one source of information about environmental health nor is there a single resource to which a public health nurse can refer an individual or community should an environmentally related problem be suspected. As mentioned earlier, the NLM's ToxTown is a great starting place, and it allows the interested browser to dig deeply into environmental health content. The EPA is another rich source of information. With the advent of the Internet, information is widely accessible, but finding an actual person to assist you or the communities you serve may not be as easy. One starting point may be the environmental epidemiology unit or toxicology unit of the state health department or department of environmental quality. Another local or state resource may be environmental health experts in nursing or medical schools or schools of public health. The Association of Occupational and Environmental Clinics (http://www.aoec.org) is a national network of specialty clinics and individual practitioners available for consultation and sometimes for provision of educational programs for health professionals. The federal government is supporting Pediatric Environmental Health Specialty Units around the country to provide education and consultation.

Local resources include local health and environmental protection agencies; poison control centers; agricultural extension offices; and occupational and environmental departments in schools of medicine, nursing, and public health. Some local and state agencies have developed topical directories to assist in accessing the appropriate staff for specific questions. Many of the resources have websites that allow ready access through the Internet and can be located by using any of the popular search methods. (Box 10-14 presents an extensive list of environmental health agency resources.)

ROLES FOR NURSES IN ENVIRONMENTAL HEALTH

Nurses can be involved in many environmental health roles, in full-time work, as an adjunct to existing roles, and as an informed citizen. Nurses who are passionate about this issue can develop research expertise, sit on commissions, write articles, and take national leadership roles. Other nurses can include environmental exposures in their history taking; consider the environmental impacts of the products they select for their clinics, hospitals, and other settings; and promote recycling. Each type and level of engagement is important. The following are some ways in which nurses can get involved both professionally and as informed citizens:

- *Community involvement/public participation.* Organizing, facilitating, and moderating; making public notices effective and public forums accessible; welcoming input. Making information exchange understandable and problem solving acceptable to culturally diverse communities are valuable assets a nurse contributes. Skills in community organizing and mobilizing can be essential for a community to have a meaningful voice in decisions that affect them.

- *Individual and population risk assessment.* Using nursing assessment skills to detect potential and actual exposure pathways and outcomes for clients cared for in the acute, chronic, and healthy communities of practice.

- *Risk communication.* Interpreting, applying principles to practice. Nurses may serve as skilled risk communicators within agencies, working for industries or working as independent practitioners. Amendments to the Clean Air Act require major industrial sources of air emissions to have risk

management plans and to inform their neighbors of specifics of the risks and plans (Clean Air Act, 1996).

- *Epidemiological investigations.* Nurses need to have the skills to respond in scientifically sound and humanely sensitive ways to community concerns about cancer, birth defects, and stillbirths that citizens fear may have environmental causes.

- *Policy development.* Proposing, informing, and monitoring action from agencies, communities, and organization perspectives.

The assimilation of the concepts of environmental health into a nurse's daily practice gives new life to traditional public health values of prevention, community building, and social justice. Box 10-15 presents the work of three nurses currently working in environmental health.

As nurses learn more about the environment, opportunities for integration into their practice, education programs, research, advocacy, and policy work will become evident and will evolve. Opportunities abound for those pioneering spirits within the nursing profession who are dedicated to creating healthier environments for their clients and communities.

BOX 10-14 INFORMATION AND GUIDANCE SOURCES FOR REFERRALS

The websites for each of these agencies can be accessed directly through the WebLinks feature on the book's website at http://evolve.elsevier.com/Stanhope.

Federal Agencies
- Agency for Toxic Substances and Disease Registry
- Centers for Disease Control and Prevention
- Consumer Product Safety Commission
- Environmental Protection Agency
- Office of Children's Environmental Health
- Food and Drug Administration
- National Institute for Occupational Safety and Health
- National Institute of Environmental Health Sciences
- National Institutes of Health
- National Cancer Institute
- National Institute of Nursing Research
- Occupational Safety and Health Administration
- National Library of Medicine—ToxNet

State Agencies
- State Health Departments
- State Environmental Protection Agencies

Associations and Organizations
- American Association of Poison Control Centers
- American Association of Occupational Health Nurses
- Association of Occupational and Environmental Clinics
- Beyond Pesticides
- Center for Health and Environmental Justice
- Children's Environmental Health Network
- Environmental Defense
- Environmental Working Group
- Health Care Without Harm
- National Environmental Education Foundation
- Natural Resources Defense Council
- Pediatric Environmental Health Specialty Units
- Society for Occupational and Environmental Health

BOX 10-15 EXAMPLES OF THREE MODERN-DAY ENVIRONMENTAL HEALTH NURSING PIONEERS

In Baltimore, MD, Dr. Claudia Smith (a nurse who is on the faculty at the University of Maryland) directed a project in which nurses worked with community members to address a variety of health problems associated with poor housing conditions. For this project, which was funded by the U.S. Department of Housing and Urban Development, Dr. Smith hired and trained community members to assess and reduce unhealthy conditions caused by lead-based paint, high levels of carbon monoxide, and asthma triggers (e.g., dust mites, pet dander, and pests); she taught community members about safer choices for pest control using the least toxic approach to pest management by using an integrated pest management approach.

After Denise Choiniere, a graduate student in community health who was working in the cardiac care unit (CCU) at the University of Maryland Medical Center,

learned about the health effects associated with heavy metals, she was very uncomfortable with simply throwing away the batteries that were used in the many small devices, like Holter monitors. Instead, she developed a recycling program for the CCU and the telemetry unit. She then discovered that her hospital purchased 97,000 small batteries every year. Each of these small batteries contains a heavy metal—mercury, lithium, cadmium, or lead. She was the driving force in developing a hospital-wide, small battery recycling program. This activity created a whole new career trajectory for Ms. Choiniere, who was recently appointed to the executive position of Sustainability Coordinator for the whole hospital. She has since addressed green cleaning products, promoted the recycling of "blue wrap" that is used in the operating rooms, and organized a farmers' market that

Continued

BOX 10-15 EXAMPLES OF THREE MODERN-DAY ENVIRONMENTAL HEALTH NURSING PIONEERS—cont'd

meets weekly in front of the hospital, thus bringing locally grown and sustainably farmed products to hospital employees and the surrounding community.

Dr. Robyn Gilden is a nursing faculty who worked for 5 years with communities that knew or suspected that they were living near a hazardous waste site. She learned about the many laws and agencies involved in hazardous waste site assessments and clean-ups. Hazardous wastes can affect soil, water, and air. Sources of contamination may come from old, unlined landfills; uncontrolled dump sites; spills or discharges from industry; leaking underground storage tanks (like gasoline tanks); or runoff from fields. The Agency for Toxic Substances and Disease Registry (ATSDR), a federal agency responsible for documenting the health hazards associated with environmental exposures, maintains a listing of the most problematic contaminants found at polluted sites. They include a wide range of highly toxic chemicals including arsenic, lead, mercury, vinyl chloride, benzene, polychlorinated biphenyls (PCBs), and cadmium. These toxic chemicals top the list because they are the most commonly found contaminants and pose a significant threat to human health based on routes of exposure and level of toxicity. Dr. Gilden learned about the resources that are available for the best

and most current toxicological information. The National Library of Medicine's Toxnet and ATSDR's websites, including their ToxFAQs, are some of the best sources of navigable information.

In working with communities, Dr. Gilden met with government officials, including mayors of small towns, as well as concerned parents, people from local governments, health departments, educational institutions, businesses, developers, bankers, realtors, and other community members. She has also learned about the many statutes that cover hazardous waste sites, such as the Superfund legislation (which covers the most polluted waste sites) and Brownfield's legislation (which covers contaminated sites where economic development is involved). Both these pieces of legislation mandate community involvement, which is where Dr. Gilden's community health and risk communication skills are used. Regardless of who is responsible for or in charge of a contaminated site, the nurse understands that the community must be an active and equal participant. It is the community members who will be impacted by decisions and have to live with the results of clean-up and redevelopment. As is true of most nurses, Dr. Gilden quickly became a trusted person to the community members.

CHAPTER REVIEW

■ PRACTICE APPLICATION

Below are two case scenarios related to exposure pathways. The first involved lead poisoning and the second, gasoline contamination of groundwater.

At the county health department, a 3-year-old boy named Billy presents with gastric upset and behavior changes. These symptoms have persisted for several weeks. Billy's parents report that they have been renovating their home. They had been discouraged from routinely testing their child because their insurance does not cover lead paint testing, and they could not find information on where to have the test done. Their concern has heightened with these new symptoms.

You test Billy's blood lead level and determine it is 45 mcg/dL, which is very high. You research lead poisoning and discover that there are many potential health effects of lead exposure and that children are at great risk because their bodies, especially their nervous system, are still developing. You also find that chronic lead poisoning may lead to long-term effects, such as developmental delays and impaired learning ability. You refer Billy's parents to his primary care health professional, inform the health professional of Billy's blood lead levels, and let the health professional know about the lead poisoning specialists in the nearby children's hospital. On further investigation, you find that Billy's home was built before 1950 and is still under renovation. Billy should not return to the

home. At this point, the sanitarian from the local health department tests the dust in the home and finds high lead levels. Because of Billy's age and associated behaviors, such as hand-to-mouth activities, you determine that the lead dust in the home is the probable exposure. However, you must also consider multiple sources of exposure.

A. What other sources of exposure might exist?

B. What would you include in an assessment of this situation?

C. What prevention strategies would you use to resolve this issue? At the individual level? At the population level?

A citizen calls the local health department to report that his drinking water, from a private well, "smells like gasoline." A water sample is collected, and analysis reveals the presence of petroleum products. A nearby rural store with a service station has removed its old underground gasoline storage tanks and replaced them, as required by law. Contaminated soil from the old leaking tank has been removed, and a well to monitor groundwater contamination is scheduled for installation. Sandy soil has allowed more rapid movement of the contamination through the groundwater, and the plume has reached the neighbor's drinking water well in levels that exceed the drinking water standard.

What are some possible responses?

Answers can be found on the Evolve site.

■ KEY POINTS

- Nurses need to be informed professionals and advocates for citizens in their community regarding environmental health issues.
- Models describing the determinants of health acknowledge the role of the environment in health and disease.
- For most chemical compounds in our homes, work, schools, and communities, no research has been completed to determine whether or not they will cause health effects.

- Prevention activities include education, reduction/elimination of exposures, waste minimization, energy policies, and land use planning.
- Control activities include use of technologies; environmental permitting; environmental standards, monitoring, compliance, and enforcement; and clean-up and remediation.

KEY POINTS—cont'd

- Each nursing assessment should include questions and observations concerning potential and existing environmental exposures.
- Useful environmental exposure data are difficult to acquire. Those data that exist can be used to aid in the assessment, diagnosis, intervention, and evaluation of environmentally related health problems.
- Both case advocacy and class advocacy are important skills for nurses in environmental health practice.
- Risk communication is a critical skill and must acknowledge the outrage factor experienced by communities with environmental hazards.

- Federal, state, and local laws and regulations, as well as international treaties, exist to protect the health of people from environmental hazards.
- Environmental health practice engages multiple disciplines, and nurses are important members of the environmental health team.
- Environmental health practice includes principles of health promotion, disease prevention, and health protection.
- *Healthy People 2020* objectives address both targets for the reduction of risk factors and diseases related to environmental causes.

CLINICAL DECISION-MAKING ACTIVITIES

1. Explain why the source of drinking water is important to investigate in the assessment of an unusually high number of infertility cases in a community; in increased lead levels in children from a certain school; and in an outbreak of a gastrointestinal epidemic in an agricultural community.
2. Discuss the use of the epidemiological triangle in explaining the determinants of health.

3. Discover if your jurisdiction has a law or regulation for the disclosure of lead-based paint or radon levels for personal property as part of the act of sale for real estate. If your community does not, investigate with the government officials of the community the reasons for the lack of disclosure requirement.

REFERENCES

Agency for Healthcare Research and Quality: *Focus on research: children with chronic illness and disabilities*, AHRQ Publication No. 02-M025, Rockville, MD, 2002, U.S. Department of Health and Human Services, AHRQ Publications Clearing House.

Alberg AJ, Brock MV, Samet JM: Epidemiology of lung cancer: looking to the future, *J Clin Oncol* 23:3175–3185, 2005.

Aldrich T, Griffith J: *Environmental epidemiology and risk assessment*, New York, 1993, Van Nostrand Reinhold.

American Cancer Society: *Cancer facts and figures*, 2010. Available at http://www.cancer.org. Accessed December 29, 2010.

Anney R, Hawi Z, Sheehan K, et al: Epigenetic effects in ADHD: parent-of-origin effects in image sample, *Am J Med Genet B Neuropsychiatr Genet* 141(7):736–737, 2006.

Bassil KL, Vakil C, Sanborn M, et al: Cancer health effects of pesticides: systematic review, *Can Fam Physician* 53(10):1704–1711, 2007.

Brown RC: Windows of exposure to pesticides and childhood leukemia: an analysis of the current literature, *Birth Defects Res A Clin Mol Teratol* 70(5):301, 2004.

Bucubalis JD, Balisitreri WF: The neonatal gastrointestinal tract. In Fanaroff AA, Marin RJ, editors: *Neonatal-perinatal medicine: diseases of the fetus and infant*, ed 6, New York, 1997, Mosby, pp 1288–1344.

Burkholder JM, Gordon AS, Moeller PD, et al: Demonstration of toxicity to fish and to mammalian cells by *Pfiesteria* species: comparison of assay methods and strains, *Proc Natl Acad Sci USA* 102:3471–3476, 2005.

Butterfield P, Postma J, ERRNIE research team: The TERRA framework: conceptualizing rural environmental health inequities through an environmental justice lens, *ANS Adv Nurs Sci* 32(2):107–117, 2009.

Cassens BJ: *Preventive medicine and public health*, ed 2, New York, 1992, John Wiley & Sons.

Centers for Disease Control and Prevention: *Health topics: childhood obesity*, 2008. Available at http://www.cdc.gov/HealthyYouth/obesity/. Accessed December 15, 2010.

Centers for Disease Control and Prevention: *Third national report on human exposure to environmental chemicals*, 2005. Available at http://www.cdc.gov/exposurereport/3rd/pdf/thirdreport_summary.pdf. Accessed May 23, 2006.

Clean Air Act: Risk management programs, Section 112(7), Federal Register, Part III EPA, 40 CFR, Part 68, June 20, 1996.

Clean Air Act 1970. http://www.epa.gov/lawsregs/laws/caa.html. Accessed February 25, 2010.

Collins RS: Contemplating the end of the beginning, *Genome Res* 11:641–643, 2001.

Congress of the United States, Office of Technology Assessment: *Screening and testing chemicals in commerce*, Publication No. OTA-BP-ENV-166, Washington, DC, 1995, Office of Technology Assessment. Available at http://www.wws.princeton.edu/ota/disk1/1995/9553_n.html. Accessed May 23, 2006.

Costello EJ, Mustillo S, Erkanli A, et al: Prevalence and development of psychiatric disorders in childhood and adolescence, *Arch Gen Psychiatry* 60(8):837–844, 2003.

Council on Linkages Between Academic and Public Health Practice: Core competencies for public health professionals. Washington DC, 2010. Public Health Foundation/Health Resources and Services Administration.

Dietert RR, Etzel RA, Chen D, et al: Workshop to identify critical windows exposure for children's health: immune and respiratory systems work group summary, *Environ Health Perspect* 108(suppl 3):483–490, 2000.

Environmental Genome Project, 2005. Available at http://www.niehs.nih.gov/research/supported/programs/egp/. Accessed December 15, 2010.

Environmental Protection Agency: *General fact sheet: 2008 national listing of fish advisories*, 2009. Available at http://www.epa.gov/waterscience/fish/advisories/fs2008.html. Accessed December 15, 2010.

Environmental Working Group: *Body burden—the pollution in newborns: a benchmark investigation of industrial chemicals, pollutants and pesticides in umbilical cord blood*, July 14, 2005.

Faber DR, Krieg EJ: Unequal exposure to ecological hazards: environmental injustices in the Commonwealth of Massachusetts, *Environ Health Perspect* 110(suppl):277–288, 2002.

Federal Insecticide, Fungicide, and Rodenticide Act (1972). http://www.epa.gov.ocecaagct/lfra.html. Accessed December 29, 2010.

Goldman DA: Thalidomide use: past history and current implications for practice, *Oncol Nurs Forum* 28:471–479, 2001.

Goldman LR: Chemicals and children's environment: what we don't know about risks, *Environ Health Perspect* 106:875–879, 1998.

Goldman LR: Environmental health and its relationship to occupational health. In Levy BS, Wegman DH, editors: *Occupational health: recognizing and preventing work-related disease and injury*, Philadelphia, 2000, Lippincott, Williams & Wilkins.

Goldman LR, Koduru SH: Chemicals in the environment and developmental toxicity in children: a public health and policy perspective, *Environ Health Perspect* 108:S443–S448, 2000.

Gulf Oil Spill: BP ruined the Gulf: http://www.fulf-oil-spill.us/. Accessed December 29, 2010.

Hill WG, Butterfield PG: Environmental risk reduction for rural children. In Lee HJ, Winters CA, editors: *Rural nursing: concepts, theory, and practice*, ed 2, New York, 2006, Springer.

Hough RL, Breward N, Young SD, et al: Assessing potential risk of heavy metal exposure from consumption of home-produced vegetables by urban populations, *Environ Health Perspect* 112:215–225, 2004.

Hunter DJ: Gene-environment interactions in human disease, *Nat Rev Genet* 6:287–298, 2005.

Infante-Rivard C, Labuda D, Krajinovic M, et al: Risk of childhood leukemia associated with exposure to pesticides and with gene polymorphisms, *Epidemiology* 10(5):481–487, 1999.

Jemal A, Siegel R, Xu J, Ward E: Cancer statistics 2010. American Cancer Society. http://caonline.amcancersoc.org/cgi/content/full/caac.2007.3vl. Accessed December 29, 2010.

Landrigan PJ, Suk WA, Amler RW: Chemical wastes, children's health, and the Superfund Basic Research Program, *Environ Health Perspect* 107:423–427, 1999.

Levy B, Wegman D: *Occupational health: recognizing and preventing work-related disease and injury*, ed 4, Philadelphia, 2000, Lippincott, Williams & Wilkins.

Louv R: *No child left inside: saving our children from nature-deficit disorder*, Chapel Hill, NC, 2005, Algonquin Books.

Ma X, Buffler PA, Gunier RB, et al: Critical windows of exposure to household pesticides and risk of childhood leukemia, *Environ Health Perspect* 110(9):955–960, 2002.

McKeown RE, Weinrich SP: Epidemiologic applications. In Stanhope M, Lancaster J, editors: *Community and public health nursing*, St Louis, 2000, Mosby.

Mood LH: Environmental health policy: environmental justice. In Mason DJ, Leavitt JK, editors: *Policy and politics in nursing and health care*, ed 4, Philadelphia, 2002, Saunders.

Myths-Dreams-Symbols, 2006. Available at http://www.mythsdreamssymbols.com/seattle.html. Accessed December 15, 2010.

National Cancer Institute: *National Cancer Institute research on childhood cancers*, 2002. Available at http://cis.nci.nih.gov/fact/6_40htm. Accessed June 23, 2005.

O'Brien M: *Making better environmental decisions: an alternative to risk assessment*, Cambridge, MA, 2000, MIT Press.

Pope AM, Snyder MA, Mood LH, editors: *Nursing, health and environment*, Washington, DC, 1995, Institute of Medicine, National Academy Press.

Powell DL, Stewart V: Children: the unwitting target of environmental injustices, *Pediatr Clin North Am* 48:1291–1305, 2001.

President's Cancer Panel: *Reducing environmental cancer risk: what can we do now*, Annual report 2008-2009. Released 2010. http://deainfo.nci.nih.gov/advisory/pcp/annualReports/pcp08-09rpt/PCP_Report_08_09_509.pdf

Previc FH: Prenatal influences on brain dopamine and their relevance to the rising incidence of autism, *Med Hypotheses* 68(1):46–60, 2007.

Quad Council of Public Health Nursing Organizations. Competencies for Public Health Nursing Practice. Washington DC, 2003, ASTDN, revised 2009. Accessed December 15, 2010.

Rawn DF, Roscoe V, Krakalovich T, Hanson C: *N*-methyl carbamate concentrations and dietary intake estimates for apple and grape juices available on the retail market in Canada, *Food Addit Contam* 21(6):555–563, 2004.

Ries LA, Eisner MP, Kosary CL, et al: *SEER cancer statistics review, 1975-2001*, Bethesda, MD, 2004, National Cancer Institute.

Ross JA, Olshan AF: Pediatric cancer in the United States: the Children's Oncology Group Epidemiology Research Program, *Cancer Epidemiol Biomarkers Prev* 13:1552–1554, 2004.

Sandman PM, Chess C, Hane BJ: *Improving dialogue with communities*, New Brunswick, NJ, 1991, Rutgers University.

Sattler B, Lipscomb L, editors: *Environmental health and nursing practice*, New York, 2002, Springer.

Schettler T, Stein J, Reich F, et al: *In harm's way: toxic threats to development, a report by Greater Boston Physicians for Social Responsibility, prepared for a joint project with Clean Water*, Cambridge, MA, 2000, PSR. Available at http://www.igc.org/psr/pubs.htm.

Schmidt CW: Childhood cancer: a growing problem, *Environ Health Perspect* 106:18–23, 1998.

Silbergeld EK, Patrick TE: Environmental exposures, toxicologic mechanisms, and adverse pregnancy outcomes, *Am J Obstet Gynecol* 192:S11–S21, 2005.

Suk WA, Davis EA: Strategies for addressing global environmental health concerns, *Ann N Y Acad Sci* 1140:40–44, 2008.

Tickner JA, Hoppin P: Children's environmental health: a case study in implementing the precautionary principle, *Int J Occup Environ Health* 6(4):281–288, 2000.

Turner MC, Wigle DT, Krewski D: Residential pesticides and childhood leukemia: a systematic review and meta-analysis, *Environ Health Perspect* 118(1):33–41, 2010.

University of Newcastle upon Tyne, School of Population and Health Sciences: *Barriers to effective risk communication: study of the role of a local public health department in a controversial environmental investigation—2001-2002*. Available at http://www.ncl.ac.uk/pahs/research/project/811. Accessed December 15, 2010.

U.S. Public Health Service: *Mental health: report of the surgeon general's conference on children's mental health: a national action agenda*, Washington, DC, 2000, U.S. Department of Health and Human Services.

U.S. Department of Health and Human Services: *Healthy People 2020*. Available at http://www.healthypeople.gov/2020topicsobjectives/default.aspx. Accessed January 1, 2011.

Van den Hazel P, Zuurbier M, Babisch W: Today's epidemics in children: possible relations to environmental pollution and suggested preventative measures, *Acta Paediatr Suppl* 95(453):18–25, 2006.

Wigle DT, Turner MC, Krewski D: A systematic review and meta-analysis of childhood leukemia and parental occupational pesticide exposure, *Environ Health Perspect* 117(10):1505–1513, 2009.

Wingspread Statement on the Precautionary Principle, Racine, WI, 1998. Available at http://www.gdrc.org/u-gov/precaution-3.html. Accessed December 15, 2010.

World Health Organization: *Protection of the human environment*, 2006. Available at http://www.who.int/phe/en/. Accessed December 15, 2010.

Yang KD: Asthma management issues in infancy and childhood, *Treat Respir Med* 4(1):9–20, 2005.

Yoshida T, Yamauchi H, Sun GF: Chronic health effects in people exposed to arsenic via the drinking water: dose-response relationships in review, *Toxicol Appl Pharmacol* 198:243–252, 2004.

CHAPTER 11

Genomics in Public Health Nursing

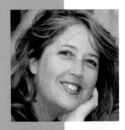

Elke Jones Zschaebitz, MSN, FNP

Elke Jones Zschaebitz has been a nurse practitioner since 1998 and has worked in the fields of school health, pediatrics and women's health, as well as telehealth practice in primary care. She has also been involved in issues of rurality, poverty, and primary care. A former instructor of nursing at the University of Virginia. School of Nursing and the UVA College at Wise for the Healthy Appalachia Institute, Zschaebitz was also in clinical practice at UVA High Risk Breast and Ovarian Cancer Center, working closely with families with a genetic or familial predisposition to breast and ovarian cancer.

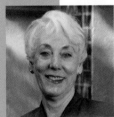

Jeanette Lancaster, PhD, RN, FAAN

Jeanette Lancaster has co-edited the previous seven editions of this textbook with Dr. Marcia Stanhope. This edition adds some new and timely chapters, including this one on genomics and its role in nursing, particularly public health nursing. Dr. Lancaster is the Medical Center Professor of Nursing at the University of Virginia, Charlottesville, VA.

ADDITIONAL RESOURCES

evolve WEBSITE
http://evolve.elsevier.com/Stanhope
• *Healthy People 2020*
• WebLinks

• Quiz
• Case Studies
• Glossary
• Answers to Practice Application

OBJECTIVES

After reading this chapter, the student should be able to do the following:

1. Define key terms related to genetics and genomics.
2. Discuss the history of genomics and its integration into public health nursing.
3. Describe the relationship between genomics, genetics, and nursing.
4. Explain the core competencies related to genomics that nurses and selected other public health professionals should integrate into their practice.
5. Describe at least three potential implications of persons knowing their genetic information on clients, families, and communities.

KEY TERMS

DNA, p. 244
family health history, p. 249
genes, p. 244
genome, p. 242

genomics, p. 242
genetics, p. 242
genetic susceptibility, p. 249
Human Genome Project, p. 243

multifactorial diseases, p. 246
mutations, p. 244
—*See Glossary for definitions*

Special thanks are given to Gia Mudd, RN, MPH, PhD, Assistant Professor, College of Nursing, University of Kentucky for reviewing the manuscript, providing public health nursing input, and providing two of the case examples.

"Mapping the human genome is the outstanding achievement not only of our lifetime but in human history. This code is the essence of mankind, and as long as humans exist, this code is going to be important and will be used."

T. Michael Dexter

THE HUMAN GENOME AND ITS TRANSFORMING EFFECT ON PUBLIC HEALTH

The mapping of the human **genome** was a strategic inflection point in the history of health care that created a massive shift in how all health professionals deliver care and how public health will be approached. The understanding of the fundamental role genetics and genomics will play in shaping the practice of public health nurses in the twenty-first century is in its early stages, although the rate of new knowledge is incredible. This chapter discusses the history of the field of genetics and genomics, what we know about genetics and genomics now, their impact on current nursing practice, and the prospects for significant changes in how nursing care is delivered. Clearly, nursing will be dramatically altered by new discoveries in molecular genetics. Examples of the effect on nursing include: (1) how nursing students will be educated, (2) how nurses will collect and use health histories, (3) how nurses will learn and apply innovative biotechnology, (4) the role genetics and genomics will play in traditional nursing arenas such as prevention and health education, (5) the administration of new therapies, and (6) in public health debates including the moral, ethical, legal, and social issues around this powerful new field of knowledge.

It is important to recognize that the fields of genetics and genomics are emerging, extremely complex, and ever changing. They have enormous implications for the detection, prevention, and treatment of human disease, not to mention educational and economic development. There is an explosion of new possibilities, such as in the prevention and treatment of human maladies ranging from cancer to cystic fibrosis and from autism to Alzheimer's disease. To understand the effects of this knowledge in public health and in nursing, it is important to pull key snapshots from this highly detailed landscape in order to begin to describe this new territory that nursing practice occupies. This chapter provides an overview of the history of the development of this new science and briefly discusses the current state of the science of genetics and genomics in relation to the role of the nurse and the future implications for care of individuals,

families, and populations. What is clear is that every nurse needs to rapidly become knowledgeable about genetics and genomics and their effects on populations.

In this chapter, the term **genetics** refers to the study of the function and effect of single genes that are inherited by children from their parents. **Genomics** is the study of all of a person's genes including their interaction with one another, as well as the interaction of a person's genes with the environment. Genomics examines the molecular mechanisms and the interplay of genetic and environmental, and of cultural and psychosocial, factors in disease. Genomics deals with the functions and interactions of all genes in an organism and is the study of the total DNA structure (Perry, 2011).

A BRIEF HISTORY OF THE SCIENCE

"The problem [with genetic research] is we're just starting down this path, feeling our way in the dark. We have a small lantern in the form of a gene, but the lantern doesn't penetrate more than a couple of hundred feet. We don't know whether we're going to encounter chasms, rock walls or mountain ranges along the way. We don't even know how long the path is…"

Francis Collins

It is important to understand the evolution of genetic and genomic knowledge. The concept of this hereditary information began with agriculture in the eighteenth century by Gregor Mendel, an Austrian monk who is usually considered to be the father of genetics. At about the same time, Charles Darwin expounded on these theories of evolution, and Darwin's cousin, Francis Galton, performed family studies using twins in an effort to understand the influence of heredity on various human characteristics.

A major breakthrough occurred on February 28, 1953 in Cambridge, England when James Watson and Francis Crick announced that they had figured out the structure of deoxyribonucleic acid (DNA), and that this double-helix structure could unzip to make copies of itself—thus confirming that

DNA carries life's hereditary information, or the secret to life (McKusick, 2007). H.J. Muller later demonstrated the genetic consequences of ionizing radiation on the fruit fly, and the theoretical basis of population genetics was developed by three prominent individuals: Ronald Fisher, J.B.S. Haldane, and Sewall Wright. Genetic diseases and their mode of inherited anomalies such as phenylketonuria, sickle cell disease, Huntington's disease, and cystic fibrosis were established. In the same decade that Watson and Crick discovered DNA, the correct specification of the number of human chromosomes was determined. Because of this 1956 discovery, for instance, one of the new findings in genetics included the discovery in 1959 that Down syndrome is caused by an extra copy of chromosome 21. The scientific revolution was underway.

To date, the Human Genome Project (HGP), an international research project funded by the U.S. Congress in 1988 and completed in 2003, has mapped all of the approximately 25,000 genes in human DNA. This enormous project reflects the work of scientists from 20 research centers in six countries: China, France, Germany, Japan, the United Kingdom, and the United States (Feetham, Thompson, and Hinshaw, 2005). The stated goals of the HGP were: *determining* the sequences of the 3 billion chemical base pairs that make up human DNA; *storing* this information in databases; *improving* tools for data analysis; *transferring* related technologies to the private sector; and *addressing* the ethical, legal, and social issues (ELSI) that may arise. The director of the Project was Francis Collins, MD. Dr. Collins and his team developed a conceptual vision for their work that had three overarching themes:

1. Genomes to biology to look at how the study of genomics would affect the future understanding of biology.
2. Genomes to health to help explain the underlying mechanisms for human health and disease including the gene-gene, gene-environment, and their interactions.
3. Genomes to society to provide the foundation for research to improve the use and interpretation of genetic and genomic information and technologies (Collins et al, 2003).

Interestingly, two key findings from early work to sequence the human genome were that all humans are 99.9% identical at the DNA level and nearly 25,000 genes make up the human genome (Perry, 2011). Most of the 0.1% genetic variations are found within and not among populations. These findings have implications for public health with its emphasis on population health.

> **DID YOU KNOW?** *Francis Collins, who directed the HGP, compared the project to a book that had many different uses. He said, "It's a history book: a narrative of the journal of our species through time. It's a shop manual, with an incredibly detailed blueprint for building every human cell. And it's a transformative book of medicine, with insights that will give healthcare providers immense new powers to treat, prevent, and cure disease" (Collins, 2006, p 1).*

Many implications for health care have emerged from this project, including ethical and moral dilemmas that continue to be challenging. As health information advances, genomics has influenced the availability of genetic tests. Many of these tests have implications for families and it is in nursing's best interest that individuals and communities understand the purpose, limitations, potential benefits, and potential risks of a test before submitting samples for analysis. The issues of genetic screening and prophylactic treatments alone are staggering and will require the full resources of the nursing profession to find answers.

> **WHAT DO YOU THINK?**
> 1. *What are some potential implications of genetic information for individuals and families?*
> 2. *What elements of genetics information need to be taken into consideration?*
> 3. *Who decides whether the test will be done?*
> 4. *Who decides what to do with the results?*

> **WHAT DO YOU THINK?**   *A Case Example: Screening for Breast or Ovarian Cancer Risk*
> During an initial visit to the High Risk Breast and Ovarian Cancer Clinic, a 37-year-old, Ms. Brown, reports that she had found a mass during a self-breast examination in 2006. She subsequently had the mass inspected by a clinician and underwent a mammogram, which showed a suspicious finding. A breast core-biopsy was performed and the pathology report indicated that she had atypical ductal hyperplasia. Ms. Brown then had a breast lumpectomy, and the lump was benign. In 1996, she had undergone a total abdominal hysterectomy and bilateral salpingo-oophorectomy for endometriosis. Ms. Brown briefly took hormone replacement therapy but stopped in 2006 when the breast mass was identified. She initiated Evista therapy as a breast cancer reduction measure, but after 6 months she stopped the medication because of the side effects. Ms. Brown reports that she is not entirely opposed to considering using Evista again. Her family history indicated that a paternal grandmother likely had a type of "female cancer." This grandmother died in her middle 30s to early 40s. There were also three cousins on the paternal side of the family who had unilateral breast cancer when they were in their 30 and 40s.
> On the maternal side of the family, her grandmother was diagnosed with breast cancer when she was in her 40s. She is alive and doing well at age 72. One of the grandmother's sisters had lymphoma and died in her late 60s. A maternal great-aunt who was a sister to her maternal grandfather, not maternal grandmother, died in her 70s of ovarian cancer. A sister to her maternal great-aunt (another maternal great-aunt) died in her 70s or 80s of a primary brain cancer.
> Reflect on these questions and see what implications they have for nursing action and for public health concerns:
> 1. *What are some possible issues that could arise if Ms. Brown has a positive test? What legal and ethical issues would you consider? What considerations would you take into account if she has a teenage daughter?*
> 2. *What effect would the client's literacy level have on how you would handle this case?*
> 3. *If you were caring for a family with multiple family members who obtain genetic testing and some members are found to be genetic mutation carriers while others are not, what would you anticipate might occur in relation to family dynamics? What actions might you take? Consider the referrals you might make.*

Over 180,000 new cases of breast cancer are diagnosed annually, and between 5% and 10% of them have an inherited susceptibility. It is important for the nurse to take a brief family pedigree as done above to identify inherited risk factors. If Ms. Brown were to have had a BRCA-1 or BRCA-2 mutation, many more implications for decision making would arise, including prophylactic surgery for prevention of breast and/or ovarian cancer. In addition, men with a BRCA-1 mutation are at increased risk to develop prostate cancer or colorectal cancer. Men who have the BRCA-2 mutation are at risk for male breast cancer and pancreatic cancer. For women, both BRCA-1 and BRCA-2 mutation carriers have the greatest risk for breast and ovarian cancer. It is important when interpreting genetic information to be sensitive to the many issues involved, including emotional, socioeconomic, lifestyle, and environmental issues that may affect the onset of disease (Calzone et al, 2010).

DNA AND ITS RELATIONSHIP TO GENOMICS AND GENETICS

At the core of the issues related to genetics and genomics is deoxyribonucleic acid (DNA). The structure of DNA is a nucleic acid that contains the genetic instructions used in the development and functioning of all known living organisms and some viruses. DNA is the chemical inside the nucleus of a cell that has the genetic instructions for making living organisms. DNA can be compared to a long-term storage or a blueprint or code to construct other components of cells such as proteins and ribonucleic acid (RNA) molecules. The DNA segments that carry the genetic information are called genes. Within cells, DNA is organized into long structures called chromosomes. These chromosomes are duplicated before cells divide, in a process called DNA replication. DNA is comprised of four bases: adenine (A), guanine (G), cytosine (C), and thymine (T). Genes are comprised of specific sequences of these bases.

Alterations in the usual sequence of bases that form a gene or changes in DNA or chromosomal structures are called muta-tions. A large number of agents are known to cause mutations (Jorde, Carey, and Bamshad, 2010). These mutations, which are attributed to known environmental causes, can be contrasted with spontaneous mutations, which arise naturally during the process of DNA replication. Approximately 3 billion DNA base pairs must be replicated in each cell division, and considering the large number of mutagens to which we are exposed, DNA replication is fascinatingly accurate (Jorde, Carey, and Bamshad, 2010). A key reason for this accuracy is a mechanism called DNA repair, which occurs in all normal cells of higher organisms. It is estimated that repair mechanisms correct at least 99.9% of initial errors.

> **DID YOU KNOW?**   *For a person living in a developed country, a typical lifetime exposure to ionizing radon is about 7 Radon Environmental Monitoring (REM), a standard unit for measuring radiation exposure. About one third to one half of this amount is thought to originate from medical and dental x-ray procedures.*

Hundreds of chemicals are now known to be mutagenic in laboratory animals. Among these are nitrogen mustard, vinyl chloride, alkylating agents, formaldehyde, sodium nitrite, and saccharin. In addition, ionizing radiation, such as those produced by x-rays and from nuclear fallout, can promote chemical reactions that change DNA bases or break the bonds of double-stranded DNA.

So what does an understanding of DNA and the science of genetics have to do with public health nursing? In essence, this brief history of the field of genetics shows that human disease comes from the collision between genetic variations and environmental factors. As knowledge has evolved with the mapping of the human genome, our understanding of this interaction continues to advance. This has increased knowledge about disease prevention and new methodologies for the practice of public health. We are learning to integrate more effectively our understanding of biological determinism within a social context.

> **DID YOU KNOW?**
> - *Most hereditary cancer syndromes are inherited in an autosomal dominant pattern with variable expression and incomplete penetrance, which means:*
>   - *Genes exist as pairs.*
>   - *A gene pair member can occur as either the normal, unaltered form or as a mutation.*
>   - *A mutation in one member of the pair is associated with an increased risk to develop certain types of cancer. If a person has a mutation in a hereditary cancer syndrome–related gene, she or he has both a normal form and an altered form of that gene in each of the cells.*
> - *Both men and women carry, pass on to children, and inherit these mutations.*
> - *For mutation carriers, the hereditary cancer syndrome can be mild or more severe.*
> - *Whether cancer ever develops, the site at which it develops, or the seriousness of the cancer can vary among different people with the same mutation, even within the same family.*
>
> *(See http://www.cancer.gov/cancertopics/factsheet/Risk/BRCA.)*

The Challenges of Genetic and DNA Testing

Tests are now available to evaluate for more than 1600 genetic disorders ranging from single-gene disorders, such as cystic fibrosis, to more complex disorders, such as diabetes (Calzone, Cashion, and Feetham, 2010). As will be discussed in a later section of the chapter, taking a family history is a useful place to begin when considering a genetic connection and prior to the onset of testing.

DNA testing was first used in the late 1970s; today, the indications for a DNA test have expanded to include predicting the development of genetic disorders, screening populations, confirming clinical diagnoses, prenatal testing, and DNA testing to develop and apply individualized medical treatment. The next few years will see an explosion in the number of DNA tests driven by information generated from the HGP. Improved technology will make DNA testing more accessible. These advances in genetics/genomics will necessitate that nurses continue to learn about this area of science in order to respond effectively to the challenges of this new knowledge.

An example of this challenge is that of genetic testing for mutations associated with a hereditary cancer syndrome. The best way to identify whether there is a mutation in a family where a hereditary cancer syndrome is suspected is to test the person who displays the most evidence of being a mutation carrier. This is usually a relative who has had a cancer that occurs typically as part of the hereditary cancer syndrome (e.g., breast or ovarian) that is suspected in the family.

The above example could present a difficulty because family members who have had cancer may not agree to being tested for genetic mutations. This refusal presents challenges to the person who desires information that might affect decision making and his or her health. An additional difficulty is that some individuals do not have an insurance carrier that reimburses for genetic testing, or they may have a high deductible in the insurance policy. Some individuals also think that testing will decrease the quality of their life and make them anxious about the future if they were to discover they have a mutation. Other people fear a positive test result may lead to feelings of guilt about passing along a disease to children and grandchildren.

Case 1

K.N. is a 42-year-old mother with three daughters, ages 16, 18, and 22. She has an extensive family history of ovarian cancer. Because of her family history, K.N. is regularly screened per current treatment guidelines. K.N.'s mother, who was diagnosed with ovarian cancer at age 55, underwent genetic testing and was discovered to be a carrier of the *BRCA-2* gene mutation predisposing to breast and ovarian cancer. Despite undergoing frequent screening, several of K.N.'s aunts have died of ovarian cancer at an early age. K.N.'s husband wants her to be tested for the *BRCA-2* gene and, if positive, has encouraged her to undergo a prophylactic salpingo-oophorectomy. K.N. is concerned that a positive genetic test may result in loss of insurance coverage. She is also concerned that this will have a negative psychological impact on her children.

Joan Akins is a public health nurse at the county health department serving the area where K.N. resides. Ms. Akins has recently conducted a cancer awareness campaign that included public health education on hereditary cancer syndromes. K.N. contacts Ms. Akins to request advice on whether to undergo genetic testing. Ms. Akins actively listens to K.N.'s concerns and provides general information on genetic testing and the implications of the test results for K.N. and for her children. She also discusses the newly enacted Genetic Information Non-discrimination Act (GINA) legislation that protects the public from genetic discrimination by employers and insurers. Ms. Akins encourages K.N. to talk with her gynecologist about her concerns and to make an appointment for genetic counseling, providing names and contact information for local genetic counselors who specialize in cancer genetics.

As mentioned, genetic testing decisions are personal and complex and can be controversial, leading to dissonance in families. It is important for public health nurses to respect individuals' and family members' decision-making processes. They must, at the same time, be well informed about genetic testing to provide accurate education to members of the public in order to support appropriate decision making.

Also, current methods of testing do not detect all of the mutations that can occur in some diseases, including hereditary cancer syndrome-related genes. If a mutation is detected during DNA testing, this would not confirm an absolute risk for cancer, but rather would indicate that a person is at increased risk to develop the cancers that are part of the particular hereditary cancer syndrome and may need high-risk management. Such a finding has implications for family members who might have inherited the same mutation, enabling them to undergo DNA testing specific to the identified mutation. Such focused testing is more accurate and cost-effective than testing for multiple potential mutations (NCI, 2010). In contrast, if DNA testing in a cancer-effected relative is negative, this does not indicate family members are not at risk. There might be a mutation in a different hereditary cancer syndrome gene than those tested. It is important to remember that many mutations associated with cancer susceptibility and familial syndromes have yet to be identified.

For these reasons, family history must also be considered. However, caution is needed in interpreting family history for several reasons: an inherited syndrome may not be evident for someone with a small family; not everyone is informed of their family's history of disease; death of a family member may be unrelated to cancer, such as early accidental death; or members may have been adopted and this may not be known to others in the family. Finally, because most cancers are not hereditary, family history should be accompanied by assessment of shared familial environments.

Case 2

Sickle cell anemia is an autosomal recessive disease in which a gene mutation results in the production of structurally abnormal hemoglobin, called hemoglobin S. Gene carriers have one normal form of the hemoglobin gene and one mutation, a condition called sickle cell trait. The highest rates of disease are among African Americans, with sickle cell anemia affecting approximately 1 in 500 African Americans and 8% of the population being carriers (anemia, sickle, National Center for Biotechnology Information [n.d.] (See http://www.ncbi.nlm.nih.gov/books/NBK22238.)

Marge Covington is a public health nurse employed by a non-profit, community-based organization that provides health care education and outreach services to members of the African American community in a large metropolitan area. The rate of sickle cell anemia among members of the community is higher than the national average. In response, Ms. Covington has implemented a program with the projected outcome to reduce disease rates among African Americans in the community. The program objectives are to: (1) increase awareness of the disease in the community, and (2) increase rates of carrier testing to support informed decision making regarding childbearing. To meet these objectives, Ms. Covington has initiated monthly educational sessions on sickle cell anemia and sickle cell trait at community centers throughout the area. She has also collaborated with a local hospital system to provide free bi-annual genetic counseling sessions with optional carrier screening at community health clinics.

Continuing education is important for public health nurses during this time of rapid integration of new genetic tests into health care practice. Only through ongoing education will public health nurses have the basis from which to appropriately educate the public regarding genetic testing. In addition, recognition of the role of gene-environment interactions in susceptibility to cancer and many other diseases underscores the importance of assessing risk from an environmental perspective. Public health nurses offer this perspective as part of the larger interprofessional team needed to address the complex issues involved in genetic testing.

CURRENT ISSUES IN GENOMICS AND GENETICS

Many issues are involved in the growing field of genetics/genomics. Selected issues will be briefly discussed here. Currently the public is not fully aware of the importance of having a family medical history. Also, many health care providers are not entirely clear about how to interpret family history of a client who has had the initiative to collect it. In addition, many clients are still reluctant to disclose this family history for fear that it would affect their health insurance status or eligibility despite current laws in place designed to protect these clients.

Another issue is a key one for public health nurses. If clients are expected to make lifestyle changes based on information about their genetic risk factors, the appropriate support and education should be available to clients and families. Nurses play an important role in answering questions and assisting in challenges these clients and families face with making decisions when there is any suspicion of increased risk for genetically based diseases. To make things more confusing, many pharmaceutical companies have begun to market their tests and advertise directly to the public. This type of marketing has implications for nurses and other health care providers who need to provide the appropriate counseling about the implications and indications for such testing. For example, marketing on the Internet complicates client decision making since it can provide consumers with easy access to genetic tests without involving a health care professional in the testing process. Even the clinically available genetic tests, which may provide legitimate test results, are difficult to interpret without genetic counseling. Currently, the Centers for Disease Control and Prevention (CDC), the Centers for Medicare Services (CMS), and the Federal Drug Administration (FDA) have oversight of genetic tests and products, whereas the Federal Trade Commission (FTC) has oversight of the advertising of these tests and products. The National Institutes of Health (NIH), Health Resources and Services Administration (HRSA), and Agency for Healthcare Research and Quality (AHRQ) support research related to genetic tests and products.

Many factors acting together typically influence disease risk, health conditions, and the therapies used to treat disease. These risks, conditions, and diseases often have a genetic/genomic element that is influenced by the environment, lifestyle, and other factors. These are considered multifactorial influences. Multifactorial disorders tend to occur in families (Perry, 2011). For example, "common congenital malformations, such as cleft lip and palate and neural tube defects, result from multifactorial inheritance, a combination of genetic and environmental factors" (Perry, 2011, p 147). Box 11-1 presents examples of

BOX 11-1 EXAMPLES OF MULTIFACTORIAL DISORDERS

- Neural tube disorders
- Cleft lip, palette
- Congenital heart disease
- Coronary artery disease
- Type I diabetes
- Type II diabetes
- Breast cancer
- Colon cancer
- Lung cancer
- Rheumatic heart disease
- Alcoholism
- Multiple sclerosis
- Asthma
- Allergies
- Autoimmune disorders
- Bipolar disorder
- Schizophrenia
- Kidney stones
- Gallstones
- Obesity
- Peptic ulcer disease
- Gout

multifactorial diseases, or those caused by gene and environment interaction.

The issue of multifactorial interactions that lead to disease is becomingly increasingly recognized in occupational health. According to the CDC, advances in technology in the last few decades have increased our knowledge of the role that genetics plays in occupational diseases. In occupational health, one of the key issues relates to genetic changes that are acquired during a lifetime as a result of exposures and the interaction between genes and environmental factors. However, the use of genetic information in occupational safety and health research and practice presents both potential benefits and concerns and raises medical, ethical, legal, and social issues that are emerging in policy and procedure and have an impact on society and individuals (CDC, 2010).

Ethical and Legal Considerations

Discoveries in genetics, including those associated with the HGP, present complicated ethical issues for consumers, providers, and health care policy-makers. All humans have a right to be deeply concerned about genetic science and its effect on their well-being. Therefore, in the face of this biotechnological revolution, nurses need to carefully review the ethical and legal implications of genetic science. GINA is a good place to begin the study of the ethical concerns associated with genetics/genomics.

WHAT DO YOU THINK? *Logan Karns, a certified genetics counselor working in the prenatal genetics department at the University of Virginia Health System, describes many ethical dilemmas as medical science moves forward: "Our technological advances have always outpaced our ethical thinking about the consequences of what we're doing. We need to have a measured thoughtfulness about everything." She describes genetic knowledge as unique: "a window from the past and a glimpse into the future."*

Karns L, Genetics Counselor UVA Health System (2010). Interview by E. J. Zschaebitz (phone interview). Accessed May 5, 2010.

On November 21, 2009, GINA took effect through an act of the U.S. Congress. It was designed to prohibit the improper use of genetic information in health insurance and employment. This act prevents group health plans and health insurers from denying coverage to a healthy individual or charging higher premiums based solely on genetic predisposition to disease. This legislation also prohibits employers from using individuals' genetic information when making hiring, firing, job placement, or promotion decisions.

GINA does the following: (1) prohibits employers from discriminating against an employee based upon genetic information, (2) places broad restrictions on an employer's deliberate acquisition of genetic information, (3) mandates confidentiality for genetic information that employers lawfully collect, (4) strictly limits disclosure of such information, and (5) prohibits retaliation against employees who complain about genetic discrimination (USDHHS, 2009).

In accordance with GINA, genetic information is defined as information about the following:

- An individual's genetic tests (including genetic tests done as part of a research study)
- Genetic tests of an individual's family members (defined as dependents and up to and including fourth-degree relatives)
- Genetic tests of any fetus of an individual or family member who is a pregnant woman, and genetic tests of any embryo legally held by an individual or family member using assisted reproductive technology
- The manifestation of a disease or disorder in an individual's family members (family history)
- Any request for, or receipt of, genetic services or participation in clinical research that includes genetic services (genetic testing, counseling, or education) by an individual or an individual's family members (USDHHS, 2010)

DID YOU KNOW? *Patenting genetic material has been a controversial issue relevant to the BRCA-1 and BRCA-2 genes, in which mutations are shown to cause a significant risk of breast and/or ovarian cancer in women. This is highlighted by recent legal action against Myriad Genetics, Inc. which, in collaboration with the University of Utah, sequenced the BRCA-1 gene and applied for patent protection in 1995. This particular case demonstrated how grounds of patentability also act as important safeguards of the public interest, aimed at ensuring that patents are granted on genuine advances in knowledge, and are "not used to exclude access to material in the public domain."*

(See http://www.wipo.int/wipo_magazine/en/2006/04/article_0003.html.)

There are many other ethical issues to consider related to genetics/genomics, and several are integrated throughout the remainder of the chapter.

PERSONALIZED HEALTH CARE

The importance of genetic developments to public health nursing practice is underscored by current national initiatives to improve population health through use of genetic and genomic information. These include the Personalized Health Care Initiative instituted by the U.S. Department of Health and Human Services. The goal of this initiative is to improve the safety, quality, and effectiveness of health care for every client in the United States. By using *genomics,* or the identification of genes and how they relate to drug treatment, personalized health care will enable medicine to be tailored to each person's needs. The initiative includes the following goals:

- *Goal 1:* Link clinical and genomic information to support personalized health care.
- *Goal 2:* Protect individuals from discrimination based on unauthorized use of genetic information.
- *Goal 3:* Ensure the accuracy and clinical validity of genetic tests performed for medical application purposes.
- *Goal 4:* Develop common policies for access to genomic databases for federally sponsored programs

Also reflecting the integration of genetics into public health are the proposed objectives for *Healthy People 2020,* which include two objectives focused on genetics. Interestingly, there were no genetic-specific objectives in *Healthy People 2010.*

♥ HEALTHY PEOPLE 2020

The objectives for *Healthy People 2020* include two new objectives that relate to genomics:

- G-2: (Developmental) Increase the proportion of persons with newly diagnosed colorectal cancer who receive genetic testing to identify Lynch syndrome (or familiar colorectal cancer syndromes).
- G-1: Increase the proportion of women with a family history of breast and/or ovarian cancer who receive genetic counseling.

GENOMIC COMPETENCIES FOR THE PUBLIC HEALTH WORKFORCE

Knowledge of genetics and applications to the health of individuals, families, and communities is critical for public health professionals. Several significant health care professions groups have developed competencies for members of their workforces that include knowledge of genetics and genomics. The development of such competencies has grown considerably since the mapping of all human genes in the HGP. The CDC developed "Genomic Competencies for the Public Health Workforce" in 2001. The CDC's contention is that all public health workers need to be aware of the advances in the science of genomics and incorporate the appropriate competencies into their work. They developed seven sets of competencies that related to the work of the individual public health worker. The competencies that are discussed here are those designed for *all* public health professionals and are intended to be used in educational and training programs for public health professionals. According to the CDC (2006), a public health worker should be able to perform the following:

- Demonstrate basic knowledge of the role that genomics plays in the development of disease
- Identify limits of his or her genomic expertise
- Make appropriate referrals to those with more genomic expertise

The CDC goes on to list eight specific competencies for public health professionals. They are not listed here since they are consistent with those that have been developed more recently that are specific to nursing. The public health competencies can be found online at http://www.cdc.gov/genomics/public.

Similar to the set of competencies developed by the CDC are those developed by the National Coalition of Health Professional Education in Genetics (NCHPEG) to be included in all health professional education (NCHPEG, 2007). NCHPEG recommends that at a minimum, health care professionals should be able to do the following:

1. Examine their competence of practice regularly in order to identify areas of strength and areas where professional development related to genetics and genomics would be helpful.
2. Understand that health-related genetic information can have social and psychological implications for individuals and families.
3. Know how and when to make a referral to a genetics professional.

NCHPEG goes on to group their competencies into the following areas: knowledge, skills, and attitudes. Their competencies are congruent with those developed by the CDC and the ones that will be discussed in more depth in the following section that pertains specifically to nursing. NCHPEG has also developed core principles in genetics related to: (1) biological variation, (2) cell biology, (3) classical (Mendelian) genetics, (4) molecular genetics, (5) development, and (6) new genetic technology (NCHPEG, 2004).

It is well established that new health technologies driven by the knowledge of human genetics can improve the safety, quality, and effectiveness of health care for every client in the United States (USDHHS, n.d.) (myhealthcare.com). This perspective of health care is proactive, focused on wellness by managing gene-based information to understand each individual's requirements for the maintenance of his or her health, prevention of disease, and therapy tailored to each individual's genetic uniqueness. An approach to health care that is inclusive of a genetic profile of each individual enables nurses and other health care professionals to design care highly customized to match individual needs. An approach to health care, built on the knowledge of genetics and genomics, also incorporates knowledge of environment, health-related behaviors, culture, values, and the impact of social conditions such as poverty. In other words, genetic science emphasizes a fundamental public health nursing issue: the importance of understanding both biological predisposition to disease and the impact of behavior and social conditions on overall community health and well-being.

INCORPORATING GENOMICS AND GENETICS INTO PUBLIC HEALTH NURSING PRACTICE

Public health nursing has long been concerned with environmental or social determinants of health and disease and has only recently become engaged in genomic variations within populations. The advances brought about by genomics, however, are changing our perceptions, since this knowledge will enable health promotion and disease prevention programs to be specifically directed at susceptible individuals and families, or at subgroups of the population, based on their unique genomic risk profile. In short, it is becoming clear that personalized health care based on a broad cultural and social context, a core value of public health nursing, can therefore be more predictive and preventative in nature. The public is beginning to expect that all nurses will use emerging genetic information and technology in their practice, in research, and in all forms of health education.

> **CUTTING EDGE** *Although there is an inherited genetic propensity for obesity, physical exercise can reduce this predisposition. For this reason, it is important for nurses to encourage clients and families to engage in regular physical exercise. Nurses need also to help communities develop areas and facilities that support exercise.*

Interestingly, nurses began applying genetic concepts to their practice in the 1970s. Some of the early nurses who worked in the genetics area served as genetic clinic coordinators and provided genetic counseling to persons with genetic diseases or risk factors for such disorders (Williams, 2002). Many of these early genetic nurses were advanced practice nurses who practiced as clinical nurse specialists or nurse practitioners. Before the 1990s, most genetic health care dealt with the diagnosis and management of "relatively uncommon conditions with specific patterns of inheritance" (Williams, 2002, p 492). The scope of the work for nurses in genetics changed in the early 1990s when the *BRCA-1* gene for familial breast cancer was mapped and cloned. This moved the scope of genetic work from diagnosis and management to that of risk identification. As discussed earlier in the chapter in a case example, the discovery of the *BRCA-1* gene made it possible to offer predictive genetic testing to persons with a strong history of breast or ovarian disease and to begin investigating possibly beneficial gene-based therapies (Williams, 2002).

> **NURSING TIP** *Clients should meet with a genetic nurse before being tested for mutations in BRCA genes. The nurse can counsel the patients about BRCA-1 and BRCA-2 mutations and also about the influence of environmental factors such as diet, smoking, alcohol use and exercise and their relationship to cancer susceptibility.*

In 2000, an expert panel was convened by the Health Resources and Services Administration (HRSA). This panel described the importance of integrating genetics content into the nursing curriculum. However, not much action was taken in this regard for many years. In 2004, the National Human Genome Research Institute (NHGRI) and the National Cancer Institute (NCI) collaborated to develop a genetic and genomic training program for the U.S. nursing workforce. Their work continued for several years and was carried out by a well-informed group of nurses with review by members of other health professional groups. The work led to the development of what is discussed later in the chapter: genomic competencies for nurses (Jenkins and Calzone, 2007).

The Codes of Ethics developed by both the International Council of Nurses and the American Nurses Association emphasize the responsibility of nurses to work with other health care professionals to meet the social and health care needs of the public. They include in this mandate, the right that people have to seek and receive genomic health care that is non-discriminatory, confidential, and private and that enables those served to make informed decisions (ICN, 2000; ANA, 2001). Similarly, the International Society of Nurses in Genetics (ISONG) advocates for nurses at both the basic and advanced practice levels to be able to deliver genetic nursing care. ISONG goes on to say that the genetic nurse at the basic level of preparation carries out this responsibility by identifying genetic risk factors, providing nursing interventions, making referrals, and providing health promotion education. The advanced practice nurse provides genetic counseling and case management for patients with or at risk for a disease that arises from a genetic susceptibility (ISONG, 1998).

> **DID YOU KNOW?** *From the study of the human genome it has been learned that "genes not only cause disease, but they also affect disease susceptibility and resistance, prognosis and progression and responses to illness and their treatments" (Feetham, Thomson, and Hinshaw, 2005, p 102).*

More recently, 48 professional nursing and consumer organizations have endorsed a set of competencies identified as needing to be included in nursing program curricula and in nursing continuing education. A knowledgeable advisory group developed the competencies that were initially published in 2006. They were revised in 2008 to incorporate outcome indicators (Consensus Panel on Genetic/Genomic Nursing Competencies, 2009). These essential competencies apply to all registered nurses. Copies are available without charge at http://www.nursingworld.org/ethics/genetics.

The competencies are organized into professional responsibilities and a professional practice domain that includes: (1) nursing assessment: applying/integrating genetic and genomic knowledge, (2) identification, (3) referral activities, (4) provision of education, care, and support, and (5) outcome indicators. Examples of competencies that have application to public health nursing are listed below.

Professional Practice Domain: Nursing Assessment: Applying/Integrating Genetic and Genomic Knowledge

The registered nurse:
- Demonstrates an understanding of the relationship of genetics and genomics to health, prevention, screening, diagnostics, prognostics, selection of treatment, and monitoring of treatment effectiveness.
- Demonstrates ability to elicit a family health history (minimum of three generations).
- Constructs a pedigree from collected family history information using standardized symbols and terminology.
- Collects personal, health, and developmental histories that consider genetic, environmental, and genomic influences and risk factors.
- Critically analyzes the history and physical assessment findings for genetic, environmental, and genomic influences and risk factors.
- Assesses clients' knowledge, perceptions, and responses to genetic and genomic information.
- Develops a plan of care that incorporates genetic and genomic assessment information.

> **HOW TO** **Help Families Complete a Family Health History**
> 1. *Inform the family that a family history is a written or graphic record of diseases or health conditions present in their family.*
> 2. *Encourage the family to develop a three-generation history of biological relatives, their age of diagnosis of a chronic disease, and the age and cause of death of any deceased family members.*
> 3. *Explain to the family that this type of history is a useful tool to help them know about their health risks and to prevent disease in themselves and their close relatives.*
> 4. *Tell the family that the health history is not a static document, and that it should be updated regularly.*
> 5. *Suggest that the family consider using the CDC online tool "My Family Health Portrait" to collect and organize their family health history. The tool is available free at https://familyhistory.hhs.gov in both English and Spanish.*

Identification

The registered nurse:
- Identifies clients who may benefit from specific genetic and genomic information and/or services based on assessment data.
- Identifies credible, accurate, appropriate, and current genetic and genomic information, resources, services, and/or technologies specific to given clients.
- Identifies ethical, ethnic/ancestral, cultural, religious, legal, fiscal, and societal issues related to genetic and genomic information and technologies.
- Defines issues that undermine the rights of all clients for autonomous, informed genetic- and genomic-related decision making and voluntary action.

Referral

The registered nurse:
- Facilitates referral for specialized genetic and genomic services for clients as needed.

Provision of Education, Care, and Support

The registered nurse:
- Provides clients with interpretation of selective genetic and genomic information or services.
- Provides clients with credible, accurate, appropriate, and current genetic and genomic information, resources, services, and/or technologies that facilitate decision making.
- Uses health promotion/disease prevention practices that:
  - Consider genetic and genomic influences on personal and environmental risk factors
  - Incorporate knowledge of genetic and/or genomic risk factors
  - Use genetic- and genomic-based interventions and information to improve clients' outcomes
  - Collaborate with health care providers in providing genetic and genomic health care
  - Collaborate with insurance providers and payers to facilitate reimbursement for genetic and genomic health care services

EVIDENCE-BASED PRACTICE

Following the completion of the HGP, Kenner, Gallo, and Bryant (2005) conducted a literature review to identify the most common childhood diseases that are linked to genetic causes. Their goal was to describe the effects of genetics and genomics on children's health care. They thought that the work done in the HGP would enable practitioners to more effectively deal with children with chronic illness in terms of prevention, disease prediction, and treatment. To accomplish their goal, they looked at 48 childhood chronic conditions that had a genetic basis. They then used two diseases—Usher syndrome and sickle cell disease—to illustrate how advances in genetics can influence screening and expanded testing beyond the newborn period. They concluded that increased knowledge of the interaction of a person's genetic profile as well as knowledge of the person's lifestyle, work environment, and family context will provide greater scope and depth of family health history information.

Nurse Use

Public health nurses who gather genetic information will be able to advise families on ways to tailor their health promotion and health care in order to deal more effectively with potential interactions between a person's genetic makeup and the environment. The nurse can make more informed referrals for screening, testing, and follow-up.

Kenner C, Gallo AM, Bryant KD: Promoting children's health through understanding of genetics and genomics. *J Nurs Scholarsh* 35(4): 308-314, 2005.

🌐 LINKING CONTENT TO PRACTICE

In addition to the organizations previously discussed who state that all nurses and public health professionals should have some level of competence in genetics and genomics, there is broader endorsement of this competency in terms of basic public health and public health nursing skills. Specifically, the Quad Council Competencies, which build on those of the Council on Linkages of the Public Health Foundation, state in Domain #6, under Public Health Sciences Skills, that nurses define, assess, and utilize the understanding of the health status of populations, determinants of health and illness, factors contributing to health promotion and disease prevention, and factors influencing the use of health services. This group also points out in Domain #8, Leadership and Systems Thinking Skills, that nurses should be able to utilize ethical standards of public health nursing practice as the basis of all interactions with organizations, communities, and individuals (Quad Council, 2009). This recommended skill would directly pertain to nursing practice that incorporates genetic and genomic competencies.

- Performs interventions and treatments appropriate to clients' genetic and genomic healthcare needs.
- Evaluates impact and effectiveness of genetic and genomic technology, information, interventions, and treatments on clients' outcomes.

Although the public health nurse will not always use each of these competencies, the ones used will depend on the nature of the role of the nurse. Nurses work at all three levels (individual, family, and community) in providing care, services, and referrals as well as advocating for policy changes and for laws that protect the right to health. Nurses also promote assurance for access to care including genetic screening, privacy of health information, and certainty that no discrimination will be allowed. The NCHPEG has developed a tool called "genetic red flags" that provides quick tips for risk

assessment related to genetics. These tips can serve as a guide to help nurses provide careful and consistent assessments. See the Did You Know? box for a summary of the genetic red flags (National Coalition of Health Professional Education in Genetics, n.d.).

DID YOU KNOW?   *Tips for Risk Assessment*

The "genetic red flags" developed by the National Coalition of Health Professional Education in Genetics provide an excellent tool to determine if an individual or family might be at risk. The group says that the primary red flag for most common diseases is a large number of affected relatives who are closely related. Some of the red flags include the following:

1. *Family history of multiple affected family members with the same or related disorders, which may or may not follow an identifiable pattern in the family*
2. *Onset at an earlier age than expected. Condition occurrence in the gender that is least expected to have it*
3. *Disease occurrence in the absence of known risk factors*
4. *Ethnic predisposition to certain genetic disorders*
5. *Close biological relationship existing between parents*

From www.nchpeg.org, accessed September 10, 2010.

📋 LEVELS OF PREVENTION

Applying the Three Levels of Prevention to Genetics and Genomics

Primary Prevention

Since family members share genes, behaviors, lifestyles, and environments with one another that may influence their health, help people complete a family health history.

Secondary Prevention

When you review the health history, observe for any diseases that may have a genetic basis; if found, immediately refer the person or family to the appropriate health care provider. The goal of screening is to detect or define risk in low-risk groups and identify those people who should have diagnostic testing.

Tertiary Prevention

If a genetic link to an early or a probable disease is found, guide the family in changing any behaviors in order to minimize the effect of the disease.

THE FUTURE

In this environment of rapid discoveries in genetics, nurses have a vital role in translating this new knowledge into improved health outcomes. Knowing which populations have genetic risk for various diseases will help nursing science to develop and apply public health interventions that will improve health outcomes and community well-being as well as reduce costs. Nurses will increasingly provide guidance on policy discussions and decisions to ensure confidentiality, provide protection against discrimination based on genetic information, and regulate commercialized genetics products and services.

As the American Academy of Nursing (AAN) has asserted, public health nurses must be well positioned to incorporate this new knowledge into practice. In order for people to benefit from widespread genetic and genomic discoveries, nurses must be competent to obtain comprehensive family histories, identify family members at risk for developing a genomic-influenced condition and genomic-influenced drug reactions, help people make informed decisions about and understand the results of their genetic and genomic tests and therapies, and refer at-risk people to appropriate health care professionals and agencies for specialized care (AAN, 2009).

In summary, "all healthcare and public health professionals will be expected to have the knowledge, skills, and abilities to integrate genomics into their research, education, and practice" (Feetham, Thomson, and Hinshaw, 2005, p 107). Conley and Tinkle (2007) associated genomic research with the research themes that were developed by the National Institute of Nursing Research in 2003. Of the five themes, Conley and Tinkle thought that two themes could be especially affected by genomics; interestingly, both of these themes are integral aspects of public health nursing. They are related to changing lifestyle behaviors in order to promote and improve health and managing chronic illness to improve health and reduce the burden caused by these diseases to individuals, families, communities, and societies. They further note that future research can examine the interactions between genetic susceptibility, environment, and lifestyle and their effect on susceptibility to chronic illness. Feetham, Thomson, and Hinshaw (2005) say that nurses will be involved increasingly in genomic research that deals with "biologic, family, ethical, legal and social implications" (p 103). Population-based research is very interested in the biobanks that are being developed in many countries to collect and store data and biological samples from a large cohort of people. According to Conley and Tinkle (2007), "Biobanks can be population-based or disease-oriented and are extremely valuable for genomic research, particularly research for complex, common conditions that require large sample sizes" (p 20). They recommend looking at the disease-oriented biobank of CONCOR, which is based in the Netherlands. Iceland and the United Kingdom also have biobanks (Feetham, Thomson, and Hinshaw, 2005). Data from countries that have "more homogenous populations and national health programs that provide infrastructure to these 'bio banks' can be useful information to nurses in other countries about the complex challenges including privacy, interpretation of genetic testing, and disease management" (Feetham, Thomson, and Hinshaw, 2005, p 104).

Nurses bring a biobehavioral perspective that includes an emphasis on prevention and health promotion for individuals, families, and communities. This enables nurses to bring considerable expertise to policy-making groups who are working in the area of genetics/genomics (Calzone, Cashion, and Feetham, 2010).

CHAPTER REVIEW

PRACTICE APPLICATION

T.S., a 4-year-old with hemophilia B, is attending his Head Start Program this fall. His mother brought all of his medical supplies and needles so that staff could start an emergency IV infusion if the need arose. The possibility of needing to start an IV concerned the staff who were teachers, not health care workers. The mother was also anxious about her son being away from home and attending preschool for the first time. As the public health nurse who is responsible for providing health care for Head Start programs in your community, how do you manage the health care for this child while also ensuring safety and making sure that adequate plans are in place for this facility?

A. Let T.S.'s mother know that she needs a note from T.S.'s physician before he can bring any medications to the facility.

B. Notify all of the student's parents/guardians of T.S.'s condition in order to set the guidelines and prevent possible bleeds. The children at the center should be aware of the condition, and the parents also need to educate their children to ensure extra precaution around T.S.

C. Organize a meeting between staff, educators, and parents of T.S. to educate about hemophilia. The aim is to educate key people to ensure the safety of T.S. while at Head Start.
Answers can be found on the Evolve site.

KEY POINTS

- Genetics is the study of the function and effect of single genes that are inherited by children from their parents. Genomics is the study of individual genes in order to understand the interplay of genetic, environmental, cultural, and psychosocial factors in disease.
- DNA is a nucleic acid that contains genetic information called genes.
- Genetic mutations can be caused by the environment or can be spontaneous and arise naturally during the process of DNA replication.
- Human disease comes from the collision between genetic variations and environmental factors.

- Genetic testing decisions are personal and complex and can be controversial, leading to challenging situations in families.
- The Genetic Information Nondiscrimination Act (GINA) in 2009 was designed to prohibit the improper use of genetic information in health insurance and employment.
- The use of genomics and how it relates to drug treatment will enable personalized health care and medicine to be tailored to each person's needs; health, therefore, can be predictive and preventive in nature.

KEY POINTS—cont'd

- According to the International Society of Nurses in Genetics (ISONG), the genetic nurse carries out the responsibility for identifying genetic risk factors, providing nursing interventions, making referrals, and providing health promotion education. The advanced practice nurse can provide genetic counseling or refer to a genetic counselor and act as case manager for a person with or at risk for a disease that arises from a genetic susceptibility.

- Nurses can promote assurance for access to care, including genetic screening, the privacy of health information, and certainly that no discrimination will be allowed in treatment or screening for disease.
- The field of genetics/genomics is growing rapidly and will require nurses to continue to learn and to be aware of advances in research in this area.
- Genomics affects individuals, families, and communities.

CLINICAL DECISION-MAKING ACTIVITIES

1. Choose a disorder that has a genetic basis. Look at three sites on the Internet to see what information is available for clients, families, and health professionals. Then evaluate the sites according to these criteria:
   - Who wrote the information on the site? Is it written by a health professional? Is it sponsored by a government organization that is a reliable source of health information such as the CDC? Is it peer reviewed?
   - Is the information written at the literacy level that a client could understand?
   - How would you improve the usefulness of these three sites based on the clients, families, and communities with whom you work?

2. Since public health nurses often identify groups within a community who are considered high risk for illness and then provide care to them as individuals, or to their families or in groups, choose a group in your community. Then develop a plan of care including appropriate referrals to other agencies and a comprehensive plan for follow-up.
3. Identify parent support groups in your community and inquire about attending a meeting.

REFERENCES

American Academy of Nursing: Nurses transforming health care using genetics and genomics, revisions submitted to American Academy of Nursing Board of Directors, January 22, 2009. Available at http://www.aannet.org/files/public/Genetic_White_Paper_1-22-09.pdf. Accessed May 20, 2010.

American Nurses Association: *Code of ethics for nurses with interpretive statements*, Kansas City, MO, 2001, ANA.

Calzone KA, Cashion A, Feetham S, et al: Nurses transforming health care using genetics and genomics, *Nurs Outlook* 58(1):26–35, 2010.

Centers for Disease Control and Prevention: *Genomics and disease prevention, genomic competencies for the public health workforce*, 2006. Available at www.cdc.gov/genomics/public. Accessed December 17, 2010.

Centers for Disease Control and Prevention: *Genetics in the workplace*. http://www.cdc.gov/niosh/topics/genetics/, 2010. Accessed October 5, 2010.

Collins FS, Green E, Guttmacher AE, Guyer MS: A vision for the future of genomic research, *Nature* 422:835–847, 2003.

Collins FS: *An overview of the human genome project*, 2006. Available at http://www.genome.gov/12011238. Accessed December 17, 2010.

Conley YP, Tinkle MB: The future of genomic nursing research, *J Nurs Scholarsh* 39(1):17–24, 2007.

Consensus Panel on Genetic/Genomic Nursing Competencies: *Essentials of genetic and genomic nursing: competencies, curricula guidelines, and outcome indicators*, ed 2, Silver Spring, MD, 2009, ANA.

Feetham S, Thomson EJ, Hinshaw AS: Nursing leadership in genomics for health and society, *J Nurs Scholarsh* 37(2):102–110, 2005.

International Council of Nurses: *The ICN code of ethics for nurses*, Geneva, Switzerland, 2000, ICN.

International Society of Nurses in Genetics, Inc: *Statement on scope and standards of genetics clinical nursing practice*, Washington DC, 1998, ANA.

Jenkins J, Calzone KA: Establishing the essential nursing competencies for genetics and genomics, *J Nurs Scholarsh* 39(1):10–16, 2007.

Jorde LB, Carey JC, Bamshad MJ, editors: *Medical genetics*, ed 4, Philadelphia, 2010, Elsevier.

Karns L, Genetics Counselor UVA Health System (2010). Interview by E. J. Zschaebitz (phone interview). Accessed May 5, 2010.

Kenner C, Gallo AM, Bryant KD: Promoting children's health through understanding of genetics and genomics, *J Nurs Scholarsh* 35(4):308–314, 2005.

McKusick VA: History of medical genetics. In Rimoin DL, Connor JM, Pyertiz RE, Korf BR, editors: *Emery and Rimoin's principles and practice of medical genetics*, ed 5, vol 1, London, 2007, Churchill Livingstone, pp 3–32.

National Cancer Institute: *BRCA1 and BRCA2: Cancer Risk and Genetic Testing* Available at http://www.cancer.gov/cancertopic/factsheet/Risk/BRCA. Accessed September 17, 2010.

National Center for Biotechnology Information: *Anemia, sickle cell*, n.d. Available at http://www.ncbi.nlm.nih.gov/books/NBK22238. Accessed December 17, 2010.

National Coalition of Health Professional Education in Genetics: *Core competencies for all health professionals*, September 2007. Available at www.nchpeg.org. Accessed September 10, 2010.

National Coalition of Health Professional Education in Genetics: *Core principles in genetics*, 2004. www.nchpeg.org. Accessed September 10, 2010.

National Coalition of Health Professional Education in Genetics: *Genetic red flags*. Available at www.nchpeg.org. Accessed September 10, 2010.

Perry SE: Genetics, conception and fetal development. In Lowdermilk DL, Perry SE, editors: *Maternity nursing*, ed 8, St Louis, 2011, Mosby, pp 135–167.

Quad Council of Public Health Nursing Organizations: *Public health nursing competencies*, Wheat Ridge, CO, 2009, QCPHNO.

U.S. Department of Health and Human Services: Guidance on the Genetic Information Nondiscrimination Act: implications for investigators and institutional review boards, 2009. Available at http://www.hhs.gov/ohrp/humansubjects/guidance/gina.html. Accessed December 17, 2010.

U.S. Department of Health and Human Services: *Healthy People 2020*, Washington, DC, 2000, U.S. Government Printing Office.

U. S. Department of Health and Human Services: *Personalized health care*, n.d. Available at http://www.hhs.gov/myhealthcare/. Accessed December 17, 2010.

Williams JK: Education for genetics and nursing practice, *AACN Clin Issues* 13(4):492–500, November 2002.

CHAPTER 12

Epidemiology

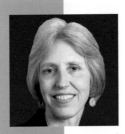

DeAnne K. Hilfinger Messias, PhD, RN, FAAN

Dr. DeAnne K. Hilfinger Messias is an international community health nurse, educator, and researcher. She spent more than two decades in Brazil, where she directed a primary health care project on the lower Amazon, taught women's health and community health nursing, and organized women's health initiatives among poor urban populations. The primary focus of her current community-based participatory research is women's work and health, immigrant women's health, language access, and community empowerment. Dr. Messias was a fellow with the International Center for Health Leadership Development at the School of Public Health, University of Illinois at Chicago (2002–2004) and a Fulbright Senior Scholar in Global/Public Health at the Federal University of Goiás, Brazil, in 2005. She is a professor at the University of South Carolina, with a joint appointment in the College of Nursing and the Women's and Gender Studies Program.

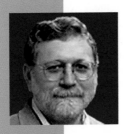

Robert E. McKeown, PhD, FACE

Dr. Robert E. McKeown is an epidemiologist with doctoral degrees in epidemiology and theology. He is a fellow and President of the American College of Epidemiology (ACE) and has served as chair of the Epidemiology Section of the American Public Health Association and of the Ethics Committee of ACE. His research focuses on psychiatric epidemiology, especially in children and adolescents, perinatal epidemiology, women's health, public health ethics, and public health and the faith community. He is professor of epidemiology and chair of the Department of Epidemiology and Biostatistics in the Arnold School of Public Health, University of South Carolina. He is also director of the Health Sciences Research Core and Interim Director of the Institute for Advancement of Health Care. He is a recipient of the Arnold School's Excellence in Teaching Award, Faculty Service Award, Faculty Research Award, and Distinguished Alumni Award. In 2010 the Epidemiology Section of the American Public Health Association honored him with the Abraham Lilienfeld Award for excellence in teaching epidemiology across a career.

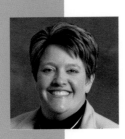

Swann Arp Adams, PhD

Dr. Swann Arp Adams has over 14 years of experience in clinical epidemiology. She holds a PhD in epidemiology and an MS in biomedical sciences. Dr. Adams has previous experience in a variety of research fields including physical activity, bone marrow transplantation, diabetes, breast cancer, and cancer disparities. She is the Associate Director of the Cancer Prevention and Control Program and is an assistant professor with a joint appointment in the College of Nursing and the Department of Epidemiology and Biostatistics at the University of South Carolina. Her current research work focuses on reducing the burden of breast cancer mortality experienced by African-American women. Past honors include the Doctoral Achievement Award (2004) and the Gerry Sue Arnold Alumni Award (2008) from the Arnold School of Public Health of the University of South Carolina.

ADDITIONAL RESOURCES

ℯvolve WEBSITE
http://evolve.elsevier.com/Stanhope
- *Healthy People 2020*
- WebLinks
- Quiz
- Case Studies

- Glossary
- Answers to Practice Application

APPENDIX
- Appendix H: Focus on Quality and Safety Education for Nurses

OBJECTIVES

After reading this chapter, the student should be able to do the following:

1. Define epidemiology and describe its essential elements and approach.
2. Describe current and historical contexts of the development of the field of epidemiology.
3. Identify key elements of the epidemiologic triangle and the ecological model and describe the interactions among these elements in both models.
4. Explain the relationship of the natural history of disease to the three levels of prevention and to the design and implementation of community interventions.
5. Interpret basic epidemiologic measures of morbidity (disease) and mortality (death).
6. Discuss descriptive epidemiologic parameters of person, place, and time.
7. Describe the key features of common epidemiologic study designs.

OBJECTIVES—cont'd

8. Describe essential characteristics and methods of evaluating a screening program.
9. Identify the most common sources of bias in epidemiologic studies.
10. Evaluate epidemiologic research and apply findings to nursing practice.
11. Discuss the role of the nurse in epidemiologic surveillance and primary, secondary, and tertiary prevention.

KEY TERMS

OUTLINE

Epidemiology is considered the basic science of public health. Like public health nursing, epidemiology is a complex and continually evolving field with a common focus: the optimal health for all members of all communities, local and global. Nurses use epidemiologic frameworks, methods, and data to better understand factors that contribute to health and disease; to develop health promotion and disease prevention interventions and measures; to identify the presence of infectious agents in individuals and groups; to design, implement, and evaluate community health programs; and to develop and evaluate public health policies. Since nurses care for individuals and families, it is important that they consider the broader context in which these individuals live and the complex interplay of social and environmental factors that affect individual and collective well-being. Basic knowledge of epidemiology is essential to the practice of nursing across all settings and populations.

DEFINITIONS OF HEALTH AND PUBLIC HEALTH

Health is the core concept in nursing and epidemiology. In 1978 the World Health Organization (WHO) affirmed that "health, which is a state of complete physical, mental and social well-being, and not merely the absence of disease or infirmity, is a fundamental human right and the attainment of the highest possible level of health is a most important world-wide social goal" (WHO, 1978, p 1). As defined by the American Nurses Association (ANA), "Nursing is the protection, promotion, and optimization of health and abilities, prevention of illness and injury, alleviation of suffering through the diagnosis and treatment of human response, and advocacy in the care of individuals, families, communities, and populations" (ANA, 2004, p 7). This definition reflects the WHO goal and coincides with epidemiologic principles. A holistic approach to health, including the incorporation of epidemiologic principles, is particularly appropriate for nurses. Nurses incorporate concepts of health into their nursing practice on a daily basis.

Public health has been described as a system and social enterprise; a profession; a collection of methods, knowledge, and techniques; governmental health services, especially medical care for the poor and underserved; and the health status of the public (Turnock, 2008). In the early twentieth century, C.E.A. Winslow defined public health as "the science and art of preventing disease, prolonging life and promoting physical health and efficiency through organized community effort." The Institute of Medicine (IOM) report *The Future of Public Health* drew upon Winslow's definition in stating the mission of public health is to fulfill "society's interest in assuring conditions in which people can be healthy" (IOM, 1988, p 40). This mission statement clearly indicates a societal interest in the health of all its members. More specifically, the mission of the public health enterprise is to *ensure conditions* that promote health and well-being. From both public health and nursing perspectives, *health* encompasses much more than the presence or absence of a physical disease or disability; it involves optimal functioning across a broad range of systems—physiological, somatic, psychological, social, and environmental. The authors of the 1988 IOM report caution that this broad view of health and the role of public health professionals and agencies forces "practitioners to make difficult choices about where to focus their energies and raises the possibility that public health could be so broadly defined so as to lose distinctive meaning" (IOM, 1988, p 40). Nurses are especially well suited to address this concern because of their holistic view of health and broad, interprofessional approach to intervention.

The practice of public health nursing is based on definitions of health and public health that go beyond a narrow biomedical model of individual health. Ensuring the public's health includes delivery of specific services to individuals, but also includes the establishment and implementation of public policies and programs. Public health and public health nursing activities focus on community prevention, disease control, and personal and community health services. The IOM report, *The Future of the Public's Health in the 21st Century* (IOM, 2002) highlights the importance of intersectoral collaborations to accomplish the mission of public health. There is further emphasis on an ecological approach to research and practice (discussed below). Interprofessional collaboration between nurses and other health professionals, including epidemiologists, is critical to efforts to create and sustain the conditions necessary for health promotion, health maintenance, and overall improvements in public health.

❤ HEALTHY PEOPLE 2020

Examples of new epidemiologic objectives included in *Healthy People 2020*
- AH-2: Increase the percentage of adolescents who participate in extracurricular and out-of-school activities.
- AOCBC-4: Reduce the proportion of adults with doctor-diagnosed arthritis who find it "very difficult" to perform specific joint-related activities.
- C-9: Reduce invasive colorectal cancer.
- D-16: Increase prevention behaviors in persons at high risk for diabetes with pre-diabetes.
- FS-5: Increase the proportion of consumers who follow key food safety practices.
- HAI-2: Reduce invasive methicillin-resistant *Staphylococcus aureus* (MRSA) infections

From U. S. Department of Health and Human Services. *Healthy People 2020*. Available at www.healthypeople2020. Accessed January 14, 2011.

DEFINITIONS AND DESCRIPTIONS OF EPIDEMIOLOGY

Epidemiology has been defined as "the study of the occurrence and distribution of health-related states or events in specified populations, including the study of the determinants influencing such states, and the application of this knowledge to control the health problems" (Porta, 2008, p 81). The word *epidemiology* comes from the Greek words *epi* (upon), *demos* (people), and *logos* (thought), and it originally referred to the spread of diseases of infectious origin. In the past century the definition and scope of epidemiology have broadened and now include the examination of the occurrence of chronic diseases, such as cancer and cardiovascular disease; mental health and health-related events, such as accidents, injuries, and violence; occupational and environmental exposures and their effects; and positive health states.

Epidemiologists investigate the distribution or patterns of health events in populations in order to characterize health outcomes in terms of *what, who, where, when, how,* and *why*: What is the outcome? Who is affected? Where are they? When do events occur? This focus is called descriptive epidemiology, because it seeks to describe the occurrence of a disease in terms of person, place, and time (Koepsell and Weiss, 2003). The *how* and *why*, or determinants of health events, are those factors, exposures, characteristics, behaviors, and contexts that determine (or influence) the patterns: How does it occur? Why are some affected more than others? Determinants may be individual, relational or social, communal, or environmental. This focus on investigation of causes and associations is called analytic epidemiology, in reference to the goal of understanding the etiology (or origins and causal factors) of disease; the broad consideration of many levels of potential determinants is called the *ecological approach* (IOM, 2002). The results of these investigations are used to guide or evaluate policies and programs that improve the health of the community. The differentiation between *descriptive* and *analytic* epidemiologic studies is not clear-cut: analytic studies rely on descriptive comparisons, and descriptive comparisons shed light on determinants.

LINKING CONTENT TO PRACTICE

It is important that nurses understand the relationship between population health concepts and clinical practice. Within the field of epidemiology, the definition of *population* is not necessarily confined to large groups of people, such as the population of the United States. Population health concepts also apply to other types of groups, such as the collective group of clients at one clinical practice site. In this case, the clinical epidemiologic application of population health concepts is evident in questions such as: What are the factors that contribute to the health and illness issues among clients that I see in my clinic? Why do some of my clients fare better than others with the same disease conditions? Are there alternative clinical practices that might positively impact the health of my clients? All of these very clinical questions incorporate epidemiologic concepts of describing the *burden of disease* in a population, identifying and understanding *determinants of health,* and examining possible *root causes* of health outcomes. Two important nursing documents recently highlighted ways in which epidemiologic knowledge and skills are essential to nursing practice. *The Council on Linkages Between Academia and Public Health Practice* (2009) outlined essential analytic/assessment and public health science skills, and *The Quad Council of Public Health Nursing Competencies* (2009) provided details and examples of ways to implement these skill sets in nursing practice.

The first step in the epidemiologic process is to answer the "what" question by defining a health outcome. The case definition usually refers to cases of disease, but also may include instances of injuries, accidents, or even wellness (Koepsell and Weiss, 2003). Epidemiology has played an important role in the refinement of the case definition for acquired immunodeficiency syndrome (AIDS) and other emerging infectious diseases and in the development of more precise diagnostic criteria for psychiatric disorders. Epidemiologic methods are used to quantify the frequency of occurrence and characterize both the case group and the population from which they come. The aim is to describe the distribution (i.e., determine who has the disease and where and when the disease occurs) and to search for factors that explain the pattern or risk of occurrence (i.e., answer the questions of why and how the disease occurs).

An epidemic occurs when the rate of disease, injury, or other condition exceeds the usual (endemic) level of that condition. There is no specific threshold of incidence that indicates the existence of an epidemic. Because of the virtual eradication of smallpox globally, any occurrence of smallpox could be considered an epidemic. In contrast, given the high rates of ischemic heart disease in the United States, an increase of many cases would be needed before an epidemic was noted. Some would argue the current high rates compared with earlier periods already indicate an epidemic. The rising rates of obesity in the United States have led the Centers for Disease Control and Prevention (CDC) to consider adult obesity as an epidemic (CDC, 2008). Recent epidemiologic data show that 34% of U.S. adults 20 years of age and older—more than 70 million people—are obese. Approximately 19% of the population ages 6 to 12 and 17% of those 12 to 19 years old are considered overweight. Obesity contributes to increased risk for heart disease, hypertension, diabetes, arthritis-related disabilities, and certain cancers.

Epidemiology builds on and draws from other disciplines and methods, including clinical medicine and laboratory sciences, social sciences, quantitative methods (especially biostatistics), and public health policy, among others. Epidemiology differs from clinical medicine, which focuses on the diagnosis and treatment of disease in individuals. Epidemiology is the study of populations in order to: (1) monitor the health of the population, (2) understand the determinants of health and disease in communities, and (3) investigate and evaluate interventions to prevent disease and maintain health. Effective nursing practice bridges the disciplines of clinical medicine and epidemiology, incorporating a focus on both individual and collective strategies. Nurses working in the community provide clinical services to individuals as they also tend to the broader context in which these individuals live and the complex interplay of social and environmental factors that affect their well-being. Nurses apply epidemiologic methods in their daily practice, as they note trends in specific illnesses (e.g., sexually transmitted infections) or conditions (e.g., accidents) and in designing, implementing, and evaluating community health programs.

> **DID YOU KNOW?**   *The AIDS epidemic was first identified because clinicians, using basic epidemiology methods, realized that much higher numbers of Pneumocystis jiroveci (carinii pneumonia) were being diagnosed than had ever been seen previously.*

HISTORICAL PERSPECTIVES

The roots of epidemiology have been traced to ancient Greece (Merrill and Timmreck, 2006). In the fourth century BC, Hippocrates maintained that to understand health and disease in a community, one should look to geographic and climatic factors, the seasons of the year, the food and water consumed, and the habits and behaviors of the people. Yet modern epidemiology did not emerge until the nineteenth century and it was only in the twentieth century that the field developed as a discipline with a distinctive identity (Susser, 1985).

Two refinements in research methods in the eighteenth and nineteenth centuries were critical for the formation of epidemiologic methods: (1) use of a comparison group, and (2) the

TABLE 12-1 HOUSEHOLD CHOLERA DEATH RATES BY SOURCE OF WATER SUPPLY IN JOHN SNOW'S 1853 INVESTIGATION

COMPANY	NO. OF HOUSES	DEATHS FROM CHOLERA	DEATHS PER 10,000 HOUSEHOLDS
Southwark and Vauxhall	40,046	1263	315
Lambeth	26,107	98	37
Rest of London	256,423	1422	59

From Snow J: On the mode of communication of cholera. In *Snow on cholera*, New York, 1855, The Commonwealth Fund.

development of quantitative techniques (numerical measurements, or counts). One of the most famous studies using a comparison group is the pivotal mid-nineteenth century investigation of cholera by John Snow, who is often credited with being the "father of epidemiology" (Merrill and Timmreck, 2006). By mapping cases that clustered around a single public water pump in one London cholera outbreak, Snow demonstrated a connection between water supply and cholera. He later observed that cholera rates were higher among households supplied by water companies whose water intakes were downstream from the city than among households whose water came from further upstream, where it was subject to less contamination (Table 12-1). Snow realized that his investigation was an example of what epidemiologists call a *natural experiment* and his findings added credibility to his argument that foul water was the vehicle for transmission of the agent that caused cholera (Rothman, 2002; Koepsell and Weiss, 2003).

DID YOU KNOW? *Lung cancer has now surpassed breast cancer as the leading cause of cancer mortality among women. The rapidly increasing rate of lung cancer deaths in women mirrors the patterns of increased rates of smoking among women and increased cigarette advertising directed toward women.*

Development and application of epidemiologic methods in the twentieth century were stimulated by dramatic changes in society and population dynamics (the combined effects of birth rates, death rates, life expectancy, and patterns of illness and causes of death) (McKeown, 2009). Contributing factors included improved nutrition, new vaccines, better sanitation, the advent of antibiotics and chemotherapies, and declining infant and child mortality and birth rates. Societal changes also resulted from large-scale events including the Great Depression and World War II, followed by a rising standard of living for many but continued deep poverty for others. These changes led to increasing longevity and significant shifts in the age distribution of the population, resulting in increases in age-related diseases, such as coronary heart disease (CHD), stroke, cancer, and senile dementia (Susser, 1985; IOM, 2002). However, disparities remain among population subgroups in life expectancy and risk of many acute and chronic diseases. Figure 12-1 shows the 10 leading causes of death in the United States in 1900, 1950, and 2006, with the percentage of all deaths attributed to each cause. The top three causes of death have not changed since 1950, whereas the composition of the remaining seven leading causes *has* changed.

With the increase in chronic disease, epidemiologists realized the necessity of looking beyond single agents (e.g., the infectious agent that causes cholera) toward a multifactorial etiology (i.e., many factors or combinations and levels of factors contributing to disease, such as the complex set of factors that cause cardiovascular disease), referred to as an **ecological model** (IOM, 2002). Researchers and practitioners also recognized the contribution of behavioral and environmental causes to some chronic conditions formerly considered to be degenerative diseases of aging. This understanding prompted new thinking about the possibility of preventing or delaying the onset of certain chronic diseases (Susser, 1985). In addition, the development of genetic and molecular techniques (such as genetic markers for increased risk of breast cancer and sophisticated tests for antibodies to infectious agents or for other biological markers of exposures to environmental toxins, such as lead or pesticides) has increased the ability to identify and classify persons in terms of exposures or inherent susceptibility to disease.

BASIC CONCEPTS IN EPIDEMIOLOGY

Measures of Morbidity and Mortality

Proportions, Rates, and Risk

The distribution of health states and events is an important focus of epidemiology. Because people differ in their probability or risk of disease, a primary concern is the identification of how they differ. Today, epidemiologists use tools such as geographic information systems (GISs) to study health-related events to identify disease distribution patterns, similar to John Snow's mapping of cholera cases in London in the nineteenth century. However, mapping cases is limited in what it can reveal. A higher number of cases may simply be the result of a larger population with more people who are potential cases, or of a longer period of observation. Any description of disease patterns should take into account the size of the population at risk for the disease. That is, we should look not only at the numerator (the number of cases), but also at the denominator (the number of people in the population at risk) and at the length of time the population was observed. For example, 50 cases of influenza in a month might be viewed as a serious epidemic in a population of 250 but would indicate a low rate in a population of 250,000. On the other hand, even in a small population, one might observe 50 cases over a period of several years. Using rates and proportions instead of simple counts of cases takes the size of the population at risk into account (Koepsell and Weiss, 2003). How time is considered differs according to the measure being used.

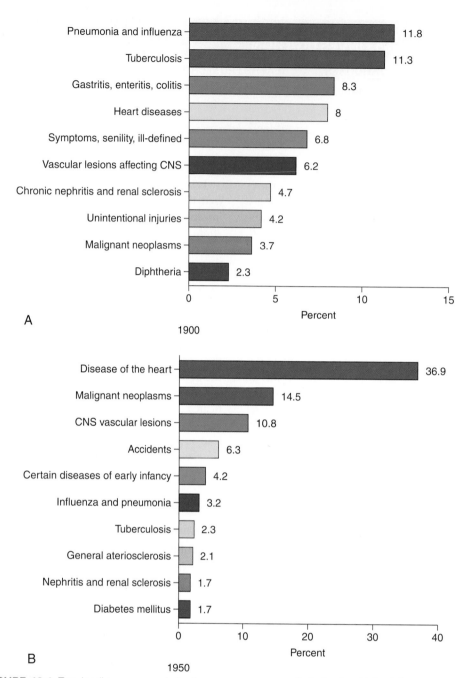

FIGURE 12-1 Ten leading causes of death as a percentage of all deaths, United States. **A,** 1900. **B,** 1950. **C,** 2006. (**B,** Data from Anderson RN: Deaths: leading causes for 2000, *Natl Vital Stat Rep* 50:16, 2002; Brownson RC, Remington PL, Davis JR: *Chronic disease epidemiology and control,* ed 2, Washington, DC, 1998, APHA; U.S. Department of Health, Education, and Welfare: *Vital statistics of the United States: 1950,* vol 1, Washington, DC, 1954, USDHEW, Public Health Service.)

Epidemiologic studies rely on proportions and rates. A **proportion** is a type of ratio in which the denominator includes the numerator. For example, in 2006 there were 2,426,264 deaths recorded in the United States, of which 631,636 were reported as caused by heart disease; so the proportion of deaths attributable to heart disease in 2006 was 631,636/2,426,264 = 0.260, or 26.0%. Because the numerator must be included in the denominator, proportions can range from 0 to 1. Proportions are often multiplied by 100 and expressed as a percent, literally meaning per 100. In public health statistics, however, if the proportion is very small, we use a larger multiplier to avoid small fractions; thus the proportion may be expressed as a number per 1000 or per 100,000.

A **rate** is a measure of the frequency of a health event in "a defined population, usually in a specified period of time" (Porta, 2008, p 207). A rate is a ratio, but it is not a proportion because the denominator is a function of both the population size and the dimension of time, whereas the numerator is the

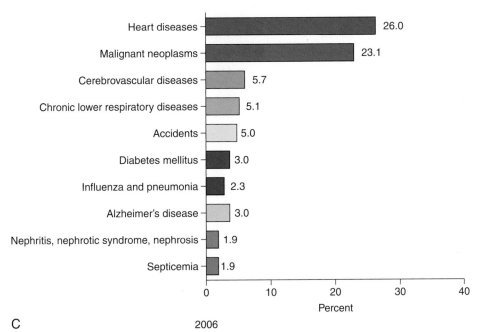

C   2006

FIGURE 12-1, cont'd Ten leading causes of death as a percentage of all deaths, United States. **C,** Data from Heron MP, Hoyert DL, Murphy SL, et al: Deaths: Final data for 2006. *Natl Vital Stat Rep,* vol 57, no 14. Hyattsville, MD, 2009, National Center for Health Statistics; Martin JA, Hamilton BE, Sutton PD, et al: Births, final data for 2006, *Natl Vital Stat Rep* 57:7, 2009.)

number of events (Rothman, 2002; Koepsell and Weiss, 2003; Gordis, 2009). Furthermore, depending on the units of time and the frequency of events, a rate may exceed 1. As its name suggests, a rate is a measure of how rapidly something is happening: how rapidly a disease is developing in a population or how rapidly people are dying. Conceptually, a rate is the instantaneous change in a continuous process. Notice the use of the words *event* and *happening*. Rates deal with change over time, as individuals move from one state of being to another (e.g., from well to ill, alive to dead, or ill to cured). In observing a population over time to observe such changes in status, we typically exclude from the population being followed those persons who have already experienced the event.

Using the same health event of death from heart disease detailed above, we can also compute a rate. To calculate the death rate, the denominator will be the number of individuals in the population *during the year in which the deaths occurred*, rather than total number of deaths. For example, in 2006, the U.S. population estimate was 299,398,484. Since rates are commonly expressed per 100,000 or per 1000, we will divide this total population figure by 100,000, to get 2993.98484. The resulting calculation of the rate of death from heart disease in the U.S. in 2006 would be 631,636/2993.98484 = 211 per 100,000.

Risk refers to the probability that an event will occur within a specified time period. A population at risk is the population of persons for whom there is some finite probability (even if small) of that event. For example, although the risk of breast cancer in men is small, a few men do develop breast cancer and therefore could be considered part of the population at risk. There are some outcomes for which certain people would never be at risk (e.g., men cannot be at risk of ovarian cancer, nor can women be at risk of testicular cancer). A high-risk population,

on the other hand, would include those persons who, because of exposure, lifestyle, family history, social or environmental context, or other factors, are at greater risk for disease than the population at large. Although anyone may be susceptible to HIV infection, the degree of susceptibility does vary. Everyone in the population is at risk for HIV and AIDS, but persons who have multiple sexual partners without adequate protection or who use intravenous drugs are in the high-risk population for HIV infection. However, others who do not fit these categories may unknowingly be at high risk. An example is women who consider themselves to be in monogamous relationships but are unaware that their partners have sexual relations with other women or men. As proportions, risk estimates have no dimensions, but they are a function of the length of time of observation. Given a continuous rate, increasing time will mean that a larger proportion of the population will eventually become ill.

Epidemiologists and other health professionals are interested in measures of morbidity, especially incidence proportions, incidence rates, and prevalence proportions (Gordis, 2009). These measures provide information about the risk of disease, the rate of disease development, and the levels of existing disease in a population, respectively.

| HOW TO   **Quantify a Health Problem in the Community**

Planning for resources and personnel often requires quantifying the level of a problem in a community. For example, to know how different districts compare in the rates of very-low-birth-weight (VLBW) infants, one would calculate the prevalence of VLBW births in each district:

1. Determine the number of live births in each district from birth certificate data obtained from the vital records division of the health department.

2. *Use the birth weight information from the birth certificate data to determine the number of infants born weighing less than 1500 g in each district.*
3. *Calculate the prevalence of VLBW births by district as the number of infants weighing less than 1500 g at birth divided by the total number of live births.*
4. *If the number of VLBW births in each district is small, use several recent years of data to obtain a more stable estimate.*

Measures of Incidence

Measures of incidence reflect the number of *new* cases or events in a population at risk during a specified time. An incidence rate quantifies the rate of development of new cases in a population at risk, whereas an incidence proportion indicates the proportion of the population at risk who experience the event over some period of time, for example, the proportion of the population who develop influenza during a given year (Rothman, 2002). The population at risk is considered to be persons without the event or outcome of interest but who are at risk of experiencing it. Note that existing (or prevalent) cases are excluded from the population at risk for this calculation, since they already have the condition and are no longer at risk of developing it. (Calculations of incidence measures for events that can recur are more complicated.) The incidence proportion is also referred to as the cumulative incidence rate (and erroneously simply as the incidence rate) because it reflects the cumulative effect of the incidence rate over the time period, whether it is a month, a year, or several years. A constant incidence rate operating over a period of time results in an increasing proportion of the population who is affected, that is, the incidence rate may stay constant while the cumulative incidence rate increases with time. An incidence proportion can be interpreted as an estimate of risk of disease in that population over that period—that is, as a probability with limits from 0 to 1. The risk of disease is a function of both the rate of new disease development and the length of time the population is at risk. The interpretation can be for an individual (i.e., the probability that the person will become ill) or for a population (i.e., the proportion of a population expected to become ill over the specified period). In epidemiology, we often calculate proportions on the basis of population frequencies. These frequencies are then translated into personal risk statements for people representative of the population on which the estimates are based.

As an example, suppose a local health department and community hospital have a joint comprehensive screening program in a specific geographic area characterized by overcrowded housing, low-income families, limited access to services, and underutilization of preventive health practices. The outreach program includes conducting health histories and physical examinations; tuberculin skin tests with follow-up chest radiography where indicated; cardiovascular, glaucoma, and diabetes screening; and mammography for women and prostate screening for men more than 45 years of age. Of 8000 women screened through the program, 35 were previously diagnosed with breast cancer; through the screening efforts, 20 with no prior breast cancer diagnosis are identified as having cancer of

the breast. Subsequently, the remaining 7945 women in whom no breast cancer was detected could be followed over the next 5 years to identify the number of new cases of breast cancer detected. Assuming no losses to follow-up (e.g., moved away or died from other causes), if 44 women were diagnosed over the 5-year period, the 5-year incidence proportion of breast cancer in this population would be as follows:

$$\frac{44}{7945} = 0.005538, \text{ or } 553.8 \text{ per } 100,000$$

Note the multiplication by 100,000, so that the number of cases is expressed as per 100,000 women. An incidence proportion estimates the risk of developing the disease in that population during that time. Also, as a proportion, each event in the numerator must be represented in the denominator, and only those persons at risk of the event counted in the numerator may be included in the denominator.

We estimate incidence rates by counting events relative to the total amount of time that persons in a population are observed *(person-time)*. This measure is called *incidence density*. For many calculations, it is generally assumed that rates are constant over the period of observation. The numerator consists of the number of new events. In calculating the person-time denominator, we count the amount of time each person contributes from the time that observation of that person begins until the person: (1) experiences the event, (2) is lost to follow-up, dies from some other cause, or otherwise is no longer at risk, or (3) reaches the end of observation. Incidence density is an estimate of the true instantaneous rate (or *hazard*) of the event. It is an indication of how rapidly a disease is developing in a population. Conceptually, a rate is the instantaneous change in a continuous process. Note that incidence density does have dimensions; it is not bounded by 1 (as risk is); its value depends on the units of time chosen. It may be interpreted as the reciprocal of the average time until disease onset, assuming there are no competing risks and there is a fixed or steady-state population with complete follow-up (Rothman, 2002).

To continue the previous example, suppose the 7945 women we follow for 5 years accumulate a total of 39,615 person-years of observation. (Person-time, such as person-years, is the sum of the time observed for all the people under observation.) Remember, the assumption was that there was no loss to follow-up or deaths from other causes. Note that the total person-time is not equivalent to 5 × 7945 (or 39,725), because we stop counting time for the 44 women who developed breast cancer at the time of diagnosis. (Note that determining the exact time of disease onset is often a problem in epidemiologic studies. The use of time of diagnosis may be biased because diagnosis occurs at different stages of disease in different populations.) Consequently, the incidence rate for breast cancer diagnosis in this population, after 5 years of observation, would be estimated as 44 newly diagnosed cases per 39,615 person-years of observation, or 0.0011107; we could express this as 11.1 cases per 10,000 person-years.

We are often concerned about the risk—that is, the probability of disease occurring over some defined period of time, such as a year or several years. Earlier we estimated the risk directly as the number of new cases over a 5-year period in a population at risk. That was straightforward because we had no losses, and observation began at the same time for all the women. A more common situation is that people come under observation at different times and there are losses attributable to attrition or competing risks (i.e., other events or deaths). We can handle those easily by counting the amount of time that is observed and calculating the incidence density as an estimate of the incidence rate. By calculating the incidence rate of an event (e.g., diagnosis of breast cancer) in a population, we then can estimate the risk of the event in that population, both in terms of the expected proportion of the population who would experience the event and in terms of the risk to a representative member of the population. When certain assumptions are met, primarily a constant rate, the average incidence density over a period of time is related to the cumulative risk for that period by the following equation:

$$Risk = 1 - e^{(-I \times T)}$$

where I is the mean per-person-time incidence rate, T is the period of observation in the same units of time, and e is the base of the natural logarithm. Again, to return to the example, suppose we observed the 44 new cases in 39,615 person-years of follow-up, but there were losses to follow-up, and women entered and left the population at different times. Assuming that the rate of new breast cancer is fairly constant over that 5-year period, the cumulative risk over 5 years is estimated as follows:

$$Risk = 1 - e^{(-0.0011107 \times 5)} = 0.005538,$$

which is the same as the risk we calculated for the simpler situation.

Note that the rate used is *not* the incidence proportion but the mean incidence densities for intervals of time comprising the total period, and the formula assumes that the rates do not vary over the period. Also, risk is a probability whose value depends on both the incidence rate and the period of observation but whose range is restricted to between 0 and 1. For example, the longer a person is at risk for an event, the greater the probability (or risk) the event will occur at some point. If the risk of being hit crossing the street is 0.01, then the risk that I will be hit at some point if I cross the street 100 times is very much greater than if I cross the street only once. The value of incidence density, on the other hand, does depend on the units of time and, because it is not a probability, is not restricted to the 0 to 1 range. Furthermore, when the incidence rate is low or the period of observation short—so that, relative to the size of the population, few people are removed from the population at risk by disease—the product of the per-person-time rate and the period of observation approximates the risk for the period (Rothman, 2002; Szklo and Nieto, 2007).

A ratio can be used as an approximation of a risk. For example, the infant mortality rate (IMR) is the number of deaths in infants less than 1 year of age that occur in a given year divided by the number of live births in that same year. The IMR approximates the risk of death in the first year of life for live-born infants in a specific year. Some of the infants who die that year were born in the previous calendar year, and some of the infants born that year may die in the following calendar year before their first birthday. However, because about two thirds of infant deaths occur within the first 28 days of life, the number of infants in the numerator (deaths in a given year) but not in the denominator (live births in that same year) will be small. It can be assumed that current year deaths from the previous year's cohort approximately equal the deaths from the current year's cohort occurring in the following year. Although technically a ratio, this is an approximation to the true proportion and, therefore, an estimate of the risk. In some publications, readers may notice that the rate of infant death is not equivalent to the number of deaths divided by the number of live births. These rates take into account the changes in the rate of death over the first year of life—that is, they use a person-time denominator.

HOW TO Use Epidemiologic Concepts in Nursing

Epidemiologic concepts and data are used in ongoing assessments of both community and individual health problems. An initial component of a community health assessment is the collection of incidence, morbidity, and mortality rates for specific diseases. Health service data, such as immunization rates, causes of hospitalization, and emergency department visits, are also obtained. Additional areas for community assessment are outlined in the How To boxes on pages 262 and 264. Individual health problems should incorporate evaluations of health risk based on lifestyle patterns along with the standard history and clinical examinations.

Prevalence Proportion

The **prevalence proportion** is a measure of existing disease in a population at a particular time (i.e., the number of existing cases divided by the current population). One can also calculate the prevalence of a specific risk factor or exposure. When used alone, the term *prevalence* typically refers to the prevalence proportion, although the term is sometimes used to refer to the count of existing cases (i.e., the numerator of the prevalence proportion). In the breast cancer example described previously, suppose the screening program discovered 35 of the 8000 women screened had previously been diagnosed with breast cancer, and 20 women with no history of breast cancer were diagnosed as a result of the screening. The prevalence proportion of current and past breast cancer events in this population of women would be as follows:

$$\frac{55}{8000} = 0.006875, \text{ or } 687.5 \text{ per } 100,000$$

A prevalence proportion is not an estimate of the risk of developing disease because it is a function of both the rate at which new cases of the disease develop and how long those cases remain in the population. In this example, the prevalence of breast cancer in this population of women is a function of how many new cases develop and how long women live after breast cancer diagnosis. One might see a fairly constant prevalence, for example, if improved survival after diagnosis was offset by an increasing incidence rate. The duration of a disease is affected by case fatality and cure. (For simplicity, in this example, women with a history of the disease are counted in the prevalence proportion even though they may have been cured.) A disease with a short duration (e.g., an intestinal virus) may not have a high prevalence proportion even if the rate of new cases is high, because cases do not accumulate (see Point Epidemic later in this chapter). A disease with a long course (e.g., Crohn's disease) will have a higher prevalence proportion than a rapidly fatal disease that has the same rate of new cases.

Incidence and Prevalence Compared

The prevalence proportion measures existing cases of disease. The prevalence odds ($P/[1 - P]$) are roughly proportional to the incidence rate multiplied by the average duration of disease (Rothman, 2002). The prevalence proportion is, therefore, affected by factors that influence risk (incidence) and by factors that influence survival or recovery (duration). For that reason, prevalence measures are less useful when looking for factors related to disease etiology. Because prevalence proportions reflect duration in addition to the risk of getting the disease, it is difficult to sort out what factors are related to risk and what factors are related to survival or recovery. In mathematical notation:

$$P/(1 - P) \approx I \times D, \text{ or, when } P \text{ is small } (< 0.1), P \approx I \times D,$$

where P = prevalence, I = incidence rate, and D = average duration.

For example, the 5-year survival rate for breast cancer is about 85%, but the 5-year survival rate for lung cancer in women is only about 15%. Even if the incidence rates of breast and lung cancer were the same in women (and they are not), the prevalence proportions would differ because, on average, women live longer with breast cancer (i.e., it has a longer duration). Incidence rates and incidence proportions, on the other hand, are the measure of choice to study etiology because incidence is affected only by factors related to the risk of developing disease and not to survival or cure. Prevalence proportions are useful in planning health care services because they indicate the level of disease existing in the population and therefore the size of the population in need of services. At the level of a local health department, epidemiologists and nurses would rely on both incidence and prevalence data in planning services focused on the prevention and control of tuberculosis (TB). They would examine the existing level of TB within the community (prevalence) to plan services and direct prevention and control measures, and they would take into consideration the rate of new TB cases (incidence) to study risk factors and evaluate the effectiveness of prevention and control programs.

| HOW TO | **Assess Health Problems in a Community** |

1. *Examine local epidemiologic data (e.g., incidence, morbidity, and mortality rates) to identify major health problems.*
2. *Examine local health services data to identify major causes of hospitalizations and emergency department visits. Consult with key community leaders (e.g., political, religious, business, educational, health, and cultural leaders) about their perceptions of identified community health problems.*
3. *Mobilize community groups to elicit discussions and identify perceived health priorities within the community (e.g., focus groups, neighborhood forums, or community-wide forums).*
4. *Analyze community environmental health hazards and pollutants (e.g., water, sewage, air, toxic waste).*
5. *Examine indicators of community knowledge and practices of preventive health behaviors (e.g., use of infant car seats, safe playgrounds, lighted streets, seat belt use, designated driver programs).*
6. *Identify cultural priorities and beliefs about health among different social, cultural, racial, or national origin groups.*
7. *Assess community members' interpretations of and degrees of trust in federal, state, and local assistance programs.*
8. *Engage community members in conducting surveys to assess specific health problems.*

Attack Rate

Another measure of morbidity, often used in infectious disease investigations, is the attack rate. This form of incidence proportion is defined as the proportion of persons who are exposed to an agent and develop the disease. Attack rates are often specific to an exposure; food-specific attack rates, for example, are the proportion of persons becoming ill after eating a specific food item.

Mortality Rates

Mortality rates are key epidemiologic indicators of interest to nurses (Table 12-2). Although measures of mortality reflect serious health problems and changing patterns of disease, they are limited in their usefulness. Mortality rates are informative only for fatal diseases and do not provide direct information about either the level of existing disease in the population or the risk of contracting any particular disease. Also, it is not uncommon for a person who has one disease (e.g., prostate cancer) to die from a different cause (e.g., stroke).

Note that many commonly used mortality rates in Table 12-2 are in fact proportions, not true rates (Rothman, 2002; Gordis, 2009). Because the population changes during the course of a year, we typically take an estimate of the population at midyear as the denominator for annual rates, because the midyear population approximates the amount of person-time contributed by the population during a given year. Using the approximation noted previously for small rates when the period of observation is a single unit of time, the annual mortality rate is an estimate of the risk of death in a given population for that year. These rates are multiplied by a scaling factor (usually 100,000) to avoid small fractions. The result is then expressed as the number of deaths per 100,000 persons. Although a crude mortality rate is calculated easily and represents the actual death rate for the total population, it has certain limitations. It does not reveal specific causes of death, which change in relative importance over time (see Figure 12-1). Also, it is affected by the age distribution of the population because older people are at much greater risk of death than younger people. For example, in 2005 the U.S. crude mortality rate for African Americans was 749.4 per 100,000, compared with a rate of 873.7 per 100,000 for white Americans, even though the mortality rate was higher for

TABLE 12-2 COMMON MORTALITY RATES

RATE/RATIO	DEFINITION AND EXAMPLE
Crude mortality rate	Usually an annual rate that represents the proportion of a population who die from any cause during the period, using the midyear population as the denominator Example: In 2006 there were 2,426,264 deaths in a total population of 299,398,484, or 810.4 per 100,000: $$\frac{2,426,264}{299,398,484} = 810.4 \text{ per } 100,000$$
Age-specific rate	Number of deaths among persons of given age group per midyear population of that age group Example: 2006 age-specific mortality rate for 20- to 24-year-olds: $$\frac{21,148}{21,111,240} = 100.2 \text{ per } 100,000$$
Cause-specific rate	Number of deaths from a specific cause per midyear population Example: 2006 cause-specific rate for accidents: $$\frac{121,599 \text{ deaths from accidents}}{299,398,484 \text{ midyear population}} = 40.6 \text{ per } 100,000$$
Case-fatality rate	Number of deaths from a specific disease in a given period divided by number of persons diagnosed with that disease Example: If 87 of every 100 persons diagnosed with lung cancer die within 5 years, the 5-year case fatality rate is 87%. The 5-year survival rate is 13%.
Proportionate mortality ratio	Number of deaths from a specific disease per total number of deaths in the same period Example: In 2006 there were 631,636 deaths from diseases of the heart, and 2,426,264 deaths from all causes: $$\frac{631,636}{2,426,264} = 0.26 \text{ or } 26\% \text{ of all deaths in 2006 were attributable to heart disease}$$
Infant mortality rate	Number of infant deaths before 1 year of age in a year per number of live births in the same year Example: In 2006 there were 28,527 infant deaths and 4,265,555 live births: $$\frac{28,527}{4,265,555} = 668.79 \text{ per } 100,000 \text{ live births or } 6.69 \text{ per } 1000 \text{ live births}$$
Neonatal mortality rate	Number of infant deaths under 28 days of age in a year per number of live births in the same year Example: In 2006 there were 18,989 neonatal deaths and 4,265,555 live births: $$\frac{18,989}{4,265,555} = 445.17 \text{ per } 100,000 \text{ or } 4.45 \text{ per } 1000 \text{ live births}$$
Postneonatal mortality rate	Number of infant deaths from 28 days to 1 year in a year per number of live births in the same year Example: In 2006 there were 9538 postneonatal deaths and 4,265,555 live births: $$\frac{9538}{4,265,555} = 223.61 \text{ per } 100,000 \text{ or } 2.24 \text{ per } 1000 \text{ live births}$$

From Heron MP, Hoyert DL, Murphy SL, et al: Deaths: Final data for 2006, *Natl Vital Stat Rep* 57(14), Hyattsville, MD, National Center for Health Statistics, 2009; Martin JA, Hamilton BE, Sutton PD, et al: Births: Final data for 2006, *Natl Vital Stat Rep* 57(7), Hyattsville, MD, National Center for Health Statistics, 2009.

African Americans than for whites in every age group up to age 85 (Heron et al, 2009).

Mortality rates are also calculated for specific groups (e.g., age-, sex-, or race-specific rates). In these instances, the number of deaths occurring in the specified group is divided by the population at risk, now restricted to the number of persons in that group. This rate may be interpreted as the risk of death for persons in the specified group during the period of observation.

The cause-specific mortality rate is an estimate of the risk of death from some specific disease in a population. It is the number of deaths from a specific cause divided by the total population at risk, usually multiplied by 100,000. Two related measures should be distinguished from the cause-specific mortality rate. The case fatality rate (CFR) is usually a proportion: the proportion of persons diagnosed with a particular disorder (i.e., cases) that die within a specified period of time. The CFR may be interpreted as an estimate of the risk of death within that period for a person newly diagnosed with the disease (e.g., the proportion of persons with breast cancer who die within 5 years). Because the CFR is the proportion of diagnosed persons who die within the period,

1 minus the CFR yields the survival rate. For example, if the 5-year CFR for lung cancer is 86%, then the 5-year survival rate is only 14% (Remington, Brownson, and Wegner, 2010). Persons diagnosed with a particular disease often want to know the probability of survival. These rates provide an estimate of that probability.

The second measure to be distinguished from the cause-specific mortality rate is the **proportionate mortality ratio (PMR)**—the proportion of all deaths that are attributable to a specific cause. The denominator is not the population at risk of death but the total number of deaths in the population; therefore, the PMR is not a rate nor does it estimate the risk of death. The magnitude of the PMR is a function of both the number of deaths from the cause of interest and the number of deaths from other causes. If deaths from certain causes decline over time, the PMR for deaths from other causes that remain fairly constant (in absolute numbers) may increase. For example, motor vehicle accidents accounted for 3.3 deaths per 100,000 persons 5 to 14 years of age in the United States in 2006, which is 21.8% of all deaths in this age group (the PMR). By comparison, motor vehicle accidents caused 22.3 deaths per 100,000 persons 75 to 84 years of age in 2006, which was less than 0.5% of all deaths in this older age group (Heron et al, 2009). This demonstrates that, although the risk of death from a motor vehicle accident was almost 6.8 times greater in the older group (based on the rates), such accidents accounted for a far greater proportion of all deaths in the younger group (based on the PMR). The reason is that there is a much greater risk of death from other causes in the older group.

Measures of infant mortality are used around the world as an indicator of overall health and availability of health care services. The most common measure, the infant mortality rate (IMR), is the number of deaths to infants in the first year of life divided by the total number of live births. Because the risk of death declines rather dramatically during the first year of life, neonatal and postneonatal mortality rates are also of interest (see Table 12-2). To effectively plan and evaluate community health interventions, nurses need to be able to understand and interpret these key epidemiologic indicators. One of the benefits of epidemiologic studies is that the results may demonstrate which disease prevention and control interventions are more useful and effective.

HOW TO Assess Health Problems in an Individual

1. *Obtain history of physical and mental health problems.*
2. *Ask the individual to identify major health problems. Always start interventions with what the individual views as important.*
3. *Obtain family history of diseases. Identify possible genetic link based on early age of onset of disease or multiple family members with disease.*
4. *Perform clinical examination, including laboratory work.*
5. *Evaluate health risk based on lifestyle. Include smoking status, dietary patterns of fiber and fat, exercise patterns, stress factors, and risk-taking behaviors.*
6. *Identify immediate and long-range safety concerns.*
7. *Assess individual's cultural beliefs about health.*
8. *Assess social support.*
9. *Examine knowledge and practice of preventive health care.*
10. *Provide appropriate age-based screening (e.g., cancer screening, hypertension screening).*

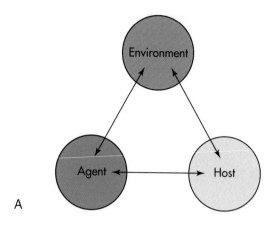

A

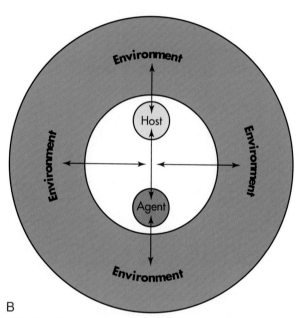

B

FIGURE 12-2 Two models of the agent-host-environment interaction (the epidemiologic triangle).

Epidemiologic Triangle, Web of Causality, and the Ecologic Model

Epidemiologists understand that disease results from complex relationships among causal agents, susceptible persons, and environmental factors. These three elements—agent, host, and environment—are traditionally referred to as the epidemiologic triangle (Figure 12-2, A). This model was originally developed as a way of identifying causative factors, transmission, and risk related to infectious diseases. Changes in one of the elements of the triangle can influence the occurrence of disease by increasing or decreasing a person's risk for disease. As illustrated in Figure 12-2, B, specific characteristics of agent and host, as well as the interactions between agent and host, are influenced by the environmental context in which they exist, and may in turn influence the environment. Examples of these three components are listed in Box 12-1.

Although the interactions of host, environment, and agent are clearly key elements in disease causation, causal relationships are often more complex than implied by the concept of

BOX 12-1 EXAMPLES OF AGENT, HOST, AND ENVIRONMENTAL FACTORS IN THE EPIDEMIOLOGIC TRIANGLE

Agent
- Infectious agents (e.g., bacteria, viruses, fungi, parasites)
- Chemical agents (e.g., heavy metals, toxic chemicals, pesticides)
- Physical agents (e.g., radiation, heat, cold, machinery)

Host
- Genetic susceptibility
- Immutable characteristics (e.g., age, sex)
- Acquired characteristics (e.g., immunological status)
- Lifestyle factors (e.g., diet and exercise)

Environment
- Climate (e.g., temperature, rainfall)
- Plant and animal life (e.g., agents or reservoirs or habitats for agents)
- Human population distribution (e.g., crowding, social support)
- Socioeconomic factors (e.g., education, resources, access to care)
- Working conditions (e.g., levels of stress, noise, satisfaction)

the epidemiologic triangle. The concept of a web of causality reflects the more complex interrelationships among the numerous factors interacting, sometimes in subtle ways, to increase (or decrease) risk of disease. Furthermore, associations are sometimes mutual, with lines of causality going in both directions. More recently, some epidemiologic researchers have advocated a new paradigm that goes beyond the two-dimensional causal web to consider multiple levels of factors that affect health and disease (Krieger, 1994; Macintyre and Ellaway, 2000). Krieger (1994) has suggested that in addition to research on the relationships within the web, we need to look for "the spider"—that is, focus on those larger factors and contexts that influence or create the causal web itself. This is consistent with the ecologic model for population health advocated by the Institute of Medicine's report (IOM, 2002), illustrated in Figure 12-3. This approach expands epidemiologic studies both upward to broader contexts (such as neighborhood characteristics and social context) and downward to the genetic and molecular level.

Like the web of causality model, the ecologic model recognizes multiple determinants of health and treats them as interrelated and acting synergistically (or antagonistically), rather than as a list of discrete factors. The ecologic model spans a broader spectrum of systems and etiological factors than the more traditional web of causality model, and it encompasses determinants at many levels: biological, mental, behavioral, social, and environmental factors, including policy, culture, and economic environments. Another way of thinking of this is that the ecologic model moves from a two-dimensional perspective to a multi-dimensional perspective. The IOM's vision of "healthy people in healthy communities" requires such a model that reflects the recognition that healthy communities are more than a collection of healthy individuals and that the characteristics of communities impact the health of their populations. Similarly, we need to recognize the impact of populations on the environment.

Social Epidemiology

A renewed interest in social epidemiology is attributed in part to the recognition of persistent social inequalities in health. Social epidemiology is the branch of epidemiology that studies the social distribution and social determinants of health and disease (Berkman and Kawachi, 2000; Krieger, 2000; Kawachi and Berkman, 2003). Social epidemiologists focus on the roles and mechanisms of specific social phenomena (e.g., socioeconomic stratification, social networks and support, discrimination, work and employment demands) in the production of health and disease states. Social epidemiologists examine social inequalities and data related to neighborhoods, communities, employment, and family conditions in order to analyze health issues and design appropriate and feasible public health interventions. Public health professionals are concerned with relationships between social conditions and patterns of health and disease in individuals, families, groups, and populations.

The complex factors that influence or lead to social inequalities in health are being increasingly examined or "rediscovered" through the lens of epidemiology. Berkman and Kawachi (2000) identified several key concepts within the subfield of social epidemiology. These include a population perspective (IOM, 2002), the social context of behavior, contextual and multilevel analysis (Sampson, Raudenbush, and Earls, 1997; Diez-Roux, 2002), a developmental and life-course perspective, and general susceptibility to disease. The aim of social epidemiology is to identify ways in which the structure of society influences the public's health, through the interactions of social context, environmental factors, biological mechanisms, and the timing and accumulation of risk, as represented by the ecological model and the life span perspective. Social epidemiologists have called for further research to examine the impact of extra-individual factors (institutions, communities, macroeconomic conditions, and economic and social policy) on exposure to resources (Lynch and Kaplan, 2000).

Levels of Preventive Interventions

The goal of epidemiology is to identify and understand the causal factors and mechanisms of disease, disability, and injuries so that effective interventions can be implemented to prevent the occurrence of these adverse processes before they begin or before they progress. The natural history of disease is the course of the disease process from onset to resolution (Porta, 2008). The three levels of prevention provide a framework commonly used in public health practice (see the Levels of Prevention box later in the chapter). As practicing epidemiologists, nurses working in the community are involved in primary, secondary, and tertiary prevention of communicable and noncommunicable diseases.

Primary Prevention

In their daily practice, nurses are often involved in activities related to all three levels of prevention (see Levels of Prevention box). Primary prevention refers to interventions aimed at preventing the occurrence of disease, injury, or disability. Interventions at this level of prevention are aimed at individuals and

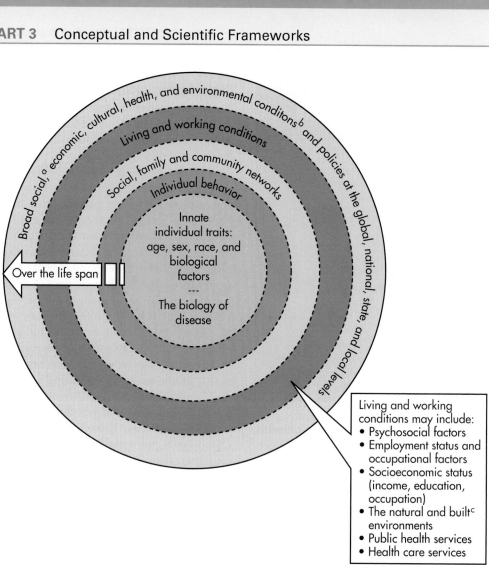

Living and working
conditions may include:
- Psychosocial factors
- Employment status and
  occupational factors
- Socioeconomic status
  (income, education,
  occupation)
- The natural and built[c]
  environments
- Public health services
- Health care services

FIGURE 12-3 Determinants of population health. This is a guide to thinking about the determinants of population health. (Reprinted with permission from The Future of the Public's Health in the 21st Century, Copyright 2002 by the National Academy of Sciences, courtesy of the National Academies Press, Washington, DC)

[a] Social conditions include, but are not limited to: economic inequality, urbanization, mobility, cultural values, attitudes and policies related to discrimination and intolerance on the basis of race, gender, and other differences.

[b] Other conditions at the national level might include major sociopolitical shifts, such as recession, war, major environmental disasters, and governmental collapse.

[c] The built environment includes transportation, water and sanitation, housing, and other dimensions of urban planning.

groups who are susceptible to disease but have no discernible pathology (i.e., they are in a state of pre-pathogenesis). This first level of prevention includes broad efforts such as health promotion, environmental protection, and specific protection. Health promotion includes nutrition education and counseling and the promotion of physical activity. Environmental protection ranges from basic sanitation and food safety, to home and workplace safety plans, to air quality control. Examples of specific protection against disease or injury include immunizations, proper use of seat belts and infants' car seats, preconception folic acid supplementation to prevent neural tube defects, fluoridation of water supplies to prevent dental caries, and actions taken to reduce human exposure to agents that may cause cancer. Primary prevention occurs in homes, in community settings, and at the primary level of health care

(e.g., in public health clinics, physicians' offices, community health centers, and rural health clinics).

Examples of nurses' involvement in primary prevention include health education and promotion programs, such as nutrition education and counseling, sex education, and family planning services. Primary prevention efforts focus on both the general population and on specific vulnerable groups (e.g., the homeless, HIV-positive persons, certain immigrant groups) to improve the general health status and to reduce the incidence of specific diseases such as TB. An example of a primary prevention intervention is the provision of health education and training for day-care workers regarding health and hygiene issues, such as proper hand hygiene, diapering, and food preparation and storage. Immunizations are another example of primary prevention. In terms of environmental protection, nurses work proactively to develop and advocate for policies and legislation that lead to prevention of environmental hazards. They can also provide consultation to industries, local governments, and groups of concerned citizens as well as public education for a wide range of preventable environmental health problems.

LEVELS OF PREVENTION

Examples Related to Cardiovascular Disease

Primary Prevention
Counsel clients about low-fat diet and regular physical exercise.

Secondary Prevention
Implement blood pressure and cholesterol screening; give treadmill stress test.

Tertiary Prevention
Provide cardiac rehabilitation, medication, surgery.

Secondary Prevention

Secondary prevention encompasses interventions designed to increase the probability that a person with a disease will have that condition diagnosed at a stage when treatment is likely to result in cure. Health screenings are the mainstay of secondary prevention. Early and periodic screenings are critical for diseases for which there are few specific primary prevention strategies, such as breast cancer. (Screening programs are discussed in more detail later in the chapter.) As noted above, primary prevention is a major focus of health education. However, nurses often use health education interventions when caring for individuals with a diagnosed health problem with the aim of preventing further complications or exacerbations. For example, at the individual and family level, teaching the asthmatic child to recognize and avoid exposure to potential asthma triggers and helping the family implement specific protection strategies, such as replacing carpets, keeping air systems clean and free of mold, and avoiding contact with household pets and second-hand smoke could be considered secondary prevention.

Interventions at the secondary level of prevention may occur in community settings as well as within primary and secondary levels of health care services. Oral rehydration therapy (ORT) for infant diarrheal disease is an excellent example of secondary prevention in the community. Particularly in developing countries, when safe water can be made available, ORT is a low-cost and effective way to treat infant diarrheal disease. When mothers identify the early signs of infant dehydration and administer a homemade ORT solution of water, sugar, and salt, they are putting secondary prevention into practice. When taking a health history with clients, nurses can integrate secondary prevention into practice by asking about family history of cancer, heart disease, diabetes, and mental illness, and then providing follow-up education about appropriate screening procedures. Other examples of secondary prevention interventions include screening tests to detect breast cancer (i.e., mammography),

cervical cancer (i.e., Pap tests), colon cancer (i.e., colonoscopy), prenatal screening of pregnant women to detect gestational diabetes, routine tuberculin testing of specific groups (e.g., health care providers, child care workers), and identification and screening of persons who have had contact with an individual known to have TB. In all these examples, the aim of secondary prevention is to identify the presence of a disease or condition at an early stage and begin necessary treatment early to increase the likelihood of cure or to prevent further complications.

Tertiary Prevention

Tertiary prevention includes interventions aimed at disability limitation and rehabilitation from disease, injury, or disability. Tertiary prevention interventions occur most often at secondary and tertiary levels of care (e.g., specialized clinics, hospitals, rehabilitation centers) but may also occur in community and primary care settings. Medical treatment, physical and occupational therapy, and rehabilitation are interventions characterized as tertiary prevention. With the emergence of new drug-resistant strains of TB, nurses now face the challenge of designing and implementing programs to increase long-term compliance and provide aftercare for clients in a variety of community settings. An example of tertiary prevention is a public health nurse providing directly observed therapy (DOT) to individuals diagnosed with active TB.

An Intervention Spectrum

The standard classification of preventive measures in public health is composed of the primary, secondary, and tertiary levels of prevention. However, this standard classification has been revised and refined for application to diverse settings and health issues. In the area of mental health, three generations of prevention have been identified, ranging from pre-intervention prevention to acute care (Figure 12-4). The IOM publication on prevention research in mental disorders (Mrazek and Haggerty, 1994) reserved the term *prevention* for those interventions that occur before the onset of a disorder. The two components of *treatment interventions* include case identification and standard treatment for known disorders. Finally, the components of maintenance in an ongoing disorder are *compliance with long-term treatment* and *provision of aftercare services, including rehabilitation*. Although this classification system was designed from the perspective of mental health, it can be applied to other public health issues. For example, within the prevention domain, it classified an intervention as *universal* when it is directed to the general population and provides general benefit with little risk at low cost. When the intervention is directed toward persons or groups who are at increased risk for developing a problem, it is designated as *selective* and risks and harms associated with the intervention must be justified on the basis of the potential reduction in adverse outcomes. The third category of prevention includes *indicated* interventions, when more costly or higher-risk interventions target high-risk persons who already indicate a problem. Nurses have critical roles in prevention at all points across the intervention spectrum.

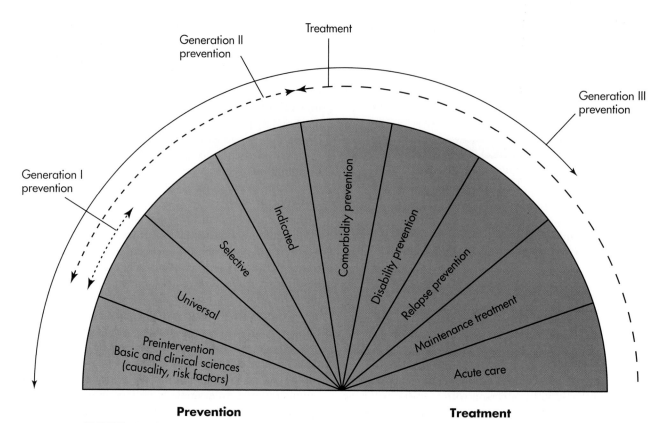

FIGURE 12-4 Health intervention spectrum. (From National Institute of Mental Health: *Priorities for prevention research at NIMH: a report by the National Advisory Health Council Workgroup on Mental Disorders Prevention Research,* Publication No. 98-4321, Washington, DC, 1998, NIH.)

SCREENING

Screening, a key component of many secondary prevention interventions, involves the testing of groups of individuals who are at risk for a certain condition but are as yet asymptomatic. The purpose is to classify these individuals with respect to the likelihood of having the disease. From a clinical perspective, the aim of screening is early detection and treatment when these result in a more favorable prognosis. From a public health perspective, the objective is to sort out efficiently and effectively those who probably have the disease from those who probably do not, again to detect early cases for treatment or begin public health prevention and control programs. A screening test is *not* a diagnostic test. Effective screening programs must have built-in referral mechanisms for subsequent diagnostic evaluation for those who screen positive, to determine if they actually have the disease and need treatment, and there must be effective protocols in place for referral to accessible and appropriate follow-up care and treatment. If there is no effective treatment, or if the individuals or groups targeted for screening experience considerable barriers in accessing appropriate treatment, the justification of the screening program must be assessed ethically as well as epidemiologically (Childress et al, 2002).

As public health advocates, nurses are responsible for planning and implementing screening and prevention programs targeted to the at-risk populations. Nurses working in schools, worksites, primary care facilities, and public health agencies

> **BOX 12-2 CHARACTERISTICS OF A SUCCESSFUL SCREENING PROGRAM**
>
> 1. *Valid (accurate):* A high probability of correct classification of persons tested
> 2. *Reliable (precise):* Results consistent from place to place, time to time, and person to person
> 3. *Capable of large group administration:*
>   a. Fast in both the administration of the test and the procurement of results
>   b. Inexpensive in both personnel required and materials and procedures used
> 4. *Innocuous:* Few, if any, side effects; minimally invasive test
> 5. *High yield:* Able to detect enough new cases to warrant the effort and expense (*yield* defined as the amount of previously unrecognized disease that is diagnosed and treated as a result of screening)
> 6. *Ethical and effective:* Meets the desired public health goal with health benefits that outweigh any moral or ethical infringements

may work together to target at-risk populations on the basis of occupational and environmental risks. Successful screening programs have several characteristics that depend on the tests and on the population screened (Box 12-2). In planning screening programs for a specific population (e.g., school, workplace, community), nurses need to take into consideration various factors. These include the characteristics of the health problem, the screening tests available, and the population (Harkness, 1995). Screening is recommended for health problems that have a high prevalence, are relatively serious, can be detected in early states, and for which effective treatment is available. The population should be easily identifiable and assessable, amenable to screening, and willing and able to seek treatment or follow-up procedures. Criteria for evaluating the suitability of screening tests include cost-effectiveness, ease and safety of administration, availability of treatment, ethics of administration or widespread implementation, sensitivity, specificity, validity, and reliability (Gordis, 2009; McKeown and Learner, 2009).

Screening procedures exist for a wide range of health conditions, including cancer (e.g., breast, cervical, testicular, colon, rectal, and skin), diabetes, hypertension, TB, lead poisoning, hearing loss, and sexually transmitted diseases (e.g., gonorrhea, chlamydia, syphilis). Nurses must keep abreast of recommended screening guidelines, which are regularly reviewed and revised on the basis of epidemiologic research results. For example, the latest U.S. Preventive Services Task Force guidelines (USPSTF, 2008) strongly recommend routine screening for lipid disorders in men 35 years and older and women 45 years and older. Screening for younger adults (men ages 20 to 35 and women ages 20 to 45) is recommended when any of the following risk factors are present: diabetes, family history of cardiovascular disease before age 50 in men or age 60 in women, family history suggestive of familial hyperlipidemia, or multiple coronary heart disease risk factors (e.g., tobacco use, hypertension). The Task Force also noted that all clients, regardless of lipid levels, should be offered counseling about the benefits of a diet low in saturated fat and high in fruits and vegetables, regular physical activity, avoidance of tobacco, and maintenance of healthy weight.

WHAT DO YOU THINK? *Genetic testing is becoming more common, but most tests for disease indicate only susceptibility to disease, not certainty. Similarly, screening tests are never perfect, so there is always some probability of misclassifying a person. How should these difficult concepts of probability and uncertainty be presented to clients when interpreting test results?*

The rationale for the current lipid screening guidelines is as follows. The clearest benefit of lipid screening is identifying individuals whose near-term risk of coronary heart disease is sufficiently high to justify drug therapy or other intensive lifestyle interventions to lower cholesterol levels. Screening men older than age 35 years and women older than age 45 years will identify nearly all individuals whose risk of coronary heart disease is as high as that of the subjects in the existing primary prevention trials. Younger people typically have a substantially lower risk, unless they have other important risk factors for coronary heart disease or familial hyperlipidemia. The primary goal of screening younger people is to promote lifestyle changes, which may provide long-term benefits later in life. The average effect of diet interventions is small, and screening is not needed to advise young adults about the benefits of a healthy diet and regular exercise because this advice is considered useful for all

age groups. Although universal screening may detect some clients with familial hyperlipidemia earlier than selective screening, it has yet to be determined if universal screening would lead to significant reductions in coronary events (USPSTF, 2008).

Reliability and Validity
Reliability

The precision, or reliability, of the measure (i.e., its consistency or repeatability) and its validity or accuracy (i.e., whether it really measures what we think it is measuring, and how exact the measurement is) are important considerations for any measurement. For example, suppose you are planning to conduct a blood pressure screening in a community setting. You will probably be taking blood pressure measurements on a large number of people and then following up with repeated measures for individuals identified as having higher levels of blood pressure. If the sphygmomanometer used for the blood pressure screening varies in its measurement so that it does not record a similar reading for the same person twice in a row, it lacks precision (or reliability). The instrument would be unreliable even if the overall mean of repeated measurements was close to the true overall mean for the persons measured. The problem would be that the readings would not be reliable for any individual, which is what a screening program requires. On the other hand, suppose the readings are reliably reproducible, but, unknown to you, they tend to be about 10 mm Hg too high. This instrument is producing precise readings, but the uncorrected (or uncalibrated) instrument lacks accuracy (or validity). In short, a measure can be *consistent* without producing *valid* results.

Three major sources of error can affect the reliability of measurement:

- Variation inherent in the trait being measured (e.g., blood pressure changes with time of day, activity, level of stress, and other factors)
- Observer variation, which can be divided into intra-observer reliability (the level of consistency by the same observer) and inter-observer reliability (the level of consistency from one observer to another)
- Inconsistency in the instrument, which includes the internal consistency of the instrument (e.g., whether all items in a questionnaire measure the same thing) and the stability (or test-retest reliability) of the instrument over time

Validity: Sensitivity and Specificity

Validity in a screening test is measured by sensitivity and specificity. Sensitivity quantifies how accurately the test identifies those *with* the condition or trait. In other words, sensitivity represents the proportion of persons with the disease whom the test correctly identifies as positive (true positives). High sensitivity is needed when early treatment is important and when identification of every case is important.

Specificity indicates how accurately the test identifies those *without* the condition or trait—in other words, the proportion of persons whom the test correctly identifies as negative for the disease (true negatives). High specificity is needed when rescreening is impractical and when reduction of false positives is important. The sensitivity and specificity of a test are determined by comparing the results from the screening test with results from a definitive diagnostic procedure (sometimes called the gold standard). For example, the Pap smear is used frequently to screen for cervical dysplasia and carcinoma. The definitive diagnosis of cervical cancer requires a biopsy with histologic confirmation of malignant cells.

The ideal for a screening test is 100% sensitivity and 100% specificity. That is, the test is positive for 100% of those who actually have the disease, and it is negative for all those who do not have the disease. In practice, sensitivity and specificity are often inversely related. That is, if the test results are such that one can choose some point beyond which a person is considered positive (a "cutpoint"), as in a blood pressure reading to screen for hypertension or a serum glucose reading to screen for diabetes, then moving that critical point to improve the sensitivity of the test will result in a decrease in specificity. In other words, an improvement in specificity can be made only at the expense of sensitivity. Table 12-3 shows how to calculate sensitivity and specificity. Some authors refer to a false-positive rate, which is 1 minus the specificity, and a false-negative rate, or 1 minus the sensitivity. These "rates" are simply the proportions of subjects incorrectly labeled as *non-diseased* and *diseased*, respectively.

A third measure associated with sensitivity and specificity is the predictive value of the test. The positive predictive value (also called predictive value positive) is the proportion of persons with a positive test who actually have the disease, interpreted as the probability that an individual with a positive test has the disease. The negative predictive value (or predictive value negative) is the proportion of persons with a negative test who are actually disease free. Although sensitivity and specificity are relatively independent of the prevalence of disease, predictive values are affected by the level of disease in the screened population and by the sensitivity and specificity of the test. When the prevalence is very low, the positive predictive value will be low, even with tests that are sensitive and specific. In addition, lower specificity produces lower positive predictive values because of the increase in the proportion of false-positive results.

In setting cutpoints, it is necessary to consider the potential human and economic costs of missing true cases by lowering the sensitivity versus the cost of falsely classifying non-cases by lowering the specificity. In making such decisions, factors to be considered include the importance of capturing all cases, the likelihood that the population will be rescreened, the interval between screenings relative to the rate of disease development, and the prevalence of the disease. A low prevalence typically requires a test with high specificity; otherwise, the screening will produce too many false positives in the largely non-diseased population. On the other hand, a disease with a high prevalence usually requires high sensitivity; otherwise, too many of the real cases will be missed by the screening (false negatives).

Two or more tests can be combined, in series or in parallel, to enhance sensitivity or specificity. In series testing, the final result is considered positive only if all tests in the series were positive, and it is considered negative if any test was negative. For example, if a blood sample were screened for HIV, a positive enzyme-linked immunosorbent assay (ELISA) might be followed up with a Western blot, and the sample would be considered positive only if both tests were positive. Series testing enhances specificity, producing fewer false positives, but sensitivity will be lower. In series testing, sequence is important; a very sensitive test is often used first to pick up all cases including false positives, and then a second, very specific test is used to eliminate the false positives. In parallel testing, the final result is considered positive if *any* test was positive and negative only if all tests were negative. To return to the example of a blood sample being tested for HIV, a blood bank might consider a sample positive if a positive result was found on either the ELISA or the Western blot. Parallel testing enhances sensitivity, leaving fewer false negatives, but specificity will be lower.

LINKING CONTENT TO PRACTICE

Nurses deal with the implications of sensitivity and specificity in everyday practice. An example is the care of clients who present with flu symptoms and are given a rapid flu test. In the case of a client with classic symptoms but a negative result from the rapid flu test, knowledge of the low sensitivity of the rapid flu test (approximately 50%-70%) may influence the decision whether or not the client should be treated with Tamiflu.

SURVEILLANCE

Surveillance involves the systematic collection, analysis, and interpretation of data related to the occurrence of disease and the health status of a given population. Surveillance systems are often classified as either active or passive (Teutsch and Churchill, 2000). Passive surveillance is the more common form used by most local and state health departments. Health care providers in the community report cases of notifiable diseases to public health authorities through the use of standardized reports. Passive surveillance is relatively inexpensive but is limited by variability and incompleteness in provider reporting practices. Active surveillance is the purposeful, ongoing search for new cases of disease by public health personnel, through personal or telephone

TABLE 12-3	CLASSIFICATION OF SUBJECTS ACCORDING TO TRUE DISEASE STATE AND SCREENING TEST RESULTS FOR CALCULATION OF INDICES OF VALIDITY

RESULT OF SCREENING TEST	DISEASE	NO DISEASE
Positive	True positive (TP)	False positive (FP)
Negative	False negative (FN)	True negative (TN)

Sensitivity = $TP/(TP + FN)$
Specificity = $TN/(TN + FP)$
False-negative "rate" = $1 -$ sensitivity = $FN/(FN + TP)$
False-positive "rate" = $1 -$ specificity = $FP/(TN + FP)$
Positive predictive value = $TP/(TP + FP)$; often multiplied by 100 and expressed as a percentage

contacts or the review of laboratory reports or hospital or clinic records. Because active surveillance is costly, its use is often limited to brief periods for specific purposes as in the emergence of a newly identified disease, a particularly severe disease, or the reemergence of a previously eradicated disease. In situations that do not require ongoing active surveillance, or where it may not be feasible to maintain a surveillance system across larger geographic areas, sentinel surveillance systems may be instituted. Representative populations may be selected and sentinel providers identified to provide information on specific diseases or conditions. Nurses engage in surveillance activities as they monitor the health status of individuals, families, and groups in their care. They use surveillance data to assess and prioritize the health needs of populations, design public health and clinical services to address those needs, and evaluate the effectiveness of public health programs.

CORE PUBLIC HEALTH FUNCTIONS

At all three levels of prevention, nurses engage in the core public health functions of *assessment, policy development,* and *assurance* (IOM, 1988). Assessment involves the regular and systematic collection, analysis, and dissemination of community health data with the aim of monitoring health status and diagnosing and investigating health problems and health hazards in the community. Policy development includes the incorporation of scientific knowledge and epidemiologic data in public health decision making and policy formulation within democratic processes. Information gathered through assessment processes provides the basis for policy development. The key processes of policy development are: (1) to inform, educate, and empower people about health, (2) to mobilize community partnerships to identify and solve health problems, and (3) to develop policies and plans that support individual and community health efforts. The third core function of public health is assurance across several domains and functions. Public health agencies are often called upon to assure that community members have equitable access to appropriate and quality health services. Public health agencies assume a regulatory role in assuring that laws and regulations that protect health and ensure safety will be enforced. Agencies also work with academic institutions and credentialing agencies to assure that the health care workforce is competent. Finally, agencies participate in broad and diverse collaborations to ensure that public health research is conducted and the resulting knowledge is applied to developing innovative solutions to health problems in the community (Turnock, 2008).

BASIC METHODS IN EPIDEMIOLOGY

Sources of Data

One of the first issues to address in any epidemiologic study is how to obtain the data (Koepsell and Weiss, 2003; Gordis, 2009). Three major categories of data sources are commonly used in epidemiologic investigations:

1. Routinely collected data, such as census data, vital records (birth and death certificates), and surveillance data as carried out by the CDC.

2. Data collected for other purposes but useful for epidemiologic research, such as medical, health department, and insurance records.

3. Original data collected for specific epidemiologic studies.

The first two types of data are often referred to as *secondary data,* and the third type is commonly considered *primary data.*

Routinely Collected Data

Vital records are the primary source of birth and mortality statistics. Although registration of births and deaths is mandated in most countries, thus providing one of the most complete sources of health-related data, the quality of specific information varies. For example, on birth certificates, sex and date of birth are fairly reliable, whereas gestational age, level of prenatal care, and smoking habits of the mother during pregnancy are less reliable. On death certificates, the quality of the cause of death information varies over time and from place to place, depending on diagnostic capabilities and custom. Vital records, readily available in most areas, are inexpensive and convenient and allow study of long-term trends. Mortality data, however, are informative only for fatal diseases or events.

Since 1790, the U.S. Census has been conducted every 10 years. The U.S. Census provides population data, including demographic distribution (e.g., age, race, sex), geographic distribution, and additional information about economic status, housing, and education. Census data are used as denominators for various rates. The American Community Survey is an ongoing survey also conducted by the U.S. Census Bureau. Data from these surveys provide important information on the status of the population and for public health planning and evaluation activities.

Data Collected for Other Purposes

Hospital, physician, health department, laboratory, and insurance records provide information on morbidity, as do surveillance systems, such as cancer registries and health department reporting systems, which solicit reports of all cases of a particular disease within a geographic region. Other information, such as occupational exposures, may be available from employer records. School and employment attendance and absenteeism records are another potential source of data that may be used in epidemiologic investigations.

Epidemiologic Data

The National Center for Health Statistics sponsors periodic health surveys and examinations in carefully drawn samples of the U.S. population. Examples are the National Health and Nutrition Examination Survey (NHANES), the National Health Interview Survey (NHIS), and several National Health Care Surveys including the National Hospital Discharge Survey (NHDS), the National Ambulatory Medical Care Survey (NAMCS), and the National Nursing Home Survey (NNHS). The CDC also conducts or contracts for surveys such as the Youth Risk Behavior Survey (YRBS), the Pregnancy Risk Assessment Monitoring System (PRAMS), and the Behavioral Risk Factor Surveillance System (BRFSS). These surveys provide information on the health status and behaviors of the population. For many studies, however, the only way to obtain the needed information is to collect the required data in a study specifically designed to investigate a particular question. The design of such studies is discussed later.

With the technological advances available through GIS, the use of cartographic data for epidemiologic studies is becoming more widespread. For example, GIS systems are now an integral component of malaria vector control in Mexico and Central America (Najera-Aguilar, Martinez-Piedra, and Vidaurre-Arenas, 2005). Local health professionals and authorities who survey their communities to identify mosquito-breeding sites now use global positioning system (GPS) and GIS technology to display and analyze their data. The resulting GIS maps are graphic illustrations of their communities, including buildings, streets, rivers, mosquito-breeding sites, and dwellings where individuals with malaria live. These maps allow the calculation of preventive treatments for dwellings located inside various radiuses, from 50 to 250 meters, around the houses with malaria cases. The standardization and integration of cartographic data collection in countries with endemic malaria are part of coordinated international efforts to strengthen malaria control. GIS technology has been used to examine other health issues, such as access to prenatal care. McLafferty and Grady (2005) compared levels of geographic access to prenatal clinics among immigrants groups in Brooklyn, New York. They used kernel estimation—a technique to depict the density of points (in this case, prenatal clinics) as a spatially continuous variable that can be represented as a smooth contour map. Then, using birth record data for the year 2000, which included the mother's country of birth, they compared clinic density levels among different immigrant groups. The authors noted the usefulness of these methods for public health departments in exploring demographic transitions and developing health service networks that are responsive to immigrant populations. GIS technology can be applied in a variety of situations, such as mapping the distribution of health exposures or outcomes, linking data with geo-coded addresses of individuals to sources of potentially toxic exposures, and mapping water quality measures in sensitive ecosystems.

THE CUTTING EDGE   *A GIS is a computer-based system of geographic, spatial, or location-based information. In public health, the advent of GIS has increased the ability of researchers to link demographic, epidemiologic, environmental, and health care system databases with spatial analysis to determine relationships between geographic patterns of disease distributions and social and physical environmental conditions. The result is that public health officials can more effectively allocate sparse public health resources in addressing health priorities.*

From McElry JA, Remington PL, Gangnon RE, et al: Identifying geographic disparities in the early detection of breast cancer using a geographic information system, Prev Chronic Dis 3(1):A10, 2006; Roche LS, Skinner R, Weinstein RB: Use of a geographic information system to identify and characterize areas with high proportions of distant stage breast cancer, J Public Health Manag Pract 3(2):26-32, 2002.

Rate Adjustment

Rates, which are of central importance in epidemiologic studies, can be misleading when compared across different populations. For example, the risk of death increases rather dramatically after

40 years of age; therefore, a higher crude death rate is expected in a population of older people compared with a population of younger people (Rothman, 2002; Koepsell and Weiss, 2003; Gordis, 2009). Because the direct comparison of the overall mortality rate in an area with a large population of older adults to the mortality rate in an area with a much younger population would be misleading, there are methods that adjust for such differences in populations. Age adjustment is based on the assumption that a population's overall mortality rate is a function of the age distribution of the population and the age-specific mortality rates. Rates for any outcome can be adjusted by the methods described here, but we focus our discussion on age adjustment of death rates because it is most common. As noted previously: as the population ages, the risk of death increases.

Age adjustment can be performed by direct or indirect methods. Both methods require a *standard population,* which can be an external population, such as the U.S. population for a given year; a combined population of the groups under study; or some other standard chosen for relevance or convenience. A direct age-adjusted rate applies the age-specific death rates from the study population to the age distribution of the standard population. The result is the (hypothetical) death rate of the study population if it had the same age distribution as the standard population.

The indirect method, as the name suggests, is more complicated. The age-specific death rates of the standard population applied to the study population's age distribution produce an index rate that is used with the crude rates of both the study and standard populations to produce the final indirect adjusted rate, which is also hypothetical. The indirect method may be required when the age-specific death rates for the study population are unknown or unstable (e.g., based on relatively small numbers). Often, instead of an indirect adjusted rate, a standardized mortality ratio (SMR) is calculated. This is the number of observed deaths in the study population divided by the number of deaths expected on the basis of the age-specific rates in the standard population and the age distribution of the study population (Szklo and Nieto, 2007; Gordis, 2009).

Although this discussion has focused on age adjustment, the process can be used to adjust for any factor that might vary from one population to another. For example, to compare infant mortality rates across populations with different birth weight distributions, these methods may be used to produce birth weight–adjusted infant mortality rates. Note that all adjusted rates are fictitious rates. They may resemble crude rates if the distribution of the study sample is similar to the distribution of the standard population. The magnitude of adjusted rates depends on the standard population used. The choice of a different standard would produce a different adjusted rate. The change from the 1940 U.S. population to the 2000 U.S. population as the standard for age-adjusted rates from the NCHS demonstrates the difference a change in standard population can make (Anderson and Rosenberg, 1998; Sorlie et al, 1999).

Comparison Groups

The use of comparison groups is at the heart of the epidemiologic approach. Incidence or prevalence measures in groups that differ in some important characteristic must be compared to gain clues about which factors influence the distribution of disease (i.e., disease determinants or risk factors). Observing the rate of disease only among persons exposed to a suspected risk factor will not show clearly that the exposure is associated with increased risk until the rate observed in the exposed group is compared with the rate in a group of comparable unexposed persons. To illustrate, one might investigate the effect of smoking during pregnancy on the rate of birth of low-birth-weight infants by calculating the rate of low-birth-weight infants born to women who smoked during their pregnancy. However, the hypothesis that smoking during pregnancy is a risk factor for low birth weight is supported only when the low-birth-weight rate among smoking women is compared with the (lower) rate of low-birth-weight infants born to non-smoking women.

The ideal approach would be to compare one group of people who all have a certain characteristic, exposure, or behavior, with a group of people *exactly* like them except they all *lack* that characteristic, exposure, or behavior. In the absence of that ideal, researchers either randomize people to exposure or treatment groups in experimental studies, or they select comparison groups that are comparable in observational studies. Advances in statistical techniques now make it possible to control for differences between groups, but these advanced techniques are effective only in reducing the bias that results from confounding by variables we have measured.

DESCRIPTIVE EPIDEMIOLOGY

Descriptive epidemiology describes the distribution of disease, death, and other health outcomes in the population according to person, place, and time, providing a picture of how things are or have been—the who, where, and when of disease patterns. Analytic epidemiology, on the other hand, searches for the determinants of the patterns observed—the how and why. That is, epidemiologic concepts and methods are used to identify what factors, characteristics, exposures, or behaviors might account for differences in the observed patterns of disease occurrence. Descriptive and analytic studies are observational, meaning the investigator observes events as they are or have been and does not intervene to change anything or introduce a new factor. Experimental or intervention studies, however, include interventions to test preventive or treatment measures, techniques, materials, policies, or drugs.

Person

Personal characteristics of interest in epidemiology include race, ethnicity, sex, age, education, occupation, income (and related socioeconomic status), and marital status. As noted previously, the most important predictor of overall mortality is age. The mortality curve by age drops sharply during and after the first year of life to a low point in childhood, then it begins to increase through adolescence and young adulthood, and after that it increases sharply (exponentially) through middle and older ages (Gordis, 2009).

There are also substantial differences in mortality and morbidity rates by sex. Female infants have a lower mortality rate than comparable male infants, and the survival advantage continues throughout life (Xu, Kochanek, and Tejada-Vera, 2009). However, patterns for specific diseases vary. For example, women have lower rates of CHD until menopause, after which the gap narrows. For rheumatoid arthritis, the prevalence among women is greater than among men (Remington, Brownson, and Wegner, 2010).

Although the concept of race as a variable for public health research has come under scrutiny (CDC, 1993; Fullilove, 1998), there are clear differences in morbidity and mortality rates by race in the United States (USDHHS, 2000; NCHS, 2009). According to the Office of Minority Health (OMH, 1999), racial and ethnic minority groups are among the fastest-growing populations in the United States, yet they have poorer health and remain chronically underserved by the health care system. Data in the OMH report *Elimination of Racial and Ethnic Disparities in Health* highlighted some of the significant health disparities within the leading categories of death in the United States. For example, in 2007 the overall infant mortality rate (IMR) was 6.8 deaths per 1000 live births, but the IMR among African Americans was 12.9 per 1000 live births (Xu, Kochanek, and Tejada-Vera, 2009), and the gap has been widening in recent years. Racial and ethnic health disparities have been observed in a wide range of diseases and health behaviors, from infant mortality to diabetes, heart disease, cancer, and HIV. Although there has been some progress toward meeting the goal of eliminating racial/ethnic disparities, with improvement in rates for most health status indicators across all racial/ethnic groups, the improvements have not been uniform across groups and "substantial differences among racial/ethnic groups persist" (Keppel, Pearcy, and Wagener, 2002). Among Native Americans and Native Alaskans, several health indicators actually worsened from 1990 to 1998. The IMR declined in all groups, but it remains 2.3 times higher for infants born to non-Hispanic African-American mothers than for those born to white non-Hispanic mothers. Similarly, the overall age-adjusted mortality rate was 22% higher in the African-American population than in the white population in 2006, and it was higher for 10 of the 15 leading causes of death (Heron et al, 2009). Although individual characteristics such as race, gender, and immigration status are of interest to epidemiologists, there has been increasing focus on social, economic, and cultural contexts and processes underlying racial and ethnic inequalities in health, such as discrimination (Krieger, 2000; Fuller et al, 2005;).

Place

When considering the distribution of a disease, geographic patterns come to mind: Does the rate of disease differ from place to place (e.g., with local environment)? If geography had no effect on disease occurrence, random geographic patterns might be seen, but that is often not the case. For example, at high altitudes there is lower oxygen surface tension, which might result in smaller babies. Other diseases reflect distinctive geographic patterns. For example, Lyme disease is transmitted from animal reservoirs to humans by a tick vector. Thus, the disease is more likely to be found in areas where there are animals carrying the disease, a large tick population for transmission to humans, and contact between the human population and the tick vectors (Heymann, 2008).

The influence of place on disease may certainly be related to geographic variations in the chemical, physical, or biological environment. However, variations by place also may result from differences in population densities, or in customary patterns of behavior and lifestyle, or in other personal characteristics. For example, geographic variations might occur because of high concentrations of a religious, cultural, or ethnic group who practice certain health-related behaviors. The high rates of stroke found in the southeastern United States are likely to be the result of a number of social, economic, cultural, and personal factors that have little to do with geographic features per se. Recent epidemiologic research has also focused on neighborhood-level variables, such as unemployment and crime rate, social cohesion, educational levels, racial segregation, and access to important services (Cohen et al, 2000; Caughy, O'Campo, and Patterson, 2001; Bradman et al, 2005; Fuller et al, 2005; McLafferty and Grady, 2005). For example, recent research on adolescent injection drug users (IDUs) found that African-American IDUs from neighborhoods with large percentages of minority residents and low adult educational levels were more likely to initiate injection use during adolescence than white IDUs from neighborhoods with low percentages of minority residents and high adult education levels. Nurses need to pay attention to this wide range of community-level variables as they assess the health of communities.

Time

Time is the third component of descriptive epidemiology. In relation to time, epidemiologists ask these questions: Is there an increase or decrease in the frequency of the disease over time? Are other temporal (and spatial) patterns evident? Temporal patterns of interest to epidemiologists include secular trends, point epidemic, cyclical patterns, and event-related clusters.

Secular Trends

Long-term patterns of morbidity or mortality rates (i.e., over years or decades) are called secular trends. Secular trends may reflect changes in social behavior or health practices. For example, the increased lung cancer mortality rates among men and women in recent years reflect a delayed effect of increased smoking in prior years. Similarly, the decline in cervical cancer deaths is primarily attributable to widespread screening with the Pap test (Remington, Brownson, and Wegner, 2010). Some secular trends may result from increased diagnostic capability or changes in survival (or case fatality) rather than in incidence. For example, case fatality from breast cancer has decreased in recent years although the incidence of breast cancer has increased. Some, although not all, of the increased incidence is a result of improved diagnostic capability. These two trends result in a breast cancer mortality curve that is flatter than the incidence curve (Remington et al, 2010). Mortality data alone do not accurately reflect the true situation. For example, changes in case definition or revisions in the coding of a disease according to the International Classification of Diseases (ICD) can produce an artificial change in mortality rates.

Point Epidemic

One temporal and spatial pattern of disease distribution is the point epidemic. This time-and-space–related pattern is important in infectious disease investigations and is a significant indicator for toxic exposures in environmental epidemiology. A point epidemic is most clearly seen when the frequency of cases is plotted against time. The sharp peak characteristic of such graphs indicates a concentration of cases in some short interval of time. The peak often indicates the response of the population to a common source of infection or contamination to which they were all simultaneously exposed. Knowledge of the incubation or latency period (the time between exposure and development of signs and symptoms) for the specific disease entity can help to determine the probable time of exposure. A common example of a point epidemic is an outbreak of gastrointestinal illness from a foodborne pathogen. Nurses who are alert to a sudden increase in the number of cases of a disease can chart the outbreak, determine the probable time of exposure, and, by careful investigation, isolate the probable source of the agent.

Cyclical Patterns

In addition to secular trends and point epidemics, there are also cyclical time patterns of disease. One common type of cyclical variation is the seasonal fluctuation seen in a number of infectious illnesses. Seasonal changes may be influenced by changes in the agent itself, changes in population densities or behaviors of animal reservoirs or vectors, or changes in human behavior that result in changing exposures (e.g., being outdoors in warmer weather and indoors in colder months). There may also be artificial seasons created by calendar events (e.g., holidays and tax-filing deadlines) that may be associated with patterns of stress-related illness. Patterns of accidents and injuries may also be seasonal, reflecting differing employment and recreational patterns. Some disease cycles, such as influenza, have patterns of smaller epidemics every few years, depending on strain, with major pandemics occurring at longer intervals (Heymann, 2008). Workers in public health can prepare to meet increased demands on resources by careful attention to these cyclical patterns.

Event-Related Clusters

A fourth type of temporal pattern is non-simultaneous, event-related clusters. These are patterns in which time is not measured from fixed dates on the calendar but from the point of some exposure or event, presumably experienced in common by affected persons, although not occurring at the same time. An example would be vaccine reactions in an ongoing immunization program. If vaccinations are given on a regular basis, one might see non-specific symptoms (e.g., fever, headaches, and rashes) fairly consistently over perhaps a year, making identification of a cluster related to the vaccinations difficult. If, however, the time of vaccination is artificially set as zero for each client, and the number of clients with symptoms is plotted against the time since time zero, the reactions are likely to show up as a peak at some period after the immunization.

ANALYTIC EPIDEMIOLOGY

Descriptive epidemiology deals with the distribution of health outcomes, whereas analytic epidemiology seeks to discover the determinants of outcomes, or the how and the why (i.e., the factors that influence observed patterns of health and disease and increase or decrease the risk of adverse outcomes). This section deals with analytic study designs and the related measures of association derived from them. Table 12-4 summarizes the advantages and disadvantages of each design.

Cohort Studies

The cohort study is the standard for observational epidemiologic studies, coming closest to the ideal of a natural experiment (Rothman, 2002). In epidemiology, the term cohort is used to describe a group of persons who are born at about the same time. In analytic studies, a cohort refers to a group of persons (generally sharing some characteristic of interest) enrolled in a study and followed over a period of time to observe some health outcome (Porta, 2008). Because they enable us to observe the development of new cases of disease, cohort study designs allow

TABLE 12-4 COMPARISON OF MAJOR EPIDEMIOLOGIC STUDY DESIGNS

STUDY DESIGN	ADVANTAGES	DISADVANTAGES
Ecologic	• Quick, easy, and inexpensive first study • Uses readily available existing data • May prompt further investigation or suggest other/new hypotheses • May provide information about contextual factors not accounted for by individual characteristics	• Ecologic fallacy: associations observed may not hold true for individuals • Problems in interpreting temporal sequence (cause and effect) • More difficult to control for confounding and "mixed" models (ecological and individual data); more complex statistically
Cross-sectional	• Gives general description of scope of problem; provides prevalence estimates • Often based on population (or community) sample, not just those who sought care • Useful in health service evaluation and planning • Data obtained at once; less expensive and quicker than cohort because no follow-up • Baseline for prospective study or to identify cases and controls for case-control study	• No calculation of risk; prevalence, not incidence • Temporal sequence unclear • Not good for rare disease or rare exposure unless large sample size or stratified sampling • Selective survival can be major source of selection bias; surviving subjects may differ from those who are not included (e.g., death, institutionalization) • Selective recall or lack of past exposure information can create bias
Case-control (retrospective, case comparison)	• Less expensive than cohort; smaller sample required • Quicker than cohort; no follow-up • Can investigate more than one exposure • Best design for rare diseases • If well designed, can be important tool for etiological investigation • Best suited to disease with relatively clear onset (timing of onset can be established so that incident cases can be included)	• Greater susceptibility than cohort studies to various types of bias (selective survival, recall bias, selection bias on choice of both cases and controls) • Information on other risk factors may not be available, resulting in confounding • Antecedent-consequence (temporal sequence) not as certain as in cohort • Not well suited to rare exposures • Gives only an indirect estimate of risk • Limited to a single outcome because of sampling on disease status
Prospective cohort (concurrent cohort, longitudinal, follow-up)	• Best estimate of disease incidence • Best estimate of risk • Fewer problems with selective survival and selective recall • Temporal sequence more clearly established • Broader range of options for exposure assessment	• Expensive in time and money • More difficult organizationally • Not good for rare diseases • Attrition of participants can bias estimate • Latency period may be very long; may miss cases • May be difficult to examine several exposures
Retrospective cohort (non-concurrent cohort)	• Combines advantages of both prospective cohort and case-control • Shorter time (even if follow-up into future) than prospective cohort • Less expensive than prospective cohort because reliant on existing data • Temporal sequence may be clearer than case-control	• Shares some disadvantages with both prospective cohort and case-control • Subject to attrition (loss to follow-up) • Relies on existing records that may result in misclassification of both exposure and outcome • May have to rely on surrogate measure of exposure (e.g., job title) and vital records information on cause of death

calculation of incidence rates and therefore estimates of disease risk. Cohort studies may be prospective or retrospective (Rothman, 2002; Szklo and Nieto, 2007; Gordis, 2009).

Prospective Cohort Studies

In a prospective cohort study (also called a longitudinal or follow-up study), subjects determined to be free of the outcome under investigation are classified on the basis of the exposure of interest at the beginning of the follow-up period. The different exposure groups constitute the comparison groups for the study. The subjects are then followed for some period of time to determine the occurrence of disease in each group. The question is the following: "Do persons with the factor (or exposure) of interest develop (or avoid) the outcome more frequently than those without the factor (or exposure)?"

For example, one might recruit a cohort of subjects classified as physically active ("exposed") or sedentary ("not exposed"). One might further quantify the amount of the "exposure" if there is sufficient information. These subjects would then be followed over time to determine the development of CHD. This study design avoids the problem of selective survival that sometimes affects other study designs (Figure 12-5). Because persons initially without the disease are followed over time, this design allows estimation of both incidence rates and incidence proportions. The cohort study can also estimate the relative risk of acquiring disease for those who are exposed compared with those who are unexposed (or less exposed). This ratio of incidence proportions is called the risk ratio (or relative risk), and a ratio incidence rate is called the rate ratio. For example, if the risk of CHD in smokers is twice as high as the risk among non-smokers, the risk ratio would be 2. If a factor is unrelated to the risk of a disease, the risk ratio will be close to 1. A value less than 1 may suggest a protective association. For example, the risk of CHD is lower among those who are physically active than among sedentary persons, so the risk ratio for the association between physical activity and CHD should be less than 1.

Suppose 1000 physically active and 1000 sedentary middle-aged men and women enroll in a prospective cohort study. All are free of CHD at enrollment. Over a 5-year follow-up period, regular examinations detect CHD in 120 of the sedentary men and women, and in 48 of the active men and women. Assuming no other deaths or losses to follow-up, the data could be presented as shown in Figure 12-5.

The incidence proportion of CHD in the active group is a/(a + b), or 48/1000, and the incidence of CHD in the sedentary group is c/(c + d), or 120/1000. The risk ratio is as follows:

$$\left(\frac{48}{1000}\right) \div \left(\frac{120}{1000}\right) = 0.4$$

Because physical activity is protective for CHD, the risk ratio is less than 1. The interpretation for this hypothetical example is that, over a 5-year period, the risk of CHD in persons who are physically active is about 0.4 as great as the risk among sedentary persons. If the risk was greater for those exposed, the risk ratio would be greater than 1. For example, if the risk ratio of CHD for overweight persons compared with normal weight is 3.5, it would be interpreted to mean that the risk of CHD among overweight persons is 3.5 times the risk of those with normal weight. The null value indicating no association is 1, because the incidence proportion and thus the risk would be equal in the two groups if there were no association.

Because subjects are enrolled before onset of disease, using the cohort design allows us to study more than one outcome, calculate incidence rates and proportions, estimate risk, and establish the temporal sequence of exposure and outcome with greater clarity and certainty. Use of the cohort design also may avoid many of the problems of the other study designs with selective survival or exposure misclassification (discussed later). On the other hand, large samples are often necessary to ensure that enough cases are observed to provide enough statistical power to detect meaningful differences between groups. This is complicated by the long period required for some diseases to develop (the latency period). In addition, the number of subjects required to observe sufficient cases makes longitudinal studies unsuitable for very rare diseases unless they are part of a larger study of a number of outcomes.

Retrospective Cohort Studies

Retrospective cohort studies combine some of the advantages and some of the disadvantages of both case-control studies and prospective cohort studies. In these studies, the epidemiologist relies on existing records, such as employment, insurance, or hospital records, to define a cohort, whose members are classified according to exposure status at some time in the past. The cohort is followed over time using the records to determine if the outcome occurred. Retrospective cohort (also called historical cohort) studies may be conducted entirely using past records or may include current assessment or additional follow-up time after study initiation. The obvious advantage of this approach is the time savings, because one does not have to wait for new cases of disease to develop. The disadvantages are largely related to the reliance on existing historical records. Retrospective cohort studies are frequently used in occupational epidemiology where industrial records are available to investigate work-related exposures and health outcomes.

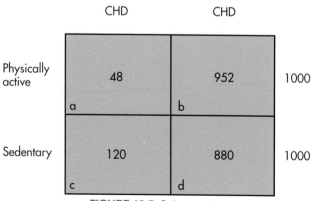

FIGURE 12-5 Cohort study.

NURSING TIP *Epidemiologic studies conducted by nurse researchers have direct application to all areas of nursing.*

Case-Control Studies

The **case-control design** can be viewed against the background of an underlying cohort. The design uses a sample from the cohort rather than following the entire cohort over time. Because it uses only samples of cases and non-cases, it is a more efficient design, although it is subject to certain types of bias (Rothman, 2002). In the **case-control study,** participants are enrolled because they are known to have the outcome of interest (cases) or they are known *not* to have the outcome of interest (controls). Case-control status is verified using a clear case definition and some previously determined method or protocol (e.g., by an examination, laboratory test, or medical chart review). Information is then collected on the exposures or characteristics of interest, frequently from existing sources, subject interview, or questionnaire (Schlesselman, 1982; Rothman, 2002; Szklo and Nieto, 2007). The question in a case-control study is the following: "Do persons with the outcome of interest (cases) have the exposure characteristic (or a history of the exposure) more frequently than those without the outcome (controls)?"

Suppose a research group wanted to study risk factors for suicide attempts among adolescents. They were able to enroll 100 adolescents who had attempted suicide, and they selected 200 adolescents from the same community with no history of suicide attempt. One of the factors they wanted to investigate is a history of substance abuse. Through a questionnaire and other medical records, they determine that 68 of the 100 adolescents who had attempted suicide had a history of substance abuse, whereas 36 of the 200 adolescents with no suicide attempt had such a history. The information could be presented as shown in Figure 12-6. The odds of a positive history of substance abuse among adolescents who attempt suicide is a/c, or 68/32, whereas the odds of substance abuse among controls (no suicide attempts) is b/d, or 36/164. The odds ratio (equivalent to ad/bc) is as follows:

$$\frac{(68 \times 164)}{(36 \times 32)} = 9.68$$

This would be interpreted to mean that the odds of a history of substance abuse are about 10 times greater among adolescents who have attempted suicide than among adolescents who have

not attempted suicide. Note that, as with the risk ratio, an odds ratio of 1 is indicative of no association (i.e., the odds of exposure are similar for cases and controls). An odds ratio less than 1 suggests a protective association (cases are less likely to have been exposed than controls).

Given the way subjects are selected for a case-control study, neither incidence nor prevalence measures can be calculated directly. However, if newly diagnosed cases are enrolled as they are found, and if case ascertainment is fairly complete and the source population well defined, an estimate of incidence may be obtained. In a case-control study, an odds ratio tells how much more or less likely the exposure is to be found among cases than among controls. The odds of exposure among cases (a/c in Figure 12-6) are compared with the odds of exposure among controls (b/d in Figure 12-6). Under certain conditions, the ratio of these two odds provides an estimate of the risk ratio or rate ratio.

Because the number of cases is known or actively sought out, case-control studies do not demand large samples or the long follow-up time that is often required for prospective cohort studies. Thus many of the influential cancer studies are of the case-control design.

Case-control studies are, however, prone to a number of biases (see further discussion under "Bias" later in this chapter). Because these studies begin with existing cases, differential survival can produce biased results. The use of recently diagnosed, or "incident," cases may reduce this bias. Also, exposure information is obtained from subject recall or past records, and there may be errors in exposure assessment or misclassification. Because participants are selected precisely because they do or do not have a specific health outcome, case-control studies are limited to a single outcome, although they may investigate a number of potential risk factors.

Cross-Sectional Studies

The **cross-sectional study** provides a snapshot, or cross-section, of a population or group (Gordis, 2009). Information is collected on current health status, personal characteristics, and potential risk factors or exposures all at once. The cross-sectional study is characterized by the simultaneous collection of information necessary for the classification of exposure and outcome status, although there may be historical information collected (e.g., on past diet or history of radiation exposure). Surveys are one common type of data collection for cross-sectional studies. They may be administered in person, over the phone, by mail, or, increasingly, on websites or through personal electronic devices. Each form of administration has its advantages and disadvantages, as does the use of surveys for epidemiologic studies, but a complete discussion of survey methodology is beyond the scope of this chapter.

Cross-sectional studies are sometimes called prevalence studies because they provide the frequency of existing cases of a disease in a population. One way cross-sectional studies evaluate the association of a factor with a health problem is by comparing the prevalence of the disease in those who have the factor (or exposure) with the prevalence in the unexposed. The ratio of the two prevalence proportions indicates an association between the factor and the outcome. If the prevalence of CHD in smokers

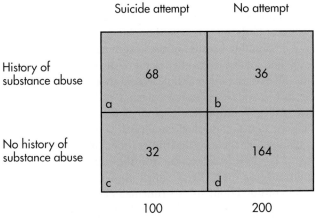

	Suicide attempt	No attempt
History of substance abuse	68 **a**	36 **b**
No history of substance abuse	32 **c**	164 **d**
	100	200

FIGURE 12-6 Case-control study.

was twice as high as the prevalence among non-smokers, the prevalence ratio would be 2. If a factor is unrelated to the prevalence of a disease, the prevalence ratio will be close to 1. A value less than 1 may suggest a protective association. For example, the prevalence of CHD is lower among those who are physically active than among sedentary persons, so the prevalence ratio for the association between physical activity and CHD should be less than 1. Prevalence ratios require caution in interpretation because the prevalence measure is affected by cure, survival, and migration and does not estimate the risk of getting the disease.

Cross-sectional studies are subject to bias resulting from selective survival (i.e., people who have survived to be in the study may be different from people diagnosed about the same time who have died and are not available for inclusion). Suppose that physical activity not only reduced the risk of CHD but also markedly improved survival among those with CHD. Sedentary persons with CHD would then have higher fatality rates than physically active persons who did develop CHD. One might observe higher rates of physical activity in a group of persons surviving with CHD than in a general population without CHD, both because of the survival advantage of those who previously were active and because of increased participation of other survivors in cardiac rehabilitation programs. It could erroneously appear that physical activity was a risk factor for CHD.

Ecologic Studies

An epidemiologic study that is a bridge between descriptive epidemiology and analytic epidemiology is the ecologic study. The descriptive component involves examining variations in disease rates by person, place, or time. The analytic component lies in the effort to determine if there is a relationship between disease rates and variations in rates for possible risk (or protective) factors. The identifying characteristic of ecologic studies is that only aggregate data, such as population rates, are used rather than data on individuals' exposures, characteristics, and outcomes. For example, information on per capita cigarette consumption might be examined in relation to lung cancer mortality rates in several countries, in several groups of people, or in the same population at different times. Other examples include comparisons of rates of breastfeeding and breast cancer, average dietary fat content and rates of CHD, or unemployment rates and levels of psychiatric disorders.

Ecologic studies are attractive because they often make use of existing, readily available rates and are therefore quick and inexpensive to conduct. They are subject, however, to ecologic fallacy (i.e., associations observed at the group level may not hold true for the individuals that make up the groups, or associations that actually exist may be masked in the grouped data). This may be the result of other factors operating in these populations for which the ecological correlations do not account. For that reason, ecologic studies may be suggestive but require confirmation in studies using individual data (Koepsell and Weiss, 2003; Gordis, 2009). However, it has been shown that ecological data can add important information to analyses even when individual-level data are available (Lynch et al, 1998; Diez-Roux, 2002). Uncertainty concerning the temporal sequence of events is a disadvantage that ecologic studies share with cross-sectional study designs. For example, in the study of unemployment rates and psychiatric disorders, it is unclear whether unemployed persons are at higher risk for psychiatric problems or whether persons with existing psychiatric problems are more likely to be unemployed. Although determining whether one event precedes or succeeds another may seem at first to be a simple matter, in practice it may be difficult to confirm.

EXPERIMENTAL STUDIES

The study designs discussed so far are called observational studies because the investigator observes the association between exposures and outcomes as they exist but does not intervene to alter the presence or level of any exposure or behavior. Studies in which the investigator initiates some treatment or intervention that may influence the risk or course of disease are called *intervention*, or *experimental, studies*. Such studies test whether interventions are effective in preventing disease or improving health. Like observational studies, experimental studies generally use comparison (or control) groups, but unlike observational studies, they are subject to the consequences of randomly allocating persons to a particular intervention group and determining the type or level of the "exposure" (the treatment or intervention). Intervention studies are of two general types: clinical trials and community trials.

Clinical Trials

In clinical trials, the research issue is generally the efficacy of a medical treatment for disease, such as a new drug or an existing drug used in a new or different way, a surgical technique, or another treatment. The preferred method of subject allocation in clinical trials is randomization (i.e., assigning treatments to clients so that all possible treatment assignments have a predetermined probability but neither subject nor investigator determines the actual assignment of any participant). Randomization avoids the bias that may result if subjects self-select into one group or the other or if the investigator or clinician chooses subjects for each group. A second aspect of treatment allocation is the use of masking, or "blinding," treatment assignments. The optimal design for most situations is the double-blind study in which neither the subject nor the investigator knows who is receiving which treatment. The aim of blinding is to reduce the bias from overestimating therapeutic benefit for the experimental treatment when it is known who is receiving it.

Clinical trials are generally thought to provide the best evidence of causality because of the assignment of treatment and the greater control over other factors that could influence outcome. Like cohort studies, clinical trials are prospective in direction and provide the clearest evidence of temporal sequence. However, clinical trials are generally conducted in a contrived situation, under controlled conditions, and with select client populations. That means that the treatment may be less effective when it is applied under more realistic clinical or community conditions in a more diverse client population. There are also ethical considerations in experimental studies that go beyond those that apply to observational studies. Also, clinical trials tend to be costly in time, personnel, facilities, and other factors.

> **WHAT DO YOU THINK?** *Epidemiologic studies are often inconclusive about causal associations. The same may be true for epidemiologic-based evaluations of prevention programs. Should there be a difference in how we interpret results for purposes of designing future research as opposed to recommending guidelines? Should there be a difference in interpretation and application of epidemiologic results for individuals and for community or public policy?*

Community Trials

Community trials are similar to clinical trials in that an investigator determines the exposure or intervention, but in this case the issue is often health promotion and disease prevention rather than treatment of existing disease. The intervention is usually undertaken on a large scale, with the unit of treatment allocation being a community, region, or group rather than individuals. Although a pharmaceutical product may be involved in a community trial (e.g., fluoridation of water or mass immunizations), community trials often involve educational, programmatic, or policy interventions. An example of community intervention is providing exercise programs and facilities and increasing the availability of healthy, fresh foods to study the effect on diabetes rates.

Although community trials provide the best means of testing whether changes in knowledge or behavior, policy, programs, or other mass interventions are effective, they are not without problems. For many interventions, it may take years for the effectiveness of the intervention to be evident. In the meantime, other factors may also influence the outcome, either positively (making the intervention look more effective than it really is) or negatively (making the intervention look less effective than it really is). Comparable community populations without similar interventions for comparative analysis are often difficult to determine. Even when comparable comparison communities are available, especially when the intervention is intended to improve knowledge or change behavior, it is difficult and unethical to prevent the control communities from making use of generally available information. Exposure to this information, however, may have the effect of making control communities more like the intervention communities. Also, because community trials are often undertaken on a large scale and over long periods, they can be expensive, requiring large staff, complicated logistics, and extensive communication resources. Although the randomized trial is often considered the "gold standard" of medical and public health research, because of the limitations noted above, there is clearly a need for other types of research designs to complement randomized control trials (Victoria, Habicht, and Bryce, 2004).

CAUSALITY

Statistical Associations

One of the first steps in assessing the relationship of some factor with a health outcome is determining whether a statistical association exists. If the probability of disease seems unaffected by the presence or level of the factor, no association is apparent. If,

on the other hand, the probability of disease does vary according to whether the factor is present, there is a statistical association. The earlier discussion of null values is pertinent at this point. When an observed measure of association (such as a risk ratio) does not differ from the null value, it may not be assumed that there is an association between the factor and the outcome under investigation.

In many studies, a great deal of emphasis is placed on tests of statistical significance. This is a judgment that the observed results are or are not likely to be attributable to chance at some predetermined level of probability (usually 0.05). However, many epidemiologists contend that much more information is provided by an estimate of the association (the ratio or difference in rates or risks) and a confidence interval that indicates the precision of the estimate (Rothman, 2002). Note that statistical significance is determined by sample size, the amount of difference between groups, and the variance in the estimates.

Bias

Although statistical testing and estimation are critical, it is important to remember that statistical testing and interval estimation generally assume that deviations from the true value are the result of chance. However, estimates may appear to be greater or less than they really are because of **bias**, a systematic error resulting from the study design, execution, or confounding. For example, if there were a gumball machine with colors randomly mixed and three red ones in a row came out, that would be a result of chance. If, however, the person loading the gumball machine had poured in a bag of red ones first, then green ones, and then yellow, it would not be surprising to get three red ones in a row because of the way the machine was loaded. In epidemiologic studies, results are sometimes biased because of the way the study was "loaded" (i.e., the way the study was designed, subjects were selected, information was collected, or subjects were classified). Three generally recognized categories are selection, classification, and confounding bias (Rothman, 2002).

Bias attributable to the way subjects enter a study is called selection bias. It has to do with selection procedures and the population from which subjects are drawn. It may involve self-selection factors as well. For example, are teenagers who agree to complete a questionnaire on alcohol, tobacco, and other drug use representative of the total teenage population?

Bias attributable to misclassification of subjects once they are in the study is information, or classification (or misclassification), bias. It is related to how information is collected, including the information that subjects supply or how subjects are classified.

Bias resulting from the relationship of the outcome and study factor with some third factor not accounted for is called *confounding*. For example, there is a well-known association between maternal smoking during pregnancy and low-birth-weight babies. There is also an association between alcohol consumption and smoking that is not attributable to chance nor is it causal (i.e., drinking alcohol does not cause a person to smoke, nor does smoking cause a person to drink alcohol). If one were to investigate the association of alcohol consumption and low birth weight, smoking would be a confounder because it is related to both alcohol consumption and low birth weight. Failure to account for smoking in the analysis would bias the observed association between alcohol use and low birth weight. In practice, one can often identify potentially confounding variables and adjust for them in analysis.

WHAT DO YOU THINK? *The concept of bias may seem difficult to grasp in the context of public health research, but is readily understood within the context of nursing practice. Understanding possible bias in a study is really about identifying how different people act in response to specific situations. Think about how accurately different individuals may self-report their levels of physical activity. What factors may contribute to their over- or under-reporting their actual level of physical activity? How might these individual biases affect the results of research in which individuals are asked to self-report their daily level of physical activity, compared with actually measuring physical activity through the use of an activity monitor?*

Assessing for Causality

The existence of a statistical association does not necessarily mean that there is a causal relationship or that causality is present (Susser, 1973). As noted previously, the observed association may be a random event (caused by chance) or may be attributable to bias from confounding or from flaws in the study design or execution. Statistical associations, although necessary to an argument for causality, are not sufficient proof. Some epidemiologists refer to *criteria for causality,* a term originally established to evaluate the link between an infectious agent and a disease but revised and elaborated to also apply to other outcomes. Although various lists of criteria have been proposed, the seven criteria listed in Box 12-3 are fairly commonly cited (Gordis, 2009; Koepsell and Weiss, 2003). Some have questioned the use of lists of criteria as misleading, especially because only temporal sequence is necessary, and none of the others really is a criterion (Rothman, 2002). Although no single epidemiologic study can satisfy all criteria, public health practitioners rely on the accumulation of evidence and the strength of individual studies to provide a basis for effective public health interventions and policies.

APPLICATIONS OF EPIDEMIOLOGY IN NURSING

Both knowledge and practical application of epidemiology are essential competencies for nurses (Gebbie and Hwang, 2000). Nurses incorporate epidemiology into their practices and take on a variety of epidemiologic roles. Nurses in diverse settings are involved in the collection, reporting, analysis, interpretation, and communication of epidemiologic data as part of their daily practice. As nurses care for persons with communicable diseases, they are implementing epidemiologic practices as they identify, report, treat, and provide follow-up on cases and contacts of TB, gonorrhea, and gastroenteritis. School nurses also function as epidemiologists, collecting data on the incidence and prevalence of accidents, injuries, and illnesses in the school population. They are also key players in the detection

---

BOX 12-3   CRITERIA FOR CAUSALITY

1. *Strength of association:* A strong association between a potential risk factor and an outcome supports a causal hypothesis (e.g., a relative risk of 7 provides stronger evidence of a causal association than a relative risk of 1.5).
2. *Consistency of findings:* Repeated findings of an association with different study designs and in different populations strengthen causal inference.
3. *Biological plausibility:* Demonstration of a physiological mechanism by which the risk factor acts to cause disease enhances the causal hypothesis. Conversely, an association that does not initially seem biologically defensible may later be discovered to be so.
4. *Demonstration of correct temporal sequence:* For a risk factor to cause an outcome, it must precede the onset of the outcome. (See Prospective Cohort Studies and Table 12-4.)
5. *Dose–response relationship:* The risk of developing an outcome should increase with increasing exposure (either in duration or in quantity) to the risk factor of interest. For example, studies have shown that the more a woman smokes during pregnancy, the greater the risk of delivering a low-birth-weight infant.
6. *Specificity of the association:* The presence of a one-to-one relationship between an agent and a disease (i.e., the idea that a disease is caused by only one agent and that agent results in only one disease lends support to a causal hypothesis, but its absence does not rule out causality). This criterion is cultivated from the infectious disease model, where it is more often, although not always, satisfied and is less applicable in chronic diseases.
7. *Experimental evidence:* Experimental designs provide the strongest epidemiologic evidence for causal associations, but they are not feasible or ethical to conduct for many risk factor–disease associations.

---

and control of local epidemics, such as outbreaks of lice. As described earlier in this chapter, nurses across practice settings are actively involved in activities related to primary, secondary, and tertiary prevention (see Levels of Prevention box on p. 267).

Some nursing job descriptions are specifically based in epidemiologic practice. These include hospital infection control nurses, nurse epidemiologists, and nurse environmental risk communicators employed by local health departments. Nurses are key members of local fetal and infant mortality review boards, which examine cases of newborn deaths for identifiable risk factors and quality of care measures. Members of these review boards may include public health and maternal child nurses as well as representatives from hospital labor and delivery and neonatal intensive care units.

Nursing documentation on client charts and records is an important source of data for epidemiologic reviews. Client demographics and health histories are often collected or verified by nurses. As nurses collect and document client information, they might not be thinking about the epidemiologic connection. However, the reliability and validity of such data can be a key factor in the quality of future epidemiologic studies. An excellent resource for the application of epidemiologic concepts and methods in practice settings can be found in Brownson and Petitti (2006).

Community-Oriented Epidemiology

Nurses are often involved in environmental health issues, where they play important roles not only as epidemiologists, but also as community liaisons (Mood, 2000). Nurses serve as important professional contacts and liaisons for people in the community who are actively investigating or concerned about the health and illness issue, such as an increase in the number of cases of cancer, asthma, or traffic accidents. The role of community liaison involves observation, data collection, consultation, and interpretation. By talking and listening to community members around their kitchen tables, at local gathering places, or at community meetings, nurses gather information from the citizens' perspectives. They can also interpret scientific information for lay persons. The liaison role also involves consultation with public health and environmental professionals and participation in environmental inspections and investigations.

Lillian Mood is a public health nurse with more than 20 years of experience in South Carolina working with communities to detect and explain the causes of illness and disability. In describing her involvement with specific communities, Mood noted that the contact often began with a telephone call of concern about a planned or existing industrial facility or a first-hand observation of illness, expressed in lay terms as "too many cases of cancer," "several people have had miscarriages," or "more respiratory problems." The citizen's reasoning behind these observations is that "'If I am seeing more health problems in my community, I ask what they have in common. The common factor may be where we live. So it must be the air or the water.' This is basic epidemiologic thinking, not irrational fear. Citizens try to make sense of what they are seeing, and they want professional help to unravel the pattern of illness" (Mood, 2000, p 24).

Popular Epidemiology

In health departments and hospitals, nurses frequently work with other professionals who have training in epidemiology. However, in the community they may encounter citizens engaged in the practice of popular epidemiology (Brown and Ferguson, 1995; Brown and Masterson-Allen, 1994). **Popular epidemiology** is a form of epidemiology in which lay people gather scientific data as well as mobilize knowledge and resources of experts to understand the occurrence and distribution of a disease or injury. Popular epidemiology is more than just adding public participation to traditional epidemiology; it also includes an emphasis on social structural factors as a component of disease etiology, as well as the involvement of social movements, political and judicial approaches to remedies, and challenges to basic assumptions of traditional epidemiology, risk assessment, and public health regulation (Brown and Ferguson, 1995, p 149). Popular epidemiology considers the physiological, psychological, and social effects of environmental hazards and attempts to show how racial, class, and gender differences are evident in the health effects of environmental toxic exposure. In contrast, many standard environmental health assessments are not designed to understand local cultures, traditions, or ethnic backgrounds (DiChiro, 1997). This lack of cultural competency can render assessment tools ineffective in terms of the ability to identify potential routes of toxic exposure.

Toxic waste activists are often women living in the community who have first-hand contact with toxic hazards and therefore have experiences and access to data that would otherwise

EVIDENCE-BASED PRACTICE

The Epidemiologic Basis for Community Health Interventions

Queso fresco, a popular Latin American fresh cheese often made from raw milk, has been implicated as a source of *Salmonella typhimurium* definitive type (DT) 104 in the United States. From 1992 to 1996, the annual incidence of *S. typhimurium* DT104 infections in Yakima County, Washington, increased from 5.4 to 29.7 cases per 100,000 population, making it one of the highest rates in the country. Between January and May 1997, 89 cases of *S. typhimurium* were reported in the county, of which 54 were culture-confirmed as DT104, a strain that is resistant to five major antibiotics. The median age of infected persons was 4 years, and 90% of the clients had Spanish surnames. A case-control investigation conducted by the CDC indicated that the most probable source of the outbreak was raw-milk *queso fresco.* The CDC investigation also indicated that street vendors were the most frequent source (70%) of *queso fresco* among those who developed the illness.

In response to the outbreak, a multiagency intervention was initiated with the goal of reducing the incidence of *S. typhimurium* infections resulting from consumption of raw-milk *queso fresco,* while maintaining the traditional, nutritious food in the local Hispanic diet. A pasteurized-milk *queso fresco* recipe developed by a local Hispanic woman was modified by dairy scientists at Washington State University to inhibit undesirable microbial growth, increase shelf life, and improve ease of preparation. The new recipe was tested by local Hispanic persons and adjusted until flavor and texture were satisfactory.

A pre-intervention survey was conducted to gather background information for use in planning the multipronged intervention, which featured safe-cheese workshops introducing the new pasteurized-milk recipe, a mass media campaign about the risk of raw-milk cheese, and newsletter articles warning dairy farmers

about the risks of selling or giving away raw milk. The safe-cheese workshops were conducted by older Hispanic women (*abuelas,* or grandmothers), who were recruited from the community and trained to make the new *queso fresco* recipe from pasteurized milk. Following the training, each abuela educator signed a contract indicating her willingness to teach at least 15 additional members of the community how to safely make *queso fresco* with pasteurized milk. They followed through on their commitment, which included returning surveys completed by the women they taught.

The incidence of *S. typhimurium* infection in Yakima County decreased rapidly to below pre-1992 levels after the multilevel intervention was initiated. Between June and December 1997, only 16 cases were reported, of which 2 were associated with consumption of *queso fresco;* in 1998 there were 18 reported cases, none of which were associated with *queso fresco.* Post-intervention surveys of Hispanic area residents who did not participate in the workshops indicated that consumption of *queso fresco* did not decrease as a result of the intervention.

Nurse Use

The *Abuela Project* is an example of a successful combination of applied epidemiology and community-based, culturally appropriate public health interventions. This activity clearly falls within the scope of good public health nursing. To be successful in seeing correlations, nurses must be vigilant, have an inquiring mind, and be able to make associations between events and characteristics (e.g., the associations between how and by whom the cheese was being made, and by whom it was being eaten).

From Bell RA, Hillers VN, Thomas TA: The Abuela project: safe cheese workshops to reduce the incidence of *Salmonella typhimurium* from consumption of raw-milk fresh cheese, *Am J Public Health* 89:1421-1424, 1999.

be inaccessible to scientists (Brown and Ferguson, 1995). Community toxic waste activists engage in a process of linking traditional scientific practices with more narrative approaches. Their health surveys often make use of sampling techniques, laboratory testing, and mapping of suspected pollutants together with experiential narratives of the effects of toxic pollutants on the body and on their local environments (DiChiro, 1997). The information gathered can be used by community activists and health professionals to lobby for health services; advocate for policy development at local, state, and federal levels; establish preventive programs; educate medical professionals about environmental illness; and work with other agencies and community groups to reduce or eliminate toxic exposures.

CHAPTER REVIEW

PRACTICE APPLICATION

You are a nurse providing health screenings at a health fair at a local community center. Mr. Greer, a 32-year-old African-American man, stops by your station and requests that you check his blood pressure. His blood pressure measurement is 135/85 mm Hg. In conducting a brief health history, you learn that Mr. Greer is single, works part time at a convenience store, often eats at fast-food establishments, and has been a smoker since age 17. His father died of a heart attack at age 48; his mother has diabetes. He does not have health insurance at this time. Which of the following would be your best choice in providing Mr. Greer recommendations related to his need for lipid disorder screening, based on the U.S. Preventive Services Task Force guidelines?

A. Do not discuss lipid screening with Mr. Greer, because he is under 35 years of age and routine screening is not recommended.
B. Suggest that Mr. Greer stop smoking and make modifications in his diet to reduce his consumption of saturated fats. Guide him to the information on local community-based resources for tobacco cessation and healthy diet programs at the health fair.
C. Discuss with Mr. Greer his increased risk for heart disease, based on his family history and status as a smoker. Provide a referral for Mr. Greer for a lipid screening, including measurement of total cholesterol and high-density lipoprotein cholesterol (HDL-C), being offered by the local hospital at the health fair.
Answers can be found on the Evolve site.

KEY POINTS

- Epidemiology is the study of the distribution and determinants of health-related events in human populations and the application of this knowledge to improving the health of communities.
- Epidemiology is a multidisciplinary enterprise that recognizes the complex interrelationships of factors that influence disease and health at both the individual level and the community level; it provides the basic tools for the study of health and disease in communities.
- Epidemiologic methods are used to describe health and disease phenomena and to investigate the factors that promote health or influence the risk or distribution of disease. This knowledge can be useful in planning and evaluating programs, policies, and services, as well as in clinical decision making.
- Epidemiologic models explain the interrelationships between agent, host, and environment (the *epidemiologic triangle)* and the interactions of multilevel factors, exposures, and characteristics (causal web) affecting risk of disease.
- A key concept in epidemiology is that of the levels of prevention, based on the stages in the natural history of disease.
- Primary prevention involves interventions to reduce the incidence of disease by promoting health and preventing disease processes from developing.
- Secondary prevention includes programs (such as screening) designed to detect disease in the early stages, before signs and symptoms are clinically evident, to intervene with early diagnosis and treatment.
- Tertiary prevention provides treatments and other interventions directed toward persons with clinically apparent disease, with the aim of lessening the course of disease, reducing disability, or rehabilitating.
- Epidemiologic methods are also used in the planning and design of community health promotion (primary prevention) strategies and screening (secondary prevention) activities, and in the evaluation of the effectiveness of these interventions.
- Basic epidemiologic methods include the use of existing data sources to study health outcomes and related factors and the use of comparison groups to assess the association between exposures or characteristics and health outcomes.
- Epidemiologists rely on rates and proportions to quantify levels of morbidity and mortality. Prevalence proportions provide a picture of the level of existing cases in a population at a given time. Incidence rates and proportions measure the rate of new case development in a population and provide an estimate of the risk of disease.
- Descriptive epidemiologic studies provide information on the distribution of disease and health states according to personal characteristics, geographic region, and time. This knowledge enables practitioners to target programs and allocate resources more effectively and provides a basis for further study.
- Analytic epidemiologic studies investigate associations between exposures or characteristics and health or disease outcomes, with a goal of understanding the etiology of disease. Analytic studies provide the foundation for understanding disease causality and for developing effective intervention strategies aimed at primary, secondary, and tertiary prevention.

CLINICAL DECISION-MAKING ACTIVITIES

1. Interview a local public health nurse or other public health professional from the local health department.
   A. Ask about the current public health priorities and how those priorities were determined.
   B. Describe the type of epidemiologic data used in determining local public health priorities.
2. Identify a current health issue in your local community (e.g., childhood lead poisoning, diabetes, HIV/AIDS).
   A. Describe primary, secondary, and tertiary prevention interventions related to this health issue.
   B. How could nurses improve the effectiveness of their prevention activities related to this health issue?
3. Look at a recent issue of the *Final Mortality Statistics* from the National Center for Health Statistics, or the most recent issue of *Health: United States*. Examine the trends in cause-specific mortality and choose one or two of the leading causes of death.
   A. On the basis of current epidemiologic evidence, explain the factors that have contributed to the following: the observed trend in mortality rates for this disease; the changes in survival; the changes in incidence.
   B. Are the changes the result of better (or worse) primary, secondary, or tertiary prevention? Are there modifiable factors, such as health behaviors, that lend themselves to better prevention efforts? What would they be?
4. Identify existing inequalities among the counties in your state, using infant mortality data.
   A. Describe the distribution of infant mortality in your state (by county), using rate ratio and population attributable risk data.
   B. Compare the infant mortality rates in your state with national and international data.
   C. Compare the characteristics of the counties (e.g., urban, rural, racial/ethnic distribution, economic indicators, distribution of health care facilities) with the highest and lowest infant mortality rates.
   D. Identify local, state, and national initiatives that are addressing infant mortality.
5. Examine the leading causes of infant death in the United States.
   A. What differences in intervention approaches are suggested by the various causes of death?
   B. How would you design an epidemiologic study to examine risk factors for specific causes of neonatal and post-neonatal death? What types of epidemiologic measures would be useful? What study design(s) would be appropriate?
   C. How would you use the information from your study to develop an intervention program and to define the target population for your intervention?
6. Find a report of an epidemiologic study in one of the major public health, nursing, or epidemiology journals. How do the findings of this study, if valid, affect your nursing practice? How do you incorporate the results of epidemiologic research into your nursing practice?

REFERENCES

American Nurses Association: *Nursing: scope and standards of practice*, Washington, DC, 2004, ANA.

Anderson RN: Deaths: leading causes for 2000, *Natl Vital Stat Rep* 50:1–85, 2002.

Anderson RN, Rosenberg HM: Age standardization of death rates: implementation of the year 2000 standard, *Natl Vital Stat Rep* 47:1–16, 1998.

Bell RA, Hillers VN, Thomas TA: The Abuela project: safe cheese workshops to reduce the incidence of *Salmonella typhimurium* from consumption of raw-milk fresh cheese, *Am J Public Health* 89:1421–1424, 1999.

Berkman LF, Kawachi I: A historical framework for social epidemiology. In Berkman LF, Kawachi I, editors: *Social epidemiology*, New York, 2000, Oxford University Press.

Bradman A, Chevier J, Tager I, et al: Association of housing disrepair indicators with cockroach and rodent infestations in a cohort of pregnant Latina women and their children, *Environ Health Perspect* 113:1795–1801, 2005.

Brown P, Ferguson FIT: "Making a big stink": women's work, women's relationships, and toxic waste activism, *Gender Society* 9:145–172, 1995.

Brown P, Masterson-Allen S: Citizen action on toxic waste contamination: a new type of social movement, *Soc Natural Res* 7:269–286, 1994.

Brownson RC, Petitti DB, editors: *Applied epidemiology: theory to practice*, ed 2, New York, 2006, Oxford University Press.

Brownson RC, Remington PL, Davis JR: *Chronic disease epidemiology and control*, ed 2, Washington, DC, 1998, American Public Health Association.

Caughy MO, O'Campo PJ, Patterson J: A brief observational measure for urban neighborhoods, *Health Place* 7:225–236, 2001.

Centers for Disease Control and Prevention: Use of race and ethnicity in public health surveillance: summary of the CDC/ATSDR workshop, *MMWR Morb Mortal Wkly Rep* 42(RR-10), 1993.

Centers for Disease Control and Prevention (CDC): *Physical activity and good nutrition: essential elements to prevent chronic diseases and obesity: at a glance*, 2008, Centers for Disease Control and Prevention, National Center for Chronic Disease Prevention and Health Promotion, Available at http://www.cdc.gov/nccdphp/publications/aag/dnpa.htm. Accessed December 23, 2010.

Childress JF, Faden RR, Gaare RD, et al: Public health ethics: mapping the terrain, *J Law Med Ethics* 30:169–177, 2002.

Cohen D, Spear S, Scribner R, et al: "Broken windows" and the risk of gonorrhea, *Am J Public Health* 90:230–236, 2000.

Council on Linkages Between Academic and Public Health Practice: Core competencies for public health professionals. Washington DC, 2010. Public Health Foundation/Health Resources and Services Administration.

DiChiro G: Local actions, global visions: remaking environmental expertise, *Frontiers* 18:203, 1997.

Diez-Roux AV: A glossary for multilevel analysis, *J Epidemiol Community Health* 56:588–594, 2002.

Fuller CM, Borrell LN, Latkin CA, et al: Effects of race, neighborhood, and social network on age at initiation of injection drug use, *Am J Public Health* 95:689–695, 2005.

Fullilove MT: Comment: abandoning "race" as a variable in public health research: an idea whose time has come, *Am J Public Health* 88:1297, 1998.

Gebbie KM, Hwang I: Preparing currently employed public health nurses for changes in the health system, *Am J Public Health* 20:716–721, 2000.

Gordis L: *Epidemiology*, ed 4, Philadelphia, 2009, Saunders.

Harkness GA: *Epidemiology in nursing practice*, St Louis, 1995, Mosby.

Heron MP, Hoyert DL, Murphy SL, et al: *Deaths: Final data for 2006. Natl Vital Stat Rep 57:14*, Hyattsville, MD, 2009, National Center for Health Statistics.

Heymann DL, editor: *Control of communicable diseases manual*, ed 19, Washington, DC, 2008, American Public Health Association.

Institute of Medicine: *The future of public health*, Washington, DC, 1988, National Academy Press.

Institute of Medicine: *The future of the public's health in the 21st century*, Washington, DC, 2002, NAP. Available at http://www.iom.edu/Reports/2002/The-Future-of-the-Publics-Health-in-the-21st-Century.aspx. Accessed December 23, 2010.

Kawachi I, Berkman LF: *Neighborhoods and health*, New York, 2003, Oxford University Press.

Keppel KG, Pearcy JN, Wagener DK: *Trends in racial and ethnic-specific rates for the health status indicators: United States, 1990-98, Healthy People statistical notes*, No. 23, Hyattsville, MD, 2002, NCHS.

Koepsell TD, Weiss NS: *Epidemiologic methods: studying the occurrence of illness*, New York, 2003, Oxford University Press.

Krieger N: Epidemiology and the web of causation: has anyone seen the spider? *Soc Sci Med* 39:887, 1994.

Krieger N: Discrimination and health. In Berkman LF, Kawachi I, editors: *Social epidemiology*, Oxford, 2000, Oxford University Press, pp 36–75.

Lynch J, Kaplan G: Socioeconomic position. In Berkman LF, Kawachi I, editors: *Social epidemiology*, New York, 2000, Oxford University Press, pp 13–35.

Lynch JW, Kaplan GA, Pamuk ER, et al: Income inequality and mortality in metropolitan areas of the United States, *Am J Public Health* 88:1074, 1998.

Macintyre S, Ellaway A: Ecological approaches: rediscovering the role of the physical and social environment. In Berkman LF, Kawachi I, editors: *Social epidemiology*, New York, 2000, Oxford University Press, pp 332–348.

Martin JA, Hamilton BE, Sutton PD, et al: Births, final data for 2006, *Natl Vital Stat Rep* 57:7, 2009.

McElry JA, Remington PL, Gangnon RE, et al: Identifying geographic disparities in the early detection of breast cancer using a geographic information system, *Prev Chronic Dis* 3(1):A10, 2006.

McKeown RE: The epidemiologic transition: changing patterns of mortality and population dynamics, *Am J Lifestyle Med* 3(S1):19S–26S, 2009.

McKeown RE, Learner RM: Ethics in Public Health Practice. In Coughlin S, Beauchamp T, Weed D, editors: *Ethics and epidemiology, ed 2*, New York, 2009, Oxford University Press, pp 147–181.

McLafferty S, Grady S: Immigration and geographic access to prenatal clinics in Brooklyn, NY: a geographic information systems analysis, *Am J Public Health* 95:638–640, 2005.

Merrill RM, Timmreck TC: *Introduction to epidemiology, ed 4*, Sudbury, MA, 2006, Jones & Bartlett.

Mood L: Toxic waste: deep in the roots of nursing comes a search for harmful sources, *Reflect Nurs Leadership* 26:21–25, 2000.

Mrazek PJ, Haggerty RJ, editors: *Reducing risks for mental disorders: frontiers for preventive intervention research*, Committee on Prevention of Mental Disorders, Institute of Medicine, Washington, DC, 1994, National Academy Press.

Najera-Aguilar P, Martinez-Piedra R, Vidaurre-Arenas M: From sketch to digital maps: a geographic information system (GIS) model and application for malaria control without the use of pesticides, *Pan Am Health Org Epidemiol Bull* 26:11, 2005.

National Center for Health Statistics: *Health, United States*, 2008 with Chartbook 2009, Hyattsville, MD.

Office of Minority Health, U.S. Department of Health and Human Services: *Elimination of racial and ethnic disparities in health: report to Congress*, Washington, DC, 1999, OMH.

Porta M: *A dictionary of epidemiology, ed 5*, New York, 2008, Oxford University Press.

Quad Council of Public Health Nursing Organizations. Competencies for Public Health Nursing Practice. Washington DC, 2003, ASTDN, revised 2009. Accessed December 15, 2010.

Remington PL, Brownson RC, Wegner MV: *Chronic disease epidemiology and control, ed 3*, Washington, DC, 2010, American Public Health Association.

Roche LS, Skinner R, Weinstein RB: Use of a geographic information system to identify and characterize areas with high proportions of distant stage breast cancer, *J Public Health Manag Pract* 3:26–32, 2002.

Rothman KJ: *Epidemiology: an introduction*, New York, 2002, Oxford University Press.

Sampson RJ, Raudenbush SW, Earls F: Neighborhoods and violent crime: a multilevel study of collective efficacy, *Science* 277:918, 1997.

Schlesselman JJ: *Case-control studies: design, conduct, analysis*, New York, 1982, Oxford University Press.

Snow J: On the mode of communication of cholera. In *Snow on cholera*, New York, 1855, The Commonwealth Fund.

Sorlie PD, Thom TJ, Manolio T, et al: Age-adjusted death rates: consequences of the year 2000 standard, *Ann Epidemiol* 9:93–100, 1999.

Susser M: *Causal thinking in the health sciences*, New York, 1973, Oxford University Press.

Susser M: Epidemiology in the United States after World War II: the evolution of technique, *Epidemiol Rev* 7:147, 1985.

Szklo M, Nieto FJ: *Epidemiology: beyond the basics, ed 2*, Boston, 2007, Jones & Bartlett.

Teutsch SM, Churchill RE: *Principles and practice of public health surveillance*, New York, 2000, Oxford.

Turnock BJ: *Public health: what it is and how it works, ed 4*, Gaithersburg, MD, 2008, Aspen.

U.S. Department of Health, Education, and Welfare: *Vital statistics of the United States: 1950*, vol 1, Washington, DC, 1954, USDHEW, Public Health Service.

U.S. Department of Health and Human Services: *Healthy People 2010: understanding and improving health, ed 2*, Washington, DC, 2000, U.S. Government Printing Office.

U.S. Preventive Services Task Force: *Screening for lipid disorders in adults: U.S. Preventive Services Task Force Recommendation Statement*, Rockville, MD, 2008, Agency for Healthcare Research and Quality.

Victoria CG, Habicht J-P, Bryce J: Evidence-based public health: moving beyond randomized trials, *Am J Public Health* 94(3):400–405, 2004.

World Health Organization: *Declaration of Alma-Ata: International Conference on Primary Health Care*, Geneva, Switzerland, 1978, WHO, p 1.

Xu J, Kochanek KD, Tejada-Vera B: Deaths: preliminary data for 2007, *Natl Vital Stat Rep* 58:1, Hyattsville, MD, 2009, National Center for Health Statistics.

CHAPTER 13

Infectious Disease Prevention and Control

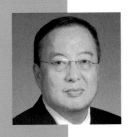

Francisco S. Sy, MD, DrPH

Dr. Francisco S. Sy is the Director of the Division of Extramural Activities and Scientific Programs at the National Center on Minority Health and Health Disparities (NCMHD) at the National Institutes of Health (NIH) in Bethesda, MD. Before joining NIH, Dr. Sy served as a Senior Health Scientist in the Division of HIV/AIDS Prevention (DHAP), National Center for HIV, STD and TB Prevention (NCHSTP), at the Centers for Disease Control and Prevention (CDC) in Atlanta, GA. Dr. Sy was a tenured professor at the University of South Carolina (USC) School of Public Health in Columbia, SC, where he taught infectious disease epidemiology for 15 years. At USC, he served as Graduate Director of the Department of Epidemiology and Biostatistics for 7 years and as Director of the school-wide Master of Public Health (MPH) program for 3 years. Dr. Sy has written several book chapters and scientific articles on various infectious and tropical diseases, HIV disease epidemiology, prevention, and program evaluation. He is the Editor of the *AIDS Education and Prevention: An Interprofessional Journal* since its inception in 1988. It is a bimonthly peer-reviewed journal published by Guilford Press in New York. Dr. Sy earned his Doctor of Public Health (DrPH) degree in Immunology and Infectious Diseases from Johns Hopkins University in 1984, Master of Science in Tropical Public Health from Harvard University in 1981, and Doctor of Medicine degree from the University of the Philippines in 1975.

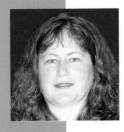

Susan C. Long-Marin, DVM, MPH

Susan C. Long-Marin developed an interest in infectious disease and public health while serving as a Peace Corps Volunteer in the Philippines in the 1970s. Training in veterinary medicine further increased her respect for the ingeniousness of microbes and the importance of primary prevention. Today she manages the epidemiology program of a county health department in Charlotte, NC, which serves a growing and rapidly changing population from a variety of racial, ethnic, and national backgrounds.

ADDITIONAL RESOURCES

ⓔvolve WEBSITE
http://evolve.elsevier.com/Stanhope
- *Healthy People 2020*
- WebLinks—Of special note, see the links for these sites
  - Centers for Disease Control and Prevention
  - *Emerging Infectious Diseases,* Centers for Disease Control and Prevention
  - *MMWR Morbidity and Mortality Weekly Report,* Centers for Disease Control and Prevention
  - World Health Organization
  - *WER/Weekly Epidemiological Record,* World Health Organization
- Quiz
- Case Studies
- Glossary
- Answers to Practice Application

OBJECTIVES

After reading this chapter, the student should be able to do the following:

1. Discuss the current impact and threats of infectious diseases on society.
2. Explain how the elements of the epidemiologic triangle interact to cause infectious diseases.
3. Provide examples of infectious disease control interventions at the three levels of public health prevention.
4. Explain the multisystem approach to control of communicable diseases.
5. Define surveillance and discuss the functions and elements of a surveillance system.
6. Discuss the factors contributing to newly emerging or reemerging infectious diseases.
7. Discuss the illnesses most likely to be associated with the intentional release of a biological agent.
8. Discuss issues related to obtaining and maintaining appropriate levels of immunization against vaccine-preventable diseases.
9. Describe issues and agents associated with foodborne illness and appropriate prevention measures.
10. Define the bloodborne pathogen reduction strategy and universal precautions.

KEY TERMS

OUTLINE

The topic of infectious diseases includes the discussion of a wide and complex variety of organisms; the pathology they may cause; and their diagnosis, treatment, prevention, and control. This chapter presents an overview of the **communicable diseases** that nurses encounter most often. Diseases are grouped according to descriptive category (by mode of transmission or means of prevention) rather than by individual organism (e.g., *Escherichia coli*) or taxonomic group (e.g., viral, parasitic). Detailed discussion of sexually transmitted diseases, human immunodeficiency virus (HIV), acquired immunodeficiency syndrome (AIDS), viral hepatitis, and tuberculosis (TB) is provided in Chapter 14. Although not all infectious diseases are directly communicable from person to person, the terms *infectious disease* and *communicable disease* are used interchangeably throughout this chapter.

> **DID YOU KNOW?** *Antibiotics are not effective against viral diseases, a fact found unacceptable to many clients looking for relief from the misery of a cold or flu. The inappropriate prescribing of antibiotics contributes to the growing problem of infectious agents that have developed resistance to once-powerful antibiotics. Healthy People 2020 calls for reducing the number of times antibiotics are prescribed for a common cold.*

HISTORICAL AND CURRENT PERSPECTIVES

In the United States, at the beginning of the twentieth century, infectious diseases were the leading cause of death. By 2000 improvements in nutrition and sanitation, the discovery of antibiotics, and the development of vaccines had put an end to infectious disease epidemics like diphtheria and typhoid fever that once ravaged entire populations. In 1900 respiratory and diarrheal diseases were major killers. For example, TB led to over 11% of all deaths in the United States and was the second leading cause of death; by the early twenty-first century, only 0.02% of all deaths were attributed to this once frequently fatal disease (CDC, 2009a). As individuals live longer, chronic diseases—heart disease, cancer, and stroke—have replaced infectious diseases as the leading causes of death.

Infectious diseases, however, have by no means vanished, and they remain a continuing cause for concern. They persist as the third-leading cause of death in the United States and the second-leading cause worldwide, where they are responsible for killing an estimated 15 million people a year (Fauci, Touchette, and Folkers, 2005). In the United States, the downward trend in mortality from infectious diseases, seen since 1900—with the exception of the 1918 influenza pandemic—reversed itself in the 1980s, with the emergence of new entities such as HIV disease and the increasing development of antibiotic resistance. Respiratory diseases in the form of pneumonias and influenza remain among the 10 leading causes of death, and new strains such as novel influenza A H1N1 and avian influenza A H5N1 test our disease control abilities and consume resources. Previously unknown causal connections between infectious organisms and chronic diseases have been recognized, such as *Helicobacter pylori* and peptic ulcer disease, and human papillomaviruses (HPVs) and cervical cancer. Also, in the twenty-first century, infectious diseases have become a means of terrorism, as illustrated by the anthrax letters of 2001.

New killers emerge and old familiar diseases take on different, more virulent characteristics. Consider the following developments from the past 30 years. HIV disease reminds us of plagues from the past and challenges our ability to control and contain infection like no other disease in recent history. Because drugs have been developed to slow the progression but there is still neither vaccine nor cure, this initially infectious disease is now a chronic condition as well. Legionnaires' disease and toxic shock syndrome, unknown at mid-twentieth century, have become part of common vocabulary. The identification of infectious agents causing Lyme disease and ehrlichiosis provided two new tickborne diseases to worry about. And, in the summer of 1993 in the southwestern United States, healthy young adults were stricken with a mysterious and unknown but often fatal respiratory disease that is now known as hantavirus pulmonary syndrome. The summer of 1994 brought public attention to a severe, invasive strain of *Streptococcus pyogenes* group A, referred to by the press as the "flesh-eating" bacteria.

In the 1990s the transmission of infectious disease through the food supply became a newsworthy concern when the consumption of improperly cooked hamburgers and unpasteurized apple juice contaminated with a highly toxic strain of E. coli (E. coli 0157:H7) caused illness and death in children across the country. In 1996 multiple states reported outbreaks of diarrheal disease traced to imported fresh berries; the implicated organism in these outbreaks, *Cyclospora cayetanensis* (a coccidian parasite), was only first diagnosed in humans in 1977.

Also in 1996, the fear that "mad cow disease" (bovine spongiform encephalopathy [BSE]) could be transferred to humans through beef consumption led to the slaughter of thousands of British cattle and a ban on the international sale of British beef. Initially seen only in Europe and Japan as well as Great Britain, the first case of BSE was diagnosed in the United States in 2003. Variant Creutzfeldt-Jakob disease (vCJD), which attacks the brain with fatal results, is the human disease hypothesized but not yet proven to result from eating beef infected with the transmissible agent causing BSE; only three acquired cases of vCJD have been seen in the United States, but these individuals were born outside of and resided in the country for only a short period (CDC, 2009b).

In 1997 vancomycin-resistant *Staphylococcus aureus* (VRSA) was first reported; previously, vancomycin had been considered the only effective antibiotic against methicillin-resistant *S. aureus* (MRSA). Although MRSA is still largely a hospital-acquired infection, community-associated disease is becoming more common with outbreaks frequently associated with school athletic programs and prison populations. Also in 1997, the first reported outbreak of avian flu affecting humans occurred in Hong Kong. No subsequent reports suggested an isolated incident, but in 2004, avian influenza A H5N1 again emerged in Southeast Asia with resulting human cases. This virus has now infected avian populations in Asia, Europe, the Near East, and North Africa, and it continues to cause sporadic human cases, especially in Southeast Asia and Egypt. Human cases are determined to largely spread through direct contact with infected poultry or infected surfaces, with human to human transmission largely ineffective and only a few rare cases thought to have occurred. In 1999 the first western hemisphere activity of West Nile virus (WNV), a mosquito-transmitted illness that can affect livestock, birds, and humans, occurred in New York City. By 2002 WNV, thought to be carried by infected birds and possibly mosquitoes in cargo containers, had spread across the United States as far west as California and was reported in Canada and Central America as well.

The viral hemorrhagic fevers Ebola and Marburg, unknown to most people 30 years ago, have become the premise of movies and books. Although caused by different viruses within the Filoviridae family, these sporadically occurring but lethal killers have similar clinical presentations. The most recent large outbreaks of Ebola have been in 2007 in the Democratic Republic of the Congo (249 cases, 183 deaths) and in Uganda (149 cases, 37 deaths). Marburg virus had only been reported five times since its recognition in 1967 before a major outbreak in Angola occurred during 2004 and 2005, affecting more than 350 people with a fatality rate of close to 90%. Since then, a much smaller outbreak occurred in Uganda in 2007 among gold miners. The source for both of these viruses is still undetermined, but there is an association with non-human primates, and evidence is also beginning to point toward a bat reservoir (Heymann, 2008).

Severe acute respiratory syndrome (SARS) was first recognized in China in February 2003. And as if in a bestselling thriller, this newly emerging infectious disease quickly achieved pandemic proportions. By the summer of 2003, major outbreaks had occurred in Hong Kong, Taiwan, Vietnam, Singapore, and

Canada. Three months after the first official news of SARS, over 8000 cases with more than 700 deaths had been reported to the World Health Organization (WHO) from 28 countries. Played out on television in pictures of people wearing face masks for protection, the rapid spread of a previously unknown disease with an initially unknown cause and no definitive treatment contributed to the creation of a perception of risk of infection far greater than actually existed. Frightened Americans canceled trips to China and Hong Kong and avoided people who had recently returned from Asia. Then, as suddenly as it began, the pandemic subsided. SARS was eventually determined to be caused by a new strain of Coronavirus, but since 2003, only a few cases, largely associated with laboratory workers, have been reported. A large number of individuals infected by SARS could be traced back to unrecognized cases in hospitals, suggesting that prompt identification and isolation of symptomatic people is the key to interrupting transmission. Global efforts continue to clarify the epidemiology of this disease as well as develop a reliable diagnostic test and vaccine. Additional information on SARS can be obtained at the WHO Global Alert and Response website (http://www.who.int/csr/sars/).

In the first decade of the twenty-first century, foodborne infections again have made headlines as *E. coli*–infected spinach sickened and killed individuals across the United States. In 2008, tomatoes were blamed for a nation-wide outbreak of salmonellosis but were ruled innocent when the green chilies that accompanied them in salsa were found to be the actual culprit. Salmonella again made the news as contaminated peanut butter forced recalls across the United States, sickened hundreds, and resulted in several deaths. Even chocolate chip cookie dough was not safe; a national recall in 2009 followed the discovery that people had been sickened after eating raw dough contaminated by *E. coli*. Perhaps the most publicized infectious disease event of 2009 was the advent of a new strain of flu, novel influenza A H1N1. First reported from Mexico and rapidly acquired by travelers to that country, H1N1 spread quickly across the world, causing the WHO to declare a pandemic and stimulate the race for a vaccine.

Worldwide, infectious diseases are the leading killer of children and young adults and are responsible for almost half of all deaths in developing countries. Of these infectious disease deaths, 90% result from six causes: acute respiratory infections, diarrheal diseases, malaria and measles among children; and TB and HIV infection among adults. Malaria alone is estimated to kill 1.2 million people a year and TB another 1.7 million (or over 4600 people per day) (Heymann, 2008). The CDC in its *Ounce of Prevention* campaign notes that in the United States as many as 160,000 people die per year with infectious diseases as an underlying cause. The economic burden of infectious diseases is staggering. In the United States, the USDA Economic Research Service estimated the cost of foodborne illnesses caused by just two organisms—salmonella and *E. coli* 0157:H7—at over $3 billion in 2008 dollars (USDA, 2009). The Produce Safety Project at Georgetown University in 2010 suggested that the total cost from foodborne illness could be more than $152 billion (Pew Charitable Trusts, 2010). CDC researchers determined that in the United States in 2000, nine million cases of sexually transmitted infections occurred among young people 15 to 24 years of age with a total estimated cost of $6.5 billion, with HIV disease and HPV accounting for 90% of the total burden (Chesson et al, 2004). Hospital-acquired infections are estimated to have killed 48,000 people and cost $8.1 billion to treat in 2006 (Eber et al, 2010).

Because of the morbidity, mortality, and associated cost of infectious diseases, the national health promotion and disease prevention goals outlined in *Healthy People 2020* list a number of objectives for reducing the incidence of these illnesses in the section on Immunization & Infectious Disease (see the *Healthy People 2020* box). Objectives for reducing salmonellosis and other foodborne infections are found in the section on Food Safety and an objective for reducing malaria cases reported in the United States may be seen under Global Health. Although infectious diseases are not currently the leading causes of death in the United States, they continue to present varied, multiple and complex challenges to all health care providers. Nurses must know about these diseases to effectively participate in diagnosis, treatment, prevention, and control.

♥ HEALTHY PEOPLE 2020

Selected Objectives Related to Immunization and Infectious Diseases

- IID-24: Reduce chronic hepatitis B virus infections in infants and young children (perinatal infections).
- IID-4: Reduce invasive pneumococcal infections.
- IID-1: Reduce, eliminate, or maintain elimination of cases of vaccine-preventable diseases.
- IID-27: Increase the percentage of persons aware they have a chronic hepatitis C infection.
- IID-12: Increase the percentage of children and adults who are vaccinated against seasonal influenza.
- IID-13: Increase the percentage of adults who are vaccinated against pneumococcal disease.

From U.S. Department of Health and Human Services: *Healthy People 2020: The Road Ahead*, 2009, USDHHS. Available at http://www.healthypeople.gov/HP2020/. Accessed January 26, 2010.

TRANSMISSION OF COMMUNICABLE DISEASES

Agent, Host, and Environment

The transmission of communicable diseases depends on the successful interaction of the infectious agent, the host, and the environment. These three factors make up the epidemiologic triangle (Figure 13-1) as discussed in Chapter 12. Changes in the characteristics of any of the factors may result in disease transmission. Consider the following examples. Antibiotic therapy not only may eliminate a specific pathological agent, but also alter the balance of normally occurring organisms in the body. As a result, one of these agents overruns another and disease, such as a yeast infection, occurs. HIV performs its deadly work not by directly poisoning the host but by destroying the host's immune reaction to other disease-producing agents. Individuals living in the temperate climate of the United States do not normally contract malaria at home, but they may become

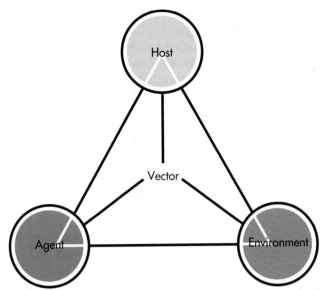

FIGURE 13-1 The epidemiologic triangle of a disease. (From Gordis L: *Epidemiology,* Philadelphia, 1996, Saunders.)

BOX 13-1 SIX CHARACTERISTICS OF AN INFECTIOUS AGENT

- *Infectivity:* The ability to enter and multiply in the host
- *Pathogenicity:* The ability to produce a specific clinical reaction after infection occurs
- *Virulence:* The ability to produce a severe pathological reaction
- *Toxicity:* The ability to produce a poisonous reaction
- *Invasiveness:* The ability to penetrate and spread throughout a tissue
- *Antigenicity:* The ability to stimulate an immunological response

---

infected if they change their environment by traveling to a climate where malaria-carrying mosquitoes thrive. As these examples illustrate, the balance among agent, host, and environment is often precarious and may be unintentionally disrupted. At present, the potential results of such disturbance require attention as advances in science and technology, destruction of natural habitats, explosive population growth, political instability, and a worldwide transportation network combine to alter the balance among the environment, people, and the agents that produce disease.

Agent Factor

Four major categories of **agents** cause most infections and infectious disease: bacteria (e.g., *Salmonella* and *E. coli*); fungi (e.g., *Aspergillus* spp. and *Candida* spp.), parasites (e.g., helminthes and protozoa) and viruses (e.g., hepatitis A and B and HIV). Less commonly seen is the prion, a transmissible agent that causes abnormal folding of normal cellular prion proteins in the brain, resulting in a family of rare progressive neurodegenerative disorders that affect both humans and animals. Variant Creutzfeldt-Jakob disease and kuru are examples of prion diseases. The individual agent may be described by its ability to cause disease and by the nature and the severity of the disease. *Infectivity, pathogenicity, virulence, toxicity, invasiveness* and *antigenicity*, terms commonly used to characterize infectious agents, are defined in Box 13-1.

Host Factor

A human or animal **host** can harbor an infectious agent. The characteristics of the host that may influence the spread of disease are host resistance, immunity, herd immunity, and infectiousness of the host. **Resistance** is the ability of the host to withstand infection, and it may involve natural or acquired immunity.

Natural immunity refers to species-determined, innate resistance to an infectious agent. For example, opossums rarely

contract rabies. **Acquired immunity** is the resistance acquired by a host as a result of previous natural exposure to an infectious agent. Having measles once protects against future infection. Acquired immunity may be induced by active or passive immunization. **Active immunization** refers to the immunization of an individual by administration of an antigen (infectious agent or vaccine) and is usually characterized by the presence of an antibody produced by the individual host. Vaccinating children against childhood diseases is an example of inducing active immunity. **Passive immunization** refers to immunization through the transfer of a specific antibody from an immunized individual to a non-immunized individual, such as the transfer of antibody from mother to infant or by administration of an antibody-containing preparation (immunoglobulin or antiserum). Passive immunity from immunoglobulin is almost immediate but short lived. It is often induced as a stopgap measure until active immunity has time to develop after vaccination. Examples of commonly used immunoglobulins include those for hepatitis A, rabies, and tetanus.

Herd immunity refers to the immunity of a group or community. It is the resistance of a group of people to invasion and spread of an infectious agent. Herd immunity is based on the resistance of a high proportion of individual members of a group to infection. It is the basis for increasing immunization coverage for vaccine-preventable diseases. Through studies, experts determine what percent coverage (e.g., >90%) of a specified group of people (e.g., children entering school) by a specified vaccine (e.g., one dose of measles vaccine) is necessary to ensure adequate protection for the entire community against a given disease and target immunization campaigns and initiatives to meet that goal. The higher the immunization coverage, the greater the herd immunity.

Infectiousness is a measure of the potential ability of an infected host to transmit the infection to other hosts. It reflects the relative ease with which the infectious agent is transmitted to others. Individuals with measles are extremely infectious; the virus spreads readily on airborne droplets. A person with Lyme disease cannot spread the disease to other people (although the infected tick can).

Environment Factor

The **environment** refers to everything that is external to the human host, including physical, biological, social, and cultural factors. These environmental factors facilitate the transmission of an infectious agent from an infected host to other susceptible hosts. Reduction in communicable disease risk can be achieved by altering these environmental factors. Using mosquito nets and repellants to avoid bug bites, installing sewage systems to prevent fecal contamination of water supplies, and washing utensils after contact with raw meat to reduce bacterial contamination are all examples of altering the environment to prevent disease.

Modes of Transmission

Infectious diseases can be transmitted horizontally or vertically. Vertical transmission is the passing of the infection from parent to offspring via sperm, placenta, milk, or contact in the vaginal canal at birth. Examples of vertical transmission are transplacental transmission of HIV and syphilis. Horizontal transmission is the person-to-person spread of infection through one or more of the following four routes: direct/indirect contact, common vehicle, airborne, or vector-borne. Most sexually transmitted infections are spread by direct sexual contact. Enterobiasis, or pinworm infection, can be acquired through direct contact or indirect contact with contaminated objects such as toys, clothing, and bedding. Common vehicle refers to transportation of the infectious agent from an infected host to a susceptible host via food, water, milk, blood, serum, saliva, or plasma. Hepatitis A can be transmitted through contaminated food and water, and hepatitis B through contaminated blood. Legionellosis and TB are both spread via contaminated droplets in the air. Vectors are arthropods such as ticks and mosquitoes or other invertebrates such as snails that transmit the infectious agent by biting or depositing the infective material near the host. Vectors may be necessary to the life cycle of the organism (e.g., mosquitoes and malaria) or may act as mechanical transmitters (e.g., flies and food).

Disease Development

Exposure to an infectious agent does not always lead to an infection. Similarly, infection does not always lead to disease. Infection depends on the infective dose, the infectivity of the infectious agent and the immunocompetence of the host. It is important to differentiate infection and disease, as clearly illustrated by the HIV disease epidemic. Infection refers to the entry, development, and multiplication of the infectious agent in the susceptible host. Disease is one of the possible outcomes of infection and it may indicate a physiological dysfunction or pathological reaction. An individual who tests positive for HIV is infected, but if that person shows no clinical signs, the individual is not diseased. Similarly, if an individual tests positive for HIV and also exhibits clinical signs consistent with AIDS (HIV stage III), that individual is both infected and diseased.

DID YOU KNOW?   *Discovered only in 1983, the infectious agent Helicobacter pylori is now recognized as the major factor in peptic ulcer disease.*

Incubation period and communicable period are not synonymous. The incubation period is the time interval between invasion by an infectious agent and the first appearance of signs and symptoms of the disease. The incubation periods of infectious diseases vary from between 2 and 4 hours for staphylococcal food poisoning to between 10 and 15 years for AIDS (HIV stage III). The communicable period is the interval during which an infectious agent may be transferred directly or indirectly from an infected person to another person. The period of communicability for influenza is 3 to 5 days after the clinical onset of symptoms. Hepatitis B–infected persons are infectious many weeks before the onset of the first symptoms and remain infective during the acute phase and chronic carrier state, which may persist for life.

Disease Spectrum

Persons with infectious diseases may exhibit a broad spectrum of disease that ranges from subclinical infection to severe and fatal disease. Those with subclinical or inapparent infections are important from the public health point of view because they are a source of infection but may not be receiving care like those with clinical disease. They should be targeted for early diagnosis and treatment. Those with clinical disease may exhibit localized or systemic symptoms and mild to severe illness. The final outcome of a disease may be recovery, death, or something in between, including a carrier state, complications requiring extended hospital stay, or disability requiring rehabilitation.

At the community level, the disease may occur in endemic, epidemic, or pandemic proportion. Endemic refers to the constant presence of a disease within a geographic area or a population. Pertussis is endemic in the United States. Epidemic refers to the occurrence of disease in a community or region in excess of normal expectancy. Although people tend to associate large numbers with epidemics, even one case can be termed epidemic if the disease is considered previously eliminated from that area. For example, one case of polio, a disease considered eliminated from the United States, would be considered epidemic. Pandemic refers to an epidemic occurring worldwide and affecting large populations. HIV disease is both epidemic and pandemic, as the number of cases continues to grow across various regions of the world as well as in the United States. SARS and novel influenza A H1N1 are both emerging infectious diseases and responsible for recent pandemics.

SURVEILLANCE OF COMMUNICABLE DISEASES

During the first half of the twentieth century, the weekly publication of national morbidity statistics by the U.S. Surgeon General's Office was accompanied by the statement, "No health department, state or local, can effectively prevent or control disease without knowledge of when, where, and under what conditions cases are occurring" (CDC, 1996a, p 531). Surveillance gathers the "who, when, where, and what"; these elements are then used to answer "why." A good surveillance system systematically collects, organizes, and analyzes current, accurate, and complete data for a defined disease condition. The resulting information is promptly released to those who need it for effective planning, implementation, and evaluation of disease prevention and control programs.

BOX 13-2 TEN BASIC DATA ELEMENTS OF SURVEILLANCE

1. Mortality registration
2. Morbidity reporting
3. Epidemic reporting
4. Epidemic field investigation
5. Laboratory reporting
6. Individual case investigation
7. Surveys
8. Utilization of biological agents and drugs
9. Distribution of animal reservoirs and vectors
10. Demographic and environmental data

Elements of Surveillance

Infectious disease surveillance incorporates and analyzes data from a variety of sources. Box 13-2 lists 10 commonly used data elements.

Surveillance for Agents of Bioterrorism

Since September 11, 2001, increased emphasis has been placed on surveillance for any disease that might be associated with the intentional release of a biological agent. The concern is that, because of the interval between exposure and disease, a covert release may go unrecognized and without response for some time if the resulting outbreak closely resembles a naturally occurring one. Health care providers are asked to be alert to: (1) temporal or geographic clustering of illnesses (people who attended the same public gathering or visited the same location), especially those with clinical signs that resemble an infectious disease outbreak—previously healthy people with unexplained fever accompanied by sepsis, pneumonia, rash, or flaccid paralysis, and (2) an unusual age distribution for a common disease (e.g., chickenpox-like disease in adults without a child source case).

Because of the heightened concern about possible bioterrorist attacks, various sorts of syndromic surveillance systems have been developed by public health agencies across the country. These systems incorporate factors such as the previously mentioned temporal and geographic clustering and unusual age distributions with groups of disease symptoms or syndromes (e.g., flaccid paralysis, respiratory signs, skin rashes, gastrointestinal symptoms) with the goal of detecting early signs of diseases that could result from a bioterrorism-related attack. Syndromic surveillance systems may include tracking emergency department visits sorted by syndrome symptoms as well as other indicators of illness including school absenteeism and sales of selected over-the-counter medications. The CDC has developed EARS (Early Aberration Reporting System), a surveillance tool that is available at no charge and used by various public health officials across the country and abroad. Although more active infectious disease surveillance is being encouraged because of the potential for bioterrorism, the positive benefit is increased surveillance for other communicable diseases as well. Such heightened surveillance can just as easily warn of a community salmonellosis or influenza outbreak. Although the benefit of syndromic surveillance as a warning system has not been proved, it has been valuable in tracking disease outbreaks such as the 2009 H1N1 pandemic. (For additional information on preparedness surveillance and EARS, see the CDC website at http://www.bt.cdc.gov/episurv/.)

Nurses are frequently involved at different levels of the surveillance system. They play important roles in collecting data, making diagnoses, investigating and reporting cases, and providing information to the general public. Examples of possible activities include investigating sources and contacts in outbreaks of pertussis in school settings or shigellosis in day care; performing TB testing and contact tracing; collecting and reporting information pertaining to notifiable communicable diseases; performing infection control in hospitals; and providing morbidity and mortality statistics to those who request them, including the media, the public, service planners, and grant writers.

List of Reportable Diseases

"A notifiable disease is one for which regular, frequent, and timely information regarding individual cases is considered necessary for the prevention and control of the disease" (CDC, 2009c, p 2). Requirements for disease reporting in the United States are mandated by state rather than federal law and as such, vary slightly from state to state. State health departments, on a voluntary basis, report cases of selected diseases to the CDC through the National Notifiable Diseases Surveillance System (NNDSS). State public health officials collaborate with the CDC to determine which diseases should be nationally notifiable. The list of nationally notifiable diseases may be revised as new diseases emerge or disease incidence declines. The diseases designated as notifiable at the national level and reported in 2010 are listed in Box 13-3. The NNDSS data are collated and published weekly in the *Morbidity and Mortality Weekly Report* (MMWR). Final reports are published annually in the *Summary of Notifiable Diseases*. (Learn more about the NNDSS at the CDC website at http://www.cdc.gov/ncphi/disss/nndss/nndsshis.htm.)

EMERGING INFECTIOUS DISEASES

Emergence Factors

Emerging infectious diseases are those in which the incidence has actually increased in the past several decades or has the potential to increase in the near future. These emerging diseases may include new or known infectious diseases. Consider the following selected examples. Identified only in 1976 when sporadic outbreaks occurred in Sudan and Zaire, Ebola virus is a mysterious killer with a frightening mortality rate that sometimes reaches 90%, has no known treatment, and has no recognized reservoir in nature. It appears to be transmitted through direct contact with bodily secretions and as such can be contained once cases are identified. Why outbreaks occur is not understood, although index cases have been associated with the handling of wild primates. Evidence is also building for a bat reservoir. Ebola and its fellow virus Marburg are examples of new viruses that may appear as civilization intrudes farther and farther into previously uninhabited natural environments, changing the landscape and disturbing ecological balances that

BOX 13-3   NATIONALLY NOTIFIABLE INFECTIOUS CONDITIONS—UNITED STATES 2010

1. Anthrax
2. Arboviral neuroinvasive and non-neuroinvasive diseases
   - California serogroup virus disease
   - Eastern equine encephalitis virus disease
   - Powassan virus disease
   - St. Louis encephalitis virus disease
   - West Nile virus disease
   - Western equine encephalitis virus disease
3. Botulism
   - Botulism, foodborne
   - Botulism, infant
   - Botulism, other (wound and unspecified)
4. Brucellosis
5. Chancroid
6. *Chlamydia trachomatis* infection
7. Cholera
8. Cryptosporidiosis
9. Cyclosporiasis
10. Dengue
    - Dengue fever
    - Dengue hemorrhagic fever
    - Dengue shock syndrome
11. Diphtheria
12. Ehrlichiosis/Anaplasmosis
    - *Ehrlichia chaffeensis*
    - *Ehrlichia ewingii*
    - *Anaplasma phagocytophilum*
    - Undetermined
13. Giardiasis
14. Gonorrhea
15. *Haemophilus influenzae*, invasive disease
16. Hansen disease (leprosy)
17. Hantavirus pulmonary syndrome
18. Hemolytic uremic syndrome, post-diarrheal
19. Hepatitis
    - Hepatitis A, acute
    - Hepatitis B, acute
    - Hepatitis B, chronic
    - Hepatitis B virus, perinatal infection
    - Hepatitis C, acute
    - Hepatitis C, chronic
20. HIV infection*
    - HIV infection, adult/adolescent (age ≥13 years)
    - HIV infection, child (age ≥18 months and <13 years)
    - HIV infection, pediatric (age <18 months)
21. Influenza-associated pediatric mortality
22. Legionellosis
23. Listeriosis
24. Lyme disease
25. Malaria
26. Measles
27. Meningococcal disease
28. Mumps
29. Novel influenza A virus infections
30. Pertussis
31. Plague
32. Poliomyelitis, paralytic
33. Poliovirus infection, non-paralytic
34. Psittacosis
35. Q fever
    - Acute
    - Chronic
36. Rabies
    - Rabies, animal
    - Rabies, human
37. Rubella
38. Rubella, congenital syndrome
39. Salmonellosis
40. Severe Acute Respiratory Syndrome–associated Coronavirus (SARS-CoV) disease
41. Shiga toxin–producing *Escherichia coli* (STEC)
42. Shigellosis
43. Smallpox
44. Spotted fever rickettsiosis
45. Streptococcal toxic-shock syndrome
46. *Streptococcus pneumoniae*, invasive disease
47. Syphilis
    - Primary
    - Secondary
    - Latent
    - Early latent
    - Late latent
    - Latent, unknown duration
    - Neurosyphilis
    - Late, non-neurological
    - Stillbirth
    - Congenital
48. Tetanus
49. Toxic-shock syndrome (other than streptococcal)
50. Trichinellosis (Trichinosis)
51. Tuberculosis
52. Tularemia
53. Typhoid fever
54. Vancomycin-intermediate *Staphylococcus aureus* (VISA)
55. Vancomycin-resistant *Staphylococcus aureus* (VRSA)
56. Varicella (morbidity)
57. Varicella (deaths only)
58. Vibriosis
59. Viral hemorrhagic fevers
    - Arenavirus
    - Crimean-Congo hemorrhagic fever virus
    - Ebola virus
    - Lassa virus
    - Marburg virus
60. Yellow fever

From Centers for Disease Control and Prevention: *Nationally Notifiable Infectious Conditions United States 2010,* 2010, CDC. Available at http://www.cdc.gov/ncphi/disss/nndss/phs/infdis2010.htm. Accessed March 25, 2010.
*AIDS has been reclassified as HIV stage III.

may have existed unaltered for hundreds of years. (Read more about the viral hemorrhagic viruses Ebola and Marburg at the CDC's special pathogens website: http://www.cdc.gov/ncidod/dvrd/spb/index.htm.)

Hantavirus pulmonary syndrome was first detected in 1993 in the Four Corner area of Arizona and New Mexico, when young, previously healthy Native Americans fell ill with a mysterious and deadly respiratory disease. The illness was soon discovered to be a variant of, but to exhibit different pathology from, a rodent-borne virus previously known only in Europe and Asia. Transmission is thought to occur through aerosolization of rodent excrement. One explanation for the outbreak in the Southwest is that an unseasonably mild winter led to an unusual increase in the rodent population; more people than usual were exposed to a virus that had until that point gone unrecognized in this country. Infection in Native Americans first brought attention to hantavirus pulmonary syndrome because of a cluster of cases in a small geographic area, but no evidence suggests that any ethnic group is particularly susceptible to this disease. Hantavirus pulmonary syndrome has now been diagnosed in sites across the United States. The best protection against this virus seems to be avoiding rodent-infested environments.

Not only is HIV disease relatively new but the resultant immunocompromise gave rise to previously rare opportunistic infections such as cryptosporidiosis, toxoplasmosis, and *Pneumocystis* pneumonia (PCP). HIV may have existed in isolated parts of sub-Saharan Africa for years and emerged, only recently, into the rest of the world as the result of a combination of factors, including new roads, increased commerce, and prostitution. TB is a familiar face turned newly aggressive. After years of decline, it has resurged as a result of infection resulting from HIV disease and the development of multi-drug resistance. New influenza viruses like A H1N1 and A H5N1 challenge scientists to rapidly develop vaccines to protect a world population with little or no immunity.

WNV, a mosquito-borne seasonal disease, was first identified in Uganda in 1937 and first detected in the United States in 1999. How WNV arrived in the United States may never be known, but the answer most likely involves infected birds or mosquitoes. Because the virus was new in this country and the outbreak of 2002 caused numerous deaths, WNV garnered a great deal of media attention. However, for the majority of people, infection with WNV results in no clinical signs (about 80%) or only mild flu-like symptoms. In a small percentage of individuals, approximately 1 of 150 cases, a more severe, potentially fatal neuroinvasive form may develop, which may leave permanent neurological deficits for those who survive. The incidence of neuroinvasive disease increases with age with the highest rates in those 70 years and older. After first appearing in New York City in 1999, the virus spent several years quietly spreading up and down the East Coast without remarkable morbidity or mortality. This situation changed abruptly in the summer of 2002 when it began moving across the country, accompanied by significant avian, equine, and human mortality. WNV has now been reported in every state except Maine, Hawaii, and Alaska and is the most common

arbovirus (virus carried by arthropods) disease in the country. The CDC estimates that during its introduction into the United States, between 1999 and 2008, WNV led to almost 30,000 confirmed and probable cases and over 1000 deaths. The number of reported cases varies widely per year. These periodic outbreaks appear to result from a complex interaction of multiple factors, including weather—hot, dry summers followed by rain, which influences mosquito breeding sites and population growth. Because the ecology of WNV is not fully understood, the future pattern and nature of the virus in the United States is uncertain. Until a human vaccine is developed (a vaccine for horses does exist), preventing human infection is dependent on mosquito control and preventing mosquito bites. Rarely, WNV has been transmitted through blood transfusions, in utero exposure, and possibly breastfeeding (CDC, 2010a). (Learn more about WNV and view maps of recent activity at the CDC website: http://www.cdc.gov/ncidod/dvbid/westnile/index.htm.)

Several factors, operating singly or in combination, can influence the emergence of these diseases (Table 13-1) (CDC, 1994). Except for microbial adaptation and changes made by the infectious agent, such as those likely in the emergence of *E. coli* 0157:H7, most of the emergence factors are consequences of activities and behavior of the human hosts, and of environmental changes such as deforestation, urbanization, and industrialization. The rise in households with two working parents

TABLE 13-1 FACTORS THAT CAN INFLUENCE THE EMERGENCE OF NEW INFECTIOUS DISEASES

CATEGORIES	SPECIFIC EXAMPLES
Societal events	Economic impoverishment, war or civil conflict, population growth and migration, urban decay
Health care	New medical devices, organ or tissue transplantation, drugs causing immunosuppression, widespread use of antibiotics
Food production	Globalization of food supplies, changes in food processing and packaging
Human behavior	Sexual behavior, drug use, travel, diet, outdoor recreation, use of childcare facilities
Environmental	Deforestation/reforestation, changes in water ecosystems, flood/drought, famine, global changes (e.g., warming)
Public health	Curtailment or reduction in prevention programs, inadequate communicable disease infrastructure surveillance, lack of trained personnel (epidemiologists, laboratory scientists, vector and rodent control specialists)
Microbial adaptation	Changes in virulence and toxin production, development of drug resistance, microbes as co-factors in chronic diseases

From Centers for Disease Control and Prevention: *Addressing emerging infectious disease threats: a prevention strategy for the U.S.*, Atlanta, 1994, CDC.

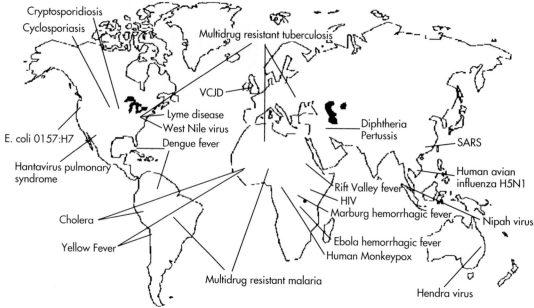

FIGURE 13-2 Examples of recent emerging and reemerging infectious diseases. (Based on Institute of Medicine: *Microbial threats to health: emergence, detection, and response,* Washington, DC, 2003, National Academy Press.)

has increased the number of children in day care and with this shift has come an increase in diarrheal diseases such as shigellosis. Changing sexual behavior and illegal drug use influence the spread of HIV disease as well as other sexually transmitted infections. Before the use of large air-conditioning systems with cooling towers, legionellosis was virtually unknown. Modern transportation systems closely and quickly connect regions of the world that for centuries had little contact. Insects and animals as well as humans may carry disease between continents on ships and planes. Immigrants, both legal and undocumented, as well as travelers bring with them a variety of known and potentially unknown diseases.

To address the challenges of emerging and reemerging diseases, the CDC published *Preventing Emerging Infectious Diseases: A Strategy for the 21st Century* first in 1994 and then updated in 1998. This plan suggests that prevention and control of emerging diseases will require education to change behaviors and the development of effective drugs and vaccines. Also, current surveillance systems must be strengthened and expanded to improve detection and tracking (CDC, 1994, 1998a). Progress in addressing infectious disease as well as current findings and topics can be found in the CDC journal *Emerging Infectious Diseases.* (The journal is published monthly and is available online at http://www.cdc.gov/ncidod/EID/about/about.htm.)

Examples of Emerging Infectious Diseases

Examples of emerging and resurgent infectious diseases around the world are shown in Figure 13-2. Selected emerging infectious diseases, including a brief description of the diseases and symptoms they cause, their modes of transmission, and causes of emergence, are listed in Table 13-2.

PREVENTION AND CONTROL OF COMMUNICABLE DISEASES

Communicable disease can be prevented and controlled. The goal of prevention and control programs is to reduce the prevalence of a disease to a level at which it no longer poses a major public health problem. In some cases, diseases may even be eliminated or eradicated. The goal of elimination is to remove a disease from a large geographic area such as a country or region of the world. Eradication is removing a disease worldwide by ending all transmission of infection through the complete extermination of the infectious agent. WHO officially declared the global eradication of smallpox on May 8, 1980 (Evans, 1985). After the successful eradication of smallpox, the eradication of other communicable diseases became a realistic challenge, and in 1987 WHO adopted resolutions for eradication of paralytic poliomyelitis and dracunculiasis (guinea worm infection) from the world by the year 2000.

These eradication goals were not reached in 2000, but substantial progress has been made. When the resolution was made in 1987 for the eradication of Guinea worm disease, there were an estimated 3.5 million cases a year in 20 countries in Asia and Africa and 120 million people were at risk for the disease. By the end of 2007 the disease was endemic only in five countries in Africa and less than 10,000 cases were reported. Of the cases occurring during the first half of 2008, 98% were reported from Sudan, Ghana, and Mali. Sporadic violence appears to be the challenge to successful eradication of endemic dracunculiasis in this region of Africa (CDC, 2008a).

By 2010 the number of polio-endemic countries had decreased from 125 to 4 (Afghanistan, India, Nigeria, and Pakistan); 1256 cases of non–vaccine-derived or wild-type polio

TABLE 13-2 EXAMPLES OF EMERGING INFECTIOUS DISEASES

INFECTIOUS AGENT	DISEASES/SYMPTOMS	MODE OF TRANSMISSION	CAUSES OF EMERGENCE
Borrelia burgdorferi	Lyme disease: rash, fever, arthritis, neurological, and cardiac abnormalities	Bite of infective *Ixodes* tick	Increase in deer and human populations in wooded areas
Cryptosporidium	Cryptosporidiosis; infection of epithelial cells in gastrointestinal and respiratory tracts	Fecal-oral, person-to-person, waterborne	Development near watershed areas; immunosuppression
Ebola-Marburg viruses	Fulminant, high mortality, hemorrhagic fever	Direct contact with infected blood, organs, secretions, and semen	Unknown, likely human invasion of virus ecological niche
Escherichia coli 0157:H7	Hemorrhagic colitis; thrombocytopenia; hemolytic uremic syndrome	Ingestion of contaminated food, especially undercooked beef and raw milk	Likely caused by a new pathogen
Hantavirus	Hemorrhagic fever with renal syndrome; pulmonary syndrome	Inhalation of aerosolized rodent urine and feces	Human invasion of virus ecological niche
Human immunodeficiency virus (HIV-1)	HIV infection; AIDS (HIV stage III); severe immune dysfunction, opportunistic infections	Sexual contact with or exposure to blood or tissues of infected persons; perinatal	Urbanization; lifestyle changes; drug use; international travel; transfusions; transplant
Human papillomavirus (HPV)	Skin and mucous membrane lesions (warts); strongly linked to cancer of the cervix and penis	Direct sexual contact, contact with contaminated surfaces	Newly recognized; changes in sexual lifestyle
Influenza A H1N1 virus (novel, pandemic)	Influenza: fever, cough, headache, myalgia, prostration, possibly GI signs	Person-to-person, airborne (droplet), and contact (direct and indirect)	Antigenic shift
Influenza A H5N1 virus (novel, avian)	Influenza: fever, cough, headache, myalgia, prostration	Direct contact with infected poultry or birds; limited person-to-person transmission	Antigenic shift
Legionella pneumophila	Legionnaires' disease: malaise, myalgia, fever, headache, respiratory illness	Air cooling systems, water supplies	Recognition in an epidemic situation
Pneumocystis jiroveci	Acute pneumonia	Unknown; possibly airborne or reactivation of latent infection	Immunosuppression
SARS	Severe and acute pneumonia	Person-to-person, airborne (droplet) and direct and indirect contact with respiratory secretions and other bodily fluid	Unknown; newly recognized coronavirus; possible animal transmission into Chinese population
West Nile virus	No clinical signs to mild flu-like symptoms to fatal neuroinvasive disease	Bite of infected mosquitoes; infected birds serve as reservoirs	International travel and commerce

Based on information from Heymann DL, editor: *Control of communicable diseases manual*, ed 19, Washington, DC, 2008, American Public Health Association; Fauci AS, Touchette NA, Folkers GK: Emerging infectious diseases: a 10-year perspective from the National Institute of Allergy and Infectious Diseases, *Emerg Infect Dis* 11(4):519-525, 2005.

virus were reported from these four polio-endemic countries in 2009, compared with 350,000 cases reported from those 125 countries in 1988; another 350 imported cases from 10 nonendemic countries were also reported. Importation of cases resulting from the ease of worldwide travel or breakdowns in coverage in a neighboring country has led to outbreaks in nonendemic countries several times in the last 10 years, the largest being spillover into adjacent countries from Nigeria beginning in 2003 and cases in far-flung countries originating from exposure during the Muslim religious pilgrimage to Mecca. Such outbreaks point to the necessity of maintaining mass vaccination campaigns in polio-free countries to protect against cases imported from endemic areas. Challenges to eradication include political instability and sporadic violence, cultural beliefs about immunization, religious fears, and distrust of immunization (CDC, 2009d).

The Americas were certified polio free in 1994 (an outbreak in Haiti and the Dominican Republic in 2000 was vaccine derived), with the western Pacific certified in 2000 and Europe in 2002 (WHO, 2002). April 2005 marked the fiftieth anniversary of the polio vaccine. In 2004 WHO released an updated Global Polio Eradication Initiative Strategic Plan, outlining activities required to: (1) interrupt global polio transmission, (2) achieve global polio eradication certification, and (3) prepare for global cessation of childhood vaccination with the oral poliovirus vaccine (CDC, 2004). With the Global Polio Eradication Initiative, WHO partnered with national governments, Rotary International, the CDC and UNICEF in what has been called the largest public health initiative the world has ever known. Since 1988, over 2 billion children around the world have been immunized against polio through the cooperation of more than 200 countries and 20 million volunteers, supported by an international investment of over \$3 billion. At the end of 2008, WHO reviewed the progress of the initiative with two independent outside agencies and concluded that the remaining technical and operational challenges to eradication could be overcome in each of the polio-endemic countries by ensuring the political commitment of all polio-affected countries to attain the highest possible coverage and enhancing routine vaccination and surveillance (CDC, 2009d). (Read more about global polio eradication efforts at http://www.polioeradication.org/.)

Primary, Secondary, and Tertiary Prevention

There are three levels of prevention in public health: primary, secondary, and tertiary. In prevention and control of infectious disease, primary prevention seeks to reduce the incidence of disease by preventing occurrence, and this effort is often assisted by the government. Many interventions at the primary level, such as federally supplied vaccines and "no shots, no school" immunization laws, are population based because of public health mandate. Nurses deliver childhood immunizations in public and community health settings, check immunization records in daycare facilities, and monitor immunization records in schools.

WHAT DO YOU THINK?   *Refusal of preventive health care to undocumented residents may prove a threat to the public's health.*

The goal of secondary prevention is to prevent the spread of infection and/or disease once it occurs. Activities center on rapid identification of potential contacts to a reported case. Contacts may be: (1) identified as new cases and treated, or (2) determined to be possibly exposed but not diseased and appropriately treated with prophylaxis. Public health disease control laws also assist in secondary prevention because they require investigation and prevention measures for individuals affected by a communicable disease report or outbreak. These laws can extend to the entire community if the exposure potential is deemed great enough, as could happen with an outbreak of smallpox or epidemic influenza. Much of the communicable disease surveillance and control work in this country is performed by nurses.

While many infections are acute, with either recovery or death occurring in the short term, some exhibit chronic courses (AIDS/HIV stage III) or disabling sequelae (leprosy/Hansen's disease). Tertiary prevention works to reduce complications and disabilities through treatment and rehabilitation. The Levels of Prevention box has examples of communicable disease prevention and control interventions at the three levels of prevention.

Role of Nurses in Prevention

Prevention is at the center of public and community health, and nurses perform much of this work. Examples include immunizations for vaccine-preventable disease, especially childhood immunization and the monitoring of immunization status in clinic, daycare, school, and home settings. Nurses work in communicable

---

LEVELS OF PREVENTION

Examples of Infectious Disease Interventions

Primary Prevention
To prevent the occurrence of disease:
- Responsible sexual behavior
- Malaria chemoprophylaxis
- Tetanus boosters, flu shots
- Rabies pre-exposure immunization
- Safe food-handling practices in the home
- Repellants for preventing vector-borne disease
- Following childhood immunizations recommendations, and "no shots, no school" laws
- Regulated and inspected municipal water supplies
- Bloodborne pathogen regulations
- Restaurant inspections
- Federal regulations protecting American cattle from exposure to bovine spongiform encephalopathy (BSE)

Secondary Prevention
To prevent the spread of disease:
- Immunoglobulin after hepatitis A exposure
- Immunization and chemoprophylaxis as appropriate in meningococcal outbreak
- Rabies post-exposure immunization
- Tuberculosis screening for health care workers
- Sexually transmitted disease (STD) partner notification
- Human immunodeficiency virus (HIV) testing and treatment
- Quarantine

Tertiary Prevention
To reduce complications and disabilities through treatment and rehabilitation:
- *Pneumocystis* pneumonia (PCP) chemoprophylaxis for people with AIDS
- Regular inspection of hands and feet as well as protective footwear and gloves to avoid trauma and infection for leprosy clients who have lost sensation in those areas

---

disease surveillance and control, teach and monitor bloodborne pathogen control, and advise on prevention of vector-borne diseases. They teach methods for responsible sexual behavior, screen for sexually transmitted infection, and provide HIV disease counseling and testing. They screen for TB, identify TB contacts, and deliver directly observed TB treatment in the community.

Multisystem Approach to Control

Communicable diseases represent an imbalance in the harmonious relationship between the human host and the environment. This state of imbalance provides the infectious agent an opportunity to cause illness and death in the human population. Given the many factors that can disrupt the agent-host-environment relationship, a multisystem approach to control of communicable diseases (Table 13-3) must be developed (Wenzel, 1998).

NURSING TIP   *When dealing with a communicable disease that has outbreak potential, include family members and close contacts as well as the sick person when developing a treatment and prevention plan.*

TABLE 13-3   A MULTISYSTEM APPROACH TO COMMUNICABLE DISEASE CONTROL

GOAL	EXAMPLE
Improve host resistance to infectious agents and other environmental hazards	Hygiene, nutrition, and physical fitness; increased immunization coverage; provision of drugs for prevention and treatment; stress control and improved mental health
Improve safety of the environment	Sanitation, clean water and air; proper cooking and storage of food; control of vectors and animal reservoir hosts
Improve public health systems	Increased access to health care; appropriate health education; improved surveillance systems
Facilitate social and political change to ensure better health for all people	Individual, organizational, and community action; legislation

Modified from Wenzel RP: Control of communicable diseases: overview. In Wallace RB, editor: *Public health and preventive medicine*, ed 14, Stamford, CT, 1998, Appleton & Lange.

AGENTS OF BIOTERRORISM

September 11, 2001, made real the specter of terrorism on American soil. The anthrax attacks that followed further highlighted the possibilities for the intentional release of a biological agent, or bioterrorism. The CDC suggests that the agents most likely to be used in a bioterrorist attack are those having both the potential for high mortality and easy dissemination—factors most likely to result in major public panic and social disruption. Six infectious agents are considered of highest concern: anthrax *(Bacillus anthracis)*, plague *(Yersinia pestis)*, smallpox (variola major), botulism *(Clostridium botulinum)*, tularemia *(Francisella tularensis)* and selected hemorrhagic viruses (filoviruses such as Ebola and Marburg; arenaviruses such as Lassa fever, Junin virus, and related viruses). The CDC urges health care providers to be familiar with the epidemiology of these diseases as well as illness patterns, possibly indicating an unusual infectious disease outbreak associated with the intentional release of a biological agent. (More information on recognition of illness associated with the intentional release of a biological agent as well as possible agents may be found at the CDC Emergency Preparedness and Response website: http://www.bt.cdc.gov.)

Anthrax

Until the fall of 2001, anthrax was more commonly a concern of veterinarians and military strategists than the general public. After September 11th, the news of deaths caused by letters deliberately contaminated with anthrax and transmitted through the postal service profoundly changed our view of this infectious disease. Anthrax is an acute disease caused by the spore-forming bacterium *B. anthracis*. It is thought that anthrax may have caused the biblical fifth and sixth plagues of Exodus as well as the Black Bane of Europe in the 1600s. In 1881 anthrax became the first bacterial disease for which immunization was available. More commonly seen in cattle, sheep, and goats, anthrax in modern times has rarely and sporadically affected humans, usually through the handling or consumption of infected animal products (Cieslak and Eitzen, 1999).

Anthrax is a clever organism that perpetuates itself by forming spores. When animals dying from anthrax suffer terminal hemorrhage and infected blood comes into contact with the air, the bacillus organism sporulates. These spores are highly resistant to disinfection and environmental destruction and may remain in contaminated soil for many years. In the United States, anthrax zones are said to follow the cattle drive trails of the 1800s. Sometimes referred to as wool handler's disease, anthrax has commonly posed the greatest risk to people who work directly with dying animals, such as veterinarians, or those who handle infected animal products such as hair, wool, and bone or bone meal or products made from these materials such as rugs and drums. Products made from infected materials may transmit this disease around the world. Person-to-person transmission is rare (Heymann, 2008).

Anthrax disease may manifest in one of three syndromes: cutaneous, gastrointestinal, and respiratory or inhalational. Cutaneous anthrax, the form most commonly seen, occurs when spores come in contact with abraded skin surfaces. Itching is followed in 2 to 6 days by the development of a characteristic black eschar, usually surrounded by some degree of edema and possibly secondary infection. The lesion itself is usually not painful. If untreated, infection may spread to the regional lymph nodes and bloodstream, resulting in septicemia and death. The fatality rate for untreated cutaneous anthrax is between 5% and 20%, but if appropriately treated, death seldom occurs. Before 2001 the last cutaneous case in the United States was reported in 1992. Gastrointestinal anthrax is considered very rare and occurs from eating undercooked, contaminated meat. Inhalational anthrax is also considered rare, typically seen in occupations with exposure to hide tanning or bone processing. Before 2001 the last case reported in the United States was in 1976. Initially, symptoms are mild and non-specific and may include fever, malaise, mild cough, or chest pain. These symptoms are followed 3 to 5 days later, often after an apparent improvement, by fever and shock, rapid deterioration, and death. Untreated cases of inhalational anthrax are fatal; treated cases may show as high as a 95% fatality rate if treatment is initiated after 48 hours from the onset of symptoms.

Because of factors such as the ability for aerosolization, the resistance to environmental degradation and a high fatality rate, inhalational anthrax has long been considered to have an extremely high potential for being the single greatest biological warfare threat (Cieslak and Eitzen, 1999). An accidental release from a biological research institute in Sverdlovsk, Russia, in 1979 resulted in the documented death of 66 individuals and demonstrated the capacity of this organism as a weapon. Manufacture and delivery of the spores have been considered a challenge because of a tendency for the spores to clump. During 1998 in the United States, more than two dozen anthrax threats (letters purporting to be carrying anthrax) were made. None of them were real. The events of the fall of 2001, when 11 people were sickened and 5 died from deliberate exposure, have shown that the threat of anthrax as a weapon of bioterror is all too real.

Any threat of anthrax should be reported to the Federal Bureau of Investigation and to local and state health departments. Anthrax is sensitive to a variety of antibiotics including the penicillins, chloramphenicol, doxycycline, and the fluoroquinolones. In cases of possible bioterrorism activity, individuals with a credible threat of exposure, with confirmed exposure, or at high risk of exposure are immediately started on antibiotic prophylaxis, preferably fluoroquinolones. Immunization is recommended as well. People who have been exposed are not contagious, so quarantine is not appropriate (Heymann, 2008).

In recent years, although no more deliberate acts of bioterrorism have been reported, England and the United States have seen rare cases of cutaneous, inhalational, and gastrointestinal anthrax associated with drumming circles using drums covered with imported animal hides. Since December 2009, in the United Kingdom, there has been an ongoing outbreak of anthrax among injecting drug users, in some cases resulting in death. The infection is believed to be caused by contaminated heroin. With no new cases after the summer Scotland declared the outbreak over in December 2010 but concluded the possibility of an ongoing risk of anthrax of heroin users supported by sporadic cases occurring in England. Ongoing national investigation continues.

Smallpox

Formerly a disease found worldwide, smallpox has been considered eradicated since 1979. The last known natural case in the United States was in 1949. The last known case of smallpox worldwide occurred in Somalia in 1977. The United States stopped routinely immunizing for smallpox in 1982. The only documented existing virus sources are located in freezers at the CDC in Atlanta and at a research institute in Novosibirsk, Russia. Controversy exists over the destruction of these viral stocks, and despite an earlier call by WHO for destruction in 2002, this date has been postponed to allow for additional research needed should clandestine supplies fall into terrorist hands.

Smallpox has been identified as one of the leading candidate agents for bioterrorism. Susceptibility is 100% in the unvaccinated (those vaccinated before 1982 are not considered protected, although they may have some immunity) and the fatality rate is estimated at 20% to 40% or higher. Immunization with a vaccinia vaccine, the immunizing agent for smallpox, can be protective even after exposure. In 2007 the U.S. Food and Drug Administration (FDA) licensed a new smallpox vaccine, derived from the only other smallpox vaccine licensed by the FDA: Dryvax, approved in 1931 and now in limited supply because it is no longer manufactured. The WHO does not recommend vaccination of the general public because currently the risk of death (1 per 1 million doses) or serious side effects is greater than that of the disease. Those who routinely are exposed to smallpox virus such as laboratory workers should be vaccinated. Because of the potential for bioterrorism and the fact that many health care providers have never seen this disease, it is important to become familiar with the clinical and epidemiological features of smallpox and how it is differentiated from chickenpox (see the How To box). Should a non-varicella, small pox–like disease

be detected, immediate contact with local and national health authorities is obligatory (FDA, 2007; Heymann, 2008).

HOW TO Distinguish Chickenpox from Smallpox

Despite the availability of a vaccine, chickenpox is still a common disease of childhood and may be seen in susceptible adults as well. Although many health care providers are familiar with chickenpox, most have never seen a case of smallpox. Because of the potential for smallpox to be used as a bioweapon, the CDC suggests that nurses and other practitioners familiarize themselves with the differences in presentation between the two diseases. The rash pattern for each disease is distinctive, but in the first 2 to 3 days of development, the two may be indistinguishable. Infectious disease texts and posters provide a pictorial description. If a smallpox infection is suspected, the local health department should be notified immediately.

CHICKENPOX (VARICELLA)	SMALLPOX (HISTORICAL VARIOLA MAJOR)
Sudden onset with slight fever and mild constitutional symptoms (both may be more severe in adults)	Sudden onset of fever, prostration, severe body aches, and occasional abdominal pain and vomiting, as in influenza
Rash is present at onset	Clear-cut prodromal illness, rash follows 2-4 days after fever begins decreasing
Rash progression is maculopapular for a few hours, vesicular for 3-4 days, followed by granular scabs	Progression is macular, papular, vesicular, and pustular, followed by crusted scabs that fall off after 3-4 weeks if client survives
Rash is "centrifugal" with lesions most abundant on the trunk or areas of the body usually covered by clothing	Rash is "centripetal" with lesions most abundant on the face and extremities
Lesions appear in "crops" and can be at various stages in the same area of the body	Lesions are all at same stage in all areas
Vesicles are superficial and collapse on puncture; mild scarring may occur	Vesicles are deep-seated and do not collapse on puncture; pitting and scarring are common

From Heymann DL, editor: Control of communicable diseases manual, ed 19, Washington, DC, 2008, American Public Health Association; Henderson DA: Smallpox: clinical and epidemiologic features, Emerg Infect Dis 5:537-539, 1999.

Plague

Plague is a vector-borne disease transmitted by rodent fleas carrying the bacterium *Y. pestis*. Portrayed vividly in the Bible and events throughout history, plague is believed responsible for the epidemic of Black Death that killed over a quarter of the population of Europe during the Middle Ages. The disease is endemic in much of South Asia, parts of South America, and the western United States, but the majority of outbreaks and cases today are reported from Africa, especially from the Democratic Republic of the Congo. Plague arrived in the United States as a consequence of a pandemic that began in China during the late 1800s and spread to the West Coast via shipboard rats. Although resulting plague in cities was largely controlled, the disease spread to and became enzootic in wild rodents. The current primary vertebrate reservoirs in the United States are usually ground squirrels rather than rats, rabbits, wild carnivores, and in some cases cats. Human plague in the western United States occurs infrequently and sporadically with fewer than 20 cases reported a year since 1970. Veterinarians have contracted the disease from infected cats. People with regular outdoor exposure such as hunters, trappers, and those living in rural areas as well as cat owners are at highest risk for natural transmission (Heymann, 2008).

Initial signs and symptoms of plague are non-specific and include myalgia, malaise, fever, chills, sore throat, and headache. As the disease progresses, lymphadenitis commonly develops in the lymph nodes, draining the area nearest the bite. This swollen node, or bubo, most frequently seen in the inguinal area, gives rise to the name bubonic plague. Whether lymphadenitis is present or not, bubonic plague may progress to septicemic plague and secondary pneumonic plague. Secondary pneumonic plague can spread through respiratory droplets, resulting in primary pneumonic plague and human-to-human outbreaks. No such transmission has been reported in the United States since 1924, but several cases of primary pneumonic plague have developed from exposure to infected cats.

Untreated cases of primary septicemic and pneumonic plague are most often fatal; the case fatality rate for untreated bubonic plague is 50% to 60%. Streptomycin is the treatment of choice; gentamicin, tetracyclines, and chloramphenicol are alternatives. Immunization may confer some protection against bubonic plague but not pneumonic. Commercial plague vaccine is no longer available in the United States. Naturally acquired plague is usually bubonic. Plague used as a means of a terrorist attack would most likely be aerosolized, resulting in pneumonic disease and human-to-human transmission (Heymann, 2008). (Read more about plague at the CDC website: http://www.cdc.gov/ncidod/dvbid/plague/index.htm.)

Tularemia

Sometimes referred to as "rabbit fever" or "deer fly fever," tularemia is a zoonotic disease caused by the bacterial agent *F. tularensis* which is carried commonly by wild animals, especially rabbits, as well as muskrats, voles, beavers, some domestic animals, and some ticks, mosquitoes, and flies. Tularemia may be transmitted by the bite of an infected arthropod; contact of eyes, skin, or mucous membranes with infected tissues, blood, or water; ingestion of inadequately cooked infected meat or contaminated water; inhalation of contaminated dust; and handling of contaminated pelts and paws. Hunters handling rabbit and rodent carcasses, lawn care workers, and those working outside in rural areas may be at higher risk. Tularemia has also been documented as occurring from running over an infected rabbit with a lawn mower and by handling sick pets including dogs, cats, hamsters, and prairie dogs. Tularemia is not transmitted from person to person (Heymann, 2008).

How tularemia presents varies depending on how the infection was acquired and the virulence of the infecting agent. There are two subspecies of *F. tularensis*—one causing few deaths even without treatment and one resulting in a 5% to 15% fatality rate without treatment, primarily from respiratory disease. Commonly the onset of tularemia is sudden and may resemble influenza with high fever, myalgia, headache, nausea, and chills. Frequently an ulcerative lesion appears at the point of inoculation accompanied by swelling of associated lymph nodes. However, lymphadenitis can occur without a primary lesion. In either case, the presence of these buboes can cause confusion with plague. Inoculation, or introduction of the organism, into the eye results in a purulent conjunctivitis accompanied by regional lymphadenitis. Ingestion of infected tissue or contaminated water produces a sore throat, abdominal pain, diarrhea, and vomiting. Infection by inhalation may cause respiratory involvement and possible sepsis. Pneumonia is a potential complication with all forms and requires prompt treatment to prevent potentially fatal complications. Aminoglycosides or ciprofloxacin are the treatment drugs of choice. There is no vaccination for tularemia currently in widespread use in the United States, although live attenuated vaccine applied intradermally by scarification is available to high-risk workers (Heymann, 2008).

Tularemia has been reported from every state except Hawaii but is not a particularly common disease, with only 120 to 130 cases documented each year (CDC, 2010b). The only two reported outbreaks of pneumonic tularemia in the United States have come from Martha's Vineyard, where the disease is endemic and cases are frequently reported in lawn care workers (Feldman et al, 2003). Because of the low incidence of naturally occurring disease, tularemia was removed from the nationally notifiable disease list in 1994 but reinstated in 2000 with the growing concern over bioterrorism. Aerosolized tularemia with resulting pneumonic disease is considered the most likely scenario for use as an agent of bioterrorism (CDC, 2005a). (Read more about tularemia at the CDC website: http://www.cdc.gov/tularemia/index.html.)

VACCINE-PREVENTABLE DISEASES

Vaccines are one of the most effective methods of preventing and controlling communicable diseases. The smallpox vaccine, which left distinctive scars on so many shoulders, is no longer in general use because the smallpox virus has been declared eradicated from the world's population. Despite threats of bioterrorism, there are no plans to reintroduce universal smallpox immunization because of potential side effects. Diseases such as polio, diphtheria, pertussis, and measles, which previously occurred in epidemic proportions, are now controlled by routine childhood immunization. They have not, however, been eradicated, so children need to be immunized against them. In the United States, "no shots, no school" legislation has resulted in the immunization of most children by the time they enter school. However, many infants and toddlers, the group most vulnerable to these potentially severe diseases, do not receive scheduled immunizations despite the availability of free vaccines. Surveys show inner-city children from minority and ethnic groups are particularly at risk for incomplete immunization, and children from religious communities whose beliefs prohibit immunization and children with parents who have philosophical objections to immunization may receive no protection at all. Studies also show low levels of vaccination against pneumonia in senior citizens and lower levels of influenza coverage in adults from minority and ethnic groups. Research also suggests that adolescents have lower rates of coverage than children or adults perhaps because they do not as frequently access preventive care (see the Evidence-Based Practice box). *Healthy People 2020* includes several objectives about obtaining and maintaining appropriate levels of immunization in all age groups. (Additional information on vaccine-preventable diseases may be found at the CDC website: http://www.cdc.gov/vaccines/.)

EVIDENCE-BASED PRACTICE

Researchers looked at data on 23,987 adolescents enrolled in a New England HMO from 1997 to 2001 with three objectives: (1) to assess the immunization rates for tetanus-diphtheria (Td), hepatitis B, and measles-mumps-rubella (MMR) vaccines among 13-year-olds, (2) to identify missed opportunities for Td immunization among adolescents 11 to 17 years of age, and (3) to evaluate the association between preventive care use and Td immunization. They found that 13-year-olds were 84%, 74%, and 67% up to date on their Td, hepatitis B, and MMR vaccinations, respectively. The finding for Td was higher than that reported nationally, but rates for hepatitis B and MMR were lower. This was surprising since most of the adolescents lived in Massachusetts, which has required two doses of MMR for school entry since 2001. One possible contributor to this finding was incomplete documentation caused by immunization records scattered among different facilities.

Missed opportunities for Td immunization occurred at 84% of all health care visits. Although many of these missed opportunities were during hospital or ER visits, there were also preventive care visits where Td was not received. Adolescents who did not seek preventive care were less likely to receive Td in a timely manner.

Nurse Use

Adolescent immunization rates lag behind rates for young children. One reason may be fewer preventive care visits. Other barriers may include the lack of awareness regarding the need for immunizations in this age group, financial concerns, and record scattering. This study finds that missed opportunities contribute to lower rates of immunization in adolescents, just as in children and adults. Nurses in public, private, school, or community-based positions can assess immunization status at every visit, ensure full documentation of complete immunization history, recommend regular preventive care, and educate on the need for and importance of immunization. Nurses who make home visits have an opportunity to ask about immunization status of all family members regardless of age and encourage age-appropriate immunization.

From Lee GM, Lorick SA, Pfoh E, et al: Adolescent immunizations: missed opportunities for prevention, *Pediatrics* 122(4):711-717, 2008.

Because many children receive their immunizations at public health departments, nurses play a major role in increasing immunization coverage of infants and toddlers. Nurses track children known to be at risk for underimmunization and call or send reminders to their parents. They help avoid missed immunization opportunities by checking the immunization status of every young child encountered, whether or not the clinic or home visit is related to immunization. In addition, they organize immunization outreach activities in the community; provide answers to parents' questions and concerns about immunization; and educate parents about why immunizations are needed, inappropriate contraindications to immunization, and the importance of completing the immunization schedule on time.

Routine Childhood Immunization Schedule

The 2010 recommended immunization schedule for children and adolescents in the United States includes routine immunization against the following 16 diseases: hepatitis B, diphtheria, pertussis, tetanus, measles, mumps, rubella, polio, *Haemophilus influenzae* type B meningitis, *Varicella* (chickenpox), *Streptococcus pneumoniae*–related illnesses, rotavirus, hepatitis A, influenza, HPV, and meningococcal disease (CDC, 2010c). The vaccine schedule is a rather complex and frequently changing document that makes continuing adjustments for the latest research and recommendations and is issued annually by the Advisory Committee on Immunization Practices (ACIP). More recent additions to the schedule include hepatitis A, rotavirus, seasonal influenza for all children ages 6 months through 18 years, and Tdap (the tetanus, reduced-strength diphtheria, and acellular pertussis vaccine licensed for older children, adolescents, and adults). Because many of these vaccines require three to four doses, the schedule begins at birth with succeeding staggered vaccinations designed to achieve recommended immunization levels by 2 years of age. Additional doses may be required before a child enters school and at adolescence or on entering college. The ACIP, the American Academy of Pediatrics and the American Academy of Family Physicians regularly update recommended immunization schedules. The ACIP also issues a recommended adult immunization schedule for those over 18 years old, by age group and immune status. The 2010 schedule includes, as appropriate, HPV, varicella, measles, mumps and rubella, pneumococcus, and zoster to prevent shingles and tetanus every 10 years with one dose given as Tdap. Other immunizations available in special circumstances include, but are not limited to, rabies, yellow fever, typhoid, smallpox, and anthrax. Recommended vaccine schedules may be viewed at http://www.cdc.gov/vaccines/recs/schedules/default.htm.

Measles

Measles is an acute, highly contagious disease that, although considered a childhood illness, may be seen in the United States in adolescents and young adults. Symptoms include fever, sneezing and coughing, conjunctivitis, small white spots on the inside of the cheek (Koplik's spots) and a red, blotchy rash beginning several days after the respiratory signs. Measles is caused by the rubeola virus and is transmitted by inhalation of infected aerosol droplets or by direct contact with infected nasal or throat secretions or with articles freshly contaminated with the same nasal or throat secretions. A very contagious nature, combined with the fact that people are most contagious before they are aware they are infected, makes measles a disease that can spread rapidly through the population. Infection with measles confers lifelong immunity (Heymann, 2008).

Measles and malnutrition form a deadly combination for many children in the developing world. Despite the introduction in 1963 of a live attenuated measles vaccine that is safe, effective, and widely available, measles is still endemic in many countries. The WHO estimates as many as 17 million measles cases and 242,000 deaths occurred in 2006, 80% of them in Southeast Asia and Africa and 85% in children under the age of 5. Much of this mortality is preventable by immunizing all infants (Heymann, 2008).

Immunization has dramatically decreased measles cases in the United States to the point that, in March 2000, a panel of experts declared measles no longer endemic in the United States. Before introduction of the vaccine in 1963, 200,000 to 500,000 cases of measles were reported yearly, but by 1983 reported cases had fallen to an all-time low of less than 1500. In the late 1980s, the incidence of measles began to climb again, with more than 55,000 cases reported between 1989 and 1991. This increase resulted from low immunization rates among preschool children and was countered with efforts to increase immunization rates and the routine use of two doses of measles vaccine for all children. Except for outbreaks in 1994 that occurred predominantly among high school and college-age persons, many of whom had not received two doses of measles vaccine, reported measles cases dropped continuously from 1991 to 2004 when only 37 confirmed cases were reported to the CDC—the lowest number since measles became a nationally reportable disease in 1912.

However, in 2005 case numbers began to slowly climb again until in the summer of 2008 the United States reported the greatest number of measles cases for that same time period since 1996. Of the 131 measles cases reported during the first 7 months of 2008, 89% were imported from or associated with importations from other countries, where outbreaks were ongoing. Of the 131 cases, 123 were U.S. residents; of these 123, 112 (91%) were not vaccinated or had an unknown vaccination status, 95 (85%) were eligible for vaccination, and 63 (66%) were not vaccinated because of religious or philosophical beliefs. These recent outbreaks in the United States highlight the ongoing risk of measles importation from other countries by people who travel. With first-dose vaccine coverage of preschool children at greater than 90% and schools in 49 states requiring two doses of vaccine, the pattern of infection has shifted from underimmunization of infants and school-age children to disease acquired from other countries. Because imported cases had not previously resulted in large outbreaks, it appeared that vaccination efforts had been successful in increasing herd immunity against measles, but groups who remained at greatest risk for infection were those who do not routinely accept immunization, such as people with religious or philosophical objections, students in schools that do not require two doses of vaccine, and infants in areas where immunization coverage is low. The exposure of these groups to an imported case could result in a major outbreak and, indeed, in the 2008 outbreaks, the increase was not the result of a greater number of imported cases but of greater viral transmission after importation into the United States, leading to a larger number of importation-associated cases. These importation-associated cases occurred largely among school-aged children who were eligible for vaccination but whose parents chose not to have them vaccinated. States vary in the ease of obtaining philosophical exemptions

and vaccination requirements for home-schooled children. The increase in importation-associated cases may result in an increase in measles morbidity, especially in communities with many unvaccinated residents (CDC, 2008b).

Healthy People 2020 calls for the sustained elimination of indigenous cases of vaccine-preventable disease. Efforts to meet this goal will require: (1) rapid detection of cases and implementation of appropriate outbreak control measures, (2) achievement and maintenance of high levels of vaccination coverage among preschool-age children in all geographic regions, (3) continued implementation and enforcement of the two-dose schedule among young adults, (4) the determination of the source of all outbreaks and sporadic infections, and (5) cooperation among countries in measles control efforts. Nurses receive reports of cases, investigate them, and initiate control measures for outbreaks. They use every opportunity to immunize adolescents and young adults who lack documentation of two doses of measles vaccine. Nurses who work in regions where undocumented residents are common, where groups obtain exemption from immunization on religious grounds or who choose not to vaccinate for philosophical reasons, where preschool coverage is low and/or where international visitors are frequent need to be especially alert for measles cases and the necessity of prompt outbreak control among particularly susceptible populations.

Rubella

The rubella (German measles) virus causes a mild febrile disease with enlarged lymph nodes and a fine, pink rash that is often difficult to distinguish from measles or scarlet fever. In contrast to measles, rubella is only a moderately contagious illness. Transmission is through inhalation of or direct contact with infected droplets from the respiratory secretions of infected persons. Children may show few or no constitutional symptoms, whereas adults usually experience several days of low-grade fever, headache, malaise, runny nose, and conjunctivitis before the rash appears. Many infections occur without a rash (Heymann, 2008).

For many years, because it caused only a mild illness, rubella was considered to be of minor importance. Then, in 1941 the link between maternal rubella and poor pregnancy outcomes was recognized and the disease suddenly assumed major public health significance. Rubella infection, in addition to causing intrauterine death and spontaneous abortion, may result in anomalies referred to as congenital rubella syndrome (CRS), affecting single or multiple organ systems. Defects include cataracts, congenital glaucoma, deafness, microcephaly, mental retardation, cardiac abnormalities, and diabetes mellitus. CRS occurs in up to 90% of infants born to women who are infected with rubella during the first trimester of pregnancy (Heymann, 2008). During the 1962 to 1965 rubella pandemic, an estimated 12.5 million cases of rubella occurred in the United States, resulting in 2000 cases of encephalitis, 11,250 fetal deaths, 2100 neonatal deaths, and 20,000 infants born with CRS. The economic impact of this epidemic was estimated at $1.5 billion (CDC, 2005b).

Since the introduction of a vaccine in 1969, cases of rubella in the United States have fallen precipitously from 57,686 to less than 25 per year since 2001. By the beginning of 2005, at the 39th National Immunization Conference, the director of the CDC announced that rubella was no longer endemic in the United States based on fewer than 10 cases a year reported in 2003 and 2004 and, as in measles, a large percentage of the cases were imported or import linked. From 2001 to 2004, four cases of CRS were reported; the mothers of three were born outside the United States. In 2007, 12 cases of rubella and no cases of CRS were reported (CDC, 2009c). Rubella remains endemic in parts of the world; in 2008 WHO estimated 110,000 cases of CRS worldwide, many of them in Asia and Africa. In 2008, WHO also reported 123 countries, or about two thirds of countries, regularly using rubella in their national immunization programs, with the highest coverage in the Americas and Western Europe. Unimmunized immigrants do not necessarily import disease, but their unimmunized status may leave them vulnerable to infection once they arrive. In addition to a focus on identifying and vaccinating foreign-born adults, the continued elimination of rubella and CRS in the United States will require: (1) maintaining high immunization rates among children, (2) ensuring vaccination among women of child-bearing age, especially those who are foreign-born, (3) continuing aggressive surveillance, and (4) responding rapidly to any outbreak.

Pertussis

Pertussis (whooping cough) begins as a mild upper respiratory tract infection progressing to an irritating cough that within 1 to 2 weeks may become paroxysmal (a series of repeated violent coughs). The repeated coughs occur without intervening breaths and can be followed by a characteristic inspiratory "whoop." Pertussis is caused by the bacterium *Bordetella pertussis* and is transmitted via an airborne route through contact with infected droplets. It is highly contagious and considered endemic in the United States. Vaccination against pertussis, delivered in combination with diphtheria and tetanus, is a part of the routine childhood immunization schedule. Treatment of infected individuals with antibiotics such as erythromycin may shorten the period of communicability but does not relieve symptoms unless given early in the course of the infection. Prophylactic treatment with antibiotics is recommended for family members and close contacts of infected individuals, regardless of immunization status and age, if there is a child in the house under the age of 1 year or a woman in the last 3 weeks of pregnancy or to prevent ongoing transmission within the family (Heymann, 2008).

Before the development of a whole-cell vaccine in the 1940s, pertussis led to hundreds of thousands of cases and thousands of deaths per year, the majority in children younger than 5 years. After vaccine licensure and the introduction of universal vaccination, reported cases in the United States steadily declined, hitting a record low of just over 1000 in 1976. However, beginning in the early 1980s, pertussis cases began to show cyclical increases every 3 to 4 years until in 2004 over 25,800 cases were reported, the highest number since 1959.

Pertussis in very young children, especially those younger than 6 months, is attributed to being too young to have received the first three of the five doses of vaccine recommended by 6 years of age. Cases in older children also result largely from inadequate or underimmunization. In adolescents and adults with histories of complete immunization, cases are thought to be the result of waning immunity. Although natural infection with pertussis results in permanent immunity, immunization through vaccination does not, and the DTaP (diphtheria, tetanus, acellular pertussis) vaccine was not licensed for use in children 7 years of age and older. In 2005, two Tdap (tetanus and reduced strength diphtheria and acellular pertussis) vaccines were licensed for the use in adults and adolescents in the United States, for the first time providing an option for boosting waning immunity in this group. Preteens are given Tdap at the age of 11 or 12 years, and adults who have never received Tdap get one dose in place of their next Td tetanus booster (CDC, 2009c).

After peaking during 2004 to 2005 at 8.9 cases per 100,000 population, the incidence of reported cases of pertussis began to decline, reaching a rate of 3.62 cases per 100,000 population in 2007. However, infants aged less than 6 months and too young to be fully vaccinated continued to show the highest reported rates of pertussis (69.9 cases per 100,000 population) while adolescents and adults contributed the greatest number of cases. Some of the continued rise in adolescents and adult cases may be attributed to increased awareness and improved reporting, but the steadiness of decline in rates of fully vaccinated younger age groups may suggest an increased pertussis circulation. Coverage with Tdap in adolescents aged 13 to 17 years increased in 2006 and 2007 from 10.8% to 30.4%; whether that increased coverage affected disease rates is not clear. Prevention efforts continue to be directed at maintaining high rates of immunization, publicizing Tdap, increasing awareness of pertussis in adolescents and adults among providers, and promptly implementing treatment and control in the face of outbreaks (CDC, 2009c).

Since pertussis does have a cyclical pattern (there are periodic outbreaks such as the California outbreak in 2010), it is important for nurses to work with the community to maintain the highest possible levels of immunization coverage to minimize these occurrences. Because of the contagious nature of pertussis, nurses play a major role in limiting transmission during outbreaks by ensuring appropriate treatment of family members and close contacts.

Influenza

Influenza is a viral respiratory tract infection often indistinguishable from the common cold or other respiratory diseases. Transmission is airborne and through direct contact with infected droplets. Unlike many viruses that do not survive long in the environment, the flu virus is thought to exist for many hours in dried mucus. Outbreaks are common in the winter and early spring in areas where people gather indoors such as in schools and nursing homes. Gastrointestinal and respiratory symptoms are common. Because symptoms do not always follow a characteristic pattern, many viral diseases that are not influenza are often called flu. The most important factors to note about influenza are its epidemic nature and the mortality that may result from pulmonary complications, especially in older adults and children less than 2 years of age (Heymann, 2008).

There are three types of influenza viruses: A, B, and C. Type A is usually responsible for large epidemics, whereas outbreaks from type B are more regionalized; type C epidemics are sporadic, less common, and usually result in only mild illness. Influenza viruses often change in the nature of their surface appearance or their antigenic makeup. Types B and C are fairly stable viruses, but type A changes constantly. Minor antigenic changes are referred to as antigenic drift, and they result in yearly epidemics and regional outbreaks. Major changes such as the emergence of new subtypes are called antigenic shift; these occur only with type A viruses. Antigenic shift and drift lead to epidemic outbreaks every few years and pandemic outbreaks every 10 to 40 years as seen with novel influenza A H1N1 in 2009. Mortality rates associated with epidemics may or may not be higher than those in non-epidemic situations.

The preparation of influenza vaccine each year is based on the best possible prediction of what type and variant of virus will be most prevalent that year. Because of the changing nature of the virus, yearly immunization is necessary and in the United States is given in early fall before the flu season begins. In recent history, if vaccine were available, immunization for seasonal flu was particularly recommended for children ages 6 months up to 19 years, pregnant women, people 50 years of age and older, people of any age with certain chronic medical conditions, people who live in nursing homes and other long-term care facilities, and people who live with or care for those at risk for complications from flu. During the 2009-2010 influenza season, pandemic novel influenza A H1N1 replaced other seasonal flu viruses as the predominantly circulating virus, and the recommended priority groups shifted from seniors to the young; high school students and pregnant women seemed particularly hard hit, whereas those over 65 appeared to perhaps have some degree of protection. For the 2010-2011 flu season, the vaccine contained novel influenza A H1N1 and the ACIP recommended universal coverage for everyone ages 6 months and older (CDC, 2010d).

Flu shots, when matched appropriately with circulating virus strains, are estimated to provide 70% to 90% protection against infection in healthy young adults; although they do not always prevent infection, they do result in milder disease symptoms. Because of small quantities of egg protein found in the vaccine, individuals with egg sensitivity should consult with their physician in determining if immunization should be administered. Although influenza is often self limiting in the healthy population, serious complications, particularly viral and bacterial pneumonias, can be deadly to older adults, children under 2 years of age, and those debilitated by chronic disease. When appropriate, it is important to couple influenza immunization of this population with immunization against pneumococcal pneumonia (Heymann, 2008).

The use of influenza antiviral drugs should be considered in the non-immunized or groups at high risk of complications. The neuraminidase inhibitors (oseltamivir, zanamivir) have activity against influenza A and B viruses, whereas the adamantanes (amantadine, rimantadine) have activity only against influenza A viruses. Since January 2006, the neuraminidase inhibitors have been the only recommended influenza antiviral drugs because of widespread resistance to the adamantanes among influenza A (H3N2) virus strains. There have been incidences, worldwide and in the United States, of H1N1 virus resistance to oseltamivir. Current guidelines indicate antiviral treatment should be guided by surveillance data on circulating viruses and confirmatory testing of viral subgroups (CDC, 2008c).

Healthy People 2020 targets increasing the proportion of the population vaccinated annually against influenza and pneumococcal disease. Nurses often spearhead influenza immunization campaigns that target older adults. Examples include conducting flu clinics at polling places during elections or at community centers and churches during "senior vaccination Sundays." Inhabitants of residences and nursing homes for older adults are at risk, since influenza can spread rapidly with severe consequences through such living arrangements. As with children, nurses should check immunization history and encourage immunization for every older adult encountered in a clinic or home visit.

Pandemic Novel Influenza A (H1N1)

Novel influenza A H1N1, a new flu virus that quickly reached pandemic proportions, was first recognized in Mexico and the United States in the spring of 2009. Originally called swine flu, the virus is of swine origins but does not spread from swine to people. Instead, it is transmitted rapidly and easily from person to person and in some cases is suspected to have spread from humans to swine as well as other animals such as dogs, cats and ferrets. Because the virus was new, the population lacked immunity and visitors to Mexico quickly became infected and carried it to people around the globe. By June of 2009 more than 70 countries had reported cases of novel H1N1 infection, and ongoing community level outbreaks of novel H1N1 occurred in multiple parts of the world, prompting the WHO to declare a global pandemic. This action was a reflection of the spread of the new H1N1 virus, not the severity of illness caused by the virus.

Although novel H1N1 appeared to spread in the same manner as seasonal influenza viruses, the groups most affected were children, young adults (especially those with underlying chronic disease), and pregnant women, as opposed to seniors who are the usual targets of seasonal flu but were thought in this case to perhaps have some degree of immunity. Initial reports made it appear that the virus inflicted a high case fatality rate, but as surveillance strengthened and expanded, this did not prove to be the case; however, by the end of the year, pediatric deaths were higher than in previous years and pediatric hospitalizations higher than other age groups. The majority of 2009 novel H1N1 deaths occurred in people between the ages of 50 and 64 years of age, 80% of whom have had an underlying health condition (CDC, 2010e).

With the identification of the virus, the scramble was on for a vaccine, which became available in the fall of 2009 in limited doses and was initially targeted to priority groups, including those 6 months to 24 years of age, caretakers, infants less than 6 months of age, pregnant women, adults 25 to 64 years of age with chronic conditions, health care providers and first responders. Initial demand for vaccine was high, but since the virus did not appear to prove overall any more frightening than seasonal flu and more vaccine came on the market, the available supply was more than enough for anyone who wished to be immunized. The delivery of the vaccine, in addition to seasonal flu vaccine, proved a planning and logistical challenge to the public health system, demanded considerable resources and provided a valuable exercise in implementation of preparedness strategies. Nurses were at the forefront of this expansive operation by planning for, scheduling, and immunizing—in a variety of community settings, schools, and clinics—a large portion of the population, including two doses to children. During the summer of 2009, novel H1N1 outbreaks extended the normal flu season far beyond the usual period and dominated reported circulating flu viruses from the Southern Hemisphere as well. Activity peaked at the end of October in the United States, but novel H1N1 continued into 2010 as the dominant circulating strain. Resistance to antiviral neuraminidase inhibitors was reported but remained low, and the vast majority of 2009 H1N1 viruses tested did not appear to change significantly, remaining related to the A/California/7/2009 H1N1 reference virus selected by WHO as the 2009 H1N1 vaccine virus. An H1N1 component was included in the 2010 seasonal vaccine (CDC, 2010e). (To learn more about novel influenza A H1N1, consult the CDC website at: http://www.cdc.gov/h1n1flu/.)

Avian Influenza A (H5N1)

In 1997 in Hong Kong, the first known cases of human illness associated with an avian influenza type A virus H5N1 were reported. Referred to in the press as Hong Kong bird flu, this virus appeared to have been transmitted to people through contact with infected poultry. As a result of this association, Hong Kong officials ordered the slaughter of all chickens in and around Hong Kong with a resulting halt in the spread of disease. No cases were reported outside Hong Kong and, despite recurring outbreaks of avian flu in poultry, no further H5N1 virus activity in humans was reported (CDC, 1998b). This situation changed dramatically in late 2003 and early 2004 when H5N1 outbreaks occurred among poultry, people, and, in some cases, other animals in nine Asian countries. And unlike the earlier situation in Hong Kong, these outbreaks have not disappeared but only subsided to again reappear. Human infections with H5N1 have been reported from Thailand, Vietnam, Cambodia, Indonesia, China, and Egypt with some fatality rates as high as 70%. An unanswered question is whether there are actually many more human cases than are identified because they are not exhibiting symptoms severe enough to cause recognition. Most of the reported cases have resulted from contact with infected poultry, but it is believed that a few cases of human-to-human transmission have occurred. So far, the documented spread from human to human has been rare and not sustained, but because influenza viruses have the ability to change, concern exists among scientists that H5N1 may modify to the point where people could easily infect each other; also, because H5N1 does not usually infect humans, they would have little immune protection. Such a change could give rise to pandemic influenza with a virus that appears to exact a high toll in human lives. Given this possibility, surveillance becomes of utmost importance and close attention is being paid to H5N1 virus activity among poultry and humans in Asia, Europe, and North Africa. Vaccine development efforts are underway and, although licensed in some countries, are not yet generally available (Heyman, 2008). Additional information and regular updates on avian influenza may be found at the CDC website (http://www.cdc.gov/flu/avian/gen-info) and the WHO website (http://www.who.int/csr/disease/en/).

FOODBORNE AND WATERBORNE DISEASES

In recent years the headlines have been full of stories related to foodborne illness associated with peanut butter, cookie dough, spinach, lettuce, tomatoes, chili peppers, strawberries, raspberries, oysters, uncooked eggs, poultry and hamburger, raw milk, unpasteurized apple cider, and so forth. Cans of beef stew suspected to be contaminated with botulism have been pulled off grocery store shelves and the term *mad cow disease* has entered the popular vocabulary. Recalls of food products have become a common occurrence. Highly centralized food production and processing systems that use food produced in far-reaching areas and distribute it through widespread distribution networks increase the potential for any contamination to result in large-scale, multistate outbreaks. One incident of contamination may affect hundreds of people across the country and result in numerous deaths. Anyone can acquire foodborne illness, regardless of socioeconomic status, race, sex, age, occupation, education or area of residence, but the very young, old, and debilitated are most susceptible and bear the highest burden of morbidity and mortality.

The CDC estimates that in the United States, as many as 76 million illnesses, 325,000 hospitalizations, and 5000 deaths occur from foodborne illnesses each year, most the result of unidentified agents (CDC, 2009e). Of the estimated 14 million illnesses in which a pathogen is identified, *Salmonella* and *Campylobacter* are most frequently implicated. About three fourths of deaths with identified agents are linked to *Salmonella, Listeria,* and *Toxoplasma* (Mead et al, 1999). Because their presentations are often not clinically distinctive and frequently self-limiting, single cases of foodborne illness may be difficult to identify. Affected individuals in single cases or in outbreak situations may not see a physician or are treated presumptively and not tested. In either case, the illness goes unreported, resulting in statistics that underestimate the true magnitude of the problem. Some public health experts believe foodborne disease may be one of the most common causes of acute illness (Heymann, 2008).

FoodNet is a CDC sentinel surveillance system targeting 10 sites across the country and collecting information from laboratories on disease caused by enteric pathogens transmitted commonly through food. It is a collaborative effort among CDC, the U.S. Department of Agriculture (USDA), and the FDA. In 2008 FoodNet reported 18,499 laboratory-diagnosed cases of infection, the majority caused by *Salmonella, Campylobacter,* and *Shigella* (CDC, 2009f).

Confirmed foodborne outbreaks are reported by states to the CDC through the Foodborne Disease Outbreak Surveillance

System; on average, 1300 outbreaks have been reported every year since 1998. In 2007, 48 states reported 1097 outbreaks. A food source was identified in less than half; of these 470 outbreaks, 50%, which were responsible for 4119 illnesses, were determined to originate from only one ingredient. Among the 235 outbreaks attributed to a single food, the most outbreaks were attributed to fish (41 outbreaks), poultry (40 outbreaks) and beef (33 outbreaks) and the most cases were attributed to poultry (691 cases), beef (667 cases) and leafy vegetables (590 cases). Of organisms paired with food sources, norovirus in leafy vegetables (315 cases), *E. coli 0157:H7* in beef (298 cases) and *Clostridium perfringens* in poultry (281 cases) were responsible for the most illnesses 2007.

The ability to identify multistate outbreaks has been greatly enhanced through technology now routinely used in public health laboratories (serotyping and pulsed-field gel electrophoresis) and the rapid sharing of this information among public health officials through PulseNet, the national molecular subtyping network for foodborne disease surveillance. In 2006, 11 multistate outbreaks were detected. These included 715 people sickened from eating *Salmonella* contaminated peanut butter, 307 from *Salmonella* in tomatoes, 359 cases attributed to *E. coli* in leafy vegetables, and 177 reported illnesses from *Vibrio parahaemolyticus* in oysters (CDC, 2009g).

A 2009 CDC report suggests that although significant declines occurred prior to 2004, progress has since slowed, making it unlikely that *Healthy People 2010* objectives for four food pathogens would be met and that this lack of progress coupled with the large multistate outbreaks seen in 2006 points to: (1) gaps in the current food safety system, and (2) the need to continue to develop and evaluate food safety practices. The report recommends three goals: (1) control or eliminate pathogens in domestic and imported food, (2) reduce or prevent contamination during growing, harvesting, and processing, and (3) continue the education of restaurant workers and consumers about risks and prevention measures. Also noted is the need for continued efforts to understand how contamination of fresh produce and processed foods occurs and to develop and implement measures that reduce it (CDC, 2009f).

Foodborne illness, or "food poisoning," as it is erroneously but commonly called, is often categorized as either food infection or food intoxication. Food infection results from bacterial, viral, or parasitic infection of food by pathogens such as *Salmonella, Campylobacter,* hepatitis A, *Toxoplasma,* and *Trichinella.* Food intoxication is caused by toxins produced by bacterial growth, chemical contaminants (heavy metals), and a variety of disease-producing substances found naturally in certain foods such as mushrooms and some seafood. Examples of food intoxications are botulism, mercury poisoning, and paralytic shellfish poisoning. Table 13-4 presents some of the most common agents of food intoxication and their incubation period, source, symptoms, and pathology. Although it is not a hard-and-fast rule, food infections are associated with incubation periods of 12 hours to several days after ingestion of the infected food, whereas intoxications become obvious within minutes to hours after ingestion. Botulism is a clear exception to this rule, with an incubation period up to several days or more in adults. Possessing a potent preformed toxin, capable of producing severe intoxication resulting in flaccid paralysis and death if not identified and treated early, *C. botulinum* is one of the organisms

TABLE 13-4 COMMONLY ENCOUNTERED FOOD INTOXICATIONS

CAUSAL AGENT	INCUBATION PERIOD	DURATION	CLINICAL PRESENTATION	ASSOCIATED FOOD
Staphylococcus aureus	30 min to 7 hr	1-2 days	Sudden onset of nausea, cramps, vomiting, and prostration, often accompanied by diarrhea; rarely fatal	All foods, especially those likely to come into contact with food-handlers' hands that may be contaminated from infections of the eyes and skin
Clostridium perfringens (strain A)	6-24 hr	1 day or less	Sudden onset of colic and diarrhea, maybe nausea; vomiting and fever unusual; rarely fatal	Inadequately heated meats or stews; food contaminated by soil or feces becomes infective when improper storage or reheating allows multiplication of organism
Vibrio parahaemolyticus	4-96 hr	1-7 days	Watery diarrhea and abdominal cramps; sometimes nausea, vomiting, fever, headache; rarely fatal	Raw or inadequately cooked seafood; period of time at room temperature usually required for multiplication of organism
Clostridium botulinum	12-36 hr, sometimes days	Slow recovery, maybe months	Central nervous system signs; blurred vision, difficulty in swallowing and dry mouth, followed by descending symmetrical flaccid paralysis in an alert person; "floppy baby" in infant; fatality <15% with antitoxin and respiratory support	Home-canned fruits and vegetables that have not been preserved with adequate heating; infants have become infected from ingesting honey

Based on information from Heymann DL, editor: *Control of communicable diseases manual,* ed 19, Washington, DC, 2008, American Public Health Association.

considered a strong candidate for a weapon of bioterrorism (Heymann, 2008).

The Role of Safe Food Preparation

Protecting the nation's food supply from contamination by virulent microbes is a multifaceted issue that is and will continue to be incredibly costly, controversial, and time consuming to address. The specter of terrorist threats to the food supply adds an additional layer of complexity. However, much foodborne illness, regardless of causal organism, can easily be prevented through simple changes in food preparation, handling, and storage. Common errors include: (1) cross-contamination of food during preparation, (2) insufficient cooking or reheating temperatures, (3) holding cooked food or storing food at temperatures that promote growth of pathogens and/or formation of toxins, and (4) poor personal hygiene. Because these measures are so important in preventing foodborne disease, *Healthy People 2020* has continued to include an objective directed toward them. WHO estimates that 2.2 million people, 1.9 million of them children, die annually from foodborne and waterborne diarrheal diseases in less-developed countries. Food safety—together with nutrition and food security—is one of WHO's 13 strategic objectives for 2008 to 2013. In 2001 WHO released a new campaign entitled *Five Keys to Safer Food*, which reduces the former *Ten Golden Rules for Food Preparation* developed in the early 1990s to five even simpler and easier to remember principles (presented in Box 13-4). A poster explaining the *Five Keys* is available in 25 languages and is accompanied by a training manual titled *Bring Food Safety Home* (Heymann, 2008). (Read more about the Five Keys at the WHO website: http://www.who.int/foodsafety/consumer/5keys/en/index.html.)

Salmonellosis

Salmonellosis is a bacterial disease characterized by sudden onset of headache, abdominal pain, diarrhea, nausea, sometimes vomiting, and almost always fever. Onset is typically within 48 hours of ingestion, but the clinical signs are impossible to distinguish from other causes of gastrointestinal distress. Diarrhea and lack of appetite may persist for several days, and dehydration may be severe. Although morbidity can be significant, death is uncommon except among infants, older adults, and the debilitated. The rate of infection is highest among infants and

---

> **BOX 13-4** **WHO FIVE KEYS TO SAFER FOOD**
>
> 1. Keep food clean.
> 2. Separate raw and cooked food.
> 3. Cook thoroughly.
> 4. Keep food at safe temperatures.
> 5. Use safe water and raw materials.
>
> From the World Health Organization: *Five Keys to Safer Food* campaign, 2009b, WHO. Available at http://www.who.int/foodsafety/consumer/5keys/en. Accessed March 25, 2010; Heymann DL, editor: *Control of communicable diseases manual*, ed 19, Washington, DC, 2008, American Public Health Association.

---

small children. It is estimated that only a small proportion of cases are recognized clinically and that only 1% of clinical cases are reported. The number of *Salmonella* infections yearly may actually be in the millions (Heymann, 2008).

> **THE CUTTING EDGE** *DNA "fingerprinting" allows the identification of once unrecognized foodborne illness outbreaks by linking cases across the country.*

Outbreaks occur commonly in restaurants, hospitals, nursing homes, and institutions for children. The transmission route is eating food derived from an infected animal or contaminated by feces of an infected animal or person. Unchlorinated municipal water supplies have also been implicated in *Salmonella* outbreaks. Raw or undercooked meat and meat products; raw or undercooked poultry; uncooked eggs; unpasteurized milk and dairy products; and contaminated produce are the foods most often associated with salmonellosis. Recent large outbreaks have been linked with eating tomatoes, jalapeño peppers, and peanut butter. Meat and poultry may be contaminated during preparation or cross-contaminate food being prepared with them. Improper food preparation temperatures (cooking and holding) and cross-contamination appear to be the biggest risk factors for food-associated outbreaks. Animals are the common reservoir for the various *Salmonella* serotypes, although infected humans may also fill this role. Animals are more likely to be chronic carriers. Reptiles such as iguanas have been implicated as *Salmonella* carriers along with pet turtles, poultry, cattle, swine, rodents, dogs, and cats. People have also been infected by handling *Salmonella*-contaminated dry dog food and treats. Person-to-person transmission is an important consideration in daycare and institutional settings (Heymann, 2008).

Enterohemorrhagic *Escherichia coli* (EHEC or *E. coli* 0157:H7)

Escherichia coli 0157:H7 belongs to the enterohemorrhagic category of *E. coli* serotypes producing a strong cytotoxin called a Shiga toxin and are collectively known as Shiga toxin–producing *E. coli* (STEC). *E. coli* serotypes in this group can cause a potentially fatal hemorrhagic colitis. This pathogen was first widely described in humans in 1992 following the investigation of two outbreaks of illness associated with consumption of hamburger from a fast-food restaurant chain. Transmission is through ingestion of food contaminated by infected feces. Ruminants, particularly cattle, are the most important reservoir, although humans may also serve as a source for person-to-person transmission. Undercooked hamburger has been implicated in several outbreaks, as have roast beef, alfalfa sprouts, melons, lettuce, uncooked spinach, unpasteurized milk and apple cider, municipal water, and person-to-person transmission in daycare centers, homes, and institutions. Recent large outbreaks have been associated with uncooked spinach and petting zoos. Infection with *E. coli* 0157:H7 causes bloody diarrhea, abdominal cramps, and, infrequently, fever. Children and older adults are at highest risk for clinical disease and complications. Hemolytic uremic syndrome (HUS) is seen in approximately 15% of cases among children and a smaller number of adults and may result in acute renal failure. The case fatality rate for infection that results in HUS can be as great as 5% (Heymann, 2008).

Hamburger often appears to be involved in outbreaks because the grinding process exposes pathogens on the surface of the whole meat to the interior of the ground meat, effectively mixing the once-exterior bacteria thoroughly throughout the hamburger so that searing the surface no longer suffices to kill all bacteria. Tracking the contamination is complicated by the fact that hamburger is often made of meat ground from several sources. The best protection against this pathogen, as with most foodborne agents, is to thoroughly cook food before eating it.

Waterborne Disease Outbreaks and Pathogens

Waterborne pathogens usually enter water supplies through animal or human fecal contamination and frequently cause enteric disease. They include viruses, bacteria, and protozoans. Hepatitis A virus is probably the most publicized waterborne viral agent, although other viruses may also be transmitted by this route (enteroviruses, rotaviruses, and paramyxoviruses). The most important waterborne bacterial diseases are cholera, typhoid fever, and bacillary dysentery. However, other *Salmonella* spp. as well as *Shigella*, *Vibrio*, and *Campylobacter* species and various coliform bacteria including *E. coli* 0157:H7 may be transmitted in the same manner. Recently, since added to surveillance in 2001, *Legionella* spp. have frequently been implicated in waterborne disease outbreaks (WBDOs) in the United States. In the past, the most important waterborne protozoans have been *Entamoeba histolytica* (amebic dysentery) and *Giardia lamblia*, but major outbreaks of cryptosporidiosis in municipal water, as seen in the diarrheal outbreak that crippled the city of Milwaukee in 1993, have pushed *Cryptosporidium* into the debate over how to best safeguard municipal water supplies. Protozoans do not respond to traditional chlorine treatment as do enteric and coliform bacteria, and their small size requires special filtration.

The CDC defines a WBDO as an incident in which two or more persons experience similar illness after consuming water that epidemiological evidence implicates as the source of that illness. Recreational water and other water not intended for drinking as well as drinking water may be involved in waterborne outbreaks. Facilities with inadequate chlorination and pools allowing diapered children pose particular risk for infection, as does drinking water without adequate disinfection while hiking and camping in the backcountry.

Since 1971, the CDC, the U.S. Environmental Protection Agency (EPA), and the Council of State and Territorial Epidemiologists have maintained a collaborative Waterborne Disease and Outbreaks Surveillance System for collecting and reporting data related to occurrences and causes of waterborne disease and outbreaks. This surveillance system is the primary source of data concerning the scope and effects of WBDOs in the United States. The CDC and the EPA, to improve timeliness and completeness of reporting, are collaborating with public health jurisdictions to implement electronic reporting through the National Outbreak Reporting System (NORS) (CDC, 2008d).

VECTOR-BORNE DISEASES

Vector-borne diseases refer to illnesses for which the infectious agent is transmitted by a carrier, or vector, which is usually an arthropod (mosquito, tick, fly), either biologically or mechanically. With biological transmission, the vector is necessary for the developmental stage of the infectious agent. Examples include the mosquitoes that carry WNV and the fleas that transmit plague. Mechanical transmission occurs when an insect simply contacts the infectious agent with its legs or mouth parts and carries it to the host. For example, flies and cockroaches may contaminate food or cooking utensils. Most vector-borne diseases involve zoonotic cycles requiring some sort of animal host or reservoir.

Vector-borne diseases commonly encountered in the United States are those associated with ticks, such as Lyme disease *(Borrelia burgdorferi)*, Rocky Mountain spotted fever *(Rickettsia rickettsii)*, ehrlichiosis *(Ehrlichia)*, and anaplasmosis *(Anaplasma phagocytophilum)*, formerly known as human granulocytic ehrlichiosis. Nurses who work with large immigrant populations or with international travelers may encounter malaria and dengue fever, both carried by mosquitoes. More recently in the news, WNV is an example of endemic mosquito-borne viruses that include St. Louis, LaCrosse, and western and eastern equine encephalitis. Plague *(Y. pestis)* is carried by fleas of wild rodents. Other more rarely seen tick-associated diseases include babesiosis *(Babesia microti)*, tularemia *(F. tularensis)*, and Q fever *(Coxiella burnetii)*. Southern tick-associated rash illness (STARI) is a newly described illness for which the causative organism has not been determined. STARI resembles Lyme disease in appearance but does not result in the neurological, arthritic, and other chronic conditions seen with Lyme disease. It is mainly found in the southeast and is associated with the bite of the Lonestar tick *(Amblyomma americanum)* (CDC, 2009k) and ticks (CDC, 2011).

Lyme Disease

Parents in Lyme, CT, concerned about the unusual incidence of juvenile rheumatoid arthritis in their children, were the first to bring attention to this tick-borne infection that now bears their town's name. First described in 1975, Lyme disease became a nationally notifiable disease in 1991 and is now the most common vector-borne disease in the United States, with over 36,000 confirmed cases and probable cases reported to CDC in 2008 (CDC, 2010f). The causative agent, the spirochete *B. burgdorferi*, was identified in 1982. Lyme disease is transmitted by ixodid ticks that are associated with white-tailed deer *(Odocoileus virginianus)* and the white-footed mouse *(Peromyscus leucopus)*. Lyme disease usually occurs in summer during tick season and it has been reported throughout the United States, with 95% of cases concentrated in rural and suburban areas of the northeast, mid-Atlantic and north-central states, particularly Wisconsin and Minnesota.

The clinical spectrum of Lyme disease can be divided into three stages. Stage I is characterized by erythema chronicum migrans, a distinctive skin lesion often called a bull's-eye lesion because it begins as a red area at the site of the tick attachment that spreads outward in a ring-like fashion as the center clears.

About 50% to 70% of infected persons develop this lesion 3 to 30 days after a tick bite. The skin lesion may be accompanied or preceded by fever, fatigue, malaise, headache, muscle pains, and a stiff neck, as well as tender and enlarged lymph nodes and migratory joint pain. Most clients diagnosed in this early stage respond well to 10 to 14 days of oral tetracycline or penicillin.

If not treated during this first stage, Lyme disease can progress to stage II, which may include additional skin lesions, headache, and neurological and cardiac abnormalities. Clients who progress to stage III have recurrent attacks of arthritis and arthralgia, especially in the knees, which may begin months to years after the initial lesion. The clinical diagnosis of classic Lyme disease with the distinctive skin lesion is straightforward. Illness without the lesion is more difficult to diagnose, because serologic tests are more accurate in stages II and III than in stage I (Heymann, 2008).

Rocky Mountain Spotted Fever

Contrary to its name, Rocky Mountain spotted fever (RMSF) is seldom seen in the Rocky Mountains and most commonly occurs in the southeast, Oklahoma, Kansas, and Missouri. The infectious agent is *R. rickettsii*. The tick vector varies according to geographic region. The dog tick, *Dermacentor variabilis,* is the vector in the eastern and southern United States. RMSF is not transmitted from person to person. It is thought that one attack confers lifelong immunity.

Clinical signs include sudden onset of moderate to high fever, severe headache, chills, deep muscle pain, and malaise. About 50% of cases experience a rash on the extremities that spreads to most of the body. Many cases of what has been referred to as "spotless" RMSF may actually be caused by recently identified forms of human ehrlichiosis, another tick-borne infection. RMSF responds readily to treatment with tetracycline. Definitive diagnosis can be made with paired serum titers. Because early treatment is important in decreasing morbidity and mortality, treatment should be started in response to clinical and epidemiologic considerations rather than waiting for laboratory confirmation (Heymann, 2008).

Prevention and Control of Tick-Borne Diseases

In *Healthy People 2020,* the *HP2010* objective for reducing Lyme disease has been archived because of lack of proven interventions to prevent transmission. A vaccine for Lyme disease, recommended for use by persons living in high-risk areas, was licensed in 1998; however, in 2002 the manufacturer withdrew it from the commercial market because of low demand and sales. Measures for preventing exposure to ticks include reducing tick populations, avoiding tick-infested areas, wearing protective clothing when outdoors (long sleeves and long pants tucked into socks), using repellants, and immediately inspecting for and removing ticks when returning indoors. The CDC reports that landscaping modifications such as removing brush and leaf litter or creating a buffer zone of wood chips or gravel between yard and forest may reduce exposure to ticks as well as appropriate pesticide application to lawns. Ticks require a prolonged period of attachment (6-48 hours) before they start blood-feeding on the host; prompt tick discovery and removal can help prevent transmission of disease. Ticks should be removed with steady, gentle traction on tweezers applied to the head parts of the tick. The tick's body should not be squeezed during the removal process to avoid infection that could be transmitted from resultant tick feces and tissue juices (Heymann, 2008). When outdoors, permethrin sprayed on clothing and tick repellents on bare skin containing 20% to 30% diethyltoluamide (DEET) can offer effective protection; use of DEET should be avoided on children less than 2 years of age because of reports of significant toxicity, including skin irritation, anaphylaxis, and seizures. Read more about tick-associated diseases at the CDC website (http://www.cdc.gov/ticks/index.html) and the prevention of tick-associated diseases on the Lyme Disease Resources CDC website, which includes handouts that can be ordered and the Handbook on Tick Management produced by the state of Connecticut (http://www.cdc.gov/ncidod/dvbid/Lyme/ld_resources.htm) (CDC, 2008c).

DISEASES OF TRAVELERS

Individuals traveling outside the United States need to be aware of and take precautions against potential diseases to which they may be exposed. Which diseases and what precautions depend on the individual's health status, the destination, the reason for travel, and the length of travel. Persons who plan to travel in remote regions for an extended period may need to consider rare diseases and take special precautions that would not apply to the average traveler. Consultation with public health officials can provide specific health information and recommendations for a given situation. Nurses often staff public health travel clinics and provide this information based on CDC recommendations.

On return from visiting exotic places, travelers may bring back with them an unplanned souvenir in the form of disease. Therefore, in a presenting client, it is important to ask about a history of travel. Even the apparently healthy returned traveler, especially one who was in a tropical country for some time, should undergo routine screening to rule out acquired infections. Likewise, refugees and immigrants may arrive with infectious disease problems ranging from helminthic infections to diseases of major public health significance, such as TB, malaria, cholera, HIV disease, and hepatitis. Nurses may find themselves dealing with these diseases, since refugees and immigrants, especially the undocumented, are often treated through the public health system.

Malaria

Caused by the bloodborne parasite *Plasmodium*, malaria is a potentially fatal disease characterized by regular cycles of fever and chills. Transmission is through the bite of an infected *Anopheles* mosquito. The word *malaria* is based on an association between the illness and the "bad air" of the marshes where the mosquitoes breed. Malaria is an old disease that appears in recorded history in 2700 BC China. Although no longer endemic in most temperate countries, worldwide, malaria is the most prevalent vector-borne disease, occurring in over 100 countries and territories. Half of the world's population is considered at risk; 90% of cases occur in Africa. Malaria is the fifth-leading cause of infectious disease death worldwide and the second-leading cause of infectious disease death (after HIV disease) in Africa. There is no vaccine available to protect against this disease, which in 2008 resulted in an estimated 243 million cases and 863,000 deaths. The WHO reports that decreases in cases and deaths have occurred since 2000. This move in a positive direction is attributed to international funding for bed net campaigns and increased access to treatment (WHO, 2009a).

Malaria prevention depends on protection against mosquitoes and appropriate chemoprophylaxis. Drug resistance is an increasing problem in combating malaria. Of the four *Plasmodium* species causing human malaria, *P. ovale* and *P. vivax* result in disease that can progress to relapsing malaria and *P. vivax* is increasingly drug resistant. *P. falciparum* causes the most serious malarial infection and is highly drug resistant. Thus decisions about antimalarial drugs must be tailored individually on the basis of the type of malaria in the specific area of the country to be visited, the purpose of the trip, and the length of the visit. The CDC and the WHO publish guides on the status of malaria and recommendations for prophylaxis on a country-by-country basis. At this time, there is no one drug or drug combination known to be safe and efficacious in preventing all types of malaria. Antimalarials are generally started a week to several weeks before leaving the country and are continued for 4 to 6 weeks after returning.

Despite appropriate prophylaxis, malaria may still be contracted. Travelers should be advised of this fact and urged to seek immediate medical care if they exhibit symptoms of cyclical fever and chills up to 1 year after returning home. Immigrants and visitors from areas where malaria is endemic may become clinically ill after entering the United States. Approximately 1500 cases of malaria in travelers and immigrants are reported in the United States every year. Also, although malaria is eliminated from the United States, the mosquito vectors are not, so local cases still can occur if these vector mosquitoes bite people infected outside the country. From the time that surveillance began in 1957 through 2009, 156 people have contracted locally transmitted malaria. And from 2003 to 2009, 67 individuals have acquired malaria through blood transfusions (CDC, 2010g). (For more information about malaria in the United States as well as worldwide, visit the malaria homepage at the CDC website: http://www.cdc.gov/malaria/.)

Foodborne and Waterborne Diseases

As in the United States, much foodborne disease abroad can be avoided if the traveler eats thoroughly cooked foods prepared with reasonable hygiene; eating foods from street vendors may not be a good idea. Trichinosis, tapeworms, and fluke infections, as well as bacterial infections, result from eating raw or undercooked meats. Raw vegetables may act as a source of bacterial, viral, helminthic, or protozoal infection if they have been grown with or washed in contaminated water. Fruits that can be peeled immediately before eating, such as bananas, are less likely to be a source of infection. Dairy products should be pasteurized and appropriately refrigerated.

Water in many areas of the world is not potable (safe to drink), and drinking this water can lead to infection with a variety of protozoal, viral, and bacterial agents including amoebae, *Giardia, Cryptosporidium,* hepatitis, cholera, and various coliform bacteria. Unless traveling in an area where the piped water is known to be safe, only boiled water (boiled for 1 minute), bottled water, or water purified with iodine or chlorine compounds should be consumed (CDC, 2009h). Ice should be avoided since freezing does not inactivate these agents. If the water is questionable, choose coffee or tea made with boiled water, carbonated beverages without ice, beer, wine, or canned fruit juices.

Diarrheal Diseases

Travelers often suffer from diarrhea, so much so that colorful names, such as Montezuma's revenge, turista, and Colorado quickstep, exist in our vocabulary to describe these bouts of intestinal upset. Some of these diarrheas do not have infectious causes; they result from stress, fatigue, schedule changes, and eating unfamiliar foods. Acute infectious diarrheas are usually of viral or bacterial origin. *E. coli* probably causes more cases of traveler's diarrhea than all other infective agents combined. Protozoan-induced diarrheas such as those resulting from *Entamoeba* and *Giardia* are less likely to be acute, and they more commonly present once the traveler returns home. Travelers need to pay special attention to what they eat and drink. (Read more about travelers' health at the CDC website: http://www.cdc.gov/travel/.)

ZOONOSES

A zoonosis is an infection transmitted from a vertebrate animal to a human under natural conditions. The agents that cause zoonoses do not need humans to maintain their life cycles; infected humans have simply managed somehow to get in their way. Means of transmission include animal bites (bats and rabies), inhalation (rodent excrement and hantavirus), ingestion (milk and listeriosis), direct contact (rabbit carcasses and tularemia), and arthropod intermediates. This last transmission route means that many vector-borne diseases are also zoonoses. For example, white-tailed deer harbor ticks that can carry Lyme disease, and rats and ground squirrels may be infested with fleas capable of transmitting plague. Other than vector-borne diseases, some of the more common zoonoses in the United States include toxoplasmosis (*Toxoplasma gondii*), cat-scratch disease (*Bartonella henselae*), brucellosis (*Brucella* species), leptospirosis (*Leptospira interrogans*), listeriosis (*Listeria monocytogenes*), salmonellosis (*Salmonella* serotypes) and rabies (family Rhabdoviridae, genus *Lyssavirus*). Many of the emerging infectious diseases such as avian influenza A H5N1, WNV, monkey pox, hantavirus pulmonary syndrome, and variant Creutzfeldt-Jakob disease are examples of zoonoses. Also, among the diseases considered best candidates for weapons of bioterrorism, anthrax, plague, tularemia, and some of the hemorrhagic fever viruses (e.g., Lassa) are all zoonoses. The CDC estimates that 75% of recently emerging infectious diseases affecting humans are diseases of animal origin and that approximately 60% of all human pathogens are zoonotic.

Rabies (Hydrophobia)

One of the most feared of human diseases, rabies has the highest case fatality rate of any known human infection, essentially 100%. Despite the availability of intensive medical care, only six individuals have been known to recover after the onset of rabies and only one survivor who did not receive pre-exposure or post-exposure prophylaxis (PEP) has been reported (CDC, 2008f). A significant public health problem worldwide with as many as 50,000 deaths a year, mostly in developing countries, rabies in humans in the United States is a rare event because of the widespread vaccination of dogs begun in the 1950s. Today, the major carriers of rabies in the United States are not dogs but wild animals—raccoons, skunks, foxes, coyotes, and bats. Small rodents, rabbits and hares, and opossums rarely carry rabies. Epidemiologic information should be consulted for information on the potential carriers for a given geographic region. When the virus spreads from wild to domestic animals, cats are often involved. Of the 28 human cases of rabies reported in the United States from 1998 to 2008, 25% were acquired outside the continental United States and 75% within the country. With a few exceptions, these domestically acquired cases have been associated with insectivorous bats; cases contracted outside the United States have most commonly resulted from the bites of infected dogs (Blanton et al, 2009).

Rabies is transmitted to humans by introducing virus-carrying saliva into the body, usually via an animal bite or scratch. Transmission may also occur if infected saliva comes into contact with a fresh cut or intact mucous membranes. Rabies is found in neural tissue and is not transmitted via blood, urine, or feces. Airborne transmission has been documented in caves with infected bat colonies. Transmission from human to human is theoretically possible but has not been documented except through transplant organs harvested from individuals who died of undiagnosed rabies. Guidelines for organ donation exist to minimize this possibility (Heymann, 2008).

The best protection against rabies remains vaccinating domestic animals—dogs, cats, cattle, and horses. If a person is bitten, the bite wound should be thoroughly cleaned with soap and water and a physician consulted immediately. Be suspicious of bites from a wild animal or an unprovoked attack from a domestic animal. Even when there is no suspicion of rabies, contact a physician since tetanus or antibiotic prophylaxis may be needed. An estimated 16,000 to 39,000 people per year require PEP after being in contact with potentially rabid animals (CDC, 2008f).

No successful treatment exists for rabies once symptoms appear, but if given promptly and as directed, PEP with human rabies immunoglobulin (RIG) and rabies vaccine can prevent the development of the disease. Three products are licensed for use as rabies vaccine in the United States: human diploid cell vaccine (HDCV), purified chick embryo cell culture vaccine (PCECV), and rabies vaccine adsorbed (RVA); only HDCV and PCECV are available for use in the United States (CDC, 2008f). In 2010, the previously recommended series of five 1-mL doses of vaccine injected into the deltoid muscle was changed to four (CDC, 2010h). Reactions to the vaccine are fewer and less serious than with previously used vaccines. Individuals who deal frequently with animals, such as zookeepers, laboratory workers, and veterinarians, may choose to receive the vaccine as pre-exposure prophylaxis. The decision to administer the vaccine to a bite victim depends on the circumstances of the bite and is made on an individual basis.

Recommendations for prevention of and vaccination for rabies in animals are found in the Compendium of Animal Rabies Prevention and Control compiled by the National Association of State Public Health Veterinarians, Inc. Recommendations for administering PEP are provided by the Advisory Committee for Recommendations on Immunization Practices and are available through local public health officials or the CDC. In general, cats and dogs that have bitten someone and have verified rabies vaccinations are confined for 10 days for observation. Treatment is initiated only if signs of rabies are observed during this period. If the animal is known or suspected to be rabid, treatment begins immediately. If the animal is unknown to the victim and escapes, public health officials should be consulted for help in deciding whether treatment is indicated. With wild animal bites, treatment is begun immediately. With bites from livestock, rodents, and rabbits, treatment is considered on an individual basis. Decisions to treat become more complicated for possible non-bite exposure to saliva from known infected animals, and again public health officials are helpful in making these treatment decisions (CDC, 2004b).

PARASITIC DISEASES

Parasites are organisms that depend on a host to survive. Endoparasites, those that live within the body, are classified into four major groups: nematodes (roundworms), cestodes (tapeworms), trematodes (flukes), and protozoa (single-celled animals). Nematodes, cestodes, and trematodes are all referred to as helminths along with acanthocephalins or thorny-headed worms, which are not as commonly involved in human infections. Table 13-5 presents examples of relatively common diseases caused by parasites from these groups. Parasites that remain on the surface of a host's body to feed rather than within it such as ticks, fleas, lice, and mites that attach or burrow into the skin are called *ectoparasites*. Many parasitic infections are vector-borne and/or zoonotic.

Parasitic diseases are more prevalent in rural areas of low-income countries than in the United States. Contributing factors are tropical climate and inadequate prevention and control measures. Poor sanitation, a lack of cheap and effective drugs, and a scarcity of funding lead to high reinfection rates even when control programs are attempted. Parasitic organisms result in a wide spectrum of diseases including leading causes of death and disability in Africa, Asia, Central America, and South America. Examples include malaria, guinea worm disease, river blindness (onchocerciasis), leishmaniasis, amoebiasis, African sleeping sickness, Chagas' disease, schistosomiasis, and lymphatic filariasis. These parasitic diseases not only cause major mortality in endemic regions—CDC suggests 500,000 deaths per year from lymphatic filariasis, onchocerciasis, and Guinea worm disease alone—but also tremendous morbidity. Debilitation from infection may result in an inability to attend school or

TABLE 13-5 EXAMPLES OF DISEASES RESULTING FROM ENDOPARASITIC INFECTION BY CATEGORY

CATEGORY	PARASITE	DISEASE
Cestodes	*Taenia saginata,*	Beef tapeworm
	Taenia solium	Pork tapeworm
Nematodes	*Ancylostoma, Necator*	Ancylostomiasis, necatoriasis (hookworm)
Intestinal	*Ascaris, Toxocara*	Ascariasis, toxocariasis (roundworm)
	Enterobius vermicularis	Enterobiasis (pinworm)
	Trichuris trichiura	Trichuriasis (whipworm)
Blood/Tissue	*Drancunculiasis medinensis*	Guinea worm
	Onchocerca volvulus	Onchoserciasis (river blindness)
	Wuchereria bancrofti	Lymphatic filariasis (elephantiasis)
Trematodes	*Schistosoma* sp.	Schistosomiasis (snail fever)
Protozoans	*Entamoeba histolytica*	Amebiasis
	Giardia lamblia	Giardiasis
	Leishmania spp.	Leishmaniasis
	Plasmodium spp.	Malaria
	Toxoplasma gondii	Toxoplasmosis
	Trichomonas vaginalis	Trichomoniasis
	Trypanosoma spp.	African sleeping sickness, Chagas' disease

Based on information from Heymann DL, editor: *Control of communicable diseases manual,* ed 19, Washington, DC, 2008, American Public Health Association.

work as well as growth retardation, developmental disabilities, and cognitive impairment in young children, all which contribute to significant economic burden for the countries affected.

Parasitic infections also affect persons living in developed countries. In the United States parasitic organisms frequently cause foodborne and waterborne diarrheal illness (*Giardia, Entamoeba, Cryptosporidia*) and sexually transmitted infections (*Trichomonas*), and they pose a particular problem for immuno-deficient individuals (*Cryptosporidia, Toxoplasma, Cyclospora*). Trichomoniasis is the most common parasitic infection in the United States, accounting for an estimated 7.4 million cases per year. *Giardia* is estimated to cause 2 million cases and *Cryptosporidium* 300,000 infections annually. Cryptosporidiosis is a frequent cause of recreational water-related disease outbreaks (CDC, 2007).

New technology for recognizing protozoan parasites, the ease of international travel, immigration from developing countries, and diseases that affect the immune system (thus leaving individuals susceptible to secondary parasitic infections such as HIV disease) all contribute to rising reports of and a

greater attention to parasitic diseases in the United States. The CDC speaks about the major neglected diseases of poverty in the United States, which it defines as diseases that disproportionately affect people in poverty, infect a significant number of people, and receive limited attention in tracking, prevention, and treatment. Five of the six are parasitic: Chagas' disease, cysticercosis, toxocariasis, toxoplasmosis, and trichomoniasis. In order to ensure an accurate diagnosis, nurses and other health professionals need to familiarize themselves with the clinical presentations and risk factors associated with these parasitic diseases.

Intestinal Parasitic Infections

Although intestinal parasites are major contributors to morbidity and mortality in developing countries, climate, improved sanitary conditions, and effective drug therapy have served to greatly reduce widespread indigenous transmission in the United States, so much so that surveillance for many of these organisms is not widely practiced. A recent CDC study reported that 14% of Americans are infected with *Toxocara*, a roundworm carried by dogs and cats that can be passed to humans. Infections were most common in young children and those under the age of 20 (Won et al, 2007). Although most people show no signs of infection, this parasite can cause systemic illness and blindness. Technological advances have allowed for improved recognition of protozoans, leading to increased reporting of organisms like *Cryptosporidium*. Cryptosporidiosis became a nationally notifiable disease in 1995, as did giardiasis in 2002 (CDC, 2005b,c).

Enterobiasis (pinworm) is the most common helminthic infection in the United States, with an estimated 40 million cases a year (CDC, 2009i). Pinworm infection is seen most often among school-aged children and is most prevalent in crowded and institutional settings. Transmission is via consumption of infected eggs found in soil contaminated by human feces. Pinworms resemble small pieces of white thread and can be seen with the naked eye. Diagnosis is usually accomplished by pressing cellophane tape to the perianal region early in the morning. Treatment with oral vermicides and concurrent disinfection is highly effective (Heymann, 2008).

Parasitic Opportunistic Infections

Opportunistic infections (OIs) are those more frequent or more severe in individuals immunocompromised by HIV infection. Before the introduction of routine prophylactic treatment and potent-combination, highly active antiretroviral therapies (ARTs), OIs were the leading cause of illness and death in this group. Some of the protozoan parasitic OIs seen in clients with HIV disease and others who are immunocompromised include PCP; cryptosporidiosis, microsporidiosis and isosporiasis, all producing diarrheal disease and transmitted by fecal–oral contact; and toxoplasmosis. With the advent of ARTs, the incidence of OIs in American HIV disease clients has dropped by 50% to 80%. Isosporiasis was always rare, but the rates for cryptosporidiosis and microsporidiosis have also declined markedly. Although no longer seen with the frequency of the past, toxoplasmosis and PCP have not disappeared. They are more likely to appear in individuals unaware of their HIV disease or without good access to health care. Guidelines for prevention and treatment of OIs in HIV-infected adults and adolescents were updated in 2009 (CDC, 2009j).

Toxoplasma gondii is a coccidial organism harbored by cats infected by ingesting other infected animals. While rodents, ruminants, swine, poultry, and other birds may have infective organisms in their muscle tissue, only cats carry this parasite in their intestinal tract, allowing the excretion of infected eggs. People contract the disease through contact with infected cat feces or eating improperly cooked meat. In most healthy people, toxoplasmosis produces a mild to inapparent infection, but in immunodeficient individuals, the disease may, in addition to rash and skeletal muscle involvement, result in cerebritis, pneumonia, chorioretinitis, myocarditis, and/or death. CNS infection is common with HIV disease. Toxoplasmosis early in pregnancy may cause fetal death or deformity. There are an estimated 1.5 million new *Toxoplasma* infections and 400 to 4000 cases of congenital toxoplasmosis in the United States each year; 1.26 million persons experience ocular involvement as part of infection; and toxoplasmosis is the third leading cause of deaths resulting from foodborne illnesses (CDC, 2007).

Control and Prevention of Parasitic Infections

Correct diagnosis by nurses and other health care workers allows the provision of early and appropriate treatment and client education for preventing and controlling parasitic infections. Diagnosis of parasitic diseases is based on history, including travel, characteristic clinical signs and symptoms, and the use of appropriate laboratory tests to confirm the clinical diagnosis. Knowing what specimens to collect, how and when to collect, and what laboratory techniques to use are all important in establishing a correct diagnosis. Effective drug treatment is available for most parasitic diseases. The high cost of the drugs, drug resistance, and toxicity are some of the common therapeutic problems. Measures for prevention and control of parasitic diseases include early diagnosis and treatment, improved personal hygiene, safer sex practices, community health education, vector control, and improvements in sanitary control of food, water, and waste disposal.

HOSPITAL-ACQUIRED INFECTIONS

Previously referred to as nosocomial infections, hospital-acquired infections (HAIs) are, as the name implies, those transmitted during hospitalization or developed within a hospital or other health care setting. They may involve clients, health care workers, visitors, or anyone who has contact with a hospital. Invasive diagnostic and surgical procedures, broad-spectrum antibiotics, and immunosuppressive drugs, along with the original underlying illness, leave hospitalized clients particularly vulnerable to exposure to virulent infectious agents from other clients and indigenous hospital flora from health care staff. In this setting, the simple act of performing hand hygiene before approaching every client becomes critical. HAIs are estimated to affect 1.7 million people every year (Klevins

et al, 2007) and to have killed 48,000 people and cost $8.1 billion to treat in 2006 (Eber et al, 2010). In addition, HAIs have a high likelihood of involving and contributing to antibiotic resistance. The CDC maintains the National Healthcare Safety Network (NHSN), a voluntary, Internet-based surveillance system managed by the Division of Healthcare Quality Promotion (DHQP) at CDC, which provides national data on the epidemiology of HAIs in the United Sates. (Read more about preventing hospital-acquired infection and antibiotic resistance at the CDC Division of Healthcare Quality Promotion website: http://www.cdc.gov/ncidod/dhqp/hai.html.)

Infection control practitioners play a key role in hospital infection surveillance and control programs. Without a qualified and well-trained person in this position, the infection control program is ineffective. A great majority of infection control practitioners are nurses. Their common job titles are infection control nurse, infection control coordinator, and nurse epidemiologist.

UNIVERSAL PRECAUTIONS

In 1985, in response to concerns regarding the transmission of HIV infection during health care procedures, the CDC recommended a universal precautions policy for all health care settings. This strategy requires that blood and body fluids from *all clients* be handled as if infected with HIV or other bloodborne pathogens. When in a situation where potential contact

---

⊕ LINKING CONTENT TO PRACTICE

Public health involves the prevention of disease, promotion of health, and protection against hazards that threaten the health of the community as reflected in the public health logo and summed up in the mission "assuring conditions in which people can be healthy." The three core functions of public health in achieving this mission as defined in 1988 by the Institute of Medicine in Recommendations for the Future of Public Health are *Assessment, Policy Development,* and *Assurance.* These three have been further divided into the "Ten Essential Services of Public Health" as a means of evaluating the effectiveness of public health efforts.

This chapter presents communicable diseases that commonly challenge the health of a community as well as prevention and control roles for public health nurses. Examples of some of the "Essential Services" under which these roles fall are presented by core function.

Assessment: (1) Monitor health/identify problems and (2) Diagnose and investigate health problems. Examples include surveillance, investigation, and identification of reportable communicable disease cases. **Policy Development:** (3) Inform, educate, and empower and (4) Mobilize community partnerships. Examples include evaluating immunization status, explaining the reason for immunizations and how to comply with the immunization schedule, organizing community partners to provide immunizations and documentation through a registry, and mounting a community campaign to inform the community of the importance of age-appropriate immunization. **Assurance:** (5) Enforce laws and regulations and (6) Link to services and provide care. Examples include assuring compliance with communicable disease control laws through treatment or prophylaxis for exposure to reportable diseases; excluding diseased students from day care or school; linking individuals without insurance to follow-up care for communicable disease treatment or exposure.

with blood or other body fluids exists, health care workers must always perform hand hygiene and wear gloves, masks, protective clothing, and other indicated personal protective barriers. Needles and sharp instruments must be used and disposed of properly (CDC, 1989). The CDC also made recommendations for preventing transmission of HIV and hepatitis B during medical, surgical, and dental procedures (CDC, 1991). Updated guidelines and recommendations for preventing HAIs including universal precautions were published in 2007 (Siegel et al, 2009).

CHAPTER REVIEW

PRACTICE APPLICATION

The rising numbers of foreign-born residents in communities that did not previously have large immigrant populations provides a challenge to those involved with communicable disease control, especially in outbreak situations. Language barriers, specific cultural practices, and undocumented status all contribute to opportunities for infection as well as presenting obstacles to prevention and control. Diseases such as TB, brucellosis, measles, hepatitis B, and parasitic infections often originate in other countries and are diagnosed only after the person(s) arrives in the United States. People coming from countries without, with newly established, or with poorly enforced vaccination programs may be unimmunized. These people are particularly susceptible to infection in outbreak situations. For example, many people coming from Latin America have not been immunized against rubella. Differences in cultural practices can lead to outbreaks of foodborne illness. Listeriosis outbreaks have been traced to the use of unpasteurized milk in cottage industry cheese production.

In the face of a single infectious disease report or an outbreak situation, when working with communities whose members speak little English, it is vital: (1) to have a means of communication, (2) to be able to provide a culturally appropriate message, and (3) to have an established level of trust. Ideally, these requirements are addressed before an outbreak occurs, allowing a prompt and efficient response when immediate action is needed.

A. What would be a useful first step in building trust with a largely non–English-speaking immigrant community?
   1. Hold a health fair in the community.
   2. Provide incentives to use health department services.
   3. Identify trusted community leaders such as religious leaders and ask their help in developing a plan.
   4. Distribute a brochure in the target community language.

B. What might best encourage undocumented residents to respond to a request to be immunized during an outbreak situation?
   1. Using an already established public health program to provide interpreter services, making it clear that proof of immigration status is not required for services
   2. Printing a request in the newspaper in the language of the targeted individuals
   3. Involving trusted community leaders in making the request
   4. Emphasizing to the individuals the severity of the consequences if immunization does not occur

C. What means of communication would work best when targeting largely non–English-speaking communities of recent immigrants?
   1. Newspaper articles in target language
   2. Radio announcements in target language
   3. Fliers in target language posted in the community
   4. Announcements from trusted community leaders

D. How would public health officials best undertake the development of information to effectively reach a largely non–English-speaking community of recent immigrants?
   1. Use the services of the local university communications department.
   2. Ask community leaders to work with translators and prevention specialists to develop messages using their own words.
   3. Hire a professional to translate an existing well-developed English-language brochure.
   4. Use brochures provided by the state health department.

Answers can be found on the Evolve site.

KEY POINTS

- The burden of infectious diseases is high in both human and economic terms. Preventing these diseases must be given high priority in our present health care system.
- The successful interaction of the infectious agent, host, and environment is necessary for disease transmission. Knowledge of the characteristics of each of these three factors is important in understanding the transmission, prevention, and control of these diseases.
- Effective intervention measures at the individual and community levels must be aimed at breaking the chain linking the agent, host, and environment. An integrated approach focused on all three factors simultaneously is an ideal goal to strive for but may not be feasible for all diseases.
- Health care professionals must constantly be aware of vulnerability to threats posed by emerging infectious diseases. Most of the factors causing the emergence of these diseases are influenced by human activities and behavior.
- Communicable diseases are preventable. Avoiding infection through primary prevention activities is the most cost-effective public health strategy.
- Health care professionals must always apply infection control principles and procedures in the work environment. They should strictly adhere to universal blood and body fluid precautions to prevent transmission of HIV and other bloodborne pathogens.
- Effective control of communicable diseases requires the use of a multisystem approach focusing on enhancing host resistance, improving safety of the environment, improving public health systems, and facilitating social and political changes to ensure health for all people.

KEY POINTS—cont'd

- Communicable disease prevention and control programs must move beyond providing drug treatment and vaccines. Health promotion and education aimed at changing individual and community behavior must be emphasized.
- Nurses play a key role in all aspects of prevention and control of communicable diseases. Close cooperation with other members of the interprofessional health care team must be maintained.

Mobilizing community participation is essential to successful implementation of programs.

- The successful global eradication of smallpox proved the feasibility of eradication of selected communicable diseases. As professionals and concerned citizens of the global village, health care workers must support the current global eradication campaigns against poliomyelitis and dracunculiasis.

CLINICAL DECISION-MAKING ACTIVITIES

1. Accompany a nurse who makes home visits. Discuss living situations and other risk factors that may contribute to the development of infectious diseases, as well as possible points at which the nurse may intervene to help prevent these diseases, such as checking the immunization status of all individuals in the household. What are realistic interventions and how much responsibility should a nurse take in attempting to affect the living situation?

2. To become familiar with the reportable diseases that are a problem in your community, look at how many cases have been reported during the past month, 6 months, and year. Contrast these numbers with national and state statistics. How is your county or city different from or similar to these larger jurisdictions? If different, what environmental, political, or demographic features may contribute to this difference?

3. Spend time with the persons who are responsible for reporting and investigating communicable disease in your community. Discuss types of surveillance conducted and outbreak procedures that may accompany the reporting of some of these diseases. If possible, attend an outbreak investigation. Would the existing surveillance systems and outbreak control policies be sufficient in the case of a bioterrorism event?

4. Review the demographic profile of your community including trends from the past 10 years and projections for the next decade. Pay special attention to growth patterns of particular populations such as racial and ethnic groups or specific age groups (e.g., children under 18, adults 65 and older). How do changes in these populations affect the delivery of interventions for infectious disease control such as immunization?

5. Visit a clinic that serves a refugee, immigrant, or migrant labor population to observe the infectious diseases commonly seen in these groups. Compare and contrast this visit with a visit to a clinic that serves an inner-city population and a visit to a clinic that serves a rural population. How are the infectious disease control issues different and/or similar for these varied populations?

6. Sit in a clinic waiting room for immunization services and talk with parents about their concerns and the barriers they may perceive in obtaining immunizations for their children. How can this information be used to better facilitate immunization services?

7. Spend time with a school nurse to see what infectious diseases are routinely encountered in the educational setting. Discuss risk factors for disease in school-age youths and the strategies used to prevent infectious diseases in this age group. Do school policies support the strategies needed for the prevention of infectious diseases in students?

8. Visit a day-care center. Observe potential situations for the communication of infectious diseases and discuss with the director the steps taken to prevent and control infection, including immunization requirements and procedures for hand hygiene and food preparation. Does the center have specific infection control policies and procedures, and does the staff appear to be following them?

REFERENCES

Blanton JD, Robertson K, Palmer D, et al: Rabies surveillance in the United States in 2008, *J Am Vet Med Assoc* 235(6):687, 2009.

Centers for Disease Control and Prevention: Guidelines for prevention of transmission of HIV and hepatitis B virus to health care and public safety workers, *MMWR Morb Mortal Wkly Rep* 37(S-6):1, 1989.

Centers for Disease Control and Prevention: Recommendations for preventing transmission of HIV and hepatitis B virus to patients during exposure-prone invasive procedures, *MMWR Morb Mortal Wkly Rep* 40(RR-8):1, 1991.

Centers for Disease Control and Prevention: *Addressing emerging infectious disease threats: a prevention strategy for the U.S,* Atlanta, 1994, CDC.

Centers for Disease Control and Prevention: Notifiable disease surveillance and notifiable disease statistics—United States, June 1946 and June 1996, *MMWR Morb Mortal Wkly Rep* 45:530, 1996a.

Centers for Disease Control and Prevention: Preventing emerging infectious diseases: a strategy for the 21st century—overview of the updated CDC plan, *MMWR Morb Mortal Wkly Rep* 47(RR15):12, 1998a.

Centers for Disease Control and Prevention: Update: isolation of avian influenza A (H5N1) viruses from humans—Hong Kong, 1997-1998, *MMWR Morb Mortal Wkly Rep* 46:1245, 1998b.

Centers for Disease Control and Prevention: Brief report: global polio eradication initiative strategic plan, 2004, *MMWR Morb Mortal Wkly Rep* 52:107–108, 2004a.

Centers for Disease Control and Prevention: Recovery of a patient from clinical rabies—Wisconsin, 2004. *MMWR Morb Mortal Wkly Rep* 53:1171–1173, 2004b.

Centers for Disease Control and Prevention: Summary of notifiable diseases—United States 2003, *MMWR Morb Mortal Wkly Rep* 52(54):1–85, 2005a.

Centers for Disease Control and Prevention: Cryptosporidiosis surveillance—United States 1999-2002, *MMWR Morb Mortal Wkly Rep* 54(SS01):1–8, 2005b.

Centers for Disease Control and Prevention: Giardiasis surveillance—United States, 1998-2002, *MMWR Morb Mortal Wkly Rep* 54(SS01):9–16, 2005c.

Centers for Disease Control and Prevention: *About parasites,* 2007, CDC. Available at http://www.cdc.gov/ncidod/dpd/aboutparasites.htm. Accessed March 25, 2010.

Centers for Disease Control and Prevention: Progress Toward Global Eradication of Dracunculiasis, January 2007-2008, *MMWR Morbid Mortal Wkly Rep* 57(43):1173–1176, 2008a.

Centers for Disease Control and Prevention: Update: Measles—United States, January-July 2008, *MMWR Morb Mortal Wkly Rep* 57(33):893, 2008b.

Centers for Disease Control and Prevention: *CDC Health Advisory: CDC issues interim recommendations for the use of influenza antiviral medications in the setting of oseltamivir resistance among circulating influenza A (H1N1) viruses, 2008-09 influenza season,* 2008c, CDC. Available at http://www2a.cdc.gov/HAN/ArchiveSys/ViewMsgV.asp?AlertNum=00279. Accessed December 26, 2010.

Centers for Disease Control and Prevention: Surveillance for waterborne disease and outbreaks associated with drinking water and water not intended for drinking—United States, 2005–2006, *MMWR Morb Mortal Wkly Rep* 57(SS09):39–62, 2008d.

Centers for Disease Control and Prevention: *Tickborne disease information*, 2008e, CDC. Available at http://www.cdc.gov/ticks/diseases/. Accessed December 26, 2010.

Centers for Disease Control and Prevention: *Human rabies prevention—United States, 2008 Recommendations of the Advisory Committee on Immunization Practices* 57:1–26, 2008f.

Centers for Disease Control and Prevention: *Reported tuberculosis in the United States, 2008*, Atlanta, 2009a, U.S. Department of Health and Human Services.

Centers for Disease Control and Prevention: Fact sheet: variant Creutzfeldt-Jakob disease, 2009b. Available at http://www.cdc.gov/ncidod/dvrd/vcjd/factsheet_nvcjd.htm#surveillance. Accessed December 26, 2010.

Centers for Disease Control and Prevention: Summary of notifiable diseases—United States 2007, *MMWR Morb Mortal Wkly Rep* 56(53):1–94, 2009c.

Centers for Disease Control and Prevention: Progress toward interruption of wild poliovirus transmission—worldwide, 2008, *MMWR Morb Mortal Wkly Rep* 58(12):308–312, 2009d.

Centers for Disease Control and Prevention: Food safety, 2009e, CDC. Available at http://www.cdc.gov/foodsafety/. Accessed December 26, 2010.

Centers for Disease Control and Prevention: Preliminary FoodNet data on the incidence of infection with pathogens transmitted commonly through food—10 States, 2008, *MMWR Morb Mortal Wkly Rep* 58(13):333–337, 2009f.

Centers for Disease Control and Prevention: Surveillance for Foodborne Disease Outbreaks—United States, 2006, *MMWR Morb Mortal Wkly Rep* 58(22):609–615, 2009g.

Centers for Disease Control and Prevention: *Water treatment methods*, 2009h, CDC. Available at http://wwwnc.cdc.gov/travel/content/water-treatment.aspx. Accessed December 26, 2010.

Centers for Disease Control and Prevention: *Parasites and health: enterobiasis*, 2009i, CDC. Available at http://www.dpd.cdc.gov/DPDx/HTML/Enterobiasis.htm. Accessed December 26, 2010.

Centers for Disease Control and Prevention: Guidelines for prevention and treatment of opportunistic infections in HIV-infected adults and adolescents, recommendations from CDC, the National Institutes of Health, and the HIV Medicine Association of the Infectious Diseases Society of America, *MMWR Morbid Mort Wkly Rep* 58(Early Release):1–198, 2009j.

Centers for Disease Control and Prevention: Southern tick-associated rash illness, 2009k. Available at http://www.cdc.gov/ncidad/dvbid/stari/. Accessed February 7, 2011.

Centers for Disease Control and Prevention: CDC estimates of foodborne illness in the United States, 2010. Available at http://www.cdc.gov/foodborneburden/trends-in-foodborne-illness.html. Accessed February 7, 2011.

Centers for Disease Control and Prevention: Surveillance for human West Nile virus disease—United States, 1999-2008, *MMWR Morb Mortal Wkly Rep* 59(2):1–17, 2010a.

Centers for Disease Control and Prevention: *Tularemia: statistics*, 2010b, CDC. Available at http://www.cdc.gov/tularemia/Tul_Statistics.html. Accessed December 26, 2010.

Centers for Disease Control and Prevention: Recommended Immunization Schedules for Persons Aged 0 Through 18 Years—United States, 2010, *MMWR Morb Mortal Wkly Rep* 58(51&52):1–4, 2010c.

Centers for Disease Control and Prevention: *CDC's Advisory Committee on Immunization Practices (ACIP) recommends universal annual influenza vaccination*, 2010d, CDC. Available at http://www.cdc.gov/media/pressrel/2010/r100224.htm. Accessed December 26, 2010.

Centers for Disease Control and Prevention: Update: Influenza Activity—United States, August 30, 2009–January 9, 2010, *MMWR Morbid Mortal Wkly Rep* 59(02):38–43, 2010e.

Centers for Disease Control and Prevention: *Reported cases of Lyme disease by year, United States, 1994-2008*, 2010f, CDC. Available at http://www.cdc.gov/ncidod/dvbid/Lyme/ld_UpClimbLymeDis.htm. Accessed December 26, 2010.

Centers for Disease Control and Prevention: *Malaria facts*, 2010g, CDC. Available at http://www.cdc.gov/malaria/about/facts.html. Accessed December 26, 2010.

Centers for Disease Control and Prevention: Use of a reduced (4-dose) vaccine schedule for postexposure prophylaxis to prevent human rabies, recommendations of the Advisory Committee on Immunization Practices, *MMWR Morb Mortal Wkly Rep Recomm Rep* 59(02):1–9, 2010h.

Centers for Disease Control and Prevention: *Nationally Notifiable Infectious Conditions United States 2010 [online notifiable conditions webpage]*, 2010i, CDC. Retrieved March 25, 2010 from http://www.cdc.gov/ncphi/disss/nndss/phs/infdis2010.htm.

Centers for Disease Control and Prevention: Surveillance for Foodborne Disease Outbreaks—United States, 2007. *MMWR*, 59(31):973–979, 2007.

Centers for Disease Control and Prevention: Ticks; webpage, last updated January 14, 2011 at http://www.cdc.gov/ticks/ [last accessed February 10, 2011].

Chesson HW, Blandford JM, Gift TL, et al: The estimated direct medical cost of sexually transmitted diseases among American youth, 2000, *Perspect Sex Reprod Health* 36(1):11–19, 2004.

Cieslak TJ, Eitzen EM Jr: Clinical and epidemiologic principles of anthrax, *Emerg Infect Dis* 5:552–555, 1999.

Eber MR, Laximaqrayan R, Perencevich EN, Malani A: Clinical and economic outcomes attributable to health care–associated sepsis and pneumonia, *Arch Intern Med* 170(4):347–353, 2010.

Evans AS: The eradication of communicable diseases: myth or reality? *Am J Epidemiol* 122:199, 1985.

Fauci AS, Touchette NA, Folkers GK: Emerging infectious diseases: a 10-year perspective from the National Institute of Allergy and Infectious Diseases, *Emerg Infect Dis [serial online]*, April 2005. Available at http://www.cdc.gov/ncidod/EID/vol11no04/04-167.htm. Accessed March 25, 2010.

Feldman KA, Stiles-Enos D, Julian K, et al: Tularemia on Martha's Vineyard: seroprevalence and occupational risk, *Emerg Infect Dis*, March 2003. Available at http://www.cdc.gov/ncidod/EID/vol9no3/02-0462.htm. Accessed December 26, 2010.

Health Protection Scotland: Scottish Anthrax Outbrek Declared Over; eWeekly Report 12 January 2011 found at http://www.hps.scot.nhs.uk/ewr/article.aspx [last accessed February 10, 2011].

Henderson DA: Smallpox: clinical and epidemiologic features, *Emerg Infect Dis* 5:537–539, 1999.

Heymann DL, editor: *Control of communicable diseases manual*, ed 19, Washington, DC, 2008, American Public Health Association.

Klevins RM, Edwards JR, Richards CL, et al: Estimating health care-associated infections and deaths in U.S. hospitals, 2002, *Public Health Rep* 122:160–166, 2007.

Lee GM, Lorick SA, Pfoh E, et al: Adolescent immunizations: Missed opportunities for prevention, *Pediatrics* 122(4):711–717, 2008.

Mead PS, Slutsker L, Dietz V, et al: Food-related illness and death in the United States, *Emerg Infect Dis* 5:607–625, 1999.

Pew Charitable Trusts: Foodborne illness costs U.S. $152 billion annually, 2010, Landmark Report Estimates. Available at http://www.pewtrusts.org/news_room_detail.aspx?id=57596. Accessed December 26, 2010.

Siegel JD, Rhinehart E, Jackson M, Chiarello L and the Healthcare Infection Control Practices Advisory Committee 2007: *Guidelines for isolation precautions: preventing transmission of infectious agents in healthcare settings*, 2009, CDC. Available at http://www.cdc.gov/hicpac/2007IP/2007isolationPrecautions.html. Accessed December 26, 2010.

U.S. Department of Agriculture: *Foodborne illness cost calculator*, 2009, USDA Economic Research Service. Available at http://www.ers.usda.gov/data/foodborneillness/. Accessed December 26, 2010.

U.S. Department of Health and Human Services: *Healthy People 2020: The road ahead*, 2009, USDHHS. Available at http://www.healthypeople.gov/HP2020/. Accessed December 26, 2010.

US Food & Drug Administration: *News release: FDA approves second-generation smallpox vaccine, FDA News, September, 2007*, FDA. Available at http://www.fda.gov/bbs/topics/NEWS/2007/NEW01693.html. Accessed December 26, 2010.

Wenzel RP: Control of communicable diseases: overview. In Wallace RB, editor: *Public health and preventive medicine*, ed 14, Stamford, CT, 1998, Appleton & Lange.

Won K, Kruszon-Moran D, Schantz P, Jones J: National seroprevalence and risk factors for zoonotic *Toxocara* spp. infection. In *Abstracts of the 56th American Society of Tropical Medicine and Hygiene*, Philadelphia, PA, Nov 4-8, 2007, CDC. Available at www.cdc.gov/ncidod/dpd/parasites/toxocara/Toxocara_announcement.pdf. Accessed December 26, 2010.

World Health Organization: *Europe achieves historic milestone as region is declared polio-free, WHO press release, Geneva, Switzerland, June 21, 2002, WHO*, 2002, WHO Information Office. Available at http://www.who.int/mediacentre/news/releases/releaseeuro02/en/index.html. Accessed March 25, 2010.

World Health Organization: *World malaria report 2009*, 2009a, WHO. Available at http://www.who.int/malaria/world_malaria_report_2009/en/index.html. Accessed December 26, 2010.

World Health Organization: *Prevention of Foodborne Disease: Five keys to safer food*, 2009b, WHO, Available at http://www.who.int/foodsafety/consumer/5keys/en. Accessed December 26, 2010.

CHAPTER 14

Communicable and Infectious Disease Risks

Patty J. Hale, RN, FNP, PhD, FAAN

Dr. Patty Hale is Professor and Graduate Program Director at James Madison University in Harrisonburg, Virginia. She has practiced public health nursing in Wisconsin and Virginia and has consulted widely with many organizations on community health and infectious diseases, most notably the World Health Organization. Dr. Hale has taught undergraduate and graduate courses in epidemiology, curriculum development and evaluation, community health, and population-focused nursing. An advocate for HIV/AIDS education and prevention, Dr. Hale developed and taught two of the first courses ever on HIV/AIDS early in the epidemic. She formerly taught at the University of Virginia in Charlottesville, Virginia and at Lynchburg College. As a family nurse practitioner, she has practiced in community health centers and, along with students, conducted clinical research. Her publications and presentations have been in the areas of HIV/AIDS, health promotion, service learning, and nursing education. She received a 2005 *American Journal of Nursing* Book of the Year Award for the CD, *Real World Community Health Nursing.* Dr. Hale was named a Carnegie U.S. Professor of the Year in 2003, and was the first nurse ever to receive this honor. Dr. Hale holds a bachelor of science from the University of Wisconsin-Milwaukee. She has a master's in community health nursing and family nurse practitioner from the University of Virginia, and a doctorate in nursing from the University of Maryland at Baltimore.

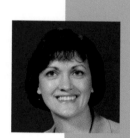

ADDITIONAL RESOURCES

evolve WEBSITE
http://evolve.elsevier.com/Stanhope
- *Healthy People 2020*
- WebLinks
- Quiz
- Case Studies

- Glossary
- Answers to Practice Application
- Resource Tool
  – Resource Tool 14.A: Resources on Sexually Transmitted Diseases

OBJECTIVES

After reading this chapter, the student should be able to do the following:

1. Describe the natural history of human immunodeficiency virus (HIV) infection and appropriate client education at each stage.
2. Explain the clinical signs of selected communicable diseases.
3. Evaluate the trends in incidence of HIV, STDs, hepatitis, and tuberculosis, and identify groups that are at greatest risk.
4. Analyze behaviors that place people at risk of contracting selected communicable diseases.
5. Evaluate nursing activities to prevent and control selected communicable diseases.
6. Explain the various roles of nurses in providing care for those with selected communicable diseases.

KEY TERMS

acquired immunodeficiency syndrome, p. 318
chlamydia, p. 324
directly observed therapy, p. 334
genital herpes, p. 325
genital warts, p. 325
gonorrhea, p. 321
hepatitis A virus (HAV), p. 326
hepatitis B virus (HBV), p. 327
hepatitis C virus (HCV), p. 328

highly active antiretroviral therapy (HAART), p. 318
HIV antibody test, p. 318
HIV infection, p. 318
human immunodeficiency virus, p. 317
human papillomavirus, p. 325
incidence, p. 321
incubation, p. 318
injection drug use, p. 319

non-gonococcal urethritis, p. 325
partner notification, p. 329
pelvic inflammatory disease, p. 324
perinatal HIV transmission, p. 319
prevalence, p. 319
sexually transmitted diseases, p. 317
syphilis, p. 324
tuberculosis, p. 328

OUTLINE

Knowledge about the risk of communicable diseases has changed dramatically in recent years. For example, in the decades following the development of antibiotics in the 1940s, sexually transmitted diseases (STDs) were considered to be a problem of the past. The recent emergence of new viral STDs and antibiotic-resistant strains of bacterial STDs has posed new challenges. Left unchecked, STDs can cause poor pregnancy outcomes, infertility, and cervical cancers. There is also the problem of co-infection, with one STD increasing the susceptibility to other STDs, such as human immunodeficiency virus (HIV).

This concern about infectious diseases has prompted the development of standards for STDs, HIV and acquired immunodeficiency syndrome (AIDS), hepatitis, and tuberculosis (TB) in the *Healthy People 2020* report. The *Healthy People 2020* box shows some objectives used to evaluate progress toward decreasing communicable diseases by the year 2020.

Several communicable diseases and all STDs are acquired through behaviors that can be avoided or changed, and thus intervention efforts by nurses have focused on disease prevention. Prevention can take the form of vaccine administration (as with hepatitis A and hepatitis B), early detection (of TB, for example), or instruction of clients about abstinence or safer sex. Individuals who live with chronic infections can transmit them to others.

This chapter describes selected communicable diseases and their nursing management. It concludes with implications for nursing care in primary, secondary, and tertiary prevention.

about HIV may lead to attitudes of blaming clients for their infections and to discrimination. These beliefs are magnified by the fact that this disease has commonly afflicted two groups who have been largely scorned by society: homosexuals and injection drug users (Fair and Ginsberg, 2010). Debates have arisen over how to control disease transmission and how to pay for related health services. An ongoing debate involves whether clean needles should be distributed to injection drug users to prevent the spread of HIV.

Economic costs of HIV/AIDS result from premature disability and treatment. The fact that nearly 75% of new HIV infections occur in persons between the ages of 30 and 49 years may result in disrupted families and lost creative and economic productivity at a period of life when vitality is the norm (CDC, 2009a). The health care delivery costs of those infected are supported primarily by Medicaid and Medicare. Many people with HIV qualify for Medicaid or Medicare because they are indigent or fall into poverty when paying for health care over the course of the illness. Lifetime cost of HIV care for one client is $618,900 (Schackman et al, 2006). The Ryan White Comprehensive AIDS Resource Emergency (CARE) Act provides services for persons with HIV infection (HRSA, 2008). This program provides funds for health care in the geographic areas with the largest number of AIDS cases. Health services that are covered include emergency services, services for early intervention and care (sometimes including coverage of health insurance), and drug reimbursement programs for HIV-infected individuals. The AIDS Drug Assistance Programs (ADAPs) are awards that pay for medications on the basis of the estimated number of persons living with AIDS in the individual state (USDHHS, 2010).

HUMAN IMMUNODEFICIENCY VIRUS INFECTION

Human immunodeficiency virus (HIV) infection and AIDS have had an enormous political and social impact on society. Controversies have arisen over many aspects of HIV. Fears

Natural History of HIV

The natural history of HIV includes three stages: the primary infection (within about 1 month of contracting the virus), followed by a period when the body shows no symptoms (clinical

HEALTHY PEOPLE 2020

The following selected objectives pertain to the communicable diseases discussed in this chapter:

- HIV-3: Reduce the rate of HIV transmission among adults and adolescents.
- HIV-5: Reduce the number of new AIDS cases among adolescents and adult heterosexuals.
- STD-8: Reduce congenital syphilis.
- STD-6: Reduce gonorrhea rates.
- IID-25: Reduce hepatitis B.
- IID-26: Reduce new hepatitis C infections.
- STD-1: Reduce the proportion of adolescents and young adults with *Chlamydia trachomatis* infections.

From U.S. Department of Health and Human Services: *Healthy People 2020 Objectives*, Washington, DC, 2010, Office of Disease Prevention and Health Promotion, USDHHS.

BOX 14-1   MODES OF TRANSMISSION OF HUMAN IMMUNODEFICIENCY VIRUS (HIV)

HIV can be transmitted in the following ways:

- Sexual contact, involving the exchange of body fluids, with an infected person
- Sharing or reusing needles, syringes, or other equipment used to prepare injectable drugs
- Perinatal transmission from an infected mother to her fetus during pregnancy or delivery, or to an infant when breastfeeding
- Transfusions or other exposure to HIV-contaminated blood or blood products, organs, or semen

From Heymann D: *Control of communicable diseases manual*, Washington, DC, 2008, APHA.

---

latency), and then a final stage of symptomatic disease (Buttaro et al, 2008).

When HIV enters the body, a person may experience a mononucleosis-like syndrome, referred to as a primary infection, which lasts for a few weeks. This may go unrecognized. The body's CD4 white blood cell count drops for a brief time when the virus is most plentiful in the body. The immune system increases antibody production in response to this initial infection, which is a self-limiting illness. Symptoms include lymphadenopathy, myalgias, sore throat, lethargy, rash, and fever (CDC, 2010e). Even if the client seeks medical care at this time, the antibody test at this stage is usually negative, so it is often not recognized as HIV.

After a variable period of time, commonly from 6 weeks to 3 months, HIV antibodies appear in the blood. Although most antibodies serve a protective role, HIV antibodies do not. However, their presence helps in the detection of HIV infection because screening tests show their presence in the bloodstream.

HIV-infected persons live several years before developing symptomatic disease. During this prolonged incubation period, clients have a gradual deterioration of the immune system and can transmit the virus to others. The use of highly active antiretroviral therapy (HAART) has greatly increased the survival time of persons with HIV/AIDS.

Acquired immunodeficiency syndrome (AIDS) is the last stage in the long continuum of HIV infection and may result from damage caused by HIV, secondary cancers, or opportunistic organisms. AIDS is defined as a disabling or life-threatening illness caused by HIV; it is diagnosed in a person with a CD4 T-lymphocyte count of less than 200/mL with documented HIV infection (CDC, 2008).

Many of the AIDS-related opportunistic infections are caused by microorganisms that are commonly present in healthy individuals but do not cause disease in persons with an intact immune system. These microorganisms proliferate in persons with HIV/AIDS because of a weakened immune system. Opportunistic infections may be caused by bacteria, fungi, viruses, or protozoa. The most common opportunistic diseases are *Pneumocystis jiroveci (carinii)* pneumonia and oral candidiasis, but also include pulmonary TB, invasive cervical cancer, or recurrent pneumonia.

In 2008 the case definition for HIV infection was revised to include the HIV classification system based on the number of CD4+ T-lymphocytes. Criteria for defining HIV infection include a positive result from the antibody screening test or a positive result from a nucleic acid test (DNA or RNA). In situations where the mother of a newborn is HIV infected, the HIV nucleic acid test (DNA or RNA) is used to identify HIV/AIDS in infants (CDC, 2008).

TB, an infection that is becoming more prevalent because of HIV infection, can spread rapidly among immunosuppressed individuals. Thus, HIV-infected individuals who live in close proximity to one another, such as in long-term care facilities, prisons, drug treatment facilities, or other settings, must be carefully screened and in some instances deemed non-infectious before admission to such settings. TB is covered in more depth later in this chapter.

Transmission

HIV is transmitted through exposure to blood, semen, transplanted organs, vaginal secretions, and breast milk (Heymann, 2008). Persons who had blood exposure or sexual or needle-sharing contact with an HIV-infected person are at risk for contracting the virus. The virus is not transmitted through casual contact such as touching or hugging someone who has HIV infection or through mosquitoes or other insects. Although HIV has been found in saliva and tears in some instances, it has not been reported to be transmitted through contact with these body fluids (Heymann, 2008). The modes of transmission are listed in Box 14-1, and the exposure categories of AIDS are shown in Figure 14-1.

Potential donors of blood and tissues are screened through interviews to assess for a history of high-risk activities and screened with the HIV antibody test. Blood or tissue is not used from individuals with a history of high-risk behavior or who are HIV infected. In addition to being screened, coagulation factors used to treat hemophilia and other blood disorders are made safe through heat treatments to inactivate the virus. Screening has significantly reduced

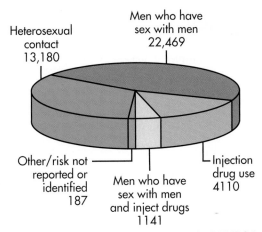

Heterosexual contact 13,180

Men who have sex with men 22,469

Injection drug use 4110

Men who have sex with men and inject drugs 1141

Other/risk not reported or identified 187

FIGURE 14-1 Estimated numbers of cases of HIV/AIDS by exposure category in 2008, United States. Note that the "other" category includes hemophilia, blood transfusion, and risk factors not reported or not identified. (Data from Centers for Disease Control and Prevention: *HIV/AIDS Surveillance Rep* 15:10, Diagnoses of HIV infection and AIDS in the United States and Dependent Areas. 2008. Available at http://www.cdc.gov/hiv/topics/surveillance/basic.htm#hivaidsexposure. Accessed January 30, 2011.)

the risk of transmission of HIV by blood products and organ donations.

When a person has an STD infection such as chlamydia or gonorrhea, the risk of HIV infection increases and HIV may also increase the risk for other STDs. This may result from any of the following: open lesions providing a portal of entry for pathogens; STDs decreasing the host's immune status, resulting in a rapid progression of HIV infection; and HIV changing the natural history of STDs or the effectiveness of medications used in treating STDs (Heymann, 2008).

The nurse serves both as an educator about the modes of transmission and as a role model for how to behave toward and provide supportive care for those with HIV infection. An understanding of how transmission does and does not occur will help family and community members feel more comfortable in relating to and caring for persons with HIV (see Box 14-1).

Epidemiology of HIV/AIDS

Worldwide 38 million persons live with HIV infection. Sub-Saharan Africa accounts for two thirds of all HIV infections (UNAIDS, 2009). The epidemic is also growing in central Asia and Eastern Europe (USAID, 2010). Women are at highest risk for infection because of unprotected sex with infected partners. However, there is some evidence that HIV prevention programs may be changing risk behavior in southern Africa. Worldwide, the treatment of HIV infection has been given higher priority, and the use of HAART has increased to 44% for those who need it. This is up from 2% in 2004 (UNAIDS, 2009).

Nurses must identify the trends of HIV infection in the populations they serve, so that they can screen clients who may be at risk and can adequately plan prevention programs and illness care resources. For example, knowing that AIDS disproportionately affects minorities helps nurses set priorities and plan services for these groups. Factors such as geographic location,

age, and ethnic distribution are tracked to more effectively target programs. It is important to identify persons infected with HIV before symptomatic AIDS develops, so that treatment can begin as early as needed.

> **THE CUTTING EDGE** *About 1 million persons in the United States are infected with HIV, but one fourth are not aware of their infections (CDC, 2006a).*

Since the first cases of AIDS were identified in 1981, the total reported number of persons living with AIDS in the United States has grown to 571,378 in 2007 (CDC, 2009a). Note that this number reflects only those who are living; it does not include those who have died. The prevalence of AIDS has increased from 2004 to 2007, reflecting increased life expectancy from the use of antiretroviral therapy (CDC, 2009a).

Figure 14-1 shows the exposure categories for persons with HIV in 2008. Men who have sex with men (MSM) make up the largest group with HIV in the United States, and the number of persons contracting HIV through heterosexual transmission is the second largest. Heterosexual transmission has surpassed injection drug use (IDU) as the primary mode of HIV transmission in women (CDC, 2006b).

The distribution of pediatric HIV infection has fallen dramatically as a result of prenatal care that includes HIV testing, antiretroviral therapy for the mother, and cesarean delivery. Perinatal HIV transmission has declined, and 92% of pediatric HIV infection results from perinatal exposure (CDC, 2007b).

As seen in Table 14-1, HIV/AIDS has disproportionately affected minority groups. African-Americans make up approximately 12% of the total U.S. population, yet they represent 49% of those reported to have AIDS (CDC, 2010b). This overrepresentation is associated with economically poor, marginalized populations composed of persons who are likely to be urban residents, may use injection drugs, and may use prostitution to obtain illicit drugs.

The geographic distribution of HIV infection is clustered in urban areas. Regionally, the southern United States and the U.S. territories of the Virgin Islands and Puerto Rico report the highest rates (CDC, 2008). States with AIDS prevalence greater than 12.5 per 100,000 population in 2008 were Florida, New York, New Jersey, Delaware, Maryland, Georgia, South Carolina, Louisiana, California, and the District of Columbia (CDC, 2008).

HIV Surveillance

Study of diagnosed cases of AIDS does not reveal current HIV infection patterns because of the interval between infection with HIV and the onset of clinical disease. Moreover, the effectiveness of antiretroviral drugs given early in the HIV infection before symptoms start provides impetus for early identification of infection. Thus in 2008 confidential reporting of HIV-positive status by name was required in all 50 States and the District of Columbia (CDC, 2010d).

TABLE 14-1	ESTIMATED NUMBERS OF NEW HIV INFECTIONS IN ADULTS AND ADOLESCENTS, 2006 (50 STATES AND THE DISTRICT OF COLUMBIA)				
RACE/ETHNICITY	MALES (NUMBER)	MALES (RATE)	FEMALES (NUMBER)	FEMALES (RATE)	TOTAL
White, non-Hispanic	16,280	19.6	3300	3.8	19,600
African American, non-Hispanic	16,120	115.7	8810	55.7	24,900
Hispanic	7420	43.1	2300	14.4	9700
Asian/Pacific Islander	1010	18.0	180	3.0	1200
Native American/Alaskan Native	150	15.5	130	12.8	290
Total	41,400	34.3	15,000	11.9	56,300

From Centers for Disease Control and Prevention, 2007. Available at http://www.cdc.gov/hiv/topics/surveillance/resources/reports/2007report/pdf/table3.pdf. Accessed December 26, 2010.

HIV Testing

The HIV antibody test is the most commonly used screening test for determining infection. This test does just as its name implies: it does not reveal whether an individual has symptomatic AIDS, nor does it isolate the virus. It does indicate the presence of the antibody to HIV. The most commonly used form of this test is the enzyme-linked immunosorbent assay (EIA). The EIA effectively screens blood and other donor products. To minimize false-positive results, a confirmatory test, the Western blot, is used to verify the results. False-negative results may also occur after infection and before antibodies are produced. Sometimes referred to as the window period, this can last from 6 weeks to 3 months.

In 2004 the use of oral fluid samples for rapid HIV antibody testing was approved. These tests (OraSure, OraQuick) are 99% accurate and provide results within 20 minutes, allowing immediate results to be given (Greenwald et al, 2006). In addition to the rapid results, this test may appeal to persons who fear having their blood drawn. If the test is positive, it requires a second specific confirmatory test. Another option for rapid test results requires blood and is available under the names Reveal Rapid HIV-1 antibody test and Uni-gold Recombigen HIV test.

Routine testing is recommended for all clients attending health department STD clinics, family planning clinics, community health centers, and primary care offices (CDC, 2006c). Voluntary screening programs for HIV may be either confidential or anonymous; the process for each is unique. Confidential testing involves reporting either by identifying the person's name and address; this information is considered protected by confidentiality. With anonymous testing, the client is given an identification code number that is attached to all records of the test results and is not linked to the person's name and address. Demographic data such as the person's sex, age, and race may be collected, but there is no record of the client's name and address. An advantage of anonymous testing may be that it increases the number of people who are willing to be tested, because many of those at risk are engaged in illegal activities. The anonymity eliminates their concern about the possibility of arrest or discrimination. However, anonymous testing does not allow for follow-up if the test is positive because the client's name and address are not available.

Perinatal and Pediatric HIV Infection

Perinatal transmission accounts for nearly all HIV infection in children and can occur during pregnancy, labor and delivery, or breastfeeding. The effectiveness of antiretroviral therapy in pregnant women and newborns in preventing transmission from mother to fetus or infant has made pediatric HIV rates decline sharply. On the basis of the effectiveness of antiviral therapy, it is recommended that HIV testing be a routine part of prenatal care and that all pregnant women be tested for HIV (CDC, 2006b). Rapid testing allows rapid results in women who are giving birth, but have not been previously tested for HIV. HIV prevention in women must remain the primary focus of efforts to reduce pediatric HIV infection.

> **DID YOU KNOW?** *Measures that prevent STDs also prevent a woman from having a baby. Current research is focused on developing products that prevent infection without killing or blocking sperm.*

If left untreated, the clinical picture of pediatric HIV infection involves a shorter incubation period than in adults, and symptoms may occur within the first year of life. The physical signs and symptoms in children include failure to thrive, unexplained persistent diarrhea, developmental delays, and bacterial infections such as TB and severe pneumonia (WHO, 2007).

Detection of HIV infection in infants of infected mothers is made through different tests from those used in children over 18 months. The EIA test is not valid because it tests for antibodies, which in the infant reflect passively acquired maternal antibodies. Thus, a diagnosis of HIV infection in early infancy requires the use of other tests that detect HIV DNA or RNA (Havens and Mofenson, 2009).

Despite having an HIV-infected mother, many children do not acquire HIV/AIDS. However, one or both parents may die from HIV infection. The families of many children with AIDS are impoverished, with limited financial, emotional, social, and health care resources. The added strain of this illness makes many individuals and families unable to provide for the emotional, physical, and developmental needs of affected children.

AIDS in the Community

AIDS is a chronic disease, so individuals continue to live and work in the community. Persons with AIDS have bouts of illness interspersed with periods of wellness when they are able to return to school or work. When ill, much of their care is provided in the home. The nurse teaches families and significant others about personal care and hygiene, medication administration, standard precautions to ensure infection control, and healthy lifestyle behaviors such as adequate rest, balanced nutrition, and exercise.

Adherence to HAART is critical for clients since administration must be consistent to be effective (Heymann, 2008). It is important for nurses to educate clients about accurate medication administration. Peer advocates and persons living with HIV infection who are trained to work with infected persons play a vital role in advocacy and teaching self-care management.

The Americans with Disabilities Act of 1990 and other laws protect persons with asymptomatic HIV infection and AIDS against discrimination in housing, at work, and in other public situations (USDJ, 2010). Policies regarding school and worksite attendance have been developed by most states and localities on the basis of these laws. These policies provide direction for the community's response when a person develops HIV infection. The nurse can identify resources such as social and financial support services and interpret school and work policies.

Mental health issues such as depression, substance abuse, and bipolar disorder are often present in someone newly diagnosed with HIV. These conditions must be addressed prior to or simultaneously with HIV treatment to be effective.

Nurses can assist employers by educating managers about how to deal with ill or infected workers to reduce the risk of breaching confidentiality or wrongful actions such as termination. Disclosing a worker's infection to other workers, terminating employment, and isolating an infected worker are examples of situations that have resulted in litigation between employees and employers. The CDC supports workplace issues through programs offered by its Business and Labor Resource Service. (See resources on the evolve website at http://evolve.elsevier.com/Stanhope.)

HIV-infected children should attend school since the benefit of attendance far outweighs the risk of transmitting or acquiring infections. None of the cases of HIV infection in the United States have been transmitted in a school setting. Decisions about educational and care needs should be made by an interprofessional team that includes the child's physician, the nurse, and the child's parent or guardian.

DID YOU KNOW? *Because of impaired immunity, children with HIV infection are more likely to get childhood diseases and suffer serious sequelae. Therefore, DPT (diphtheria, pertussis, tetanus), IPV (inactivated polio virus), and MMR (measles, mumps, rubella) vaccines should be given at regularly scheduled times for children infected with HIV. HiB (Haemophilus influenzae type B), hepatitis B, pneumococcus, and influenza vaccines may be recommended after medical evaluation.*

Individual decisions about risk to the infected child or others should be based on the behavior, neurological development, and physical condition of the child. Attendance may be inadvisable in the presence of cases of childhood infections, such as chickenpox or measles, within the school, because the immunosuppressed child is at greater risk of suffering complications. Alternative arrangements, such as homebound instruction, might be instituted if a child is unable to control body secretions or displays biting behavior.

Resources

As the number of individuals with HIV/AIDS has increased, services to meet these needs have grown. Voluntary and faith-based service organizations, such as community-based organizations or AIDS support organizations, have developed in many localities to address these needs. These services may include counseling, support groups, legal aid, personal care services, housing programs, and community education programs. Nurses collaborate with workers from community-based organizations in the client's home and may serve to advise these groups in their supportive work. The federal government and many organizations have established toll-free numbers and websites to provide information, as noted on the Evolve website at http://evolve.elsevier.com/Stanhope.

SEXUALLY TRANSMITTED DISEASES

The number of new cases (the **incidence**) of some STDs, such as gonorrhea, has been declining recently, whereas the numbers of others, such as herpes simplex and chlamydia, continue to increase. Chlamydia is the most commonly reported infectious disease; gonorrhea is the second most common. Because of the impact of STDs on long-term health and the emergence of eight new STDs since 1980, continued attention to their prevention and treatment is vital.

The common STDs listed in Table 14-2 are categorized by cause, either viral or bacterial. The bacterial infections include gonorrhea, syphilis, and chlamydia. Most of these are curable with antibiotics, with the exception of the newly emerging antibiotic-resistant strains of gonorrhea.

STDs caused by viruses cannot be cured. These are chronic diseases resulting in a lifetime of symptom management and infection control. The viral infections include herpes simplex virus and human papillomavirus (HPV), also referred to as genital warts. The hepatitis A and hepatitis B viruses, which may also be transmitted via sexual activity, are discussed later in this chapter.

Gonorrhea

Neisseria gonorrhoeae is a gram-negative intracellular diplococcal bacterium that infects the mucous membranes of the genitourinary tract, rectum, and pharynx. It is transmitted through genital–genital contact, oral–genital contact, and anal–genital contact.

Gonorrhea is identified as either uncomplicated or complicated. Uncomplicated gonorrhea refers to limited cervical or urethral infection. Complicated gonorrhea includes salpingitis, epididymitis, systemic gonococcal infection, and gonococcal

TABLE 14-2   SUMMARY OF SEXUALLY TRANSMITTED DISEASES

DISEASE/ PATHOGEN	INCUBATION	SIGNS AND SYMPTOMS	DIAGNOSIS	TREATMENT	NURSING IMPLICATIONS
Bacterial					
Chlamydia: *Chlamydia*	3-21 days	*Man:* None or non-gonococcal urethritis (NGU); painful urination and urethral discharge; epididymitis *Woman:* None or mucopurulent cervicitis (MPC), vaginal discharge; if untreated, progresses to symptoms of PID: diffuse abdominal pain, fever, chills	Nucleic acid amplification test (NAAT) of male urine and female endocervix	One of following treatments: Doxycycline 100 mg PO bid × 7 days Azithromycin 1 g PO × 1 Erythromycin 500 mg PO qid × 7 days Ofloxacin 300 mg PO bid × 7 days Doxycycline, effective and cheap Azithromycin, good because single dose is sufficient	Refer partners of past 60 days; counsel client to use condoms and to avoid sex for 7 days after start of therapy and until symptoms are gone in both client and partners; medication teaching Annual screening recommended for all sexually active women under 25, and women over 25 with new or multiple sexual partners
Gonorrhea: *Neisseria gonorrhoeae*	3-21 days	*Man:* Urethritis, purulent discharge, painful urination, urinary frequency; epididymitis *Woman:* None, or symptoms of PID	Tissue culture or NAAT	One of following treatments: Ceftriaxone 125 mg IM × 1 Ofloxacin 400 mg PO × 1 Cefixime 400 mg PO × 1 Levofloxacin 250 mg PO × 1 If chlamydial infection is not ruled out, give azithromycin 1 g PO × 1	Refer partners of past 60 days; return for evaluation if symptoms persist; counsel client to use therapy until complete and symptoms are gone in both client and partners; medication teaching
Syphilis: *Treponema pallidum*	10-90 days 6 weeks to 6 months Within 1 year of infection After 1 year from date of infection *Late active:* 2-40 years 20-30 years 10-30 years	*Primary:* usually single, painless chancre; if untreated, heals in few weeks *Secondary:* low-grade fever, malaise, sore throat, headache, adenopathy, and rash *Early latency:* Asymptomatic, infectious lesions may recur *Late latency:* Asymptomatic, non-infectious except to fetus of pregnant women *Gummas* of skin, bone, mucous membranes, heart, liver *CNS involvement:* Paresis, optic atrophy *Cardiovascular involvement:* Aortic aneurysm, aortic value insufficiency	Visualization of pathogen on darkfield microscopic examination; single painless ulcer (chancre); FTA-ABS or MHA-TP, VDRL (reactive 14 days after appearance of chancre) Clinical signs of secondary syphilis VDRL: FTA-ABS or MHA-TP Lumbar puncture, CSF cell count, protein level determination and VDRL	Penicillin G 2.4 million units, IM once If penicillin allergy: Doxycycline 100 mg PO bid × 28 days Tetracycline 500 mg daily × 28 days Tetracycline should not be administered to pregnant women or those with neurosyphilis or congenital syphilis *Early latent:* Benzathine penicillin G 7.2 million units total in three doses of 2.4 million units IM at 1-week intervals In general, penicillins are prescribed in varying doses depending on diagnosis	Counsel to be tested for HIV; screen all partners of past 3 months; re-examine client at 3 and 6 months

Viral

Organism	Incubation	Signs and Symptoms	Diagnosis	Treatment	Education/Nursing Considerations
Human immunodeficiency virus (HIV)	4-6 weeks Seroconversion: 6 weeks to 3 months AIDS: month to years (average, 11 years)	*Possible:* Acute mononucleosis-like illness (lymphadenopathy, fever, rash, joint and muscle pain, sore throat) Appearance of HIV antibody *Opportunistic diseases:* Most commonly *Pneumocystis jiroveci* pneumonia, oral candidiasis, Kaposi's sarcoma	HIV antibody test: EIA or Western blot test; OraSure (SmithKline Beecham) is an oral HIV-1 antibody testing system, test results in about 3 days CD4+ T-lymphocyte count of less than 200/µl with documented HIV infection, or diagnosis with clinical manifestation of AIDS as defined by CDC	Prophylactic administration of zidovudine (ZDV) immediately after exposure may prevent seroconversion Post-exposure prophylaxis (PEP) should begin as soon as possible. Choice of antiviral drug therapy is made based on toxicity and drug resistance. Combinations of drugs are considered such as zidovudine (ZDV) and 3TC. Drug selection is complicated and evolving.	HIV education and counseling; partner referral for evaluation; medication education; assessment and referral Men who have sex with men should be tested annually for HIV, chlamydia, syphilis, and gonorrhea
Genital warts: human papillomavirus (HPV)	4-6 weeks most common; up to 9 months	Often subclinical infection; painless lesions near vaginal openings, anus, shaft of penis, vagina, cervix; lesions are textured, cauliflower appearance; may remain unchanged over time	Visual inspection for lesions; Pap smear; hybrid capture 2 HPV DNA test; colposcopy	No cure; one third of lesions will disappear without topical treatment *Client-applied:* topical podofilix 0.5% bid × 3 days, 4 days of no therapy; or imiquimod 5% cream daily at bedtime for 16 weeks *Provider-administered:* podophyllum resin 10%-25% or trichloroacetic acid 80%-90%; repeat weekly if needed; cryotherapy with liquid nitrogen, laser, or surgical removal	Education about HPV vaccine Warts and surrounding tissues contain HPV, so removal of warts does not completely eradicate virus; examination of partners not necessary, since treatment is only symptomatic; condom use may reduce transmission; medication application
Genital herpes: herpes simplex virus 2 (HSV-2)	2-20 days; average, 6 days	Vesicles, painful ulceration of penis, vagina, labia, perineum, or anus; lesions last 5-6 weeks and recurrence is common; may be asymptomatic	Presence of vesicles; viral culture (obtained only when lesions present and before they have scabbed over)	No cure; treatment may be episodic or suppressive for frequent recurrence *Episodic treatment:* acyclovir 400 mg PO tid × 7-10 days; famciclovir 250 mg PO tid 7-10 days; or valacyclovir 1 g PO bid × 7-10 days	Refer partners for evaluation; teach client about likelihood of recurrent episodes and ability to transmit to others even if asymptomatic; condom use; annual Pap smear

From Centers for Disease Control and Prevention: Sexually transmitted diseases treatment guidelines 2006, *MMWR Morb Mortal Wkly Rep* 55:RR-11, 2006; Centers for Disease Control and Prevention: Update to CDC's sexually transmitted diseases treatment guidelines, 2006: Fluoroquinolones no longer recommended for treatment of gonococcal infections—United States, 2007, *MMWR Morb Mortal Wkly Rep* 56(14):332-336, 2007.

AIDS, Acquired immunodeficiency syndrome; *CSF,* cerebrospinal fluid; *DNA,* deoxyribonucleic acid; *EIA,* enzyme-linked immunosorbent assay; *FTA-ABS,* fluorescent treponemal antibody absorption test; *MHA-TP,* microhemagglutination–*Treponema pallidum; Pap,* Papanicolaou; *PID,* pelvic inflammatory disease; *VDRL,* Venereal Disease Research Laboratory test for syphilis.

meningitis. The signs and symptoms of infection in males are purulent and copious urethral discharge and dysuria. Symptoms in males are usually sufficient to seek treatment. Gonococcal infection in women however, is commonly asymptomatic, and treatment may not be sought. The disease will continue to be spread to others through sexual activity and may not be recognized until pelvic inflammatory disease (PID) occurs (CDC, 2006c).

Some individuals may continue to be sexually active and infect others while symptomatic. Co-infection of gonorrhea and chlamydia is common; therefore, selection of a treatment that is effective against both organisms, such as doxycycline or azithromycin, is recommended (CDC, 2006c).

Reported gonorrhea rates have stayed the same for the past decade, but the southeastern United States has consistently high rates (CDC, 2009d). The reported number of cases in the United States in 2008 was 336,742. The difference between the actual cases and reported cases occurs because gonorrhea may be unreported by health care providers, and because clients who are asymptomatic do not seek treatment and are therefore not identified. Groups with the highest incidence of gonorrhea are African Americans, persons living in the southern United States, and women 15 to 24 years of age (CDC, 2009c).

The number of antibiotic-resistant cases of gonorrhea in the United States has risen at an alarming rate. Penicillin-resistant gonorrhea was first identified in 1976 when 15 cases were reported (Phillips, 1976). By 1990, 64,972 resistant cases were reported (J. Blount, personal communication, January 18, 1991). After resistance to penicillin was identified, a strain of tetracycline-resistant *N. gonorrhoeae* developed. Antibiotics that have been effective against both penicillin- and tetracycline-resistant gonorrhea are now showing less effectiveness. Resistance to fluoroquinolones, specifically ciprofloxacin, is more common, and the only class of antibiotics effective against gonorrhea is the cephalosporin antibiotics (CDC, 2007d).

The increase in antibiotic-resistant infections is partially attributed to the indiscriminate or illicit use of antibiotics as a prophylactic measure by persons with multiple sexual partners. To ensure proper treatment and cure, those diagnosed with gonorrheal infection should return for health care if symptoms persist, have their partners of the previous 60 days evaluated for infection, and remain sexually abstinent until antibiotic therapy is completed (CDC, 2006c).

The development of PID is a risk for women who remain asymptomatic and do not seek treatment. PID is a serious infection involving the fallopian tubes (salpingitis) and is the most common complication of gonorrhea, but may also result from chlamydia infection. Its symptoms include fever, abnormal menses, and lower abdominal pain, but PID may not be recognized because the symptoms vary among women. PID can result in ectopic pregnancy and infertility related to fallopian tube scarring and occlusion. It may also cause stillbirths and premature labor (CDC, 2006c).

Syphilis

Syphilis is caused by a member of the treponemal group of spirochetes called *Treponema pallidum*. It infects moist mucous or cutaneous membranes and is spread through direct contact, usually by sexual contact or from mother to fetus. Transmission via blood transfusion may occur if the donor is in the early stages of disease (Heymann, 2008).

The highest number of cases of syphilis since 1995 occurred in 2008. Between 2007 and 2008, the number of cases of syphilis reported to the CDC increased 18% (CDC, 2009c). The highest rates are among men having sex with men, but in recent years the number of infected women has increased.

The clinical signs of syphilis are divided into primary, secondary, and tertiary infections. Latency, a period when an individual is free of symptoms but has serologic evidence, may occur early or late in the infection. Latency that occurs during the first year of infection is called early latency. Late latency may occur after this first year. During latency, the possibility of relapse remains (CDC, 2006c).

Primary Syphilis

When syphilis is acquired sexually, the bacteria produce infection in the form of a chancre at the site of entry. The lesion begins as a macula, progresses to a papule, and later ulcerates. If left untreated, this chancre persists for 3 to 6 weeks and then in most cases disappears (Heymann, 2008).

Secondary Syphilis

Secondary syphilis occurs when the organism enters the lymph system and spreads throughout the body. Signs include rash, lymphadenopathy, and mucosal ulceration. Symptoms of secondary syphilis may include skin rash, lymphadenopathy, and lesions of the mucous membranes (CDC, 2006c).

Tertiary Syphilis

Tertiary syphilis can lead to blindness, congenital damage, cardiovascular damage, or syphilitic psychoses. A further complication can be the development of lesions of the bones, skin, and mucous membranes, known as gummas. Tertiary syphilis usually occurs several years after initial infection and is rare in the United States because the disease is usually cured in its early stages with antibiotics. Tertiary syphilis is a major problem in developing countries.

Congenital Syphilis

There was a 16% increase in congenital syphilis between 2006 and 2007 (CDC, 2009e). Syphilis is transmitted transplacentally and, if untreated, can cause premature stillbirth, blindness, deafness, facial abnormalities, crippling, or death. Signs include jaundice, skin rash, hepatosplenomegaly, or pseudoparalysis of an extremity. Treatment consists of penicillin given intravenously or intramuscularly (CDC, 2006c).

Chlamydia

Chlamydia infection results from the bacterium *Chlamydia trachomatis*. It infects the genitourinary tract and rectum of adults and causes conjunctivitis and pneumonia in neonates. Transmission occurs when mucopurulent discharge from infected sites, such as the cervix or urethra, comes into contact with the mucous membranes of a non-infected person. Like gonorrhea, the infection is often asymptomatic in women, where up to 70% may experience no symptoms (Heymann, 2008). If left untreated, chlamydia can result in PID. When symptoms of chlamydial infection are present in women, they include dysuria, urinary frequency, and purulent vaginal discharge. In men, the urethra is the most common site of infection, resulting in **non-gonococcal urethritis** (NGU). The symptoms of NGU are dysuria and urethral discharge. Epididymitis is a possible complication.

THE CUTTING EDGE *The CDC recommends annual testing of all sexually active women 25 years of age or younger; older women who have a new sex partner or multiple sex partners, and all pregnant women (CDC, 2007b).*

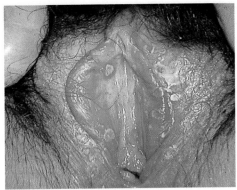

FIGURE 14-2 Herpes genitalis. (From Habif TP: *Clinical dermatology: a color guide to diagnosis and therapy,* ed 4, St Louis, 2010, Mosby.)

Chlamydia is the most common reportable infectious disease in the United States, and in 2008 a total of 1,210,523 cases of genital chlamydial infection were reported. The rate increased 9.2% between 2007 and 2008. Rates were the highest since case reporting began in the mid-1980s (CDC, 2009c). Prevention is important since chlamydia can cause PID, ectopic pregnancy, infertility, and neonatal complications. Women under 25 years of age are the most commonly infected with chlamydial infection because of inconsistent use of barrier contraceptives, multiple sexual partners, and a history of infection with other STDs (CDC, 2009c). The high frequency of chlamydial infections in individuals infected with gonorrhea requires that effective treatment for both organisms be given when a gonorrheal infection is identified (CDC, 2006c).

Herpes Simplex Virus 2 (Genital Herpes)

Herpes viruses infect genital and non-genital sites. Herpes simplex virus 1 (HSV-1) primarily causes non-genital lesions such as cold sores that may appear on the lip or mouth. Herpes simplex virus 2 (HSV-2) is the primary cause of genital herpes.

As is true for other viral STDs, there is no cure for HSV-2 infection, and it is considered a chronic disease. The virus is transmitted through direct exposure and infects the genitalia and surrounding skin. After the initial infection, the virus remains latent in the sacral nerve of the central nervous system and may reactivate periodically with or without visible vesicles.

Signs and symptoms of HSV-2 infection include the presence of painful lesions that begin as vesicles and ulcerate and crust within 1 to 4 days. The first episode is typically longer and is usually characterized by more lesions than seen in subsequent infections. Lesions may occur on the vulva, vagina, upper thighs, buttocks, and penis and have an average duration of 11 days (Figure 14-2). The vesicles can cause itching and pain and may be accompanied by dysuria or rectal pain. Although the ability to pass the infection to others is higher with active lesions, some individuals can spread the virus even when they are asymptomatic. There can be a prodromal phase up to 24 hours before lesions develop that includes tingling and paresthesia at the site (Gupta, Warren, and Wald, 2007).

HSV-2 occurs in 20% of American adolescents and adults (Gardella and Brown, 2007). Because a large number of people have no symptoms and thus HSV-2 is difficult to identify, the prevalence is likely to be underrated. The consequences of HSV-2 are of particular concern for women and their children. HSV-2 infection is linked with the development of cervical cancer. There is also an increased risk of fatal newborn infection during vaginal delivery with active lesions (Heymann, 2008). A pregnant woman who has active lesions at the time of giving birth should have a cesarean delivery before the rupture of amniotic membranes to avoid fetal contact with the herpetic lesions, whereas those who have no clinical evidence of herpes lesions should be delivered vaginally. A small number of infants are infected in utero. The clinical infection in infants may present as liver disease, encephalitis, or infection limited to the skin, eyes, or mouth (Heymann, 2008).

Human Papillomavirus Infection

Human papillomavirus (HPV) results in **genital warts.** Specific types of HPV cause cervical cancer, which is the second most common cancer worldwide (Heymann, 2008). Transmission of HPV occurs through direct contact with warts that result from HPV and can infect the mouth, genitals, and anus. Genital warts are most commonly found on the penis and scrotum in men, and on the vulva, labia, vagina, and cervix in women. They appear as textured surface lesions, with what is sometimes described as a cauliflower appearance. The warts are usually multiple and vary between 1 mm to 1 cm in diameter. They may be difficult to visualize, so careful examination is required (Buttaro et al, 2008).

A vaccine, introduced in 2006, has been widely administered and will likely reduce cervical cancer rates. The recommended age for vaccination in girls is 11 to 12 years old, but it can be given in those aged 9 to 26 years old (CDC, 2007c). The vaccine, Gardasil, stimulates the immune system to block HPV infection before it occurs. Once HPV infection occurs, the goal of therapy is to eliminate the warts. Genital warts spontaneously disappear over time, as do skin warts. However, because the condition is worrisome for the client and HPV may lead to the development of cervical neoplasia, treatment of the warts through surgical removal, laser therapy, or cytotoxic agents is often done (CDC, 2007d).

Complications of HPV infection may be especially serious for women. The link between HPV infection and cervical cancer has been established and is associated with specific types of the virus. Pap smears are vitally important because they allow for microscopic examination of cells to detect HPV, which can be surgically removed if detected early (Heymann, 2008). HPV infection is exacerbated in both pregnancy and immune-related disorders, which are believed to result from a decrease in cell-mediated immune functioning. HPV may infect the fetus during pregnancy and can result in a laryngeal papilloma that can obstruct the infant's airway. Genital warts may enlarge and become friable during pregnancy, and therefore surgical removal may be recommended.

HEPATITIS

Viral hepatitis refers to a group of infections that primarily affect the liver. These infections have similar clinical presentations but different causes and characteristics. Brief profiles of the types of hepatitis are presented in Table 14-3.

Hepatitis A Virus

Hepatitis A virus (HAV) is most commonly transmitted through the fecal–oral route. Sources may be water, food, feces, or sexual contact. The virus level in the feces appears to peak 1 to 2 weeks before symptoms appear, making individuals highly contagious before they realize they are ill (Heymann, 2008).

TABLE 14-3   VIRAL HEPATITIS PROFILES

	HEPATITIS A	HEPATITIS B	HEPATITIS C	HEPATITIS D	HEPATITIS E	HEPATITIS G
Incubation period	Average, 30 days; range, 15-50 days	Average, 75 days; range, 45-160 days	Average, 45 days; range, 14-180 days	Average, 28 days; range, 14-43 days	Average, 40 days; range, 15-60 days	Unknown
Mode of transmission	Fecal-oral, water-borne, sexual	Bloodborne, sexual, perinatal	Primarily blood-borne; also sexual and perinatal	Superinfection or co-infection of hepatitis B case	Fecal-oral	Bloodborne; may facilitate other strains of viral hepatitis to progress more rapidly
Incidence	Estimated 32,000 cases/yr in United States	Estimated 46,000 cases/yr in United States	Estimated 19,000 cases/yr in United States	7500 cases/yr in United States	Low in United States, epidemic outbreaks worldwide	0.3% of all acute viral hepatitis
Chronic carrier state?	No	Yes, 0.1%-15% of cases	Yes, 85% or more of cases	Yes, 70%-80% of cases	No	Yes, 90%-100% of cases
Diagnosis	Serologic test (anti-HAV), viral isolation	Serologic tests (HBsAg), viral isolation	Serologic tests (anti-HCV)	Serologic tests (anti-HDV), liver biopsy	Serologic tests (anti-HEV)	None currently
Sequelae	No chronic infection	Chronic liver disease; liver cancer	Chronic liver disease; liver cancer	Chronic liver disease; liver cancer	No chronic infection	Rare or may not occur
Vaccine availability	Yes, vaccination of preschool children recommended; travelers to endemic regions; men who have sex with men	Yes, vaccination of infants recommended; individuals with exposure risks; men who have sex with men	No	No	No	No
Control and prevention	Personal hygiene; proper sanitation	Pre-exposure vaccination; reduce exposure risk behaviors	Screening of blood/organ donors; reduce exposure risk behaviors	Pre-exposure or post-exposure prophylaxis for HBV	Protection of water systems from fecal contamination	Unknown

The vaccine for hepatitis A infection has been available since 1995, and since that time the incidence has declined 92% (CDC, 2009f). The vaccine makes HAV a completely preventable disease. Persons most at risk for HAV infection are travelers to countries with high rates of the disease, children living in areas with high rates of HAV infection, injection drug users, MSM, and persons with clotting disorders or chronic liver disease. Since routine childhood vaccination was recommended in 1996, the overall hepatitis A rate has declined to 2979 cases reported in 2007 (CDC, 2009f).

Hepatitis A is found worldwide. In developing countries where sanitation is inadequate, epidemics are not common because most adults are immune from childhood infection. In countries with improved sanitation, outbreaks are common in daycare centers whose staff must change diapers, among household and sexual contacts of infected individuals, and among travelers to countries where hepatitis A is endemic. In many outbreaks, one individual is the source of an infection that may spread in the community. In other cases, hepatitis A is spread through food contaminated by an infected food-handler, contaminated produce, or contaminated water. The source of infection may never be identified in many outbreaks (Heymann, 2008).

The clinical course of hepatitis A ranges from mild to severe and often requires prolonged convalescence. Onset is usually acute, with fever, nausea, lack of appetite, malaise, and abdominal discomfort followed by jaundice after several days.

Vaccination and appropriate sanitation and personal hygiene remain the best means of preventing infection. The HAV vaccine is recommended for those who travel frequently or who spend long periods in countries where the disease is endemic. In cases of exposure through close contact with an infected individual or contaminated food or water, an injection of prophylactic immunoglobulin (IG) is indicated. IG should be given as soon as possible, but can be given within 2 weeks of exposure. Candidates for Hepatitis A vaccine are listed in Box 14-2 (Heymann, 2008).

Hepatitis B Virus

The number of new cases of hepatitis B virus (HBV) has steadily declined since the use of HBV vaccination became available. In 2007 a total of 4519 acute hepatitis B cases were reported, down from 26,107 cases reported in 1986 (CDC, 2009f). The groups with the highest prevalence are users of injection drugs, persons with STDs or multiple sex partners, immigrants and

refugees and their descendants who came from areas where there is a high endemic rate of HBV, health care workers, clients on hemodialysis, and inmates of long-term correctional institutions.

The HBV is spread through blood and body fluids and, like HIV, is a bloodborne pathogen. It has the same transmission properties as HIV, and thus individuals should take the same precautions to prevent spread of both HIV and HBV. A major difference is that HBV remains alive outside the body for a longer time than does HIV and thus has greater infectivity. The virus can survive for at least 1 week dried at room temperature on environmental surfaces, and thus infection control measures are paramount in preventing transmission from client to client (Heymann, 2008).

Infection with HBV results in either acute or chronic HBV infection. The acute infection is self-limited, and individuals develop an antibody to the virus and successfully eliminate the virus from the body. They subsequently have lifelong immunity against the virus. Symptoms range from mild, flu-like symptoms to a more severe response that includes jaundice, extreme lethargy, nausea, fever, and joint pain. Any of these more severe symptoms may result in hospitalization. A second possible outcome from infection is chronic HBV infection, which more likely occurs in persons with immunodeficiency (Heymann, 2008). Chronically infected individuals are unable to rid their bodies of the virus and remain lifelong carriers of the hepatitis B surface antigen (HBsAg). As carriers, they are able to transmit the HBV to others. They may develop hepatic carcinoma or chronic active hepatitis. The signs and symptoms of chronic hepatitis B include anorexia, fatigue, abdominal discomfort, hepatomegaly, and jaundice (Heymann, 2008).

Strategies for preventing HBV infection include immunization, prevention of nosocomial occupational exposure, and prevention of sexual and injection drug–use exposure. Vaccination is recommended for persons with occupational risk, such as health care workers, and for infants. The series of vaccines required for protection from HBV consists of three intramuscular injections, with the second and third doses administered 1 and 6 months after the first (Heymann, 2008). Pregnant women should be tested for HBsAg; if the mother is positive, newborns require hepatitis B immune globulin in addition to the hepatitis B vaccine at birth, and then at 1 and 6 months thereafter (CDC, 2010f). In instances in which the individual is not protected by vaccination and exposure to HBV occurs, hepatitis B immune globulin is given as soon as possible (within 24 days is optimal) and the HBV started (CDC, 2010a).

OSHA Regulations

The Occupational Safety and Health Administration (OSHA) mandates specific activities to protect workers from HBV and other bloodborne pathogens. Potential exposures for health care workers are needlestick injuries and mucous membrane splashes. The OSHA standard requires employers to identify the risk of blood exposure to various employees. If employees perform work that involves a potential exposure to others' body fluids, employers are mandated to offer the HBV vaccine to the employee at the employer's expense, and to offer annual

---

BOX 14-2 RECOMMENDATIONS FOR ADMINISTRATIONS OF HEPATITIS A VACCINE

- All household and sexual contacts of persons with HAV
- All staff of daycare centers if a case of HAV occurs among children or staff
- Household members whose children attend a daycare center where two or more families are infected
- Food-handlers who have a co-worker infected with HAV; patrons in unhygienic situations or involvement where food is not heated

educational programs on preventing HBV and HIV exposure in the workplace. Employees have the right to refuse the vaccine. Employees may decline the vaccine for a variety of reasons including thinking they are not at risk since they are married or in a monogamous relationship, that the vaccine is too new to have adequate information about it, or that there may be side effects to the vaccine.

Hepatitis C Virus

Hepatitis C virus (HCV) infection is the most common chronic bloodborne infection in the United States (CDC, 2006c). The HCV is transmitted when blood or body fluids of an infected person enter an uninfected person. Those groups at highest risk include health care workers and emergency personnel who are accidentally exposed; infants who are born to infected mothers; and injection drug users who share needles or other drug-use equipment. Risk is greatest for persons exposed to infected blood. Others at risk include hemodialysis patients (from dialysis equipment shared with infected persons) and recipients of donor organs and blood products before 1992 (CDC, 2006c).

During the 1980s, HCV spread rapidly. It is estimated that 2.7 million people are infected in the United States, and they are a source of HCV transmission to others (CDC, 2006c). Chronic liver disease from hepatitis C is the twelfth leading cause of death among adults in the United States and is the most common reason for liver transplantation (ALF, 2010).

The clinical signs of hepatitis C may be so mild that an infected individual does not seek medical attention. The incubation period ranges from 2 weeks to 6 months. Clients may experience fatigue and other non-specific symptoms. Although some have spontaneous resolution of the infection, 50% to 80% develop chronic liver disease. HCV infection may lead to cirrhosis or hepatocellular carcinoma (Heymann, 2008).

Primary prevention of HCV infection includes screening of blood products and donor organs and tissue; risk reduction counseling and services, including obtaining IDU history; and infection control practices. Secondary prevention strategies include testing of high-risk individuals, including those who seek HIV testing, and appropriate medical follow-up of infected clients. HCV testing should be offered to persons who received blood or an organ transplant before 1992; persons who have been on dialysis for many years; persons with signs and symptoms of liver disease; and persons who received clotting factor before 1987. Routine testing for HCV is not recommended for health care workers, pregnant women, household contacts of HCV-positive persons, or the general population (CDC, 2006c).

TUBERCULOSIS

Tuberculosis is a mycobacterial disease caused by *Mycobacterium tuberculosis*. Transmission usually occurs through exposure to the tubercle bacilli in airborne droplets from persons with pulmonary tuberculosis who talk, cough, or sneeze. Common symptoms are cough, fever, hemoptysis, chest pains, fatigue, and weight loss. The incubation period is 4 to 12 weeks. The most critical period for development of clinical disease is the first 6 to 12 months after infection. About 5% of those

TABLE 14-4 U.S. TUBERCULOSIS (TB) CASE RATES BY ETHNICITY AND SEX, 2008

ETHNICITY/SEX	NEW TB CASES PER 100,000
Asian	25.6
Native Hawaiian/Pacific Islanders	15.9
African American	8.8
Hispanic/Latino	8.1
Native American/Alaskan Native	6.0
White	1.1
Female	3.2
Male	5.3
Total population	4.2

From Centers for Disease Control and Prevention: *Reported tuberculosis in the United States, 2008,* Atlanta, 2009b, USDHHS, CDC.

initially infected may develop pulmonary tuberculosis or extra-pulmonary involvement. The infection in about 95% of those initially infected becomes latent, but in about 10% of otherwise healthy individuals, it may be reactivated later in life. The chance of reactivation of latent infections increases in immunocompromised persons, substance abusers, underweight and undernourished persons, and persons with diabetes, silicosis, or gastrectomies (Heymann, 2008).

Epidemiology

The WHO (2009) estimates that one third of the world's population is infected with TB. Worldwide, Asia accounts for 55% of the cases, and Africa accounts for 31%. The TB infection in Africa reflects the infection with HIV. In the United States, the incidence of TB increased between 1985 and 1992, but since then has shown a steady rate of decline (CDC, 2009b). Of the new cases, 59% are foreign-born persons living in the United States, with Hispanics and Asians being the most common ethnic groups. Nearly half of all new cases are concentrated in four states: New York, Florida, Texas, and California (CDC, 2009b). Table 14-4 shows TB case rates in the United States by race/ethnicity.

To prevent TB, the CDC works with public health agencies in other countries to improve screening and reporting of cases and to improve treatment strategies. This includes coordination of treatment for infected individuals who migrate to the United States. This coordination is particularly significant between Mexico and the United States.

Diagnosis and Treatment

The most effective tuberculin skin test (TST) is the Mantoux test. The TST, previously referred to as purified protein derivative (PPD) test, is used for initial screening. It can be followed by chest radiography for persons with a positive skin reaction and pulmonary symptoms. Persons who are immunosuppressed by drugs or who have diseases such as advanced tuberculosis, AIDS, or measles may not have the ability to mount an immune response to the TST, so the result may be a false-negative skin test reaction resulting from anergy (non-reaction). A second issue with the TST is that a positive result may come from an earlier TST boosting their ability to respond to the infection, and not a recent infection. Therefore, it is difficult to determine if the infection is old or recent. A blood test (in vitro gamma release interferon assays or IVGRA) is available and is increasingly used for providing clinical care (Heymann, 2008). One example is the QuantiFeron-TB blood test to detect *M. tuberculosis* infection. Diagnosis can also be made through stained sputum smears and other body fluids to determine the presence of acid-fast bacilli (for presumptive diagnosis), and culture of the tubercle bacilli for definitive diagnosis. The How To box describes how to read a TST.

| **HOW TO** Perform a Tuberculin Skin Test (TST)

APPLY AND READ THE TST

- *For the Mantoux test, inject 0.1 mL containing 5 tuberculin units of PPD tuberculin.*
- *Read the reaction 48 to 72 hours after injection.*
- *Measure only induration.*
- *Record results in millimeters.*

INTERPRET THE TST

Test is positive if the induration is greater than or equal to 5 mm in the following:

- *Immunosuppressed clients*
- *Persons known to have HIV infection*
- *Persons whose chest radiograph is suggestive of previous TB that was untreated*
- *Close contacts of a person with infectious TB*
- *Organ transplant recipients*

Test is positive if the induration is greater than or equal to 10 mm in the following:

- *Persons with certain medical conditions, such as diabetes, alcoholism, or drug abuse*
- *Persons who inject drugs (if HIV negative)*
- *Foreign-born persons from areas where TB is common*
- *Children under 4 years old*
- *Residents and staff of long-term care facilities, jails, and prisons*

Test is positive if the induration is greater than or equal to 15 mm in the following:

- *All persons more than 4 years of age with no risk factors for TB*

From Heymann D: Control of communicable diseases manual, *Washington, DC, 2008, American Public Health Association.*

Clients with TB should be treated promptly with the appropriate combination of multiple antimicrobial drugs. Effective drug regimens used in the United States include isoniazid, and in some instances, rifampin. Treatment regimens for persons with active symptomatic infection may be different from the regimens used for persons with latent TB infection or with HIV (CDC, 2009g). Treatment failure may be due to clients' poor adherence in taking the medication, which can result in drug resistance. Nurses usually administer TSTs and provide education on the importance of compliance to long-term therapy. They may also be involved in directly observed therapy (DOT) and contact investigations of cases in the community.

NURSE'S ROLE IN PROVIDING PREVENTIVE CARE FOR COMMUNICABLE DISEASES

From prevention to treatment, the nurse functions as a counselor, educator, advocate, case manager, and primary care provider. Appropriate interventions for primary, secondary, and tertiary prevention are reviewed (see Levels of Prevention box). In the following discussion of primary prevention, the nursing process is applied to the care of clients with communicable diseases. Nurses are in an ideal position to affect the outcomes of communicable diseases, and their influence begins with primary prevention.

LEVELS OF PREVENTION

Primary Prevention
- Provide community education about prevention of communicable diseases to well populations.
- Vaccinate for hepatitis A virus (HAV) or hepatitis B virus (HBV).
- Provide community outreach for education and needle exchange.

Secondary Prevention
- Administer tuberculin skin test (TST).
- Test and counsel for human immunodeficiency virus (HIV).
- Notify partners and trace contacts.

Tertiary Prevention
- Educate caregivers of persons with HIV about standard precautions.
- Maintain long-term directly observed therapy (DOT) for tuberculosis treatment.
- Identify community resources for providing supportive care (e.g., funds for purchasing medications).
- Set up support groups for persons with herpes simplex virus 2.

Primary Prevention

Primary prevention consists mainly of activities to keep people healthy before the onset of disease. This begins with assessing for risk behavior and providing relevant intervention through education on how to avoid infection, mostly through healthy behaviors.

Assessment

To assess the risk of acquiring an infection, the nurse takes a history that focuses on risk behaviors and potential exposure, which varies with the specific organism by its mode of transmission. The specific questions that must be asked can be especially challenging when STDs are the object of the study. In these situations, the nurse should obtain a sexual and IDU history for clients and their partners. The sexual history provides information that leads to the need for specific diagnostic tests, treatment modalities, and partner notification. It also facilitates evaluation of risk factors and is necessary for the nurse to be able to provide relevant education for the client's lifestyle.

| **DID YOU KNOW?** *Assessing a client's risk of acquiring an STD should be done with all sexually active individuals. Such risk assessments should be included as baseline assessment data for those attending all clinics and those who receive school health, occupational health, public health, and home nursing services.*

A thorough sexual history requires obtaining personal and sensitive information. It includes information about the types of relationships, the number of sexual partners and encounters, and the types of sexual behaviors practiced. The confidential nature of the information and how it will be used should be shared with the client to establish open communication and goal-directed interaction. Most clients feel uneasy disclosing such personal information. The nurse can ease this discomfort by remaining supportive and open during the interview to facilitate honesty about intimate activities. The nurse serves as a model for discussing sensitive information in a candid manner. When discussing precautions, direct and simple language should be used to describe specific behaviors. This encourages the client to openly discuss sexuality during this interaction and with future partners.

EVIDENCE-BASED PRACTICE

The purpose of this study was to learn young people's emotions and cognitive understanding of sexually transmitted infections (STIs) and treatment. Using a qualitative focus group methodology, the researchers interviewed five groups, totaling 30 health providers who were experienced in caring for those with STIs. The groups were comprised of public health nurses, nurse practitioners, and peer educators. Focus group participants were asked for information about clients' understanding and emotional response to STIs. The Common Sense Model was used as an organizing framework, which identifies three main sources that provide information when people make inferences about illnesses. These are the current culture, social contacts (e.g., family, friends and health providers), and personal experience. Participants reported that clients thought that STIs were caused by infidelity by a partner and intoxication resulting in unprotected intercourse. Furthermore, clients may not know that oral sex can result in an STI, nor is it commonly known that condoms may not protect against genital warts and herpes. Other misconceptions include a belief that STIs may be transmitted by toilet seats, and that only women transmit STIs and men cannot. Issues surrounding antibiotic use, such as quitting the drug before taking the entire amount or a belief that antibiotics will prevent future STIs, were identified. Embarrassment and anger were the most common emotions elicited by STIs. Embarrassment surrounded having to visit a clinic for testing, talking with providers and partners about STIs, and admitting their lack of knowledge about STIs to their provider. Anger results from the mandatory reporting of some STIs and follow-up with partners. Anger also results when infidelity occurs. This study reveals areas that require additional emphasis in client education, as well as providing insight into beliefs and emotions. Public health nurses and other providers can show sensitivity when communicating about these issues.

Nurse Use
This research can help nurses anticipate client needs for education and provide care in a sensitive manner.

From Royer H, Zahner S: Providers experiences with young people's cognitive representations and emotion related to the prevention and treatment of sexually transmitted infections, *Public Health Nurs* 26(2): 161-172, 2009.

Nurses who are uncomfortable discussing topics such as sexual behavior or sexual orientation are likely to avoid assessing risk behaviors with the client. They will, consequently, be ineffective in identifying risks and helping clients modify risky behaviors. Nurses need to be adept at helping clients prevent

and control STDs. Nurses can gain confidence in conducting sexual risk assessments by understanding their own values and feelings about sexuality and realizing that the purpose of the interaction is to improve the client's health. The nurse's comfort in discussing sexual behavior can be improved by using role playing to practice assessments of sexual and IDU behavior, and by contracting with clients to make behavior changes.

Identifying the number of sexual and injection drug–using partners and the number of contacts with these partners provides information about the client's risk. The chance of exposure decreases as the number of partners decreases, so people in mutually monogamous relationships are at low risk for acquiring STDs. You can gather this information by asking, "How many sex (or drug) partners have you had over the past 6 months?" Try to avoid basing assumptions about the sexual partner or partners on the client's sex, age, ethnicity, or any other factor. Stereotypes and assumptions about who people are and what they do are common problems that keep interviewers from asking the questions that lead to obtaining useful information. For example, it should not be taken for granted that a homosexual man always has more than one partner. Be aware also that the long incubation of HIV and the subclinical phase of many STDs lead some monogamous individuals to assume erroneously that they are not at risk.

It is important to identify whether the person has sexual contact with men, women, or both. This information can be obtained by simply asking, "Do you have sex with men, women, or both?" This lets the client know that the nurse is open to hearing about these behaviors, and thus the nurse is more likely to obtain information that is relevant to sexual practices and risk. Women who are exclusively lesbian are at low risk for acquiring STDs, but bisexual women may transmit STDs between male and female partners. In addition, it is possible for men to have sexual contact with other men and not label themselves as homosexual. Therefore, education to reduce risk that is aimed at homosexual men will not be heeded by men who do not see themselves as homosexual. In such situations the nurse can ask, "When was the last time you had sex with another man?"

Certain sexual practices are more likely to result in exposure to and transmission of STDs. Dangerous sexual activities include unprotected anal or vaginal intercourse, oral–anal contact, and insertion of finger or fist into the rectum. These practices introduce a high risk of transmission of enteric organisms or result in physical trauma during sexual encounters. The nurse can obtain information about sexual encounters by asking, "Can you tell me the kinds of sexual practices in which you engage? This will help determine what risks you may have and the type of tests we should do." Clients who engage in genital–anal, oral–anal, or oral–genital contact will need throat and rectal cultures for some STDs as well as cervical and urethral cultures.

NURSING TIP *To be most effective, the nurse obtaining a client's sexual history should do the following:*
- *Remain supportive and open to facilitate honesty.*
- *Use terms the client will understand (be prepared to suggest multiple terms).*

- *Speak candidly so the client will feel comfortable talking.*
- *Ask questions in a non-threatening and non-judgmental manner.*
- *Acknowledge that many people are uneasy disclosing personal information.*

Drug use is linked to STD transmission in several ways. Drugs such as alcohol put people at risk because they can lower inhibitions and impair judgment about engaging in risky behaviors. Addictions to drugs may cause individuals to acquire the drug or money to purchase the drug through sexual favors. This increases both the frequency of sexual contacts and the chances of contracting STDs. Thus, the nurse should obtain information on the type and frequency of drug use and the presence of risk behaviors.

The administration of immunizations is another example of primary prevention, because they prevent infection. Of the diseases presented here, vaccines are available for human papillomavirus and hepatitis A and B.

HOW TO **Use a Condom**

Correct use of a latex condom requires the following:
- *Use a new condom with each act of intercourse.*
- *Carefully handle the condom to avoid damaging it with fingernails, teeth, or other sharp objects.*
- *Put the condom on the penis after it is erect and before any genital contact with the partner.*
- *Ensure no air is trapped in the tip of the condom.*
- *Ensure adequate lubrication during intercourse, possibly requiring use of exogenous lubricants.*
- *Use only water-based lubricants (e.g., K-Y Jelly or glycerin) with latex condoms; oil-based lubricants (e.g., petroleum jelly, shortening, mineral oil, massage oils, body lotions, or cooking oil) that can weaken latex should never be used.*
- *Hold the condom firmly against the base of the penis during withdrawal, and withdraw while the penis is still erect to prevent slippage.*
- *Store condoms in a cool, dry place out of direct sunlight. Do not use after the expiration date. Condoms in damaged packages or condoms that show obvious signs of deterioration (e.g., brittleness, stickiness, or discoloration) should not be used regardless of their expiration date.*

Modified from Centers for Disease Control and Prevention: Update: barrier protection against HIV infection and other sexually transmitted diseases, MMWR Morb Mortal Wkly Rep 42:520, 1993.

Interventions

Interventions to prevent infection are aimed at preventing specific infections. These interventions can take several forms and include things such as education on how to prevent infection or the availability of vaccines. For example, on the basis of the information obtained in the sexual history and risk assessment just described, the nurse can identify specific education and counseling needs of the client. The nursing interventions focus on contracting with clients to change behavior and reduce their risk in regard to sexual practice.

DID YOU KNOW? *Most agency protocols recommend the use of latex condoms. Some may be lubricated with nonoxynol-9, a spermicide. If used frequently, nonoxynol-9 may result in genital lesions, which may provide openings for viruses to enter the body.*

Sexual Behavior. Sexual abstinence is the best way to prevent STDs. However, for many people, sexual abstinence is not realistic and providing instruction about how to make sexual behavior safer is critical. Safer sexual behavior includes masturbation, dry kissing, touching, fantasy, and vaginal and oral sex with a condom.

If used correctly and consistently, condoms can prevent both pregnancy and most STDs because they prevent the exchange of body fluids during sexual activity. Condom failure may occur from incorrect use rather than condom failure. Thus, information about proper use and how to communicate about them with a partner is also necessary. The nurse has many opportunities to convey this information during counseling. Instructions for the use of condoms are presented in the How To box.

Condom use may be viewed as inconvenient, messy, or decreasing sensation. Moreover, alcohol consumption may accompany sexual activity, which may also decrease condom use. The nurse can help clients become more skilled in discussing safer sex through role modeling and practicing communication skills through role play. Role-playing scenarios with partners who are reluctant to use condoms can help individuals prepare for situations before they occur.

Female condoms can also be a barrier to body fluid contact and therefore protect against pregnancy and STDs. The main advantage of the female condom is that its use is controlled by the woman. Since it is made of polyurethane, it is also useful if a latex sensitivity develops to regular male condoms. Symptoms of latex allergy include penile, vaginal, or rectal itching or swelling after use of a male condom or diaphragm. The female condom consists of a sheath over two rings, with one closed end that fits over the cervix. The condoms are often free at public health clinics, or costs range from $2.50 to $5.00 per condom. Figure 14-3 provides instructions on its insertion.

Clients should understand the importance of knowing the risk behavior of their sexual partners, including a history of IDU and STDs, bisexuality, and any current symptoms. Each sexual partner is potentially exposed to all the STDs of all the persons with whom the other partner has been sexually active.

Drug Use. IDU is risky because the potential for injecting bloodborne pathogens, such as HIV and HBV, exists when needles and syringes are shared. During IDU, small quantities of drugs are repeatedly injected. Blood is withdrawn into the syringe and is then injected back into the user's vein. Individuals should be advised against using injectable drugs and sharing needles, syringes, or other drug paraphernalia. If equipment is shared, it should be in contact with full-strength bleach for 30 seconds, and then rinsed with water several times to prevent injecting bleach (CDC, 2010c).

People who inject drugs are difficult to reach for health care services. Effective outreach programs include using community peers, increasing accessibility of drug treatment programs

1 Use your thumb and middle finger, and squeeze the ring toward the bottom so that it becomes thin and narrow. If you squeeze the inner ring near the top, when you insert it, your hand will be in the way.

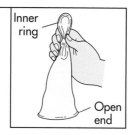

2 Push the inner ring into your vaginal canal, behind your pubic bone. You will feel the female condom slide into place. IF you can feel the inner ring, or IF it causes any pain or discomfort, the ring is not up high enough near the cervix. Don't worry, you can't push it too far inside.

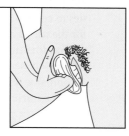

3 Next, take your index finger, put it inside the condom, and push the condom up higher into the vagina. This way, the outer ring will be closer to the outside of your vagina. YES, it has to be on the outside of you, because HE has to go inside the condom.

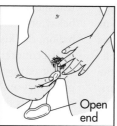

4 The condom is in place. Be sure that:
- Your partner puts his penis inside of the female condom
- Enough lubricant so the penis slips easily inside and out
- A new female condom for each sex act

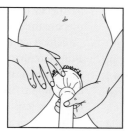

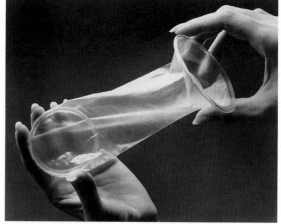

FIGURE 14-3 Insertion and positioning of the female condom. (Reproduced from The Female Health Company, Chicago, IL.)

combined with HIV testing and counseling, and encouraging long-term repeat contacts after completion of the program.

Community Outreach. Because of the illegal nature of injectable drugs and the poverty associated with HIV, many people at risk have neither the inclination nor the resources to seek health care. Nurses may work to establish programs within communities because the opportunities for counseling on the prevention of HIV and other STDs are increased by bringing services into the neighborhoods of those at risk. Workers go into communities to disseminate information on safer sex, drug treatment programs, and discontinuation of drug use or safer drug use practices (e.g., using new needles and syringes with each injection). Some programs provide sterile needles and syringes, condoms, and literature about testing services.

Community Education. Education of well populations about prevention of communicable diseases by a nurse educator is an example of primary prevention. Relevant information about the modes of transmission, testing, availability of vaccines, and early symptoms can be provided to groups in the community. Providing accurate health information to large numbers of people is vital

for preventing the spread of STDs. Nurses can provide educational sessions to community groups about HIV and other STDs. Such educational sessions are most effective in settings where groups normally meet and may include schools, businesses, and churches.

When addressing groups about HIV infection, it is important to discuss the number of people infected with HIV, the number of people living with AIDS, modes of transmission of the virus, how to prevent infection, testing services, common symptoms of illness, the need for a compassionate response to those afflicted, and available community resources. Teaching about other STDs can be incorporated into these presentations because the mode of transmission (sexual contact) is the same. Other information on these diseases can include the distribution and incidence in society, and the consequences of the infection for individuals and families.

Evaluation

Evaluation is based on the extent of vaccination within a population, whether risky behavior has changed to safe behavior, and, ultimately, whether illness is prevented. Condom use

BOX 14-3 WHO SHOULD BE ADVISED TO RECEIVE HIV TESTING AND COUNSELING?

For clients in all health care settings:
- HIV screening is recommended for clients in all health care settings after the client is notified that testing will be performed unless the patient declines (opt-out screening).
- Persons at high risk for HIV infection should be screened for HIV at least annually.
- Separate written consent for HIV testing should not be required; general consent for medical care should be considered sufficient to encompass consent for HIV testing.
- Prevention counseling should not be required with HIV diagnostic testing or as part of HIV screening programs in health care settings.

For pregnant women:
- HIV screening should be included in the routine panel of prenatal screening tests for all pregnant women.
- HIV screening is recommended after the client is notified that testing will be performed unless the client declines (opt-out screening).
- Separate written consent for HIV testing should not be required; general consent for medical care should be considered sufficient to encompass consent for HIV testing.
- Repeat screening in the third trimester is recommended in certain jurisdictions with elevated rates of HIV infection among pregnant women.

From Centers for Disease Control and Prevention: Revised recommendations for HIV testing of adults, adolescents, and pregnant women in health-care settings, *MMWR Morbid Mortal Wkly Rep* 55(RR-14), 2006.

BOX 14-4 RESPONSIBILITIES OF PERSONS WHO ARE HIV INFECTED

- Have regular medical evaluations and follow-ups.
- Do not donate blood, plasma, body organs, other tissues, or sperm.
- Take precautions against exchanging body fluids during sexual activity.
- Inform sexual or injection drug–using partners of the potential exposure to HIV, or arrange for notification through the health department.
- Inform health care providers of the HIV infection.
- Consider the risk of perinatal transmission and follow up with contraceptive use.

can be evaluated for consistency of use if the client is sexually active. Other behaviors, such as abstinence or monogamy, can be evaluated for their implementation. At the community level, behavioral surveys can be done to measure reported condom use and condom sales, and measures of disease incidence and prevalence can be calculated to evaluate the effectiveness of intervention.

Secondary Prevention

Secondary prevention includes screening for diseases to ensure their early identification, treatment, and follow-up with contacts to prevent further spread. In general, client teaching and counseling should include education about avoiding self-reinfection, managing symptoms, and preventing the infection of others.

Testing and Counseling for HIV

Testing for HIV infection should be routine for all clients aged 13 to 64 years (CDC, 2006b). Clients can decline or "opt out" of HIV testing, but the benefits of testing are considerable. For persons who have engaged in high-risk behavior, the nurse should recommend annual HIV testing (Box 14-3). Individuals with the following characteristics are considered at risk and should be offered HIV testing: those with a history of STDs (which are transmitted through the same behavior and may decrease immune functioning), multiple sex partners, or IDU; those who have intercourse without using a condom; those who have intercourse with someone who has another partner and

those who have had sex with a prostitute; men with a history of homosexual or bisexual activity; and those who have been a sexual partner to anyone in one of these groups.

Testing enables clients to benefit from early detection and treatment, as well as risk reduction education. If HIV infection is discovered before the onset of symptoms, early monitoring of the disease process and CD4 lymphocyte counts or viral loads is indicated. In addition, prophylactic therapy with antiretroviral therapy and/or antibiotics may begin in order to delay the onset of symptomatic illness.

Posttest Counseling. Persons who have a negative test should be counseled about risk reduction activities to prevent any future transmission. Clients should understand that the test may not be truly negative because it does not reveal infections that may have been acquired within the several weeks before the test. As noted earlier, evidence of HIV antibody takes from 6 to 12 weeks. Clients must be aware of the ways viral transmission occurs, and how to avoid infection.

All clients who are antibody positive should be counseled about the need to reduce their risks and notify partners. If the client is unwilling or hesitant to notify past partners, partner notification (or contact tracing, as will be described) is often done by the nurse. Clients should seek treatment from their primary health care provider so physical evaluation can be performed and, if indicated, antiviral or other therapies begun. Box 14-4 describes the responsibilities of individuals who are HIV positive.

Psychosocial counseling is indicated when positive HIV test results precipitate acute anxiety, depression, or suicidal ideation. The client should be informed about available counseling services. The person should be cautioned to consider carefully who should be informed of the test results. Many individuals have told others about their HIV-positive test, only to experience isolation and discrimination. Plans for the future should be explored, and clients should be advised to avoid stress, drugs, and infections in order to maintain optimal health.

Partner Notification and Contact Tracing

Partner notification, also known as contact tracing, is an example of a population-level intervention aimed at controlling communicable diseases. Partner notification programs usually occur in conjunction with reportable disease requirements and are carried out by most health departments. It involves confidentially identifying and notifying exposed individuals of clients who are found to have reportable diseases. This could

LINKING CONTENT TO PRACTICE

This chapter emphasizes the epidemiology and prevention of selected communicable diseases, as well as the public health nursing services provided to clients. The Council on Linkages Domains and Core Competencies are addressed through activities in caring for clients with communicable diseases. Examples of how these eight domains are used in providing nursing care to clients with communicable disease are as follows:

Domain #1, Analytic Assessment Skills, is achieved through the review of the incidence and prevalence rates of communicable diseases to determine population health status.

Domain #3, Communication Skills, is applied when PHNs teach how to prevent and treat infections.

Domain #4, Cultural Competency Skills, is met through understanding the various social and behavioral factors that make health care acceptable to diverse populations.

From Public Health Foundation, Council on Linkages: *Core competencies for public health professionals,* 2008. Available at http://www.phf.org/link/corecompetencies.htm. Accessed March 2010.

result in, for example, family members and close contacts of individuals with TB being given a TST, which may be administered in the home.

Individuals diagnosed with a reportable STD are asked to provide the names and locations of all partners so that these individuals can be informed of their exposure and obtain the necessary treatment. Clients may be encouraged to notify their partners and to encourage them to seek treatment. If the client agrees to do so, suggestions on how to tell partners and how to deal with possible reactions may be explored. In some instances, clients may feel more comfortable if the nurse notifies those who are exposed. If clients contact their partners about possible infection, the nurse contacts health care providers or clinics to verify examination of exposed partners.

If the client prefers not to participate in notifying partners, the nurse contacts them—often by a home visit—and counsels them to seek evaluation and treatment. The client is offered literature regarding treatment, risk reduction, and the clinic's location and hours of operation. The identity of the infected client who names sexual and injection drug–using partners cannot be revealed. Maintaining confidentiality is critical with all STDs but particularly with HIV, because discrimination may still occur.

Tertiary Prevention

Tertiary prevention can apply to many of the chronic viral STDs and TB. For viral STDs, much of this effort focuses on managing symptoms and maintaining psychosocial support. Many clients report feeling contaminated and thus feel lower self-worth. Support groups may be available to help clients cope with chronic STDs, such as genital herpes or genital warts.

Directly Observed Therapy

In **directly observed therapy** (DOT) programs for TB medication nurses observe and document individual clients taking their TB drugs. When clients prematurely stop taking TB

medications, there is a risk of the TB becoming resistant to the medications. This can affect an entire community of people who are susceptible to this airborne disease. Health professionals share in the responsibility of adhering to treatment, and DOT ensures that TB-infected clients have adequate medication. Thus, DOT programs are aimed at the population level to prevent antibiotic resistance in the community and to ensure effective treatment at the individual level. Many health departments have DOT home health programs to ensure adequate treatment. Directly observed treatment, short course (DOTS) is a variation applied in specific countries of the world to combat multidrug-resistant TB (CDC, 2009h).

The management of AIDS in the home may include monitoring physical status and referring the family to additional care services for maintaining the client in the home. Case management is important in all phases of HIV infection. It is especially important to ensure that clients have adequate services to meet their needs. This may include ensuring that medication can be obtained through identifying funding resources, maintaining infection control standards, reducing risk behaviors, identifying sources of respite care for caretakers, or referring clients for home or hospice care. Nursing interventions include teaching families about managing symptomatic illness by preventing deteriorating conditions such as diarrhea, skin breakdown, and inadequate nutrition.

Standard Precautions

It is important to teach caregivers about infection control in the home. Clients, families, friends, and others may express concerns about the transmission of HIV. Whereas fear may be expressed by some, others who are caring for loved ones with HIV may not take adequate precautions, such as glove wearing, because of concern about appearing as though they do not want to touch a loved one. Others may believe myths that suggest they cannot be infected by someone they love.

Standard precautions must be taught to caregivers in the home setting. All blood and articles soiled with body fluids must be handled as if they were infectious or contaminated by bloodborne pathogens. Gloves should be worn whenever hands might touch non-intact skin, mucous membranes, blood, or other fluids. A mask, goggles, and gown should also be worn if there is potential for splashing or spraying of infectious material during any care. All protective equipment should be worn only once and then disposed. If the skin or mucous membranes of the caregiver come in contact with body fluids, the skin should be washed with soap and water, and the mucous membranes should be flushed with water as soon as possible after the exposure. Thorough handwashing with soap and water—a major infection control measure—should be conducted whenever hands become contaminated and whenever gloves or other protective equipment (e.g., mask, gown) is removed. Soiled clothing or linen should be washed in a washing machine filled with hot water using bleach as an additive and dried on a hot-air cycle of a dryer.

CHAPTER REVIEW

PRACTICE APPLICATION

Yvonne Jackson is a 20-year-old woman who visits the Hopetown City Health Department's maternity clinic. Examination reveals she is at 14 weeks' gestation. She is single but has been in a steady relationship for the past 6 months with Ramone. She states that she has no other children. A routine test taken during the initial prenatal visit is an HIV test; the results are positive.

Ms. Jackson is shocked and emotionally distraught about the positive test results. Understanding that the client will not be able to concentrate on all of the questions and information that need to be covered, the nurse prioritizes essential information to obtain and provide during this visit.

A. List the relevant factors to consider on the basis of this information.

B. What questions do you need to ask with regard to controlling the spread of HIV to others?

C. What information is most important to give to Ms. Jackson at this time?

D. What follow-up does the nurse need to arrange for this client? Answers can be found on the Evolve site.

KEY POINTS

- Nearly all communicable diseases discussed in this chapter are preventable because they are transmitted through specific, known behaviors.
- STDs are among the most serious public health problems in the United States. Not only is there an increased incidence of drug-resistant gonococcal infection, but other STDs, such as HPV (genital warts), HIV, and HSV (genital herpes), are associated with cancer.
- STDs affect certain groups in greater numbers. Factors associated with risk include being less than 25 years of age, being a member of a minority group, living in an urban setting, being poor, and using crack cocaine.
- The increasing incidence, morbidity, and mortality of specific communicable diseases highlight the need for nurses to educate clients about ways to prevent communicable diseases.
- Many STDs do not produce symptoms in clients.
- Aside from death, the most serious complications caused by STDs are pelvic inflammatory disease, infertility, ectopic pregnancy, neonatal morbidity and mortality, and neoplasia.
- Hepatitis A is often silent in children, and children are a significant source of infection to others; thus, the use of the vaccination in children has caused a reduction in the number of cases.

- The emergence of multidrug-resistant TB has prompted the use of directly observed therapy (DOT) to ensure adherence with drug treatment regimens.
- Early detection of communicable diseases is important because it results in early treatment and prevention of additional transmission to others. Treatment includes effective medications, stress reduction, and proper nutrition.
- Partner notification, or contact tracing, is done by identifying, contacting, and ensuring evaluation and treatment of persons exposed to sexual and injectable drug using partners. Contact tracing is also conducted with TB and HAV.
- HIV infection has created an entirely new group of people needing health care. This rapidly growing population is straining a health care system that is already unable to meet the needs of many.
- Most of the care (both home and outpatient) that is provided for HIV is done within the community setting, which reduces direct health care costs but increases the need for financial support of home and community health services.

CLINICAL DECISION-MAKING ACTIVITIES

1. Identify sources of TB treatment in your community. Is there a DOT program available through the health department or home health agency? What factors make TB infection a difficult problem?

2. To whom does one report communicable diseases, such as HAV, in your community? How is this information given?

3. Identify the number of reported cases of AIDS and the number of reported cases of HIV infection within your state and locale (if reportable in your state). How are the cases distributed by age, sex, geographic location, and ethnicity?

4. Identify the location(s) of HIV testing services in your community. Are the test results anonymous or confidential? Describe how and to whom the results are reported.

5. Form small groups and role play a nurse–client interaction involving risk assessment and counseling regarding safer sex and injection drug using practices.

REFERENCES

American Liver Foundation: *Hepatitis C*, 2010. Available at http://www.liverfoundation.org/education/info/hepatitisc. Accessed June 2, 2010.

Buttaro T, Trybulski J, Polgar Bailey P, Sandberg-Cook J: *Primary care: a collaborative practice*, ed 3, St Louis, 2008, Mosby.

Centers for Disease Control and Prevention: Update: Barrier protection against HIV infection and other sexually transmitted diseases, *MMWR Morb Mortal Wkly Rep* 42:520, 1993.

Centers for Disease Control and Prevention: Updated U.S. Public Health Service guidelines for the management of occupational exposures to HIV and recommendations for postexposure prophylaxis, *MMWR Morb Mortal Wkly Rep* 54, RR-9, 1–17.

Centers for Disease Control and Prevention: Revised recommendations for HIV testing of adults, adolescents, and pregnant women in health-care settings, *MMWR Morb Mortal Wkly Rep* 55(RR-14):1–17, 2006a. Available at http://www.cdc.gov/mmwr/preview/mmwrhtml/rr5514a1.htm. Accessed December 26, 2010.

Centers for Disease Control and Prevention: *HIV/AIDS statistics and surveillance, Slide sets, HIV incidence 2006, slide no. 6*, 2006b. Available at http://www.cdc.gov/hiv/topics/surveillance/resources/slides/incidence/print/index.htm. Accessed December 26, 2010.

Centers for Disease Control and Prevention: Sexually transmitted diseases treatment guidelines 2006, *MMWR Morb Mortal Wkly Rep* 55(RR-11), 2006c. Available at http://www.cdc.gov/std/treatment/default.htm. Accessed June 2, 2010.

Centers for Disease Control and Prevention: *HIV/AIDS statistics and surveillance, Slide sets, HIV incidence, Pediatric HIV/AIDS surveillance (through 2007), slide no. 1*, 2007a. Available at http://www.cdc.gov/hiv/topics/surveillance/resources/slides/pediatric/slides/pediatric_1.pdf. Accessed December 26, 2010.

Centers for Disease Control and Prevention: *Chlamydia-CDC fact sheet*, 2007b. Available at http://www.cdc.gov/std/chlamydia/STDFact-Chlamydia.htm#prevented. Accessed June 2, 2010.

Centers for Disease Control and Prevention: Quadrivalent human papillomavirus vaccine: recommendations of the Advisory Committee on Immunization Practices (ACIP), *MMWR Morb Mortal Wkly Rep* 56(RR-2):1–24, 2007c. Available at http://www.cdc.gov/mmwr/preview/mmwrhtml/rr5602a1.htm?s_cid=rr5602a1_e. Accessed December 26, 2010.

Centers for Disease Control and Prevention: Update to CDC's sexually transmitted diseases treatment guidelines, 2006: fluoroquinolones no longer recommended for treatment of gonococcal infections, *MMWR Morb Mortal Wkly Rep* 56(14):332–336, 2007d. Available at http://www.cdc.gov/mmwr/preview/mmwrhtml/mm5614a3.htm?s_cid=mm5614a3_e. Accessed December 26, 2010.

Centers for Disease Control and Prevention: Revised surveillance case definitions for HIV infection among adults, adolescents, and children aged < 18 months and for HIV infection and AIDS among children aged 18 months to <13 years—United States, 2008, *MMWR Morb Mortal Wkly Rep* 57(RR-10), 2008.

Centers for Disease Control and Prevention: *HIV/AIDS Surveillance Report, 2007*, vol 19, Atlanta, 2009a. Available at http://www.cdc.gov/hiv/topics/surveillance/resources/reports/2007report/pdf/2007SurveillanceReport.pdf. Accessed December 26, 2010.

Centers for Disease Control and Prevention: *Reported tuberculosis in the United States, 2008*, Atlanta, 2009b, USDHHS, CDC. Available at http://www.cdc.gov/tb/statistics/reports/2008/pdf/2008report.pdf. Accessed December 26, 2010.

Centers for Disease Control and Prevention: *Sexually transmitted diseases in the United States, 2008, National surveillance data for chlamydia, gonorrhea, and syphilis—CDC factsheet*, 2009c. Available at http://www.cdc.gov/std/stats08/2008survFactSheet.pdf. Accessed December 26, 2010.

Centers for Disease Control and Prevention: *Sexually transmitted disease surveillance, 2008, Gonorrhea*, Atlanta, 2009d, USDHHS, CDC. Available at http://www.cdc.gov/std/stats08/gonorrhea.htm. Accessed June 2, 2010.

Centers for Disease Control and Prevention: *Sexually transmitted disease surveillance, 2008, Syphilis*, Atlanta, 2009e, USDHHS, CDC. Available at http://www.cdc.gov/std/stats08/syphilis.htm. Accessed June 2, 2010.

Centers for Disease Control and Prevention: Surveillance for Acute Viral Hepatitis—United States, 2007, *MMWR Morb Mortal Wkly Rep* 58(SS-3), 2009f. Available at http://www.cdc.gov/mmwr/pdf/ss/ss5803.pdf. Accessed December 26, 2010.

Centers for Disease Control and Prevention: *Treatment for latent TB infection (LTBI)*, 2009g. Available at http://www.cdc.gov/tb/topic/treatment/ltbi.htm. Accessed December 26, 2010.

Centers for Disease Control and Prevention: *Tuberculosis: TB: Self Study Modules 6-9: Module 9: Patient adherence to tuberculosis treatment*, 2009h. Available at http://www.cdc.gov/tb/education/ssmodules/module9/ss9reading2.htm. Accessed December 26, 2010.

Centers for Disease Control and Prevention: *Hepatitis B information for health professionals, Overview and Statistics*, 2010a. Available at http://www.cdc.gov/hepatitis/HBV/HBVfaq.htm#overview. Accessed June 2, 2010.

Centers for Disease Control and Prevention: *HIV/AIDS and African Americans*, Atlanta, 2010b, USDHHS, CDC, Available at http://www.cdc.gov/hiv/topics/aa/index.htm. Accessed December 26, 2010.

Centers for Disease Control and Prevention: *HIV/AIDS topics, Basic information*, 2010c. Available at http://www.cdc.gov/hiv/topics/basic/print/index.htm. Accessed December 26, 2010.

Centers for Disease Control and Prevention: *HIV infection reporting*, Atlanta, 2010d, USDHHS, CDC. Available at http://www.cdc.gov/hiv/topics/surveillance/reporting.htm. Accessed December 26, 2010.

Centers for Disease Control and Prevention: *HIV/AIDS: questions & answers: how can I tell if I'm infected with HIV? What are the symptoms?* Atlanta, 2010e, USDHHS, CDC. Available at http://www.cdc.gov/hiv/resources/qa/qa5.htm. Accessed December 27, 2010.

Centers for Disease Control and Prevention: *Vaccines and Immunizations, Immunization schedule*, 2010f. Available at http://www.immunize.org/catg.d/p4030.pdf. Accessed December 26, 2010.

Centers for Disease Control and Prevention: HIV Surveillance Report, 2008, Vol 20, 2010g. Available at http://www.cdc.gov/hiv/topics/surveillance/resources/reports. Accessed January 29, 2011.

Centers for Disease Control and Prevention: HIV/AIDS Surveillance Report: Diagnoses of HIV infection and AIDS in the United States and Dependent Areas. 2008. Available at http://www.cdc.gov/hiv/topics/surveillance/basic.htm#hivaidsexposure. Accessed January 30, 2011.

Fair C, Ginsburg B: HIV-related stigma, discrimination, and knowledge of legal rights among infected adults, *J HIV/AIDS Social Serv* 9(1):77–79, 2010. Available at http://dx.doi.org/10.1080/15381500903583470. Accessed December 26, 2010.

Gardella C, Brown ZA: Serologic testing for herpes simplex virus: Ready for prime time? *Contemp OB/GYN* 52(10):54–58, 2007.

Greenwald JL, Burstein GR, Pincus J, Branson B: A rapid review of rapid HIV antibody tests, *Curr Infect Dis Rep* 8(2):125–131, 2006. Available at http://www.cdc.gov/hiv/topics/testing/resources/journal_article/pdf/rapid_review.pdf. Accessed December 26, 2010.

Gupta R, Warren T, Wald A: Genital herpes, *Lancet* 370(9605):2127–2137, 2007.

Habif TP: *Clinical dermatology: a color guide to diagnosis and therapy*, ed 4, St Louis, 2010, Mosby.

Havens P, Mofenson L: Evaluation and management of the infant exposed to HIV-1 in the United States, *Pediatrics* 123(1):175–187, 2009.

Health Resources and Services Administration: *AIDS drug assistance program (ADAP)*, 2008. Available at http://hab.hrsa.gov/treatmentmodernization/partb.htm#ADAP. Accessed December 26, 2010.

Heymann D: *Control of communicable diseases manual*, ed 19, Washington, DC, 2008, American Public Health Association.

Phillips I: Beta-lactamase producing penicillin-resistant gonococcus, *Lancet* 2:656, 1976.

Public Health Foundation: Council on Linkages: *Core competencies for public health professionals*, 2008. Available at http://www.phf.org/link/corecompetencies.htm. Accessed March 2010.

Royer H, Zahner S: Providers experiences with young people's cognitive representations and emotion related to the prevention and treatment of sexually transmitted infections, *Public Health Nurs* 26(2):161–172, 2009.

Schackman B, Gebo KA, Walensky RP, et al: The lifetime cost of current human immunodeficiency virus care in the United States, *Med Care* 44(11):990–997, 2006.

UNAIDS: *AIDS Epidemic update 2009*, UNAIDS fact sheet, UNAIDS publication 09.36E/JC 1700E, 2009. Available at http:www.unaids.org/en/media/unaids/contentassets/dataimport/pub/factsheet/2009/20091124_fs_ssa_en.pdf. Accesssed January 29, 2011.

United States Department of Health and Human Services: *Healthy People 2020*. http://www.healthypeople.gov/2020/default.aspx. Accessed January 15, 2011.

U.S. Department of Health and Human Services, Health Resources and Services Administration: *The HIV/AIDS program: Legislation*, Washington, DC, 2010. Available at http://hab.hrsa.gov/law/leg.htm. Accessed December 26, 2010.

U.S. Department of Justice: *Questions and answers: the Americans with disabilities act and persons with HIV/AIDS*, Washington, DC, 2010, USDJ, Available at http://www.ada.gov/pubs/hivqanda.txt. Accessed December 26, 2010.

USAID Health: *HIV/AIDS, News/Info, Frequently asked questions,* Washington, DC, 2010. Available at http://www.usaid.gov/our_work/global_health/aids/News/aidsfaq.html. Accessed December 26, 2010.

World Health Organization: *WHO case definitions of HIV for surveillance and revised clinical staging and immunological classification of HIV-related disease in adults and children*, Geneva, 2007, WHO Press. Available at http://www.who.int/hiv/pub/vct/hivstaging/en/index.html. Accessed December 26, 2010.

World Health Organization: *10 facts about tuberculosis,* 2009. Available at http://www.who.int/features/factfiles/tuberculosis/en/index.html. Accessed December 26, 2010.

CHAPTER 15

Evidence-Based Practice

Marcia Stanhope, RN, DSN, FAAN

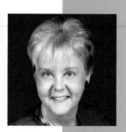

Dr. Marcia Stanhope is currently employed at the University of Kentucky College of Nursing, Lexington, Kentucky. She holds the Good Samaritan Foundation Chair and Professorship in Community Health Nursing. She has taught evidence-based practice courses, community health, public health, epidemiology, policy, primary care nursing, and administration courses. Dr. Stanhope formerly directed the Doctorate of Nursing Practice program of the College of Nursing at the University of Kentucky. In this role she developed evidence-based practice courses and implemented such practice in two nurse-managed centers. She has been responsible for both undergraduate and graduate courses in population-centered nursing. She has also taught at the University of Virginia and the University of Alabama, Birmingham. Her presentations and publications have been in the areas of home health, community health and community-focused nursing practice, and primary care nursing, including evidence-based practice.

ADDITIONAL RESOURCES

OBJECTIVES

After reading this chapter, the student should be able to do the following:
1. Define evidence-based practice.
2. Understand the history of evidence-based practice in health care.
3. Analyze the relationship between evidence-based practice and the practice of nursing in the community.
4. Provide examples of evidence-based practice in the community.
5. Identify barriers to evidence-based practice.
6. Apply evidence-based resources in practice.

KEY TERMS

evidence-based medicine, p. 339
evidence-based nursing, p. 339
evidence-based practice, p. 339

evidence-based public health, p. 339
grading the strength of evidence, p. 344
meta-analysis, p. 343

randomized controlled trial (RCT), p. 341
research utilization, p. 340
systematic review, p. 343
—*See Glossary for definitions*

Emphasis on evidence-based practice (EBP) is a recent development in health care delivery in the United States. It is a relevant approach to providing the highest quality of health care in all settings, which will result in improved health outcomes. EBP is important for all professionals who work in social and health care environments, regardless of the client or the setting with which professionals are dealing, including public health nurses who work with populations. Emphasis on EBP has resulted from increased expectations of consumers, changes in health care economics, increased expectations of accountability, advancements in technology, the knowledge explosion fueled by the Internet, and the growing number of lawsuits occurring when there is injury or harm as a result of practice decisions that are not based on the best available evidence (Leufer and Cleary-Holdforth, 2009). Nurses at all levels have an opportunity to improve the practice of nursing and client outcomes. The Institute of Medicine has set a goal that by 2020, the best available evidence will be used to make 90% of all health care decisions, yet most nurses continue to be inconsistent in implementing EBP. An even greater concern in public health is that the field is lagging behind in developing evidence-based guidelines for the community setting. It is important to recognize that regardless of the level of education, undergraduate or graduate, nurses can be involved in the development, implementation, and evaluation of the effects of EBP (Green, 2006; Melnyk, 2009; Olsen et al, 2007; Pravikoff, 2005; Vanhook, 2009).

> **DID YOU KNOW?** *Comprehensive databases are available through various Internet sites to assist nurses in applying the most recent best evidence to their clinical practice, like the Cochrane Library Database, the Centers for Disease Control and Prevention: Guide to Community Preventive Services, and others. See the WebLinks for this chapter on the book's Evolve website.*

DEFINITION OF EVIDENCE-BASED PRACTICE

The term *evidence-based* was first attributed to Gordon Gyatt, a Canadian physician at McMaster University in 1992 (Evidence Based Medicine Working Group, 1992). The term was first applied in medicine to begin the development of new ways of guiding professional decision making by using the best available

evidence. Because the concept was developed in medicine, some of the first definitions focused on evidence-based medicine.

The definition of evidence-based medicine by Sackett and associates (Sackett et al, 1996) became the industry standard. Sackett et al (1996) defined evidence-based medicine as "the conscientious, explicit, and judicious use of current best evidence in making decisions about the care of individual clients" (p 71). Without current best external evidence, they said, "practice risks become rapidly out of date, to the detriment of clients" (Sackett et al, 1996, p 72). A more succinct definition was proposed as the conscientious use of the current best evidence in making decisions about patient care (Sackett et al, 2000).

Adapting the definition by Sackett et al (1996), Rychetnik et al (2003) defined evidence-based public health as "a public health endeavor in which there is an informed, explicit, and judicious use of evidence that has been derived from any of a variety of science and social science research and evaluation methods" (p 538). Brownson et al (2009) recently expanded the definition of evidence-based public health to include "making decisions on the basis of the best available evidence, using data and information systems, applying program planning frameworks, engaging the community in decision making, conducting evaluations, and disseminating what has been learned" (p 175).

In a position statement on EBP, the Honor Society of Nursing, Sigma Theta Tau International, defined evidence-based nursing as "an integration of the best evidence available, nursing expertise, and the values and preferences of the individuals, families, and communities who are served" (Honor Society of Nursing, Sigma Theta Tau International, 2005). The definition continues to be broadened in scope and now includes a lifelong problem-solving approach to clinical practice, integrating both external and internal evidence to answer clinical questions and to achieve desired client outcomes (Melnyk and Fineout-Overholt, 2011). *External evidence* includes research and other evidence, whereas *internal evidence* includes the nurse's clinical experiences and the client's preferences.

Applied to nursing, evidence-based practice includes the best available evidence from a variety of sources including research studies, nursing experience and expertise, and community leaders. Culturally and financially appropriate interventions need to be identified when working with communities. The use of evidence to determine the appropriate use of interventions that are culturally sensitive and cost-effective is essential.

EVIDENCE-BASED PRACTICE

Chronic diseases are considered a major disease burden in the United States, accounting for 75% of all medical care costs, and 7 of 10 deaths per year. Diabetes is one of the chronic diseases considered to have a major public health impact. To meet the *Healthy People 2010* goal of eliminating racial and ethnic disparities, the CDC created a demonstration project called REACH. Community projects were funded to develop, implement, and evaluate community action plans to improve health care and outcomes for racial and ethnic groups. One funded project was the Charleston and Georgetown, South Carolina Diabetes Coalition. The coalition is described as a community campus partnership with the Medical College of South Carolina and community agencies, organizations, and neighborhoods. The project serves about 12,000 African-Americans with diabetes.

To implement the project, the coalition looked at the Chronic Care Model, and after a systematic review of the literature, decided to expand the model and developed the Community Chronic Care Model. The goals of the project were to use community-based participatory actions to decrease disparities, improve health systems using the continuous quality improvement process, educate and empower communities, and build and sustain interpersonal and interorganizational links among communities and health professionals to improve diabetes outcomes and eliminate disparities. Local coalitions were developed, funds were provided to sustain diabetes activities, two new health facilities were opened in areas of need, and free medications were offered as samples.

One of the specific health outcomes was to reduce amputations among African-American males. The University's college of nursing participated by developing and marketing a self-paced foot care educational program to train professionals in foot care. Lay educators were trained and health professionals provided patient care to the uninsured. A center for community health partnerships was established in the college of nursing and is a part of the ongoing plans for the college.

Nurse Use

Nurses can be active in establishing small groups of partners in the community to develop a plan to meet a health care need, or participate in larger coalitions like this one. The focus on developing projects to meet needs and improve health care outcomes must be based on the evidence that shows these partnerships are needed to solve the health care need and improve health care outcomes (Jenkins et al, 2010).

Jenkins C, Pope C, Magwood G: Expanding the chronic care framework to improve diabetes management: The REACH Case Study, *Prog Community Health Partnersh* 4(1):65-79, Spring 2010.

HISTORY OF EVIDENCE-BASED PRACTICE

During the mid to late 1970s, there was growing consensus among nursing leaders that scientific knowledge should be used as a basis for nursing practice. During that time, the Division of Nursing in the U.S. Public Health Service began funding research utilization projects. **Research utilization** has been defined as "the process of transforming research knowledge into practice" (Stetler, 2001, p 272) and "the use of research to guide clinical practice" (Estabrooks, Winther, and Derksen, 2004, p 293).

Three projects funded by the Division of Nursing received the most attention and were the most influential in shaping nursing's view of using research to guide practice: the Nursing Child Assessment Satellite Training Project (NCAST) (Barnard and Hoehn, 1978; King, Barnard, and Hoehn, 1981), the Western Interstate Commission for Higher Education (WICHE) Regional Program for Nursing Research Development (WICHEN) (Krueger, 1977; Krueger, Nelson, and Wolanin, 1978; Lindeman and Krueger, 1977), and the Conduct and Utilization of Research in Nursing Project (CURN) (Horsley, Crane, and Bingle, 1978; Horsley et al, 1983). Using very different approaches and methods, each project tested interventions to facilitate research use in practice.

Although nursing continued to focus on research utilization projects, medicine also began to call for physicians to increase their use of scientific evidence to make clinical decisions. In the late 1970s, David Sackett, a medical doctor and clinical epidemiologist at McMaster University, published a series of articles in the *Canadian Medical Association Journal* describing how to read research articles in clinical journals. The term *critical appraisal* was used to describe the process of evaluating the validity and applicability of research studies (Guyatt and Rennie, 2002). Later, Sackett proposed the phrase "bringing critical appraisal to the bedside" to describe the application of evidence

from medical literature to client care. This concept was used to train resident physicians at McMaster University and evolved into a "philosophy of medical practice based on knowledge and understanding of the medical literature supporting each clinical decision" (Guyatt and Rennie, 2002, p xiv).

With Gordon Guyatt as Residency Director of Internal Medicine at McMaster, the decision was made to change the program to focus on "this new brand of medicine" that Guyatt eventually called *evidence-based medicine* (Guyatt and Rennie, 2002, p xiv). Guyatt and Rennie described the goal of evidence-based medicine as being "aware of the evidence on which one's practice is based, the soundness of the evidence, and the strength of inference the evidence permits" (2002, p xiv).

In 1992 the Evidence-Based Medicine Working Group published an article in the *Journal of the American Medical Association* expanding the concept of evidence-based medicine and calling it a *paradigm shift*. A paradigm shift simply means a change from old ways of knowing to new ways of knowing and practicing. Ways of knowing in nursing have included the empirical knowledge, or the science of nursing; the aesthetic knowledge, or the art of nursing; personal knowledge, or interpersonal relationships and caring; and ethical knowledge, or moral and ethical codes of conduct usually established by professional organizations (Bradshaw, 2010). Nursing practice has often focused less on science and more on the other four ways of knowing described here.

According to the Working Group (Evidence-Based Medicine Working Group, 1992), the old paradigm viewed unsystematic clinical observations as a valid way for "building and maintaining" knowledge for clinical decision making (p 2421). In addition, principles of pathophysiology were seen as a "sufficient guide for clinical practice" (p 2421). Training, common sense, and clinical experience were considered sufficient for evaluating clinical data and developing guidelines for clinical practice. The Working Group cited developments in research over the past

30 years as providing the foundation for the paradigm shift and a "new philosophy of medical practice" (p 2421).

The new paradigm, evidence-based medicine, acknowledged clinical experience as a crucial, but insufficient, part of clinical decision making. Systematic and unbiased recording of clinical observations in the form of research will increase confidence in the knowledge gained from clinical experience. Principles of pathophysiology were seen as necessary but not sufficient knowledge for making clinical decisions. The Working Group emphasized that physicians needed to be able to critically appraise the research literature in order to appropriately apply research findings in practice. Knowledge gained from authoritative figures was also deemphasized in the new paradigm (Working Group, 1992).

In the years since the Working Group began, the term *evidence-based practice* has been proposed as a term to integrate all health professions. The underlying principle was that high-quality care is based on evidence rather than on tradition or intuition (Beyers, 1999).

Nurses have always used various resources for problem solving. Intuition, trial and error, tradition, authority, institutional standards, prior knowledge, and clinical experience have often been used as the basis for decision making in clinical settings. However, not all of these resources are reliable and all have not consistently produced desired outcomes (Bradshaw, 2010). A procedure performed based on intuition or trial and error might be performed successfully sometimes and not at other times. For example, tradition and authority, which comes from texts and policy and procedure manuals, can lead to faulty clinical decision making. Institutional standards are developed by accrediting agencies (e.g., The Joint Commission), by licensing agencies, and by professional organizations. These standards have been developed in the past primarily by expert opinion and past experiences. The standards may not reflect the best practices in the current environment or from the literature. Although prior knowledge gained in educational programs, through continuing education, or through experience can be a good teacher, it can also contain bias and quickly become outdated unless a nurse participates in constantly refreshing knowledge. For example, just because a nurse has experience in successfully performing an intervention a certain way today does not mean it is the best way or that it will be successful every time and in the future unless practices are changed based on the most current data.

When EBP was first emphasized in medicine, the focus was on the answer to clinical questions concerning an individual client problem in order to provide the best diagnosis to implement the best treatment. When nursing became involved in EBP, the focus seemed to shift to answering a clinical question about a health problem experienced by a group of clients (Levin et al, 2010).

The current nursing literature on EBP is primarily associated with applications in the acute and primary care settings and little is reported about its use in community settings. However, the basic principles of EBP can be applied at the individual level or at the community level. Although definitions of EBP vary widely in the literature, the common thread across disciplines is the application of the best available evidence to improve practice (Leufer and Cleary-Holdforth, 2009).

> **NURSING TIP** *Systematic reviews of research evidence can potentially overcome barriers to putting evidence into practice. Systematic reviews, also known as evidence summaries and integrative reviews, have been called the heart of EBP (Stevens, 2001).*

EBP has been described as both a process and a product (Bradshaw, 2010; Scott and McSherry, 2009). The product is the use of evidence to make practice changes, whereas the process is a systematic approach to locating, critiquing, synthesizing, translating, and evaluating evidence upon which to base practice changes. Scott and McSherry (2009) engaged in a process using an extensive literature review to arrive at a definition of evidence-based nursing and to differentiate the definition from evidence-based practice. Based on their review they arrived at the following definition: evidence-based nursing is a process whereby evidence, nursing theory, and the nurse's clinical expertise, are evaluated and used in conjunction with the client's involvement, to make critical decisions about the best care for the client. Continuous evaluation of the implementation of care is essential to make clinical decisions about client care for the best possible outcomes.

TYPES OF EVIDENCE

No matter which definition of EBP is supported, what counts as evidence has been the issue most hotly debated. A hierarchy of evidence, ranked in order of decreasing importance and use, has been accepted by many health professionals. The double-blind randomized controlled trial (RCT) generally ranks as the highest level of evidence followed by other RCTs, non-randomized clinical trials, quasi-experimental studies, case-controlled reports, qualitative studies, and expert opinion (Russell-Babin, 2009). Some nurses would argue that this hierarchy ignores evidence gained from clinical experience. However, the definition of evidence-based nursing presented above indicates that clinical expertise as evidence, when used with other types of evidence, is used to make clinical decisions. Also in the hierarchy of evidence, expert opinion can be gained from non-research–based published articles, professional guidelines, national guidelines, organizational opinions, and panels of experts, as well as the nurse's clinical expertise. Since it is difficult to find or perform RCTs in the community, other types of evidence have been highlighted as the best evidence in public health literature upon which to base evidence-based public health practice: scientific literature found in systematic reviews, scientific literature used or quoted in one or more journal articles, public health surveillance data, program evaluations, qualitative data obtained from community members and other stakeholders, media/marketing data such as the results of a media campaign to reduce smoking, word of mouth, and personal/professional experience (Brownson et al, 2009).

FACTORS LEADING TO CHANGE OR BARRIERS TO EVIDENCE-BASED PRACTICE

EBP represents a cultural change in practice. It provides an environment to improve both nursing practice and client outcomes. Nursing is known for providing care based on environmental and client assessments, critical observations, development of questions or hypotheses to be explored, the collecting of data from the environment through community or organizational assessments, or the client through history, physical assessment, and review of past heath records, analyzing the data to develop plans of care, whether for the individual client, family, group or community, and drawing conclusions upon which to base care for the purpose of improving client outcomes (Vanhook, 2009). However, several factors have been identified in the literature that support implementation of EBP or that will need to be overcome for nursing and other disciplines to successfully implement EBP. These factors include the following:

- Knowledge of research and current evidence
- Ability to interpret the meaning of the evidence
- Individual professional's characteristics, such as a willingness to change, or personal viewpoints about the quality and credibility of evidence
- Commitment of the time needed to implement EBP and to engage in education and directed practice
- The hierarchy of the practice environment and the level of support of managers and the ability to engage in autonomous practice,
- The philosophy of the practice environment and the willingness to embrace EBP
- The resources available to engage in EBP, such as amount of work, proper equipment, computer-based EBP programs, and information systems
- The practice characteristics, such as leadership and colleague attitudes
- Links to outside supports such as teaching facilities like a teaching health department or a university
- Political constraints and the lack of relevant and timely public health practice research (Asadoorian et al, 2010; Brownson et al, 2009; Vanhook, 2009)

Although a community agency may subscribe in theory to the use of EBP, actual implementation may be affected by the realities of the practice setting. Community-focused nursing agencies may lack the resources needed for its implementation in the clinical setting, such as time, funding, computer resources, and knowledge. Nurses may be reluctant to accept findings and feel threatened when long-established practices are questioned. Cost can also be a barrier if the clinical decision or change will require more funds than the agency has available. Compliance can be a barrier if the client will not follow the recommended intervention. Public health departments are moving toward EBP and are seeking accreditation through the national public health accreditation board. The accreditation process will be ready in 2011.

STEPS IN THE EVIDENCE-BASED PRACTICE PROCESS

EBP is a philosophy of practice that respects client values. Melnyk and Fineout-Overholt (2010) have described a seven-step EBP process:

0. Cultivating a spirit of inquiry
1. Asking clinical questions
2. Searching for the best evidence
3. Critically appraising the evidence
4. Integrating the evidence with clinical expertise and client preferences and values
5. Evaluating the outcomes of the practice decisions or changes based on evidence
6. Disseminating EBP results

Yes, their first step is step zero. This process was initially described as a five-step process by others (Dawes et al, 2004; Dicenso et al, 2005; Craig and Smyth, 2007). The unique features of the Melnyk et al model is the emphasis on the spirit of inquiry and the sharing of the results of the process.

Step zero involves a curiosity about the interventions that are being applied. Do they work, or is there a better approach? In public health nursing, for example, are there better parenting outcomes if the parents attend classes at the health department? Or are home visits to new mothers and babies more effective for achieving a healthy baby? Step one requires asking questions in a "PICOT" format. Although Melnyk et al have developed a specific process for the PICOT, the process was first described by Sackett (1996), who discussed the need to define the *(P)opulation* of interest, the *(I)ntervention* or practice strategy in question, the population or intervention to be used for *(C)omparision*, the *(O)utcome* desired, and the *(T)ime frame*. Step two involves searching for the best evidence to answer the question. This step involves searching the literature. In the case of the example above, a literature search would focus on a search of key terms like *public health nursing, parenting of new babies, parenting classes,* and *home visits*. Step three requires a critical appraisal of the evidence found in step two. To appraise the literature found, Melnyk suggests asking three questions about each of the articles found in the literature search: (1) the validity, (2) the importance, and (3) whether or not the results of the article will help you as a nurse provide quality care for your clients. Step four is the step in which the evidence found is integrated with clinical expertise and client values. Institutional standards and practice guidelines, as well as cost of care and support of the health care environment to implement the findings, are all factors considered in this step. Step five requires an evaluation of the outcomes of practice decisions and changes that were based on the answers to the first four steps. The goal in evaluation is a positive change in quality of care and health care outcomes. In the example of group parenting classes versus home visits to new mothers and babies, current literature suggests improved quality and health care outcomes with home visits (The Pew Center, 2010).

Step six is disseminating outcomes of the results to others, to colleagues, to the employing agency's administration, to faculty and other students, and through a poster or podium presentation of the student nurse organizations, or professional organizations. Professional organizations often sponsor student presentations for undergraduates as well as graduate students. Sharing of information is most important because it prevents each individual nurse from trying to find the best answer to the same question answered by someone else, and it gives us the basis for asking new questions. Sharing makes practice more efficient and improves quality and health care outcomes.

In a busy community practice setting, it is often difficult for nurses to access evidence-based resources. Using evidence-based clinical practice guidelines is one way for nurses to provide evidence-based nursing care in an efficient manner. Clinical practice guidelines are usually developed by a group of experts in the field who have reviewed the evidence and made recommendations based on the best available evidence. The recommendations are usually graded according to the quality and quantity of the evidence. The Public Health Practice Reference is an example of practice guidelines developed for population-centered nurses' use.

APPROACHES TO FINDING EVIDENCE

Returning to the previous example, the clinical question has been stated and the population has been defined as new mothers and babies. Two interventions will be compared. The outcome is stated as healthy babies and the time frame may be 6 months or 1 year, or another time at which the outcomes of the interventions will be evaluated.

Four approaches are described that allow the nurse to read research/non-research evidence in a condensed format. The first, a systematic review, is "a method of identifying, appraising, and synthesizing research evidence. The aim is to evaluate and interpret all available research that is relevant to a particular research question" (Rychetnik et al, 2003, p 542). A systematic review is usually done by more than one person and describes the methods used to search for the evidence and evaluate the evidence. Systematic reviews can be accessed from most databases, such as Medline and CINAHL. The Cochrane Library is an electronic database that contains regularly updated evidence-based health care databases maintained by the Cochrane Collaboration, a not-for-profit organization (http://www.cochrane.org). The Cochrane Library is composed of three main branches: systematic reviews, trials register, and methodology database. The Cochrane Library publishes systematic reviews on a wide variety of topics. Systematic reviews differ from traditional literature review publications in that systematic reviews require more rigor and contain less opinion of the author. Systematic reviews for public health can be found in the Guide to Community Preventive Services, the Cochrane Public Health Group, the Center for Reviews and Dissemination, and the Campbell Collaboration (Box 15-1).

The second approach, meta-analysis, is "a specific method of statistical synthesis used in some systematic reviews, where the results from several studies are quantitatively combined and summarized" (Rychetnik et al, 2003, p 542). A well-designed systematic review or meta-analysis can provide stronger evidence than a single randomized controlled trial.

The integrative review is a form of a systematic review that does not have the summary statistics found in the meta-analysis because of the limitations of the studies that are reviewed (e.g., small sample size of the population). Narrative review is a review done on published papers that support the reviewer's particular point of view or opinion and is used to provide a general discussion of the topic reviewed. This review does not often include an explicit or systematic review process.

Undergraduate students often perform narrative reviews. However, it is important to learn the process for systematic reviews, especially the use of the results of systematic reviews. Reading systematic reviews that have been completed is helpful in answering the question related to the EBP process.

What counts as evidence has also been argued in the public health literature (Victora and Habicht, 2004). RCTs, which are the highest level of evidence used to make clinical decisions, are appropriate for evaluating many interventions in medicine, but are often inappropriate for evaluating public health interventions. For example, an RCT can be designed ethically to test a new medication for diabetes, but not for a smoking cessation intervention. In a smoking cessation intervention, subjects could not be assigned randomly to smoking or non-smoking groups because a smoking cessation intervention is not appropriate for someone who does not smoke. In this situation, a case-control study would be most appropriate (see Chapter 12). Today there are many community-based clinical trials assisting in finding answers to the questions of which population level intervention has the best outcomes. (Visit the CDC website to review these trials.)

HOW TO Develop an Evidence-Based Practice Guide to a Community Preventive Service

- *Form a development team, preferably an interprofessional team, to choose a topic based on a community issue that needs to be addressed.*
- *Develop a structured approach to organize, group, select, and evaluate the interventions from the literature that work to address the issue.*
- *Select the interventions the group wishes to evaluate for use.*
- *Assess the quality of the evidence found in the literature.*
- *Summarize the findings.*
- *Make recommendations.*
- *Write a protocol or step-by-step guide to resolving the community issue.*

From Task Force on Community Prevention Services: National Center for Chronic Disease Prevention and Health Promotion. Available at http://www.cdc.gov. Accessed December 26, 2010.

HOW TO Develop an Evidence-Based Protocol

Evidence-based protocols are a recognized approach to providing quality client care. Such protocols enhance the abilities of providers and can reduce health care errors. The following are steps to developing a protocol:
- *Identify the problem.*
- *Identify stakeholders*
- *Form a team of others to help develop the protocol*
- *Develop an action plan with project goals and a timeline.*
- *Review the available evidence.*
- *Examine current practice and identify gaps as well as best practices.*
- *Develop the protocol focusing on gaps.*
- *Initiate the approval process with the setting.*
- *Evaluate current practices and modify as needed.*
- *Educate others who will use the protocol.*
- *Implement the protocol.*
- *Evaluate protocol for safety, effectiveness, and adherence.*

From McEuen JA, Gardner KP, Barnachea DF, et al: An evidence-based protocol for managing hypoglycemia, AJN 110(7): 40-45, 2010.

BOX 15-1   RESOURCES FOR IMPLEMENTING EVIDENCE-BASED PRACTICE

The following resources can assist nurses in developing evidence-based nursing practice:

1. The *Evidence-Based Practice for Public Health Project* at the University of Massachusetts Medical School Library has developed a website for evidence-based practice in public health (http://library.umassmed.edu/ebpph/). Many bibliographical databases, such as Medline, do not list all the journals of interest to public health workers. The project provides access to numerous databases of interest concerning public health. From the project's website, nurses can access free public health online journals and databases.

2. The *Agency for Healthcare Quality and Research (AHRQ)* developed clinical guidelines based on the best available evidence for several clinical topics, such as pain management. The guidelines are accessible via the agency's website (http://www.ahrq.gov) and serve as a resource to nurses involved in individual client care.

3. The *National Guideline Clearinghouse* (http://www.guideline.gov/), an initiative of the AHRQ, is an online resource for evidence-based clinical practice guidelines. AHRQ also supports Evidence-Based Practice Centers, which write evidence reports on various topics.

4. *PubMed* (http://www.pubmed.gov/) is a bibliographic database developed and maintained by the National Library of Medicine. Bibliographical information from Medline is covered in PubMed and includes references for nursing, medicine, dentistry, the health care system, and preclinical sciences. Full texts of referenced articles are often included. Searches can be limited to type of evidence (e.g., diagnosis, therapy) and systematic reviews.

5. The *Cochrane Database of Systematic Reviews* is a collection of more than 1000 systematic reviews of effects in health care internationally. These reviews are accessible at a cost via the website (http://www.cochrane.org). Nurses may also have free access from a medical library.

6. The *Evidence-Based Nursing Journal* (http://ebn.bmjjournals.com/) is published quarterly. The purpose of the journal is to select articles reporting studies and reviews from health-related literature that warrant immediate attention by nurses attempting to keep pace with advances in their profession. Using predefined criteria, the best quantitative and qualitative original articles are abstracted in a structured format, commented on by clinical experts, and shared in a timely fashion. The research questions, methods, results, and evidence-based conclusions are reported. The website for the journal is http://www.evidencebasednursing.com.

7. The Honor Society of Nursing, Sigma Theta Tau International, sponsors the online peer-reviewed journal *Worldviews on Evidence-Based Nursing* that publishes systematic reviews and research articles on best evidence that supports nursing practice globally. The journal is available by subscription (http://www.nursingsociety.org/).

8. The *Task Force on Community Preventive Services* is an independent, non-federal task force appointed by the director of the Centers for Disease Control and Prevention. Information about the Task Force may be found at the website http://www.thecommunityguide.org. The Task Force is charged with determining the topics to be addressed by the CDC's Community Guide and the most appropriate means to assess evidence regarding

population-based interventions. The Task Force reviews and assesses the quality of available evidence on the effects of essential community preventive services. The multidisciplinary Task Force determines the scope of the Community Guide that will be used by health departments and agencies to determine best practices for preventive health in populations.

9. The *U.S. Preventive Services Task Force (USPSTF)* is an independent panel of private-sector experts in prevention and primary care. The USPSTF conducts rigorous, impartial assessments of the scientific evidence for the effectiveness of a broad range of clinical preventive services, including screening, counseling, and preventive medications. Its recommendations are considered the "gold standard" for clinical preventive services. The mission of the USPSTF is to evaluate the benefits of individual services based on age, gender, and risk factors for disease; make recommendations about which preventive services should be incorporated routinely into primary medical care and for which populations; and identify a research agenda for clinical preventive care. Recommendations of the USPSTF are published as the *Guide to Clinical Preventive Services*. The guide is available online at http://www.ahrq.gov/clinic/uspstfix.htm.

10. The *Centers for Disease Control and Prevention* (www.cdc.gov) publishes guidelines on immunizations and sexually transmitted diseases. Guidelines are developed by experts in the field appointed by the U.S. Department of Health and Human Services and the CDC.

11. *Cochrane Public Health Group (PHRG)*, formerly the health promotion and public health field, aims to work with contributors to produce and publish Cochrane reviews of the effects of population-level public health interventions. The PHRG undertakes systematic reviews of the effects of public health interventions to improve health and other outcomes at the population level, not those targeted at individuals. Thus, it covers interventions seeking to address macroenvironmental and distal social environmental factors that influence health. In line with the underlying principles of public health, these reviews seek to have a significant focus on equity and aim to build the evidence to address the social determinants of health. (Visit http://www.ph.cochrane.org/.)

12. *Center for Reviews and Dissemination (CRD)* is part of the National Institute for Health Research and is a department of the University of York. CRD, which was established in 1994, is one of the largest groups in the world engaged exclusively in evidence synthesis in the health field. CRD undertakes systematic reviews evaluating the research evidence on health and public health questions of national and international importance. (Visit http://www.york.ac.uk/inst/crd/index.htm.)

13. *Campbell Collaboration*, named after Donald Campbell, was founded on the principle that systematic reviews on the effects of interventions will inform and help improve policy and services. The collaboration strives to make the best social science research available and accessible. Campbell reviews provide high-quality evidence of what works to meet the needs of service providers, policy makers, educators and their students, professional researchers, and the general public. Areas of interest include crime, justice, education, and social welfare. (Visit http://www.campbellcollaboration.org/.)

APPROACHES TO EVALUATING EVIDENCE

One approach used in evaluating evidence is **grading the strength of evidence**. When evidence is graded, the evidence is assigned a "grade" based on the number and type of well-designed studies, and the presence of similar findings in all of the studies. Grading evidence has been debated so strongly that in 2002 the Agency for Healthcare Research and Quality

(AHRQ) commissioned a study to describe existing systems used to evaluate the usefulness of studies and strength of evidence. The report reviewed 40 systems and identified three domains for evaluating systems for the grading of evidence: quality, quantity, and consistency. The *quality* of a study refers to the extent to which bias is minimized. *Quantity* refers to the number of studies, the magnitude of the effect, and the sample size. *Consistency* refers to studies that have similar findings,

TABLE 15-1	TYPOLOGY FOR CLASSIFYING INTERVENTIONS BY LEVEL OF SCIENTIFIC EVIDENCE		
TYPE/CATEGORY	**STRENGTH/HOW ESTABLISHED**	**CONSIDERATIONS FOR THE LEVEL OF SCIENTIFIC EVIDENCE — QUALITY**	**QUANTITY/CONSISTENCY DATA SOURCE EXAMPLES**
Evidence-based I	Peer review via systematic or narrative review	Based on study design and execution External validity Potential side benefits or harms Costs and cost-effectiveness	*Community Guide* Cochrane reviews Narrative reviews based on published literature
Effective II	Peer review	Based on study design and execution External validity Potential side benefits or harms Costs and cost-effectiveness	Articles in the scientific literature Research-tested intervention programs (123) Technical reports with peer review
Promising III	Written program evaluation without formal peer review	Summative evidence of effectiveness Formative evaluation data Theory-consistent, plausible, potentially high-reach, low-cost, replicable	State or federal government reports (without peer review) Conference presentations
Emerging IV	Ongoing work, practice-based summaries, or evaluation works in progress	Formative evaluation data Theory-consistent, plausible, potentially high-reaching, low-cost, replicable Face validity	Evaluability assessments Pilot studies NIH CRISP database Projects funded by health foundations

From Brownson RC, Fielding JE, Maylahn CM: Evidence-based public health: a fundamental concept for public health practice, *Annu Rev Public Health* 30:175-201, 2009.

using similar and different study designs (West et al, 2002). An example of how the U.S. Preventive Services Task Force graded the strength of evidence for the *Guidelines for Clinical Preventive Services* can be found at the website at the end of this chapter.

As indicated, many frameworks exist for evaluating the strength and the usefulness of the evidence found in the literature and other sources, such as professional standards. A popular framework was developed by the Agency for Healthcare Quality. Fineout-Overholt et al (2010) have also developed an approach for evaluating evidence. Although these approaches vary in the factors they evaluate, the best approach to choose is one that not only evaluates the strength, but also the usefulness of the evidence. Table 15-1 provides an example of an approach for evaluating evidence.

The strength of the literature is measured by the type of evidence it represents. For example, the RCT is the evidence that has the greatest strength upon which to make a clinical decision. In contrast opinion articles, descriptive studies and professional reports of expert committees have less strength. The usefulness of the evidence is measured by whether the evidence is valid, whether it is important, and whether it can be used to assist in making practice decisions or changes in the community environment and with the population of interest to improve outcomes (Scott and McSherry, 2009). The best RCT conducted in a hospital setting, using an intervention to prevent falls, may not be applicable at all in a community setting. Therefore, although it may be a strong study with outcomes that improve health, it may not have the usefulness for applicability in the community because of the setting in which it was conducted.

Shaughnessy, Slawson, and Bennett (1994) proposed criteria for evaluating the usefulness of evidence, calling the process *patient oriented evidence that matters* (POEM). In general, the reader should ask the following questions: "What are the results? (Are they important?) Are the results valid? How can the

results be applied to client care?" (p 489). Application of POEM can be found at www.essentialevidenceplus.com. Brownson et al (2009) proposed that the following questions be asked for EBP (plus suggested application examples):

- What is the size of the public health problem? What is the need for improved health outcomes for new mothers and babies in our community?
- Can interventions be found in the literature to address the problem (e.g., home visits or parenting classes)?
- Is the intervention useful in this community, with this population, or with populations at risk (e.g., the low income or uninsured)?
- Is the intervention the best one or are there other ways to address the problem considering cost and potential health outcomes for the population? (Assess cost and health outcomes of both of the interventions before choosing, including the nurses available to make home visits or who have the skills to teach the parenting class.)

Several variables are considered important in determining the quality of evidence used to make clinical decisions (Polit and Beck, 2009):

- *Sample selection:* Sample selection should be as unbiased as possible. For example, a sample is randomly selected when each subject has an equal chance of being selected from the population of interest. Random selection offers the least bias of any type of sample selection. Other types of sample selection such as convenience sampling contain researcher or evaluator bias.
- *Randomization:* When testing an intervention, randomly assign participants to either the intervention or control group. This type of assignment is less biased than if participants are allowed to choose the group they want to join.
- *Blinding:* The researcher or evaluator should not know which participants are in the experimental (treatment) group or

which are in the control group. The researcher or evaluator is "blinded" as to who is receiving the treatment and who is not receiving the treatment.

- *Sample size:* The sample size should be large enough to show an effect of the intervention. In general, the larger the sample size, the better.
- *Description of intervention:* The intervention should be described in detail and explicitly enough that another person could duplicate the study if desired.
- *Outcomes:* The outcomes should be measured accurately.
- *Length of follow-up:* Depending on the intervention, the participants should be followed for a long enough period of time to determine if the intervention continued to work or if the results just happened by chance.
- *Attrition:* Few subjects should have dropped out of the study.
- *Confounding variables:* Variables that could affect the outcome should be accounted for either by statistical methods or by study measurements.
- *Statistical analysis:* Statistical analysis should be appropriate to determine the desired outcome.

DID YOU KNOW? *It can take 16 to 20 years for research to change practice.*

APPROACHES TO IMPLEMENTING EVIDENCE-BASED PRACTICE

The first step toward implementing EBP in nursing is recognizing the current status of one's own practice and believing that care based on the best evidence will lead to improved client outcomes (Melnyk et al, 2010). Since EBP is a relatively new concept, many practicing nurses are not familiar with the application of EBP and may lack computer and Internet skills necessary to implement EBP. Also, implementation will be successful only when nurses practice in an environment that supports evidence-based care. Public health nurses consider EBP as a process to improve practice and outcomes and use the evidence to influence policies that will improve the health of communities.

THE CUTTING EDGE *Many clinical practice guidelines of interest to nurses working in the community can be easily downloaded to a handheld device for easy access in the community without having a computer available.*

CURRENT PERSPECTIVES

Cost Versus Quality

Much of the pressure to use EBP comes from third-party payers and is a response to the need to contain costs and reduce legal liability. Nurses must question whether the current agenda to contain health care costs creates pressure to focus on those research results that favor cost saving at the expense of quality outcomes for clients. Outcomes include client and community satisfaction and the safety of care. Costs can be weighed against outcomes when EBP is used to show the best practices

EVIDENCE-BASED PRACTICE

This study used a population-based descriptive survey design to describe access to health care services and perceived health care needs of people who live in coal-producing counties in southwest Virginia. A researcher-developed survey was mailed to a random sample of people who lived in the area. One person in the household was asked to complete the survey about household demographics, health insurance coverage, and needs such as prescription and health care services, family health problems, and health behaviors. A total of 922 surveys were completed. The average age of respondents was 54 years, with an annual income range of $25,000 to $29,000. Most of the respondents were employed and had health insurance, usually Medicare or Medicaid; however, 80% of other people in the households did not have health insurance.

The top 10 health problems in order of prevalence were hypertension, arthritis, obesity, back problems, tooth cavities, depression, loss of many teeth, diabetes, heart disease, and asthma. Most did not see a health care provider or dentist regularly. About half of the respondents had problems paying for health needs not covered by insurance, such as prescription medications and dental, vision, and preventive care. Family members often shared medications. There was also concern about the costs, lack of specialty providers, and long waits for appointments. About one third of the respondents thought they had fair or poor health, and 50% smoked cigarettes.

Nurse Use
Nurses can screen for depression and work with pharmacists in the community to develop educational programs to explain the dangers of medication sharing. They can also work with community leaders to overcome problems with transportation.

Huttlinger K, Schaller-Ayers J, Lawson T: Health care in Appalachia: a population-based approach, *Public Health Nurs* 21(2):103-110, 2004.

WHAT DO YOU THINK? *For EBP to be fully implemented, an organization must value EBP. What factors do you think support the development of an environment for nurses to implement EBP in the community?*

LEVELS OF PREVENTION

Using Evidence-Based Practice

According to evidence collected and averaged by the Task Force on Community Preventive Services, the following are interventions supported by the literature at each level of prevention:

Primary Prevention
Extended and extensive mass media campaigns reduce youth initiation of tobacco use.

Secondary Prevention
Client reminders and recalls via mail, telephone, e-mail, or a combination of these strategies are effective in increasing compliance with screening activities such as those for colorectal and breast cancer.

Tertiary Prevention
Diabetes self-management education in community gathering places improves glycemic control.

From Task Force on Community Prevention Services: National Center for Chronic Disease Prevention and Health Promotion. Available at http://www.cdc.gov. Accessed September 6, 2010.

available to reduce possible harm to clients (Leufer and Cleary-Holdforth, 2009; Asadoorian et al, 2010).

Individual Differences

EBP cannot be applied as a universal remedy without attention to client differences. When EBP is applied at the community level, best evidence may point to a solution that is not sensitive to cultural issues and distinctions and thus may not be acceptable to the community. Ethical practice in communities requires attention to community differences.

Appropriate Evidence-Based Practice Methods for Population-Centered Nursing Practice

Gaining a number of perspectives in a situated community is important for nurses using EBP. Nursing has a legitimate role to play in interprofessional community-focused practice and can contribute to its evidence base. Nurses are obliged to ensure that the evidence applied to practice is acceptable to the community. Establishing an EBP culture depends on the use of both qualitative and quantitative research approaches, or the best evidence available at the time. For example, a quantitative research study of a community health center could provide information about patterns of client use, the cost of various services, and the use of different health care providers. However, when quantitative research is combined with qualitative research, the nurse can gain an understanding of *why* clients use or do not use the services and help the health center be both clinically effective and cost effective. Evidence from multiple research methods has the potential to enrich the application of evidence and improve nursing practice (Wittemore, 2005).

The rising cost of health care will demand a more critical look at the benefits and costs of EBP. Finding resources to implement EBP will continue to be a challenge requiring creative strategies. An emphasis on quality care, equal distribution of health care resources, and cost control will continue. Implementing EBP can assist nurses in addressing these issues in the clinical setting. However, EBP can save money by providing the best care possible.

As nurses implement EBP in an environment focused on cost savings, the potential for governments, managed care organizations, or other health care agencies to endorse reimbursement of health care options solely on the basis of cost, without allowing for individual variation or considering environmental issues, will continue to be a concern. Nurses must use caution in adopting EBP in a prescriptive manner in different community environments. One aspect of the new health care reform act (PL 111-148) addresses the development of task forces on preventive services and community preventive services to develop, update, and disseminate EBP recommendations of the use of community preventive services. In addition, grant programs to support EBP delivery in the community are addressed in the Health Care Reform Act of 2010.

Although the Internet is one source of evidence data (see Box 15-1), there may be a lack of quality indicators to evaluate the myriad of websites claiming to contain evidence-based information. It is essential to evaluate the quantity of the information on the website, whether it comes from a reputable agency or scholar,

LINKING CONTENT TO PRACTICE

It is important for nurses to acknowledge and understand EBP. They can participate by applying EBP or they can add to the research base for public health through active programs of research, participating in systematic reviews, or reviewing the best evidence available to them by reading published systematic reviews. Nurses can demonstrate leadership in supporting EBP by becoming change agents, fostering a cultural change in the practice environment, and assisting nurses who do not know how to use EBP to make a difference in practice.

For example, nurses who have recently graduated are knowledgeable about the use of evidence in practice. The new nurses can assist nurses who have been out of school for awhile to find sources of evidence upon which to base their practice, such as referring them to the *Guide to Community Preventive Services*. Using evidence in practice will demonstrate its value, but implementation can be difficult because of the sheer volume of evidence and increasing population needs. Sharing knowledge and engaging in teamwork can help to overcome these barriers.

Nurses have an important role to play in developing and using clinical guidelines for community practices. Use of a community development model and engaging in community partnerships will ensure that the community's perspective is included (see Chapter 18).

Nurses active in EBP can devote attention to understanding how best to incorporate the guidelines into practice demonstrating practice excellence. EBP offers the opportunity for shared decision making because it can help nurses focus their thinking, observe process outcomes, and thus improve care for clients by communicating with leaders and other nurses what they have observed. Participation in EBP offers continuing professional growth and a feeling of value, recognition for contributions, and respect from peers and administrators (Bradshaw, 2010).

and whether the source of the website has a financial interest in the acceptance of the evidence presented. (Refer to Chapter 16 on health education, which discusses the Internet as a source of data and how to evaluate its usefulness and reliability.)

HEALTHY PEOPLE 2020 OBJECTIVES

Healthy People 2020 objectives offer a systematic approach to health improvement. See the *Healthy People 2020* box for the most recent objectives to improving clients' understanding of EBP and how they can contribute to health care decisions.

EXAMPLE OF APPLICATION OF EVIDENCE-BASED PRACTICE TO PUBLIC HEALTH NURSING

Chapter 9 describes The Intervention Wheel, a population-based practice model for public health nursing. The model consists of three levels of practice at the community, systems, and individual/family levels. It also consists of 17 public health interventions for improving population health. The model was originally developed using a qualitative grounded theory process but did not include a systematic review of evidence to support the interventions or their application to practice. Initially, the model was developed from an extensive analysis of the actual work of 200 practicing public health nurses working in a variety of settings. The 17 interventions grew out of this analysis, as did the three levels of practice. The authors indicated that the original intent was to provide a

♥ HEALTHY PEOPLE 2020

Information access is important to assure clients and communities have the correct information to make EBP health care decisions. The *Healthy People 2020* objectives related to providing resources are as follows:

- HC/HIT-6.3: Increase the proportion of persons who use electronic personal health management tools.
- HC/HIT-4: Increase the proportion of patients whose doctor recommends personalized health information resources to help them manage their health.
- HC/HIT-12: Increase the proportion of crisis and emergency risk messages, intended to protect the public's health, that demonstrate the use of best practices.
- HC/HIT-11: Increase the proportion of meaningful users of health information technology.
- HC/HIT-13: Increase the social marketing in health promotion and disease prevention.

From U.S. Department of Health and Human Services: *Healthy People 2020: Roadmap to Improving All American's Health,* Washington, DC, 2010, U.S. Government Printing Office.

description of the scope and breadth of public health nursing practice. Because of the positive response to the Intervention Wheel, the decision was made to complete a systematic review of the evidence supporting the use of the Intervention Wheel. The goal was to examine the evidence underlying the interventions and the levels of practice. The systematic review involved answering six questions, a comprehensive search of literature, a survey of 51 BSN programs in five states, and a critique (by five graduate students) of the 665 pieces of evidence found in the literature review for rigor (strength and usefulness). After limiting the final review to 221 sources of evidence, each source was independently rated by at least two members of a 42-member panel of practicing public health nurses and educators. The 42-member panel met to reach consensus on the outcomes of the reviews. The outcomes were field-tested with 150 practicing nurses, then critiqued by a national panel of 20 experts. The Intervention Wheel presented in Chapter 9 is the result of this systematic review and

TABLE 15-2	CORE PUBLIC HEALTH FUNCTIONS AND RELATED EVIDENCE-BASED NURSING INTERVENTIONS
CORE FUNCTIONS	**RELATED NURSING INTERVENTIONS**
Assessment	Diagnose and investigate health problems and hazards in the community.
	Mobilize community partnerships to identify and solve health problems.
	Link people to needed health services.
	Use evidence-based practice for new insights and innovative solutions to health problems.
Policy development	Inform, educate, and empower communities about health issues.
	Develop policies and plans using evidence-based practice that supports individual and community health efforts.
Assurance	Monitor health status to identify community health problems.
	Enforce laws and regulations that protect health and ensure safety.
	Ensure the provision of health care that is otherwise unavailable.
	Ensure a competent public health and personal health care workforce.
	Use evidence-based practice to evaluate effectiveness, accessibility, and quality of personal and population-based services.

critique (Keller et al, 2004). Although this critique may appear overwhelming, the undergraduate or graduate student may be involved in such a systematic critique as one of many participants contributing to the outcome of such a review. Table 15-2 applies some of the interventions to the core functions of public health.

CHAPTER REVIEW

PRACTICE APPLICATION

A nurse who is the director of a public health clinic is in the process of analyzing how best to expand services to operate as a full-time clinic in the most cost-effective and clinically effective manner. The director gathers evidence from the literature on public health clinics in rural settings to evaluate cost and clinical effectiveness of various models. The nurse also considers evidence from the following sources in the decision-making process: client satisfaction research data, knowledge of clinic staff, expert opinion of community advisory board members, evidence from community partners, and data on service needs in the state. Having examined the evidence, the nurse decides that incremental (step-by-step) growth toward full-time status is warranted. Evidence of needs in the community and analysis of statistical data indicate that the addition of wellness

services for children is a priority and a pediatric nurse practitioner is hired as a first step to assist the public health nurses while planning for full-time status continues.

A. Evaluation of the evidence gathered demonstrates which of the following?
 1. Effectiveness of the intervention in communities
 2. Application of the data to populations and communities
 3. Existence of positive or negative health outcomes
 4. Economic consequences of the intervention
 5. Barriers to implementation of the interventions in communities
B. Explain how this example applies principles of EBP.
 Answers can be found on the Evolve site.

KEY POINTS

- Evidence-based practice was developed in other countries before its use in the United States.
- The Institute of Medicine has indicated that by 2020, 90% of all health care should be evidence based.
- EBP is a paradigm shift in health care and nursing.
- EBP is both a process and a product.
- Application of EBP in relation to clinical decision making in population-centered nursing concentrates on interventions and strategies geared to communities and populations rather than to individuals.
- Nurses at all levels have an opportunity to improve the practice of nursing and client outcomes.
- The EBP process has seven steps.
- Approaches to EBP include systematic review, meta-analysis, integrative review, and narrative review.
- Evaluating the strength and usefulness of evidence is essential to finding the best evidence on which to make practice decisions.
- Cost and quality of care are issues in EBP.
- EBP includes interventions based on theory, expert opinions, provider knowledge, and research.
- Use of a community development model and community partnership model involves community leaders in making decisions about best practices in their community.
- The Intervention Wheel is an example of a result of EBP.
- Health Care Reform supports EBP.

CLINICAL DECISION-MAKING ACTIVITIES

1. Give an example of how undergraduates can be involved in EBP.
2. Explain how the nurse's knowledge of the community relates to EBP. Give examples.
3. What are the barriers to implementing EBP? How can these barriers be resolved?
4. Is the cost or quality of care more important in EBP? Debate this issue with classmates.
5. When working with a community to improve its health, is it more important to consider the perspectives of the community or those of the provider when defining health problems? Elaborate.
6. Invite the director of nursing from the local health department to speak to your class. Ask if evidence is used to develop nursing policies and practice guidelines. If not, why not?
7. Explain how you can apply evidence to your practice.

REFERENCES

Asadoorian J, Hearson B, Satyanarayana S, Ursel J: Evidence-based practice in healthcare: an exploratory cross-discipline comparison of enhancers and barriers, *J Healthcare Qual* 32(3):15–22, 2010.

Barnard K, Hoehn R: *Nursing child assessment satellite training: final report*, Hyattsville, MD, 1978, DHEW, Division of Nursing.

Beyers M: About evidence-based nursing practice, *Nurs Manag* 30:56, 1999.

Bradshaw WG: Importance of nursing leadership in advancing evidence-based nursing practice, *Neonatal Network* 29(2):117–122, 2010.

Brownson RC, Fielding JE, Maylahn CM: Evidence-based public health: a fundamental concept for public health practice, *Annu Rev Public Health* 30:175–202, 2009.

Craig JV, Smyth RL: *The evidence-based practice manual for nurses*, ed 2, Edinburgh, 2007, Churchill Livingstone Elsevier.

Dawes M, Davies P, Gray A, et al: *Evidence-based practice: a primer for health care professionals*, ed 2, London, 2004, Churchill Livingstone Elsevier.

Dicenso A, Guyatt G, Ciliska D, editors: *Evidence-based nursing: a guide to clinical practice*, St Louis, 2005, Elsevier Mosby.

Estabrooks CA, Winther C, Derksen L: Mapping the field: a biliometric analysis of the research utilization literature in nursing, *Nurs Res* 53:293–303, 2004.

Evidence-Based Medicine Working Group: Evidence-based medicine: a new approach to teaching the practice of medicine, *JAMA* 268:2420–2425, 1992.

Fineout-Overholt E, Malnyk B, Stillwell SB, Wiliamson KM: Critical appraisal of the evidence: part 1: an introduction to gathering, evaluating, and recording the evidence, *AJN* 110(7):47–52, 2010.

Green ML: Evaluating evidence-based practice performance, *ACP Journal Club* 143(2):Suppl. A-8, A-9, A-10.

Guyatt G, Rennie D, editors: *Users' guides to the medical literature: a manual for evidence-based clinical practice*, Chicago, 2002, AMA.

Honor Society of Nursing, Sigma Theta Tau International: *Position statement on evidence-based nursing*, Indianapolis, IN, 2005. Available at http://www.nursingsociety.org. Accessed December 26, 2010.

Horsley JA, Crane J, Bingle JD: Research utilization as an organizational process, *J Nurs Admin* 8:4–6, 1978.

Horsley JA, Crane J, Crabtree MK, et al: *Using research to improve nursing practice: a guide*, San Francisco, 1983, Grune & Stratton.

Jenkins C, Pope C, Magwood G: Expanding the chronic care framework to improve diabetes management: The REACH Case Study, *Prog Community Health Partnersh* 4(1):65–79, Spring 2010.

Keller L, Strohschein S, Lia-Hoagbert B, Schaffer MA: Population-based public health interventions: practice-based and evidence-supported. Part I, *Public Health Nurs* 21(5):453–468, 2004.

King D, Barnard KE, Hoehn R: Disseminating the results of nursing research, *Nurs Outlook* 29:164–169, 1981.

Krueger JC: Utilizing clinical nursing research findings in practice: a structured approach, *Commun Nurs Res* 9:381–394, 1977.

Krueger JC, Nelson AH, Wolanin MO: *Nursing research: development, collaboration and utilization*, Germantown, MD, 1978, Aspen.

Leufer T, Cleary-Holdforth J: Evidence-based practice: improving patient outcomes, *Nurs Standard* 23(32):35–39, 2009.

Levin RF, Keefer JM, Marren J, et al: Evidence-based practice improvement: merging 2 paradigms, *J Nurs Care Qual* 25(2):117–126, 2010.

Lindeman CA, Krueger JC: Increasing the quality, quantity, and use of nursing research, *Nurs Outlook* 25:450–454, 1977.

Melnyk BM, Fineout-Overholt E, Stillwell SB, Williamson KM: Igniting a spirit of inquiry: an essential foundation for evidence-based practice, *AJN* 109(11):49–52, 2009.

Melnyk B, Fineout-Overholt E, Stillwell SB, Williamson KM: The seven steps of evidence-based practice, *AJN* 110(1):51–53, 2010.

Melnyk BM, Fineout-Overholt E: *Evidence-based practice in nursing and healthcare: a guide to best practice*, ed 2, Philadelphia, 2011, Lippincott. Williams & Wilkins.

Olsen L, et al: *The learning health care system: workshop summary*, Washington, DC, 2007, National Academies Press.

Polit DF, Beck CT: *Nursing research principles and methods*, ed 7, New York, 2009, Lippincott, Williams & Wilkins.

Pravikoff DS, Pierce ST, Tanner A: Evidence based practice readiness study supported by academy nursing informatics expert panel, *Nurs Outlook* 53(1):49–50, 2005.

Russell-Babin K: Seeing through the clouds in evidence-based practice, *Nurs Manag* 40(11):26–32, 2009.

Rychetnik L, Hawe P, Waters E, et al: A glossary for evidence-based public health, *J Epidemiol Community Health* 58:538–545, 2003.

Sackett DL, Rosenberg WMC, Gray J, et al: Evidence-based medicine: what it is and what it isn't, *Br Med J* 312:71–72, 1996.

Sackett DL, Straus SE, Richardson WS, et al: *Evidence-based medicine: how to practice and teach EBM*, London, 2000, Churchill Livingstone.

Scott K, McSherry R: Evidence-based nursing: clarifying the concepts for nurses in practice, *J Clin Nurs* 18:1085–1095, 2009.

Shaughnessy AF, Slawson DC, Bennett JA: Becoming an information master: a guidebook to the medical information jungles, *J Fam Pract* 39:489–499, 1994.

Stetler CB: Updating the Stetler model of research utilization to facilitate evidence-based practice, *Nurs Outlook* 49:272–279, 2001.

Stevens KR: Systematic reviews: the heart of evidence-based practice, *AACN Clin Issues* 12:529–538, 2001.

Task Force on Community Preventive Services: *Guide to community preventive services, July 27, 2007.* Available at http://www.thecommu nityguide.org/diabetes/default.htm. Accessed September 26, 2010.

Task Force on Community Preventive Services: National Center for Chronic Disease Prevention and Health Promotion, 2010. Available at www.cdc.gov. Accessed August 6, 2010.

The Pew Center on the States: *The case for home visiting, May 2010.* Available at www.pewcenteronthestates.org. Accessed September 17, 2010.

Titler MG, Steelman VJ, Budreau G, et al: The Iowa model of evidence-based practice to promote quality care, *Crit Care Nurs Clin North Am* 13:497–509, 2001.

U.S. Department of Health and Human Services: *Healthy People 2020: ROADMAP TO IMPROVING ALL AMERICAN'S HEALTH*, Washington, DC, 2010, U.S. Government Printing Office.

U.S. Preventive Services Task Force: *Task force ratings: strength of recommendations and quality of evidence, 2000-2003.* Available at http://www.ahrq.gov/clinic/preve nix.htm.

Vanhook PM: Overcoming the barriers to EBP, *Nurs Manag* 40(9):9–11, 2009.

Victora CG, Habicht JP: Evidence-based public health: moving beyond randomized trials, *Am J Public Health* 94:400–405, 2004.

West S, King V, Carey TS, et al: *Systems to rate the strength of scientific evidence, Evidence Report/ Technology Assessment No. 47*, AHRQ Publication No. 02-E016, Rockville, MD, 2002, Agency for Healthcare Research and Quality.

Wittemore R: Combining evidence in nursing research: methods and implications, *Nurs Res* 54:56–62, 2005.

CHAPTER 16

Using Health Education and Groups to Promote Health

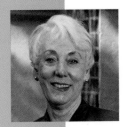

Jeanette Lancaster, PhD, RN, FAAN

Dr. Lancaster is the Medical Center Professor of Nursing at the University of Virginia. She has edited this book with Dr. Marcia Stanhope through its previous seven editions. Appreciation is extended to Professor Lisa Onega, Radford University and Assistant Professor Edie Devers Barbero, University of Virginia, who authored this chapter in the previous edition.

ADDITIONAL RESOURCES

ⓔvolve WEBSITE
http://evolve.elsevier.com/Stanhope
- *Healthy People 2020*
- WebLinks
- Quiz
- Case Studies

- Glossary
- Answers to Practice Application

APPENDIX
- Appendix H: Focus on Quality and Safety Education for Nurses

OBJECTIVES

After reading this chapter, the student should be able to do the following:
1. Describe three domains of learning.
2. Identify the steps and principles that guide community health education.
3. Describe how group purpose, member interaction, cohesion, conflict, and leadership affect group effectiveness.

4. Describe how nurses can work with groups to promote the health of individuals and communities.
5. List the five steps of the educational process.
6. Describe the importance of evaluating the educational product.

KEY TERMS

A major goal of health care reform is to reduce costs, and one way to do so is to help people stay healthy and to reduce illness and disability. Nurses can play a key role in this aspect of health care reform by teaching individuals, families, groups, and communities how to promote better health. Nurses are ideal health care practitioners to lead in health promotion through health education since: (1) they educate clients across all three levels of prevention: primary, secondary, and tertiary (see Levels of Prevention box), and (2) they work with individuals, families, groups, and communities. The goal is to enable clients to attain optimal health, prevent health problems, identify and treat health problems early, and minimize disability. Education allows individuals to make knowledgeable health-related decisions, assume personal responsibility for their health, and cope effectively with alterations in their health and lifestyles.

an educational program, selected models of health promotion, and the important topic of literacy, especially health literacy. The role of groups in health promotion is also presented. Many of the objectives of *Healthy People 2020* address the importance of health promotion, and selected objectives are cited in this chapter.

HEALTHY PEOPLE 2020 OBJECTIVES FOR HEALTH EDUCATION

As mentioned previously, the document *Healthy People 2020* lists national health needs and outlines goals and objectives designed to improve health. The *Healthy People 2020*

📋 LEVELS OF PREVENTION

Related to Community Health Education

Primary Prevention
Provide education at health fairs about diet, exercise, or environmental hazards.

Secondary Prevention
Provide both education and health screenings at health fairs for such health issues as early diagnosis and treatment of diabetes and hypercholesterolemia in order to shorten the duration and severity of the disease.

Tertiary Prevention
Provide education in rehabilitation centers to teach individuals who have been in an accident that left them with either an amputation or some paralysis ways to increase their functioning.

This chapter discusses ways to develop individual, group, and community health promotion programs. Specific content in the chapter includes information about how people learn, the sequence of actions that a nurse follows when developing

---

♥ HEALTHY PEOPLE 2020

Selected examples of *Healthy People 2020* are provided here.

- ECBP-2: Increase the proportion of elementary, middle, and senior high schools that provide comprehensive school health education to prevent health problems in the following areas: unintentional injury; violence; suicide; tobacco use and addiction; alcohol or other drug use; unintended pregnancy, HIV/AIDS, and STDs; unhealthy dietary patterns; and inadequate physical activity.
- ECBP-3: Increase the proportion of college and university students who receive information from their institution on each of the priority health-risk behavior areas listed above.
- ECBP-8: Increase the proportion of worksites that offer a comprehensive employee health promotion program to their employees.
- ECBP-9: Increase the proportion of employees who participate in employer-sponsored health promotion activities.
- ECBP-11: Increase the proportion of local health departments that have established culturally appropriate and linguistically competent community health promotion and disease prevention programs.

From U.S. Department of Health and Human Services: *Healthy People 2020: understanding and improving health promotion and disease prevention objectives*, Washington, DC, 2010, U.S. Government Printing Office.

educational objectives emphasize the importance of educating various populations (based on age and ethnicity) about health promotion activities in the priority areas of unintentional injury; violence; suicide; tobacco use and addiction; alcohol or other drug use; unintended pregnancy, HIV/AIDS, and STD infection; unhealthy dietary patterns; and inadequate physical activity (USDHHS, 2010).

In designing, implementing, and evaluating health education activities, it is useful to understand the primary health problems in the community as well as education principles related to both learning and teaching. Also, effective educational programs are built upon the premise that the best approach is to teach what people think they want to learn and in ways that facilitate their learning. For this reason, a core public health principle relates to asking the learners to participate in identifying their learning needs. Then health education programs are designed to meet the health need or problem in that population. Generally these programs involve educating individual members of the population about health promotion, illness prevention, and treatment. For example, in a community where childhood and adolescent asthma is a problem, a community-based asthma education and training program can be developed. If childhood obesity is a major health concern, a program to educate children in their schools about healthy eating, cooking, and exercise may be useful.

EDUCATION AND LEARNING

When we think about helping people change their behavior, it is important to remember that people can most easily change their own level of knowledge. The next step is to help people change their attitudes, and the most difficult area to change is behavior. For this reason, nurses provide people with health information so they can improve their decision-making abilities and thereby decide if they will change their behavior. There is a difference between education and learning and between knowing and doing. Education is an activity "undertaken or initiated by one or more agents that is designed to effect changes in the knowledge, skill and attitudes of individuals, groups, or communities" (Knowles, Holton, and Swanson, 2005, p 10). Education emphasizes the provider of knowledge and skills. In contrast, learning emphasizes the recipient of knowledge and skills and the person(s) in whom a change is expected to occur. Remember that learning involves change.

HOW PEOPLE LEARN

People learn in a variety of ways. Many people learn best through active involvement in their learning, which contrasts with the belief that learners are like sponges who simply soak up the information that is presented. Learners accept information based on many factors including what they already know, what they believe, the culture in which they have been raised, as well as how well they can understand and relate to the information that they receive. What a person hears is filtered through his past experiences, the social groups to which he belongs, assumptions, values, level of attention and knowledge,

and the esteem with which he holds the person communicating the information. In some cultures, elders are considered to be valued sources of information. In other cultures, people value individuals with more education than they have. Also, since social groups play a critical role in the development of understanding or learning, concepts related to groups will be discussed later in the chapter (Wilson and Peterson, 2006). Effective health education is a competency that is included in many documents that describe the role of public health professionals, including nurses. The Linking Content to Practice box illustrates the relationship between health education and selected standards, expectations, and competencies in public health.

🌐 LINKING CONTENT TO PRACTICE

Just as objectives in *Healthy People 2020* recommend that health education and promotion be used to provide public health care, so do other key documents such as the American Nurses Association's *Scope & Standards of Practice: Public Health Nursing*. Standard 5b, labeled "Health Education and Health Promotion," says that the "public health nurse employs multiple strategies to promote health, prevent disease, and ensure a safe environment for populations," (ANA, 2007, p 23). Similarly, the *Core Competences for Public Health Professionals* of the Council on Linkages Between Academia and Public Health Practice (2010) lists six competencies related to communication skills; five of them relate directly to this chapter. These competencies, listed below, are discussed and illustrated throughout the chapter:

1. Assesses the health literacy of populations served
2. Communicates in writing and orally, in person, and through electronic means, with linguistic and cultural proficiency
3. Solicits input from individuals and organizations
4. Uses a variety of approaches to disseminate public health information
5. Applies communication strategies in interactions with individuals and groups

---

A variety of educational principles can be used to guide the selection of health information for individuals, families, communities, and populations. Three of the most useful categories of educational principles include those associated with the nature of learning, the educational process, and the skills of effective educators.

The Nature of Learning

One way to think about the nature of learning is to examine the cognitive (thinking), affective (feeling), and psychomotor (acting) domains of learning. Each domain has specific behavioral components that form a hierarchy of steps, or levels. Each level builds on the previous one. Understanding these three learning domains is crucial in providing effective health education (Bloom et al, 1956). First, consider assumptions about how adults learn. Specifically, adults are motivated to learn when: (1) they think they need to know something, (2) the new information is compatible with their prior life experiences, (3) they value the person(s) providing the information, and (4) they believe they can make any necessary changes that are implied by the new information (Knowles, Holton, and Swanson, 2005).

Cognitive Domain

The **cognitive domain** includes memory, recognition, understanding, reasoning, application, and problem solving and is divided into a hierarchical classification of behaviors. Learners master each level of cognition in order of difficulty (Bloom et al, 1956; Dembo, 1994). Start by assessing the cognitive abilities of the learners. This is especially important when learners have a limited level of literacy either of the language used in the instruction or of the content that is presented. A later section will talk both about literacy in general and health literacy in particular. Teaching above or below a person's level of understanding can lead to frustration and discouragement. It is therefore important to be sensitive to the value of the cognitive domain in learning. The cognitive domain consists of these components (Bloom et al, 1956):

1. *Knowledge:* requires recall of information
2. *Comprehension:* combines recall with understanding
3. *Application:* new information taken in and used in a different way
4. *Analysis:* breaks communication down into parts in order to understand both the parts and their relationships to one another
5. *Synthesis:* builds on the first four levels by assembling them into a new whole
6. *Evaluation:* learners judge the value of what has been learned

Affective Domain

The **affective domain** includes changes in attitudes and the development of values. For affective learning to take place, nurses consider and attempt to influence what learners feel, think, and value. Because the attitudes and values of nurses may differ from those of their clients, it is important to listen carefully to detect clues to feelings that learners have that may influence learning. It is difficult to change deeply rooted attitudes, beliefs, interests, and values. To make such changes, people need support and encouragement from those around them. Affective learning, like cognitive learning, consists of a series of steps that the learner takes:

1. *Knowledge:* receives the information
2. *Comprehension:* responds to the information received
3. *Application:* values the information
4. *Analysis:* makes sense of the information
5. *Synthesis:* organizes the information
6. *Evaluation:* adopts behaviors consistent with new values

Psychomotor Domain

The **psychomotor domain** includes the performance of skills that require some degree of neuromuscular coordination and emphasizes motor skills (Bloom et al, 1956). Clients are taught a variety of psychomotor skills including bathing infants, changing dressings, giving injections, measuring blood glucose levels, taking blood pressures, walking with crutches, as well as many skills related to health promotion exercises.

In teaching a skill, first show clients how to do the skill, whether through pictures, a model, or a device, or via a live demonstration, video, CD, or the Internet. Next, allow clients to practice, which is a repeat demonstration approach to validate that what was being taught was actually learned. Also, if the teaching is being done in a class, participants may learn by observing one another master a task. Psychomotor learning is dependent on learners meeting the following three conditions (Bloom et al, 1956; Dembo, 1994):

- The learner must have the *necessary ability.* This will include both cognitive and psychomotor ability. For example, you may find that a person with Alzheimer's disease can follow only one-step instructions. Thus, you need to tailor your education plan to that person.
- The learner must have a *sensory image* of how to carry out the skill. For example, when teaching a group of women how to cook in a more heart-healthy manner, ask the women to describe their kitchen and how they would actually go about the cooking process.
- The learner must have *opportunities to practice* the new skills. Provide practice sessions during the program to help the client adapt the skill to the home or work environment where the skill will be performed.

In assessing a client's ability to learn a skill, be sure to evaluate intellectual, emotional, and physical ability, and then teach at the level of the learner's ability. Some clients do not have the intellectual ability to learn the steps that make up a complex procedure. Others may have cultural beliefs that conflict with healthy behaviors. Another client may be a tremulous person and have poor eyesight, making him incapable of learning insulin self-injection.

THE EDUCATIONAL PROCESS

The educational process builds on an understanding of education, learning and how people learn. The five steps of the educational process (identify educational needs, establish educational goals and objectives, select appropriate educational methods, implement the educational plan, and evaluate the educational process) are discussed next.

Identify Educational Needs

To learn about the health education needs of clients, begin by conducting a systematic and thorough needs assessment (Bartholomew et al, 2000). The steps of such an assessment are listed in Box 16-1. Once needs have been identified, they are prioritized. The goal of the prioritization is to meet the most critical educational needs first (Wolf, 2001).

BOX 16-1   STEPS OF A NEEDS ASSESSMENT

1. Identify what the client wants to know. (Consider *Healthy People 2020* educational objectives.)
2. Collect data systematically to obtain information about learning needs, readiness to learn, and barriers to learning.
3. Analyze assessment data that have been collected and identify cognitive, affective, and psychomotor learning needs.
4. Think about what will increase the client's ability and motivation to learn.
5. Assist the client to prioritize learning needs.

As has been discussed, many factors influence a person's learning needs and the ability to learn. These factors include demographic, physical, geographic, economic, psychological, social, and spiritual characteristics of the learners (Bartholomew et al, 2000). It is also important to consider the learner's knowledge, skills, and his or her motivation to learn, as well as what resources are available to support and possibly prevent learning. Resources include printed, audio or visual materials, equipment, agencies, and other individuals. Barriers for the presenter include lack of time, skill and/or confidence, money, space, energy, and organizational support.

> **NURSING TIP** *Consider the target audience carefully when developing a community health education project. Determine educational needs, educational and literacy levels, cultural backgrounds, and health beliefs. Consider also your skills and the type of program or project you can most effectively deliver.*

Establish Educational Goals and Objectives

Goals and objectives to guide the educational program are identified once you identify the learners' needs. Goals are broad, long-term expected outcomes such as, "Each child in the third-grade class will participate in 30 minutes of daily physical exercise, 4 days per week for 2 months." Your program goals should deal directly with the clients' overall learning needs. In regard to the third graders, their learning need is to know how important exercise is to their health and level of fitness.

Objectives are specific, short-term criteria that need to be met as steps toward achieving the long-term goal such as, "Within 2 weeks, each of the children will be able to demonstrate at least two exercises that they have learned." Objectives are written statements of an intended outcome or expected change in behavior and should define the minimum degree of knowledge or ability needed by a client. Objectives must be stated clearly and defined in measurable terms, and they typically imply an action (Knowles, Holton, and Swanson, 2005).

Select Appropriate Educational Methods

Educational methods should be chosen to facilitate the efficient and successful accomplishment of program goals and objectives. The methods should also be appropriately matched to the client's strengths and needs as well as those of the presenter. Choose the simplest, clearest, and most succinct manner of presentation and avoid complex program designs. Try to vary the methods in order to hold the attention of the learners and to meet the needs of different learners. Some people learn best by being actively involved in the program. Others learn by a more solitary approach such as watching a video and reflecting on how he or she might apply the content to his health situation. A few examples of strategies that may be used to enhance learning are listed in Box 16-2.

Educators also need to be able to deliver presentations, lead group discussions, organize role plays, provide feedback to learners, share case studies, use media and materials, and, where indicated, administer examinations. You will want to think

---

BOX 16-2   STRATEGIES TO ENHANCE LEARNING

- Audiovisual materials including videos, CDs, DVDs, personal digital assistants or the Internet
- Brainstorming
- Case studies
- Demonstrations
- Field trips
- Games
- Group participation
- Guest speakers
- Peer presentations, counseling, and tutoring
- Printed materials
- Role plays
- Simulation

BOX 16-3   HOW TO EFFECTIVELY TEACH CLIENTS

Use the TEACH mnemonic:

Tune in. Listen before you start teaching. Client's needs should direct the content.

Edit information. Teach necessary information first. Be specific.

Act on each teaching moment. Teach whenever possible. Develop a good relationship.

Clarify often. Make sure your assumptions are correct. Seek feedback.

Honor the client as a partner. Build on the client's experience. Share responsibility with the client.

Modified from Hansen M, Fisher J: Patient-centered teaching from theory to practice, *Am J Nurs* 98:56-60, 1998.

---

about what content to include, how to organize and sequence the information, what your rate of delivery will be, whether or not you need to include repetition, how much practice time should be included, how you will evaluate the effectiveness of the teaching, and ways that you can provide reinforcement and rewards (Knowles, Holton, and Swanson, 2005) (Box 16-3).

When choosing educational methods, consider age, gender, culture, developmental disabilities or special learning needs, educational level, knowledge of the subject, and size of the group. For example, clients with a visual impairment need more verbal description than those with no impairment in sight. Persons who have hearing impairments or language deficits need more visual material and speakers or translators who can use sign language or speak their native language. Also, when the learners have limitations in attention and concentration, the educator will need to use creative methods and tools to keep them focused. For example, you might include frequent breaks; simple surroundings with few or no distractions; use of small-group interactions to keep learners involved and interested; and the use of hands-on equipment such as mannequins, models, interactive games, and other materials and devices that the learner can physically manipulate. Try to involve the learner appropriately, actively, and creatively in learning. Interactive educational programs may be more effective than non-interactive ones. Interactive strategies include discussion, small

BOX 16-4 EXAMPLES OF LEARNING FORMATS

Presentation: This method can be used when the group is large and you want to be consistent in the message that is delivered to all participants. Remember, people tend to have a short attention span, so what can you do to keep them engaged? You might ask them to spend some time talking with one another in small groups and then have the group respond to questions or ask attendees to write answers to questions and invite several to share their answers.

Demonstration: This technique is often used to show attendees how to perform a task. For example, insulin injection demonstration, heart-healthy food preparation, and breastfeeding may be demonstrated.

Small Informal Group: Since learners often learn as much from one another as from the instructor, small groups can be valuable. This is especially true when the content lends itself to members sharing their own experiences. For example, in working with women in a shelter for abused women, participants may be able to share with one another actions they took to remove themselves safely from the violent environment. They might also be able to jointly plan how each might move to the stage of independent living outside the shelter.

Health Fair: See the How To box below on ways to plan, implement, and evaluate a health fair. For example, you might offer a health fair in a Senior Center and have displays such as posters; videos; live demonstrations; handouts on such topics as reducing fat in selected recipes (including samples) and age-appropriate exercises for flexibility; as well as screenings for elevated blood pressure, glucose, or cholesterol or for osteoporosis and vision.

Non-native Language Sessions: You could adapt the health fair approach for a Hispanic group by holding the session in Spanish and providing all of the materials in Spanish. Then ask Spanish-speaking nurses to staff each of the stations for health learning.

---

group work, games, and role playing, whereas non-interactive strategies are lectures, videos, or demonstrations. Box 16-4 details descriptions of learning formats.

The goal of nurses who use *Healthy People 2020* as a guide in educating clients is to foster healthy communities mainly through primary and secondary prevention. Health fairs are a popular way to provide primary and secondary health education. The objectives of holding health fairs are to increase awareness by providing health screenings, activities, information and educational materials, and demonstrations. A health fair can target a specific population or focus on a specific health issue, as well as target a range of groups and cover a variety of health education and health promotion topics. The fair can be held in many locations and can be either inside or outside. The How To box lists guidelines to assist nurses who chair, co-chair, or serve on a planning committee for a health fair.

HOW TO Plan, Implement, and Evaluate a Health Fair

1. *Form a planning committee:* 2-12 people who represent the groups who will be part of the health fair. Possibilities: health professionals, representatives from health agencies, schools, churches, employers, the media, and the target audience.
2. *Identify the target group. Develop a theme.*
3. *Establish goals, expected outcomes, and screening activities consistent with the needs and wishes of the target group. Your primary goal might be to improve the health of a specific*

population such as workers at one plant or children in one school. You might have secondary goals such as for the workers to reduce health care costs and for the children to reduce absenteeism.

4. *Develop a timeline and schedule.*
5. *Choose a site and consider the site logistics:* Do this about 1 year ahead. Think about the size of the site you will need and the traffic flow from one booth or demonstration to another, whether parking is available and free or low cost, and whether there are toilets and places to get food and drinks. If the site is inside, consider adequate exits; the possible risks to children, the elderly, or handicapped people; and other safety and security issues. You may need to create a map both for how to get to the fair and another one to help attendees get from one table, exhibit, or screening station to another. Be sure to include on the map the location of amenities like toilets and food vendors.
6. *Plan for supplies that you will need:* tables, chairs, electronic equipment, and accessories such as extension cords, office supplies, sign-in sheets (and what information should be included), release forms for screenings, name tags, bags for attendees to gather the educational information, and evaluation forms. Set your budget. Obtain these supplies in advance.
7. *Recruit and manage exhibitors:* Do this about 4 months ahead. Develop a list of possible exhibitors, sponsors, and contact them via letter, fax, e-mail, telephone, or in person. Follow up with a confirmation letter (or fax) that outlines the details of the health fair.
8. *Publicize the health fair:* the planning committee will have many good ideas about how to publicize in the specific community. Examples might be: fliers/posters, memos, brochures, e-mail blasts, local print, or radio/television.
9. *On the day of the fair:* greet health care professionals, agency representatives, sponsors, and members of the population being served.
10. *Evaluate the health fair:* by exhibitors, participants and volunteers. You will need a specific form for each of these groups.
11. *Between 1 week and 1 month after the fair:* send thank-you letters to health care professionals, sponsors, and agencies, and pay bills associated with the fair.

From Rice CA, Pollard JM: Health fair planning guide, AgriLIFE EXTENSION Texas A&M System, September 16, 2009. Available at http://fcs. tamu.edu/health/health_fair_planning_guide/index.php. Accessed January 22, 2011; United HealthCare: Health fair planning guide: wellness toolkit, 2005. Available at www.uhctool.com. Accessed January 27, 2010.

Skills of the Effective Educator

The educator needs to understand the basic sequence of instruction. The following nine steps are useful in planning an educational program (Driscoll, 2005; Knowles, Holton, and Swanson, 1998):

1. *Gain attention.* Begin by gaining the learner's attention and helping the learner believe that the information being presented is important and beneficial to him.
2. *Inform the learner of the objectives of instruction.* Discuss the major goals and objectives of the instruction so learners can develop expectations about what they are supposed to learn.

3. *Stimulate recall of prior learning.* Ask learners to recall previous knowledge related to the topic of interest. This assists them to link new knowledge with prior knowledge.

4. *Present the material.* Present the essential elements of the topic in a clear, organized, and simple manner and in a way congruent with the learner's strengths, needs, and limitations.

5. *Provide learning guidance.* Help the learner store information in long-term memory. You can help the learner transform general information that has been presented into meaningful information for that specific learner to facilitate later recall. You can do this by providing ways in which the learner can apply the information to his or her life and situation.

6. *Elicit performance.* Encourage learners to demonstrate what they have learned. This will help you correct any errors and improve skills.

7. *Provide feedback.* Provide feedback to help learners improve their knowledge and skills. They can then modify their thinking patterns and behaviors on the basis of the feedback.

8. *Assess performance.* Evaluate the learning by assessing if the knowledge has been gained and if the skills can be performed.

9. *Enhance retention and transfer of knowledge.* Once a baseline level of knowledge and skills is reached, help learners apply this information to new situations.

By using these steps, nurses may help clients to maximize learning experiences. If steps of this process are omitted, superficial and fragmented learning may occur. The Did You Know box includes principles to guide the educator through these steps. The next phase of the educational process is to design, deliver, and evaluate a program tailored to the needs of the learners.

DID YOU KNOW? Six Principles that Guide the Educator

1. *Message: Send a clear message to the learners*
2. *Format: Select the best learning format for the learners*
3. *Environment: Create a positive learning environment*
4. *Experience: Organize positive and meaningful learning experiences*
5. *Participation: Engage learners in their learning*
6. *Evaluation: Evaluate and give clear and objective feedback to learners*

Developing Effective Health Education Programs

The program should include a clear message conveyed in a format appropriate to the learners and in an environment that is free from distractions and consistent with the message. In regard to the message, it is important to remember that emotions such as anxiety, stress, anger, or fear can interfere with the listener actually hearing the message being sent. Also, provide information that is understandable to the listener. Use plain language and avoid jargon and complex medical terms. Use words that the listener will know and recognize. For example, some people are more familiar with terms like *high blood pressure* and *high blood sugar levels* rather than *hypertension* and *increased glucose levels.* On the other hand, be careful not to oversimplify

your terms if your audience is knowledgeable about health care. You want to avoid "talking down" or "over the head" of your listeners.

The type of learning format that you select will depend on the learners. If they are young, you will want an interactive format and many of your options will include the use of technology. You could use a game such as developing a bingo game with food groups to teach about healthy eating. The old adage "A picture is worth a 1000 words" still holds true. People tend to remember what they see or hear; a lively format rather than a passive one encourages learning. Most people have a short attention span, so you need to make your point quickly and directly. It may help to provide take home written materials or a CD for further reminders and follow-up of what is taught. Since people often learn better when they are actively engaged in the learning, having small group discussion, role playing, and question-and-answer sessions may reinforce learning. Figure 16-1 shows a community group being educated, and Box 16-5 lists ways to design clear educational programs.

HOW TO Develop Print Materials

- *Use active voice and conversational tone*
- *Make the material personal*
- *Eliminate jargon, technical terms, or slang words*
- *Use simple terms and avoid multi-syllable words*
- *Use easily readable print size: 12 point for most people; 14 point for older people*
- *Use upper and lower case; all capital letters are hard to read*
- *Use examples to show the desired behavior*
- *Have plenty of white space on the page*
- *Choose ink that markedly contrasts with the color of the background*

From Health Literacy Innovations: *10 tips for print materials, press release,* May 8, 2007. Available at http://www.HealthLiteracyInnovation. com. Accessed February 22, 2008.

EDUCATIONAL ISSUES

There are three important educational issues to consider when you are planning educational programs. First, different populations of learners require different teaching strategies. Second, be prepared to overcome barriers to learning. And third, consider the appropriateness of using technology in the programs.

Population Considerations Based on Age, Cultural and Ethnic Backgrounds

Nurses are an important source of health education in the community. The increase in populations of varying cultural and ethnic backgrounds and the aging of baby boomers require that community health education crosses age and cultural boundaries.

In terms of age, children, adults, and older adults have different learning needs and respond to different educational strategies. In each age group, learners vary also in their cognitive ability, personality, and prior knowledge. Some people learn better with more direct instruction, supervision, and encouragement than do other people.

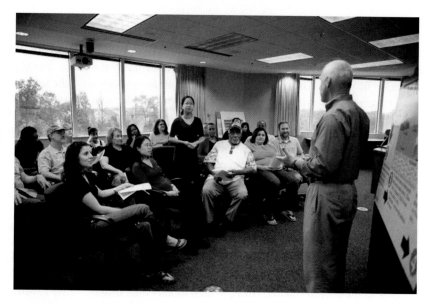

FIGURE 16-1 Educating a community group about environmental health issues and gathering their concerns. (From Centers for Disease Control and Prevention, 2009, courtesy Dawn Arlotta.)

BOX 16-5   DESIGNING CLEAR EDUCATIONAL PROGRAMS

1. Develop the content for your message.
2. Identify the most appropriate format and location for your program, taking into account your budget, location, and other available resources and constraints. See Box 16-4 for examples of formats.
3. Organize the learning experience that will suit the audience; consider how to engage the learners in the process.
4. Plan how you will deliver the material using the following points:
   - Limit the number of points that you wish to cover to the most important ones.
   - Begin with a strong opening and close with a strong ending; people remember most what is said first and last.
   - Fit your use of language to the learners; use an active voice and emphasize the positive. For example, "Many people are able to lose weight by reducing their intake by 500 calories a day and exercising 45 minutes at least four times a week."
   - Use examples, stories, and other vivid messages. Limit statistics and complex terminology.
   - Refer to trustworthy sources. In general, government, educational, or professional association sources are peer reviewed by professionals and dependable. The Centers for Disease Control and Prevention, National Cancer Institute, American Association of Public Health, and the American Academy of Pediatrics are four examples of sites that offer useful information.
   - Use aids to highlight your message. For example, you might have posters, handouts, or CDs to give to attendees. You might also incorporate a clip from a website such as www.YouTube.com to emphasize your point.
5. Don't forget to plan the evaluation when you are initially planning the program.

Learning strategies for children and individuals with little knowledge about a health-related topic are characterized as **pedagogy.** In the pedagogical model of learning, the teacher assumes full responsibility for making decisions about what will be learned, and how and when it will be learned. This form of learning is teacher directed. Learning strategies for adults, older adults, and individuals with some health-related knowledge about a topic are called **andragogy.** In the andragogical model, learners play an important role in deciding what they need and want to learn. Andragogy is a more transactional way of learning than is the pedagogical model. Each model has useful elements (Knowles, Holton, and Swanson, 2005). For example, when learners are dependent and entering a totally new content area, they may require more pedagogical experiences. In addition to considering the age of the population to be educated, think about the learning needs of the population and use the pedagogical and andragogical principles that will best meet these needs. In educational programs for children, provide information that matches the developmental abilities of the group. The following age-specific strategies may help the nurse tailor educational programs for children (Whitener, Cox, and Maglich, 1998).

- *The younger the child, the more concrete the examples and word choices will need to be.* You might tell a group of 3-year-old children that it is good to brush their teeth two times a day. With 10-year-olds, you can explain to them the benefits of brushing their teeth and the risks of not brushing and talk about issues such as the care of their teeth with braces.
- *Using objects or devices, as opposed to discussion of ideas, will increase attention.* When teaching a group of children with asthma how to use inhalers, it is better to hand out inhalers to each participant and have them practice proper technique with the inhalers rather than just giving them a handout with instructions or demonstrating how to use an inhaler while they watch you.
- *Incorporating repetitive health behaviors into games will help children retain knowledge and acquire skills.* Singing songs while acting out healthy activities such as washing hands before eating helps children get in the habit of washing their hands and makes this health promotion behavior fun. For example, the time a child should wash his or her hands is about the same amount of time it takes to sing "Twinkle, Twinkle Little Star."

In thinking about culture, it is important to know that by 2050 approximately 50% of the U.S. population will consist of ethnic minorities such as Asians, African Americans, Hispanic Americans, Native Americans, and Pacific Islanders. Culture influences family structure and interactions as well as views about health and illness. These demographic changes present new challenges to nurse educators. Nurses need to understand the health belief systems of the ethnic populations being served and be familiar with populations who are prone to develop certain health problems. When presenting seminars or providing written, audio, or visual information, make sure that the information is provided in a culturally competent manner.

For example, in a rural farming area, there might be a large population of Mexican migrant crop workers in the area. Knowing that this Spanish-speaking group is more likely to have tuberculosis than other segments of the community, nurses may visit the migrant worker camp to present information on tuberculosis such as prevention, symptom identification, early diagnosis, and treatment. An interpreter may accompany the nurses and provide oral content in Spanish. Written handouts can be in Spanish and designed to be read and understood on a second- or third-grade reading level.

Barriers to Learning

Barriers to learning fall into two broad categories: one concerning the educator and the other concerning the learner.

Educator-Related Barriers

Some common educator-related barriers to learning, together with strategies to minimize them, follow (Knowles, Holton, and Swanson, 2005):

- *Fear of public speaking.* Be well prepared; use icebreakers; recognize and acknowledge the fear; practice in front of a mirror or video camera or with a friend.
- *Lack of credibility with respect to a certain topic.* Increase your confidence by carefully preparing for the talk so you believe that you have included useful information and that you understand the information; avoid apologizing for lack of expertise, and instead convey the attitude of an expert by briefly sharing your personal and professional background.
- *Limited professional experiences related to a health topic.* You may want to describe personal experiences (brief ones), share experiences of others, or use analogies, illustrations, or examples from movies, current news, or famous people.
- *Unable to deal with difficult people who need to learn health-related information.* One strategy that may help with handling difficult learners is to confront the problem learner directly. Other strategies include using humor, using small groups to foster participation of timid people, asking disruptive people to give others a chance to speak, or, if this does not work, asking them to leave.
- *Lack of knowledge about how to gain participation.* You can foster participation by asking open-ended questions, inviting participation, and planning small-group activities whereby a person responds based on the group rather than presenting his own information.

- *Lack of experience in timing a presentation so that it is neither too long nor too short.* Strategies to help determine if the length of the presentation is appropriate include planning well and practicing the presentation and trying to speak during the practice at the same pace that you will speak to the group.
- *Feel uncertain about how to adjust instruction.* You can more easily adjust instruction when you know the participants' needs, request feedback, and redesign the presentation during breaks based on what you have learned about the participants.
- *Is uncomfortable when learners ask questions.* Try to anticipate questions, concisely paraphrasing questions to be sure that you correctly understood the question, and recognizing that it is appropriate to admit that you do not know the answer to a question.
- *Want to obtain feedback from learners.* Solicit informal feedback during the program and at the end with program evaluation.
- *Is concerned about whether media, materials, and facilities will function properly.* It is good to test the equipment before the program to make sure it runs and also that you know how to use it. You could either go in advance or arrive early to do so. You might also have back-up plans for how to get help if you have a problem.
- *Have difficulty with openings and closings.* Strategies to foster successful openings and closings include developing several examples of openings and closings, memorizing the opening and closing, concisely summarizing information, and thanking participants for attending.
- *Is overly dependent on notes.* You may wish to use note cards or visual aids as prompts, and practicing in advance is a proven way to increase skill at presenting.

Learner-Related Barriers

Two of the most important learner-related barriers are low literacy and lack of motivation to learn information and make needed behavioral changes.

Low Literacy Levels. Nurses often deal with individuals and populations who are illiterate or who have low literacy levels. These individuals may be embarrassed to admit this deficit to health care providers and educators and may try to appear to understand when they really do not. Specifically, they may not ask questions to clarify information even when they do not understand it. As society becomes more multicultural, the problem of low literacy can increase due to limited use of the primary language as well as limited education. One of the *Core Competencies for Public Health Professionals* listed in the 2009 revisions by the Council on Linkages Between Academia and Public Health Practice is to "assess the health literacy of populations served" (Council on Linkages, 2010). In the next paragraphs, you will read about the significance of this problem and the need for nurses to address health literacy.

The National Assessment of Adult Literacy (NAAL) is the largest literacy assessment study done in the United States. This assessment was first conducted in 1992. At that time, out of five levels in the assessment, 50% of American adults were in the top two levels and 50% were in the bottom three levels of literacy. The minimal standard needed to function in the workplace is that of level 3 proficiency. In 2003, the tool measured literacy in four levels: *Below Basic*, *Basic*, *Intermediate*, and *Proficient*. The literacy scales used in 2003 were: prose literacy, document literacy, and quantitative literacy. Prose examples include searching, comprehending, and using information from editorials, news stories, brochures, and instructional materials. Document literacy refers to searching, comprehending, and using information from documents such as job applications, payroll forms, transportation schedules, maps, tables, and drug and food labels. Quantitative literacy is the ability to identify and perform computations such as balancing a checkbook, completing an order form, or determining the interest on a loan from an advertisement. The 2003 test is more than just a survey and actually asks the test takers to perform tasks to demonstrate their literacy (Kutner et al, 2006). The 2003 NAAL included information about health literacy, which is an important topic for nurses. The 2003 NAAL used the Institute of Medicine's definition of health literacy: "The degree to which individuals have the capacity to obtain, process, and understand basic health information and services needed to make appropriate health decisions" (Ratzan and Parker, 2000). Kutner et al (2006), in their report on the 2003 NAAL survey, found that the majority of participants had Intermediate (53%) literacy; 12% were Proficient; 22% were Basic; and 14% had Below Basic levels of literacy. The assessment was given to over 19,000 adults in households or prisons. Interestingly, women had higher literacy than men, and white and Asian/Pacific Islander adults had higher scores than African American, Hispanic, American Indian/Alaska Native, and multiracial adults; adults 65 years of age or older and persons living below the poverty level had lower average literacy than others surveyed. One out of every five Americans reads below the fifth-grade level, and one out of every three lacks the literacy needed to understand health care providers (Roberts, 2004). Typically, individuals read three to five grade levels below the last year of school completed.

Individuals with limited literacy may be unable to understand instructions on prescription bottles, interpret health appointment cards, fill out health insurance forms, and read and understand self-care or hospital discharge instructions. What happens when someone has health illiteracy? A person with limited literacy may:

a. Have a limited vocabulary and general knowledge and does not ask for clarification
b. Focus on details and deal in literal or concrete concepts versus abstract concepts
c. Select responses on a survey or questionnaire without necessarily understanding them
d. Be unable to understand math (which is important in calculating medications)

Consequences of health illiteracy at the national level include $73 billion per year of preventable health care costs if individuals are unable to understand their health care treatment, increased numbers of hospitalizations and health care complications resulting from those hospitalizations, poorer health care outcomes, and decreased life expectancy (Kleinbeck,

2005). Although illiteracy is a challenge for nurses, one program designed to address health literacy in a population of poor, undereducated, primarily Spanish-speaking individuals created easy-to-use, health-related books for this population and found that emergency department visits decreased by 7% and that 94% found the books helpful (Roberts, 2004). It is also possible to develop CDs or videos with health information for people with low literacy.

WHAT DO YOU THINK? *Which of the following best provides information that takes into account the fact that many people are not proficient in health literacy?*
A. *"Even though your hypertension is stable, you are at risk for a myriad of complications and you need to regularly take antihypertensive medication."*
B. *"Even though the level of your blood pressure has not increased since your last visit, it is still important for you to take the medicine that you were given that will control your blood pressure. The medicine is _____."*

Nurse educators may incorporate pictures including comic books, slide and video presentations, and models in educating clients with low literacy while continuing to focus on individual learning capacity. Some people learn better via a series of educational sessions. For example, at the first session, identify learning capacity and provide a small amount of foundational information. During subsequent sessions, new information that builds on existing knowledge and skills is provided and evaluated. Give additional information when you believe that the information has been understood and can be incorporated into learners' lives. In order to evaluate if a person has limited health literacy, listen for the following clues: "I forgot my reading glasses," "I can read this when I get home," or "I will talk about this with my family—may I take the instructions home?" These comments may be quite straightforward or be a clue that the person actually cannot read the material.

Some people do not engage in learning because they have low levels of motivation to do so. Although adults respond to some external motivators, the most powerful motivators are internal. People are motivated to learn if they value and feel that they will benefit from the outcome of the learning, if they think they can follow through on what is being taught, and if it will improve their situation in life or increase their self-esteem (Ota et al, 2006).

As discussed in Chapter 17, models can be used to structure health education and health promotion plans. One model, the Health Belief Model (HBM) is an individual-level model. This model can be useful in planning programs in which the motivation of learners might be a concern. Specifically, the HBM was one of the first theories of health behavior. It began in an interesting way that is still applicable to the behavior of people today. In the 1950s the U.S. Public Health Service sent mobile X-ray units to communities to provide free chest X-rays as a way to screen for tuberculosis. The X-rays were free, convenient, and painless, yet people did not come to get them done. A group of social psychologists were asked to try to explain the failure to use this screening. Specifically, what would motivate people to seek health care?

The HBM includes six components that attempt to answer the question of what motivates an individual to do something. These components are: (1) perceived susceptibility ("Will something happen to me?"), (2) perceived severity ("If something does happen to me, will it be a big problem?"), (3) perceived benefits ("If I do what is suggested, will it really help me?"), (4) perceived barriers ("Assuming I do what is suggested, will there be barriers that will be unpleasant, costly, and so forth?"), (5) cues to action ("What might motivate me to actually do something?"), and (6) self-efficacy ("Can I really do this?"). This model has been applauded and criticized. It does offer guidance in planning health education programs in that it reminds nurses to think carefully about what motivates people to change. To understand motivation, it is important to learn: (1) how the people involved feel about the health problem, (2) if they think it is serious, (3) do they believe that action on their part will make a difference, and (4) do they think that they can both manage the barriers and actually perform the action?

Consider the following example of how the HBM might be applied to a person in the community who has recently been diagnosed with diabetes. The person, June, is 25 years old and was diagnosed 2 months ago with diabetes mellitus. She has found it hard to follow the recommendations of the public health nurse who has seen her in the community clinic. When the nurse asked June what seemed to be getting in her way of complying, June said that she had asked herself these questions:

1. If I do not follow the nurse's advice about diet, exercise, and taking my insulin, will something really happen to me?
2. If I do not follow the advice and something does happen, will it really be a problem?
3. On the other hand, if I take my medicine, eat a diet that will keep my diabetes under control, exercise as recommended by the nurse, and take my insulin according to the nurse's directions, will I really reduce the seriousness of my disease?
4. How much will it cost me to purchase the foods in order to follow the diet? How much time will it take each week to exercise as recommended? Will it hurt me to give myself insulin injections?
5. I did see that my friend, Sue, who was diagnosed about 2 years ago with diabetes was careful about what she ate at the party, and she did talk about her exercise program where she walks 50 minutes 5 days a week. Sue did look better than she did when I saw her last year.
6. Is it possible for me to take care of myself like Sue does?

A second set of models are also presented. The selection of these three models—the HBM, the Transtheoretical Model (TTM), and Precaution Adoption Process Model (PAPM)—does not imply that they are the best or only models. They are, however, useful models in health promotion. The TTM and the PAPM are discussed together since they both deal with change that occurs in stages and over time. The TTM has six stages:

1. Pre-contemplation, in which the person does not plan to change; this may be because the person does not know there is a problem or does not want to do anything about it (USD-HHS, 2005). For example, the person may not know that it is not good to cook food in lard.

2. Contemplation, in which the person begins thinking about making a change in the future and examines the pros and cons of doing so. The person may have gone to a class where he learned that it is better to cook food in canola oil rather than in lard and is beginning to wonder if his food would taste as good if he made that change.
3. Preparation, in which the person intends to do something. In the cooking example, the person might put canola oil on the shopping list.
4. Action, whereby the person actually buys the canola oil and cooks a chicken with it instead of the lard.
5. Maintenance, when the person decides that he can get used to eating chicken cooked in oil and begins preparing his food in that way on a regular basis.
6. The person terminates the change process since he is able to continue the new, more health-conscious way of cooking.

Although the terms used are slightly different, the intent of the PAPM is much like the TTM. The stages are: (1) unaware of the issue, (2) unengaged by the issue, (3) deciding about acting, (4) deciding not to act, (5) deciding to act, (6) acting, and (7) maintenance. You can apply the cooking example above to these stages as well.

EVIDENCE-BASED PRACTICE

Extensive research has been done on the hazardous effects of tobacco use. More recently, attention has focused on the harmful effects of second-hand smoke (SHS). A growing body of research supports best practices for eliminating SHS. Cramer, Roberts, and Xu (2007) described the evaluation and outcomes of a community-based coalition in the Midwest that used such practices to educate the public and change attitudes about SHS, thereby promoting social policy change for tobacco-free environments. The evaluation model used in the study incorporated evidence-based indicators as measures for coalition goal achievement and found the best practices program to be effective for eliminating exposure to SHS.

Nurse Use

This study brought together a number of different elements to create a conceptual framework that could evaluate the community coalition's efforts to combat SHS. The use of local data coupled with this framework created a roadmap for researchers to follow as they continue to evaluate the program and examine issues such as SHS-related health effects and the economic outcomes associated with SHS. This unique approach could be a useful model for other researchers seeking to evaluate similar programs. Even when clients have limited literacy and little to no computer skills, nurses may successfully incorporate interactive multimedia methods in their population-based educational programs.

From Cramer M, Roberts S, Xu L: Evaluating community-based programs for eliminating secondhand smoke using evidence-based research for best practices, *Fam Community Health* 30:129-143, 2007.

Use of Technology in Health Education

Many kinds of technologies such as computer games and programs, videos, CDs, and Internet resources can increase learning. These technologies may enable the learner to control the pace of instruction, offer flexibility in the time and location of learning, present an appealing form of education, and provide immediate feedback. You may want to use a variety of technological applications in your teaching. It is also important to be aware that people increasingly are using the Internet as a source of health information. In the Pew Internet & American Life Project, the top three choices from which Americans sought health information included health care professionals (86%), family and friends (68%), and the Internet (60%). Why do people use the Internet? A major benefit is its convenience: It is available 24 hours a day, 7 days a week, and there is no need to drive there, take public transportation, or find a parking place.

> **WHAT DO YOU THINK?** *Is the Internet a reliable and valid source of health information? All the time? Some of the time? Do you use the Internet for your health information?*

Educating people through the Internet has been shown to be more effective in fostering treatment adherence than in-person counseling, telephone counseling, or self-directed learning (Dauz et al, 2004). Clients may ask nurses to provide them with information about ways to evaluate the quality and reliability of this information. The following list provides some criteria for assessing the quality of Internet health information (AHRQ, 1999; VanBiervliet and Edwards-Schafer, 2004):

- *Authorship.* Are the authors and contributors listed with their credentials and affiliations?
- *Caveats.* Does the site clarify whether its function is to provide information or to market products?
- *Content.* Is the information accurate and complete, and is an appropriate disclaimer provided?
- *Credibility.* Does the site include the source, currency, relevance, and editorial review process for the information?
- *Currency.* Are dates listed for when the content was posted and updated?
- *Design.* Is the site accessible, capable of internal searches, easy to navigate, and logically organized?
- *Disclosure.* Is the user informed about the purpose of the site and about any profiling or collection of information associated with using the site?
- *Interactivity.* Does the site include feedback mechanisms and opportunities for users to exchange information?
- *Links.* Have the links been evaluated according to back-linkages, content, and selection?

Evaluate the Educational Process

Evaluation is as important in the educational process as it is in the nursing process. Evaluation provides a systematic and logical method for making decisions to improve the educational program (Babcock and Miller, 1994). You will need to evaluate the educator, the process and the product. Educator and process evaluation are described next, and product evaluation is described in the Educational Product section.

Educator Evaluation

Feedback to the educator provides an opportunity for the educator to modify the teaching process and enables the educator to better meet the learner's needs. The learner's evaluation of the educator occurs continuously throughout the educational program. The educator may receive written feedback from learners such as via an evaluation sheet. The educator may also ask for verbal feedback, as well as get non-verbal feedback by using return demonstrations to see what learners have mastered and by observing facial expressions when feedback is being given (Babcock and Miller, 1994; Knowles, 1990; Palazzo, 2001).

The educator should assume that inadequate learner responses reflect an inadequate program, not an inadequate learner. If the evaluation reveals that the learning objectives are not being met, the nurse must determine why the instruction is not effective. At this point, the educator will want to present the material creatively and meaningfully in new ways that will increase learner retention and the learner's ability to apply the new knowledge (Knowles, 1990). Ultimately, the educator must assume responsibility for the success or failure of the educational process and the development of learner knowledge, skills, and abilities.

Process Evaluation

Process evaluation examines the dynamic components of the educational program. It follows and assesses the movements and management of information transfer and attempts to make sure that the objectives are being met. Process evaluation is necessary *throughout* the educational program to determine whether goals and objectives are being met and the time required for their accomplishment. Ongoing evaluation also allows the teacher to correct misinformation, misinterpretation, or confusion (Babcock and Miller, 1994; Palazzo, 2001).

Goals and objectives should also be periodically reconsidered. It is important to often ask oneself if the desired health behavior change is really necessary. Such a question inevitably leads back to the original learning objectives and enables the nurse to rethink the practicality and merit of each of the objectives. Finally, factors that influence learner readiness and motivation should be reassessed if teaching seems to be ineffective. Process evaluation uses information gathered from the educator as well as from learner evaluations and assesses the dynamics of their interactions (Knowles, 1990).

THE EDUCATIONAL PRODUCT

The educational product is the outcome of the educational process. The product is measured both qualitatively and quantitatively (Krathwohl, Bloom, and Masia, 1964). For example, a qualitative assessment should answer the question, "How well does the learner appear to understand the content?" A quantitative assessment should answer the question, "How much of the content does the learner retain?" Thus, the quality of the product is measured by improvement and increase, or the lack thereof, in the learner's knowledge, skills, and abilities related to the content of the educational program. Selected outcomes for the population of interest need to be identified when the educational program is conceived. Measurement of changes in these outcomes determines the effectiveness of the program (Babcock and Miller, 1994). In nursing, the educational product is assessed as a measurable change in the health or behavior of the client.

Evaluation of Health and Behavioral Changes

A variety of approaches, methods, and tools can be used to evaluate health and behavioral changes. These include questionnaires, rating scales, surveys, checklists, skills demonstrations, testing, subjective client feedback, and direct observation of improvements in client mastery of materials (Babcock and Miller, 1994). Qualitative or quantitative strategies may be used, depending on the nature of the expected educational outcome. Evaluation of outcomes measured includes changes in knowledge, skills, abilities, attitudes, behavior, health status, and quality of life. Approaches to evaluating health education effects will vary, depending on the situation. For example, when considering a client's ability to perform a psychomotor skill such as changing a dressing, observing the client doing the skill is the most appropriate means of evaluation.

If evaluation of the educational product shows positive changes in health status and health-related behaviors, the educator can expect good results in similar health educational programs. If evaluation of the educational product shows that no changes or negative changes in health status and health-related behaviors resulted, then various components of the educational process can be examined and modified to produce better results in the future (Babcock and Miller, 1994).

Short-Term Evaluation

It is important to evaluate short-term health and behavioral effects of health education programs and to determine if they are really caused by the educational program. Short-term objectives are often easy to evaluate (Babcock and Miller, 1994). For example, a short-term evaluation of whether a client can perform a return demonstration of breast self-examination requires minimal energy, expense, or time; skill mastery can be determined within a matter of minutes. If the short-term objective is not met, the nurse determines why and identifies possible solutions so that successful learning can occur. If the short-term objective is met, the nurse can then focus on long-term evaluation designed to assess the lasting effects of the education program—in this case, that of ongoing monthly breast self-examinations performed by the learner independently at home.

Long-Term Evaluation

The ultimate goal of health education is to help clients make lasting behavioral changes that will improve their overall health status (Babcock and Miller, 1994). Long-term follow-up with clients is a challenging task. Long-term evaluation is geared toward following and assessing the status of an individual, family, community, or population over time. The tools of evaluation are designed to assess whether specific goals and objectives were met. Also, the extent and direction of changes in health status and health behaviors that the client has experienced are monitored (Babcock and Miller, 1994; Kleinpell and Mick, 2001).

Often, for nurse educators, the goal of long-term evaluation is an analysis of the effectiveness of the education program for the entire community, not the health status of a specific client. Nurses track the achievement of community objectives over time but not that of the individual community members. Thus, in a changing population, long-term evaluation of the results of an education program is still possible. The percentage of objectives and goals met by sampling the target population gives valid statistics for program assessment, even though the population of individuals may have experienced a complete turnover (Kleinpell and Mick, 2001).

For example, a nurse notes that according to annual health department data, 60% of all pregnant women in the nurse's catchment area received some prenatal care. Wanting to increase this percentage to 100%, the nurse tries an educational intervention in which radio and television stations make public service announcements about the importance and availability of prenatal services.

After 1 year, the nurse discovers that 80% of all pregnant women now receive prenatal care. The nurse continues to use public service announcements the following year because good results are evident. However, the long-term goal of the education program to influence the behavior of 100% of the pregnant women in the community has not yet been met. Therefore, the nurse enlists volunteers to put informational posters in shopping malls, grocery stores, public transportation stops, laundries, and public transportation vehicles. In the second year after implementing the revised educational program, again using the statistics from the health department, the nurse finds that 95% of all pregnant women in the target area now receive prenatal care. The nurse can thus evaluate and modify a community educational program over time to increase the rate, range, and consistency of progress made toward meeting the long-term goals of the project.

One issue related to long-term evaluation concerns keeping track of the clients; some will move, and others will lose interest and fail to keep appointments or return calls or e-mails.

A considerable amount of health education is carried out in the community in groups rather than provided to one person at a time. For this reason, the following section discusses how groups can be used as a tool for health education and the promotion of health.

GROUPS AS A TOOL FOR HEALTH EDUCATION

Nurses often provide health education to groups. People live in a social structure that may include family, co-workers, classmates, friends, and acquaintances. Health behavior is influenced by the groups to which people belong, and groups may support either beneficial or poor health practices. For example, a young person may be part of a group that abuses substances. Another youth might be part of a group who runs marathons. The health-oriented goals of each of these two groups are different. Groups are an effective and powerful medium to initiate and implement changes for individuals, families, organizations, and the community. People naturally form groups in the home, and groups in the community dramatically influence the community's health. Groups form for various reasons. They may form for a clearly stated purpose or goal, or they may form naturally as shared values, interests, activities, or personal characteristics attract individuals to each other.

Community groups represent the collective interests, needs, and values of individuals; they provide a link between the individual and the larger social system. Throughout life, membership in groups influences thoughts, choices, behaviors, and values as people socialize and interact. Through groups, people may express personal views and relate them to the views of others. Groups serve as communication networks and can help organize various aspects of communities.

Community groups may be informal or formal. **Formal groups** have a defined membership and a specific purpose. They may or may not have an official place in the community's organization. In **informal groups**, the ties between members are multiple, and the purposes are unwritten yet understood by members. These groups often form spontaneously when participants have a common interest or need. You can find out about what formal and informal groups exist in a community by reading the local newspaper, listening to public service information on the radio or television, and by asking residents about the groups to which they belong. Nurses often serve as a catalyst for forming new groups or by creating linkages among groups that currently exist (Schulte, 2000).

Group support often helps people make needed changes for health that they are unable to accomplish on their own or with the help of just one individual. Skillful use of group methods can help a person analyze the problem, sustain motivation for change, experience support during vulnerable periods, and receive quick interpersonal feedback. The discomfort associated with change can be reduced through the relationships with others in beneficial groups. Many of the *Healthy People 2020* priorities can be addressed in health promotion and disease prevention groups where individuals learn healthier behaviors and gain support from others in changing from risky to healthy lifestyle choices. For example, groups may support physical activity and fitness, sound nutrition, and safe sexual practices. Through group support, individuals may conquer smoking, drug abuse, or abusive relationships. They may identify and reduce exposure to environmental hazards and promote safer physical settings for all. Also, one of the core competencies for public health professionals is to "use group processes to advance community involvement" (Council on Linkages, 2010, p 10).

Group: Definitions and Concepts

An understanding of several group concepts facilitates group work in the community. Some of the core concepts include: (1) what is a group, (2) what is the purpose, (3) how do groups develop and function, (4) what are their stages, and (5) what roles do members typically play in the group.

Definitions

A **group** is a collection of interacting individuals who have common purposes. To some extent, each member influences and is in turn influenced by every other member. Key elements in this definition of group are **member interaction** and **group purpose.** Groups form for a variety of reasons. Families are an example of a community group. Families share kinship bonds, living space, and economic resources. They have many purposes such as teaching their members as well as providing psychological support and socialization.

Groups also form in response to community needs, problems, or opportunities. For example, community residents may form a neighborhood association to protect their health and welfare. Community groups occur spontaneously because of mutual attraction between individuals and obvious and keenly felt personal needs such as those for socialization and recreation. Health-promoting groups may form when people meet in community and health care settings and discover common challenges to their physical and emotional well-being. Health-promoting groups such as Alcoholics Anonymous, Weight Watchers, and La Leche League improve members' health and deal with specific threats to health just as do many groups that meet for exercise.

Concepts

Groups need to identify a clear purpose. Having a clear purpose helps in establishing criteria for member selection and determining the action plan. A clear statement of purpose proved valuable in forming a new group in one city's housing development. The local department of social services had received numerous reports of child abuse and neglect. Routine home visits for well-child care documented high stress between parents and their offspring, and some parents requested teaching and guidance from the nurse in child discipline. The nurse proposed that a parent group address this community need, and she chose this purpose for the group: *dealing with kids for child and parent satisfaction.* The purpose indicated both the process (to help parents deal with children) and the desired outcome (satisfaction for parents and children). As potential members were approached, this statement of group purpose helped them decide if they wanted to join.

Cohesion is the attraction between individual members and between each member and the group. Individuals in a highly cohesive group identify themselves as a unit, work toward common goals, endure frustration for the sake of the group, and defend the group against outside criticism. Attraction increases when members feel accepted and liked by others, see similar qualities in one another, and share similar attitudes and values. Group effectiveness also improves as members work together toward group goals while still satisfying the needs of individual members (Brandler, 1999).

Members' traits that increase group cohesion and productivity include the following:
- Compatible personal and group goals
- Attraction to group goals
- Attraction to other selected members
- Appropriate mix of leading and following skills
- Good problem-solving skills

Groups have both task and maintenance functions. A **task function** is anything a member does that deliberately contributes to the group's purpose. Members with task-directed abilities become more attractive to the group. These traits include strong problem-solving skills, access to material resources, and skills in directing. Of equal importance are abilities to affirm and support individuals in the group. These functions are called **maintenance functions** because they help other members stay with the group and feel accepted. Other maintenance functions are the ability to help people resolve conflicts and create social and environmental comfort. Both task and maintenance functions are necessary for group progress. Naturally, those members who provide these functions are attractive, and an abundance of such traits within the membership tends to increase group cohesion.

The following group members' traits may decrease cohesion and productivity:

- Conflicts between personal and group goals
- Lack of interest in group goals and activities
- Poor problem-solving and communication abilities
- Lack of both leadership and supporter skills
- Disagreement about types of leadership
- Aversion to other members
- Behaviors and attributes that are poorly understood by others

Usually, the more alike group members are, the stronger a group's attraction, whereas differences tend to decrease attractiveness. Members' perceptions of differences can create marked competition and jealousy. At the same time, personal differences can increase group cohesion if they support complementary functioning or provide contrasting viewpoints necessary for decision making. Cohesive factors are complex and many factors influence member attraction to each other and to the group's goal. High group cohesion positively affects productivity and member satisfaction. The following example illustrates factors that influence group cohesion:

A nurse initiated a group for clients who had been treated for burns. Ten residents, all from one town, had been discharged after a month in the local burn unit. The stated purpose for the group was to teach coping skills to assist members in the difficult transition from hospital to home. Each person had been treated for extensive burns in an intensive care treatment center; each had relied heavily on health care workers for physical, social, and emotional rehabilitation; and each had faced the challenge of resuming work and family roles. Individuals shared some similar experiences and hopes for the future but varied in the amount of trauma and stress experienced. They also differed widely in psychological readiness for return to ordinary daily routines. One woman in the group was able to return quickly to her job as a cashier in a large supermarket. The strength of her determination to overcome public reaction to her scars, coupled with an ability to "use the right words" and an empathy for others, distinguished her from others in the group. These differences proved attractive to other members, inspiring them to work toward a return to their own roles in life. These members saw her differences as attainable.

This group's cohesion was provided by the members' attraction to the common purpose of returning to successful life patterns and managing relationships with others. Members also believed that interaction with others with similar burn experiences could help them reach that goal. This example shows that certain member experiences such as crises or traumas may help individuals identify with each other and may increase member attraction.

Being different from the general population and similar to the other group members is, for some, a compelling force for membership in the group. Others are repelled by the group because they do not want to be identified by an aversive characteristic

such as disfigurement. Empathy for another's pain, learned only through mutual experience, may provide each individual with a required perspective for problem solving or affirming another's view. This nurse helped members use common experiences and learn from their differences. The group was effective.

Members' attraction to the group also depends on the nature of the group. Factors include the group programs, size, type of organization, and position in the community. Attraction to the group is increased when individuals perceive goals clearly and see group activities as effective.

The concept of cohesion helps to explain group productivity. Some cohesion is necessary for people to remain with a group and accomplish the set goals. Attractiveness positively influences members' motivation and commitment to work on the group task. Group cohesion may be increased as members better understand the experiences of others and identify common ideas and reactions to various issues. Nurses facilitate this process by pointing out similarities, contrasting supportive differences, or helping members redefine differences in ways that make those dissimilarities compatible.

Norms are standards that guide, control, and regulate individuals and communities. Group norms set the standards for group members' behaviors, attitudes, and perceptions. Group norms suggest what a group believes is important, what it finds acceptable or objectionable, or what it perceives as of no consequence. This commonly held view of what ought to be motivates members to use the group for their mutual benefit (Northen and Kurland, 2001). All groups have norms and mechanisms to accomplish conformity. Group norms serve three functions:

1. They ensure movement toward the group's purpose or tasks.
2. They maintain the group through various supports to members.
3. They influence members' perceptions and interpretations of reality.

Even though certain norms keep the group focused on its task, a certain amount of diversion is permitted as long as members respect central goals and feel committed to return to them. The **task norm** is the commitment to return to the central goals of the group. The strength of the task norm determines the group's ability to adhere to its work.

Maintenance norms create group pressures to affirm members and maintain their comfort. Individuals in groups seem most productive and at ease when their psychological and social well-being is nurtured. Maintenance behaviors include identifying the social and psychological tensions of members and taking steps to support those members at high-stress times. For example, maintenance norms often refer to things like scheduling meetings at convenient times and in an accessible and comfortable space with parking as well as seating, refreshments, and toilets.

Groups also have **reality norms,** whereby members reinforce or challenge and correct their ideas of what is real. Groups can examine the life situations confronting individuals and help to make sense of them. As individuals gather information, attempt to understand that information, make decisions, and consider the facts and their implications, they can take responsible action, not only in relation to themselves and their group, but also for the community. Group (task, maintenance, and reality) norms combine to form a group culture. Although working with a group does not mean dictating its norms, the nurse can support helpful rules, attitudes, and behaviors. Norms form when these rules, attitudes, and behaviors become part of the life of the group, independent of the nurse. Reality norms influence each member to see relevant situations in the same way the other members see them. For example, suppose a group of individuals with diabetes defines an uncontrolled diet as harmful; members may try to influence one another to maintain diet control. The nurse's role in this group is to provide accurate information about diet and the disease process while continually displaying a belief that health through diet control is attainable and desirable.

When group members have similar backgrounds, their scope of knowledge may be limited. For example, female members in a spouse abuse group may believe that men are exploitive and harmful on the basis of common childhood and marriage experiences. Such a stereotypical view of men could be reinforced by similar perceptions in other members; this might lead to continuing anger, fear of interactions with men, and a hostile or helpless approach to family affairs. Nurses or group members who have known men in loving, helpful, and collaborative ways can describe their different and positive perceptions of men, thereby adding information and challenging beliefs. The health and condition of members improve as their perceptions of reality are based on a more complete range of data. Nurses bring an important perspective to groups in which similar backgrounds limit the understanding and interpretation of personal concerns.

> **WHAT DO YOU THINK?** *Think about the last informal group in which you were a member. What was the most important benefit that you gained from the group? What did you contribute? If you could rejoin that group, are there things you would change about your participation?*

The role structure of a group refers to the expected ways in which members behave toward one another. The role that each person assumes serves a purpose in the group. Examples of roles are leader, follower, task specialist, maintenance specialist, evaluator, peacemaker, and gatekeeper. Box 16-6 includes descriptions of each of these group roles. Since leadership is an especially complex role, it will be discussed in greater detail.

Stages of Group Development

Tuckman (1965) developed a model of the stages of group development that has remained useful over time. He contended that any group, regardless of its type or setting, went through four stages: forming, storming, norming, and performing. In 1977 Tuckman and Jensen determined that there was actually a fifth stage: adjourning. This model can be used for health-related groups to identify in what stage the group is and what may be the next stage. Specifically, in the "forming" stage, members become acquainted with one another and the leader,

---

BOX 16-6 EXAMPLES OF GROUP ROLE BEHAVIOR

(There are many examples; this is a representative list of the types of roles members may use.)

- **Follower:** Seeks and accepts the authority or direction of others
- **Gatekeeper:** Controls outsiders' access to the group
- **Leader:** Guides and directs group activity
- **Maintenance specialist:** Provides physical and psychological support for group members, thereby holding the group together
- **Peacemaker:** Attempts to reconcile conflict between members or takes action in response to influences that disrupt the group process and threaten its existence
- **Task specialist:** Focuses or directs movement toward the main work of the group

---

become oriented to the group, and try to determine what their behaviors should be in relation to one another and to the goal of the group. In the "storming" stage, members begin to express their own individuality, which may run counter to that of others, and they often express hostility to one another and polarize because of interpersonal issues. In the third, or "norming," stage, members start to accept one another; develop some cohesion, norms, and roles; and become comfortable in expressing their opinions and offering ideas. Members begin to trust one another and their interaction takes on more depth. In the fourth stage, "performing," the group uses its interpersonal structure to accomplish its goals, and group energy is directed toward the tasks. In the fifth stage, "adjourning," the group engages in separating from one another.

Leadership is a complex concept. It consists of behaviors that guide or direct members and determine and influence group action. Positive leadership defines or negotiates the group's purpose, selects and helps implement tasks that accomplish the purpose, maintains an environment that affirms and supports members, and balances efforts between task and maintenance. An effective leader pays attention to communications and interactions among the members. Attention is paid to both spoken words and body language, and this information provides continuous feedback about the members and the group process. By paying close attention to communications and interactions, members detect changing group needs, and they can take responsibility and pride in their own involvement. One or more members may lead the group or leadership may be shared by many. Generally, shared leadership increases productivity, cohesion, and satisfying interactions among members.

After initiating or establishing a group, nurses may facilitate leadership within and among members, frequently relinquishing central control and encouraging members to determine the ultimate leadership pattern for their group. In some settings and circumstances, a single authority seems necessary (e.g., when members have limited skills or limited time, or when groups claim discomfort with shared responsibility for leading). A leadership style that shares leading functions with other group members is effective when there are many alternatives and when issues of values and ethics are involved in the group's action. Examples of leadership behaviors are shown in

BOX 16-7   EXAMPLES OF LEADERSHIP BEHAVIORS

- **Advising:** Introducing direction on the basis of knowledgeable opinion
- **Analyzing:** Reviewing what has occurred as encouragement to examine behavior and its meaning
- **Clarifying:** Verifying the meanings of interaction and communication through questions and restatement
- **Confronting:** Presenting behavior and its effects to the individual and group to challenge existing perceptions
- **Evaluating:** Analyzing the effect or outcome of action or the worth of an idea according to some standard
- **Initiating:** Introducing topics, beginning work, or changing the focus of a group
- **Questioning:** Generating analysis of a view or views by questions that support examination
- **Reflecting behavior:** Providing feedback on how behavior appears to others
- **Reflecting feelings:** Naming the feelings that may be behind what is said or done
- **Suggesting:** Proposing or presenting an idea to a group
- **Summarizing:** Restating discussion or group action in brief form, highlighting important points
- **Supporting:** Giving the kind of emotionally comforting feedback that helps a person or group continue ongoing actions

Box 16-7. Leadership can be described as patriarchal, paternal, or democratic. Each of these styles has a particular effect on members' interaction, satisfaction, and productivity. Groups may reflect one or a combination of styles.

A patriarchal or paternal style is seen when one person has the final authority for group direction and movement. A person using patriarchal leadership may control members through rewards and threats, often keeping them in the dark about the goals and rationale behind prescribed actions. Paternal leaders win the respect and dependence of their followers by parent-like devotion to members' needs. The leader controls group movement and progress through interpersonal power. Patriarchal and paternal styles of leadership are authoritarian. These styles are effective for groups such as a disaster team in which immediate task accomplishment or high productivity is the goal. Group morale and cohesiveness are typically low under sustained authoritarian styles of leadership, and members may not learn how to function independently. Also, issues of authority and control may disrupt productivity if the group members challenge the power of the leader.

Democratic leadership is cooperative in nature and promotes and supports members' involvement in all aspects of decision making and planning. Members influence each other as they explore goals, plan steps toward the goals, implement those steps, and evaluate progress.

Choosing Groups for Health Change

Nurses choose the type of group that will be used after studying the overall needs of the community and its people. Such a study is based on client contacts, expressed concerns from various community spokespersons, health statistics for the area, available health resources, and the community's general well-being. These data point to the community's strengths and critical needs.

The nurse can identify goals for the community and for various groups through media reports, from community informants, and from community colleagues. These goals may include visions for change as perceived by the people living and working in the local community. Data may be organized according to the opinions and behaviors of the identified groups. Such information about community groups and assessment data are used with community representatives to plan desired interventions. Community working alliances or coalitions unite diverse interest groups who share a common interest in perceived threats to community health. Nurses and other professionals are active in groups formed to address community issues. Groups are both units of community analysis and vehicles for change.

Nurses may work with existing groups or form new groups. Deciding whether to work in established groups or to begin new ones is based on the clients' needs, the purpose of existing groups, and the membership ties in existing groups. There are advantages to using established groups for individual health change. Membership ties already exist, and the existing structure can be used. It is not necessary to find new members because compatible individuals already form a working group. Established groups usually have operating methods that have proved successful; an approach for a new goal is built on this history. Members are aware of each other's strengths, limitations, and preferred styles of interaction and may be comfortable working with and may be able to influence one another. If you choose to work with an established group, be sure to determine if the new focus is compatible with the existing group purposes. Figure 16-2 shows a breakout session during a community forum.

When conducting a community assessment, nurses can use existing community groups as a source of information. Many community groups such as health-planning groups, better business clubs, women's action groups, school boards, and neighborhood councils are excellent resources for information since part of their purpose is to determine and respond to community needs. In addition, they are already established as part of the community structure. When a group representing one community sector is selected for community health intervention, the total community structure is studied. Groups reflect existing community values, strengths, and norms.

How might nurses help established groups to work toward community goals? The same interventions recommended for groups formed for individual health change can be used for groups focused on community health. Such interventions include the following:

- Building cohesion through clarifying goals and individual attraction to groups
- Building member commitment and participation
- Keeping the group focused on the goal
- Maintaining members through recognition and encouragement
- Maintaining member self-esteem during conflict and confrontation
- Analyzing forces affecting movement toward the goal
- Evaluating progress

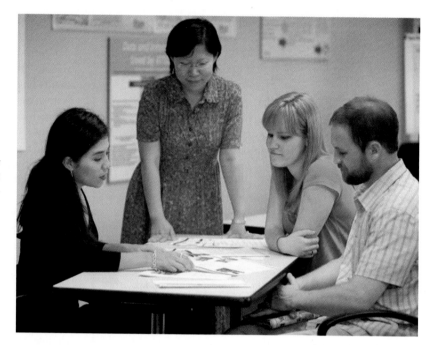

FIGURE 16-2 Breakout session in a community forum on environmental health concerns. (From Centers for Disease Control and Prevention, 2009, courtesy Dawn Arlotta.)

When nurses enter established groups, they need to assess the leadership, communications, and normative structures. This facilitates group planning, problem solving, intervention, and evaluation. The steps for community health changes parallel those of decision making and problem solving in other methodologies.

A nurse was asked to meet with a neighborhood council to help them study and "do something about" the number of homeless living on the streets. Residents knew this nurse from a local clinic and from his consulting work at a shelter for the homeless in an adjacent community. When the council invited him, they stated that "our intent is to be part of the solution rather than part of the problem." The nurse accepted the invitation to visit. He learned that the neighborhood council had addressed concerns of the neighborhood for 20 years—protecting zoning guidelines, setting up a recreational program for teens, organizing an after-school program for latchkey children, and generally representing the homeowners of the area. The neighborhood was composed of low-income families who took great pride in their homes. After meeting with the council and listening to their description of the situation, the nurse agreed to help, and he joined the council.

As the first step in addressing the problem, the council conducted a comprehensive problem analysis on the homeless situation. All known causes and outcomes of homeless persons on the street were identified, and the relationships between each factor and the problem were documented from literature and from the local history. The nurse brought expertise in health planning and knowledge of the homeless and their health risks. He suggested negotiation between the council and the local coalition for the homeless, recognizing that planning would be most relevant if homeless individuals participated. The council was cohesive and committed to the purpose, had developed working operations, and did not need help with group process.

They made adjustments in their usual group operation to use the knowledge and health-planning skills of the nurse. Interventions for the homeless included establishing temporary shelters at homes on a rotating basis, providing daily meals through the city council or churches, and joining the area coalition for the homeless.

This example shows how an established, competent group addressed a new goal successfully by building on existing strengths in partnership with the nurse. Community groups, because of their interactive roles, are logical and natural ways for people who work together for community health change. As the decision-making and problem-solving capabilities of community groups are strengthened, the groups become more able representatives for the whole community. Nurses improve the community's health by working with groups toward that goal.

How can the nurse enter existing groups and direct their attention to individual health needs? One nurse employed by an industrial firm noted the harmful effect of managerial stress on several individuals. They had elevated blood pressure, stomach pain, and emotional tension. The nurse learned that the employees with stress were all members of a jogging team that met weekly for conversation in addition to regular workouts. High-level health had been a value shared by all team members, but although jogging was seen as an enjoyable and health-promoting activity, they had never talked about a shared purpose for improved health. The nurse saw a need for stress reduction, thought that the individuals at risk could achieve stress reduction if supported through a group process from valued friends, and proposed that a new purpose be added to the jogging team's activities. All in the group readily accepted.

When it is neither desirable nor possible to use existing groups, the nurse can initiate a selected membership group. Choose members who have common health needs or concerns. For instance, individuals with diabetes can meet to discuss diet management and physical care and to share problem-solving remedies; community residents can meet for social support and rehabilitation after treatment for mental illness; or isolated older adults can meet to socialize, eat nutritious meals, and exercise.

Consider members' attributes when composing a new group. Members are attracted to others from similar backgrounds, with similar experiences, and with common interests and abilities. Individual behavior is influenced by the membership, purpose, attraction, norms, leadership, and group structure, as well as memories from prior groups. It is important to select members so that common ties or interests balance out dissimilar traits. It helps to have in the group people with expressive and problem-solving skills and others who serve in supportive roles; try to have a mix of people with both task and maintenance functions, and others who can develop these skills.

The size of the group influences effectiveness; generally, 8 to 12 is a good number for group work focused on individual health changes. Groups of up to 25 members may be effective when their focus is on community needs. Large groups often divide and assign tasks to the smaller subgroups, with the original large groups meeting less frequently for reporting and evaluation. Setting member criteria can facilitate recruitment and selection of the most appropriate members for any group. The criteria usually suggest a mixture of member traits, allowing for balance for the processes of decision making and growth.

> **NURSING TIP**   *Groups are more valuable to members when the purpose of the group is clearly stated and agreed on.*

Beginning Interactions

Work on the stated purpose begins as soon as the group forms. It is important to help members interact with a degree of satisfaction. This requires close attention to maintenance tasks of attending, eliciting information, clarifying, and recognizing contributions of members. Begin by talking about what brought each member to the group. Encourage each person to participate; recognize and support them as they take on leadership functions. The new group begins to take shape in the early sessions as members try out familiar roles and test their individual abilities. The core competency skills for communication recommended by the Public Health Foundation (Council on Linkages, 2010) are useful to nurses engaged in group work in the community. Box 16-8 lists these competencies. Subsequent steps are then planned not only according to the nurse's skill and preference, but also according to the group composition and the skills brought by members.

Conflict

Conflict occurs normally in all human relations. However, people generally see conflict as the opposite of harmony and try to guard against it. This is an unfortunate view because the tensions of difference and potential conflict actually help groups work toward their purposes. It is important to understand common causes of conflict and conflict management and resolution approaches.

BOX 16-8   CORE COMPETENCIES FOR COMMUNICATION SKILLS OF EDUCATORS

Communication Skills
- Communicates effectively both in writing and orally, including via e-mail
- Solicits input from individuals and organizations
- Advocates for public health programs and resources
- Leads and participates in groups to address specific issues
- Uses the media, varied technologies, and community networks to convey information
- Effectively presents accurate demographic, statistical, programmatic, and scientific information for professional and lay audiences

Attitudes
- Listens to others in an unbiased manner
- Respects points of view of others
- Promotes the expression of diverse opinions and perspectives

---

Conflict occurs when members feel obstructed or irritated by one or more other group members (Northen and Kurland, 2001). Conflict signals that antagonistic points of view must be considered and that one must reexamine beliefs and assumptions underlying relationships. Some people are concerned about security, control of self and others, respect between parties, and access to limited resources. In groups, members may express frustrations about trust, closeness and separation, and dependence and independence. These themes of interpersonal conflict operate to some extent in all interactions and are not unique to groups.

People tend to repeat the same patterns of behavior in conflicts. Sometimes the pattern works; other times it does not. The best approach is to match the response style to the situation (Sportsman and Hamilton, 2007), which requires personal awareness and awareness of others. Specifically, when you respond with avoidance, forcing with power, capitulation, and exclusion of a member, the behaviors fail to satisfy the concerns of participants. Assertiveness (attempting to satisfy one's own concerns) and cooperativeness (attempting to satisfy the concerns of others) can be positive responses to conflict. Behaviors that reflect either assertiveness or cooperativeness and that may satisfy the frustrated parties include confrontation, competition, compromise, reconciliation, and collaboration. Resolving conflict within groups depends on open communication among all parties, diffusion of negative feelings and perceptions, concentration on the issues, and use of fair procedures and a structured approach to the process.

Conflict can be overwhelming, especially when members view the expression of controversy as unacceptable or unremitting. Conflict suppressed over time tends to build up and finally explode out of proportion to the current frustration. A group that repeatedly avoids expressing conflict becomes fragile, unable to adapt, and helpless to face challenges. Conflict may be destructive if contentious parties fail to respect the rights and beliefs of others.

Approaches for conflict-acknowledging and problem-solving that respect others and represent self-concerns are first learned in families and other small groups. These lessons teach people to embrace conflict as a natural occurrence that supports growth and change. Other people learn to avoid conflict or to disregard others in the promotion of self. Teams that embrace a united desire for harmony to the extent of avoiding conflict in interactions may hinder collaboration and personal growth (Gerow, 2001). However, individuals may evaluate conflict management styles and refine skills in collaborative groups that support expression and resolution of conflict. Examination of conflict and resolution in supportive groups results in enhanced working relationships, stress reduction, and better coping.

Evaluation of Group Progress

It is important to evaluate individual and group progress toward health goals. Early in the planning, specify the action steps that should be taken to meet the goals. These small steps may be responses to learning objectives (listed as action steps designed to support facilitative forces and deal with resistive forces), or they may reflect the group's problem-solving plan. The action steps and the indicators of achievement are discussed and written in a group record. Recognition of accomplishments in the group and of the group is built into the group's evaluation system. Recognition may include concrete rewards such as special foods and drinks, or it may be the personal expression of joy and member-to-member approval. Celebration for group accomplishments marks progress, rewards members, and motivates each person to continue.

Implement the Educational Plan

Once educational methods have been selected, they should be implemented through management of the educational process. Implementation entails the following (Knowles, 1990):

- Control over starting, sustaining, and stopping each method and strategy in the most effective and appropriate time and manner
- Coordination and control of environmental factors, the flow of the presentation, and other contributory facets of the program
- Keeping the materials logically related to the core theme and overall program goals

In addition, administrative and political support is essential to successful program implementation.

Educators must be flexible. They must modify educational methods and strategies to meet unexpected challenges that may confront both the educator and the learner. External influences (such as time limitations, expense, and administrative and political factors) and learner needs require an ongoing evaluation of their impact on the educational program (Babcock and Miller, 1994; Knowles, 1990). Thus implementation is a dynamic element in the educational process.

CHAPTER REVIEW

PRACTICE APPLICATION

Kristi, a BSN student, is having her community health practicum at a local health department. The health department has gotten many calls from people wanting information about H1N1 virus. For Kristi's community health intervention project, she decides to do a community educative piece on this topic. What is her best course of action?

A. Develop a poster presentation to have on display at the health department.

B. Assemble an educative pamphlet to mail to anyone calling with questions.
C. Work with the health department staff to develop a community forum–style presentation and information brochures on this virus.
D. Develop an in-service program for health department staff on potential spread of the virus and ways to prevent its spread.
Answers can be found on the Evolve site.

KEY POINTS

- Health education is a vital component of nursing because the promotion, maintenance, and restoration of health rely on clients' understanding of health care topics.
- Nurse educators identify learning needs, consider how people learn, examine educational issues, design and implement educational programs, and evaluate the effects of the educational program on learning and behavior.
- Nurses often use the *Healthy People 2020* educational objectives as a guide to identifying community-based learning needs.
- Education and learning are different. Education is the establishment and arrangement of events to facilitate learning. Learning is the process of gaining knowledge and expertise and results in behavioral changes.

- Three domains of learning are cognitive, affective, and psychomotor. Depending on the needs of the learner, one or more of these domains may be important for the nurse educator to consider as learning programs are developed.
- Nine principles associated with community health education are gaining attention, informing the learner of the objectives of instruction, stimulating recall of prior learning, presenting the stimulus, providing learning guidance, eliciting performance, providing feedback, assessing performance, and enhancing retention and transfer of knowledge.
- Often theory can guide the development of health education programs. Two useful ones are the Health Belief Model and the

■ KEY POINTS—cont'd

Transtheoretical Model (TTM), which is discussed in connection with the Precaution Adoption Process Model (PAPM).

- Principles that guide the effective educator include message, format, environment, experience, participation, and evaluation.
- Educational issues include population considerations, barriers to learning, and technological issues.
- Two important learner-related barriers are low literacy, especially health literacy, and lack of motivation to learn information and make the needed changes.
- The five phases of the educational process are identifying educational needs, establishing educational goals and objectives, selecting appropriate educational methods, implementing the educational plan, and evaluating the educational process and product.
- Evaluation of the product includes the measurement of short- and long-term goals and objectives related to improving health and promoting behavioral changes.
- Working with groups is an important skill for nurses. Groups are an effective and powerful vehicle for initiating and implementing healthful changes.
- A group is a collection of interacting individuals with a common purpose. Each member influences and is influenced by other group members to varying degrees.
- Group cohesion is enhanced by commonly shared characteristics among members and diminished by differences among members.

- Cohesion is the measure of attraction between members and the group. Cohesion or the lack of it affects the group's function.
- Norms are standards that guide and regulate individuals and communities. These norms are unwritten and often unspoken and serve to ensure group movement to a goal, to maintain the group, and to influence group members' perceptions and interpretations of reality.
- Some diversity of member backgrounds is usually a positive influence on a group.
- Groups also go through a set of stages in order to form, operate, and adjourn.
- Leadership is an important and complex group concept. Leadership is described as patriarchal, paternal, or democratic.
- Group structure emerges from various member influences, including members' understanding and support of the group purpose.
- Conflicts in groups may develop from competition for roles or member disagreement about the roles ascribed to them.
- Health behavior is greatly influenced by the groups to which people belong and for which they value membership.
- An understanding of group concepts provides a basis for identifying community groups and their goals, characteristics, and norms. Nurses use their understanding of group principles to work with community groups toward needed health changes.

■ CLINICAL DECISION-MAKING ACTIVITIES

1. Think about an educational interaction that you had with each type of client (individual, family, community, and population) that did not seem to go well. For each type of client and on the basis of how people learn, identify what might have been the problem. Develop a plan for ways in which the interaction could have been improved based on how people learn.

2. Recall a learning experience in which the message, format, environment, experience, participation, or evaluation was unsatisfactory. Then develop a plan for how the problem could have been overcome and turned from a negative or neutral learning situation into a positive one.

3. Review the phases of the educational process. Apply this process to a population of individuals with hypertension, a community in which tuberculosis is on the rise, and families with a child who has attention deficit disorder.

4. Select one of the *Healthy People 2020* educational objectives and design a population-specific education program to meet that objective. Include how people learn, educational issues, educational process including teaching strategies, and evaluation procedures that you would use.

5. Consider three groups of which you are a member. What is the stated purpose of each group? Are you aware of unstated but clearly understood purposes? What is the nature of member interaction in each group? How do purpose and interaction differ in the three groups?

6. Observe two working groups in session, from the community, a health care agency, or a school. Notice the attractiveness of each group through the eyes of its members.

7. List actions that nurses may take to assist groups in various aspects of their work, such as member selection, purpose clarification, arrangements for comfort in participation, and group problem solving.

8. Observe a nurse working with a health promotion group. Does the nurse function in the way you anticipated? What nursing behavior facilitates the group process? List the areas of skill and knowledge that groups consisting of community residents would most likely expect of the nurse.

REFERENCES

Agency for Healthcare Research and Quality: *Assessing the quality of internet health information, 1999.* Available at http://www.ahcpr.gov/data/infoqual.htm. Accessed March 12, 2011.

American Nurses Association: *Scope & standards of practice: public health nursing,* Silver Springs, MD, 2007, ANA.

Babcock DE, Miller MA: *Client education: theory and practice,* St Louis, 1994, Mosby.

Bartholomew LK, Shegog R, Parcel GS, et al: Watch, discover, think, and act: a model for patient education program development, *Patient Educ Couns* 39:253–268, 2000.

Bloom BS, Englehart MO, Furst EJ, et al: *Taxonomy of educational objectives: the classification of educational goals—handbook 1: cognitive domain,* White Plains, NY, 1956, Longman.

Brandler S: *Group work: skills and strategies for effective intervention,* ed 2, New York, 1999, Haworth Press.

Council on Linkages Between Academia and Public Health Practice: *Core competencies for public health professionals,* Washington, DC, 2010, Public Health Foundation. Available at www.phf.org. Accessed March 2010.

Cramer M, Roberts S, Xu L: Evaluating community-based programs for eliminating secondhand smoke using evidence-based research for best practices, *Fam Community Health* 30:129–143, 2007.

Dauz E, Moore J, Smith CE, et al: Installing computers in older adults' home and teaching them to access a patient education web site: a systematic approach, *Comput Inform Nurs* 22:266–272, 2004.

Dembo MH: *Applying educational psychology*, ed 5, White Plains, NY, 1994, Longman.

Driscoll MP: *Psychology of learning for instruction*, ed 3, Boston, 2005, Allyn and Bacon.

Gerow SJ: Teachers in school-based teams: contesting isolation in schools. In Sockett HT, DeMulder EK, DePage PC, Wood DR, editors: *Transforming teacher education: lessons in professional development*, Westport, CT, 2001, Bergin & Garvey.

Hanson M, Fisher J: Patient-centered teaching from theory to practice, *Am J Nurs* 98:56–60, 1998.

Health Literacy Innovations: *10 tips for print materials*, press release, May 8, 2007. Available at http://www.HealthLiteracyInnovation.com. Accessed February 22, 2008.

The Joint Commission: *What did the doctor say? Improving health literacy to protect patient safety*, February 7, 2007. Available at http://www.jointcommission.org.INR/rdonlyres/F53D5t. Accessed February 24, 2010.

Kleinbeck C: Reaching positive diabetes outcomes for patients with low literacy, *Home Healthcare Nurse* 23(1):16–22, 2005.

Kleinpell RM, Mick DJ: Evaluating outcomes. In Fulter TT, Foreman MD, Walker M, editors: *Critical care nursing of the elderly*, ed 2, New York, 2001, Springer, pp 179–196.

Knowles M: *The adult learner: a neglected species*, ed 4, Houston, 1990, Gulf.

Knowles MS, Holton EF III, Swanson RA: *The adult learner: the definitive classic in adult education and human resource development*, ed 5, Houston, 1998, Gulf.

Knowles MS, Holton EF III, Swanson RA: *The adult learner: the definitive classic in adult education and human resource development*, ed 6, London, 2005, Elsevier/Butterworth Heinemann.

Krathwohl DR, Bloom BS, Masia BB: *Taxonomy of educational objectives: the classification of educational goals—handbook 2: affective domain*, New York, 1964, David McKay.

Kutner M, Greenberg E, Jin Y, Paulsen C: *The health literacy of America's adults. Results from the 2003 National Assessment of Adult Literacy*, (NCES 2006-483), 2006, U.S. Department of Education, Washington DC Center for Education. Available at http://www.edpubs.org. Accessed March 2010.

Northen H, Kurland R: *Social work with groups*, ed 3, New York, 2001, Columbia University Press.

Ota C, DiCarlo C, Burts D, et al: Training and the needs of adult learners, *J Extension* 44(6), 2006. Available at www.joe.org/joe/2006december/tt5.shtml:Accessed December 31, 2010.

Palazzo M: Teaching in crisis: patient and family education in critical care, *Crit Care Nurs Clin North Am* 13:83–92, 2001.

Pew Charitable Trusts: *Pew Internet and American Life Project, 2008*, Philadelphia. Available at www.pewinternet.org. Accessed March 2010.

Ratzan SC, Parker RM: Introduction. In Selden CR, Zorn M, Ratzan SC, Parker RM, editors: *National Library of Medicine current bibliographies in medicine: health literacy*, NLM Pub No CBM 2000-1, Bethesda MD, 2000, National Institutes of Health, U.S. Department of Health and Human Services.

Rice CS, Pollard JM: *Health fair planning guide, AgriLIFE EXTENSION*, September 16, 2009, Texas A&M System. Available at http://fcs.tamu.edu/health/health-fair-planning-guide/index.php. Accessed February 16, 2009.

Roberts K: Simplify, simplify: tackling health literacy by addressing reading literacy, *AJN* 104:118–119, 2004.

Schulte JA: Finding ways to create connections among communities: partial results of an ethnography of urban public health nurses, *Public Health Nurs* 17:3, 2000.

Sportsman S, Hamilton P: Conflict management styles in the health professions, *J Prof Nurs* 23(3):157–166, 2007.

Tuckman BW: Developmental sequence in small groups, *Psychol Bull* 63(6):384–399, 1965.

Tuckman BW, Jensen MAC: Stages of small-group development revisited, *Group Organization Stud* 2(4):419–427, 1977.

United HealthCare: *Health fair planning guide: wellness toolkit*. Available at http://www.uhctool.com. Accessed February 16, 2010.

U.S. Department of Health and Human Services: *Healthy People 2020*. Available at http://www.healthypeople.gov/2020/default.aspx. Retrieved January 3, 2011.

U.S. Department of Health and Human Services: *Theory at a glance: a guide for health promotion*, ed 2, 2005, NIH publication No. 05-3896. Available at www.cancer.org. Accessed March 2010.

VanBiervliet A, Edwards-Schafer P: Consumer health information on the web: trends, issues, and strategies, *Dermatol Nurs* 16:519–523, 2004.

Whitener LM, Cox KR, Maglich SA: Use of theory to guide nurses in the design of health messages for children, *Adv Nurs Sci* 20:21–35, 1998.

Wilson SM, Peterson PL: *Theories of learning and teaching, what do they mean for educators?* Washington DC, July 2006, National Education Association.

Wolf MS: Patient education. In Fulmer TT, Foreman MD, Walker M, editors: *Critical care nursing of the elderly*, ed 2, New York, 2001, Springer, pp 162–178.

CHAPTER 17

Promoting Healthy Communities Using Multilevel Participatory Strategies

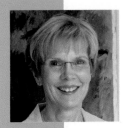

Pamela A. Kulbok, DNSc, RN, PHCNS-BC, FAAN

Pamela A. Kulbok earned her doctorate at Boston University and did postdoctoral work in psychiatric epidemiology at Washington University in St. Louis. She was a U.S. Navy nurse; has worked in a visiting nurse service; and has directed a hospital-based home health agency. She is presently Professor of Nursing and Chair of the Department of Family, Community, and Mental Health Systems at the University of Virginia, School of Nursing. Dr. Kulbok is the Principal Investigator of an interprofessional, cross-institution, community-based participatory research project to design a substance use prevention program with youth, parents, and community leaders in a rural tobacco-growing county of Virginia. This study builds on a series of externally funded studies of youth non-smoking behavior. She has taught undergraduate and graduate courses in public health nursing, health promotion research, and nursing knowledge development. Dr. Kulbok has been a leader of public health nursing professional organizations. She was president of the Association of Community Health Nursing Educators (2004-2006) and Chair of the Quad Council of Public Health Nursing Organizations (2004-2005). She recently completed a 4-year term as a member of the American Nurses Association (ANA)—Congress on Nursing Practice and Economics. She was a contributor to the *Nursing Social Policy Statement: Essence of the Profession* (ANA, 2010). She is an inaugural faculty and faculty fellow, Healthy Appalachia Institute, the University of Virginia's College at Wise, National Network of Public Institutes, in recognition of contributions to the health of the residents of Southwest Virginia (2009-2011).

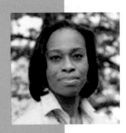

Nisha Botchwey, PhD, MCRP

Nisha Botchwey specializes in community development and neighborhood planning emphasizing local religious and secular institutions and public health promotion. She teaches undergraduate and graduate community development and health courses including *Healthy Communities*, a seminar exploring the connections between the built environment and health, and available as an online curriculum resource (http://www.builtenvironmentandpublichealthcurriculum.com). She is presently Associate Professor of Urban End Environmental Planning and Public Health Sciences at the University of Virginia. She discussed her focus on approaches to revitalize unhealthy communities, places where the physical and social environments do not enable people to maximize their lives, on the Centers for Disease Control and Prevention's 2007 National Broadcast of Public Health Grand Round titled "Healthy Places Leading to Healthy People: Community Engagement Improves Health for All." Her funded research involves three multidisciplinary collaborations with scholars from the Schools of Nursing, Medicine and Engineering, and with support from the National Institutes of Health and other public and private sources. Dr. Botchwey's publications are found in a variety of planning, public health, and nursing journals. She serves on local and national advisory boards including the Governing Board for the Association of Collegiate Schools of Planning and is a recipient of numerous awards including Annie E Casey Foundation Junior Scholar (2004), NIH Health Disparities Scholar (2005, 2006), Seven Society as an Outstanding Teacher (2007), and Rockefeller-Penn Fellow (2010).

ADDITIONAL RESOURCES

evolve WEBSITE
http://evolve.elsevier.com/Stanhope
- *Healthy People 2020*
- WebLinks—Of special note see the links for these sites:
  - Healthier People Network
  - National Wellness Institute

- Quiz
- Case Studies
- Glossary
- Answers to Practice Application

OBJECTIVES

After reading this chapter, the student should be able to do the following:

1. Describe health promotion, illness prevention, and illness care in the context of the ecological model and social determinants of health (SDOH).
2. Analyze participatory approaches and the interrelationships among communities, populations, and interprofessional health care providers in the application of health promotion strategies.
3. Describe evidence-based practice at multiple levels of the client system: individual, family, aggregate, and community.
4. Analyze nursing and interprofessional roles that are essential to health promotion, illness prevention, and illness care.

KEY TERMS

built environment, p. 376
client system, p. 377
community, p. 382
community-based participatory research (CBPR), p. 374
community health, p. 384
ecological approach, p. 374

focus of care, p. 377
health, p. 377
health behavior, p. 380
health maintenance, p. 381
health promotion, p. 381
illness care, p. 377
illness prevention, p. 381

lifestyles, p. 374
multilevel intervention, p. 374
Photovoice, p. 387
risk appraisal, p. 381
social determinants of health (SDOH), p. 374
—*See Glossary for definitions*

OUTLINE

The pursuit of long, healthy lives through participation in population-focused health programs is essential to achieve the national health vision and goals proposed in *Healthy People 2020* (USDHHS, 2009a). Interest in healthy lifestyles is obvious in the accruing epidemiological evidence linking lifestyle and health, and notably in the emphasis on public health programs that address the social determinants of health (SDOH) and healthy lifestyles in populations (Freudenberg, 2007). Virtually all people recognize the need to exercise regularly, maintain their weight at recommended levels, and manage stress in their lives. Despite increased interest in healthy lifestyles, modifiable health-related behaviors are the major contributors to deaths in the United States (NCHS, 2010). For example, tobacco use remains the leading cause of premature deaths with 443,000 deaths annually attributed to cigarette smoking (NCHS, 2010). Nurses, other health professionals, and the public recognize that initiating and maintaining a healthy lifestyle is complex and requires different approaches directed toward individuals, families, communities, populations, and the environments in which they live.

In this chapter, we describe an ecological approach to community health promotion, which integrates multilevel interventions to promote the health of the public. The integrative model of community health promotion (Laffrey and Kulbok, 1999)

can help nurses plan care for clients including communities and populations. The model synthesizes knowledge from public health, nursing, and the social sciences. In this chapter, we also define some of the basic concepts that concern nurses and their interprofessional health care partners. We describe the historical underpinnings of these concepts, including definitions of health and health promotion for communities and populations including the SDOH. The concepts of health maintenance, illness prevention, and community are also discussed. These concepts and their linkages determine the direction and methods for nursing practice with communities and populations. The chapter describes studies that illustrate community-based participatory research (CBPR) and multilevel interventions. Applications of the integrative model of community health promotion show that the way nurses view these concepts is important in their approach to practice.

THE ECOLOGICAL APPROACH TO COMMUNITY HEALTH PROMOTION

Nurses have long recognized the importance of an emphasis on wellness and health promotion in health care. In public health nursing (PHN) practice, it is clear that many factors, beyond illness, affect the health of individuals, communities, and populations. The biomedical model, in which health is defined as absence of disease, does not explain why some populations exposed to illness-producing stressors remain healthy, whereas others, who appear to be in health-enhancing situations, become ill. Viewing clients from the perspective of the biomedical model alone makes it difficult to identify health potential beyond the absence of disease. For example, most at-risk populations such as the frail elderly have at least one diagnosed chronic disease. Limiting the definition of health potential to the absence of disease, nurses would never perceive this population as healthy. Defining health as the absence of disease is a pessimistic definition; nursing actions can help older and chronically ill persons become healthier if a broader definition of health is used. Nurses can assist clients in identifying their health potential and in planning measures that enhance their health.

Studies show that there is no better way to promote health and improve the quality of life of individuals than through basic healthy habits such as exercising regularly, maintaining a balanced and healthy diet, developing a positive and optimistic outlook, and refraining from smoking (Chowdhury et al, 2010). Directing health care toward helping communities and populations to identify their health potential, and providing care and resources that move communities and populations toward their health potential, are important goals. These actions can improve the health of the overall population and thus decrease the burden of disease in vulnerable populations at the fringe of health care.

Laffrey, Loveland-Cherry, and Winkler (1986) described two perspectives from which the key concepts of nursing science (e.g., person, health, environment) and nursing can be viewed. The disease-oriented perspective views health objectively and defines it as the absence of disease. This perspective assumes that humans are composed of organ systems and cells; health care focuses on identifying what is not working properly with a given system and repairing it. In this context, how clients comply with the recommendations of health professionals forms the basis for health behavior. The second perspective defines health subjectively as a process. Humans are complex and interconnected with the environment. They are different from and greater than the sum of their parts. Health behavior within the health-oriented perspective involves a holistic view of lifestyle and interaction with the environment and is not simply compliance with a prescribed regimen.

Both perspectives support the aims and processes of population-focused nursing. The disease-oriented approach directs nursing toward illness prevention, risk appraisal, risk reduction, prompt treatment, and disease management, whereas the health-oriented approach directs nursing practice toward promotion of greater levels of positive health. Defining health broadly as the life process, taking into account the mutual and simultaneous interaction of humans and their environment, views illness as a potential manifestation of that interaction. Because positive health does not exclude any part of the life process (it includes illness prevention and illness care), it goes beyond the disease perspective to include positive and holistic health (Laffrey and Kulbok, 1999).

Ecological Perspectives on Population Health

Because individuals ultimately make decisions to engage in healthy or risky behaviors, lifestyle improvement efforts have focused typically on the individual as the target of care. Following the health belief model (Rosenstock, 1974), individuals generally concentrate on immediate personal rewards or threats when deciding whether to engage in specific behaviors; in this context, they may convince themselves that their immediate personal risks from certain behaviors such as smoking are low, or that the immediate rewards outweigh the risks. However, from a public health perspective, smoking in the United States has resulted in more than 443,000 deaths annually during 2000 to 2004, and the annual health-related economic losses were approximately 5.1 million years of potential life lost and $96.8 billion in productivity losses (CDC, 2008). Therefore, it is clear that health behaviors extend beyond the individual or the intrapersonal and the interpersonal levels, having multiple determinants both internal and external to individuals and communities, as well as determinants within the society.

For example, adolescents' decisions not to smoke are associated with their individual attributes (e.g., positive self-image), family characteristics (e.g., parent–child connectedness), aggregate characteristics (e.g., peer influence), and community factors (e.g., living in a tobacco-growing region) (Kulbok et al, 2008b). As a result, interventions to initiate or maintain healthy behaviors have greater potential for success when directed systematically toward the multiple targets of the individual, family, group, community, and society—that is, when they use an ecological approach to community health promotion.

The Social Determinants of Health

Current trends in public health and health promotion emphasize the ecological perspective with interaction between individuals and the environment. The ecological approach also addresses the SDOH (McQueen, 2009) through social networks, organizations, neighborhoods, and communities (Navarro, Voetsch, and Liburd et al, 2007). According to the World Health Organization (WHO), SDOH "are the conditions in which people are born, grow up, live, work and age, including their health. These circumstances are in turn shaped by a wider set of forces: economics, social policies, and politics" (2010, p 1). The WHO is an important contributor to defining and developing strategies to address the SDOH. They outlined ten components of SDOH. (Box 17-1 lists the 10 components.)

There is increasing awareness that to achieve lasting gains in population health, assessments and interventions must be directed to multiple levels of the client system like those outlined in the SDOH. For example, a multilevel analysis of depressive symptoms in a national sample of 18,473 adolescents in the United States (Wight et al, 2005) showed that individual, family, aggregate, and community characteristics accounted for significant differences in adolescent depression. The American Academy of Pediatrics (2005) issued a statement urging pediatricians to increase their partnerships with communities in developing programs to improve child health. Examples of pediatrician-community partnerships (Sanders et al, 2005) include establishing a child health consultant program, working with a

BOX 17-1   THE SOCIAL DETERMINANTS OF HEALTH

1. *The Social Gradient:* Life expectancy is shorter and most diseases are more common further down the social ladder in each society.
2. *Stress:* Stressful circumstances—Making people feel worried, anxious, and unable to cope—are damaging to health and may lead to premature death.
3. *Early Life:* The health impact of early development and education lasts a lifetime.
4. *Social Exclusion:* Hardship and resentment, poverty, social exclusion, and discrimination cost lives.
5. *Work:* Stress in the workplace increases the risk of disease. People who have more control over their work have better health.
6. *Unemployment:* Job security increases health, well-being, and job satisfaction. Higher rates of unemployment cause more illness and premature death.
7. *Social support:* Friendship, good social relations, and strong supportive networks improve health at home, at work, and in the community.
8. *Addiction:* Individuals turn to alcohol, drugs, and tobacco and suffer from their use, but use is influenced by the wider social setting.
9. *Food:* Because global market forces control the food supply, healthy food is a political issue.
10. *Transport:* Healthy transport means less driving and more walking and cycling, backed up by better public transport.

From World Health Organization: *Social determinants of health,* Geneva, 2010. Available at http://www.who.int/social_determinants/thecommission/finalreport/key_concepts/en/index.html. Accessed January 2, 2010.

community to repair and fund sites to facilitate safe physical activity for children, developing dance programs for overweight and obese adolescent girls, and arranging a program for community leaders to learn about the Medicaid enrollment process. Traditional interventions that target only an individual's risk or illness are not as effective as interventions and programs developed using an ecological approach that can affect all levels of the client system that contribute to good or ill health (Navarro et al, 2007). More studies are needed to design and test these ecological, multilevel community health interventions.

Farley and Cohen (2005) introduced the curve-shifting principle. This principle complements the ecological model and calls for targeting health interventions at the population level. They built upon representations of the relationship between individual and group behavior (Rose, 1992), with individual behavior being the foundation of the total population distribution. The median of this normal distribution represents prevailing social norms that govern health behavior. Traditional approaches to health behavior interventions for public health problems like obesity focus on the intrapersonal and interpersonal levels for high-risk populations—people at the extremes of the population curve. Although treating high-risk populations may be effective for selected individuals and may move them closer to the center or the prevailing social norm, this approach does little to prevent others from becoming the extremes of the distribution. Therefore, a focus on the total population, not just the high-risk group, with efforts to change the social norm so that everyone is consuming less sugar or participating in more

hours of moderate to vigorous physical activity, exemplifies the curve-shifting principle.

Consider another example of the curve-shifting principle involves the built environment. The built environment includes the physical parts of the environment where we live and work (e.g., homes, buildings, streets, open spaces, and infrastructure) (CDC, 2006). Prentice and Jebb (1995) were among the first to report the association between obesity and the built environment by measuring inactivity, car ownership, and television viewing.

Instead of simply teaching children the importance of walking and biking to school, the Safe Routes to Schools initiative improved the environment and the walkability of areas near schools, which correlates with increased local resident walking (Owen et al, 2004). Increased walking among local adult residents is evidence that "…increasing neighborhood walkability may affect people in the larger community, not just schoolchildren" (Watson et al, 2008, p 5). As a result, the population living nearest to walkable areas will walk more, thereby shifting the population social norms about walking and biking, including to school. People's behavior will change based on targeted interventions to the environment in which they live, a concept advanced by B.F. Skinner, a behavioral psychologist in the 1950s (Skinner, 1978). In following this curve-shifting principle in health promotion and illness prevention, the ecological model works at the population level to shift social norms governing health behavior and ultimately health outcomes.

An Integrative Model for Community Health Promotion

Laffrey and Kulbok (1999) developed a model for community health promotion to guide nursing and health care. The original intent of the model was threefold. First, the model assists nurses to see the continuity of care at multiple levels. Second, it helps nurses describe their own areas of expertise within the complex health care system. Third, the model provides a basis for collaboration and partnership among nurses, other health care providers, and the population. Each of these collaborators brings expertise to the client system. Important assumptions underlying the model include the need for integration of care in the complex health care system; the inseparable nature of individuals, families, aggregates, and community systems; and the maximization of health potential through health promotion interventions. In addition, the model builds upon complementary health and disease perspectives described previously (Figure 17-1). The health perspective focuses on promoting health as a dynamic and positive quality of life and includes the promotion of physical, mental, emotional, functional, spiritual, and social well-being. The disease perspective includes both the care and prevention of illness (disease and disability) and focuses on reducing risks and threats to health. Although some clinical strategies may be similar in the two perspectives, their ultimate goals differ fundamentally. The difference in these two perspectives is seen in the specific purpose of nursing and health care, as it is applied to health promotion, illness prevention, or illness care.

The integrative model (Laffrey and Kulbok, 1999) includes two major dimensions: client system and focus of care. The

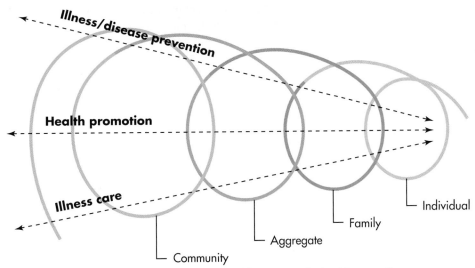

FIGURE 17-1 An integrative model for community health promotion.

client system is multidimensional with nursing and health care targeting the multiple levels of clients. The simplest level of the client system is its most delimited target, the individual. When the individual is the client, the environment includes the family, the broader aggregate, and the community of which the individual is a part. The nurse and health care provider are concerned with how these environments affect the individual as well as his or her health.

Each succeeding level of the client system is more complex, since the client can also be the family, an aggregate, or the community. The aggregate and community make up the environment for the family, and the community is the environment for the aggregate. Examples of different types of assessments and interventions appropriate at each level of client within the system are discussed later in this chapter. It is important to remember that community-oriented care is holistic in nature and is population focused in that it addresses multiple levels of clients and multiple levels of care within the total system. The integrative model of community health promotion is consistent with the ecological approach described earlier, which addresses SDOH through social networks, organizations, neighborhoods, and communities (Navarro et al, 2007).

Focus of care in the integrative model includes health promotion, illness (disease or disability) prevention, and illness care. Each focus is appropriate for some aspects of nursing and health care. It is even more important to remember that the goal of health care is a healthier community, achieved through health promotion interventions. No matter where care begins, it ultimately leads to health promotion of the community. It underscores the need for nurses and health care providers to have a good understanding of care requirements at all of the client levels. The individual, family, aggregate, and community each have characteristics, strengths, and health needs that are unique and that differ from those at the other levels.

The integrative community health promotion model reflects the basic beliefs and values of holistic nursing and health care practice. The model depicts continuity and expansiveness of the client systems and foci of care. Health promotion is the central

axis, or core, of the model. At its narrowest focus, individuals receive illness care. According to the model, at the broadest level of care, nurses work with community leaders, other community residents, and health professionals to plan programs to promote optimal health for the community and its people. The goals of nursing and health care actions in the integrative model, at any client level from the individual to the community, are to identify health potential and achieve maximal health. To achieve these goals it is essential to have an active partnership between the nurse, health care providers, and the client system. By facilitating an active partnership with the client system, whether the focus of care is health promotion, illness prevention, or illness care, nurses involve clients in each step of the process of managing care from the assessment of their health needs and resources to implementation and evaluation of outcomes.

NURSING TIP *Facilitate active partnerships with clients and other health care professionals through ongoing collaboration and involve clients in every step of the process of managing health care from assessment of their clinical and associated ecological needs to planning, implementing, and evaluating outcomes. The public health practice of forming active partnerships to solve community or population problems is also applicable in public health research, commonly called community-based participatory research (CBPR).*

HISTORICAL PERSPECTIVES, DEFINITIONS, AND METHODS

Health and Health Promotion

Historical Perspectives on Health

Health is the key term in an ecological approach to community health promotion. Beginning with Florence Nightingale's efforts to discover and use the laws of nature to enhance humanity, nursing has always taken an active role in promoting the health of communities and populations. The way one defines health shapes the process of nursing and health care, including

EVIDENCE-BASED PRACTICE

Laffrey and Kulbok's Integrative Model for Community Health Promotion (1999) was used to promote the health and wellness of people at Old Town Clinic. At the community clinic, nurses applied the foci of care (i.e., health promotion, illness prevention, and/or illness care) to provide health care that serves individuals, families, and the community. Seventy-three clients who received integrated services and seven staff members who provided services were surveyed between January and February 2003. Clients indicated high levels of satisfaction with the clinic's location, ease of accessing care, and health promotion and illness prevention education. The staff indicated moderate levels of satisfaction related to accessibility, response time, communication, support, treatment, completeness of care, and education.

Nurse Use

Nurses can use the integrative model for community health promotion to effectively guide quality improvement of services for the population in a community clinic setting.

Krautscheid L, Moos P, Zeller J: Patient & staff satisfaction with integrated services at Old Town Clinic, *J Psychosocial Nurs* 42:1-9, 2004.

BOX 17-2 HEALTH PERSPECTIVES OVER TIME

Ancient Greek View
- Health was the totality of environmental forces influencing human well-being.
- Ways of living were essential to maintain health.

1700s to 1800s
- Scientific discoveries were opposed (e.g., germ theory of disease and principle of antisepsis).
- An increasing emphasis on medical science was associated with a decreasing emphasis on self-care.

Early to Mid-1900s
- Holistic view of health was reintroduced as an antidote to the medical science model.
- Scientific and biological view of disease dominated.
- Self-care was deemphasized.

Late 1900s
- Reemergence of the ideal of self-care was accelerated by the climate of political activism.
- It was recognized that people produce health by what they do and do not do for themselves.
- Collaboration existed between consumers and providers, and renegotiation of professional roles in health care emerged.

Early 2000s
- There is renewed focus on assuring conditions for the public's health.
- There is emphasis on ecological models and interaction of multiple social determinants of health.

making decisions about what to assess, with what level of client, and how to evaluate the outcomes of care. Health, defined as alleviating an individual's illness symptoms, involves assessment of the duration, intensity, and frequency of specific symptoms. Intervention focuses on symptom relief and treatment of the cause of symptoms. Evaluation consists of determining the extent of symptom alleviation. On the other hand, health defined as maximizing a community's physical recreation opportunities, involves assessment of existing recreation facilities, accessibility to the population, and beliefs and knowledge related to recreation and land use in the community.

The holistic view of health is not new. The ancient Greeks viewed health as the influence of environmental forces such as living habits; climate; the quality of air, water, and food on human well-being; and healing from illness. As such, they represented health in two sisters, *Hygeia* and *Panacea*, symbolizing opposite approaches to the attainment of health; *Hygeia*, referring to hygiene, cleaned people and the world to protect health, whereas *Panacea* magically restored mortals to health one at a time. Certain activities of daily living, such as exercise, were essential to the maintenance of health. Box 17-2 lists health perspectives as they emerged over time. Scientific medicine emerged slowly, and resistance to scientific discoveries, such as to the germ theory of disease, hindered the application of these discoveries to medical practice. With the development of the scientific approach toward disease in the twentieth century, professional care took precedence over self-care. During the last five decades, the idea of self-care as derived from a positive idea of health has reemerged to compete with professional care. Some proponents of self-care emphasize lay diagnosis and self-treatment, whereas others focus on teaching people how to work with their health care providers. As a result, health care system changes include the renegotiation of roles and emphasize collaboration between consumers and providers.

Many health professionals contend that individuals are in a position to produce health. Fuchs (1974) suggested that the

"greatest potential for improving health lies in what we do and don't do for and to ourselves" (p 55). In the political arena, LaLonde introduced a similar conclusion in *A New Perspective on the Health of Canadians* (1974). LaLonde identified four major determinants of health: human biology, environment, lifestyle, and health care. In 1976, policy makers in the United States echoed these ideas and supported efforts to improve health habits and the environment as the best hope of achieving any significant extension of life expectancy (USDHEW, 1976, p 69). Box 17-3 lists some landmark initiatives in health promotion and disease prevention.

The U.S. Public Health Service established the first national objectives involving disease prevention, health protection, and health promotion strategies in the surgeon general's *Healthy People* report (USDHEW, 1979). Disease prevention strategies focused on services such as family planning and immunizations delivered in clinical settings. Health protection strategies included environmental measures to "significantly improve health and the quality of life for this and future generations of Americans" (USDHEW, 1979, p 101), such as occupational health and accidental injury control. Health promotion strategies focused on achieving well-being through community and individual lifestyle change measures. The *Healthy People* report (USDHEW, 1979) also described inherited biological factors, the environment, and behavioral factors as the three categories

BOX 17-3 LANDMARK HEALTH PROMOTION/DISEASE PREVENTION INITIATIVES

- 1974—LaLonde's *A New Perspective on the Health of Canadians*
- 1976—*Forward Plan for Health*, FY 1978-1982
- 1979—*Healthy People: The Surgeon General's Report on Health Promotion and Disease Prevention*
- 1989—*Guide to Clinical Preventive Services* (USPSTF, 1989)
- 1990—*Healthy People 2000*
- 1994—*Put Prevention into Practice* (PPIP)
- 2000—*Healthy People 2010: Understanding and Improving Health and Objectives for Improving Health*, ed 2 (supersedes Jan 2000 conference edition)
- 2002—Progress reviews of *Healthy People 2010* initiated
- 2005—Guide to Community Preventive Services: What Works to Promote Health? (TFCPS, 2005)
- 2009—*Healthy People 2020* Framework
- 2010—*Healthy People 2020* Objectives
- 2010—*Guide to Clinical Preventive Services*, 2010-2011 (USPSTF, 2011)

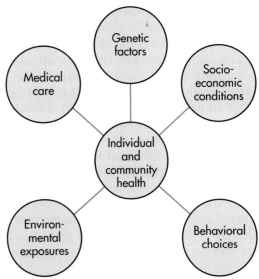

FIGURE 17-2 Interaction of multiple determinants of health. (Modified from Hernandez LM, editor: *Implications of genomics for public health: workshop summary,* Committee on Genomics and the Public's Health in the 21st Century, 2005, Institute of Medicine of the National Academies. Available at http://www.nap.edu/catalog/11260.html. Accessed January 3, 2011.)

of risks to health, which are identical to LaLonde's first three major determinants of health.

As described in Chapter 2, the health objectives for the nation outlined in *Healthy People 2010* built on initiatives that have been pursued since 1980. Designed for use by individuals, communities, states, and professional organizations, these health objectives provided a guide for programs to improve health. Nursing organizations participated in the development of the national health objectives and priorities. These organizations included the Quad Council of Public Health Nursing Organizations: the Association of State and Territorial Directors of Nursing (ASTDN), the American Nurses Association (ANA) Council on Nursing Practice and Economics, the Association of Community Health Nursing Educators (ACHNE), and the PHN Section of the American Public Health Association (APHA).

The release of the *Healthy People 2020* Framework in 2009 included a national vision, mission, and overarching goals. The four overarching goals emphasized prevention, health equity, environments conducive to health for all, and healthy development across the lifespan. This *Healthy People 2020* Framework preceded the release of the *Healthy People 2020* goals, objectives, and action plans for the nation in 2010. Information on the development process and launch of *Healthy People 2020* is available at http://www.healthypeople.gov/2020/default.aspx.

The idea that the health of communities and populations is shaped by multiple determinants has been reinforced in the national (IOM, 2002, 2006) and international (CSDH, 2008; McQueen, 2009) health policy literature. The major determinants of health have been expanded (Figure 17-2) to include ". . .interactions among genes, socioeconomic circumstances, behavioral choices, environmental exposures, and medical care" (Hernandez, 2005, p 64). Although recent trends reveal improvement in SDOH such as healthier living conditions and a decrease in smoking, these positive trends are associated with persistent socioeconomic disparities worldwide (CSDH, 2008).

♥ HEALTHY PEOPLE 2020

Tobacco Use

Selected objectives from *Healthy People 2020* that pertain to tobacco use:
- TU-1: Reduce tobacco use by adults.
- TU-2: Reduce tobacco use by adolescents.
- TU-3: Reduce the initiation of tobacco use among children, adolescents, and young adults.
- TU-6: Increase smoking cessation during pregnancies.
- TU-7: Increase smoking cessation by adolescent smokers.
- TU-11: Reduce the proportion of nonsmokers exposed to secondhand smoke.

From U.S. Department of Health and Human Services: *Healthy People 2020.* Available at http://www.healthypeople.gov/2020/default.aspx. Accessed January 15, 2011.

Definitions of Health

The WHO (1958) reflected a holistic perspective in its classic definition of health as a state of complete physical, mental, and social well-being, and not merely the absence of disease and infirmity. In 1975, Terris noted that epidemiologists considered the WHO definition to be "vague and imprecise with a Utopian aura" (p 1037). Terris expanded the definition: "Health is a state of physical, mental and social well-being and the ability to function and not merely the absence of illness and infirmity" (Terris, 1975, p 1038). In deleting the word "complete" and adding "ability to function," Terris placed the WHO definition in a more realistic context, providing a useful framework for health promotion.

Smith (1981) suggested that the "idea of health" directs nursing practice, education, and research. She observed that health was a comparative concept, allowing for "more" or "less" health along a health-illness continuum. Smith proposed four models of health, ordered from narrow and concrete to broad and abstract: clinical health, or the absence of disease; role performance health, or the ability to perform one's social roles satisfactorily; adaptive health, or flexible adaptation to the environment; and eudaemonistic health, or self-actualization and the attainment of one's greatest human potential.

Population health is a term widely used in IOM reports on the future of the public's health (IOM, 2002) and on educating public health professionals (IOM, 2003). Population health is defined as "the health of the population as measured by health status indicators and as influenced by social, economic, and physical environments, personal health practices, individual capacity and coping skills, human biology, early childhood development and health services" (Federal, Provincial, Territorial, Advisory Committee on Population Health, 1999, cited in IOM, 2002, pp xii-xiii). This definition of population health is consistent with the ecological approach to community health promotion and the SDOH.

It is important for nurses and health care providers to reflect on their own definition of health and recognize how their health definition influences the care they provide. Likewise, it is equally important for nurses to assess clients' personal health definitions. Only through knowledge of one's own health definition, together with assessment of clients' health definitions, can nurses create interventions tailored to achieve the clients' health goals. Nurses and health care providers who emphasize health promotion and population health that is congruent with the beliefs, health definitions, and goals of the population acknowledge the importance of illness prevention. Moreover, nurses must strive to understand health policies and the consequences of these policies on vulnerable populations whose living conditions may include few determinants of good health. (See Box 17-1.)

Definitions of Health Promotion

Health promotion is an accepted aim of nursing and health care, although explicit definition of health promotion and differentiation from disease prevention or health maintenance is rare. Leavell and Clark (1965) strongly influenced the evolution of health promotion and disease prevention strategies through their classic definitions of primary, secondary, and tertiary levels of prevention that were rooted in the biomedical model of health and epidemiology. The application of preventive measures, according to Leavell and Clark, corresponds to the natural history or stages of disease (see Table 12-3). Primary preventive measures apply to "well" individuals in the prepathogenesis period to promote their health and to provide specific protection from disease. Secondary preventive measures apply to diagnose or to treat individuals in the period of disease pathogenesis. Tertiary prevention addresses rehabilitation and the return of people with chronic illness to a maximal ability to function (see Levels of Prevention box).

Even though primary, secondary, and tertiary levels of prevention had their origins in the medical model, Leavell and Clark (1965) moved beyond the medical model. They conceptualized primary prevention as two distinct components: health promotion and specific protection. Health promotion focuses on positive measures such as education for healthy living and

---

LEVELS OF PREVENTION

Diabetes

Primary Prevention
For a person with identified risk factors for diabetes, the goal is to maintain a normal weight, to exercise regularly, and to reduce the intake of carbohydrates.

Secondary Prevention
Have regular blood glucose level testing done and be alert for any symptoms of the onset of diabetes.

Tertiary Prevention
If the blood glucose level indicates that the client has diabetes, begin treatment, which might include a diabetic diet, regular exercise, and medication.

---

promotion of favorable environmental conditions as well as periodic examinations including, for example, well-child developmental assessment and health education. Specific protection includes measures to reduce the threat of specific diseases, such as hygiene, immunizations, and the elimination of workplace hazards.

Health promotion and specific protection, when used as subconcepts of primary prevention, appear to stem from a definition of health as the absence of disease. However, differences in health promotion and specific protection strategies suggest that they are not the same. Some terms used to describe health promotion are linked to a positive view of health (e.g., *health habits*), whereas other terms are linked to the negative view of the absence of disease (e.g., *disease* or *illness prevention*). Using the terms *health promotion, health protection,* and *disease prevention* interchangeably, as indicators of preventive behavior, increases the confusion in terminology (Kulbok et al, 1997).

The WHO described health promotion as "the process of enabling people to increase control over, and improve their health" (WHO, 1984, p 3). According to the Ottawa Charter, health promotion combines both individual-level and community-level strategies including "building healthful public policy, creating supportive environments, strengthening community action, developing personal skills, and reorienting health services" (Bracht, 1990, p 38). Health is a resource for daily living. For individuals or communities to realize physical, mental, and social well-being, they must become aware of and learn to use the social and personal resources available within their environment.

Kulbok (1985) proposed a resource model of health behavior, which viewed social and health resources as correlates of positive **health behaviors.** Two major findings in studies to test this model (Kulbok, 1985; Kulbok et al, 1997) were: (1) health behavior is multidimensional, and there are several categories of health behavior including positive behaviors (e.g., a nutritious diet, exercise) and avoidance behaviors (e.g., non-user of tobacco, alcohol, or drugs), and (2) different health and social resources are associated with different health behaviors. Strategies to promote well-being focus on practicing new healthy behaviors or changing unhealthy behaviors. Successful intervention is more likely when nurses and health care providers understand how social and health resources relate to health behaviors of communities and populations, what social and health resources are available to communities and populations, and how these resources may affect behavior choices.

Laffrey (1990) differentiated between the terms *health promotion, illness prevention,* and *health maintenance.* Health promotion is behavior directed toward achieving a greater level of health. Illness prevention is behavior directed toward reducing the threat of illness, and health maintenance focuses on keeping a current state of health. Applying these definitions requires that nurses and health care providers assess not only behavior, but also the basis for choosing to perform a given behavior. In a study of men and women with and without chronic diseases living in a community, Laffrey (1990) asked subjects to identify their five most important health behaviors; for each behavior reported, subjects indicated three reasons for performing the behavior. For example, subjects exercised because regular, vigorous exercise produced a more energetic feeling and the ability to function at a higher level (a health promotion behavior); they exercised because of risk factors for coronary artery disease (an illness-preventing behavior); and they exercised regularly to maintain weight (a health maintenance behavior). The participants in this study characterized their health behaviors according to all three constructs, thereby demonstrating the complexity of health and illness behavior.

In 1997, Kulbok et al reported a content validity study of five national health promotion experts and found differences between the terms *health promotion* and *health promotion behavior.* The group of experts defined *health promotion* as activities undertaken by health professionals to promote health in their clients, and the term included health education and counseling. *Health promotion behavior,* on the other hand, is behavior that an individual performs to promote his or her health and well-being. Kulbok et al (2003) subsequently developed and tested the *Multidimensional Health Behavior Inventory* based on this broad definition of health and health promotion behavior.

Pender, Murdaugh, and Parsons (2011) also differentiated between health-protecting and health-promoting behaviors. Health protection refers to behaviors that decrease one's probability of becoming ill, whereas health promotion refers to behaviors that increase well-being of either an individual or a group. According to Pender et al (2011) although health protection and health promotion are complementary, health promotion is a broader concept that encompasses individuals, communities, and populations.

In summary, there is considerable evidence of agreement regarding a positive view of health underlying health promotion activities directed toward individuals, communities, and populations. For example, the WHO's definition of health promotion as a process, the resource model of health behavior (Kulbok, 1985; Kulbok et al, 2003), the notion of health behavior choices by Laffrey (1990), the definition of health promotion by Pender et al (2011), and the 10 components of the SDOH (WHO, 2010) are all grounded in the perspective of positive health. In each of these models or approaches, health promotion activities involve a broad, holistic view of lifestyle as a process as well as simultaneous interaction with the social and physical environments.

BOX 17-4	HEALTH ASSESSMENT APPROACHES

- The health hazard appraisal and its many versions
- Clinical guidelines and recommendations for preventive services
- Wellness appraisals or inventories

Modified from U.S. Department of Health and Human Services: *Healthy people in healthy communities,* Washington, DC, 2001, U.S. Government Printing Office.

Clearly, health promotion and population health are consistent with the goals of PHN and health care.

Assessing Health within Health and Illness Frameworks

Illness Prevention

Risk appraisal is widely used to help individuals and populations improve their health practices, thereby reducing their risk of disease. In a health risk appraisal, individuals supply information about their health practices, demographic characteristics, and personal and family medical history for comparison with data from epidemiologic studies. These comparisons are then used to predict individuals' risks of morbidity and mortality and to suggest areas in which disease risks may be reduced. Thus, risk appraisal is a type of secondary prevention used for screening to prevent or detect disease in its earliest stages and is one of several approaches to health assessment (Babor, Sciamanna, and Pronk, 2004). The evidence base for risk appraisal is the relationship of risk factors, disease, and the effectiveness of interventions to reduced mortality and risks of mortality. Box 17-4 lists the three most common types of health risk appraisal approaches used to assess individuals. Each type of risk appraisal is complex, and we describe only the basic concepts and selected procedures in this chapter. The references cited at the end of the chapter provide explanations that are more complete. Refer to Appendix D for an example of a risk appraisal tool.

HOW TO Profile Client Risk

1. *Assess the total risks to a client's health on the basis of knowledge of the client.*
2. *Assess the history of certain diseases and major causes of mortality for aggregates of the client's age, sex, race, and family history.*
3. *Help the health provider to initiate lifestyle changes in the client to avoid health threats or to prevent complications.*
4. *Institute treatment or lifestyle changes early in the course of disease.*
5. *To accomplish these objectives, collect data with a self-administered questionnaire, basic laboratory tests, and clinical examination.*
6. *The questionnaire asks about personal characteristics and behaviors known to predict disease.*
7. *These data are compared with data compiled from the 10 major causes of death of an aggregate of the same age, sex, and race as the client.*
8. *On the basis of the comparison, the client's appraisal age and achievable age are calculated.*

9. *The appraisal age is the health age of the average person in the client's age, sex, and race aggregate with a similar risk profile. For example, a 20-year-old white woman might have an appraisal age of 15 years if she has good health habits and no family history of chronic disease. Another 20-year-old white woman might have an appraisal age of 26 years if she smokes, fails to wear a seat belt, does not perform regular breast self-examinations, and has a family history of hypertension. The second woman's achievable age could be lowered if she were to modify her behavior.*

10. *Achievable age is the health age the client could achieve by modifying health threats.*

Guidelines for Clinical Preventive Services

Gradual acceptance of scientific evidence of the benefits associated with key preventive measures led to the development of clinical practice guidelines in the late 1970s. In 1989 the U.S. Preventive Services Task Force published the first *Guide to Clinical Preventive Services* based on review of the scientific evidence on 169 clinical preventive services for 60 target conditions. The USPSTF evaluated clinical research and assessed the merits of preventive measures, including screening tests, counseling, immunizations, and chemoprophylaxis. The USPSTF's more recent (2009) *Guide to Clinical Preventive Services* provides recommendations for preventive interventions including screening tests, counseling, immunizations, and chemoprophylaxis regimens for numerous illness conditions. Many of these preventive measures are routine nursing interventions. The abridged version of the guide is available at http://www.ahrq.gov/clinic/pocketgd.htm. Full recommendation statements or recommendation statements published after 2009 are available at http://www.preventiveservices.ahrq.gov/. These websites are accessible directly through the WebLinks section of this book's website.

> **DID YOU KNOW?** *Many of the preventive measures in the Guide to Clinical Preventive Services (USPSTF, 2009) are routine nursing interventions and have both individual-focused and population-focused applications.*

Health Risk Appraisal (HRA) Instruments

HRA instruments are convenient tools that determine individual health risks. The Carter Center at Emory University and the CDC developed one of the most comprehensive HRAs: the Healthier People Network (HPN) Health Risk Appraisal. Current information on the HPN Health Risk Appraisal program is available from http://www.thehealthierpeoplenetwork.org/. (See this book's Evolve website for a direct link to this site.) The Lifestyle Assessment Questionnaire (LAQ) from the National Wellness Institute (NWI) includes the Healthier People Questionnaire (HPQ), a wellness inventory, and a personal growth section. Users receive a personal wellness report, which summarizes their LAQ results and provides them with a sample action plan for increasing wellness behaviors. In addition, the NWI offers age-specific risk appraisals and wellness inventories. (Their website [http://www.nationalwellness.org] can be accessed directly from this book's Evolve website).

Wellness Inventories

Wellness inventories differ from HRA instruments and guidelines for preventive services by defining health risks more broadly and leading to health promotion as well as disease prevention and risk reduction. The wellness inventory of the LAQ described previously covers six dimensions: physical, social, emotional, intellectual, occupational, and spiritual.

Advantages and Disadvantages of Health Risk Appraisals

Risk appraisals support the adoption of health promotion and illness prevention behaviors by individuals and provide direction for nurses to counsel and educate clients about healthy lifestyles. Multilevel program participation, based on increased health risk awareness, has been shown to be associated with decreased worksite sickness absences (Pai et al, 2009) and decreased health risk (Rand Corporation, 2003). In addition, HRAs measure the outcomes and economic costs of risk reduction interventions (Schultz and Edington, 2009). By completing HRAs, individuals and groups receive immediate feedback about how their behavior changes can influence their health risks and life expectancy.

Despite these advantages, it is important to know the limitations of risk appraisal tools. Disadvantages of HRAs include the following: (1) validity and reliability of instruments may be limited to a specific population, (2) there may be overemphasis on lifestyle and minimal attention to other risks such as environmental hazards and inadequate health care, and (3) there may be lack of cultural sensitivity (Rand, 2003). In addition, HRAs provide less incentive to the young to change poor health practices, because they do not detect the effects of lifestyle on health and illness until middle to late adulthood. Living conditions that restrict participation in decision-making, economic, and educational opportunities, or that encourage risk-taking that is not conducive to good health, limit an individual's ability to change lifestyle.

Community
Historical Perspectives

Another major concept in an integrative and ecological approach to community health promotion is community. The emphasis on community as the target of practice has gained increased attention since the mid-1970s when the U.S. and Canadian governments and private health researchers attributed declining mortality and morbidity rates to better standards of living, such as sanitation, clean air and water, and wider availability of healthy foods. The Institute of Medicine's (IOM's) seminal report on the future of public health highlighted the importance of community in its statement that the "mission of public health is to assure conditions in which people can be healthy by generating organized community effort to prevent disease and promote health" (IOM, 1988, p 7).

As discussed previously, national health goals (USDHHS, 1979, 2000, 2009a) emphasize that environment and community are central to achieving health. *Healthy People in Healthy Communities* (USDHHS, 2001) is a community planning guide based on *Healthy People 2010* (Box 17-5). The guide outlines practical recommendations for coalition building, creating a

BOX 17-5 HEALTHY PEOPLE 2010: A STRATEGY FOR CREATING A HEALTHY COMMUNITY

To achieve the goal of improving health, a community must develop a strategy supported by many individuals who are working together. The MAP-IT technique helps you to map out the path toward the change you want to see in your community. This guide recommends that you MAP-IT—that is, **m**obilize, **a**ssess, **p**lan, **i**mplement, and **t**rack.

- Mobilize individuals and organizations that care about the health of your community into a coalition.
- Assess the areas of greatest need in your community, as well as the resources and other strengths that you can tap into to address those areas.
- Plan your approach: start with a vision of where you want to be as a community; then add strategies and action steps to help you achieve that vision.
- Implement your plan using concrete action steps that can be monitored and will make a difference.
- Track your progress over time.

From U.S. Department of Health and Human Services: *A strategy for creating a healthy community: MAP-IT.* In *Healthy people in healthy communities: A community planning guide using* Healthy People 2010, Washington, DC, 2001, U.S. Government Printing Office.

BOX 17-6 MILIO'S PROPOSITIONS FOR IMPROVING HEALTH BEHAVIOR

- Health status of populations is a function of the lack or excess of health-sustaining resources.
- Behavior patterns of populations are related to habits of choice from actual or perceived limited resources and related attitudes.
- Organizational decisions determine the range of personal resources available.
- Individual health-related decisions are influenced by efforts to maximize valued resources in both the personal and societal domains.
- Social change is reflective of a change in population behavior patterns.
- Health education will impact behavior patterns minimally without new health-promoting options for investing personal resources.

Modified from Milio N: A framework for prevention: changing health-damaging to health-generating life patterns, *Am J Public Health* 66:435, 1976.

vision, and measuring outcomes to improve the health of communities. Communities can tailor these recommendations to their own local needs, and health professionals in public and private organizations can work together with community members to develop programs that fit the needs and resources of their own communities. Nurses participate in this collaborative and interprofessional process through community assessments, community development activities, and identification of key persons in the community with whom to build partnerships for health programs. One of the four overarching goals of the *Healthy People 2020* Framework is to create social and physical environments that promote good health for all (USDHHS, 2009a). Community-wide program planning provides a strategy to achieve this goal. In Implementing *Healthy People 2020*, a community framework called MAP-IT was developed as a guide to using *Healthy People 2020* in your community (see http://healthy people.gov/2020/implementing/default.aspx). MAP-IT stands for Mobilize, Assess, Plan, Implement and Track and is used in communities to evaluate public health interventions designed to implement the goals of *Healthy People 2020.*

Nurses and interprofessional health care providers have many opportunities to participate in community-wide health care. To address community problems, these professionals need to integrate concepts of health and illness, individual and population, public health and health care, and health promotion and disease prevention. This integration means that nurses must consider the complex relationship between personal and environmental forces that affect health. Over 35 years ago, Milio (1976) offered a set of propositions for improving health behavior by considering personal choices in the context of available societal resources. These propositions (Box 17-6) remain relevant today. They constitute a fitting model for health promotion that addresses both personal and societal resources for this and future decades.

Therefore, it is important to realize that family and peers often affect individuals' perceived freedom to make personal choices within their immediate environment as well as their norms and values within the community. For example, a survey of rural communities in Missouri, Tennessee, and Arkansas (Deshpande et al, 2005) found that 37% of respondents with diabetes reported no leisure physical activity. Reasons for engaging in physical activity were the availability of nearby places to walk in the community, the presence of shoulders on the roads, and the community being a pleasant environment for physical activities. A similar study (Martin et al, 2004) on traffic safety and African Americans highlighted the importance of engaging respected institutions within their community, such as churches and schools, to effectively confer health messages and realize behavior change. These studies show that, in addition to targeting individuals within the environment, strategies to promote behavior change must include interventions targeted to the community environment.

Community Models and Frameworks

Although theoretical frameworks developed within nursing and other health disciplines are traditionally oriented toward individuals, there is increasing recognition of the importance of community and person—environment interactions that goes beyond social cognitive theory and other interpersonal frameworks (NCI, 2005) in promoting health. PHN defined community as "...persons in interaction, being and experiencing together, who may or may not share a sense of common purpose" (ANA, 2007, p 41). Nurses realize that the community is more than the sum of the individuals, families, aggregates, and organizations within it and that interaction is essential for any real change to occur.

Chopoorian (1986) was among the first to acknowledge that nurses could strengthen their position with communities by focusing on the social, economic, and political structures that make up the community, as well as the social relations and patterns of everyday life in the community. Within this perspective, interventions targeted to public health policy can have far-reaching health benefits. Shuster and Goeppinger (2008) asserted that definitions of *community* vary widely and that nurses working with communities learn quickly that there are many different types. They define community as locality-based, composed of formal systems reflecting society's institutions and informal groups or aggregates. Shuster and Goeppinger included person, place, and function, as well as interaction among systems within a community, as part of their definition. Nurses must examine the complexity inherent in community definitions and the process of community building, rather than viewing the community as a static geographic, racial, or cultural group.

Despite the ideal, it is not easy to integrate the concept of the community as client into practice. Consequently, the provision of care to individuals *in the community* may still overshadow nursing practice and health promotion directed *to the community*. Bekemeier and Jones (2010), in a study of local public health agency (LPHA) functions, leadership, and staffing, reported that the proportion of nursing staff in an LPHA related strongly to provision of services involving individual level care. These findings confirmed the work of Grumbach et al (2004), who found that the staff nurses were most likely to perform individual-family interventions, and that both the staff nurses and the managers rated individual-family interventions as more important than community- or system-level interventions. These findings suggest that there is an ongoing need to expand "…education and outreach to nurses regarding their roles and responsibilities to assure environmental health protection, community assessment, and health improvement planning" (Bekemeier and Jones, 2010, p E16).

Nursing authors have described community from a systems perspective (Anderson and McFarlane, 2000, 2008; Salmon, 1993, 2009; Smith and Bazini-Barakat, 2003). In the systems perspective, humans are part of a hierarchy of natural systems, and health is a function of harmonious interrelationships among the levels of the hierarchy. Movement in one level of the hierarchy has a corresponding movement in all other levels. Thus, individual, family, aggregate, community, and society are levels of the systems hierarchy. Any change that occurs in one level has a corresponding change in all other levels.

Anderson and McFarlane (2000, 2008) and Salmon (1993, 2009) developed a model based on the assumption that assessing the various components of the system facilitates a healthy community. Anderson and McFarlane's community-as-partner model includes eight major community subsystems. The basic core of the community, according to these authors, is its people, described by demographics and their values, beliefs, culture, religion, laws, and more. Within the community system, the people interact with the other subsystems. A **community health** assessment must include information about the subsystems and the pattern of interactions among the subsystems and of the total community with the systems external to it. The model of Salmon (1993, 2009) focused on the public health mission of organized efforts to protect, promote, and restore health. It embraces multiple determinants of health and is consistent with the Canadian Framework for Health (LaLonde, 1974). According to this model, nursing includes illness prevention, health protection, and health promotion strategies. Systems models provide important guidance for assessing community and

indicate that system-level interventions require participation with relevant subsystems. The strength of these system models is that they can be used to guide assessments, but they cannot easily be used to guide interventions. Two other models (Keller et al, 2004; Smith and Bazini-Barakat, 2003) specifically address PHN interventions. These are described below.

Keller et al (1998, 2004) proposed a population-based intervention model based on the scope of PHN practice that crosses multiple levels of care; this model defines the population-focused underpinning of PHN practice and provides guidance for PHN interventions at the individual, community, and system levels. The model was later termed the "intervention wheel" (Keller et al, 2004, p 453). The intervention wheel includes community, systems, and individual/family levels of practice. It is population based and identifies 17 public health interventions. Similar to the integrated model of community health promotion, the intervention wheel delineates multiple levels of nursing interventions.

The Los Angeles County Public Health Nursing (LACPHN) practice model, developed by the Los Angeles County Department of Health Services, built upon five assumptions (Smith and Bazini-Barakat, 2003, p 43):

1. The model incorporates the concept of the interprofessional public health team.
2. The individual, family, or community is an active participant in all steps.
3. The model is population-based practice.
4. PHN participates in and contributes to the core public health functions: assessment, policy development, and assurance.
5. The Minnesota Public Health Nursing Interventions (PHI) model (Keller et al, 1998) describes the universe of interventions that public health nurses can use while carrying out the action component of the nursing process.

The LACPHN practice model used nationally recognized components of the PHN standards of practice; the 10 essential public health services; the 10 leading health indicators of *Healthy People 2010*; additional local indicators; and the intervention wheel (Smith and Bazini-Barakat, 2003).

The models proposed by Anderson and McFarlane (2000, 2008), Keller et al (2004), Salmon (1993, 2009), and Smith and Bazini-Barakat (2003) focus on stability and equilibrium, by protecting the community from specific disease risks; less attention is directed toward factors that promote an optimally healthy community.

The social ecological model is another model used to guide nursing intervention (USDHHS, 2005). The social ecological model guides health promotion as well as illness prevention interventions. According to this model, health care and health-related behavior are a function of individual, interpersonal, organizational, community, and population factors. Thus, interventions are specific to each of these levels. Resnick et al (2009) used the social ecological model to guide implementation and testing of a restorative care program in assisted living. They hypothesized that residents who were exposed to the program would maintain or improve physical activity, physical status, functional performance, resilience, self-efficacy (SE) and outcome expectations (OE) for exercise, functional performance, and quality of life. In addition, they believed that residents would increase social support for exercise and maintain or report decreased fear of falling 4 months after program initiation. Resnick et al (2009) provided preliminary evidence of the feasibility and effectiveness of a nurse-led, restorative care–assisted, living intervention. Participants showed improvement in functional status and time spent in physical activity.

The Healthy Hawaii Initiative (Nigg et al, 2005) was aimed at improving healthy nutrition and physical activity and reducing tobacco use. Interventions were developed for schools and community groups, and there were environmental and policy changes, health and physical education instruction for teachers, and education of the medical community as well as public education. The evaluation of this initiative led the developers to conclude that targeting various levels of the client system produced a synergistic effect that was greater than the sum of the individual levels. Several other major community-wide studies have drawn on concepts such as those presented in these models. These community and epidemiological studies are described next.

Influential Multilevel Community Studies: A Chronological Review

Two significant community studies of health risks, morbidity, and mortality are the Framingham Heart Study, initiated in 1949, and the Human Population Laboratory's longitudinal survey in Alameda County, California, initiated in the early 1970s. In the Framingham Heart Study (Liao et al, 1999), 5209 adults were followed over their life span to identify factors contributing to coronary heart disease (CHD). Periodic health assessments were done, and morbidity and mortality data were collected. Major risk factors associated with CHD mortality were identified in the original cohort (e.g., elevated systolic blood pressure, elevated serum cholesterol level, and cigarette smoking). The investigators proposed predictive models (e.g., health risk appraisals) to relate the risk factors identified among well individuals in the Framingham population to the probability of future cardiovascular disease. These complex predictive models have evolved since the 1960s. They have been widely used to document the multifactorial nature of cardiovascular disease and the interrelationships among major risk factors. The Framingham study is still in progress today (see http://www.framinghamheartstudy.org/); in fact, Framingham scientists are currently using new technologies to search for the molecular basis of disease and new cardiovascular risk factors (Lieb et al, 2009).

The Alameda County study was designed to measure the relationship of health and social behaviors to mortality in a community sample of 6928 individuals over 4 years. The behaviors included eating three meals daily, eating breakfast, sleeping 7 to 8 hours a night, using alcohol moderately, exercising regularly, not smoking, maintaining a desirable weight-to-height ratio, and maintaining social networks. Smoking and excessive alcohol use were positively related to mortality (Berkman and Breslow, 1983). Physical exercise, 7 to 8 hours of sleep, optimal weight in relation to height, and social networks

(e.g., contact with friends and relatives, church and group membership) were inversely related to mortality. These findings led to the current emphasis on social and environmental variables, in addition to personal behaviors, illness prevention, and health promotion strategies. Findings from these early large-scale surveys prompted a number of public health multilevel intervention programs. Examples were the Stanford Heart Disease Prevention program (Farquhar et al, 1990), the North Karelia study (Puska et al, 1983), the Pawtucket Heart Health program (Lasater et al, 1984), the Minnesota Heart Health program (Luepker et al, 1994), and the Dutch Heart Health Community Intervention (Ronda et al, 2005).

The Stanford Five-City project began in 1979 with a 6-year community health education program aimed at reducing cardiovascular (CV) risk factors. The program was delivered through multiple channels (Winkleby et al, 1996). Two treatment cities received a low-cost, comprehensive program based on social learning theory, communication theory, behavior change theory, community organization, and social marketing. The population of these treatment cities reported improvements in serum cholesterol levels, blood pressure measurements, smoking rate, and resting heart rate immediately after the program and sustained for two decades (Farquhar et al, 1990; Winkleby et al, 1996). Although CV and all-cause death rates stabilized or improved in the treatment cities, they leveled out or worsened in the comparison cities (Winkleby et al, 1996).

The North Karelia Project also found positive changes in CV health (Puska et al, 1983). Citizens of North Karelia, a rural province in Finland, experienced a high death rate from CV disease in the early 1970s. More than half of the North Karelia men smoked, consumed large amounts of animal fat, and had elevated serum cholesterol levels. In addition, many had untreated hypertension. The government directed the multilevel program to individual and the larger community levels to help the citizens modify their high-risk behaviors. Strategies included retraining health professionals, reorganizing public health services, increasing the availability of low-fat and low-salt dairy products and meat, and providing community health education. Follow-up studies demonstrated that the three major risk factors for CV disease decreased much more in North Karelia than in a comparison county (Puska et al, 1983). After 36 years, the death rate from CHD and lung cancer in men 35 to 64 years of age had declined by 85% and 80%, respectively (North Karelia Project, 2009). This study, which initially aimed to reduce cardiovascular risk factors, has expanded to include an emphasis on health promotion lifestyles (North Karelia Project, 2009).

The Pawtucket Heart Health program (PHHP) was a community-based research and demonstration project in a Rhode Island community that traditionally demonstrated high rates of CV disease. Interventions were designed to help individuals adopt new behaviors and to create a supportive and health-promoting community environment (Carleton et al, 1995). Churches, social groups, the business community, and volunteers provided the education intervention. The food industry offered "heart healthy" food items and menus, and media campaigns informed citizens about their cholesterol levels and other CV risk factors (Carleton et al, 1995). Results 8.5 years after the beginning of the program, indicated lower obesity levels for the Pawtucket residents as compared with the comparison city (Carleton et al 1995). There were no differences in blood pressure, cholesterol levels, or smoking prevalence. The authors concluded that possible national media exposure, high levels of unemployment, and stress during the time of the study might have contributed to the lack of difference in these risk factors between the two cities.

During the peak time of the PHHP intervention, the Pawtucket population experienced a significant increase in heart-healthy behaviors, such as physical activity, suggesting that community interventions can reach a large number of people (Levin et al, 1998). Eaton et al (1999) reported on outcomes of 7 years of physical activity interventions with 4498 individuals, from fall 1983 through spring 1991. Most of the exercise participants were women (87%) and were under 35 years of age (62%). Although the PHHP intervention community did not show measurable decreases in physical inactivity from the comparison community, there was a sharp increase in vigorous physical activity among women and young men. Eaton and colleagues recommended that future community-based clinical trials of physical activity interventions should target a broad, diverse range of the population in a variety of community and clinical settings.

The Minnesota Heart Health program (Luepker et al, 1994) was initiated in 1980 with 400,000 persons in six Midwestern communities. Three communities received the program and three served as controls. There were improvements in risk factors in all six communities, but there were only modest differences between the treatment and control cities. Favorable health risk changes were found for both males and females across age and education groups. Future programs must combine public policy initiatives and community-wide health education strategies with interventions directed to specific high-risk populations (Luepker et al, 1994).

The Dutch Heart Health Community Intervention (Ronda et al, 2005) targeted both individuals and organizations. The overall purpose was to prevent cardiovascular disease. Local health committees focused on nutrition, physical activity, and smoking cessation activities within organizations (e.g., worksites; schools; supermarkets; civic, social, and sports clubs; libraries; and resident associations). After 3 years, significantly more intervention activities had been implemented in the project community than in a comparison community. Schuit et al (2006) conducted a 5-year evaluation of risk factors between the intervention and comparison group. There were significant differences in risk factors for men and women for body mass index (BMI), waist circumference, and systolic blood pressure. Significant differences existed for women only in total cholesterol and serum glucose.

These programs provided beginning scientific evidence for the implementation of community-level risk reduction programs. Although the outcomes of risk reduction interventions were in the expected direction, the relative effectiveness of specific interventions remains unclear. The results of these large programs were modest and often not statistically significant (Winkleby, Feldman, and Murray, 1997; Eaton et al, 1999;

Schuit et al, 2006). However, these studies have made major contributions to both theory and practice in building community partnerships, establishing social marketing, developing behavior change strategies, and evaluating health programs. Results of these studies make it clear that multiple levels of intervention are necessary to reach the community in a meaningful way. Nurses have close relationships with individuals, families, high-risk groups, organizations such as schools, congregations and workplaces, and other health care professionals. They are positioned to contribute to health promotion and disease and illness prevention by participating in community projects such as the ones described here. It is important that nurses develop health programs and document improved outcomes for high-risk groups with whom they interact.

> **DID YOU KNOW?** *"The Behavioral Risk Factor Surveillance System (BRFSS) obesity and diabetes maps have been widely credited for identifying the epidemics of obesity and diabetes in the United States. Thousands of articles have cited BRFSS data and/or methods focusing on different topics such as aging, depression, cardiovascular diseases, disability, alcohol consumption, immunization, language barriers, firearms, and air pollution"* (Mokdad, 2009, p 45).

INTERPROFESSIONAL APPLICATION TO NURSING AND PUBLIC HEALTH

Community-Based Participatory Research (CBPR)

The aim of PHN is to create partnerships with individuals, families, groups, and communities to promote their health. CBPR, grounded in epistemology and critical social theories (Minkler and Wallerstein, 2003), provides the philosophical and theoretical basis for forming partnerships and for collaboration with the community. CBPR has been used to conduct ecological, community, and environmental assessments. This approach to community assessment allows understanding of sociocultural contexts, systems, and meaning through a collaborative research process. In CBPR, partnerships are active and community members are involved in assessing, planning, implementing, and evaluating change. Both professionals and community residents determine health needs and plan interventions. As residents increase their awareness, they are better able to determine what they want for themselves, their families, and their community, and they are more likely to take leadership roles in program development, using health professionals as consultants.

The Community Health Advisor (CHA) program is a participatory health promotion program that builds community capacity through volunteer CHAs. This program identifies and trains natural helpers ". . .to improve the health of individuals and their communities" (Hinton et al, 2005, p 20). Through the training, CHAs link with local service providers and community leaders to increase awareness of and responsiveness to community health needs. The community is strengthened through the efforts of the CHAs, such as the successful Deep South Network for Cancer Control (Hinton et al, 2005). Public health nurses work to promote active partnerships in which community members determine their own needs and develop health programs relevant to their community. Some examples of community participatory studies, which address multiple levels of client systems and foci of care, are described in the following paragraphs.

The Cottage Community Care Pilot Project (CCCPP) was a volunteer support program to prevent child abuse and neglect among high-risk families in Sydney, Australia (Kelleher and Johnson, 2004). Nurses collaborated with other health professionals and community residents to develop the program and participated in educating volunteers to provide support and education to high-risk families. In an evaluation of the CCCPP, Kelleher and Johnson (2004) found that after 1 year, 25 first-time mothers who received the program showed significantly greater improvement in access to social support and responsiveness to their infants' needs, in comparison to 24 first-time mothers who did not receive the program. Although improvements were also seen in the other five aspects of family functioning (ability to cope with stress, self-esteem, confidence as a parent, expectations of the infant, and positive interactions with the infant), these improvements were not statistically significant. The lack of statistical significance is a function of the small sample size. This project supports the effectiveness of volunteer support programs and shows the importance of public health nurses in developing programs that have a positive impact on growth and development of children in the community.

The community residents of the East Side Village Health Worker Partnership (ESVHWP) on Detroit's East Side developed a community-based participatory program titled Healthy Eating and Exercising to Reduce Diabetes (HEED) (Schulz et al, 2005). The purpose was to increase community awareness about diabetes and prevention. Community groups and individuals with expertise in diabetes served as the project steering committee. They developed training protocols and recruited and trained community advocates. After training completion, the HEED advocates developed activities to promote healthy diets and physical activity. The advocates and other community residents identified important barriers to healthy dietary choices, such as lack of access to grocery stores and fresh produce. Members of the HEED project established a monthly mini-market at a community site with a few retail outlets carrying high-quality produce. The project was successful in fostering a strong interest among participants in healthy cooking demonstrations and cooking techniques. Subsequently, the HEED project joined forces with another community initiative to obtain funding to expand the mini-markets and food demonstrations.

The Physical Activity and Neighborhood Resources in High School Girls study (Pate et al, 2008) followed an ecological model based on the social cognitive theory for adolescent females in urban, suburban, and rural communities. Researchers hypothesized that physical activity is influenced by a comprehensive set of personal, social, and physical environmental factors. Using a geographical information system (GIS), mixed regression models on BMI, and environmental variables, as well as 3-day physical activity recall, they found that the physical environment explained less than 5% of the variance in physical activity among adolescent girls. However, after adjusting for race, BMI, socioeconomic status (SES), and household income, there was an association between churches and vigorous physical activity. An additional study by Botchwey (2007) showed that up to 80% of congregations and faith-based organizations offer health services to their community, with a greater variety of services than secular non-profit organizations. Therefore, as nurses work with communities, it is important to consider the social and physical components of the environment, especially those actively engaged in health promotion.

Photovoice Method and Projects

Photovoice is a novel method used in CBPR projects that integrates the strengths of social support and engagement, building local capacity to identify and address community concerns. Wang and Burris (1997) developed this methodology in 1997 by expanding the use of "photo novella" (Wang and Burris, 1994) as a means to empower communities while gathering qualitative data. It is a grassroots community method of gathering information by using photography. By using Photovoice participants photograph, contemplate, and then verbalize stories or simple descriptions about their photo(s) taken in response to a particular prompt, thereby allowing their voices to be heard. This process prevents written text from hindering communication and is effective in a society that uses oral tradition to preserve its culture (Riley et al, 2004). Health care researchers have used Photovoice as an assessment tool (Lacson, 2007; Strecher, 2004; Thompson et al, 2008).

THE CUTTING EDGE   *This study by Kulbok et al (2008) addressed gaps in the youth tobacco prevention literature. The purpose was to identify attitudes, beliefs, values, strategies, and shared meanings associated with tobacco-free behaviors of rural-dwelling male adolescents and their parents. This study examined differences in the meaning attached to non-smoking and non-use of smokeless tobacco among groups of African-American and white male adolescents and their parents from two tobacco-growing counties in Virginia. In addition, the study assessed whether a modified Photovoice method would enhance the contribution of male adolescent participants and parents in individual and group interviews. Photovoice is a qualitative approach that uses images to promote effective ways of sharing beliefs about a specific topic. Researchers have used Photovoice to facilitate group conversations and to encourage participants to share their thoughts among themselves. In this study, Photovoice was a concrete way for youth and parents to express their perceptions about being tobacco-free, amplified through photographs that respond to questions about this topic. This approach was particularly effective with the male adolescents, who were hesitant to share their thoughts and feelings, and had a hard time articulating their thoughts.*

From Kulbok PA, Meszaros PS, Hinton I, et al: Tobacco-free boys and parents use Photovoice to tell their stories: issues and solutions [Abstract], Proceedings of the 136th American Public Health Association, Annual Meeting, October 2008a, San Diego, CA.

The Ngudo Nga Zwinepe (NNZ) Learning through Photos projects use Photovoice to understand water perceptions and innovations as well as health in the Limpopo Province of rural South Africa where water resources are scarce and frequently contaminated (Cunningham et al, 2009). In one Photovoice project, community members took pictures documenting their perception of water and their water system. In contrast to the researchers' expectations, there was very little mention of the deleterious health effects of contaminated water. Instead, the participants listed infrastructure/storage, community, money, and food as their top priorities, with health/hygiene ranked fifth overall. Photovoice provided data to characterize the water priorities of this community and to implement an intervention that meets the community's primary concerns in the shorter-term while developing educational strategies regarding the health risks of contaminated water.

The projects described in the previous paragraphs show the importance of multiple approaches to reaching the population. A multilevel approach to community-oriented programs requires that one attend to all client levels (i.e., individual, family, aggregate, and community). For example, in nutritional programs, it is important to address the individual, the household, grocery store accessibility and environment, the community, and the food environment. No one individual can address all of these levels, but there is increasing emphasis on working in teams and in developing partnerships consisting of residents, health providers, and other professionals outside the health field. In addition, it is important to frame and initiate interventions based on participants' priorities, not the priorities of experts. This approach promotes increased buy-in to projects and the necessary compliance by community participants to adhere to healthy behaviors. Nurses have many opportunities to work with and to lead these multidisciplinary teams to conduct assessments, develop strategies with the community and its populations, and facilitate the empowerment of community residents and recommended change. It is increasingly important that nurses integrate these intervention strategies with the epidemiological evidence base for practice (see Evidence-Based Practice box).

EVIDENCE-BASED PRACTICE

A systematic review of literature published from 1985 to 2003 provided evidence of behavioral determinants of healthy aging. Specifically, eight studies were identified that addressed "healthy" or "successful aging" among adults 60 years of age or older. Refraining from smoking, being physically active, maintaining weight within normal ranges, and consuming moderate amounts of alcohol were health practices associated with healthy aging. The combination of high physical activity and not smoking improved the likelihood of healthy aging. Epidemiological evidence such as this provides a strong foundation for planning innovative health promotion programs to promote well-being among the elderly.

Nurse Use

It is important for nurses to encourage people who are 60 years or older to refrain from smoking, drink only moderate amounts of alcohol, be physically active, and maintain a normal weight.

From Peel NM, McClure RJ, Bartlett HP: Behavioral determinants of healthy aging, *Am J Prevent Med* 28:298-304, 2005.

APPLICATION OF THE INTEGRATIVE MODEL FOR COMMUNITY HEALTH PROMOTION

In the previous sections, we described the importance of multiple levels of nursing and health care aimed at health promotion and illness prevention of individuals, families, aggregates, and the total community. In the remainder of this chapter, we present some examples of the integrative model that apply these concepts.

Infant Mortality

Illness Care

One example of nursing care that reflects the four client systems and multiple foci of care is shown in Table 17-1. The health problem that the public health nurse addresses in this example is a high rate of infant mortality in a small southern city. The nurse initiates care at the individual level with a goal of reducing infant mortality and complications of high-risk pregnancy through early prenatal care and health education. High-risk pregnancy and infant mortality may be due to factors related to the mother (e.g., age of the mother [<15 or >35]), history of complications during previous pregnancy, or factors related to the fetus (e.g., exposure to infection or to addictive substances such as tobacco, alcohol, or drugs). The nurse assesses and monitors the mother's health, nutrition, and risk factors and he or she teaches anticipatory guidance for child care, including proper nutrition, feeding, and positioning of the infant for sleep in a crib. At the family level, the nurse assesses family dynamics, poor nutrition, and access to care within the family and refers family members for care as needed. In addition, the nurse assesses for the presence of risk factors such as low SES and unemployment. The family is referred for counseling to relieve the stress related to high-risk pregnancy. At the aggregate level, the nurse assesses the community for prevalence of infant mortality or teaches classes to raise awareness in the community about teen pregnancy prevention and to educate groups about culturally appropriate referral for family planning. At the community level, the nurse works with key leaders and citizens to assess the prevalence of high-risk pregnancies and infant mortality in the community. The nurse may participate in designing community programs to enhance awareness and prevention of causes of infant mortality such as sudden infant death syndrome (SIDS) among community members.

Illness Prevention

At the individual level, the nurse teaches well-balanced nutrition and child care to the high-risk pregnant woman or teen to promote healthy development and growth of the fetus and infant. A health risk appraisal and recommendations from the *Guide to Clinical Preventive Services* (USPSTF, 2009) provide direction for age-specific periodic health examination, assessment, and counseling interventions for family members. In addition, the nurse selects an appropriate health risk appraisal tool for use with clinical observation and assessment. The nurse teaches the high-risk family the importance of early and routine prenatal care and nutrition principles. The nurse helps the

TABLE 17-1   COMMUNITY HEALTH LEVELS OF CARE: INFANT MORTALITY

FOCUS OF CARE	CLIENT SYSTEM			
	INDIVIDUAL	FAMILY	AGGREGATE	COMMUNITY
Illness care	Monitor the health status of high-risk pregnant women and infants Teach mother importance of healthy lifestyle and routine prenatal care during pregnancy to promote the birth of a healthy infant	Teach signs and symptoms of risk factors and complications during pregnancy to family members Teach family about basic health practices and prenatal care to prevent health problems in mother and infant	Assess prevalence of infant mortality in the community Teach classes at local health department and community hospital to address needs of aggregate of high-risk pregnant women	Assess community for accessibility and adequacy of care providers to treat high-risk maternal and infant populations in the community
Illness/ disease prevention	Teach high-risk pregnant women the importance of early prenatal care, healthy lifestyle, and proper nutrition to promote development of a healthy infant and prevent infant mortality	Teach family members to encourage early prenatal care and model healthy lifestyles and proper nutrition	Assess community for prevalence of high-risk teen pregnancy and infant mortality Develop classes about reducing risks of infant mortality and causes such as SIDS	Participate in providing community-wide multimedia education for prevention of teen pregnancy Lobby for legislation to promote resources to ensure early prenatal care for high-risk women
Health promotion	Support individual efforts to adopt health promotion lifestyle, including avoidance of smoking and drug and alcohol abuse	Plan with family to adopt a healthy lifestyle and incorporate substance use avoidance and healthy dietary patterns	Educate school personnel regarding healthy lifestyles and early prenatal care	Work with health care providers, community leaders, and citizens to establish early and continuous prenatal care and to identify conditions and behavior that can result in low-birth-weight babies

family to incorporate healthy food into their diets to prevent nutrition-related problems. Using an aggregate approach, the nurse assesses the community for aggregates at risk for infant mortality (e.g., pregnant teens, minority, and/or poor women), analyzes health-risk data, and works with others to institute programs to reduce their risk, thereby preventing infant mortality. Community approach examples include multimedia education for teen pregnancy prevention, early prenatal care, and lobbying for legislation to promote resources for access to care and prevention services within the community. An excellent resource for community level preventive interventions is the Fetal Infant Mortality Review (FIMR) Manual (NFIMR, 2008). At the local level, the FIMR Manual is useful for assessing, planning, improving, and monitoring services and resources that promote the health and well-being of women, infants, and families.

Health Promotion

At the individual level, the nurse helps the pregnant woman or teen adopt a healthy lifestyle as appropriate to age, culture, and resources. For a high-risk pregnancy, this includes anticipatory education and support to provide a health-enhancing environment for infant growth and development. Using the perspective of the family as client, the nurse includes the entire family and

plans how to adopt healthy lifestyle activities with the family. These activities range from understanding balanced nutrition to planning for relaxation activities for the family. A wellness inventory helps the nurse and family design an intervention targeted to their awareness of personal self-care. At the aggregate level, the nurse educates high school personnel about evidence-based pregnancy prevention programs and resources for students. Regardless of the level of health need or the client system at which care begins, the nurse's ultimate goal is health promotion of the total community and its constituents. Examples of a community-level approach include participating with community leaders and citizens to establish education for teen pregnancy prevention and awareness of the need for early prenatal care for all pregnant women. Nurses should also emphasize the avoidance of tobacco, alcohol, and drugs; the importance of nutritious foods; and safe child-rearing practices available to all community members. As mentioned for illness prevention, the FIMR Manual provides numerous examples of community actions to decrease infant mortality and to promote the health of women, infants, and families.

Although an important starting point is the care of the high-risk pregnant teen or older pregnant woman, the nurse must recognize that solving the immediate problem is not sufficient. The causes of infant mortality are complex and occur within

TABLE 17-2   COMMUNITY HEALTH LEVELS OF CARE: OBESITY AND THE BUILT ENVIRONMENT

FOCUS OF CARE	CLIENT SYSTEM			
	INDIVIDUAL	FAMILY	AGGREGATE	COMMUNITY
Illness care	Administer medications Monitor weight as well as adherence to nutrition and physical activity recommendations of individual client in the home setting	Teach family members about nutrition and physical activity practices to lose weight and prevent the onset of obesity-related diseases	Assess prevalence of obesity in the community Teach obesity classes community wide in settings that high-risk groups frequent	Assess community for accessibility and adequacy of healthy food and safe physical activity venues in the local environment
Illness/disease prevention	Teach nutrition, progressive exercise, and lifestyle techniques to prevent additional weight gain	Teach nutrition and importance of regular exercise to all family members to prevent additional cases of obesity	Develop classes about obesity risk reduction for targeted high-risk groups and their community	Participate in community-wide multimedia education for obesity risk reduction
Health promotion	Empower individual to adopt a less sedentary and more active health promotion lifestyle	Plan with family to incorporate health promotion activities into lifestyle	Provide group education (classes) regarding benefits of regular exercise and healthy eating	Work with community leaders and citizens to establish safe physical activity space and healthy food options

the broader context of family, community, and society. This approach necessitates that the nursing interventions move beyond solving the immediate problem toward interventions that promote optimal health for the high-risk pregnant woman, her family, the aggregate of high-risk women and infants, and the total community.

Obesity and the Built Environment

Illness Care

A second example (Table 17-2) describes a referral of a young woman recently diagnosed with obesity. The nurse's immediate goal is to provide care that will help this client resolve her illness. Obesity rates have doubled over the last 20 years, with 33.8% of U.S. adults considered obese (Flegal et al, 2010). These rates are the result of a built environment that promotes increased unhealthy food consumption and decreased physical activity. Our built environment includes all of the places we live, work, learn, worship, and play and that are created or modified by people. According to the CDC, in order for people to make healthy choices to combat obesity, both policy and environmental changes are needed to assure affordable healthy food and safe places for activities (CDC, 2011). Therefore, teaching the client about the effects and side effects of her medications, and how to monitor her weight, nutrition, and physical activity at home, are important interventions. Since predisposing genetic, lifestyle, and environmental factors related to obesity exist, it is important to give family members information about this illness, including early recognition of signs and symptoms for themselves. Other important aspects of illness care include assessing the prevalence of obesity among high-risk aggregates in the community and teaching obesity prevention and

treatment classes in community-wide settings that high-risk groups frequent. An example is providing cooking classes in churches to African-American women in the community. At the community level, it is important to assess whether there are adequate and available providers and resources for healthy food and safe physical activity in the community.

Illness/Disease Prevention

Prevention care is also addressed at the individual level by teaching measures, such as healthy nutrition, progressive exercise, and lifestyle techniques to prevent additional weight gain. Healthy nutrition and regular moderate to vigorous exercise are important preventive measures for all family members. Aggregate-level preventive interventions include providing showers at workplaces to encourage exercise before or during the workday. Community intervention examples include year-long multimedia campaigns to provide intensive education to the community about prevention of obesity.

Health Promotion

Health promotion can motivate a person to adopt a less sedentary and more active lifestyle. Health promotion includes encouraging individuals to adopt a health-promoting lifestyle and helping them to become aware of their own power to do so. Nurses can encourage families to make health-promoting activities a part of their daily lives. This might include taking walks, swimming together, or joining an intergenerational baseball or bowling team in which families compete with other families. Aggregates can also benefit from heart-healthy classes or activities that are culturally specific to particular subgroups, such as older Hispanic women or African-American teenage girls. These activities can include stress management, well-balanced nutrition, exercise, dance classes, sports, or any other topic that can promote heart health. When looking at the total community, an example of a health promotion intervention is participating in a coalition to plan for supermarkets and parks or recreation areas within the community that are safe and accessible to the population.

In summary, the concepts of health, health promotion, and community are inextricably linked; it is difficult to discuss one without including the others. It is also important that nurses examine their definitions and beliefs about each concept as the basis for their practice. The essence of public health is the ability to see the totality of community while addressing its component parts and, at the same time, to see the total needs for health promotion, health protection, illness and disease prevention, and illness care and management. The integrative relationship among these components distinguishes public health nursing from nursing in more circumscribed settings, such as hospitals and clinics.

LINKING CONTENT TO PRACTICE

In this chapter, we describe the origins of the integrative model of community health promotion (Laffrey and Kulbok, 1999) and its application in public health nursing practice. The integrative model is one of five models, described in the *Public Health Nursing: Scope and Standards of Practice* (ANA, 2007), which address the multiple determinants of population health and are consistent with the ecological framework (IOM, 2003) and social determinants of health (SDOH) (CSDH, 2008; WHO, 2010). The ecological approach provides a basis for understanding population health. It emphasizes that multiple social determinants of health influence the conditions that promote health on multiple levels (i.e., individual, family, aggregate, community, and society). The central focus of public health nursing practice is health promotion. Health promotion is also central and dominant in the integrative model of community health promotion. Public health nurses strive to improve the health status of communities and populations. Whether the client system is the family or a vulnerable population, and the focus of care is illness prevention or illness care, health promotion remains the central goal. No matter where public health nursing care begins, it ultimately leads to health promotion of the community and population health.

CHAPTER REVIEW

PRACTICE APPLICATION

A rural health outreach program serves migrant workers, their families, and other vulnerable populations in the local community. The program's goals include increased knowledge about risk factors, services, and self-care; improved community health; increased access and affordability of individual- and community-level health promotion services; and reduced barriers to health services. The program offers health promotion and disease prevention educational materials and classes in English and Spanish throughout the region in churches, schools, community centers, fire departments, and migrant camps. In addition, clinics in eight local sites across the county provide services. Clinic services include health risk appraisal, disease screening, immunizations, health education, counseling, and referral. The program staff trained community health workers from the migrant community to deliver basic health education and resource information. Funding from a variety of public and private sources supports the program. It is essential that the program show effective outcomes if it is to sustain funding.

Mary Ann Jones, a nurse with a bachelor of science in nursing degree, works for the outreach program. She is a member of a group asked to evaluate whether the outreach program (including the eight clinics) is effective in meeting the stated objectives.

A. Using the integrative model for community health promotion as a guide, how might you organize a comprehensive approach to assessment and data collection?
B. What are sources of data you might use for assessing individual, aggregate, and community health indicators?
C. What is the value of interviewing rural residents, migrant workers, and clinic participants about their perceptions of health and the value of health services?
D. Who else can you interview to elicit important information about the usefulness of the outreach program?
E. How can you best use community health workers to increase participation and partnership among concerned health professionals, community residents, and migrant families and to sustain the program?

Be creative and comprehensive in your approach, and consider the ecological perspective, the social determinants of health, and cultural factors associated with rural and migrant populations in the United States. Current spending limits on federal and state programs for health promotion and disease prevention require that nurses deal effectively with issues of outreach, sustainability, and success of community health programs.

Answers can be found on the Evolve site.

KEY POINTS

- The idea of health shapes the process of population-focused nursing practice, from assessment of health-related needs of individuals, families, aggregates, and communities to evaluation of health outcomes.
- The greatest benefits in public health are likely to come from efforts to improve individual and family lifestyles through community and population interventions that address the social determinants of health including social conditions and the physical environment.
- Public health nurses have a history of commitment to primary health care and to enhancing levels of wellness in communities and populations.

KEY POINTS—cont'd

- When nurses examine their own definition of health, they recognize how this health definition directs the nursing care they provide.
- When nurses examine the client's definition of health, they are more likely to tailor care to the client's culture, needs, lifestyle, and social and physical environment.
- The goal of risk appraisal and reduction is the prevention or early detection of disease.
- The knowledge base for risk appraisal and risk reduction is the scientific evidence regarding the relationship between risk factors and mortality and the effectiveness of planned interventions in reducing both risks and mortality.
- Clinical preventive guidelines use clinical and epidemiological data to identify specific individual health risks, and they provide a detailed list of recommendations for preventive measures appropriate to different age groups.
- Health risk appraisal tools are used to assess the total risks to an individual's health, and resulting knowledge of health risks may be used to initiate health-promoting and disease-preventing lifestyle changes.

- Wellness inventories define health risks more broadly and emphasize empowerment of individuals to achieve health.
- Clinical observation, assessment, and nursing interventions used in conjunction with health risk appraisals are essential to obtain the best health outcomes for communities and populations.
- The Stanford Heart Disease Prevention program, the North Karelia Project, the Pawtucket Heart Health program, and the Minnesota Heart Health program contributed to the scientific knowledge base for the design, implementation, and evaluation of community and population level risk-appraisal and risk-reduction programs.
- The Framingham Heart Study has provided more than 50 years of research about risk factors and lifestyle habits; Framingham researchers are currently studying how genes contribute to common disorders such as obesity, hypertension, and diabetes.
- Public health nurses function beyond resolving a specific illness to preventing the illness and promoting optimal health for the individual, the family, the aggregate, and the total community. All of these levels are important to promote the health of the community and populations.

CLINICAL DECISION-MAKING ACTIVITIES

1. Write your own definition of health, and interview a nurse, client, and physician about their definitions of health. Use Smith's four models of health as a frame of reference to contrast different perspectives.
2. What are some difficulties encountered when you consider definitions of health promotion, disease prevention, and health maintenance? Illustrate these difficulties with examples of strategies that are health promoting, disease preventing, and/or health maintaining.
3. Discuss the importance of the built environment in community health promotion, and provide examples of environmental health promotion indicators for a specified community.
4. Develop a nursing care plan for addressing childhood obesity using the propositions of Milio (1976) as a frame of reference.
5. Use the integrative model for community health promotion and social determinants of heath to identify the most important strategies in a community-wide plan for childhood obesity.
6. Consider the role of partnerships with the community from the perspectives of school health, public health, occupational health, and home health.
7. Illustrate community health levels of care including the client system and the focus of care:
    A. For teenage pregnancy: begin with community level health promotion
    B. For childhood obesity: start with community level illness prevention

REFERENCES

American Academy of Pediatrics, Committee on Community Health Services: The pediatrician's role in community pediatrics, *Pediatrics* 115:1092–1094, 2005.

American Nurses Association: *Public health nursing: scope and standards of practice*, Washington, DC, 2007, ANA.

Anderson ET, McFarlane J: *Community-as-partner: theory and practice in nursing*, ed 4, Philadelphia, 2000, Lippincott Williams & Wilkins.

Anderson ET, McFarlane J: *Community-as-partner: theory and practice in nursing*, ed 3, Philadelphia, 2008, Lippincott Williams & Wilkins.

Babor TF, Sciamanna CN, Pronk NP: Assessing multiple risk behaviors in primary care: screening issues and related concepts, *Am J Prevent Med* 27:42–53, 2004.

Bekemeier B, Jones M: Relationships between local public health agency functions and agency leadership and staffing: a look at nurses, *J Public Health Manag Pract* 16:E8–E16, 2010.

Berkman LF, Breslow L: *Health and ways of living, the Alameda County Study*, New York, 1983, Oxford University Press.

Botchwey N: The religious sector's presence in local community development, *J Plan Educ Res* 27(1):36–48, 2007.

Bracht N, editor: *Health promotion at the community level*, Newbury Park, CA, 1990, Sage.

Carleton RA, Lasater TM, Assaf AR, et al: The Pawtucket Heart Health Program: community changes in cardiovascular risk factors and projected disease risk, *Am J Public Health* 85:777, 1995.

Centers for Disease Control and Prevention: *Centers for Disease Control and Prevention: Impact of the built environment on health, 2006.* CDC environmental health fact sheet. Available at http://www.cdc.gov/nceh/publications/factsheets/ImpactoftheBuiltEnvironmentonHealth.pdf. Accessed January 3, 2011.

Centers for Disease Conrol and Prevention: *Overweight and obesity.* Available at http://www.cdc.gov/obesity. Accessed Janaruy 25, 2011.

Centers for Disease Control and Prevention: Smoking-attributable mortality, years of potential life lost, and productivity losses—United States, 2000–2004, *MMWR Morb Mortal Wkly Rep* 57(45):1226–1228, 2008.

Chopoorian TL: Reconceptualizing the environment. In Moccia P, editor: *New approaches to theory development*, Pub. No. 15-1992, New York, 1986, National League for Nursing.

Chowdhury P, Balluz L, Town M, et al: Surveillance of certain health behaviors and conditions among states and selected local areas—Behavioral Risk Factor Surveillance System, United States, 2007, *MMWR. Surveill Summ* 59(1):1–220, 2010.

Commission on Social Determinants of Health: *Closing the gap in a generation: final report*, Geneva, 2008, World Health Organization.

Cunningham T, Botchwey N, Dillingham R, et al: Understanding water perceptions in Limpopo Province: a Photovoice community assessment, *Environ Poll Public Health IEEE*, 2009.

Deshpande AD, Baker EA, Lovegreen SL, et al: Environmental correlates of physical activity among individuals with diabetes in the rural Midwest, *Diabetes Care* 28:1012–1018, 2005.

Eaton CB, Lapane KL, Garber CE, et al: Effects of a community-based intervention on physical activity: the Pawtucket Heart Health Program, *Am J Public Health* 89:1741–1744, 1999.

Farley T, Cohen W: *Prescription for a healthy nation: a new approach to improving our lives by fixing our everyday world*, Boston, 2005, Beacon Press, Chapter 4.

Farquhar JW, Maccoby N, Wood PD, et al: Effects of community-wide education on cardiovascular disease risk factors: the Stanford Five-city Project, *JAMA* 264:359, 1990.

Flegal KM, Carroll MD, Ogden CL, et al: Prevalence and trends in obesity among U.S. adults, 1999-2008, *JAMA* 303:253–241, 2010.

Freudenberg N: From lifestyle to social determinants: new directions for community health promotion research and practice, *Prev Chronic Dis*, July 2007:[serial online]. Available at http://www.cdc.gov/pcd/issues/2007/jul/06_0194.htm. Accessed January 3, 2011.

Fuchs V: *Who shall live?* New York, 1974, Basic Books.

Grumbach K, Miller J, Mertz E, et al: How much public health in public health nursing practice? *Public Health Nurs* 21:266–276, 2004.

Hernandez LM, editor: *Implications of genomics for public health: workshop summary*, Committee on Genomics and the Public's Health in the 21st Century, 2005, Institute of Medicine of the National Academies. Available at http://www.nap.edu/catalog/11260.html. Accessed January 3, 2011.

Hinton A, Downey J, Lisovicz N, et al: The community health advisor program and the deep south network for cancer control: health promotion programs for volunteer community health advisors, *Fam Community Health* 28:20–27, 2005.

Institute of Medicine: *The future of public health*, Washington, DC, 1988, The National Academies Press.

Institute of Medicine: *The future of the public's health in the 21st century*, Washington, DC, 2002, The National Academies Press. Available at http://www.nap.edu/catalog/10548.html. Accessed January 3, 2011.

Institute of Medicine: *Who will keep the public healthy? Educating public health professionals for the 21st century*, Washington, DC, 2003, The National Academies Press. Available at http://books.nap.edu/catalog/10542.html. Accessed January 3, 2011.

Institute of Medicine: The impact of social and cultural environment on health. Defining the social and cultural environment. In *Genes, behavior, and the social environment: moving beyond the nature/nurture debate*, Washington, DC, 2006, The National Academies Press.

Kelleher L, Johnson M: An evaluation of a volunteer-support program for families at risk, *Public Health Nurs* 21:297–305, 2004.

Keller LO, Strohschein S, Lia-Hoagberg G, et al: Population-based public health nursing interventions: a model for practice, *Public Health Nurs* 15:207, 1998.

Keller LO, Strohschein S, Lia-Hoagberg B, et al: Population-based public health nursing interventions: practice-based and evidence-supported. Part 1, *Public Health Nurs* 21:453–468, 2004.

Krautscheid L, Moos P, Zeller J: Patient & staff satisfaction with integrated services at Old Town Clinic, *J Psychosoc Nurs* 42:1–9, 2004.

Kulbok PA: Social resources, health resources, and preventive health behavior: patterns and predictors, *Public Health Nurs* 2:67, 1985.

Kulbok PA, Baldwin JH: From preventive health behavior to health promotion: advancing a positive construct of health, *Adv Nurs Sci* 14:50, 1992.

Kulbok PA, Baldwin JH, Cox CL, et al: Advancing discourse on health promotion: beyond mainstream thinking, *Adv Nurs Sci* 20:12, 1997.

Kulbok PA, Carter K, Baldwin J, et al: The multidimensional health behavior inventory. In Strickland O, DiLorio C, editors: *Measurement of nursing outcomes: focus on patient/client outcomes*, New York, 2003, Springer.

Kulbok P, Meszaros P, Hinton I, et al: Tobacco-free boys and parents use Photovoice to tell their stories: issues and solutions [Abstract], San Diego, CA, October 25-29, 2008, Proceedings of the 136th American Public Health Association, Annual Meeting.

Kulbok P, Rhee H, Hinton I, et al: Factors influencing adolescents' decisions not to smoke, *Public Health Nurs* 25:505–515, 2008b.

Lacson RS: *tb. Tuberculosis. pv. Photovoice*, 2007. Available at http://tbphotovoice.org/tbpv2/. Accessed June 30, 2008.

Laffrey SC: An exploration of adult health behaviors, *West J Nurs Res* 12:434, 1990.

Laffrey SC, Kulbok PA: The integrative model for community health nursing: a conceptual guide to education, practice, and research, *J Holist Nurs* 17:88–103, 1999.

Laffrey SC, Loveland-Cherry CJ, Winkler SJ: Health behavior: evolution of two paradigms, *Public Health Nurs* 3:92–97, 1986.

LaLonde M: *A new perspective on the health of Canadians*, Ottawa, 1974, Government of Canada.

Lasater T, Abrams T, Artz L, et al: Lay volunteer delivery of a community-based cardiovascular risk factor change program: the Pawtucket experiment. In Matarazzo JD, et al, editors: *Behavioral health: a handbook of health enhancement and disease prevention*, Silver Spring, MD, 1984, Wiley.

Leavell HR, Clark EG: *Preventive medicine for the doctor in his community: an epidemiological approach*, ed 3, New York, 1965, McGraw-Hill.

Levin S, Gans KM, Carleton RA, et al: The evolution of a physical activity campaign, *Fam Community Health* 21:65–77, 1998.

Liao Y, McGee DL, Cooper RS, et al: How generalizable are coronary risk prediction models? Comparison of Framingham and two national cohorts, *Am Heart J* 137:837, 1999.

Lieb W, Pencina ML, Lanier KJ, Tofler GH, Levy D, Fox CS, Wang TJ, D'Agostina RB Sr, Vasan RS: Association of parental obesity with concentrations of select systemic biomarkers in nonobese offspring: The Framingham Heart Study, *Diabetes* 58(1):134–137, 2009.

Luepker RV, Murray DM, Jacobs JN, et al: Community education for cardiovascular disease prevention: risk factor changes in the Minnesota Heart Health Program, *Am J Public Health* 84:1383, 1994.

Martin M, Leonard M, Allen S, et al: Using culturally competent strategies to improve traffic safety in the black community, *Ann Emerg Med* 44:414–418, 2004.

McQueen DV: Three challenges for the social determinants of health pursuit, *Int J Public Health* 54:1–2, 2009.

Milio N: A framework for prevention: changing health-damaging to health-generating life patterns, *Am J Public Health* 66:435, 1976.

Minkler M, Wallerstein N, editors: *Community-based participatory research for health*, San Francisco, 2003, John Wiley & Sons.

Mokdad AH: The behavioral risk factor surveillance system: past, present, and future, *Annu Rev Public Health* 30:43–54, 2009.

National Cancer Institute: *Theory at a glance: a guide for health promotion practice*, ed 2, NIH Pub. No. 05-3896, Washington, DC: 2005. Available at http://www.cancer.gov/PDF/481f5d53-63df-41bc-bfaf-5aa48ee1da4d/TAAG3.pdf. Accessed January 3, 2011.

National Center for Health Statistics: *Health, United States, 2009: with special feature on medical technology*, Hyattsville, MD, 2010. Available at http://www.cdc.gov/nchs/data/hus/hus09.pdf. Accessed January 3, 2011.

National Fetal and Infant Mortality Program: *Fetal Infant Mortality Review Manual*, ed 2, Washington, DC, 2008. Available at http://www.acog.org/departments/nfimr/CommunityGuide.pdf. Accessed January 3, 2011.

Navarro AM, Voetsch KP, Liburd LC, et al: Charting the future of community health promotion: recommendations from the National Expert Panel on Community Health Promotion, *Prev Chronic Dis*, July 2007:[serial online]. Available at http://www.cdc.gov/pcd/issues/2007/jul/07_0013.htm. Accessed January 3, 2011.

Nigg C, Maddock J, Yamauchi J, et al: The healthy Hawaii initiative: a social ecological approach promoting healthy communities, *Am J Health Promot* 19(4):310–313, 2005.

North Karelia Project, 2009. Available at http://www.ktl.fi/portal/english/research_people_programs/health_promotion_and_chronic_disease_prevention/projects/training_seminar/ncd_seminar/north_karelia_project. Accessed January 3, 2011.

Owen N, Humpel N, Leslie E, et al: Understanding environmental influences on walking: review and research agenda, *Am J Prev Med* 27:67–76, 2004.

Pai CW, Mullin J, Payne GM, et al: Factors associated with incidental sickness absence among employees in one health care system, *Am J Health Promot* 24:37–48, 2009.

Pate RR, Colabianchi N, Porter D, et al: Physical activity and neighborhood resources in high school girls, *Am J Prev Med* 34:413–419, 2008.

Peel NM, McClure RJ, Bartlett HP: Behavioral determinants of healthy aging, *Am J Prevent Med* 28:298–304, 2005.

Pender NJ, Murdaugh CL, Parsons MA: *Health promotion in nursing practice*, ed 6, Upper Saddle River, NJ, 2011, Prentice Hall.

Prentice AM, Jebb SA: Obesity in Britain; gluttony or sloth? *Br Med J* 311:437–439, 1995.

Puska P, Salonen JL, Nissinen JT, et al: Change in risk factors for coronary heart disease during 10 years of a community intervention programme (North Karelia Project), *Br Med J* 287:1840, 1983.

Rand Corporation: *Evidence report and evidence-based recommendations: health risk appraisals and Medicare*, Baltimore, 2003, USDHHS.

Resnick B, Galik E, Gruber-Baldine AL, Zimmerman S: Implementing a restorative care philosophy of care in assisted living: pilot testing of Res-Care-AL, *J Am Acad Nurse Pract* 21(2):123–133, 2009.

Riley RG, Manias E: The uses of photography in clinical nursing practice and research: a literature review, *J Adv Nurs* 48:397–405, 2004.

Ronda G, Van Assema E, Ruland E, et al: The Dutch heart health community intervention 'Hartslag Limburg': results of an effect study at organizational level, *Public Health* 119:353–360, 2005.

Rose G: *The strategy of preventive medicine*, New York, 1992, Oxford University Press.

Rosenstock I: Historical origins of the health belief model, *Health Educ Monog* 2(4), 1974.

Salmon M: Editorial: Public health nursing: the opportunity of a century, *Am J Public Health* 83:1674–1675, 1993.

Salmon M: An open letter to public health nursing, *Public Health Nurs* 26:483–485, 2009.

Sanders LM, Robinson TN, Forster LQ, et al: Evidence-based community pediatrics: building a bridge from bedside to neighborhood, *Pediatrics* 115:1142–1147, 2005.

Schuit A, Wendel-Vos G, Verschuren W, et al: Effect of 5-year community intervention Hartslag Limburg on cardiovascular risk factors, *Am J Prev Med* 30:237–242, 2006.

Schultz AB, Edington DW: The association between changes in metabolic syndrome and changes in cost in a workplace population, *J Occup Environ Med* 51:771–779, 2009.

Schulz BJ, Zenk S, Odoms-Young A, et al: Healthy eating and exercising to reduce diabetes: exploring the potential of social determinants of health frameworks within the context of community-based participatory diabetes prevention, *Am J Public Health* 95:645–651, 2005.

Shuster G, Goeppinger J: Community as client: assessment and analysis. In Stanhope M, Lancaster J, editors: *Public health nursing: population-centered health care in the community*, ed 7, St Louis, 2008, Mosby.

Skinner BF: *Why I am not a cognitive psychologist in reflections on behaviorism and society*, Englewood Cliffs, NJ, 1978, Prentice-Hall.

Smith JA: The idea of health: a philosophical inquiry, *Adv Nurs Sci* 3:43, 1981.

Smith K, Bazini-Barakat N: A public health nursing practice model: melding public health principles with the nursing process, *Public Health Nurs* 20:42–48, 2003.

Strecher VJ: *Photovoice for tobacco, drug, and alcohol prevention among adolescents in South Africa [Abstract], 2004*. Available at http://apha.confex.com/apha/132am/techprogram/paper_84002.htm. Accessed January 3, 2011.

Task Force on Community Preventive Services: *The guide to community preventive services—what works to promote health*, New York, 2005, Oxford University Press.

Terris M: Approaches to an epidemiology of health, *Am J Public Health* 65:1037–1038, 1975.

Thompson NC, Hunter EE, Murray L, et al: Experience of living with chronic mental illness: a photovoice study [Abstract], *Perspec Psych Care*, 2008. Available at http://findarticles.com/p/articles/mi_qa3804/is_200801/ai_n21279836/pg_10. Accessed January 3, 2011.

U.S. Department of Health, Education, and Welfare: *Forward plan for health*, FY 1978-82, DHEW Pub. No. (OS) 76-50046, Washington, DC, 1976, U.S. Government Printing Office.

U.S. Department of Health, Education, and Welfare: *Healthy People: the surgeon general's report on health promotion and disease prevention*, DHEW Pub. No. 79-55071, Washington, DC, 1979, U.S. Government Printing Office.

U.S. Department of Health and Human Services: *Healthy People 2010: understanding and improving health and objectives for improving health*, ed 2, Washington, DC, 2000, U.S. Government Printing Office.

U.S. Department of Health and Human Services: *Healthy People 2020 framework*, 2009a. Available at http://www.healthypeople.gov/2020/default.aspx. Accessed January 3, 2011.

U.S. Department of Health and Human Services: *HP 2020 proposed objectives*, 2009b. Available at http://www.healthypeople.gov/2020/default.aspx. Accessed January 3, 2011.

U.S. Department of Health and Human Services: *Healthy people in healthy communities: a community planning guide using Healthy People 2010*, Washington, DC, 2001, U.S. Government Printing Office.

U.S. Department of Health and Human Services: *Theory at a glance: a guide for health promotion practice*, ed 2, NIH Pub. No. 05-3896, Washington, DC, 2005, National Cancer Institute, National Institutes of Health (revised).

U.S. Preventive Services Task Force: *Guide to clinical preventive services: report of the U.S. Preventive Services Task Force*, Baltimore, 1989, Lippincott, Williams & Wilkins.

U.S. Preventive Service Task Force: *The guide to clinical preventive services 2010-2011*. Available at http://www.uspreventiveservicestaskforce.org/recommentatios.htm. Accessed January 3, 2011.

U.S. Preventive Services Task Force: *Guide to clinical preventive services*, AHRQ Pub. No. 09-IP006, Rockville, MD, September 2009, Agency for Healthcare Research and Quality. Available at http://www.ahrq.gov/clinic/pocketgd.htm. Accessed January 3, 2011.

Wang C, Burris A: Photovoice: concept, methodology, and use for participatory needs assessment, *Health Educ Behav* 24:369–387, 1997.

Wang C, Burris M: Empowerment through photo novella: portraits of participation, *Health Educ Q* 21:171–186, 1994.

Watson M, Dannenberg AL: Investment in Safe Routes to School projects: public health benefits for the larger community, *Prev Chronic Dis* 5:1–7, 2008. Available at http://www.ncbi.nlm.nih.gov/pmc/articles/PMC2483559/pdf/PCD53A90.pdf. Accessed January 3, 2011.

Wight RG, Aneshensel CS, Botticello AL, et al: A multilevel analysis of ethnic variation in depressive symptoms among adolescents in the United States, *Soc Sci Med* 60:2073–2084, 2005.

Winkleby MA, Feldman HA, Murray DM: Joint analysis of US three community intervention trials for reduction of cardiovascular disease risk, *J Clin Epidemiol* 50(6):645–658, 1997.

Winkleby MA, Taylor CB, Jatulis D, et al: The long-term effects of a cardiovascular disease prevention trial: the Stanford Five-city Project, *Am J Public Health* 86:1773–1779, 1996.

World Health Organization: *The first ten years of the World Health Organization*, New York, 1958, WHO.

World Health Organization: *Health promotion: a discussion document on the concept and principles*, Copenhagen, 1984, WHO Regional Office for Europe.

World Health Organization: *Social determinants of health*, Geneva, 2010, WHO. Available at http://www.who.int/social_determinants/p 1. Accessed March 13, 2011.

PART 4

Issues and Approaches in Population-Centered Nursing

The primary orientation of health care delivery has been toward care and cure of the individual. There is increasing evidence that lifestyle and personal health habits influence the health of individuals, families, populations, aggregates, and communities.

Although it is necessary to identify health risk factors among individuals and groups in the community, it is of paramount importance that nurses learn to identify and work with health problems of a defined population or the total community. This may be referred to as an aggregate approach or a population-focused approach to health care delivery. Healthy communities provide greater resources for growth and nurturing of individuals and families than do the communities that ignore the need for an emphasis on the health of their populations.

Certainly, nurses can use a public health approach to work with individuals and families in promoting health, intervening in disease onset or progression, and assisting with rehabilitation. Likewise, nurses often find that strategies used to introduce health behaviors directed at illness prevention and lifestyle changes are applicable to groups in the community and the community at large. Concepts for promoting health behaviors through groups, identifying community groups and their contributions to community life, and helping groups work toward community health goals are essential to population-centered nursing practice.

Healthy communities/healthy cities is an approach to helping communities organize and strive to provide environments for healthful living for their populations. In this approach, health is described as encompassing the physical and mental health of individuals and families plus the social, political, economic, educational, cultural, and environmental settings of the total community.

Nurses can help communities attain their health goals by understanding the organization of communities, the effects of rural versus urban settings on health issues, how and why programs are managed, and how to evaluate programs for quality and effectiveness. A community assessment provides the basis for helping communities establish their goals. The use of a nurse-managed clinic is one approach nurses have found to be successful in meeting the needs of aggregates, or vulnerable at-risk populations. These needs must be considered when trying to improve the health of a community. Case management is an approach that has been used by nurses since its inception to match the most appropriate services and health care delivery interventions to population needs.

Although all communities strive to protect their populations and provide a safe living environment, natural and man-made disasters may occur; nurses can play a significant role in helping a community through such crises as the terrorist events of September 11, 2001, and other acts of terrorism as well as natural disasters such as Hurricane Katrina and the devastating landslides of 2011. The chapters in this section help nurses learn how to work with aggregates and to develop healthy communities and to provide quality health care in the community.

CHAPTER 18

Community as Client: Assessment and Analysis

George F. Shuster, RN, DNSc

Dr. George F. Shuster started as a community volunteer nurse in one of the Seattle Neighborhood Free Clinics in 1981. Since that time, he has practiced as a home-health nurse in San Francisco, California, and later in Charlottesville, Virginia. In Virginia he was involved with the American Lung Association in community-wide smoking cessation programs. In New Mexico he continues to teach public health at the undergraduate and graduate levels and also has been involved in the development of a community-focused health promotion program for older Hispanic women.

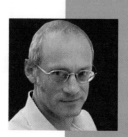

ADDITIONAL RESOURCES

evolve WEBSITE

http://evolve.elsevier.com/Stanhope
- *Healthy People 2020*
- WebLinks—Of special note see the link for these sites:
    - Centers for Disease Control and Prevention (provides numerous .pdf files for download)
    - Websites of the chapter author's home community: Bernalillo County, New Mexico
    - Behavior Risk Factor Surveillance System (BRFSS) data
    - American Public Health Association: *The Guide to Implementing Model Standards*
    - The Community Guide
- Quiz
- Case Studies
- Glossary
- Answers to Practice Application
- Resource Tool
    - Resource Tool 18.A: Community-Oriented Health Record (COHR)

APPENDIX
- Appendix C.1

OBJECTIVES

After reading this chapter, the student should be able to do the following:
1. Decide whether nursing care can be delivered in the community.
2. Illustrate concepts basic to nursing practice: community, community client, community health, and partnership for health.
3. Discuss the relevance of the nursing process to nursing practice in the community.
4. Analyze the importance of community assessment in nursing practice.
5. Decide which methods of assessment, intervention, and evaluation are most appropriate in given community situations.
6. Develop a nursing care plan for a community problem.

KEY TERMS

Although in the past, nurses have sometimes viewed the community as a client, many nurses have come to consider the community their most important client and, more recently, their partner (Anderson and McFarlane, 2008; Butterfoss, 2009). This chapter clarifies community concepts and provides a guideline for nursing practice with the community client. The core functions of public health nursing (PHN) include assessment, policy development, and assurance. A public and private group partnership called the Council on Linkages Between Academia and Public Health Practice (2009) has defined competencies for the core functions of public health practice (see Chapter 1 for more details). In the area of assessment, 11 competencies for the nurse and other health providers working in the community are listed (Box 18-1).

The nursing process from assessment through evaluation is used to promote a community's health. This process begins with community assessment—one of the core functions—which involves getting to know the community. It is a logical, systematic approach to identifying community needs, clarifying problems, and identifying community strengths and resources. This chapter provides the nurse with the knowledge necessary to develop the community assessment core competencies.

COMMUNITY DEFINED

Definitions of the meaning of community vary widely. The World Health Organization (WHO) includes this definition: "A group of people, often living in a defined geographical area, who may share a common culture, values and norms, and are arranged in a social structure according to relationships which the community has developed over a period of time. Members of a community gain their personal and social identity by sharing common beliefs, values and norms which have been

developed by the community in the past and may be modified in the future" (WHO, 2004, p 16). Other theorists and writers present typologies (lists of types), which involve classifying communities by category rather than single definitions. One such typology of community was described by Blum in 1974. This typology is still used today. The categories, or types of communities, include communities defined by geopolitical boundaries, by their interactions (such as between schools, social services, and governmental agencies), and by their ability to solve problems. Some types of communities are listed in Box 18-2.

Nurses working in communities quickly learn that society consists of many different types of communities. Some of the communities listed in Box 18-2 are *communities of place*. In this type of community, interactions occur within a specific geographic area. Neighborhood and face-to-face communities are two examples of this type of community. Other communities, such as *communities of special interest* or *resource communities*, cut across geographic areas. Common concerns and interests, which can be long term or short term in nature, bring their members together (e.g., a group to support a smoke-free environment). Another type of community is a *community of problem ecology,* which is created when environmental problems such as water pollution affect a widespread area. For example, a problem such as water pollution can bring people together from areas that would not otherwise share a common interest. Nurses also may work in partnership with *communities defined by geographic and political boundaries,* such as school districts, townships, or counties. Because the type of community varies, nurses planning community interventions must take into account each community's specific characteristics. Each community is unique, and its defining characteristics will affect the nature of the partnership.

In most definitions, the community includes three factors: people, place, and function. The *people* are the community

BOX 18-1 CORE COMPETENCIES FOR PUBLIC HEALTH PROFESSIONALS

Public health professionals should be able to do the following:
- Define a problem.
- Determine appropriate uses and limitations of both quantitative and qualitative data.
- Select and define variables relevant to the defined public health problems.
- Identify relevant and appropriate data and information sources.
- Evaluate the integrity and comparability of data and identify gaps in data sources.
- Apply ethical principles to the collection, maintenance, use, and dissemination of data and information.
- Partner with communities to attach meaning to collected quantitative and qualitative data.
- Make relevant inferences from quantitative and qualitative data.
- Obtain and interpret information regarding risks and benefits to the community.
- Apply data collection processes, information technology applications, and computer systems storage and retrieval strategies.
- Recognize how the data illuminate ethical, political, scientific, economic, and overall public health issues.

From Council on Linkages Between Academia and Public Health Practice: *Core competencies for public health professionals*, Washington, DC, 2009, USDHHS and Public Health Foundation. Available at http://www.phf.org/link/competenciesinformation.htm. Accessed January 4, 2011.

BOX 18-2 TYPES OF COMMUNITIES

- Face-to-face community
- Neighborhood community
- Community of identifiable need
- Community of problem ecology
- Community of concern
- Community of special interest
- Community of viability
- Community of action capability
- Community of political jurisdiction
- Resource community
- Community of solution

From Blum HL: *Planning for health*, New York, 1974, Human Sciences.

members or residents. *Place* refers both to geographic and to time dimensions, and *function* refers to the aims and activities of the community. Nurses regularly need to examine how the people, place, and function dimensions of community shape their nursing practice. They can use both a definition and a set of measures for the community in their practice.

In this chapter, the following definition is used: Community is a locality-based entity, composed of systems of formal organizations reflecting society's institutions, informal groups, and aggregates. As defined in Chapter 1, an aggregate is a collection of individuals who have in common one or more personal or environmental characteristics. The parts of a community are interdependent, and their function is to meet a wide variety of collective needs. This definition of community includes place and function dimensions and recognizes interaction among the

systems within a community. Measures of the dimensions for this definition are listed in Table 18-1.

If the community is where nurses practice and apply the nursing process, and the community is the client of that practice, then nurses will want to analyze and synthesize information about the boundaries, parts, and dynamic processes of the client community. The next section describes the community as client: it is both the setting for practice and the target of practice (i.e., the client) for the nurse.

COMMUNITY AS CLIENT

Nurses who have a community orientation have often been considered unique because of their target of practice. The idea of health-related care being provided within the community is, however, not new. At the turn of the century, most persons stayed at home during illnesses. As a result, the practice environment for all nurses was the home rather than the hospital. As the range of nursing services expanded into the community, many different kinds of agencies were started, and their services often overlapped. For example, both privately owned voluntary agencies and official or governmental local health agencies worked to control tuberculosis. The nurses employed by these agencies were called *community health nurses*, *public health nurses*, and *visiting nurses*. They practiced in clients' homes and not in the hospital. Today, these three types of nurses are nurses working to improve the public's health.

Early PHN textbooks in the 1940s included lengthy descriptions of the home environment and tools for assessing the extent to which that environment promoted the health of family members. Health education about the home environment was often a major part of home nursing care.

By the 1950s, schools, prisons, industries, and neighborhood health centers, as well as homes, had all become settings of practice for nurses. Many of these new nurses did not consider the environments in which they practiced. Although their practices took place within the community, they focused on the individual client or the family seeking care. The care provided was not population centered; rather, it was oriented toward the individual or family who lived in the community, and this is now called community-*based* nursing practice. This commitment to direct, hands-on, clinical nursing care delivered to individuals or families in community settings remains a more popular approach to nursing practice than recognizing the whole community as the target of nursing practice. This remains true today with the American Public Health Association: Public Health Nursing Section (APHA: PHN) statement that "Public health nurses integrate community involvement and knowledge about the entire population with personal, clinical understandings of the health and illness experiences of individuals and families within the population"(APHA: PHN, 2009, www.apha.org/membersgroups). When the location of the practice is the community and the focus of the practice is the individual or family, the client remains the individual or family, and the nurse is practicing in the community as the setting; this is an example of community based nursing practice.

The community is the client only when the nursing focus is on the collective or common good of the population

TABLE 18-1	THE CONCEPT OF COMMUNITY SPECIFIED	
DIMENSIONS	**MEASURES**	**EXAMPLES OF DATA SOURCES**
Place	Geopolitical boundaries	Maps
	Local or folk name for area	Local newspaper
	Size in square miles, acres, blocks, or census tracts	Census data
	Transportation avenues, such as rivers, highways, railroads, and sidewalks	Chamber of commerce
		City, county, or township government
	History	Library archives and local histories
	Physical environment such as land use patterns and condition of housing	Local housing office
People or person	Population: number and density	Census data
	Demographic structure of population, such as age, race, socio-economic, and racial distributions; rural and urban character; and dependency ratio	Census data
		Churches, senior centers, civic groups
	Informal groups such as block clubs, service clubs, and friend-ship networks	Local newspaper
		Telephone directory
		United Way
		Social service agencies
	Formal groups such as schools, churches, businesses, indus-tries, governmental bodies, unions, and health and welfare agencies	Chamber of commerce
		Tourist bureau
		Local or state officials
	Linking structures (intercommunity and intracommunity contacts among organizations)	Chamber of commerce
Function	Production, distribution, and consumption of goods and services	State departments
		Business and labor
		Local library
	Socialization of new members	Social and local research reports
	Maintenance of social control	Police station
	Adapting to ongoing and expected change	Social and local research reports
	Provision of mutual aid	United Way
		Welfare agencies
		Churches and religious organizations

instead of on individual health. **Population-centered practice** seeks healthful change for the whole community's benefit (Radzyminski, 2007). Although the nurse may work with individuals, families or other interacting groups, aggregates, or institutions, or within a population, the resulting changes are intended to affect the whole community. For example, an occupational health nurse's target might be preventing illness and injury and maintaining or promoting the health of an entire company workforce. Because of this focus, the nurse would help an individual disabled worker become independent in activities of daily living. The nurse would also become involved with promoting vocational rehabilitation services in the community and seek reasonable employment policies for all disabled workers through the community government.

WHAT DO YOU THINK? *Many nurses believe that hospice and home-health nursing are focused on the individual and it therefore should not be considered a part of population-centered nursing. Other nurses argue that hospice and home-health nursing both focus on the family, take place in the community, and should be considered a part of population-centered nursing. Are hospice and home-health nursing focused on the individual, family, or community or on all three? Are hospice and home-health nursing a part of population-centered nursing? Why or why not?*

Community Client and Nursing Practice

Population-focused health care is experiencing a rebirth, and the community as client is important to nursing practice for several reasons. When focusing on the community as client, direct clinical care can be a part of population-focused community health practice (Radzyminski, 2007). For example, sometimes direct nursing care is provided to individuals and family members because their health needs are common community-related problems. Changes in their health will affect the health of their communities (O'Donnell et al, 2009).

In such cases, decisions are made at the individual level because the individual's health is related to the health of the population as a whole. Improved health of the community remains the overall goal of nursing intervention. Interventions to stop spousal or elder abuse are two examples of nursing interventions done primarily because of the effects of abuse on society and therefore on the population as a whole. Also, the treatment of a client for tuberculosis reduces the risk to other community members. This care reduces the risk of an epidemic in the community.

The community client also highlights the complexity of the change process. Change for the benefit of the community client must often occur at several levels, ranging from the individual to society as a whole. For example, health problems caused by lifestyle, such as smoking, overeating, and speeding, cannot be solved simply by asking individuals to choose health-promoting habits. Society must also provide healthy choices. Most individuals cannot change their habits alone; they require the support of family members, friends, community health care systems, and relevant social policies. Individuals who have lifestyle health problems are often blamed for their illness because of their choices (e.g., to smoke). In his classic work, Ryan (1976) points out that the "victim" cannot always be blamed and expected to correct the problem without changes also being made in the helping professions and public policy. Some communities have no-smoking areas in restaurants to prevent second-hand smoke from harming others. This is an example of a community-level policy to change behavior.

Commitment to the health of the community client requires a process of change at each of these levels. One nursing role emphasizes individual and direct personal care skills, another nursing role focuses on the family as the unit of service, and a third focuses on the community as a unit of service. Collaborative practice models involving the community and nurses in joint decision making and specific nursing roles are required (Bencivenga et al, 2008). Ndirangu et al (2008) note that nurses must remember that collaboration means shared roles and a cooperative effort in which participants want to work together. These participants must see themselves as part of a group effort and share in the process, beginning with planning and including decision making. This means sharing not only the power but also the responsibility for the outcomes of the intervention. Viewing the community as client and thus as the target of service means a commitment to two key concepts: (1) community health and (2) partnership for community health. These two concepts form not only the goal (community health), but also the *means* of population-centered practice (partnership).

WHAT DO YOU THINK?   *In 2007 Radzyminski asked several related questions: What is population health? Are the terms "population health," "community health," and "public health" interchangeable? And what is nursing's role in population health? In presenting parameters for each of these three terms, Dr. Radzyminski argues that these three terms are related but different. In examining the parameters for each concept and how a nurse would apply each of these three approaches to the same problem, a case is made for how nursing interventions would differ based upon which perspective the nurse used to approach the problem.*

Take Dr. Radzyminski's three defining parameters: overall goal, health management view, and necessary elements. Make a list comparing and contrasting the components of population health, community health, and public health. Based on your own list, would you argue that population health, community health, and public health are interchangeable concepts, or would you argue they are related but different concepts?

From Radzyminski S: The concept of population health within the nursing profession, J Prof Nurs *23(1):37-46, 2007.*

GOALS AND MEANS OF PRACTICE IN THE COMMUNITY

In population-centered practice, the nurse and the community seek healthy change together (Kruger et al, 2010). Their common goal of community health involves an ongoing series of health-promoting changes rather than a fixed state. The most effective means of completing healthy changes in the community is through this same partnership. Specific examples of partnership between the nurse and the community (Bernalillo County) are provided throughout this chapter and in the tables at the end of the chapter.

Community Health

Like the concept of community, community health has three common characteristics, or dimensions: status, structure, and process. Each dimension reflects a unique aspect of community health (Cottrell, 1976).

Status

Community health in terms of *status*, or outcome, is the most well-known and accepted approach; it involves biological, emotional, and social parts. The biological (or physical) part of community health is often measured by traditional morbidity and mortality rates, life expectancy indexes, and risk factor profiles. The question of exactly which risk factors are most important has been a matter of ongoing disagreement. In an effort to help resolve this question, *Morbidity and Mortality Weekly Report (1991)* published the work of a consensus committee involving representatives from a number of community health–related organizations. This committee identified by consensus 18 community health status measures and risk factors (Box 18-3). More recently the CDC in partnership with a number of public health organizations has relaunched the Community Health Status Indicators (CHSI) project to provide an overview of key health indicators for local communities such as those identified by the *MMWR* (1991). Health status indicator data on thousands of communities can be found at http://www.communityhealth.hhs.gov.

The emotional part of health status can be measured by consumer satisfaction and mental health indexes. Crime rates and functional levels reflect the social part of community health. Other status measures, such as worker absenteeism and infant mortality rates, reflect the effects of all three parts.

Structure

Community health, when viewed as the *structure* of the community, is usually defined in terms of services and resources. Measures of community health services and resources include service use patterns, treatment data from various health agencies, and provider-to-client ratios. These data provide information, such as the number of available hospital beds or the number of emergency department visits to a particular hospital. The problems that can be found when structure measures are used are serious. For example, problems related to access to care and quality of care are well-known through stories reported in local newspapers. Less well-known, but of equal concern, is the

BOX 18-3 CONSENSUS SET OF INDICATORS FOR ASSESSING COMMUNITY HEALTH STATUS*

Indicators of Health Status Outcome

1. Race/ethnicity-specific infant mortality, as measured by the rate (per 1000 live births) of deaths among infants less than 1 year of age

Death Rates (per 100,000 Population)† for the Following:

2. Motor vehicle crashes
3. Work-related injury
4. Suicide
5. Lung cancer
6. Breast cancer
7. Cardiovascular disease
8. Homicide
9. All causes

Reported Incidence (per 100,000 Population) of the Following:

10. Acquired immunodeficiency syndrome
11. Measles
12. Tuberculosis
13. Primary and secondary syphilis

Indicators of Risk Factors

14. Incidence of low birth weight, as measured by percentage of total number of live-born infants weighing less than 2500 g at birth
15. Births to adolescents (girls 10-17 years of age) as a percentage of total live births
16. Prenatal care, as measured by percentage of mothers delivering live infants who did not receive prenatal care during first trimester
17. Childhood poverty, as measured by the proportion of children less than 15 years of age living in families at or below the poverty level
18. Proportion of persons living in counties exceeding U.S. Environmental Protection Agency standards for air quality during previous year

From Consensus set of health status indicators for the general assessment of community health status—United States, *MMWR Morbid Mortal Wkly Rep* 40:449, 1991 (updated 8/01).
*Note: Position of the indicator in the list does not imply priority.
†Age-adjusted to the 1940 standard population.

false belief that simply *providing* health care improves health. Such problems require cautious use of health services and resources as measures of community health.

A structural viewpoint also defines the characteristics of the community structure itself. Characteristics of the community structure are commonly identified as social measures, or correlates, of health. Measures of community structure include demographics, such as socioeconomic and racial distributions, age, and educational level. Their relationships to health status have been thoroughly documented. For example, studies have repeatedly shown that health status decreases with age and improves with higher socioeconomic levels.

Process

The view of community health as the *process* of effective community functioning or problem solving is well established. However, it is especially appropriate to nursing because it directs the study of community health for community action.

Community competence, defined originally in a classic work by Cottrell (1976), provides a basic understanding of the process dimension of community health. Community competence is a process whereby the parts of a community—organizations, groups, and aggregates—"are able to collaborate effectively in identifying the problems and needs of the community; can achieve a working consensus on goals and priorities; can agree on ways and means to implement the agreed-on goals; and can collaborate effectively in the required actions" (Cottrell, 1976, p 197).

The conditions of community competence are listed and defined in Table 18-2. Ruderman (2000) further expanded upon Cottrell's definition by indicating that community competence indicates the capacity of a community to implement change by assessing the need or the demand for change. Once

change is indicated, then the community must define and make available the resources for the change to occur.

The term community health as used in this chapter is the meeting of collective needs by identifying problems and managing behaviors within the community itself and between the community and the larger society. This definition emphasizes the process dimension but also includes the dimensions of status and structure. Measures for all three dimensions are listed in Table 18-3. The use of status, structure, and process dimensions to define community health, as shown in Table 18-3, is an effort to develop a broad definition of community health, involving measures that are often not included when discussions focus only on risk factors as the basis for community health. Nevertheless, epidemiological data related to health risks of aggregates and populations, commonly expressed as rates and confidence intervals, are vital measures of health status (Goodman et al, 2009).

Consideration of health risks guides us to think upstream—to identify risks that could be prevented to make and keep people healthy. Most community- and population-oriented approaches to health are grounded in the notion that the earlier in the causal process (or more upstream) interventions occur, the greater the likelihood of improved health. Frequently, prevention or upstream action requires community-wide intervention directed toward social, economic, and environmental conditions that correlate with low health status (Minkler et al, 2008). Examples of such interventions are presented under "Implementing in the Community" later in this chapter.

Healthy People 2020

One important guideline that is available for nurses working to improve the health of the community is *Healthy People 2020,* a publication from the U.S. Department of Health and Human

TABLE 18-2   THE 10 ESSENTIAL CONDITIONS OF COMMUNITY COMPETENCE

CONDITION	DEFINITION
Commitment	The affective and cognitive attachment to a community "that is worthy of substantial effort to sustain and enhance" (Cottrell, 1976, p 198)
Awareness of self and others and clarity of situational definitions	The clear and realistic view of one's own and other persons' community components, identities, and positions on issues
Articulateness	The technical aspects of formulating and stating one's views in relation to other persons' views
Effective communication	The accurate transmission of information based on the development of common meaning among the communicators
Conflict containment and management of accommodation	The inventive and effective assimilation and management of true or realistically perceived differences
Participation	Active, population-centered involvement
Management of relations with larger society	Adeptness at recognizing, obtaining, and using external resources and supports and, when necessary, stimulating the creation and use of alternative or supplementary resources
Machinery for facilitating participant interaction and decision making	Flexible and responsible procedures (formal and informal), participant interaction and facilities, interaction, and decision making
Social support	Perceptions of community competency
Leadership development	Degree to which community competence has changed since community organization efforts

From Cottrell LS: The competent community. In Kaplan BH, Wilson RN, Leighton AH, editors: *Further explorations in social psychiatry,* New York, 1976, Basic Books; Goeppinger J, Lassiter PG, Wilcox B: Community health is community competence, *Nurs Outlook* 30:464, 1982.

Services (DHHS, 2010). It offers a vision of the future for public health and specific objectives to help attain that vision. The *Healthy People 2020* vision recognizes the need to work collectively, in **community partnerships,** to bring about the changes that will be necessary to fulfill this vision. *Healthy People 2020* provides the foundation for a national health promotion and disease-prevention strategy built on the two goals of increasing the "quality and years of healthy life" and eliminating "health disparities." In Section IV of the Advisory Committee Findings and Recommendations for The Role and Function of *Healthy People 2020*, there is direct discussion about the relationship between individuals and their communities. It states, "The Advisory Committee believes *Healthy People 2020* can best be described as a national health agenda that communicates a vision and a strategy for the nation. *Healthy People 2020* should provide overarching, national-level goals. On a practical level, it is a road map showing where we want to go as a nation and how we are going to get there." "Indeed, the underlying premise of *Healthy People 2020* is that the health of the individual is almost inseparable from the health of the larger community."

In the section titled, *Healthy People 2020: The Road Ahead,* the direction for *Healthy People 2020* is stated: "The *Healthy People* process is inclusive; its strength is directly tied to collaboration." The development process strives to maximize transparency, public input, and stakeholder dialogue to ensure that *Healthy People 2020* is relevant to diverse public health needs and seizes opportunities to achieve its goals. This process is inherent for community partnerships, particularly when they reach out to non-traditional partners; these community partnerships can be among the most effective tools for improving health in communities. Because *Healthy People 2020* is dynamic

rather than static, the Public Health Service (PHS) will continue to review the progress of meeting the goals.

Community Partnerships

The executive summary written by the advisory committee for *Healthy People 2020* identifies a model for action that will require community partnership as key to meeting program goals. Community partnership is necessary because when there is a community partnership, lay community members have a vested interest in the success of efforts to improve the health of their community. Lay community members who are recognized as community leaders also possess credibility and skills that health professionals often lack. Therefore, successful strategies for improving community health must include community partnerships as the basic means, or key, for improvement (Adams and Canclini, 2008). Community partnership is a basic focus of such population-centered approaches as **Mobilizing for Action through Planning and Partnerships (MAPP)** (NACCHO, 2008).

Most changes must aim at improving community health through active partnerships between community residents and health workers from a variety of disciplines. Unfortunately, community residents are often viewed only as sources of information and receivers of interventions. This form of partnership is called *passive participation*. Passive participation is the opposite of the partnership approach in which all are involved in assessing, planning, and implementing needed community changes (Ndirangu et al, 2008; Timmerman, 2007).

The community member–professional partnership approach specifically emphasizes active participation. Power is shared among lay and professional persons throughout the assessment, planning, implementation, and evaluation processes.

TABLE 18-3   CONCEPT OF COMMUNITY HEALTH SPECIFIED

DIMENSION	MEASURES	EXAMPLES OF DATA SOURCES
Status	Vital statistics (live births, neonatal deaths, infant deaths, maternal deaths)	Census data State health department annual vital statistics
	Incidence and prevalence of leading causes of mortality and morbidity	Census data State health department
	Health risk profiles of selected aggregates	Local health department Support groups Local non-profit organizations
	Functional ability levels	Census data U.S. Department of Labor
Structure	Health facilities such as hospitals, nursing homes, industrial and school health services, health departments, voluntary health associations, categorical grant programs, and prepaid health plans	Local chamber of commerce United Way
	Health-related planning groups	Local newspapers Local magazines Local government
	Health manpower, such as physicians, dentists, nurses, environmental sanitarians, social workers	Telephone directory State and local labor statistics Professional licensing boards
	Health resource use patterns, such as bed occupancy days and client/provider visits	Medicare and Medicaid databases (federal and state governments) Annual reports from hospitals, HMOs, non-profit agencies
Process	Commitment to community health	Local government Real estate agencies (e.g., turnover/vacancy rates)
	Awareness of self and others and clarity of situational definitions	Local history Neighborhood help organizations
	Effective communication	Local/neighborhood newspapers and radio programs Local government
	Conflict containment and accommodation	Social services department
	Participation	Existence of and participation in local organizations
	Management of relationships with society	Windshield survey: observation of interactions
	Machinery for facilitating participant interaction and decision making	Notices for community organizations and meetings in public places (supermarkets, newspapers, radio)

Partnership means the active participation and involvement of the community or its representatives in healthy change (O'Donnell, 2009). For example, breast cancer is an issue for rural Native American women, and an active community partnership involving the Native American women helped develop and ensure an effective, ongoing program (Christopher et al, 2008) (Box 18-4).

Partnership, as defined here, is a concept that is as essential for nurses to know and use as are the concepts of community, community as client, and community health. Experienced nurses know that partnership is important because health is not a static reality. Rather, it is continuously generated through new and increasingly effective means of community member–professional collaboration. However, such changes also require other active professional service providers, such as school teachers, public safety officers, and agricultural extension agents. Partnership in identifying problems and setting goals is especially important because it brings commitment from all persons involved, which is essential to successful change (Biel et al, 2009).

A growing body of literature supports the significance and effectiveness of partnership in improving community health.

BOX 18-4   PARTNERSHIPS

The three main characteristics of a successful partnership are the following:
- *Being informed.* Community member and professional partners must be aware of their own and others' perceptions, rights, and responsibilities.
- *Flexibility.* Community member and professional partners must recognize the unique and similar contributions that each can make to a given situation. For example, professionals often contribute important knowledge and skills that laypersons lack. On the other hand, laypersons' definitions of community health problems are often more accurate than those of professionals.
- *Negotiation.* Because contributions vary and each situation is different, the distribution of power must be negotiated at every stage of the change process.

From Jackson EJ, Parks CP: Recruitment and training issues from selected lay health advisor programs among African Americans: a 20-year perspective [review], *Health Educ Behav* 24:418-431, 1997.

Studies document the use of partnership models for a wide range of outcomes such as diabetes prevention, environmental justice, exercise, in data analysis, and as a proposed model for international development (Cashman et al, 2008; Merriam et al, 2009; Powell et al, 2010; Yoo et al, 2009). The roles of

FIGURE 18-1 The rural area of Valle Caldera, north of the small town of Jemez Springs, New Mexico. (Courtesy George Shuster.)

these partners-in-health have included listening sympathetically, offering advice, making referrals, and starting programs among a wide range of communities. These include urban Hispanics and rural Hispanic migrant farm workers (Connor et al, 2007; Mendelson et al, 2008). They include partnerships with older adults in retirement communities as well as smaller, more rural communities (Christopher et al, 2008; Davies et al, 2008) (Figure 18-1). There are also examples of community partnerships for at-risk students at the grade school or middle school level; for promoting policies to strengthen early childhood development; or for disaster planning (Adams and Canclini, 2008; Horsley and Ciske, 2005; Powell et al, 2010; Sangster, Eccleston, and Porter, 2008; Schwartz and Laughlin, 2008). Powell et al (2010) propose the continuing use of partnership models for "transforming and sustaining international development." In international health, partnership models are generally viewed as empowering people, through their lay leaders, to control their own health destinies and lives. In the United States, partnership models have often involved informal community leaders, organizations such as churches, and communities.

Partnerships involving nurses working with community organizations offer one of the most effective means for interventions because they actively involve the community and build on existing community strengths. Nurses working with community groups and organizations fulfill many different roles. These roles include media advocacy, political action, "grass roots health communication and social marketing," and outreach facilitation to get more community members involved, for example, in a school health fair. Regardless of what roles nurses fulfill as their contribution to the partnership, they must remember to "start where the people are" (Severance and Zinnah, 2009).

Shoultz et al (2006) looked at the challenges and possible solutions in developing partnerships with communities. Community partnerships involve both influence and power. Nurses

must focus on where and how health professionals and the lay community can work together on an equal power basis. This requires equally respected inputs and voices that are equally heard. This approach requires nurses to do "with" rather than "to" the partner, while the partner's role throughout the process is active and empowered, not passive. Goal setting and the plan of action are mutually determined. Roles and responsibilities are negotiated and the partners become more effective at working independently to solve their own problems and make decisions for themselves, even if they do not solve the problems identified by the nursing diagnosis. In the language of community empowerment advocates, community participants must have an active role in the change process. The public health nurses must work hard to include members of a setting, neighborhood, or organization while developing trust and providing the community with a say and a central role throughout the process (Christopher et al, 2008; Hanks, 2006).

DID YOU KNOW? *The Healthy People 2020 website can be accessed through the WebLinks on this book's website (http://evolve.elsevier.com/Stanhope). From the Healthy People 2020 website (http://www.healthypeople.gov), information can be obtained about focus priority areas, the lead agencies, fact sheets, progress reviews, publication lists, and the Healthy People 2020 databases. Other valuable Internet sites include the following:*

- *The Behavior Risk Factor Surveillance System (BRFSS) was developed and conducted to monitor state-level prevalence of the major behavioral risks among adults associated with premature morbidity and mortality; conducted through Chronic Disease Prevention and Health Promotion (NCCDPHP, 2010) (http://www.cdc.gov/brfss/).*
- *In addition, The National Center for Health Statistics (NCHS) provides a health statistics portal site that offers information and Internet links to all types of national survey data, vital statistics, and .pdf files containing recent health-related data and reports (http://www.cdc.gov/nchs/).*

HEALTHY PEOPLE 2020

Healthy People 2020 and Community Consortium and Partners

Healthy People provides science-based, 10-year national objectives for improving the health of all Americans. For 3 decades, *Healthy People* has established benchmarks and monitored progress over time in order to:
- Encourage collaborations across sectors.
- Guide individuals toward making informed health decisions.
- Measure the impact of prevention activities.

For the implementation of *Healthy People 2020* the development of a consortium is occurring. The Consortium is a diverse, motivated group of **agencies and organizations** committed to achieving *Healthy People 2020* goals and objectives. Any agency or organization that supports *Healthy People 2020* is a welcome partner. Examples of partners includes:
- Health care providers
- State and local public health professionals
- Educators
- Community members
- Businesses
- Environmental health professionals
- Housing professionals

From USDHHS: *Healthy People 2020: A roadmap for health,* Washington, DC, 2010, U.S. Government Printing Office.

EVIDENCE-BASED PRACTICE

The purpose of this intervention was to increase the use of mammogram screening among rural Appalachian women. This effort by local agencies and organizations making up the Indiana County Cancer Coalition (ICCC) involved working with the Indiana County Community Action Program, an organization providing low-cost food to low-income county residents through a network of 18 food pantries. The intervention involved the use of volunteers and multiple tailored approaches, including the evidence-based "Tell a Friend" intervention to reach county residents.
- Measured outcomes of the intervention included the number of residents who were reached, the number of mammograms that were done, and the number of cancers detected
- The intervention was judged a success at both the individual level (a number of women were screened for the first time) and at the community level because the intervention demonstrated that multiple community agencies could successfully partner for a community wide intervention.

Nurse Use

Evaluation of the intervention indicated that both the agency and the community were affected by this effort. The use of volunteers by the ICCC was intensive for both time and labor.

From Bencivenga M, DeRubis S, Leach P, et al: Community partnerships, food pantries, and an evidence-based intervention to increase mammography among rural women, *J Rural Health* 24(1):91-95, 2008.

Strategies to Improve Community Health

Healthy People 2020 has stimulated a number of joint efforts to develop strategies for achieving its goals. These efforts have involved such organizations as the Centers for Disease Control and Prevention (CDC), the American Public Health Association (APHA), the Association of State and Territorial Health Officials (ASTHO), and the National Association of County and City Health Officials (NACCHO). The results of these efforts are a number of publications and guidelines that provide detailed strategies for achieving the objectives in the **Assessment Protocol for Excellence in Public Health (APEXPH)**, the **Planned Approach to Community Health (PATCH)**, and, more recently, MAPP. Each of these approaches offers step-by-step guidelines for community planning and interventions (see Chapter 25). A comparison of these different approaches, prepared in 2007 by the NACCHO, is available at http://www.naccho.org/topics/infrastructure/mapp/upload/MappPaceApex.pdf. (Readers interested in contacting these organizations can refer to Box 18-5.) Most recently, the CDC's Healthy Communities Program has developed the Community Health Assessment and Group Evaluation (CHANGE) Tool, which is designed to help assess for community change and establishing community priorities. It is available for free at http://www.cdc.gov/healthycommunitiesprogram/tools/change.htm.

In addition to these approaches, there have been efforts to apply the evidence-based practice approach to community-level interventions. The *Community Guide* provides recommendations for population-based interventions to promote health and to prevent disease, injury, disability, and premature death, and it is appropriate for use by communities and health care systems. The initial *Community Guide* was a result of the work of the Task Force on Community Preventive Services

---

BOX 18-5   INFORMATION FOR STRATEGIES TO IMPROVE COMMUNITY HEALTH

APEXPH and MAPP
National Association of County Health Officials
1100 17th Street, NW, 2nd Floor
Washington, DC 20036
1-202-783-5550
http://www.naccho.org/topics/infrastructure/

PATCH
National Center for Chronic Disease Prevention and Health Promotion
Centers for Disease Control and Prevention
1600 Clifton Road, NE
Atlanta, GA 30333
1-404-639-3311
1-800-311-3435
http://www.cdc.gov

(2005), which has been updated and continues to systematically review published scientific studies, weigh the evidence, and determine the effectiveness of interventions in a particular area (2009). Although it does not use the term *evidence-based practice (EBP)*, the *Community Guide* really is a guide to EBP for the community. Interventions are: (1) strongly recommended, (2) recommended, or (3) labeled as having insufficient evidence to make a recommendation. For instance, in regard to physical activity promotion, the Task Force strongly recommends community-wide campaigns, individually adapted health behavior change programs, school-based physical education, social support interventions in community contexts, and creating or improving access to places for physical activity combined with informational outreach. The work of this Task Force is ongoing, and updates as well as publications on a wide range of public health areas can be found at http://www.thecommunityguide. org/library/default.htm.

The National Center for Chronic Disease Prevention and Health Promotion website (which can be accessed through the chapter WebLinks of this book's website) includes links to CDC-supported public health programs that have been found to be effective. Links to guides and kits for the programs can also be found. Examples include the following:

- 5-A-Day for Better Health (healthy eating)
- ACEs: Active Community Environments (activity)
- KidsWalk-to-School (activity)
- National Bone Health Campaign (healthy eating, activity)
- Well-Integrated Screening and Evaluation for Women Across the Nation—WISEWOMAN (lifestyle intervention programs addressing cardiovascular and other chronic disease risk factors)
- Ready, Set, It's Everywhere You Go (physical activity) (site also in Spanish)

The WHO's Healthy Cities initiative offers yet another approach to population-centered health promotion. First initiated in Europe during the mid-1980s, Healthy Cities has become a global movement with hundreds of Healthy Cities initiatives. Healthy Cities initiatives are based on the belief that the health of the community is affected by political, economic, environmental, and social factors. The Healthy Cities approach emphasizes community development through community involvement to address local problems (Goepel, 2007). Healthy Cities efforts focus on social change, including developing supportive environments and reorienting health care services, health policy, and community collaboration and action (Goepel, 2007; Simard, 2007). An example of an organization that incorporates the Healthy Cities philosophy in California is "Healthy City" with resources at http://www.healthycity.org. For additional information, see Chapter 20.

Several different population-centered health promotion approaches have been noted here. Regardless of what approach is taken, specific strategies to improve community health often depend on whether the status, structure, or process dimension of community health is being emphasized. If the emphasis is on the status dimension, the best strategy is usually at the level of primary or secondary prevention because the objective is either to prevent a disease or to treat it in its early stages. Immunization programs are an example of a nursing intervention at the primary prevention level.

Nursing intervention strategies focused on the structural dimension are directed to either health services or demographic characteristics. Interventions aimed at altering health services might include program planning. Interventions aimed at affecting demographic characteristics might include community development.

When the emphasis is on the process dimension, the best strategy is usually health promotion, which is also a primary prevention strategy. For example, if family-life education is lacking in a community because of ineffective communication among families, children, school board members, religious leaders, and health professionals, then the most effective strategy may be to open discussion among these groups and help community members develop education programs.

COMMUNITY-FOCUSED NURSING PROCESS: AN OVERVIEW OF THE PROCESS FROM ASSESSMENT TO EVALUATION

Most nurses are familiar with the nursing process as it applies to individually focused nursing care. Using it to promote community health makes this same nursing process community focused (Minkler et al, 2008). The phases of the nursing process that directly involve the community as client begin at the start of the contract or partnership and include assessing, diagnosing, planning, implementing, and evaluating.

The use of the nursing process with the community as client is presented in the following sections with a case study based on a broader maternal infant–focused community assessment that followed the process presented in the flowchart found in Figure 18-3. Although the example here focuses on only one of the identified problems—infant nutrition—in reality, several different community health problems were identified by the partnership, including infant nutrition, a lack of prenatal care, low infant immunization rates, and a need for normal growth and development knowledge among new mothers. The relative importance of each was examined, and infant malnutrition was selected as the most important problem by the process illustrated later in this chapter from among all of the identified problems. For the purpose of clarity, infant malnutrition is the only community health problem from among four noted earlier in this paragraph that is used to show how the nursing process is applied in this case study example.

THE CUTTING EDGE   *The U.S. Department of Health and Human Services has established a search engine called "healthfinder.gov" to help link you to all kinds of recent health-related initiatives and information, including public health, at: http://www.healthfinder. gov/scripts/SearchContext.asp?topic=718&super=112/.*

Community Assessment

Community assessment is one of three core functions of PHN and is the process of critically thinking about the community. This involves getting to know and understand the community as client (Figure 18-2). Nurses start an assessment by clearly defining their client in terms of the three dimensions of place, people, and function presented in Table 18-1. Before data are collected in the assessment phase, the nurse must be able to answer questions such as the following: What are the geographic boundaries of this community? Which people are members of this community? What characteristics do they have in common? For example, homebound older adults in a particular city are a community of special interest with shared needs, who are defined by their age and homebound status. Once the nurse is clear about the boundaries of the community as client, the community assessment phase can be continued.

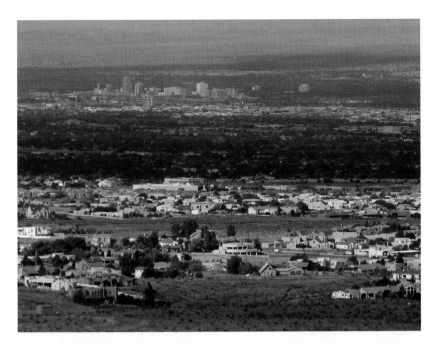

FIGURE 18-2 Downtown Albuquerque, New Mexico from a nearby mountain ridge. (Courtesy of George Shuster.)

BOX 18-6   STEPS TO ASSESSING COMMUNITY HEALTH

Step 1. Gathering relevant existing data and generating missing data
Step 2. Developing a composite database
Step 3. Interpreting the composite database to identify community problems and strengths
Step 4. Analyzing the problem

The community assessment phase itself involves a logical, systematic approach. Community assessment helps identify community needs, clarify problems, and identify strengths and resources. There are different types of community assessment. The longer and more complex process of a *comprehensive community assessment* is described here. This assessment process reflects the public health competencies essential for analysis and assessment in public health. Comprehensive community assessment is the necessary initial phase of the community nursing process with the community as client (Box 18-6).

Assessment data must be systematically collected, organized, and placed into assessment categories (see Tables 18-1 and 18-3). The database form provided in Resource Tool 18.A on the Evolve website is a useful means for entering and organizing these different types of data. Gathering the data and initial interpretation of the data are the first steps in the assessment phase of the nursing process. Figure 18-3 provides an overview of the nursing process with the community as client.

Data Collection and Interpretation

The primary goal of data collection is to obtain usable information about the community and its health. The systematic collection of data about community health requires gathering or compiling existing data and generating missing data. These data are then interpreted, and community health problems and community abilities are identified.

LINKING CONTENT TO PRACTICE

In this chapter, the focus is placed on the partnership between the public health nurse and the community throughout the process of community assessment, problem identification, planning, intervention, and evaluation. One of the Institute of Medicine's (IOM) three core functions of public health is assessment. The process of community assessment outlined and described in this chapter closely follows The Council on Linkages' *Core Competencies for Public Health* (adopted June 11, 2009). This includes the need for public health nurses to "maintain partnerships with key stakeholders." Among other identified competencies for public health providers, including public health nurses, is the ability to "assess the health status of populations and their related determinants of health and illness." This chapter presents the means by which public health nurses can construct a composite database containing assessment data from a wide variety of sources. This initial community assessment phase also directly links with The Quad Council Domains of Public Health Practice: Domain #1: Analytic Assessment Skills; Domain #5: Community Dimensions of Practice Skills; and Domain #6: Basic Public Health Sciences Skills. The Council on Linkages: Core Competencies for Public Health also emphasizes the public health nurse's ability to describe "the characteristics of a population-based health problem." Development of goals and objectives along with their problem correlates as part of the community health assessment directly relates to this competency; whereas another Council on Linkages competency—"Develops a plan to implement policy and programs"—directly relates to the development of intervention actions described in this chapter.

DID YOU KNOW?   *A complete set of blank forms for use in the different steps of the assessment process, including the database form, is available in Resource Tool 18.A on the Evolve website. These blank data forms are identical to the forms completed throughout the chapter as part of the Bernalillo County community assessment example. They can be used in steps of the community assessment presented in Box 18-6, regardless of the type of community that is being assessed.*

Data Gathering. Data gathering is the process of obtaining existing, readily available data. These data already exist. They usually describe the demography of a community: age,

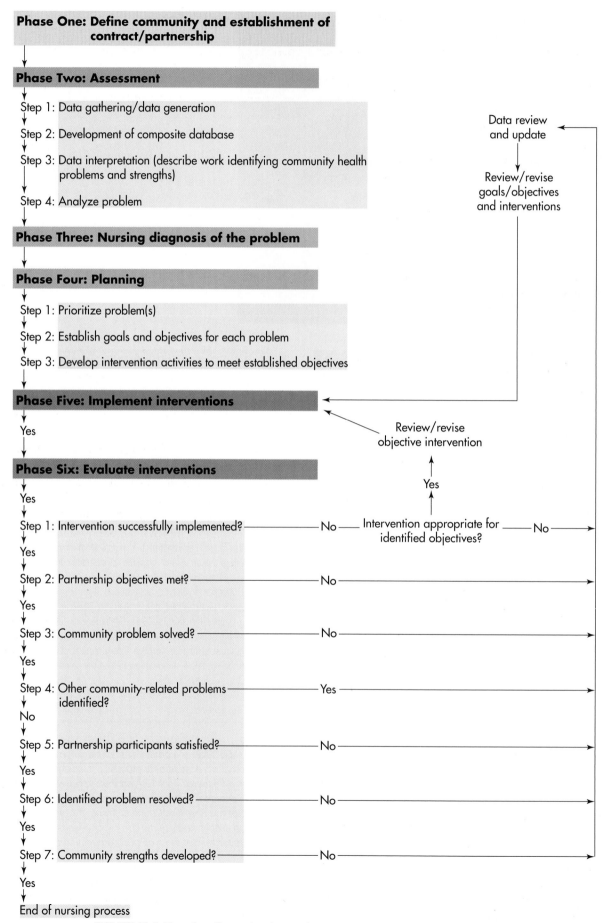

FIGURE 18-3 Flowchart illustrating the nursing process with the community as client.

sex, socioeconomic, and racial distributions. They include vital statistics, such as selected mortality and morbidity data. Another source is surveys, such as the Behavior Risk Factor Surveillance System (BRFSS) developed and conducted to monitor state-level prevalence of the major behavioral risks associated with premature morbidity and mortality in adults (see the Did You Know box on p 404 for the BRFSS website). Conducted by the National Center for Chronic Disease Prevention and Health Promotion (NCCDPHP), these survey data, from sources such as the BRFSS, are important because they also provide data about trends. Trends are important because they show whether a community problem has existed for a long time or whether it is new. Other resources include data from community institutions, including health care organizations and the services they provide, and the characteristics of health care personnel. Often these data have been collected by others via structured interviews, questionnaires, or surveys and are available in published reports. State health departments gather extensive epidemiological data in the form of rates, which are generally published at both county and state levels in the form of vital health statistics. Table 18-4, shown on p 420, provides an example of existing epidemiological data gathered as part of the Bernalillo County assessment.

The USDHHS Health Resources and Services Administration has placed its Community Health Status Indicators project on the Internet (accessible through the WebLinks on this book's Evolve site). This site provides an excellent example of how data can be gathered to provide this part of the community assessment composite database. It also provides county-level data as well as a list of peer counties for almost every county in the United States.

Data Generation. Data generation is the process of developing data that do not already exist through interaction with community members or groups. This type of information is harder to obtain and is generally not statistical in nature. Data that often must be generated include information about a community's knowledge and beliefs, values and sentiments, goals and perceived needs, norms, problem-solving processes, power, leadership, and influence structures. These data, called *qualitative data,* are more likely to be collected by interviews and observation.

Several methods to generate or collect data are needed. Methods that encourage the nurse to consider the community's perception of its health problems and abilities are as important as methods structured to identify knowledge that the nurse considers essential. Methods of collecting data rely either on what is directly observed *by* the data collector or on what is reported *to* the data collector (Richards et al, 2008; Severance and Zinnah, 2009).

Informant interviews, focus groups, participant observation, and windshield surveys are four methods of generating direct data. All four methods require sensitivity, openness, curiosity, and the ability to listen, taste, touch, smell, and see life as it is lived in a community (Cashman et al, 2008; Severance and Zinnah, 2009). Either informant interviews (see the How To Identify a Key Informant box) or focus groups, which consist of directed talks with selected members of a community about community members or groups and events are basic to effective data generation (Adams and Canclini, 2008; Levine et al, 2008; Severance and Zinnah, 2009). Also basic is participant observation, the deliberate sharing in the life of a community, to the extent that conditions permit. Informant interviews, focus groups, and participant observation are good ways to generate information about community beliefs, norms, values, power and influence structures, and problem-solving processes. Such data can seldom be reported in numbers, so they are often not collected. Even worse, conclusions that are based on intuition and unchecked are sometimes used to replace these types of data. People providing information should confirm their conclusions from direct data-generation methods.

HOW TO **Identify a Key Informant**

Talking to key informants is a critical part of the community assessment.

- *Key informants are not always people who have a formal title or position.*
- *Key informants often have an informal role within the community.*
- *County health department nurses and church leaders are often key informants. They also know many community members and can identify other key informants.*

In the example of the community with the infant malnutrition problem, informant interviews with social workers and religious leaders provided data indicating a community with well-defined clusters of persons with low incomes, concerns about adolescent pregnancy, and worries about the health of the community's babies. These data, which reflect the concerns and worries of the Bernalillo County community, would have been difficult to acquire without personal interviews (see Table 18-4).

HOW TO **Obtain a Quick Assessment of a Community**

- *One way to get a quick, initial sense of the community is to do a windshield assessment using a format like the one provided as an example in Table 18-5, p 420.*
- *Nurses interested in conducting a windshield assessment need to take public transportation, have someone else drive while they take notes, or plan to stop frequently to write down what they see.*
- *The windshield survey example is organized into 15 elements with specific questions related to each element.*
- *Nurses who use this approach will have an initial descriptive assessment of the community when they are finished.*
- *If interventions are planned, the more thorough and more comprehensive process described in this chapter will be necessary.*

Windshield surveys are the motorized equivalent of simple observation (Table 18-5). They involve the generation of data that helps to define the community, the trends, stability, and changes that all serve to define the health of the community

(Stanhope and Knollmueller, 2000). The nurse, driving a car or riding public transportation, can observe many dimensions of a community's life and environment through the windshield. Common characteristics of people on the street, neighborhood gathering places, the rhythm of community life, housing quality, and geographic boundaries can be observed readily (see the How To Obtain a Quick Assessment of a Community box). Again, using the infant malnutrition example, the windshield survey suggested that the community had a large unemployed population because adults were observed "hanging out" during the day. A windshield survey can be used by itself for a short and simple assessment. However, it is used here as one part of the longer, more complex comprehensive community assessment.

> **NURSING TIP**   *If you do a windshield survey as part of your community assessment, go twice: once during the day when people are at work and children are at school, and a second time in the evening after work is done and school is out.*

Collection of Reported Data. Three methods of generating reported data are secondary analysis of data collected by someone else, surveys, and community reconnaissance. In second-ary analysis, the nurse uses previously gathered data, such as minutes from community meetings. This type of analysis is extremely valuable because it saves time and effort. Many sources of data are readily available and useful for secondary analysis, such as public documents, health surveys, minutes from meetings, and statistical data (e.g., census and health records). In the Bernalillo County infant malnutrition example, birth records noting low birth weights and health department clinic records of low-weight-for-height children provided information that showed a higher-than-average rate of infant malnutrition.

Surveys report data from a sample of persons. They are equally useful, but they take more time and effort than observational methods and secondary analyses. They require time-consuming and costly data generation. Thus, the survey method is rarely used by the nurse. However, surveys are necessary for identifying certain community problems (Severance and Zinnah, 2009). For example, a lack of accessible personal health services cannot be documented readily and reliably in any other way.

Community Reconnaissance. Community reconnaissance, that is, surfing the Web, requires a computer and access to the Web instead of the automobile commonly used in windshield surveys noted in the previous section. However, both windshield surveys and community reconnaissance require superb detective skills.

What can you learn about a community by surfing the Web? Many counties and municipalities have their own websites. Many are represented in state-wide and national databases. (See starter websites for the home communities developed by the author of this chapter and found under additional chapter resources.) You can often find the address of a website (URL) for a community by using the county format noted in the Bernallilo County, New Mexico example (http://bernalillo.nmgen web.us/) and substituting the name of the county and state in which a particular community is located, or by browsing several websites identified by a search engine.

Local and state sites are, for example, very revealing of community economics and civic engagement. These sites typically advertise their communities to potential residents and businesses. They seldom disclose data about community issues, however, although they may include links to community newspapers and radio and television stations that will report issues (refer to Clinical Decision-Making Activities #4 and 5 at the end of the chapter). Small communities, however, may lack resources to develop their own websites.

An assessment guide is a useful tool for a community reconnaissance. A guide structures Web browsing and allows the community assessor (you!) to recognize the strengths and limitations of Web data. Demographic data and vital statistics about the populations living in the community, and data about the eight community systems delineated by Anderson and McFarlane (2008) are one possible guide, although many students have found it helpful to add a ninth system to their assessment guide, called *Religion and Faith* (see the italicized term in the Did You Know box).

> **DID YOU KNOW?**   *Community Systems*
>
> *The following is a list of system categories found within a community:*
>
> 1. *Politics and Government*
> 2. *Safety and Transportation*
> 3. *Education*
> 4. *Physical Environment*
> 5. *Recreation*
> 6. *Economics*
> 7. *Communication*
> 8. *Health and Social Services*
> 9. *Religion and Beliefs*
>
> *From Anderson ET, McFarlane J, editors:* Community as partner, *ed 5, Philadelphia, 2008, Lippincott.*

Data about the health status of a community's residents (people or populations) are often available by accessing state-wide databases via the Web. Data from the CDC-sponsored BRFSS, for example, are collected and reported by states participating in the BRFSS. Prevalence data for selected risk factors are reported by state. Information on health risks for selected local areas is also available. (Additional local data may be available at locality-specific URLs.) BRFSS prevalence data for all states can be found for a variety of categories (including activity limitations, alcohol consumption, asthma, cardiovascular disease, diabetes, injury control, tobacco use, weight control, and women's health). See the WebLinks on the book's Evolve site to access these sites.

In addition, many states have health system–specific websites. In North Carolina, for example, community assessors can review http://www.nchealthinfo.org. This website has information about the health care services in all 100 North Carolina counties, including the following: (1) professional health care providers (chiropractors, dentists, midwives, psychologists, and more), (2) health programs and facilities (birth centers, hospitals, and support groups), and (3) services specific to a disease or health issue (e.g., Alzheimer's disease, breast cancer, diabetes, and fibromyalgia).

Health status data are reported for the counties participating in the state-wide effort at the Healthy Carolinians site (http://www.healthycarolinians.org). Click on the County Profiles link on the left side of the home page and enter the name of the North Carolina county that is the focus of the community assessment. An extensive set of WebLinks to additional health data are also included. Similar sites exist for every U.S. state.

When Web data are used to introduce a community, the information source must be evaluated. Looking at the last part of a website's URL (or the extension), you will generally see .com, .edu, .gov, or .org. This will give you a clue about who owns the URL. A college or university will have the ".edu" extension at the end of their address. The URL for the University of New Mexico, for example, is http://www.unm.edu/. A non-profit organization will usually end in ".org." The Healthy Carolinians website mentioned earlier (http://www.healthycarolinians.org/) is an example of this. A governmental agency will have a ".gov" extension. Community assessments often rely heavily on data collected and made available by the CDC on its governmental website (http://www.cdc.gov/). A commercial website will have ".com" as its extension. Although there are many outstanding commercial websites that give trustworthy information, in general the assessor needs to scrutinize their data very carefully. URLs with .edu, .gov, and .org usually report information reliably. In addition, the absence of Web data about a community is important. Small communities, rural areas, and economically disadvantaged communities may not be represented on the Web, and this lack of representation may be meaningful.

NURSING TIP *Questions to ask about websites before using the data:*

1. *How current is the reported information?*
2. *When was the site last updated?*
3. *How credible is the data source?*
4. *Is an author identified?*
5. *Are demographic data reported about the people?*
6. *Are data reported about different community systems?*
7. *Is there any obvious bias in the reporting of data?*
8. *Is the community voice or voices represented?*

Composite Database. When new data that have just been collected or generated are combined with already-existing data (previously gathered by the nurse), the result is a composite database. Data analysis is used to make sense of the data in this composite database. First, data are analyzed and synthesized, and themes or trends are noted. For example, trends identified by comparing several years of epidemiological data can identify certain kinds of problems. The analysis of data generated by interviews with key informants or focus groups can identify other kinds of problems. Community health problems, or

needs for action, and community health strengths, or abilities, are determined. Problems are indicated by differences between: (1) the community health goals of the nurse and community, and (2) the themes or findings revealed by the data analysis. Strengths, on the other hand, are suggested by similarities between the nurse's and community's concepts of community health and the supporting data. The nurse and community, working in partnership, identify problems.

Problem Analysis

Problem analysis seeks to clarify the nature of the problem. The nurse identifies the origins and effects of the problem, the points at which intervention might occur, and the parties that have an interest in the problem and its solution. Analysis often requires the development of a problem matrix, in which the direct and indirect factors that contribute to the problem and to the outcomes of the problem are identified and mapped. Relationships among the factors are noted. The map or matrix is important because the nurse can anticipate that several of the same factors that contribute to a problem and that affect the outcomes of a problem may also *cause* the problem. The problem of highest priority may share factors that also contribute to other problems and affect their outcomes as well.

Problem analysis should be conducted for each identified problem. This often requires organizing a special group composed of the nurse, persons whose areas of expertise relate to the problem, persons whose organizations are capable of intervening, and representatives of the community experiencing the problem. Both content and process specialists must participate. Together they can identify the problem correlates, defined as factors contributing to the problem, and explain the relationships between each factor and the problem.

An example of problem analysis appears in Table 18-6 (see p 421). Problem correlates (factors that contribute to or result from the problem) for infant malnutrition are listed in the first column. Correlates are from all areas of community life. Social or environmental correlates are as appropriate as those oriented to the individual. For example, teenage pregnancy is a social correlate of infant malnutrition, and high unemployment is an environmental correlate. In the second column, the relationships between each correlate and the problem are noted. The third column contains data from the community and the literature that support the relationship, using the suspected infant malnutrition example and a few of its correlates. Infant malnutrition is thought to be correlated with inadequate diet, community norms, poverty, disturbed mother–child relationships, and teenage pregnancy. Active community participation is critical for the data-interpreting process, particularly in identifying problems.

The program planning model, first proposed by Delbecq and Van De Ven (1971), continues to be widely used to structure lay participation in defining problems. The model shows how to use active community participation in problem definition and program planning. It makes the most of the contributions by various groups with diverse interests, skills, and knowledge. This model depends heavily on nominal groups—"groups in which individuals work in the presence of one another but do not interact" (Delbecq and Van De Ven, 1971, p 467); the separation of individual from collective (or group) problems; and a round-robin process for listing problems without evaluating or elaborating on them at the same time. This model is popularly known as the nominal group process.

Other consensus methods, such as the Delphi technique, are also used to define the extent of agreement among content experts, policy makers, and community members about the presence and importance of certain health problems. Experience shows that consensus methods produce useful results if the following conditions are met (Goodman et al, 2009; Yoo et al, 2009):

1. Problems are carefully selected.
2. Participants in the process are deliberately selected and closely monitored.
3. Justified and reasonable levels of consensus are expected.
4. Findings are used as guides to decisions.

HOW TO   **Gain Community Trust**

Often the nurse can gain entry to the community by doing the following:

- *Taking part in community events*
- *Looking and listening with interest*
- *Visiting people in formal leadership positions*
- *Using an assessment guide*
- *Using a peer group for support*

Assessment Guides

Nursing assessment of community health—both data collecting and interpreting—must be focused. Focus, or perspective, can be provided by detailed assessment guides that are built on a conceptual framework of definitions of community and community health.

Concepts that can be measured in behavioral or observable terms can serve as assessment guides. Community and community health have already been defined in such terms. The concept of community has been specified (see Table 18-1). The definition previously given includes three dimensions: people, place, and function. Several measures specify each of these dimensions.

A detailed description of community health—its status, structure, and process dimensions—is presented in Table 18-3. In the infant malnutrition example, status dimension data were gathered from morbidity and mortality data; structural dimension data were gathered from vital statistics and from informant interviews with social workers; and process dimension data were gathered from informant interviews with community religious leaders. In this way, the concepts of community and community health provide the framework for the assessment guide in Resource Tool 18.A on this book's Evolve website. Together, the concepts and assessment guide constitute the community health assessment model, the basis of the community-oriented health record (COHR). Data, problems, and abilities are all organized by using the community health assessment model.

The community-as-partner model is another example of an assessment guide developed to show that nurses can work with communities as partners (Anderson and McFarlane, 2004).

This model shows how communities change and grow best by full involvement and self-empowerment. The heart of this model is an assessment wheel that shows that the people actually are the community. Surrounding the people, and integral to the community, are eight identified subsystems: housing, education, fire and safety, politics and government, health, communication, economics, and recreation. These subsystems both affect and are affected by the people who make up the community (see Table 18-6).

Assessment Issues

Gaining entry or acceptance into the community is perhaps the biggest challenge in assessment. The nurse is usually an outsider and often represents a health care agency that is neither known nor trusted by community members. Community members may therefore react with indifference or even active hostility to the nurse. In addition, nurses may feel insecure about their skills as a community worker, and the community may refuse to acknowledge its need for those skills. Because the nurse's success largely depends on the way he or she is viewed, entry into the community is critical.

Once the nurse gains entry at an initial level, **role negotiation** often becomes an issue. Role involves the values, behaviors, or goals that govern an individual's interactions with others. The nurse must decide how long to separate the roles of data collector and intervenor. Effective implementation of the nursing process requires an adequate database. The danger of a premature response to health needs and social injustice is great. Nurses can assist in negotiating roles by presenting thoughtful and consistent reasons for their presence in the community and by sincere demonstrations of their commitment to the community. Keeping appointments, clarifying community members' views of health needs, and respecting an individual's right to choose whether to work with the nurse are often useful approaches.

Maintaining confidentiality is also important. Nurses must be very careful to protect the identity of community members who provide sensitive or controversial data. In some cases, the nurse may consider withholding data; in other situations, the nurse may be legally required to disclose data. For example, nurses are required by law to report child abuse.

Small-area analysis can create difficulties of a less personal nature. Potential problems of small-area analysis include the mistakes made when conclusions are based on data gathered from small areas. For example, calculations of mortality rates in a rural county may be skewed when the denominator is as small as 5000. This issue often raises questions about the validity of the identified health problems. It is useful to look at the same problem by comparing similar health problems at the state and national levels. Then the nurse can be more confident of the validity of the data.

Remember, a community assessment will identify multiple community health problems. Each of these problems must be analyzed and given a priority score to determine which are the most serious. Under the following headings, the infant malnutrition example is used to show how an identified problem generates a community-focused nursing diagnosis, which is analyzed and assigned a priority score.

Community Nursing Diagnosis

Creating a community assessment composite database will result in a list of community health problems. Each problem needs to be identified clearly and stated as a community health diagnosis. The statement of the problem in a community health diagnosis format is the third phase of the community-as-client process. Developing the community health diagnosis in this phase of the process helps clarify the problem and is an important first step to planning. In the planning phase, where each diagnosis is analyzed, priorities are established and community-focused interventions are identified. Community diagnoses clarify who receives the care (the community as opposed to an individual), provide a statement identifying problems faced by who is receiving the care (i.e., the community), and identify the factors contributing to the identified problem.

Although the North American Nursing Diagnosis Association International (NANDA-I) provides a taxonomy of nursing diagnoses familiar to most students, NANDA-I's focus has been on the individual rather than the community level. However, more recent NANDA-I work has also developed community-level diagnoses such as ineffective community coping (Newfield et al, 2007). Furthermore, ongoing work with Nursing-sensitive Outcomes Classification (NOC) is an effort to produce a standard language across health care settings, including the community (Carlson, 2006; Gec, 2006). NANDA-I is only one accepted system of nursing diagnosis; for example, home-health nurses are familiar with the Omaha System classification system of nursing diagnosis (Martin and Monsen, 2009).

In this chapter, a version of the nursing diagnosis format presented by Newfield et al (2007) with three parts is used:

1. Risk of
2. Among
3. Related to

"Risk of" identifies a specific problem or health risk faced by the community. "Among" identifies the specific community client with whom the nurse will be working in relation to the identified problem or risk. "Related to" describes characteristics of the community, including motivation, knowledge, and skills of the community and its environment. Environmental characteristics include physical, cultural, psychosocial, and political characteristics (Richards et al, 2008). These data were identified in the composite database of the assessment phase and provide the basis for the community-level nursing diagnosis. Each community has its own unique characteristics. Some of these characteristics are strengths that the nurse can build on, but other characteristics contribute to the problem identified in the community health diagnosis. The characteristics, or factors, related to the identified problem are listed after the "related to" statement as the third part of the community health diagnosis.

Community nursing diagnosis language must describe at the aggregate level—in other words, the community level—responses to actual and potential illnesses and life processes. This also means that the defining characteristics for community diagnoses must be observable and measurable at the aggregate level. To do this, community-level data must be used. Epidemiological data or community survey data are two examples of community-level data. The comparison of local data with state, regional, or national data, as rates and across multiple years, is one key means of identifying community-level problems, as well as patterns and trends. Newfield et al (2007) provide a detailed example about their community-level diagnoses involving "ineffective community coping" and "risk for adverse human health effects" that were related to violence in the local community. The example being used for illustration in this chapter is infant malnutrition. On the basis of assessment data, the community diagnosis for infant malnutrition using this format would be the following:

1. *Risk of* infant malnutrition
2. *Among* families in Bernalillo County
3. *Related to* lack of regular developmental screening; lack of an outreach program to identify at-risk infants; knowledge deficit among families about infant-related nutrition and about WIC (special supplemental nutrition program for women, infants, and children); and confusion among families about WIC program enrollment criteria

Frequently, a number of community health diagnoses are made on the basis of the different problems identified during the assessment phase. The problems are stated in a community-focused nursing diagnosis format. In the next phase, planning for community health, weighting is done and priorities are established among these problems.

Planning for Community Health

The planning phase includes analyzing the community health problems identified in the community nursing diagnoses and establishing priorities among them, establishing goals and objectives, and identifying intervention activities that will accomplish the objectives. Figure 18-4 shows the relationship between the prioritized problem, goals, objectives, and intervention activities in the fourth phase of the planning process.

Problem Priorities

Infant malnutrition represents only one of several community health problems identified by the community assessment. The other community health problems included health concerns such as a low infant immunization rate. While this community assessment focused on maternal–infant health, a more general community assessment could have identified a mortality rate from cardiovascular disease that was higher than the national norm and, as expressed by many residents, a desire to quit smoking.

Each problem identified as part of the assessment process must be put through a ranking process to determine its importance. This ranking process, in which problems are evaluated and priorities established according to predetermined criteria, is termed problem prioritizing. It takes into account information provided by community members, content experts, administrators, and others who can provide resources (Box 18-7).

Using the example of infant malnutrition again, the six criteria in Box 18-7 are listed in the first column of Table 18-7 (see p 421).

Given an acceptable and comprehensive set of criteria and a list of community health problems, the process of assigning priorities is rather simple. Each problem is considered

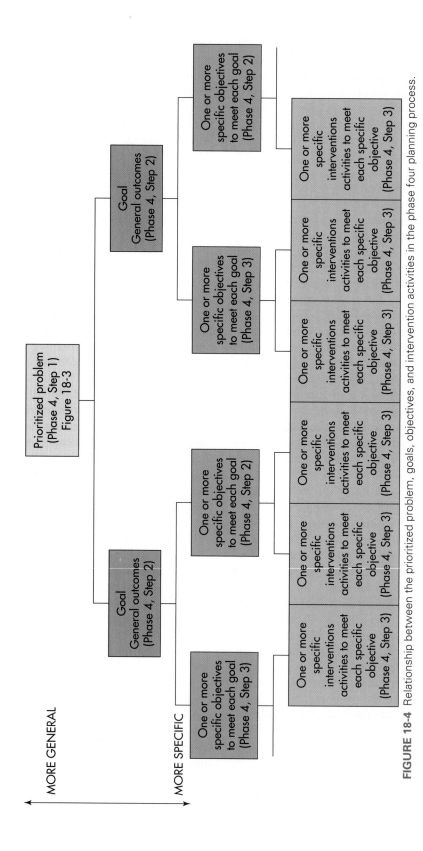

FIGURE 18-4 Relationship between the prioritized problem, goals, objectives, and intervention activities in the phase four planning process.

BOX 18-7   PROBLEM PRIORITY CRITERIA

Criteria that have been helpful in ranking identified problems include the following:

1. Community awareness of the problem
2. Community motivation to resolve or better manage the problem
3. Nurse's ability to influence problem solution
4. Availability of expertise to solve the problem
5. Severity of the outcomes if the problem is unresolved
6. Speed with which the problem can be solved

independently, and an overall priority score is calculated. This calculation involves two separate but related weighted factors: the first factor involves criteria related to the problem itself, and the second factor involves the same criteria but is weighted on the basis of the partnership's ability to make a change in each of the criteria in the first factor.

Each of the six criteria listed in Table 18-7 is considered separately and independently and then assigned a weight. The criteria are weighted on a scale ranging from a low score of 1 to a high score of 10. Listed in the second column of Table 18-7, these criteria are weighted jointly by the members of the partnership on the basis of the perceived importance of each criterion to the identified community health problem. For example, when members of the partnership assigned a weight to the first criterion listed in Table 18-7, they had to ask each other, "How important is community awareness of infant malnutrition in Bernalillo County so the problem can be solved?"

A second factor is related to the partnership's ability to resolve the problem. This factor, called the rating, is in the third column of Table 18-7. In deciding the rating to be given, the members of the partnership consider their ability to influence or change the situation. In the infant malnutrition example, they first ask each other to identify the extent of the community's awareness of the problem. After they talk about the criterion's importance and agree on its rating, the score is recorded. To understand the difference between the criterion weight and problem rating, consider that although a criterion might be weighted as extremely important, it might receive a low rating because the members of the community partnership believe that it would be difficult to influence or change things.

To understand the process of establishing a total score for a problem, or problem prioritizing, let us focus on the second criterion in Table 18-7: community motivation to resolve the problem of suspected infant malnutrition. The weighting of this criterion, 10, shows that it is considered a very important problem to resolve. However, most community residents believe that the problem cannot be solved because of the poverty of those affected. Partnership members do not believe they can actually have an impact on the poverty, so they give their ability to intervene the low rating of 3. The resulting problem ranking, obtained by multiplying the criterion weight by the criterion rating, was 30, a low score in comparison with the problem ranking scores of the other criteria in the table.

A similar process with the remaining five criteria listed in Table 18-7 yields a total ranking score of 239 for the infant malnutrition problem. This score is less than 50% of the total score possible. Other problems in the community would be ranked by the same procedure, and their ranking scores would be compared with the ranking of the infant malnutrition problem to reveal the partners' commitment to solving the problems. If 239 were found to be the highest-ranking score among the several identified community health problems, the problem of infant malnutrition would be the logical priority for intervention.

Arriving at a problem ranking score for each identified problem may appear complicated, but recall that the criteria were set up and weighted by the people taking part in the community partnership before prioritizing began. Also, the reasons for rating and each rating score are decided and set up with active input by all members in the community partnership. Although the number scores are subjective, the active involvement of the nurse and various community representatives helps to ensure that the data used to establish the rationale are real and accurate. Community participation also helps to ensure that the significance of the score for each problem reflects its importance relative to other community health problems.

Sometimes, the perceptions of the nurse and of community members differ. For example, if the issue is smoking in public buildings, the nurse might identify smoking as a public health problem. Community members, on the other hand, might view smoking as an issue of individual choice and personal freedom.

Once infant nutrition has been established as the priority problem, what to do about infant nutrition becomes the focus of the second and third steps of phase four: step 2 is establishing goals and objectives, and step 3 is developing intervention activities to meet the established objectives.

HOW TO **Prioritize Community Health Problems**

List all community health problems defined and follow these steps for each problem:

1. *Use nominal group technique to identify problem priorities.*
2. *The nurse and community partners answer the following question: "How important is community awareness to each problem so it can be solved?"*
3. *The nurse and community partners give a number score to the question, between 1 (low) and 10 (high).*
4. *The process is repeated to get a criterion score for each of the six criteria in Box 18-7.*
5. *For each problem and each criterion, ask the following question: "Can the partners influence or change the situation?"*
6. *By consensus, the nurse and partners agree on a criterion weight and a rating for each problem.*
7. *To determine the problem ranking, multiply the weight and rating for each criterion. Total the ranking score for the six criteria for each problem.*
8. *Compare the total scores for each problem to find the priority problem for the community.*

Establishing Goals and Objectives

Once high-priority problems are identified, goals and objectives are developed. Goals are generally broad statements of desired outcomes. Objectives are the precise statements of the desired outcomes.

Table 18-8 (see p 421) shows an example of one of the goals, and the specific objectives associated with it, for the infant malnutrition problem in Bernalillo County. The goal is to reduce the incidence and prevalence of infant malnutrition. The objectives must be precise, behaviorally stated, incremental, and measurable. In this example, the specific objectives pertain to assessing infant developmental levels, determining WIC eligibility, implementing an outreach program, enrolling infants in WIC, and providing supplemental foods in existing diets.

Deciding on these goals and objectives involves collaboration between the nurse and representatives of the community groups affected by both the problem and the proposed intervention. This often requires a great deal of negotiating with everyone taking part in the planning process. One important advantage offered by the continuous active involvement of people affected by the outcomes is that they come to have a vested interest in those outcomes and therefore are supportive of and committed to the success of the intervention. Once goals and objectives are chosen, intervention activities to accomplish the objectives can be identified.

Identifying Intervention Activities

Intervention activities are the strategies used to meet the objectives, the ways change will be effected, and the ways the problem cycle will be broken. Usually, alternative intervention activities do exist, and they must be identified and evaluated. Drafting possible interventions and selecting the best set of activities to achieve the goal of documenting and reducing infant malnutrition are shown in Tables 18-9 and 18-10 on p 422.

To achieve the objective related to assessing infant developmental levels (objective 1 in Table 18-8), five intervention activities are listed in the second column of Table 18-9. Each is relevant to the first objective: 80% of infants seen by the health department, neighborhood health center, and private physicians will have their developmental levels assessed. The first two activities involve WIC personnel as the principal change agents. The last three involve the nurse, WIC personnel, and the staff of the health department, neighborhood health center, and private physicians' offices as the change partners (change agents and change partners are described in greater detail later in this chapter).

The expected effect of each activity is considered in the third and fifth columns of Table 18-9. The value, or the likelihood that the activity will help meet the objective and finally resolve the problem, is noted in the third column. Clearly, it is more valuable in the long term to educate others to assess infant development (activity 4) than to do it for them (activity 1). It is also valuable to analyze the change process necessary to complete the objective (activity 5). As a result, activities 4 and 5 have higher value scores than activity 1, in which the professional staff alone carries out the intervention.

On the other hand, the probability, or the likelihood that the means can be implemented, is highest when only the nurse is involved, because the nurse has more control over self-behavior than over the behavior of others. Therefore, activities 1 and 3 have higher probabilities than activities 2, 4, and 5, as recorded in the fifth column. Conditions explaining the numerical scores are noted briefly in the fourth column. A total score is computed by multiplying the value of the activity by the probability of implementation. These scores are listed in the last column. The activities with the highest total scores become the priority intervention activities, because it is important to be able to both achieve the objective (value) and carry out the means (probability). In this case, activities 4 and 5, with total scores of 64 and 80, respectively, would be selected.

Although the numbers assigned by the nurse to both value and probability are based on subjective judgment, their products are quite useful. When the scores in the two columns are multiplied, the products give the nurse a basis for judging which of the potential intervention activities will be most effective in meeting the objectives.

A second example of developing a plan is shown in Table 18-10. The activities relate to objective 3 of the goals and objectives (in Table 18-8), which involves starting up and carrying out an outreach program. These activities involve using lay advisors, hospital nurses, community and public health nurses, and WIC personnel. Activity 1 (with an activity ranking of 48) and activity 2 (with an activity ranking of 40) were selected. Activity 1 builds on existing informal community leaders, and activity 2 addresses needed changes in the formal health care delivery system. See the How To on p 415 about prioritizing community health problems, and use a similar process for arriving at rankings. Note that in Tables 18-9 and 18-10, there is no total score.

Sufficient resources are not always available to implement all of the intervention activities, but the ranking process illustrated in Tables 18-9 and 18-10 will show which activities should be implemented first. To effectively implement each chosen activity, the health nurse must be clear about the availability of needed resources, who will be responsible for implementing the activity, how it will be evaluated, and when it will be completed. Table 18-11 (p 423) provides a format for keeping track of these specific details.

Implementing in the Community

Implementation, the fifth phase of the nursing process, involves the work and activities aimed at achieving the goals and objectives. Implementing efforts may be made by the person or group who established the goals and objectives, or they may be shared with, or even delegated to, others. Having a central authority to oversee the efforts to start up and carry out the plan is important, and the nurse's position on this issue can be affected by a variety of factors.

Factors Influencing Implementation

Implementation is shaped by the nurse's chosen roles, the type of health problem selected as the focus for intervention, the community's readiness to take part in problem solving, and characteristics of the social change process. The nurse taking part in a population-centered intervention has knowledge and skills that the partners do not have; the question is how the nurse uses his or her position, knowledge, and skills.

Nurse's Role. Nurses can act as content experts, helping communities select and attain task-related goals. In the example of infant malnutrition, the nurse used epidemiological skills to find the incidence and prevalence of malnutrition. The nurse also serves as a process expert by fostering the community's ability to document the problem rather than by only providing help as an expert in the area.

Content-focused roles often are considered change agent roles, whereas process roles are called change partner roles. Change agent roles stress gathering and analyzing facts and implementing programs, whereas change partner roles include those of enabler-catalyst, teacher of problem-solving skills, and activist advocate.

The Problem and the Nurse's Role. The role the nurse chooses depends on the nature of the health problem, on the community's decision-making ability, and on professional and personal choices. Some health problems clearly require certain intervention roles. If a community lacks democratic problem-solving abilities, the nurse may select teacher, facilitator, and advocate roles. Problem-solving skills must be explained and modeled. A problem that involves determining the status of community health, on the other hand, usually requires fact-gatherer and analyst roles. Some problems, such as the example of infant malnutrition presented earlier, require multiple roles. In that case, managing conflict among the involved health care providers demands process skills. Collecting and interpreting the data necessary to document the problem requires both interpersonal and analytical skills.

The community's history of taking part in decision making is a critical factor. In a community skilled in identifying and successfully managing its problems, the nurse may best serve as technical expert or advisor. Different roles may be required if the community lacks problem-solving skills or has a history of unsuccessful change efforts. The nurse may have to focus on developing problem-solving capabilities or on making one successful change so that the community becomes empowered to take on the job of promoting further change on its own behalf.

Social Change Process and the Nurse's Role. The nurse's role also depends on the social change process. Not all communities are open to innovation. Ability to change is often related to the extent to which a community adheres to traditional norms. The more traditional the community, the less likely it is to change. In 1995 Rogers wrote a classic book (updated in 2003) about the diffusion of innovation, and the book provides important information for nurses. Innovation is often directly related to high socioeconomic status; a perceived need for change; the presence of liberal, scientific, and democratic values; and a high level of social participation by community residents (Rogers, 2003). Innovations with the highest adoption rates are seen as better than the other available choices. They also fit with existing values, can be started as a limited trial, and are easily explained or demonstrated. They are also simple and convenient (Rogers, 2003). For example, people living in a community might go to an immunization clinic rather than a private physician if the clinic is nearby and less expensive and if the physician is not always available when needed.

Innovations are also easier to accept when the innovation is shared in ways that fit in with the community's norms, values, and customs and when information is spread by the best communication mode (mass media for early adopters and face-to-face for late adopters, explained later in this chapter). Other factors that positively influence acceptance include the support of other communities for the change efforts, identification and use of opinion leaders, and clear, straightforward communication about the innovation (Rogers, 2003; Yoo et al, 2009).

Many complex factors combine to shape how the change process is started and maintained. Therefore, the nurse must be adaptable. The roles required to begin change may differ from those used to maintain or stabilize it. Also, the roles required to initiate, maintain, and stabilize change may vary from community to community and from one intervention to another within the same community. Thus, the nurse must be skilled in a variety of implementation mechanisms.

Implementation Mechanisms

Implementation mechanisms are the vehicles, or modes, by which innovations are transferred from the planners to the community. The nurse alone is never considered an implementation mechanism. Change on behalf of the community client requires multiple implementation mechanisms. The nurse must identify and appropriately use all of them. Some important implementation mechanisms, or aids, include small interacting groups, lay advisors, the mass media, and health policies.

Small Interacting Groups. Small interacting groups, formal and informal, are essential implementation mechanisms. *Formal* groups in the community include families, legislative bodies, health care clients, and service providers. *Informal* groups include neighborhoods and social action groups. The common tie among these diverse groups is that they are located between the community and individuals. Because of their intermediate position, they can and do act both to support and to prevent change efforts at the community and individual levels. They are potentially powerful precisely because they are mediating structures.

As a result, the nurse needs to identify which groups view the proposed change as beneficial and which do not. New small groups may need to be formed to encourage the change. Changes may be necessary in the innovation or in how the innovation is spread throughout the community to increase acceptance. At first the innovation may have to be directed to groups with a majority of early adopters (those with broad perspectives and abilities to adopt new ideas from mass media information sources) and to groups whose goals are reflected in the intervention plan (Bigbee et al, 2009; Rankins et al, 2007). Using a small group to initiate population-centered change is shown in Table 18-12 (see p 423).

Lay Advisors. Lay advisors are people who are influential in approving or vetoing new ideas and from whom others seek advice and information about new ideas. They often perform a function similar to that of early adopters. Lay advisors, or opinion leaders, can be identified by their agreement with community norms, heavy involvement in formal social groups, specific areas of skill and knowledge, and a slightly higher social status than their followers (Rogers, 2003).

Mass Media. Mass media are particularly useful in creating change among late adopters, or those who are last to embrace change. However, groups dominated by early adopters and lay advisors can also be reached through the mass media. Mass media, such as the Internet, newspapers, television, and radio, represent an impersonal and formal type of communication and are useful in providing information quickly to a large number of people. Using the mass media is efficient because the ratio of money spent to population covered is low and populations can be targeted (Bretthauer-Mueller et al, 2008). For example, information about teenage pregnancy can be efficiently provided through rock music stations. In addition to being efficient, the mass media are effective aids in intervention.

Health Policy. Health policy can also play a critical part in the adoption of healthful population-centered change (Givel, 2008; Popkin, 2009). The major intent of public policy in the health field is to address collective human needs, and it often limits individual choice in order to serve the public good. For example, drivers have been urged for several years to wear automobile seat belts. However, the incidence of automobile fatalities was not reduced until drivers were required to observe lowered speed limits and, in some states, to wear seat belts and use special restraining seats for children. Clearly, health policy can help encourage interventions that promote community health.

If public policy that will encourage or even simply allow health-generating choices is to become law, the nurse must actively lobby for it. See Chapter 8 for a more in-depth discussion.

The nurse also must use small groups, lay advisors, and the mass media as aids to getting started. Working with naturally occurring small groups, such as the family, and with lay advisors is familiar to most nurses. Working with legislators or the mass media is less familiar, yet all resources must be used to achieve healthful change in the community client. No matter what means are used, all efforts to start and maintain changes must be documented.

Evaluating, the sixth phase of this process, is also important to determine and improve the ability of population-centered nursing practice to produce the desired results. Evaluating also increases the knowledge base and improves the rate of success in competing for funds for needed programs to solve community problems.

Evaluating Community Health Intervention

Simply defined, evaluation is the appraisal of the effects of some organized activity or program. Evaluating may involve the design and conduct of evaluation research, in which social science research methods are used to determine what works, what processes are involved, and the need for indicators to measure outcomes (Butterfoss, 2009). Evaluating may also involve the more elementary process of assessing progress by comparing the objectives and the results, as discussed here.

Evaluation begins in the planning phase, when goals and measurable objectives are established and goal-attaining activities are identified. After implementing the intervention, only the meeting of objectives and the effects of intervening activities

have to be assessed. The progress notes direct the nurse to perform such appraisals during the implementing activities. In assessing the data recorded there, the nurse is requested to evaluate whether the objectives were met and whether the intervening activities used were effective.

The nurse also must decide whether the costs in money and time were worth the resulting benefits. This process is shown in the progress notes. In Table 18-12, the nurse has noted progress toward the needs assessed and the difficulties encountered in handling conflict among the group members.

Such an evaluating process is oriented to community health because the intervening goals and objectives come from the nurse's and the community's ideas about health. Simple as it appears, it is not without problems. The results must be compared with the baseline information collected on the nurse's community before the intervention, as well as to results obtained in other communities. Either of these comparisons will help reveal the success or failure of the intervention.

The lay role in evaluation is also important. Professionals have adopted partnerships in assessing and implementing more readily than in evaluating. The question of who has the power to define, judge, and institute change in professional activities is an issue. With evaluation, the entire process is open to renegotiation to achieve community health (Figure 18-5).

Role of Outcomes in the Evaluation Phase

Students using the community-as-client process presented in this chapter must recognize that in a political climate in which health resources are limited, the measurement of outcomes is a particularly important part of the evaluation process. This is one reason for emphasizing measurable objectives. Objectives must also be chosen with sensitivity to the changes that may result from the interventions. Cashman et al (2008) examined the role of community involvement in the evaluation process and how community participation can help in understanding the data better. Butterfoss (2009) recommends outcome questions about appropriate and effective interventions. To answer these and other outcome questions, many community health interventions emphasize the correct use of rates and numbers as one means of evaluating intervention outcomes in defined communities. Often, data collected over time can also provide important outcome information about health trends within the community. As indicated previously, epidemiological data and trends do not provide the only measures of success, but they do provide important information about the intervention. Nurses need to consider collecting this type of outcome data for use as part of the evaluation phase. Other types of evaluation questions focus on the intervention process itself—for example, was the process of implementing the intervention efficient, and was it acceptable to the community?

PERSONAL SAFETY IN COMMUNITY PRACTICE

Effective nursing practice starts with personal safety, and this remains important throughout the process. An awareness of the community and common sense are the two best guidelines

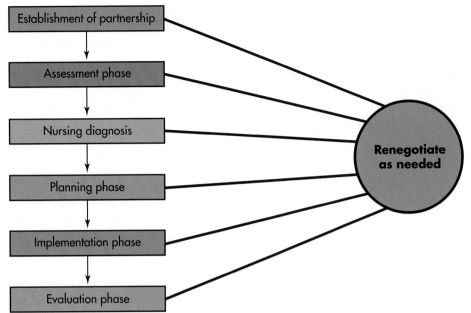

FIGURE 18-5 Summary flowchart illustrating the nursing process with the community as client. (Courtesy of George Shuster.)

for judgment. For example, common sense suggests not leaving anything valuable on a car seat and not leaving your car unlocked. Similar guidelines apply to the use of public transportation. Calling ahead to clients to schedule meetings will help prevent delays or confusion, and it gives the nurse an opportunity to lay the groundwork for the meeting. If there is no telephone and no access to a neighbor's telephone, plan to establish a time for any future meetings during the initial visit. Regardless of whether there has been telephone contact, there are rare situations when a meeting is postponed because the nurse arrives at a location where people are unexpectedly loitering by the entrance and the nurse has concerns about personal safety.

For nurses who either are just beginning their careers in the community or are just starting a new position, three clear sources of information will help answer any questions about personal safety:

1. *Other nurses, social workers, or health care providers who are familiar with the dynamics of a given community:* They can provide valuable insights into when to visit, how to get there, and what to expect, because they function in the community themselves.

2. *Community members:* The best sources of information about the community are the community members themselves, and one benefit of developing an active partnership with community members is their willingness to share their insight about day-to-day community life.

3. *The nurse's own observations:* Knowledge gained during the data collection phase of the process should provide a solid basis for an awareness of day-to-day community activity. Nurses with experience practicing in the community generally agree that if they feel uncomfortable in a situation, they should trust their instincts and leave.

EXAMPLES OF TABLES DESCRIBING THE PROCESS OF A COMMUNITY ASSESSMENT

Tables 18-4 and 18-6 through 18-12 are specific examples of the assessment of Bernalillo County. The series of tables using infant malnutrition as an identified problem provide an example of the process after data have been gathered or generated by means described earlier in the chapter. Table 18-4 illustrates how gathered data such as epidemiological rates or generated data such as numbers or percentages from key informants can be organized by the nurse for tracking and analysis.

Analysis of the community assessment data will generate a list of problems. Each of these identified problems have correlates or contributing causes in the community that combine to create the problem itself. Before going further in the community assessment process, the identification and listing of these contributing causes is crucial to understanding the nature of the problem itself (Table 18-6).

Decisions must be made about the relative importance of each problem to the community and the ability of the community partnership to successfully intervene to resolve or reduce the problem's impact in the community (Table 18-7). While the process of prioritizing involves some subjectivity by the members of the community partnership, if the same process is used for each problem and the criterion weights are assigned by the same people, then the problem rankings will be valid.

Goals are what the community partnership hopes to accomplish through their interventions, whereas *objectives* identify each of the concrete steps the community partnership wants to accomplish in order to reach each of their identified goals (Table 18-8).

Intervention activities are the means by which the identified objectives are accomplished. Tables 18-9 and 18-10 illustrate

TABLE 18-4 ASSESSMENT DATABASE

Data recording sheet page #_
Name of community: Bernalillo County
Assessment category: Community health
Subcategory status: Vital statistics

DATE	DATA SOURCE	DATA*
1/30/10	New Mexico Selected Health Statistics Annual Report Volume 1 Birth, Fetal Death, Abortion 2007	• 2007 teen birth rate was 57.7 per 1000 females ages 15-19 and 32.9 per 1000 females ages 15-17. • Proportion of infants weighing less than 2500 g was 8.7% in 2007. • The 2007 teen birth rate was 57.7 per 1000 females ages 15-19. • 2.2% of births to teen mothers (<18 years old) • Of all births, 11% of mothers had received little or no care in first trimester, with teen mothers under 19 having the highest rate at 19%.

*Noted with an asterisk are the themes identified, like teen pregnancy and meanings of the data are the rates given.

TABLE 18-5 WINDSHIELD SURVEY GUIDELINES

Each community has its own characteristics. These characteristics along with demographic data provide valuable information in understanding the population that lives within the community and the health status, strengths/limitations, risks and vulnerabilities unique to the "population-of-interest". Once you have defined a "community-of-interest" to assess, a **windshield survey** is the equivalent of a community head-to-toe assessment. The best way to conduct a windshield survey is to have a designated driver and at least one other passenger to scan the outline and take notes. Having one pair of eyes on the road, you can benefit from having several other individuals noticing the unique characteristics of the community...a shared experience provides additional insight. As you analyze your findings, it may be necessary to make a second tour to fill in any blanks. Many of us take these characteristics for granted, but they provide a rich context for understanding communities and populations and have significant impact on the health status of the community in general. You will report your findings in practicum conference and use relevant findings in your Community Problem Analysis (CPA) paper, so collect your findings and analysis in a useful format.

ELEMENTS	DESCRIPTION
Boundaries	What defines the boundary of? Roads, water, railroads? Does the area have a name? A nickname?
Housing and zoning	What is the age of the houses? What kind of materials in the construction? Describe the housing including space between them, general appearance and condition, and presence of central heating, air conditioning, and modern plumbing.
Open space	Describe the amount, condition, use of open space? Is the space used? Safe? Attractive?
Commons	Where do people in the neighborhood hang out? Who hangs out there and what hours during the day?
Transportation	How do people get from one place to another? Public transportation and if so, what kind and how effective; How timely? Personal autos? Bikes, etc?
Social service centers	Do you see evidence of recreation centers, parks, social services, offices of doctors, dentists, pharmacies
Stores	Where do residents shop? How do they get to the shops? Do they have groceries or sources of fresh produce? Is this a "food desert"?
Street people and animals	Who do you see on the streets during the day? Besides the people, do you see animals? Are they loose or contained?
Condition of the area	Is the area well kept or is there evidence of trash, abandoned cars or houses? What kind of information is provided on the signs in the area?
Race and ethnicity	What is the race of the people whom you see? What do you see about indices of ethnicity? Places of worship, food stores, restaurants? Are signs in English or other languages? (If the latter, which ones)?
Religion	What indications do you see about the types of religion residents practice?
Health indicators	Do you see evidence of clinics, hospitals, mental illness, and/or substance abuse?
Politics	What indicators do you see about politics? Posters, headquarters?
Media	Do you see indicators of what people read? If they watch television? Listen to the radio?
Business & industry	What type of business climate exists? Manufacturers? Light or heavy industry? Large employers? Small business owners? Retail? Hospitality industry? Military installation? Do people have to seek employment elsewhere?

Adapted by J. Lancaster from: Mizrahi TM: School of Social Work, Virginia Commonwealth Cniversity, Richmond VA, September 1992; Stanhope MS, Knollmueller RN: Public and Community Health Nurse's Consultant: A Health Promotion Guide, St. Louis, 1997, Mosby.

TABLE 18-6 PROBLEM ANALYSIS: INFANT MALNUTRITION

Community: Bernalillo County
Problem: Infant Malnutrition

PROBLEM CORRELATES*	RELATIONSHIP OF CORRELATE TO PROBLEM	DATA SUPPORTIVE OF RELATIONSHIPS†
1. Inadequate diet	Diets lacking in required nutrients contribute to malnutrition.	All county infants and their mothers seen by PHNs in 2008 were referred to nutritionist because of poor diets.
2. Community norms	Bottle-fed babies are less apt to receive adequate amounts of safe milk containing necessary nutrients.	Area general practitioners and nurses agree that 86% of mothers in the county bottle-feed.
3. Poverty	Infant formulas are expensive.	52% of eligible new mothers in county are receiving WIC.
4. Disturbed mother–child relationship	Poor mother–child relationship may result in infant's failure to thrive.	Data from charts of 43 nursing mothers' relationship show infants diagnosed with failure to thrive.
5. Teenage pregnancy	Teenage mothers are most apt to have inadequate diets prenatally, to bottle-feed, to be poor, and to lack parenting skills.	16% of births in 2007 for women 19 years of age or younger; 46% were to women under 24. 52% of births to single women

*These are factors that contribute to problem and outcomes.
†Refer to appropriate sections of the database and relevant research of the findings in current literature.

TABLE 18-7 PROBLEM PRIORITIZING: INFANT MALNUTRITION IN BERNALILLO COUNTY*

CRITERION	CRITERION WEIGHT (1-10)	CRITERION RATING (1-10)	RATIONALE FOR RATING	PROBLEM RANKING (WEIGHT × RATE)
1. Community awareness of the problem	5	10	Health service providers, teachers, and a variety of parents have mentioned problem.	50
2. Community motivation to resolve or better manage the problem	10	3	Most believe that this problem is not solvable because most of those affected are poor.	30
3. Nurse's ability to influence problem solution	5	8	Nurses are skilled at consciousness raising and mobilizing support.	40
4. Availability of expertise to solve the problem	7	10	WIC and nutritionists are available. A county extension agent is interested.	70
5. Severity of the outcomes if the problem is unresolved	8	5	Effects of marginal malnutrition are not well documented.	40
6. Speed with which the problem can be solved	3	3	Time to mobilize community within this area is lengthy.	9

*Note: Maximum possible problem ranking score = 600; total for Bernalillo County = 239.

TABLE 18-8 GOALS AND OBJECTIVES: INFANT MALNUTRITION

Community: Bernalillo County
Problem/Concern: Infant Malnutrition
Goal Statement: To Reduce the Incidence and Prevalence of Infant Malnutrition

PRESENT DATE	OBJECTIVE (NUMBER AND STATEMENT)	COMPLETION DATE
7/10	1. 80% of infants seen by health department, neighborhood health center, and private physicians will have developmental levels assessed.	8/11
7/10	2. WIC eligibility will be determined for 80% of infants seen by health department, neighborhood health center, and private physicians.	7/11
7/10	3. An outreach program will be implemented to identify at-risk infants presently unknown to health care providers.	10/11
7/10	4. WIC eligibility will be determined for 25% of at-risk infants.	7/11
7/10	5. 75% of all infants eligible for WIC food supplements will be enrolled in the program.	11/11
7/10	6. 50% of the mothers of infants enrolled in WIC will demonstrate three ways of incorporating WIC supplements into their infants' diets.	10/11

TABLE 18-9   PLAN: INTERVENTION ACTIVITIES TO ASSESS INFANTS' DEVELOPMENTAL LEVELS

Community: Bernalillo County
Objective 1 and Statement: 80% of Infants Seen by Health Department, Neighborhood Health Center, and Private Physicians will Have Developmental Levels Assessed

DATE	INTERVENTION ACTIVITIES/MEANS	VALUE TO ACHIEVING OBJECTIVE (1-10)	ACTIVITY/MEANS FOR SELECTED IMPLEMENTATION	PROBABILITY OF IMPLEMENTING ACTIVITY (1-10)	ACTIVITY RANKING (VALUE × PROBABILITY)
7/10	1. WIC supplies personnel to assess infant development levels.	1	Insufficient personnel and time; existing community resources (potential) are ignored.	10	10
7/10	2. WIC provides in-service education to staff on assessment of infant development.	5	Antipathy between WIC personnel and other health workers is high.	5	25
7/10	3. Community nurse (CN) provides in-service education to staff on assessment of infant development.	3	CN cannot do it alone.	10	30
7/10	4. CN helps WIC personnel identify in-service educational needs of area health care providers related to assessment of infant development.	8	Most likely to build on existing community strengths; CN skilled in needs assessment, and interpersonal approaches are needed to increase interest.	8	64
7/10	5. CN helps WIC personnel identify driving and restraining forces relative to implementation of objective.	10	Without this change, effort is likely to fail.	8	80

TABLE 18-10   PLAN: INTERVENTION ACTIVITIES TO IMPLEMENT AN OUTREACH PROGRAM

Community: Bernalillo County
Objective 3 and Statement: An Outreach Program is Implemented to Identify At-Risk Infants Presently Unknown to Health Care Providers

DATE	INTERVENTION ACTIVITIES/MEANS	VALUE TO ACHIEVING OBJECTIVE (1-10)	ACTIVITY/MEANS SELECTED FOR IMPLEMENTATION	PROBABILITY OF IMPLEMENTING ACTIVITY (1-10)	ACTIVITY RANKING (VALUE × PROBABILITY)
7/10	1. Community nurse (CN) identifies and trains lay advisors in community as case finders.	8	Lay leaders already known, proven to be effective change agents; cannot, however, be paid.	6	48
7/10	2. Local hospital administrators alter job descriptions of nurses in maternity and pediatrics to include case finding and referral.	8	Program to include all babies in Bernalillo County born in hospital since 2000. Administrator interested in community. Administration powerful and can alter nurses' job descriptions.	5	40
7/10	3. CN encourages public health nurses (PHNs) to do better job of case finding.	8	Public health nurses have historic role in case finding. CN not well-known by PHNs. PHNs reported to be overworked.	2	16
7/10	4. WIC personnel devote one evening per week to case finding.	1	One nurse (non-resident) eager to do this. Does not develop existing community resources.	10	10

the process of evaluating and ranking which intervention activities could probably be implemented if chosen by the community partnership and how much effect that specific intervention activity would have upon that particular objective if it were implemented by the community partnership.

Determining who will be responsible for completing a given intervention activity and determining specific, measurable ways for judging whether it worked are important to the process.

Specific dates for when each intervention activity will be completed are also important because together these help the community partnership to answer the question of whether the intervention worked and whether it got done on time (Table 18-11).

Community assessment is a multiphase process (see Figure 18-3) occurring over time, and progress notes are the means by which the nurse keeps track of what has been done and what needs to be done (Table 18-12).

TABLE 18-11 INTERVENTION ACTIVITY IMPLEMENTATION AND EVALUATION DETAILS

Community: Bernalillo County
Objective Number and Statement: _____

INTERVENTION ACTIVITY	RESPONSIBLE AGENCY/INDIVIDUAL	HOW INTERVENTION ACTIVITY WILL BE EVALUATED (OBSERVABLE, MEASURABLE CRITERIA)	TARGET DATE FOR COMPLETION OF INTERVENTION ACTIVITY	RESULTS/OUTCOMES OF INTERVENTION (COMPLETION DATE)
1. Community nurse (CN) identifies and trains lay advisors in community as case finders (from Table 18-9, activity 1).	Community nurse	Lay advisors will be able to verbally describe case-finding methods to CN. Number of new WIC cases will be tracked by CN on monthly basis for 1 year.	Lay advisor training completed by 5/10.	

TABLE 18-12 PROGRESS NOTES: INFANT MALNUTRITION

Community: Bernalillo County
Goal: To Reduce the Incidence and Prevalence of Infant Malnutrition

DATE	NARRATIVE, ASSESSMENT, PLAN*	BUDGET, TIME
8/22/10	Objective 1, means 4 *Narrative:* Meeting to develop needs assessment was attended by community nurse (CN), two WIC personnel, and physicians from health department, neighborhood health centers, and local medical society. Consensus rapidly achieved among 5 of 6 participants that goal, objectives, and means (especially objective 1, means 4) were appropriate. Physician representing medical society consistently objected, stating vehemently that private sector had long provided adequate medical care for area youngsters. Physician would not recommend that medical society support the effort. CN afraid that this would jeopardize entire effort. Eventually, however, physician left and plans were made to develop and conduct needs assessment and to continue seeking medical society's help. *Agenda:* CN to develop needs assessment tool with WIC personnel and health systems agency planner. Physicians to develop list of providers to be contacted. Neighborhood health center physician to get a place on medical society agenda and attempt to clarify plans. WIC personnel to contact non-physician health workers to introduce plan and develop provider list. *Assessment:* Plans made to proceed with needs assessment and partner support essential to accomplishment of objective. Group process problematic, and CN ineffective because of discomfort with conflict between physician and WIC staff member. *Plans:* Meeting scheduled for 2/28/11 to deal with agreed-on agenda. Before 2/28/11 meeting, CN will discuss ways to better handle conflict with consultation group, collaborate on drafting needs assessment, and telephone others to determine their progress. G. Shuster	$200; 2 hours of meeting and 2 hours of preparation time

*Record both objective and subjective data. Interpret these data in terms of whether the objectives were achieved and whether the intervention activities were effective. The plan depends on the assessment and may include both new or revised objectives and activities.

CHAPTER REVIEW

PRACTICE APPLICATION

Lily, a nurse in a small city, became aware of the increased incidence of respiratory diseases through contact with families in the community and the local chapter of the American Lung Association. During family visits, Lily noticed that many of the parents were smokers. Because most of the families Lily visited had small children, she became concerned about the effects of second-hand smoke on the health of the infants and children in her family caseload.

Further assessment of this community indicated that the community recognized several problems, including school safety and the risk of water pollution, in addition to the smoking problem that Lily had identified during her family visits. Talks with different community members revealed that they wanted each of these identified

problems "fixed," although these same community members were uncertain about how to start. In deciding which of the three identified problems to address first, which criterion would be most important for Lily to consider?

A. The amount of money available
B. The level of community motivation to "fix" one of the three identified problems
C. The number of people in the community who expressed a concern about each of the three identified problems
D. How much control she would have in the process
Answers can be found on the Evolve site.

KEY POINTS

- Most definitions of community include three dimensions: (1) networks of interpersonal relationships that provide friendship and support to members, (2) residence in a common locality, and (3) shared values, interests, or concerns.
- A community is defined as a locality-based entity, composed of systems of formal organizations reflecting societal institutions, informal groups, and aggregates that are interdependent and whose function or expressed intent is to meet a wide variety of collective needs.
- A community practice setting is insufficient reason for stating that practice is oriented toward the community client. When the location of the practice is in the community but the focus of the practice is the individual or family, the nursing client remains the individual or family, not the whole community.
- Population-centered practice is targeted to the community—the population group in which healthful change is sought.
- Community health as used in this chapter is defined as the meeting of collective needs through identification of problems and management of behaviors within the community itself and between the community and the larger society.
- Most changes aimed at improving community health involve, out of necessity, partnerships among community residents and health workers from a variety of disciplines.
- Assessing community health requires gathering existing data, generating missing data, and interpreting the database.

- Five methods of collecting data useful to the nurse are informant interviews, participant observation, secondary analysis of existing data, surveys, and windshield surveys.
- Gaining entry or acceptance into the community is perhaps the biggest challenge in assessment.
- The nurse is usually an outsider and often represents an established health care system that is neither known nor trusted by community members, who may react with indifference or even active hostility.
- The planning phase includes analyzing and establishing priorities among community health problems already identified, establishing goals and objectives, and identifying intervention activities that will accomplish the objectives.
- Once high-priority problems are identified, broad relevant goals and objectives are developed; the goal is generally a broad statement of the desired outcome while the objectives are precise statements of the desired outcome.
- Intervention activities, the means by which objectives are met, are the strategies that clarify what must be done to achieve the objectives, the ways change will be effected, and the way the problem will be interpreted.
- Implementation, the third phase of the nursing process, means transforming a plan for improved community health into achieving goals and objectives.
- Simply defined, evaluation is the appraisal of the effects of some organized activity or program.

CLINICAL DECISION-MAKING ACTIVITIES

1. Observe an occupational health nurse or public health nurse, school nurse, family nurse practitioner, or emergency department nurse for several hours. Determine which of the nurse's activities are population centered. Give specific examples and present your reasons for considering them population centered.
2. Using your own community as a frame of reference, develop examples illustrating the concepts of community, community client, community health, and partnership for health. What are some of the complexities of this question?
3. Read your local newspaper and identify articles illustrating the concepts of community, community client, community health, and partnership for health. How does your article specifically relate to the concept?

4. Using any two of the conditions of community competence given in the chapter, briefly analyze your own community. Give examples of each condition.
5. Search the Boone County, Iowa website (http://www.co.boone.ia.us/) for information on county festivals. Ask yourself the following question: To what extent do the county festivals depicted on the website reveal community cohesion?
6. Search the Washtenaw County, Michigan, website (http://www.ewashtenaw.org/) for information about "county conversations." Identify which issues are being addressed, and read the local newspaper for additional information. Did you find other county-wide issues when you read the newspaper? Are there positions on the issues that are not presented?

REFERENCES

Adams LM, Canclini SB: Disaster readiness: a community-university partnership, *Online J Issues Nurs* 13(3):11, 2008.

American Public Health Association: Public Health Nursing Section: *Public Health Nursing Section, 2009*. Available at http://www.apha.org/membergroups/sections/aphasections/phn/. Accessed January 8, 2011.

Anderson ET, McFarlane J, editors: *Community as partner*, ed 4, Philadelphia, 2004, Lippincott.

Bencivenga M, DeRubis S, Leach P, et al: Community partnerships, food pantries, and an evidence-based intervention to increase mammography among rural women, *J Rural Health* 24(1):91–95, 2008.

Biel M, Evans SH, Clarke P: Forging links between nutrition and healthcare using community-based partnerships, *Fam Community Health* 32(3):196–205, 2009.

Bigbee JL, Hampton C, Blanford D, Ketner P: Community health nursing and cooperative extension: a natural partnership, *J Community Health Nurs* 26(4):192–197, 2009.

Blum HL, editor: *Planning for health*, New York, 1974, Human Sciences Press.

Bretthauer-Mueller R, Berkowitz JM, Thomas M, et al: Catalyzing community action within a national campaign: VERB community and national partnerships, *Am J Prev Med* 34(6):S210–S221, 2008.

Butterfoss FD: Evaluating partnerships to prevent and manage chronic disease, *Prev Chronic Dis* 6(2):1–10, 2009.

Carlson J: Professional nursing latent tuberculosis infection standards of practice development using NANDA, NIC, and NOC, *Int J Nurs Terminol Clasif* 17(1), 2006:62–62.

Cashman SB, Adeky S, Allen AJ, et al: The power and the promise: working with communities to analyze data, interpret findings, and get to outcomes, *Am J Public Health* 98(8):1407–1417, 2008.

Christopher S, Watts V, McCormick A, Young S: Building and maintaining trust in a community-based participatory research partnership, *Am J Public Health* 98(8):1398–1406, 2008.

Connor A, Rainer LP, Simcox JB, Thomisee K: Increasing the delivery of health care services to migrant farm worker families through a community partnership model, *Public Health Nurs* 24(4):355–360, 2007.

Cottrell LS: The competent community. In Kaplan BH, Wilson RN, Leighton AH, editors: *Further explorations in social psychiatry*, New York, 1976, Basic Books.

Council on Linkages Between Academia and Public Health Practice: *Core competencies for public health professionals, 2009*. Available at http://phf.org/link/competenciesinformation.htm:Accessed February 14, 2010.

Davies J, Lester C, O'Neill M, Williams G: Sustainable participation in regular exercise amongst older people: developing an action research approach, *Health Educ J* 67(1):45–55, 2008.

Delbecq AL, Van De Ven AH: A group process model for problem identification and program planning, *J Appl Behav Sci* 62:467, 1971.

Gec T: Development of NANDA nursing diagnosis in community nursing in Slovenia, *Int J Nurs Terminol Clasif* 17(1):34, 2006.

Givel M: Policy and health implications of using the U.S. Food and Drug Administration product design approach in reducing tobacco product risk, *Curr Drug Abuse Rev* 1(2):135–141, 2008.

Goepel E: Development of Healthy Cities networks in Europe, *Promot Educ* 14(2):103–104, 2007.

Goeppinger J, Lassite PG, Wilcox B: Community health is community competence, *Nurs Outlook* 30(8):464, 1982.

Goodman M, Almon L, Bayakly R, et al: Cancer outcomes research in a rural area: a multi-institution partnership model, *J Community Health* 34(1):23–32, 2009.

Hanks CA: Community empowerment: a partnership approach to public health program implementation, *Policy Polit Nurs Pract* 7(4):297–306, 2006.

Horsley K, Ciske SJ: From neurons to King County neighborhoods: partnering to promote policies based on the science of early childhood development, *Am J Public Health* 95(4):562–567, 2005.

Jackson EJ, Parks CP: Recruitment and training issues from selected lay health advisor programs among African Americans: a 20-year perspective, *Health Educ Behav* 24(4):418–431, 1997.

Kruger BJ, Roush C, Olinzock BJ, Bloom K: Engaging nursing students in a long-term relationship with a home-base community, *J Nurs Educ* 49(1):10–16, 2010.

Levine D, McCright J, Dobkin L, et al: SEXINFO: a sexual health text messaging service for San Francisco youth, *Am J Public Health* 98(3):393–395, 2008.

Martin KS, Monsen KA: The Omaha System International Conference, *Caring Newsl* 24(2), 2009:9–9.

Mendelson SG, McNeese-Smith D, Koniak-Griffin D, et al: A community-based parish nurse intervention program for Mexican American women with gestational diabetes, *J Obstet Gynecol Neonatal Nurs* 37(4):415–425, 2008.

Merriam PA, Tellez TL, Rosal MC, et al: Methodology of a diabetes prevention translational research project utilizing a community-academic partnership for implementation in an underserved Latino community, *BMC Med Res Methodol* 9(20):1–19, 2009.

Minkler M, Vasquez VB, Tajik M, Petersen D: Promoting environmental justice through community-based participatory research: the role of community and partnership capacity, *Health Educ Behav* 35(1):119–137, 2008.

Morbidity and Mortality Weekly: Consensus set of health status indicators for the general assessment of community health status—United States, *MMWR Morb Mortal Wkly Rep* 40(27):449–451, 1991:(updated August 2001).

National Center for Chronic Disease Prevention and Health Promotion: *National Center for Chronic Disease and Health Promotion: Chronic Disease Prevention 2010*. Available at http://www.cdc.gov/nccdphp/. Accessed March 1, 2010.

National Association of Community and City Health Officials (NACCHO): *Mobilizing for action through planning and partnerships: a community approach to health improvement*, Washington, DC, 2008, NACCHO.

Ndirangu M, Yadrick K, Bogle ML, Graham-Kresge S: Community-academia partnerships to promote nutrition in the Lower Mississippi Delta: community members' perceptions of effectiveness, barriers, and factors related to success, *Health Promot Pract* 9(3):237–245, 2008.

Newfield SA, Hinz MD, Tilley DS, et al: Coping-stress tolerance pattern. In Cox HC, editor: *Cox's clinical applications of nursing diagnosis*, ed 5, Philadelphia, 2007, FA Davis, pp 739–797.

O'Donnell L, Bonaparte B, Joseph H, et al: Keep It Up: development of a community-based health screening and HIV prevention strategy for reaching young African American men, *AIDS Educ Prev* 21(4):299–313, 2009.

Popkin BM: What can public health nutritionists do to curb the epidemic of nutrition-related noncommunicable disease? *Nutr Rev* 67(Suppl 1):S79–S82, 2009.

Powell DL, Gilliss CL, Hewitt HH, Flint EP: Application of a partnership model for transformative and sustainable international development, *Public Health Nurs* 27(1):54–70, 2010.

Radzyminski S: The concept of population health within the nursing profession, *J Prof Nurs* 23(1):37–46, 2007.

Rankins J, Wortham J, Brown LL: Modifying soul food for the Dietary Approaches to Stop Hypertension (DASH) diet plan: implications for metabolic syndrome (DASH of Soul), *Ethn Dis* 17(3 Suppl 4), 2007:S4-7-12.

Richards EL, Riner ME, Sands LP: A social ecological approach of community efforts to promote physical activity and weight management, *J Community Health Nurs* 25(4):179–192, 2008.

Rogers E, editor: *Diffusion of innovations*, ed 4, New York, 2003, Free Press.

Ruderman M, editor: *Resources guide to concepts and methods for community-based and collaborative problem solving*, Johns Hopkins University, 2000, Women's and Children's Health Policy Center.

Ryan W, editor: *Blaming the victim*, New York, 1976, Free Press.

Sangster J, Eccleston P, Porter S: Improving children's physical activity in out-of-school hours care settings, *Health Promote J Aust* 19(1):16–21, 2008.

Schwartz M, Laughlin A: Partnering with schools: a win-win experience, *J Nurs Educ* 47(6):279–282, 2008.

Severance JH, Zinnah SL: Community-based perceptions of neighborhood health in urban neighborhoods, *J Community Health Nurs* 26(1):14–23, 2009.

Shoultz J, Oneha MF, Magnussen L, et al: Finding solutions to challenges faced in community-based participatory research between academic and community organizations, *J Interprof Care* 20(2):133–144, 2006.

Simard P: The Quebec Healthy Cities and Towns Network: a powerful movement faced with new challenges, *Promot Educ* 14(2):121–122, 2007.

Stanhope M, Knollmueller R, editors: *Handbook of community-based and home health nursing practice*, ed 3, St Louis, 2000, Mosby.

Task Force on Community Preventive Services: Guide to community preventive services: Systematic reviews and evidence based recommendations, 2005. Updated in 2009. Available at http://www.thecommunityguide.org/. Accessed January 8, 2011.

Timmerman GM: Addressing barriers to health promotion in underserved women, *Fam Community Health* 30(1):S34–S42, 2007.

U.S. Department of Health and Human Services: *Healthy People 2020*. Available at www. healthypeople.gov/2020/default. aspx. Accessed January 8, 2011.

World Health Organization: *Centre for health development: Ageing and health technical report: a glossary of terms for community health care and services for older persons, vol 5*, Kobe, Japan, 2004, WHO.

Yoo S, Butler J, Elias TI, Goodman RM: The 6-step model for community empowerment: revisited in public housing communities for low-income senior citizens, *Health Promot Pract* 10(2):262–275, 2009.

Population-Centered Nursing in Rural and Urban Environments

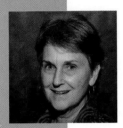

Angeline Bushy, PhD, RN, FAAN, PHCNS-BC

Dr. Angeline Bushy, Professor and Bert Fish Endowed Chair at the University of Central Florida, College of Nursing holds a BSN degree from the University of Mary in Bismarck, North Dakota; an MN degree in rural community health nursing from Montana State University in Bozeman; an MEd in adult education from Northern Montana College in Havre; and a PhD in nursing from the University of Texas at Austin. She is a Fellow in the American Academy of Nursing and a clinical specialist in public health nursing. She has worked in rural facilities located in the north-central and intermountain states; presented nationally and internationally on various rural nursing and rural health issues; published six textbooks and numerous articles on that topic; and, is a Lieutenant Colonel (Ret.) in the U.S. Army Reserve.

ADDITIONAL RESOURCES

evolve WEBSITE
http://evolve.elsevier.com/Stanhope
- *Healthy People 2020*
- WebLinks
- Quiz

- Case Studies
- Glossary
- Answers to Practice Application

OBJECTIVES

After reading this chapter, the student should be able to do the following:

1. Compare and contrast definitions of rural and urban.
2. Describe residency as a continuum, ranging from farm residency to core inner city.
3. Compare and contrast the health status of rural and urban populations on select health measures.
4. Analyze barriers to care in health professional shortage areas and for underserved populations.
5. Evaluate issues related to the delivery of public health services for rural underserved populations.
6. Describe characteristics of rural and small-town residency.
7. Examine the role and scope of public health nursing practice in rural and underserved areas.
8. Evaluate two professional-client-community partnership models that can effectively provide a continuum of health care to residents living in an environment with sparse resources.

KEY TERMS

farm residency, p. 428
frontier, p. 434
health professional shortage area (HPSA), p. 433
medically underserved, p. 443

metropolitan area, p. 429
micropolitan area, p. 429
non-core area, p. 429
non-farm residency, p. 428
rural, p. 428

rural-urban continuum, p. 429
suburbs, p. 429
urban, p. 428
—See Glossary for definitions

Access to health care is a national priority, especially in regions with an insufficient number of health care providers. Recruiting and retaining qualified health professionals can be a challenge in underserved communities, particularly inner cities and rural areas of the United States. Until recently, however, only limited research has been undertaken on the special challenges, problems, and opportunities of nursing practice—especially public health nursing in rural settings. This chapter presents major issues surrounding health care delivery in rural environments, which sometimes differs from that in urban or more populated settings. Common definitions for the term *rural* are discussed, as are its associated lifestyle, the health status of rural populations, barriers to obtaining a continuum of health care services, and public health nursing practice issues. Strategies are discussed to help nurses deliver more effective population-focused nursing services to clients who live in more isolated environments with sparser resources. This chapter describes rural public health nursing practice and can be used by students, nurses who practice in rural public health departments, and those who work in agencies located in urban areas that offer outreach services to rural populations in their catchment area.

HISTORIC OVERVIEW

Formal rural nursing originated with the Red Cross Rural Nursing Service, which was organized in November 1912. The Committee on Rural Nursing was under the direction of Mabel Boardman (Chair), Jane Delano (Vice-Chair), and Annie Goodrich along with other Red Cross leaders and philanthropists (Bigbee and Crowder, 1985). Before the formation of the Red Cross Rural Nursing Service, care of the sick in a small community was provided by informal social support systems. When self-care and family care were not effective in bringing about healing, this task was assigned to healers, who often were women who lived in the local community. Historically, the health needs of rural Americans have been numerous, and although not necessarily unique, they are different from those of urban populations. Consistent problems of maldistribution of health professionals, poverty, limited access to services,

ignorance, and social isolation have plagued many rural communities for generations.

Over the years, the history of the Red Cross Rural Nursing Service shows a consistent movement away from its initial rural focus, as demonstrated by its frequent name changes. Unfortunately, concern for rural health is similarly often temporary and replaced by other areas of greater need. It can be hoped that health care reform initiatives will ensure equitable access to care for rural and urban residents alike (NACRHHS, 2008; USDHHS, 2010a).

DEFINITION OF TERMS

Rurality: A Subjective Concept

Everyone has an idea as to what constitutes rural as opposed to urban residence. However, the two cannot be viewed as opposing entities. With the increased degree of urban influence on rural communities, the differences are no longer as distinct as they may have been even a decade ago (Bureau of the Census, 2009; Gamm et al, 2003; USDA, 2005, 2006, 2008a,b). In general, rural is defined in terms of the geographic location and population density, or it may be described in terms of the distance from (e.g., 20 miles) or the time (e.g., 30 minutes) needed to commute to an urban center.

Both urban and rural communities are highly diverse and vary in their demographic, environmental, economic, and social characteristics. In turn, these characteristics influence the magnitude and types of health problems that communities face. Urban counties, however, tend to have more health care providers in relation to population, and residents of more rural counties often live farther from health care resources (CDC, 2010; Cromartie, 2008; Mead et al, 2008).

Some equate the idea of rural with farm residency and urban with non-farm residency, whereas others consider *rural* to be a "state of mind." For the more affluent, rural may bring to mind a recreational, retirement, or resort community located in the mountains or in lake country where one can relax and participate in outdoor activities, such as skiing, fishing, hiking, or hunting. For the less affluent, the term can impose grim scenes. For example, some people may think of an impoverished Indian

BOX 19-1 TERMS AND DEFINITIONS

Farm residency: Residency outside area zoned as "city limits"; usually infers involvement in agriculture

Frontier: Regions having fewer than six persons per square mile

Large central: Counties in large (1 million or more population) metro areas that contain all or part of the largest central city

Large fringe: Remaining counties in large (1 million or more population) metro areas

Metropolitan county: Regions with a central city of at least 50,000 residents

Non-farm residency: Residence within area zoned as "city limits"

Micropolitan county: Counties that do not meet SMSA (see below) criteria

Rural: Communities having less than 20,000 residents or fewer than 99 persons per square mile

Small: Counties in metro areas with less than 1 million people

Standard metropolitan statistical area (SMSA): Regions with a central city of at least 50,000 residents

Suburban: Area adjacent to a highly populated city

Urban: Geographic areas described as non-rural and having a higher population density; more than 99 persons per square mile; cities with a population of at least 20,000 but less than 50,000

reservation as comparable to an underdeveloped country, and other people may think about a migrant labor camp with several families living in a one-room shanty with no access to safe drinking water or adequate sanitation.

Just as each city has its own unique features, it is also difficult to describe a "typical rural town" because of the wide population and geographic diversity. For example, rural towns in Florida, Oregon, Alaska, Hawaii, and Idaho are different from one another, and quite different from those in Vermont, Texas, Tennessee, Alabama, or California. Also, there can be vast differences between rural areas within one state. Still, descriptions and definitions for *rural* tend to be more subjective and relative in nature than those for urban (Cromartie, 2008).

For example, "small" communities with populations of more than 20,000 have some features that one may expect to find in a city. Then again, residents who live in a community with a population of less than 2000 may consider a community with a population of 5000 or 10,000 to be a city. Although some communities may seem geographically remote on a map, the residents who live there may not feel isolated. Those residents believe they are within easy reach of services through telecommunication and dependable transportation, although extensive shopping facilities may be 50 to 100 miles from the family home, obstetric care may be 150 miles away, or nursing services in the district health department in an adjacent county may be 75 or more miles away.

Rural-Urban Continuum

Frequently used definitions to describe rural and urban and to differentiate between them are provided by several federal agencies (Cromartie, 2008) (Box 19-1). These definitions, which in many cases are dichotomous in nature, fail to take into account the relative nature of ruralness. Rural and urban residencies are not opposing lifestyles. Rather, they must be seen as a rural-urban continuum ranging from living on a remote farm,

to a village or small town, to a larger town or city, to a large metropolitan area with a *core inner city* (Figure 19-1).

Several federal agencies classify counties according to population density, specifically, metropolitan area (1090 U.S. counties), micropolitan area (674 U.S. counties), and non-core area (1378 U.S. counties) (USDA, 2006). The terms metropolitan and micropolitan statistical areas (metro and micro areas) refer to geographic entities primarily used for collecting, tabulating, and publishing Federal statistics. Core-Based Statistical Area (CBSA) is a collective term for both metro and micro areas. A metro area contains a core urban area of 50,000 or more population. A micro area contains an urban core of at least 10,000 (but less than 50,000) population. Each metro or micro area consists of one or more counties containing the core urban area. Likewise, adjacent counties have a high degree of social and economic integration (as measured by commuting to work) with its urban core (Cromartie, 2008).

Demographically, micro areas contain about 60% of the total non-metro population, with an average of 43,000 people per county. In contrast, non-core counties, with no urban cluster of 10,000 or more residents, have on average about 14,000 residents. In general, lack of an urban core and low overall population density may place these counties at a disadvantage in efforts to expand and diversify their economic base. The designation of micro areas is an important step in recognizing non-metro diversity. The term also provides a framework to understand population growth and economic restructuring in small towns and cities that have received less attention than metro areas. Nationally and regionally, many measures of health, health care use, and health care resources among rural populations vary by the level of urban influence in a particular region.

Micro areas embody a widely shared residential preference for a small-town lifestyle—an ideal compromise between large highly populated urban cities and sparsely populated rural settings. As information about these places makes its way into government data and publications alongside metro areas in the coming years, hopefully the notion of "micropolitan" will draw increased attention from policymakers and the business community.

In the past decade there has been a notable population shift from urban to less-populated regions of the United States. The fastest growing rural counties are located in rural regions of the nation and along the edges of larger metropolitan counties. Demographers metaphorically refer to this demographic phenomenon as the "doughnut effect." That is to say, people are moving away from highly populated areas to outlying suburbs of urban centers. Most of the population growth has been in counties with a booming economy, with the geographic space to expand, and in western and southern states. Of the 10 fastest growing counties with 10,000 persons or more, 4 were located in western states, 5 in southern states, and 1 in a Midwestern state (Cromartie, 2008; USDA, 2005, 2006).

Clearly, a notable population shift will also affect the health status and lifestyle preferences of communities in which the shift occurs. As beliefs and values change over time, urban-rural differences narrow in some aspects and expand in others. Depending on the definition that is used, the actual rural

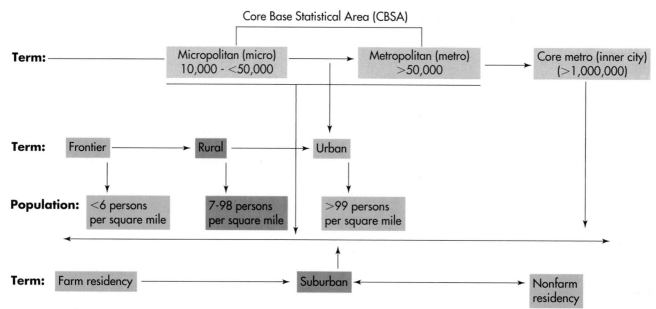

FIGURE 19-1 The continuum of rural-urban residency.

population might vary slightly. According to Bureau of the Census estimates (2009), about 25% of all U.S. residents live in rural settings. In this chapter, rural refers to areas having fewer than 99 persons per square mile and communities having 20,000 or fewer inhabitants.

CURRENT PERSPECTIVES

Population Characteristics

Adding to the confusion about what constitutes rural versus urban residency are the special needs of the numerous under-represented groups (minorities, subgroups) who reside in the United States. In general, there are a higher proportion of whites in rural areas than in urban areas. There are, however, regional variations, and some rural counties have a significant number of minorities. Little is documented on the needs and health status of special rural populations (Mead et al, 2008; USDHHS, 2010b,c). Anthropologists are quick to report that, within a group, there often exists a wide range of lifestyles. Consequently, even in the smallest or most remote town or village, a subgroup may behave differently and have different values about health, illness, and patterns of accessing health care. Also, a group's lifestyle may be associated with health problems that are different from those of the predominant cultural group in a given community. Background information on selected populations can be found in Chapters 7 and 32.

Demographically, rural communities include a higher proportion of younger and older residents. Nurses can expect to encounter more residents under the age of 18 and over 65 years of age in rural areas compared with an urban setting. Rural residents 18 years of age and older are more likely to be, or to have been, married than are their urban counterparts. As a group, rural adults are more likely to be widowed and have fewer years of formal education than urban adults (Cromartie, 2008; USDA, 2008a,b).

Although there are regional variations, rural families in general tend to be poorer than their urban counterparts. Comparing annual incomes with the standardized index established, more than one fourth of rural Americans live in or near poverty, and nearly 40% of all rural children are impoverished (Gamm et al, 2003; Rand Corporation, 2010a,b). Compared with those in metropolitan settings, a substantially smaller proportion of rural families are at the high end of the income scale. Accompanying the recent population shifts from urban to formerly rural areas, one can speculate that average income level might also change; however, no data are available at this time to substantiate this estimate. Regardless, level of income is a critical factor in whether a family has health insurance or qualifies for public insurance. Consequently rural families are less likely to have private insurance and more likely to receive public assistance or to be uninsured.

The working poor in rural areas are particularly at risk for being underinsured or uninsured. In working poor families, one or more of the adults are employed but still cannot afford private health insurance. Furthermore, their annual income is such that it disqualifies the family from obtaining public insurance. Several factors help explain why this phenomenon occurs more often in rural settings. For example, a high proportion of rural residents are self-employed in a family business, such as ranching or farming, or they work in small enterprises, such as a service station, restaurant, or grocery store. Also, an individual may be employed in part-time or in seasonal occupations, such as farm laborer and construction, in which health insurance often is not an employee benefit. In other situations, a family member may have a preexisting health condition that makes the cost of insurance prohibitive, if it is even available to them. At present it remains to be seen if this situation will change with the recent health care reform. A few rural families fall through the cracks and are unable to access any type of public assistance because of other deterrents, such as language barriers, compromised physical status, the geographic location of an agency, lack of transportation, or undocumented worker status. Insurance, or the lack of it, has serious implications for the overall health status of rural residents and the nurses who provide services to them (AHCPR, 2009; Bennett, Olatosi, and Probst, 2008; Nelson and Stover-Gingerich, 2010; USDHHS, 2010c).

Health Status of Rural Residents

Even though rural communities constitute about one fourth of the total population, the health problems and the health behaviors of the residents in them are not fully understood. This section summarizes what is known about the overall health status of rural adults and children. The health status measures that are addressed are perceived health status, diagnosed chronic conditions, physical limitations, frequency of seeking medical treatment, usual source of care, maternal-infant health, children's health, mental health, minorities' health, and environmental and occupational health risks (Bennett et al, 2008; Gamm et al, 2003; OSHA, 2010). Residents of rural areas suffer some of the same health problems as migrant farmworkers, as described in Chapter 34, including exposure to environmental factors and accidents.

DID YOU KNOW?   *Compared with urban Americans, rural residents have the following health disparities:*

- *Higher infant and maternal morbidity rates*
- *Higher rates of chronic illness, including heart disease, chronic obstructive pulmonary disease, unintentional motor vehicle traffic-related injuries, suicide, hypertension, cancer, and diabetes*
- *Unique health risks associated with occupations and the environment, such as machinery accidents, skin cancer from sun exposure, and respiratory problems associated with exposure to production chemicals*
- *Stress-related health problems and mental illness (although incidence not known)*
- *Disparities in access to health promotion and anticipatory guidance services*

Perceived Health Status

In general, people in rural areas have a poorer perception of their overall health and functional status than their urban counterparts. Rural residents over 18 years of age assess their health status less favorably than do urban residents. Studies show that rural adults are less likely to engage in preventive behavior, which ultimately increases exposure to risk. Specifically, they are more likely to use tobacco products and self-report higher rates of alcohol consumption and obesity; furthermore, they are less likely to engage in routine physical activity during leisure time, wear seat belts, have regular blood pressure checks, have Pap smears, complete breast self-examinations, and have colorectal screenings. Ultimately, failure to participate in health-promoting lifestyle behaviors affects the overall health status of rural residents, their level of function, physical limitations, degree of mobility, and level of self-care activities (American Legacy Foundation, 2009; Bennett et al, 2008; Gamm et al, 2003; NCHS, 2010; USDHHS, 2010b).

Chronic Illness

Rural adults are more likely than urban adults to have one or more of the following chronic conditions: heart disease, chronic obstructive pulmonary disease, hypertension, arthritis and rheumatism, diabetes, cardiovascular disease, and cancer. Nearly half of all rural adults have been diagnosed with at least one of these chronic conditions, compared with about one fourth of non-rural adults. Also, the prevalence of diagnosed diabetes in rural adults is about 7 out of 100 as opposed to 5 out of 100 in non-rural environments. Rural adults are more likely to have cancer (almost 7%) compared with urban adults (about 5%). Although most cases of acquired immunodeficiency syndrome (AIDS) are still found in urban areas, the rate is increasing in some rural populations (Bennett et al, 2008; Gamm et al, 2003; NCHS, 2010).

Rural-urban health disparities have been documented in health status (Box 19-2) and for health behaviors (Box 19-3). For example, there are disparities in the proportion of rural adults who receive medical treatment for both life-threatening illness, and degenerative or chronic conditions compared with urban adults. The proportion of rural residents who receive these treatments is high in rural versus urban areas. Life-threatening conditions include malignant neoplasms, heart disease,

---

BOX 19-2   DISPARITIES AMONG U.S. URBAN (METROPOLITAN) AND RURAL (MICROPOLITAN) RESIDENTS' HEALTH STATUS

Residents of fringe counties near large metro areas have the following:
- Lowest levels of premature mortality, partly reflecting lower death rates for unintentional injuries, homicide, and suicide
- Lowest levels of smoking, alcohol consumption, and child bearing among adolescents
- Lowest prevalence of physical inactivity during leisure time among women
- Lowest levels of obesity among adults
- Greatest number of physician specialists and dentists per capita
- Lowest percentage of the population without health insurance
- Lowest percentage of the population who had no dental visits

Residents in the most rural counties have the following:
- Highest death rates for children and young adults
- Highest death rates for unintentional and motor vehicle traffic–related injuries
- Highest death rates among adults for ischemic heart disease and suicide
- Highest levels of smoking among adolescents
- Highest levels of physical activity during leisure time among men
- Highest levels of obesity among adults
- Highest percentage of adults with activity limitations caused by chronic health conditions
- Fewest physician specialists and dentists per capita
- Least likely to have seen a dentist
- Highest percentage of the population without health insurance

From Centers for Disease Control and Prevention: *United States, 2001—urban and rural chartbook*, Washington, DC. Available at http://www.cdc.gov/nchs/data/hus/hus01.pdf. Accessed December 22, 2010; Gamm L, Hutchison L, Dabney B, Dorsey A: *Rural healthy people 2010: a companion document to Health People 2010 (Vol. I, II, III)*, 2003. Available at http://www.srph.tamhsc.edu/centers/rhp2010/publications.htm. Accessed June 28, 2005.

BOX 19-3 RURAL-URBAN DISPARITIES: LIFESTYLE AND HEALTH BEHAVIORS

- Residents in any rural areas are more likely to report fair to poor health status (19.5%) than were residents of urban counties (15.6%).
- Rural residents are more likely to report having diabetes (9.6%) versus urban adults (8.4%).
- Rates of diabetes are markedly higher among rural American Indians (15.2%) and Black adults (15.1%).
- Rural residents are more likely to be obese (27.4%) versus urban residents (23.9%).
- Rural black adults are particularly at risk for obesity; ranging from 38.9% in rural micropolitan counties to 40.7% in remote rural counties.
- Rural residents are less likely to meet CDC recommendations for moderate or vigorous physical activity (44%) versus urban residents (45.4%).
- Rural African-American adults are less likely to meet recommendations for physical activity than other rural residents; this difference persists across all levels of rurality.

Access to Healthcare Services

- Rural residents are more likely to be uninsured (17.8%) versus urban residents (15.3%).
- Hispanic adults are more likely to lack insurance, with uninsured rates ranging from 40.8% in rural micropolitan counties to 56.1% in small remote counties.
- Most rural residents (81%) and urban residents (79.4%) report having a personal health care provider. However, residents in remote rural counties were least likely to have a personal physician (78.7%).

- Rural white adults are more likely to have a personal health care provider than were other adults. Among Hispanic adults, the proportion with a personal provider ranged from 60.4% in rural micropolitan counties to 47.7% in remote rural counties.
- Rural adults are more likely than urban adults to defer seeking health care because of cost (15.1% vs 13.1%)
- Rural adult African Americans, Hispanics, and American Indians are more likely to report having deferred care due to cost compared with white rural residents.

Receipt of Preventive Services

- Rural women are less likely (70.7%) than urban women (77.9%) to be in compliance with mammogram screening guidelines.
- Rural women are less likely (86%) than urban women (91.4%) to have had a Pap smear within the past 3 years.
- Rural residents over age 50 years are less likely (57.7%) to have had a colorectal screening versus urban counterparts (61.4%).

Quality of Diabetes Care

- The proportion of adults with diabetes who reported receiving at least two hemoglobin A1c tests within the past year was low among both rural (33.1%) and urban residents (35%).
- White rural residents with diabetes were more likely than African-American or Hispanic residents to receive at least two hemoglobin A1c tests in the past year.
- Only 64.2% of rural and 69.1% or urban residents with diabetes reported receiving an annual dilated eye examinations.

From Bennett K, Olatosi B, Probst J: *Health disparities: a rural-urban chartbook,* 2008. Available at http://rhr.sph.sc.edu/report/(73)%20Health%20Disparities%20A%20Rural%20Urban%20Chartbook%20-%20Distribution%20Copy.pdf. Accessed December 8, 2011.

---

cardiovascular problems, and liver disorders. Degenerative or chronic diseases include diabetes, kidney disease, arthritis, and chronic diseases of the circulatory, nervous, respiratory, and digestive systems. In essence, chronic health conditions, coupled with their poor health status, limit the physical activities of a larger proportion of rural residents than of their urban counterparts (Bennett et al, 2008; Gamm et al, 2003; NCHS, 2010).

DID YOU KNOW?

- *Americans who live in the suburbs are significantly healthier on several key health measures than those who live in the most rural and most urban areas of the nation.*
- *Death rates for working-age adults are higher in the most rural and the most highly populated urban areas. The highest death rates for children and young adults exist in the most rural counties.*
- *Residents of rural areas have the highest death rates for unintentional injuries in general, and for motor vehicle injuries in particular.*
- *Homicide rates are highest in the central counties of large metro areas. Suicide rates are highest in the most rural areas.*
- *Suburban residents are more likely to exercise during leisure time and more likely to have health insurance. Suburban women are the least likely to be obese.*
- *Both the most rural and the most urban areas have a high percentage of residents without health insurance. Residents in the most rural communities have the fewest dental visits.*
- *Teenagers and adults in rural counties are more likely to smoke and use tobacco products.*

- *The AIDS rates are increasing more quickly in rural areas (30%) than in metropolitan areas (25.8%). Rural populations (fewer than 50,000) have the highest rates of increase in AIDS cases, representing 6.7% of all cases in the United States, with heterosexual contact accounting for most cases in many areas.*
- *In rural areas, gay men often are not openly gay and tend to engage in unprotected sex with strangers. Homophobia, racism, sexism, and AIDS stigma make HIV prevention efforts nearly impossible in some rural areas. Migration of people from urban to rural areas is cited as one possible contributor to the increased rates in rural areas. Among HIV-infected persons, more interstate than intrastate migration takes place from time of diagnosis until death.*

From Bennett K, Olatosi B, Probst J: Health disparities: a rural-urban chartbook, 2008. Available at http://rhr.sph.sc.edu/report/(7-3)%20Health%20Disparities%20A%20Rural%20Urban%20Chartbook%20-%20Distribution%20Copy.pdf. Accessed January 8, 2011; Gamm L, Hutchison L, Dabney B, et al: Rural Healthy People 2010: a companion document to Healthy People 2010, Vol I, II, III, College Station, TX, 2003, The Texas A&M University System Health Science Center, School of Rural Health, Southwest Rural Health Research Center. Available at http://www.srph.tamhsc.edu/centers/rhp2010/publications.htm. Accessed January 8, 2011.

Physical Limitations

Limitations in mobility and self-care are strong indicators of an individual's overall health status. Specific assessed measures on a national health survey included walking one block, walking uphill or climbing stairs, bending, lifting, stooping, feeding, dressing, bathing, and toileting. In fact, 9% of rural adults report at least three or more of these physical limitations, compared with 6% of metropolitan adults. The increased prevalence of poor health status and impaired function is not necessarily attributable to the increased number of older adults found in rural areas. Similar patterns are evident in adults 18 to 64 years of age. Rural adults under 65 years of age are more likely than urban adults to assess their health status as fair to poor, and a greater percentage have been diagnosed with a chronic health condition (Bennett et al, 2008; NCHS, 2010; USDHHS, 2010b).

Based on data from national health surveys, the overall health status of rural adults leaves much to be desired. This is attributed to a number of factors, including impaired access to health care providers and services, coupled with other rural factors. Thus nurses who practice in areas play an important role in providing a continuum of care to clients living in these underserved areas. Specifically, nurses can help clients have healthier lives by teaching them how to prevent accidents, engage in more healthful lifestyle behaviors, and reduce the risk of chronic health problems. Once clients in rural environments have been diagnosed with a long-term problem, nurses can help them manage chronic conditions to achieve better health outcomes and functioning (Nelson and Stover-Gingerich, 2010).

Patterns of Health Service Use

When the use of health care services is measured, it is found that more than three fourths of adults in rural areas received medical care on at least one occasion during a year. Despite their overall poorer health status and higher incidence of chronic health conditions, rural adults seek medical care less often than urban adults. In part, this discrepancy can be attributed to scarce resources and lack of providers in rural areas. Other reasons for this phenomenon are discussed later under Rural Health Care Delivery Issues and Barriers to Care (AHCPR, 2009; IOM, 2004; Cromartie, 2008; NACRHHS, 2008).

> **NURSING TIP** *Nurses must be especially thorough in their health assessment of rural clients who may not receive regular care for chronic health conditions.*

Availability and Access of Health Care

The ability of a person to identify a usual source of care is considered a favorable indicator of access to health care and a person's overall health status. Essentially, a person who has a usual source of care is more likely to seek care when ill and adhere to prescribed regimens. Having the same provider of care can enhance continuity of care, as well as a client's perception of the quality of that care. Rural adults are more likely than urban adults to identify a particular medical provider as their usual source of care. Rural adults are more likely to receive care from general practitioners and advanced practice registered nurses (APRNs) compared to urban adults who are more likely to seek care from a medical specialist. However, this trend may be changing with

health care reform, which emphasizes the importance of primary care (BHPR, 2007, 2009; USDHHS, 2010a,c).

Another measure of access to care is traveling time and/or distance to ambulatory care services. Rural persons who seek ambulatory care are more likely to travel more than 30 minutes to reach their usual source of care. Extended commuting time may also be a factor for residents in highly populated urban areas and those who must rely on public transportation. Once the person arrives at the clinic or physician's office, no differences between rural and urban residents are found in the waiting time to see the provider.

In general there is a maldistribution of health professionals among rural and urban counties. For instance, 1 out of 17 rural counties is reported to have no physician. Among rural respondents on national surveys, the ability to identify a usual site of care or a particular provider often stems from a community or county having only one, perhaps two, health care providers. The limited number of health care facilities is reinforced by the finding that nearly all rural residents who seek health care use ambulatory services that are provided in a physician's office as opposed to a clinic, community health center, hospital outpatient department, or emergency department (Gamm et al, 2003; IOM, 2004). One can speculate about the indicator of *usual place and usual provider*; that is to say, it suggests that rural residents are at least as well off as urban residents in regard to access to care (Woolston, 2010). However, this finding may be related to the fact that rural physicians tend to live and practice in a particular community for decades, thus providing care to multigenerational families who seek care from this particular provider.

Moreover, in a **health professional shortage area (HPSA)**, a physician or a nurse practitioner may provides services to residents who live in surrounding counties. Or, one or two nurses in a county public health department usually offer a full range of services for all residents in a catchment area, which may span more than 100 miles from one end of a county to the other. Consequently, rural physicians and nurses frequently report, "I provide care to individuals and families with all kinds of conditions, in all stages of life, and across several generations." It should not come as a surprise that rural respondents who participate in national surveys are able to identify a usual source and a usual provider of health care (BHPR, 2009; NCHS, 2010).

Maternal-Infant Health

Reports in the literature conflict regarding pregnancy outcomes in rural areas. Overall, rural populations have higher infant and maternal morbidity rates, especially counties designated as HPSAs, which often have a high proportion of racial minorities. Here one also finds fewer specialists, such as pediatricians, obstetricians, and gynecologists, to provide care to at-risk populations. There are extreme variations in pregnancy outcomes from one part of the country to another, and even within states. For example, in several counties located in the north-central and intermountain states, the pregnancy outcome is among the finest in the United States. However, in several other counties within those same states, the pregnancy outcome is among the worst. Particularly at risk are women who live on or near Indian reservations, are migrant workers, and are of African-American descent residing in rural areas in southeastern states (Mead et al, 2008; NCFH, 2010).

Public health nurses appreciate the interactive effects of socioeconomic factors, such as income level (poverty), education level, age, employment-unemployment patterns, and use of prenatal services, on pregnancy outcomes. There are other, less well-known health determinants, such as environmental hazards, occupational risks, and the cultural meaning placed on child-bearing and child-rearing practices by a community. The interaction effects of these multifaceted factors vary and often are difficult to measure.

Health of Children

Reports on the health status of rural children show regional variations and conflicting data. Comparing rural with urban children under 6 years of age on the measures of access to providers and use of services reveals the following (Bennett et al, 2008; Gamm et al, 2003):

- Urban children are less likely to have a usual provider but are more likely to see a pediatrician when they are ill.
- Like rural adults, rural children are more likely to be cared for by a general practitioner who is identified as their usual caregiver.

School nurses play an important role in the overall health status of children in the United States. The availability of school nurses in rural communities also varies from region to region. More specifically, in frontier and rural areas of the United States, school nurses usually are scarce. In part, this deficit can be attributed to limited resources associated with very low local tax revenues and shortages of health personnel in those counties. In other words, there are fewer taxpayers living in those large geographic areas. Some frontier areas have fewer than four persons per square mile and a few areas have less than two persons per square mile. Consequently, rural county commissioners, like their urban counterparts, are forced to prioritize the allocation of scarce resources, in particular for essential public services such as maintaining the infrastructures of utilities, roads, bridges, and education; supporting a financially suffering county hospital; hiring a county health nurse; and offering school health services. In rural communities there are fewer resources overall; yet, certain public services must be provided to local residents—albeit in many situations with aging and outdated infrastructures.

Clearly, creativity is required by both community residents and local public health care providers to resolve health care and school nursing needs. Partnership arrangements, for example, have been negotiated by two or more counties that agree to share the cost of a "district" public health nurse. Other county commissioners have forged partnerships with an agency in an urban setting and contracted for specific health care services. In both of these situations, it is not unusual for the nurse to provide services to all children attending schools in the participating counties. In some frontier states, schools may be situated more than 100 miles apart and as many miles or more from the district health office. Because of the number of schools and distances between them, the county nurse may be able to visit each

school only once or twice in a school term. Usually the nurse's visit is to update immunizations and perhaps teach maturation classes to students in the upper grades.

The health status of rural women, infants, and children is less than optimal. In part this can be attributed to inadequate preventive, primary, and emergency services to meet their particular health care needs. On one hand, scarce resources can pose a challenge to a nurse who provides care to rural residents, especially those in underserved areas. On the other hand, resource deficits encourage creativity and innovation; both of these behaviors are characteristic of nursing in general and of rural nurses in particular.

Mental Health

Like many other measures of health, the facts about the mental health status of rural people are also ambiguous and conflicting (Gale and Lambert, 2006; Merwin, 2008; Moore et al, 2005; USDHHS, 2010b). Stress, stress-related conditions, and mental illness are prevalent among populations who are economically deprived. The increasing regulations imposed on agriculture, timber, and marine- and mining-related industries in the last two decades led to many job losses in rural communities. The term *farm stress* is associated with the economic downturn in the agriculture industry as it impacts an individual, family, and the community. This same term or diagnosis could be applied to other communities experiencing economic recessions in their predominate enterprises, such as marine-, automobile-, and timber-related industries. Economic factors also contribute to a family's being underinsured or uninsured. Interestingly, even if mental health services are available and accessible, rural residents delay seeking care when they have an emotional problem until there is an emergency or a crisis. This behavior is reflected in the lower number of annual visits for mental health services and chronic health conditions by rural residents (Gamm et al, 2003).

Mental health professionals who serve rural populations report a persistent, endemic level of depression among residents in economically stressed rural areas. They speculate this condition is exacerbated by high levels of poverty, geographic isolation, and an insufficient number of mental health services. Depression may also contribute to the escalating incidence of accidents and suicides, especially among rural male adolescents and young men. These incidents have increased dramatically over the last decade and continue to rise within this group, to the point of being epidemic in some small communities. Likewise, the stigma associated with mental illness remains, especially in communities having fewer health care providers to educate the public about mental and behavioral health conditions (Gale and Lambert, 2006).

Reports on the prevalence of interpersonal violence and alcohol and substance use among rural populations are also conflicting. These behaviors are less likely to be reported in areas where residents are related or personally acquainted. Over time, destructive coping behaviors in small, tight-knit communities may be accepted by local residents as "business as usual" for a particular family. Family problems may also be ignored if formal social services and public health services are sparse or non-existent, or if residents do not trust the professionals who provide services at a local agency. In underserved rural areas, there are gaps in the continuum of mental health services, which, ideally, should include preventive education, anticipatory guidance, screenings, early intervention programs, crisis and acute care services, and follow-up care. As with other aspects of health care, nurses in rural areas play an important role in community education, case finding, advocacy, and case management of client systems experiencing acute and chronic emotional and behavioral health problems (Gale and Lambert, 2006; Moore et al, 2005).

Health of Minorities

As mentioned previously, a significant number of at-risk minority groups in rural America have some rather distinctive concerns (particularly children, older adults, Native Americans, Native Alaskans, Native Hawaiians, migrant workers, African Americans, and the homeless) (Gamm et al, 2003; Mead et al, 2008; NRHA, 2010; NCFH, 2010; USDHHS, 2010b). The rural homeless, for example, may be migrant farmworkers or local families whose home was foreclosed. Sometimes the family may be allowed by law to continue living in the house that once was theirs. The family no longer has a means of livelihood and often remains hidden in the community with insufficient income to purchase food or other necessary services. The particular health problems of these at-risk groups are discussed in Chapters 7 and 27 through 38. Nurses should be aware, however, that at-risk and underrepresented groups may experience some unique challenges associated with rural social structures, lifestyle, and sparse resources.

Environmental and Occupational Health Risks

A community's primary industry or industries are a determinant in the local lifestyle, the health status of its residents, and the number and types of health care services it may need. For example, four high-risk industries identified by the Occupational Safety and Health Administration (OSHA) and found in predominantly rural environments are forestry, mining, marine-related fields, and agriculture (Table 19-1). Associated health risks of these industries are machinery and vehicular accidents, trauma, selected types of cancer related to environmental factors, and allergies and respiratory conditions associated with repeated exposure to toxins, pesticides, and herbicides (NCFH, 2010; NCHS, 2010; OSHA, 2010; USDA, 2005, 2006).

For example, agriculture-production industries such as farming and ranching are often owned and operated by a family. Small enterprises with a very low number of employees do not fall under OSHA guidelines. For that reason safety standards are not enforceable on most farms and ranches, since these often are family enterprises. Moreover, small businesses, such as farms, are not covered under workers' compensation insurance. Additional concerns arise because family members participate in the farm or ranch work. This means that some adults and children may work with animals and operate dangerous machinery with minimal operating instructions on the hazards and on safety precautions. Also, it is not unusual for workers in agriculture to not be able to speak or read English.

Consequently, agriculture-related accidents result in a significant number of deaths and long-term injuries, particularly among children and women. The morbidity and mortality rates associated with agriculture vary from state to state. The rising incidence of these injuries and deaths, however, has become a national concern. Nurses in rural settings can help address this problem by including farm safety content in school and community education programs (NCHS, 2010; OSHA, 2010).

In summary, it is risky to generalize about the health status of rural Americans because of their diversity coupled with conflicting definitions of what differentiates rural from urban residences. Many vulnerable individuals and families live in rural communities across the United States, but little is known about most of them. This information deficit therefore is a potential area of research for nurses who practice in rural environments.

RURAL HEALTH CARE DELIVERY ISSUES AND BARRIERS TO CARE

Although each rural community is unique, the experience of living in a rural area has several common characteristics (Bushy, 2008a,b; AHCPR, 2009; UDSA, 2008a,b) (Box 19-4). Barriers to health care may be associated with these characteristics (e.g., whether services and professionals are available, affordable, accessible, or acceptable to rural consumers).

Availability implies the existence of health services as well as the necessary personnel to provide essential services. Sparseness of population limits the number and array of health care services in a given geographic region. Lacking a critical mass, the cost of providing special services to a few people often is prohibitive, particularly in frontier states where there are an insufficient number of physicians, nurses, and other types of health care providers. Consequently, where services and personnel are scarce, these must be allocated wisely. Accessibility implies that a person has logistical access to, as well as the ability to purchase, needed services. Affordability is associated with both availability and accessibility of care. It infers that services are of reasonable cost and that a family has sufficient resources to purchase these when needed. Acceptability of care means that a particular service is appropriate and offered in a manner that is congruent with the values of a target population. This can be hampered by a client's cultural preference and the urban orientation of health professionals (NACRHHS, 2008) (Box 19-5).

Providers' attitudes, insights, and knowledge about rural populations are also important. A patronizing or demeaning attitude, lack of accurate knowledge about rural populations, or insensitivity about the rural lifestyle on the part of a nurse can perpetuate difficulties in relating to those clients. Moreover, insensitivity perpetuates mistrust, resulting in rural clients' perceiving professionals as outsiders to the community. Some nurses in rural public health practice settings express feelings of professional isolation and community non-acceptance. To address disparate views, nursing faculty members should expose students to the rural environment and the people who live there. Clinical experiences must include opportunities to provide care to clients in their natural (e.g., rural) setting to gain accurate insight about a particular community.

TABLE 19-1   SELECT HEALTH CARE NEEDS, RISKS/CONDITIONS OF SELECT RURAL AGGREGATES

RURAL AGGREGATES	HEALTH CARE NEEDS	HEALTH RISKS/CONDITIONS
Farmers/ranchers	Advanced life support/emergency services Oral/dental care Obstetrical/perinatal/pediatric services Mental/behavioral health services Agricultural health nurses Geriatric specialists	Agricultural chemicals and environmental hazards Dermatitis Stress/depression/anxiety disorders Respiratory conditions (i.e., farmer's lung) Accidents (vehicular/machinery) Trauma-related chronic conditions Dental caries/loss Interpersonal/domestic violence
Native Americans	Advanced life support/emergency services Oral/dental care Obstetrical/perinatal/pediatric services Mental/behavioral health services Culturally appropriate substance abuse treatment programs Epidemiologists Diabetes screening and educators Community health workers/education	Infectious diseases (e.g., hepatitis, TB) Sudden infant death syndrome (SIDS) Interpersonal/domestic violence Diabetes Alcohol/substance abuse Cirrhosis of the liver Vehicular accidents Hypothermic/environmental injuries Trauma-related injuries/chronic conditions Dental caries/loss
African Americans	Community nursing health promotion and screening services Diabetes screening and educators Hypertension screening/education Prenatal and perinatal health care services Oncology services (education/screening/follow-up interventions) HIV/AIDS prevention education/screening/follow-up care Mental/behavioral health services	Diabetes Hypertension Sickle cell anemia Infectious diseases (e.g., hepatitis, HIV/AIDS) Cancer (e.g., prostate, breast) Dental caries/loss Depression Interpersonal/domestic violence
Migrant farmworkers	Environmental protection policies (safe drinking water/sanitation) Community nursing/migrant health services (primary, secondary, tertiary prevention) Diabetes screening and educators Hypertension screening/education Maternal/child services Oncology services (education/screening/follow-up interventions) Mental/behavioral health services	Infectious diseases (e.g., hepatitis, typhoid, TB, HIV/AIDS, STDs) Exposure effects of pesticides/herbicides Otitis media (children) Substance abuse (alcohol, recreational drugs, imported medicinal/herbs) Dental caries/loss Interpersonal/domestic violence
Native Alaskans	Advanced life support/emergency care services Medical transport services Oral/dental care Obstetrical/perinatal/pediatric services Mental/behavioral health services Culturally appropriate substance abuse treatment programs Epidemiologists Diabetes screening and educators	Infectious diseases (e.g., hepatitis, TB) Dental caries/loss Depression Interpersonal/domestic violence Environmental health risks (e.g., exposure to toxic substances/contaminants, hypothermia) Diabetes Alcohol/substance abuse Cirrhosis of the liver Vehicular accidents/trauma/long-term chronic residual effects
Coal miners	Occupational Safety and Health Administration policy/standards Mental/behavioral health services Emergency/advanced life support services Occupational health nurses Grief counselors	Depression/substance abuse Occupational-related accidents/trauma Respiratory conditions (e.g., black lung, chronic obstructive pulmonary disease) Interpersonal/domestic violence

Adapted from Bennett K, Olatosi B, Probst J: Health disparities: a rural- urban chartbook, 2008. Available at http://rhr.sph.sc.edu/report/(7-3)%20 Health%20Disparities%20A%20Rural%20Urban%20Chartbook%20-%20Distribution%20Copy.pdf. Accessed January 8, 2011; Gamm L, Hutchison L, Dabney B, et al: *Rural Healthy People 2010:* a companion document to *Healthy People 2010,* Vol I, II, III, College Station, TX, 2003, The Texas A&M University System Health Science Center, School of Rural Health, Southwest Rural Health Research Center. Available at http://www.srph.tamhsc.edu/centers/rhp2010/publications.htm. Accessed January 8, 2011.

To design population-focused programs that are available, accessible, affordable, and appropriate, nurses must implement interventions that mesh with clients' beliefs. This implies that a family and a community are actively involved in planning and delivering care for those who receive it. Nurses must have an accurate perspective of rural clients. Although the importance of forming partnerships and ensuring mutual exchange seems obvious, to date, most research about rural communities has been for policy or reimbursement purposes. Empirical data about rural family systems are sparse in terms of their health beliefs, values, perceptions of illness, and health care–seeking behaviors as well as what is deemed to be appropriate nursing care. Therefore, nurse scholars must assume a more active role in implementing research on the needs of rural populations for nursing services to expand the profession's theoretical base and subsequently implement community-oriented, empirically based clinical interventions (Bushy, 2009).

BOX 19-4 CHARACTERISTICS OF RURAL LIFE

- More space; greater distances between residents and services
- Cyclical/seasonal work and leisure activities
- Informal social and professional interactions
- Access to extended kinship systems
- Residents who are related or acquainted
- Lack of anonymity
- Challenges in maintaining confidentiality stemming from familiarity among residents
- Small (often family) enterprises; fewer large industries
- Economic orientation to land and nature with industries that are extractive in nature (e.g., agriculture, mining, lumbering, marine-related; outdoor recreational activities)
- More high-risk occupations
- Town as center of trade
- Churches and schools as socialization centers
- Preference for interacting with locals (insiders)
- Mistrust of newcomers to the community (outsiders)

BOX 19-5 BARRIERS TO HEALTH CARE IN RURAL AREAS

- Lack of health care providers and services
- Great distances to obtain services
- Lack of personal transportation
- Unavailable public transportation
- Lack of telephone services
- Unavailable outreach services
- Inequitable reimbursement policies for providers
- Unpredictable weather and/or travel conditions
- Inability to pay for care/lack of health insurance
- Lack of "know how" to procure publicly funded entitlements and services
- Inadequate provider attitudes and understanding about rural populations
- Language barriers (caregivers not linguistically competent)
- Care and services not culturally and linguistically appropriate

NURSING CARE IN RURAL ENVIRONMENTS

Theory, Research, and Practice

The body of literature on nursing practice in small towns and rural environments is growing, and several themes have emerged (Box 19-6). A nurse who practices in this setting can view each of these dimensions either as an opportunity or as a challenge.

Researchers from the University of Montana contend that existing theories do not fully explain rural nursing practice (Winters and Lee, 2009; Long and Weinert, 1989). These researchers examined the four concepts pertinent to nursing theory (health, person, environment, and nursing/caring) and proposed relational statements that are relevant to clients and nurses in rural environments (see the Evidence-Based Practice box). Because the focus of their research was Anglo Americans living in the Rocky Mountain area, care must be taken about generalizing those findings to other geographic regions and minorities. These researchers propose that rural residents often judge their health by their ability to work. They consider themselves healthy, even though they may suffer from several chronic illnesses, as long as they are able to continue working. For the rural person, being healthy is the ability to be productive.

BOX 19-6 CHARACTERISTICS OF NURSING PRACTICE IN RURAL ENVIRONMENTS

- Variety/diversity in clinical experiences
- Broader/expanding scope of practice
- Generalist skills
- Flexibility/creativity in delivering care
- Sparse resources (e.g., materials, professionals, equipment, fiscal)
- Professional/personal isolation
- Greater independence/autonomy
- Role overlap with other disciplines
- Slower pace
- Lack of anonymity
- Increased opportunity for informal interactions with clients/co-workers
- Opportunity for client follow-up upon discharge in informal community settings
- Discharge planning allowing for integration of formal and informal resources
- Care for clients across the life span
- Exposure to clients with a full range of conditions/diagnoses
- Status in the community (viewed as prestigious)
- Viewed as a professional role model
- Opportunity for community involvement and informal health education

From Bushy A: Conducting culturally competent rural nursing research. In Merwin B, editor: *Annual review of nursing research: focus on rural health,* 26:221-236, 2008; Hurme E: Competencies for nursing practice in a rural critical access hospital, *Online J Rural Nurs Health Care* 9(2):67-81, 2009. Available at http://www.rno.org/journal/index.php/online-journal/article/viewFile/198/256. Accessed January 8, 2011; Nelson W, editor: *Handbook for rural health care ethics,* Lebanon, NH, 2009, Dartmouth. Available at http://dms.dartmouth.edu/cfm/resources/ethics/. Accessed January 8, 2011; Winters C, Lee H: *Rural nursing: concepts, theory and practice,* ed 3, New York, 2009, Springer Publishing.

EVIDENCE-BASED PRACTICE

Nurse researchers at Montana State University proposed the following theoretical concepts and dimensions of rural nursing practice (Winters and Lee, 2009; Long and Weinert, 1999):

- **Health:** Defined by rural residents as the ability to work. Work and health beliefs are closely related for rural Montana sample.
- **Environment:** Distance and isolation are particularly important for rural dwellers. Those who live long distances neither perceive themselves as isolated nor perceive health care services as inaccessible.
- **Nursing:** Lack of anonymity, outsider versus insider, old-timer versus newcomer. Lack of anonymity is a common theme among rural nurses who report knowing most people for whom they care, not only in the nurse–client relationship, but also in a variety of social roles, such as family member, friend, or neighbor. Acceptance as a health care provider in the community is closely linked to the outsider/insider and newcomer/old-timer phenomena. Gaining trust and acceptance of local people is identified as a unique challenge that must be successfully negotiated by nurses before they can begin to function as effective health care providers.
- **Person:** Self-reliance and independence in relationship to health care are strong characteristics of rural individuals. They prefer to have people they know care for them (informal services) as opposed to an outsider in a formal agency.

Nurse Use

In working with rural residents, it is important to know how they define their health and their environment, since their definitions may differ from yours. Understand that you may not find acceptance and trust immediately; rural residents often trust informal caregivers more than those in a formal organization.

Long K and Weinert C: Rural nursing: developing a theory base, *Sch Inq Nurs Pract* 13(3):275-279, 1999; Winters C and Lee H: *Rural nursing: concepts, theory and practice,* ed 3, New York, 2009, Springer Publishing.

Chronically ill people emphasize emotional and spiritual well-being rather than physical wellness.

Distance, isolation, and sparse resources characterize rural life and are seen in residents' independent and innovative coping strategies. Self-reliance and independence are demonstrated through their self-care practices and preference for family and community support. Community networks provide support but still allow for each person's and family's independence. Ruralites prefer and usually seek help through their informal networks, such as neighbors, extended family, church, and civic clubs, rather than seeking a professional's care in the formal system of health care, including services such as those provided by a mental health clinic, social service agency, or health department.

Although nursing is generally similar across settings and populations, there are some unique features associated with practice in a geographically remote area or in small towns where most people know one another. The following paragraphs highlight a few of the variations that nurses in rural practice report (Hurme, 2009; Molinari and Monserud, 2008; Nelson, 2009; Skillman et al, 2007).

A nurse's professional and personal boundaries often overlap and are diffuse. It is not unusual for a nurse to have more than one work-related role in the community. For example, a nurse may work at the local hospital or in a physician's office and may also be actively involved in managing the family farm, a local grocery store, or pharmacy. For nurses, this means that many, if not all, clients they encounter are known also as neighbors, as friends of an immediate family member, or as part of one's extended family. Associated with social informality is a corresponding lack of anonymity in a small town. Some rural nurses say, "I never really feel like I am off duty because everybody in the county knows me through my work." In part, this can be attributed to nurses being highly respected and viewed by local people as experts on health and illness. Often rural residents informally ask a nurse's advice before seeing a physician for a health problem. Rural residents may ask health-related questions when they see a local nurse (who may be a neighbor, friend, or relative) in a grocery store, at a service station, during a basketball game, or at church functions.

Nurses in rural public health practice must make decisions about the care of individuals of all ages with a variety of health conditions. They assume many roles because of the range of services they provide in a rural health care facility and because of the scarcity of nurses and other health professionals. Nurses who work in rural areas need to have skills that include technical and clinical competency, adaptability, flexibility, strong assessment skills, organizational abilities, independence, interest in continuing education, sound decision-making skills, leadership ability, self-confidence, skills in handling emergencies, teaching, and public relations. The nurse administrator is also expected to be a jack-of-all-trades (i.e., a generalist) and to demonstrate competence in several clinical specialties in addition to managing and organizing staff within the facility for which he or she is responsible.

Rural nursing practice provides challenges, opportunities, and rewards. The way in which each factor is perceived depends on individual preferences and the situation in a given community. Challenges of rural practice sometimes include professional isolation, limited opportunities for continuing education, lack of other kinds of health personnel or professionals with whom one can interact, heavy workloads, an ability to function well in several clinical areas, lack of anonymity, and, for some, a restricted social life (Nelson, 2009; Roberge, 2009).

The most often cited opportunities and rewards in rural nursing practice are close relationships with clients and co-workers, diverse clinical experiences that evolve from caring for clients of all ages who have a variety of health problems, caring for clients for long periods of time (in some cases, across several generations), opportunities for professional development, and greater autonomy. Many nurses value the solitude and quality of life found in a rural community personally and for their own family. Others thrive on the outdoor recreational activities. Still others thoroughly enjoy the informal, face-to-face interactions coupled with the public recognition and status associated with living and working as a nurse in a small community. Disease prevention is also an important consideration in rural communities. The Levels of Prevention box shows the levels of prevention as they might be used by a nurse in a rural locale.

Although most of the publications about rural health care and nursing focus on hospital practice, much of that information is applicable to both community agencies and

LEVELS OF PREVENTION

Rural Health

Primary Prevention

The public health nurse partners with a women's organization in a faith community located in a small Midwestern town to instruct members on meal planning as a strategy to offset the tendency to develop diabetes in family members.

Secondary Prevention

The public health nurse screens congregation members of the faith community in the Midwestern town for the presence of diabetes.

Tertiary Prevention

The public health nurse collaborates with the senior center in the small community town, which provides meals on a routine basis to the elderly to reach individuals with a diagnosis of diabetes. The nurse provides consultation on diabetic nutrition, exercise habits, foot care, and, if needed, assists clients in obtaining medications through a mail-order pharmaceutical vendor.

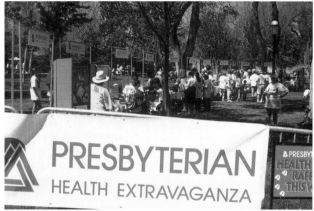

FIGURE 19-2 A hospital-sponsored health fair is one example of a community event to provide health services to individuals in a rural area.

community-focused nursing (Davis and Droes, 1993; Molinari and Monserud, 2008; Skillman et al, 2007). The work-related stressors of nursing in rural communities have received some attention in the literature. Case (1991) in the 1990s identified stressful experiences of nurses working in rural Oklahoma public health departments as including: political/bureaucratic problems and intraprofessional and interpersonal conflicts associated with inadequate communication; unsatisfactory work environment and understaffing; difficult or unpleasant nurse–client encounters, such as with relatives who refuse to deliver needed care to clients, and with clients who are hostile, apathetic, dependent, or of low intelligence; fear for personal safety; difficulty locating clients, and clients falling through the cracks of the health care system. These same stressors continue to be cited by nurses who work in rural as well as urban public health agencies. Anecdotal reports describe specific stressors associated with geographic distance, isolation, sparse resources, and other environmental factors that characterize rurality.

Nursing in rural areas is characterized by physical isolation that may lend itself to any one of the following: professional isolation; scarce financial, human, and health care resources; and a broad scope of practice. Associated with personal familiarity with local residents, nurses often possess in-depth knowledge about clients and their families. Along with the acknowledged benefits, informal (face-to-face) interactions can significantly reduce a nurse's anonymity in the community and at times be a barrier to completing an objective assessment on a client. Like urban practice, rural community nursing takes place in a variety of locations, including homes, clinics, schools, occupational settings, and correctional facilities, and at community events, such as county fairs, rodeos, civic and church-sponsored functions, and school athletic events (Figure 19-2).

Research Needs

Recent empirical studies on rural nursing practice reinforce anecdotal reports by nurses (Merwin, 2008; Graves, 2009). Specific research topics that are of importance to nursing

practice in rural environments include the following, among others:

1. Most nurses indicate that they enjoy practicing in rural areas and are proud of what they do. They believe, however, that their work deserves more recognition by professional nursing organizations. Furthermore, the retention rate of nurses in some practice settings is poor. The perspective of nurses who are dissatisfied with rural nursing is necessary to provide a more complete picture of the rural experience. This information can be useful to a variety of people: other nurses who are considering rural practice, nurse managers in need of better screening tools to assess the fit between the nurse and the environment when interviewing applicants, planners of continuing nursing education programs, and faculty members who teach public health to undergraduate and graduate students.

2. More information is needed about the stressors and rewards of rural practice, in particular public health nursing. These data could lead to the development of stress management techniques to be used by nurses and their supervisors to retain nurses and to improve the quality of their workplace environment.

3. With the increasing number of rural residents in all regions of the United States, empirical data are needed on the particular nursing needs of rural-client systems, especially underrepresented groups, minorities, and other at-risk populations that vary by region and state.

4. A need also exists for the international perspective on the health of rural populations, and on nursing practice within the rural community. Australian, New Zealand, and Canadian nurse scholars have provided some insights into rural practice in these nations. Information is needed from less-industrialized nations as well as from those that are highly industrialized.

5. Technology increasingly is used in health care and seems to hold great potential in improving access to health care in rural and underserved areas. However, research is needed to determine the most efficient and effective way to meet the needs and preferences of rural clients, and to ensure quality.

6. Communication technology increasingly is used by institutions of higher learning to deliver educational programs to nurses who live and work some distance from campus. Empirical studies are needed to measure the most effective modalities to achieve desired learning outcomes and the impact on recruitment and retention of nurses in rural settings.

7. Rural–urban disparities in health status and health behaviors need closer examination from the nursing perspective. Evidence-based practice nursing guidelines are needed that take into consideration the rural context and preferences of residents who obtain health care in these settings.

Preparing Nurses for Rural Practice Settings

Nurses in rural practice must have broad knowledge about nursing including health promotion, primary prevention, rehabilitation, obstetrics, medical-surgical specialties, pediatrics, planning and implementing community assessments, and understanding the public health risks and needs for emergency preparedness in a particular state. A community's demographic profile and its principal industry(ies) can provide a snapshot of some of its social, political, and health risks. Using demographic information, a nurse can anticipate the particular nursing skills that will be needed to care for clients in a catchment area (U.S.A. Center for Rural Health Preparedness, n.d.). In rural areas nurses use their knowledge of resources and their ability to coordinate formal and informal services in order to coordinate a continuum of services for clients even when resources are sparse and fragmentation exists in the health care delivery system.

Technology has great potential for connecting rural public health providers and consumers with resources outside of their community. The concept of *telehealth* is an expansion of the term *telemedicine*. Essentially, telemedicine more narrowly focuses on the curative aspect of health care, whereas telehealth encompasses preventive, promotive, and curative aspects of health care and can include delivery of education/information to a more distant site. Telehealth uses a variety of technology solutions such as a health care provider communicating by e-mail with clients, ordering medications from a pharmacy, consulting with other health care providers, or accessing advanced or continuing education offered by a university located some distance from the receiving site. More specifically, telecommunication technology could be as simple as nurses in two or more different public health settings consulting over the telephone or via computer video conferencing coordinating local health fairs, or as complex as nurse scholars collaborating with international peers on a community health–focused research project or a medical specialist located at a health science center completing complex robotic surgical technology on a client who is located in another country. Regardless of the practice setting, the nurse must be computer literate and be proficient in using the communication technology that is available in that community. Increasingly, the Internet is linking nurses in rural public health practice with nursing colleagues, educators, and researchers in urban-based academic settings, thereby addressing often-cited concerns associated with professional isolation (NRHA, 2007, 2008).

> **WHAT DO YOU THINK?** *There is disagreement about the manner in which rural (vs urban) is defined. Likewise, nursing scholars are debating whether or not rural nursing is a specialty practice having an empirically supported body of nursing knowledge.*

FUTURE PERSPECTIVES

It is important for all people involved in providing health care in rural areas to understand the possible problems they might encounter when trying to provide the continuum of needed services in an area with a disproportionally high number of underserved persons. Those who should be involved include residents, their elected representatives, the administrators of public and private health care agencies, and members of the media. The media need to focus on public health as well as hospital care and the lack of primary care providers in rural areas (Hurme, 2009; NRHA, 2007). As discussed later, both case management and primary health care (COPHC) have proved to be effective models for dealing with some of the care deficits and resolving rural health disparities.

Scarce Resources and a Comprehensive Health Care Continuum

The current fragmented health care system creates considerable difficulty in providing a comprehensive continuum of care to populations living in areas having scarce resources, such as money, personnel, equipment, and ancillary services. In rural communities, the most critically needed services are usually preventive services, such as health screening clinics, nutrition counseling, and wellness education (Gamm et al, 2003; Mead et al, 2008) (Box 19-7).

Although the nursing needs vary by community, there is generally a need in most rural areas for the following:
- School and parish nurses
- Family planning services
- Prenatal and postpartum services
- Resources for individuals diagnosed with HIV/AIDS and their families
- Emergency medical services
- Resources for families of children with special needs, including those who are physically and mentally challenged
- Mental and mental health services
- Resources for older adults (especially the frail elderly and those with declining mental capacity) to include a continuum of residential and respite services, including adult day care, hospice, homemaker assistance, and provision of nutritional meals along with public transportation for those who remain at home

Providing a continuum of care has been further hindered by the closure of many small hospitals in the past 2 decades. Of those that remain, many report financial problems that could lead to closure (NACRHHS, 2008; USDA, 2006). A shortage or the absence of even one provider, most often a physician or nurse, could mean that a small hospital must close its doors. Closure of the hospital has a ripple effect on the health of local residents, other health care services, recruiting and retaining

BOX 19-7   HEALTH-RELATED PRIORITIES FOR MANY RURAL COMMUNITIES

- Access to care
- Cancer (screening, early intervention, oncology services)
- Diabetes (prevention, screening, tertiary care)
- Maternal/Infant and children services
- Mental illness and behavioral health services
- Nutrition/obesity
- Drugs, alcohol, and substance abuse
- Use of tobacco products
- Education and an array of community-based programs
- Public health infrastructures
- Immunizations and infectious diseases
- Injury and violence prevention
- Family planning
- Environmental and occupational health
- Emergency medical services infrastructures
- Long-term care/assistive living facilities

From Bennett K, Olatosi B, Probst J: Health disparities: a rural- urban chartbook, 2008. Available at http://rhr.sph.sc.edu/report/(7-3)%20Health%20Disparities%20A%20Rural%20Urban%20Chartbook%20-%20Distribution%20Copy.pdf. Accessed January 8, 2011; Gamm L, Hutchison L, Dabney B, et al: *Rural Healthy People 2010:* a companion document to *Healthy People 2010,* Vol I, II, III, College Station, TX, 2003, The Texas A&M University System Health Science Center, School of Rural Health, Southwest Rural Health Research Center. Available at http://www.srph.tamhsc.edu/centers/rhp2010/publications.htm. Accessed January 8, 2011.

 HEALTHY PEOPLE 2020

These selected objectives pertain to residents of both rural and urban areas:
- AHS-3: Increase the proportion of persons with a usual primary care provider.
- IVP-13: Reduce motor vehicle crash–related deaths.
- MHMD-9: Increase the proportion of adults with mental disorders who receive treatment.
- HDS-2: Reduce coronary heart disease deaths.
- IVP-1: Reduce fatal and non fatal injuries.

From U.S. Department of Health and Human Services. *Healthy People 2020,* 2010. Available at http://www.healthypeople.gov/2020/default.aspx. Accessed January 9, 2011.

health professionals, as well as on economic development efforts in a small community (USDA, 2008a,b).

The short supply and increasing demand for primary care providers in general, and nurses in particular, will continue for some time. To help solve this problem, elected officials and policy developers need nurses, especially those in advanced practice roles, to provide vital services in underserved areas. In an effort to effectively respond to this opportunity, nurses must be creative to ensure delivery of appropriate and acceptable services to at-risk and vulnerable populations who live in rural and underserved regions. Nurses must be sensitive to the health beliefs of clients, and then plan and provide nursing interventions that mesh with the community's cultural values and preferences.

Healthy People 2020 National Health Objectives Related to Rural Health

Because the demographic profile varies from community to community, each state has variations in the health status of its population. *Healthy People 2020* has important implications for nurses in that a significant number of at-risk populations cited in that policy-guiding document live in rural areas across the United States (Gamm et al, 2003; USDHHS, 2010b,c). Consequently, priority objectives vary, depending on population mix, health risks, and health status of residents in the state.

At the local level, communities have been using *Healthy People* as a guide for action and to identify objectives and establish meaningful goals. The three-volume *Rural Healthy People 2010: A Companion Document to Healthy People 2010* focused on the particular concerns relative to vulnerable populations in rural environments (Gamm et al, 2003). It remains to be seen if a parallel rural compendium will be developed for *Healthy People 2020.*

The Center for Disease Control's (CDC, 2010) *Healthy Communities Initiative* mobilized rural as well as urban communities to focus on chronic disease prevention. Individuals and groups at the local level collaborated with state health departments, the CDC, and other organizations to implement programs that promote and support good health in their community. This CDC initiative is a useful tool for state and local officials and health care planners to use to tailor *Healthy People* objectives to fit a community's specific needs. For example, *Healthy Communities: A Rural Action Guide* (North Carolina Smart Growth Alliance, 2004) addressed features of rural communities and complements CDC's *Healthy Community Initiative*; and both promote establishing professional-community partnerships. Translating national objectives highlighted in *Healthy People 2020* (USDHHS, 2010a) into achievable community health goals requires integration of the following components to ensure that services will be acceptable and appropriate for rural clients:

- Health statistics must be meaningful and understandable, and they must include appropriate process and outcome objectives that can be readily measured.
- Strategies must be designed that involve the public, private, and voluntary sectors of the community to achieve agreed-upon local objectives.
- Coordinated efforts are needed to ensure that the community works together to achieve the goals.

Consider, for example, general objectives in developing a health plan for a rural county having a large population of young people. *Healthy People 2020* objectives for the county should target women of child-bearing age, children, and adolescents. Priority objectives should include offering accessible prenatal care programs, improving immunization levels, providing preventive dental care instructions, implementing vehicular accident prevention and firearm safety programs, and educating teachers and health professionals for early identification of cases of domestic violence. On the other hand, consider a rural county that has a higher number of residents over the age of

65 years, compared with the national average. Priority objectives in the health plan should target health risks and problems of older adults in that community. Specific objectives might include developing health-promoting programs to prevent chronic health problems, or establishing community programs to meet the needs of those having chronic illness, specifically cardiovascular disease, diabetes, hypertension, and accident-related disabilities; or, organizing a partnership to build progressive/assistive care residential facilities in the community. In general the objectives in *Healthy People 2020* are pertinent to people living in all areas and not unique to rural residents. The *Healthy People 2020* box illustrates selected objectives that fit people in rural as well as more urban areas.

When implementing community-focused health plans that emerge from *Healthy People 2020*, consideration must always be given to the rural context, such as sparse population, geographic remoteness, scarce resources, personnel shortages, and physical, emotional, and social isolation. In addition to being actively involved in empowering the community and planning and delivering care, nurses play an important role in representing their community's perspective to local, state, regional, and national health planners and to their elected officials.

THE CUTTING EDGE   *Community prevention programs require scientific evidence to demonstrate their effectiveness. Although rural public health agencies implement many such programs, often these are fettered by low budgets and small staffs, with restricted access to evaluation experts and information resources. Furthermore, community-oriented health promotion programs in rural areas may work differently from those in more populated settings. Program evaluation can be hampered by lack of control groups and the instability that is associated with small populations. An exemplary rural model was developed by the Mississippi State University Extension Service, which partnered with community leaders in Oktibbeha County Mississippi to develop the Smart Aging: Healthy Futures program. This initiative was designed to help underserved rural communities foster healthy aging among their senior population. The initiative included organizing forums that involve the community in dialogue to identify challenges that hinder healthy aging and note formal and informal resources that are supportive within a particular county. These public forums also facilitated emergence of grassroots community action groups that focused on identifying and developing local solutions addressing the concerns and health-related needs of elderly residents. Another component of the initiative was delivering health promotion programs for local elderly along with their families and support systems. The university-community partnership lead to evidence-based outcomes related to health promotion for Mississippi's rural-based elderly programs. This innovative program could serve as a model for other rural communities who have an interest in responding to the needs of the elderly.*

Adapted from Mississippi State University Extension Service: A community report of Oktibbeha County: Smart aging—healthy futures, Mississippi State, MS, 2009, MSUES. USDA Grant Award # 2007461000395608010087. Available at http://msucares.com/health/smart_aging/community_reports.html. Accessed January 8, 2011.

BUILDING PROFESSIONAL-COMMUNITY-CLIENT PARTNERSHIPS IN RURAL SETTINGS

Health care reform initiatives are focusing on cutting costs while improving access to care with equitable quality for all citizens, especially vulnerable and underserved populations. State and local grass roots organizations must be actively involved if health care reform succeeds in rural areas. Specifically, professional-client-community partnerships are essential in order to accomplish reform at the local level. As seen in the Linking Content to Practice box, nursing practice in rural areas is comprehensive and incorporates skills from nursing and public health. Two models have been found to be particularly useful for nurses in rural environments: case management and COPHC.

🌐 LINKING CONTENT TO PRACTICE

As discussed, practice in rural areas relies on excellent nursing and public health skills in assessment, communication, cultural competency, problem solving, coalition building, coordination, and policy development among others. Documents that guide the practice include the American Nurses Association Standards of Nursing Practice, the core competencies as identified by the Council on Linkages, and the Quad Council Public Health Nursing Competencies. As one example of the congruence, consider assessment. The Council on Linkages' Core Competency of "Assess the health status of populations and their related determinants of health and illness" under their analytic assessment skills is then elaborated on by the Quad Council as a public health nursing skill of "Conducts thorough health assessments of individuals, families, communities and populations" and the public health nursing practice standard under assessment of "the public health nurse collects comprehensive data pertinent to the health status of populations" (p 15). The relationship among these three sets of standards continues through all phases of the public health care provision process.

From American Nurses Association: *Public health nursing: scope and standards of practice,* Silver Spring, MD, 2007, Available at http://www.nursebooks.org; Public Health Foundation: Council on linkages: *Core competencies for public health professionals,* 2008, Washington, DC, Author. Available at http://www.phf.org/link/index.htm. Accessed June 24, 2010; Quad Council: *Public health nursing competencies,* 2009. Available at http://www.astdn.org/publications_quad_council_phn_competencies.htm. Accessed January 17, 2011.

Case Management

Case management is a client-professional partnership that can be used to arrange a continuum of care for rural clients, with the case manager tailoring and blending formal and informal resources. Collaborative efforts between a client and the case manager allow clients to participate in their plan of care in an acceptable and appropriate way, especially when local resources are few and far between. The Practice Application at the end of this chapter demonstrates how nursing case management can allow an older adult resident to stay at home in a rural environment if adequate supports can be provided. Outcomes are often remarkably different when case management is used. Additional information on case management is found in Chapter 22.

<table>
<tr><td>

BOX 19-8 COMMUNITY-ORIENTED PRIMARY HEALTH CARE (COPHC): A PARTNERSHIP PROCESS

The steps in the COPHC process include the following:
- Define and characterize the community.
- Identify the community's health problems.
- Develop or modify health care services in response to the community's identified needs.
- Monitor and evaluate program process and client outcomes.

</td></tr>
</table>

Community-Oriented Primary Health Care

COPHC is an effective model for delivering available, accessible, and acceptable services to vulnerable populations living in medically underserved areas. This model emphasizes flexibility, grassroots involvement, and professional-community partnerships. It blends primary care, public health, and prevention services, which are offered in a familiar and accessible setting. The COPHC model is interprofessional, uses a problem-oriented approach, and mandates community involvement in all phases of the process (McGinnis, 2003; Nelson, 2009) (Box 19-8).

Building professional-community partnerships is an ongoing process. At various times, nurses, other health professionals, and community leaders must assume the role of advocate, change agent, educator, expert, or group facilitator to gain both active and passive support from the community. Partnerships involve give-and-take negotiations by all participants to reach consensus. Essentially, the process begins with professionals gaining entrance into a community, establishing rapport and trust with local people, and then working together to empower the community to resolve mutually defined problems and goals. As mentioned previously and discussed also in Chapter 20, the *Healthy Communities Initiative* is an excellent resource for developing, defining, and responding to the stated goals. Because of the importance of churches and schools in a rural community, leaders from those institutions often are key players in building provider-community partnerships. The organizational phase is a priority since it forms the foundation for all other activities related to planning, implementing, and evaluating community initiatives.

As was described for case management, professional-community partnerships allow more effective identification of existing informal support systems that are accepted by rural residents. The goal is to integrate community preferences with new or existing formal services. Public input should be encouraged early in the planning process and must continue throughout the process to allow the community to feel that it has ownership in the project. This strategy can go a long way to address local

residents viewing the process as an outsider bringing another bureaucratic program into town. Strategies that nurses can use to enhance the building of partnerships in rural environments are listed in the How To Build Professional-Community-Client Partnerships box.

HOW TO Build Professional-Community-Client Partnerships

1. *Gain the local perspective.*
2. *Assess the degree of public awareness and support for the cause.*
3. *Identify special interest groups.*
4. *List existing services to avoid duplication of programs.*
5. *Note real and potential barriers to existing resources and services.*
6. *Generate a list of potential community volunteers and professionals who are willing to assist with the project.*
7. *Create awareness among target groups of a particular program (e.g., individuals, families, seniors, church and recreation groups, health care professionals, law enforcement personnel, and members of other religious, service, and civic clubs).*
8. *Identify potential funding sources needed to implement the program.*
9. *Establish the community's health care priority list, and involve many community members in considering and selecting their health care options.*
10. *Incorporate business principles in marketing the program.*
11. *Measure the health system's local economic impact.*
12. *Educate residents about the important role the local health care system plays in the economic infrastructure of the community and the consequences of a system failure.*
13. *Develop local leadership and support for the community's health system through training and providing experience in decision making.*

From McGinnis P: Rural policy development: a community leadership development approach, Kansas City, MO, 2003, National Rural Health Association.

Partnership models, such as case management and COPHC, have proven to be highly effective in areas with scarce resources and an insufficient number of health care providers. Individuals and communities who are informed, active participants in planning are more likely to develop consensus about the most appropriate solution for local problems. Subsequently, involved participants are more likely to use and support that system after it is implemented. Partnership models enhance the ability of rural communities to do what they historically have done well (i.e., assume responsibility for the services and institutions that serve their residents). Knowledge about partnership models and the skills to effectively implement them are useful for nurses who coordinate services that are accessible, available, and acceptable for rural populations in their catchment area.

PRACTICE APPLICATION

Mrs. Jones, an 89-year-old widow, was diagnosed over 10 years ago with progressive congestive heart failure. She continues to live in her beloved home of 60+ years in spite of being on continuous oxygen the last 3 years. She also has "bad knees" and gets around her house and yard with the use of a walker. Her husband of more than 60 years suddenly died 4 years ago of a heart attack while working on their farm. Their two married daughters live in California and Arkansas. The Midwestern town where she lives has about 1000 residents. The nearest hospital is more than 60 miles away from this town. Mrs. Jones's 82-year-old widowed sister, Lydia Thomas, lives a few blocks from her. Their 76-year-old brother recently entered the county nursing home located in a town 20 miles away.

Even with her dyspnea and physical limitations, Mrs. Jones is able to live alone with her dog and cat, and insists that she will not relinquish her independent lifestyle as has her brother. Yet, in the past year she has been hospitalized three times: for a bad chest cold, for a kidney infection, and after a neighbor found her lying unconscious by the picnic table in her yard. Her doctor says this episode was related to a "heart problem."

Upon being discharged from the hospital, Crystal Moore, the local home-health nurse, was assigned to visit Mrs. Jones. Ms. Moore's office is based in the County Senior Center near the nursing home where the brother is a resident. He is also a client of Ms. Moore and she visits him every Wednesday. The nurse provides outreach services to all the residents in the county referred to her by a large home-health agency located in the city 70 miles away. As a case manager, she works closely with the hospital's discharge planners to arrange a continuum of care for clients in the county. Nursing-related activities include coordinating formal and informal services for clients, including biomedical supplies, oxygenation, nutrition, hydration, pharmacological care, arranging for personal care, homemaker assistance, writing checks, home maintenance, emergency respite services, and home delivery of meals.

A. Describe the nursing roles that Ms. Moore uses in coordinating a continuum of care for Mrs. Jones in terms of nutrition, oxygenation, pharmaceutical, and biomedical equipment, transportation, and homemaker assistance.

B. Identify formal health care and support resources that can be accessed for Mrs. Jones.

C. Identify informal support resources that might be available in the small community that could help to ensure that Mrs. Jones is safe.

D. Identify three outcomes for Mrs. Jones that can be achieved by using nursing care (case) management.

E. Select a rural community in your geographic area. Create hypothetical situations, or select real clients with real health problems (e.g., an older adult with Alzheimer's disease, a middle-aged person with cancer requiring end-of-life care, a child who is dependent on technology as a result of a farm accident). Prepare a list of services and referral agencies in that community that could be used to develop a continuum of care for each of these cases. How are these the same as, or different from, the case described in this chapter?

F. How could a public or home health nurse who is new to the community learn about formal and informal resources that could be accessed to develop a continuum of care for a rural resident for whom she cares?

Answers can be found on the Evolve site.

KEY POINTS

- There is wide diversity in the demography, economy, and geography of rural communities.
- Not all rural communities are based on an agricultural economy; most are not!
- Although many are struggling, not all rural communities are suffering economically. Some rural communities only need more extensive economic development for sustainability.
- Some rural towns are located in urban counties.
- There are wide variations in the health status of rural populations, depending on genetic, social, environmental, economic, and political factors.
- There is a higher prevalence of working poor in rural America than in more populated areas.
- There are rural-urban health disparities. Rural adults 18 years and older overall are in poorer health than their urban counterparts; nearly 50% have been diagnosed with at least one major chronic condition. However, they average one less physician visit each year than healthier urban counterparts.

- More than 26% of rural families are below the poverty level; more than 40% of all rural children younger than 18 years of age live in poverty.
- General practitioners and nurse practitioners are usual providers of care for rural adults and children.
- Rural residents must often travel more than 30 minutes to access a health care provider.
- Nurses must take into consideration the belief systems and lifestyles of a rural population when planning, implementing, and evaluating community services.
- Barriers to rural health care include the lack of availability, affordability, accessibility, and acceptability of services.
- Partnership models, particularly case management and community-oriented primary health care (COPHC), are effective models to provide a comprehensive continuum of care in environments with scarce resources.

CLINICAL DECISION-MAKING ACTIVITIES

1. Compare and contrast the terms *urban, suburban, rural, frontier, farm, non-farm residency, metropolitan,* and *micropolitan areas.*
2. Describe residency as a continuum, ranging from farm residency to core metropolitan residency.
3. Discuss economic, social, and cultural factors that affect rural lifestyle and the health care–seeking behaviors of residents who live there.
4. Identify factors that affect the accessibility, affordability, availability, and acceptability of services in the health care delivery system.
5. Compare and contrast the health status and lifestyle behaviors of rural and urban residents.
6. Summarize key nursing concepts in terms of practice in the rural context.
7. Examine the characteristics of rural community nursing practice and describe how these might differ from those of practice in more populated settings.
8. Compare and contrast challenges, opportunities, and benefits of living and practicing as a nurse in the rural environment.
9. Evaluate case management and community-oriented primary care as partnership models that can help nurses enhance the continuum of care for clients living in an environment with sparse resources.
10. Propose potential areas for rural nursing research activities. Specify research questions that focus on the professional and clinical concerns of public health nurses who practice in the rural context.

REFERENCES

Agency for Health Care Policy and Research (AHCPR): *Health care in urban and rural areas combined years 2004-2006: update of Content in MEPS Chartbook No. 13,* 2009. Available at http://www.ahrq.gov/data/meps/chbook13up.htm. Accessed January 8, 2011.

American Legacy Foundation: *Tobacco control in rural America,* Washington, DC, 2009, ALF. Available at http://www.legacyforhealth.org/PDF/Tobacco_Control_in_Rural_America.pdf. Accessed January 8, 2011.

Bennett K, Olatosi B, Probst J: *Health disparities: a rural-urban chartbook,* 2008. Available at http://rhr.sph.sc.edu/report/(7-3)%20Health%20Disparities%20A%20Rural%20Urban%20Chartbook%20-%20Distribution%20-Copy.pdf. Accessed January 8, 2011.

Bigbee J, Crowder E: The Red Cross Rural Nursing Service: an innovation of public health nursing delivery, *Public Health Nurs* 2(2):109, 1985.

Bureau of the Census: *Annual estimates of the resident population for incorporated places,* 2009. Available at http://www.census.gov/compendia/statab/2008/tables/08s0028.pdf. Accessed January 8, 2011.

Bureau of Health Professions (BHPR): *Shortage designation: HPSAs, MUAs, MUPs,* Washington, DC, 2009, U.S. Department of Health and Human Services. Available at http://bhpr.hrsa.gov/shortage. Accessed June 12, 2010.

Bureau of Health Professions (BHPR): *Nurse shortage counties,* Washington, DC, 2007, U.S. Department of Health and Human Services. Available at http://bhpr.hrsa.gov/healthworkforce/nursingshortage/issues.htm#f8. Accessed January 8, 2011.

Bushy A: Conducting culturally competent rural nursing research. In Merwin B, editor: *Annual Review of Nursing Research: Focus on Rural Health,* 26:221–236, 2008a.

Bushy A: *Rural nursing: practice and issues,* American Nurses Association On-line Continuing Education Program. Available at http://www.nursingworld.org/mods/mod700/rurlfull.htm. Accessed January 8, 2011.

Bushy A: American nurses credentialing center (ANCC) pathway to excellence program: addressing and meeting the needs of small and rural hospitals, *Online J Rural Nurs Health Care* 9(1):6–10, 2009. Available at http://www.rno.org/journal/index.php/online-journal/article/viewFile/171/221. Accessed January 8, 2011.

Case T: Work stresses of community health nurses in Oklahoma. In Bushy A, editor: *Rural nursing,* vol 2, Newbury Park, CA, 1991, Sage.

Centers for Disease Control and Prevention (CDC): *Healthy communities program: an overview,* 2010. Available at http://www.cdc.gov/healthycommunitiesprogram. Accessed January 8, 2011.

Cromartie J: Defining the "rural" in rural America, *Amber waves: the economics of food, farming, natural resources, and rural America,* 2008. Available at http://www.ers.usda.gov/AmberWaves/June08/Features/RuralAmerica.htm. Accessed January 8, 2011.

Davis D, Droes N: Community health nursing in rural and frontier counties, *Nurs Clin North Am* 28:159, 1993.

Gale J, Lambert D: Mental healthcare in rural communities: the once and future role of primary care, *North Carolina Med J* 67(1):67–70, 2006. Available at http://www.ruralhealthresearch.org/centers/maine/publications_date.php. Accessed January 17, 2011.

Gamm L, Hutchison L, Dabney B, et al: *Rural Healthy People 2010: a companion document to Healthy People 2010,* Vol I, II, III, College Station, TX, 2003, The Texas A&M University System Health Science Center, School of Rural Health, Southwest Rural Health Research Center. Available at http://www.srph.tamhsc.edu/centers/rhp2010/publications.htm. Accessed January 8, 2011.

Graves B: Community-based participatory research: toward eliminating rural health disparities, *Online J Rural Nurs Health Care* 9(1):12–14, 2009. Available at http://www.rno.org/journal/index.php/online-journal/article/viewFile/173/223. Accessed January 8, 2011.

Hurme E: Competencies for nursing practice in a rural critical access hospital, *Online J Rural Nurs Health Care* 9(2):67–81, 2009. Available at http://www.rno.org/journal/index.php/online-journal/article/viewFile/198/256. Accessed January 8, 2011.

Institute of Medicine (IOM): *Quality through collaboration: the future of rural health,* Washington, DC, 2004, IOM. Available at http://www.iom.edu/report.asp?id=23359. Accessed June 12, 2010.

Long K, Weinert C: Rural nursing: developing a theory base, *Sch Inq Nurs Pract* 3:99–113, 1999.

McGinnis P: *Rural policy development: a community leadership development approach,* Kansas City, MO, 2003, National Rural Health Association.

Mead H, Cartwright-Smith L, Jones K, et al: *Racial and ethnic disparities in U.S. health care: a chartbook,* 2008. Available at http://www.commonwealthfund.org/~/media/Files/Publications/Chartbook/2008/Mar/Racial%20and%20Ethnic%20Disparities%20in%20U%20S%20%20Health%20Care%20%20A%20Chartbook/Mead_racialethnicdisparities_chartbook_1111%20pdf.pdf. Accessed January 8, 2011.

Merwin B, editor: *Annual review of nursing research: focus on rural health,* vol 26, New York, 2008, Springer.

Mississippi State University-Extension Service: *A community report of Oktibbeha County: smart aging—healthy future,* Mississippi State, MS, 2009, MSUES. Available at http://msucares.com/health/smart_aging/community_reports.html. Accessed January 8, 2011.

Molinari D, Monserud M: *Rural nurse job satisfaction,* Rural and Remote Health: The International Electronic Journal of Rural Remote Health, Research, Education, Practice and Policy, 2008. Available at http://www.rrh.org.au/articles/subviewnew.asp?ArticleID=1055. Accessed January 8, 2011.

Moore G, Mink M, Probst J, et al: *Mental health risk factors: unmet needs, and provider availability for rural children,* 2005. Available at http://rhr.sph.sc.edu/report/(4-1)%20Mental%20Health%20Risk%20Factors.pdf. Accessed January 8, 2011.

National Advisory Committee on Rural Health and Human Services (NACRHHS): *The 2008 report to the secretary: rural health and human services issues,* 2008. Available at ftp://ftp.hrsa.gov/ruralhealth/committee/NACreport2008.pdf. Accessed January 8, 2011.

National Center for Farmworkers' Health: *Fact sheets about farmworker's health*, 2010. Available at http://www.ncfh.org/?pid=5. Accessed January 8, 2011.

National Center for Health Statistics (NCHS): *Health behaviors of adults United States—2005-2007*, 2010. Available at http://www.cdc.gov/nchs/data/series/sr_10/sr10_245.pdf. Accessed January 8, 2011.

Nelson J, Stover-Gingerich B: Rural health: access to care and services. *Home Health Care Management Practice Online,* 2010. Available at http://hhc.sagepub.com/cgi/rapidpdf/1084822309353552v1. Accessed January 8, 2011.

Nelson W, editor: *Handbook for rural health care ethics*, Lebanon, NH, 2009, Dartmouth. Available at http://dms.dartmouth.edu/cfm/resources/ethics/. Accessed June 18, 2010.

National Rural Health Association (NRHA): *NRHA policy brief: Addressing the health care needs in the U.S.-Mexico Border Region*, Kansas City, MO, 2010, NRHA. Available at http://www.ruralhealthweb.org/go/left/policy-and-advocacy/policy-documents-and-statements/official-policy-positions. Accessed January 8, 2011.

National Rural Health Association (NRHA): *NRHA policy position workforce series: rural behavioral health*, Kansas City, MO, 2008, NRHA. Available at http://www.ruralhealthweb.org/go/left/policy-and-advocacy/policy-documents-and-statements/official-policy-positions. Accessed January 8, 2011.

National Rural Health Association (NRHA): *NRHA policy position workforce series: recruitment and retention of a quality workforce in rural America, #6 rural public health*, Kansas City, MO, 2007, NRHA. Available at http://www.ruralhealthweb.org/go/left/policy-and-advocacy/policy-documents-and-statements/official-policy-positions. Accessed January 8, 2011.

North Carolina Smart Growth Alliance: *Healthy rural communities: a resource and action guide for North Carolina*, Chapel Hill, NC, 2004, NCSGA. Available at http://www.activelivingbydesign.org/events-resources/resources/healthy-rural-communities-resource-and-action-guide-north-carolina. Accessed January 8, 2011.

Occupational Safety and Health Administration (OSHA): *Safety and health topics: agricultural operations*, Washington, DC, 2010, OSHA. Available at http://www.osha.gov/SLTC/agriculturaloperations/index.html. Accessed Jnuary 8, 2011.

Rand Corporation: *U.S. Health care today: coverage,* 2010a. Available at http://www.randcompare.org/us-health-care-today/coverage. Accessed January 8, 2011.

Rand Corporation: *U.S. Health care today: health,* 2010b. Available at http://www.randcompare.org/us-health-care-today/health. Accessed January 8, 2011.

Roberge C: Who stays in rural nursing practice? An international review of the literature on factors influencing rural nurse retention. *Online Journal of Rural Nursing and Health Care*, 9(1):82-93, 2009. Available at http://www.rno.org/journal/index.php/online-journal/article/viewFile/180/230. Accessed January 8, 2011.

Skillman S, Palazzo L, Hart G, Butterfield P: *Changes in the rural Registered Nurse workforce from 1980 to 2004*, 2007. WWAMI Rural Health Research Center, Available at http://depts.washington.edu/uwrhrc/uploads/RHRC%20FR115%20Skillman.pdf. Accessed January 8, 2011.

U.S.A. Center for Rural Health Preparedness: *Rural emergency preparedness toolkit (CD-ROM.)*, n.d. Available at http://www.rural-preparedness.org/index.aspx?page=3f3872b2-72dd-499f-8079-523bfd06d61f. Accessed January 8, 2011.

U.S. Department of Agriculture (USDA): *Rural America at a glance: 2009 edition*, 2008a. Available at http://www.ers.usda.gov/Publications/EIB59/EIB59.pdf. Accessed January 8, 2011.

U.S. Department of Agriculture (USDA): *What is rural?* 2008b. Available at http://www.nal.usda.gov/ric/ricpubs/what_is_rural.shtml#character. Accessed January 8, 2011.

U.S. Department of Agriculture (USDA): *Measuring rurality: 2004 County typology codes*, 2005. Available at http://www.ers.usda.gov/Briefing/rurality/Typology/. Accessed March 17, 2011.

U.S. Department of Agriculture (USDA): *Measuring rurality: what is a micropolitan area?* (2006). Available at http://www.ers.usda.gov/Briefing/Rurality/Micropolitan Areas/. Accessed March 17, 2011.

U.S. Department of Health and Human Services (USDHHS) *More choices, better coverage: health insurance reform and rural America*, 2010a. Available at http://www.healthreform.gov/reports/ruralamerica/index.html. Accessed June 12, 2010.

U.S. Department of Health and Human Services (USDHHS): *Healthy People 2020*, 2010b. Available at http://www.healthypeople.gov/2020/default.aspx. Accessed January 8, 2011.

U.S. Department of Health and Human Services (USDHHS): *Health, United States, 2009: with special feature on technology*, 2010c. Available at http://www.cdc.gov/nchs/data/hus/hus09.pdf. Accessed January 8, 2011.

Winters C, Lee H: *Rural nursing: concepts, theory and practice*, ed 3, New York, 2009, Springer Publishing.

Woolston C: Lonesome doc: Medicine in a small town, *AARP Bulletin*, June 10, 2010. Available at http://www.aarp.org/health/doctors-hospitals/info-06-2010/medicine_in_a_small_town.html. Accessed January 8, 2011.

CHAPTER 20

Promoting Health Through Healthy Communities and Cities

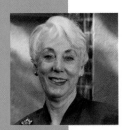

Jeanette Lancaster, PhD, RN, FAAN

Dr. Jeanette Lancaster is the Medical Center Professor of Nursing, School of Nursing at the University of Virginia. She has co-edited the first seven editions of this text with Dr. Marcia Stanhope. Gratitude is extended to Mary Beth Riner, DNS, RN who is an associate professor at Indiana University School of Nursing and who authored this chapter in the seventh edition and has contributed a case study to this edition that reflects actual healthy community practice.

ADDITIONAL RESOURCES

ⓔvolve WEBSITE
http://evolve.elsevier.com/Stanhope
- *Healthy People 2020*
- WebLinks

- Quiz
- Case Studies
- Glossary
- Answers to Practice Application

OBJECTIVES

After reading this chapter, the student should be able to do the following:
1. Discuss the history of the Healthy Communities and Cities movement.
2. Discuss the Centers for Disease Control and Prevention Healthy Communities Program.
3. Describe the core concepts and principles that guide the development of a healthy community program.
4. Describe the steps used when working with communities in the Healthy Communities and Cities process.
5. Apply the steps in working with Healthy Communities and Cities to the concepts of health promotion.
6. Explain the role nurses can assume in working with Healthy Communities and Cities.

KEY TERMS

appropriate technology, p. 449
Community Health Promotion Model, p. 455
community participation, p. 449
equity, p. 449

health promotion, p. 448
Healthy Communities and Cities (HCC), p. 448
healthy public policy, p. 451
international cooperation, p. 449

multisectoral cooperation, p. 449
primary health care, p. 449
—*See Glossary for definitions*

OUTLINE

The **Healthy Communities and Cities** (HCC) initiative or movement began with the World Health Organization (WHO) in 1986 with the signing of the Ottawa Charter for Health Promotion. The initiative has grown and changed since 1986. This initiative, originally called *Healthy Cities,* has assumed a healthy communities focus in recent years. Some locales use the term *healthy communities and cities,* whereas other locales talk about *healthy municipalities and cities,* and still others use the term *healthy communities.* The Centers for Disease Control and Prevention (CDC) in the United States initiated work in this area in 2003, and called their program the *steps program.* The CDC program is now called *Healthy Communities.* The term *healthy communities* will be used in this chapter; however, reference will be made to other terms in order to describe the history of the movement and to refer to specific programs that use a term other than *healthy communities and cities.* The goal of this movement is to promote health through community involvement in problem solving. The premise is that community citizens must be involved in identifying the need for health programs and in developing programs to meet those needs. Building healthy communities relies on broad-based citizen participation to make systems change in communities that can improve the health of the residents. The overall goals are to build community capacity, use local resources and skills, measure progress and evaluate outcomes, and to develop projects that reduce inequalities in health status and access to services.

This chapter provides an introduction to the history of the HCC movement and to the basic terminology related to the movement. It describes various models in which communities have structured their programs both in the United States and selected other countries. Key facilitators and barriers to the Healthy Communities process are discussed, as is the role for nurses in supporting the development and sustainment of Healthy Communities.

HISTORY OF THE HEALTHY COMMUNITIES AND CITIES MOVEMENT

HCC is found in many regions of the world. As noted previously, this movement began in 1986 with the WHO's Ottawa Charter. In essence, in 1986, the WHO's Ottawa Charter became the first worldwide action plan for health promotion. At that time, the delegates to the conference declared that the following broad categories were prerequisites to health: peace, shelter, education, food, income, a stable ecosystem, sustainable resources, social justice, and equity. This is a much different approach to viewing health than the individualistic approach that holds that each person is responsible for his or her own health. Although 1986 seems to be in the distant past, the areas for action that were determined by the *Ottawa Charter for Health Promotion* deserve attention today (WHO, 1986). They are:

- *Building healthy public policy:* Many countries around the world are struggling with health reform and attempting to emphasize **health promotion** and disease prevention in contrast to focusing on curative aspects of health care. What this means is that policies should focus on such areas as lowering

speed limits in residential areas or enforcing the use of helmets, seat belts, and no-smoking policies. Health must be on the agenda of policy makers at the local level as well as the state and national levels.
- *Creating supportive environments:* For example, when communities are being revitalized or developed, areas should be set aside for "green areas," with parks, walking or bike paths, and fitness facilities. Both work and leisure should be a source of health for people.
- *Strengthening community action:* The Ottawa Charter states (and this continues to hold true) that health promotion is most effective in communities when residents are fully engaged in the development and implementation of programs. This requires a "tried and true" public health approach in which nurses listen to and respond to the needs of the community. Community members need to be involved in setting priorities, making decisions, planning strategies, and implementing them in order to attain better health.
- *Developing personal skills:* This includes teaching people the skills that they need in order to be healthy, such as regular and competent hand washing, choosing the right foods, engaging in regular age-appropriate exercise, and learning to avoid risk factors and increase one's protective factors. This step increases the options available to people so they can exercise more control over their own health and their environments.
- *Reorienting health services:* This implies an emphasis on prevention whereby you work to promote health and prevent disease. The responsibility for health promotion is shared by individuals, community groups, health practitioners, health care institutions, and the government (WHO, 2010).

As discussed in Chapter 17, health promotion is a process designed to help people increase control over, and improve, their health. Health promotion is not just the responsibility of the health sector but rather includes individuals, families, groups, and communities. Strategies and programs should be customized to meet local needs and take into account different economies, customs, resources, and priorities. The original goals of the Ottawa Conference continue to be areas of concern, and work must continue to achieve the goals. Chapter 4 also addresses, from a global health perspective, the need for a healthy community approach in selected countries around the world.

HCC began in the United States in 1988, with Healthy Cities Indiana and the California Healthy Cities project. Healthy Cities Indiana adapted the European experiences to the American context. The concept of Healthy Communities was used to include localities that were not cities but rather smaller communities such as towns or counties. In recent years, many U.S. communities have initiated the HCC process with the result that thousands of communities have taken local action to promote health. Several of these communities are featured in the chapter as examples of what a focus on health promotion at the community level would look like.

In other parts of the world, HCC has different names, including Healthy Islands, Healthy Villages, and, in Latin America, Healthy Municipalities and Communities. In addition, national networks have developed in Australia, Canada, Costa Rica, Iran, and Egypt. Other regional networks have been developed in Francophone Africa, Latin America, Southeast Asia, and the western Pacific. Particular attention will be given later in the chapter to Healthy Municipalities and Communities in the Pan American Health Organization (PAHO) region, since PAHO's work is long standing and well developed and has demonstrated effective results.

Some claim that the concept of a healthy community or city is not new (Hancock, 1993). It is based on the belief that the health of the community is largely influenced by the environment in which people live and that health problems have multiple causes—social, economic, political, environmental, and behavioral. The HCC process has been applied to rural and metropolitan areas. The HCC process engages local residents in action and is based on the premise that when people have the opportunity to work out their own locally defined health problems, they will find sustainable solutions to those problems. This concept is integral to good public health practice, which is to engage those for whom programs are being developed in the identification of need for, planning, implementing, and evaluating the programs. The *Healthy People 2020* process is consistent with the way in which healthy communities and cities have developed their priorities and plans. One of the four goals of *Healthy People 2020* is to create physical and social environments that promote good health for all. This goal relies on an ecological perspective that says that health and health behaviors are determined by many influences including personal, organizational, environmental, and policy factors. Many of the goals of *Healthy People 2020* will be challenging to meet in light of the poor economic conditions in the United States and many other countries. For example, it is difficult to increase the income of low-income persons in an era in which people continue to lose their jobs. See the *Healthy People 2020* box for objectives that relate to healthy communities and cities.

♥ HEALTHY PEOPLE 2020

Selected Goals That Pertain to Healthy Communities

- ECBP-8: Increase the proportion of worksites that offer a comprehensive employee health promotion program to their employees.
- ECBP-9: Increase the proportion of employees who participate in employer-sponsored health promotion activities.
- ECBP-11: Increase the proportion of local health departments that have established culturally appropriate and linguistically competent community health promotion and disease prevention programs.
- PA-13: Increase the proportion of trips made by walking.
- PA-1: Reduce the proportion of adults who engage in no leisure-time physical activity.
- PA-4: Increase the proportion of the Nation's public and private schools that require daily physical education for all students.
- OSH-9: Increase the proportion of employees who have access to workplace programs that prevent or reduce employee stress.

From U.S. Department of Health and Human Services: *Healthy People 2020,* Washington, DC, 2010, U.S. Government Printing Office.

DEFINITION OF TERMS

There are many definitions of a healthy community. The *Healthy People 2010* document described a healthy community as one that included those elements that enable people to maintain a high quality of life and productivity (USDHHS, 2000). To expand on this definition, consider what was stated in the document, *Healthy People in Healthy Communities: A Community Planning Guide Using Healthy People 2010,* that a healthy community would include access to health care services that include both treatment and prevention for all community members; the community would be safe; and there would be adequate roads, schools, playgrounds, and other services to meet the needs of the people in the community and that the environment would be healthy and safe (USDHHS, 2001).

The CDC defines a healthy place as one that is "designed and built to improve the quality of life for all people who live, work, worship, learn, and play within their borders—where every person is free to make choices amid a variety of healthy, available, accessible, and affordable options" (CDC, Healthy Places, n.d.). The CDC also points out that a healthy community is one that continuously creates and improves both the physical and social environments and expands community resources to enable people to mutually support each other in carrying out essential life functions as well as in developing to their maximum potential. A healthy community seeks to improve the quality of life of its people and does this through collaboration, partnerships, diverse and extensive citizen ownership, and partnership in the process.

Instrumental in the development of the Healthy Cities movement were the principles of primary health care (WHO and UNICEF, 1978) and the Ottawa Charter for Health Promotion (WHO, 1986). Primary health care refers to meeting the basic health needs of a community by providing readily accessible health services. Because health problems transcend international borders, international cooperation is important to ensure health. The principles of primary health care include equity, health promotion, community participation, multisectoral cooperation, appropriate technology, and international cooperation.

Equity implies providing accessible services to promote the health of populations most at risk for health problems (e.g., the poor, the young, older adults, minorities, the homeless, and immigrants and refugees). As discussed in Chapter 17, health promotion and disease prevention focus on providing community members with a positive sense of health that strengthens their physical, mental, and emotional capacities. Individuals within communities become involved in health promotion through community participation, whereby well-informed and motivated community members participate in planning, implementing, and evaluating health programs. Multisectoral cooperation is the coordinated action by all parts of a community, from local government officials to grassroots community members. Appropriate technology refers to affordable social, biomedical, and health services that are relevant and acceptable to individuals' health, needs, and concerns.

ASSUMPTIONS ABOUT COMMUNITY PRACTICE

There are different models of community practice, and the assumptions that professionals have about communities shape the implementation of the HCC process. The classic work of Rothman and Tropman (1987) describing these different models and some of the key assumptions continue to be relevant today, as will be seen in the examples used in this chapter. The key models for community practice include the following:

1. Locality development is a process-oriented model that emphasizes consensus, cooperation, and building group identity and a sense of community.
2. Social planning stresses rational-empirical problem solving, usually by outside professional experts. Social planning does not focus on building community capacity or fostering fundamental social change.
3. Social action, on the other hand, aims to increase the problem-solving ability of the community with concrete actions that attempt to correct the imbalance of power and privilege of an oppressed or disadvantaged group in the community.

Effective models of community practice use a partnership between citizens and professionals in which there is delegated power and citizen control (Rothman and Tropman, 1987). A partnership approach, considered a bottom-up approach, incorporates the concepts of a multisectoral approach as well as community participation. A partnership approach contrasts with the top-down type in which professionals and experts tell the citizens what to do rather than involve and ask them.

> **DID YOU KNOW?** *Community participation can begin at town meetings, city council meetings, crime watch, and other settings where community members from different walks of life (including health professionals) identify the strengths and health needs of their community and plan appropriate action to address their needs. This is an example of social action—a bottom-up approach to community practice.*

A bottom-up approach uses broad-based community problem solving that includes health professionals, local officials, service providers, and other community members, including those at risk for health problems. The locality development and social action models are examples of a bottom-up approach, in which community participation is evident in all stages of community health planning and practice.

> **WHAT DO YOU THINK?** *Community participation in health decisions is more effective in promoting healthy public policy than decision making by outside professional experts.*

HEALTHY COMMUNITIES AND CITIES IN THE UNITED STATES

In the following paragraphs, HCC initiatives in various regions of the United States are discussed. These examples show the different models of community practice that are being implemented.

Specifically, the CDC's Healthy Communities Program emphasizes policy, systems, and environmental changes that focus on chronic diseases and that encourage people to be more physically active, eat a healthy diet, and not use tobacco. The rationale is based on the fact that about 50% of Americans are affected by chronic disease, and these diseases account for 7 of the 10 leading causes of death in the country. Also, there are many direct and indirect costs associated with being obese and overweight. Many chronic diseases are preventable. By preventing a chronic disease from occurring, people can enjoy a higher quality of life, communities have a decreased burden of illness, and both the state and federal governments are able to reduce the amount they spend on health care (CDC, 2009a). Using diabetes as an example, the CDC says that between 1994 and 2009, the number of people with diabetes doubled. The CDC predicts that if that trend continues, one third of the children born in 2000 will develop type 2 diabetes during their lifetime. The CDC said also that more than one third of all adults fail to meet recommendations for aerobic physical activity based on the *2008 Physical Activity Guidelines for Americans*; that tobacco is the single most preventable cause of disease, disability, and death; and that excessive alcohol use is the third leading cause of death related to lifestyle (CDC, 2009a).

These chronic disease facts support the priority that the CDC has placed on funding projects that will interrupt chronic diseases in communities around the country. Since 2003, the CDC has funded more than 240 rural, urban, and tribal communities to support their goals. Specifically, their programs include: Strategic Alliances for Health Communities, ACHIEVE (Action Communities for Health, Innovation, and EnVironmental ChangE), REACH U.S., Pioneering Healthy Communities (in collaboration with the YMCA of the USA), and Steps Communities (CDC, 2009b).

The CDC has also developed a set of "tools for community action" that can be used in developing healthy communities. The Did You Know? box includes examples of the CDC tools for community action.

> **DID YOU KNOW?** *The CDC has developed several tools to help communities improve their health. Some of these tools are:*
> 1. *Community Health Resources Database: see http://www.cdc.gov/communityhealthresources to find assistance in planning, implementing, and evaluating community health interventions and programs that address their focus on chronic disease.*
> 2. *Community Health Assessment and Group Evaluation (CHANGE) Tool: Community leaders can use this tool to see what local policy, systems, and environmental strategies are currently in place in their communities and identify areas where health strategies are needed. CHANGE assists communities to define and prioritize areas for their own improvement. See http://www.cdc.gov/healthycommunitiesprogram/tools/change/htm. Accessed January 21, 2011.*
> 3. *Action Guides: The Community Health Promotion Handbook: Action Guides to Improve Community Health (2008). In collaboration with the Partnership for Prevention program, the CDC has developed a set of "how-to" guides for five community-level health promotion strategies related to its chronic disease prevention target areas of diabetes self management,*

physical activity, and tobacco-use cessation. See http:// www.cdc.gov/healthycommunities program/tools/community healthpromotionhandbook.htm for a listing of the five specific guides. Also, see the CDC website for three additional guides to help communities develop health programs.

Given the usefulness of the CDC *Community Health Promotion Handbook*, further discussion is warranted here. The recommendations for the five guides that the CDC chose came from the Task Force on Community Preventive Services (TFCPS, 2005). The handbooks primarily target public health professionals but also can be used by community leaders. The guides build on a socioecological model that recognizes that social and physical environments affect health and health behavior. This model divides the environment into five areas that affect health behavior: individual, interpersonal, organizational, community, and policy. Using the *Handbook* relies on the same process used in the assessment of a community. In other words, before deciding which of the five areas to target in your work, follow these steps:

1. Conduct a needs assessment and set health priorities.
2. Find out what social and environmental factors may affect each health priority as well as what options are available for dealing with the chosen health priorities.
3. Think about the acceptability (to the community) and the feasibility (are resources available, etc.) to implement the project(s).

As you work with the action guides, remember to take small steps and do first things first; involve the appropriate people and do not be reluctant to make changes as you go based on what you learn and the outcomes you have (Partnership for Prevention, 2008).

HEALTHY COMMUNITIES AND CITIES AROUND THE WORLD: SELECTED EXAMPLES

As mentioned earlier, PAHO in collaboration with the WHO has a long-standing involvement in developing healthy communities that they call the Healthy Municipalities and Communities Movement. The mission of this movement is to "strengthen the implementation of health promotion activities at the local level, making health promotion a high priority of the political agenda; fostering the involvement of government authorities and the active participation of the community, supporting dialogue, sharing knowledge and experiences and stimulating collaboration among municipalities and countries" (PAHO, *Healthy Municipalities and Cities*, n.d.). Other key concepts in their approach are that of multisectoral partnerships to improve social and health conditions and advocacy for developing healthy public policy, maintaining healthy environments, and promoting healthy lifestyles. PAHO believes that creating a healthy municipality involves a process that relies on strong political commitment and support that is aligned with equally strong communities who are determined to achieve their goals and who participate actively in the process of goal achievement (PAHO *Healthy Municipalities and Cities*, n.d.).

PAHO recommends a participatory development framework in which you gain commitment from the mayor, local government (all sectors), and representatives of community groups and organizations. PAHO has found this process to be the most effective in the Americas. The phases are:

1. Aspects in the initial phase of the process
   - Meet with local government authorities and community leaders to gain their perspectives about such things as healthy spaces and health promotion and to request that they make a public statement as well as a joint declaration of their commitment.
   - Create an intersectoral, community planning committee.
   - Conduct a needs assessment including analysis of problems and needs.
   - Build consensus and decide upon priorities for action.
2. Steps in the planning process
   - Train the committee and task forces to ensure that they understand the concept of healthy community, the settings approach to health promotion, and participatory methods including needs assessment, planning, evaluation, and health education.
   - Develop an action plan.
   - Mobilize resources needed to implement the plan and develop a detailed work plan.
3. Moments in the consolidation phase of the process
   - Implement activities that are included in the plan. Examples might be establishing health-promoting schools, work places, markets, hospitals, and other healthy environments.
   - Evaluate the results as well as the quality of participation.
   - Share knowledge and experiences with others.

PAHO notes that the steps that work in its region may be somewhat different from those that have been successful in Canada, the United States, and Europe. Later in this chapter, the 20 steps that PAHO says have been used by these other countries will be cited as a way for nurses and other public health workers to develop a healthy community strategy. Interestingly, PAHO has found that it must start its process by gaining support from the mayor of the community and from other community leaders. These individuals must understand the concept of health promotion and the healthy municipalities process before they will offer their support. PAHO has also found that it must have a strong and knowledgeable support group who can envision a healthy municipality and convey that vision to opinion leaders (PAHO, *Healthy Municipalities and Communities*, n.d.).

| DID YOU KNOW? *There are many excellent examples of Healthy Communities and Cities around the world. Only a few are highlighted here with information on how to locate their websites and learn more about the work being done around the world.*

- *Ontario (Canada) Healthy Communities Coalition: Their focus in 2010 was on "What makes a healthy community." Their website, www.ohcc-ccso.ca, is filled with useful resources.*
- *Horsens Denmark: One of their key foci is on "safe community Horsens." Their website, www.sundbyhorsens.dk, is in Danish, but the button to choose English is clearly marked and they provide an overview of the work they are doing in 2010.*

- *Community Builders of New South Wales Australia: They have an interactive electronic clearinghouse for persons involved in community level, social, economic, and environmental renewal, and they include rural and regional communities (www.communitybuilders.nsw.gov.au).*
- *Association for Community Health Improvements: This organization's website has many healthy community tools and organizations in the United States and internationally. Similarly, www.hospitalconnect.com hosts a website with valuable information about healthy communities and extensive links to other sites. Selected examples of healthy communities in the United States are discussed later in this chapter.*

Also see Box 4-2 in Chapter 4 for examples of Healthy Cities Toronto, Canada, and Chengdu, China.

DEVELOPING A HEALTHY COMMUNITY

What do people want from a healthy community? We know that each community is different and their challenges, goals, resources, competencies, problem-solving skills, and practices are different. As discussed throughout the chapter, many organizations in the United States and other countries have worked to help communities become healthier (Figure 20-1). One of these organizations in the United States is the National Civic League (2007). They emphasize the complexity of developing healthy communities and have identified five principles that they think should be applied in community work if the goal is to find solutions using a broad-based inclusive process. These principles are:

- A broad definition of health that goes beyond the absence of disease to address the root problems in communities and includes economy, education, parks and recreation, arts, mental health, and community spirit and unity.
- A collaborative, consensus-based approach to problem solving that involves a diverse group of citizens from the community.

- An assets-based approach to problem solving that defines people and relationships by their skills and abilities rather than their needs and deficits.
- Addressing challenges at a systems level in the community rather than implementing just another short-term, low-impact project.
- Creating a shared vision for the future that captures the hopes and dreams of the community and that guides collaborative work.

Other principles will guide the development and implementation of a healthy community. Examples of useful principles are listed below:

- The whole is greater than the sum of the parts; in other words, most communities have limited resources, and no one agency can do all that is needed. However, if agencies work together, the outcome of the whole can be much bigger than the outcome of the aid provided by one agency.
- A change in one part of the system affects the others. For example, if the public transportation workers in a large city go on strike and there is no public transportation for many days, many areas of the community will be affected.
- Collaboration is central to the development of a healthy community.
- All systems have feedback loops whereby information from one area is fed back to the whole and provides an opportunity for change or "course correction." For example, you might establish a helping program for dependent older adults whereby daycare would be provided at low cost. This would enable the family members with whom the elder lived to provide safe care while they worked. However, if the family has no transportation of their own and the facility is not accessible by public transportation, the program would not be as helpful as hoped.

The National Civic League also asked hundreds of communities across the country "What would your community look like if it were a really healthy place to live?" The replies shown in Box 20-1 come as no surprise. You might ask yourself that same question before looking at Box 20-1 and see how close your replies are to those of the respondents.

This chapter indicates that a healthy community has involvement, inclusiveness, cooperation, and collaboration, among

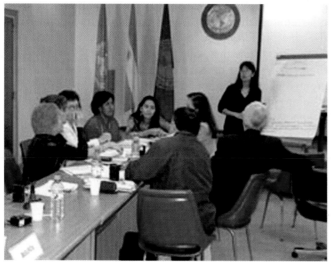

FIGURE 20-1 Community participation for developing a healthy community involves a representative community planning committee. (From CDC, Pulsenet News, 2004. Available at http://www.cdc.gov/pulsenet/newsletter/Spring_2004.htm. Accessed January 10, 2011.)

BOX 20-1 WHAT IS A HEALTHY COMMUNITY?

- A clean and safe environment
- A diverse and vibrant economy
- Good housing for all
- Good roads and good public transportation
- Parks, playgrounds and recreational facilities
- People who respect and support each other
- A place that promotes and celebrates its cultural and historical heritage
- A place where citizens and government share power and where citizens feel a sense of belonging
- A place that has affordable health care for all
- A place that has good schools
- A place that has and supports strong families

other qualities. Collaboration can help make the best use of resources, reduce duplication and competition, increase effectiveness, and develop more sustainable resources. It is like a recipe in that each agency in the collaboration brings one or more ingredients to the product. Putting all the ingredients together leads to a better product. Collaboration involves doing things differently than in the past and developing different kinds of partnerships and relationships. Organizations that work together effectively have generally achieved three things:

- High levels of trust
- Serious time commitment from the partners
- A diminished need to protect their own turf (Torres and Margolin, 2003)

Collaboration requires the same mix of behaviors and goals as those associated with the development of a healthy community—that is, a group of participants including those who are paid and volunteers who bring different skills and talents to the process and who work together to do the following:

1. Address a specific problem or opportunity
2. Work on a broad agenda of mutually beneficial goals
3. Provide a forum to discuss and respond to community concerns, interests, and resources
4. Recognize that there are roles in a partnership and they will be different from the role the person had in the parent organization.

As mentioned earlier, Indiana and California have the longest history of Healthy Communities and Cities in the United States. Healthy Cities Indiana began as a pilot program in 1988 with a grant from the W.K. Kellogg Foundation as a collaborative effort among Indiana University School of Nursing, Indiana Public Health Association, and six Indiana cities. On the basis of this project's success, the W.K. Kellogg Foundation funded the dissemination phase, called CITYNET-Healthy Cities, in cooperation with the National League of Cities through their network of 19,000 local officials (Flynn, Rider, and Ray, 1991). This was an extensive project that initially involved six cities (Gary, Fort Wayne, New Castle, Indianapolis, Seymour, and Jeffersonville). Activities in these cities focused on problems of diverse populations. For example, actions were consistent with local priorities that included problems of children, teen parents, the homeless, access to health care, crime and violence, and older adults. Action was also taken on the broader environmental policy issues, including management of solid waste and promotion of air quality. For each of these projects, the Community Health Promotion process was followed, thereby providing a broad base of community participation at all stages of community planning. This was a process developed at Indiana University School of Nursing, and it was consistent with many of the other U.S. and international processes for implementing healthy community initiatives.

An early example of the use of the Community Health Promotion process was the New Castle Healthy City community assessment. The community committee found that there were high death rates in the community from cancer, chronic obstructive pulmonary disease, and heart disease. The committee asked the following questions: Why were rates higher in this area than in the state and the nation? What were the lifestyle choices of people in the community? What in the environment supported or inhibited healthy choices?

The committee worked with the staff at Indiana University School of Nursing to develop a survey to obtain baseline data on health behaviors in the community. Staff at the University trained local volunteers in survey data collection. They distributed 1000 door-to-door surveys using a system that ensured appropriate geographic coverage in the community. The response rate of 50% demonstrated the community's interest in health concerns. They then compared their findings with the national health objectives (DHHS, 1991). They found high levels of unhealthy behaviors, such as cigarette smoking and inadequate exercise, compared with the *Healthy People 2000* national objectives.

They used the survey results to determine the focus of their Healthy City initiatives. Using the data, they testified before the county commissioners about the need for health education and to support the employment of a health educator in the local health department. The cigarette smoking results were used by the committee to testify before the city council in support of an ordinance banning smoking in city buildings. The committee also sponsored community health awareness programs including a family fitness walk, safety checks of bicycles, and presentations on healthy food preparation emphasizing reduced fat and salt in meals.

New Castle has expanded its focus and is now known as Healthy Communities of Henry County. Their latest efforts are directed toward developing a network of walking trails throughout the county on the Trans-Indiana National Road Heritage Trail (NRHT) (Figure 20-2). (See www.hchcin.org for more details on this worthy project and the implied enthusiasm for its accomplishment.) The process for the walking trails initiative, which began in 2002, is consistent with that of other successful

EVIDENCE-BASED PRACTICE

Community gardens enhance nutrition and physical activity and promote the role of public health in improving quality of life. Opportunities to organize around other issues and build social capital also emerge through community gardens.

California Healthy Cities and Communities (CHCC) promotes an inclusionary and systems approach to improving community health. CHCC has funded community-based nutrition and physical activity programs in several cities. Successful community gardens were developed by many cities incorporating local leadership and resources, volunteers, and community partners, as well as skills-building opportunities for participants.

Through community garden initiatives, cities have enacted policies for interim land and complementary water use, improved access to produce, elevated public consciousness about public health, created culturally appropriate education and training materials, and strengthened community-building skills.

Nurse Use

Nurses can advocate for more local communities to establish community gardens among inner city neighborhoods. In addition, encouraging residents to participate can improve physical, emotional, and social health.

From Twiss J, Dickinson J, Duma S, et al: Community gardens: lessons learned from California Healthy Cities and Communities, *Am J Public Health* 93:1435-1438, 2003.

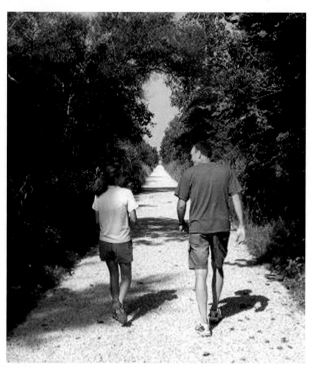

FIGURE 20-2 Walking trails in Indiana help people engage in health-promoting exercise. (From indianatrails.org, 2010. Courtesy of Beverly Matthews. Available at http://www.indianatrails.org/NRHT/photos.htm. Accessed January 12, 2011.

healthy community projects. Specifically, consultants worked with the committee to conduct a feasibility study and write a grant. Over the years, the committee obtained broad community support and cooperation, not only in defining local problems, but also in setting priorities and implementing their initiatives. Their interventions integrated individual lifestyle changes and policy changes aimed at promoting supportive environments for health.

Currently another example in Indiana is the Healthy Communities Initiative in Bartholomew County. The Initiative began in 1994 with a goal of improving health and quality of life of all residents of the county. It has remained true to its original concept of collaboration across the community. The current collaboration is between the hospital, schools, businesses, local government, churches, and others working together to meet identified health needs. They have action teams in the following areas: a medication assistance program, caring parents, domestic violence, Proyecto Salud, healthy lifestyles, tobacco awareness, volunteers in the medicine clinic, and a breastfeeding coalition (Columbus Regional Hospital, 2010).

THE CUTTING EDGE   *Because of a local influx of a Latino population, Healthy Communities of Bartholomew County, Indiana, initiated nurse-managed services in a voluntary medical clinic to provide health care to low-income, uninsured Hispanic people. Nurses are beginning to evaluate the impact of the project on the Latino community, which will provide data for future evidence-based nursing practice.*

The second state to be featured is California. They have supported over 70 cities and communities since they began

work in Healthy Cities and Communities in 1988. The California Healthy Cities and Communities Network, a membership program designed to support the healthy community work, also began in 1988. This network is built on the premise of shared responsibility among community members, local officials, and the private sector. Community participation is the cornerstone of the projects, and the mission is to reduce inequities in health status that exist among diverse populations in communities.

In 1989 Pasadena became a charter city of the California Healthy Cities project and produced a quality-of-life index with extensive input from residents, technical panels, and neighborhood groups. The index included over 50 indicators affecting community life, such as safety, education, substance abuse, recreation, economy, and housing. The index guided policy development in tobacco control, alcohol availability, and infant health education. It also assisted city and community agencies in planning, priority setting, resource development, and budgeting. In 2008, Pasadena engaged a consulting group to help them update these indicators so they might continue their growth as a healthy city.

Another example of California Healthy Cities and Communities is in Chico. A Healthy Chico Kids 2000 community-wide initiative was started, focusing on nutrition and health promotion. Nutrition education was provided for students in kindergarten through sixth grade. A dietary assessment was conducted that led the school district to reduce fat calories in school lunches. The initiative was expanded to increase awareness of cardiovascular risk factors among elementary school students, and the work is ongoing.

A new effort in California is being funded by the California Endowment called Building Healthy Communities. The California Endowment distributed $1.7 billion during its first decade of operations. The Endowment thinks that a specific focus helps them have a great impact, and they are focusing on healthy community building. Specifically, they are targeting "a nexus of community, health, and poverty to advance a 'prevention movement' in California" (California Endowment, 2010, p 1). The Endowment plans to focus on this area for the next decade in order to develop "places where children and youth are healthy, safe and ready to learn" (California Endowment, 2010, p 2). They think that the health of children is a primary indicator of the health of its communities (Figure 20-3). See www.calendow.org/healthycommunities for news and information regarding Building Healthy Communities.

There is a strong network of Healthy Communities and Cities in Massachusetts. Boston has at least 12 Healthy Communities and Cities initiatives. One example is the Chinatown Coalition, a community-based initiative involving community residents, community organizations, churches, businesses, and government agencies committed to improving the social, economic, environmental, and spiritual life of the Chinatown and Boston Asian community. The Chinatown Coalition facilitates and coordinates neighborhood-based efforts and resources to address community concerns. It also actively promotes advocacy and coordination with agencies that interact with the Asian community.

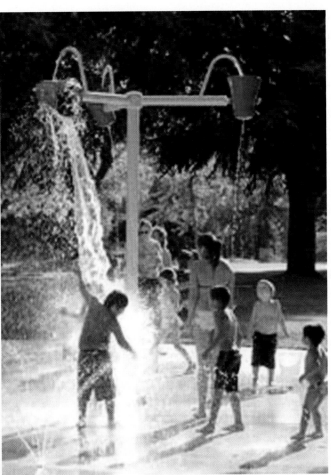

FIGURE 20-3 Supportive communities provide playgrounds where children can play and exercise in a safe location. (From Metro Regional Government, 2010. Available at http://www.oregonmetro. gov/index.cfm/go/by.web/id/149. Accessed January 10, 2011.)

THE CUTTING EDGE   *The CDC has invested in 40 programs since 2003. One of the programs is in Broome County, New York. Residents have increased fruit and vegetable consumption by 14% in all of their 46 elementary and middle schools. They have done this by using a county-consolidated bid to purchase healthy foods at lower costs. Also, over 50,000 people enrolled in an innovative walking program, and the percentage of adult participants who walked more than 30 minutes on 5 or more days per week grew from 47% to 54% in just 1 year (CDC, Chronic Disease-Healthy Communities-At a Glance, 2009).*

There are thousands of Healthy Communities and Cities programs in the United States that are seeking local solutions to complex problems. Nurses often play key roles in the work of Healthy Communities and Cities programs.

MODELS FOR DEVELOPING A HEALTHY COMMUNITY

There are many models to guide the development of a healthy community. As described earlier in this chapter, they do have a considerable amount of commonality. This section discusses how a nurse could either lead or be part of a team responsible for designing, implementing, and evaluating a healthy community. As has been seen, most of the successful healthy community or cities establish priorities that are identified after careful assessment and enormous amounts of community involvement. Nearly 20 years ago, faculty at the Indiana University School of Nursing under the leadership of Beverly Flynn developed a **Community Health Promotion Model** by adapting the European model of cities to the United States. This section discusses the key steps needed to develop a healthy community and compares them to the model developed at Indiana University. The steps of a general model that PAHO describes as common to models in the United States, Canada, and Europe are (PAHO, *Healthy Municipalities and Cities,* n.d.):

1. Build a local support group
2. Know about the Healthy Cities idea
3. Know the city or community
4. Gain financial support
5. Decide where the organization for the project will be located
6. Develop the proposal
7. Appoint a project steering committee
8. Analyze the environment in which the project will take place
9. Define clearly the work of the project
10. Set up the project office
11. Plan a long-term strategy
12. Build Project Capacity
13. Establish accountability mechanisms

WHAT DO YOU THINK?   *The support of local political officials as well as community opinion leaders who may not be in a designated leadership role in planning and implementing health and health-related programs in communities is critical to the development of a Healthy Community program as well as to that of healthy public policies.*

Now compare this 13-step model above to the nine steps in the Community Health Promotion Model (Produced by the Institute for Action Research for Community Health/Indiana University, 1994) (Flynn, 1997):

1. Orient the community to the idea of community health promotion. For example, meet with formal and informal leaders to identify persons in the community who have an interest in and the capability to support the community development process. You could hold an informational community forum, or establish a task force to plan. The key is to find people who are committed to the process.
2. Build the partnership. It is important to learn who the formal and informal community leaders are so you know who is listened to in the community. Be sure to have broad-based representation on your planning committee. Remember that people participate when they think there is a need, feel a sense of community, see their involvement as helpful and worth their time, and think the benefits outweigh possible costs (CDC, 1997). Box 20-2 describes principles of community engagement that need to be considered in the community engagement process.

BOX 20-2 PRINCIPLES OF COMMUNITY ENGAGEMENT

Before starting a community engagement effort:

- Be clear about the purposes or goals of the engagement effort, and the populations and/or communities you want to engage.
- Become knowledgeable about the community in terms of its economic conditions, political structures, norms and values, demographic trends, history, and experience with engagement efforts. Learn about the community's perceptions of those initiating the engagement activities.

For engagement to occur, it is necessary to:

- Go into the community, establish relationships, build trust, work with the formal and informal leadership, and seek commitment from community organizations and leaders to create processes for mobilizing the community.
- Remember and accept that community self-determination is the responsibility and right of all people who comprise a community. No external entity should assume it can bestow on a community the power to act in its own self-interest.

For engagement to succeed, you need to:

- Partner with the community to create change and improve health.
- Recognize and appreciate all aspects of community engagement and respect community diversity. In order to effectively design and implement approaches for community engagement, be aware of the various cultures and other areas of diversity of a community.
- Realize that you can only sustain community engagement by identifying and mobilizing community assets, and by developing capacities and resources for community health decisions and action.
- Be prepared to turn over control of actions or interventions to the community, and be flexible enough to meet the changing needs of the community.
- Make a long-term commitment to the engaging organization and its partners.

From Centers for Disease Control and Prevention: *Principles of community engagement,* Atlanta, 1997, CDC. Available at http://www.cdc.gov/phppo/pce. Accessed April 4, 2010.

BOX 20-3 DESIGNING INTERVENTIONS AND EVALUATING RESULTS OF HEALTHY MUNICIPALITIES AND CITIES

- **Health education:** Health knowledge, attitudes, motivation, intentions, behavior, personal skills, and effectiveness
- **Influence and social action:** Community participation, community empowerments, social standards, and public opinion
- **Healthy public policies and organizational practices:** Political statutes, legislation, and regulation; location of resources; organization practices, culture, and behavior
- **Healthy living conditions and lifestyles:** Use of tobacco, availability of food and food choices, physical activity, consumption of alcohol and drugs, relationship between protective factors and risk factors in the physical and social environment
- **Effectiveness of health services:** Delivery of preventive services, access to the health services, and quality of services
- **Healthy environments and spaces:** Restricted sale of tobacco and alcohol; restrictions on illicit drug use; positive environments for children, young people, and older adults; and sanctions for abuse and violence
- **Social results:** Quality of life, social support networks, positive discrimination, equity, development of life skills
- **Health outcomes:** Reduction of morbidity and mortality, disability, and avoidable mortality; psychosocial and life skills
- **Capacity building and development:** Measures of sustainability, community participation and empowerment, human-resources development

From Pan American Health Organization: *Healthy municipalities and communities: mayor's guide for promoting quality of life,* Washington, DC, n.d., World Health Organization, p 24. Available at http://www.paho.org/english/ad/sde/hs/mayors_guide.htm. Accessed January 21, 2011.

3. Develop a structure in the community for health promotion. This step is similar to the PAHO stage of assembling a steering committee that will plan and coordinate the work. Some ways to collaborate and get the work done that support the HC process are: (1) the whole local partnership deliberates and shares information, but subgroups make decisions and implement them, (2) the local partnership serves as a single advisory board for multiple agencies, and (3) the whole local partnership makes decisions, but subgroups take action together (Veazie et al, 2001). The steering group might develop and communicate a clear vision and mission that is broadly understood by all participants and not just by health professionals. The mission should define the problem and acceptable solutions in such a way as to engage (not blame) those community members most affected and not to limit the strategies and environmental changes needed to address the community-identified concern. Ongoing action planning should identify specific community and system changes that can lead to widespread behavior change and community health improvement. The committee should develop widespread leadership, engaging a broad group of members and allies in the work of the community organization, mobilization, and change (Roussos and Fawcett, 2000). The membership of the working group should be diverse and clearly reflect the community's composition.

4. Determine who will lead the health promotion work. You may need to provide some leadership development work at this stage, such as sending members to conferences or workshops or using consultants or online training programs.

5. Assess the community. The steps here follow those in the chapter on community assessment. Start by clarifying the purpose of the assessment and what you will do with the data you collect. The assessment provides the frame of reference for identifying the community's strengths, needs, and resources.

6. Plan for community-wide health. Many of the skills about working with groups that are discussed in Chapter 16 will be used in this step of the process as will models for planning in Chapter 25 that discusses program management.

7. Develop community action for health. The interventions at this stage should be designed to achieve the outcomes cited in Box 20-3. These nine areas can guide the selection of actions and provide a focus for the evaluation.

8. Provide information based on data to policy makers. Effective development of public policy relies on dialogue between those making the policies and the members of the public who will be affected by them. The aim is to link policy

makers, professionals, and citizens together to achieve commonly agreed upon health goals. Examples of healthy public policies include seat belt legislation, no-smoking policies, motorcycle helmet laws, handgun laws, and immunization policies for school-age children. Providing information is a way to serve as an advocate. Nurses may be asked to testify or assist others to prepare testimony that will give the city council, county commissioners, or other members of planning groups the information they need to promote the development of healthy public policy.

9. Monitor and evaluate the progress. This step is similar in all problem-solving processes. You must watch the progress, make sure you stay on track, or make a course correction if needed and then evaluate the outcome.

As can be seen, both models use a problem-solving approach, and the latter is clearly similar to the use of the nursing process in the community with a goal of promoting health. A brief case is offered below that illustrates how a model such as the ones above are used to guide the development of a healthy community.

HOW TO Work with a Healthy Community Initiative: a Case Example

The Crooked Creek Quality of Life Initiative (CC QOLI): A Community Development Experience took place in Indianapolis, Indiana. The purpose of the initiative was to improve the quality of life of residents of a geographically defined neighborhood in an urban Midwestern city in the United States. An advisory board provided oversight for a comprehensive assessment conducted by nursing students. The assessment results were used for developing a proposal that funded an advisory group appointed by the mayor of the city. The PAHO Healthy Cities and Municipalities model was used to bring diverse sectors of the community together to collaborate in order to address the conditions responsible for health and wellbeing. Organizations involved included a hospital, social service agency, housing development agency, and university.

The goal of the CC QOLI was to improve the quality of life of Crooked Creek residents through:

1. *Revitalization of built environments (such as in commercial and community buildings, housing, roads, and sidewalks)*
2. *New collaborations among health, education, and social service organizations*
3. *Engagement of the residents in community improvement*

Initiatives implemented to achieve these goals were investment in a housing program for low- and moderate-income residents; construction of a Family Pavilion to address the civic, social, intergenerational, cultural, and recreational needs of Crooked Creek individuals and families; and a School Health Program for area students.

Results Achieved

The Fay Biccard Glick Family Pavilion at Crooked Creek was constructed and now provides a wonderful space for community gatherings, youth and family activities, recreation, and an affordable venue for wedding receptions, family reunions, graduation ceremonies, open houses, and religious services. The School Health Program moved health care delivery beyond traditional hospital walls and is now part of a broader vision to build healthier communities. School corporations have adopted healthier school policies and are able to address chronic issues of asthma, obesity, and absenteeism. Investments in housing have resulted in completion of three congregate living homes providing a home for 12 disabled

residents, and the most recent home uses "green" building practices. Additional results have been the provision of costly repairs to the homes of 33 elderly homeowners; education of 60 potential homebuyers about the home-buying process; and down payment assistance for 12 first-time buyers who purchased homes in Crooked Creek.

Factors Affecting and/or Hindering Success

A major barrier occurred when the contractor for the Family Pavilion project walked off the job midway through the project, resulting in an 8-month delay and cost overruns. Another contractor was hired and funds were raised in order to complete the project. The School Health Program became more complex when partners realized that the unique nature of each school required that interventions be tailored for each particular school's student population. The investments in housing programs found the cost of projects were sustainable only to the degree that the organization continued to successfully compete for public and private funds to underwrite projects.

Summing Up

Lessons learned across initiatives include:

1. *Collaboration makes individual organizations stronger—a new organization without a track record benefits from partnering with an established organization, which gives others "permission" to be supportive. Established organizations benefit from the energy and entrepreneurial aspects of start-ups.*
2. *Having a good plan based on good data is crucial to securing funding and support.*
3. *Program operators need to ensure that senior leaders (senior executives and board members) stay informed and engaged over time in order to sustain initiatives over the long term. Otherwise they risk being replaced by the next new (and not necessarily better) thing.*

Author(s): Alicia Chadwick with Crooked Creek Northwest Community Development Corporation, Helen Lands with Fay Biccard Glick Neighborhood Center, Mary Beth Riner with Indiana University School of Nursing, and Marty Rugh with St. Vincent Health.

DID YOU KNOW? *The Council on Linkages Competencies Project includes a set of skills that complement the processes used in the development of healthy communities.*

Community Dimensions of Practice Skills

1. *Assess community linkages and relationships among multiple factors (or determinants) affecting health.*
2. *Collaborate in community-based participatory research efforts.*
3. *Establish linkages with key stakeholders.*
4. *Facilitate collaboration and partnerships to ensure participation of key stakeholders.*
5. *Maintain partnerships with key stakeholders.*
6. *Use group processes to advance community involvement.*
7. *Describe the role of governmental and non-governmental organizations in the delivery of community health services.*
8. *Negotiate for the use of community assets and resources.*
9. *Use community input when developing public health policies and programs.*
10. *Promote public health policies, programs, and resources.*

From Council of Linkages Competency Project: Council on Linkages between academia and public based practice, 2009, Public Health Foundation. Available at http://www.phf.org. Accessed January 11, 2011.

NURSING TIP *Because nurses naturally work with community people from different walks of life and are respected health professionals in the community, they are well suited to promote Healthy Communities. Look for opportunities within existing community partnerships that you work with and that are also interested in promoting the community's health. Plan how to introduce them to the HC process, and work together to find ways to initiate the process with your combined network of contacts to develop activities that support improved health.*

Nurses may work with the healthy community process in a variety of ways and in many stages. It is important to remember that evaluation and research are important parts of the process. Specifically, nurses may initiate, coordinate, or be part of a research team conducting program evaluation research. Providing data relevant to changes in health status through short-term impact evaluation and long-term outcome evaluation is valuable in creating the knowledge base for validating the field of community health promotion.

The Linking Content to Practice box applies many of the key public health documents to the work of developing a healthy community.

LINKING CONTENT TO PRACTICE

Health promotion using the healthy community model relies on key public health skills and core competencies. Such an approach includes the core functions of assessment, policy development, and assurance, which is making sure that there is a competent work force available to meet the needs of the community. See Chapter 1 for details on the public health core functions.

Specifically, the *Public Health Nursing: Scope and Standards* uses a community-focused problem-solving process that is consistent with the steps in developing a healthy community. For example, in the 5th implementation standard the nurse should implement the identified community plan by partnering with others (ANA, 2007). The Did You Know? box earlier in the chapter examines how the Council on Linkages project's core competencies related to community dimensions of practice complement the healthy community development process (Public Health Foundation, 2009). Throughout the Quad Council Public Health Nursing Competencies documents are competencies that also fit this process. For example, in many of the domains, there is an emphasis on collaboration with others for determining health priorities and in using the policy-making progress to achieve health goals (Quad Council, 2009). Lastly, the steps in healthy community development are congruent with the Intervention Wheel that is discussed in Chapter 9.

Remember that the ultimate goal is to promote the community's own leadership for health. In other words, the nurse must not do for the community what it can do for itself. The role of the nurse and of other health professionals in Healthy Communities is to work in partnership with community leaders (Flynn, 1997). John Ashton (1989), one of the founders of the European Healthy Cities project, summarizes the role of health professionals in Healthy Cities as being "on tap, not on top."

LEVELS OF PREVENTION

Healthy Communities

Primary Prevention
Develop a community forum to initiate communication about health promotion.

Secondary Prevention
Assess needs and strengths in the community to detect ways to address health problems.

Tertiary Prevention
Initiate community action when problems have occurred and evaluate and monitor progress of programs and policies.

HOW TO Organize a Community Meeting About Healthy Communities

1. *Identify who should be included in the community meeting. It is critical that all sectors and population groups in the community be involved?*
2. *How will they be invited to the meeting? Who will invite them? Allow at least 2 weeks so people can arrange their schedules.*
3. *Who will convene the meeting?*
4. *Set the date and time for the meeting and arrange for a neutral meeting place.*
5. *Plan the meeting agenda:*
   a. *Introduction of participants*
   b. *Introduction to Healthy Communities (HC)*
   c. *Identification of community people who should be there ("Whom did we miss?")*
   d. *Questions and discussion about HC, and about community issues that are important*
   e. *Commitment to the HC process*
   f. *Formation of the HC committee (obtain names and addresses of those interested)*
   g. *Other suggestions*

CHAPTER REVIEW

PRACTICE APPLICATION

Because nurses work in partnership with the community in Healthy Communities, the examples of outcomes of HC initiatives reflect that partnership rather than a specific nursing intervention. An example of an outcome of a HC initiative that used the Community Health Promotion process is Fort Wayne, Indiana, Healthy City.

Healthy City committee members of the Fort Wayne, Indiana, Healthy City project collaborated in a community-wide program to address the fact that only 65% of Fort Wayne preschool children were immunized. Access to immunization services was expanded to five sites throughout the city at three different times in a program called Super-Shot Saturday.

A nurse, along with other members of the Fort Wayne, Indiana, HC committee, would be using which of the following principles of health promotion to provide access to immunizations for preschool children?

A. Promoting healthy public policy
B. Creating supportive environments
C. Strengthening community action
D. Reorienting health services
E. Improving personal skills
Answers can be found on the Evolve site.

KEY POINTS

- Although Healthy Cities began in 1986 in Europe, it is now an international movement of communities and cities focused on mobilizing local resources and political, professional, and community members to improve the health of the community.
- The principles of primary health care and health promotion guide the Healthy Communities movements.
- The name used for the healthy community activity varies from one locale to another.
- The models of community practice most frequently found in the Healthy Communities movement are that of working with the local people to plan via community partnerships that will best meet their needs.
- Community participation can be gained in many ways; it is often helpful to have a local person on the planning committee to advise on how to best enlist the aid and support of the residents.
- The CDC has become involved in the Healthy Communities work in its efforts to reduce the amount of chronic illness.
- The CDC has developed a wide range of tools to help communities improve their health; these tools are available on its website at no charge.

- The concept of healthy communities is used in the United States as well as in many other nations. One region that has a well-developed set of programs is that covered by the Pan American Health Organization (PAHO). The steps that are used in PAHO countries are included in the chapter.
- The steps for developing a healthy community including the use of the PAHO model or the Community Health Promotion model developed at Indiana University School of Nursing can be used by nurses working with communities to improve their health capacity.
- The first two states to develop health community projects were Indiana and California. These two states have ongoing active and responsive programs; some are discussed in the chapter.
- The *Healthy People 2020* objectives incorporate many of the key concepts of health communities including providing access to health services; combating chronic illnesses; and providing safe food, a safe and healthy environment, opportunities for fitness, immunizations, and reduction in injuries and violence, to name a few.

CLINICAL DECISION-MAKING ACTIVITIES

1. In collaboration with a community group, conduct a community assessment. Identify the community's assets and problems.
2. Evaluate the effectiveness of a current approach to a health problem in your community (e.g., teen pregnancy). Describe how the approach would change if you were to use the steps in developing a healthy community such as the Community Health Promotion process.
3. Discuss the role of the nurse in health promotion within a healthy community model.
4. Identify city council members, the president of the chamber of commerce, the director of family services, the mayor, a religious leader, and other community leaders who are the "movers and shakers" in getting things done. Generate a list of questions that

will help these leaders describe the major assets and problems of the community. Interview several local leaders and summarize their responses.
5. You are asked by the health commissioner to organize a community coalition for orientation to the Healthy Communities process. Outline the steps you would take.
6. Describe your philosophy of community leadership development for health promotion.
7. Discuss ways in which the *Healthy People 2020* objectives can incorporate community participation. Select one topic area within *Healthy People 2020* and outline a community inclusive approach that you could use.

REFERENCES

American Nurses Association: *Scope & standards of practice*, Silver Springs, MD, 2007, Public Health Nursing, ANA.

Ashton J: *Creating healthy cities*, paper presented at Healthy Cities Indiana Network Session, Seymour, IN, May 1989.

California Endowment: *Overview strategic vision 2010-2020: Building Healthy*, 2010, author. Available at www.calendow.org/healthycommunities. Accessed January 10, 2011.

Centers for Disease Control and Prevention: *About healthy places,* n.d. Available at www.cdc.gov/healthyplaces. Accessed January 10, 2011.

Centers for Disease Control and Prevention: *Principles of community engagement* (electronic version), Atlanta, 1997. Available at http://www.cdc.gov. Accessed January 10, 2011.

Centers for Disease Control and prevention: *The Power of prevention: Chronic diseases...the public health challenge of the 21st century*, Atlanta GA, 2010, National Center for Chronic Disease Promotion, CDC.

Centers for Disease Control and Prevention: *Healthy communities: Preventing chronic disease by activating grassroots change: at a glance*, 2009b. Available at www.cdc.gov/chronicdisease/resources/publications/AAGealthy_communities.htm. Accessed January 21, 2011.

Centers for Disease Control and Prevention: *Healthy communities: at a glance report*. December 23, 2009. Available at www.cdc.gov/healthycommunitiesprogram/overview/index.htm. Accessed January 10, 2011.

Columbus Regional Hospital: *Healthy communities initiative*, 2010. Available at www.crh.org/community-involvement/healthy-communities.aspx. Accessed March 12, 2010.

Flynn BC: Partnership in Healthy Cities and Communities: a social commitment for advanced practice nurses, *Adv Pract Nurs Q* 2:1, 1997.

Flynn BC, Rider MS, Ray DW: Healthy Cities: the Indiana model of community development in public health, *Health Educ Q* 18:331, 1991.

Hancock T: The evolution, impact, and significance of the Healthy Cities/Healthy Communities movement, *J Public Health Policy* 14:5, 1993.

National Civic League: *Healthy Communities initiatives*, Denver CO, 2007, author.

Pan American Health Organization: *Healthy municipalities & communities: mayors' guide for promoting quality of life,* Washington, DC, n.d., PAHO. Available at http://www.paho.org/english/ad/sde/hs/mayors-guide.htm. Accessed January 21, 2011.

Pan American Health Organization: *Healthy municipalities and communities,* Washington, DC, n.d., PAHO. Available at www.paho.org/english/hpp/hpf/hmc/hmc_about.htm. Accessed January 10, 2010.

Partnership for Prevention: *The community health promotion handbook: action guides to improve community health,* Washington, DC, 2008, Partnership for Prevention.

Public Health Foundation: *Council on Linkages between Academia and Public Health Practice, Core competencies for public health professionals,* author. Washington DC, June 11, 2009, Public Health Foundation.

Quad Council of Public Health Nursing Organizations: *Public health nursing competencies*, Wheat Ridge, CO, 2009, Quad Council.

Rothman J, Tropman JE: Models of community organization and macro practice: their mixing and phasing. In Cox FM, Tropman ME, Rothman J, Erlich JL, editors: *Strategies of community organization*, ed 4, Itasca, IL, 1987, Peacock.

Roussos ST, Fawcett SB: A review of collaborative partnerships as a strategy for improving community health, *Annu Rev Public Health* 21:369–402, 2000.

Task Force on Community Preventive Services: *The guide to community preventive services: Social environment and health,* n.d. Available at http://www.thecommunityguide.org/social/Default.htm. Accessed January 10, 2011.

Torres GW, Margolin FS: *Collaboration primer: proven strategies, consideration, and tools to get you started*, Chicago, 2003, Health Research & Educational Trust. Available at www.hret.org.

Twiss J, Dickinson J, Duma S, et al: Community gardens: lessons learned from California Healthy Cities and Communities, *Am J Public Health* 93:1435–1438, 2003.

U.S. Department of Health and Human Services: Healthy people in healthy communities: a community planning guide using *Healthy People 2010*, Washington, DC, February 2001, U.S. Government Printing Office.

U.S. Department of Health and Human Services: *Healthy People 2000: national health promotion and disease prevention objectives*, Washington, DC, 1991, USDHHS.

U.S. Department of Health and Human Services: *Healthy People in Healthy Communities 2010*, Atlanta, 2000, USDHHS, Centers for Disease Control and Prevention, National Center for Chronic Disease Prevention and Health Promotion (electronic version). Available at http://www.healthypeople.gov/Publications/HealthyCommunities2001/default.htm. Accessed July 7, 2005.

U.S. Department of Health and Human Services: Healthy People in Healthy Communities: a community planning guide using *Healthy People 2010*, Washington, DC, U.S. Goverment Printing Office, February 2001.

U.S. Department of Health and Human Services: *Healthy People 2020*, Washington, DC, 2010, USDHHS.

Veazie MA, Teufel-Shone NI, Silverman GS, et al: Building community capacity in public health: the role of action-oriented partnerships, *J Public Health Manag Pract* 7:21–32, 2001.

World Health Organization: *About WHO. Ottawa Charter for Health Promotion, 1986*, 2010. Available at www.euro.who.int/aboutwho/policy/20010827_2. Accessed January 21, 2011.

World Health Organization: *Ottawa charter for health promotion*, Copenhagen, Denmark, 1986, WHO Regional Office for Europe.

World Health Organization: United Nations Children's Fund: *Primary health care*, Geneva, Switzerland, 1978, WHO, UNICEF.

CHAPTER 21

The Nursing Center: A Model for Nursing Practice in the Community

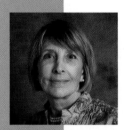

Katherine K. Kinsey, PhD, RN, FAAN

Dr. Katherine K. Kinsey is the Principal Investigator and Administrator of the Philadelphia Nurse-Family Partnership (NFP), the Mabel Morris Early Head Start Program, and the First Steps Autism Spectrum Disorder Program. Dr. Kinsey previously directed a nationally recognized academic-based nurse-managed health center. She is a past chairperson of the American Public Health Association, Public Health Nursing Section. Dr. Kinsey serves on several non-profit boards and is the president of the Kingsley Family Foundation. The foundation is dedicated to improving the well-being of vulnerable, underserved populations. Dr. Kinsey has a particular interest in advancing public health nurses and nurse-managed health centers as mainstream primary health care providers in the twenty-first century.

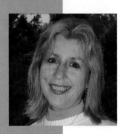

Mary Ellen T. Miller, PhD, RN

Dr. Mary Ellen T. Miller is an Assistant Professor at De Sales University School of Nursing in Center Valley, PA and teaches in the undergraduate and graduate programs. Dr. Miller serves as Co-Chair of the Wellness Center Committee of the National Nursing Center Consortium. Previously, she served as the Associate Director of Public Health Programs for an academic nursing center. Dr. Miller has published works about nurse-managed centers and presents regionally and nationally on topics related to her work, as well as about student involvement with community service and learning, and about nurse-managed wellness centers. She is a member of the American Public Health Association, the American Nurses Association, Sigma Theta Tau International, Kappa Delta Chapter, and she serves on several non-profit boards.

ADDITIONAL RESOURCES

ℯvolve WEBSITE
http://evolve.elsevier.com/Stanhope
- *Healthy People 2020*
- WebLinks
- Quiz
- Case Studies
- Glossary
- Answers to Practice Application
- Resource Tools
  - Resource Tool 21.A: Factors Influencing the Success of Collaboration
- Resource Tool 21.B: The Evolution of Nursing Centers
- Resource Tool 21.C: Nursing Center Positions
- Resource Tool 21.D: Outline of Essential Elements in Nursing Center Development
- Resource Tool 21.E: WHO Priorities for a Common Nursing Research Agenda
- Resource Tool 21.F: Principles for Nursing Center Research

OBJECTIVES

After reading this chapter, the student should be able to do the following:
1. Describe key characteristics of nursing center models.
2. Explain community collaboration.
3. Identify interventions that address *Healthy People 2020* goals.
4. Determine the feasibility of establishing and sustaining a nursing center.
5. Describe the roles and responsibilities of the advanced practice nurse in a nursing center.
6. Discuss the future of population-centered nursing practice, education, and research.

KEY TERMS

advanced practice nurses, p. 463
business plan, p. 472
community collaboration, p. 462
comprehensive primary health care, p. 465
convenient care clinics, p. 470
cost-effectiveness, p. 473
evidence-based practice, p. 474
feasibility study, p. 472

Drs. Kinsey and Miller thank Marjorie Buchanan, MS, RN for her thoughtful contributions to the development of this chapter as well as chapter co-authorship in earlier editions of *Public Health Nursing*.

Considerable data document that nursing centers improve health outcomes. The nurse-managed health center (NMHC) model increases access to care; provides a more comprehensive approach to health and illness; decreases racial, ethnic, and geographic disparities in health status; and can potentially reduce the overall costs of health care. Nurse-managed health centers, as safety net providers, reach out to and engage underserved, vulnerable populations in public health and primary health care initiatives. This chapter describes nursing centers and their origins, evolution, and future directions. Emphasis is placed on the *Healthy People 2020* framework, community collaboration, and multilevel interventions to improve access and reduce health disparities. This chapter describes nursing roles and responsibilities in delivering community-based services, managing center operations, and expanding initiatives for practice, research, and education in public health and primary care settings. Economic, social, political, national health care reform, and global factors influencing NMHC operations and population-centered nursing practice are discussed.

WHAT ARE NURSING CENTERS? (ALSO KNOWN AS NURSE-MANAGED HEALTH CENTERS OR CLINICS)

Overview and Definition

In 2011 and beyond, the terms *nursing center, nurse-managed health center,* and *nurse-managed health clinic* will be interchangeable and used to describe this model of health care. The citations in this eighth edition of *Public Health Nursing: Population-Centered Health Care in the Community* include historical references noted in earlier editions and current references regarding the evolution of NMHCs. The references frame the decades' long NMHC movement. However, the acquisition of knowledge is undergoing metamorphosis. The introduction of new Internet-based technology and communication venues regarding public health programs and NMHCs will grow exponentially (Khan et al, 2010). Access to NMHCs initiatives, public health practice examples, and career opportunities are now featured on social networking websites, wikis, and blog communities. These venues, and others still in the research and development phases, will add

---

BOX 21-1   AMERICAN NURSES ASSOCIATION NURSING CENTERS TASK FORCE: NURSING CENTER DEFINITION

Nursing centers—sometimes referred to as community nursing organizations, nurse-managed centers, nursing clinics, and community nursing centers—are organizations that give the client direct access to professional nursing services. Using nursing models of care, professional nurses in these centers diagnose and treat human responses to actual and potential health problems, and promote health and optimal functioning among target populations and communities. The services provided in these centers are holistic and client-centered and are reimbursed at the reasonable fee level. Accountability and responsibility for client care and professional practice remain with the professional nurse. Overall accountability and responsibility remain with the nurse executive. Nursing centers are not limited to any particular organizational configuration. Nursing centers can be freestanding businesses or may be affiliated with universities or other service institutions such as home-health agencies and hospitals. The primary characteristic of the organization is responsiveness to the health needs of the population.

From Aydelotte MK, Barger S, Branstetter E, et al: *The nursing center: concept and design,* Kansas City, MO, 1987, American Nurses Association, p 1.

BOX 21-2   NURSE-MANAGED HEALTH CLINIC (NMHC) INVESTMENT ACT OF 2009 DEFINITION

The term "nurse-managed health clinic" or "NMHC" means a nurse-practice arrangement, managed by advanced practice nurses, that provides primary care or wellness services to underserved or vulnerable populations and is associated with a school, college, university, or department of nursing, federally qualified health center, or an independent non-profit health or social services agency.

Source: Nurse-managed Health Clinic Investment Act of 2009. Senate Bill 1104 and House of Representatives bill 2754. For exact language see Title V, section 2512 of the House bill (HF 3962) and Title V, Subtitle c, section 5208 of the Senate bill (HR 3590).

---

rich content as NMHCs continue to transition into mainstream health care provider status.

In the past, the most frequently cited and referenced definition of *nursing centers* has been the one developed by the American Nurses Association (ANA) Nursing Centers Task Force in the mid-1980s (Box 21-1). However, the recently passed Nurse-Managed Health Clinic Investment Act of 2009 (Senate Bill 1104/House of Representatives Bill 2754) of the 111th Congress provides a more current and functional definition of nurse-managed health clinics with an amendment to Title III of the Public Health Service Act (42 U.S.C. 241 et sez.) (Box 21-2).

Nursing centers provide unique opportunities to improve the health status of individuals, families, and communities through direct access to nurses and nursing models of care (Lancaster, 1999). All nursing centers possess characteristics that reflect the values, beliefs, and scientific knowledge and skills inherent in nursing models of care. Furthermore, each is guided, managed, and primarily staffed by nurses, thus ensuring that decision making and ultimate accountability for this model of care rest with professional nurses (Kinsey and Gerrity, 2005).

The NMHC is supported by the ANA seminal position paper titled *Health Promotion and Disease Prevention* (ANA, 1995). The paper recognizes health promotion strategies as pivotal points of any health care system designed to control costs and reduce human suffering. It acknowledges nursing's scope of practice and underscores its efforts to focus on disease prevention interventions (ANA, 1995).

Nursing center models combine human caring, scientific knowledge about health and illness, and understanding of family and community characteristics, interests, assets, needs, and goals for health promotion, disease prevention, and disease management. Nursing center models de-emphasize illness-oriented and institutional care that has dominated health care

since World War II and subscribe to a holistic perspective on improving personal, community, and societal well-being.

Nursing Models of Care

Nursing centers are strategically positioned to improve the health and well-being of vulnerable populations (Kinsey, 1999), build on the core values and beliefs of the profession (Matherlee, 1999), and reduce health disparities by providing access to comprehensive primary health care and health promotion and disease prevention services (Hansen-Turton, Miller, and Greiner, 2009) (Figure 21-1). Social determinants of health (Wilensky and Satcher, 2009) as well as the integration of trust, caring, personal respect, equity, and social justice perspectives serve as the foundation from which health is viewed as a resource for everyday life (Buchanan, 1997). Efforts of the center focus on enhancing people's capacity to meet their personal, family, and community responsibilities and interests and typically include the following:

- *Community-based culturally competent care* that is accessible, acceptable, and responsive to the populations being served
- A *holistic approach* to care based upon complex and interrelated biopsychosocial factors
- *Interorganizational and interdisciplinary collaboration* that crosses health and human service systems and increases opportunities for comprehensive and seamless services among care providers, agencies, and payers
- *Multilevel interventions* that acknowledge organizational, environmental, health, economic, and social policy contributions to health, health problems, and issues of access to care
- *Community partnerships* in establishing and supporting the center's health efforts
- *Relationship-based practice* with individuals, families, organizations, and communities that fosters understanding of context, interests, and needs for health care

Nursing center models combine people, place, approach, and strategy in everyday life to develop appropriate health interventions. Advanced practice nurses (APNs) work in close partnership with the communities they serve to provide public health programs, community-wide health education, and primary health care services. They establish relationships with

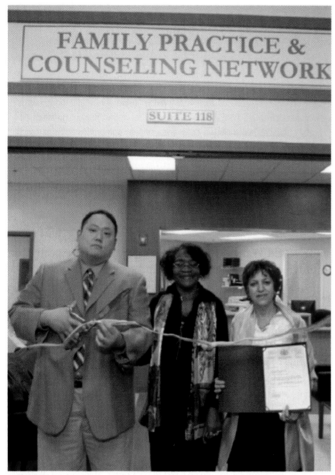

FIGURE 21-1 Donna Torrisi, MSN, Nurse-Managed Health Center Director with community leaders at the 2008 Grand Opening of the Family Practice and Counseling Health Annex, Philadelphia, PA. (From Family Practice and Counseling Network Clients, Philadelphia, PA.)

BOX 21-3   NURSING CENTER TYPOLOGIES

Service Model
- *Wellness centers:* Provide health promotion and disease prevention programs
- *Comprehensive primary care centers:* Provide health-oriented primary care and public health programs
- *Special care centers:* Provide programs targeting specific health conditions (such as diabetes) or population groups (such as the frail elderly)

Organizational Structure
- *Academic nursing center:* Housed within a school of nursing
- *Free-standing center:* Independent center with its own governing board
- *Subsidiary:* Part of larger health care systems, home-health agencies, community centers, senior centers, schools, and others
- *Affiliated center:* Legal partnership association with health, human services, or other organization

Internal Revenue Service Designation
- *501(c)3:* Non-profit business
- *Proprietary:* Incorporated as a for-profit business

Reimbursement Mechanism
- *Fee-for-service:* Payment at time of service; may include sliding-fee scale
- *HMO provider:* Payment at contracted rates by health maintenance organization
- *Federally Qualified Health Center (FQHC):* Federal designation that allows cost-based reimbursement per encounter
- *Third-party reimbursement:* Client billing to public program or commercial/private insurance
- *Contributions:* Individual donations, philanthropic gifts, fund-raising activities to support a program

---

families, community representatives, policy makers, and others in designing, implementing, and evaluating appropriate health intervention strategies, services, and programs (Zimmerman, Mieczkowski, and Wilson, 2002; Hansen-Turton, Miller, and Greiner, 2009).

A nursing center's *health* and *community* orientation builds strong connections to the population served. These strong relationships with community leaders, residents, and clients foster a deep awareness of local factors that influence daily life (Lundeen, 1999). This orientation builds on Lillian Wald's community work more than a century ago. Wald's work to establish The Henry Street Visiting Nurse Service and a cadre of public health nurses who treated social and economic problems—not just infections, diseases, and providing care to the chronically ill—is part of the nursing center legacy (Fee and Bu, 2010).

TYPES OF NURSING CENTERS

There are many types of nursing centers. Each has a "personality" of its own (Gerrity and Kinsey, 1999). A center's mission, values, goals, and strategies, as well as its commitment to community well-being, contribute to its profile (Clear, Starbecker, and Kelly, 1999). Organizational structure (academic, nonacademic), federal tax status (profit or non-profit), and **reimbursement systems** (fee for service, sliding scale fee rates, or no charge) also define centers. Other types will evolve due to the 2010 national health care reform legislation. The legislative initiatives include maximizing federally qualified health center services; increasing access to **primary health care** for people of all ages; introducing new public health, preventive health, and home visiting programs; and implementing and using electronic medical records. To date, most nursing centers fit into the types described in Box 21-3.

Wellness Centers

Wellness centers focus on health promotion, disease prevention, and management programs. APNs and others provide outreach and public awareness services, health education, immunizations, family assessment and screening services, home visiting, and social support (Evans et al, 1997; Hansen-Turton, Miller, and Greiner, 2009). Public health education and support programs may include smoking cessation (Lakon, Hipp, and Timberlake, 2010), weight management counseling, and parenting classes (Hurst and Osban, 2000). "Enabling" services help people access language translation, registration for entitlement programs, transportation vouchers, and specialty services. *Healthy People 2020* goals and objectives provide direction to services planned, implemented, and evaluated through the wellness center model.

These centers complement existing primary care services. The staff maintains strong relationships with local health care providers in community health centers, clinics, private practices, long-term care facilities, and other organizations. In general, financial support for center programs comes from public health department and other service contracts, foundation grants, fee for services, voluntary contributions, and shared resources from affiliated organizations (Oros et al, 2001). In addition, these centers often serve as venues for community service learning activities for graduate and undergraduate students from multiple disciplines. Nursing centers extend learning beyond the classroom and into the community, providing a legitimate experience whereby students apply theoretical content to a community setting (Miller and Guigliano, 2006).

Special Care Centers

Some nursing centers focus on a particular demographic group or on those with special health care needs. Special care centers are responsive and provide services and specialized health knowledge and skills to a particular group, and they are an adjunct to comprehensive primary health care models. Examples of special care centers are those that focus on the needs of people with diabetes or HIV/AIDS, adolescent mothers, the frail elderly, and support services for people with mental disorders (Alakeson, Frank, and Katz, 2010).

Comprehensive Primary Health Care Centers

In many communities, nursing centers offer comprehensive primary health care. In addition to the health and wellness programs described previously, these centers also serve as the primary care (medical) home for families in the communities where they are located. Both physical and behavioral health care services are provided by nurse practitioners, other APNs, and allied health professionals. These centers address the needs of individuals and families across the life span, ensuring access to specialized health care as indicated. Public health nurses and community workers provide outreach, social support, and an array of public health programs. The public health programs include health education, screening, immunizations, lead poisoning prevention, home visitation such as the Nurse-Family Partnership, Early Head Start, environmental health initiatives, and other preventive community-based health services (Figure 21-2).

Comprehensive primary health care centers face the challenge of establishing systems for documenting clinical care and utilization patterns. These systems include demographic profiles, accounting support, billing mechanisms, reimbursement protocols, quality improvement strategies, and client satisfaction measures (Sherman, 2005). Nursing centers must meet standards established by government, insurers, health maintenance organizations, and other payers.

Some primary health centers are designated as federally qualified health centers (FQHCs) by the Bureau of Primary Health Care (BPHC) of the U.S. Department of Health and Human Services (USDHHS). Their purposes are to (1) provide population-based comprehensive care in medically underserved

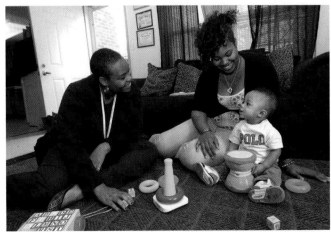

FIGURE 21-2 Investing in the future: public health nurses and programs like Nurse-Family Partnership, Early Head Start, Parents as Teachers, and others improve family health and mother-child (or maternal-child) well-being. (Used with permission of Philadelphia Inquirer Copyright © 2010. All rights reserved.)

areas and (2) maintain the appropriate mission, organizational, and governance structure according to the FQHC designation. These designations include community health center, public housing center, homeless center, or school based center.

The FQHC designation is important from a number of perspectives. Most importantly, it supports a primary care center's efforts to serve low-income and uninsured populations and remain fiscally solvent. FQHCs receive federal grant funds from the Health Resources and Services Administration (HRSA) to support operational expenses. They also receive cost-based payment for services provided to Medicare and Medicaid patients, Federal Tort Claim coverage, and 340b drug pricing, and they have the option to participate in the National Health Services Corps.

Many nursing centers need to overcome internal and external organizational hurdles to initiate the FQHC application process and receive funding approval (Torrisi and Hansen-Turton, 2005). The National Nursing Centers Consortium (NNCC), with offices in Philadelphia and Washington, DC, provides regional training for the FQHC application processes. By 2010, more nurse-managed primary care centers have achieved FQHC or "Look Alikes" status and are documenting clinical outcomes regarding chronic disease management as well as fiscal solvency that allows for site expansion. The recent passage of the Nurse-Managed Health Clinic Investment program by the 111th Congress holds great potential for additional NMHC-affiliated academic institutions to be eligible for FQHC status.

Many NMHCs are in non-profit academic settings. They are housed within or closely affiliated with schools of nursing. These NMHCs actively integrate service, education, and research in their model. They build upon public health and primary care nurse practitioner educational programs, draw upon the knowledge and skills of faculty, and provide rich learning experiences for nursing students at all levels. Furthermore, they use the knowledge, skills, and resources of other schools of health professions, business, communications, and law to expand the center's service capacity (Shiber and D'Lugoff, 2002).

One example of an academic nurse-managed health center is the Lewis and Clark Community College Nurse-Managed Health Center located in Godfrey, Illinois. The college also has a mobile health unit. This NMHC was the first to open to the public on a U.S. community college campus. The center provides non-emergency, low-cost primary care services and partners with the Southern Illinois Healthcare Foundation for referrals and specialty care. Nursing students have clinical rotations through the NMHC and its mobile unit. Students and faculty are involved in client education and illness prevention services. This model introduces students to the expanding roles and responsibilities of APNs in community settings and career options (Weller, 2010).

Other centers may be affiliated with free-standing organizations, subsidiaries of health care or other human services organizations, or sponsored by an affiliate of such entities. Each of these organizational arrangements requires carefully established legal agreements. To conduct business, these organizations must become incorporated; apply to the Internal Revenue Service (IRS) for a tax status designation; and receive a Statement of Tax Status Determination. Organizations are generally categorized as a non-profit (501(c)3) entity or some form of proprietary (for-profit) organization. The majority of nursing centers are with non-profit organizations; others fit within a proprietary business mode, and others operate as subsidiaries of established organizations. In all cases, staff must be familiar with the particular laws and regulations associated with the IRS tax status under which they operate.

Another way to describe nursing centers involves the health care system's financial reimbursement methods that support services and programs. These include fee-for-service, designated HMO provider, Medicaid provider, Medicare provider, and FQHC status. Each designation requires a center to possess certain characteristics, meet a set of standards, and possess identification numbers that allow them to participate in billing and reimbursement systems.

Regardless of the type of nursing center, a wide array of personal, social, educational, economic, and environmental concerns indicate the need for and expansion of nursing centers. Increasing population density and diversity, challenging community conditions, and long-standing and emerging health problems indicate the role such models of care can play (Kinsey, 2002). The national health reform law, The Patient Protection and Affordable Care Act, holds the potential for NMHCs to work with like entities to help improve the nation's health. The new law and other legislative changes focus on reforming the health care system, increasing disease prevention initiatives and access to services, and containing or reducing health care expenditures (Thorpe and Ogden, 2010). The national commitment to build integrated delivery systems offers nursing centers and academic health systems new opportunities to demonstrate effectiveness, efficiency, and cost savings (Dentzer, 2010).

With the anticipation of NMHC expansion grants, it is essential to work with like-minded individuals and groups to share knowledge, resources, and lessons learned. Several organizations dedicated to the promotion and sustainability of NMHCs are in place to support its members through these expansion phases. The NNCC is one nationally recognized organization

dedicated to this work. As of 2010, NNCC represents more than 200 members and is the largest national repository of member nurse–managed health centers. Its members represent organizations, programs within parent organizations, free-standing entities, and individuals invested in the nurse-managed center model. (A current membership list is available at www.nncc.us.) Members have the benefits of NNCC monthly newsletters, grant updates, current legislative and advocacy work, and its Annual National Conference. NNCC reaches out to non-profit organizations and individuals interested in establishing or expanding a nurse-managed health center (clinic) model. The Consortium often links members with potential members to share expertise and consult on program design and implementation.

Another consortium, The Michigan Academic Consortium (MAC), recently conducted a survey of all schools of nursing identified by the American Association of Colleges of Nursing. The survey found that there are approximately 138 academic NMHCs. Additional information can be found through the Institute of Nursing Centers (http://www.nursingcenters.org/) and the Nursing Centers Research Network (http://www4.uwm.edu/nursing/ncrn/). According to NNCC surveys, there are an additional 112 NMHCs operating as non-profit organizations or through community colleges.

DID YOU KNOW? *Nursing centers can be found in every region of the nation.*

⬤ LINKING CONTENT TO PRACTICE

This chapter discusses the ways in which nurses provide primary care and public health services within the context of a nursing center. The skills of assessment, planning, implementation, evaluation, and policy development are integral to this role. In order to effectively practice in a nursing center, nurses use the standards of nursing practice from many specialty areas as well as the core competencies for both public health nursing and public health. Specifically, the nurse working in this setting would incorporate the following core competencies from the Quad Council of Nursing (2009). These competencies are built on those of the Council on Linkages (PHF, 2009) and their core competencies for public health professionals. For example, Domain #1 in both documents describes analytic assessment skills and Competency #1 is "conducts thorough health assessments of individuals, families, communities and populations." There are 10 additional skills that nurses would use from this domain in nursing centers. As has been discussed throughout this chapter, nurses working in nursing centers use the policy process in providing care. Domain #2 is that of policy development/program planning skills and each of the 11 competencies/skills are used in a nursing center.

From Public Health Foundation, Council on Linkages: *Core competencies for public health professionals,* Washington DC, 2009, PHF; Quad Council: Domains of practice, 2009. Available at http:www.sphtc.org/phn_competencies_final_comb.pdf. Accessed July 29, 2010.

THE FOUNDATIONS OF NURSING CENTER DEVELOPMENT

The foundations for integrating primary care and public health services through the NMHC model include the perspective of the World Health Organization (WHO) and the *Healthy People*

2020 systematic approach to improving individual and community health.

World Health Organization

The WHO's (1978) definition of health and its framework to address global health supports an NMHC's integration of primary care and public health services in community settings.

Healthy People 2020

The *Healthy People* initiative has framed the nation's health promotion and disease prevention agenda since 1980. Its framework, vision, mission, goals, and objectives are developed to achieve better health for all by 2020. *Healthy People* represents a collaborative federal, public, and stakeholder process and accounts for global and national environmental, social, demographic changes, and trends such as the increasing older populations. *Healthy People* accommodates the escalating technological influences on personal and population health status, and incorporates anticipated changes in the U.S. sickness-oriented health system. Chapter two describes the history of *Healthy People,* and chapters throughout the text apply the objectives of *Healthy People 2020* to their content. The concept of *Healthy People 2020* builds on shared responsibility to improve the nation's health. Communities, individuals, and systems have the potential for change, yet no one person or organization can do this alone. Powerful, productive partnerships among diverse people and groups and long-term commitments to community collaboration are needed to achieve *Healthy People 2020* goals. NMHCs can help to achieve the goals and objectives of *Healthy People 2020* and would emphasize those goals and objectives that fit the target populations' needs. For example, an NMHC associated with an elementary school where more than 40% of the students are obese would select *Healthy People 2020* objectives relative to childhood nutrition, physical activity, and exercise. The NMHC would also implement communication strategies that address the need to reduce childhood obesity in school-age children.

Community Collaboration

Nursing centers and APNs are well positioned to guide and facilitate community collaboration and engagement (Keefe, Leuner, and Laken, 2000; Bechtel and Ness, 2010). Productive collaboration requires staff expertise and commitment from many to change communication patterns, professional agendas, and speak in a common voice to generate positive community transformation (Cross and Prusak, 2002). The community transformations occur through policy, legislative, and funding changes that improve the health status of many and help design the patient-centered medical homes that include NMHCs (Landon et al, 2010).

Individuals, families, groups, organizations, policy makers, and staff are involved in the process. Referred to as stakeholders, each entity offers diversity in perspective. Their particular knowledge and skills enhance the community's efforts to address critical needs, solve problems, and recognize unique strengths and resources. Stakeholders facilitate or undermine

HEALTHY PEOPLE 2020

The following objectives are examples that pertain to the work of nurses in nursing centers:
- ECBP-3.3: Advocating for personal, family and community health (skills).
- HC/HIT-2: Increase the proportion of persons who report that their health care providers have satisfactory communication skills.
- AHS-7: Increase the proportion of persons who receive appropriate evidence-based clinical preventive services.
- MICH-10: Increase the proportion of pregnant women who receive early and adequate prenatal care.
- MICH-21: Increase the proportion of infants who are breastfed.

From U.S. Department of Health and Human Services: *Healthy People 2020: understanding and improving health,* Washington, DC, 2010, U.S. Government Printing Office.

strategic efforts to improve health. It is impossible to fully know and address issues and concerns in a community without having all perspectives heard and every stakeholder respectful of different opinions and experiences (Hansen-Turton and Kinsey, 2001; Bechtel and Ness, 2010).

> **NURSING TIP** *Take the time to carefully listen to others' perspectives and experiences before taking action.*

Collaboration takes time, effort, and resources. It requires nurturing and support to make it work. Relationships among people and organizations serve as the foundation for the collaborative process and for community change. Relationships begin with introductions and open discussion to listen and learn from one another. From this, relationships grow toward a collective willingness to work together toward a common purpose, sharing *risks, responsibilities, resources,* and *rewards* along the way. The definition of collaboration developed by Mattessich and Monsey (1992) describes the work involved; they view collaboration as a relationship entered into by two or more groups to achieve common goals that are well defined and beneficial to all. There must be a respectful commitment to these goals with mutual accountability and authority that allows for shared responsibilities, resources, and successes. See Resource Tool 21.A: Factors Influencing the Success of Collaboration.

Nursing center staff require skills in networking, coordination, and cooperation in order to collaborate (Floyd, 2001). A number of basic agreements and interview strategies help set the stage for a long-term process of discussion, decision making, and action (Rollnick, Miller, and Butler, 2008). Once established, they are reviewed and rigorously adhered to throughout the life of the collaboration. These agreements are:

- Regular meetings where diverse perspectives are heard and respected
- A mutually agreed upon decision-making process
- Consistent and accurate communications so all participants have the necessary information to make decisions
- Agreement by all participants to support collaborative decisions once they are made—within the groups or organizations they represent and publicly in the community

Mattessich and Monsey (1992) have identified six critical elements that contribute to the success of a collaborative endeavor: the environment, membership characteristics, process and structure of the group, communication patterns, purpose of the collaboration, and resources within and outside the group.

Perhaps the most important feature in community collaboration is the capacity of those involved to enhance the capacity of *another* person, group, or organization in service to the common purpose. For instance, rather than the nursing center serving as the lead organization, different participating organizations will serve from time to time in the leadership role, or hold greater responsibility, or perhaps receive additional funds to achieve the common purpose to which they all have subscribed. Through this, mutual benefit is realized by all (Goffee and Jones, 2001).

Each nursing center develops its philosophy, goals, and activities through a process of community collaboration, community assessment, and strategic planning. Strategic planning recognizes multiple levels of intervention required for bringing about and sustaining change. Often, community collaboration and assessment are concurrent activities.

Community Assessment

Nurse-managed centers must conduct periodic community assessments. This chapter reemphasizes the importance of data and analysis of community needs and assets in determining the type of nursing center to establish or expand. Through the assessment process, nurses learn both the community's formal and informal infrastructure and the communication networks through which everyday life takes place (Baker, White, and Lichtveld, 2001). Neighborhood walks, bus rides, car trips, and discussions with elected officials, administrators of health care systems, public health department staff, and community members provide insight into the community's health and the many other influencing factors (Figure 21-3). Also, historical,

ethnographic multimedia news features add context to the community assessment (Anderson, 1999).

Assessment activities identify community assets and health problems. For example, there may be a rich network of block captains who serve as leaders and communication liaisons with the community. There may be a local community college that can provide space and support for meetings. If high rates of childhood asthma are discovered, there may be human service organizations that can help in disease prevention and management efforts (Kawachi and Berkman, 2003).

As nurses conduct individual interviews and focus groups, develop surveys, review health care data, and examine various indexes (social, educational, employment, economic, housing, and others), they gather detailed information about the health status of the community. These sources of information build an understanding of the community and its traditions, strengths, interests, concerns, problems, needs, and preferences. The assessment process includes sharing current health data, historical trends, and future projections with the community. Center staff can discuss the findings, share perspectives and ideas, and encourage involvement in the collaborative process. From this, the nursing center's overall direction, services, and programs emerge (Anderko, 2000).

Multilevel Interventions

As the community and the center work together for comprehensive community health, a multilevel approach is needed. Some behavioral decisions or changes occur at the individual and family level. However, for comprehensive community health improvement, strategies are needed at organizational, community, and sociopolitical levels. Nursing center staff may focus their efforts on system issues, community capacity, and family and individual health care access concurrently. Alternatively, the staff may concentrate programmatic efforts solely

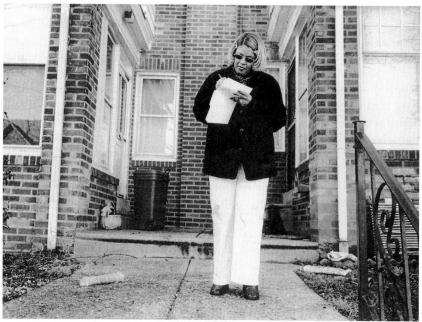

FIGURE 21-3 Neighborhood walks provide insight into the community's health.

at the individual or family level and later address system and community issues. There is no one approach. Figure 21-4 presents the "big picture" perspective that the majority of center interventions take place in community rather than institutional settings. In the twenty-first century, innovative and disruptive preventive health models are challenging the status quo of institutionally driven primary care practices (Lawrence, 2010). APNs involved in public health and nurse-managed center services are strategically positioned to communicate, adapt, and influence change to improve and support individual, population and community health outcomes (Vermeulen, Puranam, and Gulati, 2010). The multilevel intervention approach helps people enter the health care system earlier, with greater ease and confidence, and continue in care long enough to realize positive outcomes (Berkman and Lochner, 2002). This approach also recognizes that one size (static, rote services) does not meet all the needs and interests of the target population.

> **WHAT DO YOU THINK?**   *Using the multilevel approach, how could you address childhood obesity in the community served by your nursing center?*

Prevention Levels

Nurses keep in mind the prevention levels that improve the health of the public. *Primary, secondary,* and *tertiary prevention* are not terms the general population understands. In fact, the idea of prevention at different levels requires thoughtful investigation and analysis. One of multiple national resources regarding prevention levels and agendas is Partnership for Prevention (www.prevent.org). The Levels of Prevention box is one example that a NMHC might use.

History Has Paved the Way

The foundations of nursing center development are rooted in public health nursing history and the evolution of the nursing profession (Reverby, 1993; Fee and Bu, 2010). Other chapters provide historical details and factors that have influenced nursing education, practice, service, and research throughout the twentieth century.

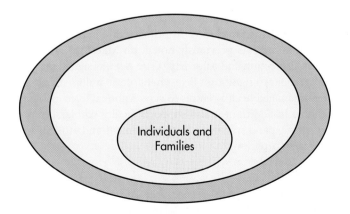

Sociopolitical systems
FIGURE 21-4 Multilevel intervention model.

> **LEVELS OF PREVENTION**
> *Nursing Center Application*
>
> **Primary Prevention**
> Assess home for lead dust; educate family on lead poisoning prevention strategies.
>
> **Secondary Prevention**
> Conduct blood lead level screenings on a regular basis for children younger than age 6.
>
> **Tertiary Prevention**
> Treat child who has an elevated blood lead level with appropriate therapies and eliminate environmental lead toxicity exposures.

The twenty-first–century nursing center model was a new and untested dimension of the health care landscape in the 1970s. Most nursing center models as currently known emerged from academic nursing programs in the 1970s through 1990s. At that time, opportunities did not exist within the traditional health care system for faculty or their nurse practitioner students to apply their knowledge and skills in a nursing framework of care. Bold ideas in the schools of nursing at the University of Wisconsin-Milwaukee, Arizona State University, Columbia University, and others established practice settings that simultaneously provided health care to the community and learning experiences for students. Many of the academic centers focused on the underserved populations in nearby communities. Over time, centers have achieved national recognition as essential safety net providers to vulnerable populations (Sherman, 2005).

> **DID YOU KNOW?**   *Most nursing centers are recognized in their communities as essential safety net providers.*

The success of these early efforts supported the establishment of other academic nursing centers across the nation. Interest in this model of practice grew rapidly among community service organizations, schools, churches, public housing facilities, and others (Bellack and O'Neil, 2000). Although there continues to be no historical or current databank regarding the absolute number of nursing centers that have been developed, NNCC surveys document that models have been developed in every state, and in urban, suburban, and rural communities. However, there are nurse-managed centers that have curtailed services or shut their doors. Factors cited include funding challenges, changes in institutional commitment, scarcity of qualified advanced practice nurses, and population losses resulting from natural catastrophes (Pohl et al, 2010).

Resource Tool 21.B highlights the evolution of nursing centers over the past century, and lists educational, political, legislative, and funding factors that have influenced the development and sustainability of nursing centers. This evolutionary trend will be altered given the Patient Protection and Affordability Care Act and committed funding to NMHCs. New opportunities for growth and secure funding are predicted. Time will tell.

THE NURSING CENTER TEAM

Nurses, including APNs, other health and allied health professionals, support staff and the community at large, comprise the nursing center team. The nursing center type and its services determine staff patterns and roles, responsibilities, and reporting lines. Every nursing center must have an organizational chart that clearly shows staffing positions and reporting responsibilities. The organizational framework may be dynamic in nature and adaptive to new community-focused initiatives.

A fundamental premise to any nursing center is that the community in which the model is placed has the most power and influence on model development and team composition. The demand for services will be community driven. A rural nursing center model may have different staff needs than one situated in a distressed urban area (Jacobson, 2002).

A center's success also relates to how well the team works together to ensure the delivery of high-quality health care to target populations (Heifetz and Linsky, 2002). Positive collegial and professional relationships set the tone for the work. Critical nursing center clinical and management positions are briefly highlighted in the following section. Resource Tool 21.C presents actual or potential nursing center positions and extensive descriptions of staff and adjunct roles.

Director: Nurse Executive

The director or nurse executive is an APN who is committed to the nursing center model. The roles and responsibilities of the nurse executive are dynamic and diverse. The director has a current knowledge of the target community, the ability and willingness to work with many community organizations and groups, and a background in organizational planning, administration, and fiscal management. The nurse executive is responsible for oversight of contracts and grants, annual reports, and development of the advisory board or board of directors. Other responsibilities include hiring and retention of highly qualified staff.

Directors are visionary leaders and planners. They constantly use data, collaborative feedback, existing resources, and partnerships to modify and adjust the overall direction of the nursing center (Salmon, 2007; Torrisi and Hansen-Turton, 2005). As NMHCs have evolved and third-party reimbursement opportunities for nurse practitioner services increase, APN practitioners have assumed leadership positions in center practices. Likewise, advanced practice public health nurses have led the nurse-managed health center movement and employed nurse practitioners as advanced practice providers. For the most part, public health nurse directors have implemented a holistic service model. This model incorporates public health service and community-based programs that complement the primary care services.

There are nurse-managed centers that started with public health programs and then established primary health care services. These public health programs include maternal-child home visitation funded by Title V federal funds, Nurse-Family Partnership (NFP), and Environmental Protection Agency (EPA) grants focusing on lead poisoning prevention, asthma triggers prevention, and many others. Other centers started with primary health care services at one location and later considered public health services.

Advanced Practice Nurses

Advanced practice nurses (APNs) have additional education and training beyond their basic nursing program and are certified or licensed in a specialty area such as women's health nurse practitioner. They provide an expanded level of health services to individuals and families. These nurses are responsible for the oversight of clinical staff as well as program services and outcome measures.

Nurses with advanced preparation in community or public health nursing are essential to the advancement of nursing center and integrated health services (Aydelotte et al, 1987; Dentzer, 2010). These nurses use nursing and public health principles to promote and sustain the health of populations in neighborhood and community settings. Their work is diverse. Nurses are responsible for assessing populations' needs and interests in health care, developing grant proposals to expand services, and managing contracts for preventive and early intervention programs in community settings. Nurses implement group health education classes and screenings, and provide individual case management in community and home settings. Health advocacy is an essential component of their work (ANA, 2007).

In comprehensive primary care centers, nurse practitioners provide on-site services. As APNs, nurse practitioners can be generalists (i.e., family nurse practitioners who provide services to people of all ages) or specialists. The specialist nurse practitioner has skills with particular age groups (e.g., pediatric, adolescent, or geriatric) or skills developed to meet the interests and needs of particular population groups such as women's health; menopausal health; and wound, ostomy, and continence management (Horrocks, Anderson, and Salisbury, 2002).

Naylor and Kurtzman's article in *Health Affairs* (2010) discusses nursing workforce issues, and the need to support the work of APNs in primary care settings. In 2004, APNs represented about 8% of the 2.9 million licensed registered nurses in the United States (DHHS, 2004). The majority of APNs practice in primary care and public health settings, including FQHCs, local and state health departments, NMHCs, and convenient care clinics (retail clinics).

National health reform legislation supports increasing the advanced practice workforce in primary care patient–centered medical homes. As previously noted, on March 23, 2010, the Patient Protection and Affordable Care Act was signed into law. The act makes a significant investment of $50 million to expand nurse-managed health centers to serve vulnerable, at-risk populations. In addition, it also supports faculty scholarship programs to expand nursing school enrollment and student loan repayment programs.

Other Staff

Community health workers are essential staff in many nursing centers. Typically, they are neighborhood residents who have completed high school or 2-year associate degree programs and who want to work with others in their community. The workers are trained in community outreach, family case management, or on-site services (Rosenthal et al, 2010).

The operations of any nursing center require support staff. Staff include a business or operations manager and data operations personnel. A parent organization may dedicate a portion of staff lines including human resources and public relations to assist the director and senior staff. The operations manager handles contracts and grant budgets, advertising for staff, personnel hires, and billing. Personnel management, staffing patterns, and site management including data collection are also responsibilities of an operations manager.

Data operations personnel are essential. Client-based and population-based outcomes are necessary for program evaluation, proposal development, and funding purposes. Rapid changes in technology related to billing and reporting requirements, and federal regulations regarding protection of information about an individual's health care status, require data operations personnel on site or as consultants. In today's litigious society, the operation of any nursing center involves ensuring privacy of client records and securing access to computerized data.

At present and into the future, information systems (IS) and technology support (TS) personnel must be in place to meet the escalating expectation to institute and effectively use a computerized client-centered database. Computerized systems require upgrades and maintenance. Also, as hardware and software programs become obsolete and new programs are introduced, staff will need training and support to adapt to new data systems.

Staff may also be needed for public relations and multimedia campaigns to gain support as the center expands. Other multidisciplinary providers are engaged in nursing center work and share responsibility in outreach and educational campaigns. Provider representation is diverse. Staff includes physician collaborators, family therapists, mental health counselors, students, faculty, administrators, and clinical social workers. Other professionals include dentists, podiatrists, lactation specialists, and clinicians with interests in holistic health (Lutz, Herrick, and Lehman, 2001).

Educators and Researchers

The education and research roles held by faculty, staff, and consultants are essential if the nursing center model is to advance in today's health care system (AACN, 2002). The opportunity for faculty involvement through clinical training of students as well as community-focused research programs is evident and promising for community collaboration and well-being (Greiner and Knebel, 2003).

Students

Nursing center programs are client and student oriented. Nursing students can learn about the intersection of health care economics, service, education, and research (Thies and Ayers, 2004). Students also have opportunities to promote social justice while engaging in community service learning activities with underserved, vulnerable populations (Hansen-Turton, Miller, and Greiner, 2009). If the nursing center is part of a school of nursing, faculty roles include clinical oversight of graduate and undergraduate students assigned to the nursing center or involved in related community projects, such as adult influenza inoculation campaigns.

Other Members

Other members include community advocates, board of directors/advisory board members, and organizational partners. Community advocates are frequently known as key stakeholders. Community voices are often the most influential and listened to by elected officials and their staff.

Every nursing center should have a board of directors or advisory board. The organizational structure of a nursing center as part of a larger institution or a free-standing entity dictates the type of board members that govern or advise staff on the direction of the center. A board of directors has oversight responsibilities, including fiscal management, for the nursing center model. An advisory board guides the work of a nursing center but holds no fiduciary or voting responsibilities. The board should represent diverse professions and occupations and be knowledgeable about the target community and its residents.

In addition, organizational partners are valued members. Nursing centers that develop and maintain organizational relationships will benefit through service agreements and contracts with one or more of the partners.

THE BUSINESS SIDE OF NURSING CENTERS: ESSENTIAL ELEMENTS

Nurses who work in nursing centers are committed to working with diverse people in non-institutional settings. The nurses use community characteristics, population profiles, health indexes, epidemiological findings, and positive working relationships with professionals and the public at large to develop the model (Gerrity and Kinsey, 1999). The model requires careful planning and structure to be a successful education, service, and business enterprise. During the planning and implementation phases, interrelated elements must be considered. Resource Tool 21.D outlines essential elements in nursing center development. These elements serve as an annual checklist to measure growth of a nursing center and guide sound decisions regarding sustainability and future planning.

Start-Up and Sustainability

In planning and establishing a nursing center (Schultz, Krieger, and Galea, 2002), nurses and others need to seek expert advice and support. This includes having financial advisors. It is important to remember that this work is a business enterprise in which the art and science of nursing is practiced. Final decisions about establishing a nursing center are made after exploration of the following essential areas:

1. Organizational goals, commitments, and resources
2. Community interests, assets, and needs
3. Feasibility study, internal and external to the parent organization
4. Strategic plan
5. Business plan
6. Information management plan and resources

7. Existing social policy and health care financing
8. Legal and regulatory considerations
9. Mission, vision, and commitment of the lead organization

The initial work of assessing the interests, resources, and capacity of an organization to undertake the nursing center model is interrelated yet separate. For example, a feasibility study may be undertaken before the development of a business plan, but elements of the feasibility study will be incorporated into the business plan. Similarly, a strategic plan must build on feasibility data as well as economic principles and practices. Planners must also consider workforce needs, personnel management, public information and outreach campaigns, community capacity, and the health care environment relative to funding streams. In 2011 and beyond, any feasibility study must analyze the national health care reform legislation, dollars committed, and funded programs. As a cautionary note, dollars committed do not guarantee funding at that level. Regardless of the federal funding level, there will be widespread competition for program support.

Feasibility Study

A **feasibility study** identifies the strengths, limitations, and capacity of an organization and the community to support the establishment and continuation of a nursing center. It requires interviews with key individuals, surveys and data collection, focus groups, and community forums. It is necessary to consider epidemiological, environmental, and other community assessments as well as data from public health agencies. Local agencies and tertiary care institutions can provide data about health needs and gaps in care for targeted groups. The study must consider legal and regulatory policies. States vary in their regulations for APNs, particularly nurse practitioners. The planners must investigate required professional credentialing, site accreditation, state Medicaid waivers, physician collaborative agreements, and any local or state requirements (Stacy, 2000; Naylor and Kurtzman, 2010). The overall processes of community collaborations, assessment, and feasibility studies support the development of business plans, strategic plans, and timelines.

A sound business plan considers all aspects of establishing a nursing center and describes the development and direction of the nursing center and how goals will be met (see the How To Develop a Business Plan box).

HOW TO Develop a Business Plan

1. *Cover page includes date, name, address, and phone number(s) of the person(s) responsible for the nursing center and any consultants to the business plan.*
2. *Executive summary. This is a one- or two-page overview of the center and the plan.*
3. *Table of contents*
4. *Description of the business plan. This details what the center is and what services it will provide.*
5. *Survey of the industry. This summarizes the past, present, and future of the local and regional health care market.*
6. *Market research and analysis. This description outlines existing competition and the potential market share and identifies target groups.*
7. *Marketing plan. This details how the center will reach its targeted clients.*
8. *Organizational chart with a description of the management team.*
9. *List of supporting professional staff (e.g., accountants).*
10. *Operations plan. This describes how and where services will be provided.*
11. *Research and development. This projects program improvement and opportunities for new initiatives.*
12. *Overall schedule. The timeline establishes the start date and development phase of the nursing center.*
13. *Critical risks and problems. This examines the internal and external threats to the center and how these will be addressed.*
14. *Financial plan. The fiscal projections for the first 3 to 5 years are presented. A budget, cash flow forecast, and break-even point are included.*
15. *Proposed funding. Specific sources are listed that can provide funding.*
16. *Legal structure of the center. This describes the status of the center, such as free standing, a corporation, or part of a larger organization.*
17. *Appendixes and supporting documents.*

A **business plan** is built on the known or more predictable sources of funding at the time the plan is developed. In today's uncertain economic health care environment, it may be necessary to modify the business plan at a moment's notice (Torrisi and Hansen-Turton, 2005). Legislative changes and reimbursement regulations can significantly alter the business plan. In addition, no grant allocation should ever be included in the business plan until the grant is awarded.

The strategic plan complements the business plan. A strategic plan looks into the future and guides the work of the nursing center in that direction. Strategic plans have a regular timeline and may change as indicated by local, national, and global events. Strategic planning meetings are periodically scheduled to review and refine the plan. The plan includes goals, objectives, and target timelines for implementation and evaluation of projected and ongoing services. The strategic plan should answer these questions: (1) What resources will the center need after start-up? (2) What economic and legislative factors may influence center productivity and sustainability? (3) What will be the center's core functions in 5, 7, and 9 years? (4) How can the staff move the center in the appropriate direction? (5) How will staff process and handle change?

Feasibility studies, business plans, and strategic plans lay the foundation for strong nursing centers. These components are crucial to the day-to-day functioning of a newly opened nursing center and reflect the abilities of the management team to build community coalitions and collaboratives. In addition, the management team must be knowledgeable about federal regulations, acts, and funding changes, especially Medicaid and Medicare reimbursement, and grant opportunities. One resource tool that should be on site for reference is the NNCC Guide: *Nurse-managed wellness centers: Developing and maintaining your center, a National Nursing Center Consortium Guide and Toolkit* (Hansen-Turton et al, 2009).

WHAT DO YOU THINK?   *How much do you think it costs a nursing center with 12 staff and 4000 enrolled clients to implement and maintain an electronic medical record?*

Once the community assessment, feasibility study, business plans, and organizational networking are completed, it is important for key people to ask the following questions:

- Why would the organization want to do this?
- What will be the immediate and long-term outcomes for the organization and the community at large?
- Can the investment (that is, staff, money, time, and space) be made?
- Does the community truly want and need a nursing center model?

The organization cannot drive the desire for the nursing center. The center must be person- and community-centric, not provider-centric. If the establishment of a nursing center is solely done from the organization's vantage point, the possibility of long-term sustainability may be jeopardized. The final question is the most critical one: Does the community truly want and need a nursing center model? No assessment, study, or plan can ignore this question. If the answer is not clear, more time must be invested to find out if there is a match in need, interest, and a center's potential capacity. For example, if the community is focused on helping young women move from public assistance into jobs and the immediate need is day care, a nursing center that offers linkages with day-care providers and on-site physical examinations and childhood immunizations will be an essential community resource. However, if the nursing center offers only senior citizen services , the immediate and expressed community need was ignored.

NURSING TIP   *There must be a match between the services wanted and needed and those offered by the center.*

The establishment of a nursing center is warranted if the model reflects the needs, interests, and strengths of the target population and is economically feasible. There should be long-term commitments by all involved in the planning process, including any parent organization. The parent organization's mission, vision, and commitment influence the viability of the nursing center model. Planners must determine the support of the parent organization before investing the time, effort, and collaborative work necessary to develop the model. If there is uncertainty at the administrative level, it is foolhardy to move forward until there is strong and documented commitment from the organization that matches the community commitment.

It is challenging for those involved in the planning process to forecast programs, determine service patterns, integrate outcome measures, and project costs. The planning process over time can be daunting. Planners may not devote sufficient time to the matter of nursing center revenue sources (Torrisi and Hansen-Turton, 2005). If money matters are not thoroughly considered, any nursing center's future will be compromised

and may not withstand the stresses of changing funding streams, political decisions, and policy changes (Kinsey and Gerrity, 2005).

The business plan provides information that forecasts the minimum funding necessary to start up a nursing center and project income 1, 3, and 5 years from inception. A break-even analysis is essential. A business plan must be periodically modified when legislation regarding Medicaid and Medicare reimbursement rates occurs. In addition, a business plan must accommodate a state's reimbursement parameters for APNs.

Potential income sources include fee-for-service, commercial reimbursement, and self-pay. Fee-for-service may be the most viable of economic strategies. Commercial reimbursement includes private health care insurers with established fee schedules. Clients without a source of health insurance are characterized as self-pay. Costs and charges for services must be established. Nursing centers located in medically underserved areas or working with medically underserved populations (migrants) have sliding-fee schedules based on published federal poverty guidelines. Managed care contracts with particular insurance companies, particularly Medicaid contractors, are other sources of income; however, the monthly Medicaid reimbursements do not cover the cost of providing health care to the most vulnerable and underserved in society (Torrisi and Hansen-Turton, 2005). Cost-effectiveness and quality care are key concerns as providers deal with the instability of reimbursement rates and the variable number of underinsured people seeking a medical home.

Financial support for nursing centers may also come from foundations, charitable contributions, private giving, and fundraising. Fund-raising can take the form of direct mailings, pledges, and events that raise money. Grants are a source of initial and ongoing funding. The funding organization generally releases guidelines of what the organization will fund. The guidelines are frequently released as a request for proposals (RFP). A proposal developed in response to the RFP specifies how the nursing center would meet the goals of the granting organization in the given timeline. The description of services and client outcomes must be presented in relation to the RFP guidelines.

Nursing centers have agreements and contracts in place for specific services. Agreements and contracts may have different language as well as reporting and fiscal management requirements; however, the basic premise is similar. The nursing center enters into a written agreement to provide services to a select population group or develop a program that targets a specific area. For example, a center may have an agreement with the American Cancer Society to develop a cancer education program for minority seniors in a low-income senior housing complex. The agreement is for a defined time period, has target goals and objectives, and outlines staff assignments and expectations, but there is no budget related to the program. A contract is a legal document that lists the purchase of services, reporting requirements, invoicing, and expected client outcomes. An example would be a city health department that issues a contract to a nursing center to immunize 100 adults against influenza for a specified sum per vaccine. Each nursing center may have one or many contracts and agreements; however, a nursing center should enter into each arrangement with clear understanding of the business side of the model. Any contract or agreement should be fiscally sound and not deplete center resources.

EVIDENCE-BASED PRACTICE MODEL

Evidence-based practice represents the clinical application of particular nursing (health care) interventions and documented client and population outcome data (Deaton, 2002). Trends in health care services, client responses, and changes in community characteristics must be documented and summarized periodically (Oros et al, 2001). Assessments of sources of ill health, including non-communicable conditions, and community influences on economic, environmental, behavioral, and physical health are conducted periodically and reported (Lancaster, 2005). Outcome measurements include client use of on-site services, childhood and adult immunizations patterns, pregnancy outcomes, emergency department and hospital use, and other health indexes including client satisfaction and quality-of-life measures.

The cost of collecting and documenting outcome measures must be included in the NMHC budget (Tudor, 2005; Bates and Bitton, 2010). Measurement instruments require technological support and staff expertise and ongoing monitoring and analyses (Garrett and Yasnoff, 2002; Browne et al, 2010). The Patient Protection and Affordable Care Act includes the prevention and wellness national strategy to fund and support evidence-based and community-based services. This act should provide support to NMHCs with defined outcome measures and electronic medical records (EMRs) in place (Forrest and Whelan, 2000).

Defined outcome measures (evidence) will enable NMHC staff to determine program effectiveness and cost savings associated with clinical outcomes. The challenge is how to define the criteria, develop measurements and collection methods, compare the evidence with broader community findings, interpret the data to funders, and disseminate findings to the wider health care community. Nursing center staff can use a variety of forums to share findings including professional conferences and publications, popular press, multimedia venues, and testimonies at public hearings (Callahan and Jennings, 2002).

Health Insurance Portability and Accountability Act (HIPAA)

Staff committed to evidence-based practice, outcome measures, EMRs, data collection, and analyses must be mindful of the Health Insurance Portability and Accountability Act (HIPAA). HIPAA, which is Public Law 104-191 passed by the 104th Congress to protect the privacy of individually identified health data referred to as protected health information (PHI). The regulations took into consideration the shift to paperless, electronic medical records. Electronic records increase the potential for individuals to access, use, and disclose sensitive personal health data. The act enables consumers to have more control over their health information, establishes boundaries about the use and release of health records, sets safeguards about provider protection of private health information and penalizes violations of

same, and enables consumers to obtain and/or make informed decisions about how their health information is used and disclosed. According to current regulations, all staff must monitor and keep secure client records, have mechanisms to transfer client information securely and appropriately, and strictly adhere to client confidentiality (Thorpe and Ogden, 2010).

Nurses in NMHCs are required to comply with HIPAA regulations, as well as be responsive to and report public health threats such as tuberculosis, disease outbreaks related to food contaminations, and influenza. Reference resources for staff include the HIPAA website of the Office for Civil Rights (http://www.hhs.gov/ocr/hipaa/) (USDHHS, 2010b) and the CDC website on Privacy Rule guidelines (http://www.cdc.gov/privacy rule) (CDC, 2010b). Other chapters further detail public health responsiveness and HIPAA documentation challenges.

Outcomes and Quality Indicators

Quality health indicators and related performance measures are priorities in any type of nursing center (Stryer, Clancy, and Simpson, 2002). These data are presented to the nursing center's board, funders, and the community at large and document the center's contributions to the health and welfare of the community. Outcome measures and quality indicators can be preset, or staff may determine that there are outcome measures that were not predetermined, but at time of review have meaningful results. For example, the nurse practitioners may have set up a call-back system that improves timely use of primary care services. This can now be documented through client satisfaction, adherence to advised health practices, and changes in health behaviors. Such outcomes can be considered quality indicators that emerged from the day-to-day practices.

Center staff must carefully consider and determine what outcome measures and quality indicators have meaning for the community and the health care system. Despite a staff tendency to want to measure everything, it is prudent to begin with particular indicators and measures and incrementally add as information is indicated. Excessive measures consume staff time and resources and valid measurements may not emerge.

The Quality Care Task Force of the NNCC has developed *Guidelines for Quality Management for Nursing Centers with Standards for Community Nursing Centers*. This publication is a vital tool for staff and can be accessed at www.nncc.us. The standards assist nursing centers to assess growth and development and areas that need improvement. The standards also include quality indicators, population groups, performance targets, and measures. The indicators are grouped into the areas of prevention, utilization, client satisfaction, functional status, symptom severity, and others.

Utilization of the standards and select indicators and associated processes enable a nursing center to document evidence-based practice. References used to develop the standards include the National Committee for Quality Assurance (NCQA) (Gingerich, 2000). An example of NMHCs evidence-based practice follows; also refer to Table 21-1.

The Philadelphia Nurse-Family Partnership (NFP) serves first-time low-income parents and their children through an

TABLE 21-1	EXAMPLES OF QUALITY HEALTH INDICATORS FOR NURSING CENTER APPLICATION		
INDICATOR	**POPULATION**	**PERFORMANCE TARGETS**	**MEASURE**
Prevention Annual influenza vaccine	High-risk groups: Age 65 or those with heart or lung disease and other chronic conditions	*Healthy People 2020* = 90% age 65+ *Healthy People 2020* = 60% high-risk ages 18-64 years	Client self-report and/or clinical records/audit
Utilization Mammogram within past 2 years	HEDIS: Women age 52-69 years *Healthy People 2020:* Women 40 years and older	HEDIS 2001 = 81% *Healthy People 2020* = 70%	Client self-report and/or clinical records/audit
Client Satisfaction Client satisfaction, annual	100 consecutive clients per quarter	Performance targets to be determined by individual nursing center and/or health care plan	Surveys
Functional Status Quality-of-life indicator	Adults age 18 years and older	Determined by individual nursing center and related to baseline indicators and improvement goals	Screen using Short Form 12 or 36

intensive public health nurse home visit model. This replication model is based on the most rigorously tested program of its kind (www.nursefamilypartnership.org). Several urban NMHCs located in economically distressed neighborhoods united to successfully respond to an RFP issued by the Philadelphia Department of Health. On July 1, 2001, the Philadelphia Nurse-Family Partnership Collaborative was formed to provide the NFP program to adolescent and adult women living in high-risk neighborhoods with the goal of reducing child abuse and neglect. Eligible low-income women are enrolled during pregnancy. Each woman receives intensive home visit services until the child reaches age 2 (program graduation). The Philadelphia NFP adheres to the national NFP model of nurse home visitation. NFP goals are to improve pregnancy outcomes, improve children's health and development, and improve families' economic self-sufficiency over time. NFP is based on the primary prevention and early intervention model developed by Dr. David Olds and colleagues (Eckenrode et al, 2010). Advanced practice public health nurses receive extensive education in NFP protocols, maternal-infant-toddler assessment measures, and motivational interviewing strategies. As of 2010, NFP replication programs are in 29 states (and more than 300 counties).

Philadelphia's NFP is the largest site in the Commonwealth of Pennsylvania with 40 sites in Pennsylvania. The local NFP is concluding its third 3-year service cycle. At any one time, 400 adolescent and adult women can be enrolled in the program. Data released in June 2010 summarize participant demographics and health and employment outcomes from 2001 to 2010 ($N = 2079$). Upon enrollment, the median age of clients was 18 years (range, 10 to 44 years). The median education was eleventh grade. Ninety-three percent of the population was unwed with 72% unemployed and median annual incomes of $10,500.

Ninety-two percent of the population was of African-American or Hispanic heritage. Cumulative data document the following outcomes: there was a 19% reduction in smoking during pregnancy, a statistically significant (63%) reduction in marijuana use, and a statistically significant (62%) reduction in domestic violence during pregnancy. Sixty percent of mothers initiated breastfeeding with 11.5% breastfeeding at 12 months of infancy. Upon graduation when children turn 2 years, 93% of the toddlers were fully immunized. Of the mothers who entered the program without high school or GED diplomas, 60% were still in school and 40% completed education, with 17% pursuing higher education. Philadelphia NFP mothers during the first year postpartum entered the workforce earlier than national counterparts and remained employed.

The Philadelphia NFP reflects NFP National Service Office findings across the nation. It is a cost-effective nurse home visit program proven to be of great benefit for low-income, first-time at-risk mothers and their first-borns (NFP, 2010). NFP demonstrates significant cost savings to the public over time according to the 2009 analysis conducted by the Pacific Institute for Research and Development (PIRE).

NFP is a nationally recognized model of what nurses can do to promote well-being and to prevent long-lasting health, social, educational, economic, and home stressors of at-risk, low-income families. Since the introduction of the NFP replication model in 1999, there has been increasing interest to implement NFPs in local communities. In fact, other NMHCs as well as children's hospitals in other states, notably Texas, have introduced NFP programs.

The momentum to support evidence-based home visitation programs will continue this decade. On July 21, 2010, Health and Human Services Secretary Kathleen Sebelius announced the Affordable Care Act Initial Funding for Maternal, Infant, and Early Childhood Home Visiting State Grants totaling $88 million. The grants will fund evidence-based home visiting programs that improve the well-being of families with young children. Forty-nine states, the District of Columbia, and five territories were awarded funds to create and support successful home visiting programs, such as Nurse-Family Partnerships. Each awardee should conduct a state and regional needs assessment, submit an approvable home visitation model, and a plan to address the needs of low income families (USDHHS, 2010a).

This is an opportune time for APNs interested in public health and prevention initiatives to participate in these assessment phases and explore employment options in NMHCs that host nurse-family partnerships and other maternal-child-family health services.

Quality Improvement

The evidence-based practice application exemplifies what nurses can do to measure outcomes, strive to improve those outcomes given particular standards, and make meaningful contributions to the public's health. Accurate data collection, measurement methods, summary statistics, and preparation of evidence practice reports are fundamental standards in any NMHC.

As the nursing center model continues to grow throughout the nation, the potential to collectively summarize data and outcomes will further strengthen this movement. Through collaboration and the pooling of data, this model will continue to move into the mainstream health care system (Christensen, Bohmer, and Kenagy, 2000; Naylor and Kurtzman, 2010). However, the staff must be as committed to data as to the provision of quality services. Data will enable the staff to clearly understand what goals are in place, and if areas are to be improved, they can develop action plans to improve services and client outcomes (Campbell, 2000). The concurrent emphasis on service and data can stress staff and the capacity of any nursing center to effectively and efficiently manage services and technology (Goetzel, 2001; Bates and Bitton, 2010).

Technology and Information Systems

Currently, technology and information systems are essential for data collection and analyses. Available technologies need to be used to collect, collate, and analyze data and to support the provision of quality health care services (Shortliffe, 2005; DesRoches, Campbell, and Vogeli, 2010). Technology and information systems will continue to change and adapt to accommodate existing health care legislation, HIPAA, *Healthy People 2020*, public health mandates, and unfolding global and national events. Continual reinforcement about the confidentiality of client records is critical (Callahan and Jennings, 2002). Transfer of information must be carefully monitored, and the use of computers and the entering and retrieval of data by staff will be delineated by role and responsibility and passwords. One resource tool that should be on site for reference is the National Nursing Center Consortium Guide: *Community and Nurse-Managed Health Centers: Getting Them Started and Keeping Them Going* (Torrisi and Hansen-Turton, 2005).

EDUCATION AND RESEARCH

There are many education and research opportunities in the nursing center model. Clinical assignments through the nursing center model enable students at all levels to work with skilled clinicians, develop positive community collaboratives, and build their skills to become professionals. These students often develop an interest in working with underserved populations in medically underserved areas of the nation. Students are assets to the nursing center model. Faculty brings skill sets that enable nursing center staff to develop and implement programs that integrate faculty-student contributions and enable the programs to engage more of the target population (Donnelly, 2005).

It is necessary to carefully coordinate, supervise, and evaluate student education in nursing centers. A faculty liaison enables students to have a resource within the educational system as well as a link with the nursing center. Student schedules must also be coordinated with nursing center timelines. A year-round nursing center that provides 24-hour coverage of services must accommodate academic schedules and students moving in and out of clinical assignments. Nursing center staff and faculty must work to maintain ongoing communication with clients and community agencies about student rotations, program assignments, and student projects. Students should be encouraged to share their work with the community because learning is a mutual exchange of goods and services. In addition, in any nursing center model nothing is done in isolation (Shiber and D'Lugoff, 2002).

Research in nursing centers provides the opportunity to gain answers to questions and to share the findings with colleagues and the public (Sherman, 2005). It is important to answer questions about individual and population health status, client outcomes over time, roles and capacities to address health promotion with the existing health system, and the value and affordability of care (Gladwell, 2005). Centers offer many opportunities for educational research.

Each center needs a research or program evaluation agenda. Resource Tool 21.E displays the WHO's priorities for a common nursing research agenda. The research focus includes identification and clarification of client needs, particularly those not engaged in an existing health system; description of nursing interventions and linkages with consumer needs and resources; demonstration of effective interventions that produce appropriate outcomes; and cost analysis and documented cost-effectiveness of services (Hirschfeld, 1998).

Over the past three decades, nursing center research has principally focused on the development and characteristics of nursing centers (Sherman, 2005). Descriptive data have been collected about clients, types of services, the financial supports, and community relationships. However, more than descriptive clinical studies are needed. Research efforts are underway to capture and name the unique features of nursing models of care and link them with health outcomes. For example, the significance of psychosocial interventions inherent in nursing practice is being examined, such as listening to, supporting, and interpreting information for clients. Client satisfaction studies document the perceived value by those who use nursing centers.

Factors associated with access to services are being examined. These include availability, timeliness, acceptability, and affordability of services. Environmental conditions, such as housing, transportation, criminal activities, and welfare-to-work transitions that influence health care access and use patterns are being examined. Resource Tool 21.F presents a template for research in nursing centers.

Program Evaluation

Program evaluation is an essential organizational practice in nursing centers, and research questions emerge from program evaluation. The evaluation process is a systematic approach to improve and account for public health and primary care actions. Evaluation is thoroughly integrated in routine program operations. The process drives community-focused strategies, allows for program improvements, and identifies the need for additional services.

Program evaluation separates what is working from what is not and enables clinicians, faculty, and students to ask difficult questions and handle pressing challenges (Schultz, Krieger, and Galea, 2002). Resources are available to nursing center staff to enhance their understanding and application of program evaluation in their particular setting. Resources include courses offered through the Centers for Disease Control and Prevention (CDC) Public Health Training Network, The Community Toolbox (http://www.cdc.gov/eval/framework.htm), and other resources updated by the CDC Evaluation Working Group (2010a). These resources enable nursing center staff to implement the six essential program evaluation steps in the context of their model and in their particular community. The essential steps are outlined in Box 21-4.

POSITIONING NURSING CENTERS FOR THE FUTURE

Emerging Health Systems

Nationally, the nursing profession is strategically placed to make significant contributions to the health of people (Buhler-Wilkerson, 1993) and achieve the *Healthy People 2020* goals. The nursing center model offers unique opportunities to develop preventive services to improve the well-being of individuals, families, and communities. Nurses working in this model will continue to build the community trust, support, and capacity necessary to move the nursing center model into the mainstream of health care by 2020 and beyond.

Opportunities exist to advance this model. The traditionalist health care system is changing. The September 11, 2001,

terrorist attack on the nation, the threat of widespread bioterrorism, and global pandemics require that primary health care providers, such as NMHCs, be prepared for unexpected public health threats (Miro and Kaufman, 2005). The need for public health workers and APNs is evident following the devastating aftermath of Hurricanes Katrina (New Orleans) and Ike (Galveston, Texas) on much of the South. Likewise, the 2010 British Petroleum (BP) gulf oil spill is an environmental catastrophe that will threaten the well-being of people and the nation's natural resources for decades.

The public health system and community models of primary health care are now in the forefront of prevention, early intervention, and community-wide education when disasters occur (Rottman, Shoaf, and Dorian, 2005). Urban, rural, and suburban NMHCs and their community counterparts must be prepared to meet the everyday needs of people as well as the precipitous, unexpected events that threaten our society's future. Participation in disaster and emergency response plans are essential.

Other threats, such as the escalating numbers of underinsured adults and children that present for care or seek no care, will continue to be a concern for health care providers and legislators (AHRQ, 2002; Fairbrother et al, 2010). Any extended economic downswings as well as devastating events can increase the number of people without health care coverage, and more public dollars will be consumed to support those in need (Lancaster, 2005).

The Great Recession of 2008 is predicted to influence American life for a decade or longer (Henig, 2010). Many people who are unemployed or underemployed, and make choices about routine medical and dental care and often deny themselves preventive services, then end up consuming more services through emergency rooms.

Another point of service option for the underinsured is the retail store convenient clinic typically staffed by nurse practitioners. The clinics are typically located in high-volume retail businesses including grocery stores and pharmacies. These clinics have a limited scope of care that includes immunizations, routine school physicals, and common acute problems.

Retail care clinics are controversial. The majority of retail clinics are owned by for-profit organizations and its management does not consider the clinics as NMHCs. In fact, there is concern that the retail clinic fragments care and threatens the viability of primary care provider services, including NMHCs (Pollack, Gidengil, and Mehrotra, 2010). In the future, market forces including the public's interest in convenient and affordable care will determine the growth of NMHCs and the demand for retail clinics as alternative sources of care.

Another underappreciated threat to community and personal well-being is social isolation, particularly in the elderly or those who are disenfranchised because of geography or a community's social anomie or the chronically unemployed (Case and Paxson, 2002). People are lonely, sad, and afraid to expose their vulnerability to providers. Since the advent of the Great Recession, more people self-report (on blogs, Facebook, etc.) confusion, pessimism, and a sense of imbalance. Social supports are fragmented and many people feel forgotten and abandoned. Established NMHCs that integrate

---

BOX 21-4   ESSENTIAL PROGRAM EVALUATION STEPS

- Engaging stakeholders
- Describing the program
- Focusing the evaluation design
- Gathering credible evidence
- Justifying conclusions
- Ensuring use and sharing lessons learned

multidisciplinary services across the life span are well positioned to engage people in need of mental and physical health services and document prevention and early intervention health outcomes over time.

National and Regional Organizations

Nursing center staff will grapple with complex health, social, and environmental issues presented by their clients and the community at large. Membership in professional organizations including nursing center consortia will enable people to organize around one or more critical health threats and strategize about what interventions work locally, regionally, and nationally. In addition, lessons learned and programmatic successes can be shared, compared, and used to build legislative support for NMHCs.

There are many professional organizations for nurses to join and contribute their skills to advance the future of nursing. Nurses choose membership in organizations based on interest, clinical and academic preparation, and employment. Nurses involved in the nurse-managed health center models have several consortiums available to advance their administrative and clinical skill base. The opportunities to unite professionally and share contributions to the public's health are offered through membership in one or more of the member consortiums. The NNCC website (www.nncc.us) provides an extensive overview of one membership organization service. Services include data warehousing, information systems, public policy development, health care advocacy, and monthly postings of relevant grant opportunities for education, service, and research initiatives. Other consortiums and professional organizations support the work of NMHCS and APNs. These include the Nursing Centers Research Network, the American Public Health Association, and others.

Expanding opportunities for far-reaching changes in primary care service models has been created by the work of these consortiums and professional organizations, including the ANA. Today, the collective national, legislative, and public interest in nurse-managed health centers and nursing as essential, mainstream providers is notable. At the federal level, millions of dollars are now committed to establishing or expanding existing nurse-managed centers. In addition, the federal government, in response to the Great Recession, has increased the federal allocation to expand FQHCs. These investments will support further growth of NMHCs across the nation.

Nursing Workforce

Much has been noted about the nursing workforce issues that confront our nation and the world in this century. The documented decline in people entering the profession over the past two decades is notable. Legislators, health care systems, the nursing profession, and educational institutions as well as the public are now examining the interrelated factors that contribute to the decline in new nursing graduates, erratic surges in nurse employment, and the number of nurses who leave the profession (Bingham, 2002; Donelan et al, 2008; Buerhaus, Auerbach, and Staiger, 2009).

National and state-wide initiatives are available to underwrite graduate study expenses (loan forgiveness, grants) so that more qualified nursing faculty can work in academic settings; this expands student enrollment and graduation rates (Donelan et al, 2010). What confounds nurse employment is the regional and national variations in hiring new nurse graduates. Unlike other decades, nurses are self-reporting lengthier job search efforts and finite employment opportunities. New graduates or those reentering the workforce indicate they are considering geographic relocation or other interim positions to secure full-time employment.

Regardless of career and employment variables, there will continue to be great need for skilled nurses who are committed and passionate about nursing regardless of the clinical setting. As people live longer and as advances in technology and drug therapies increase, the need for nurses to have current knowledge and skills to care for acutely ill people in hospitals, homes, and extended care facilities will increase. The growing demand for nurses in community settings in this decade, given static workforce numbers and the aging of the workforce, make nurses valuable workers. Salaries, benefits, and working hours have improved; however, institutional working conditions for nurses have not consistently improved. Nurses deal with mandatory overtime and a complex client mix (number of clients and acuity levels) on a daily basis. Some nurses choose public health or community-based practices so they can have more control over their work and personal lives (Bellack and O'Neil, 2000). These nurses often gravitate toward the nursing center model. Their opportunities to make meaningful differences in the lives of people served and to shape an evolving practice model are appealing. Nurses attracted to this model often discover that they can be front-line advocates for people and have more opportunity to do policy development (Drevdahl, 2002). Through the nursing center model, the voices of nurses are heard and lasting changes are made in public policy based on their work with legislators and public officials.

Policy Development and Health Advocacy

Health advocacy is an essential nursing role in nurse-managed health centers. Nurses involved in this model of care focus on health disparities and access to care for all. Nurses promote the nursing center model as a system of public health and primary care services that reduces health disparities and improves ongoing access to health care. The roles of advocate can be as diverse as working with a community group to reduce the exposure of vulnerable children to lead-based paint in older homes to testifying in the House of Representatives about the contributions of NMHCs as safety net providers. Advocates often integrate policy development work as they learn more about community needs and strengths.

Nursing centers are a disruptive and innovative approach to the delivery of health care services (Christensen, Bohmer, and Kenagy, 2000). An outcome of this approach will be the ongoing need to address policy and political issues that influence this significant and essential model of health care (Malone, 2005). Other pressing issues include: (1) lingering effects of the Great

Recession, including the consequential decline in tax dollars for needed public health programs, (2) legislative and insurance barriers that reduce access to appropriate funding resources by NMHCs, (3) the public's increasing disenchantment with health costs, (4) the double-digit gross national product (GNP) percentage spent on health care expenditures, and (5) the national emphasis on achieving *Healthy People 2020* goals and objectives despite the absence of universal health insurance.

Today's Nursing

There is no better time than the present to be a nurse and to advance the profession. The profession is undergoing change, and more nurses are needed to enter the profession to meet the needs of the people in many settings (Zysberg and Berry, 2005). Nurses in nurse-managed health centers are uniquely positioned to introduce nursing to community members, to speak on behalf of the profession, and to introduce educational opportunities to those seeking a future in health care. Nurses involved in the nurse-managed health centers are front-line advocates for social justice and equality for all, and their work is a lasting legacy for those who follow (Figure 21-5).

The authors envision the following advancements within this decade: (1) a full complement of APNs, population-focused nurses, nurse practitioners, and other nurse experts who are the backbone of primary health care providers throughout the nation, and (2) an exponential expansion of the NMHC model. The practice application at the conclusion of this chapter exemplifies the potential of nursing contributions to improve the health of one urban community.

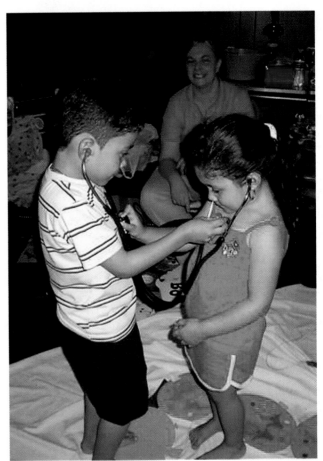

FIGURE 21-5 Preparing for their future as advanced practice nurses in a nurse-managed health clinic. (From Mabel Morris Head Start Program, Philadelphia, PA.)

CHAPTER REVIEW

■ PRACTICE APPLICATION

Annual summaries of client use patterns and program outcome data document erratic patterns of client access and ongoing use of one nursing center's services. The center, located in a public housing site, offers comprehensive primary health care to clients of all ages, a sliding-fee schedule so no one is turned away, managed care contracts, and a variety of public health and social services provided in home or community settings. The office is open 6 days a week with appointments available during day and early evening hours. The site is readily accessible by public or private transit, and it is less than a 5-minute walk for any public housing resident. A large, attractive sign is in the front of the site for advertising purposes. Monthly outreach is conducted to local businesses, schools, social service agencies, and tertiary care centers. Outreach includes information such as the center's services, hours, and location. Personal contacts, flyers, and posters advertising unique programs such as flu clinics are strategically placed within the housing complex and proximal neighborhoods.

Despite these efforts, data indicate that other strategies are needed. A focus group held with staff, public housing residents, and users of the health center services began. Client users candidly shared their need to have more flexibility in the appointment schedule. Appointments made months in advance were often not kept because of conflicting schedules (such as work or school), despite the client's best intent. Staff said that too many clients were "no-shows" and their work schedules were "too light." Public housing residents were concerned about keeping their "business private."

Consensus was reached to establish an "open access" appointment model. Clients can schedule appointments or call the day before or day of a needed visit. Nurses would reinforce the open access model and the center's confidentiality standards with clients. All staff would reinforce the option during client visits as well as prepare press releases and community presentations. Staff would review client access and use patterns quarterly. By the next quarter, client access and adherence to appointments increased by 50% and primary care staff reported greater satisfaction in their work responsibilities. Nurses noted that clients in public housing expressed positive comments on how the nursing center had helped them manage their appointment schedules better. Overall, the increased access and use of appropriate primary health care services support the center's goal to promote community well-being.

KEY POINTS

- Nursing centers provide unique opportunities to improve the health status of individuals, families, and communities through direct access to nursing care.
- Nursing center models combine people, place, approach, and strategy in everyday life to develop appropriate health care interventions.
- A nursing center's health and community orientation builds strong connections to the community served.
- A center is defined by its particular array of services and programs, such as comprehensive primary health care centers and special care centers.
- The foundations for the nursing center model include the perspective of the World Health Organization and the *Healthy People 2020* systematic approach to improving individual and community health.
- Each center develops its philosophy, goals, and activities through a process of community collaboration, assessment, and strategic planning.
- As the community and the center work together for health, a multilevel approach is used that includes individuals and expands to legislators.
- Nursing center development is rooted in public health nursing history and the evolution of the nursing profession.
- Most current nursing center models emerged from academic nursing centers in the 1970s.
- Nursing center models support the skill development of advanced practice nurses, allied health professionals, and paraprofessionals.
- Any nursing center must have a board of directors or an advisory board to guide program development, fund-raising, community networking, and other work.
- The nursing center requires careful planning and structure to be a successful education, service, and business enterprise.
- Start-up and sustainability are based on a community-focused feasibility study, a sound business and financial plan, operational support, and resource management.
- Evidence-based practice in nursing centers is essential and represents the clinical application of particular nursing interventions and documented client outcomes.
- The Health Insurance Portability and Accountability Act will increase a center's investment in administrative and oversight services.
- Available technology and systems management must be used to collect, collate, and analyze center data.
- Education, community service and learning, and research opportunities abound in this model.
- Program evaluation is an organizational practice in nursing centers; research questions are developed from program evaluation.
- Threats to the viability of nursing centers include the uninsured or underinsured, erratic funding resources, community decline, and disenfranchised high-risk populations.
- Nurses attracted to the nursing center model discover professional fulfillment in advocating for people in need and becoming involved in public policy change.
- Nursing centers represent an innovative approach to the delivery of primary health care services.
- Nurses involved in the nursing center model are front-line advocates for social justice and equality for all.

CLINICAL DECISION-MAKING ACTIVITIES

1. Discuss why a nursing center should be started or not started in your home town.
2. What is your state's position on credentialing APNs who work in an NMHC model?
3. What existing public policy might adversely affect the viability of nursing centers?
4. Why would APNs be attracted to this model of primary health care?
5. How many elected officials at the local level are familiar with the nursing center model and, if the majority is uninformed, what could you do to educate the officials?
6. Where do you envision yourself professionally in 2015?

REFERENCES

Agency for Healthcare Research and Quality: Medicaid program expansions to cover otherwise uninsured poor children appear to be relatively inexpensive, *AHRQ Res Activities*, February 2002.

Alakeson V, Frank RF, Katz RE: Specialty care medical homes for people with severe, persistent mental disorders, *Health Aff* 29:867–873, 2010.

American Association of Colleges of Nursing: *Hallmarks of the professional nursing practice movement*, Washington, DC, 2002, AACN.

American Nurses Association: *Health promotion and disease prevention: a position statement*, Kansas City, MO, 1995, ANA.

American Nurses Association: Public Health Nursing: *Scope and standards of practice*, Silver Spring, MD, 2007, ANA.

Anderko L: The effectiveness of a rural nursing center in improving health care access in a three-county area, *J Rural Health* 16:177–184, 2000.

Anderson E: *Code of the street*, New York, 1999, WW Norton & Co.

Aydelotte MK, Barger S, Branstetter E, et al: *The nursing center: concept and design*, Kansas City, MO, 1987, ANA.

Aydelotte MK, Gregory MS: Nursing practice: innovative models. In *Nursing centers: meeting the demand for quality health care*, New York, 1989, National League for Nursing.

Baker EL, White LE, Lichtveld MY: Reducing health disparities through community-based research, *Public Health Rep* 116:517–519, 2001.

Bates DW, Bitton A: The future of health information technology in the patient-centered medical home, *Health Aff* 29:614–621, 2010.

Bechtel C, Ness DL: If you build it, will they come? Designing truly patient-centered health care, *Health Aff* 29:915–920, 2010.

Bellack JP, O'Neil EH: Recreating nursing practice for a new century: recommendations and implications of the Pew health professions commission's final report, *Nurs Health Care Perspect* 21:14–21, 2000.

Berkman LF, Lochner KA: Social determinants of health: meeting at the crossroads, *Health Aff* 21:291–293, 2002.

Bingham R: Leaving nursing, *Health Affairs* 21:211–217, 2002.

Browne K, Roseman D, Shaller D, et al: Measuring patient experience as a strategy for improving primary care, *Health Aff* 29:921–925, 2010.

Buchanan M: The new system of care. In *Teaching in the community: preparing nurses for the 21st century*, New York, 1997, National League for Nursing.

Buerhaus P, Auerbach D, Staiger D: The recent surge in nurse employment: causes and implications, *Health Aff* 28:657–668, 2009.

Buhler-Wilkerson K: Bring care to the people: Lillian Wald's legacy to public health nursing, *Am J Public Health* 83:1778–1786, 1993.

Callahan D, Jennings B: Ethics and public health: forging a strong relationship, *Am J Public Health* 92:169–176, 2002.

Campbell BS: Preventive health service outcomes in three government funded health centers, *Fam Community Health* 23:18–28, 2000.

Case A, Paxson C: Parental behavior and child health, *Health Aff* 21:164–178, 2002.

Centers for Disease Control and Prevention: *Evaluation Working Group*, 2010a. Available at http://www.cdc.gov/eval/index/htm. Accessed January 22, 2011.

Centers for Disease Control and Prevention: *HIPAA privacy rules guidelines*, 2010b. Available at http://www.cdc.gov/privacyrule. Accessed January 15, 2011.

Christensen CM, Bohmer R, Kenagy J: Will disruptive innovations cure health care? *Harv Bus Rev* 78:102–112, 2000.

Clear JB, Starbecker M, Kelly DW: Nursing centers and health promotion: a federal vantage point, *Fam Community Health* 21:1–14, January 1999.

Cross R, Prusak L: The people who make organizations go—or stop, *Harv Bus Rev* 80(6):104–112, June 2002.

Deaton A: Policy implications of the gradient of health and wealth, *Health Aff* 21:13–30, 2002.

Dentzer S: Geisinger chief Glenn Steele: Seizing health reform's potential to build a superior system, *Health Aff* 29:1200–1207, 2010.

DesRoches CM, Campbell EG, Vogeli C: Electronic health records' limited successes suggest more targeted uses, *Health Aff* 29:639–646, 2010.

Donelan K, Buerhaus P, DesRoches C, et al: Public perceptions of nursing careers: The influence of the media and nursing shortages, *Nurs Econ* 26:143–150, 2008.

Donelan K, Buerhaus P, DesRoches C, et al: Health policy thought leaders' views of the health workforce in an era of health reform, *Nurs Outlook* 58:175–189, 2010.

Donnelly G: Improving the health of communities: the Drexel experience, *Emerg Trends Acad Drexel Univ*, May 2005.

Drevdahl D: Social justice or market justice? The paradoxes of public health partnerships with managed care, *Public Health Nurs* 19: 161–169, 2002.

Eckenrode J, Campa M, Luckey D, et al: Long-term effects of prenatal and infancy nurse home visitation on the life course of youths, *Arch Pediatr Adolesc Med* 164:9–15, 2010.

Evans LK, Kinsey K, Rothman N, et al: *Health care for the 21st century—greater Philadelphia style,* paper prepared for the Independence Foundation, March 28, 1997.

Fairbrother GL, Carle AD, Cassedy A, et al: The impact of parental job loss on children's health coverage, *Health Aff* 29:1343–1349, 2010.

Fee E, Bu L: The origins of public health nursing: The Henry Street Visiting Nurse Service, *Am J Public Health* 100:1206–1207, 2010.

Floyd JM: Envisioning new nursing roles and scopes of practice, *Reflect Nurs Leadership* Second Quarter, 2001.

Forrest CB, Whelan EM: Primary care safety-net delivery sites in the United States: a comparison of community health centers, hospital outpatient departments, and physicians' offices, *JAMA* 284:2077–2083, 2000.

Garrett NY, Yasnoff WA: Disseminating public health practice guidelines in electronic medical record systems, *J Public Health Manag Pract* 8:1–10, 2002.

Gerrity P, Kinsey KK: An urban nurse-managed primary health care center: health promotion in action, *Fam Community Health* 21:29–40, 1999.

Gingerich BS: National Committee for Quality Assurance, *Home Health Care Manage Pract* 14:387–388, 2000.

Gladwell M: The moral-hazard myth, *The New Yorker*, August 29, 2005, pp 44–49.

Goetzel R: The financial impact of health promotion and disease prevention programs: why is it so hard to prove value? *Am J Health Promot* 15:277–280, 2001.

Goffee R, Jones G: Followership: it's personal, too, *Harv Bus Rev* 79:147, 2001.

Greiner AC, Knebel E: *Institute of Medicine health professionals education: a bridge to quality*, Washington, DC, 2003, National Academies Press.

Hansen-Turton T, Kinsey K: The quest for self-sustainability: nurse-managed health centers meeting the policy challenge, *Policy Politics Nurs Pract* 2:304–309, 2001.

Hansen-Turton T, Miller ME, Greiner P: *Nurse-managed wellness centers: developing and maintaining your center, a National Nursing Center Consortium Guide and Toolkit*, Philadelphia, 2009, Saunders.

Heifetz RA, Linsky M: A survival guide for leaders, *Harv Bus Rev* 80(6):65–74, June 2002.

Henig R: The post-adolescent, pre-adult, not quite decided life stage, *The New York Times Magazine*, August 22, 2010.

Hirschfeld MJ: WHO priorities for a common nursing agenda, *Int Nurs Rev* 30:13–14, 1998.

Horrocks S, Anderson E, Salisbury C: Systematic review of whether nurse practitioners working in primary care can provide equivalent care to doctors, *BMJ* 324:819–823, 2002.

Hurst CP, Osban LB: Service learning on wheels: the Nightingale mobile clinic, *Nurs Health Care Perspect* 21:184–187, 2000.

Institute for Nursing Centers, 2010. Available at http://www.nursingcenters.org.

Jacobson PD: Form versus function in public health, *J Public Health Manag Pract* 8:92–94, 2002.

Kawachi I, Berkman LF: *Neighborhoods and health*, New York, 2003, Oxford University Press.

Keefe MF, Leuner JD, Laken MA: The caring for the community initiative integrating research, practice, and education, *Nurs Health Care Perspect* 21:287–292, 2000.

Khan AS, Fleischauer A, Casani J, Groseclose SL: The next public health revolution: Public health information fusion and social networks, *Am J Public Health* 100:1237–1242, 2010.

Kinsey KK: Models that work: an interview with Dorothy Harrell, Philadelphia community activist, *Fam Community Health* 21:74–79, 1999.

Kinsey KK: *La Salle neighborhood nursing center annual report*, Philadelphia, 2002, La Salle University.

Kinsey KK, Gerrity P: Planning, implementing, and managing a community-based nursing center: current challenges and future opportunities, *Handbook Home Health Care Admin* 68:872–882, 2005.

Lakon CM, Hipp JF, Timberlake DS: The social context of adolescent smoking: A systems perspective, *Am J Public Health* 100:1218–1228, 2010.

Lancaster J: From the editor, *Fam Community Health* 21:vi, 1999.

Lancaster J: From the editor, *Fam Community Health* 28:109–110, 2005.

Landon BE, Gill JM, Antonelli RC, et al: Prospects for rebuilding primary care using the patient-centered medical home, *Health Aff* 29:827–834, 2010.

Lawrence DM: How to forge a high-tech marriage between primary care and population health, *Health Aff* 29:1004–1009, 2010.

Lundeen SP: An alternative paradigm for promoting health in communities: the Lundeen community nursing center model, *Fam Community Health* 21:15–28, 1999.

Lutz J, Herrick CA, Lehman BB: Community partnership: a school of nursing creates nursing centers for older adults, *Nurs Health Care Perspect* 22:26–29, 2001.

Malone R: Assessing the policy environment, *Policy Politics Nurs Pract* 6:135–143, 2005.

Matherlee K: The nursing center in concept and practice: delivery and financing issues in serving vulnerable people, *Issue Brief Natl Health Policy Forum* 746:1–10, 2000.

Mattessich P, Monsey B: *Collaboration: what makes it work?* St. Paul, MN, 1992, Amherst H. Wilder Foundation.

Miller ME, Guigliano L: The real world: service, learning and missions, *Acad Exchange Q* 10(3):30–34, 2006.

Miro S, Kaufman S: Anthrax in New Jersey: a health education experience in bioterrorism response and preparedness, *Health Promot Pract* 6:430–436, 2005.

Naylor MD, Kurtzman ET: The role of nurse practitioners in reinventing primary care, *Health Aff* 29:893–899, 2010.

Nurse Family Partnership, 2010. Available at http://www.nursefamilypartnership.org. Accessed January 15, 2011.

Oros M, Johantgen M, Antol S, et al: Community-based nursing centers: challenges and opportunities in implementation and sustainability, *Policy Politics Nurs Pract* 2:277–287, 2001.

Pohl JM, Hanson C, Newland JA, et al: Analysis and commentary: Unleashing nurse practitioners potential to deliver primary care and lead teams, *Health Aff* 29:900–905, 2010.

Pollack CE, Gidengil C, Mehrotra A: The growth of retail clinics and the medical home: two trends in concert or conflict? *Health Aff* 29:998–1003, 2010.

Reverby S: From Lillian Wald to Hillary Rodman Clinton: what will happen to public health nursing? *Am J Public Health* 83:1662–1663, 1993.

Rollnick S, Miller WR, Butler CC: *Motivational interviewing in health care*, New York, 2008, The Guilford Press.

Rosenthal EL, Brownstein JN, Rush CR, et al: Community health workers: part of the solution, *Health Aff* 29:1338–1342, 2010.

Rottman S, Shoaf K, Dorian A: Development of a training curriculum for public health preparedness, *J Public Health Manag Pract* Suppl:S128–S131, 2005.

Salmon M: A dozen (or so) things I think I've learned about leadership. In Hansen-Turton T, Sherman S, Ferguson V, editors: *Conversations with leaders*, Indianapolis, IN, 2007, Sigma Theta Tau International.

Schultz AJ, Krieger J, Galea S: Addressing social determinants of health: community-based participatory approaches to research and practices, *Health Educ Behav* 29:287–295, 2002.

Sherman S: Nurse-managed health centers: a promising model to ensure access for the underserved. From the field, *Grant Makers Health*, July 4, 2005.

Shiber S, D'Lugoff M: A win-win model for an academic nursing center: community partnership faculty practice, *Public Health Nurs* 19:81–85, 2002.

Shortliffe E: Strategic action in health information technology: why the obvious has taken so long, *Health Aff* 25:1222–1233, 2005.

Stacy NL: The experience and performance of community health centers under managed care, *Am J Manag Care* 6:1229–1239, 2000.

Stryer D, Clancy C, Simpson L: Minority health disparities: AHRQ efforts to address inequities in care, *Health Promot Pract* 3:125–129, 2002.

Thies K, Ayers L: Community-based student practice: a transformational model of nursing education, *Nurs Leadersh Forum* 9:3–12, 2004.

Thorpe KE, Ogden LL: The foundation that health reform lays for improved payment, care coordination, and prevention, *Health Affairs* 29:1183–1187, 2010.

Torrisi D, Hansen-Turton T: *Community and nurse-managed health centers: getting them started and keeping them going*, New York, 2005, Springer.

Tudor R: Blind faith and choice, *Health Affairs* 24:1624–1628, 2005.

U.S. Department of Health and Human Services: *Affordable Care Act Initial Funding for Maternal, Infant, and Early Childhood Home Visiting Grants*, 2010a. Available at https://www.piersystem.com/go/doc/2430/799427/. Accessed January 15, 2011.

U.S. Department of Health and Human Services: *Offices for Civil Rights*, 2010b. Available at http://www.hhs.gov/ocr/hipaa. Accessed January 15, 2011.

U.S. Department of Health and Human Services: Bureau of Labor Statistics: *The registered nurse population: findings from the March 2004 National Sample survey of Registered Nurses, 2006-2007 edition*, Washington, DC, 2004, BLS.

Vermeulen F, Puranam P, Gulati R: Change for change's sake, *Harv Bus Rev?* 71–76, June 2010.

Weller LN: Nurse managed center helps students, public. *The Telegraph* , August 15, 2010. Available at http://www.thetelegraph.com/articles/health-43776-center-community.html. Accessed January 15, 2011.

Wilensky GR, Satcher D: Don't forget about the social determinants of health, *Health Aff Millwood*: w194–w198, January 16, 2009.

World Health Organization: *Primary health care: report of the International Conference on Primary Health Care*, Alma-Ata, September 6-12, 1978, USSR.

Zimmerman RK, Mieczkowski TA, Wilson SA: Immunization rates and beliefs among elderly patients of inner city neighborhood health centers, *Health Promot Pract* 3:197–206, 2002.

Zysberg L, Berry D: Gender and students' vocational choices in entering the field of nursing, *Nurs Outlook* 53:193–198, 2005.

CHAPTER 22

Case Management

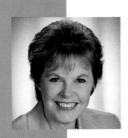

Ann H. Cary, PhD, MPH, RN, A-CCC

Dr. Ann H. Cary began practicing public health nursing in the 1970s as a home-health nurse in New Orleans, Louisiana, where she executed case management functions daily. She has served on national workgroups that established the standards of practice for case managers, created certification examinations for case managers, authored numerous articles on case management issues, taught baccalaureate and graduate-level courses in case management, and directed graduate programs in case management and continuity of care. She is the Director of the School of Nursing at Loyola University New Orleans. In New Orleans, she also serves on a variety of foundation and community boards whose missions are to increase access, coordinated care, and quality delivery for their clients.

ADDITIONAL RESOURCES

evolve WEBSITE
http://evolve.elsevier.com/Stanhope
- *Healthy People 2020*
- WebLinks
- Quiz
- Case Studies

- Glossary
- Answers to Practice Application

APPENDIX
- Appendix H: Focus on Quality and Safety Education for Nurses

OBJECTIVES

After reading this chapter, the student should be able to do the following:
1. Define continuity of care, care management, case management, and advocacy.
2. Describe the scope of practice, roles, and functions of a case manager.
3. Compare and contrast the nursing process with processes of case management and advocacy.
4. Identify methods to manage conflict, as well as the process of achieving collaboration.
5. Define and explain the legal and ethical issues confronting case managers.

KEY TERMS

advocacy, p. 495
affirming, p. 497
allocation, p. 498
amplifying, p. 496
assertiveness, p. 499
autonomy, p. 502
beneficence, p. 502
brainstorming, p. 498
care management, p. 485
care maps, p. 491
case management plans, p. 490
case manager, p. 491
clarifying, p. 496

collaboration, p. 499
cooperation, p. 499
coordinate, p. 487
critical pathways, p. 485
demand management, p. 485
disease management, p. 485
distributive outcomes, p. 499
information exchange process, p. 496
informing, p. 496
integrative outcomes, p. 499
justice, p. 502
life care planning, p. 492

negotiating, p. 499
nonmaleficence, p. 502
population management, p. 484
problem-purpose-expansion method, p. 498
problem solving, p. 498
risk sharing, p. 491
social mandate, p. 484
supporting, p. 497
utilization management, p. 485
veracity, p. 502
verifying, p. 497
—*See Glossary for definitions*

The health care industry comprises systems that attempt to integrate financing, management, and delivery of services. Challenges abound for clients and providers as they attempt to coordinate care, transition clients among providers and systems, access documentation about clients, communicate with each information system of the provider, and navigate the complexity of values to optimize quality and access while holding or reducing costs. Delivery of care may occur through a network of providers, such as negotiated contracts with hospitals, physicians, nurse practitioners, pharmacies, ancillary health services, and outpatient centers. Managing the health of populations served by the integrated systems is essential. **Population management** includes wellness and health promotion, illness prevention, acute and subacute care, rehabilitation, end-of-life care, and care coordination. Examples include planning strategies for adolescents in a school system or the elderly in a community (Huber, 2010). The use of integrated systems has had the following important consequences on the focus of care (AHA, 2003-2004):

- Emphasis is on population health management across the continuum, rather than on episodes of illness for an individual.
- Management has shifted from inpatient care as the point of management to primary care providers as points of entry.
- Care management services and programs provide access and accountability for the continuum of health.
- Successful outcomes are measured by systems performance and now pay for performance for providers to meet the needs of populations.

The contemporary focus of integrated health systems defines the nature of the client as a population rather than as an individual. In these systems, population management involves the following activities:

- Assessing the needs of the client population through health histories (and, in the future, genograms), claims, use-of-service patterns, and risk factors; and communicating through interoperable information systems
- Creating benefits and network designs to address these needs

- Prioritizing actions to produce a desired outcome with available resources
- Selecting programs related to wellness, prevention, health promotion, and demand management; and educating the population about them
- Instituting a care management process that coordinates care across the health continuum for a population aggregate
- Deploying case managers within a variety of delivery and insurance systems to clients and providers

Establishing a relationship between financing, managing, delivering, and coordinating services is critical to reach the goal of population management—that is, achieving healthy outcomes at the population level. The *Healthy People 2020* goals are to increase both quality of life and years of healthy life, to achieve health equity and eliminate health disparities, and to create social and physical environments as a social mandate for health care. In the second decade of the twenty-first century, case management will be an intervention of choice to positively influence the leading health indicators and focus areas of *Healthy People 2020*.

Establishing evidence-based strategies is critical to the success of case management for individuals and populations. Using the current best evidence blended with clinical expertise is a critical skill of the case manager (Allison, 2004; CMSA, 2010). In their practice, nurse case managers have the following core values: increasing the span of healthy life, reducing disparities in health among Americans, and promoting access to care and to preventive services. Many of the interventions nurses use with clients and health care systems will further the *Healthy People 2020* objectives. These include case management interventions to minimize fragmentation and promote quality transitions of care; incorporate standardized practice tools and adherence guidelines; improve safety of care; and use interprofessional teams to deliver services.

In the Intervention Wheel model for public health nursing practice, the nursing actions of case management, collaboration, and advocacy comprise 3 of 16 evidence-based interventions for individuals, families, and populations served by public health nurses (Keller et al, 2004). These three concepts and practice arenas for public health nurses are more fully described in this chapter.

HEALTHY PEOPLE 2020

Case Management Strategies Offer Opportunities for Nurses to Help Meet the Following Healthy People 2020 Objectives for Target Populations

Access to Care

- AHS-2: Increase the proportion of insured persons with coverage for clinical preventive services
- AHS-3: Increase the proportion of persons with a usual primary care provider
- AHS-6: Reduce the proportion of individuals that experience difficulties or delays in obtaining necessary medical care, dental care, or prescription medications
- ECBP-14 & 14.1: Increase the inclusion of clinical prevention and population content in undergraduate nursing including counseling training for health promotion and disease prevention
- SA-9: Increase the portion of persons who are referred for follow up for substance abuse problems

From USDHHSS: *Healthy People 2020: A roadmap for health*, Washington, DC, 2010, U.S. Government Printing Office.

DEFINITIONS

Care management is a health care delivery process that helps achieve better health outcomes by anticipating and linking clients with the services they need more quickly (CMSA, 2010). It is an enduring process in which a population manager establishes systems and processes to monitor the health status, resources, and outcomes for a targeted aggregate of the population. The population manager is the tactical architect for a population's health in the delivery system. Building blocks that are used by the manager include risk analysis; data mapping; monitoring for health processes, indicators, and unexpected illnesses; epidemiological investigation of unexpected illnesses; development of multidisciplinary action plans and programs for the population; and identifying case management triggers or events (e.g., when dramatic results are obtained by prevention or early intervention) that indicate the need for early referrals of high-risk clients (Haag and Kalina, 2005).

Care management strategies were initially developed by health maintenance organizations (HMOs) in the late 1970s to manage the care of different populations. The purpose was to promote quality and ensure appropriate use and costs of services. Typically these involved clients with reduced self-care capacity and whose diseases and treatments were intense (Michaels and Cohen, 2005). Care management strategies include utilization management, critical pathways, case management, disease management, and demand management. **Utilization management** attempts to promote optimal use of services to redirect care and monitor the appropriate use of provider care/treatment services for both acute and community/ambulatory services. Providers are offered multiple options for care with different economic implications. Through the use of utilization management, clients who have repetitive readmissions (i.e., they fail to respond to care) are often referred to care management programs. **Critical pathways** and maps, which were more popular in the early 2000s, are tools that specify activities providers may use in a timely sequence

to achieve desired outcomes for care. The outcomes are measurable, and the pathway tools strive to reduce differences in client care. Today, agencies are more likely to use clinical paths, evidence-based practice protocols or guidelines, or case management plans of care. Case management services are used for clients with specific diagnoses who may have high-use patterns, non-compliance issues, cost caps (e.g., no more than $10,000 to $20,000 can be spent on their case), or threshold expenses.

Disease management constitutes systematic activities to coordinate health care interventions and communications for populations with conditions in which client self-care efforts are significant (CMSA, 2010). For example, diabetes, asthma, and depression are typically targeted by providers and insurers. These programs have evolved largely as initiatives in managed care organizations (Huber, 2010).

Demand management seeks to control use by providing clients with correct information and education strategies to make healthy choices, to use healthy and health-seeking behaviors to improve their health status, and to make fewer demands on the health care system (Tufts Managed Care Institute, 2011).

In contrast, *case management* comprises the activities implemented with individual clients in the system. The case manager builds on the basic functions of the traditional nurse's role and adapts new competencies for managing transitions from health care facility to home, such as wellness and prevention, and interprofessional teams). Case management is the single most frequent intervention reported by 91% of staff public health nurses (Grumbach et al 2004). Case management is provided by the disciplines of nursing, social work, and rehabilitation counseling, to name a few. Research by Park, Huber, and Tahan (2009) found that common knowledge exists for case management providers from the disciplines of nursing, social work, and rehabilitation counseling: case recording and documentation, conflict resolution strategies, negotiation, ethics, relevant legislation, interpersonal communication, and roles and functions required in various settings. Figure 22-1 illustrates the unified knowledge domains for professionals in case management and emphasizes the fluidity of common knowledge used by case managers regardless of discipline. In addition, case managers in case-management programs are expanding their clinical expertise to embrace the process of disease management, a successful strategy for population outcomes. Specialty case management in advanced nursing practice is a critical role in this field (Cohen and Cesta, 2005). In implementing case management, these nurses work with clients or community aggregates as well as systems managing disease and outcomes, whereas nurses with bachelor's degrees more often focus on care at the individual level (Stanton and Dunkin, 2002).

This chapter describes the nature and process of case management for individual and family clients. Case management has a rich tradition in public health nursing and is frequently found in hospitals, transitional and long-term care, home and hospice care, and health insurance companies. Case management is at the top of the care management pyramid, reserved for a subset of the population. In Figure 22-2 Coggeshall (2008) illustrates a case management model pyramid that recognizes the tenets of risk stratification and case finding, coordination,

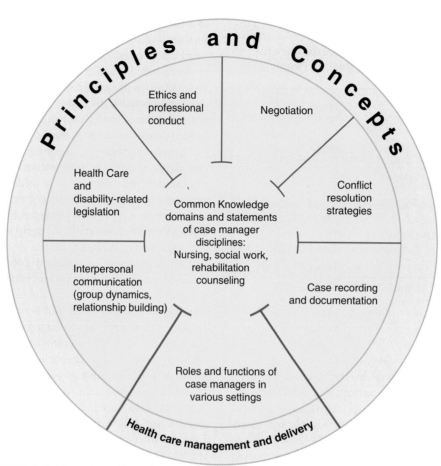

FIGURE 22-1 Evidence-based knowledge of case managers from disciplines of nursing, social work, and rehabilitation counseling. (Courtesy of Ann H. Cary.)

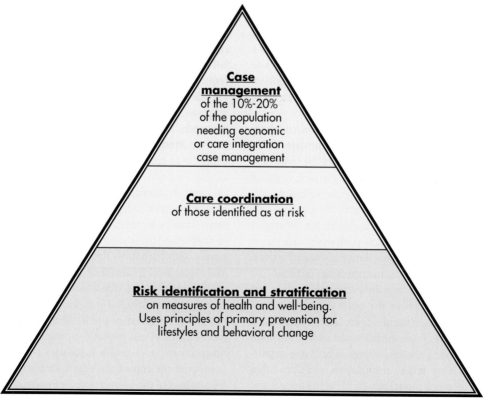

FIGURE 22-2 Case management model. (From Coggeshall Press: Case management model, Coralville, IA, 2008, author, as cited in Huber, 2010.)

and ultimately case management of a smaller proportion of clients in the population. This model recognizes the interchange of public health and populations at risk for service intensity resulting from economic or care integration needs.

CONCEPTS OF CASE MANAGEMENT

Reviewing multiple or historical definitions of case management helps to demonstrate the complex process and the concept of case management over time. Weil and Karls, in 1985, described case management as a "set of logical steps and process of interacting within a service network which ensures that a client receives needed services in a supportive, effective, efficient and cost-effective manner" (p 4). Case management was defined by the American Hospital Association (1986) as the process of planning, organizing, coordinating, and monitoring services and resources needed by clients, while supporting the effective use of health and social services. Secord (1987) defined case management as a systematic process of assessing, planning, and coordinating the service, referrals, and monitoring that meets the multiple needs of clients. Bower (1992) described the continuity, quality, and cost-containment aspects of case management as a health care delivery process, whose goals are to provide quality health care, decrease fragmentation, enhance the client's quality of life, and contain costs. A focus on collaboration is important in the National Case Management Task Force definition. The definition emphasizes a collaborative process between the case manager, the client, and representatives of other agencies and provider groups. The process includes assessments, plans, implementation, coordination, monitoring and the evaluation of the options and services to meet an individual's health needs. Effective communication is essential to identify available resources to promote quality, cost effective outcomes (CMSA, 2010; Mullahy, 2010).

As a competency, case management was defined in the public health nursing literature as the "ability to establish an appropriate plan of care based on assessing the client/family and coordinating the necessary resources and services for the client's benefit" (Muller and Flarery, 2003, p 230). Knowledge and skills required to achieve this competency include the following:

- Knowledge of community resources and financing mechanisms
- Written and oral communication and documentation
- Proficient negotiating and conflict-resolving practices
- Critical-thinking processes to identify and prioritize problems from the provider and client viewpoints
- Application of evidence-based practices and outcomes measures

In the latest *Standards of Practice for Case Management*, case management is defined as "a collaborative process of assessment, planning, facilitation, care coordination, evaluation and advocacy for options and services to facilitate an individual's and family's comprehensive health needs through communication and available resources to promote quality cost-effective outcomes" (CMSA, 2010, p 24).

Case management practice is complex as evidenced by the need to coordinate activities of multiple providers, payers, and settings throughout a client's continuum of care. For example, in a contemporary model of primary care practice, the medical home provides accessible, continuous, coordinated, comprehensive care and is managed centrally by a physician with the active involvement of non-physician practice staff. Care provided must be assessed, planned, implemented, adjusted, and evaluated on the basis of goals designed by many disciplines as well as goals of the client, the family, significant others, and community organizations. Although likely employed and located in one setting, the nurse as case manager will be influencing the selection and monitoring of care provided in other settings by formal and informal care providers. With the increased use of electronic care delivery through telehealth activities, case management activities are now handled via telephone, e-mail, and fax, and through video visits and electronic monitoring in a client's residence. Case managers may also deliver care to a global network of clients located in different countries. A challenging problem is the fragmentation of services, which can result in overuse, underuse, gaps in care, and miscommunication. This can result in costly client outcomes and quality issues in hand-offs and transitions from provider to provider.

Case management differs between urban and rural settings. In the rural setting, where the distance between populations is more expansive, there are fewer organized community-based systems and communication and distance is often a greater challenge. Furthermore, the economics, pace and style of life, values, and social organization all differ. In a study by Stanton and Dunkin (2002) and later referenced in 2009 (Stanton and Dunkin), rural residents identified four barriers to access to care that confront case managers in rural areas: lack of proximity to providers, limited services, scarcity of providers, and availability of emergency and acute care services. Transportation, both for nurses and for clients, and lack of health insurance and benefits were documented challenges to rural clients of case managers. These issues were also identified by Waitzkin, Williams, and Bock (2002) as problems for rural clients in managed care systems. In a 2009 study, Stanton and Dunkin identified the need for safety during transitional care and by the nurse case managers. Specific actions included the need for effective communication, medication reconciliation during transitions, and coordination of care among multiple providers for rural clients in a rural nurse-managed clinic. These actions are essential to support The Joint Commission's National Safety Goals (2009).

> **DID YOU KNOW?** *Although the activities in case management may differ among providers and clients, the following five goals are shared:*
> - *To promote quality case management services to populations*
> - *To reduce institutional care, fragmentation of care, and safety gaps in transition of care while maintaining quality processes and satisfactory outcomes*
> - *To manage resource utilization through the use of protocols, evidence-based guidelines, utilization, and disease management programs*

- *To control expenses by managing care processes and outcomes*
- *To improve adherence to guidelines for quality case management by clients and providers*

Modified from Flarey DL, Blancett SS: Case management: delivering care in the age of managed care. In Flarey DL, Blancett SS, editors: Handbook of nursing case management: health care delivery in a world of managed care, Gaithersburg, MD, 1996, Aspen.

| DID YOU KNOW? *Medication non-adherence (appropriate medication-taking behaviors) is at an epidemic proportion. The number one problem with treating illness today is failure to take prescriptions correctly. As an example, for the cardiac client population:*

- *12% fail to have their prescriptions filled.*
- *An additional 12% obtain initial supplies but do not take them.*
- *29% of clients stop taking their medication before they have concluded the course of therapy.*
- *Although 50% of clients continue to take their medications, 22% of these take less medication than prescribed because of missed or skipped doses.*

By following Case Management Adherence Guidelines, you can improve the benefits of medication therapy resulting from adherence with client populations.

From CMAG, Case Management Adherence Guidelines, 2006. Available at http://www.cmsa.org/portals/0/pdf/CMAG2.pdf. Accessed January 20, 2011.

Case Management and the Nursing Process

The nurse views the process of case management through the broader health status of the community. Clients and families receiving service represent the microcosm of health needs within the larger community. Through a nurse's case management activities, general community deficiencies in quality and quantity of health services are often discovered. For example, the management of a severely disabled child by a nurse case manager may uncover the absence of respite services or parenting support and education resources in a community. While managing the disability and injury claims within a corporation, the nurse may discover that alternative care referrals for home-health visits and physical therapy are generally underused by the acute care providers in the community. Through a nurse's case management of brain-injured young adults, the absence of community standards and legislative policy for helmet use by bicyclists and motorcyclists may be revealed, stimulating advocacy efforts for changing community policy. Case management activities with individual clients and families will reveal the broader picture of health services and health status of the community. *Community assessment, policy development,* and *assurance activities* that frame core functions of public health actions are often the logical next step for a nurse's practice. When observing lack of care or services at the individual and family intervention levels, the nurse can, through case management, intervene at the community level to make changes. Clearly, the core components of case management and the nursing process are complementary (Table 22-1).

Secord's (1987) classic illustration of case management remains an appropriate picture of the process that nurses use. The CMSA model (2010) is a contemporary illustration of the case manager's process in the continuum of care (Figure 22-3).

Characteristics and Roles

Case management can be labor intensive, time consuming, and costly. Because of the rapid growth in the nature of complexity in clients' problems, the intensity and duration of activities required to support the case management function may soon exceed the demands of direct caregiving. Managers and clinicians in community health are exploring methods to make case management more efficient. In an earlier effort to achieve efficiency (Weil and Karls, 1985), the characteristics desired for case manager effectiveness were described. These characteristics, which incorporated the four CMSA activities (previously noted in the Concepts of Case Management section), are used today (CMSA, 2010):

1. The technical qualifications to understand and evaluate specific diagnoses, generally requiring clinical credentials (and experience), financial resources and analyses, and risk arrangements
2. Capability in language and terminology (able to understand and then to explain to others in simple terms)
3. Assertiveness, diplomacy, and negotiation skills with people at all levels
4. The ability to *assess* situations objectively and to *plan* appropriate case management services
5. Knowledge of available clinical evidence and resources as well as their strengths and weaknesses
6. The ability to act as *advocate* for the client and payer in models relying on third-party payment
7. The ability to act as a counselor or *facilitator* to clients to provide support, understanding, information, and intervention

In 1998, Cary described the roles of case managers in the practice setting. These roles are clearly affirmed today in the work of Llewellyn and Moreo (2001) and by the CMSA (2010) (Box 22-1). The roles demanded of the nurse as case manager are greatly influenced by the forces that support or detract from the role. Figure 22-4 presents factors that demand the attention of both the nurse and the client during the case management process.

| NURSING TIP *Use the components of the nursing process when executing the functions of a case manager with clients. Incorporate your knowledge of community resources, human behavior dynamics, cultural competency, financial eligibility, health promotion, disease trajectories, and advocacy as you execute the process.*

Knowledge and Skill Requisites

Nurses are not automatically experts in the role of case manager. First, they develop and refine the knowledge and skills that are essential to implementing the role successfully. Knowledge domains useful for nurses in systems desiring to

TABLE 22-1   THE NURSING PROCESS AND CASE MANAGEMENT

NURSING PROCESS	CASE MANAGEMENT PROCESS	ACTIVITIES
Assessment	• Case finding • Identification of incentives for target population • Screening and intake • Determination of eligibility • Assessment	• Develop networks with target population • Disseminate written materials • Seek referrals • Apply screening tools according to program goals and objectives • Use written and on-site screens • Apply comprehensive assessment methods (physical, social, emotional, cognitive, economic, and self-care capacity) • Obtaining consent for services if appropriate
Diagnosis	• Identification of problem/opportunity	• Hold interprofessional, family, and client conferences • Determine conclusion on basis of assessment • Use interprofessional team
Planning for Outcomes	• Problem prioritizing • Planning to address care needs • Identify resource match	• Validate and prioritize problems with all participants • Develop goals, activities, time frames, and options • Gain client's consent to implement • Have client choose options
Implementation	• Advocate clients' interests • Frequent monitoring to assess alignment with goals and changing nature of client needs	• Contact providers • Negotiate services and price • Adjust as implementation is needed • Document processes and monitor progress
Evaluation	• Measure attainment of activities and goals of service delivery plan • Continued monitoring of client status during service • Reassessment • Bring closure to care when client needs are achieved or change • Discharge appropriately	• Ensure quality of transitional communication and coordination of service delivery • Monitor for changes in client or service status • Examine outcomes against goals • Examine needs against service • Examine costs • Examine satisfaction of client, providers, and case manager • Examine best practices and outcomes for this client

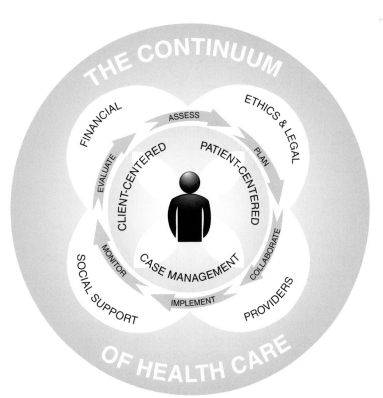

FIGURE 22-3 The continuum of care case management model. (From Case Management Society of America: *Standards of practice for case management*, Little Rock, AR, 2010, CMSA, p 5.)

BOX 22-1   CASE MANAGER ROLES

- **Broker:** Acts as an agent for provider services that are needed by clients to stay within coverage according to budget and cost limits of health care plan
- **Consultant:** Works with providers, suppliers, the community, and other case managers to provide case management expertise in programmatic and individual applications
- **Coordinator:** Arranges, regulates, and coordinates needed health care services for clients at all necessary points of services. Effectively participates on interprofessional teams
- **Educator:** Educates client, family, and providers about case management process, delivery system, community health resources, and benefit coverage so that informed decisions can be made by all parties
- **Facilitator:** Supports all parties in work toward mutual goals
- **Liaison:** Provides a formal communication link among all parties concerning the plan of care management
- **Mentor:** Counsels and guides the development of the practice of new case managers
- **Monitor/reporter:** Provides information to parties on status of member and situations affecting client safety, care quality, and client outcome, and on factors that alter costs and liability

- **Negotiator:** Negotiates the plan of care, services, and payment arrangements with providers; uses effective collaboration and team strategies
- **Client advocate:** Acts as advocate, provides information, and supports benefit changes that assist member, family, primary care provider, and capitated systems
- **Researcher:** Accesses and applies evidence-based practices for programmatic and individual interventions with clients and communities; participates in protection of clients in research studies; initiates/collaborates in research programs and studies; accesses real-time evidence for practice
- **Standardization monitor:** Formulates and monitors specific, time-sequenced critical path and care map plans (see text) as well as disease management protocols that guide the type and timing of care to comply with predicted treatment outcomes for the specific client and conditions; attempts to reduce variation in resource use; targets deviations from standards so adjustments can occur in a timely manner
- **Systems allocator:** Distributes limited health care resources according to a plan or rationale

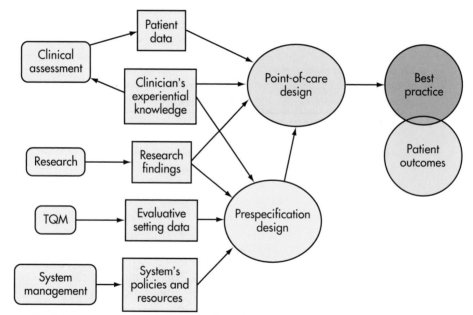

FIGURE 22-4 Factors that require the attention of the nurse and client in the case management process.

implement quality case management roles are found in Box 22-2 (Cary, 1998; Llewellyn and Moreo, 2001; Stanton and Dunkin, 2009).

When a nurse seeks a case manager position, some of the skills and knowledge will need to be acquired through academic and continuing education programs, literature reviews, and orientation and mentoring experiences. Basic nursing education may need to be updated, while practical experiences in case management may be required. In fact, professional development activities for case managers in public health have been demonstrated to contribute to job satisfaction (Schutt et al, 2010).

Tools of Case Managers

The five "rights" of case management are right care, right time, right provider, right setting, and right price. How does the nurse judge the effectiveness of case management? Three tools are useful for case management practice: case management plans, disease management, and life care planning tools. An underlying principle for use of each of these tools is the need to use robust evidence as the basis for the selection of activities.

Case management plans have evolved through various terms and methods (e.g., critical paths, critical pathways, care

BOX 22-2 KNOWLEDGE DOMAINS FOR CASE MANAGEMENT

- Standards of practice for case management
- Evidence-based practice guidelines for specific health and disease conditions and communities
- Knowledge of health care financial environment and the financial dimension of client populations managed by nurses
- Clinical knowledge, skill, and maturity to direct quality timing and sequencing of care activities
- Care resources for clients within institutions and communities: facilitating the development of new resources and systems to meet clients' needs
- Transition planning for ideal timing, sequencing, and levels of care
- Management skills: communication, delegation, persuasion, use of power, consultation, problem solving, conflict management, confrontation, negotiation, management of change, marketing, group development, accountability, authority, advocacy, ethical decision making, and profit management
- Teaching, counseling, and education skills
- Program evaluation and research
- Performance improvement techniques
- Peer consultation and evaluation
- Requirements of eligibility and benefit parameters by third-party payers
- Legal and ethical issues
- Information management systems: clinical and administrative
- Health care legislation/policy
- Technical information skills, interoperable information systems, data management, and analysis
- Outcomes management and applied research

maps, multidisciplinary action plans, nursing care plans). Regardless of the title given, standards of client care, standards of nursing practice, and clinical guidelines using evidence-based practices for case management serve as core foundations of case management plans. Likewise, in interprofessional action plans, core professional standards of each discipline guide the development of the standard process.

As early as 1985, the New England Medical Center in Boston instituted a system of critical path development to guide the case management process in the acute care setting. A *critical path* was described as a case management tool comprised of abbreviated versions of discipline-specific processes; it was used to achieve a measurable outcome for a specific client "case" (Zander, Etheredge, and Bower, 1987). The critical path detailed the essential and sequential activities in care, so that the expected progress of the client was known at a point in time. Outcomes from critical paths included satisfaction, client competency, continuity of care, continuity of information, and costs and quality of care. However, one criticism was that critical paths may not be evidence based (Renholm, Leino-Kilpi, and Suominen, 2002). The prevailing method of establishing critical paths was by internal, "expert knowledge" from a specific institution, the result being that they could not be applied generally or tested under systematic, scientific methods. In the New England model, key incidents included consults, tests, activities, treatments, medication, diet, discharge planning, and teaching. The paths showed the differences between clients' progress. However, the paths were generally not revised unless a body of evidence was found to adjust the expected actions.

Care maps became the second generation of critical pathways of care. Rather than give definitions, Brown (2001) discussed the "various types of evidence that must be accessed, interpreted, and integrated into care design." Brown (2001, p 3) proposed the Best Practice Health Care Map (BPHM) as a model for providing quality clinical care within an interprofessional practice. This model discussed all the components of knowledge development and care planning activities that must occur to have positive client outcomes. The author noted that care designed in advance takes the form of "clinical guidelines, care maps, decision algorithms, and clinical protocols for specified populations of clients" (Brown, 2001, p 3). The "Prespecification Design" of the BPHM entailed these preplanning courses of care. Brown (2001) stressed the importance of incorporating research findings and clinical experience when developing prespecified plans. Furthermore, the author emphasized that at the point of care, these prespecified plans must be adapted to the individual client or population.

The Brown BPHM was: (1) client centered, (2) scientifically based, (3) population-outcomes based, (4) refined through quality assessment and compared with other maps, (5) individualized to each client, and (6) compatible with the larger system of health care in the United States such activities are more likely referred to as case management plans, care maps, and integrated clinical pathways (Figure 22-5).

Adaptation of the case management care plan to each client's characteristics is a crucial skill for standardizing the process and outcome of care. It links multiple provider interventions to client responses and offers reasonable predictions to clients about health outcomes. Institutions report that sharing case management plans with clients empowers the clients to assume responsibility for monitoring and adhering to the plan of care. Self-responsibility by clients incorporates autonomy and self-determination as the core of case management. For the nurse employed to function as a case manager, ample opportunity exists to develop, test, and revise critical path/map prototypes for a target population experiencing acute health problems.

Disease management is an organized program of coordinated health care interventions and communications for populations with conditions in which client self-care efforts are critical (CMSA, 2010). This approach focuses on the natural progression of a disease. Disease management programs may contain many of the following components (DMAA, 2008, 2010):

- Financial and risk sharing arrangements between payers and providers
- Programs for monitoring the use of clinical paths and evidence-based guidelines to assess outcomes and costs
- Protocols for clinical and administrative processes as well as cost allocations
- Services to educate clients and promote self-management skills
- Enhanced quality through evidence-based decision support and other registry technologies
- Support for provider/client relationships and plans of care
- Evaluation of clinical, humanistic, and economic outcomes to address the goal of improving overall health

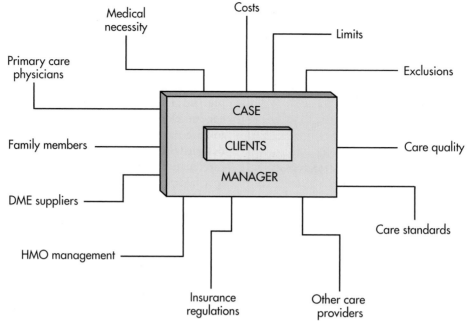

FIGURE 22-5 Forces affecting solutions in the case management process. (From Hicks LL, Stallmeyer JM, Coleman JR: *The role of the nurse in managed care,* Washington, DC, 1993, American Nurses Publishing.)

HOW TO   Apply Telehealth Interventions for Clients

To learn more about telehealth interventions for clients, case managers can do the following:

- *Make it a point to learn how telehealth works in your community and in the industry.*
- *Examine the evidence base for telehealth as an option when considering available resources.*
- *Seek continuing education courses to prepare you on the art and science of telehealth application. Read the literature on e-communication and monitoring effectiveness impact.*
- *Seek networking opportunities with professional organizations and other case managers about the uses of telehealth.*
- *Examine the clinical guidelines and practice algorithms for telehealth adoption, application, and use.*
- *Sharpen your personal interaction and program evaluation skills to better assist in decision making about the use of telehealth services.*

From Hagan L, Morin D, Lepine R: Evaluation of telenursing outcomes: satisfaction, self-care practices, and cost savings, Public Health Nurs 17:305-313, 2000.

The philosophy of disease management gives the clients the tools needed to better manage their lives (McConnell and Conyea, 2004; CMSA, 2010). Clients with chronic diseases benefit from a disease management approach. The goals are to interrupt continued development of a disease and prevent future disease and complications through secondary and tertiary prevention interventions. Promotion of wellness is necessary for success. For specific client populations that consume a disproportionate share of resources, disease management apprograms allocate the correct resources in an efficacious manner (Owen, 2004).

Disease management programs also reduce emergency department visits, result in fewer inpatient days, greater client satisfaction, and reduced school absences (McClatchey, 2001; Sidorov, 2011). As the science of disease management evolves to predict direct relationships between outcomes and protocols of care, case managers will be able to ensure cost-effective, optimal clinical care across the continuum—a goal of care management for populations. In fact, disease management is viewed as a top strategy by employers. For case managers, disease management strategies, which are part of the care management programs, shift the client interventions from specific, episodic care to holistic care functions that are proactive and population based (AHA, 2003-2004). The Joint Commission (TJC) certifies and the American Accreditation HealthCare Commission accredits disease management organizations and programs on the basis of their respective standards (see websites http://www.jointcommission.org and www.urac.org). This may influence the choice of programs a case manager selects to use with clients.

Life care planning is another tool used in case management. It assesses the current and future needs of a client for catastrophic or chronic disease over a life span. The life care plan is a customized, medically based document that provides assessment of all present and future needs (medical, financial, psychological, vocational, spiritual, physical, and social), including services, equipment, supplies, and living arrangements for a client (Llewellyn and Moreo, 2001). These plans may be used by either plaintiff or defense lawyer to analyze damages. They are also used to set financial rewards, which can be used to pay for care in the future and create a lifetime care plan. Life care plans are typically used for clients experiencing catastrophic illness or adverse events resulting from professional malpractice. Another group of life care planning beneficiaries is those who have sustained injury when younger and whose care requirements have changed as a result of aging (Demoratz, 2004). A systematic process is used and interprofessional input is required. The first phase of the plan is crafted to include a thorough assessment of the client, financial/billing agreements, an information release signed by the client, and a targeted date for report completion. Development of the plan is the second phase. Case management plans are based on a number of factors: social situation, leisure activities, educational and employment status, medical history, physical abilities, current status, and assistance required for completing activities of daily living.

HOW TO Ensure High-Quality Care

The following actions can ensure high-quality care for clients and have implications for case managers in their practice:

- *Provide access to easily understood information for each client based on their needs.*
- *The client is the source of control.*
- *Provide access to appropriate specialists with coordination and communication transparency.*
- *Ensure continuity of care for those with chronic and disabling conditions (transition care).*
- *Provide access to emergency services when and where needed.*
- *Disclose financial incentives that could influence medical decisions and outcomes.*
- *Prohibit "gag clauses" (which mean that providers cannot inform clients of all possible treatment options).*
- *Provide antidiscrimination protections.*
- *Provide internal and external appeal processes to solve grievances of clients.*
- *Decision making is evidence based.*

Modified from McClinton DH: Protecting patients, Contin Care 17:6, 1998; Institute of Medicine: Crossing the quality chasm, Washington, DC, 2001, National Academy of Science.

The plan includes projected costs and resources needed for the frequency and duration of treatments, equipment, and supplies. It also includes plans for future evaluations. The life care plan seeks to portray the needs of a client that are consistent with the changes in a client's life over the predicted life span, taking into account the injury or diagnosis (McCollom, 2002).

All of these tools/programs, in coordination, constitute population health management strategies to educate clients and promote self-management, provide nurse coaching support, promote safe care transitions, improve care management and coordination, and enhance quality (DMAA, 2010).

WHAT DO YOU THINK? *The health care benefit plan of a client may omit treatments and services that could improve health outcomes. Other complementary health services (e.g., acupuncture) may be omitted from the benefit plan because the evidence available to determine health outcomes is not available. What should the case manager's role be with the client, the insurance benefit plan administrator, and the provider when a client is not eligible for services from their health plan?*

EVIDENCE-BASED EXAMPLES OF CASE MANAGEMENT

Historical Evidence

Carondelet Health at St. Mary's Hospital in Tucson, Arizona, developed a community nursing network in which enrollees are distributed among a number of community health centers. Professional nurse case managers assisted older clients to attain healthier lifestyles and maintain themselves in the community. Nurses were successful in delivering economical services per month for Medicare enrollees. Through nurse case management services, this nursing HMO was reported to have reduced the number of inpatient days per 1000 enrollees by one third, at an average cost of $900 per day, for a savings of $300,000 for every 1000 enrollees (ANA, 1993; ANF, 1993). These strengths have been critical to allow the model to evolve to provide group and telephonic case management and automated standardized care instruments. Future endeavors will capitalize on the advances in information technology to capture clinical and cost data in a timely manner for decision support (Cohen and Cesta, 2005).

Community-based statewide programs in New Jersey used case management methods to promote early identification, selection, evaluation, diagnosis, and treatment of children who are potentially physically compromised. Local case management units provided coordinated and comprehensive care. Collaboration with existing local and regional agencies serving children supported this process. The nurse case manager: (1) provided counseling and education to parents and children about identifying problems and increasing their knowledge, (2) developed individual plans incorporating multidisciplinary services (education, social issues, medical development, rehabilitation), (3) obtained appropriate community services, (4) acted as a family resource in crises and service concerns, (5) facilitated communication between child and family, and (6) monitored services for outcomes. Interprofessional teams include nurses and social workers (with master's degrees) for larger caseloads. A recommended caseload was 300 to 350 children per case manager (Bower, 1992).

A national study of 2437 people who tested positive for human immunodeficiency virus (HIV) and who had case managers demonstrated that, regardless of the model, these clients were more likely to use life-prolonging HIV medications and meet the needs for income, health insurance, home care, and supportive emotional counseling than those without case management. Having contact with a case manager was not significantly related to use of outpatient care, hospital admission, or emergency department visits. Case managers in this study included social workers, nurses, and AIDS service organization staff (Katz et al, 2001).

Liberty Mutual Insurance Company had used case management principles for more than 30 years in workers' compensation cases and expanded services for employees whose conditions were noted as chronic or catastrophic (Box 22-3). Case managers coordinated all clients, providers, and services to reduce expenses caused by lack of coordination, failure to use beneficial alternatives, and duplication and fragmentation of services (Bower, 1992).

BOX 22-3   EXAMPLES OF CASE-MANAGED CONDITIONS

- Acquired immunodeficiency syndrome (AIDS)
- Amputations
- Cerebrovascular accident (CVA)
- Chronic diseases and disabilities (asthma, diabetes, mental illness, behavioral health)
- High-risk neonates
- Multiple fractures
- Severe burns
- Brain trauma
- Spinal cord injury
- Substance abuse
- Terminal illness
- Transplantation
- Ventilator dependency
- Work-related injuries
- Psychiatric conditions
- High utilization of services

Important guidance in developing a community-based case management program can be found in the United States. Case management is a key component of federally financed and many state-financed health delivery options. The experiences of states over the past two decades provide testimony to the importance of case management for populations at risk. For older clients, state-derived case management provides objective advice and assistance with care needs. It also provides access to interprofessional providers and services. For payers (federal, state, clients), case management serves as a way to ensure that funds are allocated appropriately to those in greatest need. Case management serves a policy assurance and accountability function for communities. The PACE (Program of All-inclusive Care for the Elderly) program addresses the needs of chronically ill seniors who wish to remain in their homes and are enrolled in a managed care model of medical and support services, case management, medications, respite, hospital, and nursing home care when necessary. PACE prevents institutionalization in nursing homes, uses a strong social model of health care delivery, and case manages transitions of clients between delivery systems and providers. The PACE model has been permanently recognized as a provider type under both Medicare and Medicaid and has grown to 72 programs operating in 30 states (NPA, 2010).

Within the states, the types of agencies designated to conduct case management are often district offices of state government, area agencies on aging, county social services departments, and private contractors. States maintain the oversight responsibilities for case management agencies to: (1) ensure they are complying with program standards, contracts, reporting, and fiscal controls, (2) identify emerging problems and issues to be resolved by additional state policies, and (3) provide on-site technical assistance and consulting to improve performance. States' payment methods for case management include daily/monthly rates, hourly/quarterly rates, capped rates for services, and capped aggregate rates to cover both case management and provider costs (HRSA, 2004; USDHHS, 2008).

The models of case management vary today as they did in the recent past. In 1999, Taylor described three models by their focus: client, system, and social service. *Client-focused models* are concerned with the relationship between case manager and client to support continuity of care and to access providers of care. *System-focused models,* in contrast, address the structure and processes of using the population-based tools of disease management and case management plans to offer care for client populations. The *social service models* provide services to clients to assist them in living independently in the community and in maintaining their health by eliminating or reducing the need for hospital admissions or long-term care.

These models offer a solution to unnecessary health care expenses by reducing costs and accessing appropriate health care services. Imagine the impact on health status if these saved resources were shifted to primary prevention and health promotion activities.

Contemporary Evidence

Reducing the rate of readmission within 30 days is a quality goal in health care. For psychiatric clients, the risk of rehospitalization is greatest and most costly during this time. Kolbasovshy (2009) replicated a model of intensive case management (ICM) in the United States that had been successful in Europe in reducing 30-day readmission rates (Burns et al, 2001, 2007) and found that ICM significantly reduced readmissions and the associated costs of 305 clients at a cost of $41.39 per member during the 30-day period. Had these persons been rehospitalized, the hospital psychiatric costs would have been $1528.14 per member. The nature of the case management activities included transitional and coordination of aftercare, monitoring of symptoms, medication and treatment adherence, education of client and families, motivational interviewing to detect barriers, linkages to community-based resources, treatment refill reminders, alcohol screening, and brief interventions.

In a randomized controlled trial of 450 clients post-cardiac bypass surgery, case management intervention by nurses using telephone-based collaborative care improved the mental and physical health of persons experiencing depression after cardiac bypass in an 8-month case management intervention. Case management activities included education about post-cardiac depression, self management skills, assessing and monitoring of treatment and medication adherence, interprofessional weekly case conferences, and routine communication with persons and primary care providers to ensure the provision of coordinated, consistent care. The case manager used ongoing telephone support, encouragement of client preferences, self-management workbooks, coaching, and electronic support for care guidelines and protocols. Outcomes included increased mental health scores, improved physical and functional status, and fewer readmissions among males with subsequent cost savings (AHRQ, 2010a).

Using a managed care model of enrollment, the CARE ONE program at the University of New Mexico Health Sciences Center provides intensive case management and care coordination to medically complex, costly clients who lack health insurance. Among the top 1% of high-cost clients, all were offered enrollment in a case management service with an interprofessional team of providers who help persons in this population to navigate the system, access available financial assistance, and use appropriate community resources. Each person meets with the entire team to assess and prioritize needs, goals, and subsequent steps, and to schedule medical appointments. Activities also include securing financial resources; counseling and assistance

EVIDENCE-BASED PRACTICE

A successful pilot program led to the execution of a randomized controlled trial—After Discharge Care Management of Low Income Frail Elderly (AD-LIFE)—for community-based elderly. The care management model uses the integration of medical and social care to improve the outcomes of low-income, and chronically and functionally impaired elderly after hospital discharge. AD-LIFE uses an interprofessional team, comprehensive geriatric assessment, and care management by a team nurse. Throughout the first year after hospital discharge, the nurse works with the area Agency on Aging social services program, performs a hospital and home assessment, uses a client goal-setting approach, creates a plan for development of self-care skills, and provides care planning for chronic illnesses and geriatric syndromes (e.g., incontinence, depression, nutrition, skin problems, and memory impairment). The interprofessional team can access specialists, and the primary care provider performs frequent evaluations and revises care plans as needed.

Ninety-two percent (92%) of the 118 clients had the need for at least one medical or social intervention. Half were taking 5 to 10 prescription drugs, 40% were living alone, 28% had congestive heart failure, 28% had diabetes, and many were unable to perform some ADLs or experienced geriatric syndrome. About 70% of clients said the care management program improved their health, allowed them to more easily access health care services, and provided them with a greater understanding of their disease(s). Hospital admissions decreased and the care cost savings were $1000 per client per month.

- As a nurse working in public health, what aspects of this program could you build on to design an interprofessional program for community-based clients with Alzheimer's disease? People living with AIDS? Chronically ill or disabled children? Clients with unstable psychiatric conditions?
- Identify the interprofessional team members that could be assembled to conduct the program with each client group.
- What measures of success could you identify for each of the programs?
- Which *Healthy People 2020* objectives could be addressed for each of these client groups?

Nurse Use

Post-discharge care management that integrates medical and social care can improve outcomes of the low-income elderly.

From Wright K, Hazelett S, Jarjoura D, Allen K: The AD-LIFE trial, *Home Healthc Nurse* 25(5):308-314, 2007.

to complete paperwork; scheduling appointments, reminders, and follow-ups; behavioral health counseling; medication management; and access to community resources to support health. Case management resulted in 80% fewer hospital admissions, a 60% decline in emergency room visits, and consistently high client satisfaction scores (AHRQ, 2010b).

ESSENTIAL SKILLS FOR CASE MANAGERS

Three skills are essential to the role performance of the case manager: advocacy, conflict management, and collaboration.

Advocacy

Case managers report that they are first and foremost client advocates (Barefield, 2003; Stanton and Dunkin, 2009; CMSA, 2010). The definition of nursing includes **advocacy:** "Nursing is the protection, promotion and optimization of health and abilities, prevention of illness and injury, alleviation of suffering through the diagnosis and treatment of human response, and advocacy in the care of individuals, families, communities and populations" (ANA, 2010, p 6). For nurses, advocacy involves a number of activities, ranging from exploring self-awareness to lobbying for health policy. Advocacy is essential for practice with clients and their families, communities, organizations, and colleagues on an interprofessional team. The functions of advocacy require scientific knowledge, expert communication, facilitating skills, and problem-solving and affirming techniques. As the *Code of Ethics for Nurses* (ANA, 2008) states, "The nurse, in all professional relationships, practices with compassion and respect…" (p 4). This means the nurse has the obligation to move beyond his or her own personal feelings of agreement or disagreement to respond compassionately. However, this goal is a contemporary one; the perspective regarding the advocacy function has shifted through time. The nurse advocate has been described in earlier writings as one who acted on behalf of or interceded for the client (Nelson, 1988). An example of the nurse interacting on behalf of the client is the nurse who calls for a well-child appointment for a mother visiting the family planning clinic when the mother is capable of making an appointment on her own.

The advocate role evolved to that of mediator and is described as a response to the complex configuration of social change, reimbursement, and providers in the health care system (Tahan, 2005). Mediating is an activity in which a third party attempts to provide assistance to those who may be experiencing a conflict in obtaining what they desire. The goal of the nurse advocate as mediator is to assist parties to understand each other on many levels so that agreement on an action is possible. In the example of a nurse as case manager for an HMO, mediating activities between an older adult client and the payer (the HMO) could accomplish the following results: the client may understand the options for community-based skilled nursing care, and the payer may understand the client's desires for a less restrictive environment for care, such as the home. The case manager as mediator does not decide the plan of action but facilitates the decision-making processes between the client and the payee so that the desired care can be reimbursed within the options available.

In contemporary practice, nurse advocates place the client's rights as the highest priority. The goal of promoter for the client's autonomy and self-determination may result in an optimal degree of independence in decision making. For example, when a group of young pregnant women is the collective "client" (the aggregate), the nurse advocate's role may be to inform the group of the benefits and consequences of breastfeeding their infants. However, if the new mothers decide on formula feeding, the nurse advocate should support the group and continue to provide parenting, infant, and well-child services. This example shows a different perspective of the nurse as advocate. It notes that the nurse's role as advocate may demand a variety of functions that are influenced by the client's physical, psychological, social, and environmental abilities. Advocacy can result in clients becoming their own "client expert" in problem-solving, decision making, maximization of resources, partnership development with providers, and ultimately appropriate interventions (Burton, Murphy, and Riley, 2010).

The nurse adapts the advocacy function to the client's dynamic capabilities as the client moves from one health state to another. Even clients who desire access to more substantial health promotion activities can benefit from a partnership with the nurse advocate. Case managers are called to mediate between client needs and payer requirements/economic constraints without becoming a barrier to quality care. Examples of advocacy in such cases might include promoting a client's (as an aggregate) access to on-site physical fitness programs in the occupational setting, or supporting parents' and students' concerns about the high-fat content of vending machine food in the school system. With the cost of health care exceeding $2 trillion annually and consumers assuming a larger financial portion of the care they choose, the promoter role of advocacy for those clients capable of autonomy is expected to increase.

| **THE CUTTING EDGE**   *Pharmaceutical companies have a program of free supplies of drugs for clients who have no health coverage or who do not qualify for other programs. Call a pharmaceutical company for information about clients' eligibility.*

Process of Advocacy

The goal of advocacy is to promote self-determination in a client. The client may be an individual, family, peer, group, or community. The classic process of advocacy has been defined by Kohnke (1982), Mallik and Rafferty (2000), and Smith (2004) to include informing, supporting, and affirming. All three activities are more complex than they may initially seem, and they require self-reflection by the nurse as well as skill development. It is often easier for the nurse to inform, support, and affirm another person's decision when it is consistent with the nurse's values. When clients make decisions within their value systems that are different from the nurse's values, the advocate may feel conflict about contributing to the process of informing, supporting, and affirming those decisions. Promoting self-determination in others demands that the nurse have a philosophy of free choice once the information necessary for decision making has been discussed.

Informing. Knowledge is essential, but it is not enough to make decisions that affect outcomes. Interpreting knowledge is affected by the client's values and the meanings assigned to the knowledge. Interpreting facts is the result of both objective and subjective processing of information. Subjective processes greatly influence client decisions.

Informing clients about the nature of their choices, the content of those choices, and the consequences to the client is not a one-way activity. The information exchange process is composed of interactions that reflect three subprocesses: amplifying, clarifying, and verifying. Amplifying occurs between the nurse and the client to assess the needs and demands that will eventually frame the client's decision. Information is exchanged from both viewpoints. Although the exchange may be initiated at the objective, factual level, it is likely to proceed to incorporate the subjective perspectives of both parties.

🌐 **LINKING CONTENT TO PRACTICE**

Advocacy: Text Link to Public Health Nursing

The focus of this chapter is the use of the clinical practice skill of advocacy as an inherent concept in the practice of case management. Of the 16 interventions by public health nurses described in the Wheel of Intervention model (see Chapter 9) both advocacy and case management are described in accordance with best practices and operational definitions of 2 of the 16 interventions. Advocacy can be applied at the community, systems, individual, or family levels. In fact, while a public health nurse advocates for any one of these clients, the source of conflict and collaboration will likely come from competing values among the client and any of these other levels of population values. While a client may want access to unlimited treatment, financial values may pose a source of conflict as the system attempts to justify the comparative effectiveness or costs. Family members may pose conflicting values for the nature of care they wish a family member to receive, even as the client refuses care. Communities can divert budget allotments to needs that are in competition for other population services such as community policing, health care access, and environmental services. The nurse as advocate must listen carefully to his or her client in order to truly represent the interest of the client and encourage "win-win" processes and outcomes for the client. Advocacy occurs at all three of the core functions of public health: assessment, policy development, and assurance.

The tone of the amplifying process can direct the remainder of the information exchange. It is important to relate with clients in a manner that reflects the advocate's endorsement of the client's self-determination. Setting aside the time necessary to listen to clients is critical. Clients will sense they are part of a mutual process if the nurse can engage them during the information exchange with a message that says, "I respect your needs and desires as I share my knowledge with you." Nonverbal behaviors, including using direct eye contact, sitting at the client's level, arriving and concluding at a prescribed time, and using verbal patterns that foster exchange (e.g., open-ended statements, questions, probes, reflections of feelings, paraphrasing), convey the nurse's desire to promote the client's ability to self-determine. Recent research indicates that clients' race and ethnicity may influence how providers and clients communicate with one another, thus contributing to disparities in health. More active participation of clients in conversations with providers has been linked to better treatment compliance and health outcomes (Johnson et al, 2004).

A client may not desire to exchange information because of lack of self-esteem, fear of the information, or inability to comprehend the content of the communication. In such a case, the focus is to understand the client's desire to be given no information and to express to the client the consequences of such inaction. The nurse may invite the client to ask for the information exchange at a later time, when the client is ready, and can periodically check with the client whether information exchange and amplifying are desired. In these cases, the nurse should document the implemented nursing actions to reflect the guidelines just discussed. This can reduce the basis for lawsuits and misunderstanding by other parties.

Clarifying is a process in which the nurse and client strive to understand meanings in a common way. Clarifying builds on the breadth and depth of the exchange developed during amplifying to determine if the nurse and client understand each other. During this process, misunderstandings and confusions are examined. The goal of clarifying is to avoid confusion between the nurse and the client. To foster clarifying, nurses can use certain verbal prompts such as the following:

- "What do you understand about . . . ?"
- "Please tell me more about how you . . ."
- "I don't think I am clear. Let me explain the situation in another way."
- "As an example, . . ."
- "What other information would be helpful so that we both understand?"

Verifying is the process used by the nurse advocate to establish accuracy and reality in the informing process. A lack of health literacy is a challenge for 90 million Americans who have difficulty understanding and acting on health information. The average U.S. client on Medicaid reads at a fifth-grade level, compared with the average American who reads at an eighth- or ninth-grade level (Wilson, 2003). If the nurse discovers that a client is misinformed, the nurse may return to the clarifying or amplifying stage and begin the process again. Verifying produces the chance for the advocate and client to examine "truth" from their points of view, which may include knowledge, intuition, previous experiences, and anticipated consequences.

Promoting a client's self-determination may take the advocate and client through the information exchange process several times, as new dimensions, or obstacles, to an issue develop. Information exchange is a critical process for advocacy and is applicable to all advocacy clients: individuals, families, groups, and communities (see the How To box).

HOW TO **Provide for Information Exchange Between Nurse and Client**

1. *Assess the client's present understanding of the situation. Have you considered your client's literacy level? Cultural and ethnic values? Age and any disabilities that would interfere with learning?*
2. *Provide correct information.*
3. *Communicate on the client's literacy level, making the information as understandable as possible.*
4. *Use a variety of media sources and teach-back methods to increase the client's comprehension.*
5. *Discuss other factors that affect the decision, such as financial, legal, and ethical issues.*
6. *Discuss the possible consequences of a decision.*

Supporting. The second major process, supporting, involves upholding a client's right to make a choice and to act on it. People who are aware of clients' decisions fall into three general groups: supporters, dissenters, and obstructers. Supporters approve and support clients' actions. Dissenters do not approve and do not support clients. Obstructers cause difficulties when clients try to implement their decisions.

In 1998, Cary noted that the nurse advocate needs to implement several actions to fulfill the supporting role. Important interventions are assuring clients that they have the right and responsibility to make decisions, and reassuring them that

NURSING PROCESS	ADVOCACY PROCESS
Assessment/diagnosis	• Information exchange • Gather data • Illuminate values
Planning/outcome	• Generate alternatives and consequences • Prioritize actions
Implementation	• Decision making • Support of client • Assure • Reassure
Evaluation	• Affirmation • Evaluation • Reformulation

TABLE 22-2 COMPARISON OF NURSING PROCESS AND ADVOCACY PROCESS

they do not have to change their decisions because of others' objections.

Affirming. The third process in the advocacy role is **affirming.** It is based on an advocate's belief that a client's decision is consistent with the client's values and goals. The advocate validates that the client's behavior is purposeful and consistent with the choice that was made. The advocate expresses a dedication to the client's mission, and a purposeful exchange of new information may occur so that the client's choice remains possible. Recognizing that a client's needs may fluctuate with changing resources, the affirming activity must encourage a process of reevaluation and rededication to promote client self-determination.

The importance of affirming activities cannot be emphasized strongly enough. Many advocacy activities stop with assuring and reassuring, but affirming is often critical in promoting a client's self-determination. Table 22-2 compares the nursing process with the advocacy process.

The advocate's role in the decision-making process is *not* to tell the client that an option is correct or right. The advocate's role is to provide the opportunity for information exchange, and to arm clients with tools that can empower them in making the best decision from their point of view. Enabling clients to make an informed decision is a powerful tool for building self-confidence. It gives clients the responsibility for selecting the options and experiencing the success and consequences of their decisions. Clients are empowered in their decision making when they recognize that although some events are beyond their control, other events are predictable and can be affected by decisions they can make.

Nurses can promote client decision making by using the information exchange process, promoting the use of the nursing process, incorporating written techniques (e.g., contracts, lists), using reflecting and prioritizing techniques, and using role playing and sculpturing to "try on" and determine the "fit" of different options and consequences for the client. By engaging clients in the information-sharing process and assisting them to recognize the progression of activities they experience as they build their informed decision-making base, the nurse advocate is providing clients the opportunity to empower themselves with skills that can strengthen their autonomy and confidence in the future.

Advocacy is a complex process that maintains a delicate balance between doing for the client and promoting autonomy. The process is influenced by the client's physical, emotional, and social capabilities. The goal of advocacy is to promote the maximum degree of client self-determination, given the client's current and potential status; for most clients, this goal can be realized. When clients are comatose, unborn, or legally incompetent, nurse advocates have unique functions. The advocate's role is usually determined by the legal system; however, in some cases, nurses must decide what roles they will play. These are areas requiring intensive self-exploration, research, and collaboration with professionals, family members, and significant others. We are reminded that every encounter with a client is an opportunity to serve in the advocacy role (Beyea, 2005).

Skill Development

Skills needed by the nurse advocate are not unique to their profession. Nursing demands scientific, technical, relationship, and problem-solving knowledge and skills. Advocacy applies nursing skills of communication and competency to promote client self-determination.

Knowledge of nursing and other disciplines as well as of human behavior is essential for the advocacy role in establishing authority, promoting authenticity, and developing skills. The capacity to be assertive for personal rights and the rights of others is essential.

Systematic Problem Solving

The nursing process—assessment, diagnosis, planning, implementing, and evaluating—is an example of a method of **problem solving** that can be used in the advocacy role. Advocates can be particularly helpful with clients in identifying values and generating alternatives.

Illuminating Values. People's values affect their behavior, feelings, and goals. In the process of amplifying, clarifying, and validating, the advocate understands a client's values. Through the process of self-revelation, an emerging value (such as environment, people, cost, or quality) may become more apparent to a client. This can have an effect in two ways. The client may be able to focus on actions on the basis of the value, or the value may confuse the decision process. The nurse can assist the client in prioritizing action and clarifying the value. Values can also change as new or relevant data are processed. The advocate's role is to assist clients in discovering their values. This process can be particularly demanding in the information exchange and affirming process.

Generating Alternatives. Clients and advocates may feel limited in their options if they generate solutions before completely analyzing the problems, needs, desires, and consequences. Several techniques can be used to generate alternatives, including brainstorming and a technique known as the problem-purpose-expansion method. In **brainstorming**, the nurse, client, professionals, or significant others generate as many alternatives as possible, without placing a value on them. Brainstorming

creates a list that can then be examined for the critical elements the client seeks to preserve (e.g., environmental preferences, degree of control). The list can be analyzed according to the consequences and the effect of the alternatives on self and others.

The classic **problem-purpose-expansion method,** as described by Volkema (1983) and later expanded upon by Heslin and Moldoveanu (2002), is a way to broaden limited thinking. It involves restating the problem and expanding the problem statement so that different solutions can be generated. For example, if the problem statement is to convince the insurance company to approve a longer length of service, the nurse and client have narrowed their options. However, if the problem statement is to improve the client's convalescence and safety, several solutions and options are available, such as the following:

- Obtaining skilled nursing facility placement
- Obtaining home-health skilled services
- Arranging physician home visits
- Paying for custodial care
- Paying for private skilled care
- Obtaining informal caregiving

Impact of Advocacy

Advocacy empowers clients to participate in problem-solving processes and decisions about health care. Clients try to understand changing opportunities in the health care system for access, use, and achieving continuity of care. Nurse advocates promote client self-determination and management of behavior as it relates to health and the adherence to therapeutic regimens. Clients are part of larger systems: the family, the work environment, and the community. Each system interacts with the client to shape the available options through resources, needs, and desires. Each system also exhibits both confirming and conflicting goals and processes that need to be understood for client self-determination to be successful. For example, the practice of advocacy among minority groups may involve the ability to focus attention on the magnitude of problems caused by diseases affecting minority clients. Whether the client is an individual, family, group, or community, the advocacy function can promote the interest of self-determination, which influences the progress of societies.

Advocacy is not without opposition. Clients and advocates may find barriers to services, vendors, providers, and resources. A community may experience a shortage in nursing home beds or providers, a childcare facility may experience staffing shortages, a family may not have the money to keep a child at home, and a client may find that the school system cannot fund a full-time nurse for its clinic. The reality of scarce resources creates a difficult barrier for advocates. However, events such as these often stimulate a community's self-determination and lead to innovative actions to correct gaps in service (see the Levels of Prevention box).

Allocation and Advocacy: Complements or Conundrum?

Whereas advocacy holds a traditional role in the nursing profession, **allocation** is a staple of market competition. Nurses perform allocation roles when they triage clients or perform the

📋 LEVELS OF PREVENTION

Case Management

Primary Prevention
Use the information exchange process to increase the client's understanding of how to use the health care system and the health promotion strategies that will maintain health.

Secondary Prevention
Use case finding to identify existing health problems in your caseload and the population served by your agency. Timely, holistic assessments and interventions can slow disease trajectories and promote healing and health.

Tertiary Prevention
Monitor and adjust the use of prescription medications and adherence to treatment to reduce the risk of complications. Use models such as the *CMAG Case Management Adherence Guidelines* at http://www.csma.org to prevent subsequent consequences of issues in medication compliance as part of the treatment plan. Institutionalize this model in your agency.

gatekeeping and rationing functions. The field of medicine has struggled with the allocation debate, as Tauber (2003) notes. Nurses often reflect that clinical judgments are influenced by their values and ethics as well as organizational demands (ANA, 2008). When working in organizations, nurses experience allocation demands at the systems level through budgetary decisions and staffing assignments. At the clinical level, demands relate to implementing treatment protocols. When nurses act as client advocates by clarifying a client's desires or needs, they can conflict with systems procedures for allocation of limited resources within these systems.

Case managers need to balance efficient use of resources by comparing costs of alternative options to care, calculating private and public costs of provider services recommended, and monitoring service expenses over time (Fraser and Strang, 2004).

Nurses who shoulder both advocacy and allocation responsibilities may benefit from a clear understanding of their personal and professional values. A systematic procedure for mediating conflict between the two competing responsibilities is also helpful (Cary, 1998; Fink-Samnick and Muller, 2010).

Conflict Management

Case managers help clients manage conflicting needs and scarce resources. Techniques for managing conflict include a range of active communication skills. These skills are directed toward learning all parties' needs and desires, detecting their areas of agreement and disagreement, determining their abilities to collaborate, and assisting in discovering alternatives and activities for reaching a goal. Mutual benefit with limited loss is a goal of conflict management.

Conflict and its management vary in intensity and energy in a number of ways. The effort needed to manage a conflict depends on different factors: the existing evidence to support facts and the objective and subjective perceptions of the parties involved.

Negotiating is a strategic process used to move conflicting parties toward an outcome. The outcome can vary from one in which one party gains benefit at the other's expense (distributive outcomes). The outcome may be one in which mutual advantages override individual gains (integrative outcomes). Integrative outcomes are usually based on problem-solving and solution-generating techniques (Bazarman, 2005).

The process of negotiating can be characterized in three stages: prenegotiating, negotiating, and aftermath. Prenegotiating activities are designed to have parties agree to collaborate. Parties must see the possibility of agreeing and the costs of not agreeing (Lowrey, 2004). Preparations must be made as to time, place, and ground rules concerning participants, procedures, and confidentiality.

The negotiation stage consists of phases in which parties must develop trust, credibility, distance from the issue (to limit the feeling of "one best way"), and the ability to retain personal dignity. Bazarman (2005) characterizes the phases as follows:

Phase 1: Establishing the issues and agenda. This is accomplished by identifying, clarifying, presenting, and prioritizing the issues.

Phase 2: Advancing demands and uncovering interests. Negotiations center on presenting parties' interests and differentiating parties' demands and positions on the conflict.

Phase 3: Bargaining and discovering new options. Debates include gathering facts based on reasoning that will generate understanding and promote relearning. Bargaining reduces differences on issues by giving or removing rewards or desired objects. Creating new solutions or options through brainstorming, reflective thinking, and problem-purpose-expansion techniques is important in achieving options that provide mutual benefits.

Phase 4: Working out an agreement. This may involve settling on some but not all points. Parties can agree to reexamine the issues later, and steps for implementing and follow-up must be clarified.

The aftermath is the period following an agreement in which parties are experiencing the consequences of their decisions. The reality of their decisions may lead to reevaluating their values. In a conflict situation, parties engage in behaviors that reflect the dimensions of assertiveness and cooperation. **Assertiveness** is the ability to present one's own needs. **Cooperation** is the ability to understand and meet the needs of others. Each person uses a primary and secondary orientation to engage in conflict (Box 22-4).

Clearly, flexibility in conflict management behavior can facilitate an outcome that meets the client's goals. Helping parties navigate the process of attaining a goal requires effective personal relations, knowledge of the situation and alternatives, and a commitment to the process.

Collaboration

In case management, the activities of many disciplines (social workers, nurses, physicians, insurers, physical therapists, etc.) are needed for success. Clients, the family, significant others, payers, and community organizations contribute to achieving the goal. **Collaboration** is achieved through a developmental process. Cary and Androwich (1989) found that collaboration occurs in a sequence and is reciprocal and can be characterized by seven stages and activities (Figure 22-6).

BOX 22-4   CATEGORIES OF BEHAVIORS USED IN CONFLICT MANAGEMENT

- **Accommodating:** Individual neglects personal concerns to satisfy the concerns of another.
- **Avoiding:** Individual pursues neither his or her concerns nor another's concerns.
- **Collaborating:** Individual attempts to work with others toward solutions that satisfy the goals of both parties.
- **Competing:** Individual pursues personal concerns at another's expense.
- **Compromising:** Individual attempts to find a mutually acceptable solution that partially satisfies both parties.

Modified from Volkema RJ, Bergmann TJ: Conflict styles as indicators of behavioral patterns in interpersonal conflicts, *J Social Psychol* 135: 5-15, 2001; CPP: History and validity of the Thomas-Kilmann Conflict Mode Instrument (TKI). Mountainview, CA, CPP, Inc. Available at http://www.cpp.com/products/tki/tki_info.aspx. Retrieved June 14, 2010.

The goal of communication in the collaborative development process is to amplify, clarify, and verify all team members' points of view. Although communication is essential in collaboration, it is not sufficient to result in or maintain collaboration. Although the collaboration model recognizes the contributions of joint decision making, one member of the team should be accountable to the system and to the client. This team member should be responsible for monitoring the entire process.

Case managers encounter conflict on a daily basis. Competing needs, resources, organizational demands, and professional role boundaries present opportunities and pitfalls for conflict management and collaboration (Box 22-5). Barriers to collaborating effectively include time restraints, lack of information, and failure to communicate essential, complete information in a timely manner (Birmingham, 2002). Providers report that in the collaborative role of serving as advocates for clients, they encounter competing expectations by other providers in the system (Corser, 2003).

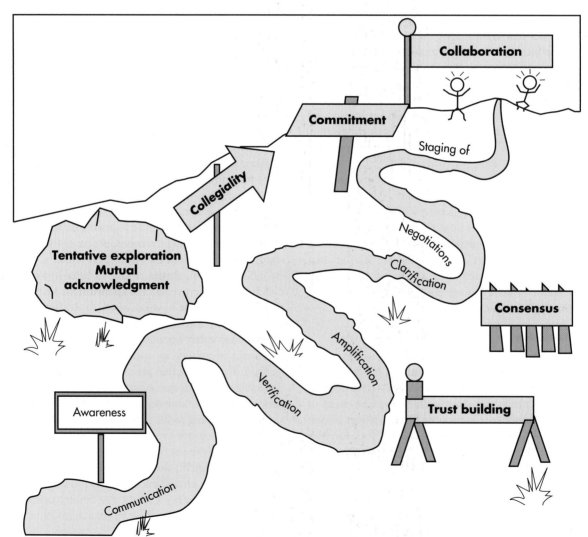

FIGURE 22-6 Collaboration is a sequential yet reciprocal process. (From Cary A, Androwich I: *A collaboration model: a synthesis of literature and a research survey,* paper presented at the Association of Community Health Nurse Educators Spring Institute, Seattle, June 1989.)

BOX 22-5   STAGES OF COLLABORATION

1. Awareness
   * Make a conscious entry into a group process; focus on goals of convening together; generate a definition of collaborative process and what it means to team members.
2. Tentative exploration and mutual acknowledgment
   * Exploration: Disclose professional skills for the desired process; disclose areas where contributions cannot be made; disclose values reflecting priorities; identify roles and disclose personal values, including time, energy, interest, and resources.
   * Mutual acknowledgment: Clarify each member's potential contributions; verify the group's strengths and areas needing consultation; clarify member's work style, organizational supports, and barriers to collaborative efforts.
3. Trust building
   * Determine the degree to which reliance on others can be achieved; examine congruence between words and behaviors; set interdependent goals; develop tolerance for ambiguity.
4. Collegiality
   * Define the relationships of members with each other; define the responsibilities and tasks of each; define entrance and exit conditions.
5. Consensus
   * Determine the issues for which consensus is required; determine the processes used for clarifying and making decisions to reach consensus; determine the process for reevaluating consensus outcomes.
6. Commitment
   * Realize the physical, emotional, and material actions directed toward the goal; clarify procedures for reevaluating commitments in light of goal demands and group standards for deviance.
7. Collaboration
   * Initiate a process of joint decision making reflecting the synergy that results from combining knowledge and skills.

Modified from Cary A, Androwich I: *A collaboration model: a synthesis of literature and a research survey,* paper presented at the Association of Community Health Nurse Educators Spring Institute, Seattle, June 1989; Mueller WJ, Kell B: *Coping with conflict,* Englewood Cliffs, NJ, 1972, Prentice Hall.

Teamwork and collaboration clearly demand knowledge and skills about clients, health status, resources, treatments, and community providers. The ability to assess clients' and families' complex needs involves knowledge of intrapersonal, interpersonal, medical, nursing, and social dimensions. Demonstrating team member and leadership skills in facilitating a goal-directed group process is essential. It is unlikely that any single professional possesses the expertise required in all dimensions. It is likely, however, that the synergy produced by all can result in successful outcomes.

ISSUES IN CASE MANAGEMENT

Legal Issues

Case managers today face pressure to control costs, to use evidence-based guidelines for practice, and to reduce risks for legal liability. They are vulnerable to legal risks because of inadequate preparation, changing legislation and policy, insufficient support, and unclear role expectations (Hendricks and Cesar, 2003). Liability concerns of case managers exist when the following three conditions are met: (1) the provider had a duty to provide reasonable care, (2) a breach of contract occurred through an act or an omission to act, and (3) the act or omission caused injury or damage to the client. Case managers must strive to reduce risks, practice wisely within acceptable practice standards, and limit legal defense costs through professional insurance coverage. Five general areas of risk are reviewed (Hendricks and Cesar, 2003; Cunningham, 2007; Llewellyn and Leonard, 2009):

1. Liability for managing care
   a. Inappropriate design or implementation of the case management system
   b. Failure to obtain all pertinent records on which case management actions are based
   c. Failure to have cases evaluated by appropriately experienced and credentialed clinicians
   d. Failure to confer directly with the treating provider (physician or nurse practitioner) at the onset and throughout the client's care
   e. Substituting a case manager's clinical judgment for that of the medical provider
   f. Requiring the client or his or her provider to accept case management recommendation instead of any other treatment
   g. Harassment of clinicians, clients, and family in seeking information, and setting unreasonable deadlines for decisions or information
   h. Claiming orally or in writing that the case management treatment plan is better than the provider's plan
   i. Restricting access to otherwise necessary or appropriate care because of cost
   j. Referring clients to treatment furnished by providers related to the case management agency without proper disclosure
   k. Connecting case managers' compensation to reduced use and access of services
   l. Inappropriate delegation of care
   m. Inappropriate use of clinical practice guidelines
2. Negligent referrals
   a. Referral to a practitioner known to be incompetent
   b. Substituting inadequate treatment for an adequate but more costly option
   c. Curtailing treatment inappropriately when treatment was actually needed
   d. Referral to a facility or practitioner inappropriate for the client's needs
   e. Transfer to another facility that lacks care requirements
3. Experimental treatment and technology
   a. Failure to apply the contractual definition of "experimental" treatment found in the client's insurance policy

b. Failure to review sources of information referenced in the applicable insurance policy (e.g., Food and Drug Administration, or published medical literature)

c. Failure to review the client's complete medical record

d. Failure to make a timely determination of benefits in light of timeliness of treatment

e. Failure to communicate coverage determined to be needed, to the insured client or participant

f. Improper economic considerations determining the coverage

4. Confidentiality/security

a. Failure to deny access to sensitive information that is awarded special protection by federal or state law

b. Failure to protect access to computerized medical records

c. Failure to adhere to regulatory provisions (e.g., Health Insurance Portability and Accountability Act provisions [http://hipaa.cms.gov]; Americans with Disabilities Act)

5. Fraud and abuse

a. Making false statements of claims or causing incorrect claims to be filed

b. Falsifying the adherance to conditions of participation of Medicare and Medicaid

c. Submitting claims for excessive, unnecessary, or poor-quality services

d. Engaging in remuneration, bribes, kickbacks, or rebates in exchange for referral

e. Upcoding intensity of care or intervention requirements

Legal citations relevant to case management and managed care include negligent referrals, provider liability, payer liability, breach of contract, denial of care, and bad faith. As in any scope of nursing practice, proactive risk management strategies can lower the provider's exposure to legal liability (Hendricks and Cesar, 2003).

Hendricks and Cesar (2003) note that court cases influence the legal considerations of case managers. When courts find that cost considerations affect medical care decisions, all parties to the decision will be liable for resulting damages. Guidelines to reduce risk exposure include the following:

1. Clear documentation of the extent of client participation in decision making and reasons for decisions

2. Records demonstrating accurate and complete information on interactions and outcomes

3. Use of reasonable care in selecting referral sources, which may include verifying of licensure of providers

4. Written agreements when arrangements are made to modify benefits other than those in the contract

5. Good communication with clients

6. Informing clients of their rights of appeal

Ethical Issues

Case managers as nursing professionals are guided in ethical practice by the *Code of Ethics for Nursing* (ANA, 2008) and *Code of Professional Conduct for Case Managers* (CCMC, 2005), by performance indicators for ethics in the *Standards of Practice for Case Management* (CMSA, 2010), and by the contract expressed in *Nursing's Social Policy Statement* (ANA, 2010).

By integrating these guidelines and philosophies, nursing practice is ideally suited to preserve the ethical principles of autonomy, beneficence, fidelity, justice, nonmaleficence, and veracity in case management processes. Hendricks and Cesar (2003), McCollom (2004), Llewellyn and Leonard (2009), and Fink-Samnick and Muller (2010) describe how case managers may confront dilemmas in these areas.

Case management may hamper a client's **autonomy,** or the individual's right to choose a provider, if a particular provider is not approved by the case management system. If a new provider must be found who can be approved for coverage, continuity of care may be disrupted.

Beneficence, or doing good, can be impaired when excessive attention to containing costs supersedes the nurse's duty to improve health or relieve suffering. Fidelity is faithfulness to the obligation of duty to the client by keeping promises and remaining loyal within the nurse–client relationship (Burkhardt and Nathaniel, 2002). Duty to clients to secure benefits on their behalf and to limit unnecessary expenditures can create dilemmas when the goals are not uniform.

Justice as an ethical principle for case managers considers equal distribution of health care with reasonable quality. Tiers of quality and expertise among provider groups can be created when quality providers refuse to accept reimbursement allowances from the managed system, leaving less-experienced or lower-quality providers as the caregiver of choice for clients being managed.

Nonmaleficence is doing no harm. When case managers incorporate outcomes measures, evidence-based practice, and monitoring processes in their plans of care, this principle is addressed.

Veracity, or truth telling, is absolutely necessary to the practice of advocacy and building a trusting relationship with clients. Clients particularly complain that in the changing health care system, payers do not seem to be able to provide comprehensive yet inexpensive options for care.

Three of the most common dilemmas are conflicts in advocacy, priorities, and duties (Hendricks and Cesar, 2003). For example, a case manager may advocate for many perspectives—clients, organizations, and society—that are not harmonious. When considering priorities in values, the case manager will ultimately be considering personal, professional, organizational, and client values. Selecting which values to honor can result in violating the values of the other, and asking the question "Whose best interests can be served?" may create a dilemma. Finally, conflicts in duties can result when placing the best interest of a client first adversely affects the other party.

Standards of practice and care, codes of ethics, licensure laws, credentialing through certification, and organizational policies and procedures (e.g., ethics committees, risk management units) offer the case manager information and support in managing ethical conflicts and dilemmas in the case management system. Maintaining familiarity with ethical issues published in the case management literature can offer specific assistance for practicing case managers (Tables 22-3 and 22-4).

TABLE 22-3 CREDENTIALING RESOURCES FOR CASE MANAGERS (INDIVIDUAL CERTIFICATION OPTIONS)

ORGANIZATION	PHONE NUMBER AND WEBSITE	CREDENTIALS AND INITIALS
American Nurses Credentialing Center	1-800-284-2378 http://www.nursecredentialing.org	Nurses, RN-BC for Case Management
Case Management Administrators	1-781-446-6980 http://www.ptcny.com	CMAC, for Case Management Administrators
Certification of Disability Management Specialist Commission	1-847-944-1335 http://www.cdms.org	Interprofessionals, CDMS for Certified Disability Management Specialist
Commission for Case Manager Certification	1-651-789-3744 http://www.ccmcertification.org	Interprofessionals, CCM for Certified Case Managers
Certification Board for Certified Nurse Life Care Planners	1-212-356-0660 http://www.ptcny.com	CNCLP, Specialty certification for nurses who are life care planners
National Academy of Certified Care Managers	1-800-962-2260 http://www.naccm.net	Interprofessionals, CCM for Certified Care Managers
National Board for Certification in Continuity of Care	1-888-776-2023 http://www.nbccc.net	Interprofessional, A-CCC for Continuity of Care Certification–Advanced Professionals
Rehabilitation Nursing Certification Board	1-800-229-7530 http://www.rehabnurse.org/certification	CRRN for Certified Rehabilitation Registered Nurses

TABLE 22-4 WEBSITES FOR CASE MANAGEMENT RESOURCES

RESOURCE	WEBSITE	DETAILS
AIDS Global Information System	http://www.aegis.com	Contains largest AIDS library
American Accreditation Healthcare Commission (URAC)	http://www.ahip.org	Accredits disease management programs and other services. Supports efforts for clinical benchmarking, quality of care, chronic care evidence-based models.
American Nurses Credentialing Center	http://www.nursecredentialing.org	Offers review course materials for case managers preparing for certification examinations by any certifying body. Certifies Case Managers.
American Medical Association	http://www.ama-assn.org	Includes continuing education unit (CEU) programs
Case Management Society of America	http://www.cmsa.org	Specialty organizations for case managers
Centers for Medicare and Medicaid Services	http://www.cms.hhs.gov	Oversees execution of rules and regulations for clients of state and federally funded services
Center Watch Clinical Trial Listing Service	http://www.centerwatch.com	Global source for clinical trials information
Centers for Disease Control and Prevention	http://www.cdc.gov	Provides education, training, and research for disease, emergency preparedness, environmental health, traveler health, workplace safety and health, population health, and healthy living
The Joint Commission (TJC)	http://www.jointcommission.org	Accredits health care–related delivery organizations
Medscape	http://www.medscape.org	Features clinical updates for professionals
National PACE Association	http://www.npaonline.org	Provides information on models and locations of PACE services for the elderly
National Committee for Quality Assurance	http://www.ncqa.org	Publishes HEDIS performance indicators for provider systems and accredits managed care organizations. Provides certification of Disease Management and Credentialing Verification Organizations (among other organizations).
National Library of Medicine	http://www.nlm.nih.gov	Global medical library
Nurseweek	http://www.nurse.com	Provides information links to other sites
Oncology	http://www.oncolink.upenn.edu	Oncology links
Online Journal of Issues in Nursing	http://www.nursingworld.org	Publication on issues in nursing
Commission on Accreditation of Rehabilitation Facilities	http://www.carf.org	Accredits services globally that may be used by case management clients such as adult day care, assisted living, behavioral health, employment and community services, and medical rehabilitation

CHAPTER REVIEW

PRACTICE APPLICATION

During her regularly scheduled visit to a blood pressure clinic in a local apartment cluster, Mrs. B., 45 years old, complained of feeling dizzy and forgetful. She could not remember which of her six medications she had taken during the last few days. Her blood pressure readings on reclining, sitting, and standing revealed gross elevation. The nurse and Mrs. B. discussed the danger of her present status and the need to seek medical attention. Mrs. B. called her physician from her apartment and agreed to be transported to the emergency department.

In the emergency department, Mrs. B. manifested the progressive signs and symptoms of a cerebrovascular accident (a CVA, or stroke). During hospitalization, she lost her capacity for expressive language and demonstrated hemiparesis and loss of bladder control. Her cognitive function became intermittently confused, and she was slow to recognize her physician and neighbors who came to visit. The utilization review nurse contacted the case manager from the health department to screen and assess for the continuum of care needs as early as possible, because Mrs. B. lived alone and family members resided out of town.

It became apparent that family caregiving in the community could only be intermittent because family members lived too far away. Mrs. B. had residual functional and cognitive deficits that would demand longer-term care.

As the case manager contracted by the plan, place the following actions in the correct sequence to construct a case management plan:
A. Discuss with the family their schedule of availability to offer care in the client's home.
B. Call the client and introduce yourself, as a prelude to working with her.
C. Obtain information on the scope of services covered by the benefit plan for your client.
D. Arrange a skilled nursing facility site visit for the client and family.

Answers can be found on the Evolve site.

KEY POINTS

- An important role of the nurse is that of client advocate.
- The goal of advocacy is to promote the client's self-determination.
- When performing in the advocacy role, conflicts may emerge about the full disclosure of information, territoriality, accountability to multiple parties, legal challenges to clients' decisions, and competition for scarce resources.
- The functions of advocacy and allocation can pose dilemmas in practice.
- Amplification, clarification, and verification are three communication skills necessary in the advocacy process.
- Additional skills important to fulfilling the role of client advocate include the helping relationship, assertiveness, and problem solving.
- Problem solving is a systematic approach that includes understanding the values of each party and generating alternative solutions.
- Brainstorming and the problem-purpose-expansion method are two techniques to enhance the effectiveness of problem-solving skills.
- During conflict, negotiations can move conflicting parties toward an outcome.
- Prenegotiation, negotiation, and aftermath are three phases of managing a conflict.
- Each individual has a predominant orientation when engaging in conflict: competing, accommodating, avoiding, collaborating, or compromising.
- Collaboration may result by moving through seven stages: awareness, tentative exploration and mutual acknowledgment, trust building, collegiality, consensus, commitment, and collaboration.
- Care management is a strategic program to maintain the health of a population enrolled in a delivery system.
- Continuity of care is a goal of nursing practice. It requires making linkages with services and information systems to improve the client's health status.

- As the structure of the health care system moves toward delivering more services in the community, the achievement of continuity of care will present a greater challenge.
- Case management is typically an interprofessional process in which the client is the focus of the plan.
- Documentation of case management activities and outcomes is essential to nursing practice.
- Case management is a systematic process of assessment, planning, service coordination, referral, monitoring, and evaluation that meets the multiple service needs of clients.
- A nurse's scope of practice includes advocacy, allocation, and case management functions.
- Nurses functioning as advocates and case managers need to be aware of the ethical and legal issues confronting these components of their practice.
- Standardization of care for predictable outcomes can be achieved through critical paths, disease management protocols, clinical guidelines, interprofessional action plans, and a caring-based practice in which processes of diagnosis and treatment are applied to the human experiences of health and illness.
- Nurses are guided by a philosophy of caring and advocacy.
- Nurses have a high regard for client self-determination, independence, and informed choice in decision making.
- Recognizing that responses to illness and disability may limit independence and self-determination, nurses focus on the rights of individuals, families, and communities to define their own health and evidence-based guidelines for practice.
- Telehealth application provides expansive alternatives within resource delivery options but must be customized for clients.

CLINICAL DECISION-MAKING ACTIVITIES

1. Observe a typical work day of a nurse working with a population, noting the types of activities that are done in coordination, transition care, case management, and documentation as well as the amount of time spent in these areas. Interview several staff members to determine whether they perceive that their time spent in case management is changing. To what degree are the staff members involved in care management activities? What are the top three legal and ethical issues they encounter in their practice? What do the nurses report as their greatest sources of satisfaction and dissatisfaction in their jobs?

2. Initiating, monitoring, and evaluating resources are essential components of nursing practice. Describe a client situation and the case management process that might occur in the following practices:
   A. A school nurse in an elementary school and one in a high school working with brain-injured students
   B. An occupational health nurse in a hospital and one in a manufacturing plant
   C. A nurse working in a well-child clinic
   D. A case manager employed by a managed care organization
   E. A care manager employed in a health benefits corporation

Explain how the case management processes affected client outcome in each of these situations.

3. The values and beliefs held by a nurse influence the nurse's ability to be an advocate for clients. Analyze your values and beliefs about rationing health care and describe how they may affect your ability to be a client advocate. How did you develop your values and beliefs?

4. Read the following article: Fink-Samnick E, Muller LS: Ethical obligations versus best practice, *Prof Case Manag* 15(3):153-156, 2010. Discuss your reactions to the mini case studies and the statement, *Allocation always works within the mixed interests of the individual and other stakeholders*. What values do you hold and how do they frame your reactions?
   A. What are the mixed values of individuals?
   B. What are the mixed values of other stakeholders (providers, policy makers, insurers)?
   C. What are the mixed values of society in the United States? What are the mixed values of society in underdeveloped nations? How are the mixed values different or similar in these three situations (A-C)? How does your answer affect client outcomes?

REFERENCES

AHRQ Health Care Innovations Exchange: *Nurse-led, telephone-based collaborative care improves mental and physical health of depressed clients after cardiac bypass surgery*, 2010a. Available at http://www.innovations.ahrq.gov. Accessed January 20, 2011.

AHRQ HealthCare Innovations Exchange: *Intensive case management reduces inpatient admissions and emergency department visits among costly, medically complex clients without insurance*, 2010b. Available at http://www.innovations.ahrq.gov. Accessed January 20, 2011.

Allison L: Evidence based practice as a tool for case management, *Case Manager* 15:62–65, 2004.

American Hospital Association: *Glossary of terms and phrases for health care coalitions*, Chicago, 1986, AHA Office of Health Coalitions and Private Sector Initiatives.

American Hospital Association: *Guide to the health care field*, Chicago, 2003-2004, AHA.

American Nurses Association: *Managed care: cornerstone for health care reform—a fact sheet*, Washington, DC, 1993, ANA.

American Nurses Association: *Guide to the code of ethics for nurses*, Silver Spring, MD, 2008, Nursing Books.

American Nurses Association: *Nursing's social policy statement*, ed 3, Silver Spring, MD, 2010, Nursing Books.

American Nurses Foundation: *America's nurses: an untapped natural resource*, Washington, DC, 1993, ANF.

Barefield F: Working case managers' views of the profession, *Case Manager* 14:69–71, 2003.

Bazarman MH, editor: *Negotiating, decision making and conflict management*, Cheltenham, UK, 2005, Edward Elgar Publishing United.

Beyea SC: Patient advocacy—nurses keeping patients safe, *AORN*, May 2005. Available at http://findarticles.com/p/articles/mi_m0FSL/is_5_81/ai_n13793213/. Accessed January 20, 2011.

Birmingham J: Managing the dynamics of collaboration, *Case Manager* 13:73–77, 2002.

Bower KA: *Case management by nurses*, Washington, DC, 1992, American Nurses Association.

Brown SJ: Managing the complexity of best practice health care, *J Nurs Care Qual* 15:1–8, 2001.

Burkhardt MA, Nathaniel AK: *Ethics and issues in contemporary nursing*, ed 2, Clifton Park, NY, 2002, Delmar.

Burns T, Catty J, Dash M, et al: Use of intensive case management to reduce time in hospital in people with severe mental illness: systematic review and meta-regression, *BMJ* 335(7615):336–342, 2007.

Burns T, Fioritti A, Holloway F, et al: Case management and assertive community treatment in Europe, *Psychiatr Serv* 52:631–636, 2001.

Burton J, Murphy E, Riley P: Primary immunodeficiency disease: a model for case management of chronic disease, *Prof Case Manag* 15(11):5–14, 2010.

Cary AH: Advocacy or allocation, *Nurs Connect* 11:1–7, 1998.

Cary A, Androwich I: *A collaboration model: a synthesis of literature and a research survey*, paper presented at the Association of Community Health Nurse Educators Spring Institute, Seattle, June 1989.

Case Management Society of America: *Standards of practice for case management*, Little Rock, AR, 2010, CMSA.

Case Management Society of America: *Case management adherence guidelines*, Little Rock, AR, 2006, CMSA. Available at http://www.cmsa.org/portals/0/pdf/CMAG2.pdf. Accessed January 20, 2011.

Coggeshall Press: *Care for the total population*, Coralville, IA, 2008, author.

Cohen EL, Cesta TG: *Nursing case management*, ed 4, St Louis, 2005, Elsevier.

Commission for Case Management Certification (CCMC): *Code of professional conduct for case managers*, St Paul, MN, 2005, CCMC.

Corser WD: A complex sense of advocacy, *Case Manager* 14:63–69, 2003.

CPP: History and validity of the Thomas-Kilmann Conflict Mode Instrument (TKI). Mountainview, CA, CPP, Inc. Retrieved June 14, 2010 at http://www.cpp.com/products/tki/tki_info.aspx.

Cunningham B: In Powell SK, Tahan HA, editors: *CMSA Core curriculum for case management*, Philadelphia, 2007, Lippincott, Williams & Wilkins.

Demoratz MJ: Incorporating life care planning concepts in case management, *Case Manager* 15:48–50, 2004.

Disease Management Association of America: *The care continuum alliance*, Washington, DC, 2008, DMAA.

Disease Management Association of America: *Organization calls for MLR to recognize population health as aspect of clinical care*, Washington, DC, 2010, DMAA. Available at http://www.dmaa.org/news_releases/2010/pressrelease_043010.asp. Accessed January 15, 2011.

Fink-Samnick E, Muller LS: Case management across the life continuum—ethical obligations versus best practice, *Prof Case Manag* 15(3):153–156, 2010.

Fraser KD, Strang V: Decision-making and nurse case management: a philosophical perspective, *Adv Nurs Sci* 27:32–43, 2004.

Grumbach K, Miller J, Mertz E, Finnochio L: How much public health in public health nursing practice? *Public Health Nurs* 21:266–276, 2004.

Haag AB, Kalina CM: How are community resources used in case management? *AAOHN J* 53:286–287, 2005.

Hagan L, Morin D, Lepine R: Evaluation of telenursing outcomes: satisfaction, self-care practices, and cost savings, *Public Health Nurs* 17:305–313, 2000.

Health Resources and Services Administration, Health Systems and Financing Group: *Medicaid case management services by state*, archived Webcast, 2004. Available at http://www.hrsa.gov/financeMC/webcast-Sept1-Case-Mgmt-by-State-040825.htm.

Hendricks AG, Cesar WJ: How prepared are you? Ethical and legal challenges facing case managers today, *Case Manager* 14:56–62, 2003.

Heslin PA, Moldoveanu M: *What's the "real" problem here? A model of problem formulation,* Conference on Complex Systems and the Management of Organizations. Toronto, Canada, 2002, heslin@cox.smu.edu. Retrieved June 14, 2010.

Hicks LL, Stallmeyer JM, Coleman JR: *The role of the nurse in managed care,* Washington, DC, 1993, American Nurses Publishing.

Huber DL: *Leadership and nursing care management,* ed 4, St Louis, 2010, Elsevier.

Institute of Medicine: *Crossing the quality chasm,* Washington, DC, 2001, National Academy of Science.

Johnson RL, Roter D, Powe NR, et al: Patient race/ethnicity and quality of patient-physician communication during medical visits, *Am J Public Health* 94:2084–2090, 2004.

Katz MH, Cunningham WE, Fleishman JA, et al: The effects of case management on unmet needs and utilization of medical care and medications among HIV-infected persons, *Ann Intern Med* 135:557–565, 2001.

Keller LO, Strohschein S, Lia-Hoagberg B, Schaffer MA: Population-based public health interventions: innovations in practice, teaching and management, Part II, *Public Health Nurs* 21:469–487, 2004.

Kohnke MF: *Advocacy risk and reality,* St Louis, 1982, Mosby.

Kolbasovsky A, Reducing: 30 day inpatient psychiatric recidivism and associated costs through intensive case management, *Prof Case Manag* 14(2):96–105, 2009.

Llewellyn A, Moreo K: *The essence of case management,* Washington, DC, 2001, American Nurses Credentialing Center.

Llewellyn A, Leonard M: *Case management review and resource manual,* ed 3, Silver Spring, MD, 2009, NursingBooks.

Lowrey S: Negotiating for successful outcomes in case management practice, *Case Manager* 15:70–72, 2004.

Mallik M, Rafferty AM: Diffusion of the concept of advocacy, *J Adv Nurs* 32(4):399–404, 2000.

McClatchey S: Disease management as a performance improvement strategy, *Top Health Inform Manag* 22:15–23, 2001.

McClinton DH: Protecting patients, *Contin Care* 17:6, 1998.

McCollom P: Guiding the way: the evolution of life care plans, *Contin Care* 21:26–28, 2002.

McCollom P: Advocate versus abdicate, *Case Manager* 15:43–45, 2004.

McConnell S, Conyea A: Member-centered disease management yields measurable results, *Case Manager* 15:48–51, 2004.

Michaels C, Cohen EL: Two strategies for managing care. In Cohen EL, Cesta TG, editors: *Nursing case management,* ed 4, St Louis, 2005, Elsevier.

Mueller WJ, Kell B: *Coping with conflict,* Englewood Cliffs, NJ, 1972, Prentice Hall.

Mullahy C: *The case manager's handbook,* ed 4, Sudbury, MA, 2010, Jones and Bartlett.

Muller LS, Flarery DL: Defining advanced practice nursing, *Lippincott's Case Manag* 8:230–231, 2003.

National PACE Association: *Who, what & where is PACE?* 2010. Available at http://www.npaonline.org/website/article.asp?id=12. Accessed January 20, 2011.

Nelson ML: Advocacy in nursing, *Nurs Outlook* 36:136–141, 1988.

Owen M: Disease management: breaking down silos to improve chronic care, *Case Manag* 15:45–47, 2004.

Park EJ, Huber DL, Tahan HA: The evidence base for case management practice, *West J Nurs Res* 31:693–714, 2009.

Renholm M, Leino-Kilpi H, Suominen T: Critical pathways: a systematic review, *J Nurs Admin* 32:196–202, 2002.

Schutt RK, Fawcett J, Gall GB, et al: Case manager satisfaction in public health, *Prof Case Manag* 15(3):124–134, 2010.

Secord LJ: *Private case management for older persons and their families,* Excelsior, MN, 1987, Interstudy.

Sidorov J: *Tricare saves taxpayers millions on chronic illness disease management,* Disease Management Care Blog. Available at http:/diseasemanagementcareblog.blogspot.com. Accessed January 15, 2011.

Smith AP: Patient advocacy: roles for nurses and leaders, *Nurs Econ,* March-April, 2004. Available at http:findarticles.com/p/articles/mi_m0FSW/is_2_22/ai_n17206874/?tag=rbxcra.2.a.44. Accessed January 20, 2011.

Stanton MP, Dunkin J: Rural case management: nursing role variations, *Case Manag* 7:48–58, 2002.

Stanton MP, Dunkin J: A review of case management functions related to transitions of care at a rural nurse managed clinic, *Prof Case Manag* 14(6):321–327, 2009.

Tahan HA: Essentials of advocacy in case management, *Lippincott's Case Manag* 10:136–145, 2005.

Tauber AI: A philosophical approach to rationing, *Med J Aust* 178:454–456, 2003.

Taylor P: Comprehensive nursing case management: an advanced practice model, *Nurs Case Manag* 4:2–10, 1999.

The Joint Commission: *2009 National Patient Safety Goals for Ambulatory Care,* Oakbrook Terrace, IL, 2009, TJC.

Tufts Managed Care Institute. Demand management: introduction and references. Available at http://jobfunctions.bnet.com/abstract.aspx?docid=102064. Accessed January 20, 2011.

U.S. Department of Health and Human Services: *Healthy People 2020: a roadmap for health,* Washington, DC, 2010, U.S. Government Printing Office.

U.S. Department of Health and Human Services: *Redefining case management,* Rockville, MD, 2008, USDHHS, HRSA, HIV/AIDS Bureau.

Volkema RJ: *Problem–purpose–expansion: a technique for reformulating problems,* 1983, University of Wisconsin (unpublished manuscript).

Volkema RJ, Bergmann TJ: Conflict styles as indicators of behavioral patterns in interpersonal conflicts, *J Social Psychol* 135:5–15, 2001.

Waitzkin H, Williams RL, Bock JA: Safety net institutions buffer the impact of Medicaid managed care, *Am J Public Health* 92:598–610, 2002.

Weil M, Karls JM: Historical origins and recent developments. In Weils M, et al, editors: *Case management in human service practice,* San Francisco, 1985, Jossey-Bass.

Wilson JF: The crucial link between literacy and health, *Ann Intern Med* 139(10):875–878, 2003.

Wright K, Hazelett S, Jarjoura D, Allen K: The AD-LIFE trial, *Home Healthcare Nurse* 25(5):308–314, 2007.

Zander K, Etheredge ML, Bower KA: *Nursing case management: blueprints for transformation,* Waban, MA, 1987, Winslow Printing Systems.

CHAPTER 23

Public Health Nursing and the Disaster Management Cycle

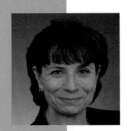

Susan B. Hassmiller, PhD, RN, FAAN

Dr. Susan Hassmiller is the Senior Advisor for Nursing at the Robert Wood Johnson Foundation in Princeton, New Jersey, and Director of the RWJF Initiative on the Future of Nursing, at the Institute of Medicine in Washington, D.C. The Foundation provides support to improve the health and health care for all Americans. Dr. Hassmiller has taught public health nursing at the university level and has dedicated her career to the care and prevention of disease in vulnerable populations. She is a former member of the National Board of Governors for the American Red Cross, having served as the Chair of Chapter and Disaster Services. She is currently on the board of the Central New Jersey Chapter of the American Red Cross. She is a 2002 recipient of both the national American Red Cross Ann Magnussen Award and the regional American Red Cross Clara Barton Award, both recognizing her outstanding leadership in the field of nursing and disaster services. She is the 2009 recipient of the Florence Nightingale Medal of Honor, the highest award in nursing presented by the International Committee of Red Cross in Geneva, Switzerland. She oversees the annual Susan Hassmiller American Red Cross Award, which provides recognition to a Red Cross chapter that has made outstanding contributions in providing disaster health services involving nurses as leaders.

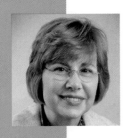

Sharon A. R. Stanley, PhD, RN, RS

Dr. Sharon Stanley is the Chief Nurse of the American Red Cross and the Director of Disaster Health Services and Mental Health. She has worked in the public health field for over 30 years, with experience as a county Health Commissioner and faculty member at private and public institutions. Her past positions in public health preparedness include Director of the Ohio Center for Public Health Preparedness, The Ohio State University, and Chief of Disaster Planning, Ohio Department of Health. Colonel Stanley retired from the U.S. Army Reserve in 2007 with 34 years of service, 12 of them active duty. Her military assignments include a three-state Brigade level command and Army Reserve Leadership Campaign Chief, assigned to the Pentagon. She is the recipient of numerous military awards, including the Order of Medical Military Merit. Dr. Stanley is a member of the Institute of Medicine Forum for Medical and Public Health Preparedness for Catastrophic Events, the Working Panel for Integration of Civilian and Military Domestic Disaster Medical Response, and the Federal Nursing Service Council, which includes the Chief Nurses of the Army, Navy, Air Force, Public Health Service, and Veterans Administration. She is a recent graduate of the Center for Homeland Security and Defense, Naval Postgraduate School, where she completed research in the field of mass fatality management.

ADDITIONAL RESOURCES

⊖volve WEBSITE
http://evolve.elsevier.com/Stanhope
- *Healthy People 2020*
- WebLinks
- Quiz
- Case Studies

- Glossary
- Answers to Practice Application

APPENDIX
- Appendix H: Focus on Quality and Safety Education for Nurses

OBJECTIVES

After reading this chapter, the student should be able to do the following:

1. Discuss types of disasters, including natural and human made.
2. Assess how disasters affect people and their communities.
3. Differentiate disaster management cycle phases to include prevention, preparedness, response, and recovery.
4. Examine the nurse's role in the disaster management cycle.
5. List sources of competencies for public health nursing practice in disaster.
6. Explain how the community and its partners work together to prevent, prepare for, respond to, and recover from disasters.
7. Identify organizations in which nurses can volunteer to work in disasters.

The authors wish to acknowledge the manuscript review and consultation of a review committee, which included Donna Jensen, PhD, RN, Professor Emeritus, Oregon Health and Science University and Disaster Health Services Manager, Oregon Trail Chapter, American Red Cross; Janice Springer, RN, PHN, MA, Nurse Manager and Recruiter for Concordia Language Villages and Disaster Health Services Advisor and State Nurse Liaison for Minnesota, American Red Cross; and Barbara J. Polivka, PhD, RN, Associate Professor, College of Nursing, The Ohio State University.

KEY TERMS

OUTLINE

"Wherever disaster calls there I shall go. I ask not for whom, but only where I am needed."

From the Creed of the Red Cross Nurse by Lona L. Trott, RN, 1953

Around the world, people are experiencing unprecedented disasters from natural causes like hurricanes and earthquakes to human-made disasters such as oil spills and terrorism.

Disasters, whether human-made or natural, are inevitable, but there are ways to help communities prepare for, respond to, and recover from disaster. This chapter describes disaster management approaches including phases of prevention, preparedness, response, and recovery. The public health nurse's role in these phases is described.

DEFINING DISASTERS

A disaster is any natural or human-made incident that causes disruption, destruction, and/or devastation requiring external assistance. Although natural incidents like earthquakes or hurricanes trigger many disasters, predictable and preventable human-made

factors can further affect the disaster. On August 30, 2005, the day after Hurricane Katrina hit New Orleans, a breach in the Lake Pontchartrain levees created a disaster within a disaster as 75% of the city filled with up to 20 feet of water (Reagan, 2005). The flooding of New Orleans has been called the largest civil engineering disaster in the history of the United States (Marshall, 2005). Box 23-1 lists examples of natural and human-made disasters.

From a health care standpoint, the disaster event type and timing predict subsequent injuries and illnesses. If there is prior warning (e.g., in hurricanes or slow-rising floods), the impact brings fewer injuries and deaths. Disasters with little or no advance notice such as terrorism events will often have more casualties because those affected have little time to make evacuation preparations. Disasters with warnings also carry their own dangers, because individuals can be injured attempting to prepare for the disaster or while evacuating. Public health disasters create pressing needs across a widespread region. In a pandemic, pressing and competing health needs occur within a close timeframe, producing a public health surge. In the recovery disaster phase, the immediate threat shifts to adjusting to a new normal in the affected community or region.

DISASTER FACTS

Disasters can affect one family at a time, as in a house fire, or they can kill thousands and result in economic losses in the millions, as with floods, earthquakes, tornadoes, hurricanes, tsunamis, and bioterrorism. The American Red Cross reports that

it responds to a disaster in the United States every 8 minutes, resulting in response to over 70,000 incidents each year (American Red Cross, 2009).

The number of reported natural and human-made disasters continues to rise worldwide. Although the number of lives lost declined over the past 20 years—800,000 people died from natural disasters in the 1990s, compared with 2 million in the 1970s—the number of people affected increased. In one decade, the number affected tripled to 2 billion (UN Office for the Coordination of Humanitarian Affairs, 2005). The increase in the number of lives saved may be explained by better forecasting and early warning systems (International Federation of Red Cross and Red Crescent Societies, 2009). Within a 1-week period in the fall of 2009, three disasters—a tsunami in the Samoa Islands, an earthquake in Indonesia, and a typhoon in the Philippines and Vietnam—collectively left over 1000 dead, hundreds of thousands homeless, and caused millions of dollars in damages (Thomson Reuters Foundation, 2009). Two disasters in 2008 accounted for 93% of all people dead or missing in disasters: Cyclone Nargis in Myanmar and the Sichuan earthquake in China took over 225,000 lives (International Federation of Red Cross and Red Crescent Societies, 2009). The Centers for Disease Control and Prevention (CDC) estimates that between 41 million and 84 million cases of H1N1 occurred between April 2009 and January 16, 2010 in the United States, with 17,000 deaths, 1800 of them children (Fox, 2010). The 2010 Haiti earthquake (Figure 23-1) claimed an estimated 230,000 lives, left 1.5 million Haitians homeless, and destroyed the nation's capital (American Red Cross, 2010d).

Disaster disproportionably strikes at-risk individuals, whether their day-to-day risk is physical, emotional, or economic. Disasters can also wipe out decades of progress in a matter of hours, in a manner that rarely happens in more developed countries. The poor, elderly, women, and children in developing communities are excessively affected and least able to rebound (Duque, 2005). Unfortunately by 2050, the percentages of

BOX 23-1   TYPES OF DISASTERS

Natural

- Hurricanes
- Tornadoes
- Hailstorms
- Cyclones
- Blizzards
- Drought
- Floods
- Mudslides

- Avalanches
- Earthquakes
- Volcanic eruptions
- Pandemics and epidemics
- Lightning-induced forest fires
- Tsunamis
- Thunderstorms and lightning
- Extreme heat and cold

Human-Made

- Conventional warfare
- Unconventional warfare (e.g., nuclear, chemical)
- Transportation accidents
- Structural collapse
- Explosions/bombing
- Fires
- Hazardous materials incident
- Pollution

- Civil unrest (e.g., riots)
- Terrorism (chemical, biological, radiological, nuclear, explosives)
- Cyber attacks
- Airplane crash
- Radiological incident
- Nuclear power plant incident
- Critical infrastructure failure
- Water supply contamination

From U.S. Department of Health and Human Services: *Healthy People 2020: a roadmap to improve all Americans health*, Washington, DC, 2010, USDHHS.

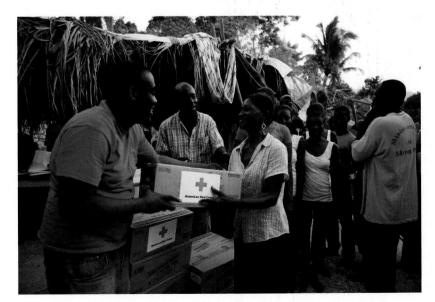

FIGURE 23-1 In the immediate aftermath of the 2010 Haiti earthquake, the American Red Cross provided thousands of Haitians with emergency supplies, food, and shelter. (Courtesy of The American Red Cross Disaster Online Newsroom, Washington, DC. Available at http://newsroom.redcross.org. Accessed August 1, 2010.)

TABLE 23-1	TOTAL AMOUNT OF DISASTER ESTIMATED DAMAGE, BY CONTINENT AND BY YEAR (2000-2009) IN MILLIONS OF U.S. DOLLARS (2009 PRICES)										
	2009	**2000**	**2001**	**2002**	**2003**	**2004**	**2005**	**2006**	**2007**	**2008**	**TOTAL**
Africa	173	1,243	805	436	6,455	1,908	38	244	782	863	12,947
Americas	13,337	6,800	15,946	15,386	25,085	74,679	189,370	7,226	16,625	64,162	428,616
Asia	15,449	27,108	15,687	15,855	27,630	75,332	30,494	24,873	35,747	117,927	386,102
Europe	10,789	22,176	2,395	40,283	21,415	2,072	17,261	2,584	22,796	4,644	146,414
Oceania	1,726	668	696	2,601	691	627	241	1,368	1,488	2,506	12,612
Very high development	24,655	39,272	16,087	60,332	50,959	122,083	192,144	11,694	46,461	64,178	627,865
High human development	2,412	2,259	3,952	3,328	2,907	7,058	14,607	2,041	11,564	6,360	56,488
Medium human development	14,234	8,370	15,421	10,842	27,178	24,878	30,641	22,557	18,922	119,537	292,579
Low human development	173	8,094	69	60	233	600	12	3	489	27	9,760
Total	41,474	57,995	35,528	74,561	81,277	154,619	237,404	36,295	77,436	190,102	986,691

From International Federation of Red Cross and Red Crescent Societies: *World disasters report 2010: Focus on urban risk*, Geneva, Switzerland, 2010, ATAR Roto Presse, p 167.

n.a., no data available. For more information, see section on caveats in introductory text.

Damage assessment is often unreliable. Even for existing data, the methodologies are not standardized and the financial coverage can vary significantly. Depending on where the disaster occurred and who reports it, estimations may vary from zero to billions of U.S. dollars. The total amount of damage reported in 2009 is the third lowest of the decade.

population areas more vulnerable to disasters will increase. Eighty percent of the world's population will live in developing countries, while 46% will live in tornado and earthquake zones, near rivers, and on coastlines (United Nations Development Programme, 2001; NASA, 2005).

The monetary cost of disaster recovery efforts also rose sharply. The cost in more developed countries is higher because of the extent of material possessions and complex infrastructure, including technology. In the United States, increases in population and development in areas vulnerable to natural disasters, especially coastal areas, have led to major increases in insurance payouts (see Table 23-1).

HOMELAND SECURITY: A HEALTH-FOCUSED OVERVIEW

There is a concerted national effort to provide guidance to state and local planning regions to assist with the coordinated and successful responses and recovery efforts in all-hazard disasters and catastrophes. Many documents have been written at the national level, some of which will be reviewed in this overview and chapter.

The reader may ask: "Isn't this all beyond what an individual nurse should have to know?" Actually, it matters greatly how the nation dials 911, and it matters to individuals as well as communities, regions, and the country as a whole. It also matters globally, beyond our own borders. Our national response is not just about the United States, but our international ability to assist other nations in their times of need.

As the single largest profession within the health care network, nurses must understand the national disaster management cycle. Without nursing integration at every phase,

communities and clients lose a critical part of the prevention network, and the multidisciplinary response team loses a first-rate partner.

The U.S. Department of Homeland Security was created through the Homeland Security Act of 2002 (DHS, 2008b), consolidating more than 20 separate agencies into one unified organization.

Homeland Security Presidential Directive-8 (HSPD-8) was issued in December of 2003. It established national policies to strengthen the preparedness of the United States to prevent, protect against, respond to, and recover from threatened or actual terrorist attacks and major disasters, and it included a goal for national preparedness (DHS, 2008c). The national preparedness goal resulted in the National Preparedness Guidelines (NPG) and The National Response Plan (NRP), a national doctrine for preparedness to include Emergency Support Function (ESF) 8: Public Health and Medical (DHS, 2008a). ESF 8 provides coordinated federal assistance to supplement state, local, and tribal resources in response to public health and medical care needs. The 2004 NRP, an all-discipline, all-hazards comprehensive framework for managing domestic incidents, was updated to the National Response Framework (NRF) in January 2008. The NRF remains a guide for conducting a nationwide all-hazards response, "built upon scalable, flexible, and adaptable coordinating structures to align key roles and responsibilities across the Nation, linking all levels of government, nongovernmental organizations, and the private sector" (DHS, 2008d, p i).

Homeland Security Presidential Directive-5 (HSPD-5) directed the Secretary of Homeland Security to develop and administer the National Incident Management System (NIMS), a unified, all-discipline, and all-hazards approach to domestic incident management (DHS, 2008c). The NIMS was established to provide a common language and structure enabling all those involved in disaster response the ability to communicate together more effectively and efficiently.

Two national preparedness documents specifically guide disaster health preparedness, response, and recovery: HSPD 21: Public Health and Medical Preparedness and the National Health Security Strategy (NHSS). HSPD 21 established a national strategy that enables a level of public health and medical preparedness sufficient to address a range of possible disasters. It does so through four critical components of public health and medical preparedness: (1) biosurveillance, (2) countermeasure distribution, (3) mass casualty care, and (4) community resilience (DHS, 2008c). The NHSS focuses specifically on the national goals for protecting people's health in the case of disaster in any setting. National health security is achieved when "the Nation and its people are prepared for, protected from, respond effectively to, and able to recover from incidents with potentially negative health consequences" (USD-HHS, 2009, p 2). The NHSS was directed by the Pandemic and All-Hazards Preparedness Act (PAHPA), which was enacted in 2006 to improve the nation's ability to detect, prepare for, and respond to a variety of public health emergencies (Hodge, Gostin, and Vernick, 2007).

In discussing community resiliency and impact of health care reform on public health preparedness, Vinter, Lieberman, and Levi (2010) state: "Comprehensive health reform presents a rare opportunity to further strengthen our nation. However, even with health reform, there are still major gaps in our public health preparedness. Addressing these underlying weaknesses in our health system will not be easy or cheap, but failure to address these concerns could prove extremely costly" (p 340).

It should be apparent by this point that our national system of homeland security includes public health preparedness and response as a core part of its national strategies. Some of the strategy documents introduced in this section are covered in greater detail throughout the chapter. Every aspect of disaster management involves public health nursing.

HEALTHY PEOPLE 2020 OBJECTIVES

Because disaster affects the health of people in many ways, disaster incidents have an effect on almost every *Healthy People 2020* objective. For example, although Access to Health Services and Public Health Infrastructure comprise two important *Healthy People 2020* topic areas with subsequent objectives, they become even more significant when individual and community needs escalate in disaster (USDHHS, 2010). Disasters also play a direct role in the objectives related to environmental health, food safety, immunization and infectious disease, and mental health and mental disorders. Public health professionals, such as those who work at the CDC, study the effect that disasters have on population health and continuously develop new prevention strategies. Other organizations, such as the American Psychological Association and the American Red Cross, work with communities in the preparedness, response, and recovery phases of a disaster and to revise and align the *Healthy People 2020* objectives related to mental health.

♥ HEALTHY PEOPLE 2020

Examples of Objectives Related to Disaster Mitigation

- EH-21: Improve the utility, awareness, and use of existing information systems for environmental health.
- FS-1: Reduce infections caused by key pathogens transmitted commonly through food.
- HC/HIT-12: Increase the proportion of crisis and emergency risk messages, intended to protect the public's health, that demonstrate the use of best practices.
- IID-12: Increase the percentage of children and adults who are vaccinated annually against seasonal influenza.
- IID-13: Increase the percentage of adults who are vaccinated against pneumococcal disease.

From Department of Health and Human Services (DHHS): *Healthy people 2020.* Available at http://www.healthypeople.gov/2020/default. asp. Accessed February 3, 2011.

THE DISASTER MANAGEMENT CYCLE AND NURSING ROLE

Disaster management includes four stages: prevention (or mitigation), preparedness, response, and recovery. Figure 23-2 shows the disaster emergency management cycle. Nurses have unique skills for all aspects of disaster to include assessment, priority setting, collaboration, and addressing of both preventive and acute care needs. In addition, public health nurses have a skill set that serves their community well in disaster to include health education and disease screening, mass clinic expertise, an ability to provide essential public health services, community resource referral and liaison work, population advocacy, psychological first aid, public health triage, and rapid needs assessment. Nurses have been serving in disasters for more than a century, and to this day, provide a significant resource to both the employee and the volunteer disaster management workforce, unmatched by any other profession.

The World Association for Disaster and Emergency Medicine (WADEM) includes a nursing section. The Nursing Section of WADEM serves to welcome and represent nurses from all countries with an intent and desire to strengthen and improve the practice and knowledge of disaster nursing. The Nursing Section purposes are as follows (WADEM, 2010):

- Define nursing issues for public health care and disaster health care
- Exchange scientific and professional information relevant to the practice of disaster nursing
- Encourage collaborative efforts enhancing and expanding the field of nursing disaster research
- Encourage collaboration with other nursing organizations
- Inform and advise WADEM of matters related to disaster nursing

WADEM sponsored a text entitled *International Disaster Nursing* that was edited in 2010 by Robert Powers and Elaine Daily and is available from Cambridge University Press.

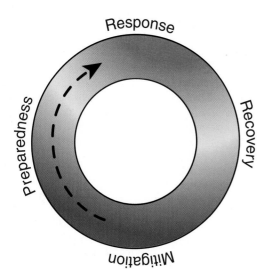

FIGURE 23-2 Disaster management cycle.

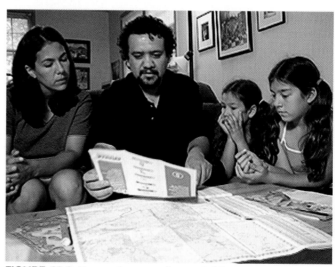

FIGURE 23-3 Personal preparedness. Public health nurses need to develop their own disaster plan as a part of their community disaster activities. (Courtesy of the Wichita Falls Health District, Texas. Available at www.cwftx.net/index.aspx?nid=1301. Accessed August 1, 2010.)

Prevention (Mitigation)

All-hazards mitigation (prevention) is an emergency management term for reducing risks to people and property from natural hazards before they occur. Prevention can include structural measures, such as protecting buildings and infrastructure from the forces of wind and water, and non-structural measures, such as land development restrictions. These primary prevention measures implemented at the local government level achieve effectiveness, in an all-hazards approach to threats. Of course, prevention also includes human-made hazards and the ability to deter potential terrorists, detect terrorists before they strike, and take decisive action to eliminate the threat (DHS, 2007b). Prevention activities may include heightened inspections; improved surveillance and security operations; public health and agricultural surveillance; and testing, immunizations, isolation, or quarantine and halting of CBRNE threats: chemical, biological, radiological, nuclear, and explosive (DHS, 2007b).

Within the community, the nurse may be involved in many roles in prevention of disaster. As community advocates, nurses partner for environmental health by identifying environmental hazards and serving on the public health team for mitigation purposes. Public health nurses in particular will be involved with organizing and participating in mass prophylaxis and vaccination campaigns to prevent, treat, or contain a disease. The nurse should be familiar with the region's local cache of pharmaceuticals and how the Strategic National Stockpile (SNS) (described later in the chapter) will be distributed. Once federal and local authorities agree that the SNS is needed, medicine delivery to any state in the United States occurs within 12 hours (CDC, 2009b). Then state and local emergency planners ensure Points of Dispensing (POD), to provide prophylaxis to the entire population within 48 hours (CDC, 2007).

In terms of human-made disaster prevention, the nurse should be aware of high-risk targets and current vulnerabilities and what can be done to eliminate or mitigate the vulnerability. Targets may include military and civilian government facilities, health care facilities, international airports and other transportation systems, large cities, and high-profile landmarks. Terrorists might also target large public gatherings, water and food supplies, banking and finance, information technology, postal and shipping services, utilities, and corporate centers.

Preparedness

Role of the Public Health Nurse in Personal and Professional Preparedness

Public health nurses play a key role in community preparedness, but they must accomplish the critical elements of personal and professional preparedness first.

Personal Preparedness

Disasters by their nature require nurses to respond quickly. Public health nurses without plans in place to address their own needs, to include family and pets, will be unable to fully participate in their disaster obligations at work or in volunteer efforts (Figure 23-3). Many first responders left their jobs to care for their homes and their families when Hurricane Katrina occurred. In addition, the nurse assisting in disaster relief efforts must be as healthy as possible, both physically and mentally. A disaster worker who does not practice self-health is of little service to their family, clients, and community (see the How To box titled Be Red Cross Ready). Disaster kits should be made for the home, workplace, and car. The Nursing Tip lists emergency supplies specific to nursing that should be prepared and stored in a sturdy, easy-to-carry container. Important documents should always be in waterproof containers. Nurses should consider several contingencies for children and older adults with a plan to seek help from neighbors in the event of being called to a disaster. Many public shelters do not allow pets inside and other arrangements must be made. Currently, local emergency management agencies include pet management in the local disaster plans (FEMA, 2009d). During Hurricane

Katrina, in Hattiesburg, MS, 2385 pets were rescued and subsequently sheltered (Reagan, 2005).

HOW TO Be Red Cross Ready

1. Get a Kit

Consider the following when assembling or restocking your kit to ensure that you and your family are prepared for any disaster:

- *Store at least 3 days of food, water, and supplies in your family's easy-to-carry preparedness kit. Keep extra supplies on hand at home in case you cannot leave the affected area.*
- *Keep your kit where it is easily accessible.*
- *Remember to check your kit every 6 months and replace expired or outdated items.*

2. Make a Plan

When preparing for a disaster, always:

- *Talk with your family.*
- *Plan.*
- *Learn how and when to turn off utilities and how to use life-saving tools such as fire extinguishers.*
- *Tell everyone where emergency information and supplies are stored. Provide copies of the family's preparedness plan to each member of the family. Always ensure that information is up-to-date and practice evacuations, following the routes outlined in your plan. Don't forget to identify alternative routes.*
- *Include pets in your evacuation plans.*

3. Get Informed

There are three key parts to becoming informed:

- *Get Info: Learn the ways you would get information during a disaster or an emergency.*
- *Know Your Region: Learn about the disasters that may occur in your area.*
- *Action Steps: Learn First Aid from your local Red Cross chapter.*

Courtesy of the American National Red Cross. All rights reserved.

NURSING TIP *Emergency Supplies That Nurses Should Have Ready*

- *Identification badge and driver's license*
- *Proof of licensure and certification (e.g., RN, CPR/AED, First Aid)*
- *Pocket-size reference books (e.g., nursing protocols and intervention standards)*
- *Blood pressure cuff (adult and child) and stethoscope*
- *Gloves, mask, other personal protective equipment (PPE) for general care*
- *First aid kit with mouth-to-mouth CPR barrier*
- *Radio with batteries and cell phone charger*
- *Cash, credit card*
- *Important papers*
- *Sun protection*
- *Sturdy shoes with socks*
- *Medical identification of allergies, blood type*
- *Medications for self*
- *Weather-appropriate clothing to include rain gear*
- *Toiletries*
- *Watch, cell phone, PDA with pre-entered emergency numbers*
- *Flashlight, extra batteries*
- *Record-keeping materials to include pencil/pen*
- *Map of area*

One way a nurse can feel assured about family member protection is by working with them to develop the skills and knowledge necessary for coping in disaster. For example, long-term benefits will occur by involving children and adolescents in activities such as writing preparedness plans, exercising the plan, preparing disaster kits, becoming familiar with their school emergency procedures and family reunification sites, and learning about the range of potential hazards in their vicinity to include evacuation routes. This strategy also offers children and adolescents an opportunity to express their feelings.

THE CUTTING EDGE *Federal Medical Stations*

State and local health resources can quickly become overwhelmed in the event of a disaster. The CDC's Division of Strategic National Stockpile (DSNS) can assist these communities by deploying Federal Medical Stations (FMSs). An FMS is a cache of medical supplies and equipment that can be used to set up a temporary non-acute medical care facility. Each FMS has beds, supplies, and medicine to treat 250 people for up to 3 days. The local community is expected to provide some operational support. A 250-bed FMS set consists of three modules: (1) Base Support: Administrative, food service, housekeeping, basic medical supplies, and personal protective equipment. There are five bed units, with 50 beds each. (2) Treatment: Medical/surgical items. (3) Pharmacy: Medications up to an additional 85 beds. The FMS debuted internationally to support the USNS Comfort in the 2010 Haiti earthquake.

From Centers for Disease Control and Prevention: Federal medical station profile, Atlanta, 2009, Division of Strategic National Stockpile. Available at http://www.texasjrac.org/documents/FMSfactsheetv3-1.pdf. Accessed February 6, 2010.

Professional Preparedness

Every state needs a qualified workforce of public health nurses for solutions for today's public health problems to include natural disasters and the threat of terrorism. Public health nurses, in turn, need "dedicated, resourceful, and visionary leaders" (ASTDN, 2008, p 4). Chief public health nurse officers at the state level develop and maintain a strong public health nursing workforce (ASTDN, 2008). Disaster management in the community is about population health: The core public health functions of *assessment, policy development, and assurance* hold as true in disaster as in day-to-day operations. Operating in the chaos of disaster surge, however, demands a flexible and proficient practice base in each of the core functions and 10 essential services.

Just like the mission of public health and its core functions and essential services does not change in disaster, neither does the practice of public health nursing. The public health nurse must be prepared to advocate for the community in terms of a focus on population-based practice. The number of public health nurses available to get the job done is small compared with those with generic or other specialty nurse preparation. Also, disaster produces conditions that demand an aggregate care approach, increasing the need for public health nursing involvement in community service during disaster and catastrophe.

The Public Health Nursing Intervention Wheel (Figure 23-4) is explained in detail in Chapter 9 and is a population-based practice model that encompasses three levels of practice (community, systems, and individual/family) and 16 public health interventions. Each intervention and practice level contributes to improving population health, providing a practice foundation. This Wheel holds true to public health nursing interventions whether the nurse is working in day-to-day or in disaster operations.

Disaster response teams need nurses with disaster and emergency management training, especially those who have served previously in disaster. Although the majority of disaster work is not high tech, the knowledge one needs for CBRNE disasters must be developed to include access to a ready cache of information related to nursing care. The following sites provide useful information:

- CDC: Emergency preparedness and response A to Z index (http://www.bt.cdc.gov/agent)
- National Library of Medicine: Disaster information management research center (http://disaster.nlm.nih.gov/)
- Unbound Medicine: Relief Central (http://relief.unbound medicine.com/relief/ub/)
- National Library of Medicine: WISER-Wireless information system for emergency responders (http://wiser.nlm.nih.gov/) (See Box 23-2 for further information.)

Depending on the job and possible volunteer assignments, it is also expected that nurses know how to use personal protective equipment (PPE), operate specialized equipment needed to perform specific activities, and safely perform duties in disaster environments.

Professional preparedness also requires that nurses become aware of and understand the disaster plans at their workplace

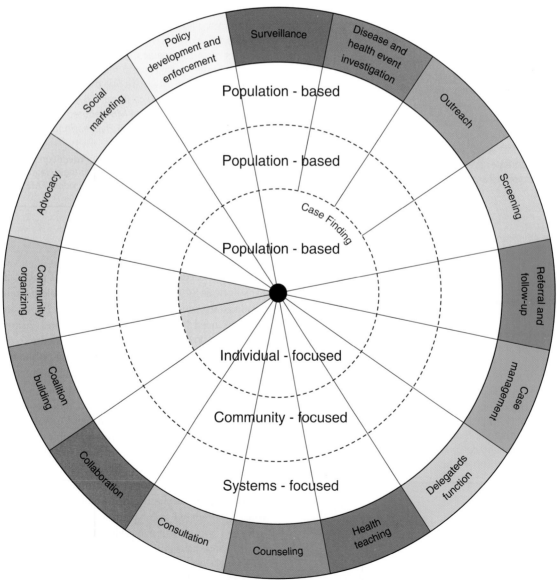

FIGURE 23-4 Public Health Nursing Intervention Wheel. Sixteen public health nursing interventions that work in daily operations or disaster. (Courtesy of Minnesota Department of Health, St. Paul, MN. Available at http://www.health.state.mn.us/divs/cfh/ophp/resources/docs/wheelbook2006.pdf. Accessed August 1, 2010.)

and community. Nurses need to review the disaster history of the community, including how past disasters have affected the community's health care delivery system. Since September 11, 2001, there has been a national emphasis for emergency responding entities to further develop their disaster preparedness and response skills. It is important for nurses to understand and gain the competencies needed to respond in times of disasters *before* disaster strikes.

Box 23-3 shows bioterrorism and emergency readiness competencies for those working in public health. Specific disaster competencies for public health nursing practice have been proposed in a set of 25 competencies categorized into preparedness, response, and recovery (Polivka et al, 2008). The preparedness competencies focus on personal preparedness and on comprehending disaster preparedness terms, concepts, and roles. The competencies also focus on becoming familiar with the health department's disaster plan and its communication equipment suitable for disaster situations, as well as on the role of the PHN in a surge event. Response phase competencies include conducting a rapid needs assessment, outbreak investigation and surveillance, public health triage, risk communication, and technical skills such as mass dispensing. Recovery competencies include participating in after-action processes, contributing to disaster plan modifications, and coordinating efforts to address the psychosocial and public health impact of the event. See Box 23-4 for additional education and training opportunities.

Nurses who seek increased participation or who seek an in-depth understanding of disaster management can become involved in any number of community organizations. The **National Disaster Medical System (NDMS)** provides nurses the

---

BOX 23-2 NURSES AND TECHNOLOGY

Hazardous Material Information Delivered via Wireless

WISER (Wireless Intervention System for Emergency Responders) is a system designed to assist first responders in hazardous material incidents. By inputting a substance's physical properties and entering an individual's symptoms, WISER can help narrow the range of substances that may be involved. It provides detailed information about hazardous substances, health effects, treatment, personal protective equipment, toxicity, the emergency resources available, and the surrounding environmental conditions. As of August 2009, WebWISER, a web browser, could be used to access the same functionality of the stand-alone applications when the Internet is available. WebWISER supports both PC- and PDA-based browsers, including BlackBerry and iPhone.

From National Library of Medicine: *WISER*, Bethesda, MD, 2005. Available at http://wiser.nlm.nih.gov/. Accessed February 6, 2010.

BOX 23-3 BIOTERRORISM AND EMERGENCY READINESS—COMPETENCIES FOR ALL PUBLIC HEALTH WORKERS

CORE COMPETENCY 1. Describe the public heath role in emergency response in a range of emergencies that might arise (e.g., "This department provides surveillance, investigation and public information in disease outbreaks and collaborates with other agencies in biological, environmental, and weather emergencies").

CORE COMPETENCY 2. Describe the chain of command in emergency response.

CORE COMPETENCY 3. Identify and locate the agency emergency response plan (or the pertinent portion of the plan).

CORE COMPETENCY 4. Describe functional role(s) in emergency response and demonstrate role(s) in regular drills.

CORE COMPETENCY 5. Demonstrate correct use of all communication equipment used for emergency communication (phone, fax, radio, etc.).

CORE COMPETENCY 6. Describe communication role(s) in emergency response:
- Within the agency using established communication systems
- With the media
- With the general public
- Personal (with family, neighbors)

CORE COMPETENCY 7. Identify limits to own knowledge/skill/authority and identify key system resources for referring matters that exceed these limits.

CORE COMPETENCY 8. Recognize unusual events that might indicate an emergency and describe appropriate action (e.g., communicate clearly within the chain of command).

CORE COMPETENCY 9. Apply creative problem solving and flexible thinking to unusual challenges within his or her functional responsibilities and evaluate effectiveness of all actions taken.

From Centers for Disease Control and Prevention: *Bioterrorism and emergency readiness: Competencies for all public health workers*, Atlanta, 2002. Available at http://www.nursing.columbia.edu/chp/pdfArchive/btcomps.pdf. Accessed February 6, 2010.

BOX 23-4 WEBSITES PROVIDING EDUCATION AND TRAINING OPPORTUNITIES

Public Health Workforce Development Centers
- Centers for Disease Control and Prevention: http://www.bt.cdc.gov/training/
- National Public Health Training Centers Network, ASPH: http://www.asph.org/phtc/search-new.cfm
- Public Health Training Centers, CDC: http://www.cdc.gov/phtrain/

Government Training Facilities and Others
- National Nurse Emergency Preparedness Initiative: http://www.nnepi.org/
- Emergency Management Institute: http://training.fema.gov/
- Federal Emergency Management Agency (FEMA) Training: http://www.fema.gov/prepared/train.shtm

Public Health Organizations
- American Nurses Association (ANA): http://www.ana.org
- American Public Health Association (APHA): http://www.apha.org
- Association of Schools of Public Health (ASPH): http://www.asph.org
- Association of State and Territorial Directors of Nursing (ASTDN): http://www.astdn.org
- National Association of County and City Health Offices (NACCHO): http://www.naccho.org
- Public Health Foundation (PHF): http://www.phf.org

BOX 23-5   VOLUNTEER OPPORTUNITIES IN DISASTER WORK

- American Red Cross (ARC): http://www.redcross.org
- Buddhist Compassion Relief (Tzu Chi): http://www.tzuchi.org/
- Certified Emergency Response Team (CERT): https://www.citizencorps.gov/cert/
- Citizen Corps: http://www.citizencorps.gov/
- Disaster Medical Assistance Team (DMAT): http://www.dmat.org/
- Medical Reserve Corps (MRC): http://www.medicalreservecorps.gov/HomePage
- National Baptists Convention, USA, Inc.: http://www.nationalbaptist.com/index.cfm?FuseAction=Page&PageID=1000000
- National Voluntary Organizations Active in Disaster (NVOAD): http://www.nvoad.org
- The Salvation Army: http://www.salvationarmyusa.org/usn/www_usn_2.nsf

opportunity to work on specialized teams such as the Disaster Medical Assistance Team (DMAT). The Medical Reserve Corps (MRC) and the Community Emergency Response Team (CERT) provide opportunities for nurses to support emergency preparedness and response in their local jurisdictions. The American Red Cross offers training in disaster health services and disaster mental health for both response in local jurisdictions and national deployment opportunities. After participation in disaster training, nurses can take the following steps: join a local disaster action team (DAT); act as a liaison with local hospitals; determine health-services support for shelter sites; plan on a multidisciplinary team for optimal client service delivery; address the logistics of health and medical supplies; and teach disaster nursing in the community. A list of opportunities is shown in Box 23-5.

The importance of being adequately trained and properly associated with an official response organization to serve in a disaster cannot be overstated. In a disaster, many untrained and ill-equipped individuals rush in to help. Spontaneous volunteer overload creates added burden on an already tense situation to include role conflict, anger, frustration, and helplessness. The World Trade Center attacks of September 11, 2001 brought many qualified but unassociated responders to the site. "Many well-intentioned local physicians in shirt sleeves and light footwear proceeded to the area and attempted to find victims, risking further injuries to themselves and getting in the way of structured rescue protocols....prohibited from participating in rescue operations within any area designated as a disaster by the Fire Department of New York" (Crippen, 2002). After the bombing of the Alfred P. Murrah building in Oklahoma City in 1995, a nurse who rushed into the building to rescue people became the only fatality who was not killed or injured in the initial blast and collapse (Devlen, 2007).

WHAT DO YOU THINK? *Trust for America's Health (TFAH): Bioterrorism and Public Health Preparedness.*

Health emergencies pose some of the greatest threats to our nation, because they can be difficult to prepare for, detect, and contain. Important progress has been made to improve emergency preparedness since September 11, 2001, the subsequent anthrax attack, and Hurricane Katrina—three events that put severe stress on our public health system. However, major problems still remain in our readiness to respond to large-scale emergencies and natural disasters. The country is still insufficiently prepared to protect people from disease outbreaks, natural disasters, or acts of bioterrorism, leaving Americans unnecessarily vulnerable to these threats.

TFAH publishes an annual report on public health preparedness titled "Ready or Not? Protecting the Public's Health from Diseases, Disasters and Bioterrorism," which examines America's ability to respond to health threats and help identify areas of vulnerability. TFAH also offers a series of recommendations to further strengthen America's emergency preparedness.

What do you think of them, and how would you apply them to the role of the public health nurse?

From Trust for America's Health: TFAH initiatives—Bioterrorism and public health preparedness, 2010. Available at http://healthyamericans.org/bioterrorism-and-public-health-preparedness/. Accessed February 7, 2010.

Community Preparedness

The Public Health Security and Bioterrorism Preparedness and Response Act of 2002 addressed the need to enhance public health and health care readiness and community health care infrastructures. It reaffirmed the public health department role on the front line of disaster prevention, preparedness, response, and recovery, to include a national need for "...emergency-ready public health and healthcare services in every community" (Office of Legislative Policy and Analysis, 2010). Public health departments throughout the country have been receiving federal government funding through the CDC, the Health Resources and Services Administration (HRSA), and the Department of Homeland Security (DHS). This funding is intended to upgrade and integrate the capacity of state and local public health jurisdictions to quickly and effectively prepare for and respond to bioterrorism, outbreaks of infectious disease, and other public health threats and emergencies. Planning and implementation require a coordinated response that involves a variety of stakeholders, including first and foremost the general public as well as all levels of government, public health agencies, hospitals, first responders, emergency management, health care providers within the community, schools and universities, the private sector, and business and non-governmental organizations (NGOs) such as the Red Cross. Mutual aid agreements establish relationships between partners prior to the incident at the local, regional, state, and national levels and ensure seamless service.

Emergency management is responsible for developing and coordinating emergency response plans within their defined area, whether local, state, federal, or tribal. The Federal Emergency Management Agency (FEMA) is a coordination entity responsible for creating a comprehensive, all-hazard plan that incorporates scenarios that illustrate plausible major incidents that may affect their community. Plans incorporate all levels of disaster management including prevention (mitigation), preparedness, recovery, and response efforts. Agency personnel

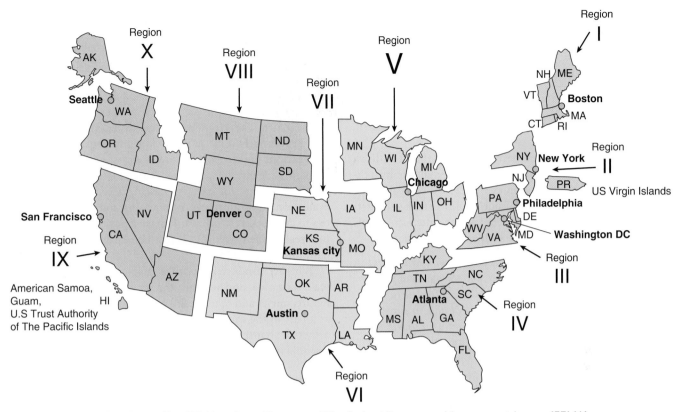

FIGURE 23-5 Ten FEMA regions. (Courtesy of The Federal Emergency Management Agency [FEMA] Map Service Center, Washington, DC. Available at http://msc.fema.gov/webapp/wcs/stores/servlet/FemaWelcomeView?storeId=10001&catalogId=10001&langId=-1. Accessed August 1, 2010.)

who work closely with their communities and community partners provide opportunities to train, exercise, evaluate, and update the plan. Stronger pre-disaster partnerships produce a more coordinated response. Respective FEMA assets are divided into regions across the nation (Figure 23-5).

Good disaster preparedness planning involves simplicity and realism with back-up contingencies because (1) plans never exactly fit the disaster as it occurs, and (2) all plans need implementation viability, no matter which key members are present at the time (DHS, 2007a).

Finally, the community must have an adequate warning system and an evacuation plan that includes measures to remove those individuals from areas of danger who hesitate to leave. Some people refuse to leave their homes over fear that their possessions will be lost, destroyed, or looted. They also do not want to leave pets behind. Also, some people mistakenly believe that experience with a particular type of disaster is enough preparation for the next one. The nurse's visibility in the community helps develop the trust and credibility needed to help in contingency planning for evacuation.

> **DID YOU KNOW?** *"For the ninth consecutive year, nurses have been voted the most trusted profession in America according to Gallup's annual survey of professions for their honesty and ethical standards. Eighty-one percent of Americans believe nurses' honesty and ethical standards are either 'high' or 'very high.' Nurses have received the highest rating every year except in 2001 when firefighters were*

noted as the most trusted. This very positive result brings with it a great deal of responsibility. Even if a nurse chooses not to formally participate in a disaster, neighbors and friends may still reach out for health guidance during a disaster. Participating in preparedness activities further supports the trust that the public puts in that service."

From Advance for Nurses: Available at http://nursing.advanceweb.com/news/national.news/nurses/nurses-rated-most-trusted-profession.Again.aspx. Accessed April 17, 2011.

Nurses should be involved in identifying and educating these vulnerable populations about what impact the disaster might have on them, including helping them set up a personal preparedness plan. In addition to identifying high-risk individuals in neighborhoods, locations of concern include schools, college campuses, residential centers, prisons, and high-rise buildings (Langan and James, 2005). Nurses can assist in community preparedness with their knowledge of the community's diversity such as non–English-speaking groups, immunocompromised clients, children, and the physically challenged.

The National Health Security Strategy (NHSS)

The purpose of the NHSS is to reconnect public health and medical preparedness, response, and recovery strategies to ensure the nation's resilience in the face of health threats or incidents with potentially negative health consequences. Outcomes of the NHSS include community strengthening, integration of response and recovery systems, and seamless coordination between all levels of the public health and medical system (USDHHS, 2009).

The 2006 PAHPA directed the Secretary of the Department of Health and Human Services (DHHS) to develop a National Health Security Strategy, presented to Congress in December 2009, with revision scheduled every 4 years afterward (ASPR, 2007).

Community resilience has become a central theme in disaster planning. The NHSS is built on the premise that healthy individuals, families, and communities with access to health care and knowledge become some of our nation's strongest assets in disaster incidents. In an open letter to the American people introducing the NHSS, Secretary Kathleen Sebelius stated:

Community resilience is not possible without strong and sustainable public health, health care, and emergency response systems. This means that the health care infrastructure is capable of meeting anticipated needs and able to surge to meet unanticipated ones; ready to prevent or mitigate the spread of disease, morbidity and mortality; able to mobilize people and equipment to respond to emergencies; capable of accommodating large numbers of people in need during an emergency; and knowledgeable about its population—including people's health needs, culture, literacy, and traditions—and therefore able to communicate effectively with the full range of affected populations, including those most at risk, during an emergency (DHS, 2009, p ii).

Disaster and Mass Casualty Exercises

Although practice will not ensure a perfect response to disaster, disaster and mass casualty drills and exercises are extremely valuable components of preparedness. After the exercise, the lessons learned through after-action reports are used to update disaster plans and subsequent operations. Exercise categories include discussion-based simulations or "tabletops" and operations-based events such as drills, functional, and full-scale exercises (Gebbie and Valas, 2006). The latter operations-types involve escalating scope and scale testing of the disaster preparedness and response network using a specific plan.

National Level Exercise 2009 (NLE09), conducted July 27-31, 2009, was the first major exercise conducted by the U.S. government that focused exclusively on terrorism prevention and protection, as opposed to incident response and recovery. NLE09 was designated as a Tier I National Level Exercise. Tier I exercises (formerly known as the Top Officials exercise series [TOPOFF]) occur annually in accordance with the National Exercise Program (NEP) (FEMA, 2009b). This program serves as the nation's over-arching exercise program for planning, organizing, conducting, and evaluating national level exercises and provides the opportunity to prepare for catastrophic crises ranging from terrorism to natural disasters. The NLE09 full-scale exercise began in the aftermath of a terrorism event outside the United States, with subsequent efforts by the terrorists to enter the United States and carry out additional attacks. The activities took place at command posts, emergency operation

centers, intelligence centers, and potential field locations to include federal headquarters facilities in the Washington DC area, and in federal, regional, state, tribal, local, and private sector facilities in the states of Arkansas, California, Louisiana, New Mexico, Oklahoma, and Texas.

Most exercises conducted in hospitals, communities, colleges, counties, or regions are much smaller in scope and scale than NLE09. The Homeland Security Exercise and Evaluation Program (HSEEP) was developed to help states and local jurisdictions improve overall preparedness with all natural and human-made disasters. It provides a standardized methodology and terminology for exercise design, development, conduct, evaluation, and improvement planning and assists communities to create exercises that will make a positive difference prior to a real incident (FEMA, 2010). HSEEP is the national standard for all exercises.

Whether conducted as drills, tabletops, functional, or full-scale scenarios, and whether the scope is local or national in nature, nurses and other health care providers must be included as a part of the exercise's planning, response, and after-action activities. Nurses, as client and community advocates, are essential players in the exercise and preparedness arena.

Response

The first level of disaster response occurs at the local level with the mobilization of responders such as the fire department, law enforcement, public health, and emergency services. If the disaster stretches local resources, the county or city emergency management agency (EMA) will coordinate activities through an emergency operations center (EOC). Generally, local responders within a county sign a regional or state-wide mutual aid agreement to allow the sharing of needed personnel, equipment, services, and supplies.

The initial scope of disaster assessment is usually measured in dollars, health risk and injury, and/or lives lost. The more destruction and lives at risk, the greater the degree of attention and resources provided at the local, regional, and state levels. When state resources and capabilities are overwhelmed, governors may request federal assistance under a Presidential disaster or emergency declaration. If the event is considered an incident of national significance (a potential or high-impact disaster), appropriate response personnel and resources are provided.

National Response Framework (NRF)

The NRF was written to approach a domestic incident in a unified, well-coordinated manner, enabling all emergency responding entities the ability to work together more effectively and efficiently. The on-line component, the NRF Resource Center (http://www.fema.gov/emergency/nrf/), contains supplemental materials including annexes, partner guides, and other supporting documents and learning resources. This information is dynamic and is designed to change with lessons learned from real-world events (DHS, 2008d).

The second part of the NRF includes Emergency Support Functions (ESFs). The 15 ESFs provide a mechanism to bundle federal resources/capabilities to support the nation. Examples of functions include transportation, communications, and energy.

Each ESF includes a coordinator function, and both primary and support agencies that work together to coordinate and deliver the full breadth of federal capabilities. Specifically, the ESFs provide the structure for coordinating federal interagency support for a federal response to an incident. The NRFs also include support annexes, incident specific annexes, and partner guides.

ESF 8 (described previously) is Public Health and Medical Services. It provides guidance for medical and mental health personnel, medical equipment and supplies, assessment of the status of the public health infrastructure, and monitoring for potential disease outbreaks. The ESF 8 primary agency is the DHHS; supporting agencies include the DHS, the American Red Cross, the Department of Defense, and the Department of Veterans Affairs.

The NDMS is part of ESF 8 and includes the DMATs. These teams of specially trained civilian physicians, nurses, and other health care personnel can be sent to a disaster site within hours of activation (USDHHS, n.d.).

National Incident Management System (NIMS)

The NIMS is the nation's common platform for disaster response, to include universal protocols and language. "The [NIMS] provides a systematic, proactive approach to guide departments and agencies at all levels of government, nongovernmental organizations, and the private sector to work seamlessly…to reduce the loss of life and property and harm to the environment" (FEMA, 2009c). No matter what type of nursing practice or which agency a nurse chooses, they will most likely come into direct contact with NIMS, to include the Incident Command System (ICS). Figure 23-6 lays out how ICS operates at the basic level. The

NIMS includes varying levels of education and training, with many organizations requiring a base level of familiarization to comply with federal funding requirements. A well-developed training program promotes nation-wide NIMS implementation. The training program also grows the number of adequately trained and qualified emergency management/response personnel. The How To Be Incident Command Ready box demonstrates a basic NIMS training plan for nurse responders.

| HOW TO **Be Incident Command Ready**

Five-Year NIMS Training Plan

A critical tool in promoting the nationwide implementation of NIMS is a well-developed training program that facilitates NIMS training throughout the nation, growing the number of adequately trained and qualified emergency management/response personnel. The Five-Year NIMS Training Plan compiles the existing and ongoing development of NIMS training and guidance for personnel qualification. The National Training Program for the NIMS will develop and maintain a common national foundation for training and qualifying emergency management/response personnel. To accomplish this, the Five-Year NIMS Training Plan describes a sequence of goals, objectives, and action items that translates the functional capabilities defined in the NIMS into positions, core competencies, training, and personnel qualifications.

Emergency Management Institute

The Emergency Management Institute (EMI), located at the National Emergency Training Center in Emmitsburg, MD, offers a broad range of NIMS-related training, including the following online courses:

- *IS-100.HC—Introduction to the Incident Command System for Healthcare/Hospitals*
- *IS-200.HC—Applying ICS to Healthcare Organizations*

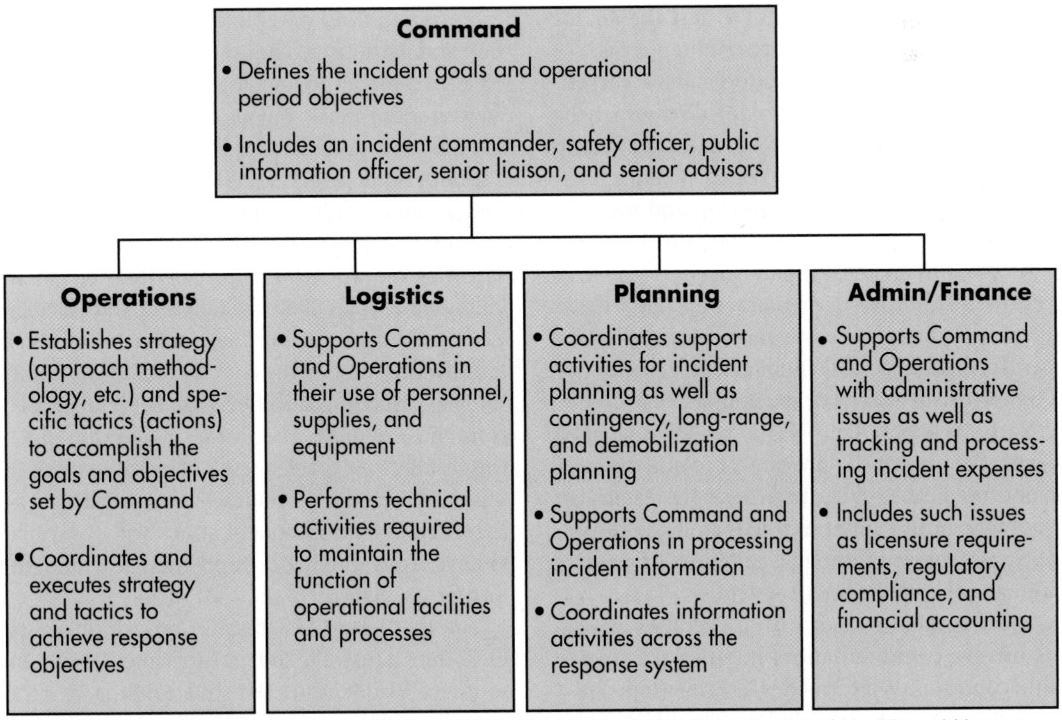

Command
- Defines the incident goals and operational period objectives
- Includes an incident commander, safety officer, public information officer, senior liaison, and senior advisors

Operations
- Establishes strategy (approach methodology, etc.) and specific tactics (actions) to accomplish the goals and objectives set by Command
- Coordinates and executes strategy and tactics to achieve response objectives

Logistics
- Supports Command and Operations in their use of personnel, supplies, and equipment
- Performs technical activities required to maintain the function of operational facilities and processes

Planning
- Coordinates support activities for incident planning as well as contingency, long-range, and demobilization planning
- Supports Command and Operations in processing incident information
- Coordinates information activities across the response system

Admin/Finance
- Supports Command and Operations with administrative issues as well as tracking and processing incident expenses
- Includes such issues as licensure requirements, regulatory compliance, and financial accounting

FIGURE 23-6 Incident Command System (ICS). (Courtesy of U.S. Department of Health and Human Services, Washington, DC. Available at http://www.phe.gov/Preparedness/planning/mscc/handbook/chapter1/Pages/emergencymanagement.aspx. Accessed August 1, 2010.)

- *IS-700.A—National Incident Management System (NIMS), An Introduction*
- *IS-701—NIMS Multiagency Coordination System*
- *IS-800.B—National Response Framework, An Introduction*

From Federal Emergency Management Agency, NIMS Resource Center, 2010. Available at http://www.fema.gov/emergency/nims/NIMS TrainingCourses.shtm and www.training.fema.gov. Accessed August 1, 2010.

Response to Bioterrorism

The twenty-first century has experienced threats not addressed by the public health philosophy of the twentieth century, "where adversaries may use biological weapons agents as part of a long-term campaign of aggression and terror" (The White House, 2004, p 2). Results of a biological release can be difficult to recognize because many biological agent symptoms mimic influenza or other viral syndromes. Pathogens such as bacteria, viruses, and toxins can be used to create biological weapons. While an aerosol release may be a likely vehicle for dissemination, certain biological agents could also be released through the water and food supply. Only about a dozen pathogens pose a major threat, even though there are thousands of pathogens, some highly contagious. Quarantine of those exposed to contagious agents may be considered in some instances. A few vaccines have been developed to combat bacterial pathogens. The CDC provides an excellent source of biological agent information to include the latest agent fact sheets for health practitioners (CDC, n.d.). Biodefense programs help public health professionals mount a proactive response (TFAH/RWJF, 2009):

- **BioWatch** is an early warning system for biothreats that uses an environmental sensor system to test the air for biological agents in several major metropolitan areas.
- **BioSense** is a data-sharing program to facilitate surveillance of unusual patterns or clusters of diseases in the United States. It shares data with local and state health departments and is a part of the BioWatch system.
- **Project BioShield** is a program to develop and produce new drugs and vaccines as countermeasures against potential bioweapons and deadly pathogens.
- **Cities Readiness Initiative** is a program to aid cities in increasing their capacity to deliver medicines and medical supplies during a large-scale public health emergency such as a bioterrorism attack or a nuclear accident.
- **Strategic National Stockpile (SNS)** is a CDC-managed program with the capacity to provide large quantities of medicine and medical supplies to protect the American public in a public health emergency to include bioterrorism. The SNS is deployed through a combination of state level request and the public health system.

Some of the most common lessons from exercises as well as live incidents involve communication. In an effort to keep the public health community informed, CDC developed the Public Health Information Network (PHIN). The PHIN is "is a national initiative to improve the capacity of public health to use and exchange information electronically by promoting the use of standards and defining functional and technical requirements" (CDC, 2010a, p 530). The PHIN focuses on six components that help ensure information access and sharing: early event detection, outbreak management, connecting laboratory systems, countermeasure and response administration, partner communications and alerting, and cross-functional components. Table 23-2 describes the components.

How Disasters Affect Communities

"When things are lost, disasters are measured in dollars. When people are killed, distant observers rate the toll in numbers of lives" (Pigott, 2005, p 1). Although both benchmarks make for easy comparisons, the pain and suffering of those in and on the fringes of the impact zone cannot be dismissed. People in a community will be affected physically and emotionally, depending on the type, cause, and location of the disaster; its magnitude and extent of damage; the duration; and the amount of pre-warning provided.

The first goal of any disaster response is to re-establish sanitary barriers as quickly as possible (Veenema, 2009). Water, food, waste removal, vector control, shelter, and safety are basic needs. Difficult weather conditions such as extreme heat or cold can hamper efforts, especially if electricity is affected. Continuous monitoring of the environment proactively addresses potential hazards. Disease prevention is an ongoing goal, especially if there is an interruption in the public health infrastructure. Infectious disease outbreaks occur in the recovery phase of disasters, and occasionally disaster workers introduce new organisms into the area.

Although the immediate response to a disaster by civilians may be unpredictable, the response is not always a negative one. For example, the terrorist attacks of September 11, 2001, created extreme anger and grief but also led to a huge increase in compassion and patriotism. Thousands of people helped, from donating blood and money to rescuing individuals from the buildings. Four days after the attack, buying an American flag was nearly impossible, as most stores had sold out (Associated Press, 2001). Within 1 month of the attack, an estimated $757 million in cash contributions and hundreds of truckloads of goods had been donated to help the families of victims and rescue workers (Yates, 2001). This was the worst human-made disaster in American history, killing more than 2500 civilians and 460 emergency responders. Yet, the terrorist attacks of September 11 will also be remembered for how they unified the country (Rand Corporation, 2004).

The psychological effects of September 11 were different from those of more contained, single-event disasters. The attack was totally unexpected and of great magnitude, with much uncertainty and fear about what might happen next. Not knowing when or if a subsequent attack will occur may prevent individuals from moving beyond their fear and anger (American Red Cross, 2002).

Another recent U.S. disaster raises similar issues. At 7:10 AM EDT on August 29, 2005, Hurricane Katrina made landfall in southern Plaquemines Parish, Louisiana, as a Category 3 hurricane. Starting as a natural disaster, its consequences were compounded by a human-made disaster caused by flooding from levee failure. Later joined by Hurricane Rita, Hurricane Katrina

TABLE 23-2   PUBLIC HEALTH INFORMATION NETWORK (PHIN) COMPONENTS

EARLY EVENT DETECTION	OUTBREAK MANAGEMENT	LABORATORY RESPONSE NETWORK (LRN)	COUNTERMEASURE AND RESPONSE ADMINISTRATION	PARTNER COMMUNICATION AND ALERTING	CROSS-FUNCTIONAL COMPONENTS
Creates a national health surveillance system that signals a public health emergency. Provides a consistent manner in which data are collected, managed, transmitted, analyzed, retrieved, and disseminated. Detects subsequent cases of the health event. Localizes the population affected and tracks the health changes over time. Evaluates the effectiveness of the response activities. Provides ongoing investigation and management of the event.	Provides consistency in the capture and management of activities associated with the investigation and containment of a disease outbreak or public health emergency, including: • Case investigation • Tracing and monitoring • Exposure source investigation and linking of cases and contacts to exposure sources • Data collection, packaging, and shipment of clinical and environmental specimens • Integration with early detection and countermeasure administration capabilities; ability to link laboratory test results with outbreak information	Connects a wide variety of laboratories to detect biological and chemical terrorism and other public health emergencies, including: • State and local public health • Agriculture • Water and food testing • Veterinary • Federal • Military • International (The CDC has set the standard for development of secure communication networks between laboratories and establishment of a standard way of naming/sharing laboratory test results.)	Enables partners to meet the needs of managing the administration of countermeasures and response activities. It includes such capabilities as single and multiple dose delivery of countermeasure, adverse events monitoring, follow-up of clients, isolation and quarantine management, and links to distribution vehicles such as the Strategic National Stockpile to provide traceability between distributed and administered products.	Health Alert Network (HAN) enables secure, high-speed, two-way communication among the federal agencies, states, local public health officials, and health-related institutions to reference new and emerging infectious diseases, chronic disease epidemics, environmental health dangers, bioterrorist attacks, and other epidemiological and laboratory data. It provides: • Health alerts/updates • Advisories • Secure collaboration among designated public health professionals involved in an outbreak or event • Sharing of information with the public The network also includes a redundancy of communication devices to include: e-mail; voice mail; texting; faxing; Web capability.	Provides the infrastructure for all other components to ensure that systems can remain available and dependable, exchange data, protect private information, and support national standards. Components include: • Secure message transport • Public health directory and directory exchange • Message addressing • Vocabulary standards • Operational policies and procedures • System security and availability • Privacy requirements

Modified from Centers for Disease Control and Prevention: *Public health information network*, 2010. Available at http://www.cdc.gov/phin/resources/phin-facts.html. Accessed February 27, 2010.

affected the Gulf Coast and the nation in ways that will be felt for generations to come. It is the costliest U.S. disaster ever, with economic estimates of more than $125 billion (NOAA, 2007). The hurricane, floods, and more than 1800 confirmed deaths created traumatic stress that rose to unbearable levels in New Orleans, resulting in a tense and sometimes violent aftermath (Reagan, 2005). New Orleans was typically described as a warzone in the weeks following the disaster, as was the Gulfport-Biloxi coastline in Mississippi where 90% of the buildings were demolished. Hundreds of thousands of people lost access to their homes and their jobs as a result of Hurricane Katrina. Although the response and recovery efforts eventually superseded any natural recovery efforts in the history of the country, many residents of both Louisiana and Mississippi believed that the help was too little, too late. Despite the enormous efforts of people and the vast amounts of money spent to help the area recover, there is much work to be done and more funds will be needed in order to restore the area (ISS, 2009).

Stress Reactions in Individuals. A traumatic event can cause moderate to severe stress reactions. Individuals react to the same disaster in different ways depending on their age, cultural background, health status, social support structure, and general ability to adapt to crisis. Symptoms that may require assistance are listed in Table 23-3.

TABLE 23-3	COMMON RESPONSES TO A TRAUMATIC EVENT		
COGNITIVE	**EMOTIONAL**	**PHYSICAL**	**BEHAVIORAL**
• Poor concentration	• Shock	• Nausea	• Suspicion
• Confusion	• Numbness	• Lightheadedness	• Irritability
• Disorientation	• Feeling overwhelmed	• Dizziness	• Arguments with friends and
• Indecisiveness	• Depression	• Gastrointestinal problems	loved ones
• Shortened attention span	• Feeling lost	• Rapid heart rate	• Withdrawal
• Memory loss	• Fear of harm to self and/or	• Tremors	• Excessive silence
• Unwanted memories	loved ones	• Headaches	• Inappropriate humor
• Difficulty making decisions	• Feeling nothing	• Grinding of teeth	• Increased/decreased eating
	• Feeling abandoned	• Fatigue	• Change in sexual desire or
	• Uncertainty of feelings	• Poor sleep	functioning
	• Volatile emotions	• Pain	• Increased smoking
		• Hyperarousal	• Increased substance use or
		• Jumpiness	abuse

From Centers for Disease Control and Prevention: *Coping with a traumatic event: information for health professionals,* 2005. Available at http://www.bt.cdc.gov/masscasualties/copingpro.asp. Accessed March 6, 2010.

People who are affected by a disaster often have an exacerbation of an existing chronic disease. For example, the emotional stress of the disaster may make it difficult for people with diabetes to control their blood glucose levels. Grief results in harmful effects on the immune system. It reduces the function of cells that protect against viral infections and tumors. Hormones produced by the body's flight-or-fight mechanism also play a role in mediating the effects of grief.

Older adults' reactions to disaster depend a great deal on their physical health, strength, mobility, independence, and income (Ellen, 2001) (Figure 23-7). They can react deeply to the loss of personal possessions because of the high sentimental value attached to the items and their irreplaceable value. Their need for relocation depends on the extent of damage to their home or their compromised health. They may try and conceal the seriousness of their health conditions or losses if they fear loss of independence. Box 23-6 lists other populations at higher risk for serious disruption post-disaster, many of them the same populations at risk for adverse health affects pre-disaster as well.

The effect of disasters on young children can be especially disruptive (FEMA, 2009a) (Figure 23-8). Regressive behaviors such as thumb sucking, bedwetting, crying, and clinging to parents can occur. Children tend to re-experience images of the traumatic event or have recurring thoughts or sensations, or they may intentionally avoid reminders, thoughts, and feelings related to disaster events. Children may have arousal or heightened sensitivity to sights, sounds, or smells and may experience exaggerated responses or difficulty with usual activities. Children not immediately impacted by a disaster can also be affected by it. The constant bombardment of disaster stories on television can cause fear in children. They may believe that the event could happen to them or their family, to believe someone will be injured or killed, or to think they will be left alone. It is best to turn off the television news and engage in activities with family, friends, and neighbors (FEMA, 2009a). The parents' reaction to a disaster greatly influences children.

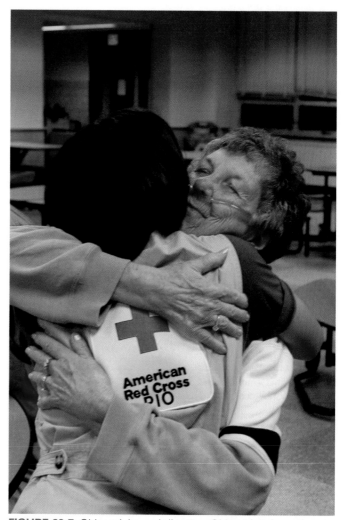

FIGURE 23-7 Older adults and disaster. Older adults' reactions to a disaster depend on a variety of pre-disaster factors. (Courtesy of the American Red Cross Disaster Online Newsroom, Washington, DC. Available at http://www.flickr.com/photos/americanredcross/page4/. Accessed October 7, 2010.)

Public health nurses should help those in the affected community talk about their feelings, including anger, sorrow, guilt, and perceived blame for the disaster or the outcomes of the disaster. Community members should be encouraged to engage in healthy eating, exercise, rest, daily routine maintenance, limited demanding responsibilities, and time with family and friends.

Stress Reactions in the Community. Communities reflect the individuals and families living in them, both during and after a disaster incident (Figure 23-9). Four community phases are commonly recognized: (1) Heroic, (2) Honeymoon, (3) Disillusionment, and (4) Reconstruction (USDHHS, 2000). The first two phases, the Heroic and Honeymoon phases, are most often associated with response efforts. The latter two phases, Disillusionment and Reconstruction, are most often linked with recovery. For purposes of continuity, all phases will be discussed in this Response section.

During the Heroic phase, there is overwhelming need for people to do whatever they can to help others survive the disaster. First responders, who include health and medical personal, will work

hours on end with no thought of their own personal or health needs. They may fight needed sleep and refuse rest breaks in their drive to save others. Moreover, imported responders may be unfamiliar with the terrain and inherent dangers. Those with oversight responsibilities may need to order helpers to take necessary breaks and attend to their health needs. Exhausted, overworked responders present a danger to themselves and the community served.

In the Honeymoon phase, survivors may be rejoicing in that their lives and the lives of loved ones have been spared. Survivors will gather to share experiences and stories. The repeated telling to others creates bonds among the survivors. A sense of thankfulness over having survived the disaster is inherent in their stories.

The Disillusionment phase occurs after time elapses and people begin to notice that additional help and reinforcement may not be immediately forthcoming. A sense of despair results and exhaustion starts to takes its toll on volunteers, rescuers, and medical personnel. The community begins to realize that a return to the previous normal is unlikely and that they must make major changes and adjustments. Nurses need to consider the psychosocial impact and the consequent emotional, cognitive, and spiritual implications. Public health nurses should identify groups/population segments particularly at risk for burn out and exhaustion, to include responders and volunteers involved in rescue efforts. They may need breaks and reminders for nourishment. In addition, those in shock and those consumed by grief related to loss of loved ones will need compassionate care, with possible referrals to mental health counseling resources.

The last phase, Reconstruction, is the longest. Homes, schools, churches, and other community elements need to be rebuilt and reestablished. The goal is to return to a new state of normalcy. Because the scope of human need may still be extensive, the nurse will continue to function as a member of the interprofessional team to provide and assure provision of the best possible coordinated care to the population.

BOX 23-6   POPULATIONS AT GREATEST RISK FOR DISRUPTION AFTER DISASTER

- Seniors
- Vision and/or hearing impaired
- Women
- Children
- Individuals with chronic disease
- Individuals with chronic mental illness
- Non–English-speaking
- Low income
- Homeless
- Tourists; persons new to an area
- Persons with disabilities
- Single-parent families
- Substance abusers
- Undocumented residents

From National Institutes of Health, National Library of Medicine: *Special populations: emergency and disaster preparedness,* 2010. Available at http://sis.nlm.nih.gov/outreach/specialpopulationsand disasters.html. Accessed January 25, 2011.

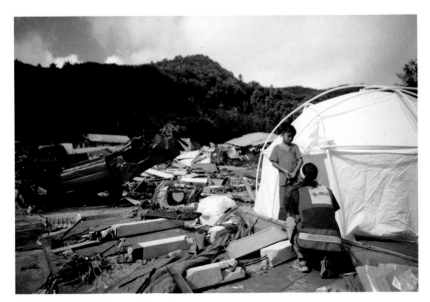

FIGURE 23-8 Children and disaster. The effects of a disaster on young children can be especially disruptive. (Courtesy of the American Red Cross Disaster Online Newsroom, American Samoa, 2009, credit to Talia Frenkel. Available at http://www.flickr.com/photos/americanredcross/sets/72157622497666858/. Accessed August 1, 2010.)

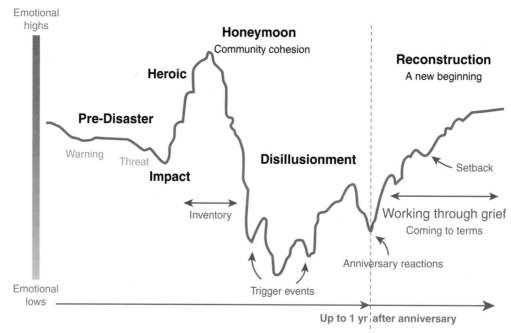

FIGURE 23-9 Community phases of disaster. (Courtesy of U.S. Department of Health and Human Services, Substance Abuse and Mental Health Services Administration [SAMHSA]: *Training manual for mental health and human services workers in major disasters,* ed 2, Washington, DC, 2000, SAMHSA. Available at http://mentalhealth.samhsa.gov/dtac/CCPtoolkit/Phases_of_disaster.htm. Accessed August 1, 2010.)

Role of the Public Health Nurse in Disaster Response

The role of the public health nurse during a disaster depends a great deal on the nurse's experience, professional role in a community disaster plan, and prior disaster knowledge to include personal readiness. Public health nurses bring leadership, policy, planning, and practice expertise to disaster preparedness and response (ASTDN, 2008). One thing is certain about disasters: continuing change. Public health nursing roles in disaster are generally consistent with the scope of public health nursing practice, but the nurses provide that practice in chaotic surge. That said, there is ongoing demand for flexibility in disaster, especially during the response (Stanley et al, 2008).

Nursing Role in First Responder. Although valued for their expertise in community assessment, case finding and referring, prevention, health education, and surveillance, there may be times when the nurse is the first to arrive on the scene. In this situation, it is important to remember that life-threatening problems take priority. Once rescue workers begin to arrive at the scene, plans for triage should begin immediately. Triage at the individual level is the process of separating casualties and allocating treatment on the basis of the individuals' potentials for survival. Highest priority is always given to those who have life-threatening injuries but who have a high probability of survival once stabilized (Chames, 2007).

A type of triage called public health triage also exists, which is a population-based approach for use in an incident undefined by a geographical location. Public health triage involves the sorting or identification of populations for priority interventions (Stanley et al, 2008). In epidemics, for example, the public health triage focus becomes the prevention of secondary infection (Burkle, 2006).

Nursing Role in Epidemiology and Ongoing Surveillance. Health care providers and public health officers are the first line of defense. A comprehensive public health response to outbreaks of illness consists of five components. These components do not vary from normal operations in epidemiological investigation; they simply become "field expedient" (Polivka et al, 2008). They include detecting the outbreak, determining the cause, identifying factors that place people at risk, implementing measures to control the outbreak, and informing the medical and public communities about treatments, health consequences, and preventive measures (Rotz et al, 2000).

Ongoing assessments or surveillance reports are just as important as initial assessments. Surveillance reports indicate the continuing status of the affected population and the effectiveness of ongoing relief efforts. Surveillance continues into the recovery phase of a disaster.

Nursing Role in Rapid Needs Assessment. The traditional model of community assessment presents the foundation for the rapid community assessment process. The acute needs of populations in disaster turn the community assessment into rapid appraisal of a sector or region's population, social systems, and geophysical features. Elements of a rapid needs assessment include: determining the magnitude of the incident, defining the specific health needs of the affected population, establishing priorities and objectives for action, identifying existing and potential public health problems, evaluating the capacity of the local response including resources and logistics, and determining the external resource needs for priority actions (Stanley et al, 2008). Noji (1997) points out that disaster assessment priorities relate to the type of disaster. Sudden-impact disasters such as tornadoes and earthquakes involve ongoing hazards, injuries and deaths, shelter requirements, and clean water. Gradual-onset disasters such as famines produce concerns with mortality rates, nutritional status, immunization status, and environmental health.

THE CUTTING EDGE *Illness Surveillance and Rapid Needs Assessment Among Hurricane Katrina Evacuees: Colorado, September 1-23, 2005*

After Hurricane Katrina struck the U.S. Gulf Coast on August 29, 2005, approximately 200,000 evacuees were sent to shelters in 18 states (CDC, 2006). On September 3, 2005, Colorado was asked to assist in sheltering some of the evacuees; the next day the first evacuees were airlifted into the Denver area, where they were housed at the former Lowry Air Force Base. During the next 4 weeks, 3600 evacuees registered at Lowry, with an average of 400 persons in residence per day. Other persons self-evacuated to other parts of the state, including approximately 2000 who went to Colorado Springs. In all, an estimated 6000 evacuees were living throughout Colorado in the weeks after Hurricane Katrina. As a result of the influx of evacuees, the Colorado Department of Public Health and Environment (CDPHE) and the Tri-County Health Department (TCHD) established surveillance systems to provide early detection of outbreaks and determine the scope of medical conditions of evacuees. A rapid needs assessment was also conducted at the local level to assess acute medical and other needs of evacuees. Results indicated that many evacuees had chronic conditions and approximately half planned to remain in the area, suggesting a long-term need for increased health-related and other services. In addition, the most common acute symptoms were related to altitude sickness, requiring education of incoming Gulf Coast evacuees regarding the effects of the mile-high altitude in Denver.

From Centers for Disease Control and Prevention: Illness Surveillance and Rapid Needs Assessment Among Hurricane Katrina Evacuees— Colorado, September 1-23, 2005; MMWR Weekly 55(9):244-247, March 2006. Available at http://www.cdc.gov/mmwr/preview/mmwr html/mm5509a7.htm. Accessed March 13, 2010.

Nursing Role in Disaster Communication. Nurses working as members of an assessment team need to return accurate information to relief managers to facilitate rapid rescue and recovery. A part of that communication is involved with the rapid and ongoing needs assessment just described. Lack of or inaccurate information regarding the scope of the disaster and its initial effects can contribute to a mismatched resource supply. After Hurricane Andrew in 1992, a well-meaning public continued to ship thousands of pounds of clothing to South Florida. Much of the clothing eventually was burned because there were inadequate on-site personnel to sort and distribute the clothing, and the piles eventually became a public health nuisance.

Times of crisis or great uncertainty call for great skills in communication. The community needs accurate information transmitted in a timely manner. Health care personnel are the best sources for essential health information that is technical in nature. Disaster incidents also use public affairs spokespersons

for formal communication. The Public Information Officer (PIO) is an individual with the authority and responsibility to communicate information to the public at large. Still, nurses are considered trustworthy sources of information and may be approached for an interview. The nurse should refer the media to the PIO representing the agency. If the public approaches the nurse for information, however, that health information should be conveyed. It is entirely within public health nursing scope of practice to provide health education.

Finally, although there are official spokespersons in all major disasters, there may be an occasion for the nurse to serve as a member of the risk communications' team. **Risk communication** is the "science of communicating critical information to the public in situations of high concern. The objectives in emergency communication are to identify and respond to the barriers of fear, panic, distrust, and anger: build or re-establish trust; resolve conflicts; and coordinate between stakeholders so that the necessary messages can be received, understood, accepted and acted on" (AHRQ, 2005, p 55).

EVIDENCE-BASED PRACTICE

A variety of ethical challenges are presented at the time of public health emergencies due to the fact that the stakes are often high since many people may be affected at once; there is little time to deliberate and problem solve; and the emergency may have affected essential resources such as roads, electrical power and so forth. Thomas, MacDonald, and Wenink (2009) interviewed 13 responders in the Epidemiology Section of the North Carolina Division of Public Health to learn how they identified and addressed ethical issues in public health emergencies. What they learned is that the responders were aware of the issues and able to address them in a group interaction. However, few of the study participants had any training in public health ethics. The researchers found in their interviews with the 13 responders that they were able to describe the types of ethical issues they had experienced, the patterns of decision making they engaged in and possible improvements that could be made to improve their skills in these areas.

The potential improvements can be applied to the use that nurses could make to them. Specifically, this study concluded that potential improvements could be made in the areas of identifying a wider range of ethical issues to consider; by discussion and training, developing a deeper understanding of the ethical issues; identifying and using resources to aid in identifying the issues and making decisions about them; assigning roles to designated persons and providing training for these people; reducing the vulnerability of the ethics environment when leadership turnover occurred and evaluating action taken in public health emergencies after they are over.

Nurse Use

The potential improvements that these authors identified for their epidemiology section responders could easily be applied to the work of public health nurses. For example, nurses could have training including role playing, case studies and scenario development in order to identify the ethical dilemmas and work through possible solutions prior to a disaster. Nurses could also identify issues and possible responses, assign roles, design a care path that is not vulnerable to leadership changes and evaluate their actions in the face of a real or mock disaster so they would be better prepared to deal with the actual ethical challenges as they might arise.

Modified from Thomas, JC, MacDonald PDM, and Wenink E: Ethical decision making in a crisis: a case study of ethics in public health emergencies, *J Pub Health Manag Pract* 15(2):E16-E21, 2009.

Nursing Role in Sheltering. General population shelters are often the responsibility of the local Red Cross chapter under the ESF 6 partner function. In massive disasters, however, "mega shelters" with the capability to house thousands may be initiated in partnership with the local, regional, or state government for the masses needing temporary shelter. ESF 6 provides both short- and long-term care. This responsibility includes the plan for structure, operations, management, and staffing of mass care sites. Each person arriving at a shelter is assessed by a nurse to determine the type of facility that is appropriate. Nurses, because of their comfort with delivering aggregate health promotion, disease prevention, and emotional support, make ideal shelter managers and team members. Nurses in shelter functions are involved in providing assessment and referral, health care needs (e.g., prescription glasses, medications), first aid, and appropriate dietary adjustment; keeping client records; ensuring emergency communications; and providing a safe environment (American Red Cross, 2010c). The Red Cross provides training for shelter support and use of appropriate protocols and partners with other agencies such as the Medical Reserve Corps (MRC) and local public health agencies to ensure adequate health delivery capacity to the shelter community.

Common-sense approaches work best when dealing with the shelter community. Basic measures that can be taken by the shelter nurse include the following: listen to shelter residents tell and retell their disaster story and current situation; encourage residents to share their feelings with one another if it seems appropriate to do so, especially those suffering from similar circumstances; help residents make decisions; delegate tasks (e.g., reading, crafts, and playing games with children) to teenagers and others to help combat boredom; provide the basic necessities (e.g., food, clothing, rest); attempt to recover or gain needed items (e.g., prescription glasses or medication); provide basic compassion and dignity (e.g., privacy when appropriate and if possible); and refer to a mental health counselor or other sources of help as the situation warrants (American Red Cross, 2010c).

Although general population shelters can accommodate a variety of functional needs for individuals (e.g., assistance with activities of daily living), there may be circumstances where another type of shelter can provide a more supportive environment for the individual. President Bush marked the anniversary of the Americans with Disabilities Act in 2004 with an executive order that charged federal agencies to fully integrate people with disabilities into the national emergency preparedness effort (DHS, 2006). Based on lessons learned from Hurricanes Katrina and Rita, the DHS charged emergency planners to ensure that the needs of special populations are being addressed through the provision of appropriate information and assistance. The updated DHS plan established the emergency planning category of special needs shelters. These shelters are designed for those individuals who have pre-existing conditions resulting in medical impairments and who have been able to maintain activities of daily living in a home environment prior to the disaster or emergency situation. Special medical needs shelters provide special/supervised housing to individuals whose physical or mental condition exceeds the general population shelter level but do not require inpatient care.

Nurses need awareness of the surrounding medical facilities and services provided in their area, including alternate care sites and medical shelters. The federal government provides assistance to medical needs shelters through ESF 8 by assessing public health and medical needs, offering health surveillance, and supplying health care personnel. Special needs shelters reduce the surge demands on hospitals and long-term care facilities that generally occur during disasters. Although helpful in reducing surge, too many referrals can create tension between the special needs shelters, the general population shelters, and the health care facilities as roles and responsibilities become blurred and overall resources are drained. Careful preplanning for a community's special needs populations is essential.

Psychological Stress of Disaster Workers

Disaster relief work can be rewarding because it provides an opportunity to have a profound and positive impact on the lives of those who may be experiencing their greatest time of need. However, the work can also be challenging and stressful. During an assignment, responders may be exposed to chaotic environments, long hours, rapidly changing information and directives, long wait times before getting to work, noisy environments, and living quarters that are less than ideal (American Red Cross, 2010a).

Nurses who work with survivors of disasters may be at risk for vicarious traumatization. "Vicarious traumatization occurs in response to listening to survivors' stories of the traumatic event" (McLaughlin, Murray, and Benbenishty, 2005, p 73). The degree of workers' stress depends on the nature of the disaster, their role in the disaster, individual stamina, and other environmental factors. Environmental factors include noise, inadequate workspace, physical danger, and stimulus overload, especially exposure to death and trauma. Other sources of stress may emerge when workers do not think that they are doing enough to help, from the burden of making life-and-death decisions, and from the overall change in living patterns (Bryce, 2001). Disaster nurses who live in the community where disaster strikes and who are also directly affected by the disaster will experience additional stress. Anger and resentment may occur since their disaster work demands time away from their own personal situations created by the disaster.

Symptoms that may signal a need for stress management assistance include the following: being reluctant or refusing to leave the scene until the work is finished; denying needed rest and recovery time; feelings of overriding stress and fatigue; engaging in unnecessary risk-taking activities; difficulty communicating thoughts, remembering instructions, making decisions, or concentrating; engaging in unnecessary arguments; having a limited attention span; and refusing to follow orders (Bryce, 2001). Physical symptoms such as tremors, headaches, nausea, and colds or flu-like symptoms can also occur.

The nurse should understand that everyone reacts differently following a disaster assignment. Most reactions are considered normal and are temporary, resolving in days to a few weeks (American Red Cross, 2010c). For some workers, disasters bring forth strong thoughts and emotions, both positive and negative. Other workers may experience mild reactions or hardly any reaction at all. There are some common strategies that will help individuals returning from the incident: rest and recovery time, focusing on accomplishments, using calming strategies such as relaxation techniques or working on hobbies, and concentrating on self-care to include healthy food and drink, exercise, and sleep (American Red Cross, 2010c).

Recovery

In recovery, the immediate response actions to address initial consequences subside. Recovery is about returning to the new normal, a community balance of infrastructure and social welfare that is near the level that it would have had if the event had not occurred (Leonard and Howitt, 2010). The recovery phase is often the hardest part of a disaster. It involves ongoing work beyond the preparedness and the rush to response. Although the initial response phase to a disaster generally provides an onslaught of relief aid, impatience and the loss of momentum toward seeking normalcy is soon felt (see Figure 23-9). During the recovery phase for a large-scale incident, the federal government provides assistance with rebuilding property, restoring lifelines, and restoring economic institutions with the assistance of individuals, the private sector, and non-governmental entities.

An incident that creates a need for a public health surge response is not a transitory event. Recovery involves a shift from short-term aid to long-term support for communities: sustainment of effort. Long-term support should include the disaster-affected population representation in the recovery effort, using local knowledge and skills to prioritize use of resources, personnel, and surviving systems and infrastructure. Assisting relief organizations incorporate and build on the existing community resilience.

Role of the Public Health Nurse in Disaster Recovery

The role of the public health nurse in the recovery phase of a disaster is as varied as in the preparedness and response phases. Flexibility remains important for a successful recovery operation. Community clean-up and rebuilding efforts can cause many physical and psychological problems. Nurses need awareness of the potential public health challenges specific to the disaster area and should monitor the physical and psychosocial environment. Disruption of the public health infrastructure—water and food supply, sanitation system, vector control programs, and access to primary and mental health care—can lead to increased disease and community dysfunction.

Nursing Role in Ongoing Community Assessment. The reality of the recovery effort is that the rapid needs assessment continues into an ongoing community needs assessment. To determine effective interventions to ensure the best possible outcomes, it is essential to have ongoing accurate data about the population. Some conditions are manifest only after time elapses. A major advantage of the recovery community assessment efforts is that they can be more in-depth, with a better sense and confidence in the result. Some examples of community data points in the recovery phase include: ongoing

illnesses and injuries related to the disaster; disease and acute respiratory infections related to disruption of environmental or health services; health facility infrastructure in terms of adequate personnel, beds, medical and pharmaceutical supplies; and environmental health assessment to include water quantity and quality, sanitation, shelter, solid waste disposal, and vector populations (Landesman, 2006).

A realistic perspective is most useful to the community recovery effort. It will take months or perhaps years to achieve the new sense of normalcy, which may be significantly different from the normal pre-disaster state. The health care system and related resources will continue to be taxed, probably beyond abilities for adequate response.

Nurses should also be aware that post-disaster cleanup creates opportunities for unintentional injury and hazards, including those occurring from falls, contact with live wires, accidents with cutting devices, heart attacks from overexertion and stress, and auto accidents resulting from road conditions and missing traffic controls (e.g., stoplights). Nurses should also educate the public of the hazards related to carbon monoxide poisoning stemming from using lanterns, gas ranges, or generators or from burning charcoal for a heat source in enclosed areas.

The Nursing Role in Psychosocial Support. Acute and chronic illnesses can become worse by the prolonged effects of disaster. The psychological stress of cleanup and/or moving can cause feelings of severe hopelessness, depression, and grief in the disillusionment phase (see Figure 23-9). Recovery can be impeded by short-term psychological effects that eventually merge with the long-term results of living in adverse circumstances (Bryce, 2001). Although the majority of individuals will eventually recover from disasters, mental distress may persist for months to come. Especially at risk are the members of vulnerable populations who continue to live in chronic adversity.

Shehab, Anastario, and Lawry (2008) describe a community assessment of a Mississippi manufactured-home population conducted 2 years after Katrina. The researchers surveyed the displaced population for health care needs and access to care as well as identified barriers to and gaps in health care services. At the time of the study, there were about 17,800 trailers in 20 Mississippi counties. Manufactured home parks were included in the survey if they contained 10 or more trailers. There were 69 parks sampled, and homes were selected using random sampling methods. Data gathered included demographic data, displacement information, self-reported health status, types of health services needed and accessed during displacement, depression, suicidal ideation and attempts, and reproductive child health.

Key findings from the 610 respondents included: 80% of households had at least one adult with a chronic condition, and 58% of households had a child with a chronic condition. Sixty-two percent (62%) of respondents indicated their health was fair or poor since displacement. Fifty-seven percent (57%) of respondents were clinically depressed, 72% had depressive symptoms, 24% had suicidal ideation, and 5% had attempted suicide. Ninety-four percent (94%) noted that health care services were not available in their community, and 75% reported no access to counseling or support services since displacement (Shehab et al, 2008).

Referrals to mental health professionals should continue throughout the recovery phase and as long as the need exists. The role of the nurse in case finding and referral remains critical during this phase. In the end, it is the concept of community resilience that will return the community back to its new normal. The public health nurse is the community and client advocate that ensures resilience is enabled in partnership with the population.

LEVELS OF PREVENTION

Primary Prevention
Participate in community disaster exercises; assist in development of the disaster management plan for the agency/community; pre-identify vulnerable populations.

Secondary Prevention
Assess disaster survivors; conduct rapid needs assessment; use individual and population-based triage for care.

Tertiary Prevention
Ensure that community service linkages are available to individuals and families; conduct community outreach; participate in planning efforts for the community's "new normal."

FUTURE OF DISASTER MANAGEMENT

In the last several years, the terrorist events of 9/11, Hurricane Katrina, the H1N1 pandemic, and the Haiti earthquake of 2010 continued to underscore the need for nursing involvement at every step of the disaster management cycle. To fully participate in this mission, nurses must continue to plan and train in an all-hazards environment, regardless of their specialty practice. Public health nurses are especially critical members of the multidisciplinary disaster health team given their population-based focus and specialty knowledge in epidemiology and community assessment. Although sophisticated technology and surveillance will continue to advance in response to both human-made and natural disasters, the nature of disasters will retain the element of unpredictability. That unpredictability and the medical and public health surge requirements in disaster makes prevention and preparedness activities on the part of individuals and communities even more important. Disaster information changes rapidly because of the learning that occurs during and after each incident, producing progressive best practices. Staying current in disaster training requires the public health nurse's commitment in community planning activities, exercise participation, and actual disaster work.

LINKING CONTENT TO PRACTICE

Throughout this chapter, how nurses work in disaster management is applied to standards of public health nursing, core competencies of health professionals in disaster work, and the public health nursing intervention wheel. Other applicable areas include discussion about the continuous processes of assessment, planning, implementation, evaluation, collaboration and cooperation. The role of the nurse in disaster management relates to both standards of nursing and public health practice. Specifically, the nurse must first assess, then plan, implement, and evaluate while simultaneously working with a variety of other concerned and involved agencies and individuals.

CHAPTER REVIEW

PRACTICE APPLICATION

You are a public health nurse working at the local health department when a level 7.4 earthquake strikes with the epicenter 40 miles away. You have two children in grade school across town, a husband downtown at his place of business, and older parents who live 10 miles out of town, toward the epicenter.

You are not hurt and the health department is not extensively damaged, although neither cell phone nor landline phones are working. Emergency auxiliary electricity is activated, but the computer system is down. A rapid damage assessment and visual survey within the immediate neighborhood reveals some structural damage, and 18 individuals with injuries have already approached the health department clinic for assistance. Three of the clients' injuries are serious but not life threatening, with the remainder of the clients experiencing minor injuries and varying stress levels.

An hour passes and there is no word about damage outside of the immediate health department area. Health department workers are very worried and concerned about their homes and family. Two staff members have already left on foot to check on their homes, which are within 3 miles of the department.

What are your priorities in this situation? List them in order and defend your position. Discuss the concepts of prevention and preparedness and how they relate to this disaster situation to include home, community, and workplace.

Answers can be found on the Evolve site.

KEY POINTS

- The number of disasters, both human made and natural, continues to increase, as do the number of people affected by them.
- Professional preparedness involves personal planning as well as an understanding of the disaster plan at work and in the community.
- *Healthy People 2020* objectives are linked in many ways to the disaster management cycle, since a disaster incident affects the health of a community in many areas.
- For effectiveness in disaster prevention, preparedness, response, and recovery, nurses must get involved in their community's disaster plan, preferably through their workplace and partnering community agencies.
- Nurses must be adequately trained and properly associated with an official response organization to serve communities during a disaster.
- Becoming knowledgeable about available community resources prior to a disaster incident, to include vulnerable population assets, ensures a more coordinated response and recovery.
- Flexibility is a key attribute in providing nursing care during disaster.
- The *Public Health Intervention Wheel* is appropriate for daily operations as well as during disaster chaos.
- With any disaster it is always best to use the resources, personnel, and infrastructure of the community itself to promote self-reliance and resilience.
- The National Response Framework and National Incident Management System work together to ensure a unified, well-coordinated national response by public and private entities.
- The public health nursing role in the disaster management cycle includes helping clients maintain a safe environment and advocating for environmental safety measures in the community; risk communication and client education; community assessment to include rapid needs assessment; public health triage; and surveillance and field epidemiology.
- Triage in a disaster setting involves both individual and population-based approaches.
- People in a community react differently to a disaster depending on the type, cause, and location of the disaster; its magnitude and extent of damage; its duration; and the amount of warning that was provided.
- Individual variables that cause people to react differently include their age, cultural background, health status, social support structure, and general adaptability to crisis.
- The affected community experiences four stages of stress during disaster: honeymoon, heroic, disillusionment, and reconstruction.
- The nurse assisting in disaster relief efforts must maintain self-health, both physically and mentally, to be of service to his or her family and clients.
- Ongoing community assessment is just as important as initial rapid needs assessment. Surveillance reports indicate the continuing status of the affected population and the effectiveness of ongoing relief efforts.

CLINICAL DECISION-MAKING ACTIVITIES

1. Select a vulnerable population within your community and determine what special needs the group would have in time of disaster. What community resources are currently available to help this group? Where is the gap in services?
2. Describe the role of the public health nurse across the disaster management cycle: prevention (mitigation), preparedness, response, and recovery. How do you sustain your nursing practice across these stages?
3. Interview a nurse who has responded to a disaster. What role did the nurse play? Were his or her interventions provided at the individual or aggregate level or both? Ask the nurse to give you specific examples.
4. Conduct an interview with an official from the Emergency Management Agency, American Red Cross, Medical Reserve Corps, or other agency involved with disaster management. What is your community's plan for response to a disaster? What agencies are involved?
5. Discuss the advantages and disadvantages of serving on a disaster team in your own community. Are you a good candidate to serve on a disaster team? Have you examined your ability to be flexible? What about your personal preparedness?
6. Contact your local public health department to determine its role in a local disaster, including the role of the nurses who work there. How could you determine a specific nurse's role in disaster management?
7. Determine what the disaster plan is where you work; get specific details.
8. Identify community response mechanisms and facilities with the capacity to provide medical care for trauma, burns, and chemical, biological, nuclear, and radiological exposure.

REFERENCES

Agency for Healthcare Research and Quality: *Health emergency assistance line and triage hub (HEALTH) model*, Rockville, MD, 2005. Available at http://www.ahrq.gov/research/health. Accessed January 25, 2011.

Advance for Nurses: Available at http://nursing.advanceweb.com/news/national.news/nurses/rated-most-trusted-profession.Again.aspx. Accessed April 17, 2011.

American Red Cross: *Disaster mental health services: an overview*, ARC Publication No. 3077-2A, Washington, DC, 2002, Disaster Mental Health.

American Red Cross: *About us, 2009*. Available at http://www.redcross.org/en/aboutus. Accessed January 25, 2011.

American Red Cross: *Coping with disaster—returning home from a disaster assignment*, Washington DC, 2010a, Disaster Mental Health.

American Red Cross: *Coping with disaster—preparing for deployment*, Washington, DC, 2010b, Disaster Mental Health.

American Red Cross: *Disaster health services guidance*, Washington, DC, 2010c, Disaster Health Services.

American Red Cross: *Haiti assistance program disaster response report 17*, Washington, DC, 2010d.

Assistant Secretary for Preparedness and Response: *Pandemic and All-Hazards Preparedness Act (PAHPA) progress report*, Washington, DC, 2007, USDHHS. Available at http://www.hhs.gov/aspr/conference/pahpa/2007/pahpa-progress-report-102907.pdf. Accessed February 7, 2010.

Associated Press: As patriotism soars, flags are hard to come by, *USA Today*, September 16, 2001.

Association of State and Territorial Directors of Nursing: *The role of public health nurses in emergency preparedness and response*, Washington, DC, 2007, ASTDN. Available at http://www.astdn.org/downloadablefiles/ASTDN%20EP%20Paper%20final%2010%2029%2007.pdf. Accessed January 25, 2011.

Association of State and Territorial Directors of Nursing: *Every state health department needs a public health nursing leader, 2008*. Available at http://www.astdn.org/downloadablefiles/2008_ASTDN_Bro_web.pdf. Accessed February 3, 2011.

Bryce CP: *Stress management in disasters*, Washington, DC, 2001, Pan American Health Organization. Available at http://www.paho.org/English/ped/stressmgn1.pdf. Accessed April 17, 2011.

Burkle FM: Population-based triage management in response to surge-capacity requirements during a large-scale bioevent disaster, *Acad Emerg Med* 13(11):1118–1129, 2006.

Centers for Disease Control and Prevention: *Bioterrorism*, Atlanta, n.d. Available at http://www.bt.cdc.gov/bioterrorism/. Accessed February 27, 2010.

Centers for Disease Control and Prevention: *Bioterrorism and emergency readiness: Competencies for all public health workers*, Atlanta, 2002. Available at http://www.nursing.columbia.edu/chp/pdfArchive/btcomps.pdf. Accessed January 25, 2011.

Centers for Disease Control and Prevention: *Coping with a traumatic event: information for health professionals*, 2005a. Available at http://www.bt.cdc.gov/masscasualties/copingpro.asp. Accessed January 25, 2011.

Centers for Disease Control and Prevention: Illness Surveillance and Rapid Needs Assessment Among Hurricane Katrina Evacuees—Colorado, September 1-23, 2005b, *MMWR Weekly* 55(09):244–247, March 2006. Available at http://www.cdc.gov/mmwr/preview/mmwrhtml/mm5509a7.htm. Accessed January 25, 2011.

Centers for Disease Control and Prevention: *Mass antibiotic dispensing: taking the guesswork out of POD design*, Atlanta, 2007, CDC. Available at http://www2.cdc.gov/phtn/poddesign/default.asp. Accessed January 25, 2011.

Centers for Disease Control and Prevention: *Federal medical station profile*, Atlanta, 2009b, Division of Strategic National Stockpile. Available at http://www.texasjrac.org/documents/FMSfactsheetv3-1.pdf. Accessed February 6, 2010.

Centers for Disease Control and Prevention: *Strategic National Stockpile (SNS)*, Atlanta, 2009a, CDC. Available at http://www.bt.cdc.gov/stockpile/. Accessed February 5, 2010.

Centers for Disease Control and Prevention: *Public Health Information Network (PHIN)*, Atlanta, 2010a. Available at http://www.cdc.gov/phin/index.html. Accessed January 25, 2011.

Centers for Disease Control and Prevention: *2009 H1N1 flu, 2010b*. Available at http://www.cdc.gov/H1N1FLU/. Accessed February 6, 2010.

Chames V: *S.T.A.R.T. disaster triage: when 911 can't come, 2007*. Available at http://ezinearticles.com/?S.T.A.R.T.-Disaster-Triage-When-911-Cant-Come&id=433812. Accessed January 25, 2011.

Crippen DW: *Disaster management: lessons from September 11, 2001*, Sydney, Australia, 2002, presented at the 8th World Congress of Intensive and Critical Care Medicine.

Department of Homeland Security: *Individuals with disabilities in emergency preparedness: executive order 13347*, Washington, DC, 2006. Available at http://www.preventionweb.net/files/8223_emergencypreparednessprogressreport.pdf. Accessed January 25, 2011.

Department of Homeland Security: *National preparedness guidelines*, Washington, DC, 2007a. Available at http://www.dhs.gov/files/publications/gc_1189788256647.shtm. Accessed January 25, 2011.

Department of Homeland Security: *Target capabilities list: Version 2.0*, Washington, DC, 2007b. Available at http://www.fema.gov/pdf/government/training/tcl.pdf. Accessed January 25, 2011.

Department of Homeland Security: *Emergency support function #8 (ESF 8-1–8-16): Public health and medical, national response framework*. Washington, DC, 2008a. Available at http://www.fema.gov/pdf/emergency/nrf/nrf-esf-08.pdf. Accessed January 25, 2011.

Department of Homeland Security: *Homeland Security Act of 2002: Title 1 – Department of Homeland Security*, Washington, DC, 2008b. Available at http://www.dhs.gov/xabout/laws/law_regulation_rule_0011.shtm. Accessed January 25, 2011.

Department of Homeland Security: *Homeland security presidential directives*, Washington, DC, 2008c. Available at http://www.dhs.gov/xabout/laws/editorial_0607.shtm. Accessed January 25, 2011.

Department of Homeland Security: *National response framework*, Washington, DC, 2008d. Available at http://www.fema.gov/pdf/emergency/nrf/nrf-core.pdf. Accessed January 25, 2011.

Department of Homeland Security: *National infrastructure protection plan*, Washington, DC, 2009. Available at http://www.dhs.gov/files/programs/editorial_0827.shtm. Accessed January 25, 2011.

Devlen A: *Evolution of incident command in healthcare: an implementation of HICS IV in a multi-hospital healthcare system*, Toronto, Canada, 2007, presented at the Canadian Centre for Emergency Preparedness at the 17th World Conference on Disaster Management. Available at http://www.bcpwho.org/presentations/100a.htm. Accessed January 25, 2011.

Duque PP: Disaster management and critical issues on disaster risk reduction in the Philippines, *International Workshop on Emergency Response and Rescue*, November 2005. Available at http://www.docstoc.com/docs/15486261/disaster-management-and-critical-issues-on-disaster-risk-reduction. Accessed January 25, 2011.

Ellen EF: The elderly may have advantage in natural disasters, *Psychiatric Times* 18, 2001. Available at http://www.psychiatrictimes.com/display/article/10168/50581?verify=0. Accessed March 6, 2010.

Federal Emergency Management Agency: *Helping children cope with disaster*, 2009a. Available at http://www.fema.gov/rebuild/recover/cope_child.shtm. Accessed January 25, 2011.

Federal Emergency Management Agency: *National level exercise 2009(NLE09)*, 2009b. Available at http://www.fema.gov/media/fact_sheets/nle09.shtm. Accessed February 26, 2010.

Federal Emergency Management Agency: *NIMS resource center*, 2009c. Available at http://www.fema.gov/emergency/nims/. Accessed January 25, 2011.

Federal Emergency Management Agency: *Ready America: pet items, 2009d*. Available at http://www.ready.gov/america/getakit/pets.html. Accessed January 25, 2011.

Federal Emergency Management Agency: *HSEEP mission, 2010*. Available at https://hseep.dhs.gov/pages/1001_HSEEP7.aspx. Accessed January 25, 2011.

First International Conference on Disaster Management and Human Health Risk: *Post conference report*, New Forest, UK, September 2009. Available at http://www.wessex.ac.uk/09-conferences/disaster-management-2009.html. Accessed January 25, 2011.

Fox M: *Swine flu has killed up to 17,000 in US report*, February 12, 2010, *Reuters*. Available at http://www.reuters.com/article/idUSN1223579720100212. Accessed January 25, 2011.

Gebbie KM, Valas J: *Public Health Emergency Exercise Toolkit*, New York, 2006, Columbia University, Available at http://www.nursing.columbia.edu/pdf/PublicHealth Booklet_060803.pdf. Accessed January 25, 2011.

Hodge JG, Gostin LO, Vernick JS: The Pandemic and All-Hazards Preparedness Act: improving public health emergency response, *JAMA* 297:1708–1711, 2007. Available at http://jama.ama-assn.org/cgi/content/extract/297/15/1708. Accessed January 25, 2011.

Institute for Southern Studies: *Grading the Katrina recovery: how Gulf Coast leaders rate the President and Congress four years after the storm*, Durham, NC, August/September 2009, ISS. Available at http://www.southernstudies.org/ISSKatrina%204YearReport.pdf. Accessed January 25, 2011.

International Federation of Red Cross and Red Crescent Societies: *World disaster reports: introduction—building the capacity to bounce back, 2004.* Available at http://www.icrc.org/eng. Accessed January 25, 2011.

International Federation of Red Cross and Red Crescent Societies: *World disaster report 2009: Focus on early warning, early action*, Geneva, Switzerland, 2009, ATAR Roto Presse. Available at http://www.ifrc.org/Docs/pubs/disasters/wdr2009/WDR2009-full.pdf. Accessed January 25, 2011.

Landesman L: *Public health management of disasters: the pocket guide*, Washington, DC, 2006, American Public Health Association.

Langan JC, James DC, editors: *Preparing nurses for disaster management*, Upper Saddle River, NJ, 2005, Pearson Prentice Hall. Available at http://www.disaster-center.com/Rothstein/cd798.htm. Accessed January 25, 2011.

Leonard HB, Howitt AM: Acting in time against disasters: a comprehensive risk-management framework. In Howard K, Michael U, editors: *Learning from catastrophes: strategies for reaction and response*, Upper Saddle River, NJ, 2010, Wharton School Publishing. Available at http://www.hks.harvard.edu/programs/crisisleadership/publications/articles. Available at Accessed January 25, 2011.

Marshall B: Levee engineers faulted for missing obvious problem. *The Times-Picayune* , December 1, 2005. Available at http://www.chron.com/disp/story.mpl/front/3494775.html. Retrieved January 25, 2011.

McLaughlin DE, Murray RB, Benbenishty J: Promoting mental health: predisaster and postdisaster. In Langan JC, James DC, editors: *Preparing nurses for disaster management*, Upper Saddle River, NJ, 2005, Pearson Prentice Hall.

National Aeronautics and Space Administration (NASA): Natural disaster hotspots: a global risk analysis. *Earth Observatory*, 2005. Available at http://earthobservatory.nasa.gov/Newsroom/view.php?id=26455. Accessed January 25, 2011.

National Institutes of Health, National Library of Medicine: *Special populations: emergency and disaster preparedness*, 2010. Available at http://sis.nlm.nih.gov/outreach/specialpopulationsanddisasters.html. Accessed January 25, 2011.

National Oceanic and Atmospheric Administration (NOAA): *Hurricane Katrina*, 2007. Available at http://www.katrina.noaa.gov/. Accessed January 25, 2011.

Noji EK: *The public health consequences of disasters*, New York, 1997, Oxford University Press.

Office of Legislative Policy and Analysis: *Linking the National Institutes of Health and Congress, 2010.* Available at http://olpa.od.nih.gov/legislation/107/publiclaws/publichealthsecurity.asp. Accessed January 25, 2011.

Pigott I: In the news: Red Cross Mental Health Services play key role in drill, 2005 *American Red Cross.*

Polivka B, Stanley S, Gordon D, et al: Public health nursing competencies for public health surge events, *Public Health Nursing* 25(2):159–165, 2008.

Rand Corporation: *Compensating the victims of 9/11*, Santa Monica, CA, 2004, RAND. Availble at http://www.rand.org/pubs/research_briefs/RB9087/index1.html. Accessed March 6, 2010.

Reagan M: *Editor in Chief: CNN reports: Katrina state of emergency*, Kansas City, MO, 2005, Andrews McMeel Publishing.

Rotz LD, Koo D, O'Carroll PW, et al: Bioterrorism preparedness: planning for the future, *J Public Health Manag Pract* 6:45, 2000.

Shehab N, Anastario MP, Lawry L: Access to care among displaced Mississippi residents in FEMA travel trailer parks two years after Katrina, *Health Aff* 27(5):w416–429, 2008.

Stanley S, Polivka B, Gordon D, et al: The ExploreSurge trail guide and hiking workshop: discipline specific education for public health nurses, *Public Health Nursing* 25(2):166–175, 2008.

Thomson Reuters Foundation: Typhoons in the Philippines and Vietnam, earthquake in Indonesia, tsunami in Samoa, Reuters AlertNet, September 2009. Available at http://www.alertnet.org/thenews/fromthefield/219563/f7ee4aef9b6e28cc2db650b258c777a0.htm. Accessed January 9, 2010.

Trust for America's Health: *TFAH initiatives—Bioterrorism and public health preparedness, 2010.* Available at http://healthyamericans.org/bioterrorism-and-public-health-preparedness/. Accessed January 25, 2011.

Trust for America's Health (TFAH) and Robert Wood Johnson Foundation (RWJF): *Ready or Not: protecting the public's health from diseases, disasters, and bioterrorism*, Washington, DC, 2009, TFAH. Available at http://healthyamericans.org/reports/bioterror09/pdf/TFAHReadyorNot200906.pdf. Accessed January 25, 2011.

United Nations Development Programme: *Disaster profiles of the least developed countries,* Third UN Conference on Least Developed Countries, Brussels, May 2001. Available at http://www.undp.org/cpr/disred/documents/publications/dpldc.pdf. Accessed January 25, 2011.

United Nations Office for the Coordination of Humanitarian Affairs: In-depth: disaster reduction and the human cost of disaster. *IRIN-Online*, June 2005. Available at http://www.irinnews.org/IndepthMain.aspx?IndepthId=14&ReportId=62446. Accessed January 25, 2011.

U.S. Department of Health and Human Services: *National Disaster Medical System*, n.d. Available at http://www.hhs.gov/aspr/opeo/ndms/index.html. Accessed March 31, 2010.

U.S. Department of Health and Human Services: *Training manual for mental health and human services workers in major disasters*, ed 2, Washington, DC, 2000, Substance Abuse and Mental Health Services Administration (SAMHSA). Available at http://mentalhealth.samhsa.gov/dtac/ccptoolkit/phases_of_disaster.htm. Accessed January 25, 2011.

U.S. Department of Health and Human Services: *National Health Security Strategy of the United States of America*, Washington DC, 2009, USDHHS, Available at http://www.hhs.gov/aspr/opsp/nhss/index.html. Accessed January 22, 2010.

U.S. Department of Health and Human Services: *Healthy People 2020: a roadmap to improve all Americans Health*, Washington, DC, 2010, US Government Printing Office. Available at http://www.healthypeople.gov. Accessed February 26, 2010.

Veenema TG: *Ready RN: The healthcare technology readiness source for disaster and emergency preparedness staff*, New York, 2009, Tener Consulting Group LLC, Elsevier Publishing, and MC Strategies. Available at http://www.readyrn.com/. Accessed March 6, 2010.

Vinter S, Lieberman DA, Levi J: Public health preparedness in a reforming health care system. *Harv Law Policy Rev* 4:339–360, 2010. Available at http://healthyamericans.org/assets/files/HLPR_TFAH.pdf. Accessed August 2, 2010.

White House: *Biodefense for the 21st century*, Washington, DC, 2004, Office of the Press Secretary. Available at http://www.fas.org/irp/offdocs/nspd/hspd-10.html. Accessed January 25, 2011.

World Association for Disaster and Emergency Medicine: *Nursing Section Overview*. Available at http://www.wadem.org/nursing_section.html. Accessed January 25, 2011.

Yates J: Gifts, letters piling up at N.Y. relief centers, *Chicago Tribune*, October 6, 2001, p A1.

CHAPTER 24

Public Health Surveillance and Outbreak Investigation

Marcia Stanhope, RN, DSN, FAAN

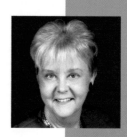

Dr. Marcia Stanhope, as Chair and board member of the local board of health, has been involved in developing policy, processes, and responses for community surveillance and outbreak investigations in her local community. She is also involved in the development of a course on this topic for the doctorate of nursing practice program at the University of Kentucky. The Lexington community, through the health department incident command center, responded to the Hurricane Katrina disaster by establishing shelters for New Orleans residents who had to leave their homes and who came to Kentucky. Dr. Stanhope had an opportunity to participate with the American Red Cross and Dr. Susan Hassmiller (author of Chapter 23) in the past to consider nursing education curricular ideas related to the topic.

ADDITIONAL RESOURCES

OBJECTIVES

After reading this chapter, the student should be able to do the following:
1. Define public health surveillance.
2. Analyze types of surveillance systems.
3. Identify steps in planning, analyzing, interviewing, and evaluating surveillance.
4. Recognize sources of data used when investigating a disease/condition outbreak.
5. Relate the role of the nurse in surveillance and outbreak investigation to the national core competencies for public health nurses.

KEY TERMS

Disease surveillance has been a part of **public health protection** since the 1200s during the investigations of the bubonic plague in Europe. During the 1600s John Grant developed the fundamental principles of public health including surveillance and outbreak investigation, and in the 1700s Rhode Island passed the first public health laws to provide for the protection of health and care of the population of the state. In the eighteenth century, Farr introduced the modern version of surveillance and, along with the United States, Italy, and Great Britain, began required reporting systems for infectious diseases. By 1925 the United States began national reporting of morbidity causes. By 1935 the first national health survey had been conducted, and in 1949 the National Office of Vital Statistics published weekly mortality and morbidity statistics in the *Journal of Public Health Reports*. This activity was later transferred to the Centers for Disease Control and Prevention, who began publishing the *Morbidity and Mortality Weekly Report* in 1961. Laws, regulations, reporting mechanisms, and data collections are all essential to surveillance and disease outbreak investigations.

> **DID YOU KNOW?** *In 1901, the United States began the requirement for reporting cases of cholera, smallpox, and tuberculosis.*

The Constitution of the United States provides for "police powers" necessary to preserve health safety as well as other events (see Chapter 8). These powers include public health surveillance. State and local "police powers" also provide for surveillance activities. Health departments usually have legal authority to investigate unusual **clusters of illness** as well (CDC, 2009a).

> **WHAT DO YOU THINK?** *Florence Nightingale first demonstrated the nurses' role in responding to disasters. Public health nurses bring specific skills to events that require emergency responses. They are prepared to focus on the population that is affected in order to develop policies and comprehensive plans for conducting and evaluating disaster response drills, exercises, and trainings. Public health nurses are first responders in emergency situations in the community, they can lead and manage in the field and in the incident command center, and they are able to collaborate with others to sustain the emergency infrastructure (ASTDN, 2007).*
>
> *Is it important for you to be prepared to lead and be a team member if an unusual occurrence or event strikes your community?*

DISEASE SURVEILLANCE

Definitions and Importance

Disease surveillance is the ongoing systematic collection, analysis, interpretation and dissemination of specific health data for use in public health (Lee et al, 2010; Webster's, 2008). Surveillance provides a means for nurses to monitor disease trends in order to reduce morbidity and mortality and to improve health (Veenema and Toke, 2006).

Surveillance is a critical role function for nurses practicing in the community. A comprehensive understanding and knowledge of the surveillance systems and how they work will help nurses improve the quality and the usefulness of the data collected for making decisions about needed community services, community actions, and public health programming (Box 24-1).

BOX 24-1   FEATURES OF SURVEILLANCE

- Is organized and planned
- Is the principle means by which a population's health status is assessed
- Involves ongoing collection of specific data
- Involves analyzing data on a regular basis
- Requires sharing the results with others
- Requires broad and repeated contact with the public about personal health issues
- Motivates public health action as a result of data analyses to:
  - Reduce morbidity
  - Reduce mortality
  - Improve health

Surveillance is important because it generates knowledge of a disease or event outbreak patterns (including timing, geographic distribution, and susceptible populations). The knowledge can be used to intervene to reduce risk or prevent an occurrence at the most appropriate points in time and in the most effective ways. Surveillance is built on understanding of epidemiological principles of agent, host, and environmental relationships and on the natural history of disease or conditions (see Chapter 12). Surveillance systems make it possible to engage in effective continuous quality improvement activities within organizations and to improve quality of care (Veenema, 2007).

Surveillance focuses on the collection of process and outcome data. Process data focus on what is done (i.e., services provided or protocols for health care delivery). Outcome data focus on changes in health status. The activities generated by analyses of these data aim to improve public health response systems. An example of process data is collection of data about the proportion of the eligible population vaccinated against influenza in any one year. Outcome data in this case are the incidence rates (new cases) of influenza among the same population in the same year.

Although surveillance was initially devoted to monitoring and reducing the spread of infectious diseases, it is now used to monitor and reduce chronic diseases and injuries, and environmental and occupational exposures (Veenema and Toke, 2007) as well as personal health behaviors. Surveillance systems help nurses and other professionals monitor emerging infections and bioterrorist outbreaks (Pryor and Veenema, 2007). Bioterrorism is one example of an event creating a critical public health concern that involves environmental exposures that must be monitored. This event also requires serious planning in order to be able to respond quickly and effectively. Biological terrorism is defined as "the deliberate release of viruses, bacteria, or other germs (agents) used to cause illness or death in people, animals, or plants" (http://www.bt.cdc.gov/bioterrorism) (CDC, 2007). Chemical terrorism is the intentional release of hazardous chemicals into the environment for the purpose of harming or killing (CDC, 2006). In the event of a bioterrorist attack, imagine how difficult it would be to control the spread of biological agents such as botulism or anthrax or chemical agents such as sarin or ricin if no data were available about these agents, their resulting diseases or symptoms, and their usual incidence (new cases) patterns (new cases) in the community. (See Box 24-1 for a summary of the features of surveillance.)

THE CUTTING EDGE   *The United States spent approximately $60 billion since 2001 to assist states in preparing for bioterrorist incidents. Roughly one half of that money has funded detection systems, dramatically expanded research on bioweapon agents, and the development, procurement, and stockpiling of vaccines and other medical countermeasures against these agents.*

From Scientists Working Group on Biological and Chemical Weapons: Biological threats: a matter of balance, 2010, Bulletin of the Atomic Scientists, electronic edition. Available at http://www.thebulletin.org/web-edition/op-eds/biological-threats-matter-of-balance. Accessed September 27, 2010.

BOX 24-2   PURPOSES OF SURVEILLANCE

- Assess public health status
- Define public health priorities
- Plan public health programs
- Evaluate interventions and programs
- Stimulate research

From Koo D: *Overview of public health surveillance,* 2010. Epidemiology Program Office, Centers for Disease Control and Prevention. Available at http://www.cdc.gov/ncphi/disss/nndss/phs/overview.htm. Accessed January 27, 2011.

Uses of Public Health Surveillance

Public health surveillance can be used to facilitate the following (CDC, 2010c):

- Estimate the magnitude of a problem (disease or event)
- Determine geographic distribution of an illness or symptoms
- Portray the natural history of a disease
- Detect epidemics; define a problem
- Generate hypotheses; stimulate research
- Evaluate control measures
- Monitor changes in infectious agents
- Detect changes in health practices
- Facilitate planning

Purposes of Surveillance

Surveillance helps public health departments identify trends and unusual disease patterns, set priorities for using scarce resources, and develop and evaluate programs for commonly occurring and universally occurring diseases or events (Box 24-2).

Surveillance activities can be related to the core functions of public health: assessment, policy development, and assurance. Disease surveillance helps establish baseline (endemic) rates of disease occurrence and patterns of spread. Surveillance makes it possible to initiate a rapid response to an outbreak of a disease or event that can cause a health problem. For example, surveillance made it possible to respond quickly to the anthrax outbreak that occurred shortly after the September 11th attack on the World Trade Centers. Surveillance also made it possible to respond early to the H1N1 outbreak that initially began in Mexico in 2009 (CDC, 2010a).

Surveillance data are analyzed, and interpretations of these data analyses are used to develop policies that better protect the public from problems such as emerging infections, bioterrorist biological and chemical threats, and injuries from problems such as motor vehicle accidents. In 2006 a lot of emphasis was placed on developing disaster management policies in health care organizations, industries, and homes so the U.S. population could be prepared in the event of an emergency. Surveillance within individual organizations, such as infection control systems in hospitals, can be used to establish policies related to clinical practice that are designed to improve quality of care processes and outcomes. An example is documented by Ergaz et al (2010), where a policy of weekly fecal cultures for vancomycin-resistant enterococci (VRE) was instituted following the investigation of an outbreak of VRE in the neonatal intensive care unit.

Surveillance makes it possible to have ongoing monitoring in place to ensure that disease and event patterns improve rather than deteriorate. They can also make it possible to study whether the clinical protocols and public health policies that are in place can be enhanced based on current science so disease rates actually decline. For example, the ongoing monitoring of obesity in children in a community may show that new clinical and effective protocols need to be developed to be used in school-based clinics to reduce the prevalence of obesity among the school populations.

Surveillance data are very helpful in determining whether a program is effective. Such data make it possible to determine whether public health interventions are effective in reducing the spread of disease or the incidence of injuries. By determining the change in the number of cases at the beginning of a program (baseline) with the number of cases following program implementation, it is possible to estimate the effectiveness of a program. One could then compare the effectiveness of different approaches to reducing the problem or to improving health. Johns et al (2010) investigated whether prior seasonal influenza vaccination was effective against the pandemic strain of H1N1 (pH1N1) virus among military personnel. Their findings indicated that with the seasonal influenza vaccines of 2004 to 2009, moderate protection against H1N1 was associated with the vaccines of these years. The protection seemed to have a greater association with severe disease rather then a mild case regardless of age of the ill person.

Collaboration Among Partners

A quality surveillance system requires collaboration among a number of agencies and individuals: federal agencies, state and local public health agencies, hospitals, health care providers, medical examiners, veterinarians, agriculture, pharmaceutical agencies, emergency management, and law enforcement agencies, as well as 911 systems, ambulance services, urgent care and emergency departments, poison control centers, nurse hotlines, schools, and industry. Such collaboration promotes the development of a comprehensive plan and a directory of emergency responses and contacts for effective communication and information sharing. The type of information to be shared includes the following:

- How to use **algorithms** to identify which events should be investigated (i.e., using a precise step-by-step plan outlining a procedure that in a finite number of steps helps to identify the appropriate event)
- How to investigate
- Whom to contact
- How and to whom information is to be disseminated
- Who is responsible for appropriate action

Nurses are often in the forefront of responses to be made in the surveillance process whether working in a small rural agency or a large urban agency; within the health department, school, or urgent care center; or on the telephone performing triage services during a disaster. It is the nurse who sees the event first (ASTDN, 2007).

EVIDENCE-BASED PRACTICE

A study was conducted to identify pediatric age groups for influenza vaccination using a real-time regional surveillance system. Evidence has shown that vaccination of school-age children significantly reduces influenza transmission. To explore the possibility of expanding the recommended target population for flu vaccination to include preschool-age children, the researchers sought to determine which age groups within the pediatric population develop influenza the earliest and are most strongly linked with mortality in the population.

Using a real-time regional surveillance system, client visits for respiratory illness were monitored in six Massachusetts health care settings. Data from a variety of health monitoring systems were used: the Automated Epidemiologic Geotemporal Integrated Surveillance System, the National Bioterrorism Syndromic Surveillance Demonstration Project, and the CDC's U.S. Influenza Sentinel Providers Surveillance Network. Data were retrospectively identified and included clients seen between January 1, 2000, and September 30, 2004.

Study findings indicate that client age significantly influences timeliness of presenting at the health care facility with influenza symptoms ($p = .026$), with pediatric age-groups arriving first ($p < .001$); children ages 3 to 4 years are consistently the earliest ($p = .0058$). Age also influences the degree of prediction of mortality ($p = .036$). Study findings support the strategy to vaccinate preschool-age children. Furthermore, monitoring respiratory illness in the ambulatory care and pediatric emergency department populations using syndromic surveillance systems was shown to provide even earlier detection and better prediction of influenza activity than the current CDC's sentinel surveillance system.

Nursing Use

It is important to offer the flu vaccine to high-risk populations, such as young children, as recommended by the CDC's Advisory Committee on Immunization Practices. Influenza vaccination is the primary method for preventing influenza and its severe complications.

From Brownstein JS, Kleinman KP, Mandl KD: Identifying pediatric age groups for influenza vaccination using a real-time regional surveillance system, *Am J Epidemiol* 162:686-693, 2005.

Nurse Competencies

The national core competencies for public health nurses were developed from the work of the Council on Linkages Between Academia and Public Health Practice (Core Competencies for Public Health Professionals, 2010) and by the Quad Council of Public Health Nursing Organizations (2009). These competencies are divided into eight practice domains: analytical assessment skills, policy/program development, communication, cultural competency, community dimensions of practice, basic public health sciences, financial planning/management, and leadership.

To be a participant in surveillance and investigation activities, the staff nurse must have the following knowledge related to the core competencies:

1. Analytical assessment skills
   - Defining the problem
   - Determining a cause
   - Identifying relevant data and information sources
   - Partnering with others to give meaning to the data collected
   - Identifying risks

2. Communication
   - Providing effective oral and written reports
   - Soliciting input from others and effectively presenting accurate demographic, statistical, and scientific information to other professionals and the community at large
3. Community dimensions of practice
   - Establishing and maintaining links during the investigation
   - Collaborating with partners
   - Developing, implementing, and evaluating an assessment to define the problem
4. Basic public health science skills
   - Identifying individual and organizational responsibilities
   - Identifying and retrieving current relevant scientific evidence
5. Leadership and systems thinking
   - Identifying internal and external issues that have an effect on the investigation
   - Promoting team and organizational efforts
   - Contributing to developing, implementing, and monitoring of the investigation

While the staff nurse participates in these activities, the nurse clinical specialist should be proficient in applying these competencies. In addition, the nurse applies the nursing process in preparedness as illustrated in Table 24-1.

The Minnesota Model of Public Health Interventions: Applications for Public Health Nursing Practice (2001, pp 15-16) suggests that surveillance is one of the interventions related to public health nursing practice. The model gives seven basic steps of surveillance for nurses to follow:

1. Consider whether surveillance as an intervention is appropriate for the situation.
2. Organize the knowledge of the problem, its natural course of history, and its aftermath.
3. Establish clear criteria for what constitutes a case.
4. Collect sufficient data from multiple valid sources.
5. Analyze data.
6. Interpret data and disseminate to decision makers.
7. Evaluate the impact of the surveillance system.

Data Sources for Surveillance

Clinicians, health care agencies, and laboratories report cases to state health departments. Data also come from death certificates and administrative data such as discharge reports and billing records (Pryor and Veenema, 2007). The following are select sources of mortality and morbidity data:

1. Mortality data are often the only source of health-related data available for small geographic areas. Examples include the following:
   - Vital statistics reports (e.g., death certificates, medical examiner reports, birth certificates)
2. Morbidity data include the following:
   - Notifiable disease reports
   - Laboratory reports
   - Hospital discharge reports
   - Billing data
   - Outpatient health care data
   - Specialized disease registries
   - Injury surveillance systems
   - Environmental surveys
   - Sentinel surveillance systems

A good example of a process in place to collect morbidity data is the National Program of Cancer Registries. This program provides for monitoring of the types of cancers found in a state and the locations of the cancer risks and health problems in the state.

Each of the data sources has the potential for underreporting or incomplete reporting. However, if there is consistency in the use of surveillance methods, the data collected will show trends in events or disease patterns that may indicate a change needed in a program or a needed prevention intervention to reduce morbidity or mortality. Underreporting or incomplete reporting may occur for the following reasons: social stigma attached to a disease (such as HIV/AIDS); ignorance of required reporting system; lack of knowledge about the case definition, procedural changes in reporting, or changes in a database; limited diagnostic abilities; or low priority given to reporting (CDC, 2010a).

Mortality data assist in identifying differences in health status among groups, populations, occupations, and communities; monitor preventable deaths; and help to examine cause-and-effect factors in diseases. Vital statistics can be used to plan programs and to monitor programs to meet *Healthy People 2020* goals.

The notifiable disease laboratory as well as hospital discharge and billing data provide mechanisms for classifying diseases and events and calculating rates of diseases within and across groups, populations, and communities.

The sentinel surveillance system provides for the monitoring of key health events when information is not otherwise

TABLE 24-1 PHASES OF NURSING PROCESS LINKED TO PREPAREDNESS

DEFINITION OF PREPAREDNESS	ASSESSMENT	PLANNING	IMPLEMENTATION	EVALUATION
Assure capacity to respond effectively to disasters and emergencies	Assess the populations at risk for special needs during a disaster	Develop plans to care for special needs populations during a disaster	Conduct training, drills, and exercises related to care of special needs persons	Evaluate plans for serving populations with special needs

Excerpted from ASTDN: *The role of public health nurses in emergency preparedness and response*, 2007, The Association, Table 1, Phases of Disaster Linked to the Nursing Process.

available or in vulnerable populations to calculate or estimate disease morbidity. Registrations monitor chronic disease in a systematic manner, linking information from a variety of sources (health department, clinics, hospitals) to identify disease control and prevention strategies. Surveys then provide data from individuals about prevalence of health conditions and health risks. Such surveys allow for monitoring changes over time and assessing the individual's knowledge, attitudes, and beliefs. This information can be used for health education and other planned interventions (CDC, 2009a).

❤ HEALTHY PEOPLE 2020

Surveillance Objectives

- EH-5: Reduce waterborne disease outbreaks arising from water intended for drinking among persons served by community water systems.
- FS-1: Reduce outbreaks of infections caused by key foodborne bacteria.
- FS-2: Reduce infections associated with foodborne outbreaks due to pathogens commonly transmitted through food.
- GH-1: Reduce the number of cases of malaria reported in the United States.
- IID-16: (Developmental) Increase the scientific knowledge on vaccine safety and adverse events.
- PHI-2: Increase the proportion of tribal, state, and local public health agencies that incorporate core competencies for public health professionals into the job.
- PHI-7: Increase the proportion of population-based *Healthy People 2020* objectives for which national data are available for all population groups identified for the objective.

NOTIFIABLE DISEASES

Before 1990 state and local health departments used many different criteria for identifying cases of reportable diseases. Using different criteria made the data less useful than it could have been because it could not be compared across health departments or states. For this reason some diseases may have been underreported and others may have been overreported. In 1990 the CDC and the Council of State and Territorial Epidemiologists assembled the first list of standard case definitions. This list was revised in 1997, and more information may be found at the CDC Division of Public Health Surveillance and Informatics website (CDC, 1997). This site contains information about the National Notifiable Disease Surveillance System (CDC-NNDSS, 2010d), and the definitions remain the same today.

National Notifiable Diseases

Box 24-3 shows the national notifiable infectious diseases. Reporting of disease data by health care providers, laboratories, and public health workers to state and local health departments is essential if trends are to be accurately monitored. "The data provide the basis for detecting disease outbreaks, for identifying person characteristics, and for calculating incidence, geographic distribution, and temporal trends. They are used to initiate prevention programs, evaluate established prevention and control practices, suggest new intervention strategies, identify areas for research, document the need for disease control funds, and help answer questions from the community" (http://www.ced.

BOX 24-3 INFECTIOUS DISEASES DESIGNATED AS NOTIFIABLE AT THE NATIONAL LEVEL DURING 2008*

- Acquired immunodeficiency syndrome (AIDS)
- Anthrax
- Domestic arboviral diseases, neuroinvasive and non-neuroinvasive
- California serogroup virus
- Eastern equine encephalitis virus
- Powassan virus
- St. Louis encephalitis virus
- West Nile virus
- Western equine encephalitis virus
- Botulism
- Foodborne, infant
- Foodborne, other (wound and unspecified)
- Brucellosis
- Chancroid
- Chlamydia trachomatis infections
- Cholera
- Coccidioidomycosis[†]
- Cryptosporidiosis
- Cyclosporiasis
- Diphtheria
- Ehrlichiosis/Anaplasmosis[†]
- *Ehrlichia chaffeensis*
- *Ehrlichia ewingii*
- *Anaplasma phagocytophilum*
- Undetermined
- Giardiasis

- Gonorrhea
- *Haemophilus influenzae,* invasive disease
- Hansen disease (leprosy)
- Hantavirus pulmonary syndrome
- Hemolytic uremic syndrome, post-diarrheal
- Hepatitis, viral, acute
- Hepatitis A, acute
- Hepatitis B, acute
- Hepatitis B, chronic
- Hepatitis B virus, perinatal infection
- Hepatitis C, acute
- Hepatitis, viral, chronic
- Hepatitis C virus infection (past or present)
- Human immunodeficiency virus infection, adult (age ≥13 yr)
- Human immunodeficiency virus infection, pediatric (age <13 yr)
- Influenza-associated pediatric mortality
- Legionellosis
- Listeriosis
- Lyme disease[†]
- Malaria
- Measles
- Meningococcal disease
- Mumps[†]
- Novel influenza A virus infections
- Pertussis
- Plague

Continued

BOX 24-3   **INFECTIOUS DISEASES DESIGNATED AS NOTIFIABLE AT THE NATIONAL LEVEL DURING 2008*—cont'd**

- Poliomyelitis, paralytic
- Poliovirus infection, non-paralytic
- Psittacosis
- Q fever,† acute
- Q fever,† chronic
- Rabies, animal
- Rabies, human
- Rocky Mountain spotted fever†
- Rubella
- Rubella, congenital syndrome
- Salmonellosis
- Severe acute respiratory syndrome–associated coronavirus
- SARS-CoV disease
- Shiga toxin-producing *Escherichia coli* (STEC)
- Shigellosis
- Smallpox
- Streptococcal disease, invasive, Group A

- Streptococcal toxic-shock syndrome
- *Streptococcus pneumoniae*, drug resistant, all ages, invasive disease
- *S. pneumoniae*, invasive disease non-drug resistant in children aged <5 years
- Syphilis
- Syphilis, congenital
- Tetanus
- Toxic-shock syndrome (other than streptococcal)
- Trichinellosis
- Tuberculosis
- Tularemia
- Typhoid fever
- Vancomycin-intermediate *Staphylococcus aureus* infection (VISA)
- Vancomycin-resistant *Staphylococcus aureus* infection (VRSA)
- Varicella (morbidity)
- Varicella (mortality)
- Vibriosis
- Yellow fever

From Centers for Disease Control and Prevention: Summary of notifiable diseases—United States, 2008, *MMWR Morbid Mortal Wkly Rep* 57(54):1-94, 2010. Available at http://www.cdc.gov/mmwr/PDF/wk/mm5754.pdf. Accessed September 27, 2010.
*Position Statements the Council of State and Territorial Epidemiologists approved in 2007 for national surveillance were implemented beginning in January 2008. No new conditions were added to the Notifiable Disease list in 2008.
† Revised national surveillance case definition.

---

gov/epo/dphsi/phs/infdis2010.htm) (CDC, 2010e). The CDC and the Council of State and Territorial Epidemiologists have a policy that requires state health departments to report selected diseases to the CDC's NNDSS. The data for nationally notifiable diseases from 50 states, the U.S. territories, New York City, and the District of Columbia are published weekly in the *Morbidity and Mortality Weekly Report (MMWR)*. Data collection about these diseases is ongoing and revision of statistics is ongoing. Annual updated final reports are published in the CDC *Summary of Notifiable Diseases—United States* (CDC, 2010d).

State Notifiable Diseases

Requirements for reporting diseases are mandated by law or regulation. Although each state differs in the list of reportable diseases, the usefulness of the data depends on "uniformity, simplicity, and timeliness." Because state requirements differ, not all nationally notifiable diseases are legally mandated for reporting in a state. For legally reportable diseases, states compile disease incidence data (new cases) and transmit the data electronically (weekly) to the CDC through the National Electronic Telecommunications System for Surveillance (CDC-NETSS, 2011) (www.cdc.gov/surveillance).

Ongoing analysis of this extensive database has led to better diagnosis and treatment methods, national vaccine schedule recommendations, changes in vaccine formulation, and the recognition of new or resurgent diseases. Selected data are also reported in documents such as *Epidemiologic Notes and Reports* (CDC, 2011). Adverse health data for the calendar year are documented on the reportable disease form titled EPID to the local health department or the state department for public health. Local health department surveillance personnel investigate case reports and proceed with recommended public health

measures, requesting assistance from the state's department assigned to monitor the reports when needed. Reports are forwarded by mail or fax or, in urgent circumstances, by telephone 24 hours a day, 7 days a week. When reports are received, they are scrutinized carefully and, when appropriate, additional steps are initiated to assist local health departments in planning interventions.

NURSING TIP   *To determine which of the national notifiable diseases are reportable in your state, go to your state health department website.*

CASE DEFINITIONS

Criteria

Criteria for defining cases of different diseases are essential for having a uniform, standardized method of reporting and monitoring diseases. A case definition provides understanding of the data that are being collected and reduces the likelihood that different criteria will be used for reporting similar cases of a disease. Case definitions may include clinical symptoms, laboratory values, and epidemiological criteria (e.g., exposure to a known or suspected case). Each disease has its own unique set of criteria based on what is known scientifically about that particular disease. Cases may be classified as *suspected, probable,* or *confirmed,* depending on the strength of the evidence supporting the case criteria.

While some diseases require laboratory confirmation, although clinical symptoms may be present, other diseases do not have laboratory tests to confirm the diagnosis. Other cases are diagnosed based on epidemiological data alone, such as exposure to contaminated food. If a case definition has been established by the CDC or another official source, it should be used for reporting purposes. The case definition should not be used as the only criteria for clinical diagnosis, quality assurance, standards for reimbursement, or taking public health action. Action to control a disease should be taken as soon as a problem is identified, although there may not be enough information to meet the case definition. For example, following the September 11, 2001, terrorist attacks and subsequent crises, when white powder substances were found in the offices of Congress and select post offices, the offices were shut down and evacuated for safety until the final determination of the presence or absence of anthrax (Wills et al, 2008).

Case Definition Examples

Many examples of case definitions exist in the literature and in government documents. The case definition for a *confirmed* case of anthrax was given by the CDC (2010a) as: "(1) a clinically compatible case of cutaneous, inhalational, or gastrointestinal illness that is laboratory confirmed by isolation of *B. anthracis* from an affected tissue or site, or (2) other laboratory evidence of *B. anthracis* infection based on at least two supportive laboratory tests." A *suspected* case was defined as "an illness suggestive of one of the known anthrax clinical forms. No definitive, presumptive, or suggestive laboratory evidence of *B. anthracis*, or epidemiologic evidence relating it to anthrax" (http://www.cdc.gov).

Kuo et al (2009) reported on the first *Shigella sonnei* outbreak in Austria in July 2008. They provided case definitions for confirmed cases as follows: a cluster of 22 laboratory-confirmed cases of infection with *S. sonnei*, which was restricted to public health district X in the province of Salzburg. All cases had attended a youth-group trip to a small village in the province of Tyrol from July 7 to July 9. An outbreak case among the trip participants was a person who: (1) attended the trip, and (2) fell ill with diarrhea in the period between July 8 and July 12. Among the 61 trip participants, 42 fit the outbreak case definition, including 31 culture-confirmed cases. A household outbreak case was a person who: (1) did not participate in the trip, (2) fell ill with diarrhea not before July 10, and (3) had household contact with an outbreak case between 1 and 3 days before onset of illness.

Dauner et al (2007) provided a case definition for a non-infectious disease, streptococcal pneumonia, as "the isolation of the bacterium from a normally sterile site (blood or spinal fluid) from a resident in a defined geographic surveillance area" (p 14). This case definition relies on laboratory data and the geographic location (epidemiological place) of the resident to confirm antibiotic non-susceptibility to the disease.

TYPES OF SURVEILLANCE SYSTEMS

Informatics is essential to the mission of protecting the public's health. Surveillance systems are designed to assist public health professionals in the early detection of disease/event outbreaks in order to intervene and reduce the potential for morbidity or mortality, or to improve the public's health status (CDC, 2010b;

Koo, 2010). Surveillance systems in use today are defined as *passive, active, sentinel,* and *special.*

Passive System

In the passive system, case reports are sent to local health departments by health care providers (e.g., physicians, public health nurses), or laboratory reports of disease occurrence are sent to the local health department. The case reports are summarized and forwarded to the state health department, national government, or organizations responsible for monitoring the problem, such as the CDC or an international organization such as the World Health Organization.

The National Notifiable Disease Surveillance System (NNDSS) is a voluntary system monitored by the CDC and includes a total of 52 infectious diseases or conditions with case definitions that are considered important to the public's health. In the list of 52 reportable conditions, 7 critical biological agents have potential use in a terrorist attack. Each state determines for itself which of the diseases and conditions are of importance to the state's health and legally requires the reporting of those diseases to the state health department by health care providers, health care agencies, and laboratories. The passive system may not provide an accurate picture of the problem because of delayed reporting by providers and laboratories and incomplete reporting across providers and laboratories. This system, however, has the ability to provide disease-specific demographic, geographic, and seasonal trends over time for reported events. An example is a cancer registry system in which cases are required to be reported to the state on the basis of the type of cancer, the demographics of the client, and the geographic location. Because the system has limits, a disease outbreak may be occurring before all reports are received by the state health department (Veenema, 2007; CDC, 2010b).

Active System

In the active system, the public health nurse, as an employee of the health department, may begin a search for cases through contacts with local health providers and health care agencies. In this system, the nurse names the disease/event and gathers data about existing cases to try to determine the magnitude of the problem (how widespread it is).

A recent example would be a search for existing cases of severe acute respiratory syndrome (SARS) within a geographic area or a foodborne outbreak of gastroenteritis, or H1N1 at the local school. An ongoing tracking system within an occupational setting to monitor work-related injuries/illnesses and symptoms is a process that includes occupational health and infection control personnel in interviewing workers, collecting laboratory data and demographics of workers, and seeking potential agents of exposure (Dall'Era et al, 2008). The active system is costly and requires a lot of personnel. Because the nurse is actively looking for a case, this system offers a more complete picture of the number of existing cases. Because of limits, the active system is often used on a limited basis for investigation after a disease outbreak has been recognized (Gordis, 2008; Veenema, 2007).

Sentinel System

In the sentinel system, trends in commonly occurring diseases or key health indicators are monitored (*Healthy People 2020*, 2010; US AID Health, 2009). A disease/event may be the sentinel, or a population may be the sentinel. In this system a sample of health providers or agencies is asked to report the problem. Some of the questions that may be asked include the following: What really happened? What are the consequences? What was different in this event? What was the outcome? Could the occurrence have been prevented? Did providers follow procedures? Did providers know what to do? Has this happened before? If so, how was it fixed? Who reported the event? What might prevent it from happening again (CDC, 2009)?

For example, certain providers/agencies in a community may be asked to report the number of cases of influenza seen during a given time period in order to make projections about the severity of the "flu season." Another example would be monitoring the population of children in the local elementary school to determine the rate of obesity among school-age children. A previously used example referred to an evaluation of laboratory surveillance of the prevalence of antibiotic-resistant pneumonia (sentinel) in communities (Dauner et al, 2007). Although much may be learned about diseases and conditions using the sentinel system, because the system data are based on a sample of a problem or a specific population, they cannot be used to follow specific clients, or to initiate prevention and control interventions for individuals. The system is useful because it helps monitor trends in commonly occurring diseases/events.

Special Systems

Special systems are developed for collecting particular types of data and may be a combination of active, passive, and/or sentinel systems. An example of a special system is the **PulseNet** system developed by the CDC, the Association of Public Health Laboratories, and federal food regulatory agencies to "fingerprint" foodborne bacteria. This system is designed to provide data for early recognition and investigation of foodborne outbreaks in all 50 states. Similarly, **BioNet** is a system developed by the PulseNet Partners and the **Laboratory Response Network (LRN)** to detect and determine links between disease agents during terrorist attacks. As a result of bioterrorism, newer systems called **syndromic surveillance systems** are being developed to monitor illness syndromes or events. For example, data showing increased medication purchases, physician or emergency department visits, or culture orders as well as increased school or work absenteeism may indicate that an epidemic is developing hours or days before disease clusters are recognized or specific diagnoses are made and reported to public health agencies (Buehler et al, 2008, 2009). This approach requires the use of automated data systems to report continued (real time) or daily (near real time) disease outbreaks (Tokars et al, 2010) (Box 24-4).

Another example of a special system designed to help assess unusual patterns of diseases or conditions is the CDC's **Enhanced Surveillance Project (ESP)**. The ESP monitors

---

BOX 24-4	BIOTERRORISM AND RESPONSE NETWORKS

Integrating of training and response preparedness can be supported by the following networks:
- Health Alert Network
- Emergency Preparedness Information Exchange (EPIX)
- The Emerging Infections program
- Epidemiology and Laboratory Capacity program
- Assessment initiatives
- Hazardous substances
- Emergency events surveillance
- Influenza surveillance
- Local metropolitan medical response systems

From Koo D: *Overview of Public Health Surveillance*, 2010, Epidemiology Program Office, Centers for Disease Control and Prevention. Available at http://www.cdc.gov/ncphi/disss/nndss/phs/overview.htm. Accessed September 27, 2010.

---

emergency department data to detect unusual patterns (or aberrations) so quick epidemiological case confirmation and follow-up can be initiated. More information on this system can be found at the WebLinks website. Although useful, these systems are designed to be used for disease case detection, case management, and outbreak management; they require good timing. False alarms occur. The systems provide national data to detect, diagnose, and handle disease and the effects of biological and chemical agents resulting from bioterrorism. The systems are intended to be used with more traditional systems. In epidemics or terrorist attacks, there is a network of links for foodborne (PulseNet), chemical (LRN), and biological genetic patterns of disease (BioNet). New systems are being developed and tested to predict epidemics, as in bioterrorism, before they have occurred (CDC, 2010b; Veenema, 2007). The new syndromic systems may also predict naturally occurring epidemics. (See Box 24-4 for a list of special systems available to assess data in the case of a terrorist event.)

Although all of the systems are important, the public health nurse is most likely to use the active or passive systems. An example of when one might use a passive system is the use of the state reportable disease system to complete a community assessment or MAPPS (see Chapters 18 and 25). The active system is used when several school children become ill after eating lunch in the cafeteria or at the local hot dog stand, to investigate the possibility of food poisoning, or following up on contacts of a newly diagnosed tuberculosis or sexually transmitted disease (STD) client at the local homeless shelter (CDC, 2009b).

THE INVESTIGATION

Investigation Objectives

Any unusual increase in disease incidence (new cases) or an unusual event in the community should be investigated. The system used for investigation depends on the intensity of the event, the severity of the disease, the number of people/communities affected, the potential for harm to the community or the spread of disease, and the effectiveness of available interventions (Sistrom and Hale, 2006). The objectives of an investigation are as follows:

- To control and prevent disease or death
- To identify factors that contribute to the disease outbreak/event occurrence
- To implement measures to prevent occurrences

Defining the Magnitude of a Problem/Event

The following definitions provide a way to describe the level of occurrence of a disease/event for purposes of communicating the magnitude of the problem. A disease/event that is found to be present (occurring) in a population is defined as endemic if there is a persistent (usual) presence with low to moderate disease/event cases. The endemic levels of a disease/event in a population provide the baseline for establishing a public health problem. For example, foodborne botulism is endemic to Alaska. One would need to know the baseline to determine the existence of a change or increase in the number of cases from the baseline. If a problem is considered hyperendemic, there is a persistently (usually) high number of cases. An example is the high cholera incidence rate among Asians/Pacific Islanders. Sporadic problems are those with an irregular pattern with occasional cases found at irregular intervals. Epidemic means that the occurrence of a disease within an area is clearly in excess of expected levels (endemic) for a given time period. This is often called the outbreak. Pandemic refers to the epidemic spread of the problem over several countries or continents (such as the SARS and most recently the H1N1 influenza outbreak). Holoendemic implies a highly prevalent problem found in a population commonly acquired early in life. The prevalence of this problem decreases as age increases (Stich et al, 2006). Outbreak detection, or identifying an increase in frequency of disease above the usual occurrence of the disease, is the function of the investigator (Tokars et al, 2010).

Patterns of Occurrence

Patterns of occurrence can be identified when investigating a disease or event. These patterns are used to define the boundaries of a problem to help investigate possible causes or sources of the problem. A common source outbreak refers to a group exposed to a common noxious influence such as the release of noxious gases (e.g., ricin in the Japanese subway system several years ago and more recently in a water system in the United States) (Sobel and Watson, 2009). A point source outbreak involves all persons exposed becoming ill at the same time, during one incubation period. A mixed outbreak (which was described by Kuo et al [2009] while investigating a foodborne gastroenteritis caused by a *Shigella sonnei* virus) is a common source followed by secondary exposures related to person-to-person contact, as in the spreading of influenza. Intermittent or continuous source cases may be exposed over a period of days or weeks, as in the recent food poisonings at a restaurant chain throughout the United States as a result of the restaurant's purchase of contaminated green onions. A propagated outbreak does not have a common source and spreads gradually from person to person over more than one incubation period, such as the spread of tuberculosis from one person to another.

> ### BOX 24-5   CLASSIFICATION OF AGENTS
>
> - **Infectivity:** Refers to the capacity of an agent to enter a susceptible host and produce infection or disease
> - **Pathogenicity:** Measures the proportion of infected people who develop the disease
> - **Virulence:** Refers to the proportion of people with clinical disease who become severely ill or die

> ### BOX 24-6   TYPES OF AGENT FACTORS
>
> 1. Biological
>   - Bacteria (e.g., tuberculosis, salmonellosis, streptococcal infections)
>   - Viruses (e.g., hepatitis A, herpes)
>   - Fungi (e.g., tinea capitis, blastomycosis)
>   - Parasites (protozoa causing malaria, giardiasis; helminths [roundworms, pinworms]; arthropods [mosquitoes, ticks, flies, mites])
> 2. Physical
>   - Heat
>   - Trauma
> 3. Chemical
>   - Pollutants
>   - Medications/drugs
> 4. Nutrients
>   - Absence
>   - Excess
> 5. Psychological
>   - Stress
>   - Isolation
>   - Social support

WHAT DO YOU THINK?   *In today's environment of tight budgets, how would nurses know which programs should be developed and continued without good data to indicate what are the most commonly occurring public health problems? How would one know if programs were effective without a source of valid and reliable ongoing data?*

Causal Factors from Epidemiologic Triangle

Factors that must be considered as causes of outbreak are categorized as agents, hosts, and environmental factors (see Chapter 12). The belief is that these factors may interact to cause the outbreak and therefore the potential interactions must be examined. Box 24-5 presents definitions used to classify agents in an attack. Box 24-6 lists the type of agent factors that may be present. The host factors associated with cases may be age, sex, race, socioeconomic status, genetics, and lifestyle choices (e.g., cigarette smoking, sexual practices, contraception, eating habits). The environmental factors that may be related to a case are physical (e.g., weather, temperature, humidity, physical surroundings) or biological (such as insects that transmit the agent). Some of the socioeconomic factors that might affect development of a disease/event are behavior (e.g., terrorist behaviors), personality, cultural characteristics of group, crowding, sanitation, and availability of health services.

BOX 24-7 EPIDEMIOLOGICAL CLUES THAT MAY SIGNAL A COVERT BIOTERRORISM ATTACK

- Large number of ill persons with similar disease or syndrome
- Large number of unexplained disease, syndrome, or deaths
- Unusual illness in a population
- Higher morbidity and mortality than expected with a common disease or syndrome
- Failure of a common disease to respond to usual therapy
- Single case of disease caused by an uncommon agent
- Multiple unusual or unexplained disease entities coexisting in the same person without other explanation
- Disease with an unusual geographic or seasonal distribution
- Multiple atypical presentations of disease agents
- Similar genetic type among agents isolated from temporally or spatially distinct sources
- Unusual, atypical, genetically engineered, or antiquated strain of agent
- Endemic disease with unexplained increase in incidence
- Simultaneous clusters of similar illness in non-contiguous areas, domestic or foreign
- Atypical aerosol, food, or water transmission
- Ill people presenting at about the same time
- Deaths or illness among animals that precedes or accompanies illness or death in humans
- No illness in people not exposed to common ventilation systems, but illness among those people in proximity to the systems

When to Investigate

An unusual increase in disease incidence should be investigated. The amount of effort that goes into an investigation depends on the severity or magnitude of the problem, the numbers in the population who are affected, the potential for spreading the disease, and the availability and effectiveness of intervention measures to resolve the problems. Most of the outbreaks of diseases (or increased incidence rates) occur naturally and/or are predictable when compared with the consistent patterns of previous outbreaks of a disease, like influenza, tuberculosis, or common infectious diseases. When a disease/event outbreak occurs as a result of purposeful introduction of an agent into the population, the predictable patterns may not exist. Sobel and Watson (2009) provide clues to be used when trying to determine the existence of bioterrorism. These clues are simplified and appear in Box 24-7 (CDC, 2009b).

Steps in an Investigation

In determining whether a real disease/condition outbreak exists or if there has been a false alarm, first confirm that an occurrence/outbreak exists. Review the information available about the situation. Determine the nature, location, and severity of the problem. Verify the diagnosis and develop a case definition to estimate the magnitude of the problem; this may change as new information is made available. Compare current incidence (number of new cases) with usual or baseline incidence. Use local data if available and compare them to the literature, or call the state health department. Assess the need for outside consultation. Report the situation to state public health authorities if required. Check the state reportable disease list. Early and continuing changing control measures should be used on the basis of the magnitude and nature of the condition (infectious disease, chronic disease,

injuries, personal behaviors, environmental exposure). Control measures may include eliminating a contaminated product, modifying procedures, treating carriers, or immunizing those who might contract the infectious disease. A request should be made that laboratory specimens be saved until the investigation is completed (if applicable to the case definition).

HOW TO **Conduct an Investigation**

- *Confirm the existence of an outbreak.*
- *Verify the diagnosis/define a case.*
- *Estimate the number of cases.*
- *Orient the data collected to person, place, and time.*
- *Develop and evaluate a hypothesis.*
- *Institute control measures and communicate findings.*

Excerpted from Centers for Disease Control and Prevention: Summary of notifiable diseases—United States, 2004, MMWR Morbid Mortal Wkly Rep 53:1-5, 2006.

As the investigation continues, seek additional cases and collect critical data and specimens. Encourage immediate reporting of new cases from laboratory reports (e.g., radiology in cases of pneumonia) and physicians/other health care providers, including public health nurses, health care agencies, and others in the community as appropriate. In addition, search for other cases that may have occurred in the past or are now occurring by reviewing laboratory reports, medical records, and client charts and questioning physicians, other health providers and agencies, and others in the community. Use a specific data collection form such as a questionnaire or a data abstract summary form. Characterize the cases by person, place, and time. Evaluate the client characteristics (i.e., age, sex, underlying disease, geographic location) and possible exposure sites. The place the outbreak occurs provides clues to the population at risk. Did the problem occur in a community, school, or homes? Drawing tables or spot maps helps to visualize the clusters of the disease condition in specific areas of the community. The exact time period of the outbreak/occurrence is important (be sure to go back to the first case or first indication of outbreak/occurrence activity). Given the diagnosis, describe what appears to be the period of exposure. Record the date of onset of morbidity/mortality cases and draw an epidemic curve. Determine whether the outbreak/condition originates from a common source or is propagated. Table 24-2 suggests factors to monitor and explains the reasons for their use. It provides clues to the use of time, place, and person.

As the investigation continues, develop a tentative hypothesis (the best guess about what is happening). Do a quick evaluation of the outbreak by assessing previous findings. Record, tabulate, and review data collected from the previously described activities to summarize common agent, environment, host factors, and exposures. On the basis of this analysis (and literature review if necessary), develop a hypothesis (best guess) on (a) the likely cause, (b) the source(s), and (c) the mode of transmission of the disease. The hypothesis should explain the majority of cases. Frequently there will be concurrent cases not explained by the hypothesis that may be related to endemic or sporadic cases, a different disease or condition (similar symptomatology), or a different source or mode of transmission.

TABLE 24-2 POTENTIAL EPIDEMIOLOGICAL FACTORS THAT CALL FOR INCREASED INVESTIGATION OR MONITORING

FACTORS	REASON
Disease located in one geographic area	Might indicate a point source of a disease agent that can be discovered and controlled
Severe symptoms/diagnoses such as encephalitis or death	Indicates disease process that needs rapid investigation because of severity
Rapid rise to very high numbers of illness two to three times normal baseline with steep epidemic curve	Potential for continuing rapid rise in numbers; requires immediate investigation to institute control measures
Outbreak detected and confirmed in multiple data sources	Unlikely to be attributable to error; possibly widespread
Outbreak occurring at an unusual time or place (e.g., respiratory/influenza-like symptoms in summer)	Might indicate targeted population or early signs in a susceptible population (e.g., very young or very old)
Outbreak confined to one age or gender group	Might indicate targeted population or early signs
Number of cases continuing to rise over time	Indicates sustained outbreak that might continue to grow

From Pavlin J: Investigation of disease outbreaks detected by "syndromic" surveillance systems, *J Urban Health:* Bulletin of the New York Academy of Medicine, 80(2):107-110, 112, 2003.

Test your hypothesis with other public health team members (e.g., epidemiologists). Many investigations do not reach this stage because of lack of available personnel, lack of severity of the problem, and lack of resources available. Situations that should be studied include disease/events associated with a commercial product, disease/events associated with considerable morbidity and/or mortality, and disease/events associated with environmental exposures (e.g., terrorist attack). Analyze data collected to determine sources of transmission and risk factors associated with disease/condition. Determine how this problem differs in incidence or exposure for other population groups. Refine the hypothesis (best guess) and carry out additional studies if necessary.

Evaluate the effects of control measures. Cases may cease to occur or return to endemic (normal) level. If the control interventions do not produce change, return to the beginning and start the investigation over or reevaluate cases. Use the opportunity of an outbreak to review and correct practices related to the current situation that may contribute to an outbreak in the future.

Communicate findings to those who should be notified. Communication of findings may take two forms: an oral briefing for local authorities or a written report. Describe the problem, the data collected, the case definition with verification of the diagnosis, data sources, the hypothesis, and testing of the hypothesis. Present only the facts of the situation, the data analysis, and the conclusions.

Displaying of Data

Reporting of data in an investigation needs to be valid: Does the event reported reflect the true event as it occurs? It must also be reliable: Is the same event reported consistently by different observers? A number of tools can be used to display data according to time, place, or person. The spatial map shows where the event is occurring and allows prevention resources to be targeted. Figure 24-1 provides a map of the location of reported cases of hepatitis A in the United States. From looking at this map, priority prevention target areas appear to be Georgia, the District of Columbia, California, New Mexico, Kansas, and Florida. Table 24-3 shows the number of cases of an

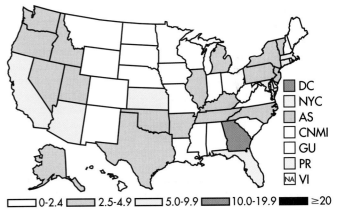

		DC
		NYC
		AS
		CNMI
		GU
		PR
		VI

0-2.4	2.5-4.9	5.0-9.9	10.0-19.9	≥20

FIGURE 24-1 Hepatitis A cases reported in United States and U.S. territories in one year.

TABLE 24-3 EXAMPLE OF WAYS TO DISPLAY DATA*

Number of Clients with Hepatitis A, by Month, for 4 Years

	YEAR 1	YEAR 2	YEAR 3	YEAR 4
January	12	20	21	16
February	14	19	26	19
March	7	21	8	27
April	12	10	11	13
May	5	0	11	0
June	4	11	1	6
July	5	5	9	8
August	5	9	12	7
September	6	7	13	8
October	15	8	10	70
November	?	8	11	0
December	0	11	20	0
Total	75	129	153	174

Modified from Centers for Disease Control and Prevention: Summary of notifiable diseases—United States, *MMWR Morbid Mortal Wkly Rep* 53:1-5, 2006.

*This table shows the number of persons who match a case definition of a select infectious disease over a 4-year period. Note that for year 4, there were overall more cases, especially in March and October, with a serious outbreak in October.

infectious disease compared by month and year over 4 years. In this table, cases have increased by year with a serious outbreak in October of year 4. When cases are reported by person, they are usually reported by a person's characteristic. Data displays are a step in analysis that shows graphically what is happening. It reduces the assumptions made about the event and provides a means for describing the event using quantitative data. Data help in stating your hypothesis or your best guess about what is happening.

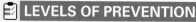

LEVELS OF PREVENTION

Surveillance Activities

Primary Prevention

Develop an approach for mass immunizations of citizens to prevent the occurrence of H1N1 in the community.

Secondary Prevention

Investigate an outbreak of flu-like illness in a local school.

Tertiary Prevention

Provide health care and treatment for those infected by H1N1.

LINKING CONTENT TO PRACTICE

Remember that disease and event surveillance systems exist to help improve the health of the public through the systematic and ongoing collection, distribution, and use of health-related data. A nurse can contribute to such systems and best use the data collected through such systems to help manage endemic health problems and those that are emerging, such as evolving infectious diseases and bioterrorist (human-made) health problems. Functions of surveillance and investigation are detecting cases, estimating the impact of disease or injury, showing the national history of a health condition, determining the distribution and spread of illness, generating hypotheses, evaluating prevention and control measures, and facilitating planning (CDC, 2010b). Response to bioterrorism or large-scale infectious disease outbreak may require the use of emergency public health measures such as quarantine, isolation, closing public places, seizing property, mandatory vaccination, travel restrictions, and disposal of the deceased. In 2008 in preparation for a projected H1N1 flu epidemic, information was distributed about the use of several of these interventions, including isolation and closure of public places (see Appendix D-3).

Suggestions for protecting health care providers from exposure include use of standard precautions when coming in contact with broken skin or body fluids, use of disposable non-sterile gowns and gloves followed by adequate hand washing after removal, and use of a face shield (CDC, 2010b).

The Robert Wood Johnson Foundation (RWJF) funded a project initiative focusing on the development of competencies and resources to enhance the ability of nursing professionals to deliver high-quality and safe nursing care. The Quality Safety Education for Nurses collaboration identified and defined six quality and safety competencies for nursing. In addition, the project allowed for the development of proposed targets for the knowledge, skills, and attitudes of students for each of the six competencies that were identified by the Institute of Medicine as: client-centered care, teamwork and collaboration, evidence-based practice, quality improvement, safety, and informatics. The overall goal for the Quality and Safety Education for Nurses (QSEN) project is to meet the challenge of preparing future nurses who will have the knowledge, skills, and attitudes (KSAs) necessary to continuously improve the quality and safety of the health care systems within which they work. This chapter focuses on the importance of using informatics to identify, monitor, and intervene with unusual occurrences and events to protect the public and to keep communities safe. (See Chapter 26 for further discussion.) Informatics in the QSEN project is defined as the use of information and technology to communicate, manage knowledge, mitigate error, and support decision making. The knowledge requirement for the public health nurse and student is to explain why information and technology skills are essential for safety. The skill to be developed is the seeking of education about how information is managed in the setting before providing an intervention. This chapter applies this by looking at trends of occurrences and events before investigating the situation and deciding on an intervention. It is also important to be able to use the databases and the tools of investigation to ensure safe processes of care. The attitude of engaging in continuous learning and the development of new technology skills is essential. In the case of an influenza pandemic and to assist clients in being safe during such an outbreak, the How to Plan for Pandemic Flu Using a Planning Checklist for Individuals and Families box provides steps for assisting individuals and families in preparation for such an occurrence.

From Centers for Disease Control and Prevention: *National Electronic Telecommunications System for Surveillance,* 2011. Available at http://www.cdc.gov/surveillance. Accessed June 1, 2011.

HOW TO Plan for Pandemic Flu Using a Planning Checklist for Individuals and Families

Nurses are responsible for assisting clients by providing them the means for safety. One of the roles of the nurse, to assure safety, is to assist clients in being prepared for an occurrence or an event in emergent and urgent situations that could compromise their health status or health outcomes. Below is a checklist to assist individual and family clients to prepare for a pandemic. Although this presents a process in preparation for pandemic flu, this process may be used in other communicable disease outbreaks that may reach pandemic proportions.

Use this as a guide to educate clients if an epidemic or pandemic is forecasted:

Prepare for an influenza pandemic as soon as it is forecasted. Prepare clients with the knowledge of both the magnitude of what can happen during a pandemic outbreak and what actions can be taken to help lessen the impact of an influenza pandemic on the client(s). This checklist helps to gather the information and resources needed in case of a flu pandemic.

1. To plan for a pandemic: the client(s) will want to:
- *Store a 2-week supply of water and food.*
- *During a pandemic, if clients cannot get to a store, or if stores are out of supplies, it will be important to have extra supplies on hand.*
- *This can be useful in other types of emergencies, such as power outages and disasters.*
- *Periodically check regular prescription drugs to ensure a continuous supply at home.*
- *Have non-prescription drugs and other health supplies on hand, including pain relievers, stomach remedies, cough and cold medicines, fluids with electrolytes, and vitamins.*

The nurse may want to:
- Talk with clients about preparation for family members and loved ones regarding care if they get sick, or what will be needed to care for them in the home.
- Volunteer with local groups to prepare and assist with emergency response.
- Get involved in the community as it works to prepare for an influenza pandemic.
- Encourage clients to be involved in community activities as well.

2. To limit the spread of germs and prevent infection:
- Teach children to wash hands frequently with soap and water, and suggest that family members model the current behavior.
- Teach children to cover coughs and sneezes with tissues, and be sure to model that behavior in families.
- Teach children to stay away from others as much as possible if they are sick.
- Encourage family members to stay home from work and school if sick.

3. Items to have on hand for an extended stay at home:

Examples of food and non-perishables
- Ready-to-eat canned meats, fish, fruits, vegetables, beans, and soups
- Protein or fruit bars
- Dry cereal or granola
- Peanut butter or nuts
- Dried fruit

- Crackers
- Canned juices
- Bottled water
- Canned or jarred baby food and formula
- Pet food

Examples of medical, health, and emergency supplies
- Prescribed medical supplies such as glucose and blood-pressure monitoring equipment
- Soap and water, or alcohol-based (60%-95%) hand wash
- Medicines for fever, such as acetaminophen or ibuprofen
- Thermometer
- Antidiarrheal medication
- Vitamins
- Fluids with electrolytes
- Cleansing agent/soap
- Flashlight
- Batteries
- Portable radio
- Manual can opener
- Garbage bags
- Tissues, toilet paper, disposable diapers

Excerpted and adapted from the U.S. Department of Health and Human Services: Plan for pandemic flu using a planning checklist for individuals and families, 2006. Available at www.flu.gov. Accessed October 28, 2010.

CHAPTER REVIEW

PRACTICE APPLICATION

As a clinical project, the health department asked the public health nursing class at the university to develop a community service message to air on local radio about the potential of a pandemic flu.

What does the message need to contain to help the community prepare?

Answers can be found on the Evolve site.

KEY POINTS

- Disease surveillance has been a part of public health protection since the 1200s during the investigations of the bubonic plague in Europe.
- By 1925 the United States began national reporting of morbidity causes.
- Surveillance provides a means for nurses to monitor disease trends in order to reduce morbidity and mortality and to improve health.
- Surveillance is a critical role function for nurses practicing in the community.
- Surveillance is important because it generates knowledge of a disease or event outbreak patterns.
- Surveillance focuses on the collection of process and outcome data.
- Although surveillance was initially devoted to monitoring and reducing the spread of infectious diseases, it is now used to monitor and reduce chronic diseases and injuries, and environmental and occupational exposures.
- Surveillance activities can be related to the core functions of public health of assessment, policy development, and assurance.

- A quality surveillance system requires collaboration among a number of agencies and individuals.
- The Minnesota Model of Public Health Interventions: Applications for Public Health Nursing Practice (2001) suggests that surveillance is one of the interventions related to public health nursing practice.
- Clinicians, health care agencies, and laboratories report cases to state health departments. Data also come from death certificates and administrative data such as discharge reports and billing records.
- Each of the data sources has the potential for underreporting or incomplete reporting. However, if there is consistency in the use of surveillance methods, the data collected will show trends in events or disease patterns that may indicate a change needed in a program or a needed prevention intervention to reduce morbidity or mortality.
- The notifiable disease laboratory, hospital discharge data, and billing data provide mechanisms for classifying diseases and events and calculating rates of diseases within and across groups, populations, and communities.

KEY POINTS—cont'd

- The sentinel surveillance system provides for the monitoring of key health events when information is not otherwise available or in vulnerable populations to calculate or estimate disease morbidity.
- In 1990 the CDC and the Council of State and Territorial Epidemiologists assembled the first list of standard case definitions.
- Reporting of disease data by health care providers, laboratories, and public health workers to state and local health departments is essential if trends are to be accurately monitored.
- Requirements for reporting diseases are mandated by law or regulation.
- Criteria for defining cases of different diseases are essential for having a uniform, standardized method of reporting and monitoring diseases. A case definition provides understanding of the data that are being collected and reduces the likelihood that different criteria will be used for reporting similar cases of a disease.

- Surveillance systems in use today are defined as *passive, active, sentinel,* and *special.*
- Any unusual increase in disease incidence (new cases) or an unusual event in the community should be investigated.
- Patterns of occurrence can be identified when investigating a disease or event. These patterns are used to define the boundaries of a problem to help investigate possible causes or sources of the problem.
- Factors that must be considered as causes of outbreak are categorized as agents, hosts, and environmental factors.
- An unusual increase in disease incidence should be investigated.
- Functions of surveillance and investigation are detecting cases, estimating the impact of disease or injury, showing the national history of a health condition, determining the distribution and spread of illness, generating hypotheses, evaluating prevention and control measures, and facilitating planning.

CLINICAL DECISION-MAKING ACTIVITIES

1. Call the local health department and attend an emergency response team planning meeting. How many agencies are involved? Determine the roles of each agency. Does the nurse have a role on the team? Explain.

2. Go to the Health Hazard Evaluation program website (see WebLinks). What is the purpose of this program? How would information from the website be used in a disease investigation?

3. Explain the purpose of applying the sentinel system to improve population health outcomes.

REFERENCES

Association of State and Territorial Directors of Nursing, Public Health Preparedness Committee: *The role of public health nurses in emergency preparedness and response position paper, 2007.* Available at http://www.astdn.org. Accessed January 27, 2011.

Bloom RM, Buckeridge DL, Cheng KE: Finding leading indicators for disease outbreaks: filtering, cross-correlation, and caveats, *J Am Med Informatics Assoc* 14(1):76–85, 2007.

Brownstein JS, Kleinman KP, Mandl KD: Identifying pediatric age groups for influenza vaccination using a real-time regional surveillance system, *Am J Epidemiol* 162:686–693, 2005.

Buehler JS, Sonricker A, Paladini M, et al: Syndromic surveillance practice in the United States: findings from a survey of state, territorial and selected local health departments, *Int Soc Dis Surveill* 6(3):1–20, 2008. Available at http://www.syndromic.org. Accessed September 27, 2010.

Buehler JW, Whitney EA, Smith D, et al: Situational uses of syndromic surveillance, *Biosecur Bioter* 7(2):1–13, 2009. Available at http://www.liebertonline.com. Accessed September 27, 2010.

Centers for Disease Control and Prevention: Case definitions for infectious conditions under public health surveillance, *MMWR Morbid Mortal Wkly Rep* 46(RR-10):2, 1997.

Centers for Disease Control and Prevention: *Chemical emergencies overview, 2006.* Available at http://www.bt.cdc.gov. Accessed September 27, 2010.

Centers for Disease Control and Prevention: *Bioterrorism overview, 2007.* Available at http://www.bt.cdc.gov/bioterrorism. Accessed September 27, 2010.

Centers for Disease Control and Prevention: Summary of notifiable diseases—United States, 2008, *MMWR Morbid Mortal Wkly Rep* 57(54):1–94, 2008.

Centers for Disease Control and Prevention: *Joint Public Health—Law Enforcement Investigations: Model Memorandum of Understanding (MOU), 2009a.* Available at http://info.publicintelligence.net. Accessed September 27, 2010.

Centers for Disease Control and Prevention: Preliminary FoodNet data on the incidence of infection with pathogens transmitted commonly through food—10 states, 2008, *MMWR Morbid Mortal Wkly Rep* 58(13):333–337, 2009b. Available at http://www.medscape.com. Accessed September 25, 2010.

Centers for Disease Control and Prevention: *Anthrax (Bacillus anthracis) 2010 case definition, 2010a.* Available at http://www.cdc.gov. Accessed September 27, 2010.

Centers for Disease Control and Prevention: *National Program of Cancer Registries (NPCR)—about the program, 2010b.* Available at http://www.cdc.gov. Accessed September 27, 2010.

Centers for Disease Control and Prevention: *Public health preparedness: strengthening the nation's emergency response state by state, 2010c.* Available at http://emergency.cdc.gov. Accessed September 27, 2010.

Centers for Disease Control and Prevention: *An overview of the national electronic disease surveillance system (NEDSS) initiative, 2010d.* Available at http://www.cdc.gov/nedss. Accessed July 27, 2010.

Centers for Disease Control and Prevention: *Nationally notifiable infectious diseases—United States, 2010e.* Available at http://www.ced.gov/epo/dphsi/phs/infdis2010.htm. Accessed September 27, 2010.

Centers for Disease Control and Prevention: *National Electronic Telecommunications System for Surveillance, 2011.* Available at http://www.cdc.gov/surveillance. Accessed June 1, 2011.

Council on Linkages Between Academia and Public Health Practice: *Tier 1, tier 2 and tier 3 core competencies for public health professionals, 2010.* Available at http://www.phf.org. Accessed September 27, 2010.

Dall'Era MA, Cooperberg MR, Chan JM, et al: Active surveillance for early-stage prostate cancer, *Cancer* 112(8):1650–1659, 2008.

Dauner DG, Roberts DF, Kotchmar GS: Statewide Sentinel Surveillance for antibiotic nonsusceptibility among *Streptococcus pneumoniae* isolates in South Carolina, 2003-2004, *South Med J* 100(1):14–19, 2007.

Ergaz Z, Arad I, Bar-Oz B, et al: Elimination of vancomycin-resistant enterococci from a neonatal intensive care unit following an outbreak, *J Hosp Infect* 74(4):370–376, 2010.

Gordis L: *Epidemiology,* ed 4, New York, 2008, Saunders.

Johns MC, Eick AA, Blazes DL, et al: Seasonal influenza vaccine and protection against pandemic (H1N1) 2009-associated illness among US military personnel, *PLoS ONE [Electronic Resource]* 5(5):e10722, 2010.

Koo D: *Overview of public health surveillance,* 2010, Epidemiology Program Office, Centers for Disease Control and Prevention. Available at www.cdc.gov/ncphi/disss/nndss/phs/overview.htm. Accessed September 27, 2010.

Kuo HW, Kasper S, Jelovcan S, et al: A food-borne outbreak of *Shigella sonnei* gastroenteritis, Austria, 2008, *Wiener Klinische Wochenschrift* 121(3-4):157–163, 2009.

Lee LM, Michael L, Teutsch SM, Thacker SB: *Principles and practice of public health surveillance*, ed 3, New York, 2010, Oxford University Press.

Minnesota Model of Public Health Interventions: applications for public health nursing practice, 2001, pp 15–16.

Pryor ER, Veenema TB: Surveillance systems for bioterrorism. In Veenema TG, editor: *Disaster nursing and emergency preparedness for chemical, biological, and radiological terrorism and other hazards*, New York, 2007, Springer, pp 330–353.

Quad Council of Public Health Nurse Organizations: *Quad Council PHN Competencies*, 2009. Available at http://www.sphtc.org. Accessed September 27, 2010.

Scientists Working Group on Biological and Chemical Weapons: *Biological threats: a matter of balance*, 2010, Bulletin of the Atomic Scientists, electronic edition. Available at http://www.thebulletin.org/web-edition/op-eds/biological-threats-matter-of-balance. Accessed January 27, 2011.

Sistrom M, Hale P: Outbreak investigations: community participation and role of community and public health nurses, *Public Health Nurs* 23:256–263, 2006.

Sobel J, Watson JC: *Intentional terrorist contamination of food and water*. In Lutwick SM, Lutwick LI, editors: *Beyond anthrax: the weaponization of infectious diseases*, New York, 2009, Springer.

Stich A, Oster N, Abdel-Aziz IZ, et al: Malaria in a holoendemic area of Burkina Faso: a cross-sectional study, *Parasitology Research* 98(6):596–599, 2006.

Tokars JI, English R, McMurray P, Rhodes B: Research article of data reported to CDC's national automated biosurveillance system, 2008. *BMC Medical Informatics and Decision Making* 10:30, 2010. Available at http://www.biomedcentral.com. Accessed September 27, 2010.

USAID Health: *Sentinel surveillance*, 2009. Available at http://www.usaid.gov. Accessed September 27, 2010.

U.S. Department of Health and Human Services: *Healthy People 2020: a roadmap to improve all Americans Health*, Washington, DC, 2010, U.S. Government Printing Office. Available at http://www.healthypeople.gov. Accessed September 27, 2010.

Veenema TG: *Disaster nursing and emergency preparedness for chemical, biological, and radiological terrorism and other hazards*, New York, 2007, Springer.

Veenema TG, Toke J: Early detection and surveillance for biopreparedness and emerging infectious diseases, *Online J Issues Nurs* 11(1):3, 2006. Available at http://www.nursingworld.org. Accessed September 24, 2010.

Webster's New World Medical Dictionary, ed 3, 2008, Webster's New World (Publisher).

Wills B, Leikin J, Rhee J, Saeedi B: Analysis of suspicious powders following the post 9/11 anthrax scare, *J Med Toxicol* 4(2):93–95, 2008.

CHAPTER 25

Program Management

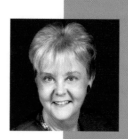

Marcia Stanhope, RN, DSN, FAAN

Dr. Marcia Stanhope has been involved in program management since 1967, both in clinical practice and in education. She has written numerous program grants, and developed, implemented and evaluated a number of educational program initiatives. She has consulted about program management and has spoken and published on the topic many times. The program she manages, and is extremely devoted to is the Good Samaritan Nurse Managed Center at the University of Kentucky.

ADDITIONAL RESOURCES

evolve WEBSITE
http://evolve.elsevier.com/Stanhope
- *Healthy People 2020*
- WebLinks—Of special note see the link for these sites:
  - Turning Point Program
  - Centers for Disease Control and Prevention
  - National Association of County & City Health Officials

- Quiz
- Case Studies
- Glossary
- Answers to Practice Application

APPENDIX
- Appendix B: Program Planning and Design

OBJECTIVES

After reading this chapter, the student should be able to do the following:
1. Compare and contrast the program management process and the nursing process.
2. Analyze the application of the program planning process to nursing.
3. Critique a program planning method to use in nursing practice.
4. Analyze the components of program evaluation methods, techniques, and sources.
5. Compare different types of cost studies applied to program management.

KEY TERMS

case registers, p. 568
community assessment, p. 552
community health planning, p. 549
cost accounting, p. 569
cost–benefit, p. 569
cost effectiveness, p. 569
cost efficiency, p. 570
cost studies, p. 569
evaluation, p. 550
evidence-based practice, p. 556

formative evaluation, p. 549
grant writing, p. 570
health program planning, p. 553
outcome, p. 568
planning, p. 550
planning process, p. 552
population needs assessment, p. 553
process, p. 568
program, p. 549

program effectiveness, p. 550
program evaluation, p. 550
program management, p. 549
projects, p. 549
quality assurance, p. 560
strategic planning, p. 552
structure, p. 568
summative evaluation, p. 549
tracer, p. 568
—*See Glossary for definitions*

OUTLINE

Program management consists of assessing, planning, implementing, and evaluating a program. This chapter focuses primarily on planning and evaluation. Although presented in separate discussions, these factors are related and interdependent processes that work together to bring about a successful program. This chapter does not address implementing programs because other chapters in this text focus on implementation.

The program management process is parallel to the nursing process. One process is applied to a program that addresses the needs of a specific population, whereas the other process is applied to individuals or families. The process of program management, like the nursing process, consists of a rational decision-making system designed to help nurses know when to make a decision to develop a program (through the needs assessment and defining the problem), where they want to be at the end of the program (goal setting), how to decide what encompasses a successful program (planning), how to develop a plan to go forward so they will know where they want to be (implementing), how to know that they are getting there (formative evaluation), and what to measure to know that the program has successful outcomes (summative evaluation).

Today there is a greater need for the nurse to be accountable for nursing actions and client outcomes. Prospective payment systems, pay for performance, health care reform, and integrated care delivery models have changed the focus of nursing. Planning for nursing services is necessary today if the nurse is to survive in the health care delivery field. Nurses are expected to demonstrate leadership in addressing community-based health problems.

This chapter examines how nurses can act, instead of react, by planning programs that can be evaluated for their effectiveness. The discussion focuses on the historical development of health planning and evaluation, a general program planning and evaluation method, the benefits of planning and evaluation, the elements of planning and evaluation, how cost studies are applied to program evaluation, and how programs may be funded. Some sections of this chapter can be used by undergraduate students, whereas other sections are more appropriately used by graduate students.

DEFINITIONS AND GOALS

Community health planning is population focused, and it positions the well-being of the public above private interests (Steen, 2008). A program is an organized approach to meet the assessed needs of individuals, families, groups, populations, or communities by reducing the effect of or eliminating one or more health problems. Community health programs are planned to meet the needs of designated populations or subpopulations in a community. Many programs exist as specific efforts within the umbrella of large, complex organizations such as state health departments, universities, health systems, and private organizations such as insurance companies. Unlike these complex organizations, smaller programs are endeavors that focus on more specific services and communities or groups. Specific examples in population-focused nursing are home health, immunization and infectious disease programs, health-risk screening for industrial workers, and family planning programs. These are usually conducted under the direction of the total plan of a local health department, a managed care agency, or, in some instances, an insurance company. Examples of more complex broadly based group and community programs are the community school health, occupational health and safety, environmental health, and community programs directed at preventing specific illnesses through special-interest groups (e.g., American Heart Association, American Cancer Society, March of Dimes). Disaster preparedness is a type of program that may be conducted through collaborative efforts of several community organizations or agencies.

Programs are ongoing organized activities that become part of the continuing health services of a community or organization, whereas projects are smaller, organized activities with a limited time frame. A health fair and a blood pressure screening day at the mall are examples of projects that nurses may implement.

Planning is defined as the selecting and carrying out of a series of activities designed to achieve desired improvements (Issel, 2008). The *goal* of planning is to ensure that health care services are acceptable, equal, efficient, and effective. Planning provides a blueprint for coordination of resources to achieve these goals. Evaluation is determining whether a service is needed and can be used, whether it is conducted as planned, and whether the service actually helps people in need (Royse, 2010). Evaluation is a process of accountability. Evaluation for the purpose of assessing whether objectives are met or planned activities are completed is referred to as *formative* or *process evaluation.* This type of evaluation begins with an assessment of the need for a program and involves ongoing monitoring of the activities conducted by the program. Evaluation to assess program outcomes or as a follow-up of the results of the program activities is called *summative* or *impact evaluation.*

Program evaluation is an ongoing process from the beginning of the planning phase until the program ends. It is used to make judgments about improving, managing, and continuing programs. The major goals of program evaluation are to determine the relevance, adequacy, progress, efficiency, effectiveness, impact, and sustainability of program activities (Veney and Kaluzny, 2008).

HISTORICAL OVERVIEW OF HEALTH CARE PLANNING AND EVALUATION

As the health care delivery system has grown during the last century, emphasis on health planning and evaluation has increased. Factors that have intensified interest in planning and evaluation are advances in health care technology and consumer education, escalating health care costs, increased consumer expectations, third-party payers, focus on health care as a business, personnel shortages, unionizing of health care workers, professional conflicts, focus on preventive care, recognition of increasing health disparities, and the threats from terrorism, natural disasters, and emerging infectious diseases. From the 1920s to the 1940s, specific actions were initiated that related to health planning. Table 25-1 outlines the development of health planning.

The post–World War II era brought an interest in evaluating program effectiveness. As government and third-party payers began to finance health care services and money became more plentiful, public demand for health services grew. As a result, numbers and kinds of health care agencies increased; laws were passed to increase the scope of and control over health care, and the health care delivery system began to be held accountable for its actions. During this time, legislation was passed to require health care providers and consumers to work together in groups to address issues in health care.

Through the 1970s, laws were passed to provide more comprehensive structure and more power over federal program funds. In 1974 Congress enacted the National Health Planning and Resources Development Act. This legislation had the goal of reducing the growth of health care costs by ensuring that only needed services and facilities would be added to the health care system. Under this legislation, health care providers were required to obtain a certificate of need (CON) in order to add services or facilities. However, very little authority existed to carry out some of the more critical tasks of improving the health of clients, increasing access and quality of services, restraining costs, and preventing the duplication of unnecessary services. Power over the private health care sector continued to be absent.

As "the new federalism" became the catch phrase of the 1980s and emphasis was placed on shifting costs, reducing costs, and providing more competition within the health care system, President Ronald Reagan proposed eliminating the federal government's role in health planning. In 1981, with cutbacks in federal spending, states began the takeover or dismantling of their own health planning systems. The national health planning system came to a halt. The federal, state, and consumer partnership for health care was ended.

In 1993, with President Bill Clinton's emphasis on health care reform, the decision was made that the government would continue to not be involved in health planning. It would use its power to set limits on health insurance costs and limit overall health care spending. In this way, it would influence health planning decisions made by the private health care agencies and providers (Sparer, 2008). Although national health care reform did not occur, many states engaged in reforming their systems.

Today, in the early years of the twenty-first century, the process of health planning was not coordinated but is for the most part in the control of different interests in the health care industry. The health care system has been mainly shaped by decisions of hospitals, physicians, pharmaceutical companies, equipment companies, insurance companies, and managed care organizations, which determine where, how, and for whom health care will be delivered. Although the federal health planning legislation is no longer in effect, some states continue to have health system agencies (HSAs), even though these organizations have much less authority than when they were established in the 1970s. In some states, the HSA must approve the planned expanding of agencies or services, and a CON must be issued by the state before these plans may proceed. The primary purpose of such health planning is to improve the health of local communities by increasing available and accessible services, preventing the duplication of services, and controlling health care costs.

The political party in power often influences the outcome of the national and state health planning efforts. To impact the direction of health care reform, nurses must be involved in all aspects of health planning for the community in which they live. An example of this is the recent passage of the Patient Protection and Affordable Care Act, led by President Obama and the Democratic party in March 2010, which addresses planning at national, state, and local levels (PL 111-148). The American Nurses Association (March 2010) reports numerous activities nurses participated in related to the health care reform effort (see http://www.nursingworld.com/healthcarereform).

In addition to health planning in the external environment, internal health care agency planning is necessary to meet the

TABLE 25-1   HISTORICAL DEVELOPMENT OF HEALTH PLANNING AND EVALUATION

YEAR	INITIATOR	ACTION-PURPOSE
Late 1800s	Lumber, railroad, mining, and other industry	Contract with providers for health care to maintain health of workers.
1920	Committees on administrative practice and evaluation of American Public Health Association	Called for public health officers to engage in better program planning. Reduced haphazard methods used to develop public health programs.
1920s	Committee on costs of medical care	Studied social and economic aspects of health services. Cited the need for comprehensive health care planning because of rising costs and unequal health care services to target populations.
1921	Congress	Sheppard Towner Act on Maternity and Infancy provided first continuing program of federal grants-in-aid for state health departments to provide direct care. States established maternal-child divisions with the funding.
1930s	Federal government, Congress	Blue Cross Insurance founded for provision of prepayment for hospital services in response to Great Depression and increased cost of health care.
1935	Federal government, Congress	Social Security Act passed. This was an early movement to provide resources for the elderly and impoverished.
1944	American Hospital Association	Established committee on post-war planning.
1946	Federal government, Congress	Passed the Hospital Survey and Construction Act (Hill-Burton Act) to legislate health planning, which resulted in increase in number of hospitals.
1963	Federal government, Congress	Community Mental Health Centers Act (PL 88-464) passed to provide mental health programs in the states; defined the role of consumers in making decisions and of professionals as advisors in the planning process.
1965	U.S. Department of Health and Human Services	Office of Health Planning opened; no direct authority for health planning given.
1965	Federal government, Congress	Passed regional medical program legislation (PL 89-239); upgraded quality of tertiary health care services for the leading causes of death. Coined the term *Partnership for Health*.
1966	Federal government, Congress	Passed the Comprehensive Health Planning (CHP) and Public Health Services amendments (Public Law 89-749). Developed a national health planning system.
Late 1960s to early 1970s	Individual state legislation	Certificate of Need established as a check against duplication of services. Limited new construction, plant modernization, and major technology.
1973	President Nixon	Government encouragement for health maintenance organizations (HMOs) for prepaid health insurance with emphasis on preventive health efforts.
1974	Federal government, Congress	Passed National Health Planning and Resources Development Act (Public Law 93-641), which provided specific directions for developing the structure, process, and functions of a national health planning system.
1980	U.S. Department of Health and Human Services	Began *Healthy People* initiative. Support for national level assessment, data collection, analysis, goal setting, and evaluation for the U.S. population.
1982	Congress	Tax Equity and Fiscal Responsibility Act (TEFRA) imposed financial cuts to Medicare and Medicaid and directed the Department of Health and Human Services (DHHS) to instill a prospective payment system for hospitals. Capitation through prospective payment was created with diagnosis-related groups (DRGs).
1993	President Clinton	Introduced Health Security Act to provide for health care reform and planning based on population needs (not passed).
2000	Congress	Home Health Prospective Payment System placed capitation on Medicare home health expenses based on clinical assessment of recipients using the Outcome and Assessment Information Set (OASIS).
2001	Congress	Creation of Department of Homeland Security following the terrorist attacks of September 11, 2001. Consolidated selected government departments into one entity for providing national security.
2004	CDC	Development of guidelines for distribution of flu vaccine to the U.S. population following flu vaccine recall.
2005	Hurricane Katrina	This natural disaster on the Gulf Coast and New Orleans shed light on deficiencies of government for emergency planning at local, state, and national levels.
2010	President Obama	Passage into law of the Patient Protection and Affordable Health Care Act (Public Law 111-148).

goals and objectives of providing efficient, effective health care services to clients at a reasonable cost. Health care planning within the community and national health care planning affect health planning within an agency. For example, following the attack on the World Trade Center in 2001, there was much emphasis on developing national and community health plans for emergency preparedness and to prevent terrorism. In a comprehensive reorganization of the federal government, President George W. Bush created the Department of Homeland Security. This reorganization consolidated 22 federal agencies into a single department with the goal of protecting America from terrorism. In addition, states and communities have been given federal monies to develop their own plans. Agencies within communities have been asked to develop emergency preparedness plans and to be a part of community plans.

Public health personnel have a responsibility to participate in internal planning and evaluation to solve the problems of a client population and to ensure the delivery of health services that are accessible, acceptable, and affordable.

BENEFITS OF PROGRAM PLANNING

Systematic planning for meeting the health needs of populations in a community has benefits for clients, nurses, employing agencies, and the community. It ensures that available resources are used to address the actual needs of people in the community, and it focuses attention on what the organization and health provider are attempting to do for clients. Planning assists in identifying the resources and activities that are needed to meet the objectives of client services. It also reduces role ambiguity (uncertainty) by giving responsibility to specific providers to meet program objectives.

Furthermore, planning reduces uncertainty within the program environment and increases the abilities of the provider and the agency to cope with the external environment. Everyone involved with the program can anticipate what will be needed to implement the program, what will occur during the implementation process, and what the program outcomes will be. Planning helps the provider and the agency anticipate events. Also, planning allows for quality decision making and better control over the actual program results by setting specific goals, examining those goals regularly to determine whether the agency continues with the existing programs or makes changes based on the needs of the population they serve. Today, this type of planning is referred to as **strategic planning,** and it involves the successful matching of client needs with specific provider strengths and competencies and agency resources. Managers of programs engage in *management planning*. This type of planning assists managers to determine whether the resources of the agency are used properly to actually implement the agency programs. The type of planning emphasized in this chapter is the program planning process (Kettner et al, 2008). This **planning process** shifts from a focus on the agency as a unit to one aspect of the agency. Program planning reflects the desires to implement a reality-based program that can be readily evaluated and can reduce the number of unexpected events that occur in a defined population. There can be numerous programs within

an agency, and each needs to engage in program planning and evaluation.

> **THE CUTTING EDGE**   *A major national program to assist communities to plan, organize, and develop programs specific to their needs is called Turning Point. Visit http://www.turningpointprogram.org for more information.*

ASSESSMENT OF NEED

Planning for effective and efficient programs must be based on identifying the needs of populations within a community. Identification of at-risk groups and documentation of the health needs of the targeted population provide the basic justification and rationale for the proposed program plan. Such documentation of need is essential if funding will be required to implement the plan. Funding is always required either from the agency or the community at large unless the program is totally voluntarily. An assessment of health needs may be approached as either a community assessment or a population needs assessment.

Community Assessment

A thorough assessment of a community is necessary to provide a clear understanding of the overall health status of a community, to identify populations at risk, and to document health needs. Public health agencies, health planners, nurses, and agencies wishing to address the true needs of a community benefit from accurate and thorough community assessment data.

A **community assessment** is comprehensive. It is a population-focused approach that views the entire community as the client. Community assessment considers all of the people in a community for the purpose of identifying the most vulnerable populations and determining unmet health needs. All of the services of a community are examined to assess their effect on the health of the population, and the environment is assessed for its impact on the health of the people. For example, some vulnerable groups may lack access to existing services because of lack of transportation, or there may be a high prevalence of asthma because of air pollution from a particular industrial source.

Community assessment begins with the collection of existing data (secondary data). Variables related to the characteristics of the population in the community include demographic data such as age, sex, ethnic group/race, income, occupation, education, and health status. Such data, which for most communities are readily available on the Internet, are derived from census data and morbidity and mortality statistics. Much can be learned about a community through use of secondary data found on the Internet (UNC, 2009). In addition, data about communities may be found in local libraries, courthouse records, service agencies, newspapers, the phonebook, and other local resources. Public health departments are also good sources of secondary data.

New data about the community may be collected through surveys or interviews with community members and key informants. When community members have a voice in clarifying

BOX 25-1 EXAMPLE OF A REAL-TIME COMMUNITY ASSESSMENT

Public Health Assessments in Three Communities after Hurricane Ike: Liberty, Brazoria, and Galveston Counties, Texas, September 25-30, 2008

Community assessment data can help social groups and the government understand residents' needs on a regular basis as well as in times of crises. Specific reports were prepared based on the assessment of each community identifying the need for expediting restoration of electricity, trash and debris removal services, housing, vector control, and the potential need for tetanus vaccine. The results assisted the Health District to gain local and state support for needed public health outreach activities. The assessment provided insight to citizens' concerns that the Health District used in answering questions received at the local phone bank. In addition, a one-page flyer to address community issues was developed and consisted of quick reference information (which included contact numbers) such as medical care sources, utilities, vaccination sites, transportation, mosquito prevention techniques, garbage collection, mold prevention, safety guidelines for use of generator or charcoal/gas grills, and local availability of services. About 6000 flyers were distributed door to door and at identified sites within a week throughout the island.

The assessment was valuable because it provided quantifiable information that was used to educate local emergency and elected officials of the health hazards related to lack of basic utilities and health care in the community. The nurse can be essential to the answering of questions and monitoring the phone bank and assisting residents to locate needed supplies and other services. Nurses are valuable in establishing programs and services based on the assessment such as mass immunization clinics for vaccinations needed as well as assisting in providing health care services at temporary shelters, or temporary clinics.

Adapted and excerpted from information provided by the Texas Department of State Health Services, Galveston County Health District, Brazoria County Health Department, Centers for Disease Control and Prevention, and the U.S. Public Health Service Applied Public Health Team 3 (2008); Rodenbeck S: Essential environmental services provided by USPHS applied public health teams after disasters, CDC, 2008, Atlanta, GA, USPHS.

norms and values of their community, in identifying needs, and in planning programs, community acceptance and use of that program are likely to be increased.

Variables related to people, resources, and the environment of a community may be determined by using existing models that provide an organizing framework for the collection and analysis of data (Box 25-1). (For more information about community assessment and the community-as-partner model, see Chapter 18.)

Population Needs Assessment

Agencies or health care providers are frequently interested in providing a specific service in a community and want to assess the need for that service in a target population. In this case, an assessment may be focused on determining the needs of a specific population in a community. The *assessment of need* is defined as a systematic appraisal of type, depth, and scope of problems as perceived by clients or health providers, or both.

A population needs assessment focuses on the characteristics of a specific population, its health needs, and the resources available to address those needs. For example, a nurse may want to initiate a health education program for older adults with diabetes, to establish an immunization program for children of a certain age, or to provide health services for migrant workers. In each case, assessment would focus on the characteristics and health status of the target population and the resources available to address the identified need for that group. When assessing a population, the same types of data collected for community assessment are collected and entered for the population, such as demographic data.

It is important to avoid planning services that do not focus on the health needs of the target population and services already provided by other agencies. A needs assessment determines gaps in or duplication of needed services (i.e., their availability), examines the quality of existing resources to meet the identified needs (i.e., their adequacy), and identifies barriers to the use of existing resources (i.e., their acceptability).

A number of needs assessment tools exist to assist the nurse in the needs assessment process. The major sources of information used for needs assessment, summarized in Table 25-2, are census data, key informants, community forums, surveys of existing community agencies with similar programs, surveys of residents of the community to be served (client population), and statistical indicators (Kettner et al, 2008).

DID YOU KNOW? *Nurses working in community agencies who identify unmet needs among vulnerable populations can initiate program development and find funding to provide needed services and modify health disparities. For example, staff public health nurses in one community identified a need for schools to have more school health nurses, especially to meet the needs of unserved children in poverty. The nurses held a series of meetings with key informants, surveyed health departments of surrounding counties, and found an unknown source of funds through the state Medicaid program that would reimburse public health nurses for providing school health services. The result was the development of a program to increase the numbers of school health nurses in the community.*

PLANNING PROCESS

Health program planning is affected by government control over licensure and funding by political forces, and by the culture and belief system of the population in which the program must function. Program planning is required by federal, state, and local governments; by philanthropic organizations; and by the employing agency. Planning programs and planning for the evaluation of programs are two very important activities, whether the program being planned is a national health insurance program such as Medicare, a state health care program such as an early childhood development screening program, or a local program such as vision screening for elementary school children. Regardless of the type of program, the planning process is the same.

Nutt (1984) describes a basic planning process that is reflected in the steps of most planning methods and remains a great influence on strategic planning for population health and

TABLE 25-2   SUMMARY OF NEEDS ASSESSMENT TOOLS

NAME	DEFINITION	ADVANTAGES	DISADVANTAGES
Community forum	Community, group, organization, open meeting	Low cost Learn perspectives of large number of persons	Limited data Limited expression of views Discourages less powerful Becomes arena to discuss political issues
Focus groups	Open discussion with small representative groups	Low cost Clients participate in identification of need Initiates community support for the program	Time consuming Allows focus on irrelevant or political issues
Key informant	Identify, select, and question knowledgeable leaders	Provides picture of services needed	Bias of leaders Community characteristics may be incorrectly perceived by informants
Indicators approach	Existing data used to determine problem	Excellent data on problems and characteristics of client groups	Growth and change in population may make data outdated
Survey of existing agencies	Estimates of client populations via services used at similar community agencies	Easy method to estimate size of client group Know extent of services offered in existing programs	Records and data may be unreliable All cases of need may not be reported Exaggeration of services may occur
Surveys	Measurement of total or sample client population by interview or questionnaire	Direct and accurate data on client population and their problems	Expensive Technically demanding Need many interviews or observations Interviews may be biased

health programs today (Issel, 2008). The process includes five planning stages: formulating, conceptualizing, detailing, evaluating, and implementing (Table 25-3).

Basic Program Planning Model Using a Population-Level Example

Formulating

The initial and most critical step in planning a health program is defining the problem and assessing client need. This stage in the planning process can be *preactive,* projecting a future need; *reactive,* defining the problem based on past needs; *inactive,* defining the problem on the basis of the existing health state of the population to be served; or *interactive,* describing the problem using past and present data to project future population needs.

Needs assessment is a key component of the planning process in the formulating stage. The target population or client to be served by any program must be identified and involved in every stage of designing the program. To avoid duplication or gaps in services, program planners must verify that a current health problem exists and is being either ignored or unsuccessfully treated in a client group. Data provide the rationale to establish a new program or revise existing programs to meet the needs of the client group. The client population should be defined specifically by its demographic and psychosocial characteristics, by geographic location, and by problems to be addressed (Figure 25-1).

For example, in a community with a large number of preschool children who require immunizations to enter school, the client population may be described as all children between 4 and 6 years of age residing in Central County who have not had

TABLE 25-3   BASIC PLANNING PROCESS

BASIC PLANNING	ELEMENTS
1. Formulating	Client identifies problems.
2. Conceptualizing	Provider group identifies solutions.
3. Detailing	Client and provider analyze available solutions.
4. Evaluating (the plan)	Client, providers, and administrators select best plan.
5. Implementing	Best plan is presented to administrators for funding.

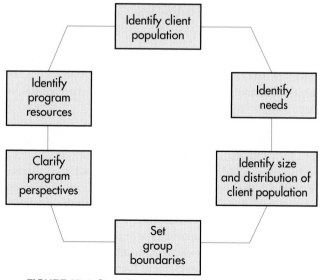

FIGURE 25-1 Steps in the needs assessment process.

up-to-date immunizations. A health education program may be necessary to alert the population to the existing need. In the example of the need for immunizing preschool children, public service announcements on television and radio and in newspapers may be used to alert parents to laws requiring immunizations, to the continuing problems with communicable diseases, and to the outcomes of successful immunizing programs, such as vaccination programs that have been successful in eliminating smallpox worldwide. A good example of the use of media was seen when an outbreak of rubella occurred in Los Angeles. Local and national television was used to bring attention to the problem, to encourage parents to have children immunized, and to encourage other communities to launch campaigns to prevent additional outbreaks.

Specifying the size and distribution of a client population for a program involves more than counting the number of persons in the community who may be eligible for the program. It involves determining the number of persons with the problem who are not being served by existing programs and the numbers of eligible persons who have and who have not taken advantage of existing services. For example, consider again the community need for a preschool immunization program. In planning the program, the size of the population of preschool children in the county may be obtained from census data or state vital statistics. The nurse then must determine the number of children unserved and the number of children who have not used services for which they are eligible. Today there are many opportunities to locate the unserved children through early start programs for preschool children.

Boundaries for the client population are primarily established by defining the size and distribution of the client population. The boundaries will stipulate who is included in and who is excluded from the health program. If the fictional immunization program were designed to serve only preschool children of low-income families, all other preschool children would be excluded.

Perspectives on the program, or what people think about the need for a program, might differ between health providers, agency administrators, policy makers, and potential clients. These groups are considered the stakeholders in the program. Collecting data on the opinions and attitudes of all persons, whether directly or indirectly involved with the program, is necessary to determine if the program is feasible, if there is a need to redefine the problems, or if a new program should be developed or an existing program should be expanded or modified. If a new or changed program is to be successful, it must not only be *available,* but also be *accessible* and *acceptable* to the people who will use it. For example, policy makers in the 1970s decided that neighborhood health clinics were the answer to providing services for low-income residents. They discovered that their perspective was not the same as those of most health providers and clients, who did not support development of neighborhood clinics. The neighborhood health clinics were unsuccessful because the clients would not use them. If the policy makers had explored the perspectives of the clients when planning the program, they might have chosen another type of service to offer. Today community health centers have replaced the concept of

the neighborhood health centers, and these centers are being supported and increased in number by health care reform.

Before implementing a health program, the nurse must also identify available resources. *Program resources* include financing, personnel, facilities, and equipment and supplies. The source and amount of funds must be adequate to support the program. The number and kinds of personnel required and available must be determined. There must be a place for the program to operate, and up-to-date equipment and supplies are essential. If any one of the four categories of resources is unavailable, the program is likely to be inadequate to meet the needs of the client population. If planners consider the problem to be a critical one, funding may be sought by seeking donations or by writing a proposal for grant funds to support the program. A well-done assessment provides direction and suggests strategies for appropriate interventions (see the Evidence-Based Practice box).

NURSING TIP *The needs to be met for the client population must be identified by both the client and the health provider if the program is to be accepted by the client population. If the client population does not recognize the need, the program will usually be unsuccessful.*

Conceptualizing

The need and demand for a program are determined through the formulating process. The conceptualizing stage of planning creates options for solving the problem and considers several solutions. Each option for program solution is examined for its uncertainties (risks) and consequences, leading to a set of *outcomes.*

EVIDENCE-BASED PRACTICE

In *Healthy People 2020*, one of the overarching goals aims to achieve health equity, eliminate disparities, and improve the health of all groups. A thorough community assessment was used as the basis for the development of a program that addresses health education needs related to cardiovascular disease for deaf individuals. A community development approach was used, and the deaf community was involved through each step of the program. A 14-member multidisciplinary coalition was created that included 9 non-deaf and 5 deaf (lay) community members. The group focused on data gathering using two interview guides: A General Health Interview Guide and The Heart Health Risk Interview. Individuals fluent in sign language conducted the interviews. The coalition analyzed the results of the interviews, determined a community diagnosis, and decided on a program for implementation based on the assessment and community diagnosis. The Deaf Heart Health Intervention (DHHI) uses social cognitive theory as the conceptual foundation for the intervention. The intervention is 8 weeks long with classroom and home assignments. The intervention uses a train-the-trainer, community health worker model.

Nurse Use

The nurse can use this study to find effective strategies to work with groups with disabilities and to plan services that are acceptable and useful.

From Jones EG, Renger R, Firestone R: Deaf community analysis for health education priorities, *Public Health Nurs* 22:27-35, 2005.

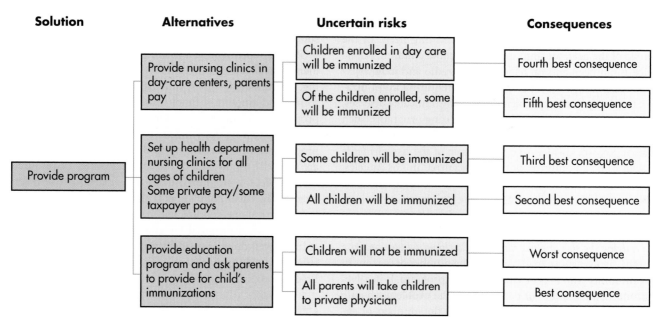

FIGURE 25-2 Ranking of solutions to a problem: providing a preschool immunization program to low-income children using a decision tree.

A first step in the conceptualizing process is a review of the literature to determine what approaches have been used in other places with similar problems, and with what success. Such review can assist nurses to improve the quality, effectiveness, and appropriateness of health programs by synthesizing the evidence and translating it into practice (evidence-based practice). Review of the literature should be guided by the following question: What can be learned from the experience of others in similar circumstances?

Some alternative solutions to the problem will have more risks or uncertainties than others. The nurse must decide between a solution that involves more risk and a solution that is free of risk. A "do nothing" decision is always the decision with the least risk to the provider. When choosing a solution, the nurse looks at whether the desired outcome can be achieved. After careful thought about each possible solution to the problem, the nurse rethinks the solutions. The assessment data compiled during the formulation stage should be used to develop alternative solutions.

Decision trees are useful graphic aids that give a picture of the solutions and the risks of each solution. Such a picture graph of the process of identifying a solution helps clients and administrators rank the consequences of a decision. Figure 25-2 shows an example of a decision tree.

As shown in Figure 25-2, the best consequence would be for each low-income child to be given flu immunization by their private physician. One must consider the value of this action to the person, the odds that immunizations will be obtained, the cost to families as opposed to the taxpayer, and the cost to the community. Costs to the community include the possibility of increased incidence of communicable disease or mortality and increased need for more expensive services to treat the diseases if vulnerable people

are not immunized. Conversely, if families self-pay for the immunizations, costs to the taxpayer and to the community are low.

Detailing

In this phase, the provider, with client input, considers the possibilities of solving a problem using one of the solutions identified. The provider details (or is specific about) the costs, resources, and program activities needed to choose one of the solutions from the conceptualizing phase. For each of the three proposed alternatives shown in the immunization scenario in Figure 25-2, the program planner lists the activities that would need to be implemented. Using the proposed solution of encouraging families to see their private physicians for the vaccine (the best consequence), examples of activities include developing a script for a health education program and implementing a television program to encourage parents to see a physician. If an alternative that produced the second, third, fourth, or fifth best consequence was chosen, offering a clinic at the health department or providing a mobile clinic to each day care center to provide the immunizations would be possible activities.

For each alternative, the nurse lists the resources needed to implement each activity. The resources to be considered include all costs of personnel, supplies, equipment, and facilities, and the potential acceptance by the clients and the administrators of the program. In the example, personnel could include nurses, volunteers, and clerks; supplies might include handouts, Band-Aids, vaccines, records, and consent forms; equipment might include syringes, needles, stethoscopes, and blood pressure cuffs; and facilities might include a television studio for a media blitz on the education program and a room with examination tables, chairs, and emergency carts. The total costs of each

TABLE 25-4 COMPARISON OF THE NURSING PROCESS AND PROGRAM PLANNING

NURSING PROCESS	BASIC PLANNING PROCESS
Assessment Subjective and objective data are systematically collected.	**Formulation** Assess the client's need and define the problem.
Nursing Diagnosis Client's problem is defined by using the assessment data to guide the nurse in looking for similar patterns in the systematically collected subjective and objective data.	**Conceptualization** Provider group identifies solutions; each solution is examined for its risks, consequences, and expected outcomes.
Nursing Intervention Any direct care treatment or nursing action based on the nursing diagnosis is performed by a nurse and includes rationale that justifies the treatment or nursing action. Treatment or action is evaluated by the nurse for its appropriateness and acceptability to the client before implementation.	**Detailing** Client and provider analyze solutions proposed in the conceptualizing phase for costs, resources, and program activities.
Implementation Direct care treatment or nursing action established in the intervention is implemented.	**Evaluation of the Plan** Client, providers, and administrators select best plan based on costs, benefits, and acceptability of the plan to the client and provider.
Evaluation Implementation of the nursing intervention is evaluated.	**Implementation** Best plan (solution) based on input from the client and provider is presented to administration and implemented.
	Program Evaluation Implemented best plan (solution) is evaluated.

solution must be considered. As indicated, clients should review each solution for acceptance.

Evaluating

In the evaluation phase of the plan, each alternative is weighed to judge the costs, benefits, and acceptance of the idea to the client population, community, and providers. The information outlined in the detailing phase would be used to rank the solutions for choice by the client population and provider on the basis of cost, benefit, and acceptance. Consideration must be given to the solution that will provide the desired outcomes. Review of the literature or interviews might disclose whether someone else had previously tried each of the options in another place, and what costs and outcomes occurred. The experience of others in similar circumstances is helpful in deciding whether a chosen solution would be useful.

Implementing

In the planning process, the clients, providers, and administrators selected the best plan to solve the original problem. Providing reasons why a particular solution was chosen will help the provider get the approval of the agency administration for the plan. Once approved, the plan is implemented.

Implementation requires obtaining and managing the resources required to operationalize the program in a way that is consistent with the plan. Program implementation requires accountability and responsibility (Issel, 2008). Change theory

can be useful to help create an environment in which the program is supported.

Community members may participate in implementing the program either as volunteers or as paid staff. Program success will be increased if community residents are included in the work of the program and if they are on advisory boards and participate in program evaluation. The greater the participation of community members in developing a program, the greater the sense of ownership of that program by members of the target population, and therefore the greater the probability that the program will achieve its objectives and result in positive changes in health (Issel, 2008). The planning process may be compared with the nursing process (Table 25-4).

Formulating Objectives

The most important step in the planning and evaluation process is the writing of program objectives. The objectives provide direction for conducting the program, and they provide the mechanism for evaluating specific activities and the total program. The following discussion addresses the development of well-written objectives. Development of program objectives begins with the initial phases of program planning.

Specifying Goals and Objectives. A program may begin with a mission statement. This is a broad general statement of the overall conceptual framework or philosophy of the program. The mission statement clarifies the values and overall purpose of the program and provides a framework for the goals and objectives that follow.

BOX 25-2 LEVELS OF PROGRAM PLAN

- Mission—statement of values
- Goal—overall aim
- Objectives—specific measurable outcomes
- Action steps—explicit actions to accomplish objectives

A goal is a statement that describes the general direction of logical response to a demonstrated need. One or two goals are often sufficient for a program to state how it will resolve or lessen the problem defined in the need statement. The goals should be consistent with the values and overall intent set forth in the mission statement. Their purpose is to focus on the major reason for the program (Box 25-2).

Objectives are concise statements describing in measurable and time-bound terms precisely what specific outcome is to be accomplished. *Measurable* means that the objective contains the specific outcome anticipated that could be documented with collectable data. *Time-bound* means that the objective contains the target date when the specific outcome will be accomplished. Objectives should be realistic and attainable means to meet the program goal.

Clear, concise, and measurable objectives help with evaluating the program. If the objectives are too general, program evaluation becomes impossible. The objectives must be specific and stated so that anyone reading them could conduct the program without further instruction. The document *Healthy People 2020* (USDHHS, 2010) may be used as a template to guide the development of more specific objectives that are tailored to address the needs of a given community.

Useful program objectives include a statement of the specific behaviors that the program will accomplish, and success criteria, or expected results, for the program. Each program objective requires a *strong, action-oriented verb* to specify the behavior; *a statement of a single purpose; a statement of a single result;* and *a time frame for achieving the expected result.*

For example, a general program goal may be to reduce the incidence of low-birth-weight babies in Center County by 2020 by improving access to prenatal care. Several specific objectives are required to meet a general program goal. A specific objective for this program may be to open (action verb) a prenatal clinic in each health department within the county by January 2015 (time frame) to serve the population within each census tract of the county (purpose) to improve pregnancy outcomes (result).

As objectives are developed, an *operational indicator* for each objective should be considered so the evaluator knows when and if the objective has been met. For instance, an operational indicator for the previous objective would be a 10% to 25% increase in the use of prenatal care by women in Center County. Such indicators provide a target for persons involved with implementing programs. A review of *Healthy People 2020* health objectives will give the reader examples of objectives that include all the elements just listed.

Action steps are written for each program objective. An action step is defined as a concise statement describing precisely how (by what method), when, and by whom each activity will

BOX 25-3 PLANNING PROGRAMS FOR ELDERS IN THE COMMUNITY

The Jefferson Area Board for Aging (JABA) has created a vision for the one-city, five-county planning district. In concert with 85 public and private organizations and more than 500 individuals, they developed a comprehensive community plan, known as the "2020 Community Plan on Aging." The plan started with a comprehensive community assessment that addressed the livability for elders in the community. The "2020 Community Plan on Aging" has been an asset for the community in providing guidance for specific programs at JABA and throughout the community. In September 2005 the city of Charlottesville and the surrounding counties were honored when presented with the U.S. Department of Health and Human Services, Administration on Aging (AOA), "Livable Communities for All Ages" award. Seven communities received the award for their model efforts to make their communities more supportive places to live and grow for seniors and all populations. The competition was administered by the Center for Home Care and Policy Research, Visiting Nurse Service of New York, with the participation of the American Planning Association and the International City/County Management Association.

Excerpted from Jefferson Area Board of Aging: What we do and who we are, *JABA Facts,* 2010. Available at http://www.jabacares.org/. Accessed January 31, 2011.

be accomplished in order to achieve the objective for which it was written. These activities address resources, such as number of nurses, equipment, supplies, and location. A time frame is planned for each activity. It is assumed that as each specific objective is met, progress is made toward achieving the general program objective (or goal) (Box 25-3).

HOW TO Develop a Program Plan

A. Define the problem
B. Formulate the plan
  1. Assess population need
    a. Who is the program population?
    b. What is the need to be met?
    c. How large is the client population to be served?
    d. Where are they located?
    e. How does the target population define the need?
    f. Are there other programs addressing the same need? (Describe.)
    g. Why is the need not being met?
  2. Establish program boundaries
    a. Who will be included in the program?
    b. Who will not be included? Why?
    c. What is the program goal?
  3. Program feasibility
    a. Who agrees that the program is needed (stakeholders: administrators, providers, clients, funders)?
    b. Who does not agree?
  4. Resources (general)
    a. What personnel are needed? What personnel are available?
    b. What facilities are needed? What facilities are available?
    c. What equipment is needed? What equipment is available?
    d. Is funding available to support the project? Is additional funding needed?

e. Are resources being donated (space, printing, paper, medical supplies)?
  (1) Type
  (2) Amount
5. Tools used to assess need
  a. Census data
  b. Key informants
  c. Focus groups
  d. Community forums
  e. Existing program surveys
  f. Surveys of client population
  g. Statistical indicators (e.g., demographic and morbidity/mortality data)
C. Conceptualize the problem
1. List the potential solutions to the problem.
2. What are the risks of each solution?
3. What are the consequences?
4. What are the outcomes to be gained from the solutions?
5. Draw a decision tree to show the problem-solving process used.
D. Detail the plan
1. What are the objectives for each solution to meet the program goal?
2. What activities will be done to conduct each of the alternative solutions listed under C1 and based on objectives?
3. What are the differences in the resources needed for each of the alternative solutions?
4. Which of the alternative solutions would be chosen if the resources described under B4 were the only resources available?
5. Who would be responsible or accountable for implementing the plan?
E. Evaluate the plan
1. Which of the alternative solutions is most acceptable to the following:
  a. The client population
  b. The agency administrator
  c. You
  d. The community
2. Which of the alternative solutions appears to have the most benefits to the following:
  a. The client population
  b. The agency administrator
  c. You
  d. The community
3. On the basis of cost, which alternative solution would be chosen by the following:
  a. The client population
  b. The agency administrator
  c. You
  d. The community
F. Implement the program plan
1. On the basis of data collected, which of the solutions has been chosen?
2. Why should the agency administrator approve your request? Give a rationale.
3. Will additional funding be sought?
4. When can the program begin? Give date.

Developed by Marcia Stanhope and based on the Basic Program Planning Model (Nutt, 1984; Issel, 2008).

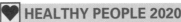

HEALTHY PEOPLE 2020

Example of Healthy People 2020 Goals for Program Planning

FOCUS AREA	OVERALL GOAL	OBJECTIVE	MEASURING THE OBJECTIVE
IID-23: Immunization and infectious diseases	Attain high-quality, longer lives free of preventable disease, disability, injury, and premature death.	IID-11: Increase routine vaccination coverage levels for adolescents.	IID: 11-1: Increase (action verb) to one dose of tetanus-diphtheria-acellular pertussis (Tdap) booster vaccine by 13 to 15 years (Purpose) for 80% of this age group (operational indicator) by 2020 (timeframe).

From USDHHS: *Healthy People 2020: a roadmap for health,* Washington, DC, 2010, U.S. Government Printing Office.

PROGRAM EVALUATION

Benefits of Program Evaluation

Program evaluation is a method of ensuring that a program has met its goals. It is a means of documenting accountability by the program managers to the clients and the funding sources. The major benefit of program evaluation is that it shows whether the program is fulfilling its purpose. It should answer the following questions:

1. Are the needs for which the program was designed being met?
2. Are the problems it was designed to solve being solved?

This is critical information for program managers, funding agencies, top-level decision makers, program accreditation reviewers, health providers, and the community. Evaluation data are used to make judgments about a program and may be used to justify sustaining the program, making adjustments in the program, expanding or reducing the program, or even discontinuing it.

Process evaluation, also referred to as formative evaluation, occurs during the program implementation and makes it possible to do mid-program corrections to ensure achievement of program goals. Designing the evaluation during the planning phase of the program allows the evaluation to be guided by the program goals (Issel, 2008). Brownson, Fielding, and Maylahn (2009) describe process evaluation as an ongoing function of examining, documenting, and analyzing the progress of a program. Changes are required when there is an unacceptable difference between what was observed and what was anticipated from the implementation of program activities. Corrective action may then be taken to get the program back on track. This description of process evaluation is consistent with what Veney and Kaluzny (2008) refer to as program monitoring. Three critical questions are addressed when monitoring a program (Veney and Kaluzny, 2008): (1) Does the program reach the target population? (2) Were activities to reach the goals carried out as planned? (3) What was the resource use in implementing the program?

Quality assurance programs are prime examples of program evaluation in health care delivery. Evaluation data are used to justify continuing programs in public health. Program evaluation focuses on whether goals were met and the efficiency and effectiveness of program activities. Many methods of program evaluation are described in the literature. One of the primary methods of evaluation used in health care today is Donabedian's (1982; updated in 2003) classic evaluative framework, which examines the structure, process, and outcomes of a program. Other models and frameworks have been developed using this approach. The tracer method and case register are examples of other methods applied to program evaluation. (See Chapter 26 for further discussion.)

Program records and a community index serve as the major source of information for program evaluation. Surveys, interviews, observations, and diagnostic tests are ways to assess client and community responses to health programs. Cost studies help identify program benefits and objectiveness.

As financial resources become scarce, nursing and the health care system must be able to justify their existence, prove that their services are responsive to client needs, and show their concern for being accountable. Planning and evaluation will assist in meeting these objectives.

Planning for the Evaluation Process

Planning for the evaluation process is an important part of program planning. When the planning process begins, the plan for evaluating the program should also be developed. All persons to be involved in implementing a program should be a part of the plan for program evaluation. Assessment of need is one component of evaluation. The basic questions to be answered, after carefully considering the data collected from a census, key informants, community forums, surveys, or health statistics indicators, are as follows:

1. Will the objectives and resources of this program meet the identified needs of the client population?
2. Is the program relevant?

Once need has been established and the program is designed, the nurse must continue plans for program evaluation. As a part of the planning process, Posavac and Carey (2006) described six steps to use for continuing program evaluation (Figure 25-3):

1. Identify the key people for evaluation. Program personnel, program funders, and the clients of the program should be included in planning for evaluation.
2. Arrange preliminary meetings to discuss the question of how the group wants to evaluate the program and where to start. If the program planners and others agree on an evaluation, the resources needed to do the evaluation must be identified. Evaluation is necessary even though some may not be interested in it. Nurses can help others see that without evaluation, money to support programs will not be available, or the need for a new nurse to help with the work cannot be justified. In health care today, there is great emphasis on outcomes of care. The only way to see outcomes is through evaluation.
3. After the key people have met and considered the questions in the previous steps, they are ready to begin the evaluation

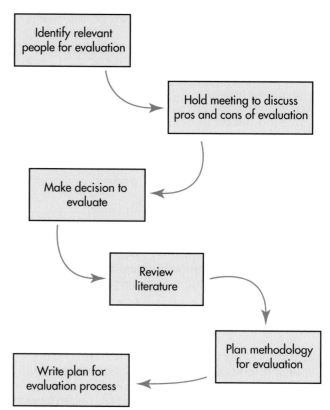

FIGURE 25-3 Six steps in planning for program evaluation.

process. Even though evaluation may be desired, the decision to conduct the evaluation may be an administrative one, based on available resources and existing circumstances. For example, if a program evaluation were attempted in a situation in which program personnel wanted it but clients chose to be uncooperative, evaluation efforts would be unsuccessful.

4. Examine the literature for suggestions about the appropriate methods and techniques for evaluation and their usefulness in program evaluation. If an agency has chosen to use an external evaluator, this person may make suggestions about the questions to be answered in the evaluation process. These questions are based on the program goals. Nurses who have reviewed the literature and communicated with others affected by the evaluation can determine whether the evaluation suggestions are appropriate for the situation.
5. Plan the method to be used, including decisions about what goals and objectives will be measured, how they will be measured, and for what population.
6. Write a plan that outlines the mission and goals of the overall program, the type of evaluation to be done, the operational measures to be used to evaluate the program goals, the choice of who will do the evaluation (i.e., internal or external personnel), the available resources for conducting the evaluation, and the readiness of the organization, personnel, and clients for program evaluation.

WHAT DO YOU THINK?   *Nurses at all levels of education and preparation can participate in program planning and evaluation.*

CDC Framework

Engage **stakeholders**

↓

Describe the program

↓

Focus the evaluation design

↓

Gather credible evidence

↓

Justify conclusions

↓

Ensure use and share lessons learned

Rossi et al. Framework

Goal setting

↓

Determining goal measurement

↓

Identifying goal-attaining activities

↓

Making the activities operational

↓

Measuring the goal effect

↓

Evaluating the program

FIGURE 25-4 The evaluation process.

Evaluation Process

A framework for evaluation in public health has been developed by the Centers for Disease Control and Prevention (CDC) to guide understanding about program evaluation and to facilitate integration of evaluation in the public health system. Royse (2010) further expands this approach. This framework defines program evaluation as a systematic way to improve and to account for public health actions by using methods that are useful, feasible, ethical, and accurate. Six interdependent steps are identified that must be part of an evaluation process (CDC, 1999; Royse, 2010) (Figure 25-4):

1. *Engage stakeholders*—This includes those who are involved in planning, funding, and implementing the program, those who are affected by the program, and the intended users of its services.
2. *Describe the program*—The program description should address the need for the program and should include the mission and goals. This sets the standard for judging the results of the evaluation.
3. *Focus the evaluation design*—Describe the purpose for the evaluation, the users who will receive the report, how it will be used, the questions and methods to be used, and any necessary agreements.
4. *Gather credible evidence*—Specify the indicators that will be used, sources of data, quality of the data, quantity of information to be gathered, and the logistics of the data gathering phase. Data gathered should provide credible evidence and should convey a well-rounded view of the program.
5. *Justify conclusions*—The conclusions of the evaluation should be validated by linking them to the evidence gathered and then appraising them against the values or standards set by the stakeholders. Approaches for analyzing, synthesizing, and interpreting the evidence should be agreed on before data collection begins to ensure that all needed information will be available.

6. *Ensure use and share lessons learned*—Use and dissemination of findings require deliberate effort so that the lessons learned can be used in making decisions about the program.

It should be noted that the steps are very similar to the steps in the planning process:

1. *Goal setting*—The values and beliefs of the agency, the providers, and the clients provide the basis for establishing a mission statement and setting goals, and should be considered at every step of the evaluation process. In the preschool immunization example, the fact that children should not be exposed to early childhood diseases would lead to a program goal to decrease the incidence of early childhood diseases in the county where the program is planned.
2. *Determining goal measurement*—In the case of the previous goal, reduced disease incidence would be an appropriate goal measurement.
3. *Identifying goal-attaining activities*—These activities include, for example, media presentations urging parents to have their children immunized.
4. *Making the activities operational*—This involves the actual administration of the immunizations through the health department clinics.
5. *Measuring the goal effect*—This consists of reviewing the records and summarizing the incidence of early childhood disease before and after implementation of the program.
6. *Evaluating the program*—This involves determining whether the program goal was achieved. Keep in mind that only one program goal is used in this example. Most programs have multiple goals.

Sources of Program Evaluation

Both quantitative and qualitative methods may be used to conduct an evaluation; however, the strongest evaluation designs combine both qualitative and quantitative methods. Major sources of information for program evaluation are the program clients, program records, and community indexes.

Qualitative methods such as site visits, structured observations of interventions, or open-ended interviews may be used (Farquhar et al, 2006). The program participants, or clients of the service, have a unique and valuable role in program evaluation. Whether the clients, for whom the program was designed, accept the services will determine to a large extent whether the program achieves its goal. Thus, their reactions, feelings, and judgments about the program are very important to the evaluation. For example, to garner feedback from participants in a program, an evaluator may use a written survey in the form of a questionnaire or an attitude scale. Interviews and observations are other ways of obtaining feedback about a program. Attitude scales are probably used most often, and they are usually phrased in terms of whether the program met its objectives. The client satisfaction survey is an example of an attitude scale often used in the health care delivery system to evaluate the program objectives (Hsieh, 2006). Client input into the development of evaluation tools ensures that the questions and approaches are more acceptable to the clients and that the tools effectively elicit the information needed.

The second major source of information for program evaluation is program records, especially clinical records. Clinical records provide the evaluator with information about the care given to the client and the results of that care. To determine whether a program goal has been met, one might summarize the data from a group of records. For example, if one overall goal were to reduce the incidence of low-birth-weight babies through prenatal care, records would be reviewed to obtain the number of mothers who received prenatal care and the number of low-birth-weight babies born to them. Records would be reviewed from the beginning of the program and at the end of a specific time frame, such as at the end of each year. Care must be taken to ensure that any review and use of clinical records complies with HIPAA regulations. (For details about HIPAA compliance, see http://aspe.hhs.gov/admnsimp/index.shtml.)

The third major source of evaluation is epidemiological data. Mortality and morbidity data measuring health and illness are probably cited more frequently than any other single index for program evaluation. These health and illness indicators are useful in evaluating the effects of health care programs on the total community. Incidence and prevalence data are valuable indexes for measuring program effectiveness and impact, and these data are readily available on the Internet. Useful sites for such data include vital statistics available at state department of health sites, the CDC, and the U.S. census site. Most counties and communities have their own sites, and many of these contain very useful demographic and health data.

An example of a national program based on a needs assessment of the U.S. population is the national health objectives program *Healthy People 2020* (USDHHS, 2010). *Healthy People* documents have been published every 10 years since 1980. The data gathered from each 10-year period have been used to evaluate the population needs met and the assessment of needs for the next *Healthy People* document.

The Healthy Communities Program (USDHHS, 2010) suggests activities to evaluate national health objectives related to communities. The example shown in the *Healthy People 2020* box on p. 563 highlights injury and violence prevention. This box shows that objectives include an action verb, a result, an operational indicator, and a time frame for implementing the objective (10 years, begun in 2010).

The Levels of Prevention box provides examples of applying levels of prevention to program planning and evaluation.

♥ HEALTHY PEOPLE 2020

Objectives Focus Areas

1. Access to Health Services	22. HIV
2. Adolescent Health	23. Immunization and Infectious Diseases
3. Arthritis, Osteoporosis, and Chronic Back Conditions	24. Injury and Violence Prevention
4. Blood Disorders and Blood Safety	26. Maternal, Infant, and Child Health
5. Cancer	27. Medical Product Safety
6. Chronic Kidney Diseases	28. Mental Health and Mental Disorders
7. Dementias, including Alzheimer's	29. Nutrition and Weight Status
8. Diabetes	30. Occupational Safety and Health
9. Disability and Health	31. Older Adults
10. Early and Middle Childhood	32. Oral Health
11. Educational and Community-Based Programs	33. Physical Activity and Fitness
12. Environmental Health	34. Preparedness
13. Family Planning	35. Public Health Infrastructure
14. Food Safety	36. Respiratory Diseases
15. Genomics	37. Sexually Transmitted Diseases
16. Global Health	38. Sleep Health
17. Healthcare-Associated Infections	40. Substance Abuse
18. Health Communication and Health IT	41. Tobacco Use
20. Hearing and Other Sensory or Communication Disorders (Ear, Nose, Throat—Voice, Speech, and Language)	42. Vision
21. Heart Disease and Stroke	Three other objectives are under development—numbers 19, 25, 39.

From USDHHS: *Healthy People 2020: a roadmap for health,* Washington, DC, 2010, U.S. Government Printing Office.

HEALTHY PEOPLE 2020

Example of a Measurable National Health Objective

In the *Healthy People* focus area of injury and violence prevention, one objective is:

- IPV-5: Increase (action verb) the number of States and the District of Columbia where 90% of deaths of children aged 17 years and under (operational indicator) due to external causes are reviewed by a child fatality review team (purpose), by 2020 (time frame).

From USDHHS: *Healthy People 2020: A roadmap for health,* Washington, DC, 2010, U.S. Government Printing Office.

 LEVELS OF PREVENTION

Program Planning and Evaluation

Primary Prevention
Plan a community-wide program with the local school system and health department to serve healthy meals and snacks in all schools to promote good childhood nutrition.

Secondary Prevention
Develop screening programs for all school children to determine the incidence/prevalence of childhood obesity before implementing the program.

Tertiary Prevention
Evaluate the incidence/prevalence of obesity among school children after the implementation of the program and provide programs to reduce complications from the condition.

Aspects of Evaluation

The aspects of program evaluation include the following (Veney and Kaluzny, 2008):

1. *Relevance*—Need for the program
2. *Adequacy*—Program addresses the extent of the need
3. *Progress*—Tracking of program activities to meet program objectives
4. *Efficiency*—Relationship between program outcomes and the resources spent
5. *Effectiveness*—Ability to meet program objectives and the results of program efforts
6. *Impact*—Long-term changes in the client population
7. *Sustainability*—Enough resources to continue the program

The How To box suggests questions that may be asked about program evaluation using this process.

HOW TO Do a Program Evaluation

To do a program evaluation, first choose the type of evaluation you wish to conduct. Second, identify the goal and objectives for the evaluation. Third, decide who will be involved in the evaluation. Fourth, answer the questions related to the type of evaluation as follows:

A. Program relevance: needs assessment (formative)
  1. Use answers to all questions listed in section B of How To Develop a Program Plan.
  2. On the basis of the needs assessment, was the program necessary?

B. Adequacy
  1. Is the program large enough to make a positive difference in the problem/need?
  2. Are the boundaries of the services defined so that the problem/need can be addressed for the target population?

C. Program progress (formative)
  1. Monitor activities (circle which this reflects: daily, weekly, monthly, annually).
    a. Name the activities provided.
    b. How many hours of service were provided?
    c. How many clients have been served?
    d. How many providers are there?
    e. What types of clients have been served?
    f. What types of providers were needed?
    g. Where have services been offered (e.g., home, clinic, organization)?
    h. How many referrals have been made to community sources?
    i. Which sources have been used to provide support services?
  2. Budget
    a. How much money has been spent to carry out activities?
    b. Will more/less money be needed to conduct activities as outlined?
    c. Will changes to objectives and activities be needed to sustain the program?
    d. What changes do you recommend and why?

D. Program efficiency (formative and summative)
  1. Costs
    a. How do costs of the program compare with those of a similar program to meet the same goal?
    b. Do the activities outlined in C1 compare with the activities in a similar program?
    c. Although this program costs more/less than expected, is it needed? Why?
  2. Productivity (may use national or state averages for comparison)
    a. How many clients does each type of staff see per day (e.g., registered nurses, clinical nurse specialists, nurse practitioners)?
    b. How does this compare with similar programs?
    c. Although the productivity level of this program is low/high, is the program needed? Why?
  3. Benefits
    a. What are the benefits of the program to the clients served?
    b. What are the benefits to the community?
    c. Are the benefits important enough to continue the program? Why? (Look at cost, productivity, and outcomes of care.)

E. Program effectiveness (summative)
  1. Satisfaction
    a. Is the client satisfied with the program as designed?
    b. Are the providers satisfied with the program outcomes?
    c. Is the community satisfied with the program outcomes?
  2. Goals
    a. Did the program meet its stated goal?
    b. Are the client needs being met?
    c. Was the problem solved for which the program was designed?

F. Impact (summative)
  1. Long-term changes in health status (1 year or more)

a. *Have there been changes in the community's health?*
b. *What are the changes seen (e.g., in morbidity or mortality rates, teen pregnancy rates, pregnancy outcomes)?*
c. *Have there been changes in individuals' health status?*
d. *What are the changes seen?*
e. *Has the initial problem been solved or has it returned?*
f. *Is new or revised programming needed? Why?*
g. *Should the program be discontinued? Why?*

G. Sustainability
   1. *Was the program funded as a demonstration or by an external agency?*
   2. *Can money and resources be found to continue the program after the initial funding is gone?*

Depending on the answers to the questions, the program can be found to be successful or unsuccessful.

Developed by Marcia Stanhope using the framework in Veney A, Kaluzny J: Evaluation and decision making for health service programs, Englewood Cliffs, NJ, 2008, Prentice Hall.

The following paragraphs provide an explanation of each step in program evaluation.

Relevance. Evaluation of relevance is an important component of the initial planning phase. As money, providers, facilities, and supplies for delivering health care services are more closely monitored, the needs assessment done by the nurse will determine whether the program is needed.

Adequacy. Evaluation of adequacy looks at the extent to which the program addresses the entire problem defined in the needs assessment. The magnitude of the problem is determined by vital statistics, incidence, prevalence, and expert opinion.

Progress. The monitoring of program activities, such as hours of services, number of providers used, number of referrals made, and amount of money spent to meet program objectives, provides an evaluation of the progress of the program. This type of evaluation is an example of formative or process evaluation, which occurs on an ongoing basis while the program exists. This provides an opportunity to make effective day-to-day management decisions about the operations of the program. Progress evaluation occurs primarily while implementing the program. The nurse who completes a daily or weekly log of clinical activities (e.g., number of clients seen in clinic or visited at home, number of phone contacts, number of referrals made, number of community health promotion activities) is contributing to progress evaluation of the nursing service.

Efficiency. If the reason for evaluation is to examine the efficiency of a program, it may occur on an ongoing basis as formative evaluation or at the end of the program as a summative evaluation. The evaluator may be able to determine whether the program provides better benefits at a lower cost than a similar program, or whether the benefits to the clients, or number of clients served, justify the costs of the program.

Effectiveness and impact. An evaluation of program effectiveness may help the nurse evaluator determine both client and provider satisfaction with the program activities, as well as whether the program met its stated objectives. However, if evaluation of impact is the goal, long-term effects such as changes in morbidity and mortality must be investigated. Both effectiveness and impact evaluations are usually *summative evaluation* functions primarily performed as end-of-program activities.

Sustainability. A program can be continued if there are resources for the program. Ongoing evaluation of sustainability is important!

WHAT DO YOU THINK? *The combination of prenatal care programs delivered by nurses and the supplemental nutritional program for women, infants, and children (WIC) produces better pregnancy and postnatal outcomes for mothers and babies than traditional medical care.*

ADVANCED PLANNING METHODS AND EVALUATION MODELS

After a need and a client demand for a program have been determined through the needs assessment process, the next step in the development of the program is to choose a procedural method that will assist the nurse in planning the program to be offered. The following is offered for students who are more advanced in their career and need to consider several methods of program planning plus more extensive evaluation models for program management.

Five planning methods are discussed in this section:
1. Program planning method (PPM)
2. Multi-attribute utility technique (MAUT)
3. Planning Approach to Community Health (PATCH)
4. Assessment Protocol for Excellence in Public Health (APEXPH)
5. Mobilizing for Action through Planning and Partnership (MAPP)

PPM is a more general approach to program planning, whereas MAUT offers guidelines for identifying and tracking specific program activities essential to program success. PATCH, APEXPH, and MAPP are PPMs that were designed by the CDC and the National Association of County Health Officials with input from local and state health departments. All of these approaches establish the basis for program evaluation.

Program Planning Method

PPM is a technique using the nominal group technique described by Delbecq and Van de Ven in 1971. The nurse can use this method to involve clients more directly in the planning process. PPM is a five-stage process to identify program needs. It focuses on three levels of planning groups composed of clients, providers, and administrators. The client or consumer group relays a list of problems to the provider group, who in turn aids the client group by presenting the solutions to the problems to the administrative group (Issel, 2008).

The stages of PPM are compared with MAUT's planning process in Table 25-5. The five stages are as follows:
1. *Problem diagnosis.* Each client in the group works with all other members of the group to develop a written problem list, one problem at a time. After all problems have been

TABLE 25-5 PLANNING METHODS COMPARED WITH BASIC PLANNING PROCESS

BASIC PLANNING	PPM	PATCH	APEXPH	MAUT	MAPP
Formulating	Problems identified by client.	Community members identify health priorities.	Assess community capacity to address health problems.	Identify target populations and program objectives.	Assess community themes and strengths, health status, and strategic issues.
Conceptualizing	Provider group identifies solution.	Stakeholders use data to develop program activities.	Assess with community the strengths and health problems.	Identify alternative problem solutions.	Formulate goals and strategies.
Detailing	Analyze available solutions.	Design comprehensive program to meet identified health priorities.	Choose plan based on community capacity resources.	Identify criteria for choice; rank and weight; calculate value.	Develop plan for action; engage in visioning.
Evaluating	Clients, providers, and administrators select best plan.	Use process evaluation to improve program.	Support recommendations for program change.	Choose best alternatives.	Evaluate the plan.
Implementing	Best plan presented to administrators for funding.		Partners implement the plan.		Assess community ability to change and implement the plan.

shared and recorded, they are discussed by the total client group. After the discussion, clients select the problems with the highest priority by voting on the ranking of each problem.

2. *Expert provider group identifies solutions for each of the problems identified by the clients.*
3. *Client and provider groups present their problems and suggested solutions* to the administrative group to determine the possibilities of developing a program to resolve one or more of the problems using one or more of the solutions. In this phase, clients and providers are seeking acceptance from the administrators who control the program resources.
4. *Alternative solutions to the problem are identified,* and the pros and cons of each are analyzed.
5. *Clients, providers, and administrators select the best plan* for program implementation. In this phase, the link between the planned solutions and the problem is evaluated, pointing out strengths and limitations of the proposed program plan.

A nurse might use this technique for developing school health services within the total community or in one school. A nurse working with a senior citizens group might use this method to identify the priority needs for nursing clinic services at the health department. It is important to note that this method is used to obtain consensus among all persons involved in the program: clients, providers, and administrators. Consensus is most helpful in having a successful program. The process may also be used in a community decision-making activity in which community representatives come together to decide health care service needs for the entire community.

Multi-Attribute Utility Technique

MAUT is a planning method based on decision theory (Brennan and Anthony, 2000; Kabassi and Vroom 2006). This method can be adapted for making decisions about the care of a single client or about national health care programs. Recently it has been used to evaluate nursing practice. The purpose of MAUT is to separate all elements of a decision and to evaluate each element separately for its effects on the overall decision, considering available options.

If money is no object, then the option with the highest use value is the best decision. However, if this option exceeds the budget, the next best option may be the alternative to choose. The steps of MAUT (listed in Box 25-4) relate closely to the basic planning process described by Nutt (1984) as shown in Table 25-5.

Steps 1 and 2 of MAUT relate to problem formulating. Step 3 involves conceptualizing the program alternatives, and steps 4 through 9 focus on detailing and the implications of each option. Step 10 involves the evaluating phase of planning or the choice of the best solution as identified in steps 4 through 9. Placing quantitative values on solutions to meet program needs is most helpful in the implementing phase of planning (e.g., convincing administrators of the need for such a program). However, caution must be taken in using all planning methods, because the best solution reflects the bias of the planner.

Planning Approach to Community Health (PATCH)

The PATCH model was developed in the 1980s by the CDC with input from state and local health departments. The model was developed using as a framework the PRECEDE model developed by Laurence Green in the 1970s. The PRECEDE model

BOX 25-4 TEN BASIC STEPS OF THE MULTI-ATTRIBUTE UTILITY TECHNIQUE METHOD

1. Identify the person or aggregate for whom a problem is to be solved. Who is the client for whom the program is being planned?
2. Identify the issue(s) or decision(s) that is (are) relevant. This step involves the identification of the program objectives.
3. Identify the options to be evaluated. The program planner identifies the available options or action alternatives to accomplish the program goals.
4. Identify the relevant criteria related to the value of each option. The program planner places a value on competing options or alternatives or identifies criteria to be considered in making a choice between them.
5. Rank the criteria in order of importance. The program planner decides which of the criteria are most important and which are least important for meeting program goals.
6. Rate criteria in importance. In this step the program planner assigns an arbitrary rating of 10 to the least important criterion. In considering the next least important criterion, the planner decides how many times more important it is than the least important criterion. If it is considered twice as important, the dimension will be assigned a 20. If it is only considered half as important, it will be assigned a 15. If it is considered four times as important, it will be assigned a 40. The process is continued until all criteria have been rated.
7. Add the importance rate, divide each by the sum, and multiply by 100. This process is called *normalizing* the weights. It is recommended that the number of criteria be kept between 6 and 15. Therefore, in this initial process, the planner can be concerned with only general criteria for choosing action alternatives.
8. Measure the location of the option being evaluated by each criterion. The planner may ask a colleague or expert to estimate on a scale of 0 to 100 the probability that a given option from step 3 will maximize the value of the criterion from step 4.
9. Calculate the use of options. The program planner will obtain the usefulness of each identified action alternative by multiplying the weight for each criterion (step 7) by the rating of an option for each criterion (step 8) and adding the products. The sum of the products for each action is termed the *aggregate utility.*
10. Decide on the best alternative to meet the program objective. The action alternative with the highest aggregate use is considered the best decision for meeting the program objectives.

was used originally for planning health education programs (Glanz and Bishop, 2010).

Although this model was originally developed to strengthen health promotion activities, the PATCH model is used by communities and agencies to plan, develop, implement, and evaluate both health promotion and disease prevention programs. Application of PATCH emphasizes community participation and ownership by all who are involved. The PATCH process includes the following:
- Mobilizing the community
- Collecting and analyzing data to support local health issues
- Choosing health priorities
- Setting objectives and standards to denote progress and success
- Developing and implementing multiple intervention strategies to meet objectives
- Evaluating the process to detect the need for change

- Securing support of the public health infrastructure within the target community

These elements are essential to the success of any community-based program:
- Participation in the planning process by community members (stakeholders)
- Use of data to help stakeholders select health priorities and develop and evaluate program activities
- Development by stakeholders of a comprehensive approach to design the program to meet the identified health needs
- Use of process (formative) evaluation to improve the program and provide feedback to the stakeholders
- Increase in the capacity of the community to address a variety of health priorities by improving the health program planning skills of the stakeholders

The PATCH model is useful in developing programs to address *Healthy People 2020* goals (http://www.cdc.gov). PATCH materials are available online at the CDC.

Assessment Protocol for Excellence in Public Health (APEXPH)

Following the development of the PATCH model in 1987, the CDC, partnering with the National Association of City and County Health Officers (NACCHO) and other organizations, developed its APEXPH model. The model was introduced for use in 1999.

The APEXPH model incorporates the three core functions of public health in assessment, assurance, and policy development. Although the model was developed for use by local health departments, it can be adapted to fit other situations and resources. The model framework includes the following:
- Process for assessing agency organization and management
- Process for working with communities to assess the health of a community as well as a community's strengths and health problems
- Process for integrating plans for resolving health problems based on the capacity, resources, and community members partnering to implement the plan

This model uses the strategic planning process of Nutt (1984) and has three elements:
- Assessing internal organization capacity to address the community's health problems
- Assessing and priority setting for the community's health problems
- Implementing the plan to address these problems

Application of the APEXPH process is useful for the following:
- Supporting recommendations for change in programs/services
- Highlighting the need for improvements in program functions

If APEXPH is applied along with the project budget process, key stakeholders may unite to discuss health and program priorities and options for providing services as well as to make plans for the year (http://www.cdc.gov). Workbooks and other resources are available through NACCHO at their website (http://www.naccho.org).

Mobilizing for Action through Planning and Partnership (MAPP)

The strategic planning model MAPP can be applied at the community level to improve the community's health. Application of this model helps to identify public health issues and priorities and to identify resources to address the priorities.

As with PATCH and APEXPH, it is important that the community feels ownership of the process. The community's strengths, needs, and wishes are integral to the process.

Two figures (Figures 25-5 and 25-6) show the MAPP process and the community roadmap to a healthier community. The phases of the MAPP process are as follows:

- Organize for success/partnership development.
  1. Organize agencies.
  2. Recruit partners.
  3. Prepare to implement MAPP.
- Visioning
  1. Work toward long-range goals through a shared vision and common values.
- Engage in four assessment processes:
  1. Assess community themes and strengths.
     a. Identify issues.
     b. Identify interest to community.
     c. Explore quality of life perceptions.
     d. Identify community assets.
  2. Assess local public health system.
     a. Identify all agencies and other partners who contribute to the public's health.
     b. Measure each partner's capacity to participate; what can each partner contribute?
     c. Measure the performance of each partner; how have they addressed issues in the past?
  3. Assess the health status of the community.
     a. Assess available data.
     b. Assess quality of life.
     c. Assess community risk factors.
  4. Assess ability of community to change.
     a. Identify forces for change.
     b. Identify forces against change.
- Identify strategic issues.
  1. What are the health issues that need to be addressed?
  2. Which are the most important?
  3. Where should the community begin?

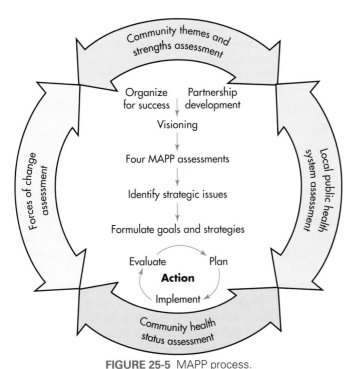

FIGURE 25-5 MAPP process.

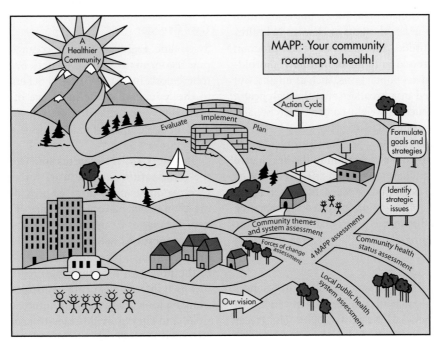

FIGURE 25-6 MAPP roadmap to community's health.

- Formulate goals and strategies.
  1. Which goals will be met?
  2. Which strategies will be used to meet the goals?
- Act
  1. Participants develop plan for action.
  2. Implement the plan.
  3. Evaluate the implementation.

Two products are available to assist in implementing the MAPP process (Figure 25-5): the NACCHO website (see the WebLinks on this book's Evolve site) and the MAPP toolbox (http://www.naccho.org).

The five models of program planning presented here may be adapted to use with a single program or with a community.

Evaluation Models and Techniques

Structure-Process-Outcome Evaluation

The method for evaluation of programs by Donabedian (1982) was initially directed primarily toward medical care but is applicable to the broader area of health care. He describes three approaches to assessment of health care: structure, process, and outcome.

- **Structure** refers to settings in which care occurs. It includes materials, equipment, qualification of the staff, and organizational structure (Donabedian, 1982). This approach to evaluation is based on the assumption that, given a proper setting with good equipment, good care will follow. However, this assumption is not strongly supported.
- **Process** refers to whether the care that was given was "good" (Donabedian, 1982), competent, or preferred. Use of process in program evaluation may consist of observing practice but more likely consists of reviewing records. The review could focus on whether documentation of preventive teaching was on the clinical record. Audits using specific criteria are examples of the use of process.
- **Outcome** refers to results of client care and restoration of function and survival (Donabedian, 1982), but is also used in the sense of changes in health status or changes in health-related knowledge, attitude, and behavior. Thus program outcomes may be expressed in terms of mortality, morbidity, and disability for given populations, such as infants, but they could be expressed in a broader sense through health promotion behaviors such as weight control, exercise, and abstinence from tobacco and alcohol.

Donabedian's model of evaluating program quality is a popular model and is widely used for evaluation in the health care field. It can be useful in evaluating program effectiveness. The Center for Medicare and Medicaid Services and other third-party payers are currently placing more emphasis on outcome evaluation. It is essential that nurses begin to develop outcome criteria for client interventions.

Tracer Method

The Board of Medicine of the National Academy of Sciences developed a program to evaluate health service delivery called the **tracer** method (Veney and Kaluzny, 2008). The tracer method of evaluation of programs is based on the premise that health status and care can be evaluated by viewing specific

---

BOX 25-5   EXAMPLES OF QUESTIONS ASKED ABOUT CASES FOR CASE REGISTER

1. What is the incidence of disease? What is the prevalence? What differences in incidence and prevalence are there between one community and another?
2. What percentage of clients recover? What percentage die?
3. Where does death occur?
4. How long do clients wait before contacting a health care provider?
5. How long is it before they are seen by a health care provider?
6. How many cases are associated with other major risk factors?
7. How many cases are associated with environmental factors such as water hardness or air pollution?
8. What happens after clients leave the hospital and when they return to work? Are there rehabilitation programs?
9. How many clients had been seen by a health care provider shortly before the problem occurred?
10. What prevention measures are taken for persons considered susceptible?

---

health problems called tracers. Just as radioactive tracers are used to study the thyroid gland, specific health problems are selected to evaluate the delivery of health and nursing services. Examples of conditions selected as tracers are cardiovascular disease, diabetes, obesity, smoking patterns, and breast and cervical cancer. This approach can be used to compare the following:

- Health status among different population groups and in different geographical locations
- Health status in relation to social status, economic level, medical care, nursing care, and behavioral variables
- Various arrangements for health care delivery

The tracer method is a useful technique for looking at the efficiency, effectiveness, and effect of a program.

Case Register

Systematic registration of a contagious disease has been a practice for many years. Denmark began a national register of tuberculosis in 1921 (Friis and Sellers, 1999). Its contribution to the reduction in the incidence of contagious diseases has been widely recognized. **Case registers** (Issel, 2008) are also used for acute and chronic diseases (e.g., cancer and myocardial infarction).

Registers collect information from defined groups, and the information may be used for evaluating and planning services, preventing disease, providing care, and monitoring changes in patterns and care. The method is described here because of its use in evaluation of services. The answers to the questions listed in Box 25-5, asked before and after implementing a program, give information about the effects of the program. A tuberculosis register indicates the degree to which infection is being controlled. Cancer registers make state, regional, national, and international comparisons possible, and they provide clues to causes of disease. They are also used to direct the development of programs specific to population needs.

COST STUDIES APPLIED TO PROGRAM MANAGEMENT

Although cost must be considered in planning and evaluating, it is particularly significant in programs involving nursing services. The major types of cost studies primarily applied to the health care industry are cost accounting, cost–benefit, cost efficiency, and cost effectiveness. A discussion of the types of cost studies is presented to give the reader an idea of the kinds of questions that can be answered with such studies. Nurses must be willing to answer these questions to help show the actual costs of nursing programs and the relevance of the programs to the clients they have served. Note that regardless of the type of method used, all methods require a comparison to another program.

Cost Accounting

Cost-accounting studies are performed to find the actual cost of a program. A question answered by this method could be the following: "What is the cost of providing a family planning program in Anytown, USA?" To answer the question, the total costs of equipment, facilities (rental), personnel (salaries and benefits), and supplies used over a period are calculated. The total program costs are divided by the number of clients participating in the program during that time. The total program cost per client is the end product. Thus a cost-accounting study can provide data about total program costs and about total cost per client, which makes program management easier. A simple example of cost accounting is the monthly balancing of a personal checkbook. One looks at the costs of providing food, shelter, and clothing for a family and relates these costs to the family income.

Cost–Benefit

Cost–benefit studies are a way of assessing the desirability of a program by placing a specific dollar amount on all costs and benefits. If benefits outweigh the costs, the program is said to have a *net positive impact*. The major problem with cost–benefit analysis is placing a quantifiable value on all benefits of the program. Can a dollar value be placed on human life, on safety, on the relief of pain and suffering, or on prevention of illness? These are all program benefits. If an attempt is made to perform cost–benefit analysis of a hospice program, can a dollar amount be placed on the family and client support and comfort provided or on the relief of pain of the terminally ill client? Can such benefits be weighed against costs to justify continuing the program? Should the program be continued despite costs?

Public health programs are recognized as having net positive impacts because preventing morbidity with illness prevention programs such as hypertension screening reduces the future cost of chronic long-term illnesses such as cerebrovascular accident (stroke) or cardiovascular disease. To do a cost–benefit study for a program, it must be decided which costs and which benefits are to be included, how the costs and benefits are to be valued, and what constraints are to be considered legal, ethical, social, and economic. For example, in a home health care program funded by the state health department to offer care

---

BOX 25-6   STEPS IN COST-EFFECTIVENESS ANALYSIS

1. Identify the program goals or client outcomes to be achieved.
2. Identify at least two alternative means of achieving the desired outcomes.
3. Collect baseline data on clients.
4. Determine the costs associated with each program activity.
5. Determine the activities each group of clients will receive.
6. Determine the client changes after the activities are completed.
7. Combine the costs (step 4), the amount of activity (step 5), and outcome information (step 6) to express costs relative to outcomes of program goals.
8. Compare cost–outcome information for each goal to that in a similar program to present cost-effectiveness analysis.

---

to clients with acquired immunodeficiency syndrome (AIDS), the mortality would continue to be high because a cure is not available. Would the program be considered to have a low cost-to-benefit ratio *(a negative impact)* because clients cannot be cured? The program would be considered to have a high cost-to-benefit ratio *(a positive net impact)* if the cost of home health care services was less expensive than providing similar care in the hospital. The benefits of the program would include reducing the costs to the client and reducing the hospital services (Issel, 2008). The cost per client to use the intervention is considered a negative net impact because the nation has had to spend money on illness that could be prevented and there have been lost work productivity and lost lives (increased mortality rate) as a result of preventable illness.

Cost Effectiveness

Cost-effectiveness analysis, which measures the quality of a program as it relates to cost, is the most frequently used analysis in nursing. Cost effectiveness is a subset of cost–benefit analysis and is designed to provide an estimate of costs to achieve an outcome. A cost-effectiveness study can answer several questions (Veney and Kaluzny, 2008): Did the program meet its objectives? Were the clients and nurses satisfied with the effects of the interventions? Are things better as a result of the interventions? In cost–benefit analysis, both costs and outcomes are quantitative, whereas in cost-effectiveness analysis, the outcomes are qualitative and quantitative. Outcome measures addressed by cost effectiveness might identify the increase in client knowledge after health teaching, a change in the client's condition after treatment, the difference in graduates of two nursing programs with similar goals, and the ability of two screening programs to detect hearing loss.

A cost effectiveness study requires collecting baseline data on clients before the program is implemented and evaluated. This occurs after the program is completed. Box 25-6 shows the procedure for completing such a study. There are several potential outcomes of a cost-effectiveness study. For example, a nurse is interested in comparing two methods for implementing a program to teach diabetic clients self-care techniques. The nurse chooses self-teaching modules and a group instruction program for comparison. There are several potential outcomes of comparing the two teaching methods. Of the potential outcomes in a cost-effectiveness study, the program of choice would be the

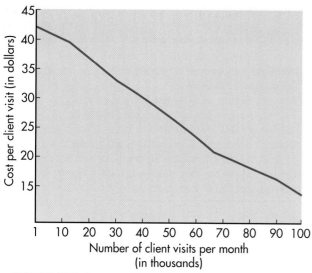

FIGURE 25-7 Cost per client visit at a home health agency.

more effective teaching method for the lesser cost. However, if the more costly program demonstrates superior outcomes, it may be chosen. If the less costly program is of poor quality, the more costly program would be appropriate.

Cost Efficiency

Cost-efficiency analysis is the actual cost of performing a number of program services. To determine the cost efficiency of a program, its productivity must be analyzed. Productivity is the relationship between what the nurse does and how much it costs to do it.

To determine the nurse's activities with a group of clients, a nurse's workload is of primary concern. This includes direct client care and indirect care activities such as charting, making phone calls, attending client care conferences, and travelling. The functions are then related to the client load, client need, and the number of nurses available to meet the needs of all clients served by a program.

Figure 25-7 shows an example of the cost efficiency of a home health agency. The graph indicates that as the number of client visits per year increases, the cost per client visit decreases. The graph assumes that the number of nurses from the beginning to the end of the period is the same, that the nurses' workloads were necessary to provide home health services, that caseloads were assigned on the basis of staff mix and client need, and that the organizational structure helped nurses be highly productive.

All cost studies have three major tasks: financial, research, and statistical. The financial tasks involve identifying total program costs and breaking them down into smaller parts. To identify the costs of a nurse's participation in a teaching program, the costs for facilities, equipment, supplies, and salaries would have to be examined. All costs associated with the program, such as the nurse's time and use of facilities, equipment, and supplies, should be compared with the total program costs. The statistical tasks involve the identification of appropriate quantifiable measures for analyzing data, and the research tasks involve setting up an appropriate study design to answer the questions of benefit, efficiency, or effectiveness.

Nurses with various educational backgrounds may be involved in cost studies with the assistance of people knowledgeable in research statistics and accounting techniques. Nurses with undergraduate degrees may be involved in the actual implementation of a cost study, whereas nurses with graduate degrees may be involved in planning, designing, implementing, analyzing, and evaluating study results as they relate to program management.

Cost studies are essential to show the worth of nursing in the marketplace of the future, and nurses should be familiar with the results of cost studies so that sound decisions can be made about future program management. Nurses must be ready to identify appropriate program outcomes, client outcomes, graduate roles in health care delivery, and requirements needed to perform nursing procedures so that appropriate decisions about program management will be made on the basis of adequate information.

PROGRAM FUNDING

Providing adequate funding for programs to meet the needs of populations can be a challenge to nurse managers in communities. When money is not available to support endeavors that serve the public good, non-profit organizations may seek funding from outside the organization. Such funding may be in the form of gifts, contracts, or grants.

Gifts are philanthropic contributions from individuals, foundations, businesses, religious or civic organizations, or voluntary associations. Many organizations engage in extensive development efforts to solicit monetary gifts that support the agency's goals. Contracts are awarded for the performance of a specific task or service, usually to meet guidelines specified by the organization making the award. Contracts are frequently used by the government to purchase services of others to perform certain services. Grants are awards to non-profit organizations to allow recipients to implement activities of their own design that address the interests of the funding agency. Grants are given by the government, foundations, and corporations.

Nurse leaders working in non-profit agencies may write grants to fund community programs that meet the needs of at-risk populations. Development of a proposal is guided by concepts and principles of program planning and evaluation that have been discussed in this chapter. Successful grant writing meshes the plan for the envisioned program of the applying organization with the criteria set forth by the funding agency. A grant proposal is a means of recording plans for establishing, managing, and evaluating a program into a written document. Funding agencies provide guidelines for grant applications, and it is essential to follow those specific guidelines if grant funding is to be acquired. In general, however, most grant proposals include certain essential components.

First, it is important to identify the target population and define the problem(s) that the project intends to address. Specific data, conditions, or circumstances that illustrate the problem and that document the need (e.g., environmental characteristics, economic conditions, population characteristics, and health status indicators) should be included and discussed. Health services should be discussed in relationship to availability, accessibility, and acceptability to the target population within both the public and private sectors. Identification of duplication or gaps in services that result in unmet needs should be addressed.

The second component is the description of the program that is being proposed. The program description should provide details about what is planned, how it will be done, where it will be done, and by whom. This section should present the reviewer with a clear understanding of the details of the program structure and function. It should be apparent that the program is realistic and can be accomplished. This section includes goals, objectives, action steps, and anticipated outcomes that describe how, when, and by whom each activity will be accomplished to achieve the outcome of the objective for which it was written.

Plans for evaluation address the method that will be used to ensure ongoing and timely review of the specific action steps and objectives involved in achieving the stated goal (formative) and to assess program outcomes (summative).

Applicants for grant funds should develop a realistic operating budget that is appropriate to the requirements of the project. The budget represents the plan for how the program will be implemented and reflects the project's proposed spending plan.

LINKING CONTENT TO PRACTICE

Program planning skills and knowledge are essential for public health nurses. In *Public Health Nursing: Scope and Standards of Practice* (ANA, 2007), the first standard is that of assessment. This addresses the issue of conducting needs assessments and having the ability to collect multiple sources of data, analyze population characteristics, problem solve, and set priorities based on the data collected. Standard speaks to using the assessment data to diagnosis health problems with input from the client population. Standards 3 through 5 address the nurses' roles in identifying health status outcomes, planning and implementing processes to address the health problem, and directing strategies to meet the outcomes. Standard 6 discusses the nurses' role in evaluation including participating in process and outcome evaluation by monitoring activities in programs.

The four professional organizations dedicated to public health nursing—The Association of State and Territorial Directors of Nursing, The Association of Community Health Nursing Educators, The Public Health Nursing section of the APHA, and the American Nurses Association—have banned together to form an organization call the Quad Council. This council developed a document identifying the domains of practice for public health nurses. One of the domains is Policy Development and Program Planning Skills. The competencies the nurse needs for this domain of practice related to program management are:

- Manages public health programs consistent with public health laws and regulations.
- Develops a plan to implement policy and programs.
- Develops mechanisms to monitor and evaluate programs for their effectiveness and quality (Quad Council, 2003).

New baccalaureate nurses will want to be knowledgeable and be able to participate in program management; graduate nurses will want to be able to direct programs. Appendix B describes a Program Planning and Design process to use for practicing the content from this chapter. Try out this process on the development of a small program of interest to you and the client population you want to serve and the community level health problem of interest to you.

CHAPTER REVIEW

PRACTICE APPLICATION

The following is a real-life example of the application of the program management process by an undergraduate nursing student. This activity resulted in the development and implementation of a nurse-managed clinic for the homeless. This example shows how students as well as providers can make a difference in health care delivery. It also illustrates that no mystery surrounds the program management process.

Eva was listening to the radio one Sunday afternoon and heard an announcement about the opening of a soup kitchen within the community for the growing homeless population. She was beginning her public health nursing course and wanted to find a creative clinical experience that would benefit herself as well as others. The announcement gave her an idea. Although it mentioned food, clothing, shelter, and social services, nothing was said about health care.

Eva was interested in finding a way to provide nursing and health care services at the soup kitchen. Which of the following should she do?

A. Talk with key leaders to determine their interest in her idea.
B. Review the literature to find out the magnitude of the problem.
C. Survey the community to determine if others were providing services.
D. Discuss the idea with members of the homeless population.
E. Consider potential solutions to the health care problems.
F. Consider where she would get the resources to open a clinic.
G. Talk with church leaders and nursing faculty members to seek acceptance for her idea.

Answers can be found on the Evolve site.

KEY POINTS

- Planning and evaluation are essential elements of program management and vital to the survival of the nursing discipline in health care delivery.
- The program management process is population focused and is parallel to the nursing process. Both are rational decision-making processes.
- The health care delivery system has grown in the past century, making health planning and evaluation very important.
- Comprehensive health planning grew out of a need to control costs.
- A program is an organized approach to meet the assessed needs of individuals, families, groups, populations, or communities by reducing or eliminating one or more health problems and addressing health disparities.
- Planning is defined as selecting and carrying out a series of actions to achieve a stated goal.
- Evaluation is defined as the methods used to determine if a service is needed and will be used, whether a program to meet that need is carried out as planned, and whether the service actually helps the people it intended to help.
- To develop quality programs, planning should include four essential elements: assessment of need and problem diagnosis, identification of problem solutions, analysis and comparison of alternative methods, and selection of the best plan and planning methods.
- The initial and most critical step in planning a health program is assessment of need. Assessment focuses on the needs of the population who will use the services planned.
- Some of the major tools used in needs assessment are census data, community forums, surveys of existing community agencies, surveys of community residents, and statistical indicators about demographics, morbidity, and mortality of the population.
- The major benefit of program evaluation is to determine whether a program is fulfilling its stated goals. Quality assurance programs are prime examples of program evaluation.
- Plans for implementing and evaluating programs should be developed at the same time.
- Program records and community indexes and health data serve as major sources of information for program evaluation.
- Planning programs and planning for their evaluation are two of the most important ways in which nurses can ensure successful program implementation.
- Cost studies help identify program benefits, effectiveness, and efficiency.
- Program planning helps nurses and agencies focus attention on services that clients need.
- Planning helps everyone involved understand their role in providing services to clients.
- The assessment of need process provides an evaluation of the relevance that a new service may have to clients.
- A decision tree is a useful tool to choose the best alternative for solving a problem.
- Setting goals and writing objectives to meet the goals are necessary to evaluate program outcomes.
- *Healthy People 2020* is an example of a national program based on needs assessment that has stated goals and objectives on which the program can be evaluated.
- Cost-accounting studies (which are similar to balancing a checkbook) help to determine the actual cost of a program.
- Cost-benefit studies are used to assess the desirability of a program by examining costs and benefits, such as the value of human life.
- Cost-effectiveness studies measure the quality of a program as it relates to cost.
- Cost-efficiency studies examine the actual cost of performing program services and focus on productivity versus cost.
- Program planning models include PPM, MAUT, PATCH, APEXPH, and MAPP.
- Program evaluation includes assessing structure, process, and outcomes of care.
- Grant writing is a tool used by nurse managers to provide resources for needed services.
- Grant proposals are documents that incorporate principles of program planning and evaluation.

CLINICAL DECISION-MAKING ACTIVITIES

1. Choose the definitions that best describe your concept of a program, of planning, and of evaluation. Explain how each of these definitions can help you in accomplishing planning and evaluation.
2. Apply the program planning process to an identified clinical problem for a client group with whom you are working in the community. Give specific examples.
   A. Assess the client needs and existing resources.
   B. Choose tools appropriate to the assessment of unmet needs.
   C. Analyze the overall planning process of arriving at decisions about implementing a program.
   D. Summarize the benefits for program planning that apply to your situation.
3. Given the situation just described, choose three or four of your classmates to work with you on the following projects:
   A. Plan for evaluation of the program in activity 2.
   B. Apply the evaluation process to the situation.
   C. Identify the measures you will use to gather data for evaluating your program.
   D. Identify the sources you will tap to gain information for program evaluation.
   E. Analyze the benefits of program evaluation that apply to your situation.
   F. Talk with a nurse or an administrator working in the community about the application of program planning and evaluation processes at the local agency. Compare their answers to your research. What are some of the difficulties that your group and the agency had in evaluating a program?

REFERENCES

American Nurses Association: *Public health nursing: scope and standards of practice*, Silver Springs, MD, 2007, American Nurse Association.

American Nurses Association: *ANA's Nurses' Efforts Pay off in Historic Health Care Bill Signing*, March 2010. Available at www.nurseworld.com\healthcarereform. Accessed February 18, 2011.

Brennan PF, Anthony MK: Measuring nurse practice models using multi-attribute utility theory, *Res Nurs Health* 23:372–382, October 2000.

Brownson RC, Fielding JE, Maylahn CM: Evidence-based public health: a fundamental concept for public health practice, *Annu Rev Public Health* 30:175–201, 2009.

Centers for Disease Control and Prevention: Framework for program evaluation in public health, *MMWR* 48(RR-11), 1999.

Delbecq A, Van de Ven A: A group process model for problem identification and program planning, *J Appl Behav Sci* 7:466, 1971.

Donabedian A: *Explorations in quality assessment and monitoring*, vol 2, Ann Arbor, MI, 1982, Health Administration Press.

Donabedian A: *An introduction to quality assurance in health care*, New York, 2003, Oxford University Press.

Farquhar SA, Parker EA, Schulz AJ, Israel BA: Application of qualitative methods in program planning for health promotion interventions, *Health Promot Pract* 7(2):234–242, 2006.

Friis R, Sellers T: *Epidemiology for public health practice*, Gaithersburg, MD, 1999, Aspen.

Glanz K, Bishop DB: The role of behavioral science theory in development and implementation of public health interventions, *Annu Rev Public Health* 31:399–418, 2010.

Hsieh C: Using client satisfaction to improve case management services for the elderly, *Res Social Work Pract* 16(6):605–612, 2006.

Issel LM: *Health program planning and evaluation: a practical, systematic approach for community health*, Boston, 2008, Jones and Bartlett.

Jefferson Area Board of Aging: What we do and who we are, *JABA facts*, 2010. Available at http://www.jabacares.org/. Accessed January 31, 2011.

Jones EG, Renger R, Firestone R: Deaf community analysis for health education priorities, *Public Health Nurs* 22:27–35, 2005.

Kabassi K, Vroom M: MAUT and adaptive techniques for web based educational software, *Instruct Sci* 34(2):313–358, 2006.

Kettner P, Moroney R, Martin L: *Designing and managing programs: an effectiveness based approach*, Thousand Oaks, CA, 2008, Sage.

Nutt P: *Planning methods for health and related organizations*, New York, 1984, Wiley.

Posavac EJ, Carey RG: *Program evaluation: methods and case studies*, Englewood Cliffs, NJ, 2006, Prentice Hall.

Quad Council of Public Health Nursing Organization: *Competencies for public health nursing practice*, 2003, revised 2009, ASTDN, Washington, D.C.

Rodenbeck S: *Essential environmental services provided by USPHS applied public health teams after disasters*, Atlanta, GA, 2008, USPHS, CDC.

Royse D, Thyer BA, Padgett DK: *Program evaluation: an introduction*, ed 5, Belmont, CA, 2010, Wadsworth.

Sparer MS: The role of government in U.S. health care. In Kovner A, Knickman J, editors: *Jonas and Kovner's health care delivery in the United States*, New York, 2008, Springer.

Steen J: *Community Health Planning*, 2008, American Health Planning Association. Available at http://www.ahpanet.org/files/Community_Health_Planning_09.pdf. Accessed January 31, 2011.

Texas Department of State Health Services: *Community assessment for public health response (CASPER)*, 2008. Available at http://www.dshs.state.tx.us/comprep/rna/Intro.shtm. Accessed January 31, 2011.

University of North Carolina Health Services Library: *Finding information for a community health assessment*, 2009. Available at http://www.hsl.unc.edu/services/guides/communityHealth.cfm. Accessed January 31, 2011.

USDHHS: *Healthy People 2020: a roadmap for health*, Washington, DC, 2010, U.S. Government Printing Office.

Veney J, Kaluzny A: *Evaluation and decision making for health service programs*, Englewood Cliffs, NJ, 2008, Prentice Hall.

CHAPTER 26

Quality Management

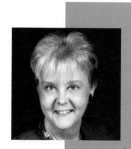

Marcia Stanhope, RN, DSN, FAAN

Marcia Stanhope has been involved in the development and evaluation of quality management in public health through her role as former chair and continuing member of the local board of health. She teaches quality management processes to public health and executive management students and has been a director of continuous quality improvement in home health.

ADDITIONAL RESOURCES

evolve WEBSITE
http://evolve.elsevier.com/Stanhope
- *Healthy People 2020*
- Quiz
- WebLinks
- Case Studies
- Glossary

- Answers to Practice Application
- Resource Tools
  - Resource Tool 46.A: Core Competencies and Skills Levels for Public Health Nursing

APPENDIX
- Appendix H: Focus on Quality and Safety Education for Nurses

OBJECTIVES

After reading this chapter, the student should be able to do the following:

1. Explain differences in total quality management/continuous quality improvement (TQM/CQI).
2. State the goals of TQM/CQI in a health care system.
3. Define quality assurance/quality improvement (QA/QI).
4. Evaluate the role of QA/QI in CQI.
5. Analyze the historical development of the quality process in nursing and describe the changes developing under managed care.
6. Evaluate approaches and techniques for implementing CQI.
7. Examine how managed care is changing the way quality is ensured in health care.
8. Plan a model QA/QI program.
9. Identify the purposes for the types of records kept in community and public health agencies.
10. Evaluate a method for documentation of client care.

KEY TERMS

Although the concept of quality assurance has been a part of the health care arena for a number of years, it is only in the last few years that major movement to improve health care quality has begun in the United States. The Institute of Medicine (IOM, 2001), not confident of the current health care systems' ability to deliver the quality of care expected, set forth a series of recommendations to transform current systems to meet American's expectations. Very little is known about quality of care in this country for two reasons: (1) a variety of definitions of *quality* are used, and (2) it is difficult to obtain comparable data from all providers and health care agencies.

However, in the Healthcare Research and Quality Act of 1999 (PL 106-129), Congress mandated that the Agency for Healthcare Research and Quality (AHRQ) produce an annual report on health care quality in the United States beginning in fiscal year 2003. This National Healthcare Quality Report (NHQR) is a collaborative effort among the agencies of the U.S. Department of Health and Human Services (USDHHS) and includes a broad set of performance measures that will be used to monitor the nation's progress toward improved health care quality. The NHQR represents the broadest examination of quality of health care, in terms of number of measures and number of dimensions of care, ever undertaken in the United States. The report represents progress toward improving quality as well as recommendations for how to improve quality outcomes (USDHHS, 2007).

The NHQR is intended to serve a number of purposes, such as demonstrating the validity (or lack) of concerns about quality, documenting whether health care quality is stable, improving, or declining over time and providing national benchmarks against which specific states, health plans, and providers can compare their performance (AHRQ, 2002; NCQA, 2009).

In a changing health care market, the demand for quality has become a rallying point for health care consumers. All consumers, including private citizens, insurance companies, industry, and the federal government, are concerned with the highest quality outcomes at the lowest cost (Wakefield and Wakefield, 2008). In addition to the demand for higher quality and lower cost, the public wants health care delivered with greater access, and health care that is accountable, efficient, and effective. Moreover, consumers want information about quality. Information is empowering to the consumer. With the expanded use of the Internet, access to information about quality in health care is readily available in topics ranging from talking to consumers about quality health care (http://www.talkingquality.gov) to clinical practice guidelines that promise to improve care for all (http://www.guideline.gov). **Total quality management** (TQM) is a management philosophy that includes a focus on client, **continuous quality improvement (CQI),** and teamwork (Kelly, 2007). Although relatively new in public health care, the concepts of TQM/CQI has been tried and proven in industry at large. The terms *total quality management, continuous quality improvement, total quality,* and *organization-wide quality improvement* are often used interchangeably. However, they have different meanings. As indicated, TQM refers to a management philosophy that focuses on the statistical processes by which to assess work done with the goal of organization-wide quality effectiveness. The term for TQM is often referred to as TQ, and both acronyms have the same meaning. CQI, while different from the other three terms, can be implemented not only to address system problems, but also to maintain and enhance good performance through the use of differing techniques. Everyone in the public health or community-based organization is involved in CQI, the leaders, the staff, and the client. By obtaining facts about work processes (e.g., all the steps in certifying a child for the women, infants, and children nutritional program [WIC]), it is possible to discover which steps are unnecessary (i.e., non–value adding) and to eliminate those steps to produce better health outcomes for individuals and communities (Carmichael, 2005). Box 26-1 presents several abbreviations that are commonly used in health care and quality management.

Both consumers and providers have a vested interest in the quality of the health care system.

1. Improving safety of care saves lives
2. Costs reduction by using effective interventions
3. Increases in client confidence in health care delivery regardless of setting (NQF, 2009)

Kovner and Jonas state that in health care there is a direct link between doing a good job and individual and professional survival. Health care providers pride themselves on individual achievement and responsibility for good client outcomes (Kovner and Knickman, 2008). Health care organizations are natural extensions of health care providers and thus can

BOX 26-1	**COMMONLY USED ABBREVIATIONS**
AACN	American Association of Colleges of Nursing
ACHNE	Association of Community Health Nursing Educators
AHRQ	Agency for Healthcare Research and Quality (formerly AHCPR)
ANA	American Nurses Association
APHA	American Public Health Association
CCNE	Commission on Collegiate Nursing Education
CHAP	Community Health Accreditation Program
CMS	Centers for Medicare and Medicaid Services (formerly HCFA)
CQI	Continuous Quality Improvement
HEDIS	Health Plan Employer Data and Information Set
IOM	Institute of Medicine
JCAHO	Joint Commission on Accreditation of Healthcare Organizations
MCO	Managed Care Organization
NCQA	National Committee for Quality Assurance
NHQR	National Healthcare Quality Report
NLN	National League for Nursing
NPHPSP	National Public Health Performance Standards Program
OCQI	Outcomes-Based Quality Improvement
PRO	Professional Review Organization
QA	Quality Assurance
QI	Quality Improvement
TQI	Total Quality Improvement
TQM	Total Quality Management

demonstrate their responsibility for optimal outcomes through a rigorous **quality improvement** process. The application of quality improvement strategies through six areas of performance could affect both process and outcomes of health care:

1. Consistently providing appropriate and effective care
2. Reducing unjustified geographic variation in care
3. Eliminating avoidable mistakes
4. Lowering access barriers
5. Improving responsiveness to clients
6. Eliminating racial/ethnic, gender, socioeconomic, and other disparities and inequalities in access and treatment (Mead et al, 2008)

In the 1990s the United States entered a new era of population-centered, community-controlled delivery of care in which **managed care** organizations (MCOs) played an integral role. MCOs are agencies such as health maintenance organizations (HMOs) and preferred provider organizations (PPOs) designed to monitor and deliver health care services within a specific budget. Currently, providers, clients, payers, and policy makers all have input into the quality measurement process. The Health Plan Employer Data and Information Set (HEDIS), a data collection arm of the National Committee for Quality Assurance (NCQA), provides performance information, or **report cards,** for MCOs. In 2009, 702 HMOs and 277 PPOs reported audited HEDIS data to show the level of quality performance. These MCOs covered 116 million, or 2 in 5 Americans in that year (NCQA, 2009).

Although introduced in the 1990s, report cards for public health agencies are currently being developed and promoted to measure quality health care in communities. The term *community health report card* refers to different types of reports, community health profiles, needs assessments, scorecards, quality of life indicators, health status reports, and progress reports. All of these reports are critical components of community-based approaches to improving the health and quality of life of communities.

An example at the national level is the Community Health Status Indicator (CHSI) Project, which is a collaborative effort between the Health Resources and Services Administration (HRSA), the Association of State and Territorial Health Officials (ASTHO), the National Association of County and City Health Officials (NACCHO), and the Public Health Foundation. In 2000, the project published and disseminated community health status reports for all U.S. counties. These reports provided county-level data, including peer county and national comparisons, for every county in the country. The goal of CHSI is to provide an overview of key health indicators for local communities and to encourage dialogue about actions that can be taken to improve a community's health. The CHSI report was designed not only for public health professionals, but also for members of the community who are interested in the health of their community. They are designed to support health planning by local health departments, local health planners, community residents, and others interested in community health improvement. The CHSI report contains over 200 measures for each of the 3141 United States counties. Although CHSI presents indicators like deaths resulting from heart disease and cancer, it is imperative to understand that behavioral factors such as tobacco use, diet, physical activity, alcohol and drug use, and sexual behavior substantially contribute to these deaths (Metzler et al, 2008).

These community health improvement initiatives have grown out of three major trends: (1) an increasing recognition of the importance of local community action to solve local problems, (2) an increasing emphasis on outcomes and accountability, and (3) the Healthy Cities/Healthy Communities movement (see Chapter 20). The Healthy Cities/Healthy Communities movement views community health and its determinants broadly, and they use a set of indicators (to track their progress) that reflects this broad definition. These indicators might include the following:

- Physical and mental health status
- Educational achievement
- Economic prosperity
- Public safety
- Adequate housing and transportation
- A clean and safe physical environment
- Recreational and cultural opportunities (Encyclopedia of Public Health, 2002)

Community health report cards can be a useful tool in efforts to help identify areas where change is needed, to set priorities for action, and to track changes in population health over time. The report card may be used to track leading causes of morbidity and mortality in a community, looking at trends over time to see if public health interventions have improved health care outcomes. The card may also be used to assess a specific chronic disease, like diabetes, to determine the health status of the community for this particular disease (CDC, 2010). The report card may be used as an internal measure of public health program outcomes and CQI measures within the agency (Gunzenhauser et al, 2010).

In 2009, HEDIS measures of care included several that address public health issues, including breast and cervical cancer screening, childhood immunization status, comprehensive diabetes care, flu shots for adults, lead screening in children, physical activity in older adults, and prenatal and postpartum care, to name a few (NCQA, 2009).

As a part of a movement to provide quality health care in communities, health departments are increasingly examining their place in promoting quality (USDHHS, 2005b). McLaughlin and Kaluzny (2006) state that public health and CQI are connected because of the use of systems approaches that public health takes in identifying problems and developing interventions. Aspects of planning, implementing, and evaluating by TQM fall under each of the core public health functions of assessment, assurance, and policy development. However, it is with the assurance core function, related to ensuring available access to the health care services essential to sustain and improve the health of the population, that TQM programs must be undertaken. Public health cannot ensure services that improve health if those services lack quality. Public health will want to maintain quality in its workforce and continually evaluate the effectiveness of its services whether service is delivered to the individual, the community, or the population.

DID YOU KNOW? *At least four documents provide report cards on how well the United States is performing on improving safety of health care delivery, quality of and access to care across population groups, progress and opportunities for improving health care quality, and the state of health care quality. These reports are published regularly by the Agency for Health Care Research and Quality, the National Quality Forum, and the National Committee for Quality Assurance.*

Nurses are in a perfect position to implement strategies to improve population-centered health care. Community assessments, identification of high-risk individuals, use of targeted interventions, case management, and management of illnesses across a continuum of care are strategies suggested as part of the focus in improving the health of communities (Quad Council of Public Health Nursing Organizations, 2009). These strategies have long been used by nurses.

The growth of the managed care industry has changed the face of health care in the United States, both in how health care is delivered and in how it is received by consumers. Consumers are forming **partnerships** in communities to counteract the power of MCOs by holding them accountable for health outcomes in relation to costs. Partnerships are using data-based community assessments to improve health and to ensure that communities receive quality services (Keyser et al, 2009).

Because of managed care agencies and consumer demands for quality nursing, objective and systematic evaluation of nursing care is a priority for the nursing profession. Since organized nursing is committed to direct individual **accountability,** is evolving as a scientific discipline, and is concerned about how

BOX 26-2	THE AREAS OF PUBLIC HEALTH NURSING INTERVENTIONS FOR QUALITY POPULATION-CENTERED HEALTH CARE

INTERVENTIONS	CHAPTER
Advocacy	5, 6, 10, 16, 22, 30, 32, 34, 37, 46
Case finding	22, 32, 33, 42
Case management	19, 22, 30, 32, 33, 42, 46
Coalition building	8, 18, 20
Collaborating	21, 22, 26, 32, 39, 41, 45
Community organizing	18, 20
Consulting	40, 41
Counseling	9, 14, 30, 32, 36, 39, 42, 45, 46
Delegated functions	40, 41
Disease and health event investigation	12, 13, 14, 23, 24
Health teaching	9, 13, 14, 16, 17, 20, 36, 38, 39, 40, 42, 43, 44, 45
Outreach	33, 35, 46
Policy development and enforcement	1, 8, 10, 18, 27, 30, 33
Referral and follow-up	10, 22, 27, 28, 32, 46
Social marketing	13, 18, 34, 38
Survey	18, 24

From Minnesota Department of Health, Division of Community Health Services: *Public health interventions: applications for public health nursing practice,* St Paul, MN, March 2001, p 1, Public Health Nursing Section.

costs of health services limit access, it demands delivery and evaluation of quality service aimed at superior client outcomes (ANA, 1999, 2010; Brownson, Fielding, and Maylahn, 2009). In the public health arena, the Quad Council of Public Health Nursing Organizations (2009) has identified competencies for public health nursing based on the Council on Linkages Between Academia and Public Health Practice document of 2008 with the most recent update on these competencies occurring in 2010 (Council on Linkages). Other states have developed models to document outcomes attributable to nursing interventions and are adding methods for evaluating total quality (Minnesota Department of Health, 2001; Keller et al, 2004a,b; Sakamoto and Avila, 2004; Smith and Bazini-Barakat, 2004; University of Wisconsin-Madison, 2010). Box 26-2 is a list of the areas of nursing interventions that nurses will want to be able to use. The chapters that discuss the interventions are noted. (See Chapter 9 for the most recent updates on the Keller et al. model of the Intervention Wheel.)

The competencies for public health leadership developed by the Council on Linkages (2001, updated 2010) are crucial to ensure the quality and performance of the public health workforce (Rowitz, 2009). (See Resource Tool 46.A on the Evolve website for a list of the competencies.)

Records are maintained on all health care system clients to provide complete information about the client and to show the quality of care being given to the client within the system. Records are a necessary part of a CQI process, as are the tools and methods for evaluating quality. Electronic medical records are becoming more common and are aiding in decreasing errors, increasing quality, and monitoring interventions.

DEFINITIONS AND GOALS

The IOM definition of quality is "the degree to which health services for individuals and populations increase the likelihood of desired health outcomes and are consistent with current professional knowledge" (2001, p 1000). The AHRQ defines quality health care as doing the right thing, for the right client, and having the best possible results (2007). Quality in public health is defined as "the degree to which policies, programs, services, and research for the population increase desired health outcomes and conditions in which the population can be healthy" (USDHHS, 2008, p 2).

However, a definition of quality rests largely on the perception of the client, the provider, the care manager, the purchaser, the payer, or the public health official. Whereas the physician views quality in a more technical sense, the client may look at the personal outcome; the manager, purchaser, or payer may consider the cost-effectiveness; and the public health official will look at the appropriate use of health care resources to improve population health (Mead et al, 2008).

According to the AHRQ (2002), problems with quality of care were divided into five groups: variation of service, underuse of service, overuse of service, misuse of service, and disparities in quality. Variation in service refers to the lack of standards of practice continuity. This variation is often seen between regional, state, and local health care services and stems from lack of evolutionary health care practice and not keeping abreast of the constant changes taking place in health care (evidence-based practice) (NCQA, 2009). Underuse of service refers to conservative treatment practices. As an example, there is a lack of immunizations for pneumonia given to Asians 65 years or older as a preventive measure as compared with immunization levels of whites (AHRQ, 2008). Overuse of service refers to the over-ordering of unnecessary tests, surgeries, and treatments. This overuse drives up the cost of already expensive health care. Misuse of service refers to client safety issues and how disability and mortality can be reduced. With diligent care by health care providers, client injury and death can be avoided (NQF, 2009). Disparities in quality refer to racial, ethnic, and socioeconomic disparities in accessibility and affordability of health care (AHRQ, 2008).

The term *health services* applies to a wide range of health delivery institutions. Of particular interest to public health is the question of access to appropriate and needed services, a well-prepared workforce, and improvement in the status of the population's health. Client satisfaction and well-being and the processes of client–provider interaction should be considered as well.

TQM is a process-driven, customer-oriented management philosophy that includes leadership, teamwork, employee empowerment, individual responsibility, and continuous improvement of system processes to yield improved outcomes (Carmichael, 2005). Under TQM, quality is defined as customer satisfaction. **Quality assurance/quality improvement (QA/QI)** is the promise or guarantee that certain standards of excellence are being met in the delivery of care. Godfrey et al (2007) discuss what is called the *Juran trilogy*. This consists of quality planning, quality control, and quality improvement. This trilogy combines components of QA as well as CQI to improve client outcomes in health care delivery.

QI is defined as a structured approach to improving performance (Lotstein et al, 2008). QI in public health is the use of a deliberate and defined improvement process, such as plan-do-check-act (PDCA), which is focused on activities that are responsive to community needs and improving population health. It refers to a continuous and ongoing effort to achieve measurable improvements in the efficiency, effectiveness, performance, accountability, outcomes, and other indicators of quality in services or processes that achieve equity and improve the health of the community (Bialek et al, 2010).

QA is concerned with the accountability of the provider and is only one tool in achieving the best client outcomes. Accountability means being responsible for care and answerable to the client (McLaughlin and Kaluzny, 2006). Under QA/QI, quality may have a variety of definitions. According to the National Health and Medical Research Council (NHMRC) (2003), QA should consist of peer review leading to QI to improve health care delivery. Client standards of care and safety issues are the core of QA.

The AHRQ has indicated that the assurance of quality is organized around four dimensions: effectiveness, client safety, timeliness and client centeredness and is assessed using four stages of care: staying healthy (primary prevention), getting better (secondary prevention), living with illness or disability, and coping with end of life (tertiary prevention) (AHRQ, 2008).

Quality traditionally has been an important issue in the delivery of health care. QA programs historically have ensured this accountability. The goals of QA and QI are on a continuum of quality, and in public health they are: (1) to continuously improve the timeliness, effectiveness, safety, and responsiveness of programs, and (2) to optimize internal resources to improve the health of the community (Riley et al, 2010).

Under a CQI philosophy, QA and QI are but two of the many approaches used to ensure that the health care agency fulfills what the client thinks are the requirements for the service. QA focuses on finding what providers have done wrong in the past (e.g., deviations from a standard of care found through a chart audit). CQI operates at a higher level on the quality continuum but requires the commitment of more organization resources to move in a positive direction. CQI focuses on the sources of differences in the ongoing process of health care delivery and seeks to improve the process (Kelly, 2007; Varkey et al, 2007).

The process of health care includes two major components: technical interventions (e.g., how well procedures are accomplished, accurate assessments, and effective interventions) and interpersonal relationships between public health practitioner and client. Both contribute to quality care, and both can be evaluated (Donabedian, 2003). Several approaches and techniques are used in quality programs. *Approaches* are methods used to ensure quality, and *techniques* are tools for measuring differences in quality (Kovner and Knickman, 2008).

Traditional approaches to quality focus on assessing or measuring performance, ensuring that performance conforms to standards, and providing remedial work to providers if those standards are not met. Such a definition of quality is too narrow in health care systems that try to meet the needs of many clients, both internal and external to the agency (Donabedian, 2003). CQI requires constant attention and should involve surveillance of all records while there is still the opportunity to intervene in both the client's care and the practitioner's actions. Comprehensive data analysis is necessary to detect process failure. Many agencies use some of the TQM/CQI concepts, such as client satisfaction questionnaires, but have not adopted the entire management philosophy. However, because QA/QI methods have traditionally been used and are still in use in many agencies, the QA/QI concepts will be covered.

 HEALTHY PEOPLE 2020

Goal of Improving Access to Comprehensive, High-Quality Health Care, and Examples of Objectives to Eliminate Health Disparities

- AHS-1: Increase the proportion of persons with health insurance.
- AHS-5: Increase the proportion of persons who have a specific source of ongoing care.
- AHS-7: Increase the proportion of persons who receive evidence-based clinical preventive services.

From U.S. Department of Health and Human Services: *Healthy People 2020,* Washington, DC, 2010, U.S. Government Printing Office.

HISTORICAL DEVELOPMENT

Improving the quality of care has been a part of nursing since the days of Florence Nightingale. In 1860 Nightingale called for the development of a uniform method to collect and present hospital statistics to improve hospital treatment. Nightingale was a pioneer in setting standards for nursing care. The movement to establish nursing schools in the United States came in the late 1800s from a desire to set standards that would upgrade nursing care. In the early 1900s efforts were begun to set similar standards for all nursing schools. From 1912 to 1930 interest in quality nursing education led to the development of nursing organizations involved in accrediting nursing programs. Licensure has been a major issue in nursing since 1892. By 1923 all states had permissive or mandatory laws directing nursing practice.

After World War II, the attention of the emerging nursing profession focused on establishing a scientific method of practice. The nursing process was the chosen method and included evaluation of how nursing activities helped clients (Maibusch, 1984). QA/QI was the evaluative steps in the nursing process.

The 1950s brought the development of QA measurement tools. One of the first tools was Phaneuf's nursing audit method (1965), which has been used extensively in population-centered nursing practice.

In 1966, the American Nurses Association (ANA) created the Divisions on Practice. As a result, in 1972, the Congress for Nursing Practice was charged with developing standards to institute QA programs. The Standards for Community Health Nursing Practice were distributed to ANA Community Health Nursing Division members in 1973. In 1986, 1999, and in 2005, with updates in 2007, the scope and standards were again revised with a change in focus from community health nursing to public health nursing.

In 1972, the Joint Commission on Accreditation of Hospitals (JCAH) clearly stated the responsibilities of nursing in its description of standards for nursing services. The JCAH called on the nursing industry to clearly plan, document, and evaluate nursing care provided. In the mid-1980s, the JCAH became the Joint Commission on Accreditation of Healthcare Organizations (JCAHO) and began developing quality control standards for hospital and home health nursing. JCAHO is now known as The Joint Commission (TJC) and presently incorporates CQI principles in its standards.

Also in 1972, the Social Security Act (PL 92-603) was amended to establish the Professional Standards Review Organization (PSRO) and to mandate the process review of the delivery of health care to clients of Medicare, Medicaid, and maternal and child health programs. The PSRO program later became the Professional Review Organization (PRO) under the 1983 Social Security amendments. The purpose of the PROs was to monitor the implementation of the prospective reimbursement system for Medicare clients (the diagnosis-related groups [DRGs]). Although PSROs were intended for physicians, PROs have made QI a primary issue for all health care professionals.

In response to increasing charges of malpractice, the government passed the National Health Quality Improvement Act of 1986. Although it was not funded until 1989, its two major goals were to encourage consumers to become informed about their practitioner's practice record and to create a national clearinghouse of information on the malpractice records of providers. The emphasis of this act continued to be on the structure of care rather than the process or outcomes of care (Dlugacz, Restifo, and Greenwood, 2004; NAHQ, 1993). (See Chapter 25 for discussion of structure, process, and outcome.)

Efforts to strengthen nursing practice in the community have been carried out by several nursing organizations, including the ANA, the Public Health Nursing Section of the American Public Health Association (APHA), the Association of State and Territorial Directors of Nursing (ASTDN), and the Association of Community Health Nursing Educators (ACHNE). As mentioned previously, these organizations are called the Quad Council for Public Health Nursing. The quality of nursing education is a major concern of the ACHNE, which was established in 1978. In 1993, 2000, and 2003, four reports published by this organization identified the curriculum content required to prepare nursing students for practice in the community (ACHNE, 1993, 2000a,b, 2003). In 2005, and again in 2007, the Quad Council reviewed scopes and standards of population-focused (public health) and community-based nursing practice and developed new standards to guide the profession in obtaining the best health outcomes for the populations they serve. QA/QI programs remain the enforcers of standards of care for many agencies that have not elected to engage in a program of CQI. These activities are called *assurance activities* because they make certain that those policies and procedures are followed so that appropriate quality services are delivered.

The Council on Linkages Between Academia and Public Health Practice (the Council) is a coalition of representatives from 17 national public health organizations. Since 1992, the Council has worked to further academic/practice collaboration to ensure a well-trained, competent workforce and a strong, evidence-based public health infrastructure. The Council is funded by the CDC and staffed by the Public Health Foundation. The most recent core competencies were updated in 2010. These competencies are used in QA/QI as performance measurements of providers to ensure quality of services (Council on Linkages, 2010). In 2003 and using the work of the Council on Linkages, the Quad Council of Public Health Nursing developed a set of core competencies for public health nurses. This was updated in 2009 and can be used as a performance measure for public health nursing practice.

APPROACHES TO QUALITY IMPROVEMENT

Two basic approaches exist in QI: *general* and *specific*. The general approach involves a large governing or official body's evaluation of a person's or an agency's ability to meet criteria or standards. Specific approaches to QI are methods used to manage a specific health care delivery system in an attempt to deliver care with outcomes that are acceptable to the consumer. QA/QI programs that evaluate provider and client interaction through compliance with standards historically have been used alone to monitor quality care. In a TQM approach, CQI with QA/QI methods are an integral, but not the only, tool for ensuring quality or customer satisfaction.

General Approaches

General approaches to protect the public by ensuring a level of competency among health care professionals are *credentialing, licensure, accreditation, certification, charter, recognition,* and *academic degrees*. Although there has been a long history of public oversight of quality in the United States, this public oversight increasingly involves the private sector. Public oversight for quality emerged when the private market failed to focus on health care quality. Previously mentioned reports about quality on p 576 are indicators of public sector involvement in public oversight of quality.

Credentialing is generally defined as the formal recognition of a person as a professional with technical competence, or of an agency that has met minimum standards of performance. These mechanisms are used to evaluate the agency structure through which care is provided and the outcomes of care given by the provider. Credentialing can be mandatory or voluntary. Mandatory credentialing requires laws. State nurse practice acts are examples of mandatory credentialing. Voluntary credentialing is performed by an agency or an institution. The certification examinations offered by the ANA through the American Nurses Credentialing Center are examples of voluntary credentialing. Licensing, certification, and accreditation are all examples of credentialing.

Licensure is one of the oldest general QA approaches in the United States and Canada. Individual licensure is a contract between the profession and the state. Under this contract, the profession is granted control over entry into, and exit from, the profession and over quality of professional practice.

The licensing process requires that written regulations define the scope and limits of the professional's practice. Job descriptions based on these regulations set minimum and maximum limits on the functions and responsibilities of the practitioner. Licensure of nurses has been mandated by law since 1903. Today all 50 states have mandatory nurse licensure, which requires all individuals who practice nursing, whether it be for money or as a volunteer, be licensed. A new approach to interstate practice requires a pact between states so that nurses can practice across state borders. Although reciprocity (which means nurses can have their license accepted through an application process if there is agreement between the states requiring application) exists among states for nursing licensure, interstate practice without approval is an issue for state boards of nursing. The states' compact agreements were to reduce the barriers for interstate practice. The mutual recognition model of nurse licensure allows a nurse to have one license (in his or her state of residency) and to practice in other states (both physical and electronically when giving advise through programs like 'ask a nurse'), subject to each state's practice law and regulation. Under mutual recognition, a nurse may practice across state lines unless otherwise restricted. This is referred to as a multistate nurse licensure model, specifically referred to as the Nurse Licensure Compact (NLC). All states that currently belong to the NLC also operate the single state licensure model for those nurses who do not reside legally in an NLC state or do not qualify for multi-state licensure. In order to achieve mutual recognition, each state must enact legislation or regulation authorizing the NLC. States entering the compact also adopt administrative rules and regulations for implementation of the compact.

Once the compact is enacted, each compact state designates a Nurse Licensure Compact Administrator to facilitate the exchange of information between the states relating to compact nurse licensure and regulation. On January 10, 2000, the **Nurse Licensure Compact Administrators (NLCA)** were organized to protect the public's health and safety by promoting compliance with the laws governing the practice of nursing in each party state through the mutual recognition of party state licenses (NCSBN, 2010).

WHAT DO YOU THINK?   *Historically, licensure has protected the public by ensuring at least a beginning level of competence. Nurses are licensed by state government, even though all nurses take the same licensing examination. What do you think about allowing nurses to practice across state lines without registering in each state?*

Accreditation, a voluntary approach to QC, is used for institutions. Since 1954 the National League for Nursing (NLN), a voluntary organization, has had established standards for inspecting nursing education programs. In 1997 the NLN board established an accrediting body as an independent organization: the NLN Accrediting Commission (NLNAC). In 1997 the American Association of Colleges of Nursing (AACN), also a voluntary organization supporting baccalaureate and higher degree programs, established an affiliate—the Collegiate Commission on Nursing Education (CCNE)—to accredit baccalaureate and higher degree nursing programs. In 1966 community health/home health program standards were established by the NLN for the purpose of accrediting these programs through their Community Health Accreditation Program (CHAP). In addition, state boards of nursing accredit basic nursing programs so that their graduates are eligible for the licensing examination. In some states, state boards of nursing accredit graduate programs.

The accreditation function is quasi-voluntary. Although accreditation appears to be a voluntary program, it is often linked to government regulation that encourages programs to participate in the accrediting process. Examples include the federal Medicare regulations restricting payments only to accredited public health and home health care agencies.

Accreditation, whether voluntary or required, provides a means for effective peer review and an opportunity for an in-depth review of program strengths and limitations. Accreditation applies external pressure and places demands on institutions to improve quality of care. In the past, the accreditation process primarily evaluated an agency's physical structure, organizational structure, and personnel qualifications. However, beginning in 1990, more emphasis was placed on evaluation of the outcomes of care and on the educational qualifications of the person providing the care.

In the past there has not been a mechanism for accrediting public health agencies. In 2007 the Public Health Accreditation Board (PHAB) was incorporated, after public health leaders explored the feasibility of a national accreditation program. The field saw the need for, and value of, public health accreditation, and advocated for the implementation of a national voluntary program. The PHAB was developed in accordance with the recommendations generated by the Exploring Accreditation Steering Committee. The Steering Committee was comprised primarily of state and local public health officials, including boards of health. The committee called on the expertise from other specialty areas engaged in accreditation. The PHAB is a non-profit organization and is developing and testing national standards and processes that will be used to assess the strengths and areas for improvement in public health.

The PHAB mission is to promote and protect the health of the public by advancing the quality and performance of *all* public health departments in the United States. The PHAB works in pursuit of creating a high-performing public health system that will make the United States the healthiest nation.

The CDC and the Robert Wood Johnson Foundation are funders, and partners, of PHAB. The goal is for the accreditation program to be self-sustaining, and the accrediting process which began in 2011 (PHAB, 2010).

Certification, another general approach to quality, combines features of licensure and accreditation. Certification is usually a voluntary process within professions. Educational achievements, experience, and performance on an examination determine a person's qualifications for functioning in an identified specialty area. The American Nurses Credentialing Center provides certification in several areas of nursing. Many other professional nursing specialty credentialing organizations also provide for individual certification.

Although usually a voluntary process, certification can also be a quasi-voluntary process. For example, to function as a nurse practitioner in some states, one must show proof of educational credentials and take an examination to be certified to practice within the boundaries of the state.

Major concerns exist about certification as a QA mechanism. Data are lacking about the clinical competence of the practitioner at the time of certification because clinical competency is usually not measured by a written test. Although better data exist about the quality of the practitioner's work after the certification process, the American Nurses Credentialing Center conducted a research program to look at how certification is related to the work of the certified nurse (Cary, 2000; Damberg et al, 2008). Except for occupational health nurses and nurse anesthetists, certification has not been recognized by employers as an achievement beyond basic preparation, so financial rewards are few (Keefe, 2010).

Although the nursing profession has accepted the certification process as a mechanism for recognizing competence and excellence, certifying bodies must help nurses communicate the importance of certified nurses to the public.

Charter, recognition, and academic degrees are other general approaches to QA. **Charter** is the mechanism by which a state government agency, under state laws, grants corporate status to institutions with or without rights to award degrees (e.g., university-based nursing programs).

Recognition is a process whereby one agency accepts the credentialing status of and the credentials conferred by another. For example, some state boards of nursing accept nurse practitioner credentials that are awarded by the American Nurses Credentialing Center or by one of the specialty credentialing agencies. Academic degrees are titles awarded to individuals recognized by degree-granting institutions as having completed a predetermined plan of study in a branch of learning. There are four academic degrees awarded in nursing, with some variety at each degree level: Associate of Arts/Sciences; Bachelor of Science in Nursing; master's degrees, such as Master of Science in Nursing and Master of Nursing; and doctoral degrees, such as Doctor of Philosophy and Doctor of Nursing Practice.

Although these general quality management methods are important and should continue, newer and better approaches must be devised. If performance in the area of quality health care is to advance, better diagnosis of performance problems and corrective strategies that are effective will be necessary (Mead et al, 2008).

A recent approach to recognition is the Magnet nursing services recognition status given by the American Nurses Credentialing Center to agency nursing services that, after an extensive review, are considered excellent. This program began with recognition of excellent hospital nursing services. Although the Magnet program has expanded to include nursing home and home health agencies, approximately 6% (372 of 5815) of the nation's hospitals had qualified for Magnet designation as of 2010. Reapplication for Magnet status must occur every 4 years to ensure that Magnet organizations stay at the top of their games (ANCC, 2010).

Specific Approaches

Historically, QA programs conducted by health care agencies have measured or assessed the performance of individuals and how they conformed to standards set forth by accrediting agencies. TQM as a management philosophy uses CQI methods that incorporate many tools, including QA, to increase customer satisfaction with quality care. According to the AHRQ, quality health care means doing the right thing, at the right time, in the right way, for the right people—and having the best possible results (AHRQ, 2001, 2008). To the Institute of Medicine (IOM, 2001, p 3), quality health care is care that is:

- *Effective*—Providing services based on scientific knowledge to all who could benefit and refraining from providing services to those not likely to benefit
- *Safe*—Avoiding injuries to clients from the care that is intended to help them
- *Timely*—Reducing waits and sometimes harmful delays for both those who receive and those who give care
- *Client-centered*—Providing care that is respectful of and responsive to individual client preferences, needs, and values and ensuring that client values guide all clinical decisions
- *Equitable*—Providing care that does not vary in quality because of personal characteristics such as gender, ethnicity, geographic location, and socioeconomic status
- *Efficient*—Avoiding waste, including waste of equipment, supplies, ideas, and energy

QA seeks to eliminate errors before negative outcomes can occur rather than waiting until after the fact to correct individual performance.

Health care agencies have only recently paid heed to the tenets of TQM, although Donabedian's early concepts of quality bear a striking similarity to writings of the industry's TQM leaders. This management philosophy has been used in Japanese industry since the post–World War II era when W. Edwards Deming was invited to Japan to help rebuild its broken economy. In addition to Deming, people associated with the total quality concept are Walter Stewart (who first published on the subject), Joseph M. Juran, Armand F. Feigenbaum, Phillip B. Crosby, Genichi Taguchi, and Kaoru Ishikawa. Unlike traditional QA programs, the focus of CQI is the *process*

of delivering health care. This focus on process avoids placing personal blame for less-than-perfect outcomes. Applying TQM in health care allows management to look at the contribution of all systems to outcomes of the organization.

Deming's (1986, p 23) guidelines are summarized by his 15-point program:

1. Create, publish, and give to all employees a statement of the aims and purposes of the company or other organization. The management must demonstrate constantly their commitment to this statement.
2. Learn the new philosophy, top management, and everybody.
3. Understand the purpose of inspection, for improvement of processes and reduction of costs.
4. End the practice of awarding business on the basis of price tag alone.
5. Improve constantly and forever the system of production and service.
6. Institute training.
7. Teach and institute leadership.
8. Drive out fear. Create trust. Create a climate for innovation.
9. Optimize toward the aims and purposes of the company the efforts of teams, groups, and staff areas.
10. Eliminate exhortations for the work force.
11. Eliminate numerical quotes for production. Instead, learn and institute methods for improvement.
12. Eliminate management by objective. Instead, learn the capabilities of processes and how to improve them.
13. Remove barriers that rob people of pride of workmanship.
14. Encourage education and self-improvement for everyone.
15. Take action to accomplish the transformation.

Deming's first point emphasizes that an organization must have purpose and values. Health care providers have a clear idea of their values and have been committed to quality in the past, as demonstrated by codes of ethics and standards of care. However, successful TQM and CQI processes rely on a cultural change within an organization and the full support of management. With respect to providing quality health care, a paradigm shift from individual provider responsibility to team responsibility must occur (McLaughlin and Kaluzny, 2006). A guiding principle is a customer orientation focused on positive health outcomes and perceived satisfaction. Customer (client) satisfaction surveys must be done for both internal and external users of services.

Personnel policies that are motivating as well as continuous training/learning opportunities are crucial to any CQI program. Deming's eighth point addresses driving out fear. Fear in this context means the fear of being fired for being innovative or taking risks. In the CQI process, individuals are not blamed for failures in the system and therefore are motivated through the group to continually look for problems and improve system performance.

TQM works best in a flat organizational structure. This means there are very few supervisors between the staff and the director. This organization operates with a multidisciplinary team approach and a separate but parallel management quality council that monitors strategy and implementation. Teams are empowered to solve problems and locate opportunities for system improvement. Shewhart's plan-do-check-act cycle serves as a guideline for the team approach to problem solving. Steps include the following (Deming, 1986, p 88):

1. PLAN: Ask questions, such as: What could be the most important accomplishments of this team? What changes might be desirable? What data are available? Are new observations needed? If yes, plan a change or implement a test. Decide how to use the observations.
2. DO: Carry out the change or test decided upon.
3. CHECK: Observe the effects of the change. Study the results. What did we learn? What can we predict?
4. ACT: Repeat the cycle, if the changes worked, or implement a different strategy if the first plan was flawed, or revise the initial strategy based on the changes needed.

A suggested way to start the problem-solving process with a team in step 1 is brainstorming (Simon, n.d.). Brainstorming is getting everyone's input about a possible process situation with no team member criticizing the suggestion. Because TQI organizations are data driven, moving to step 2 requires that ongoing statistics be collected. Differences from the mean or norm are detected through consistent use of tools, such as the flow chart, the Pareto chart (used to compare the importance of differences between groups of data), cause-and-effect diagrams, check sheets (see p 590 for a client satisfaction check sheet), histograms, control charts, regression, and other statistical analyses (e.g., QA data and techniques, risk management data, risk-adjusted outcome measures, and cost–effectiveness analysis) (McLaughlin and Kaluzny, 2006). Steps 3, 4, and 5 are self-explanatory.

Joseph Juran built on Deming's initial quality work and became a supporter of building quality into all processes. The *Juran trilogy* provides an effective way to compare the tasks of quality planning, QC, and QI. Quality planning involves determining who the clients are, the needs of those clients, the service that fulfills the needs, and the process to produce that service. QC evaluates the performance of that service, compares it with the service goals, and then makes corrections if necessary. QI makes sure the infrastructure exists to enable individuals to identify improvement projects. Management of QI establishes project teams and provides those teams with the resources needed to carry out improvement projects (Juran and Godfrey, 2010).

TQM/CQI IN COMMUNITY AND PUBLIC HEALTH SETTINGS

Guidelines provided by the 1991 APHA *Model Standards* linked standards to meeting the health goals for the nation in the year 2000 (McLaughlin and Kaluzny, 2006). *Healthy People 2000* and APHA *Model Standards* (APHA, 1991) provided not only lists of priority health objectives for the nation and a way for public health to implement TQM/CQI, but also the most current statistics and scientific knowledge about health promotion and disease prevention. *Healthy People in Healthy Communities* (USDHHS, 2001) provided the objectives with their stated targets, measurement tools, and reflected intended performance expectations.

Healthy People 2010 built on *Healthy People 2000* and contained modified and additional objectives for promoting health and preventing disease (USDHHS, 2000). An important part of the framework of *Healthy People 2010* was eliminating health disparities and ensuring access to quality health care for all. After extensive review of the *Healthy People 2010* objectives, new goals and objectives were developed for *Healthy People 2020*. The goals for *Healthy People 2020* are as follows:

- Attain high-quality, longer lives free of preventable disease, disability, injury, and premature death.
- Achieve health equity, eliminate disparities, and improve the health of all groups.
- Create social and physical environments that promote good health for all.
- Promote quality of life, healthy development, and healthy behaviors across all life stages.

Although all of the goals speak to quality of life and health, goal two specifically addresses issues related to quality of health care delivery.

In addition, the *Planned Approach to Community Health* (PATCH) (CDC, 1995 with update in 2010); the Assessment Protocol for Excellence in Public Health (APEXPH), *APEXPH in Practice* (NACCHO, 1995); and most recently the *Mobilizing for Action through Planning and Partnerships* (MAPP) process (NACCHO, 2001) provide methods of assessing community needs to see how well health departments are operating to meet existing standards (see Chapter 25).

As health care reform continues, especially with the implementation of the Patient Protection and Affordable Care Act public health agencies face competition and are trying to reform themselves. A promising outcome of reform is how private health care and public health can come together in a community-level effort to monitor performance and improve health.

Recognizing the many factors that cause health problems and the fragmenting that continues to exist in the health care system, the public-private collaborative framework supported by the *Healthy People* documents involves many stakeholders, including public health, in monitoring the health of entire communities. Performance monitoring is defined as "a continuing community-based process of selecting indicators that can be used to measure the process and outcomes of an intervention strategy for health improvement (making the results available to the community as a whole) to inform assessments of an effective intervention and the contributions of accountable agencies to this." (*Healthy People,* 2011) These indicators would measure processes or states that contribute to health, and thus the processes are potentially alterable. As previously noted, there are four documents that monitor the quality and safety of health care including the contributions of public health. Box 26-3 provides highlights from each of these reports.

Home health care agencies have increasingly adopted QI programs because of the competition that exists. Congruent with the TQM philosophy, meeting customer expectations is essential for home health care agencies. Models for QA/QI in home health care have been developed to improve the quality

BOX 26-3 NATIONAL QUALITY AND SAFETY REPORTS

NAME OF REPORT	MOST RECENT RESULTS
The National Health Care Quality Report, Agency for Healthcare Research and Quality, began publication in 2003	Assesses four dimensions of quality effectiveness, client safety, timeliness and client centeredness. Between 2003-2007: • Health care quality improved but the rate has slowed • Variation in quality across states is decreasing but not for all of the quality measures • The safety of health care improved but not enough
The State of Health Care Quality, 2009; The National Committee for Quality Assurance	Has been published annually for 13 years. Assesses HEDIS to determine Quality Improvement across third-party payers. • Reports after more than a decade of progress in quality of care, there is a plateau in progress • Found there is no link between cost and quality • For years, quality of performance in behavioral health and some preventive measures like screening for colon cancer are deemed unacceptable • Quality of care varies among geographic locations, with New England having the highest quality and the South Atlantic states having the lowest
National Healthcare Disparities Report, 2007; The Agency for Healthcare Research and Quality	Published since 2000. Assesses four dimensions of quality effectiveness, client safety, timeliness, and client centeredness. Assesses four stages of care: staying healthy, getting better, living with illness/disability, and coping with end of life • Findings indicate disparities in quality and access are not getting smaller • Persistent lack of insurance is a major barrier to reducing disparities • Some select improvements in preventive care, chronic care management, and access have eliminated disparities for priority populations, like low-income compared with high-income persons. • Being insured and high-quality care go hand in hand
Safe Practices for Better Healthcare, 2009; The National Quality Forum	Published first in 2003, then in 2006 and 2009 The report presents 34 safe practices with descriptions of their safety impact. • Adverse health care events continue to be a leading cause of death and injury • Evidence indicates that the 34 safe practices identified are effective in improving safety • Although many of the 34 practices can be adapted to public health, two can be specifically applied in public health: a quality workforce and influenza prevention

of care in TQM frameworks emphasizing processes, empowerment, collaboration, consumers, data and measurement, and standards and outcomes (Carmichael, 2005). Datasets of clinical information, such as those developed through the Omaha System (see Chapter 40) and the OASIS toolkit from the National Association of Home Care and Hospice (NAHC) (NAHC, 2010), are useful in measuring quality of care. In 2003 the Home Health Care Quality Initiative (HHQI) was developed by the USDHHS to provide consumers with data on the quality of home health services. *Home Health Compare,* posted on the Medicare website, is a home health report card available to consumers nationwide (USDHHS, 2010).

Finally, in the area of standards and guidelines, Mead et al (2008) addresses six areas of performance that need improvement. One of these areas is consistently providing appropriate and effective care. This area is applicable to all health care practitioners, including nurses. Evidence-based practice guidelines are one way to deliver consistent, up-to-date care and to improve outcomes for individuals, communities, and populations. In 2001, five Minnesota health plans, covering most of the state's insured population, endorsed standard treatment and prevention guidelines for 50 common diseases (Varkey et al, 2007). The use of guidelines helps gather data on the effectiveness and outcomes of nurse interventions (Keller et al, 2004a). The AHRQ, formerly the Agency for Healthcare Policy and Research (AHCPR), has played a major role in developing clinical practice guidelines.

Guidelines are protocols or statements of recommended practice developed by governmental and health care agencies, and by professional organizations; they are based on the distilling of scientific evidence and expert opinion that guide a clinician in decision making. Guidelines provide research-based evidence for interventions and promote improved health outcomes. Using research findings as guidelines or frames of reference can improve nurses' awareness of new or better ways to practice, allow for documentation of nurse interventions, and improve outcomes at all levels of public health nursing practice (Keller et al, 2004b) (see Chapter 9). Keystones of evidence-based practice guidelines arise from client concerns, clinical experience, best practices, and clinical data and research (Malloch and Porter-O'Grady, 2006). Clinical practice guidelines are systematically developed statements to assist practitioner and client decisions about appropriate health care for specific clinical circumstances (as discussed in Chapter 15). An example of criteria for clinical practice guidelines are those set forth by the AHRQ and available on the Internet at the National Guideline Clearinghouse (NGC) website (http://www.guideline.gov/) (NGC, 2010):

• The practice guideline contains systematically developed statements that include recommendations, strategies, or information that assists health care practitioners and clients make decisions about appropriate health care for specific health care circumstances.

• The practice guideline was produced under the auspices of specialty associations; relevant professional societies, public or private organizations, government agencies at the federal, state, or local level; or health care organizations or plans. A practice guideline developed and issued by an individual not officially sponsored or supported by one of the above types of organizations does not meet the inclusion criteria for the NGC.

- Corroborating documentation can be produced and verified that a systematic literature search and review of existing scientific evidence published in peer-reviewed journals was performed during the guideline development. A guideline is not excluded from the NGC if corroborating documentation can be produced and verified detailing specific gaps in scientific evidence for some of the guideline's recommendations.
- The full text guideline is available upon request in print or electronic format (for free or for a fee) in English. The guideline is current and the most recent version produced. Documented evidence can be produced or verified that the guideline was developed, reviewed, or revised within the last 5 years (http://www.guideline.gov/contact/coninclusion. aspx).

Primary care practice guidelines are available in the *Guide to Clinical Preventive Services* (AHRQ, 2010) and the population-based *Guide to Community Preventive Services* available on the CDC website. This guide is an ongoing process of the Taskforce on Community Preventive Services that offers information on changing risk behaviors; reducing specific diseases, injuries and impairments, and environmental concerns; and state-of-the-art public health activities. Nurses need guidelines to reduce differences in care practices, to improve outcomes on the basis of the best research available, and to deliver effective care to individuals, communities, and populations.

Using QA/QI in CQI

QA/QI methods and tools help agencies conform to standards required by external accrediting agencies. QA/QI provides a way to identify examples of substandard care and to improve that care when standards are not met. QA is focused on problem detection, whereas CQI is focused on problem prevention and continuous improvement. In QA, little attention is paid to preventing errors or problems and finding out who owns the quality issues. Furthermore, the QA process may stop unless another problem is found. McLaughlin and Kaluzny (2006) point out differences in traditional management models that use performance standards versus those that use TQM (Table 26-1). The most important difference is in the emphasis on QA, or simply identifying the problem in the traditional management model versus the emphasis on CQI in the total quality management model. In TQM the problem is identified and measures are implemented to correct the problem. The TQM model is required in health care delivery because of the standards set by the national accrediting agencies like TJC. Public health, through the public health accrediting process, begun in 2011, will also be required to emphasize TQM.

Positive steps of a known QA program can be integrated into a CQI approach. Strengths of QA include a history of expertise in developing evaluation of structure, identifying high-priority

TABLE 26-1	TRADITIONAL MANAGEMENT MODEL COMPARED WITH TOTAL QUALITY MANAGEMENT (TQM) MODEL
TRADITIONAL MODEL	**TQM MODEL**
Legal or professional authority	Collective or managerial responsibility
Specialized accountability	Process accountability
Administrative authority	Participation
Meeting standards	Meeting process and performance expectations
Longer planning horizon	Shorter planning horizon
Quality assurance	Continuous improvement

problems, and developing knowledge in QA and information systems (Vogt et al, 2004). These strengths can be used advantageously in a CQI effort.

Traditional Quality Assurance

Traditional QA programs can fit well with the CQI process. The overall goal of specific QA approaches is to monitor the process and outcomes of client care. The goals of CQI are as follows:

1. To identify problems between provider and client through QA methods
2. To intervene in problem cases
3. To provide feedback regarding interactions between client and provider
4. To provide documentation of interactions between client and provider

Specific approaches are often implemented voluntarily by agencies and provider groups interested in the quality of interactions in their setting. However, state and federal governments require mandatory programs within public health agencies. For example, periodic utilization review, peer reviews (audits), and other QA measures are required in public health agencies that receive funds from state taxes, Medicaid, Medicare, and other public funding sources. Examples of specific approaches to QA are agency **staff review committees** (peer review), utilization review committees, research studies, PRO monitoring, client satisfaction surveys, risk management, and malpractice lawsuits.

Staff Review Committee

Staff review committees are the most common specific approach to QA in the United States. Staff review committees are designed to monitor client-specific aspects of certain levels of care. The audit is the major tool used to evaluate quality of care.

The **audit process** (Figure 26-1) consists of six steps:

1. Select a topic for study.
2. Select explicit criteria for quality care.
3. Review records to determine whether criteria are met.
4. Do a peer review for all cases that do not meet criteria.
5. Make specific recommendations to correct problems.
6. Follow up to determine whether problems have been eliminated.

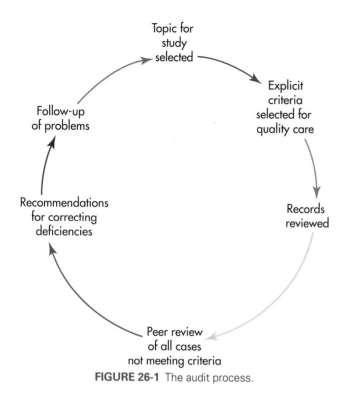

FIGURE 26-1 The audit process.

Two types of audits are used in nursing peer review: concurrent and retrospective. The **concurrent audit** is a process audit that evaluates the quality of ongoing care by looking at the nursing process. Concurrent audit is used by Medicare and Medicaid to evaluate care being received by public health/home health clients. The audit data look at the group, population, or community served. The advantages of this method are as follows:

- Identification of problems at the time care is given
- Provision of a mechanism for identifying and meeting client needs during the intervention
- Implementation of measures to fulfill professional responsibilities
- Provision of a mechanism for communicating on behalf of the client

The disadvantages of the concurrent audit are as follows:

- It is time consuming
- It is more costly to implement than the retrospective audit
- Because the intervention is ongoing, it does not present the total picture of the outcomes of the intervention that the client ultimately will receive

The **retrospective audit,** or outcome audit, evaluates quality of care through evaluation of the nursing process at the end of a program or as an audit of the long-term impact of a program within the health care system. The advantages of the retrospective audit are that it provides the following:

- Comparison of actual practice to standards of care
- Analysis of actual practice findings
- A total picture of care given to a population or group of clients
- More accurate data for planning corrective action

- Disadvantages of the retrospective audit method are as follows:
  - The focus of evaluation is directed away from ongoing care
  - Client problems (group or population or community) are identified after care is offered through the program; thus corrective action can be used only to improve the care of future clients

Currently in public health, program record audits are done to determine the processes and outcomes of care, such as family planning audits, WIC audits, breast and cervical cancer screening audits, billing coding (to audit costs) and registration audits. Programs regarding physical activity, nutrition, obesity, arthritis, smoking cessation, and others are all designed to address the major causes of morbidity and mortality locally, statewide, and nationwide. The audits assist in determining the progress being made in reducing morbidity and mortality.

Utilization Review

The purpose of **utilization review** is to ensure that care is needed and that the cost is appropriate. Utilization review is more likely used in HMOs and other MCOs, including Medicaid or Medicare state-level managed care programs. There are three types of utilization review:

1. *Prospective:* An assessment of the necessity of care before giving service
2. *Concurrent:* A review of the necessity of services while care is being given
3. *Retrospective:* An analysis of the necessity of the services received by the client after the care has been given

Each of these reviews assesses the appropriate cost of care. Prospectively, care can be denied and money saved. Concurrently, services can be cut if they are not found to be essential. Retrospectively, payment can be denied to the provider if the care was not necessary.

Utilization review began in the middle part of the twentieth century out of concern for increasing health care costs. The first committees were developed by insurance companies and professional groups. Utilization review committees became mandatory under the 1965 Medicare law as a way to control hospital costs.

The utilization review process includes development of explicit criteria regarding the need for services and the length of service. Utilization review has been used primarily in hospitals to establish the need for client admission and to determine the length of hospital stay. In community and public health, especially home health care, utilization review establishes criteria for admission to agency service, the number of visits a client may receive, the eligibility for client services (e.g., a nursing aide or physical therapist), and discharge.

Utilization review has several advantages:

- It helps clients avoid unnecessary care.
- It may encourage clients to consider alternative care options, such as home health care rather than hospital care.

- It can provide guidelines for staff and program development.
- It provides for agency accountability to the consumer.

The major disadvantage of utilization review is that not all clients fit the classic picture presented by the explicit criteria used to determine approval or denial of care. For example, an older adult client was admitted to a home health care agency for management after hospital discharge. The client was paraplegic as a result of a cerebrovascular accident. After several weeks of physical and speech therapy, the client showed little sign of progress. The utilization review committee considered the client's condition to be stable and did not recognize the continued need for management to prevent future complications; therefore, Medicare payment was denied.

Appeal mechanisms have been built into the utilization review process used by Medicare and Medicaid. The appeal allows providers and clients to present additional data that may help to reverse the original decision to deny payment.

EVIDENCE-BASED PRACTICE

Home visiting has been a mainstay in the repertoire of the public health nurse for decades. Randomized clinical trials have shown the effectiveness of home visiting, particularly with high-risk clients. Home visiting can be considered as a population-based activity when it meets the criteria that service is rendered to individuals because they are members of an identified population and because those services will improve the health status of that population. This article describes another approach, other than the randomized control trial, to continuous quality improvement: the focus group.

Nurses' experience of home visits for new mothers in a health service region of Western Australia is reported in this QI article. Nurses recognized the benefits of home visits as improvement in maternal and child health status, resulting in better parenting skills which led to positive maternal–child interaction. Although nurses supported home visits and saw the positive outcomes, agency factors such as costs, lack of resources, and staffing made it difficult to continue home visits as a part of the community health nurses' responsibilities.

Twelve nurses in the agency, who worked in child health, participated in a focus group–taped interview to explore the nurses' experience in the home visits for new mothers. The purpose of the focus groups was to evaluate and improve home visits. Data were transcribed verbatim and content analyzed to identify the themes emerging from the discussion.

Three themes were identified. These were: (1) determining how nurses managed home visits, such as scheduling first home visits and making the first phone call, (2) staying safe during home visits while managing high-risk clients and scheduling subsequent visits, and (3) building positive partnerships with clients during home visits. The findings indicated that nurses followed a defined process, or protocol for successfully completing home visits.

Nurse Use
Such a QI approach is important for better describing the population being served and determining the effect of home visitation on client outcome. This is an international article, which can provide insights into how public health nurses in the United States can use QI approaches to improve practice. The article points out how the nurse who is delivering care can make a difference in promoting services that work to improve health status.

Modified from Henderson S: Community Child Health (CCH) nurses' experience of home visits for new mothers: a quality improvement project, *Contemp Nurse* 34(1):66-76, 2009.

Risk Management

Risk management committees are often a part of the CQI program of a community agency. Risk management seeks to reduce the agency's liability because of grievances brought against them. The risk management committee reviews all risks to which an agency is exposed. It reviews client and personnel safety policies and procedures and determines whether personnel are following the rules. Examples of problems reviewed by a risk management committee in public health clinics include administering incorrect vaccination dosage, pediatric client injury caused by a fall from an examination table, or injury to the nurse from a needlestick in the sexually transmitted diseases clinic at the health department or as a result of an accident while making a home visit. Incident reports are reviewed by the risk management committee for appropriate, accurate, and thorough documentation of any problem that occurs relating to clients or personnel. In addition, patterns are identified from looking at program data that may require changes in policy or staff development to correct the problem. As a part of risk management, grievance procedures are established for both clients and personnel.

Professional Review Organizations

The **Professional Standards Review Organization (PSRO)** was established in 1972 in an amendment to the Social Security Act (PL 92-603) as a publicly mandated utilization and peer review program. This law provided that medical, hospital, and nursing home care under Medicare, Medicaid, and Title V Maternal and Child Health Programs would be reviewed for appropriateness and necessary care to be reimbursed.

In 1983 Congress passed the Peer Review Improvement Act (PL 97-248), creating PROs. PROs replaced PSROs and are directed by the federal government to reduce hospital admissions for procedures that can be performed safely and effectively in an ambulatory surgical setting on an outpatient basis. The goal was to reduce inappropriate or unnecessary admissions or invasive procedures by specific practitioners or hospitals. Quality measures include reducing unnecessary admissions caused by previous substandard care, avoidable complications and deaths, and unnecessary surgery or invasive procedures (Varkey et al, 2007).

Institutions contract with PROs for quality reviews. PROs are local (usually state) organizations that establish criteria for care on the basis of local patterns of practice, and they can be for-profit or not-for-profit organizations. They have access to physicians or may include physicians in their membership. PROs must define their operational objectives and are required to consult with nurses and other non-physician health care providers when reviewing the activities of those professionals. PROs monitor access to care and cost of care. Professionals working under the regulation of PROs should develop accurate and complete documenting procedures to ensure compliance with the criteria of the PRO.

Debate has occurred over the limits and benefits of the federally mandated quality review process. Limits include jeopardizing professional autonomy because decision making regarding care includes professionals, consumers, and government representatives. Another limitation of this process is the development of a costly control mechanism whereby client care activities may be determined by cost rather than by professional criteria. The benefit of the PSRO/PRO system has been the development of standards and the peer review mechanisms to increase accountability for care provided. In 1985 PRO authority was expanded to include review of services offered by HMOs and competitive medical plans. In addition, the Medicare Quality Assurance Act was passed to strengthen QA programs and to improve access to care after hospitalization. This act required hospitals receiving Medicare payments to provide to Medicare beneficiaries written forms of discharge planning supervised by registered nurses and social workers.

> **DID YOU KNOW?** *TQM provides direction for managing a system of care, whereas CQI using QA/QI focuses on the care a client receives within the system.*

Evaluative Studies

Evaluative studies for quality health care increased during the twentieth century. Studies demonstrate the effect of nursing and health care interventions on client populations. Three key models have been used to evaluate quality: Donabedian's structure-process-outcome model, the tracer method, and the sentinel method.

Donabedian's model (1981, 1985, 2003) introduced three major methods for evaluating quality care:

1. **Structure:** Evaluating the setting and instruments used to provide care; examples of structure are facilities, equipment, characteristics of the administrative organization, client mix, and the qualifications of health providers
2. **Process:** Evaluating activities as they relate to standards and expectations of health providers in the management of client care
3. **Outcome:** The net change or result that occurs as a result of health care

The three methods may be used separately to evaluate a part of care. However, to get an overall picture of quality of care, they should be used together.

The tracer method described by Kessner and Kalk (1973) is a measure of both process and outcome of care and is used today. This method is more effective in evaluating health care of groups than of individual clients. It is also more effective in evaluating care delivered by an institution than care delivered by an individual provider. The following are essential characteristics for implementing the tracer method (Neuhauser, 2004; Kelly, 2007):

1. A tracer, or a problem, that has a definite impact on the client's level of functioning
2. Well-defined and easily diagnosed characteristics
3. Population prevalence high enough to permit adequate data collection
4. A known variation resulting from use of effective health care
5. Well-defined management techniques in prevention, diagnosis, treatment, or rehabilitation

6. Understood (documented) effects of non-medical factors on the tracer

Groups are selected for tracer outcome studies in nursing. The client groups would have the following:

1. A shared health problem
2. Receiving a similar intervention
3. Sharing similar needs
4. Located in the same community
5. Having a similar lifestyle
6. Being at the same illness stage

The tracer method provides nurses with data to show the differences in outcomes as a result of nursing care standards.

The sentinel method of quality evaluation is based on epidemiological principles. This method is an outcome measure for examining specific instances of client care (Kelly, 2007). Changes in the sentinel indicate potential problems for others. For example, increases in encephalitis in certain communities may result from increases in mosquito populations. Data may be collected at the health department through a state or local required disease reporting system. The health department would be notified and an immediate mosquito control strategy would be put into place. Such an intervention would include, for example, nurses notifying the population to remove standing water around the outside of homes, such as animal water bowls, rain barrels, and gutter down spout water collection pools. Flyers may be sent home with school children or given to clients visiting the public health clinics, and media announcements may be used. In addition, the environmental office at the health department may inspect local swimming pools and may also implement a nighttime mosquito spraying program throughout the community.

> **HOW TO** **Conduct a Sentinel Evaluation**
> - *Identify cases of unnecessary disease, disability, and complications (for example, tuberculosis (TB).*
> - *Count the deaths from these causes.*
> - *Examine the circumstances surrounding the unnecessary event (or sentinel), in detail.*
> - *Review morbidity and mortality rates as an index for comparison; determine the critical increase in the untimely event, which may reflect changes in quality of care. Example: Compare the incidence and prevalence of TB cases before the increased population occurred.*
> - *Explore health status indicators, such as changes in social, economic, political, and environmental factors that may have an effect on health outcomes. Example: Overcrowding in the shelter where migrant workers stay (environmental) and the inability to follow up on testing because of the transient nature of the population (social).*

CLIENT SATISFACTION

Client satisfaction is another approach to measuring quality of care. Client satisfaction can be assessed using in-person or telephone interviews and mailed questionnaires. Satisfaction surveys are used to assess care received during an admission to

Please mark the following questions using the scale.

Domain	Example	Strongly Agree	Somewhat Agree	Agree	Somewhat Disagree	Strongly Disagree
Affective support	1. The visiting nurse was understanding of my health concerns.					
	2. The nurse gave me encouragement in regard to my health problems.					
Health information	3. I got my questions answered in an individual way.					
	4. The information I received from the nurse helped me to take care of myself at home.					
Decision control	5. I was included in decision making.					
	6. I was included in the planning of my care.					
Technical competencies	7. The care I received was of high quality.					
	8. Decisions regarding my health care were of high quality.					
Accessibility	9. The nurse was available when I needed help.					
	10. The nurse was on time.					
Overall satisfaction	11. Overall, I was satisfied with my health care.					
	12. The care I received was of high quality.					

FIGURE 26-2 Client satisfaction tool domains and examples.

a specific agency, to assess a client's personal nursing care, or to assess the total care that the client received from all services.

Satisfaction surveys may measure the interventions used for client care, attitudes about the care received and the providers of care, and perceptions of the situation (environment) in which the care was received. Clients are often more critical of interpersonal and situational components of care than of the interventions of care.

Satisfaction surveys are an essential aspect of QA. Survey data provide clues to reasons for client compliance or noncompliance with plans of care. Although consumers may not view quality in the same light as the health professional, surveys provide data about health-seeking behaviors, the probability of

malpractice litigation, and the likelihood of continuing client-provider-agency relationships—always an important measure for community based and public health agencies (Carmichael, 2005) (Figure 26-2).

Malpractice Litigation

Malpractice litigation (i.e., a lawsuit) is a specific approach to QA imposed on the health care delivery system by the legal system. Malpractice litigation typically results from client dissatisfaction with the provider and with the content of the care received. Nursing is not immune from malpractice litigation. Nursing must continue to have a sound QA program that ensures quality care. This will reduce the risk of quality control

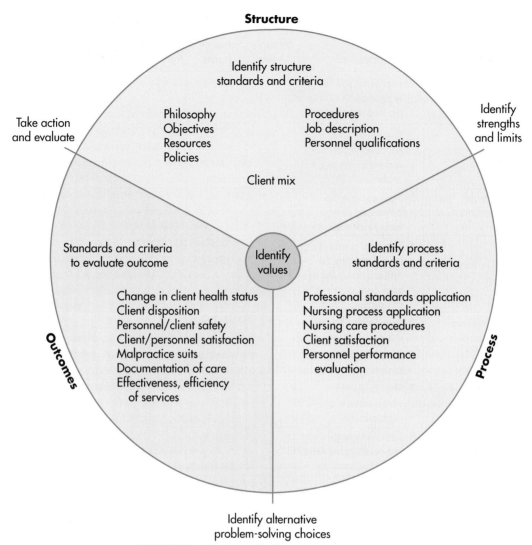

Structure

Identify structure
standards and criteria

Take action
and evaluate

Philosophy
Objectives
Resources
Policies

Procedures
Job description
Personnel qualifications

Identify
strengths
and limits

Client mix

Standards and criteria
to evaluate outcome

Identify
values

Identify process
standards and criteria

Change in client health status
Client disposition
Personnel/client safety
Client/personnel satisfaction
Malpractice suits
Documentation of care
Effectiveness, efficiency
of services

Professional standards application
Nursing process application
Nursing care procedures
Client satisfaction
Personnel performance
evaluation

Outcomes

Process

Identify alternative
problem-solving choices

FIGURE 26-3 Model quality improvement programs.

measures being imposed by an external source, such as the legal system. As a true example, a public health nurse was individually sued by a new family to the community because the nurse repeated an immunization the child had already received prior to moving to the community. The result was Guillain-Barré syndrome. The nurse was found at fault even though the parents did not provide the physician's record of immunizations to the nurse. It was the nurse's responsibility to follow standard guidelines and to obtain the essential records prior to proving the immunization. The public health department was dismissed from the lawsuit because of immunity granted to state agencies.

MODEL CQI PROGRAM

The primary purpose of a QA/QI program is to ensure that the results of an organized activity are consistent with the expectations. All personnel affected by a QI program should be involved in its development and implementation. Although administration and management are responsible for the quality of services, the key to that quality is in the personnel who deliver the service: their knowledge, skills, and attitudes.

Figure 26-3 shows a model that identifies the basic components of a QI program. QI programs answer the following questions about health care services and nursing care:

1. What is being done now?
2. Why is it being done?
3. Is it being done well?
4. Can it be done better?
5. Should it be done at all?
6. Are there improved ways to deliver the service?
7. How much does it cost?
8. Should certain activities be abandoned or replaced?

As a part of answering the questions and determining changes that can improve services, public health is adopting the PDCA model. The steps of the model are shown in Figure 26-4.

The PDCA is a model for continuous improvement and can be used after an audit of a program, for example to begin a new improvement project or when developing a new or improved design of a process, product, or program.

It can also be used to define a repetitive work process or for planning data collection and analysis in order to verify and prioritize problems or root causes, which are actually the system

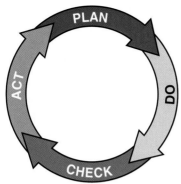

FIGURE 26-4 The plan-do-check-act (PDCA) model of continuous quality improvement. The concept of the PDCA cycle was originally developed by Walter Shewhart, the pioneering statistician who developed statistical process control in the Bell Laboratories in the United States during the 1930s. It is often referred to as the "Shewhart Cycle." It was adopted in the 1950s by W. Edwards Deming, and is often referred to as the "Deming Wheel."

problems that lead to the problem. It is also used to implement change.

The PDCA procedure involves the following steps:
1. Plan. Recognize an opportunity and plan a change.
2. Do. Test the change. Carry out a small-scale study.

3. Check. Review the data, analyze the results, and identify what you've learned.
4. Act. Take action based on what you learned in the check/study step: If the change did not work, go through the cycle again with a different plan. If you were successful, incorporate what you learned from the test into wider changes. Use what you learned to plan new improvements, and begin the cycle again. Beginning the cycle again defines the 'continuous' program of CQI. This is also referred to as a rapid cycle improvement process in health care.

Donabedian's framework for evaluating health care programs using the components of structure, process, and outcome can be used in developing a QI program. *Outcome* is the most important ingredient of a program because it is the key to evaluating providers and agencies by accrediting bodies, by insurance companies, and by Medicare and Medicaid through PROs, report cards, and other accrediting agencies.

Structure

The vision, values, philosophy, and objectives of an agency serve to define the structural standards of the agency. Evaluation of structure is a specific approach to looking at quality. In evaluating the structure of an organization, the evaluator determines whether the agency is adhering to the stated philosophy and

LINKING CONTENT TO PRACTICE

The PDCA model is being used in public health to promote CQI. A brief example of how to apply this model is given below.

This approach was designed to improve new mother and baby outcomes by improving nurse/client communication processes. This model for improvement includes four components recommended by the Institute of Healthcare Improvement: (1) aims and goals, (2) performance measures, (3) strategies and ideas for changes, and (4) the use of PDCA cycles.
1. The goal of the project is to improve health outcomes for at-risk new mothers and babies involved in the nurse home visiting program by offering a daily telephone consultation to answer questions and provide support up to 3 months after the baby's birth.
2. The performance measures include:
   A. An assessment of the numbers of nurses on the home visiting team who could successfully answer the questions of the mothers who received the daily consultation.
   B. The second measure is a retrospective record audit at 6 months to assess the progress of the mothers who had access to the daily call as compared with mothers who were involved in the program prior to the daily phone consult.
3. The strategies include:
   A. A work session of the nurses to review their knowledge about parenting and caring for a new baby up to 3 months using a simple pretest.
   B. An update on what new mothers need to know to bond with their babies and to provide for the new babies' needs followed by a post-test of the nurses' knowledge.
   C. The development of the process for the daily phone consultation including a check list of assessment questions the nurse might ask and time built in to respond to parent's questions.
Plan: Plan a mock "daily consult" call to a public health nurse (or a fellow student) with her first baby.

Develop different scenarios for the public health nurse to respond to in order to assess each home visiting nurse's ability to respond to the mother's questions, such as feeding techniques, bathing, crying, and holding the baby.
Do: Engage each of the home visiting nurses in participating in the mock calls.
Check: Assess the abilities of each of the nurses to respond to the questions from the new mother by having the public health nurse use a simple yes/no check list of prepared questions.

Assess how efficient the nurse is in completing the consultation. Can she answer the questions immediately, or does she need to seek help from others prior to answering the mother's question? Use a checklist to identify the time on the call, and ability to independently answer the questions.
Act: If the nurses were able to provide the consultation without assistance and efficiently, implement the process with new mothers and babies. Use PDCA for the implementation to identify any problems with the process.

If the nurses were unable to efficiently provide the consult, provide additional education and tools to increase their efficiency. Use the PDCA process until the nurses are able to efficiently provide the consult.

The PDCA cycle is continuously repeated until the administration, the nurses, and the clients are satisfied that the process is working.

Data from these small tests will provide realistic estimates of the percentage of the nurses who can successfully engage in consultation via phone. The purpose in the initial assessment and education of the nurses is to ensure faster consults so more mothers and babies can be contacted in a short period without adding to the nurses' workload, while potentially reducing the amount of time for the home visit because the mother may be better prepared to care for the baby's needs with this support. The improvement process may enlist the support of all nursing staff and administration and create a change in the work environment through the development of a planned phone consultation process for all clients who may receive home visits.

As students develop questions, they also develop a PDCA approach to answering those questions.

From Cronenwett L, Sherwood G, Barnsteiner J, et al: Quality and safety education for nurses, *Nurs Outlook* 55(3):122-131, 2007.

objectives and to its vision and stated values. Is the agency providing services to populations across the life span? Are primary, secondary, and/or tertiary preventive services offered? Standards of structure are defined by the licensing or accrediting agency (e.g., the Community Health Accreditation Program's [CHAP's] standards for accrediting home health agencies).

Identifying values, the first step in a QA program, serves to define the beliefs of the agency about humanity, nursing, the community, and health. The beliefs of the community, the population to be served, and the providers of care are equally important to the agency, and all need to be considered to provide quality service.

Identifying standards and criteria for QA begins with writing the philosophy and objectives of the organization. Program objectives define the intended results of nursing care, descriptions of client behaviors, and/or change in health status to be demonstrated on discharge.

Once objectives are formulated, the resources needed to accomplish the objectives should be identified. The personnel, supplies and equipment, facilities, and financial resources that are needed should be described. Once resources are determined, policies, procedures, and job descriptions should be formed to serve as behavioral guides to the employees of the agency. These documents should reflect the essential nursing and other health provider qualifications needed to implement the services of the agency.

Standards of structure are evaluated internally by a committee composed of administrative, management, and staff members for the purpose of doing a self-study. Standards of structure are also evaluated by a utilization review committee, often composed of an external advisory group with community representatives for all services offered through an agency, such as a nurse, a public health physician, an environmental engineer, a sanitation engineer, a health educator, a board member, and an administrator from a similar agency. The data from these committees identify the strengths and weaknesses of the agency structure.

Process

The evaluation of process standards is a specific look at the quality of care being given by agency providers, such as nurses. Agencies use a variety of methods to determine criteria for evaluating provider activities: conceptual models; the standards of care of the provider's professional organization, such as the ANA's *Scope and Standards of Public Health Nursing Practice* (ANA, 2007) (see Chapter 1); or the nursing process. The activities of the nurse are evaluated to see whether they are the same as the nursing care procedures defined by the public health agency.

The primary approaches used for process evaluation include the peer review committee and the client (often community) satisfaction survey. The techniques used for process evaluation are direct observation, focus groups, questionnaire, interview, written audit, and video or digital recordings of client and provider encounters.

Once data are collected to evaluate nursing process standards, the peer review committee reviews the data to identify strengths and weaknesses in the quality of care delivered. The peer review committee is usually an internal committee composed of representatives of the nursing staff who are trained to administer audit instruments and conduct client interviews.

NURSING TIP *Know the standards of care for your agency and for your practice area (e.g., ANA's Scope and Standards of Practice for Public Health Nursing). Keep your eyes open for recurring practices that are not up to the quality standards of your agency. (For example, the population complains that there are not enough nurses to meet the needs of the WIC clients.) Chances are that these same practices may be occurring in other areas of the agency, and knowing this helps the agency improve quality.*

Outcome

The evaluation of outcome standards, or the result of nursing care, is one of the more difficult tasks facing nursing today. Identifying changes in the client's health status that result from nursing care provides nursing data that demonstrate the contribution of nursing to the health care delivery system. Research studies using the tracer or sentinel method to identify client outcomes and client satisfaction surveys can be used to measure outcome standards. Measures of outcome standards include client data about the changes in the community in low-birth-weight babies as a result of improved prenatal care and client compliance with care through the WIC program.

From these data, strengths and weaknesses in nursing care delivery can be determined. The most common measurement methods are direct physical observations and interviews. Instruments have also been developed to measure general health status indicators in home health. The Omaha Visiting Nurse Association problem classification system includes nursing diagnosis, protocols of care, and a problem-rating scale to measure nursing care outcomes. In addition, the ANA has developed 10 areas for data collection of outcome criteria in community-based, non–acute care settings, including pain management, consistency of communication, staff mix, client satisfaction, prevention of tobacco use, cardiovascular disease prevention, caregiver activity, identification of primary caregiver, activities of daily living, and psychosocial interactions (Rowell, 2001). Nursing has been involved primarily in evaluating program outcomes to justify program expenses rather than in evaluating client outcomes.

Outcome evaluation assumes that health care has a positive effect on client status. The major problem with outcome evaluation is determining which nursing care activities are primarily responsible for causing changes in client status. Recently, studies have been conducted on nurse-sensitive indicators, such as failure to rescue, that show the importance of nurse staffing in adverse client outcomes (Aiken et al, 2008; Kane et al, 2007). In nursing, many uncontrolled factors in the field, such as environment, community services, and family relationships, have an effect on client status. Often it is difficult to determine whether these factors are the cause of changes in client status or whether nursing interventions have the most effect.

Types of problems studied in a QA program include reasons for the following:

- Client death (population mortality)
- Client injury (population morbidity)
- Personnel and client safety
- Agency liability

TABLE 26-2 QUALITY ASSURANCE MEASURES

STRUCTURE	PROCESS	OUTCOME
Internal agency	Peer review committees	Internal agency committees
Self-study	Prospective audit	Evaluative studies
Review agency documents	Concurrent audit Retrospective audit	Survey health status
External agency	Client	Client
Regulatory audit	Satisfaction survey	Malpractice suits
	Utilization review	Satisfaction survey

- Increased costs
- Denied reimbursement by third-party payers (decreased program funding by government)
- Client complaints
- Inefficient service
- Staff non-compliance with standards of structure
- Lack of resources
- Unnecessary staff work and overtime
- Documenting of care
- Client health status (population health status)

Table 26-2 summarizes QA measures.

Evaluation, Interpretation, and Action

Interpreting the findings of a quality care evaluation is an important part of the process. It allows differences between the quality care standards of the agency and the actual practice of the nurse or other health providers to be identified. These patterns reflect the total agency's functioning over time and generate information for decisions to be made about the strengths and limits of the agency. Regular intervals for evaluation should be established within the agency, and periodic reports should be written so that the combined results of structure, process, and outcome efforts can be analyzed and health care delivery patterns and problems can be identified. These reports should be used to establish an ongoing picture of changes that occur within an agency to justify nursing services.

Identifying choices of possible courses of action to correct the weaknesses within the agency should involve both the administration and the staff. The courses of action chosen should be based on their importance, cost, and timeliness. For example, if there is a nursing problem in the recording of client health education, the agency administration and staff may analyze the problem to see why it is occurring. Reasons for lack of record-keeping given by the nurses include a lack of time to do paperwork properly, workloads that reduce the amount of time spent with clients, and lack of available resources for health education. If such reasons are given, it would not be appropriate for management to deal with the problem by providing a staff development program on the importance of doing and recording health education; it would be more important to assess how to provide the time and resources necessary for the nurses to offer health education to the clients. Economically, it may be more beneficial to provide personal data assistants or laptop computers and clerical assistance so that nurses can make notes at the point of implementation, thereby providing more client contact time, or it may be more beneficial economically to employ an additional nurse and reduce workloads.

Taking action is the final step in the QA/QI model. Once the alternative courses of action are chosen to correct problems, actions must be implemented for change to occur in the overall operation of the agency. Follow-up and evaluation of actions taken must occur to improve quality of care. Although health provider evaluation will continue to be included in a QI effort, the focus of a CQI effort emphasizes the process and not the person. The assumption here is that health care professionals and other employees customarily want to do the best job possible for the client, and problems or differences in a process should not be automatically attributed to their behavior. Although frequent feedback should be given to all employees, the hallmark of QI is continuous learning. Staff development must be ongoing for all employees. (The Levels of Prevention box shows prevention levels related to quality management.)

LEVELS OF PREVENTION

Quality Management

Primary Prevention
The nurse participates in a parent education program to improve the immunization level of children in the local elementary school and develops a strategy for follow-up.

Secondary Prevention
Agency evaluation, using a retrospective audit of records of the immunization program, determines that the vaccine preventable infectious disease rates have declined in the elementary school after the implementation of the parent education program.

Tertiary Prevention
A review of the public health report card indicated that community incidence of complications from vaccine preventable diseases have declined over a 2-year period after the implementation of the parent education program.

Documentation is essential to evaluating quality care in any organization. The following text focuses on the kinds of documentation that normally occur in a community agency.

RECORDS

Records are an important part of the communication structure of the health care organization. Accurate and complete records are required by law and must be kept by all government and non-government agencies. In most states, the state departments of health stipulate the kinds of records to be kept and their content requirements for community agencies.

Records provide complete information about the client (whether a family, group, population or community), indicate the extent and quality of services being given, resolve legal issues in malpractice suits, and provide information for education and research.

Community and Public Health Agency Records

Within the community or public health agency, many types of records are kept and used to predict population trends in a community, to identify health needs and problems, to prepare and justify budgets, and to make administrative decisions. The kinds of records kept by the agency may include reports of accidents, births, census, chronic disease, communicable disease, mortality rates, life expectancy, morbidity rates, child and spouse abuse, occupational illness and injury, and environmental health.

Other types of records kept within the agency are those used to maintain administrative contact and control of the organization. Three types of records make up this category: clinical, provider service, and financial. The *clinical record* is the client health record. The *provider service records* include information about the number of clinic clients seen daily, the immunizations given, home visits made daily, transportation and mileage, the provider's time spent with the client, and the amount and kinds of supplies used. The service record is completed on a daily basis by each provider and is summarized monthly and annually to indicate trends in health care activities and costs related to personnel time, transportation, maintenance, and supplies. The provider service records are used to compare with the agency's *financial records* of salaries, overhead, and transportation costs, and they serve as the basis for the cost accounting system (see Chapter 25). These records are basic to peer review and audit.

Three additional kinds of service records seen in the community agency are the central index system, the annual implementation plan, and the annual summary of agency activities. The *central index system* is a data-filing system that indicates the services requested, services offered, active and inactive clients of the agency, and a profile of the agency's clients.

The *annual implementation plan* (often referred to as the strategic plan or tactical plan) is developed at the beginning of each fiscal year to define the short- and long-term goals of the agency. The annual implementation plan serves as the basis for the agency's annual summary. The *annual summary* reflects the success of the agency in meeting the annual objectives, the changes in population trends and health status during the year, the actual versus the projected budget requirements, the number of services offered, the number of clients served, and the plans and changes recommended for the future. This plan serves as the basis for the evaluation of agency structure.

As an outgrowth of QA efforts in the health care system, comprehensive methods are being designed to document and measure client progress and client outcome from agency admission through discharge. An example of such a method is the client classification system developed at the Visiting Nurses Association of Omaha, Nebraska (Martin, 2005; The Omaha System 2010). This comprehensive method for evaluating client care has several components: a classification system for assessing and categorizing client problems, a database, a nursing problem list, and anticipated outcome criteria for the classified problem. Such schemes are viewed as having the potential to improve the delivery of nursing care, documentation of care, and the descriptions of client care. Briefly, implementing a comprehensive documentation method improves nursing assessment, planning, implementing, and evaluating of client care; it also allows the organization of important client information for more effective and efficient nurse productivity and communication (see Figure 26-2).

LINKING CONTENT TO PRACTICE

The Robert Wood Johnson Foundation (RWJF) funded a project initiative focusing on the development of competencies and resources to enhance the ability of nursing professionals to deliver high-quality and safe nursing care. The Quality Safety Education for Nurses collaboration identified and defined six quality and safety competencies for nursing. In addition, the project allowed for the development of proposed targets for the knowledge, skills, and attitudes of students for each of the six competencies identified by the Institute of Medicine as: client-centered care, teamwork and collaboration, evidence-based practice, quality improvement, safety, and informatics. The overall goal for the Quality and Safety Education for Nurses (QSEN) project is to meet the challenge of preparing future nurses who will have the knowledge, skills, and attitudes (KSAs) necessary to continuously improve the quality and safety of the healthcare systems within which they work. The following are the definitions for each of the six competencies and examples of the chapters in the text where content can be found and related to the competency:

Client-centered care: Recognize the client or designee as the source of control and full partner in providing compassionate and coordinated care based on respect for client's preferences, values, and needs. (Chapters 4, 6, 7, 9, 12, 14, 15, 19)

Teamwork and Collaboration: Function effectively within nursing and interprofessional teams, fostering open communication, mutual respect, and shared decision-making to achieve quality client care. (Chapters 5, 6, 8, 10, 16, 18, 20, 21, 22, 26, 27, 28, 30, 32, 33, 34, 35, 37, 39, 41, 45, 46)

Evidence-Based Practice (EBP): Integrate best current evidence with clinical expertise and client/family preferences and values for delivery of optimal health care. (All chapters with emphasis in Chapters 15 and 26)

Quality Improvement (QI): Use data to monitor the outcomes of care processes and use improvement methods to design and test changes to continuously improve the quality and safety of health care systems. (Chapters 3, 8, 10, 12, 14, 18, 20, 24, 25, 26)

Safety: Minimizes risk of harm to clients and providers through both system effectiveness and individual performance. (Chapters 12, 13, 14, 23, 24, 28, 39-46)

Informatics: Use information and technology to communicate, manage knowledge, mitigate error, and support decision making. (Chapters 23, 24, 25, 26)

All of these competencies are addressed in this text as the competencies relate to public health nursing practice. The knowledge, skills and attitudes related to QI are addressed in this chapter and one area of the QI competency appears in the following table.

KNOWLEDGE	SKILLS	ATTITUDES
Describe approaches for changing processes of care	Design a small test of change in daily work (using an experiential learning method such as PDCA) Practice aligning the aims, measures and changes involved in improving care Use measures to evaluate the effect of change	Value local change (in individual practice or team practice on a unit) and its role in creating joy in work Appreciate the value of what individuals and teams can to do to improve care

From Institute of Medicine: *Health professions education: a bridge to quality,* Washington, DC, 2003, National Academies Press.

CHAPTER REVIEW

PRACTICE APPLICATION

Oscar, a nursing student, has been working in the migrant farm-worker clinic and has noted that each practitioner uses a different educational method for teaching good nutrition practices to newly diagnosed diabetic clients. The clinic has seen a substantial increase in the number of new diabetic clients in the Hispanic farm-worker population. Oscar knows that practice guidelines for teaching nutrition practices exist in his clinical facility and that charts have an area to note nutrition education information. He also knows that for nurses to be most effective and ensure quality client outcomes, research-based practice guidelines should be used by all nurses in the health department.

As part of his course, Oscar must prepare a teaching plan and conduct a class on a health care problem. He obtains permission from his instructor and the director of the clinic to conduct an in-service program. The purpose of Oscar's in-service program is to instruct the nursing staff how to teach newly diagnosed diabetic clients good nutrition practices. He obtains and studies the guidelines about teaching good nutrition practices, from the National Guideline Clearinghouse titled Diabetes Type 1 and 2 Evidence-based Nutrition Practice Guideline for Adults (2010), and he researches the methodological background for development of the guidelines. Oscar's native language is Spanish, so this will help him in determining whether brochures for newly diagnosed diabetic clients regarding good nutrition convey the appropriate message.

As part of his in-service program, Oscar keeps demographic records on attendees and conducts before-and-after tests of knowledge, adding questions about the present use of the guidelines. He plans to follow up with the nurses in 6 months with a further test and questions about use of the guidelines. The director will help him determine an outcome measure that can be used with the client population to show effective use of the guidelines.

A. What outcome measure would be useful in this project?
B. How will this help in the overall assessment of quality in the nursing service?

Answers can be found on the Evolve site.

KEY POINTS

- The health care delivery system is the largest employing industry in the United States; society is demanding increased efficiency and effectiveness from the system.
- The actual quality and safety of care in the United States are being assessed regularly and reported in four reports.
- Because of varying definitions, logistics, and data collection methods, quality is difficult to assess accurately.
- Responding to the quality of care question, the federal government has instituted several quality improvement programs. Among these are the National Healthcare Quality Report (NHQR) that is used to monitor the nation's progress toward improved health care quality; the Center for Medicare and Medicaid Services (CMS) Outcomes Based Quality Improvement (OBQI) for home health; and the National Committee for Quality Assurance (NCQA), which provides performance information, or report cards, for health care agencies.
- Quality improvement is the tool used to ensure effective and efficient care.
- The managed care industry is changing the face of the American health care delivery system and how quality is defined and measured.
- Objective and systematic evaluation of nursing care has become a priority within the profession for several reasons, including the effects of cost on health care access, consumer demands for better quality care, and increasing involvement of nurses in formulating public and health agency policy.
- Total quality management is a management philosophy new to the public health care arena. It is prevention oriented and process focused. Its primary focus is to deliver quality health care. One measure of quality is customer satisfaction.
- Public and private sectors are forming partnerships to monitor the performance of all players in health care delivery to improve the health of communities. The different players in the health care system have different perceptions of quality.
- Quality assurance/quality improvement (QA/QI) is the monitoring of client care activities to determine the degree of excellence attained in implementing activities.
- Quality assurance has been a concern of the profession since the 1860s, when Florence Nightingale called for a uniform format to gather and disseminate hospital statistics.
- Licensure has been a major issue in nursing since 1892.
- Two major categories of approaches exist in QA/QI today: general and specific.
- Accreditation is an approach to quality control used for institutions, whereas licensure is used primarily for individuals.
- Certification combines features of both licensing and accreditation.
- Three major models have been used to evaluate quality: Donabedian's structure-process-outcome model, the sentinel model, and the tracer model.
- A fourth model to evaluate quality—the PDCA model—has been adopted by the public health system.
- Seven basic components of a quality improvement program are: (1) identifying values, (2) identifying structure, process, and outcome standards and criteria, (3) selecting measurement techniques, (4) interpreting the strengths and weaknesses of the care given, (5) identifying alternative courses of action, (6) choosing specific courses of action, and (7) taking action.
- Records are an integral part of the communication structure of a health care organization. Accurate and complete records are by law required of all agencies, whether governmental or nongovernmental.
- QA/QI mechanisms in health care delivery are the mechanisms for controlling the system and requesting accountability from individual providers within the system. Records help establish a total picture of the contribution of the agency to the client community.
- Delivering quality care to individuals, communities, and populations falls under the 10 essential services of public health.
- Evidence-based practice guidelines can help population-centered nurses document the outcomes and effectiveness of their interventions.

CLINICAL DECISION-MAKING ACTIVITIES

1. Write your own definition of TQM; compare your definition with the one given in the text. Are they the same or different? Give justification for your answer.
2. How does traditional QA/QI fit with the CQI effort? Explain the relative importance of a continuing QA/QI effort.
3. Interview a nurse who is a coordinator of or is responsible for QA/QI in a local health agency. Ask the following questions and add your own. Do the answers to the questions relate to what you have learned about QA/QI? Explain.
   A. Does the agency subscribe to the TQM approach to management?
   B. If not, is the agency incorporating elements of the TQM process as outlined by Deming (1986) in his 14 points?
   C. Is a traditional method of management used to ensure quality?
   D. Describe the components of the QA/QI program.
   E. How are records used in your QA/QI effort?
   F. Discuss the approaches and techniques that are used to implement the QA/QI program.
   G. How has the QA/QI program changed in the health agency over the past 20 years?
   H. What influence has the QA/QI program had on decreasing problems attributable to process? To provider accountability?
   I. List and describe the types of records usually kept in a community health agency. Explain the purpose of each type of record.
4. Identify partnerships necessary to ensure quality health outcomes for your community from data gathered in a community assessment. Explain why these partners are necessary.
5. Find the *Guide to Community Preventive Services* on the CDC website, and look for the segments on smoking cessation or tuberculosis control. How could you use this information in your practice in health?
6. Explain the nurse's responsibilities and role in the CQI program.

REFERENCES

Agency for Healthcare Research and Quality: *Improving healthcare quality,* Rockville, MD, 2002, U.S. Department of Health and Human Services.

Agency for Healthcare Research and Quality: *Your guide to choosing quality health care,* Rockville, MD, 2001, AHRQ.

Agency for Healthcare Research and Quality: *Your guide to choosing quality health care,* Rockville, MD, 2007, AHRQ. Available at http://archive.ahrq.gov/consumer/qnt/. Accessed February 5, 2011.

Agency for Healthcare Research and Quality: *Guide to clinical preventive services,* 2010, Publication No. 10-05145. Rockville, MD, 2010, AHRQ. Available at http://www.ahrq.gov/clinic/pocketgd.htm.

Agency for Healthcare Research and Quality: *2007 National Healthcare Disparities Report,* Rockville, MD, February 2008, USDHHS, AHRQ Pub. No. 08–0041.

Aiken LH, Clarke SP, Sloane DM, et al: Effects of hospital care environment on patient mortality and nurse outcomes, *J Nurs Adm* 38(5):223–229, 2008.

American Nurses Association: *The scope and standards of public health nursing practice,* Washington, DC, 1999, The Association.

American Nurses Association: *Public health nursing: scope and standards of practice,* Silver Springs, MD, 2007, The Association.

American Nurses Association: *Public health nursing: scope and standards of practice,* Silver Springs, MD, 2009, The Association.

American Nurses Association: *Code of ethics for nurses with interpretive statements,* Washington, DC, 2010, ANA.

American Nurses Credentialing Center: *Magnet recognition program,* 2010. Available at http://www.nursingworld.oRG. Accessed September 12, 2010.

American Public Health Association: *Healthy communities 2000: model standards, guidelines for community attainment of the year 2000 national health objectives,* ed 3, Washington, DC, 1991, APHA.

Association of Community Health Nursing Educators: *Perspectives on doctoral education in community health nursing,* Lexington, KY, 1993, ACHNE.

Association of Community Health Nursing Educators: *Essentials of baccalaureate nursing education for entry level community health nursing practice,* Chapel Hill, NC, 2000a, ACHNE.

Association of Community Health Nursing Educators: *Graduate education for advanced practice education in community/public health nursing,* Chapel Hill, NC, 2000b, ACHNE.

Association of Community Health Nursing Educators: *Graduate education for advanced practice in community public health nursing,* New York, 2003, ACHNE.

Bialek R, Carden J: Supporting public health departments' quality improvement initiatives: lessons learned from the Public Health Foundation, *J Public Health Manag Pract* 16(1):14–18, 2010.

Brownson RC, Fielding JE, Maylahn CM: Evidence-based public health: a fundamental concept for public health practice, *Annu Rev Public Health* 30:175–201, 2009.

Carmichael S: Total quality management and outcomes based quality improvement: revisiting the basics, *Home Health Care Manag Pract* 17:119–124, 2005.

Cary AH: Data drives policy: the case for certification research, *Pol Polit Nurs Pract* 1:165–171, 2000.

Centers for Disease Control and Prevention: *Planned approach to community health: guide for local coordinators,* Atlanta, 1995, CDC, National Center for Chronic Disease Prevention and Health Promotion. and updated 2010.

Council on Linkages Between Academia and Public Health Practice: *The core competencies for public health professionals,* Washington, DC, 2010, The Public Health Foundation.

Damberg CL, Ridgely MS, Shaw R, et al: Adopting information technology to drive improvements in patient safety: lessons from the Agency for Healthcare Research and Quality health information technology grantees, *Health Serv Res* 44(2):2, 2008.

Deming WE: *Out of the crisis,* Cambridge, MA, 1986, Massachusetts Institute of Technology, Center for Advanced Engineering Study.

Dlugacz YD, Restifo A, Greenwood A: *The quality handbook for health care organizations: a manager's guide to tools and programs,* Hoboken, NJ, 2004, Jossey-Bass.

Donabedian A: *Explorations in quality assessment and monitoring,* vol 2, Ann Arbor, MI, 1981, Health Administration Press.

Donabedian A: *Explorations in quality assessment and monitoring,* vol 3, Ann Arbor, MI, 1985, Health Administration Press.

Donabedian A: *An introduction to quality assurance in health care,* New York, 2003, Oxford University Press.

Encyclopedia of Public Health, 2002: *The Gale Group, Inc.* Available at www.gale.comgage.com. Accessed September 20, 2010.

Godfrey AB, Kenett RS, Joseph M: Juran, a perspective on past contributions and future impact, *Qual Reliab Engng Int* 23:653–663, 2007.

Gunzenhauser JD, Eggena ZP, Fielding JE, et al: *J Public Health Manage Pract* 16(1):39–48, 2010.

Healthy People 2020: Implementing *Healthy People 2020* MAP-IT: A guide to using *Healthy People 2020* in your community, February 2011. Available at www.healthypeople2002.gov. Accessed June 17, 2011.

Henderson S: Community Child Health (CCH) nurses' experience of home visits for new mothers: a quality improvement project, *Contemp Nurse* 34(1):66–76, 2009.

Institute of Medicine: *Crossing the quality chasm,* Washington, DC, 2001, National Academy Press.

Juran JM, Godfrey AB: *Juran's quality handbook,* New York, 2010, McGraw-Hill.

Kane RKL, Shamlayan T, Mueller C, et al: The association of registered nurse staffing levels and patient outcomes: systematic review and meta-analysis, *Medical Care* 45(12):1195–1204, 2007.

Keefe S: *Advance: nurses salary survey: results in! Many hospitals don't need to increase salaries to be competitive—for now,* March 1, 2010. Available at www.advanceweb.com.

Keller LO, Strohschein S, Lia-Hoagberg B, et al: Population-based public health interventions: practice-based and evidence-supported. Part I, *Public Health Nurs* 21:453–468, 2004a.

Keller LO, Strohschein S, Schaffer MA, et al: Population-based public health interventions: innovations in practice, teaching and management. Part II, *Public Health Nurs* 21:469–487, 2004b.

Kelly D: *Applying quality management in health care: a systems approach*, ed 2, Washington, DC, 2007, AAUPHA Press.

Kessner DM, Kalk CE: Assessing health quality—the case for tracers, *N Engl J Med* 288:189, 1973.

Keyser DJ, Dembosky JW, Kmetik K, et al: Using health information technology–related performance measures and tools to improve chronic care, *Jt Comm J Qual Patient Saf* 35(5):248–255, 2009.

Kovner A, Knickman JR, editors: *Jonas and Kovner's health care delivery in the United States*, New York, 2008, Springer.

Lotstein D, Seid M, Ricci K, et al: Using quality improvement methods to improve public health emergency preparedness: PREPARE for pandemic influenza, *Public Health* 27(5):328–339, 2008.

Maibusch RM: Evolution of quality assurance for nursing in hospitals. In Schroder PS, Maibusch RM, editors: *Nursing quality assurance*, Rockville, MD, 1984, Aspen.

Malloch K, Porter-O'Grady T: *Evidence-based practice in nursing and health care*, Sudbury, MA, 2006, Jones and Bartlett.

Martin S: *The Omaha System: a key to practice, documentation, and information management*, ed 2, St. Louis, 2005, Mosby.

McLaughlin CP, Kaluzny AD, editors: *Continuous quality improvement in healthcare: theory, implementation and applications*, ed 3, Boston, 2006, Jones and Bartlett.

Mead H, Cartwright-Smith L, Jones K, et al: *Racial and ethnic disparities in U.S. health care: a chartbook*, Pub. No. 1111, New York, 2008, Commonwealth Fund.

Metzler M, Kanarek N, Highsmith K, et al: Community Health Status Indicators Project: the development of a national approach to community health, *Prev Chronic Dis* 5(3):A94, 2008.

Minnesota Department of Health, Division of Community Health Services: *Public health interventions: applications for public health nursing practice*, St Paul, MN, March 2001, Public Health Nursing Section.

National Association of City and County Health Officials: *APEXPH in practice*, Washington, DC, 1995, NACCHO.

National Association of City and County Health Officials: *Mobilizing for action through planning and partnerships: web-based tool*, Washington, DC, 2001, NACCHO. Available at http://mapp.naccho.org. Accessed September 25, 2005.

National Association for Healthcare Quality: *Risk management: NAHQ guide to quality management*, Skokie, Ill, 1993, NAHQ Press.

National Association of Home Care: *Uniform data set for home care and hospice*, 2010. Available at http://www.nahc.org/NAHC/Research/unidata.html. Accessed February 5, 2011.

National Committee for Quality Assurance: *HEDIS: health plan for employee and data information set*, Washington, DC, 2009, NCQA.

National Committee on Quality Assurance: *National healthcare quality report*, Rockville, MD, 2009, Agency for Healthcare Quality and Research, USDHHS.

National Council of State Boards of Nursing: *Nurse licensure compact*, 2010. Available at www.nursecompact.ncsbn.org. Accessed September 20, 2010.

National Guideline Clearinghouse: *Fact sheet*, Rockville, MD, 2010, Agency for Healthcare Research and Quality, USDHHS.

National Health and Medical Research Council (NHMRC): *When does quality assurance in health care require independent ethical review? Advice to institutions, human research ethics committees, and health care professionals*, Canberra, 2003, NHMRC.

National Quality Forum: *Safe practices for better healthcare*, 2009. Available at http://www.ahrq.gov/qual/nqfpract.htm. Accessed February 5, 2011.

National Training Institute for Child Care Health Consultation. Available at http://www.sph.unc.edu/courses/childcare/. Accessed September 25, 2010.

Neuhauser D: Assessing health quality: the case for tracers, *J Health Serv Res Policy* 9:246–247, 2004.

Phaneuf M: A nursing audit method, *Nurs Outlook* 5:42, 1965.

Public Health Accreditation Board: *National voluntary accreditation program for public health agencies*, Washington, DC, 2010, PHAB.

Quad Council of Public Health Nursing Organizations: Public health nursing competencies, *Public Health Nurs* 219:443–452, 2009.

Riley WJ, Moran JW, Corso LC, et al: Defining quality improvement in public health, *J Public Health Manage Pract* 16(1):5–7, 2010.

Rowell PA: Beyond the acute care setting: community-based nonacute care nursing-sensitive indicators, *Outcomes Manag Nurs Pract* 5:24, 2001.

Rowitz L: *Public health leadership: putting principles into practice*, ed 2, Sudbury, MA, 2009, Jones & Bartlett.

Sakamoto SD, Avila M: The public health nursing practice manual: a tool for public health nurses, *Public Health Nurs* 21:179–182, 2004.

Simon K: *Effective brainstorming iSixSigma*, n.d. Available at http://www.isixsigma.com/library/content/c010401a.asp. Accessed April 12, 2007.

Smith K, Bazini-Barakat N: A public health nursing practice model: melding public health practice with the nursing process, *Public Health Nurs* 20:42–48, 2004.

The Omaha System: *Omaha system overview*. Available at http://www.omahasystem.org/overview.html. Accessed September 15, 2010.

University of Wisconsin-Madison, School of Nursing: *Wisconsin Public Health Nursing Practice Model, companion notes*, 2010, Linking Education and Practice for Excellence in Public Health Nursing (LEAP). Available at http://www.son.wisc.edu/LEAP/pdfs/WPHN_companion_2010_07.pdf. Accessed February 5, 2011.

U.S. Department of Health and Human Services: *Healthy people in healthy communities*, Washington, DC, February 2001, U.S. Government Printing Office.

U.S. Department of Health and Human Services: *Consensus statement on quality in the public health system*, 2008. Available at http://www.hhs.gov/ophs/programs/initiatives/phqf-consensus-statement.html. Accessed February 5, 2011.

U.S. Department of Health and Human Services: *Home health compare: Medicare*, 2010. Available at http://www.hhs.gov. Accessed September 20, 2010.

U.S. Department of Health and Human Services: *Healthy People 2010: understanding and improving health*, ed 2, Washington, DC, 2000, U.S. Government Printing Office.

U.S. Department of Health and Human Services: *National public health performance standards program*, 2005. Available at http://www.cdc.gov/od/ocphp/nphpsp/. Accessed February 5, 2011.

U.S. Department of Health and Human Services: *Healthy People 2020*, Washington, DC, 2010, U.S. Government Printing Office.

U.S. Department of Health and Human Services: *2006 National Health Care Quality Report*, Rockville MD, 2007, Agency For Health Care Quality and Research.

Varkey P, Reller K, Resar RK: Basics of quality improvement in health care, *Mayo Clin Proc* 82(6):735–739, 2007.

Vogt TM, Aickin M, Faruque A, et al: The prevention index: using technology to improve quality assessment, *Health Serv Res* 39:511–529, 2004.

Wakefield DS, Wakefield BJ: The complexity of health care quality. In Kovner AR, Knickman JR, editors: *Jonas and Kovner's health care delivery in the United States*, ed 9, New York, 2008, Springer.

PART 5

Health Promotion with Target Populations Across the Life Span

CHAPTER 27

Family Development and Family Nursing Assessment

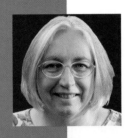

Joanna Rowe Kaakinen, PhD, RN

Dr. Joanna Rowe Kaakinen has been a family nurse scholar for the last 20 years. She has written extensively about family nursing. She is a reviewer for the *Journal of Family Nursing, the Journal of Family Relations,* a member of the International Association of Family Nurses, and a member of the National Council of Family Relations. She has presented nationally and internationally on family nursing. Dr. Kaakinen is a Professor in the School of Nursing at the University of Portland in Portland, Oregon, where she teaches undergraduate and graduate family nursing courses.

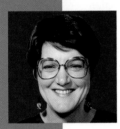

Linda K. Birenbaum, PhD, RN

Dr. Linda K. Birenbaum has been practicing and teaching family nursing for over 30 years since she first developed a family nursing theory course at Oregon Health Sciences University. Dr. Birenbaum has presented nationally and internationally on families with cancer. She was a professor at the University of Portland and taught undergraduate and graduate students community health nursing. Dr. Birenbaum currently is the Public Health Program Supervisor for Washington County Health and Human Services Public Health Department in Hillsboro, Oregon, where she manages three public health clinics providing services in family planning, sexually transmitted infections, immunizations, and prophylaxis for latent tuberculosis.

ADDITIONAL RESOURCES

Evolve WEBSITE
http://evolve.elsevier.com/Stanhope
- *Healthy People 2020*
- Quiz
- Case Studies
- WebLinks
- Glossary
- Answers to Practice Application
- Resource Tools
  - Resource Tool 5.A: Schedule of Clinical Preventive Services

- Resource Tool 27.A: Family Systems Stressor-Strength Inventory
- Resource Tool 27.B: Case Example of Family Assessment
- Resource Tool 27.C: List of Family Assessment Tools

APPENDIXES
- Appendix E: Freidman Family Assessment Model (Short Form)

OBJECTIVES

After reading this chapter, the student should be able to do the following:
1. Explain the multiple ways public health nurses work with families and communities.
2. Identify barriers to family nursing.
3. Describe family function and structure.
4. Describe family demographic trends and demographic changes that affect the health of families.
5. Compare and contrast four social science theoretical frameworks nurses use when working with the family.
6. Assess family needs to develop family action plans.
7. Discuss implications for social and family policy.

The health of communities is directly related to the health of the families (ANA, 2007; APHA, 2010; Eddy and Doutrich, 2010). Public health nurses must have skills to move competently between working with individual families, bridge relationships between families and the community, and advocate for family and community legislation and influence policies that promote and protect the health of populations. Therefore, public health nurses must integrate knowledge and practice of family nursing and community health nursing (APHA, 2010) in meeting the needs of families.

Family nursing is a philosophy and a science that is based on the following assumptions: health and illness are family events; what affects one family member affects the whole family; and health care practices, decisions, and behaviors are made within the context of the family (Kaakinen, Hanson, and Denham, 2010).

The definition of *community health nursing practice* used in this book states that it is a "synthesis of nursing theory and public health theory applied to promoting, preserving and maintaining the health of populations through the delivery of personal health care services to individuals, families, and groups. The focus of practice is the health of individuals, families and groups and the effect of their health status on the health of the community as a whole" (refer to Chapter 1).

LINKING CONTENT TO PRACTICE

In this chapter the core functions with the essential services below are applied to family nursing.

Assessment
- Monitor health status to identify community health problems.
- Diagnose and investigate health problems and health hazards in the community.
- Evaluate effectiveness, accessibility, and quality of personal and population-based health services.

Policy Development
- Develop policies and plans that support individual and community health efforts.
- Enforce laws and regulations that protect health and ensure safety.
- Research for new insights and innovative solutions to health problems.

Assurance
- Link people to needed personal health services and assure the provision of health care when otherwise unavailable.
- Assure a competent public health and personal health care workforce.
- Mobilize community partnerships to identify and solve health problems.

♥ **HEALTHY PEOPLE 2020**

New Objectives Specific to Families and Family Nursing

- EMC-2: Increase the proportion of parents who use positive parenting and communicate with their health care providers about positive parenting.
- FP-13: Increase the proportion of adolescents who talked to a parent or guardian about reproductive health topics before they were 18 years old.
- MHMD-11: Increase depression screening by primary care providers.
- MICH-11: Increase the abstinence from alcohol, cigarettes, illicit drugs among pregnant women.
- MICH-30: Increase the proportion of children, including those with a special need, who have a medical home.
- MICH-31: Increase the proportion of children with special health care needs who receive their care in family-centered, comprehensive, coordinated systems.
- NWS-4: (Developmental) Increase the proportion of Americans who have access to a food retail outlet that sells a variety of foods that are encouraged by the dietary guidelines for Americans.
- FN-12: Increase the proportion of sexually active women who receive instruction on reproductive health before they are age 18 years.
- IVP-39: (Developmental) Reduce violence by current or former intimate partners.
- OA-9: (Developmental) Reduce the proportion of unpaid caregivers of older adults who report an unmet need for caregiver support services.

NOTE: The term-developmental-means the objective continues to be worked on to set targets, additional subobjectives and timelines. From the U.S. Department of Health and Human Services: *Healthy People 2020,* Washington, DC, 2010, U.S. Government Printing Office.

Community health nurses use the core competencies for public health professionals (PHF, 2009) and the core public health functions of assessment, assurance, and policy development to promote the interconnectedness of individual health with the health of families and communities (Eddy and Doutrich, 2010). The Linking Content to Practice box shows the applications of public health nursing practice from a family perspective. The *Healthy People 2020* box highlights new objectives proposed for the upcoming *Healthy People 2020* initiatives. Community health nurses who practice with a family nursing philosophy and theory base will improve the health of families, their members, and the community.

CHALLENGES FOR NURSES WORKING WITH FAMILIES IN THE COMMUNITY

Numerous challenges exist that affect the practice of family nursing in a community setting. Many of the following challenges have been recognized in the family nursing literature for a long time, yet they persist in the current health care system. One role for the community health nurse would be to advocate that the following challenges be addressed in federal and state health care policies and programs.

Definition of Family

Now more than ever, the definition of *family* is being challenged. There is still no universally agreed upon definition of family (Kaakinen, Hanson, and Denham, 2010). Community health nurses and family nurses struggle on a daily basis with the conflict between the narrow traditional legal definition of family used in the health care system and by social policy makers and the broader term used by the family. Family, as defined and implemented in the health care system, has traditionally been based on using the legal notions of relationships such as biological/genetic blood ties, and contractual relationships such as adoption, guardianship, or marriage. However, the family system and family nurses use the following broader definition of family: Family refers to two or more individuals who depend on one another for emotional, physical, and/or financial support. The members of the family are self-defined" (Hanson, 2005).

Today more than ever, nurses need to adopt the open definition described above because the families they work with have a wide variety of family structures. Nurses who work with the people in the individual's every day world have a higher likelihood of helping them to achieve better health outcomes.

DID YOU KNOW? *Most nursing students tend to have a narrow view of family based on their own experiences with their family of origin. Therefore, their greatest challenge is to be non-judgmental when working with a family that functions in ways outside of their personal experience.*

Communication Difficulties

A common pitfall of the home health care system is the lack of communication and information in the transfer of clients between agencies that often occurs in interventions and health outcomes (Daily and Newfield, 2005) that frequently result in hospital admission or readmission. Nationally, the number of home health care clients who were admitted to the hospital between 2002 and 2006 was 28.3% (AHCRQ, 2008). The majority of these hospital admissions in home health care clients occurred within 7 days of admission to the home health agency (Vasquez, 2008). Approximately 18% of all Medicare hospitalizations result in readmissions within 30 days of discharge (Hackbarth, 2009). These hospital readmissions accounted for $15 billon, $12 billion of which was estimated to be preventable (Hackbarth, 2009).

In addition to a lack of communication between health care systems, there are communication issues between health care providers within the community agencies, such as incomplete or missing documentation that result from rushed assessments. Rushed procedures and failure to follow the plan of action and standards of care are known causes of hospital readmissions (Vasquez, 2008). It is crucial that home health care staff have current updates on evidence-based practice, standards of care (Hogue and Fairnot, 2006), and interventions to ensure quality health outcomes. Community health nurses have a significant role in working with multiple health care systems to improve communication and design protocols that are evidence-based to improve the quality of care and the health of the home health population (Ventura et al, 2010).

Nurses must develop and hone excellent negotiation skills because they spend a significant amount of time arranging for limited services for their underinsured and uninsured clients and families. In working with families, communication and teaching would be more effective if hours of service matched the times of day when family members, specifically the family care provider, can attend appointments. Bringing a companion to office visits benefits communication (Wolff et al, 2009; Wolff and Roter, 2008) enhances shared decision making (Clayman et al, 2005) and improves the sharing of information (Eggly et al, 2006). Involving family in the care of the client improves self management of health care, results in fewer medication errors (Kinnersley et al, 2007; Wolff et al, 2009), and improves health outcomes (Weinberg et al, 2007).

Uninsured, Underinsured, and Limited Services

Nurses must be adept at working among health care systems to find resources and services for the large population of uninsured clients and families. As of 2008, there were 46.6 million Americans without health insurance (U.S. Census Bureau, 2009). Although the number of uninsured children is the lowest since 1987, the fastest growing group of uninsured is young adults (U.S. Census Bureau, 2009). In addition, for those who have health care insurance, these companies traditionally base reimbursement and coverage on the individual's disease or health problem and not the family unit or for informal family caregiving (Kaakinen, Hanson, and Denham, 2010).

The lack of insurance makes finding adequate services for clients and families difficult. In some areas federal and state funding for care in health clinics is free or available for a minimal fee. However, because the number of primary health care clinics is limited, care is provided on a lottery based solely on the number of volunteer health care providers working that day in the clinic. Many clinics are program based, such as family planning clinics, sexually transmitted disease (STD) clinics, and immunizations clinics. Thus, it is difficult to meet the needs of the uninsured or underinsured populations.

EVIDENCE-BASED PRACTICE

Kub et al (2009) hypothesized that in addition to sociodemographic variables and life events, chronic stressors would be related to maternal depression symptoms. Specifically they hypothesized that asthma management and exposures to community violence would be related to maternal depression. They studied 201 mothers of children with asthma between the ages of 6 and 12 years recruited from community pediatric practices and emergency departments of two urban university hospitals. They found that 25% of the mothers had high depressive symptoms. In a statistical method called multiple logistic regression, they found that education or unemployment was positively associated with the use of quick-relief asthma medications.

Nurse Use

Although this is a single study and needs further collaboration, it indicates that public health nurses should consider assessing mothers of children with asthma for depression in order to improve the asthma management for low-income urban children. Refer to the Levels of Prevention box for Asthma in Children.

From Kub J, Jennings JM, Donihan M, et al: Life events, chronic stressors, and depressive symptoms in low-income urban mothers with asthmatic children, *Public Health Nurs* 26(4):297-306, 2009.

LEVELS OF PREVENTION

Asthma in Children

Primary Prevention
Educating parents about smoking in the home and children developing asthma

Secondary Prevention
Testing children for asthma whose parent smokes in the home
Testing mothers for depression

Tertiary Prevention
Obtaining appropriate ongoing medication for childhood asthma early before the disease becomes severe
Obtaining appropriate health care services for a mother who scored high on the depression assessment instruments

These challenges are pervasive and serious. Nurses help clients and families negotiate and maneuver through the health care system. They must work closely with the family to remove barriers and provide services and resources that enhance the families' abilities to provide quality care to family members. To successfully address these challenges, the community health nurses must integrate principles of family nursing with those of community/public health (see Evidence-Based Practice and Levels of Prevention boxes).

FAMILY FUNCTIONS AND STRUCTURES

Knowledge of family functions and structures is essential for understanding how families influence health, illness, and well-being. Nurses who understand family functions and structures can use this knowledge to empower families through evidence-based interventions.

Family functions are the ways in which families meet the needs of (a) each family member, (b) the family as a whole, and (c) their relationship to society. Throughout history, the following functions have been performed by families (Kaakinen, Hanson, and Denham, 2010):

1. *Economic function:* Family income is a substantial part of family economics, but it is also related to family consumerism, money management, housing decisions, insurance choices, retirement, and savings. Family economics affect and reflect the nation's economy.

2. *Reproductive function:* The survival of a society is linked to patterns and rates of reproduction. The family has been the traditional structure in which reproduction was organized. Today, the reproductive function of family has become more separated from traditional family structure as more children are born outside of marriage and into non-traditional family structures.

3. *Socialization function:* A major expectation of families is that they are responsible for raising their children to fit into society and take their place in the adult world. In addition, families disseminate their culture, including religious faith and spirituality.

4. *Affective function:* Families provide boundaries and structure that provide a sense of belonging and identity of who the

family members are individually and to their family. The purpose of the affective function is to learn about intimate reciprocal caring relationships, to learn about dependency and how to nurture future generations.

5. *Health care function:* It is in the family that one learns the concepts of health, health promotion, health maintenance, disease prevention, and illness management. Family members provide informal caregiving to ill family members and are primary sources of support.

WHAT DO YOU THINK?   *All families have secrets. Some information gleaned from families may be exaggerated, minimized, or withheld.*

Family structure refers to the characteristics and demographics (e.g., sex, age, number) of individual members who make up family units. More specifically, the structure of a family defines the roles and the positions of family members (Box 27-1).

Family structures have changed over time to meet the needs of the family and society. The great speed at which changes in family structure, values, and relationships are occurring makes working with families at the beginning of the twenty-first century exciting and challenging. According to Kaakinen, Hanson, and Denham (2010, p 22), the following aspects need to be addressed when determining the family structure:

1. The individuals that compose the family
2. The relationships between them
3. The interactions between the family members
4. The interactions with other social systems

As social norms have become more tolerant of a range of choices in relation to managing one's life, there is no longer a general consensus that the traditional nuclear family model, consisting of father, mother, and children, is the "best" model. There is no "typical" family model or family structure. For example, the single-mother household may be represented by the unmarried teenage mother with an infant (unplanned pregnancy), the divorced mother with one or more children, or the career-oriented woman in her late 30s who elects to have a baby and remain single.

The family structure changes and modifies over time. An individual may participate in a number of family life experiences over a lifetime (Figure 27-1). For example, a child may spend the early, formative years in the family of origin (mother, father, siblings); experience some years in a single-parent family

---

BOX 27-1   FAMILY AND HOUSEHOLD STRUCTURES

Married Family
- Traditional nuclear family
- Dual-career family
- Spouses reside in same household
- Commuter marriage
- Husband/father away from family
- Stepfamily
- Stepmother family
- Stepfather family
- Adoptive family
- Foster family
- Voluntary childlessness

Single-Parent Family
- Never married
- Voluntary singlehood (with children, biological or adopted)
- Involuntary singlehood (with children)
- Formerly married
- Widowed (with children)
- Divorced (with children)
- Custodial parent
- Joint custody of children
- Binuclear family

Multi-Adult Household (with or without children)
- Co-habitating couple
- Communes
- Affiliated family
- Extended family
- Newly extended family
- Home-sharing individuals
- Same-sex partners

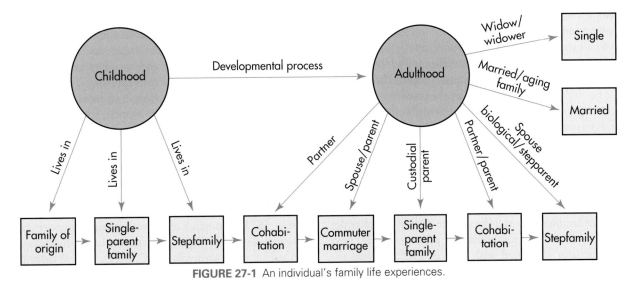

FIGURE 27-1 An individual's family life experiences.

because of divorce; and participate in a stepfamily relationship when the single parent who has custody remarries.

This same child as an adult may experience several additional family types: cohabitation while completing a desired education, and then a commuter marriage while developing a career. As an adult, the individual may divorce and become a custodial parent. The adult may eventually cohabitate with another partner and finally marry a different partner who also has children. As couples age, they have to address issues of the aging family, and subsequently the woman may become an older single widow. Thus, nurses work with various families representing different structures and living arrangements.

Prospects for families in the twenty-first century are numerous. New family structures that are currently experimental will emerge as everyday "natural" families (e.g., families in which the members are not related by blood or marriage, but who provide the services, caring, love, intimacy, and interaction needed by all persons to experience a quality life).

At times it is helpful to understand families through a narrow framework of family function and structure. However, a family is a system within itself as well as the basic unit of a society. Some would argue that the traditional concept of family is disintegrating based on how the structure and functions of the family have changed over time. On the other side of that debate, families change in response to the societal changes and are ever evolving and thriving as they seek different ways of interconnectedness (Kaakinen, Hanson, and Denham, 2010).

| **WHAT DO YOU THINK?** *Is the American family in trouble?* |

FAMILY DEMOGRAPHICS

Historically, family demographics can be analyzed by looking at data about the families and household structures and the events that alter these structures. Nurses draw on family demographic data to forecast and predict family community needs, such as family developmental changes, stresses, and ethnic issues affecting family health, as they formulate possible solutions to identified family community problems. In this chapter, family demographic trends valuable to community health nurses are presented.

In 2007 in the United States, there were over 11.2 million households with 67% being family households and the remaining 33% being non-family households. Family households include a householder and at least one other member related by birth, marriage, or adoption; whereas a non-family household is either a person living alone or a householder who shares the house only with non-relatives, such as boarders or roommates (Krieder and Elliot, 2007).

Family demographic trends have continued in the direction of fewer married couples with children households (currently 71% compared with 93% in 1970). Children living in single parent families have stabilized since 2002 at 9% (Krieder and Elliot, 2009). Large households (five people or more) have decreased to 10% compared with 21% in 1970; whereas the small households (one to two people) increased from 46% to 60% over this same time period (Krieder and Elliott, 2007). The average household size remains at 2.6, but the average household has been affected by changes in us demographics (Krieder and Elliot, 2009; Grieco, 2007). Immigration and modest differences in natural increases have resulted in an increased racial and ethnic diversity, which is reflected in the white, non-Hispanic population declining 17% to 66% of the total population in 2007 (Grieco, 2010). Of the non-family households, 31 million were individuals living alone; 35% of the non-family households are 65 years of age or older.

Marriage and Cohabitation

Marriage, although still a popular American ideal, has assumed a forerunner: cohabitation. Cohabitation is a couple living together who are having a sexual relationship without being married. The probability that Americans will marry by age 40 is over 80% (Goodwin, McGill, and Chandra, 2009); however, cohabitation has become commonplace with a majority of young people projected to cohabitate at least once (Bumpass and Lu, 2000). Currently cohabitation rates are reported to be about 9% for men and women between the ages of 15 and 44 (Goodwin, Mosher, and Chandra, 2010).

Casper, Hagga, and Jayasundera (2010) suggest that people cohabitate for three reasons: some cohabitants would marry but do not for economic reasons; others seek a more equalitarian relationship; and others use cohabitation as a trial period to negotiate and assess whether to marry. Younger cohabitants are more likely to view their relationship as a prelude to marriage (King and Scott, 2005). This view is common, with a 65% chance of cohabitation transitioning to marriage within the first 5 years (Goodwin, Mosher, and Chandra, 2010). Phillips and Sweeney (2005) suggest that there is an ethnic factor in the meaning of cohabitation, with whites viewing cohabitation as a trial marriage and African Americans and Hispanic Americans viewing cohabitation as a substitute for marriage. In 2000 Seltzer suggested that, with the aging of the population, cohabitation may be of increasing importance among older persons. In 2005 King and Scott found that older adults enjoy relationships of higher quality and perceived stability despite having fewer plans to marry and are more likely than younger cohabitants to view their relationship as an alternative to marriage.

Different factors were associated with duration of marriage and cohabitation. Duration of marriage was associated with two factors: age of first marriage and timing of first child. Marriage at a younger age had a lower probability of the marriage lasting 10 years. Women who gave birth 8 months or more after the marriage began compared with women who had no first birth during the marriage had a 79% chance versus a 34% chance of the marriage lasting 10 years. Education was a factor in both men and women's duration of cohabitation, with lower education being associated with longer cohabitation (Goodwin, McGill, and Chandra, 2010).

As cohabitation increases, ensuring sexually transmitted disease (STD) reduction and family planning services becomes essential. The most frequently reported infectious disease in the United States is chlamydia (CDC, 2010). In 2008 more than 1.2 million cases of chlamydia were reported. Women between the ages of 15 and 19 years of age and minority women are at the highest risk (CDC, 2010). Untreated chlamydia can cause severe and costly reproductive health problems. A model collaborative program is the Region X Infertility Prevention Project (2000), which aims to control chlamydia through collaborative efforts of STD and family planning providers and public health laboratories. A comprehensive approach to STD prevention that includes screening, treatment of infected partners, and behavioral interventions with a focus on reducing racial disparities is an important aspect of providing community health (CDC, 2010). See the *Healthy People 2020* boxes on Family Planning and Sexually Transmitted Diseases.

Effects of Cohabitation on Children

Most children are born into families with married couples (64.5%), but 28.4% are born to mothers who had never married, and the remaining 7% are born to mothers who were divorced, separated, or widowed (Dye, 2008a). Since "never married" has the second highest ranking, attempts have been made to examine the effects of cohabitation on children. Poverty, income expenditures, and maternal parenting have been examined. DeLeire and Kalil (2005) found relatively high rates of poverty in cohabitating families with children compared with the national average (18.2%-22.4%, compared with 12.1% overall and 5.3% among married couples). They also found that cohabitating-parent families spend a greater share of their budgets on alcohol and tobacco than do married, divorced, and never-married single-parent families (DeLeire and Kalil, 2005). Nurses must ensure that these families have access to health insurance such as the Medicaid S-CHIP program. Teaching cohabitating families with children about the implications of second-hand smoke becomes a priority, since these children are at risk for health problems such as increased lower respiratory tract infections and asthma. Because poverty rates are higher, assisting these families in gaining access to resources such as food stamps and budget management skills is the work of nurses in the community. In 2001, Thomson et al found that although mothers yell and spank or hit their children less when cohabitating or remarrying, they provide less supervision. Spending more on alcohol and providing less child supervision place these children at risk for abuse or neglect, so nurses need to be vigilant in assessing these children and their families to prevent such unhealthy environments. These children are further endangered by the short-lived duration of cohabitation (DeLeire and Kalil, 2005).

Additional Trends in Marriage

Two additional trends in marriage are worth noting: increased age for first marriage and increased number of interracial marriages. The mother's age at first birth has increased by 3.6 years between 1970 and 2006, making the average age 25 rather than 21.4 (Mathews and Hamilton, 2009). This may be influenced by educational attainment. Although men have a higher rate of attaining college degrees than women, that number is narrowing as data on younger cohorts show higher attainment for women than men, suggesting that the majority of people with college degrees may be women in the future (Crissey, 2009).

Later marriages can lead to older women becoming pregnant along with all the joys and complications attributed to these pregnancies in later life, such as infertility, STDs, and an increase in all obstetrical complications. Interracial marriage is another growing phenomenon in the United States. Lee and Edmonston (2005) report that interracial marriages increased from less than 1% of all married couples in 1970 to more than 5% in 2000.

Since 1965 when the Immigration Act abolished the national origins quota, the United States has become more diversified. In 1960, 75% of foreign-born people living in the United States were born in Europe; by 2007, 80% of foreign-born were born either in Latin America or Asia (Grieco, 2010). The current emphasis in family demographics is the race or ethnicity of the American family, which has weighty implications for community health nursing (Crissey, 2009; Davis and Bauman, 2009; Dye, 2008a,b). Of the 281.4 million counted in the 2000 Census, 75.1% were white, 12.1% were Black or African American, 0.9% were American Indian and Alaska Native, 3.6% were Asian, and 0.1% were Native Hawaiian and other Pacific Islander. The Hispanic population was 12.5%. For the first time, Hispanics outnumbered African Americans in this country; the Hispanic population reached 41.3 million people as of July 1, 2004 (Bernstein, 2005).

Race and ethnicity has implications for American women's fertility, educational attainment, and participation in government assistance programs. Family Planning and Women, Infants, and Children (WIC) are two federally funded public health programs that require community health nurses to understand the implications of race and ethnicity on public health services. For example, in some instances a woman attending a public health clinic for family planning services may be accompanied by her husband who is the only adult family member who speaks English. If adequate interpretative services are not available, the husband may attempt to complete the medical history form and it may or may not be accurate, thus impacting the services provided. This requires community health nurses being knowledgeable about the race and ethnic composition of their community and providing adequate staffing for the major languages spoken in that community.

Births

Fertility rates differ by race and ethnicity. Hispanic women have the highest fertility rates with 74 births per 1000; American Indian and Alaska Native women were next with 68 births per 1000, followed by African-American women with 58 births per 1000; Asian women had 54 births per 1000 and white non-Hispanic women had the lowest rates of 50 births per 1000 (Dye, 2008a). Foreign-born Hispanic women who were not citizens had statistically higher fertility rates than their native naturalized counterparts between 20 and 29 years of age.

Not all cultures value limiting the number of children in a family, and nurses may be challenged to understand these values and to provide services where the woman assumes the value of limiting the number of children where the husband does not. For example, a Hispanic woman comes to the public health clinic for family planning services. It is not uncommon for the husband to come in at the end of the week to pay for those services. If the wife is on birth control, such as Depo, but does not want her husband to know, itemizing services on the receipt would present a problem. The nurse needs to understand these changing values and facilitate the family planning services requested by the woman without violating her confidentiality.

Divorce or Dissolution of Cohabitation

Divorce can be said to be increasing, declining, or remaining stable, depending on the time referent. Divorce rates in the 1970s and into the mid-1980s climbed to 5.0 per 1000, but around 1985 through 2000 they began to decline to 4.0 per 1000 (U.S. Census Bureau, 2008). In 2001 the median length of a marriage for divorcing couples was 8 years for men and women overall (Kreider, 2005). Lowenstein (2005) identified the following factors that lead to divorce: women's independence in the marriage, money issues, poor education and social skills, inability to manage conflict, sexual incompatibility, alcohol and substance abuse, risk-taking behaviors, and religious issues. Lowenstein summarized the following effects on the divorced family:

- Diminishment of the father's role in the family
- Negative impact on the children
- Emotional problems for a number of persons involved
- Reduced living standard

The economic hardships of divorce and cohabiting dissolution are similar (Avellar and Smock, 2005). These economic hardships of cohabiting dissolution are unequally distributed, with white women faring better than African-American or Hispanic women (Avellar and Smock, 2005).

The characteristics of people who divorce vary by race, religion, and educational level. The divorce rate for African Americans is higher than for whites, Hispanic Americans, or Asian and Pacific Islander Americans (Kreider, 2005; Teachman, Tedrow, and Scanzioni, 2000). Protestants have a higher divorce rate than Catholics. Women and men with at least a bachelor's degree are less likely to divorce than those who have a high school degree or less (Kreider, 2005). Phillips and Sweeney (2005) found that whites who cohabitated with their spouse before marriage were at a greater risk of divorce than African Americans or Hispanic Americans. Premarital conception was a risk factor for divorce in African Americans who cohabitated before marriage. Nativity (American born) was a risk factor for divorce in Mexican Americans who cohabitated before marriage.

Divorce and dissolution of cohabitation come to the attention of the nurse mostly with respect to the 40% of children projected to live in parent-cohabiting families before they reach adulthood. Since women are still the dominant custodial parent, the economic adverse effects they suffer are also experienced by the children. Nurses need to ensure that health care services are available for these families.

Remarriage

Until the 1970s, bereavement, the leading cause of remarriage, was replaced with divorce (Coleman, Ganong, and Fine, 2000). More than 50% of divorced people remarry (Kreider, 2005). Whereas gender was previously a leading factor in remarriage rates, the person who initiated the divorce has been found to be a more significant factor (Sweeney, 2002). That is, women who

initiate divorce are more likely to remarry than women who were the non-initiators. The probability of remarriage for white women is 58%, for Hispanic women is 44%, and for African-American women is 32% (CDC, 2002).

For middle-aged families, this results in more blended families and issues of childcare. Although some persons remarry more than once, remarriages by adults more than 40 years of age may be more stable than first marriages (Coleman, Ganong, and Fine, 2000).

It is imperative that the nurse keep informed and up to date about demographic trends pertaining to families and all types of households. Such knowledge is essential so that nurses can identify high-risk populations, such as children living in poverty, children of working mothers who care for themselves (latch-key children), and older adult women living alone. Changing demographics have implications for planning health, developing community resources, and becoming politically active, so that scarce funds and resources can be made available for health services needed by the growing and diverse population. Demographic data are usually updated every 5 years. In 2010 a new census was taken of the U.S. population.

FAMILY HEALTH

The meaning of family health is not precise and lacks consensus, despite the increased focus on family health within the nursing profession. The term *family health* is often used interchangeably with the concepts of family functioning, healthy families, and familial health. Hanson (2005, p 7) defines family health as "a dynamic changing relative state of well-being which includes the biological, psychological, spiritual, sociological, and cultural factors of the family system."

This holistic approach refers to individual members as well as the family unit as a whole entity and in turn the family within the community context. An individual's health (the wellness and illness continuum) affects the functioning of the entire family, and in turn, the family's functioning affects the health of individuals. Thus assessment of family health involves simultaneous assessment of individual family members, the family system as a whole, and the community in which the family is imbedded.

Health professionals have tended to classify clients and their families into two groups: healthy families and non-healthy families, or those in need of psychosocial evaluation and intervention. The term *family health* implies mental health rather than physical health. A popular term for *non-healthy families* is dysfunctional families, also called non-compliant, resistant, or unmotivated—phrases that label families who are not functioning well with each other or in the world.

> **NURSING TIP** *The labeling of a family as dysfunctional does not, however, allow for families to change, and it obstructs any kind of intervention; this and similar terms need to be dropped from nursing language.*

Families are neither all good nor all bad; rather, all families have both strengths and difficulties. All families have seeds of

BOX 27-2 CHARACTERISTICS OF HEALTHY FAMILIES

1. The family tends to communicate well and listen to all members.
2. The family affirms and supports all of its members.
3. Teaching respect for others is valued by the family.
4. The family members have a sense of trust.
5. The family plays together, and humor is present.
6. All members interact with each other, and a balance in the interactions is noted among the members.
7. The family shares leisure time together.
8. The family has a shared sense of responsibility.
9. The family has traditions and rituals.
10. The family shares a religious core.
11. Privacy of members is honored by the family.
12. The family opens its boundaries to admit and seek help with problems.

From Hanson SMH: Family health care nursing: an introduction. In Hanson SMH, Gedaly-Duff V, and Kaakinen JR, editors: *Family health care nursing: theory, practice & research*, ed 3, Philadelphia, 2005, FA Davis, p 9.

resilience and strengths upon which the nurse should work with the family to build interventions and design plans of action. Nurses should view family behavior on a continuum of need for intervention.

Families with strengths, functional families, and *balanced families* are terms often used to refer to *healthy families* that are doing well. Studies have identified traits of healthy families as well as family stressors that are useful for nurses to include in their assessment (Driver et al, 2003; Olson and Gorall, 2003). Box 27-2 shows characteristics of families who are healthy and functioning well in society.

The most recent concept described in the family literature pertains to ways families function across the family life cycle. Balanced families are those that have the ability to adapt to situations; therefore, they demonstrate family flexibility in leadership, relationships, rules, control, discipline, negotiation, and role sharing (Olson and Gorall, 2005). Balanced families have the ability to allow family members to be independent from the family yet remain connected to the family as a whole, which is termed family cohesion (Olson and Gorall, 2005).

FOUR APPROACHES TO FAMILY NURSING

Central to the practice of family nursing is conceptualizing and approaching the family from four perspectives. All have legitimate implications for family nursing assessment and intervention (Figures 27-2 and 27-3). The approaches that nurses use are determined by many factors, including the issues for which the individuals or families as a whole are seeking help, the environment in which they coexist with other family members and the community, the interaction among all of these factors, and of course the nursing resources available to deal with all of these factors (Hanson, 2005).

Family as Context. The family has a traditional focus that places the individual first and the family second. The family as context serves as either a strength or a stressor to individual health and illness issues. The nurse is most interested in the individual and realizes that the family influences the health of the individual. A nurse using this focus might ask an individual client the following questions: "Is your family available to help you get to your doctor appointments?" "Can your wife help you with your insulin injections?" or "Perhaps your son could help you up and down the stairs since your mother is so much smaller than you and your Dad."

Family as Client. The family is the primary focus and individuals are secondary. The family is seen as the sum of individual family members. The focus is concentrated on how the family as a whole is reacting to the event when a family member experiences a health issue. In addition, the nurse looks to see how each family member is affected by the health event. From this perspective, a nurse might say the following to a family member who has recently become ill: "How is the family reacting to your mother's recent diagnosis of liver cancer?" "How have you experienced your mother's recent diagnosis of liver cancer?" "How has your diagnosis of insulin-dependent diabetes affected your family?" "Will your need for medication at night be a problem for your family?"

Family as a System. The focus is on the family as client, and the family is viewed as an interactional system in which the whole is more than the sum of its parts. This approach focuses on individual members and the family as a whole at the same time. The interactions among family members become the target for nursing interventions (e.g., the interactions among both parents and children, and between the parental hierarchy). The systems approach to families always implies that when something happens to one family member, the other members of the family system are affected, and vice versa. Questions nurses ask when approaching the family as a system are the following: "What has changed between you and your spouse since your child's head injury?" "How do you feel about the fact that your son's long-term rehabilitation will affect the ways in which the members of your family are functioning and interact with one another?"

Family as a Component of Society. The family is seen as one of many institutions in society, along with health, education, and religious and financial institutions. The family is a basic or primary unit of society, as are all the other units, and they are all a part of the larger system of society. The family as a whole interacts with other institutions to receive, exchange, or give services. Nurses who work with families have derived many of their tenets of practice from this component of society, because they focus on the interface between families and community agencies. Nurses using this approach see families as a population. Questions the nurse might ask using this lens are "How should we talk with Somali refugee women about birth control given what we know about their culture?" or "What plan should we develop to increase the H1N1 immunization rates in the families living in the lower-income housing developments?" This is the approach used by public health nurses as they implement population-centered strategies to improve the health of the overall community.

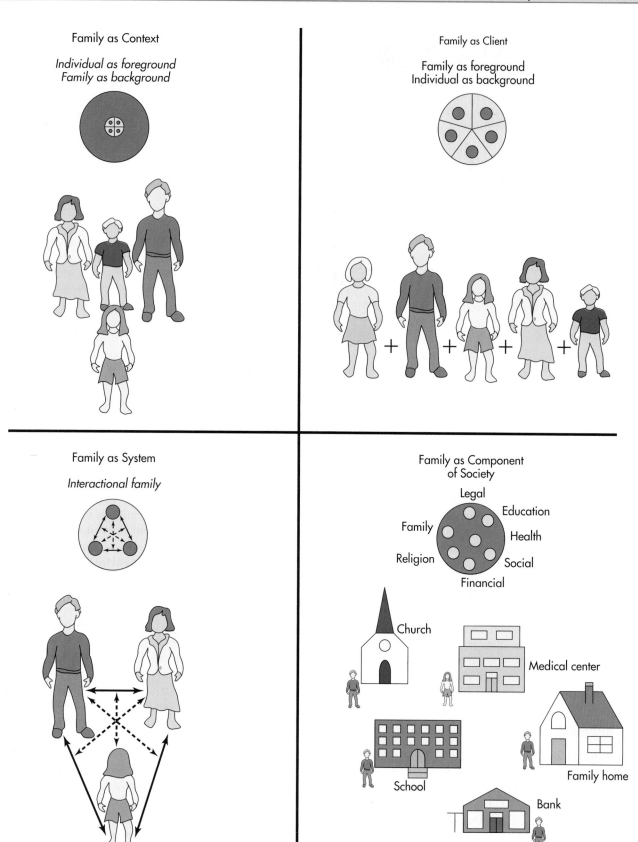

FIGURE 27-2 Approaches to family nursing. (From Hanson SMH, Gedaly-Duff V, Kaakinen JR, editors: *Family health care nursing: theory, practice and research,* ed 3, Philadelphia, 2005, FA Davis.)

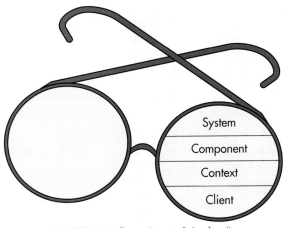

FIGURE 27-3 Four views of the family.

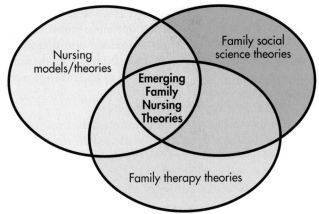

FIGURE 27-4 Theory-based family nursing. (Modified from Hanson SMH, Kaakinen JR: Theoretical foundations for family nursing. In Hanson SMH, Gedaly-Duff V, Kaakinen JR, editors: *Family health care nursing: theory, practice and research,* Philadelphia, 2005, FA Davis.)

THEORIES FOR WORKING WITH FAMILIES IN THE COMMUNITY

There is no single theory or conceptual framework that fully describes the relationships and dynamics and can be used to understand and intervene with families. Thus, an integrated theoretical approach is necessary because one theoretical perspective does not provide nurses with enough knowledge to work effectively with families. Community/public health nurses must also blend family nursing theories with public health theories and frameworks to work both with individual families and populations of families.

Family nursing theory is an evolving synthesis of the scholarship from three different traditions: family social science, family therapy, and nursing (Figure 27-4). Of the three categories of theory, the family social science theories are the most well-developed and informative with respect to how families function, the environment-family interchange, interactions within the family, how the family changes over time, and the family's reaction to health and illness. Therefore, in this chapter, three family social science theories that blend well with community/public health nursing are reviewed. These social science theories are the family systems theory, family developmental and life cycle theory and the bioecological systems theory.

Family Systems Theory

Families are social systems and much can be learned from the systems approach. A system is composed of a set of organized, complex, interacting elements. Nurses use **family systems theory** to understand how a family is an organized whole as well as composed of individuals (Kaakinen and Hanson, 2010). The purpose of the family system is to maintain stability through adaptation to internal and external stresses that are created by change (Kaakinen and Hanson, 2010; White and Klein, 2008). Assumptions of the family systems theory include the following:

- Family systems are greater than and different from the sum of their parts.
- There are many hierarchies within family systems and logical relationships between subsystems (e.g., mother–child, family–community).

- Boundaries in the family system can be open, closed, or random.
- Family systems increase in complexity over time, evolving to allow greater adaptability, tolerance to change, and growth by differentiation.
- Family systems change constantly in response to stresses and strains from within and from outside environments.
- Change in one part of a family system affects the total system.
- Family systems are an organized whole; therefore, individuals within the family are interdependent.
- Family systems have homeostatic features to maintain stable patterns that can be adaptive or maladaptive.

An excellent way to understand family systems theory is to visualize a mobile that consists of different members of a family suspended from each arm of the mobile; this represents the family as a whole. The parts of the mobile move about in response to changes in the balance. The amount of movement and length of time it takes to achieve a calm, balanced state depends on the severity of the imbalance. The family is a system similar to that of the mobile. When one member is affected by a health event, the whole family and each member of the family is affected differently by this change in balance. Imagine what would happen to the mobile if one of the parts was cut off as in the death of a family member, an additional part was added as in the birth or adoption of an infant, an arm of the mobile was extended such as a child moving out of the family home, or one part is yanked really hard and held down for an extended period of time and then suddenly released such as when a family member experiences a life-limiting illness and recovers or proceeds to a chronic illness.

The family systems theory encourages nurses to view both the individual clients as participating members of a whole family. The goal is for nurses to help families maintain balance and stability as they maintain the ability to function and adapt (Kaakinen and Hanson, 2010). Nurses using this theory determine the effects of illness or injury on the entire family system. Emphasis is on the whole rather than on individuals. Nursing assessment of family systems includes assessment of individual members, subsystems, boundaries, openness, inputs and outputs, family interactions, family processing, and adapting or changing abilities. Examples of assessment questions nurses could ask a family based on a family systems theory would include the following:

- Who are the members of your family?
- How has one member's illness affected the family?
- Who in the family is or will be affected the most?
- What has helped your family in the past when you have had a similar experience?
- Who outside of your family do you see as being able to help?
- How would your family react to having someone from outside the family come to help?
- How do you think the children, spouse, or parents are meeting their needs?
- What will help the family cope with the changes?

Interventions need to build on the strengths of the family in order to improve or support the functioning of the individual members and the whole family. Some nursing strategies based on a family systems theory include establishing a mechanism for providing families with information about their family members on a regular basis, helping the family maintain routines and rituals, and discussing ways to provide for everyday functioning when a family member becomes ill.

The major strength of the systems framework is that it views families from both a subsystem and a suprasystem approach. That is, it views the interactions within and between family subsystems as well as the interaction between families and the larger supersystems, such as the community and the world. The major weakness of the systems framework is that the focus is on the interaction of the family with other systems rather than on the individual, which is sometimes more important.

Family Developmental and Life Cycle Theory

Family developmental and life cycle theory provides a framework for understanding normal predicted stresses that families experience as they change and transition over time. In the original theory of family development, Duvall and Miller (1985) applied the principles of individual development to the family as a unit. The stages of family development are based on the age of the eldest child. Overall family tasks are identified that need to be accomplished for each stage of family development. Table 27-1 shows the stages of the family life cycle and some of the family developmental tasks. One developmental concept of this theory is that families as a system move to a different level of functioning, thus implying progress in a single direction. Family disequilibrium and conflicts occur during these expected transition periods from one stage of family development to another. The family begins as a married couple. Then the family becomes more complex with the addition of each new child until it becomes simpler and less complex as the younger generation begins to leave the home. Finally, the family comes full circle to the original husband–wife pair. Recognizing that families of today are different in structure, function, and processes, Carter and McGoldrick

TABLE 27-1	TRADITIONAL FAMILY LIFE CYCLE STAGES AND FAMILY DEVELOPMENTAL TASKS
STAGES OF FAMILY LIFE CYCLE	**FAMILY DEVELOPMENTAL TASKS**
Married couple	Establish relationship as a family unit, role development
	Determine family routines and rituals
Childbearing families with infants	Adjust to pregnancy and then birth of infant
	Learn new roles as mother and father
	Maintain couple time, intimacy, and relationship as a unit
Families with preschool children	Understand growth and development, including discipline
	Cope with energy depletion
	Arrange for individual time, family time, and couple time
Families with school-aged children	Learn to open family boundaries as child increases amount of time spent with others outside of the family
	Manage time demands in supporting child's interest and needs outside of the home
	Establish rules, new disciplinary actions
	Maintain couple time
Families with adolescents	Adapt to changes in family communication, power structure and decision making as teen increases autonomy
	Help teen develop as individual and as a family member
Families launching young adults	As young adult moves in and out of the home allocate space, power, communication, roles
	Maintain couple time, intimacy, and relationship
Middle-aged parents	Refocus on couple time, intimacy, and relationship
	Maintain kinship ties
	Focus on retirement and the future
Aging parents	Adjust to retirement, death of spouse and living alone
	Adjust to new roles (i.e., widow, single, grandparent)
	Adjust to new living situations, changes in health

(2005) expanded the work of Duvall and Miller (1985) to have the family developmental and life cycle theory include different family structures such as divorced families and blended families.

Traditional Family Life Cycle Stages and Family Developmental Tasks

Family developmental and life cycle theory explains and predicts the changes that occur to families and its members over time. Achievement of family developmental tasks helps individual family members to accomplish their tasks. Two of the major assumptions of this theory are:

- Families change and develop over time based on the age of the family members and the social norms of the society. Families have predictable stressors and changes based on changes in the family development and family structure. For example, when a family has their first child, there are predictable stresses and goals to accomplish. Also, families who experience a divorce have some predictable stresses based on when in the life cycle of the family the divorce occurs.
- Families experience disequilibrium when they transition from one stage to another stage. These transitions are considered "on time" or "off time." For example, a couple in their late 20s having their first child would be considered "on time," whereas a teenager having a child or a 30-year-old wife and mother dying from breast cancer would be considered "off-time" transitions.

This theory assists nurses in anticipating stresses families may experience based on the stage of the family life cycle and if the family is experiencing these changes "on time" or "off time." Nurses can also use these predictable stresses to identify family strengths in adaptation to the changes. In conducting an assessment of families, the following are examples of the types of questions nurses can ask based on the family developmental and life cycle theory.

- How has time that the family spends together been affected?
- How has communication among and between the family members been altered?
- Has physical space in the home been changed to meet the needs of the evolving family?
- In what ways have the informal roles of the family been changed?
- What changes are being experienced in family meals, recreation, spirituality, or sleep habits?
- How are the family finances affected as the family members age?
- Who should be included in the family decision making?

Nursing intervention strategies that derive from the family developmental and life cycle theory help individuals and families understand the growth and development stages and to manage the normal transition periods between developmental periods (e.g., tasks of the school-age family member versus tasks of the adolescent family member) with the least amount of stress possible. Family nurses must recognize that in every family there are both individual and family developmental tasks that need to be accomplished for every stage of the individual or family life cycle that are unique to that particular family.

The major strength of this approach is that it provides a basis for forecasting normative stresses and issues that families will experience at any stage in the family life cycle. The major weakness of the model is that it was developed at a time when the traditional nuclear family was emphasized and that some theory development has been conducted on how family life cycles or stages are affected in divorced families, step-parent families, and domestic-partner relationships (Carter and McGoldrick, 2005).

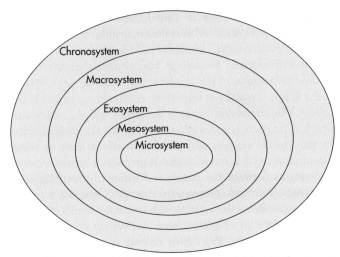

FIGURE 27-5 Bioecological family systems model: levels of systems.

Bioecological Systems Theory

The **bioecological systems theory** was developed by Urie Bronfenbrenner (1972, 1979, 1997) to describe how environments and systems outside of the family influence the development of a child over time. Even though this theory was designed around how both nature and nurture shape the development of a child, the same underlying principles can be applied when the client is the family. This theory is very useful for community/public health nurses since it helps identify the stresses and potential resources that can affect family adaptation. Figure 27-5 depicts the four systems in this theory at different levels of engagement that can affect family development and adaptation. The family as the client is at the center of the concentric circles. Each of the levels contains roles, norms, and rules that influence the current situation of the family.

Microsystems are composed of the systems and individuals that the family directly interacts with on a daily basis. These systems vary for each family, but could include their home, their neighborhood, place of work, school systems, extended family, health care system, community/public health system, or close friends.

Mesosystems are the systems that the family interacts with frequently but not on a daily basis. These systems vary based on the situation in which the community/public health nurse is working with a family. Some ideas for systems at this level could be a home health aide who comes to the home twice a week, a hospice nurse who comes to the home once a week, a social worker, church members who come to deliver food to the family, the transportation system, the school system, specialty physicians, pharmacy, or extended family.

Exosystems are external environments that have an indirect influence on the family. For example, some of these systems could be the economic system, local and state political systems, religious system, the school board, community/health and welfare services, the social security office, or protective services.

Macrosystems are broad overarching social ideological and cultural values, attitudes, and beliefs that indirectly influence the family. Examples include a Jewish religious ethic, a cultural value of autonomy in decision making, or ethnicity.

Chronosystems refer to time-related contexts in which changes that have occurred over time may influence any or all of the other levels/systems. Examples include the death of a young parent, a divorce and remarriage, war, or natural disasters.

One assumption of this model is that what happens outside of the family is equally as important as what happens inside the family. The interaction between the family and the systems in which it interacts is bidirectional in that the family is affected by the outside systems and the family affects these systems. The strength of this model is that it provides a holistic view of interactions between the family and society. In working with the family, a critical intervention strategy is drawing a family ecomap that shows the systems with which the family interacts, including the flow of energy from that system into the family or out of the family. The family ecomap is explained in more detail later in the chapter. The weakness of this model is that it does not address how families cope or adapt to the interaction with these systems.

WORKING WITH FAMILIES FOR HEALTHY OUTCOMES

Family nurses should transcend the traditional nursing approach as a service model and change their practice to a capacity-building model (Bomar, 2004). In a capacity-building model nurses assume the family has the most knowledge about how their health issues affect the family, supports family decision making, empowers the family to act, and facilitates actions for and with the family. The goal of family nursing is to focus care, interventions, and services to optimize the self-care capabilities of families and to achieve the best possible outcomes.

Nurses work with all types of family structures in a variety of settings. Each family is unique in how it responds to the stresses that evolve when a family member experiences a health event. Community/public health nurses are in a unique position to help families by providing direct care, removing barriers to needed services, and improving the capacity of the family to take care of its members (Kaakinen, 2010).

Pre-encounter Data Collection

Using excellent communication skills, nurses help families determine the priority of issues they are confronting, identify their needs, and develop a plan of action. Family members are experts in their own health. They know the family health history, their health states, and their health-related concerns (Smith, 2009).

Nurses gather information about the family from a myriad of sources as well as directly from the family. Data collection begins when an actual or potential problem is identified by a source, which may be the family, the physician, a school nurse, or a caseworker. Several examples follow:

1. A family is referred to the home health agency because of the birth of the newest family member. In that district, all births are automatically followed up with a home visit.
2. A family calls hospice to request assistance in providing care to a family member with a terminal illness.
3. A school nurse is asked to conduct a family assessment by a teacher who noticed that the student has frequent absences and has demonstrated significant behavior changes in the classroom.
4. A physician requests a family assessment for a child who has failure to thrive.
5. An individual seeks health care in a primary care county clinic or a program-specific clinic such as family planning or STD clinic.

The assessment process and data collection begin as soon as the referral occurs or the appointment is made. Sources of pre-encounter data the nurse gathers include the following:

- *Referral source.* The information collected from the referral source includes data that lead to the identification of a problem for this family. Demographic information and subjective and objective information may be obtained from the referral source.
- *Family.* A family may identify a health care concern and seek help. During the initial intake or screening procedure, valuable information can be collected from the family. Information is collected during phone interaction with the family member, even when calling to set up the initial appointment. This information might include family members' views of the problem, surprise that the referral was made, reluctance to set up the meeting, avoidance in setting up the interview, or recognition that a referral was made or that a probable health care concern exists.
- *Previous records.* Previous records may be available for review before the first meeting between the nurse and the family. Often, a record release for information is necessary to obtain family or individual records.

Determine Where to Meet the Family

Before contacting the family to arrange for the initial appointment, the nurse decides the best place to meet with the family, which might be in the home, clinic, or office. The How To Plan for Family Assessment box identifies reflection questions nurses need to address before meeting the family. Often the decision about the place of the family meeting will be determined by the type of agency with which the nurse works (e.g., home health is conducted in the home and mental health agencies meet the family in the clinic).

HOW TO Plan for Family Assessment

Assessment of families requires an organized plan before you see the family. This plan includes the following:
1. *Why are you seeing the family?*
2. *Are there any specific family concerns that have been identified by other sources?*
3. *Is there a need for an interpreter?*
4. *Who will be present during the interview?*
5. *Where will you see the family and how will the space be arranged?*
6. *What are you going to be assessing?*
7. *How are you going to collect the data?*
8. *What services do you anticipate the family will need?*
9. *What are the insurance sources for the family?*

One major advantage to meeting in the family home is seeing the everyday family environment. Family members are likely to feel more relaxed in their home, thereby demonstrating typical family interactions. Meeting with a family in their home emphasizes that the problem is the responsibility of the whole family and not one family member. Conducting the interview in the home may increase the probability of having more family members present. There are two important disadvantages of meeting in the family home: (1) the family home may be the only sanctuary or safe place for the family or its members to be away from the scrutiny of others, and (2) meeting with a family on their ground requires the nurse to be highly skilled in communication by setting limits and guiding the interaction.

Conducting the family appointment in the office or clinic allows easier access to other health care providers for consultation. An advantage of using the clinic may be that the family situation is so intense that a more formal, less personal setting may be necessary for the family to begin discussion of emotionally charged issues. A disadvantage of not seeing the everyday family environment is that it may reinforce a possible culture gap between the family and the nurse.

Making an Appointment with the Family

After the decision is made regarding where to meet the family, the nurse contacts the family. It is important to remember that the family gathers information about the nurse from this initial phone call to arrange a meeting, so the nurse should be confident and organized. After the introduction, the nurse concisely states the reason for requesting the family visit and encourages all family members to attend the meeting. The How To Make an Appointment with the Family box reviews steps for making an appointment with the family. Determine if you need an interpreter with you or if you need to arrange to have one available by phone during the visit. Several possible times for the appointment can be offered, including late afternoon or evening, which allows the family to select the most convenient time for all members to be present. It is important to remember that families ultimately retain control of the situation and they do not have to let the nurse enter their home (Smith, 2009).

HOW TO **Make an Appointment with the Family**

Data collection starts immediately upon referral to the nurse. The following are suggestions that will make the process of arranging a meeting with the family easier:

1. *Remember that the assessment is reciprocal and the family will be making judgments about you when you call to make the appointment.*
2. *Introduce yourself and the purpose for the contact.*
3. *Do not apologize for contacting the family. Be clear, direct, and specific about the need for an appointment.*
4. *Arrange a time that is convenient for all parties and allows the most family members to be present.*
5. *If appropriate, ask if an interpreter will be needed during the meeting.*
6. *Confirm place, time, date, and directions.*

Planning for Your Own Safety

It is critical to plan for your own safety when you make a home visit. Learn about the neighborhood you will be visiting, anticipate needs you may have, and determine if it is safe for you to make the home visit alone or if you need to arrange to have a security person with you during the visit. Always have your cell phone fully charged and readily available. In addition, the following strategies will help to ensure your own safety when you visit families in their homes (Smith, 2009, p 316).

1. Leave a schedule at your office.
2. Plan the visit during safe times of day.
3. Dress appropriately, bringing little jewelry or money.
4. Avoid secluded places if you are by yourself.
5. Obtain an escort; take a co-worker or neighborhood volunteer.
6. Sit between the client and the exit.
7. If you feel unsafe, do not visit or leave immediately.
8. Check in with your work at the end of the day.

Interviewing the Family: Defining the Problem

One of the underlying central tenets of family nursing is to build a trusting family–nurse relationship. Working with families requires nurses to use therapeutic communication efficiently and skillfully by moving between informal conversation and skilled interviewing strategies. Prepare your family questions before your interview based on the best family theory given what is known about the family situation.

Although it seems commonplace, it is important for nurses to introduce themselves to the family and to initiate conversation with each member present. Spending some initial time on informal conversation helps put the family at ease, allows them time to assess the person/nurse, and disperses some of the tension surrounding the visit (Tabacco, 2010). Involving each family member in the conversation, including children, elderly, or any disabled family member, demonstrates respect and caring and sends the message that the purpose of the visit is to help the whole family and not just the individual family member.

NURSING TIP *Too much disclosure during the early contacts between the family and nurse may scare the family away. Slow down the process and take time to build trust.*

Shifting the conversation into a more formal interview can be accomplished by asking the family to share their story about the current situation. If the nurse focuses only on the medical aspect or illness story, much valuable information and the priority issue confronting the family may be missed in the data collection. The purpose of the interview is to gather information and help the family focus on their problem and determine solutions. The following specific therapeutic questions have been found to provide important family information (Leahey and Svavarsdottir, 2009, p 449):

- What is the greatest challenge facing your family now?
- Who in the family do you think the illness has the most impact on?
- Who is suffering the most?

BOX 27-3 FAMILY INTERVIEW QUESTIONS

- What do you believe is the most important or pressing issue right now?
- What have you done to improve the situation?
- Share with me your primary goal in the immediate situation.
- What are the main problems you are having related to ____?
- What is causing you the most stress?
- How has this stress affected you and the members of your family?
- How are the everyday needs of the family getting done (e.g., cooking, shopping, cleaning, laundry, transportation, sleeping)?
- How well is your family managing this stress?
- What results or outcomes do you hope for?
- What do you feel you need to help solve this situation?
- What can your family do for you?
- Who do we need to involve in this situation?
- What information do you need to know?
- Walk me through a typical 24-hour day in your home.

- During times of need, where can you go for support and resources?
- What do you think would help me better understand what you are experiencing?
- How does your family anticipate caring for ____?
- How does this situation affect you financially?
- Where, how, and from whom do you receive your support, inspiration, and energy to maintain the responsibilities required of you?
- What has been the biggest surprise to you about all of this?
- How do you think your family roles and routines are going to change in this situation?
- How have you and your family prepared to provide care for ____?
- What are your family plans for when you have to return to work?
- What does your family do to feel relief or take a break?
- What are some specific changes that you and your family members have had to make?
- What do you fear the most about ____?

- What has been most and least helpful to you in similar situations?
- If there is one question you could have answered now, what would that be?
- How can we best help you and your family?
- What are your needs/wishes for assistance now?

Box 27-3 lists a variety of additional interview questions that will help uncover the family story. Encourage several members of the family to provide input into the discussion. One strategy is to ask the same question of several different family members. It is critical for the nurse to not take sides in the family discussion and to focus on guiding them in their decision making. In addition to the family story, the nurse will likely need to ask specific assessment questions about the family member who is in need of services.

Assessment Instruments

One quick way for nurses to gather information from a family is to use reliable and valid short assessment instruments that are specifically focused on the relevant family situation. Well over 1000 different family assessment instruments exist (Touliatos, Perlmutter, and Straus, 2001); therefore, it is critical that the following criteria be used to help determine the most appropriate assessment tool (Kaakinen, 2010, p 109):

- Written in uncomplicated language at a fifth-grade level
- Only takes 10 to 15 minutes to complete
- Relatively easy and quick to score
- Offers valid data on which to base decisions
- Sensitive to gender, race, social class, and ethnic background

Families should always be asked their permission to use an assessment instrument and informed of how the information will be used by the nurse in helping to plan their care. Nurses should review the results or interpretation of the information with the family.

Genograms and ecomaps are both assessment instruments that actively engage the family in their care. In addition, they both provide visual diagrams of the current family story and offer ideas about the plan of action, solutions, and resources

(Kaakinen, 2010; Rempel, Neufeld, and Kushner, 2007; Ray and Street, 2005). The genogram and ecomap are essential components of any family assessment, and they should be used concurrently with any other specific assessment tools used in the interview.

Genogram

The genogram displays pertinent family information in a family tree format that shows family members and their relationships over at least three generations (McGoldrick, Schellenberger, and Petry, 2008). The genogram shows family history and patterns of health-related information, which is a rich source of information for planning interventions. The identified client and his or her family are highlighted on the genogram. Genograms enhance nurses' abilities to make clinical judgments and connect them to family structure and history.

The diagramming of the genogram must adhere to a specific format to ensure that all parties understand the information. A form that can be used for developing genograms is depicted in Figure 27-6, and the symbols most often used in a genogram are shown in Figure 27-7.

An outline for gathering information during the genogram interview is presented in Box 27-4, and genogram interpretive categories are found in Box 27-5. The health history for all family members (morbidity, mortality, onset of illness) is important information for family nurses and can be the focus of analysis of the family genogram. The more information that can be added to the family genogram, the more the family and nurse understand the family situation. Most families are cooperative and interested in completing the genogram, which does not have to be completed in one sitting. The genogram becomes a part of the ongoing health care record.

Ecomap

The ecomap is a visual diagram of the family unit in relation to other units or subsystems in the community. The ecomap serves as a tool to organize and present factual information and thus allows the nurse to have a more holistic and integrated perception of the family situation. The ecomap shows the nature

Date _____   Completed by _____

Family Name _____

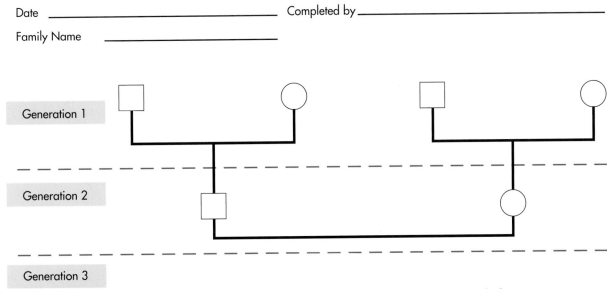

FIGURE 27-6 Genogram form. (Modified from McGoldrick M, Gerson R, Schellenburger S: *Genograms: assessment and intervention,* ed 2, New York, 1999, Norton.)

BOX 27-4   OUTLINE FOR A GENOGRAM INTERVIEW

For each person on the genogram, the nurse should determine which of the following pieces of information to include on the genogram. The information should be relevant to the issues the family is facing.

- First name
- Age
- Date of birth
- Occupation
- Health problems
- Cause of death
- Dates of marriages, divorces, separations, commitments, cohabitations, and remarriages
- Education level
- Ethnic or religious background

Modified from McGoldrick M, Gerson R: *Genograms in family assessment,* New York, 1985, Norton.

BOX 27-5   GENOGRAM INTERPRETIVE CATEGORIES

The following areas are important to note in the family genogram:

- Family structure: nuclear, blended, single-parent household, gay/lesbian relationship, cohabitation, divorces, and separations
- Sibling subsystem group: birth order, sex, distance between ages of children
- Patterns of repetition: patterns across the generations related to family structure, behaviors, health problems, relationships, violence, abuse, poverty
- Life events: repeated similar events across generations, such as transitions, traumas

---

of the relationships among family members, and between family members and the community; it is an overview of the family, picturing both the important nurturing and the important stress-producing connections between the family and its environment. The nurse starts with a blank ecomap, which consists of a large circle with smaller circles around it (Figure 27-8). The identified client and his or her family are placed in the center of the large circle. The outer smaller circles around the family unit represent significant people, agencies, or institutions in the family's environment that interact with the family members (Kaakinen, 2010). The nature and quality of the relationships and the direction of energy flow between the family members and the subsystems are shown by different connecting lines.

The ecomap serves as a tool to organize and present information, allowing the nurse and family to have a more holistic and integrated perception of the current situation. Not only does it portray the present situation, but it can also be used to set goals for the future by encouraging connection and exchange with

individuals and agencies in the community. A more detailed discussion of ecomapping can be found in Kaakinen (2010) and McGoldrick et al (2008).

Family Health Literacy

In order for the family or its members to be actively involved in their care, they must be able to understand the information in order to make appropriate health care decisions, accurately carry out their plan of action, and successfully advocate for their family in the complex health care systems in which they receive care (Kaakinen, 2010). Those with poor health literacy skills have been strongly associated with lower health outcomes (Hibbard et al, 2007; Wolff et al, 2009).

Functional health literacy includes the ability to read and understand numbers in order to use this health information to make informed decisions (DeWalt, Boone, and Pignone, 2007) and to understand the consequences when instructions or plans of action are not followed (Speros, 2005).

Nurses can assess for health literacy in conversations and when completing genograms and ecomaps. Rather than spend time determining the extent of the health literacy in a family, it is most important that nurses use the following techniques when writing out plans of care, listing directions, discussing

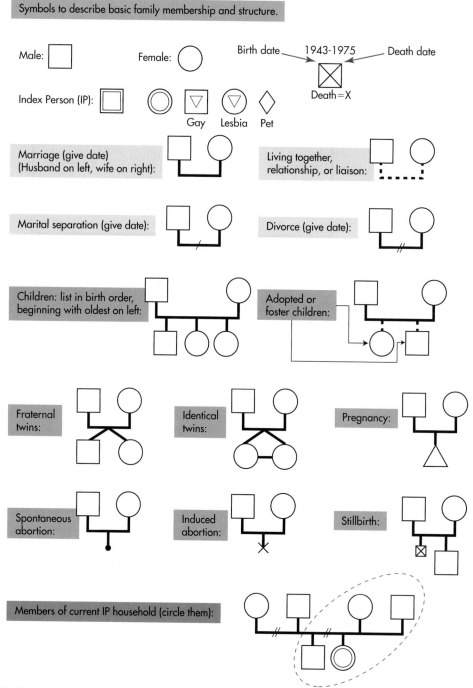

FIGURE 27-7 Genogram symbols. (Modified from McGoldrick M, Shellenberger S, Petry SS: *Genograms: assessment and intervention,* ed 3, New York, 2008, Norton.)

medication management, or writing telephone numbers (Kaakinen, 2010; Peters et al, 2007).

- Use black ink on white paper
- Use short sentences
- Use bullets no longer than seven items
- Information should be written at the fifth-grade level
- Remove all extra words
- Print in upper- and lower-case letters
- If using a computer, use 14-point font with high contrasting Arial or Sans Serif print
- Have plenty of white space

Families retain more information when nurses use a variety of communication methods (Bass, 2005), including both visual materials and visual language (Peters et al, 2007). Families need direct, clear information to assist in their decision making and carrying out the plans of action (Salmond, 2008).

Designing Family Interventions

Nurses will be challenged to help families identify the primary problem confronting them and to step aside and accept the family priority as they work in partnership with the family to keep their interventions simple, specific, timely, and realistic.

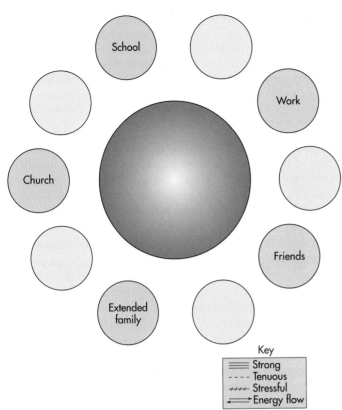

Key
≡ Strong
- - - Tenuous
+++ Stressful
← → Energy flow

FIGURE 27-8 Ecomap form. (Modified from Kaakinen JR, Hanson SMH: Family nursing assessment and intervention. In Hanson SMH, Gedaly-Duff V, Kaakinen JR, editors: *Family health care nursing: theory, practice and research,* ed 3, Philadelphia, 2005, FA Davis.)

It is essential that the family participate in determining the primary need and in designing interventions.

It is important to view the family with an open approach, since the central issue identified by the referral source may not be the actual problem the family is experiencing. See the following case study:

> The Raggs family is referred to the home health clinic by a physician for medication management. Sam, the 73-year-old husband, has been a diabetic for 13 years and has developed insulin-dependent diabetes mellitus (NIDDM). He is being discharged from the hospital. The potential area of concern that prompted the referral was the administration of insulin. After the initial meeting with the family, the primary problem the family uncovers is really not the administration of the medication, but managing his nutrition. The inference of the referral source was that the family knew how to manage the dietary aspects of diabetes because Sam has had a form of diabetes for 13 years.

If the primary family issue is not accurately identified, the family and the nurse will collect data, design interventions, and implement plans of care that do not meet the most pressing family needs. The importance of identifying the family issue of concern and accurately making the family nursing diagnosis is demonstrated by comparing the following two scenarios:

Scenario #1: The hypothesized central issue for the Raggs family was identified by the referral source: Is insulin being administered correctly? Based on this question from the referral source, the nurse asked only for information pertaining to this specific problem. The nurse asked questions that elicited information about (1) concerns of giving injections, (2) difficulty drawing up the accurate amount of insulin, and (3) the storage of insulin. The nurse focused on the interventions on: (1) the psychomotor skills of family members necessary to give the insulin injection, (2) the correct amount of insulin to give according to blood glucose level, and (3) the correct storage and handling of the medication and the equipment. By not looking at the whole family, the care was based on the nurse's perception of the problem confronting the family.

Scenario #2: The central question asked by a nurse who knows how to integrate family theory into practice was, "What is the best way to ensure that the Raggs family understands how to manage the new diagnosis of insulin-dependent diabetes?" By asking the family to share their story of the situation together, they determined that the primary issue was not medication administration but rather a lack of family knowledge related to health care management of a family member who has been newly diagnosed with insulin-dependent diabetes.

Asking broader-based questions uncovers the whole picture of the family dealing with this specific health concern and directs a more comprehensive holistic data-collection process. More evidence was collected in this case scenario because more options for possible interventions were considered concurrently. Areas of data collection based on the whole family story were: (1) administration of medication, (2) nutritional management, (3) blood glucose monitoring, (4) activity exercise, (5) coping with a changed diagnosis, and (6) knowledge of pathophysiology of diabetes. Out of all these problems, the nurse worked with the family to help them identify that their major concern centered on nutritional management, which ultimately affects the administration of medication.

The major difference between the two scenarios presented here was the way in which the nurse framed questions while listening to the family story. In the first scenario the nurse asked questions that allowed for consideration of only one aspect of family health. This type of step-by-step nurse-lead linear problem-solving process is tedious and time consuming, and will likely cause errors in the identification of the most pressing family concern (Figure 27-9). In the second scenario, the nurse asked questions that allowed for critical thinking about the family view of their challenges (Figure 27-10). The nurse gathered information from the referral source, conducted an assessment of the impact of the new diagnosis on the whole family, and collaboratively the nurse and family identified the critical family issue that had a more far-reaching effect on the health of the whole family.

The nurse works with the family to help them design realistic steps or a plan of action based on their ability to successfully adapt to the health issue given the strengths of the family. Working with the family, the following action plan approach helps focus the family on things they can immediately do to help address the problem:

1. We need the following type of help.
2. We need the following information.
3. We need the following supplies.
4. We need to involve or tell the following people.
5. To make our family action plan happen we need to... (list 5 things in the order they need to have happen).

Using knowledge and evidence-based practice, the nurse guides the family in outlining ways to prevent a potential problem, minimize the problem, stabilize the problem, or help the family recognize it as a deteriorating problem. The following scenario shows how nurses work with families to determine their strengths, identify the problem, and design interventions.

Scenario #3: The home hospice nurse has been working with the Brush family for 3 weeks. The Brush family consists of the members outlined in Figure 27-11.

Family story: Beatrice was diagnosed with terminal liver cancer 4 weeks ago. The Brush family—Bernice, Dylan, Myra, William and Jessica—agreed that Bernice should live with them and be cared for until her death in their home. Bernice has other children who live in the same city. The hospice nurse in collaboration with the Brush family identified that the primary problem is that Myra is experiencing role stress, strain, and overload in her new role as the family caregiver. Myra showed her role conflict by stating, "Sometimes I do not know who I am—daughter, nurse, mother, or wife." As Myra took a family leave from her job to stay home to care for her mother, some members of the family were surprised by her statement as they did not realize she was so overwhelmed. The family worked with the nurse to find ways to minimize her role strain by spreading the caregiver role among the extended family members.

By understanding the family systems theory, the nurse knows that what affects one member of the family, affects all members of the family. One of the strengths this family has is the shared belief that caring for the dying grandmother in their home is the "right" ethical choice for them. The nurse brings knowledge and evidence into this situation because he or she knows that the disruption to the family and their expected roles will be short term because the grandmother will probably not live for more than 4 months. However, experience with families also supports this nurse's knowledge that Myra's role conflict may likely increase as her caregiver role becomes more intense as her mother's health declines. By conducting a family genogram, another strength of this family is uncovered: it has a strong internal and external support system. The family determines that the extended family is willing to be involved in the care of Bernice. The intervention is aimed at mobilizing resources to minimize Myra's role conflict. Using the simple action plan outlined previously, the family determined that:

1. We need the following type of help:
   - Other family members to come every day to relieve Myra
   - Every other weekend, one of Bernice's other daughters will provide care through the night to relieve Myra
   - Jobs in the family will be shared to relieve Myra. Dylan will do the shopping, William will clear the table and put dishes in the dishwasher, and Jessica will help fold the clothes and put them away. William and Jessica agreed to help by spending some time each evening with Bernice, such as reading to her or watching TV with her.

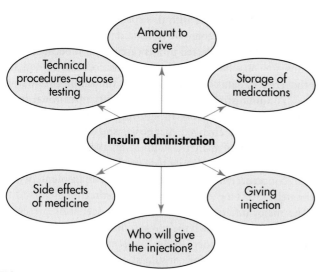

FIGURE 27-9 Scenario 1: Nurse-lead linear problem-solving identification process.

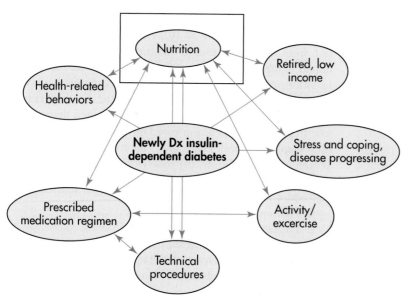

FIGURE 27-10 Scenario 2: An example of complex relationships between issues affecting the whole family because of the new diagnosis.

2. We need the following information:
   - How to call the hospice nurse when Bernice gets worse or they need immediate help
   - A list of who to call when an emergency occurs
   - A list and numbers of Bernice's health care team
3. We need the following supplies: None at this time
4. We need to involve or tell the following people: Sally and Peggy
5. To make our family action plan happen we need to... (list 5 things in the order they need to happen):
   - Invite Sally and Peggy over for a family meeting, and include the home hospice nurse.
   - Make a list of what weekends Sally and Peggy will help with Bernice.
   - Make a calendar with whose turn it is to spend time with Bernice every evening, which will relieve Myra of the care.

Based on the family story just described, as viewed through the frame of family systems theory, the following interventions were implemented: (1) assisting the family in the role negotiation of tasks and who performs them, (2) educating family members so they can safely care for Bernice now and when she enters the stage of active dying, and (3) determining what additional resources the family needs. After a plan is put into place, it needs to be evaluated periodically.

Evaluation of the Plan

In evaluating the outcome, nurses engage in critical thinking to determine if the plan is working, if it is working fast enough to address the problem, if it is addressing only part of the problem, or if the plan needs to be revised based on changes. When the plan is not working, the nurse and the family work together to determine the barriers interfering with the plan or figure out if something changed in the family story. Family apathy and indecision are known to be barriers in family nursing (Friedman, Bowden, and Jones, 2003). Friedman, Bowden, and Jones (2003) also identified the following nurse-related barriers that can affect achievement of the outcome: (1) nurse-imposed ideas, (2) negative labeling, (3) overlooking family strengths, and (4) neglecting cultural or gender implications. Family apathy may occur because of value differences between the nurse and the family, because the family is overcome with a sense of hopelessness, because the family views the problems as too overwhelming, or because family members have a fear of failure. Additional factors to be considered are that the family may be indecisive because they cannot determine which course of action is better (because they have an unexpressed fear or concern) or because they have a pattern of making decisions only when faced with a crisis.

An important part of the judgment step in working with families is the decision to terminate the relationship between the nurse and the family. Termination is phasing out the nurse from family involvement. When termination is built into the interventions, the family benefits from a smooth transition process. The family is given credit for the outcomes of the interventions that they helped design. Strategies often used in the termination component are decreasing contact with the nurse, extending invitations to the family for follow-up, and making referrals when appropriate. The termination should include a summative evaluation meeting, in which the nurse and family put a formal closure to their relationship.

When termination with a family occurs suddenly, it is important for the nurse to determine the forces bringing about the closure. The family may be initiating the termination prematurely, which requires a renegotiating process. The insurance or agency requirements may be placing a financial constraint on the amount of time the nurse can work with a family. Regardless of how termination comes about, it is important to recognize the transition from depending on the family nurse on some level to having no dependence. Strategies that help with the termination are to: (1) increase time between the nurse's visits, (2) develop a plan for the transition, (3) make referrals to other resources, and (4) provide a written summary to the family.

SOCIAL AND FAMILY POLICY CHALLENGES

Social and family policy challenges are part of the nurse's practice. As professionals, public health nurses are accountable for participating in the three core public health functions: assessment, policy development, and assurance.

Family policy is government actions that have a direct or indirect effect on families. The range of social policy decisions that affect families is vast, such as health care access and coverage, low-income housing, social security, welfare, food stamps, pension plans, affirmative action, and education. Although all government polices affect families in both negative and positive ways, the United States has little overall explicit family policy (Gebbie and Gebbie, 2005). Most government policy indirectly affects families. The Family Medical Leave legislation passed in 1993 by the U.S. Congress is an example of a type of family policy that has been positive for families. A family member may take a defined amount of leave for family events (e.g., births, deaths) without fear of losing his or her job. The Health Care Reform Act of 2010 is a long-awaited example of family policy (see the Cutting Edge box). Many programs that do exist for families, such as Social Security and Temporary Assistance to Needy Families, are not available to all families. State assistance for families varies by state.

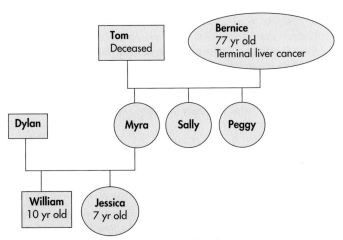

FIGURE 27-11 The Brush Family genogram.

The challenges of social policy for families are numerous. Given the ongoing debate as to what constitutes a family, social policies may specify a definition that is not consistent with the family's own definition. Examples include same-sex partnerships and/or marriage, legal definition of parents, reproductive and fertility issues (e.g., a surrogate mother decides she wants to keep the baby), or issues involving care of older adults (e.g., a niece wants to institutionalize an older aunt with dementia because her children are not available). Besides how families define themselves, governments define health care services that affect families.

Teen pregnancy prevention is a monitored health status throughout the United States and a good example of the challenges of family health policy. In some states, any child who is sexually active may have access to reproductive health services. This is a family policy to which some families object, yet the sexually active teenager is protected by a number of laws, both state and federal. The teenager who requests confidential services is protected by Title X and HIPPA federal regulations given the state law allowing access to services. Providers can encourage the teen to talk with his or her parents, but ultimately it is the teen's decision. Nurses need to be knowledgeable about these policies since they participate in carrying out family policy and have a responsibility to inform state policy regarding the services they provide.

WHAT DO YOU THINK? *Do you think teens should have access to family planning services without their parents' consent?*

Nurses participate in enforcing laws and regulations that affect the family such as state immunization laws. Most states have some school immunization laws that exclude children from school who are not vaccinated. If the child does not have that particular set of immunizations and the parents do not want the child vaccinated, two sets of laws are in conflict: the immunization laws and the school attendance laws. The state could provide a mechanism for a waiver, or the child could be excluded from school, thus making home schooling the only option.

WHAT DO YOU THINK? *What would you say to the mother who brings her child for school immunizations, but complains in front of her child that she is only there because she needs her child to be in school so that she can go to work, but does not see the need for the immunizations?*

Health care insurance is a social and family policy issue. Ensuring that health services are available or providing those services is problematic for many states and county health departments. Medicare and Medicaid, enacted in 1965, provide some health care for the elderly and low-income families. Insuring the elderly has proven to be beneficial, yet is fraught with numerous problems. Both living wills and durable power of attorney for health care, legal contracts that designate a person to make health care decisions when the individual is incapacitated, are more commonplace today than in the past. However, without these legal instruments, families are faced with making end-of-life decisions for their loved ones. Although Medicare and Medicaid provide health care to many, a significant population is still uninsured. For the uninsured, often the only access to health care is through the emergency department. Using the emergency department for primary care results in charity care that frequently gets relegated to the insured through higher premiums.

The Affordable Health Care Act (2010) signed into law by President Obama has been reported to have many benefits for families (see the Cutting Edge Box). Public health nurses now have a responsibility to participate at the state level in developing these insurance exchanges and in assessing, developing policy, and ensuring that the preventive care for better health becomes a reality for more Americans.

The H1N1 pandemic was an excellent example of mobilizing community partnerships to solve health problems. In one county health department, space for storing vaccines was insufficient in the county health clinics, so arrangements were made with the law enforcement departments to store vaccines in their secure evidence refrigerators. Other examples of partnering included collaboration with Health and Human Service departments and homeless programs to get at-risk populations and the homeless vaccinated. County health departments and pediatricians worked together to get family members who had infants under 6 months of age vaccinated, since these infants were too young to receive the H1N1 vaccine.

These are only a few examples of social and family policy in which nurses are involved. Population-focused nurses need to be involved in making policy at the local, state, and national level that affects families. Using the core public health functions as a framework allows the population-focused nurse to view the broad spectrum of activities that improve the lives of communities, families, and the individuals within those families.

CHAPTER REVIEW

PRACTICE APPLICATION

One of the most notable changes in the twenty-first century is women and mothers working outside of the home. The difference can be seen the following statistic: In 1960 only 19% of married mothers with children under 6 years of age worked outside the home, compared with 60% in 2005 (U.S. Census Bureau, 2008).

A. In what ways does this influence family socialization and affective functions?
B. In what ways does this situation affect the family health care function?
C. How does this impact family nursing?
   Answers can be found on the Evolve site.

KEY POINTS

- Families are the context within which health care decisions are made. Nurses are responsible for assisting families in meeting health care needs.
- Family nursing is practiced in all settings.
- Family nursing is a specialty area that has a strong theoretical base and is more than just common sense.
- Community health nurses must integrate both family theory and public health theory in their practice.
- Family demographics is the study of structures of families and households as well as events that alter the family, such as marriage, divorce, births, cohabitation, and dual careers.
- Demographic trends affect the family.
- Traditionally, families have been defined as nuclear: mother, father, and young children. There are a variety of family definitions, such as a group of two or more, a unique social group, and two or more persons joined together by emotional bonds.
- The five functions performed by families are economic, reproduction, socialization, affective, and health care.
- Family structure refers to the characteristics, sex, age, and number of the individual members who make up the family unit.
- Family health is difficult to define, but it includes the biological, psychological, sociological, cultural, and spiritual factors of the family system.
- There are four approaches to viewing families: family as context, family as client, family as a system, and family as a component of society.

- Systems theory describes families as a unit of the whole composed of members whose interactional patterns are the focus of attention, in that what affects one member affects all the others.
- Family developmental and life cycle theory emphasizes how families change over time and focuses on interactions and relationships among family members.
- Bioecological family theory helps community/public health nurses identify the stresses and potential resources that can affect family adaptation.
- Nurses should ask clients whom they consider to be family and then include those members in the health care plan.
- Families want to be involved in identifying their major problem and designing solutions that are family focused.
- It is important for the nurse to recognize that the family has the right to make its own health decisions.
- The goal of family nursing is to focus care, interventions, and services to optimize the self-care capabilities of families and to achieve the best possible outcomes.
- One of the underlying central tenets of family nursing is to build a trusting family–nurse relationship.
- Working with families requires nurses to use therapeutic communication efficiently and skillfully by moving between informal conversation and skilled interviewing strategies.
- Genograms and ecomaps are essential components of any family assessment.
- All government actions, whether at the local, county, state, or national level, affect the family.

CLINICAL DECISION-MAKING ACTIVITIES

1. Select six or more health professionals and ask them to define family. Analyze the responses for common points and differences. Write your own definition of family.
2. Characterize the different family structures and household arrangements represented in your community. This information may be available from various sources, such as the health department, schools, other social and welfare agencies, and census data. Be specific.
3. Draw your own family genogram and ecomap. Discuss how they are used in family nursing.
4. Discuss the role of nursing related to family policy. Be specific about issues related to family culture.
5. Break into small groups and have students discuss the Brush family presented in the chapter in terms of the three family social science theories. What questions would they ask the family from the different theoretical perspectives? Examine different situations when one theory might be more appropriate to use than another.
6. How might you go about obtaining services for a Hispanic woman who tests positive for diabetes who is uninsured or underinsured?
7. Break into small groups to discuss how you have found judging or reacting to family structure situations that are different from those you personally bring to practice. What helps you try to reframe this situation in order to practice family nursing?
8. You are working with a lesbian family with three children. What barriers or problems do you anticipate with social policies while trying to access resources?

REFERENCES

Agency for Health Care Research and Quality: *National health care quality report,* 2008, USDHHS. Available at http://www.ahrq.gov/qual/nhqr08/Chap2c.htm. Accessed February 10, 2011.

American Nurse Association: *Public health nursing: scope and standards of practice,* Silver Spring, MD, 2007, ANA.

American Public Health Association: *The role of public health nurses,* 2010. Available at http://www.apha.org/membergroups/sections/aphasections/phn/about/phnroles.htm. Accessed February 10, 2011.

Avellar S, Smock PJ: The economic consequences of the dissolution of cohabiting unions, *J Marriage Family* 67:315–327, 2005.

Bass L, guest editor: *Sociological studies of children and youth,* vol 10, New York, 2005, Elsevier Science.

Bernstein R: *Hispanics Population Surpasses 40 Million,* 2005. Available at usa.usembassy. de/etexts/soc/ff_hispanicheritage2005.pdf. Retrieved March 30, 2011.

Bomar P: *Nurses and family health promotion: concepts, assessment, and interventions,* ed 3, Philadelphia, 2004, Saunders.

Bronfenbrenner U: *Influences on human development,* Hinsdale, IL, 1972, Dryden Press.

Bronfenbrenner U: *The ecology of human development,* Cambridge, MA, 1979, Harvard University Press.

Bronfrenbrenner U: Ecology of the family as a context for human development: research perspectives. In Paul JL, Churton M, Rosselli-Kostoryz H, et al, editors: *Foundations of special education,* Pacific Grove, CA, 1997, Brooks/Cole.

Bumpass L, Lu H: Trends in cohabitation: an implication for childrens' family content in the United States, *Population Studies* 54:29–41, 2000.

Carter B, McGoldrick M, editors: *The expanded family life cycle: individual, family and social perspectives,* ed 3, New York, 2005, Allyn & Bacon.

Casper LM, Hagga JG, Jayasundera RR: Demography and family health. In Kaakinen JR, Gedaly-Duff V, Coehlo DP, Hanson SMH, editors: *Family health care nursing: theory, practice & research,* ed 4, Philadelphia, 2010, FA Davis, pp 103–130.

Centers for Disease Control and Prevention: *New report sheds light on trends and patterns in marriage, divorce, and cohabitation,* 2002. Available at http://www.cdc.gov/nchs/pressroom/02news/div_mar_cohab.htm. Accessed February 10, 2011.

Centers for Disease Control and Prevention: *Chlamydia and gonorrhea — two most commonly reported notifiable infectious diseases in the United States,* 2010. Available at http://www.cdc.gov/Features/dsSTDData/. Accessed February 10, 2011.

Clayman M, Roter D, Wissow I, Baudeen-Rocher K: Autonomy-related behaviors of patient companions and their effect on decision-making activity in geriatric primary care visits, *Soc Sci Med* 60(7):1583–1591, 2005.

Coleman M, Ganong L, Fine M: Reinvestigating remarriage: another decade of progress, *J Marriage Family* 62:1288–1307, 2000.

Crissey SR: Educational attainment in the United States: 2007. *Current population reports,* 20–560, Washington, DC, January 2009, U.S. Census Bureau.

Daily M, Newfield J: Legal issues in home care: Current trends, risk-reduction strategies, and opportunities for improvement, *Home Health Care Manag Pract* 17(2):93–100, 2005.

Davis JW, Bauman KJ: School enrollment in the United States: 2006, *Current population reports,* 20-559, Washington, DC, 2009, U.S. Census Bureau.

DeLeire T, Kalil A: How do cohabiting couples with children spend their money? *J Marriage Family* 67:286–295, 2005.

DeWalt DA, Boone RS, Pignone MP: Literacy and its relationship with self-efficacy, trust and participation in medical decision making, *Am J Health Behav* 31(suppl 3):S27–S35, 2007.

Driver J, Tabares A, Shapiro A, Nahm EY, Gottman J: Interactional patterns in marital success and failure: Gottman laboratory studies. In Walsh F, editor: *Normal family process: growing diversity and complexity,* ed 3, New York, 2003, Guilford Press, pp 493–513.

Duvall EM, Miller BC: *Marriage and family development,* ed 6, New York, 1985, Harper & Row.

Dye JL: Fertility of American women: 2006, *Current population reports,* 20-558, Washington, DC, 2008a, U.S. Census Bureau.

Dye JL: *Participation of mothers in government assistance programs:* 2004, *Current population reports,* 70-116, Washington, DC, 2008b, U.S. Census Bureau.

Eddy LL, Doutrich D: Families and community/public health nursing. In Kaakinen JR, Gedaly-Duff V, Coehlo DP, Hanson SMH, editors: *Family health care nursing: theory, practice & research,* ed 4, Philadelphia, 2010, FA Davis, pp 470–489.

Eggly S, Penner I, Greene M, et al: Information seeking during "bad news" oncology interactions: question asking by patients and their companions, *Soc Sci Med* 63(11):2974–2985, 2006.

Friedman MM, Bowden VR, Jones EG: *Family nursing: research, theory and practice,* ed 5, Upper Saddle River, NJ, 2003, Prentice Hall.

Gebbie K, Gebbie E: Families, nursing, and social policy. In Hanson SMH, Gedaly-Duff V, Kaakinen JR: *Family health care nursing,* ed 3, Philadelphia, 2005, FA Davis.

Goodwin P, McGill B, Chandra A: *Who marries and when? Age at first marriage in the United States:* 2002, NCHS Data Brief, No. 19, Hyattsville, MD, 2009, National Center for Health Statistics.

Goodwin PY, Mosher WD, Chandra A: *Marriage and cohabitation in the United States: a statistical portrait based on cycle 6 (2002) of the National Survey of Family Growth,* Vital and Health Statistics Series 23, No 28, 2010, National Center for Health Statistics.

Grieco EM: *Race and Hispanic origin of the foreign-born population in the United States, 2007, American community survey reports,* Washington, DC, 2010, U.S. Census Bureau. 2007.

Hackbarth GM: Reforming America's health care system: *Medicare payment advisory commission: statement to Senate Finance Committee,* 2009. Available at http://www.medpac.gov/documents/Hackbarth%20Statement%20SFC%20Roundtable%204%2021%20FINAL%20with%20header%20and%20footer.pdf. Accessed February 10, 2011.

Hanson SMH: Family health care nursing: an overview. In Hanson SMH, Gedaly-Duff V, Kaakinen JR, editors: *Family health care nursing: theory, practice and research,* ed 3, Philadelphia, 2005, FA Davis.

Hibbard JH, Peters E, Dixon A, Tusler M: Consumer competencies and the use of comparative quality information: it just isn't about literacy, *Med Care Res Rev* 64(4):379–394, 2007.

Hogue EE, Fairnot DC: Home health care nurses should follow case management standards to achieve patient outcomes, *Caring* 25(6):50–53, 2006.

Kaakinen JR: Family nursing process: family nursing assessment models. In Kaakinen JR, Gedaly-Duff V, Coehlo DP, Hanson SMH, editors: *Family health care nursing: theory, practice & research,* ed 4, Philadelphia, 2010, FA Davis, pp 103–130.

Kaakinen JR, Hanson SMH: Theoretical foundations for the nursing of families. In Kaakinen JR, Gedaly-Duff V, Coehlo DP, Hanson SMH, editors: *Family health care nursing: theory, practice & research*, ed 4, Philadelphia, 2010, FA Davis, pp 63–102.

Kaakinen JR, Hanson SMH, Denham SA: Family health care nursing: an introduction. In Kaakinen JR, Gedaly-Duff V, Coehlo DP, Hanson SMH, editors: *Family health care nursing: theory, practice & research*, ed 4, Philadelphia, 2010, FA Davis, pp 3–33.

King V, Scott ME: A comparison of cohabiting relationships among older and younger adults, *J Marriage Family* 67:271–285, 2005.

Kinnersley P, Edwards A, Hood K, et al: Interventions before consultations for helping patients, address their information needs. *Cochrane Database Systematic Review*, 3, CD004565. PMID: 17636767.

Krieder RM, Elliot DB: American's families and living arrangements: 2007, *Current population reports*, P 20-561, Washington, DC, 2007, U.S. Census Bureau.

Kreider RM: Number, timing and duration of marriages and divorces: 2001. *Current population reports*, P 70–97, Washington DC, 2005, U.S. Census Bureau.

Leahey M, Svavarsdottir EK: Implementing family nursing: how do we translate knowledge into clinical practice? *J Fam Nurs* 15(4):445–460, 2009.

Lee SM, Edmonston B: New marriages, new families: U.S. racial and Hispanic intermarriage, *Population Bull* 60:3–36, 2005.

Lowenstein LF: Causes and associated features of divorce as seen by recent research, *J Divorce Remarriage* 42:153–171, 2005.

Mathews TJ, Hamilton BE: *NCHS brief, no. 21*, Hyattsville, MD, 2009, National Center for Health Statistics.

McGoldrick M, Shellenberger S, Petry SS: *Genograms: assessment and interventions*, ed 3, New York, 2008, W.W. Norton.

Olson DH, Gorall DM: Circumplex model of marital and family systems. In Walsh F, editor: *Normal family processes*, ed 3, New York, 2003, Guilford, pp 514–517.

Peters DJ, Dieckann N, Dixon A, et al: Less is more in presenting quality information to consumers, *Med Care Res Rev* 64(2):169–190, 2007.

Phillips JA, Sweeney MM: Premarital cohabitation and marital disruption among white, black and Mexican American women, *J Marriage Family* 67:296–314, 2005.

Public Health Foundation: *Core competencies for public health professionals*, June 2009. Available at http://www.phf.org/link/core-061109.htm. Accessed March 8, 2010.

Ray RA, Street AF: Ecomapping: an innovative research tool for nurses, *J Adv Nurs* 50(5):545–552, 2005.

Region X: *IPP Committee: Infertility prevention project: program guidelines and data collection*, 2000. Available at http://www.oregon.gov/DHS/ph/std/ipp/overview.shtml. Accessed February 10, 2011.

Rempel GR, Neufeld A, Kushner KE: Interactive use of genograms and ecomaps in family care giving research, *J Fam Nurs* 13(4):403–419, 2007.

Salmond S: Who is family? Family and decision making. In Lewenson SB, Truglio-Londrigan M, editors: *Decision-making in nursing: thoughtful approaches for practice*, Sudbury, MA, 2008, Jones and Bartlett, pp 89–104.

Seltzer JA: Families formed outside of marriage, *J Marriage Family* 62:1247–1268, 2000.

Smith CM: Home visit: opening the doors for family health. In Maurer FA, Smith CM, editors: *Community public health nursing practice: health for families and populations*, ed 4, St Louis, 2009, Saunders, pp 302–326.

Speros C: Health literacy: concept analysis, *J Adv Nurs* 50(6):633–640, 2005.

Sweeney MM: Remarriage and the nature of divorce, *J Family Issues* 33:410–440, 2002.

Tabacco A: Nursing assessment of the family. In Votroubek W, Tabacco A, editors: *Pediatric home care for nurses: a family-centered approach*, ed 3, Boston, 2010, Jones & Bartlett, pp 59–80.

Teachman JD, Polonko KA, Scanzioni J: Demography of the family. In Sussman MB, Steinmetz SK, editors: *Handbook of marriage and the family*, New York, 2000, Plenum Press, p 17.

Thomson E, Mosley J, Hanson T, et al: Remarriage, cohabitation, and changes in mothering behavior, *J Marriage Family* 63:370–380, 2001.

Touliatos J, Perlmutter B, Straus M: *Handbook of family measurement techniques*, Newbury Park, CA, 2001, Sage.

U.S. Census Bureau: *Employment status of women, by marital status and presence and age of children: 1960 to 2005*, 2008. Available at http://www/census/gov/compendia. Accessed April 8, 2010.

U.S. Census Bureau: *Income, poverty, and health insurance coverage in the United States: 2008*, 2009. Available at http://www.census.gov/Press-Release/www/releases/archives/income_wealth/014227.html. Accessed March 9, 2010.

Vasquez MS: Preventing rehospitalization through effective home health nursing care, *Home Health Nurse* 26(2):75–81, 2008.

Ventura MS, Brown D, Archibald T, et al: *Improving care transitions and reducing hospital readmissions: establishing the evidence for community-based implementation strategies through the care transitions theme, The Remington Report*. Available at http://www.cfmc.org/caretransitions/files/Care_Transition_Article_Remington_Report_Jan_2010.pdf. Accessed February 10, 2011.

Weinberg DB, Lusenhop RW, Gittell JH, Kautz CM: Coordination between formal providers and informal caregivers, *Health Care Manag Rev* 32(2):140–149, 2007.

White JM, Klein DN: *Family theories: an introduction*, ed 3, Thousand Oaks, CA, 2008, Sage.

Wolff J, Roter D: Hidden in plain sight: medical visit companions as a resource for vulnerable older adults, *Arch Int Med* 168(13):1409–1415, 2008.

Wolff JL, Roter DL, Given B, Gitlin LN: Optimizing patient and family involvement in geriatric home care, *J Healthcare Qual* 31(2):24–33, 2009.

CHAPTER 28

Family Health Risks

Debra Gay Anderson, PhD, PHCNS, BC

Dr. Debra Gay Anderson is currently an associate professor of nursing at the University of Kentucky's College of Nursing in Lexington. She is certified as a clinical specialist in public/community health nursing and has provided health care for the homeless and other vulnerable populations. Dr. Anderson has taught public health, epidemiology, leadership, and research courses at both the graduate and undergraduate levels. The focus of her program of research, publications, and presentations is vulnerable populations, primarily women who are statistically at greater risk of experiencing domestic violence or workplace violence. Dr. Anderson has also completed a family nursing postdoctoral fellowship at Oregon Health Sciences University in Portland, Oregon. Dr. Anderson is an active member of the American Public Health Association (APHA) and has served in various leadership capacities, including Chair of the Public Health Nursing Section of APHA.

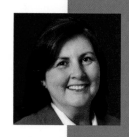

Amanda Fallin, RN, MSN

Amanda Fallin graduated from the University of Kentucky in 2009 with a Master of Science in Nursing degree. She is currently working on her PhD at the University of Kentucky's College of Nursing. While in graduate school, Ms. Fallin has worked as a research assistant to Drs. Anderson and Ellen Hahn, participating in grant and manuscript preparation and poster presentations at the national conference of the American Public Health Association and the Southern Nursing Research Society.

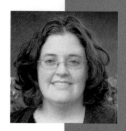

ADDITIONAL RESOURCES

ⓔvolve WEBSITE
http://evolve.elsevier.com/Stanhope
- *Healthy People 2020*
- Quiz
- Case Studies
- WebLinks
- Glossary
- Answers to Practice Application

- Resource Tools
  - Resource Tool 5.A: Schedule of Clinical Preventive Services
  - Resource Tool 27.A: Family Systems Stressor-Strength Inventory
  - Resource Tool 27.B: Case Example of Family Assessment

APPENDIX
- Appendix E: Friedman Family Assessment Model (Short Form)

OBJECTIVES

After reading this chapter, the student should be able to do the following:

1. Evaluate the various approaches to defining and conceptualizing family health.
2. Analyze the major risks to family health.
3. Analyze the interrelationships among individual health, family health, and community health.
4. Explain the relevance of knowledge about family structures, roles, and functions for family-focused nursing in the community.
5. Discuss the implications of policy and policy decisions, at all governmental levels, on families.
6. Explain the application of the nursing process (assessment, planning, implementation, evaluation) to reducing family health risks and promoting family health.

The family as a client unit is basic to the practice of population-centered nursing, and nurses are responsible for promoting healthy families in society. As such, families are described as a unique population in public health. The purpose of this chapter is to make the reader aware of influences, both individual and societal, that place families at risk for poor health outcomes, and to discuss how positive outcomes for diverse families can be accomplished through appropriate nursing interventions.

The expanding definition of the family unit presents today's nurse with an array of challenges and opportunities to address the health needs of families. First, it is essential to place the family in the context of the twenty-first century. Many Americans tend to idealize *family* and wish for a return to family values of the past and a golden time for families. However, historical demographic statistics reveal that this prevalence of the idealized family that has often been portrayed in the media never actually existed. Rather than arguing for a return to the "traditional family" (male breadwinner and woman at home), serious discussions are needed about how to help today's diverse families succeed. A focus on all family structures is a moral and ethical imperative in the promotion of the health of individuals as well as the health of the community (Nightingale et al, 1978; Wright and Leahey, 2009).

The varying family structures of today need to be recognized and examined in order to better understand both the strengths and weaknesses associated with each. Only by doing this will we be able to help all families live healthy and productive lives.

Nurses can play an active role in leading and facilitating this learning process. This facilitation can enable better-informed health care policy decisions that have a positive effect on single-parent families, remarried and stepfamilies, gay and lesbian families, grandparent-headed families, and ethnically diverse families, as well as "traditional" families.

A nation's family health care **policy** is a primary determinant of **family health**. Family policy means anything that is done by the government that directly or indirectly affects families. Family health policy and its relative effectiveness demonstrates a government's understanding of families and its role in promoting their health, with an important desired outcome being that families derive a sense of empowerment and are able to take responsibility for their own health (Chinn, 2008). The responsibility for family health programs is shared by the federal government with state and local governments. Each state, as well as regions within states, has programs and laws related to family services. The United States is one of the richest and most technologically advanced countries in the world today and yet, despite the profusion of technological advances and the continually growing proportion of the national budget spent on health care, the disparities in health status between different populations of families has continued to grow (Families USA, 2009). These disparities have resulted, at least in part, from previous attempts to develop and implement "family policies" that either directly or indirectly affect specific issues related to family health but which have failed to take a comprehensive system-wide approach. An example of this is the recent Health Care and Education Reconciliation Act of 2010 that aims to help families who are currently uninsured or underinsured to obtain insurance coverage. Although well intended, it may well turn out to be just one more piece in an incomplete patchwork of existing legislation that is struggling to effectively improve family health.

Evidence to date suggests that the United States could benefit from a cohesive family policy designed to enhance the well-being of all families. Such a policy would go a long way to prevent future crises in vulnerable family populations, such as those in or on the verge of poverty, or families overwhelmed with abuse and neglect, by providing a structural safety net to help families to maintain their health in times of disaster, economic downturns, unemployment, health crises, and other situations. An effective family health policy may consider as its foundational element an infrastructure of programs designed to provide access to primary and preventive health care. The building of this foundation requires a multi-professional process in which nurses can be actively involved. Nurses are educated in community assessment, planning, development, and evaluation activities that emphasize and address issues crucial to promoting and sustaining primary family health. Nurses looking to positively influence family health will want to be aware of and actively participate in the ongoing national debate and dialogue on family health policy that embraces their role as principal constituents in building healthy families.

In establishing health objectives for the nation, an emphasis has been placed on both health promotion and risk reduction. Reducing the risks to segments of the population is a direct way to improve the health of the general population. Specific objectives have been identified related to specific health risks for families. The family is an important environmental factor that affects the health of individuals as well as a social unit whose health is basic to that of the community and the larger population. It is within the family that health values, health habits, and health risk perceptions are developed, organized, and carried out. Individuals' health behaviors are affected by and acted out within the family environment, the larger community, and society. Family health habits are developed in the same manner in the context of community norms and values, and on the basis of availability and accessibility. For example, in a television commercial for an over-the-counter stimulant, a man is featured who is able to coach his child's basketball team, work at a rehabilitation center, and work as a borough inspector for the city, all while pursuing a college degree at night. The commercial credits the drug for providing the man with the energy needed to be successful in all of these areas. The message is clear: you can, and must, do it all, and taking drugs to succeed is a viable option. The health risks to individual and family health are affected by the societal norms—in this example, the norm is increasing productivity through drugs.

To intervene effectively and appropriately with families to reduce their health risk and thereby promote their health, nurses need to understand not only family structure and functioning, but also family theory, nursing theory, and models of health risk (see Chapters 9, 17, and 27). In addition, the effective nurse needs to look beyond the individual and the family in order to understand the complex environment in which the family exists. Increasing evidence of the effects of social, biological, economic, and life events on health requires a broader approach to addressing health risks for families. Nurses and the communities they serve have a vital interest in exploring new and appropriate options for structuring nursing interventions with families to decrease health risks and to promote health and well-being for all families. It is important for the nurse to focus on families who share similar health risks as a population. Working and planning interventions to reduce health risks in family populations provides a mechanism for shared communication and support among families as well as efficient and effective health care interventions that will not only make the families, but the community as a whole, healthier.

EARLY APPROACHES TO FAMILY HEALTH RISKS

Health of Families

Historically, the study of the family relative to health and illness focused on three major areas: (1) the effect of illness on families, (2) the role of the family in the cause of disease, and (3) the role of the family in its use of services. In his classic review of the family as an important unit, Litman (1974) pointed out the important role that the family (as a primary unit of health care) plays in health and illness and emphasized that the relationship between health, health behavior, and family "is a highly dynamic one in which each may have a dramatic effect on the other" (p 495). At about this same time, Mauksch (1974) proposed the idea of distinguishing between family health and individual health. Pratt's (1976) examination of the role of the family in health and illness included the role of family health in the promotion of healthy or unhealthy behavior. Pratt proposed and described the *energized family* as being an ideal family type that was most effective in meeting health needs. The energized family is characterized as promoting freedom and change, active contact with a variety of other groups and organizations, flexible role relationships, equal power structure, and a high degree of autonomy in family members. Doherty and McCubbin (1985) proposed a family health and illness cycle consisting of six phases, beginning with family health promotion and risk reduction and continuing through the family's vulnerability to illness, their illness response, their interaction with the health care system, and finally their ways of adapting to illness.

Health of the Nation

In recent years, increased attention has been given to improving the health of everyone in the United States. As a result of major public health and scientific advances, the leading causes of morbidity and mortality have shifted from infectious diseases to chronic diseases, accidents, and violence, all of which have strong lifestyle and environmental components. A classic population-focused study in Alameda County, California (Belloc and Breslow, 1972) demonstrated the relationships between seven lifestyle habits and decreased morbidity and mortality. These habits were: (1) sleeping 7 to 8 hours daily, (2) eating breakfast almost every day, (3) never or rarely eating between meals, (4) being at or near recommended height-adjusted weight, (5) never smoking cigarettes, (6) moderate or no use of alcohol, and (7) regular physical activity. These same lifestyle health habits are still important for improved health in the twenty-first century.

A growing body of literature supports the notion that lifestyle and the environment interact with heredity to cause disease. In response to these findings and to the limited effect of medical interventions on the growing incidence and prevalence of injuries and chronic disease, the government launched a major effort to address the health status of the population. Part of this effort was a report by the Division of Health Promotion and Disease Prevention of the Institute of Medicine that examined the critical components of the physical, socioeconomic, and family environments related to decreasing risk and promoting health (Nightingale et al, 1978). *The Surgeon General's Report on Health Promotion and Disease Prevention* (Califano, 1979) described the risks to good health in the United States at that time. As a result of these reports, health objectives for the nation were established and then evaluated and restated for the year 2000 and again for 2010 (USDHHS, 2000). The *Healthy People 2020* objectives extend the work of the three past documents. An innovative part of this latest *Healthy People* update has been a move to become more creative and inclusive. The focus challenges health care providers with a national goal of improving health and will provide the necessary background for future policy initiatives to reduce risk in all populations. Of the four goals, three are particularly important to families:

- Achieve health equity, eliminate disparities, and improve the health of all groups.
- Create social and physical environments that promote good health for all.
- Promote quality of life, healthy development, and healthy behaviors across all life stages.

With the notion of **risk,** any factor resulting in a predisposition toward or an increased likelihood of ill health takes on increased importance. Specific attention is being paid to those environmental and behavioral factors that lead to ill health with or without the influence of heredity. Reducing health risks is a major step toward improving the health of the nation. Although the family is considered an important environment related to achieving important health objectives, limited attention and research have been directed at family health risks and the role of society in promoting healthy families.

♥ HEALTHY PEOPLE 2020

Objectives Related to Family and Home Health

- EH-18: Decrease the number of U.S. homes that are found to have lead-based paint or related hazards.
- MICH-11: Increase abstinence from alcohol, cigarettes, and illicit drugs among pregnant women.
- NWS-12: Eliminate very low food security among children in U.S. households.
- TU-14: Increase the proportion of smoke-free homes.

From U.S. Department of Health and Human Services: *Healthy People 2020,* Washington, DC, 2010, U.S. Government Printing Office.

CONCEPTS IN FAMILY HEALTH RISK

Pender's Health Promotion Model (2010), described in the latest edition of her textbook, continues to be useful in research that is done with families. This health promotion model states there are two factors that motivate individuals to participate in positive health behaviors. One is a desire to promote one's own health, using behaviors that have been determined to increase the individual, family, community and society's well-being, and in the process, actually moving toward not only individual self actualization, but a society actualization as well. The second factor is a desire to protect health, using those same behaviors in an effort to decrease the probability of ill health and provide active protection against illness and dysfunction in families (Pender, 2010). Understanding family health risk requires an examination of several related concepts: family health, family health risk, risk appraisal, risk reduction, life events, lifestyle, and family crisis. These concepts will be defined and discussed here. It important to remember that *health* can be defined in a number of ways, and it is defined by individuals and families within their own culture and value system.

Family Health

Family theorists refer to healthy families but generally do not define family health (White and Klein, 2009). Based on the variety of perspectives of family (see Chapters 9, 17, and 27), definitions of healthy families can be derived within the guidelines of the framework associated with that perspective. For example, within the perspective of the developmental framework, family health can be defined as possessing the abilities and resources to accomplish family developmental tasks. Thus, the accomplishment of stage-specific tasks is one indicator of family health.

Because the family unit is a part of many societal systems, the systems perspective will be discussed in more detail. Using the Neuman Systems Model (Nursing Theory Network, 2005; Neumann University, 2010), family health is defined in terms of system stability as characterized by five interacting sets of factors: physiological, psychological, sociocultural, developmental, and spiritual. The client family is seen as a whole system with the five interacting factors. The Neuman Systems Model is a wellness-oriented model in which the nurse uses the strengths and resources of the family to keep the system stable while adjusting to stress reactions that lead to health change and wellness. In other words, this model focuses on family wellness in the face of change. Because change is inevitable in every family, the Neuman Systems Model proposes that families have a flexible external line of defense, a normal line of defense, and an internal line of resistance. When a life event is big enough to contract the flexible line of defense (a protective mechanism) and breaks through the normal line of defense, the family feels stress. The degree of wellness is determined by the amount of energy it takes for the system to become and remain stable. When more energy is available than is being used, the system remains stable. Examples of energy-building characteristics in this system are social support, resources, and prevention (or avoidance) of stressors. Nurses can use preventive health care both to reduce the possibility that a family encounters a stressor and to help strengthen the family's flexible line of defense. The following clinical example applies the Neuman Systems Model to one family's situation:

> The Harris family consists of Ms. Harris (Gloria), 12-year-old Kevin, 8-year-old Leisha, and Ms. Harris's mother, 75-year-old Betty. Kevin was recently diagnosed with insulin-dependent diabetes mellitus, and the family was referred by the endocrinology clinic to the nursing service at the local health department to work with the family in adjusting to the diagnosis.

The focus of the Neuman Systems Model would be to assess the family's ability to adapt to this stressful change and then focus on their strengths in the stabilizing process. The *five interacting variables* would compose an important component of the assessment:

- *Physiological:* Is the Harris family physically able to deal with Kevin's illness? Is everyone else in the family currently healthy? Are there current health stressors?
- *Psychological:* How well will the family be able to deal with the illness psychologically? Are their relationships stable and healthy? Are there any memories of other family members with diabetes?
- *Sociocultural:* How will the sociocultural variable come into play in Kevin's illness? Does the family have social support? Are the treatment and diagnosis culturally sensitive? Can family members support each other?
- *Developmental:* How will Kevin's development as a preadolescent be affected by diabetes? How will the family's development change? How will Kevin's diagnosis affect Leisha?
- *Spiritual:* How will the family's spiritual beliefs be affected by the diagnosis? What effect will they have on his treatment and willingness to adhere to therapy?

Health Risk

Several factors contribute to the development of healthy or unhealthy outcomes. Clearly, not everyone exposed to the same event will have the same outcome. The factors that determine or influence whether disease or other unhealthy results occur are called *health risks*. Controlling health risks is done through disease prevention and health promotion efforts. Health risks can be classified into general categories: inherited **biological risk** (including age-related risks), social and physical environmental risks and **behavioral risk** as well as health care risks. The first three of these categories of risk is discussed later in terms of family health risk, under Major Family Health Risks and Nursing Interventions *Healthy People 2020* (USDHHS, 2010).

Although single risk factors can influence outcomes, the combined effect of accumulated risks is greater than the sum of the individual effects. For example, a family history of cardiovascular disease is a single biological risk factor that is affected by smoking (a behavioral risk that is more likely to occur if other family members also smoke) and by diet and exercise. Diet and exercise are influenced by family and society's norms. Although the demographics may be changing, residents of the Northwest and West have historically been more likely to eat heart-healthy diets and to exercise compared

with people who live in the Midwest and South; thus, communities in the Northwest and West are often more supportive of exercise programs, bicycle paths, and diets lower in fat than communities in other parts of the United States. The combined effect of a family history, family behavioral risks, and society's influences is greater than the sum of the three individual risk factors (smoking, diet, and exercise). Thus, working with populations of families and intervening within a community is more likely to reduce the effects of the health risks overall and produce a healthier community as well as a healthier family unit.

Health Risk Appraisal

Health risk appraisal refers to the process of assessing for the presence of specific factors in each of the categories that have been identified as being associated with an increased likelihood of an illness, such as cancer, or an unhealthy event, such as an automobile accident. Several techniques have been developed to accomplish health risk appraisal, including computer software programs and paper-and-pencil instruments. One technique is the Youth Behavioral Health Risk Appraisal instrument of the Centers for Disease Control and Prevention (CDC, 2010). The general approach is to determine whether and to what degree a risk factor is present. On the basis of scientific evidence, each factor is weighted, and a total score is derived. This appraisal method provides an individual score that can be examined as a whole within the family being assessed, thus appraising the health risks that are likely to be experienced by other members of the family. Additional research is needed to determine if the individual appraisals can be used to determine family risk.

DID YOU KNOW? *Adolescents from families that have close, supportive interactions, clearly set and enforced rules, and parents who are involved with their children are at decreased risk for alcohol use or misuse. These family patterns can be enhanced through family-focused intervention sessions in the home, in the schools, and at other community levels.*

Health Risk Reduction

Health risk reduction is based on the assumption that decreasing the number of risks or the magnitude of risk will result in a lower probability of an undesired event occurring. For example, to decrease the likelihood of adolescent substance abuse, family behaviors such as parents not drinking, alcohol not available in the home, and family contracts related to alcohol and drug use may be useful. Health risks can be reduced through a variety of approaches, such as those just described. It is important to note the specific risk and the family's tolerance of it. Pender (2010) provides examples of different kinds of risks:

- Voluntarily assumed risks are better tolerated than those imposed by others.
- Risks over which scientists debate and as a result have some level of uncertainty as to their magnitude are more feared than risks on which scientists agree.

- Risks of natural origin are often considered less threatening than those created by humans.
- Thus, risk reduction is a complex process that requires knowledge of the specific risk and the family's perceptions of the nature of the risk.

> **WHAT DO YOU THINK?**   *Would governmental priority for funding health risk reduction and health promotion programs, including assistance programs, have greater benefit to the population's health than funding for illness treatment activities?*

Family Crisis

A **family crisis** occurs when the family is not able to cope with an event or multiple events and becomes disorganized or dysfunctional. When the demands of the situation exceed the resources of the family, a family crisis exists. When families experience a crisis or a crisis-producing event, they attempt to gather their resources to deal with the demands created by the situation. McKenry and Price (2005) differentiate between family resources and family coping strategies. The former are the resources, such as money and extended family, that a family has available to them. The latter are the family's efforts to manage, adapt, or deal with the stressful event in order to achieve balance in the family system (McKenry and Price, 2005). Thus, if a family were to experience an unexpected illness of the primary wage earner, family resources might include financial assistance from relatives or emotional support. Family coping strategies, in contrast, would include whether the family was able to ask a relative to loan them emergency funds or was able to talk with relatives about the worries they were experiencing. On the basis of the existing literature, Friedman et al (2003) developed a system of coping strategies (Table 28-1).

It is important to note that the amount of support available to families in times of crisis from government and nongovernment agencies varies in different regions, states, and locales. In addition, the rules and conditions of support often differ and may inhibit families from seeking support, particularly if the conditions are demeaning. Nurses must be aware and sensitive to these differences in assessing the accessibility of support resources to families.

MAJOR FAMILY HEALTH RISKS AND NURSING INTERVENTIONS

As mentioned earlier, risks to a family's health arise in three major areas: biological, environmental, and behavioral. In most instances, a risk in one of these areas may not be enough to threaten family health, but a combination of risks from two or more categories could threaten health. For example, a family history of cardiovascular disease by itself may not indicate an increased risk, but the health risk is often increased by an unhealthy lifestyle. An understanding of each of these categories provides the basis for a comprehensive perspective on family health risk assessment and intervention.

Healthy People 2020 targets areas in health promotion, health protection, preventive services, and surveillance and data systems to describe age-related objectives (USDHHS, 2010a). Included in the area of health promotion are physical activity and fitness, nutrition, tobacco use, use of alcohol and other drugs, family planning, mental health and mental disorders, and violent and abusive behavior. Health protection activities include issues related to unintentional injuries, occupational safety and health, environmental health, food and drug safety, and oral health. Preventive services, designed to reduce risks of illness, include maternal and infant health, heart disease and stroke, cancer, diabetes and other chronic disabling conditions, human immunodeficiency virus (HIV) infection, sexually transmitted diseases, immunization for infectious diseases, and clinical preventive services. The interrelationships among the various groups of risk are clear when the objectives for the nation are considered. Most of the national health objectives are based on risk factors of groups or populations in a variety of categories like age, gender, and health problems. However, it is important to recognize that some of these factors also relate to and have potential effects on the individuals' families, work, school, and communities.

Family Health Risk Appraisal

Assessment of family health risk requires many approaches. As in any assessment, the first and most important task is to get to know the family, their strengths, and their needs (see Chapter 27).

TABLE 28-1	FRAMEWORK OF COPING STRATEGIES
INTERNAL STRATEGIES (FROM WITHIN FAMILY)	**PROCESSES FOR COPING**
1. Cognitive	1. Be accepting of the situation and others.
	2. Gain useful knowledge. Use of Internet helpful.
	3. Collaborate in problem solving (reframe the situation).
2. Relationships	4. Increase cohesion (togetherness).
	5. Increase flexibility.
	6. Share feelings and thoughts.
	7. Increase family structure.
3. Communication	8. Be open and honest.
	9. Listen to one another.
	10. Be sensitive to non-verbal communication.
	11. Use humor when appropriate.
EXTERNAL STRATEGIES	**PROCESSES FOR COPING**
4. Community links	12. Maintain links in organizations.
5. Spiritual	13. Be more involved in religious activities.
	14. Increase faith or seek help from God.
6. Social support	15. Seek help and support from others.

From Friedman M, Bowden V, Jones E: *Family nursing: research, theory & practice*, ed 5, Upper Saddle River, NJ, 2003, Prentice Hall.

BOX 28-1 **DEFINITIONS RELATED TO FAMILY HEALTH**

Determinants of health: An individual's biological makeup influences health through interaction with social and physical environments as well as behavior.
Behaviors: These may be learned from other family members.
Social environment: This includes the family, and it is where culture, language, and personal and spiritual beliefs are learned.
Physical environment: Hazards in the home may affect health negatively, and a clean and safe home has a positive influence on health.

This section focuses on appraisal of family health risks in the areas of biological and age-related risk, social and physical environmental risk, and behavioral risk. Box 28-1 provides some definitions related to family health.

Biological and Age-Related Risk

The family plays an important role in both the development and the management of a disease or condition. Several illnesses have a family component that can be accounted for by either genetics or lifestyle patterns. These factors contribute to the biological risk for certain conditions. Patterns of cardiovascular disease, for example, can often be traced through several generations of a family. Such families are said to be at risk for cardiovascular disease. How or whether cardiovascular disease is found in a family is often influenced by the lifestyle of the family. Research evidence consistently supports the positive effects of diet, exercise, and stress management on preventing or delaying cardiovascular disease. The development of hypertension can be managed by following a low-sodium diet, maintaining a normal weight, exercising regularly, and using effective stress management techniques, such as meditation. Diabetes mellitus is another disease with a strong genetic pattern, and the family plays a major role in the management of the condition. Family patterns of obesity increase the risk in individuals for a number of conditions, including heart disease, hypertension, diabetes, some types of cancer, and gallbladder disease (USDHHS, 2010a). The role of genetics is becoming increasingly important. Box 28-2 discusses two examples of adult-onset hereditary diseases and offers caution about the importance of fully understanding the implications of the disease and the action to be taken. It is often difficult to separate biological risks from individual lifestyle factors.

Transitions (movement from one stage or condition to another) are times of potential risk for families. Age-related or life-event risks often occur during transitions from one developmental stage to another. Transitions present new situations and demands for families. These experiences often require that families change behaviors, schedules, and patterns of communication; make new decisions; reallocate family roles; learn new skills; and identify and learn to use new resources. The demands that transitions place on families have implications for the health of the family unit and individual family members and can be considered as life-event risks. How well prepared families are to deal with a transition depends on the nature of the event. If the event is normative, or anticipated, then it is possible for families to identify needed resources, make plans, learn new skills, or otherwise prepare for the event and its consequences. This kind of anticipatory preparation can increase the family's coping ability and lessen stress and negative outcomes. If, on the other hand, the event is non-normative, or unexpected, families have little or no time to prepare and the outcome can be increased stress, crisis, or even dysfunction. Table 28-2 lists family stages and the developmental tasks associated with each stage.

Several normative events have been identified for families. The developmental model organizes these events into stages and identifies important transition points. It provides a useful framework for identifying normative events and preparing families to cope successfully with related demands. The developmental tasks associated with each stage identify the types of skills families need. The kinds of normative events families experience are usually related to the addition or loss of a family member, such as the birth or adoption of a child, the death of a grandparent, a child moving out of the home to go to school or take a job, or the marriage of a child. There are health-related responsibilities associated with each of these tasks. For example, the birth or adoption of a child requires that families learn about human growth and development, parenting, immunizations, management of childhood illnesses, normal childhood nutrition, and safety issues.

Non-normative events present different kinds of issues for families. Unexpected events can be either positive or negative. Getting a job promotion or inheriting a substantial sum of money may be unexpected but are usually positive events. More often, non-normative events are unpleasant, such as a major illness, divorce, death of a child, or loss of the main family income.

Both normative and non-normative life events pose potential risks to the health of families. Even events that are generally viewed as being positive require changes and can place stress on a family. The normative event of the birth of a child, for example, requires considerable changes in family structures and roles. Furthermore, family functions are expanded from previous levels, requiring families to add new skills and establish additional resources. These changes can in turn result in strain and, if adequate resources are not available, stress. Therefore, to adequately assess life risks, both normative and non-normative events occurring in the family need to be considered. Regardless of whether a life event is normative or non-normative, it is often a source of stress for families. Several theoretical frameworks have been developed to examine the processes of family stress and coping. Perhaps the most widely used is the ABC-X model. The model was originally developed by Hill (1949) and was based on work with families separated by war. In the model, crisis (X) was proposed to be a product of the nature of the event (A), the family's definition of the event (B), and the resources available to the family (C). Doherty and McCubbin (1985) extended the model to the Double ABC-X model to encompass the period after the initial crisis and introduced the idea of a pile-up of stressors. Adaptation or maladaptation by the family is proposed to be determined by the pile-up of stressors (Aa), the family's perception of the crisis (Bb), and new resources and coping strategies (Cc).

BOX 28-2 GENETICS AND FAMILY HEALTH RISKS

Population studies of health outcomes resulting from community approaches often show important trends but fail to reach statistical significance. Discovery of single gene variants associated with adult-onset disorders often leads to commercial development of "predictive" genetic tests for the disorders. The hope and hype are that these tests will identify individuals for whom specific health promotion and disease prevention strategies can be targeted. However, the sensitivity of these genetic tests is often quite low when used in the general population because the gene variants were discovered by studying families in which the adult-onset disorder was clearly hereditary. Two examples of adult-onset disorders for which gene variant discoveries resulted in early excitement and later caution about population genetic screening are hereditary hemochromatosis and factor V Leiden–related thrombophilia.

Hereditary Hemochromatosis

Since the mid to late 1990s, there have been ongoing debates about whether or not to use genetic testing to screen the population for the autosomal recessive *HFE* form of hereditary hemochromatosis. This disorder can lead to irreversible liver cirrhosis, diabetes, and/or cardiovascular disease. The associated morbidity and mortality are considered preventable when hereditary hemochromatosis is recognized early and treatment is started before overt symptoms emerge. Treatment is relatively benign: therapeutic phlebotomy for the purpose of depleting iron stores.

The gene most commonly associated with hereditary hemochromatosis in people with northern European ancestry is *HFE*. Approximately 1 in 10 people of northern European ancestry are heterozygotes (have 1 *HFE* gene with a disease-associated mutation) and approximately 1 in 200 are homozygotes (have a disease-associated mutation in both of their *HFE* genes). The genetic test to determine the presence of disease-associated mutations in the *HFE* gene is technically routine and relatively inexpensive. However, the penetrance of the two disease-associated *HFE* mutations is low. In population studies, people have been identified who have two disease-associated *HFE* mutations but no biochemical signs of iron overload (elevated fasting transferrin saturation and serum ferritin levels). Furthermore, population studies have identified individuals with biochemical signs of iron overload who show no other clinical signs of the disorder in their seventh and eighth decades of life. The penetrance of *HFE* mutations is modified by other genes responsible for iron absorption, transport, and metabolism and by environmental factors such as diet, alcohol consumption, and use of supplements.

Guidelines regarding population screening for hereditary hemochromatosis were published in 2005 by the American College of Physicians (Qaseem et al, 2005, p 517). The first recommendation states, "There is insufficient evidence to recommend for or against screening for hereditary hemochromatosis in the general population." The use of biochemical testing for case identification and the use of genetic testing in clients with a positive family history are two alternative approaches for reducing the disease burden of hereditary hemochromatosis.

Factor V Leiden–Related Thrombophilia

Each year in the United States, approximately 200,000 new cases of deep vein thromboembolism (VTE) are recognized. Factor V Leiden (FVL) is associated with a specific mutation in the clotting *factor V* gene. FVL heterozygotes are at approximately seven-fold greater risk for VTE, and FVL homozygotes are at about an 80-fold increased risk for VTE by the age of 70. Approximately 6% of whites and 1% of African Americans in the United States have FVL. The mutation has not been found in Native Americans, Asians, or Africans. In addition to VTE risk, women with FVL have an increased risk for recurrent pregnancy loss and complications.

Vandenbroucke et al (1994) found that women with FVL who used oral contraceptives were at further risk for VTE. Women without FVL who used oral contraceptives were found to have a four-fold increased risk for VTE, whereas women with one *factor V* mutation who used oral contraceptives were at a 30-fold increased risk for VTE. The investigators estimated that FVL homozygotes who used oral contraceptives were at a 100-fold increased risk for VTE. The results from this study stimulated much discussion about screening all females for the *factor V* mutation before prescribing oral contraceptives. Yet, similar to the *HFE* mutations, the *factor V* mutation has incomplete penetrance. Not all FVL homozygotes who use oral contraceptives develop VTE.

Consensus recommendations from two different organizations (Press et al, 2002; Spector et al, 2005) agree that universal screening before use of oral contraceptives would be cost prohibitive and could result in a significant number of asymptomatic women being labeled with a genetic disorder and being denied the most effective form of contraception. It has been suggested that FVL testing may be considered for women with a family history of thrombosis, particularly in first-degree relatives (e.g., parents, siblings). In addition to counseling about alternative contraceptives, such asymptomatic FVL-positive women could also benefit from education about the importance of maintaining appropriate weight, exercising, avoiding prolonged sitting periods, and smoking cessation.

Summary

Hereditary hemochromatosis and FVL demonstrate that despite being relatively common conditions with potentially significant health consequences, it is not yet time for universal genetic testing. It is true that *HFE* mutations contribute to iron overload and associated morbidity and mortality, but the evidence is also convincing that iron overload is multigenic and significantly influenced by environmental factors. Likewise, FVL is a significant contributor to thrombophilia, but there are many other clotting factors—each factor with its own corresponding gene—that contribute to overall risk. In addition, inherited VTE risk factors are moderated by lifestyle behaviors and other environmental factors. Recognizing the multigenic nature of these and other common disorders, companies are developing and testing chip technology that enables the simultaneous testing of relevant mutations in many different genes associated with a specific disorder. As this technology becomes less expensive and predictive, universal testing or at least testing of large targeted segments of the population will become more likely.

References

Press RD, Bauer KA, Kujovich JL, et al: Clinical utility of factor V Leiden (R506Q) testing for the diagnosis and management of thromboembolic disorders, *Arch Pathol Lab Med* 126:1304–1318, 2002.

Qaseem A, Aronson M, Fitterman N, et al: Screening for hereditary hemochromatosis: a clinical practice guideline from the American College of Physicians, *Ann Intern Med* 143:517–521, 2005.

Spector EB, Grody WW, Matteson CJ, et al: Technical standards and guidelines: venous thromboembolism (Factor V Leiden and prothrombin 20210G >A testing): a disease-specific supplement to the standards and guidelines for clinical genetics laboratories, *Genet Med* 7(6):444–453, 2005.

Vandenbroucke JP, Koster T, Briet E, et al: Increased risk of venous thrombosis in oral-contraceptive users who are carriers of factor V Leiden mutation, *Lancet* 344:1453–1457, 1994.

For Further Reading

Horne MK III, McCloskey DJ: Factor V Leiden as a common genetic risk factor for venous thromboembolism, *J Nurs Schol* 38:19–25, 2006.

Khoury MJ, McCabe LL, McCabe ER: Population screening in the age of genomic medicine, *N Engl J Med* 348:50–58, 2003.

Powell LW, Dixon JL, Ramm GA, et al: Screening for hemochromatosis in asymptomatic subjects with or without a family history, *Arch Intern Med* 166:294–301, 2006.

Developed by Cynthia A. Prows, MSN, CNS, Cincinnati Children's Hospital Medical Center, Division of Human Genetics, Cincinnati, Ohio.

TABLE 28-2 FAMILY LIFE CYCLE STAGES

FAMILY LIFE CYCLE STAGES	KEY PRINCIPLES FOR EMOTIONAL TRANSITION PROCESS	SECOND-ORDER CHANGES IN FAMILY STATUS REQUIRED TO PROCEED DEVELOPMENTALLY
Leaving home; single young adults	Accepting emotional and financial responsibility of self	Differentiation of self in relation to family of origin Development of intimate peer relationships Development of self as related to work and financial independence
Joining of families through marriage; the new couple	Commitment to new system	Formation of marital system Realignment of relationships with extended families and friends to include spouse
Families with young children	Accepting new members into system	Adjusting marital system to make space for child(ren) Joining in child rearing, financial matters, and household tasks Realignment of relationships with extended family to include parenting and grandparenting roles
Families with adolescents	Increasing flexibility of family boundaries to include children's independence and grandparents' frailties	Shifting of parent–child relationships to permit adolescent to move in and out of system Refocus on midlife marital and career issues Begin shift toward caring for older generation
Launching children and moving on	Accepting a multitude of exits from and entities into the family system	Renegotiation of marital system as a dyad Development of adult-to-adult relationship between grown children and their parents Realignment of relationships to include in-laws and grandchildren Dealing with disabilities and death of parents (grandparents)
Families in later life	Accepting the shifting of generational roles	Maintaining own and couple functioning and interests in face of physiological decline; exploration of new familiar and social role options Support for a more central role of middle generation Making room in the system for the wisdom and experience of the older generation, and supporting them without overfunctioning for them Dealing with loss of spouse, siblings, and other peers and preparing for own death Life review and integration by the older adult

From McGoldrick M, Carter B, Garcia-Preto N: *The expanded family life cycle,* ed 4, New York, 2011, Pearson.

Lorenz, Wickrama, and Conger (2004) challenged this step-by-step view of families and stress and coping. They advocated a more systems-oriented concept of family stress. They pointed out that families develop a series of processes to manage or transform inputs to the system (e.g., energy, time) to outputs (e.g., cohesion, growth, love) known as *rules of transformation.* Over time, families develop these patterns in enough quantity and variety to handle most changes and challenges; this is referred to as *requisite variety of rules of transformation.* However, when families do not have an adequate variety of rules to allow them to respond to an event, the event becomes stressful. Rather than being able to deal with the situation, they fall into a pattern of trying to figure out what it is they need to do, and the usual tasks of the family are not adequately addressed. Rules that were implicit in the family are now reconsidered and redefined.

Furthermore, the family stress theory of Lorenz et al (2004) proposes three levels of stress: level I is change "in the fairly specific patterns of behavior and transforming processes" (e.g., change in who does which household chores); level II is change "in processes that are at a higher level of abstraction" (e.g., change in what are defined as family chores); and level III is changes in highly abstract processes (e.g., family values)

(Lorenz et al, 2004). Coping strategies can be identified to address each level of stress that families go through in sequence, if necessary (see the Evidence-Based Practice box).

Biological Health Risk Assessment

One of the most effective techniques for assessing the patterns of health and illness in families is the genogram (see Chapter 27 for further discussion and an example). Briefly, a genogram is a drawing that shows the family unit of immediate interest and includes several generations using a series of circles, squares, and connecting lines. Basic information about the family, relationships in the family, and patterns of health and illness can be obtained by completing the genogram with the family. As shown in Figure 28-1, a square indicates a male, a circle indicates a female, and an "X" through either a square or a circle indicates a death. Marriage is indicated by a solid horizontal line and offspring/children by a solid vertical line. A broken horizontal line indicates a divorce or separation. Dates of birth, marriage, death, and other important events can be indicated where appropriate. Major illness or conditions can be listed for each family member. Patterns can be quickly assessed and provide a guide for the health interviewer about health areas that need further exploring.

EVIDENCE-BASED PRACTICE

Building the evidence-based case for the effectiveness of a nursing intervention program is not a goal that can be accomplished quickly. Rather, such a case requires many years of testing and refining interventions, as well as the ongoing and arduous task of obtaining funding from federal and state entities. It is also dependent on the intense advocacy involved in influencing legislators to achieve health and social policy reform necessary to enable lasting change. The Nurse Family Partnership (NFP) is one such program that was begun in the late 1970s by a social and behavioral sciences major, who focused on psychology, specifically with early infant attachment (Goodman, 2006). Dr. David Olds would later complete his doctoral studies under the mentoring of Dr. Urie Bronfenbrenner, a professor at Cornell University, and continued his research with the goal of improving the lives of children. Using nurses only for the intervention study, Olds set out to study the impact that home visitation to new mothers by nurses would have on social and health outcomes of both mother and baby. The home visitation began during pregnancy. Olds conducted randomized control studies in diverse locations and diverse populations. He also completed a study that compared the use of nurses with the use of paraprofessionals and determined that the use of nurses had more positive outcomes than did the use of paraprofessionals.

Outcomes of these studies have demonstrated that new mothers receiving nurse home visits, beginning during pregnancy and continuing for 2 years, exhibit improvements to maternal health, decrease in childhood injuries, lower rates of child abuse, and greater spacing of subsequent pregnancies when compared with new mothers not receiving nurse home visits. The results have also shown that these mothers are more likely to enter the workforce, and longitudinal data have demonstrated that the nurse-visited families are more economically self-sufficient and that criminal behavior has been less in both mothers and children., The Olds model in 2004 became the Nurse Family Partnership (NFP), a non-profit organization, in an effort to make it more accessible as well as to ensure quality control, educate nurses, and monitor existing programs. NFP is currently operating in 32 states. Criteria have been established to keep the program true to Olds' fundamental principles outlined here in order to ensure consistent quality and positive outcomes.

Of his model, Olds says, "It reduces injuries to children. It helps families plan future pregnancies and create better spacing between the birth of the first and second children. It helps women find employment. It helps improve prenatal health. It improves children's school readiness."

Nurse Use

The NFP developed by Dr. Olds and his team provides the ultimate example of the effects of nursing on the individual, family, and community. From care of the pregnant woman, to the care of her newborn and family, to the policy implications that provide for healthier families and healthier communities, the NFP makes a difference in outcomes. The NFP is nursing at its very best—it provides evidence-based early nursing interventions that result in the positive outcomes listed above rather than the poor societal outcomes often described with teen pregnancies and single parenting. The evidence-based NFP model should continue to be tested in other populations and environments, such as in foster and adoptive homes early in the foster or adoption process, thus allowing the benefits of the program to have an even broader reach.

References

Eckenrode J, Campa M, Luckey DW, et al: Long-term effects of prenatal and infancy nurse home visitation on the life course of youths: 19-year follow-up of a randomized trial, *Archiv Pediatr Adolesc Med* 164(1):9–15, 2010.

Goodman A: *The story of David Olds and the Nurse Home Visiting program*, Princeton, NJ, 2006, Robert Wood Johnson Foundation.

Olds DL, Henderson CR, Tatelbaum R, Chamberlin R: Improving the delivery of prenatal care and outcomes of pregnancy: a randomized trial of nursing home visitation, *Pediatrics* 77:16–28, 1986.

Olds DL, Robinson J, Pettitt LM, et al: Effects of home visits by paraprofessionals and by nurses: age four follow-up results of a randomized trial, *Pediatrics* 114(6):1560–1568, 2004.

The genogram in Figure 28-1 was completed for the fictional Graham family. Some of the interesting health patterns that can be seen from the genogram are the repetition of hypertension, adult-onset diabetes, cancer, and hypercholesterolemia. Completing a genogram requires interviews with as many family members as possible. A family chronology—a timeline of family events over three generations—can be completed to extend the genogram.

A more intensive and quantitative assessment of a family's biological risk can be achieved through the use of a standard family risk assessment. Because such assessments involve other areas in addition to biological risk, one will be described later, after the description of assessment of other types of risk.

Community-level support groups (e.g., Families Anonymous, Bereaved Parents, Parents and Friends of Lesbian and Gay Persons, Single Parents) have been successful in assisting families in dealing with a variety of stressful situations and crises that arise from both life events and age-related events. Nurses have been instrumental in developing and moderating such groups. These are examples of intervening with families as a specific population.

Environmental Risk

The importance of social risks to family health is gaining increased recognition (see Chapters 7 and 18). Living in high-crime neighborhoods, in communities without adequate recreation or health resources, in communities that have major noise pollution or chemical pollution, or in other high-stress environments increases a family's health risk. One social stress is discrimination, whether racial, cultural, or other. The psychological burden resulting from discrimination is itself a stressor, and it adds to the effects of other stressors. The implication of these examples of risky social situations is that they contribute to the stressors experienced by the families. If adequate resources and coping processes are not available, breakdowns in health can occur.

The poor are at greater risk for health problems (see Chapter 33). Economic risk, which is related to social risk, is determined by the relationship between family financial resources and the demands on those resources. Having adequate financial resources means that a family is able to purchase the necessary commodities related to health. These include adequate housing, clothing, food, education, and health or illness care. The amount of money that a family has available is relative to situational, cultural, and social factors. A family may have an income well above the poverty level, but because of a devastating illness in a family member, they may not be able to meet financial demands. Likewise, families from ethnic populations or families with same-sex parents frequently experience discrimination in finding housing. Even if they find housing, they may not be welcome and may be harassed, resulting in increased stress.

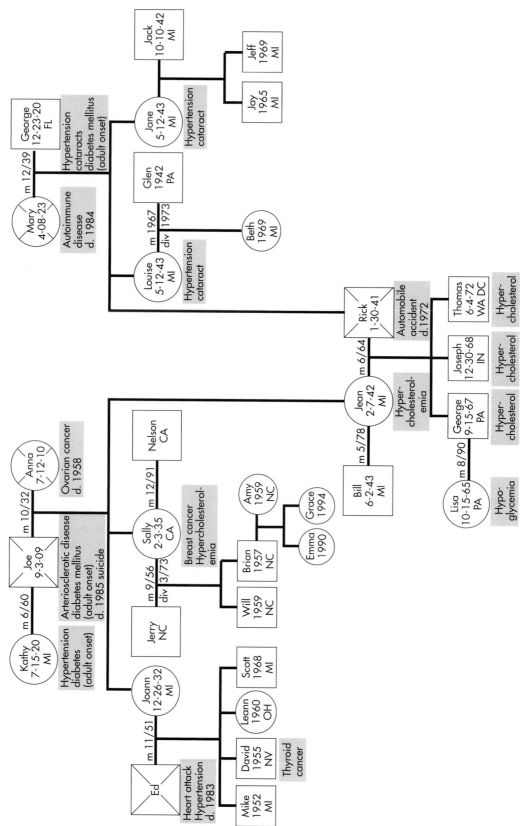

FIGURE 28-1 Family genogram of the Graham family. (Developed by Carol Loveland-Cherry for the fifth edition of this book.)

Unfortunately, not all families have access to health care insurance. For families at the poverty level, programs such as Medicaid are available to pay for health and illness care. Families in the upper-income brackets usually have health insurance through an employer, or they can afford to either purchase health insurance or pay for health care out of pocket. An increasing number of middle-income families have major wage earners in jobs that do not have health benefits. These people often do not have enough income to purchase health care but earn too much money to qualify for public assistance programs. Consequently, many families have financial resources that allow them to maintain a subsistence level but that limit the quality of their purchasing power. Illness care may be available, but preventive care may not; food high in fat and calories may be affordable, whereas fresh fruit and vegetables are not. Nutritious diets are important in preventing illness and promoting health. Devaney (2007) presents an analysis of the first 35 years of the Women, Infants, and Children (WIC) program and the relationship of participation in WIC to Medicaid costs and use of health care services and found that children who participated in WIC were more linked to the health care system than children who were not. Children in WIC were more likely to receive both preventive and curative care more often than children not participating in WIC (Devaney, 2007).

Environmental Risk Assessment

Assessment of environmental health risk is less well-defined and developed. Information on relationships that the family has with others (e.g., relatives and neighbors), their connections with other social units (e.g., church, school, work, clubs, and organizations), and the flow of energy (positive or negative) can be assessed through the use of an ecomap (see Chapter 27 for further discussion and an example).

An ecomap represents the family's interactions with other groups and organizations, accomplished using a series of circles and lines. The family of interest (the Graham family in Figure 28-2) is represented by a circle in the middle of the page; other groups and organizations are then indicated by other circles. Lines, representing the flow of energy, are drawn between the family circle and the circles representing other groups and organizations. An arrowhead at the end of each line indicates the direction of the flow of energy (into or out of the family), and the darkness of the line indicates the intensity of the energy. The Graham family ecomap indicates that much of the family energy goes into work (also a source of stress for the parents). Major sources of energy for the Grahams are their immediate and extended families and friends.

In addition to the support network shown by the ecomap, other aspects of social risk include characteristics of the neighborhood and community where the family lives. A nurse who has worked in the general geographic area may already have performed a community assessment (see Chapter 18) and have a working knowledge of the neighborhood and community. It is important, however, for the nurse to obtain information from the family to understand their perceptions of the community.

Information about the origins of the family is useful to understand other social resources and stressors. Information about how long the family has lived in their current location and the immigration patterns of the family and their ancestors provides insight into the pressures they experience.

Economic risk is one of the foremost predictors of health. Families often consider financial information private, and both the nurse and the family may be uncomfortable when discussing finances. It is not necessary to know actual family income except in certain instances when it is necessary to determine whether families are eligible for programs or benefits. It is useful to know whether the family's resources are adequate to meet their needs, and it is important to understand that the family may be quite comfortable with their finances and standard of living, which may be different from those of the health care provider. The provider should not try to push financial values onto the family. In terms of health risk, it is important to understand the resources that families have to obtain health/illness care; adequate shelter, clothing, and food; and access to recreation. Families with limited resources may qualify for programs such as Medicaid, WIC, or Maternal Support Systems/Infant Support Systems. Families with wage earners with medical benefits and those with enough income are usually able to afford adequate health care. Unfortunately, in a growing number of families, the main wage earner is employed but receives no medical benefits and the salary is not sufficient for health promotion or illness-related care. This is a policy issue for which nurses are very capable of drafting legislation and providing testimony related to the stories of families in their caseloads. (See Chapter 8 for a discussion of policy involvement by nurses.)

Behavioral (Lifestyle) Risk

Personal health habits continue to contribute to the major causes of morbidity and mortality in the United States (see Chapter 17). The pattern of personal health habits and behavioral risk defines individual and family lifestyle risk. The family is the basic unit within which health behavior—including health values, health habits, and health risk perceptions—is developed, organized, and performed. Families maintain major responsibility for determining what food is purchased and prepared, setting sleep patterns, planning family activities, setting and monitoring norms about health and health risk behaviors, determining when a family member is ill, determining when health care should be obtained, and carrying out treatment regimens. In 2006 more than half of all deaths in the United States were attributed to heart disease or cancer, both of which identify diet as a causative factor (NCHS, 2009). General guidelines from the U.S. Department of Health and Human Services and the U.S. Department of Agriculture include eating a variety of foods; maintaining healthy weight; choosing a diet low in fat and cholesterol, including plenty of vegetables, fruits, and grain products; limiting use of sugars, salt, and sodium; and consuming alcohol only in moderation.

Multiple health benefits of regular physical activity have been identified; regular physical exercise is effective in promoting and maintaining health and preventing disease. Physical activity can help to prevent obesity, diabetes, heart disease, cancer, osteoporosis, and depression (Mayo Clinic, 2010).

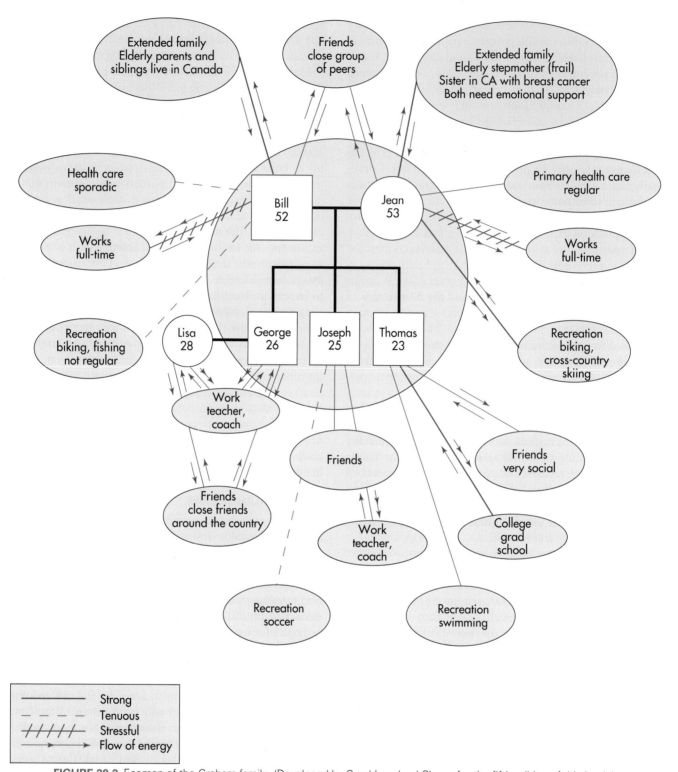

FIGURE 28-2 Ecomap of the Graham family. (Developed by Carol Loveland-Cherry for the fifth edition of this book.)

Among the benefits of regular physical activity are increased muscle strength, endurance, and flexibility; management of weight; prevention of colon cancer, stroke, and back injury; and prevention and management of coronary heart disease, hypertension, diabetes, osteoporosis, and depression (USD-HHS, 2010a). Families can structure time and activities for family members. It is helpful when the community in which they live promotes exercise by having accessible parks and walking or biking paths that help families select activities that provide moderate, regular physical exercise, rather than sedentary activities in the home setting.

Substance use and abuse, such as the use of drugs, alcohol, or tobacco, is a major contributor to morbidity and mortality in the United States. Drug use is a major social and health problem. Drug use is associated with transmission of human immunodeficiency virus (HIV), fetal alcohol syndrome, liver disease, unwanted pregnancy, delinquency, school failure, violence, and crime source (NIDA, 2010). Drunk driving is also a public health hazard. It is well known that tobacco use increases morbidity and mortality. When caring for families with a smoking member, nurses can consider not only smoking cessation, but also education regarding second-hand smoke. Passive smoking has been associated with several types of cancer, heart disease, chronic obstructive pulmonary disease, low birth weight, premature births, and sudden infant death syndrome (USDHHS, 2010a).

Although violence and abusive behavior are well known health risks for individuals, the extent of their prevalence within families is not well understood. The amount of intrafamilial violence is thought to be underestimated. It is difficult to collect data and obtain accurate statistics on family violence because the issue is so sensitive for families. There is evidence, however, to support the intergenerational nature of violence and abuse—that is, abusers were often abused as children.

Behavioral (Lifestyle) Health Risk Assessment

Families are the major source of factors that can promote or inhibit positive lifestyles. They regulate time and energy and the boundaries of the system. A number of tools exist for assessing individuals' lifestyle risks, but few are available for assessing family lifestyle patterns. Although assessment of individual lifestyle contributes to determining the lifestyle risk of a family, it is important to look at risks for the family as a unit. One approach is to identify family patterns for each of the lifestyle components included in *Healthy People 2020*. In the areas of health promotion, health protection, and preventive services, lifestyle can be assessed in several dimensions. From the literature on health behavior research, the critical dimensions include the following:

- Value placed on the behavior
- Knowledge of the behavior and its consequences
- Effect of the behavior on the family
- Effect of the behavior on the individual
- Barriers to performing the behavior
- Benefits of the behavior

It is important to assess the frequency, intensity, and regularity of specific behaviors. It also is important to evaluate the resources available to the family for implementing the behaviors. Thus, items for assessment of physical activity include the value that a family places on physical activity, the hours that a family spends in exercise, the kinds of exercise in which the family participates, and resources available for exercise.

NURSING APPROACHES TO FAMILY HEALTH RISK REDUCTION

Home Visits

Nurses work with families in a variety of settings, including clinics, schools, support groups, and offices. However, an important aspect of the nurse's role in reducing health risks and promoting the health of populations has been the tradition of providing services to families in their homes.

Purpose

Home visits, as compared with clinical visits, give a more accurate assessment of the family structure, the natural or home environment, and behavior in that environment. Home visits also provide opportunities to identify both barriers and supports for reaching family health promotion goals. The nurse can work with the client directly to adapt interventions to match resources. Visiting the family in their home may also contribute to the family's sense of control and active participation in meeting their health needs. The majority of historical studies evaluating home visits have focused on the maternal-child population (Fraser et al, 2000; Hammond-Ratzlaff and Fulton, 2001; Koniak-Griffin et al, 2003; Wagner et al, 2004). Studies of home visits are often conducted for maternal/child health (Donovan, 2007; Nurse Family Partnership, 2010; Olds, 2007).

Home visiting programs are receiving increased attention and provide a broad range of services to achieve a variety of health-related goals. Long-term effects of home visits are positive and are shown to be cost effective for society. As a result, several states have reinstituted home visits for high-risk families. If the home visit is to be a valuable and effective intervention, careful and systematic planning must occur (Pew Center, 2010).

> **NURSING TIP** *A home visit is more than just an alternative setting for service; it is an intervention.*

Advantages and Disadvantages

The effectiveness of health promotion services in the home has been critically reexamined by agencies such as health departments and visiting nurses associations. Advantages include client convenience, client control of the setting, availability of an option for those clients unwilling or unable to travel, the ability to individualize services, and a natural, relaxed environment for the discussion of concerns and needs. Costs are a major disadvantage; the cost of pre-visit preparation, travel to and from the home, time spent with one client, and post-visit preparation is high. Many agencies have actively explored alternative modes of providing service to families, particularly group interventions. The important issue is determining which families would benefit the most and how home visits can most effectively be structured and scheduled. With increasing demands for home health care, the home visit is again becoming a prominent mode for delivery of nursing services. When looking at cost versus effectiveness, it is not always the least costly service that is the most effective. The references cited in the Purposes section show that home visits for certain services are more effective in family health outcomes then visits to the health department or clinic, even though they are more costly.

Process

The components of a home visit are summarized in Table 28-3. The phases include the initiation phase, the pre-visit phase, the in-home phase, the termination phase, and the post-visit phase. Building a trusting relationship with the family client is the

TABLE 28-3	**PHASES AND ACTIVITIES OF A HOME VISIT**
PHASE	**ACTIVITY**
I. Initiation phase	Clarify source of referral for visit.
	Clarify purpose for home visit.
	Share information on reason and purpose of home visit with family.
II. Pre-visit phase	Initiate contact with family.
	Establish shared perceptions of purpose with family.
	Determine family's willingness for home visit.
	Schedule home visit.
	Review referral and/or family record.
III. In-home phase	Introduce self and professional identity.
	Interact socially to establish rapport.
	Establish nurse–client relationship.
	Implement nursing process.
IV. Termination phase	Review visit with family.
	Plan for future visits.
V. Post-visit phase	Record visit.
	Plan for next visit.

From Whitley DM, Kelley SJ, Sipe TA: Grandmothers raising grandchildren: are they at increased risk of health problems? *Health Soc Work* 26:105-114, 2001.

cornerstone of successful home visits. Five skills are fundamental to effective home visits: observing, listening, questioning, probing, and prompting. The need for these skills is evident in all phases of the home visit process.

Initiation Phase. Usually, a home visit is initiated as the result of a referral from a health or social agency. However, a family may request services, or the nurse may initiate the home visit as a result of case-finding activities. The initiation phase is the first contact between the nurse and the family. It provides the foundation for an effective therapeutic relationship. Subsequent home visits should be based on need and mutual agreement between the nurse and the family. Frequently, nurses are not sure of the reason for the visit. This carries with it the potential for the visit to be compromised and to come aimlessly or abruptly to a premature halt. Regardless of the reason for making a home visit, it is necessary that the nurse be clear about the purpose for the visit and that this purpose or understanding be shared with the family.

Pre-visit Phase. The pre-visit phase has several components. For the most part, these are best accomplished in order, as presented in the How To box.

HOW TO Prepare for the Home Visit: Pre-Visit Phase

- *First, if at all possible, the nurse should contact the family by telephone before the home visit to introduce self, to identify the reason for the contact, and to schedule the home visit. A first telephone contact should be a maximum of 15 minutes. The nurse should give name and professional identity. For example, the nurse might say, "This is Karen Smith. I'm a community health nurse from the Fayette County Health Department."*

- *The family should be informed of how they came to the attention of the nurse—for example, as the result of a referral, or a contact from observations, or records in the school setting. If a referral has been received, it is important and useful to ascertain whether the family is aware of the referral.*

- *A brief summary of the nurse's knowledge about the family's situation will allow the family to clarify their needs. For example, the nurse might say, "I understand that your baby was discharged from the hospital yesterday and that you requested some assistance with learning more about how to care for your baby at home."*

- *A visit should be scheduled as soon as possible. Letting the family know agency hours available for visits, the approximate length of the visit, and the purpose of the visit are helpful to the family in determining when to set the visit. Although the length of the visit may vary, depending on circumstances, approximately 30 to 60 minutes is usual.*

- *If possible, the visit should be arranged when as many family members as possible will be available for the entire visit. It is also important for the nurse to tell the client about any fee for the visit and subsequent visits and possible methods for payment.*

- *The telephone call can terminate with a review by the nurse of the time, place, and purpose for the visit and a means for the family to contact the nurse in case they need to verify or change the time for the visit or to ask questions. If the family does not have a telephone, another method for setting up the visit can be used. A note can be dropped off at the family home or sent by mail informing the family of when and why the home visit will occur and providing a way for the family to contact the nurse if necessary.*

The possibility exists that the family may refuse a home visit. Less-experienced nurses or students may mistakenly interpret this as a personal rejection. Families make decisions about when and which outsiders are allowed entry into their homes. The nurse needs to explore the reasons for the refusal; there may be a misunderstanding about the reason for a visit, or there may be a lack of information about services. The contact may be terminated as requested if the nurse determines either that the situation has been resolved or that services have been obtained from another source, and if the family understands that services are available and how to contact the agency if desired. There are instances when the nurse will be mandated to persist in requesting a home visit because of legal obligations, such as follow-up of certain communicable diseases.

Before visiting a family, the nurse should review the referral or, if this is not the first visit, the family record. If there is a time lapse between the contact and the visit, a brief telephone call to confirm the time often prevents the nurse from finding no one at home.

Personal safety is an issue that may arise either while approaching the family home or when the family has opened the door to the nurse. Nurses need to evaluate personal fears and objective threats to determine if safety is indeed an issue. Certain precautions can be taken in known high-risk situations. Agencies may provide escorts for nurses or have them visit in pairs; readily identifiable uniforms may be required; or a sign-out process indicating timing and location of home visits may be used routinely. Home visits are generally very safe; however, as with all worksites, the possibility of violence exists. Therefore, the nurse needs to use caution. If a reasonable question exists about the safety of making a visit, the visit should not be made.

The nurse should be aware that families may feel that they are being scrutinized, that they are seen as being inadequate or dysfunctional, or that their privacy is being intruded upon. Nursing services, especially those from health departments, have been perceived by the public as being "public services" for needy families or those with inadequate funds to pay for care. These potential areas of concern underlie the need for sensitivity on the part of the nurse, the need for clarity in information regarding the reason for visits, and the need to establish collaborative, trusting relationships with the family.

Another factor that may affect the nature of the home visit is whether the visit is viewed as voluntary or required. A *voluntary* home visit (visit requested by the client) is characterized by easier entry for the nurse, client-controlled interaction, an informal tone, and mutual discussion of frequency of future visits. An example of a voluntary visit is a new mother who has requested the nurse come to the home and assist her with learning how to care for the infant. In contrast, the client may feel little need for *required* home visits that often may be legally mandated. In these instances, entry may be difficult for the nurse; the interaction may be nurse-controlled; there may be a more formal, investigatory tone to the visit with distorted nurse–client communication; and there may be no mutual discussion of scheduling or frequency of future visits. Two examples of a required home visit are: (1) when a family member has been diagnosed with tuberculosis and the nurse needs to make certain that the client is taking medications regularly, and (2) when there is known child abuse and a new baby has arrived. The nurse may need to visit the home to observe the interaction between the parents and the child.

The changing nature of the American family can make it difficult to schedule visits during what have been traditional agency hours. The number of working single-parent or dual-income, two-parent families is increasing, which means that families have more demands on their time. Even if one parent is at home during the usual workday, the ideal is to work with the entire family unit. This often is not possible because of conflict between agency hours and school or work schedules. It may be possible to schedule a visit at the beginning or end of a day to meet with working or school-age members. In some parts of the country, agencies are reconsidering traditional hours and Monday through Friday visits. These issues are important to assess and address during the pre-visit phase so the nurse and the family will be better prepared for the visit.

Culture influences a person's interpretation of and response to health care (Shi and Singh, 2008). It is impossible, given the diversity of the United States and the diversity within cultural groups, to cover every group extensively. Instead, practitioners need to take the responsibility to learn about their client's culture as they prepare for visits with families or communities.

In-Home Phase. The actual visit to the home constitutes the in-home phase and affords the nurse the opportunity to assess the family's neighborhood and community resources, as well as the home and family interactions. The actual home visit includes several components. Once at the family home, the nurse provides personal and professional identification and tells the client the location of the agency. Then, a brief social period allows the client to assess the nurse and establish rapport. The next step is a description by the nurse of his or her role, responsibilities, and limitations. Another important component of the home visit is to determine the client's expectations.

The major portion of the home visit is concerned with establishing the relationship and implementing the nursing process. Assessment, intervention, and evaluation are ongoing. What then occurs in the home visit is determined by the reason for the visit. Keller et al (2004a,b) recommend using the Intervention Wheel to guide nursing practice during home visits. The Intervention Wheel provides appropriate guidelines for the purpose of the home visit. Some reasons for visits are listed in Box 28-3.

A nurse must be flexible and anticipate that families may or may not be able to control interruptions during the visit. Telephones ring, pets join in the visit, people come and go, and televisions may be left on. The nurse can ask that televisions be turned off for a limited time or that other disruptive activities be limited. Families may be so accustomed to the background noises and routine activities that they do not recognize them as being potentially disruptive.

It is important that the nurse be realistic about what can be accomplished in a home visit. In some situations, one visit may be all that is possible or appropriate. In this instance, needs and the resources available to meet them are explored with the family, and it is determined whether further services are desired or indicated. If further services are indicated and the nurse's agency is not appropriate, the nurse can assist the family in identifying other services available in the community and can help in initiating referrals. Although it is not unusual to

BOX 28-3 REASONS FOR THE HOME VISIT

Nursing interventions may include some or all of the 17 resources identified by the Minnesota Department of Health, Section of Public Health Nursing:
- Advocacy
- Case management
- Coalition building
- Collaboration
- Community organizing
- Consultation
- Counseling
- Delegated medical treatment and observations
- Disease and other health investigation
- Health teaching
- Outreach
- Policy development and enforcement
- Case finding
- Referral and follow-up
- Screening
- Social marketing
- Surveillance

From Keller LO, Strohschein S, Lia-Hoagberg B, Schaffer MA: Population-based public health interventions: practice-based and evidence-supported. Part I, *Public Health Nurs* 21:453-468, 2004a.

have only one home visit with a family, multiple visits are often made. The frequency and intensity of home visits vary not only with the needs of the family, but also with the eligibility of the family for services as defined by agency policies and priorities. It is realistic to expect an initial assessment and at least the beginning of building a relationship to occur on a first visit.

Termination Phase. When the purpose of the visit has been accomplished, the nurse reviews with the family what has occurred and what has been accomplished. This is the major focus of the termination phase, and provides a basis for planning further home visits. Ideally, termination of the visit and, ultimately, termination of service begin at the first contact with the establishment of a goal or purpose. If communication has been clear to this point, the family and nurse can now plan for future visits, specifically the next visit. Planning for future visits is part of another issue: setting goals and planning service. Contracting is a constructive approach to working with clients to specify and achieve agreed-on goals and is receiving increasing attention by health professionals. The purpose and components of contracting with clients are discussed in more detail later.

Post-visit Phase. Even after the nurse has concluded the home visit and left the client's home, responsibility for the visit is not complete until the interaction has been recorded. A major task of the post-visit phase is documenting the visit and services provided. Agencies may organize their records by families. That is, the basic record may be a "family" folder with all members included. However, this often does not occur, although it is useful for the family history and background. More often, each family member has a separate record, and other family members' records are cross-referenced. This is because the focus often shifts from the family to the individual. Consequently, nursing diagnoses, goals, and interventions are directed toward individual family members rather than the family unit. This approach has its shortcomings and it is important for the nurse to recognize these. Chapter 41 provides an approach for offering nursing diagnoses, stating goals, and identifying interventions for the individual. It is important for the nurse to focus on the continuing assessment of the individual behaviors, responses, or health status and the impact on the family. Interventions at the family level may become necessary, such as educating all family members on hygiene and cleanliness or on the appropriate disposal of supplies of the tuberculosis client in the home.

Record systems and formats vary from agency to agency. The nurse needs to become familiar with the particular system used in the agency. All systems should include a database; a nursing diagnosis and problem list; a plan, including specific goals; actual actions and interventions; and evaluation. These are the basic elements needed for legal and clinical purposes. The format may consist of narratives; flow sheets; problem-oriented medical records (POMRs); subjective, objective, assessment plans (SOAP); or a combination of formats. It is important that recording be current, dated, and signed.

The nurse should be sure to use theoretical frameworks that are appropriate to the family-centered nursing process. For example, a nursing diagnosis of *ineffective mothering skill,* related to lack of knowledge of normal growth and development, is an individual-focused nursing diagnosis. The *inability*

for family to accomplish stage-appropriate tasks of providing a safe environment for a preschooler related to lack of knowledge and resources is a family-focused nursing diagnosis based on knowledge of the developmental approach to families. At times, it may be necessary to present information for a specific family member. However, the emphasis should be on the individual as a member of, and within the structure of, the family.

Contracting with Families

Increasingly, health professionals are looking at working with clients in an interactive, collaborative style. This approach is consistent with a more knowledgeable public and the recent self-care movement in the United States. However, it may not be consistent with other cultures that look to health care providers for more direct guidance; therefore, it is important to determine the family's value system before assuming that contracting will work.

Contracting is a strategy aimed at formally involving the family in the nursing process and jointly defining the roles of both the family members and the health professional. Contracting involves making an agreement between two or more parties and seeks to create a shift in responsibility and control toward a shared effort by client and professional as opposed to an effort by the professional alone. This active involvement of the client is reflected in several nursing models, such as that of Orem (1995). The motivational premise of contracting is family control. It is assumed that when the family has legitimate control, their ability to make healthful choices is increased.

Purposes

The nursing contract is a working agreement that is continuously renegotiable and may or may not be written. It may be either a contingency or a non-contingency contract. A *contingency contract* states a specific reward for the client after completion of the client's portion of the contract; a *non-contingency contract* does not specify rewards. The implied rewards are the positive consequences of reaching the goals specified in the contract.

For family health risk reduction, it is essential that the contract be made with all responsible and appropriate members of the family. Involving only one individual is not sufficient if the goal is family health risk reduction, which requires a total family system effort and change. Scheduling a visit with all family members present may require extra effort. If meeting with the entire family is not possible, each family member can review a contract, give input, and sign it. This allows active participation by all family members without the necessity of finding a time when everyone involved can be present.

Process of Contracting

Contracting is a learned skill on the part of both the nurse and the family. All persons involved need to know the purpose and process of contracting. There are three general phases: beginning, working, and termination. The three phases can be further divided into eight sets of activities, as summarized in Table 28-4.

The first activity is collection and analysis of data, and it involves both the family and the nurse. An important aspect of

TABLE 28-4   PHASES AND ACTIVITIES IN CONTRACTING

PHASE	ACTIVITY
I. Beginning phase	Mutual data collection and exploration of needs and problems
	Mutual establishment of goals
	Mutual development of a plan
II. Working phase	Mutual division of responsibilities
	Mutual setting of time limits
	Mutual implementation of plan
	Mutual evaluation and renegotiation
III. Termination phase	Mutual termination of contract

this step is obtaining the family's view of the situation and its needs and problems. The nurse can present his or her observations, validate them with the family, and obtain the family's view.

It is important that goals be mutually set and be realistic. A pitfall for nurses and clients who are new to contracting is to set overly ambitious goals. The nurse should recognize that there may be discrepancies between their professional priorities and those of the client and determine whether negotiating is required. Because contracting is a process characterized by renegotiation, the goals are not static.

Throughout the process, the nurse and family continually learn and recognize what each can contribute to meeting health needs. The exploring of resources allows both parties to become aware of their own and one another's strengths and requires a review of the nurse's skills and knowledge, the family support systems, and community resources.

Developing a plan to meet the goals involves specifying activities, prioritizing goals, and selecting a starting point. Next, the nurse and the family need to decide who will be responsible for which activities. Setting time limits involves determining the frequency of contacts for evaluating progress toward accomplishing goals and deciding on a deadline for accomplishing the goal. At the agreed-on time or times, the nurse and family together evaluate progress both in terms of process and outcome. The contract can be modified, renegotiated, or terminated on the basis of the evaluation.

Advantages and Disadvantages of Contracting

Contracting takes time and effort and may require the family and nurse to reorient their roles. Increased control on the part of the family also means increased responsibility. Some nurses may have difficulty relinquishing the role of the controlling expert professional. Contracts are not always successful, and contracting is neither appropriate nor possible in some cases. Some clients do not want to have this kind of involvement; they prefer to defer to the "authority" of the professional. Included in this group are individuals with minimal cognitive skills, those who are involved in an emergency situation, those who are unwilling to be more active in their care, and those who do not see control or authority for health concerns as being within their domain. Some of these clients may learn to contract; others never will.

The nursing process does not necessarily provide an active role for the family as a client; the assumption that a need exists is based on professional judgment only, and it is also assumed that changes can and should be made within the family unit. Contracting is one alternative approach that depends on the value of input from both nurse and family, on the competency of the family, on the family's ability to be responsible, and on the dynamic nature of the process. This not only allows for but requires continual renegotiating. Although it may not be appropriate in all situations or with all families, contracting can give direction and structure to health risk reduction and health promotion in families.

Empowering Families

Approaches for helping individuals and families assume that an active role in promoting their health care should be characterized by **empowerment** rather than enabling or providing help (Chinn, 2008). Interventions in which help is given do not always have positive outcomes for clients. If families do not perceive a situation as a problem or need, offers of help may cause resentment. Providing help also may have negative consequences if there is not a match between what is expected and what is offered. A nurse's failure to recognize a family's competencies and to define an active role for them can lead to the family's dependency and lack of growth. This can be frustrating for both the nurse and the family. For families to become active participants, they need to feel a sense of personal competence and a desire for and willingness to take action. Definitions of empowerment reflect three characteristics of the empowered family seeking help:

- Access and control over needed resources
- Decision-making and problem-solving abilities
- The ability to communicate and to obtain needed resources

The last characteristic refers to the fact that families may need to learn how to identify sources of help, how to contact agencies, how to ask critical questions, and how to negotiate with agencies to meet family needs. These characteristics generally reflect a process by which people (individuals, families, organizations, or communities) take control of their own lives. The outcomes of empowerment are positive self-esteem, the ability to set and reach goals, a sense of control over life and change processes, and a sense of hope for the future (Koelen and Linstrom, 2005). The Levels of Prevention box shows prevention strategies applied to families.

LEVELS OF PREVENTION

Strategies Applied to Families

Primary Prevention
Completing a family genogram and assessing health risks with the family to contract for family health activities to prevent diseases from developing.

Secondary Prevention
Using a behavioral health risk survey and identifying the factors leading to obesity in the family.

Tertiary Prevention
Developing a contract with the family to change nutritional patterns to reduce further complications from obesity.

Empowerment requires a viewpoint that often conflicts with the views of many helping professions, including nursing. Empowerment's underlying assumption is one of a partnership between the professional and the client as opposed to one in which the professional is dominant. Families are assumed to be either competent or capable of becoming competent. This implies that the professional is not an unchallenged authority who is in control. Empowerment promotes an environment that creates opportunities for competencies to be used. Finally, families need to identify that their actions result in behavior change. A nursing intervention that incorporates the principles of empowerment is directed toward the building of nurse–family partnerships that emphasize health risk reduction and health promotion. The nurse's approach to the family should be positive and focused on competencies rather than on problems or deficits. The interventions need to be consistent with family cultural norms and the family's perception of the problem. Rather than making decisions for the family, the nurse supports the family in primary decision making and bolsters their self-esteem by recognizing and using family strengths and support networks. Interventions that promote desired family behaviors increase family competency and decrease the need for outside help, resulting in families viewing themselves as being actively responsible for bringing about desired changes. The goal of an empowering approach is to create a partnership between the nurse and the family characterized by cooperation and shared responsibility.

COMMUNITY RESOURCES

Families have varied and complex needs and problems. The nurse is often involved in mobilizing several resources to effectively and appropriately meet family health promotion needs. Although the specific resources vary from community to community, general types can be identified. Government resources such as Medicare, Medicaid, Aid to Families with Dependent Children, Supplementary Security Income, Food Stamps, and WIC are available in most communities. These programs primarily provide support for basic needs (e.g., illness/health care, nutritional needs, funds for housing and clothing), and funds are based on meeting eligibility criteria.

In addition to government agencies providing health-related services to families, most communities have voluntary (nongovernmental) programs. Local chapters of such organizations as the American Cancer Society, the American Heart Association, the American Lung Association, and the Muscular Dystrophy Association provide education, support services, and some direct services to individuals and families. These agencies provide primary prevention and health promotion services, as well as screening programs and assistance after the disease or condition is diagnosed. Local social service agencies, such as Catholic Social Services, provide direct services such as counseling to families. Other voluntary organizations provide direct service (e.g., shelters for homeless or battered individuals, substance abuse counseling and treatment, Meals on Wheels, transportation, clothing, food, furniture).

Health resources in the community may be proprietary, voluntary, or public. In addition to private health care providers, nurses should be aware of voluntary and public clinics, screening programs, and health promotion programs.

Identifying resources in a community requires time and effort. One valuable source is the telephone book. Often community service organizations, such as the local chamber of commerce and health department, publish community resource listings. These resources may be listed on the organizations' websites. Regardless of how the resource is identified, the nurse must be familiar with the types of services offered and any requirements or costs involved. If this information is not available, the nurse can contact the resource.

Locating and using these systems often requires skills and patience that many families lack. Nurses work with families to identify community resources, and as client advocates they help families learn to use resources. This may involve sharing information with families, rehearsing with families what questions to ask, preparing required materials, making the initial contact, and arranging transportation. The appropriateness and effectiveness of resources should be evaluated with families afterward. Navigating the maze of resources is often difficult, even for the nurse. It is important to remember that if a family is in crisis or does not have a phone or a home base from which to call or receive return calls, this process is even more difficult, and their sense of helplessness may be increased. Therefore, the nurse's assistance, while promoting the family's sense of empowerment, is both necessary and often complex.

Telehomecare

Telehomecare (also referred to as telehealth or telemedicine) is an emerging practice that allows clients to communicate with and transfer health information to providers from home. Bowles and Baugh (2007) reviewed the literature on the use of telehomecare interventions from 1995 to 2005. These authors found that the practice had improved certain health outcomes, such as reducing the duration of hospitalization. Telehomecare monitoring requires less time per client interaction, so it allows nurses to feasibly care for more clients per day. In addition, clients (including elderly individuals), as well as their caregivers, report few technological problems (Bowles and Baugh, 2007). Considering these results, nurses may increasingly rely on this technology to assist with home visits to families. Telehomecare can be a particularly useful option in situations where ongoing and frequent monitoring of a family member's condition is necessary; however, it should be recognized that it is not a substitute for the in-home trust and relationship building and assessment of both family and community resources that can only be accomplished by an attentive and engaged nurse spending time with the family in their home environment.

Family Policy

This chapter ends where it began, with a discussion of the nurse's role in policy development and implementation. Florence Nightingale, Lillian Wald, and Mary Breckenridge were all strongly committed and involved nurses who advocated for families and influenced policy to improve the health of families and consequently the health of communities. Building on the gains made possible by these influential women is essential.

Families are affected by the rules and values of their surrounding society in general. If families—all families—are valued, the community will be strong and connected. If any family is neglected and not supported, the community will be weak and disconnected. One current national policy passed to strengthen and support the family is the Family Medical Leave Act (FMLA).

On February 5, 1993, President Clinton signed the FMLA (PL 103-3). This act allows covered employees to take up to 12 weeks of leave each year for certain family and medical reasons (Office of Compliance, 2003). Many states have added more leave time and benefits for employees in their state (National Conference of State Legislatures, 2002). Under the FMLA, employees may take a leave of absence for many reasons: for their own serious illness; for the illness of their child, parent, or spouse; and for the birth or adoption of a child (PL 103-3). While on leave, employees still receive their medical benefits and are guaranteed that their position or one similar to it will be available to them upon returning to work.

The FMLA was needed to help Americans meet the needs of their families while maintaining employment. Women in particular were experiencing hardship in keeping a job while having a family. In 1990 only 37% of all working women in firms with 100 employees or more were eligible for unpaid maternity upon the birth of a child (USBLS, 2005). Without national family and medical legislation, thousands of Americans were forced to choose between a career and a family. Seven years after the FMLA was signed into law, a survey was conducted to evaluate the FMLA (Waldfogel, 2001). Findings from this survey indicated that the FMLA had no adverse effect on more than two thirds of businesses, and that employees are using the FMLA in increasing numbers (see Chapter 8 for additional information) (Waldfogel, 2001). A relatively recent emerging family policy issue is paid leave for fathers. Internationally, paternity leave policies vary greatly from country to country. Family policy such as this reflects a growing recognition and valuing of the healthy family unit as a key factor and contributor to the health of not only individuals, but our communities and society at large (USDHHS-B).

THE CUTTING EDGE   *Government initiatives to strengthen families include empowering families by giving tax breaks to increase financial independence, thus decreasing the family's dependence upon federal assistance to survive.*

Vulnerable Populations: LGBT Families at Risk

Lesbian, gay, bisexual and transgendered (LGBT) families are another vulnerable group. Over the past decade, there has been an explosion of visibility for this population. Debates and legal battles centering on LGBT rights have taken place nationally and in states all across the country. Notable examples include same-sex marriage, adoption, and anti-discrimination laws.

As noted in the introduction to this chapter, nurses have an ethical obligation to provide culturally competent care to LGBT families. To begin, nurses should provide a safe environment for clients to discuss their sexual orientation. Some nurses may

---

⬤ LINKING CONTENT TO PRACTICE

Vulnerable Populations: Teenage Parent Families at Risk

Although endless hours have been spent researching ways to help parents of teenagers, it is also important to remember the teenagers who *are* parents. This family structure faces multiple health-related and social challenges, the most prominent being affordable and accessible health care. A closely related challenge is the recruitment and development of mentors to help teen parents acquire this health care, as it is uncharted water for nearly all teenagers. The humiliation teens experience when visiting doctors and agencies is a pain analyzed and discussed incessantly, and yet little has been done for the teenage parents.

The most common issue raised by teenage parents is their uncertainty and low self-confidence in handling adult responsibilities *other* than actual parenting. There is a great need for more teenage-instructional literature on family health policy information and health care service accessibility written from the perspective of teenagers. Single teenage parents need to be able to understand welfare and how to apply, as well as to find support communities. Teenage parents who decide not to be involved in a child's life must be able to understand child support, adoption, and legal visitation and involvement issues.

The rising numbers of teenagers giving birth must be met with stronger and more extensive plans for families led by teens. Education, vocational opportunity, and social acceptance are "luxuries" often missed by adolescent parents. While the last of these issues can only be solved by eventual cultural assimilation, schooling and careers should be made possible.

Although it is not advisable to simply hand out opportunities to teenagers with children, it is definitely necessary to offer assistance, not only so that they may have a second chance at a successful life, but for their children as well. It is recognized that the children of teenage parents often make the same mistakes as their parents, due to factors of poor living conditions, low socioeconomic status, and a rough childhood. Without adequate family care, there will be no end to the cycle of child parents. Today, many people are advocating for sex education and prevention, but it is also time *now* for post-pregnancy programs, which accept that there is a child born to two teenagers; although they may have made a poor choice, these teenagers now have *no* choice but to accept parental responsibility and be shown the tools to do so.

Contributed by Marylynne Anderson-Cooper, age 17. She can be contacted through the author of the chapter.

---

feel a degree of discomfort discussing sexual orientation with their clients. However, it is important to overcome this barrier to care for LGBT families.

Nurses should assess LGBT family dynamics. Just as there is great variation among heterosexual families, all LGBT families are not the same. In addition, same-sex couples have historically had special barriers within the health care system. Some problems may stem from the lack of legal recognition for LGBT relationships in most areas of the country. Same-sex marriage laws vary widely from state to state. Certain states (e.g., Massachusetts) have legalized same-sex marriage, whereas others have constitutional amendments defining marriage as a union between one man and one woman. Similarly, there is great variation in LGBT adoption rights across the nation.

These legal barriers present challenges for LGBT families in the health care system. For example, it may be difficult for LGBT couples living in states without same-sex marriage to make medical decisions or visit their partners in the hospital.

There are similar barriers for same-sex households with children. Consider this case example:

> Sarah and Maria have been in a long-term relationship for 10 years. Five years ago, the couple decided to have a baby. Sarah is the child's biological mother, but the couple has raised Mark together since he was born. The couple lives in a state that does not recognize same-sex marriage or adoption. One day, Sarah and Mark were in a serious car accident. When Maria arrived at the hospital, she learned she was unable to make decisions or access medical information for her partner and child.

On April 15, 2010, President Obama signed a directive instructing hospitals that accept Medicaid and Medicare to allow adult clients the right to designate specific individuals that can visit them in the hospital or make medical decisions on their behalf. This will help alleviate some issues that LGBT partners face when interacting with the healthcare system. (See http://www.whitehouse.gov/the-press-office/presidential-memorandum-hospital-visitation for more information.)

Nurses are in an optimal position to fulfill a vital role in helping LGBT families achieve equitable access to health care.

Nurses can assist with assessing the implementation of President Obama's directive. In addition, nurses can help to advocate for more policies designed to reduce barriers within the health care system for LGBT families.

Another type of family at risk is the more "traditional" families with a non-heterosexual member. After a family member declares his or her sexual preferences, families may need initial support to process the information. Nurses may be in a position to provide support during this time. Nurses may also refer families to community resources, such as Parents and Friends of Lesbians and Gays (www.pflag.org). Check within your local community for other appropriate resources.

In addition to providing support for the family unit as a whole, nurses may also be in a position to assess LGBT individuals. As in all family units, the health of individual members of a family affects the entire family unit. Sexual minorities face a higher risk for depression, anxiety, substance abuse, thoughts of suicide, and suicide. Addressing mental health issues in this population may help reduce the mental health disparities the LGBT population faces.

CHAPTER REVIEW

■ PRACTICE APPLICATION

The initial contact between a nursing service and a family provides limited information, and the situation that develops may be much more complex than originally anticipated. The following example, based on an actual case, illustrates the issues and approaches outlined in this chapter.

The Local County Health Department was notified that Amy C., age 16, had been referred by the school counselor at the local high school for prenatal supervision. Amy was 4 months pregnant, apparently in good health, and in the tenth grade. She lived at home with her mother, stepfather, and younger sister. The family lived in a rural area outside of a small farming community. The father of

the baby also lived in the community and continued to see Amy on a regular basis. The referral information provided the nurse with a beginning, but limited, assessment of the family situation.

A. What would you do first as the nurse assigned to this family?
B. How would you help this family empower themselves to take responsibility for this situation?
C. After the initial contact, how would you extend the assessment to the entire family system?
D. Would you contract with this family? How? On what terms?
Answers can be found on the Evolve site.

■ KEY POINTS

- The importance of the family as a major client system for nurses in reducing health risks and promoting the health of individuals and populations is well documented.
- The family system is a basic unit within which health behavior, including health values, health habits, and health risk perceptions, is developed, organized, and performed.
- Knowledge of family structure and functioning, family theory, nursing theory, and models of health behavior is fundamental to implementing the nursing process with families in the community.
- Nurses need to go beyond the individual and family, and to understand the complex environment in which the family functions, to be effective in reducing family health risks. Categories of risk factors that are important to family health are biological risk, environmental risk (including economic factors), and behavioral risk.

- Several factors contribute to the experience of healthy/unhealthy outcomes. Not everyone exposed to the same event will have the same outcome. The factors that influence whether disease or other unhealthy results occur are called health risks. The accumulated risks are synergistic; their combined effect is more than the sum of the individual effects.
- An important aspect of nursing's role in reducing health risk and promoting the health of populations has been the tradition of providing services to individual families in their homes.
- Home visits afford the opportunity to gain a more accurate assessment of the family structure and behavior in the natural environment. Home visits also provide opportunities to make observations of the home environment and to identify both barriers and supports to reducing health risks and reaching family health goals.

KEY POINTS—cont'd

- Health professionals increasingly have come to look toward working with clients in a more interactive, collaborative style.
- Contracting, which is making an agreement between two or more parties, involves a shift in responsibility and control, from the professional alone to a shared effort by client and professional.
- Families have varied and complex needs and problems. The nurse often mobilizes several resources to effectively and appropriately meet family health needs.
- Policy development and implementation is an important skill that the nurse uses to improve the health of families and thus improve the health and livability of communities.

CLINICAL DECISION-MAKING ACTIVITIES

1. Select one of the *Healthy People 2020* objectives and identify how biological risk (including age-related risk), environmental risk (including economic risk), and behavioral risk contribute to family health risks for that objective. Give examples.
2. Select three to four families (hypothetically or from actual situations) that represent different ethnic and socioeconomic backgrounds. Complete a family genogram and ecomap for each family, and identify and compare major health risks. Summarize your findings.
3. Select one or more agencies in which nurses work, and examine the agency and nursing philosophies and objectives with emphasis on individual care, family care, illness care, risk reduction, and health promotion. If you were to accept a position with this agency, what approach to family risk reduction would you be required to use? Is there a better way?
4. Identify three public health problems in your community, and discuss the implications of these problems for the health of families. How did you arrive at your conclusions?
5. Identify three health problems common to families in your community, and discuss the implications of the problems for the health and/or health care resources of the community. What strategies might you use to address the health problems?

REFERENCES

Belloc NB, Breslow L: Relationship of physical health in a general population survey, *Am J Epidemiol* 93:329, 1972.

Bowles KH, Baugh AC: Applying research evidence to optimize telehomecare, *J Cardiovasc Nurs* 22(1):5–15, 2007.

Califano JA Jr: *Healthy People: the surgeon general's report on health promotion and disease prevention*, Washington, DC, 1979, U.S. Government Printing Office.

Centers for Disease Control and Prevention: *Behavioral risk factor surveillance system*, 2010. Available at www.cdc.gov. Accessed November 15, 2010.

Chinn PL: *Pease and power: creative leadership for building community*, ed 7, Sudbury, MA, 2008, Jones & Bartlett.

Devaney B: *WIC turns 35: Program effectiveness and future directions*, Minneapolis, MN, December 7, 2007, Mathematica Policy Research National Invitational Conference of the Early Childhood Research Collaborative.

Doherty WJ, McCubbin HI: Family and health care: an emerging arena of theory, research and clinical intervention, *Family Relat* 34:5, 1985.

Eckenrode J, Campa M, Luckey DW, et al: Long-term effects of prenatal and infancy nurse home visitation on the life course of youths: 19-year follow-up of a randomized trial, *Arch Pediatr Adolesc Med* 164(1):9–15, 2010.

Families USA: *Too great a burden: Americans face rising health care costs*, April 2009. Available at www.families usa.com.

Fraser JA, Armstrong KL, Morris JP, et al: Home visiting intervention for vulnerable families with newborns: follow-up results of a randomized controlled trial, *Child Abuse Neglect* 24:1399–1429, 2000.

Friedman M, Bowden V, Jones E: *Family nursing theory and practice*, ed 5, Upper Saddle River, NJ, 2003, Prentice Hall.

Goodman A: *The story of David Olds and the Nurse Home Visiting program*, Princeton, NJ, 2006, Robert Wood Johnson Foundation.

Hammond-Ratzlaff A, Fulton A: Knowledge gained by mothers enrolled in a home visitation program, *Adolescence* 36:435–442, 2001.

Hill R: *Families under stress*, New York, 1949, Harper.

Horne MK III, McCloskey DJ: Factor V Leiden as a common genetic risk factor for venous thromboembolism, *J Nurs Schol* 38:19–25, 2006.

Keller LO, Strohschein S, Lia-Hoagberg B, Schaffer MA: Population-based public health interventions: practice-based and evidence-supported, Part I, *Public Health Nurs* 21:453–468, 2004a.

Keller LO, Strohschein S, Schaffer MA, Lia-Hoagberg B: Population-based public health interventions: innovations in practice, teaching, and management, Part II, *Public Health Nurs* 21:469–487, 2004b.

Khoury MJ, McCabe LL, McCabe ER: Population screening in the age of genomic medicine, *N Engl J Med* 348:50–58, 2003.

Koelen MA, Linstrom B: Making healthy choices easy choices: the role of empowerment, *Eur J Clin Nutr* 59:10–15, 2005.

Litman TJ: The family as a basic unit in health and medical care: a social behavioral overview, *Soc Sci Med* 8:495, 1974.

Lorenz F, Wickrama KAS, Conger R, editors: *Family Research Consortium Summer Institute (1996), continuity and change in family relations: theory, methods, and empirical findings (Advances in Family Research)*, Mahwah, NJ, 2004, Lawrence Erlbaum Associates.

Mauksch HO: A social science basis for conceptualizing family health, *Soc Sci Med* 8:521, 1974.

Mayo Clinic: *Exercise: 7 benefits of regular physical activity*, July 2010. Available at www.mayoclinic.com. Accessed November 15, 2010.

McGoldrick M, Carter B, Garcia-Preto N: *The expanded family life cycle*, ed 4, New York, 2011, Pearson.

McKenry P, Price S: *Families and change*, ed 3, Thousand Oaks, CA, 2005, Sage.

National Center for Health Statistics: *Health, United States, 2009*, Hyattsville, MD, 2010, NCHS.

National Conference of State Legislatures: *State family and medical leave laws*, 2002. Available at http://www.ncsl.org/programs/employ/fmlachart.htm. Accessed February 15, 2011.

National Institute on Drug Abuse: *Addiction and health*. Washington, DC, 2010, USDHHS. Available at www.drugabuse.com. Accessed November 15, 2010.

Neumann University: *The Neuman Systems Model*, 2010. Available at www.neumann.edu. Accessed February 15, 2011.

Neuman B: *The Neuman Systems Model*, ed 4, Norwalk, CT, Appleton & Lange. Available at www.nursingtheory.net.

Neumann University: *The Neuman Systems Model*, 2010. Available at www.neumann.edu. Accessed February 15, 2011.

Nightingale EO, Cureton M, Kalmar V, Trudeau MB: *Perspectives on health promotion and disease prevention in the United States*, Washington, DC, 1978, Institute of Medicine, National Academy of Sciences.

Nurse Family Partnership: *Evidentiary foundations of nurse family partnership*, 2010. Available at http://www.nursefamilypartnership.org/assets/PDf/Policy/. Accessed April 7, 2010.

Nursing Theory Network, Neuman B: *The Neuman Systems Model*, ed 4, Norwalk, Cenn, Appleton & Lange. Accessed at www.nursingtheory.net.

Office of Compliance: *The Family and Medical Leave Act fact sheet*, Washington, DC, 2003. Available at www.compliance.gov. Accessed February 15, 2010.

Olds DL, Henderson CR, Tatelbaum R, Chamberlin R: Improving the delivery of prenatal care and outcomes of pregnancy: a randomized trial of nursing home visitation, *Pediatrics* 77:16–28, 1986.

Olds D, Kitzman H, Cole R, et al: Effects of nurse home-visiting on maternal life course and child development: age 9 follow-up results of a randomized trial, *Pediatrics* 120:e832–e845, 2007.

Olds DL, Robinson J, Pettitt LM, et al: Effects of home visits by paraprofessionals and by nurses: age four follow-up results of a randomized trial, *Pediatrics* 114(6):1560–1568, 2004.

Orem DE: *Nursing: concepts of practice*, ed 5, St Louis, 1995, Mosby.

Pender NJ: *Health promotion in nursing practice*, ed 6, Stamford, CT, Upper Saddle River, NJ, 2010, Pearson/Prentice-Hall.

Pew Center on the States: *The case for home visiting*, May 2010. Available at http://www.pewcenteronthestates.org. Accessed February 15, 2011.

Powell LW, Dixon JL, Ramm GA, et al: Screening for hemochromatosis in asymptomatic subjects with or without a family history, *Arch Intern Med* 166:294–301, 2006.

Pratt L: *Family structure and effective health behavior*, Boston, 1976, Houghton-Mifflin.

Press RD, Bauer KA, Kujovich JL, et al: Clinical utility of factor V Leiden (R506Q) testing for the diagnosis and management of thromboembolic disorders, *Arch Pathol Lab Med* 126:1304–1318, 2002.

Qaseem A, Aronson M, Fitterman N, et al: Screening for hereditary hemochromatosis: a clinical practice guideline from the American College of Physicians, *Ann Intern Med* 143:517–521, 2005.

Shi L, Singh DA: *Delivering health care in America: a systems approach*, Sudbury, MA, 2008, Jones and Bartlett.

Spector EB, Grody WW, Matteson CJ, et al: Technical standards and guidelines: venous thromboembolism (Factor V Leiden and prothrombin 20210G >A testing): a disease-specific supplement to the standards and guidelines for clinical genetics laboratories, *Genet Med* 7(6):444–453, 2005.

U.S. Bureau of Labor Statistics: *Percent of workers participating in selected employee benefit plans, private industry and state and local government, 1989-99. Compensation and working conditions*, 2005. Available at http://www.bls.gov.

U.S. Department of Health and Human Services: *Healthy People 2010: understanding and improving health*, ed 2, Washington, DC, 2000, USDHHS, Public Health Service.

U.S. Department of Health and Human Services: *Healthy People 2020*, Washington, DC, 2010, U.S. Government Printing Office (USDHHS-A).

U.S. Department of Health and Human Services (USDHHS-B) Administration for Children and Families: *A celebration of family, principles of family policy, n.d.* Available at http://www.acf.hhs.gov/programs/family_celebration.htm.

Vandenbroucke JP, Koster T, Briet E, et al: Increased risk of venous thrombosis in oral-contraceptive users who are carriers of factor V Leiden mutation, *Lancet* 344:1453–1457, 1994.

Wagner KA, Lee FW, Bradford WD, et al: Qualitative evaluation of South Carolina's postpartum/infant home visit program, *Public Health Nurs* 21:541–546, 2004.

Waldfogel J: *Family and medical leave: evidence from the 2000 surveys, Monthly labor review*, September 2001. Available at http://www.bls.gov/opub/mlr/2001/09/art2exc.htm. Accessed February 15, 2011.

White JM, Klein DM: *Family theories*, ed 3, Thousand Oaks, CA, 2009, Sage Publications.

Wright LM, Leahey M: *Nurses and families: a guide to family assessment and intervention*, Philadelphia, 2009, FA Davis.

CHAPTER 29

Child and Adolescent Health

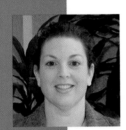

Cynthia Rubenstein, RN, PhDc, CPNP-PC

Cynthia Rubenstein is currently a faculty member at James Madison University in the Department of Nursing. She has over 18 years of experience in pediatric nursing, from NICU to ER to home health, and she has been a practicing pediatric nurse practitioner for 13 years. She is active in developing childhood obesity prevention educational programs. Dr. Rubenstein works collaboratively with a multidisciplinary team to develop expert nutritional content for an interactive Web-based educational program for the Virginia WIC program.

ADDITIONAL RESOURCES

evolve WEBSITE

http://evolve.elsevier.com/Stanhope

- *Healthy People 2020*
- Quiz
- Case Studies
- WebLinks
- Glossary
- Answers to Practice Application
- Resource Tools
  - Resource Tool 5.A: Schedule of Clinical Preventive Services
  - Resource Tool 29.A: Vision and Hearing Screening Procedures
  - Resource Tool 29.B: Screening for Common Orthopedic Problems

  - Resource Tool 29.E: Common Concerns and Problems of the First Year (Neonate)
  - Resource Tool 29.F: Common Concerns and Problems of the Toddler and Preschool Years
  - Resource Tool 29.I: Feeding and Nutrition Guidelines for Infants
  - Resource Tool 29.J: Health Problems of the School-Age Child and Adolescent

APPENDIXES

- Appendix D.2: 2009 State and Local Youth Risk Behavior Survey
- Appendix E: Friedman Family Assessment Model (Short Form)
- Appendix F.4: Motivational Interviewing

OBJECTIVES

After reading this chapter, the student should be able to do the following:

1. Describe significant physical and psychosocial developmental factors characteristic of the child and adolescent population.
2. Examine the role of the nurse and discuss appropriate nursing interventions that promote and maintain the health of children and adolescents as individuals, as members of their family, and as members of the community.

3. Discuss the built environment and how it relates to major health issues of children and adolescents.
4. Explain the current status of children and their physical, emotional, behavioral, and environmental health issues.
5. Differentiate between the models for delivery of health care to the pediatric populations in the community and other settings.

KEY TERMS

abusive head trauma, p. 661
body mass index, p. 656
built environment, p. 654
child feeding practices, p. 656
child maltreatment, p. 661
Children's Health Insurance Plan, p. 649

cognitive development, p. 651
development, p. 651
developmental screening, p. 652
environmental tobacco smoke (ETS), p. 667
family-centered medical home, p. 668

food deserts, p. 655
food landscape, p. 655
growth, p. 651
H1N1, p. 663
human ecology theory, p. 652
immunization, p. 653

KEY TERMS—cont'd

CHAPTER OUTLINE

Walt Disney identified the greatest natural resource of any nation as the minds of its children. The future of the world depends on how well it cares for its youth. If this population is to thrive, it must be nurtured in an appropriate environment. Focusing on the health needs and health promotion of children increases the chances that they will become adults who value and practice healthy lifestyles. Population-focused nurses have two major roles in the area of child and adolescent health:

1. The nurse provides direct services to children and their families: assessing, managing care, educating, and counseling.
2. Nurses are involved in the assessment of the community and the establishment of programs to ensure a healthy environment for this population.

The population-focused nurse has the opportunity to teach healthy lifestyles to children and caregivers and to provide family-centered care in the community setting. This chapter provides information on the assessment of children and adolescents as well as activities to promote their health. The content includes basic principles of childhood growth and development and major health problems seen in this population. The concept of evaluating child health and implementing health education and models of health behavioral change will be explored within the context of the child's built environment. The family-centered medical home, motivational interviewing, and the use of interactive health communication are discussed in this chapter as strategies to promote improved health behaviors within families. *Healthy People 2020* objectives (USDHHS, 2010) are used as a framework for focusing on needs of children in the community.

STATUS OF CHILDREN

Poverty Status

There were 73.9 million children through age 17 in the United States in 2008, representing slightly more than 25% of the population (Federal Interagency Forum on Child and Family Statistics, 2008a; USCB, 2009b). Approximately 40% of them live in low-income families, with one out of every five children living below poverty levels and 8% of America's children living in extreme poverty with a family income of half of the federal poverty level. The federal poverty level for 2009 was defined as a family income of less than $22,050 for a family of four whereas low income (the amount of income necessary to provide for the family's basic needs) is two times the federal poverty level.

Minority children, most notably black and Hispanic children, have higher proportions of living at poverty or low-income

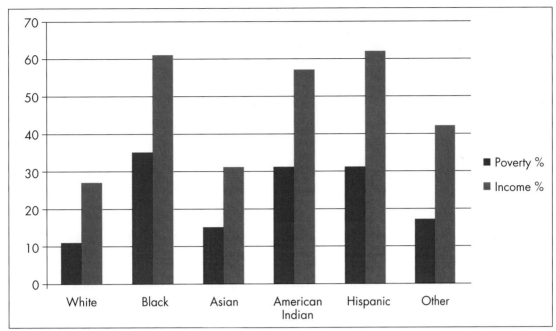

FIGURE 29-1 Percentage of children living in poverty and low income by ethnicity, 2008. (From National Center for Children in Poverty, *Basic facts about low income children, 2009,* Available at http://www.nccp.org/publications/pub_892.html. Accessed February 19, 2011.)

levels (Figure 29-1). About 60% of children born to immigrant parents live in low-income families compared with 37% of native-born parents (Wight and Chau, 2009). Characteristics that put children at risk for living in low-income families are parents without a high school degree, having a lack of parental employment, and living in a single-parent household. Children's ability to learn in school and reach their full cognitive ability is affected by low-income status. Children living in poverty experience a higher incidence of behavioral, social, and emotional problems (Wight, Chau, and Aratani, 2010).

In addition, U.S. children face other challenges. More than 20% of American households with children experience low food security. Low food security, a lack of available food and access to food on a regular basis, affects children's physical health, development, and school performance. Homelessness is increasing for American children and is highly correlated to poverty status (Wight and Chau, 2009; Wight, Chau and Aratani, 2010). It is estimated that over 10 million children each year are witnesses to or victims of violence, and this exposure to violence is linked to physical, emotional, and behavioral problems.

Access to Care

Access to quality health services is one of the focus areas of *Healthy People 2020* (USDHHS, 2010). Children with health care coverage are more likely to have a regular and accessible source of health care. In 2007, 11% (8.1 million) of all children had no health insurance. For children living in poverty, in 2007 the uninsured rate for children was 17.6% (DeNavas-Walt, Proctor, Smith, 2008). The number of children covered by government health insurance programs has been climbing since then.

The Medicaid program, established by the Social Security Act in 1965, is a state-administered health insurance program financed jointly by the federal and state governments. Children under 18 years of age living in a household with an income level at or below 133% of the federal poverty level or children meeting disability requirements qualify for this program. The program provides health services at no cost to participants and includes outpatient visits, hospitalization, laboratory testing, immunizations, well care/preventive services, and dental care (CMMS, 2010). In June 2009, 24.8 million children under the age of 18 years were enrolled in the Medicaid program, which is a 12.1% increase from the previous year (KFF, 2010).

The Children's Health Insurance Plan (CHIP) was the result of federally mandated legislature passed in 1997 to expand health insurance to the nation's uninsured children. The Children's Health Insurance Program Reauthorization Act of 2009 has continued to provide insurance to over 5 million American children. CHIP is a federal and state partnership that is directed toward uninsured children and pregnant women in families with incomes too high to qualify for state Medicaid programs but usually too low to afford private coverage. Following federal guidelines, each state determines the model of its particular CHIP program, which includes the eligibility parameters, benefit package, payment levels for coverage, and administrative process. The program is jointly financed by the federal and state governments, and administered by the states (CMMS, 2009) (Box 29-1).

CHIP enrollment has steadily increased annually since its inception, and 7.3 million children were enrolled in the program in 2008. The lowest enrolling eligible groups are Hispanic and non-English-speaking families (Division of State Children's Health Insurance, 2008). Over 5 million children remain who likely qualify for CHIP but are without health insurance (USCB, 2009a). This is an area of outreach opportunity for

> ### BOX 29-1 CHILDREN'S HEALTH INSURANCE PROGRAM (CHIP) GUIDELINES
>
> **CHIP Eligibility**
> - Family income too high for Medicaid qualification (up to $44,100 for family of 4)
> - Uninsured children under 19 years of age in the home
>
> **CHIP Coverage**
> - Primary care provider/specialist visits
> - Immunizations
> - Hospitalizations and ED visits

nurses to identify potential families eligible for CHIP and provide appropriate referrals to state agencies.

With the passage of federal health care reform in 2010 (HR 3590), changes to both the Medicaid and CHIP programs will be forthcoming with the beginning of states' health insurance exchanges. The full impact will not be noted until complete implementation of health care reform occurs later in the decade. With the anticipated health insurance coverage of all children, health outcomes and preventive services for children in the United States should improve dramatically.

Infant Mortality

Promotion of healthy pregnancies is a focus of *Healthy People 2020*. The *Healthy People 2020* target goal for the U.S. infant mortality rate is 4.5 infant deaths per 1000 live births. The U.S. infant mortality rate steadily declined over the past decades and is currently 6.2 per 1000 live births. Although infant death rates have decreased, the United States has a higher infant mortality rate than 44 other nations (CIA, 2009) and its position in a global ranking has consistently fallen over past years.

Infant mortality rates are critical indicators of a country's overall health. Infant mortality rates are associated with a variety of factors such as maternal health, socioeconomic circumstances, quality and access to medical care, and community health practices. The infant mortality rate for specific ethnic groups in the United States is significantly higher for non-Hispanic black (13.63 per 1000 live births), Puerto Rican (8.30 per 1000 live births), and American Indian or Alaska Native (8.06 per 1000 live births) (MacDorman and Mathews, 2008).

Risk-Taking Behaviors

Risk behaviors are any behaviors that place early and middle adolescents at risk for physical, emotional, or psychological harm. Much progress has been made through health promotion and education to decrease risk factors in adolescents. There have been consistent declines in the number of teens who smoked tobacco (20%), used marijuana (17.9%), and rode in the car with a driver who drank alcohol (29.1%). Increasingly, drugs of abuse are inhalants. Nationally, 13.3% of high school students have breathed the contents of aerosol spray cans, sniffed glue, or inhaled any paints or sprays to get high one or more times (NCDPHP, 2010).

There are still unchanged rates of adolescents engaging in sexual activity (47.8%), using condoms during intercourse (61.5%), and currently using alcohol (44.7%) (NCDPHP, 2010). From the 1990s through 2005, adolescent birth rates dropped steadily to approximately 42 per 1000 15- to 19-year-old adolescents. This number remains a significant concern for public health nurses since teen pregnancy has a significant socioeconomic burden on society and the family (CDC, 2010b).

Nurses should be aware of the factors associated with increased adolescent risk-taking behaviors: poor academic performance, poor parental role models, low self esteem, lack of a supportive social environment, and poverty. Individual assessment of an adolescent's risk-taking behavior can provide the direction to focus education and interventions. Providing afterschool extracurricular activities, identifying a positive adult role model, and engaging teens in support systems to build self-esteem can reduce risk-taking behaviors in at-risk adolescents.

A recent concern has emerged about the misuse and abuse of prescription stimulant medication to treat attention-deficit hyperactivity disorder (ADHD). Misuse of these drugs occurs in 5% to 9% of children and adolescents. Misuse ranges from selling or trading the prescription stimulant, taking a prescription stimulant with no ADHD symptoms, taking more than the recommended dose, or taking it by a route other than the prescribed route (i.e., inhaling an oral medication) (Wilens et al, 2008). It is vital to promote community and family awareness of this problem and educate children and adolescents on the dangers of taking others' prescription medications.

■ WHAT DO YOU THINK? *Most states have enacted laws allowing health care providers to treat adolescents in certain situations without parental consent. These include emergency care, substance abuse, pregnancy, and birth control. All 50 states recognize the mature minors' doctrine. This allows youths 15 years of age and older to give informed medical consent if it is apparent that they are capable of understanding the risks and benefits and if the procedure is medically indicated.*

If a minor can give consent, is there also an obligation to maintain confidentiality when providing health care? Three principles guide health care providers: (1) It is thought that adolescents may not seek health care if they think that their parents will be notified, (2) many providers note that the client is the adolescent, not the parent, and (3) federal and state statutes and professional ethical standards support confidentiality for adolescents. In most situations it is important to provide confidentiality. At certain times, release of information should occur despite the adolescent's desire for confidentiality. These include legal situations (e.g., physical abuse) or if the minor poses a danger to self or others.

Emily, a 15-year-old, has revealed to the nurse that she has become sexually active with her boyfriend. She has no interest in any form of birth control. The nurse wants to involve her parents, but Emily does not want them to know. What are the issues? What are Emily's rights? What strategies could the nurse use in this situation?

CHILD DEVELOPMENT

Growth and Development

Growth is the measurable aspect of the individual's size and follows a predictable pace that is evaluated at regular intervals to determine if a child is growing based on standard parameters. Development involves the observable changes in the individual and relates to physical, psychosocial, and cognitive achievements. Growth and development in children is an ongoing, dynamic process that results in physical, cognitive, and emotional changes (Figure 29-2). Health visits or well-child check-ups are scheduled at key ages to monitor these processes and provide anticipatory guidance to families. Nursing assessments include growth and health status, developmental level, and the quality of the parent–child relationship. (See Tables 29-2, 29-3, 29-4, and 29-5 for considerations and issues to address at each stage.) The recommendations for preventive pediatric health care (see Resource Tool 5.A on the Evolve site) list components of well-child assessments. Further tools and specific interventions are included in Appendixes D and E.

Developmental Theories

Many developmental theories provide perspectives on children's growth and development. The work of Erik Erikson on psychosocial development emphasizes that personality development culminates in the achievement of ego identity, which involves accepting oneself and having the skills for healthy functioning in society (Figure 29-3). According to Erickson, development is a continual process that occurs in distinct stages with a developmental crisis needing resolution at each stage and some degree of mastery being achieved before proceeding successfully to the next stage. All new development is rooted in prior experiences, and difficulty resolving the crisis will cause problems progressing through the subsequent stages.

The work of Jean Piaget is widely used to understand the process of cognitive development. According to Piaget, learning results from actively manipulating objects and information,

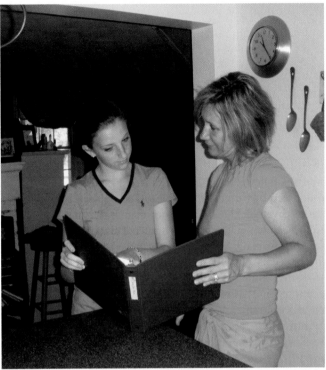

FIGURE 29-2 Conflict between parents and teenagers is normal as teenagers experience physical and emotional growth processes.

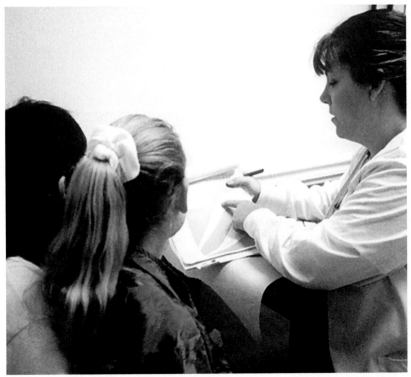

FIGURE 29-3 A nurse explains the growth patterns on a growth chart to a child and her mother.

TABLE 29-1	DEVELOPMENTAL SCREENING TOOLS
TOOL	**PURPOSE**
Denver II	Domain specific development (gross and fine motor, social, language)
Ages and Stages Questionnaire	Social and emotional development
Parents' Evaluation of Developmental Status (PEDS)	General developmental and behavioral screening
Modified Checklist for Autism in Toddlers (M-CHAT)	Autism spectrum disorder
Pediatric Symptom Checklist	Coping and mental health concerns

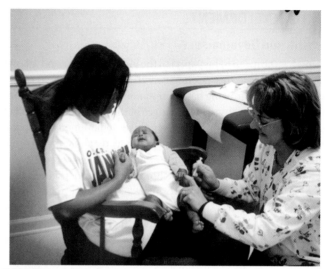

FIGURE 29-4 An infant receives a regularly scheduled immunization.

which is followed by a mental processing of the event. As the child interacts with the environment, new objects and problems are discovered. The child creates mental schemes or thought patterns to understand the encounter. This permits the child to receive information from the world, make sense of it, and predict future events. Development occurs as the schemes increase in scope and complexity. Piaget identified four stages of cognitive development that represent increasing problem-solving ability. As one will remember from pediatric courses, these stages are sensorimotor, preoperational, concrete and formal operations.

Bronfenbrenner's **human ecology theory** emphasizes the complex relationship between the growing child and his/her immediate environment. Children are greatly influenced by the environments in which they spend time and one of the most important environments in affecting growth is the family environment. Educational programs, communities, and other environmental factors also influence the child's development. Children learn to accommodate to their environment and alter themselves based on environmental interactions. This theory explains that individuals do not develop in isolation but in relation to their home and family, school, community, and society.

Developmental Screening

Developmental screening is a process designed to identify children who should receive more intensive assessment or diagnosis of potential developmental delays. These delays may be in any of the developmental domains—gross motor, fine motor, language, or social skills. Developmental screening promotes early detection of delays and improves child health and well-being for identified children. In the United States, 17% of children have a developmental disability such as autism, attention-deficit disorder, or a language delay; yet only 50% of these children were diagnosed prior to school entry. Nurses are critical to early screening and identification of developmental delays in young children and appropriately initiating referrals to maximize school readiness and maximum achievement. Multiple screening tools are available and are selected based on the nurse's role in the community (Table 29-1).

Children with delayed skills or other disabilities may qualify for special services that provide individualized education programs in public schools that are free of charge to families. Nurses can be effective health advocates for these children within educational settings. The passage of the updated version of the Individuals with Disabilities Education Act (IDEA, 2004) promotes a collaborative focus on meeting the needs of children with disabilities. Parents, educators, administrators, nurses, and other team members collaboratively develop a plan—the individualized education plan (IEP)—to help children succeed in school. The IEP explains the goals the team sets for a child during the school year as well as any special support needed to help achieve these goals.

> **NURSING TIP** *The three clinical findings for children diagnosed with autism spectrum disorder, which is a neurodevelopmental disorder, are: (1) impaired reciprocal social interaction, (2) impaired communication, and (3) restricted, repetitive, or stereotypical behaviors. Symptoms are apparent in the first 3 years of life.*

IMMUNIZATIONS

Increasing immunization coverage for children remains a significant focus of the *Healthy People 2020* objectives. Currently, 93% of the nation's 19- to 35-month-old children have received all of the polio and hepatitis B vaccinations in the recommended series but only 44% have received the complete hepatitis A series (CDC, 2010c). For adolescents, although rates continue to rise steadily, vaccination rates remain low overall for this age group. For those aged 13 to 17 years, 40% received the recommended tetanus-diphtheria-acellular pertussis vaccine (Tdap) and the meningococcal conjugate vaccine (MCV4). Lowest immunization rates are noted for the human papillomavirus vaccine (HPV4) series, with 37% of girls receiving one dose and only 18% receiving the full three-dose series (CDC, 2009d). Routine immunization of children is very successful in the prevention of selected diseases. The ultimate challenge is making sure that children receive immunizations (Figure 29-4).

Barriers

There are several barriers to successful immunizations. These include vaccine cost, vaccine refusal by parents, vaccine shortages, and changes in vaccine scheduling and recommendations. Health disparities in vaccinations continue to exist. Children living in poverty have lower immunization rates than their peers, and African-American adolescents have lower immunization rates compared with white adolescents (Burns, Walsh, and Popovich, 2010). It is important to educate parents to obtain immunizations for their children and to focus on the issue at every encounter with families.

Parental fears about vaccines prevent children from getting immunized. Parents readily access the Internet for information about vaccines, and disreputable sites provide parents with incorrect vaccine information. It is critical for nurses to educate families on the safety and efficacy of vaccinations. Scientific studies have not found a relationship between immunizations and autism, sudden infant death syndrome, diabetes, neurological disabilities, deafness, or cancer. Parents question the need to vaccinate because the incidence of vaccine-preventable diseases is low. However, Japan, Great Britain, and Sweden stopped the use of the pertussis vaccine, and within 5 years there were epidemic levels of the disease and rising death rates (CDC, 2007b). When a parent chooses not to vaccinate their child, this puts the child and others at risk.

Shortages of vaccines have periodically occurred as a result of manufacturing problems, and the U.S. Department of Health and Human Services (USDHHS) has focused on maintaining adequate manufactured supplies of vaccines. When a shortage does occur, the CDC provides priority administration guidelines for highest-risk clients. When the immunization schedule is revised, there can be delays in practitioners implementing the new recommended vaccination schedules. Nurses will want to continually review the CDC recommendations for any changes to implement within the public health and community settings.

Vaccines and vaccine administration costs are high and those families without health insurance often find following the vaccination recommendations financially prohibitive. A federal program established in 1995, Vaccines for Children (VFC), provides free vaccines to eligible children, including those without health insurance coverage, children enrolled in Medicaid, American Indians and Alaskan Natives, and children whose health insurance does not cover vaccines. Identifying children who qualify for VFC is a primary prevention strategy of population-focused nurses.

Immunization Theory

The goal of immunization is to protect by using immunizing agents to stimulate antibody formation (see Chapter 13 for types of immunity). Immunizing agents for active immunity are in the form of toxoids and vaccines. A toxoid is a bacterial toxin (e.g., from the bacteria that cause tetanus and diphtheria) that has been heated or chemically treated to decrease virulence but not antibody-producing ability. Vaccines are suspensions of attenuated (live) or inactivated (killed) microorganisms. Examples include pertussis (inactivated bacteria); measles,

---

EVIDENCE-BASED PRACTICE

A literature review evaluated home-based community health interventions to reduce environmental exposures to children with asthma. Studies provided education to families on how to reduce environmental triggers in their homes. Overall, the studies resulted in reductions in asthma symptoms, daytime activity limitations, and emergency and urgent care use for the children.

Nurse Use

Environmental triggers are a primary cause of asthma exacerbations. Having a nurse provide a home visit, complete a home environmental assessment, and provide specific education for a family to make environmental changes can greatly improve the health of children with asthma. This can result in much lower need for emergency care and sick days. This can result in cost savings for the family and improved health and school attendance for the child. Public health nurses are capable of making significant differences in the pediatric asthma health burden in their community.

From Postma J, Karr C, Kieckhefer G: Community health workers and environmental interventions for children with asthma: a systematic review, *J Asthma* 46(6):564-576, 2009.

mumps, and rubella (live attenuated viruses); and hepatitis B (inactivated virus).

The neonate receives placental transfer of maternal antibodies. This natural passive immunity lasts for about 2 months. Protection is temporary and is only to diseases to which the mother has adequate antibodies. The immune system of both term and preterm infants is capable of adequate antibody response to immunizations by 2 months of age. Generally, this is the recommended age to start immunizations; the exception is the hepatitis B series, which begins at birth.

The interval between immunizations is important to the immune response. After the first injection, antibodies are produced slowly and in small concentrations (the primary response). When subsequent injections of the same antigen are given, the body recognizes the antigen and antibodies are produced much faster and in higher concentration (the secondary response). Because of this secondary response, once an initial immunization series has been started, it does not need to be restarted if interrupted, regardless of the length of time elapsed. Once the initial series is completed, boosters are required at appropriate intervals to maintain an adequate concentration of antibodies. Further information about immunizing agents is available on the Evolve website.

Recommendations

Immunization recommendations rapidly change as new information and products are available. Two major organizations are responsible for guidelines: the American Academy of Pediatrics (AAP, 2009a) and the U.S. Public Health Service's Advisory Committee on Immunization Practices (ACIP). Current recommendations for children and adolescents can be found on the Evolve website. The main goal of the guidelines is to provide flexibility to ensure that the largest number of children will be immunized. All health care providers are urged to assess immunization status at every encounter with children and to update immunizations whenever possible.

DID YOU KNOW? *For 2007 to 2008, infants younger than 6 months of age continued to have the highest reported rate of pertussis with 79.41 cases per 100,000 and had the highest rate of associated morbidity and mortality with pertussis (MMWR, 2010).*

Contraindications

There are relatively few contraindications to giving immunizations. Minor acute illness is not a contraindication. Immunizations should be deferred with moderate or acute febrile illnesses because the reactions may mask the symptoms of the illness. The side effects of the immunization may be accentuated by the illness.

People with the following conditions are not routinely immunized and require medical consultation: pregnancy, generalized malignancy, immunosuppressive therapy or immunodeficiency disease, sensitivity to components of the agent, or recent administration of immune serum globulin, plasma, or blood.

Legislation

The National Childhood Vaccine Injury Act became effective in 1988. It requires providers to counsel parents and clients about the risks and benefits of the immunizing agent as well as possible side effects. Informed consent is recommended. Vaccine information statements (VISs) are used for this purpose. The VISs are information sheets produced by the CDC that explain both the benefits and risks of a vaccine. Federal law requires that a VIS be given to parents or legal guardians before each vaccine dose is given.

The Vaccine Adverse Event Reporting System (VAERS) is a national safety surveillance program. It requires providers and vaccine manufacturers to report any adverse effects following the administration of routinely recommended vaccinations. The program has been effective in tracking and identifying adverse effects associated with vaccinations. In 1999, VAERS detected reports of intussusception above what would be expected to occur by chance alone after the administration of the RotaShield rotavirus vaccine. Subsequently, this vaccine was pulled from manufacturing and the vaccine formulation was redeveloped.

THE BUILT ENVIRONMENT

A built environment is simply defined as the person's human-made or modified surroundings in which they live, work, and partake in recreation (Renalds, Smith, and Hale, 2010). This is the actual physical environment in which children live and includes neighborhood access to recreation opportunities, grocery stores, the home environment, and the consideration of general safety for children in their physical environments. A child's built environment is influential in the managing of risk factors for obesity, amount and type of physical activity, risk for injuries, and exposure to environmental toxins. Therefore, as nurses, assessing a child's built environment provides a foundation for identifying interventions and education to promote health and prevent injuries and diseases.

TABLE 29-2	CENTERS FOR DISEASE CONTROL AND PREVENTION CLASSIFICATION OF BODY MASS INDEX (BMI) FOR CHILDREN AGE 2 YEARS AND ABOVE
PLOTTED PERCENTILE FOR AGE AND GENDER	**BMI INTERPRETATION**
<5th percentile	Underweight
5th-85th percentile	Normal
85th-95th percentile	Overweight
>95th percentile	Obese

From Centers for Disease Control and Prevention: Classification of body mass index, 2009. Available at http://www.cdc.gov/

Obesity

Obesity rates in American children have risen to epidemic levels over the past few decades. These increases are noted for all children aged 2 to 18 years regardless of gender or ethnicity. The CDC defines overweight as a body mass index (BMI) at or above the 85th percentile and lower than the 95th percentile, and obesity is defined as a BMI at or above the 95th percentile for children of the same age and sex when plotted on the CDC growth charts (Table 29-2) (CDC, 2010d).

The prevalence of the overweight and the obese combined is 38% in children ages 2 to 5 years, 69% for children ages 6 to 11 years, and 65% for adolescents 12 to 19 years. The prevalence of obesity in children is approximately 17% for ages 2 to 5 years, 34% for ages 6 to 11 years, and 31% for ages 12 to 19 years (Ogden et al, 2010) (Figure 29-5). Comparing these 2008 National Health and Nutrition Examination Survey (NHANES) findings with 1974 NHANES results demonstrates that prevalence rates for obesity have more than quadrupled for most children over the past 30 years (Ogden et al, 2002, Ogden et al, 2010).

LEVELS OF PREVENTION

Childhood Obesity

Primary Prevention
Offer healthy cooking classes for families in the community.

Secondary Prevention
Conduct child body mass index screenings in community daycares and preschools.

Tertiary Prevention
Develop individualized weight loss plans and counsel children identified as obese on lifestyle changes.

The physiological consequences of childhood obesity are extensive and significantly impact the health status of American children. Research has clearly identified strong relationships between being obese as a child and increased disease risk and disease burden in the cardiovascular, metabolic, musculoskeletal,

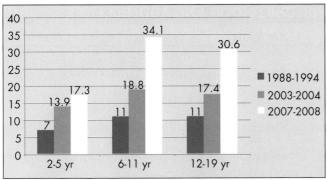

FIGURE 29-5 Obesity prevalence for 2 to 19 years. (Data from Ogden C & Carroll M (2010, June). Health E-Stat: Prevalence of obesity among children and adolescents: United States, trends 1963-1965 through 2007–2008. Centers for Disease Control and Prevention: National Center of Health Statistics. Available at http://www.cdc.gov/nchs/data/hestat/obesity_child_07_08/obesity_child_07_08.html#table1. Accessed March 15, 2011.)

respiratory, and renal systems (Freedman et al, 2001; Viner et al, 2005; Miller et al, 2006;). Another critical consequence for children is the negative psychological and social impact of obesity with decreased self-esteem; higher incidence of depression, sadness, and anxiety; problems with social relationships; and higher reports of being the victim of bullying (Cornette, 2008; Gable, Britt-Rankin, and Krull, 2008; Wang et al, 2009).

Multiple factors contribute to the likelihood that a child will become overweight or obese. Genetics is certainly a contributing component, although the genetic composition of the population has been stable over time, thereby failing to account for a sudden rise in obesity in recent years (Lawrence and Chowdhury, 2004). Within the literature, three modifiable risk factors for the development of childhood obesity have been identified. These risk factors are monitor viewing hours (including television, computer, and video game monitors), physical activity engagement, and dietary intake/eating behaviors (AAP, 2003; Bowman et al, 2004; Kranz, Siega-Riz, and Herring, 2004; Taveras et al, 2007).

A rising co-morbidity for childhood obesity is type 2 diabetes mellitus. Currently, about 151,000 U.S. children and adolescents have type 2 diabetes. Children and adolescents diagnosed with type 2 diabetes are usually between 10 and 19 years old, are obese with a strong family history for type 2 diabetes, and have insulin resistance. Most children and adolescents with type 2 diabetes have poor glycemic control with hemoglobin A1C levels between 10% and 12%. Type 2 diabetes affects all ethnic groups but occurs more frequently in non-white groups (Nader and Kumar, 2008).

Screening for type 2 diabetes is recommended for children with a BMI of 85th to 95th percentile with two risk factors of family history of diabetes, belonging to a racial minority group, or with signs of insulin resistance; all children with a BMI above the 95th percentile; and at age 10 years or onset of puberty (ADA, 2000). In addition, these children should be screened for hypercholesterolemia and hypertension, which are also associated with childhood obesity. Nurses can be instrumental in the management of type 2 diabetes in children by educating and counseling families on lifestyle changes related to dietary habits and physical activity.

DID YOU KNOW? *If current trends continue, one in three American children will develop diabetes sometime in their lifetime, and those diagnosed with diabetes will lose an average of 10 to 15 years of their life.*

Built Food Environments

A discussion on the risk factors for childhood obesity should be considered within the context of a child's environment. The emerging research on the relationship of built environments and obesity evaluates the factors within an individual's environment that may contribute on a macro- or micro-level to the development of obesity. The current literature focuses on the role of the built environment in increasing energy consumption while decreasing energy expenditure and looks at the interaction of the individual with his or her environment that influences health (Papas et al, 2007).

For children, the built environment as it relates to nutrition includes both macro- and micro-level considerations. On the community, or macro level, the factors of the built environment that influence nutrition and risk factors for obesity include a greater reliance on convenience foods and fast foods, increasing portion sizes, and the food landscape (Sallis and Glanz, 2006). The food landscape evaluates the accessibility and availability of healthy foods, and it is clear that low-income neighborhoods have limited access to stores offering fruits and vegetables (Rosenkranz and Dzewaltowski, 2008).

Close proximity to fast food restaurants and convenience stores are negatively correlated with daily fruit and vegetable consumption for school age children (Timperio et al, 2008). Many urban and rural Americans live in areas termed as food deserts, which are defined as having limited access to affordable and nutritious foods. The inability to easily obtain nutritious foods has been identified as a contributing factor to the development of obesity and obesity-related diseases (USDA, 2009). About 2.2% of American households live more than 1 mile from a supermarket and do not have access to a car.

The factors on the macro level interact closely with those factors on the micro level. For children, the micro-level factors of the built environment that influence nutrition include the home food environment. The home food environment factors include home availability and accessibility of fruits and vegetables, parent role modeling, child feeding practices, and general parenting style (Galvez, Pearl, and Yen, 2010; Rosenkranz and Dzewaltowski, 2008).

Obesity Prevention

A united national movement is underway to reduce risk factors for developing obesity in children. The current White House administration is promoting the "Let's Move!" campaign as a comprehensive and coordinated initiative to prevent childhood obesity. The initiative emphasizes four primary components: healthy schools, access to affordable and healthy food, raising children's physical activity levels, and empowering families to make healthy choices (White House, 2011). The CDC's Health Protection Goal of *Healthy People in Every Stage of Life* for preschool-age children emphasizes early identification,

TABLE 29-3   DAILY DIETARY RECOMMENDATIONS: CHILDHOOD AND ADOLESCENCE

FOOD GROUP*	2-3 YEARS	4-8 YEARS	9-13 YEARS	14-18 YEARS
Milk Try to select low-fat sources of milk, cheese, yogurt	2 cups	2 cups	3 cups	3 cups
Meat and Beans Lean meats, beans, eggs, seafood	2 oz	3-4 oz	5 oz	5-6 oz
Vegetables Fresh vegetables best choice	1 cup	1-1½ cups	1½ cups	2 cups
Fruits Limit fruit juices	1 cup	1-1½ cups	1½ cups	2 cups
Grains Half of grains should be whole grains Cooked pasta or rice, bread, cereals	3 oz	4-5 oz	5-6 oz	6-7 oz

Adapted from U.S. Department of Agriculture: Daily Food Plan, MyPyramid.gov, 2009.
*Recommendations are per day for each group.

tracking, prevention, and follow-up treatment of chronic diseases including obesity (CDC, 2007a). In addition, the *Healthy People 2020* priority focus areas of prevention include a direct focus on achieving the goals of reducing the proportion of children who are overweight or obese, increasing the proportion of daily servings of fruits for children, and increasing the proportion of daily servings of vegetables for children.

Promoting good nutrition and dietary habits is a key to maintaining child health. The first 6 years are the most important for developing sound lifetime eating habits. Parents as primary caregivers are most influential in teaching children specific eating behaviors through their own child-feeding practices. Child feeding practices are a primary factor in the development of eating behaviors for children and include the level of control the parent or caregiver exerts over the type and amount of food the child eats, the role modeling of eating behaviors, the feeding cues given to the child, and the actual mealtime environment and routine. The resulting learned eating behaviors then follow an individual through adolescence and into adulthood.

THE CUTTING EDGE   *Health insurance coverage for pediatric obesity management and counseling has been almost non-existent in recent years, making obesity management difficult in the community setting. Recently, the private insurer Anthem announced a joint collaboration with Alliance for a Healthier Generation to combat childhood obesity. The insurer will provide coverage for children with a BMI >85th percentile for age/gender to receive four primary care provider educational sessions and four individualized educational sessions with a dietitian. The Alliance will provide webinar training for health care providers counseling families.*

Nutrition Assessment

Physical growth serves as an excellent measure of adequacy of the diet. Measurements of height and weight, plotted on appropriate growth curves at regular intervals, allow assessment of growth patterns. Head circumference is followed until age 3. For children 2 years and older, the body mass index (BMI) should be calculated (kilograms/[meters]^2) based on the weight and height measurements. BMI for age and gender is plotted on the standardized BMI-for-age charts available through the CDC. Children falling outside the expected growth patterns can then be identified and interventions implemented (ADA, 2008).

A 24-hour diet recall by the parent is a helpful screening tool to assess the amount and variety of food intake. If the recall is fairly typical for the child or adolescent, the nurse can compare the intake with basic recommendations for the child's or adolescent's age. It is important to ask about parent's concerns regarding diet. It is also helpful to look at the family's meal patterns. Other important parts of the nutrition assessment include amount of physical activity and any behavior problems that occur during meals. Table 29-3 offers guidelines to daily requirements for all ages.

DID YOU KNOW?   *The current consumption of fruits and vegetables by preschool children fails to meet national guidelines or recommendations (ADA, 2008) with only 45% of children ages 2 to 5 years consuming two or more fruits per day and only 49% consuming three or more vegetables daily.*

Physical Activity

Physical activity levels contribute significantly to the overall health of children, particularly related to their risk for obesity. Fewer children are meeting the recommended physical activities levels today compared with previous generations. There are several contributing factors including the physical built environment, changes in school practices for physical education, and increased time spent in monitor viewing.

Some children are at higher risk for not getting enough physical activity, particularly those children living in poverty in urban neighborhoods that are unsafe for outdoor playtime and have

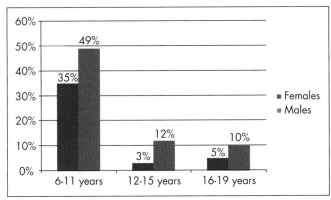

FIGURE 29-6 Prevalence of daily moderate physical activity, 2004, NHANES. (From Troiano RP, Berrigan D, Dodd KW, et al: Physical activity in the United States measured by accelerometer, *Med Sci Sports Exercise* 40[1]:181-188, 2008.)

limited access to playgrounds and parks. Even in suburban areas, parents are wary of allowing their children to play unsupervised outdoors. Few families live in locations where they can regularly walk or bike to school or for errands. As a society, Americans have become increasing sedentary, which contributes greatly to obesity and the development of many chronic diseases.

The AAP recommends that every child and adolescent gets 60 minutes of moderate, aerobic physical activity daily. This can be accumulated throughout the day with smaller increments of activity, those obtained during school, at home, and while engaged in leisure or sports activities (AAP, 2006). It is important to encourage families to be active together since this promotes greater physical activity levels in children. It also provides family time for promoting family engagement, connection, and communication. Figure 29-6 shows developmental guidelines for physical activity promotion.

According to the most recent NHANES data, all age groups are failing to meet recommended daily activity levels. For children 6 to 11 years of age, 42% get 60 minutes of moderate activity daily; this drops to 8% for 12- to 15-year-olds and just 7.6% for 16- to 19-year-old adolescents (Troiano et al, 2008). Of significant note, girls are much more sedentary than boys, with the disparity increasing with age (Table 29-4).

Schools

Children and adolescents spend much of each weekday in school. Based on the results of a school health survey, 79.1% of elementary schools provided daily recess for students in all grade levels while only 11.8% of states require elementary schools to provide students with regularly scheduled recess. For the recommended minutes per week of daily physical education (150 minutes per week in elementary schools and 225 minutes per week in middle schools and high schools), only 3.8% of elementary schools, 7.9% of middle schools, and 2.1% of high schools provided the recommended daily physical education or its equivalent for the entire school year (36 weeks) for students in all grades in the school (National Center for Chronic Disease Prevention and Health Promotion, 2006).

Schools have a vital ability to influence student health through federal and state school policies. Quality physical

TABLE 29-4	PHYSICAL ACTIVITY RECOMMENDATIONS BY AGE GROUP
AGE GROUP	**RECOMMENDATIONS**
Infants and toddlers (0-2 years)	• Safe, minimally structured play environment • Promote outdoor activities and exploration under supervision of a responsible adult • No television viewing • Organized exercise classes are not recommended
Preschoolers (2-6 years)	• Encourage free play and exploration under proper supervision • Provide unorganized play with opportunity for running, swimming, tumbling, throwing, catching with supervision • Take short walks with family member; limit use of strollers for transportation • Limit television viewing to <2 hours/day
Elementary school age (6-9 years)	• Encourage free play with emphasis on basic skills acquisition • Promote walking, dancing, jumping rope • Organized sports (soccer, baseball) can be started but should be flexible with rules, allowing free time in practice • Take walks, short bike rides together as a family • Limit television viewing, video games to <2 hours/day
Middle school age (10-12 years)	• Encourage physical activities enjoyed with families and friends • Emphasize skills acquisition with increased focus on strategies • Participation in complex sports (football, basketball) is appropriate • Weight training can begin with good supervision and small weights • Limit television viewing, video games to <2 hours/day
Adolescents	• Encourage physical activities that are enjoyed with friends and considered fun to the teen • Promote personal fitness—running, yoga, dance, swimming • Encourage active transportation—biking and walking • Weight training is safe for this age • Limit television viewing, video games to <2 hours/day

From American Academy of Pediatrics: Policy statement: active healthy living: prevention of childhood obesity through increased physical activity, *Pediatrics* 117(5):1834-1842, 2006.

education requires adequate time (per week, at least 150 minutes for elementary schools and 225 minutes for secondary schools), teacher preparation and professional support, and adequate facilities and class size. Recommendations to meet high levels of physical activity in schools include strategies that integrate physical activity into structured classroom activities, encouraging more unstructured play, expanding extracurricular activities promoting physical activity, and guiding adolescents in developing their own personal fitness goals and plans.

> **DID YOU KNOW?** *The WIC Reauthorization Act of 2004 required that all schools that received federal funding must develop wellness policies targeted towards the reduction of obesity (Serrano et al, 2007).*

The *Healthy People 2020* objectives include a focus on increasing the proportion of adolescents and children who engage in moderate vigorous activity on a daily basis, increasing the proportion of adolescents who spend at least 50% of school physical education class time being physically active, and increasing the proportion of adolescents who participate in daily school physical education. Nurses will want to be active in educating school administrators and school boards on the benefits of physical activity in improving children's and adolescents' physical health, cognitive performance, and behavior. Nurses should be engaged in policy revisions in the school systems to restore compulsory, quality, daily physical education classes; retain school recess; and expand extracurricular activities that promote physical activity before and after schools.

Media

The concept of "media" has changed significantly over the past couple of decades. In addition to television and movies, media now include the Internet, video and computer games, and cell phones. With the extensive incorporation of media into our society, its impact on children and adolescents is significant. Children and adolescents now spend more time engaged with media than any other activity except for sleeping; on average over 7 hours each day. More than 90% of teens are online, more than 70% have a cell phone, and 97% report playing video games via some type of media device (Strasburger, Jordan, and Donnerstein, 2010).

Research has strongly correlated increased use of media with an increased sedentary lifestyle, obesity, hypercholesterolemia, and hypertension. In addition to the negative physiological effects, exposure to such extensive media has been correlated to desensitization to violence and increased aggression, greater sexual content exposure and increased sexual activity, and lower academic performance if the child or adolescent has a television in their bedroom.

Interventions need to be based on the goal of lifestyle changes for the entire family. The AAP recommends that children and adolescents over the age of 2 years be limited to 2 hours per day of media "screen" time and that children under 2 years do not have any screen time (Strasburger, Jordan, and Donnerstein, 2010). Televisions, video game systems, and computers should be kept out of the child's or adolescent's bedroom and in open spaces in the home. Parents should engage in media viewing with their children and discuss the content, avoid exposing young children to PG-13 or R-rated movies, and role model limited media usage.

Nurses are uniquely positioned within the community to effect change in the childhood obesity rates. With the knowledge and skills to identify children as at risk or obese, nurses can develop interventions for healthy change for these families and refer to providers appropriately. Education on healthy eating, child-feeding practices, and physical activity levels are necessary for individuals, families, and groups within the community. Nurses have the abilities and knowledge to develop creative programs to provide families with the skills to grow their own gardens and cook healthy meals. Advocating for exercise trails and physical activity programs within the community will improve the health of families living in the vicinity. It is clear from obesity research that a community-based approach is most effective at reducing obesity rates and improving health. Box 29-2 highlights some guidelines on nutrition education for families.

BOX 29-2 FAMILY RECOMMENDATIONS FOR OBESITY PREVENTION

- Breastfeeding is the recommended exclusive feeding choice for infants from birth to 6 months and should be continued until 1 year of age. Breastfeeding is associated with a lower risk for developing childhood obesity.
- Parents' responsibilities are to provide healthy meals and snacks for their children. It is their child's responsibility to decide how much to eat.
- Limit 100% fruit juices and avoid all other sugary beverages. These are empty calories and fill children up so they are not hungry at meals. Appropriate beverages are milk and water.
- For toddlers and preschoolers, it sometimes takes 10 to 15 tastes of a new food before learning to like that food. Be persistent!
- Parents should role model good eating behaviors—lots of fruits and vegetables, no sugary beverages, and little to no "junk" food or "fast" food.
- Family meals are important for teaching manners, listening to hunger cues, and having quality family time together.
- Encourage children to help with food selection and preparation as appropriate to developmental skills. Allow them to select new foods to try in the produce section of the grocery store.
- Avoid using food as a punishment or reward. Do not expect your child to "clean their plate." These feeding techniques have been associated with increased risk for obesity.

- Turn off the television during meals and do not let your child eat in front of the television. Children do not listen to their cues of satiety when distracted.
- Cook meals at home. Broil, bake, stir-fry, or poach foods rather than frying.
- Modify family eating habits to include low-fat food choices. Serve calorically dense foods that incorporate the food guide pyramid: whole grains, fruits, vegetables, lean protein foods, and low-fat dairy products.
- Encourage family members to stop eating when they are satisfied. Encourage recognizing hunger and satiation cues.
- Schedule regular times for meals and snacks. Include breakfast and do not skip meals.
- Have low-calorie, nutritious snacks ready and available. Avoid having empty-calorie junk foods in the home. Plan for healthy snacks when eating "on the run"—granola, fruits, and nuts.
- Decrease salt, sugar, and fat. Increase complex carbohydrates—whole grains.
- Maintain regular activity (e.g., exercise, sports) and limit television viewing.
- Select family activities and vacations that include or focus on physical activity (hiking, bicycling, swimming).

Injuries and Accidents

Unintentional injuries are the leading cause of morbidity and mortality in the United States. Unintentional injuries are any injuries sustained by accident such as falls, drowning, or motor vehicle accidents. It is one of the most under-recognized public health problems facing the United States today, with about 20 children dying each day from a preventable injury. Reducing injuries from unintentional causes, as well as from violence and abuse, is a goal of *Healthy People 2020*. Unintentional injuries are the leading cause of death for children ages 1 through 19 years with more than 12,000 U.S. children and adolescents dying each year from unintentional injuries. It is estimated that 9.2 million children are seen in emergency departments each year for treatment from an unintentional injury, with falls being the leading non-fatal injury (Borse et al, 2008).

Motor vehicle crashes are the leading cause of death for unintentional injuries. Each day, 4 children and adolescents are killed and 504 are injured. One fourth of those deaths involved drunk drivers. One research study found that 72% of almost 3500 observed car and booster seats were mishandled in a way that could possibly increase a child's risk of injury during a

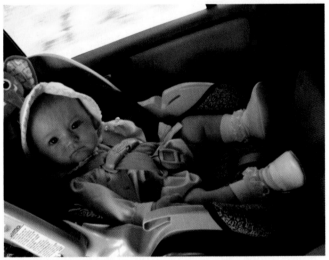

FIGURE 29-7 Children should always be restrained while riding in a vehicle.

crash. It is recommended by the National Highway Traffic Safety Administration for children to remain in booster seats until they are at least 8 years of age or 4 feet, 9 inches tall (Figure 29-7). A study found that booster seats reduced injury risk by 59% compared with seat belts alone for children 4 to 7 years. National standards recommend that all children ages 12 years and younger ride in the back seat since they are at significant risk of injury from airbag deployment, and the back seat is known as the safest part of the vehicle if a crash occurs. Even for adolescents to age 16 years, sitting in the back seat is associated with a 40% decrease in the risk of serious injury (Borse et al, 2008; CDC 2010a).

Drowning, poisonings, and burns account for most of the other deaths. For infants, the leading cause of death is suffocation (Table 29-5). To effectively implement prevention strategies, nurses need to understand the developmental factors that place this population at risk.

Developmental Considerations

Infants. Infants have the second highest injury rate of all groups of children; their small size contributes to some types of injury. The small airway may be easily occluded. The small body fits through places where the head may be entrapped. In motor vehicle crashes, small size is a great disadvantage and increases the risk for crushing or being propelled into surfaces.

The second half of infancy brings major accomplishments in gross motor activities. Rolling, sitting, pulling up, and walking bring safety concerns. Their developing motor skills remain immature, which limits their ability to escape from injury and places them at risk for drowning, suffocating, and burns.

Toddlers and Preschoolers. This population experiences a large number of non-fatal falls and being struck by or against an object. They are active and lack an understanding of cause and effect, and their increasing motor skills make supervision difficult. They are inquisitive and have relatively immature logic abilities.

School-Age Children. The school-age group has the lowest injury death rate. At this age, it is difficult to judge speed and distance, placing them at risk for pedestrian and bicycle accidents. Boys are twice as likely as girls to sustain a non-fatal bicycle injury, and the highest injury rate is 10 to 14 years of age. Universal use of bicycle helmets would prevent most deaths.

TABLE 29-5	LEADING CAUSES OF UNINTENTIONAL INJURY DEATH AMONG U.S. CHILDREN 0 TO 19 YEARS, 2000-2005				
RANK	**0-1 YEAR**	**1-4 YEARS**	**5-9 YEARS**	**10-14 YEARS**	**15-19 YEARS**
1	Suffocation (66%)	MVT-related* (31%)	MVT-related* (53%)	MVT-related* (58%)	MVT-related* (76%)
2	MVT-related* (14%)	Drowning (27%)	Other injuries (15%)	Other injuries (18%)	Other injuries (9%)
3	Drowning (7%)	Other injuries (15%)	Burns/fire (13%)	Drowning (10%)	Poisonings (7%)
4	Other injuries (6%)	Burns/fire (14%)	Drowning (13%)	Burns/fire (6%)	Drowning (5%)
5	Burns/fire (4%)	Suffocation (8%)	Suffocation (4%)	Suffocation (4%)	Falls (1%)
6	Poisonings (2%)	Falls (2%)	Falls (1%)	Poisoning (2%)	Burns/fire (1%)
7	Falls (2%)	Poisonings (2%)	Poisonings (1%)	Falls (2%)	Suffocation (1%)

From Borse NN, Gilchrist J, Dellinger AM, et al: *CDC childhood injury report: patterns of unintentional injuries among 0 -19 year olds in the United States, 2000-2006,* Atlanta, 2008, CDC, National Center for Injury Prevention and Control.
*MVT-related: Motor vehicle traffic–related includes motor vehicle injuries, pedestrian injuries, and bicycle injuries.

Peer pressure and lack of parental role modeling often inhibits the use of protective devices such as helmets and limb pads.

Adolescents. Motor vehicle–related injuries and violence are the leading causes of morbidity and mortality for adolescents. Risk-taking becomes more conscious at this time, especially among boys. The injury death rates for boys are twice as high as those for girls. Adolescents are at the highest risk of any age group for motor vehicle deaths and fatal poisonings. Use of weapons and drug and alcohol abuse play an important role in injuries in this age group. Homicides are the second leading cause of death for U.S. adolescents.

In a survey of adolescents, 35.5% reported being in a physical fight at least one time in the previous 12 months, and 5.5% reported missing school at least one day in the previous month because they felt unsafe at school or on their way to school (NCCDPHP, 2006). Suicide is the third leading cause of death among youths between the ages of 15 and 24 years. Poor social adjustment, psychiatric problems, and family disorganization increase the risk for suicide.

For all ages, families should be given anticipatory guidance in the high-risk areas for each age group to promote safety and injury prevention. Nurses can use community centers, schools, workplaces, and health centers to provide teaching to families on how to prevent injuries in their children.

Sports Injuries

Encouraging participation in team sports and individual sports and active leisure activities can increase the physical activity of children and adolescents. Children who are active in sports should have annual sports physicals, and guidelines for sports safety should be discussed (Box 29-3). About 25% of children and adolescents surveyed who played sports or exercised needed a medical evaluation for an injury within the past month (NCDPHP, 2010).

To protect children and adolescents during sports, families require education on selecting age and physically appropriate activities, using the correct safety gear, maintaining the safety gear in good condition, and practicing good body mechanics (Figure 29-8). Management of acute injuries sustained during sports should be monitored closely by coaches and primary care providers. The incidence of concussions, or brain injuries, is 3.8 million per year in the United States. Recognition of concussions and proper treatment is critical to prevent repeat concussions, which can cause long-term problems (Table 29-6).

Child Maltreatment

In 2008, 3.3 million children were reported abused or neglected with about 772,000 cases confirmed by Child Protective Services. For the same year, about 1740 U.S. children

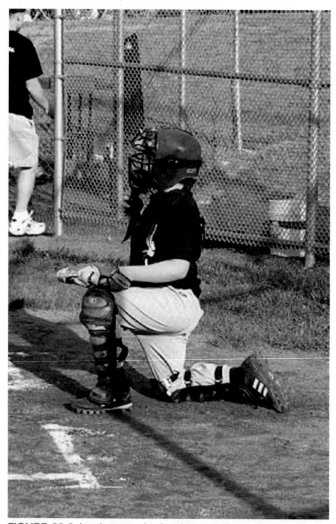

FIGURE 29-8 Involvement in developmentally appropriate sports promotes physical activity and skills acquisition.

TABLE 29-6 RECOGNIZING A CONCUSSION IN AN ATHLETE

SIGNS OBSERVED BY COACHES/PARENTS	SYMPTOMS REPORTED BY ATHLETE
Appears dazed, stunned, confused	Headache or "pressure" in head
Forgets sports plays	Nausea or vomiting
Moves clumsily	Balance problems, dizziness, double/blurred vision
Answers questions slowly	Sensitivity to light and/or noise
Loses consciousness (even briefly)	Feeling sluggish, foggy, or groggy
Shows behavior or personality changes	Concentration or memory problems
Cannot recall events prior to or after hit or fall	Confusion or does not "feel right"

From U.S. Department of Health and Human Services: Heads up, concussion in youth sports: a fact sheet for coaches, 2009. Available at www.cdc.gov.

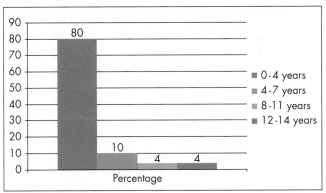

FIGURE 29-9 U.S. child deaths from maltreatment, 2008. Estimated 1,740 deaths in 2008. (U.S. Department of Health and Human Services, Administration for Children and Families, Administration on Children, Youth and Families, Children's Bureau (2010). Child Maltreatment 2008. Available from http://www.acf.hhs.gov/programs/cb/stats_research/index.htm#can.)

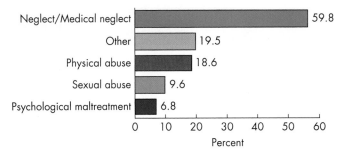

FIGURE 29-10 Child maltreatment by type, 2000.

(2.33 deaths per 100,000 children) died as a result of maltreatment (USDHHS, 2009) (Figure 29-9). **Child maltreatment** is defined as any act or series of acts of commission or omission by an adult that results in harm, potential for harm, or threat of harm to a child. Acts of commission (abuse) include physical abuse, sexual abuse, and psychological abuse; acts of omission (neglect) include failure to provide (physical neglect, emotional neglect, medical/dental neglect, educational neglect) and failure to supervise (inadequate supervision, exposure to violent environments) (Leeb et al, 2007) (Figure 29-10).

Child maltreatment occurs in all socioeconomic, racial, and ethnic groups. Yet African American, American Indian, and multiracial children experienced higher rates of victimization. Children under the age of 4 years and those children with special needs are at highest risk. Children are most likely to be maltreated by their parents, and common parental characteristics include a poor understanding of child development and children's needs, history of abuse in the family of origin, substance abuse in the household, and non-biological transient caregivers in the home (e.g., mother's boyfriend). Families at highest risk for maltreatment are those families experiencing social isolation, family violence, parenting stress, and poor parent–child relationships (CDC, 2009b).

> **DID YOU KNOW?** *More than three-quarters (75.7%) of the children who died because of child abuse and neglect were younger than 4 years old.*

The consequences of child maltreatment are often devastating. Children experience long-term physical consequences as well as negative psychological and behavioral consequences. **Abusive head trauma** (AHT), also known as shaken baby syndrome, results from violent shaking or shaking and impacting of the head of an infant or young child. Intracranial injury, subdural bleeding, retinal hemorrhages, and skull fractures can result, leading to death or survival with associated motor impairments, visual deficits, and cognitive deficits.

Preventive strategies are necessary to reduce the incidence of child maltreatment. Parental education should be started prenatally to prevent AHT. Nurses can use home visiting programs, peer mentoring programs, preschool and Head Start programs, and public health centers to identify at-risk families and provide support and education to prevent child maltreatment. Nurses can provide education to those individuals in the community who work with children on recognizing signs of abuse and how to report suspected maltreatment. Increased awareness within the community and early intervention can prevent maltreatment from occurring and rescue children from violent and unsafe abuse situations.

Injury Prevention

Health care provider offices, schools, community centers, public health centers, and daycare/preschool facilities provide opportunities to teach children, adolescents, and their families about prevention of injuries. Safety and health promotion can be incorporated into required health education courses within the school systems. Community-sponsored car seat and seat belt safety checks and safety fairs are another way to educate families. Early home visitation programs to high-risk families resulted in a reduction of 48% in child abuse. Injury prevention is a topic that should be addressed at all health visits.

Reducing Gun Violence. In 2007, 3067 (3.62 per 100,000) children and adolescents died from firearm-related injury. A survey of adolescents found that 5.2% had carried a gun on at least one day during the previous month. Witnessing gun violence or knowing the victims affects children indirectly (National Center for Injury Prevention and Control, 2007).

A recent study compared firearm-related mortality rates in urban and rural settings. The study found no significant differences in the death rates between the settings but noted a difference in the firearm intent that resulted in deaths for children and adolescents. The urban victims died from high rates of firearm homicide while the rural victims experienced high rates of firearm suicide and unintentional firearm-related accidental deaths. This study provides evidence that to reduce firearm mortality effectively, prevention strategies should be geared for the specific type of firearm injury issue within the community of interest (Nance et al, 2010).

Characteristics associated with gun violence include history of aggressive behaviors, poverty, school problems, substance

BOX 29-4   GUIDELINES FOR PLAYGROUND SAFETY

- Playgrounds should be surrounded by a barrier to protect children from traffic.
- Activity centers should be distributed to avoid crowding in one area.
- Surfaces should be finished with substances that meet Consumer Product Safety Commission (CPSC) regulations for lead.
- Durable materials should be used.
- Sand, gravel, wood chips, and wood mulch (not CCA treated) are acceptable surfaces for limiting the shock of falls.
- Equipment should be inspected regularly for protrusions that could puncture skin or entangle clothes.
- Inspect equipment for openings/angles that allow for possible head entrapment.
- Multiple-occupancy swings, animal swings, rope swings, and trampolines are not recommended.

From U.S. Consumer Product Safety Commission: *Public Playground Safety Handbook,* April 2008.

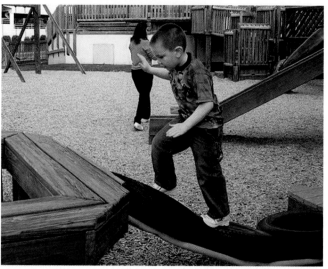

FIGURE 29-11 Playground injuries are frequent among young children.

abuse, and cultural acceptance of violent behavior. Young children are inquisitive and often imitate in play what they see in the media and on television. A significant number of accidental firearm injuries and deaths in children occur in the homes of friends and family members. Interventions must begin early and address each of these factors.

The *Healthy People 2020* objectives seek to reduce the number of high school students who carry weapons. Nurses can actively participate in efforts to reduce gun violence among young people in the following ways:

- Urge legislators to support gun control legislation.
- Collaborate with schools to develop programs to discourage violence among children.
- Encourage families to remove guns from their homes. If unable to do this, educate families to:
  - Store all firearms unloaded and uncocked in a securely locked container. Only the parents should know where the container is located.
  - Store the guns and ammunition in separate locked locations.
  - When handling or cleaning a gun, never leave it unattended, even for a moment; it should be in the parent's view at all times.
- Initiate community programs focusing on gun storage and safety at school.
- Educate parents on communicating with the homeowners of the homes their children visit regarding gun access and safety.
- Children and adolescents learning to hunt in rural areas should take gun safety courses.
- Identify populations at risk for violence and target aggression or anger management.
- Discourage mixing alcohol or drugs with guns.

Promoting Safe Playgrounds and Recreation Areas. Schools, daycare centers, families, and community groups often need guidance toward developing safe places for children to play. Each year, more than 200,000 children are treated in emergency

BOX 29-5   INJURY PREVENTION TOPICS

- Car restraints, seat belts, air-bag safety
- Preventing fires, burns
- Poison prevention
- Preventing falls
- Preventing drowning, water safety
- Bicycle safety
- Safe driving practices
- Sports safety
- Pedestrian safety
- Gun control
- Decreasing gang activities
- Substance abuse prevention

departments for injuries sustained on playgrounds and play sets. Approximately 45% of playground-related injuries are severe injuries and include fractures, internal injuries, concussions, dislocations, and amputations. Between 1990 and 2000, 147 children under the age of 14 died from playground-related injuries. These deaths were attributable to strangulation (56%) and falls (20%) to the playground surface, with most of these deaths (70%) occurring on home playgrounds (Tinsworth and McDonald, 2001; CDC, 2009c).

The U.S. Consumer Product Safety Commission has published guidelines for public and home playground safety. Guidelines cover structure, materials, surfaces, and maintenance of equipment (Box 29-4). The developmental skills of specific ages are incorporated, as well as recommendations for physically challenged children. Nurses can use these guidelines to help the community establish standards for play areas (Figure 29-11).

Nurses share responsibility in the prevention of intentional and unintentional injuries in the pediatric population. Assessment of the characteristics of the child, family, and environment identifies risk factors. Interventions include anticipatory guidance, modification of the environment, and safety education.

Education focuses on age-appropriate interventions based on knowledge of leading causes of death and risk factors. Topics to consider are listed in Box 29-5 (see also the Evolve website).

HEALTH PROBLEMS OF CHILDHOOD

Acute Illnesses

Acute illnesses are those illnesses with an abrupt onset and are usually of a short duration. For children, it is common for viruses to spread easily through daycares, preschools, and school systems. Nurses use developmental factors at each age to plan assessment and intervention strategies to prevent the spread of illnesses between children. Community-focused interventions, education, and programs can prevent many childhood illnesses.

Hand washing is a simple and reliable strategy to reduce the incidence of acute illnesses in children (Box 29-6). Infants and young children are particularly at risk for contracting viral and bacterial illnesses spread by contact because their immune systems are not yet fully developed. Focusing community education on preschools, daycare centers, and other programs that serve the families of infants and young children can reduce the occurrence of acute illnesses.

Several strategies can be used to reduce the occurrence of acute illnesses as follows: sanitizing objects such as toys that are handled by multiple children each day to prevent the spread of diseases; practicing good hand hygiene and diaper disposal techniques in daycares to prevent the spread of illnesses; and educating parents, daycares, and schools on when to keep children home to prevent putting others at risk for illness.

Influenza is a common viral illness that affects children and adolescents primarily during the winter months. It is a highly contagious acute febrile illness of the nose, throat, and lungs that leads to missed school days and can result in complications including pneumonia and infrequently death. The best prevention strategy is vaccinations for all children ages 6 months and above. It is important to educate families about the need for vaccination and home management of symptoms.

In 2009, a new influenza A strain was identified and known as **H1N1,** otherwise known as the "swine flu." This new strain of influenza virus contained a combination of swine, avian, and human influenza virus genes and cases were reported in all 50 states. For children, this particular influenza strain was noted to have more severe and frequent complications compared with other influenza types (CDC, 2009a).

Nurses can focus on preventive measures and promote high vaccination rates, good hand-washing hygiene, and early identification to prevent the spread of illness. If a child or adolescent is diagnosed with influenza, parents can be instructed to keep children at home until symptoms have improved and fever has been gone for 24 hours. Nurses can be actively involved in developing community-based policies in the event of a pandemic, and this may include plans for mass immunizations, specific flu clinics, and protocols for school closures.

Sudden infant death syndrome (SIDS) is defined as the sudden death of an infant under 1 year of age, which remains unexplained after a thorough case investigation, including performance of a complete autopsy, examination of the death

---

BOX 29-6   TEACHING FAMILIES ABOUT HAND WASHING

Always wash your hands *before*:
- Preparing foods
- Eating
- Touching someone who is sick
- Inserting or removing contact lenses

Always wash your hands *after*:
- Preparing foods, particularly raw meats or poultry
- Using the toilet
- Changing a diaper
- Touching animals, animal toys, leashes, or animal waste
- Blowing your nose, coughing, or sneezing into your hands
- Touching someone who is sick

Or anytime you feel that your hands need washing!

How to wash your hands:
- Wet your hands with warm running water
- Apply soap (liquid, bar, or powder)
- Lather your hands well
- Rub your hands vigorously for at least 20 seconds (sing the "Happy Birthday" song)—scrub all surfaces including between your fingers, under your nails, backs of your hands, and your wrist
- Rinse your hands well
- Dry your hands with a clean towel, disposable towel, or air dryer
- Use your towel to turn off the faucet if possible

---

scene, and review of the clinical history (AAP, 2005). The peak age for SIDS deaths occurs between 2 and 3 months of age, although SIDS may occur up to 1 year of age. There are specific independent risk factors for SIDS:
- Prone or side-lying sleep position
- Sleeping on a soft surface
- Maternal smoking during pregnancy
- Overheating
- Late or no prenatal care
- Young maternal age
- Preterm birth and/or low birth weight
- Male gender

There are consistently higher rates of SIDS in African-American and American Indian/Alaska Native infants—two to three times the national average. The incidence has decreased more than 50% since the "Back to Sleep" campaign was promoted in 1994. There is no test to identify infants who may die, making this a frustrating clinical problem. Nurses should teach the preventive measures found in Box 29-7.

When an infant dies from SIDS, the family requires tremendous support. The nurse provides empathetic support and assists the family as they progress through the grief process and provides guidance for siblings and other family members. Referral to support groups may be helpful.

Chronic Health Conditions

Improved medical technology has increased the number of children surviving with chronic health problems. In addition, environmental factors are leading to an increase in certain chronic health conditions. At present, it is estimated that about 26% of American children have a chronic health condition

(Van Cleave, Gortmaker, and Perrin, 2010). Some examples of common chronic conditions in children are Down syndrome, spina bifida, cerebral palsy, asthma, ADHD, diabetes, congenital heart disease, cancer, hemophilia, bronchopulmonary dysplasia, and AIDS.

Despite the differences in the specific diagnoses, all of these families have complex needs and face similar problems. Several variables exist to assess for each child and family:

- What is the actual health status? Is the condition stable or life threatening?
- What is the degree of impairment to the child's ability to develop?
- What types of treatments and therapy are required and with what frequency?
- How often are health care visits and hospitalizations required?
- To what degree are the family routines disrupted?

The common issues nurses will want to evaluate for these families include the following:

- All children and adolescents with chronic health problems need routine health care. The same issues of pediatric health promotion and acute health care need to be addressed with this group. The use of the medical home (discussed later in the chapter) is very important for this population.
- Ongoing medical care specific to the health problem needs to be provided. Examples include monitoring for complications of the health problem, medications management, dietary adjustments, and coordination of therapies. Evaluation of the effectiveness of the treatment plan is critical.
- Care is often provided by multiple specialists. There is a need for coordinating the scheduling of visits, tests, or procedures and the treatment regimen.
- Skilled care procedures are often required and may include suctioning, positioning, medications, feeding techniques, breathing treatments, physical therapy, and use of appliances.
- Equipment needs are often complex and may include monitors, oxygen, ventilators, positioning or ambulation devices, infusion pumps, and suction machines.

- Educational needs are often complex. Communication between the family, the team of health care providers, school administrators, and teachers is essential to meet the child's health and educational needs.
- Safe transportation to health care services and school must be available. Several barriers may exist, including family resources, location, and the burden of supportive equipment.
- Financial resources may not be adequate to meet the needs.
- Behavioral issues include the effect of the condition on the child's behavior as well as on other family members.

The ultimate goal is for children with chronic health conditions to achieve optimal health and functioning. Identifying barriers for individual families and overall community barriers is a focus for nurses. Developing support groups, advocating for improved community access to resources, and educating those working with these children on their conditions and needs will promote the family's functioning. Box 29-8 details a community nursing approach to supporting a child with ADHD.

WHAT DO YOU THINK? *Many children with chronic health conditions have physical limitations requiring adaptive devices and the use of wheelchairs. All children love to play, but most playgrounds are designed with equipment that is not friendly to children with physical disabilities. Should communities be required to adapt or build playgrounds with wheelchair access and swings for disabled children so that all children can enjoy outdoor play?*

Mental Health

Psychosocial stressors have increased over the years for children, and there is a current focus on pediatric mental health issues. There are many underlying causes for mental health problems

EVIDENCE-BASED PRACTICE

California has a large Hmong population. Despite having health insurance, community providers noted that the Hmong children consistently had lower than national and state levels for immunizations. The authors conducted a study to determine the primary barriers for this cultural group related to immunizing their children. The study identified two primary barriers to immunization: lower socioeconomic status and greater use of traditional Hmong health care (shamans and herbalists).

Nurse Use

We often make assumptions about the barriers to positive health decisions or behaviors. This study demonstrates that cultural differences can be influential in making health care decisions. By targeting the specific population of concern, nurses can identify the specific barriers that prevent parents from obtaining preventive health care. Public health nurses can then develop interventions and education to address those specific barriers and improve pediatric health.

From Baker D, Dang M, Diaz R: Perception of barriers to immunization among parents of Hmong origin in California, *Am J Public Health* 100:839-845, 2010.

in children, ranging from lead poisoning to exposure to violence in the home. Approximately 11% of children and adolescents have mental health problems with functional impairment. Children who live in poverty, live with a single parent, or are exposed to violence are at higher risk for developing a mental health condition. Only 20% of children with a mental health or substance abuse problem are currently receiving treatment (AACAP, 2009).

Some of the common mental health problems diagnosed in children and adolescents are anxiety disorders, autism spectrum disorders, depression, bipolar disorder, conduct disorder, oppositional defiant disorder, and substance abuse (AACAP, 2009). Each of these mental health diagnoses has a specific set of criteria for diagnosis found in the DSM-IV. Early recognition and coordinated management of pediatric mental health issues is critical to a child's functioning in school, home, and the community.

Many families can be at a loss for the behaviors or symptoms they observe in their child. A sense of embarrassment may prohibit parents from seeking help. Nurses can be instrumental in promoting community awareness about common mental health problems in children and identifying resources for families. The use of the medical home to coordinate management of mental health problems is important in the ability to provide oversight of subspecialties, medications, and therapies. A challenge for treating pediatric mental health disorders is an inadequate number of practitioners specializing in pediatric mental health, which may leave some families without adequate support and resources.

DID YOU KNOW?   *Bullying has always been an issue for children and adolescents. With the extensive use of texting, e-mails, social networking, and other means of electronic communication among tweens and adolescents, cyber bullying has become a significant problem within communities. Girls are more likely to be victims of cyber bullying, and victims report thinking about self-harm and/or suicide as a result of bullying. Cyber bullying includes sending*

hurtful messages, starting rumors, and uploading and sharing unflattering or altered photographs of the victims via an electronic means. Many cyber bullies use avatars or other ways of disguising their true identity, which makes it difficult for the victim to know who the bully is. The victims often do not report cyber bullying for fear of retaliation from the bully.

Environmental Health

The built environment that children and adolescents live in directly affects their health. Growth, size, and behaviors place the pediatric population at greater risk for damage from various toxins. Lead poisoning is one of the most common environmental health hazards. Pesticides, mercury exposure, plasticizers, and poor air quality also pose serious risks. Common toxins and sources of pediatric exposure are listed in Table 29-7.

Growing tissues absorb toxins readily. Developing organ systems are more susceptible to damage. Smaller size means increased concentration of toxins per pound of body weight. The fact that children are short exposes them to lower air spaces, where heavy chemicals tend to concentrate. Outdoor play, especially during summer months, increases the opportunity for exposure to air pollutants. Chewing and mouthing behaviors offer contact to toxins such as lead. Playing on the floor increases exposure to chemicals in rugs and flooring. Rolling and playing in grass can result in pesticide exposure and playground materials that are treated with chemicals put children at risk. Exposure risks for adolescents are similar to those for adults and are primarily through work, school, and hobbies.

It is critical to assess for these environmental health hazards during health care visits. Referral for treatment may be necessary (AAP, 2005a). Counseling families on risk reduction is important to children's health. Population-focused nurses identify environmental problems within the community and target at-risk populations with community interventions (see Table 29-8 for examples). Bringing screening programs into neighborhoods at risk may facilitate early identification and prevent complications. Lobbying efforts and education can effect public policy changes to make the environment healthier. The case presentation in Box 29-9 gives an example of how a school environment can lead to health problems.

Lead Poisoning.   Lead is a heavy metal that is absorbed into the body primarily through ingestion. Lead poisoning is defined as a serum lead level above 10 µg/dL and causes significant neurological, cardiovascular, and renal disease. A *Healthy People 2020* goal is to eliminate elevated blood lead levels in all children. More than 250,000 children ages 1 to 5 have lead poisoning, and the most common exposure is through lead-based paints and lead-contaminated soil and dust in houses built before 1987 (AAP, 2005b).

A more recent exposure risk is through imported toys and costume jewelry that are painted with a lead-based paint. Young children are exposed through their mouthing behaviors. If a piece of contaminated costume jewelry is accidentally swallowed, the high lead concentration can result in death. In 2007, the U.S. Consumer Products Safety Commission

TABLE 29-7 COMMON ENVIRONMENTAL AGENTS HAZARDOUS TO CHILDREN

TOXINS	SOURCES
Arsenic	Food, water
Asbestos	Building materials: insulation, ceilings, floor tiles
Carbon monoxide	Space heaters, woodstoves, fireplaces, engine exhaust, tobacco smoke
Lead	Paint, dust, soil, water, occupational exposure (e.g., battery plant), hobbies (e.g., stained glass)
Mercury	Water contamination, fish, thermometer/sphygmomanometer breakage
Molds	Food, ubiquitous to moist outdoor and indoor environment
Nitrites, nitrates	Water, food
Nicotine, benzene, tars	Environmental tobacco smoke
Particulate matter	Outdoor air pollution, dust mites, animal dander, roach parts
Pesticides	Food, soil, plants, water, air, topical application for lice treatment, home and school insect management
Phthalates and bisphenol (BPA)	Linings of canned foods, children's toys, vinyl flooring, hard plastics made of polycarbonate (many sports water bottles and baby bottles)
Solvents/volatile organic compounds	Furniture, carpet, building materials, solvents and degreasers, cleaning products, acetone, formaldehyde
Ultraviolet light	Outdoor sun exposure, tanning beds

TABLE 29-8 PREVENTION STRATEGIES APPLIED TO ENVIRONMENTAL HAZARDS

PREVENTION STRATEGIES	EXAMPLES
Primary	
Identification of at-risk populations	Substandard housing communities
	Pregnant women
	Children with asthma
Health education about environmental risks	Poison prevention
	Responses to poor air quality alerts
	Discontinue use of plasticizers
Formation of public health policies	Air/water quality standards
	Safety inspections: playgrounds, schools, daycare centers
	Standards for lead levels in imported products intended for children
Research to assess impact of environmental hazards on the pediatric population	Developing reference ranges/biological markers to assess toxic levels in children
	Identify long-term physiological and cognitive consequences of exposure to environmental toxins
Secondary	
Early detection, treatment, and referral for management of environmental toxins	Removal of at-risk persons when lead hazards are detected
	Assessment of lead levels of populations of at-risk children with treatment of individuals as indicated
Tertiary	
Restoration of environment and occupants to healthier state	Asbestos/lead abatement of buildings
	Radon remediation of homes
	Replacement of heating, ventilation, air conditioning, systems contaminated with mold
	Chelating agents for individuals with lead toxic levels

Modified from Burns C, Dunn A, Sattler B: Resources for environmental health problems, *J Pediatr Health Care* 16:3, 2002.

(CPSC) issued numerous recalls for these toys and passed the Consumer Product Safety Improvement Act in 2008 that requires third-party testing and certification of all imported toys and products marketed to children (Galvez et al, 2009).

Universal screening for lead poisoning of all children at ages 1 and 2 years is recommended. This screening is recommended when children receive well-child or EPSDT screening at regular intervals. In addition, families should be assessed for environmental risk factors to determine the need for screening at other ages. Specific guidelines for minimizing lead exposure through contaminated toys is included in Box 29-10.

Mercury. Mercury is a heavy metal like lead. The most common exposure for humans is the ingestion of contaminated fish. Mercury poisoning is determined with a blood mercury level of 5.8 µg/L or above. Mercury poisoning can result in significant developmental deficits, and the fetuses of pregnant women are particularly vulnerable. Screening for dietary intake and other

BOX 29-9   CASE PRESENTATION: THE BUILT ENVIRONMENT

A child's built environment includes exposure to media and the resulting influence on behavior and choices. Food and beverage corporations spend over $1.6 billion each year on advertising that specifically targets children. Much of this advertising uses licensed cartoon characters to promote food products with the majority of products being of poor nutritional value. The heart of the question is whether this advertising is effective in influencing children's food choices. A study by Roberto et al (2010) looked at the preferences of preschool children for food packaged with a licensed cartoon character. The study found that preschoolers rated the taste of the foods packaged with the licensed character over the identical food without the character packaging. The children also selected the high-density character-packaged foods more often. Nurses in the community can use this information to provide guidance to parents to limit exposure to television and media, make healthy food choices for their children, and avoid unhealthy foods packaged with licensed cartoon characters. Nurses can also advocate for stricter advertising laws for those unhealthy foods targeted to children.

From Roberto CA, Baik J, Harris JL, Brownell KD: Influence of licensed characters on children's taste and snack preferences, *Pediatrics* 126:88-93, 2010.

BOX 29-10   STEPS TO MINIMIZE LEAD EXPOSURE IN CONTAMINATED TOYS AND PRODUCTS

- Read recall notices from the CPSC (www.cpsc.gov) and do not buy recalled toys.
- Check old toys at home to make sure they have not been recalled.
- Avoid purchasing toys second hand from yard sales and flea markets.
- Check labels and recommended ages on all toy labels and follow recommendations.
- Do not purchase children's costume jewelry or allow children to play with adult costume jewelry.

possible exposures is critical to identification of risk factors. The nurses' responsibility is to educate families on how to minimize mercury exposure risks. It is recommended that families eat commercially caught fish that are low in mercury (tilapia, Alaskan salmon, herring). For pregnant women, women of child-bearing age, breastfeeding mothers, and young children, these steps are recommended:

- Avoid ingesting shark, tilefish, and king mackerel because of the high mercury levels
- Limit intake of tuna to 4 to 6 ounces each week and all other fishes to 12 ounces each week

Plasticizers. Phthalates and bisphenol (BPA) are chemicals that are commonly added to plastics to create flexibility and durability. Exposure to these products has caused significant adverse health effects in animal studies. Human studies have noted a link between BPA and cardiovascular and liver disease. The possible exposures for children are many and include the linings of canned foods (ready-to-feed formulas), children's toys, vinyl flooring, and hard plastics made of polycarbonate (many sports water bottles and baby

LEVELS OF PREVENTION

Lead Poisoning

Primary Prevention
Community education about lead exposure, lead sources in the community, and the adverse health consequences for children.

Secondary Prevention
Implement universal screening for all children ages 1 and 2 years that present to the community health centers and primary care practices.

Tertiary Prevention
Provide families with guidance and resources for lead abatement and to eliminate lead exposure for children with blood lead levels >10 µg/dL.

bottles). Increased exposure occurs when these products are exposed to high heat, which occurs with the sterilization of baby bottles. The half-life of these plasticizers is very short, which makes it difficult to thoroughly screen for exposure (Galvez, 2009).

The Consumer Products Safety Act of 2009 provided guidelines for eliminating these plasticizers nationally from children's products. Continued education of families is needed until all of these plasticizers are no longer available for purchase, and recommendations on avoiding second-hand children's products should be promoted.

Environmental Tobacco Smoke

Environmental tobacco smoke (ETS) is exhaled smoke, smoke from burning tobacco, or smoke from the mouthpiece or filter end of a cigarette, cigar, or pipe. Cigarettes have many known poisons, and both cigarettes and ETS were classified as Class A known human carcinogens in 1992 by the Environmental Protection Agency (EPA, 2009). Parents often do not understand or believe the effects of smoking on children. Children, particularly those under age 5 years and those living in poverty, have higher levels of exposure to ETS.

Children exposed to ETS experience increased episodes of middle ear infections, asthma, upper respiratory tract infections, and more missed school days. Prenatal exposure to ETS is linked to preterm births, low birth weight, and increased risk for several childhood cancers. Prenatal exposure is also linked to the fetal brain becoming sensitized to nicotine, leading to greater addiction when exposed at an older age. Children living in smoking households with a parent role modeling smoking are more likely to start smoking (AAP, 2009b).

Interventions to discourage smoking focus on the parent, the child or adolescent, and public policy. Offer educational programs for parents dealing with the negative effects of smoking on children, interventions to stop smoking, and ways to create a smoke-free environment. Anti-smoking programs directed toward children and teenagers are more successful if the focus is on short-term effects rather than on long-term effects. Developmentally, children and teenagers cannot visualize the future to imagine the consequences of smoking. Teaching social skills to resist peer pressure is critical.

BOX 29-11   COMMUNITY INTERVENTIONS TO REDUCE ETS EXPOSURE

- Collaborate with schools to provide tobacco-free environments (for all school facilities, vehicles, and events).
- Work with schools to provide prevention curricula in elementary, middle, and high schools.
- Develop or identify smoking cessation programs and provide information to health care providers and workplaces in the community.
- Provide education to families on the dangers of ETS exposure for children and adolescents.
- Partnership with community merchants to enforce minors' access laws
- Advocate for local policy change to limit smoking in public and private enterprises.

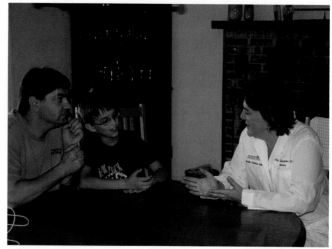

FIGURE 29-12 Motivational interviewing is an effective way for nurses to intervene with families and promote positive behavioral change in the home.

Nurses will want to become politically active in the area of smoking. Banning tobacco advertising, enforcing restrictions of sale to minors, increasing funds for anti-smoking education, and restriction of public smoking may reduce the incidence of smoking. Community-based interventions to reduce smoking and ETS exposure are included in Box 29-11.

MODELS FOR HEALTH CARE DELIVERY TO CHILDREN AND ADOLESCENTS

Nurses are in a position to work with specific populations through programs targeting the health care needs of children and particularly those at risk. In the following section, strategies for promoting the health care of children and adolescents are described.

Family-Centered Medical Home

A **family-centered medical home** is a partnership between a child or adolescent, the child or adolescent's family, and the pediatric team who oversees the child or adolescent's health and well-being within a community-based system that provides uninterrupted care to promote optimal health outcomes. The **medical home** incorporates preventive, acute, and chronic care from birth through transition to adulthood. The medical home emphasizes an integrated health system with collaboration of care from an interprofessional team of primary care physicians, specialists and subspecialists, other health professionals, hospitals and health care facilities, public health, and the community working with children and families (AMCHP, 2010).

Approximately 58% of all children have a medical home compared with 47% of children with special health care needs. It is imperative to increase the use of medical homes for all children, particularly children with special health care needs (AMCHP, 2010). A child with Down syndrome will greatly benefit from collaborative care from the primary care provider, subspecialty physicians, school system, community therapists, family support groups, and other community resources to achieve optimal health.

A successful medical home relies on the multitude of supports that are brought to the service delivery system that surrounds the family and community. Families can trust that there is a place where their child or adolescent is provided holistic care that addresses all aspects of physical, mental, and emotional health. The medical home is not a specific building, but it is a system of care that is accessible, continuous, comprehensive, coordinated, compassionate, and culturally effective. Nurses in the community play an active role as a team member of the medical home by identifying resources for families, referring families to a medical home, and participating in the health care of children in medical homes.

Motivational Interviewing

Motivational interviewing is a focused communication strategy in which the parents are encouraged to set goals, identify personal barriers, and identify potential mechanisms to overcome the barriers to make safety and health promotion changes for their child. This can be an effective intervention to promote healthy changes within the family environment. It can be easily implemented by nurses in primary care settings and public health clinics under limited time constraints (Levensky et al, 2007) and is readily incorporated into the medical home model.

Motivational interviewing emphasizes a collaborative approach to behavior change instead of a prescriptive approach (Figure 29-12). Nurses use open-ended questioning and reflection to encourage the parent or adolescent to share their identified barriers to change. When individuals demonstrate positive comments toward change, the nurse expands upon those comments and provides further support for that change. This strategy is very effective with positive health behavior changes such as smoking cessation, healthy eating, and safety behaviors. (See Appendix F.4 in the back of the book.)

Interactive Health Communication

In 1999 **interactive health communication (IHC)** was defined as the use of an electronic device or communication technology to access or transmit health information or provide health-related support to any consumer or health care professional (Science Panel on Interactive Communication and Health,

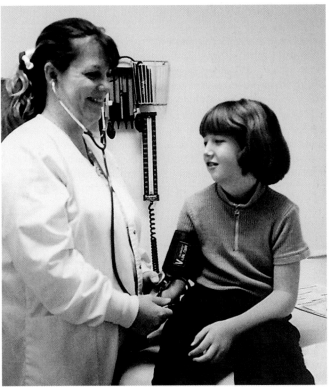

FIGURE 29-13 A child gets her blood pressure taken during a well-child care assessment. (Contributed by Cynthia Rubenstein.)

BOX 29-12 COMMUNITY RESOURCES FOR PEDIATRIC HEALTH CARE

- Children's service clinics
- Well-child clinics
- Immunization clinics
- Infectious disease clinics
- Children's Specialty Services
- Family violence/child abuse centers
- Homeless shelters
- School health programs
- Head Start
- Parents Anonymous
- Crisis hotlines
- Community education classes
- Early intervention/developmental services
- Childbirth education classes
- Breastfeeding support groups
- Parent support groups
- Family planning clinics
- Women, Infants, and Children (WIC) programs
- Medicaid and CHIP
- Youth employment/training programs

---

easy-access point for parents to find health information. While it is difficult to determine exact numbers of users, more than 60%, and up to 90%, of American adults have searched the Internet for health and disease information, with female users less than 65 years of age being the predominant group of users to search for this information (Fox, 2006; AHRQ, 2011). Of those searching online for health information, 60% report that information found online affected their health decisions (Fox and Jones, 2009).

There are many reliable, accurate health information websites available through national and state agencies as well as private corporations. Community and public health nurses can refer families to these sites for additional information on many health topics and preventive health guides. Social networking sites provide a means for online peer support groups for new mothers and parents of children with special health needs. E-mail provides a quick and simple communication method for families to communicate with partners within the medical home to get questions answered easily and accurately.

ROLE OF THE POPULATION-FOCUSED NURSE IN CHILD AND ADOLESCENT HEALTH

Population-focused nurses have the opportunity to work with families to achieve growth toward many of the *Healthy People 2020* objectives. They practice in a variety of settings, including community health centers, school-based clinics, and home health programs. They provide care through well-child clinics, immunization programs, federally mandated programs (such as the nutrition program Women, Infants, and Children [WIC]), or specific state-funded programs, such as Head Start.

With the legislation to expand national health care, strategies to implement improved access will likely include expanding the role of nurses and the settings for practice. The nursing process and a knowledge base of the factors unique to the pediatric population provide a framework of care. Nursing, through developing and coordinating community services and through formation of public policies, promotes the well-being of children and families within the community. Assessments are made to identify the needs and target populations at risk (Figure 29-13). Programs based on the needs of specific at-risk populations are developed for the delivery of health care.

The nursing plan of care includes three major components. The first is the management of actual or potential health problems. The second involves both education and anticipatory guidance. This enables families to understand what to expect in the areas of growth and development as well as social, emotional, and cognitive changes. Nurses offer information to promote healthy lifestyles and to prevent acute and chronic health problems as well as unintentional injuries. A third role is case management or coordination of care. For example, the nurse coordinates referrals to community agencies, other health care services or providers, or assistance programs. Box 29-12 lists community resources.

1999). Over the past decade, there has been a phenomenal growth in the development and use of IHC.

The purpose of IHC for families is to provide general or individualized pediatric health information and promote healthy choices and safety. The Internet provides an inexpensive,

LINKING CONTENT TO PRACTICE

In this chapter, emphasis is placed on the community health needs of children and adolescents within the context of the family. The public health core functions of disease prevention, health promotion, and the three levels of health services are directly related to the pediatric population and their specific population needs. To meet the core public health competencies, nurses must learn how to assess children and adolescents using developmental principles to determine safety risks for injury and environmental health exposures. Policy and program development for the pediatric population is geared toward improving the built environment in which a child grows and providing parents with education on health promotion strategies like smoking cessation to improve their child's

health. Nurses develop competencies in communication strategies with children of varying developmental levels and recognize the various locations in the community that need education on promoting the health of children (e.g., daycare centers, schools). Basic health services such as well-child care and immunizations are critical to the health of the pediatric population, and the nurse is poised as a leader within the medical home model of health care delivery for children and adolescents. This chapter prepares the community health nurse to provide comprehensive, developmentally appropriate education to families; deliver basic health care services in a holistic approach; and develop community programming to improve safety and environmental wellness for children and adolescents.

HEALTHY PEOPLE 2020

Objectives Focused on Children and Adolescents

Education and Community-Based Programs
- ECB-4: Increase the proportion of elementary, middle, and senior high schools that provide school health education to promote personal health and wellness in the following areas: hand washing or hand hygiene; oral health; growth and development; sun safety and skin cancer prevention; benefits of rest and sleep; ways to prevent vision and hearing loss; and the importance of health screenings and checkups.
- ECB-7: Increase the proportion of middle, junior high, and senior high schools that provide comprehensive school health education to prevent health problems in the following areas: unintentional injury; violence; suicide; tobacco use and addiction; alcohol or other drug use; unintended pregnancy; HIV/AIDS and STD infection; unhealthy dietary patterns; inadequate physical activity; and environmental health.
- ECB-11: Increase the proportion of local health departments that have established culturally appropriate and linguistically competent community health promotion and disease prevention programs for racial and ethnic minority populations.

Environmental Health
- EH-8: Eliminate elevated blood lead levels in children.
- EH-17: Increase the proportion of persons living in pre-1978 housing that have tested for the presence of lead-based paint.

Immunizations and Infectious Disease
- IID-7: Achieve and maintain effective vaccination coverage levels for universally recommended vaccines among young children.

Injury/Violence Prevention
- IVP-1: Reduce fatal and non-fatal unintentional injuries.
- IVP-16: Increase use of age appropriate child restraints in cars.

Maternal, Infant, and Child Care
- MICH-4: Reduce deaths of adolescents and young adults.

Nutrition and Weight Status
- NWS-10: Reduce the proportion of children and adolescents who are overweight or obese.

Physical Activity and Fitness
- PA-3: Increase the proportion of adolescents who meet current physical activity guidelines.
- PA-4: Increase the proportion of the nation's public and private schools that require daily physical education for all students.

Tobacco Use
- TU-15: Tobacco-free environments in schools, including all school facilities, property, vehicles, and school events.
- TU-18: Reduce the proportion of adolescents and young adults exposed to tobacco advertising and promotion.

From U.S. Department of Health and Human Services: *Healthy People 2020*, Washington, DC, 2010, U.S. Government Printing Office.

CHAPTER REVIEW

PRACTICE APPLICATION

Sam is a 4-year-old boy brought to the clinic by his mother for his 4-year well-child check and immunizations. Sam will be attending the local Head Start program in the fall. He is the oldest of three children and his siblings are 9 months and 35 months. His mother is a single parent who works at a local restaurant as a waitress. Sam and his siblings are insured by Medicaid. Mom is 24 years old and the family lives with the maternal grandparents. Sam's mother is in good health and does not smoke or abuse drugs. Sam has been watched by his grandmother since birth and is exposed to cigarette smoke in the home by both grandparents.

On the developmental exam, Sam is very cooperative, eager to please, and speaks clearly. His development is significant for failure to identify three colors, count to 5, or recognize any letters. His gross motor skills are appropriate but he only scribbles when given a crayon. Sam reports enjoying watching television with his family for fun. On physical examination, Sam has a >95th percentile BMI for age/gender but no other abnormal exam findings are noted. Hearing and vision are within normal limits for age.

Based on the above scenario, answer the following questions:
A. What additional history and assessment information should you collect based on the child's home environment?
B. What immunizations and lab tests are indicated based on his age and risk factors?
C. What education should you give this mother on changes in the home to promote development? To reduce ETS exposure? To ensure safety?
D. Based on the BMI percentile, what additional nutrition and dietary practices information should you obtain?
E. What interventions and education should you provide to this mother regarding Sam's obesity and associated risk factors?
F. In an analysis of the Medicaid child population in Sam's medical home, the population-focused nurse found that a number of children had similar risk factors. Is there a population-level intervention the nurse may want to use to reduce the risk in the future child population?

Answers can be found on the Evolve site.

KEY POINTS

- Physical growth and development is an ongoing process resulting in physical, cognitive, and emotional changes that affect health status.
- Good nutrition is essential for healthy growth and development, and it influences disease prevention in later life.
- Childhood obesity is increasing in prevalence. Modifiable risk factors include dietary intake, physical activity, and screen viewing time.
- Immunizations are successful in prevention of selected diseases. Barriers to immunizing children are parental concerns, cost, vaccine shortages, and changes in recommended vaccine scheduling.
- The built environment is influential on a child's physical, emotional, and psychosocial health. Nurses can design interventions for families and communities to improve a child's environment if improvement is indicated.
- The family is critical to the growth and development of the child. Social support has a powerful influence on successful parenting.
- Unintentional injuries are the major cause of morbidity and mortality in the child and adolescent population. Most are preventable. Nurses have a major role in anticipatory guidance and prevention.

- Population-focused nurses have a strong role in the prevention, identification, and education about child maltreatment. Child advocacy is critical to reduce the incidence of abuse and neglect in childhood.
- Minimizing complications of the major health risks to the pediatric and adolescent population follows the goals of *Healthy People 2020* initiatives.
- The pediatric population is vulnerable to environmental hazards. Decreasing exposure and identifying problems early are important areas for interventions by population-focused nurses.
- Nurses are involved in strategies to meet the needs of the pediatric population and their families in the community.
- The family-centered medical home is a successful system for coordinating health care for children and for facilitating continuous family support and health management.
- Children who are low income or live in poverty are at increased risk for violence, injuries, and environmental hazards.
- The use of motivational interviewing and IHC can facilitate positive health behavior changes for families with children.

CLINICAL DECISION-MAKING ACTIVITIES

1. Develop a plan of immunization for a 5½-year-old who has had one DTaP, Hib, and IPV. Be specific about due dates for immunizations.
2. Develop a screening program for children and adolescents who live in a low-income older neighborhood with a large percentage of Hispanic residents. What risk factors would you consider in the process? Have you examined the thoughts of others in the community that might affect the success of the screening program? Be specific.
3. Plan a survey of a school district to determine its "friendliness" to children with chronic health problems. How would you implement changes?
4. Develop a community program for smoking cessation. Identify how you will target parents and caregivers of children. Discuss how you will incorporate the concept of ETS exposure in your program.

5. Develop nutrition education programs for (1) mothers who are breastfeeding their infants, (2) a group of 5-year-olds in a kindergarten class, and (3) a group of high school sophomores. What factors do these programs have in common? How do they differ?
6. Administer a safety survey (e.g., the Injury Prevention Program [TIPP] from the American Academy of Pediatrics, or develop your own) to assess the home environment of a 6-month-old and a 5-year-old. Develop a plan of education and anticipatory guidance for the family. How would you apply this information to a larger population?

REFERENCES

AHRQ: *The CAHPS improvement guide practical strategies for improving the patient care experience. Internet access for health information and advice,* USDHHS, Rockville, Md. Available at http://www.ahrq.gov. Accessed June 17, 2011.

American Academy of Child and Adolescent Psychiatry: Committee on Health Care Access and Economics Task Force on Mental Health. Improving mental health services in primary care: reducing administrative and financial barriers to access and collaboration, *Pediatrics* 123(4):1248–1251, 2009.

American Academy of Pediatrics: Policy statement: active healthy living: prevention of childhood obesity through increased physical activity, *Pediatrics* 117(5): 1834–1842, 2006.

American Academy of Pediatrics: *Red book: 2009 Report of the Committee on Infectious Diseases,* ed 28, Elk Grove Village, IL, 2009a, AAP.

American Academy of Pediatrics: Technical report—secondhand and prenatal tobacco smoke exposure, *Pediatrics* 124:e1017–e1044, 2009b.

American Academy of Pediatrics: Policy statement: the future of pediatrics: mental health competencies for pediatric primary care, *Pediatrics* 124:410–421, 2009c.

American Academy of Pediatrics Committee on Nutrition: *Pediatric nutrition handbook,* ed 6, Elk Grove Village, IL, 2009d, AAP.

American Academy of Pediatrics: Policy statement: lead exposure in children: prevention, detection, and management, *Pediatrics* 116(4):1036–1046, 2005a.

American Academy of Pediatrics: Policy statement: the changing concept of sudden infant death syndrome: diagnostic coding shifts, controversies regarding the sleeping environment, and new variables to consider in reducing risk. *Pediatrics* 116(5):1245–1255, 2005b. doi:10.1542/peds.2005-1499.

American Academy of Pediatrics: Policy statement: prevention of pediatric overweight and obesity, *Pediatrics* 112(2):424–430, 2003.

American Academy of Pediatrics: *Children's health topics: environmental health,* 2005a. Available at http://www.aap.org/healthtopics/environmentalhealth.cfm.

American Diabetes Association: Type 2 diabetes in children and adolescents, *Pediatrics* 105:671–680, 2000.

American Dietetic Association: Position of the American Dietetic Association: Nutrition guidance for healthy children ages 2 to 11 years, *J Am Dietetic Assoc* 108(6):1038–1047. doi:10.1016/j.jada.2008.04.005.

Association of Maternal and Child Health Programs: Medical home. *Pulse Newsletter,* April 2010. Available at http://www.amchp.org/About AMCHP/Newsletters/Pulse/April2010/Documents/Pulse_April10.pdf.

Borse NN, Gilchrist J, Dellinger AM, et al: *CDC childhood injury report: patterns of unintentional injuries among 0-19 year olds in the United States, 2000-2006,* Atlanta, 2008, CDC, National Center for Injury Prevention and Control.

Bowman S, Gortmaker S, Ebbeling C, et al: Effects of fast-food consumption on energy intake and diet quality among children in a national household survey, *Pediatrics* 113(1):112–118, 2004. doi: 10.1542/peds.113.1.112.

Brown R, Arthur J, Karnon, Parnaby A: AAP Subcommittee on ADHD: treatment of ADHD: overview of the evidence, *Pediatrics* 115:749–757, 2010.

Burns C, Dunn A, Sattler B: Resources for environmental health problems, *J Pediatr Health Care* 16:3, 2002.

Burns J, Walsh L, Popovich J: Practical pediatric and adolescent immunization update, *J Nurse Practitioners* 6(4):254–266, 2010.

Centers for Disease Control and Prevention MMWR: Summary of notifiable diseases, *MMWR* 57(54):1–94, 2010.

Centers for Disease Control and Prevention: Economic and health burden of chronic disease. In Centers for Disease Control, editor: *National Center for Chronic Disease Prevention and Health Promotion,* Washington, DC, 2007a, CDC. Available at http://www.cdc.gov/nccdphp/press/. Accessed February 19, 2011.

Centers for Disease Control and Prevention: *Some common misconceptions about vaccination and how to respond to them,* 2007b. Available at http://www.cdc.gov/vaccines/vac-gen/6mishome.htm. Accessed February 19, 2011.

Centers for Disease Control and Prevention: *H1N1 flu (swine flu): general information,* 2009a, . Available at http://www.cdc.gov/h1n1flu/general_info.htm. Accessed February 19, 2011.

Centers for Disease Control and Prevention: *Injury prevention and control: child maltreatment. ,* 2009b. Available at http://www.cdc.gov/ViolencePrevention/childmaltreatment/index.html. Accessed February 19, 2011.

Centers for Disease Control and Prevention: *Playground injuries: FactSheet,* 2009c. Available at http://www.cdc.gov/HomeandRecreationalSafety/Playground-Injuries/playgroundinjuries-factsheet.htm. Accessed February 19, 2011.

Centers for Disease Control and Prevention: *Statistics & surveillance July 2007-June 2008, Table Data: Adolescents 13-17 years,* 2009d. Available at http://www.cdc.gov/vaccines/stats-surv/nisteen/data/tables_2008.htm. Accessed February 19, 2011.

Centers for Disease Control and Prevention: *Child passenger safety: fact sheet,* 2010a. Available at http://www.cdc.gov/ncipc/factsheets/childpas.htm#how big problem. Accessed February 19, 2011.

Centers for Disease Control and Prevention: *Statistics & surveillance July 2008-June 2009, Table Data: Children 19–35 months,* 2010b. Available at http://www.cdc.gov/vaccines/stats-surv/nis/data/tables_0809.htm. Accessed February 19, 2011.

Centers for Disease Control and Prevention: *Teen birth rates rose again in 2007,* 2010c. Available at http://www.cdc.gov/Features/dsTeenPregnancy/. Accessed February 19, 2011.

Centers For Disease Control and Prevention: *Defining overweight and obesity,* 2010d. Available at http://cdc.gov/obesity/defining.html. Accessed February 19, 2011.

Centers for Medicare & Medicaid Services (CMMS): *Low cost health insurance for families & children: the Children's Health Insurance Plan,* 2009. Available at http://www.cms.gov.

Centers for Medicare & Medicaid Services (CMMS): *Medicaid program: general information,* 2010. Available at www.cms.gov.

Central Intelligence Agency (CIA): *The world factbook: infant mortality rate,* 2009. Available at https://www.cia.gov/.

Cornette R: The emotional impact of obesity on children. *Worldviews on evidence-based nursing* 5(3):136–141, 2008. doi:10.1111/j.1741-6787.2008.00127.

DeNavas-Walt C, Proctor B, Smith J: *Income, poverty, and health insurance coverage in the U.S.: 2007,* 2008. Available at http://www.census.gov/prod/2008pubs/p60-235.pdf. Accessed February 19, 2011.

Division of State Children's Health Insurance: *2007 SCHIP annual reports: a review,* 2008. Available at http://www.cms.gov/NationalCHIPPolicy/downloads/Final2007CHIPAnnualReport.pdf.

English A: Understanding legal aspects of care. In Neinstein L, editor: *Adolescent health care: a practical guide,* ed 3, Philadelphia, 1996, Williams & Wilkins.

Environmental Protection Agency: *EPA designates passive smoking a class A human carcinogen,* August 2009. Available at http://www.epa.gov/history/topics/smoke/01.htm. Accessed February 19, 2011.

Federal Interagency Forum on Child and Family Statistics: *America's children in brief: key national indicators of well being,* 2008a. Available at http://www.childstats.gov/pdf/ac2008/ac_08.pdf. Accessed February 19, 2011.

Federal Interagency Forum on Child and Family Statistics: *Child population: number of children (in millions) ages 0-17 in the United States by age,* 2008b. Available at http://www.childstats.gov/americaschildren/tables/pop1.asp. Accessed February 19, 2011.

Fox S: *Pew Internet and American Life Project: online health search 2006,* 2006. Available at http://www.pewinternet.org.

Fox S, Jones S: *Pew Internet and American Life Project: the social life of health information,* 2009. Available at http://www.pewinternet.org/~/media/Files/Reports/2009/PIP_Health_2009.pdf. Accessed February 19, 2011.

Freedman D, Kettel Khan L, Dietz W, et al: Relationship of childhood obesity to coronary heart disease risk factors in adulthood: the Bogalusa Heart Study, *Pediatrics* 108(3):712–718, 2001. doi:10.1542/peds.108.3.712.

Gable S, Britt-Rankin J, Krull JL: Ecological predictors and developmental outcomes of persistent childhood overweight, USDA *Contractor and Cooperator Report, No. 42,* June 2008.

Galvez M, Graber N, Sheffield P, et al: Hot topics in pediatric environmental health, *Contemp Pediatr* 26(7):34–47, 2009.

Galvez MP, Pearl M, Yen IH: Childhood obesity and the built environment. *Curr Opin Pediatr* 22:202–207, 2010. doi:10.1097/MOP.0b013e328336eb6f.

Kaiser Family Foundation (KFF): *Medicaid enrollment: June 2009 data snapshot,* 2010. Available at http://www.kff.org/medicaid/upload/8050.pdf. Accessed February 19, 2011.

Kranz S, Siega-Riz A, Herring A: Changes in diet quality of American preschoolers between 1977 and 1998, *Am J Public Health* 94(9):1525–1530, 2004.

Lawrence VJ, Chowdhury T: The genetics of human obesity, In Barnett AH, Kumar S, editors: *Obesity and diabetes,* ed 2, West Sussex, England, 2004, John Wiley & Sons.

Leeb RT, Paulozzi L, Melanson C, et al: *Child maltreatment surveillance: uniform definitions for public health and recommended data elements, Version 1.0*, Atlanta, 2007, CDC, National Center for Injury Prevention and Control.

Levensky ER, Forcehimes A, O'Donohue WT, Beitz K: Motivational interviewing, *Am J Nurs* 107(10):50–58, 2007.

MacDorman M, Mathews T: *NCHS data brief: recent trends in infant mortality in the United States*, 2008. Available at http://www.cdc.gov/nchs/data/databriefs/db09.pdf. Accessed February 19, 2011.

Miller J, Kranzler J, Liu Y, et al: Neurocognitive findings in Prader-Willi syndrome and early-onset morbid obesity, *J Pediatr* 149:192–198, 2006. doi: 10.1016/j.jpeds.2006.04.013.

Nader N, Kumar S: Type 2 diabetes mellitus in children and adolescents: Where do we stand with drug treatment and behavioral management? *Curr Diabetes Rep* 8:383–388, 2008.

Nance M, Carr B, Kallan M, et al: Variation in pediatric and adolescent firearm mortality rate in rural and urban U.S. counties, *Pediatrics* 125(6):1112–1118, 2010. doi: 10.1542/peds.2009-3219.

National Center For Chronic Disease Prevention and Health Promotion: Youth risk behavior surveillance—United States, 2009 [pdf 3.5M], *MMWR* 59(SS-5):1–142, 2010.

National Center for Chronic Disease Prevention and Health Promotion: *School health policies and program study: physical education*. Available at http://www.cdc.gov/HealthyYouth/shpps/2006/factsheets/pdf/FS_PhysicalEducation_SHPPS2006.pdf. Accessed February 19, 2011b.

National Center for Injury Prevention & Control: *2007, U.S. Firearm deaths and rates per 100,000 for ages 0-19 years*, 2007. Available at http://webappa.cdc.gov.

Ogden CL, Carroll MD, Curtin LR, et al: Prevalence of high body mass index in U.S. children and adolescents, 2007-2008, *J Am Med Assoc* 303(3):242–249, 2010. doi:10.1001/jama.2009.2012.

Ogden C, Flegal K, Carroll M, Johnson C: Prevalence and trends in overweight among U.S. children and adolescents, 1999-2000, *J Am Med Assoc* 288(14):1728–1732, 2002.

Papas MA, Alberg AJ, Ewing R, et al: The built environment and obesity, *Epidemiol Rev* 29:129–143, 2007. doi:10.1093/epirev/mxm009.

Renalds A, Smith TH, Hale PJ: A systematic review of built environment and health, *Family Community Health* 33(1):68–78, 2010.

Roberto CA, Baik J, Harris JL, Brownell KD: Influence of licensed characters on children's taste and snack preferences, *Pediatrics* 126:88–93, 2010.

Rosenkranz RR, Dzewaltowski DA: Model of the home food environment pertaining to childhood obesity, *Nut Rev* 66(3):123–140, 2008. doi:10.1111/j.1753-4887.2008.00017.x.

Sallis JF, Glanz K: The role of built environments in physical activity, eating, and obesity in childhood, *Future Children* 16(1):89–108, 2006.

Science Panel on Interactive Communication and Health: *Wired for health and well-being: the emergence of interactive health communication*, Washington, DC, 1999, US Department of Health and Human Services, US Government Printing Office. Available at http://www.health.gov/scipich/pubs/finalreport.htm. Accessed February 19, 2011.

Serrano E, Kowaleska A, Hosig K, et al: Status and goals of local school wellness policies in Virginia: a response to the child nutrition and WIC reauthorization act of 2004, *J Nutr Educ Behav* 39:95–100, 2007. doi:10.1016/j.jneb.2006.10.011.

Strasburger V, Jordan A, Donnerstein E: Health effects of media on children and adolescents, *Pediatrics* 125:756–767, 2010.

Taveras EM, Ross-Degnan D, Goldmann DH, et al: The association of television and video viewing with fast food intake by preschool-age children, *Obesity* 14(11):2034–2041, 2007.

Timperio A, Ball K, Roberts R, et al: Children's fruit and vegetable intake: associations with the neighbourhood food environment, *Prev Med* 46(4):331–335, 2008. doi:10.1016/p.ypmed.2007.11.011.

Tinsworth D, McDonald J: *Special study: injuries and deaths associated with children's playground equipment*, Washington, DC, 2001, U.S. Consumer Product Safety Commission.

Troiano RP, Berrigan D, Dodd KW, et al: Physical activity in the United States measured by accelerometer, *Med Sci Sports Exercise* 40(1):181–188, 2008.

U.S. Department of Agriculture: Access to affordable and nutritious food: measuring and understanding food deserts and their consequences: Report to Congress, *USDA Economic Research Service*, 2009.

U.S. Department of Health and Human Services: *Heads up, concussion in youth sports: a fact sheet for coaches*, 2009.

U.S. Department of Health and Human Services: *Healthy People 2020*, Washington, DC, 2010, U.S. Government Printing Office.

U.S. Department of Health and Human Services: *Administration on Children, Youth, and Families: Child Maltreatment 2008*, 2010. Available at http://www.acf.hhs.gov/programs/cb/pubs/cm07/index.htm. Accessed June 16, 2011.

U.S. Census Bureau: *Low income uninsured by state*, 2009a. Available at http://www.census.gov/.

U.S. Census Bureau: *National and state population estimates*, 2009b. Available at http://www.census.gov/popest/states/NST-ann-est2008.html. Accessed February 19, 2011.

Van Cleave J, Gortmaker S, Perrin J: Dynamics of obesity and chronic health conditions among children and youth, *J Am Med Assoc* 303(7):623–630, 2010.

Viner R, Segal T, Lichtarowicz-Krynska E, Hindmarsh P: Prevalence of the insulin resistance syndrome in obesity. *Arch Dis Child* 90:10–14, 2005. doi:10.1136/adc.2003.036467.

Wang F, Wild TC, Kipp W, et al: The influence of childhood obesity on the development of self-esteem, *Health Reports* 20(2):21–27, 2009.

White House: *Let's Move!* Available at http://www.letsmove.gov/accessing/index.html. Accessed February 19, 2011.

Wight V, Chau M: *Basic facts about low-income children: children under age 18.*, 2009, National Center for Children in Poverty. Available at http://www.nccp.org/publications/pub_892.html. Accessed February 11, 2010.

Wight V, Chau M, Aratani Y: *Who are America's poor children? The official story*, 2010, National Center for Children in Poverty. Available at http://www.nccp.org/publications/pub_912.html. Accessed February 11, 2010.

Wilens T, Adler L, Adams J, et al: Misuse and diversion of stimulants prescribed for ADHD: a systematic review of the literature, *J Am Acad Child Adolesc Psychiatry* 41(1):21–31, 2008.

CHAPTER 30

Major Health Issues and Chronic Disease Management of Adults Across the Life Span

Monty Gross, PhD, RN, CNE

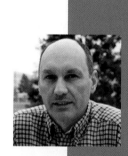

Dr. Monty Gross is Associate Professor of Nursing at James Madison University in Harrisonburg, Virginia. As a Certified Nurse Educator, he teaches in the bachelor's and master's programs. He holds a BS in communications from Clarion University of Pennsylvania and a BSN and MSN in community health from the University of Virginia. Since 1999 he has taught various nursing courses. In 2006 he completed his PhD from Virginia Tech. He has experience in both acute and critical care and continues to practice at the University of Virginia Medical Center, Charlottesville, Virginia.

Linda Hulton, PhD, RN

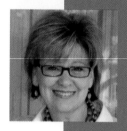

Dr. Linda Hulton is Professor of Nursing at James Madison University (JMU). She received her BSN in Nursing from Roberts Wesleyan College and her Masters and PhD in nursing from the University of Virginia. Prior to coming to JMU, she had over 20 years of clinical experience in community health. Her area of research interest is adolescent health promotion and unintended pregnancy. She has received grants for evaluation of school-based health programs and teen pregnancy prevention programs. She has served as a consultant to the Virginia State Public Health Department regarding school-based teen pregnancy prevention programs. She was named the JMU Mosier Fellow 2002-2003 for her work, "Strengthening the Safety Net: A Health Education Program for an Alternative High School." She currently serves as Project Evaluator for the Federal Office on Adolescent Pregnancy Programs grant awarded to the Office on Children and Youth. She has had her scholarly work published in *Issues in Comprehensive Pediatric Nursing, Sigma Theta Tau's Online Journal of Knowledge Synthesis in Nursing, the Journal of Gynecological and Neonatal Nursing, The Journal of School Nursing,* and *the Journal for Specialists in Pediatric Nursing.* At JMU, she teaches undergraduate courses in community health nursing and graduate courses in research and technology in nursing education.

Sharon Strang, RN, DNP, APRN, FNP-BC

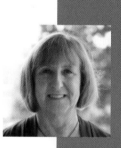

Dr. Sharon Strang is an Assistant Professor of Nursing and an Assistant Professor in the Graduate School at James Madison University. She is a Board Certified Family Nurse Practitioner who practices at a free clinic. She received her BSN from Duquesne University in Pittsburgh, PA and her Masters of Science in Nursing from the University of Pennsylvania at Edinboro. Sharon completed a Post Masters Nurse Practitioner Certificate Program at Old Dominion University and received her DNP from the University of Virginia. The focus of her doctoral studies and grant writing is chronic disease. She has presented at national nursing and education conferences and published in nursing education and nurse practitioner journals. In 2005 she received the Virginia Council of Nurse Practitioner's nurse practitioner in education award.

ADDITIONAL RESOURCES

Ⓔvolve WEBSITE
http://evolve.elsevier.com/Stanhope
- *Healthy People 2020*
- Quiz
- Case Studies
- WebLinks—Of special note see the links for these sites:
  - American Cancer Society
  - American Diabetes Association
  - American Heart Association
  - American Stroke Association
  - CDC Men's Health
  - Food and Drug Administration
  - Men's Health Network
  - National Cancer Institute
  - National Center for Complementary and Alternative Medicine
  - National Institute of Mental Health
  - National Women's Health Information Center
  - United States Department of Health and Human Services
- Glossary
- Answers to Practice Applications
- Resource Tools
  - Resource Tool 30.A: Lifestyle Assessment Questionnaire
  - Resource Tool 30.B: Health Risk Appraisal for Older Adults

OBJECTIVES

After reading this chapter, the student should be able to:

1. Define terms commonly used in the care of adults.
2. Describe historical and current perspectives of adult health and health policy.
3. Discuss sources of population-based public health data and health status indicators about adults to be used to align community resources to support adults with chronic illnesses.
4. Use appropriate assessment tools and development strategies to care for adults across the life span.
5. Discuss the concepts of self-management and the implementation of the Chronic Care Model to support adults with chronic illness.

6. Explain the dynamic forces that contribute to shared and gender specific diseases, health disparities, cultural diversity, and culturally competent care of adults in their communities.
7. Appraise the role of cultural, social, and behavioral factors in accessibility, availability, acceptability, and delivery of community-based models of care for adults.
8. Examine role opportunities for nurses in providing care in the community.

KEY TERMS

OUTLINE

This chapter provides an overview of major health issues of adults that occur at various stages of life. Nurses struggle with these numerous and complex topics. As the Baby Boomers age, the health care system will be faced with large numbers of people needing care for chronic disease (Robine, Michel, and Herrmann, 2007). Unhealthy lifestyles, environmental pollution, and politics are a sample of factors a nurse will need to consider in population-centered health care. Descriptive statistics are frequently provided to help illustrate the significance of a disease or condition. There is strong evidence that community interventions, such as those designed for disadvantaged populations to improve diabetes care, can improve health through political involvement and strategies such as implementing well-planned programs (Glazier et al, 2006; Brownson, Chriqui, and Stamatakis, 2009). Significant changes are rapidly occurring in health care and in the communities through policy changes and research. Nurses will be better prepared to practice by having a better understanding of these major health issues.

HISTORICAL PERSPECTIVES ON ADULT MEN AND WOMEN'S HEALTH

Men and women have always faced a wide array of health issues that transition over time to impact their lives and the community. Gender inequalities span throughout time and all societies, damaging the health of both genders (WHO, 2007). Social and political climates influence research and funding agendas that ultimately affect how health care is delivered in the community. A gender gap has existed where the emphasis on health issues and community focus has given priority to one gender over the other through research, policies, and funding. This has resulted in the focus of prevention and treatment being on one or the other gender, depending on social and political time period. Gender disparities are an ongoing global problem (Holdcroft, 2007).

Historically men have dominated the medical and research professions because of cultural and societal norms. Because of this, health researchers focused on issues predominately oriented toward men with the exception of mental health (Riska, 2009). At the beginning of the twentieth century, discussions of women's health focused primarily on reproduction and women's roles as mothers. In the 1920s, with the birth control movement in its initial stages, women's health expanded to address family planning and reproductive health. Women began to be empowered by the suffragette movement, winning the right to vote in 1920. As the women's rights movement gained momentum, women's health issues and the research of those issues displaced many issues of men. In the 1980s recommendations were made by the U.S. Public Health Services Task Force on Women's Health Issues to increase gender equity in biomedical research and the establishment of guidelines for including women in federally sponsored studies (Alexander et al, 2007). In 1990 the Society for Women's Research was founded. Through political action of the National Institute of Health (NIH), legislation once again included women and other minorities in research studies (NIH Revitalization Act of 1993).

As the United States prospered and scientific knowledge grew, illness and death rates from infectious diseases decreased and those of chronic diseases increased for men and women. Primary infections, for example, involving diarrhea and pneumonia shifted to chronic illnesses, such as cardiovascular disease and cancers (WHO, 2009). This transition occurred because vaccines were developed, living standards improved, and health policies and programs were implemented to reduce the spread of infections and increase life span.

HEALTH POLICY AND LEGISLATION

Health policy is action taken by public and private agencies to promote health. It is a reflection of the values held in society and can greatly influence the health of the citizens overall. Legislation consists of laws that regulate health care and promote health. Nursing practice and the care provided is impacted by policy and legislation. To be fully engaged in improving the health care from the bedside to the community level, nurses must understand how policy and legislation, along with other system factors such as social, cultural, and economic forces, can be incorporated into planning care for clients (Smith-Campbell, 2009).

The following are four examples of important federal legislation that has influenced the health of adults and their lives in communities: The Older Americans Act of 1965, the Americans with Disabilities Act of 1990, the Family and Medical Leave Act of 1993, and the Personal Responsibility and Work Opportunity Reconciliation Act of 1996.

The Older Americans Act (OAA), originally passed in 1965, established the Administration on Aging (AOA) and state agencies to provide for the social service needs of older people. The mission of the AOA is to help older adults maintain dignity and live independently in their communities through a comprehensive and coordinated network across the United States (AOA, 2010). In 2008, of the $1.9 billion funding allotted to the AOA, two thirds supported state and community grants for multiple social and nutritional service programs. Title III of the OAA authorizes funding for non-profit area agencies on aging to coordinate social services that provide supportive and nutritional services, family caregiver support, and disease prevention and health promotion activities. The services are available to all people age 60 or over, specifically targeted to those with the greatest economic or social need.

In 1990, the Americans with Disabilities Act (ADA) was passed, providing protection against discrimination to millions of Americans with disabilities. This legislation requires government and businesses to provide disabled individuals with equal opportunities for jobs, education, access to transportation and public buildings, and other accommodations for both physical and mental limitations. Although some business owners voiced concerns about the economic burden the required accommodations would cost, Travis (2009) points out that modification generally does not cost a lot of money in comparison to economic gain. Not only did the disabled, but the non-disabled and businesses themselves benefited from the changes.

The **Family and Medical Leave Act (FMLA),** initially passed in 1993, provides job protection and continuous health benefits where applicable for eligible employees who need extended leave for their own illness or to care for a family member. Frequently **caregivers** provide unpaid care for their family members, including aging parents, children, grandchildren, and partners. Often adults find themselves struggling to balance work and caring for a family member. More families find themselves in this struggle as more women enter the work force and work full time. Caregivers' multiple roles and responsibilities are frequently coupled with financial strain, which can lead them to experience **caregiver burden.** In 2008 the Act was amended to increase military family entitlements (Rogers et al, 2009).

In 1996 Congress passed the **Personal Responsibility and Work Opportunity Reconciliation Act,** commonly known as "welfare reform." This law targeted women who received public assistance and changed the previous Aid to Families with Dependent Children (AFDC) to **Temporary Assistance for Needy Families (TANF)**—a work program that mandates that women heads-of-household find employment to retain their benefits. The Administration for Children and Families (ACF), within the Department of Health and Human Services (USDHHS) is responsible for federal programs such as TANF that promote the economic and social well-being of families, children, individuals, and communities (ACF, n.d.).

The nurse serves in a unique position for advocacy and support of health legislation and policy that supports the physical, mental, and social well-being of adults. Advocacy can be accomplished in a variety of ways such as lobbying, public speaking, participating in grass roots activities, and staying abreast of proposed legislation that influences the health of men and women, their families, and communities.

> **DID YOU KNOW?** *The Office on Women's Health in the U.S. Department of Health and Human Services (USDHHS) was established in 1991 to improve the health of American women by advancing and coordinating a comprehensive women's health agenda throughout the USDHHS. Almost a decade and a half later, the Men's Health Act of 2005, which would amend the Public Health Service Act to establish an Office of Men's Health within the USDHHS, was introduced in both the U.S. House of Representatives (HR 457) and Senate (S 228) in February 2005.*

Ethical and Legal Issues and Legislation for Older Adults

Ethical issues regarding the care and treatment of older adults arise regularly. As the population continues to age and technological advances continue to be developed, complex ethical and legal questions will continue to increase. The most common of these issues involve decision making—assessment of the ability of the client to make decisions, the appropriate surrogate decision maker, disclosure of information to make informed decisions, level of care needed on the basis of function, and termination of treatment at the end of life. One often-overlooked concern of older persons is that of

abuse. The National Center on Elder Abuse (NCEA), within the Administration on Aging, notes that **abuse** encompasses physical, emotional, and sexual abuse, as well as exploitation, neglect, and abandonment. Identification of abuse consists of recognizing the following: (a) The willful infliction of physical pain or **injury,** (b) infliction of debilitating mental anguish and fear, (c) theft or mismanagement of money or resources, and (d) unreasonable confinement or the depriving of services.

Only one in six cases of elder abuse are reported, although nearly all states have enacted mandatory reporting laws and have services available to provide assistance (Halphen and Sadowsky, 2009). Although legal definitions vary from state to state, the NCEA defines **neglect** as "the refusal or failure to fulfill any part of a person's obligations or duties to an elder. Neglect may also occur if the person who has fiduciary responsibilities fails to pay for items or necessary home care services or, on the part of the in-home service provider, to provide the necessary care (NCEA, n.d., p 2). Older persons can make independent choices with which others may disagree. Their right to self-determination can be taken from them if they are declared incompetent. According to the Older Americans Act, **financial exploitation** is the "illegal or improper act or process of an individual, including a caregiver, using the resources of an older individual for monetary or personal benefit, profit or gain" (Area Agency on Aging, n.d., p 1).

During the assessment process, nurses will want to be aware of contradictions between injuries and the explanation of their cause, co-dependency issues between client and caregiver, and substance abuse by the caregiver. The local social services agency or area agency on aging can help with information on reporting requirements. Nurses can play a key role in reducing elder abuse.

The **Patient Self-Determination Act** of 1991 requires those providers receiving Medicare and Medicaid funds to give clients written information regarding their legal options for treatment choices if they become incapacitated. A routine discussion of **advanced medical directives** can help ease the difficult discussions faced by health care professionals, families, and clients (Emanuel, 2008). The nurse can help an individual complete a values' history instrument. These instruments ask questions about specific wishes regarding different medical situations (Messinger-Rapport, Baum, and Smith, 2009). "Your Life Your Choices: Planning for Future Medical Decisions: How to Prepare a Personalized Living Will" (Pearlman et al, n.d.) is a valuable resource to help people by using scenarios and information to guide people through the process of developing advance medical directives. There are two parts to the advanced directives. The **living will** allows the client to express wishes regarding the use of medical treatments in the event of a terminal illness. A **durable medical power of attorney** is the legal way for the client to designate someone else to make health care decisions when he or she is unable to do so. A **do-not-resuscitate order** (DNR) is a specific order from a physician not to use cardiopulmonary resuscitation. State laws vary widely regarding the implementation of these tools, so it is important to consult a knowledgeable source for information. It is also important to involve the family, and especially the designated decision maker or agent, in these discussions so that everyone is clear about the client's choices (Emanuel, 2008).

Environmental Impact

The environmental impact of an unhealthy environment adds significantly to the burden of disease for men and women. Men and women are often exposed to different environmental factors because of upbringing, employment, cultural, or tradition variations.

It is important to understand that the hosts (men and women) may respond differently to environmental factors. For example, Clougherty (2010) reports that women and girls are affected more than men and boys by air pollution. Both gender (a social construct) and sex (a biological construct) are factors that make identification of the impact of environmental hazards on men and women more complex. Social and environmental factors influence adults' choices of health behaviors. Understanding how these factors impact health outcomes will require additional research and policy analysis (Angel and Angel, 2006; USDHHS, *Healthy People 2020, 2010*). Conducting gender analysis as part of research would help clarify if environment is influencing separate social and biological differences between men and women.

Governmental programs are in place to improve environmental health. The Centers for Disease Control and Prevention (CDC) Environmental Hazards and Effects Program (EHEP) is designed to prevent and control disease or death and to promote health and quality of life that result from interactions between people and their environments. The program uses indicators that can be used to assess and monitor progress on goals to improve the environmental health. It is incumbent on community health nurses to decrease the burden of disease resulting from an unhealthy environment (Levin P et al, 2008).

HEALTH STATUS INDICATORS

Health status indicators are the quantitative or qualitative measures used to describe the level of well-being or illness present in a defined population or to describe related attributes or risk factors. They can be represented in the form of rates, such as mortality and morbidity, or proportions, such as percentages of a given population that receive immunizations (Community Health Status Indicators, 2008).

Over the past decade, efforts to reduce chronic disease risk factors have resulted in less-than-expected improvements. The CDC developed the *Future Initiative* (2005) as part of a major strategic planning process and developed a set of Health Protection Goals to track measure of mortality and morbidity by life stages. The goals were categorized by four themes, each with an overarching goal: Healthy People in Every Stage of Life, Healthy People in Healthy Places, People Prepared for Emerging Health Threats, and Healthy People in a Healthy World. Improvements were noted among all life stages with the exception of adults. Adults reported continued declining trends in perceived

health status and dramatic declines in healthy weight indicators (Roy et al, 2009).

> **WHAT DO YOU THINK?**   *Research has demonstrated that several factors contribute to health disparities, especially unequal access to health care. There may also be inequities in the use of online resources. Some existing minority groups are less likely to use the Internet for health information despite the relationship between healthy literacy and use of online health resources. What do you think can be done to decrease barriers to health information via the Internet (Miller, West, and Wasserman, 2007)?*

Mortality

Life expectancy is a measure that is often used to gauge the overall health of a population. Although the United States spends more money per capita on health than any other country, other developed countries have a longer life expectancy for both genders. As illustrated in Figure 30-1, in the United States, life expectancy for men (75.2 years) ranked 25th out of 37 countries and territories and 23rd for women (80.4 years) (MMWR, 2008).

In 2007, both American men and women could expect to live longer than they did in 1990. Overall, American men gained 3.5 years of life and women could expect to live 1.6 years longer. Mortality from heart disease, stroke, and cancer has continued to decline in recent years and was substantially lower in 2006 than in 1950, decreasing overall by 46%. Specifically, the age-adjusted rates for heart disease declined by 66%, cerebrovascular disease by 75%, and the overall death rates for cancer declined 16% (NCHS, 2009). However, mortality from chronic respiratory disease and unintentional injury has not seen this decline (Miniño et al, 2009; NCHS, 2009).

Life expectancy and mortality rates also vary among ethnic/racial groups in the United States. The gap in life expectancy between white adults and African-American adults persists but has narrowed since 1990 (NCHS, 2009). The age-adjusted death rate was 1.3 times greater, infant mortality rate 2.4 times greater, and maternal mortality rate 3.4 times greater for the African-American population than for the white population. Life expectancy for the white population exceeded that for the African-American population by 5.0 years (Heron et al, 2009).

Morbidity

When healthy years of life are increased, longer life spans are generally considered desirable. However, increasing prevalence of chronic diseases and other conditions associated with aging can increase functional limitations and affect quality of life. Moreover, being male or female leads to different socialization, expectations, and lifestyles that affect and interact with health in very complex ways (Azad and Nashtar, 2005; Chandra and Minkovitz, 2006; Chang et al, 2006; Brittle and Bird, 2007).

Of particular concern is the high prevalence of adults with risk factors such as tobacco use, high cholesterol, obesity, and insufficient exercise habits, which are associated with chronic disease. Cholesterol levels have been dropping, in particular for

TABLE 30-1	DEATHS CAUSED BY CANCERS*	
POPULATION	**MEN**	**WOMEN**
White	218.7	153.4
African American	278.8	176.9
Hispanic	145.4	101.4
Native American	137.0	108.9
Asian/Pacific Islander	128.2	93.3

*Rates are per 100,000.
From Centers for Disease Control and Prevention (n.d.): Rates for new cancer cases and deaths by race/ethnicity and sex. Available at www.cdc.gov.

187.1 per 100,000 is approximately a 1.7% improvement from the 2005 statistics (NCHS, 2009).

The American Cancer Society's (ACS) 2009 Cancer Facts and Figures report provides estimates by the National Institutes of Health that place the overall costs of cancer in 2008 at $228.1 billion (ACS, 2009). Of this total, $93.2 billion is for direct medical costs; $18.8 billion for indirect costs or those resulting from lost productivity related to illness; and $116.1 billion for indirect costs resulting from lost productivity because of premature death (ACS, 2009). These costs could be reduced by removing barriers to care such as lack of health insurance and improving the health literacy of Americans.

WHAT DO YOU THINK? *On March 23, 2010, President Obama signed the Patient Protection and Affordable Care Act along with the Health Care and Education Reconciliation Act. This constitutes the biggest expansion of federal health care guarantees in more than four decades. Part of the plan includes spending an estimated $940 billion to extend insurance coverage to roughly 32 million additional Americans. As time has passed since President Obama signed this legislation, are you seeing evidence of improved health care?*

Early screening and detection, promotion of healthy lifestyles, expansion of access to services, and improvement in cancer treatments will help reduce the burden of cancer and disparities. For example, the declining death rates of colorectal cancer are largely attributed to screening and to risk factor reduction (Edwards et al, 2009). Finding cancer lesions in a precancerous state, such as those found in cervical, colorectal, and breast cancer, allow for treatment while in a highly treatable stage. Obesity, physical inactivity, smoking, heavy alcohol consumption, a diet high in red or processed meats, and insufficient intake of fruits and vegetables are risk factors for colorectal cancer. Reducing these risk factors will reduce the incidence of the disease.

Public health agencies, health care providers, and communities must work together to reduce the burden of cancer on society. The *Healthy People 2020* goal is to reduce the number of overall cancer cases as well as the illness, disability, and death caused by cancer. Education on the hazards of tobacco use and second-hand smoke, eating a healthy diet and limiting daily consumption of alcohol, and exposure to ultraviolet rays are examples of topics for education programs that will reduce the burden of cancer on society.

THE CUTTING EDGE *For many years cancer treatment focused on surgery, chemotherapy, and radiation. As researchers gained more in-depth understanding of how the body fights cancer, new therapies such as vaccines have been developed. Cancer vaccines are emerging as new biological therapy to treat or prevent cancer. The human papillomavirus (HPV) most often causes cervical cancer and genital warts. It was studied in thousands of females (ages 9-26 years) around the world, and its safety continues to be monitored by the CDC and the U.S. Food and Drug Administration (FDA). The FDA approved an HPV vaccine that is routinely recommended for 11- and 12-year-old girls. It is also recommended for girls and women ages 13 through 26 who have not yet been vaccinated or completed the vaccine series. The vaccine is given in three doses over 6 months.*

From Centers for Disease Control and Prevention: HPV vaccination information for young women. Available at http://www.cdc.gov/std/hpv/STDFact-HPV-vaccine-young-women.htm#hpvvac2.

STDs/HIV/AIDS

Sexually transmitted diseases (STDs) refer to more than 25 infectious organisms transmitted primarily through sexual activity. STDs are infectious organisms, such as a virus, bacteria, or parasites typically passed through sexual contact. Some other means of transmission include lice, mother-to-child transmission during pregnancy or breastfeeding, or contaminated needles used doing drug use or surgery. The term **sexually transmitted infections** (STIs) is also used synonymously, although there are distinctions. Shuford (2008) explained that STI is a broader term meaning the body has had an invasion and multiplication of microorganisms. STDs signify that pathology or damage has occurred with or without symptoms. STDs continue to be a major burden to society and have tremendous health and economic consequences in the United States despite their relative preventive nature. The costs to the U.S. health care system related to STDs are as much as $15.3 billion annually (CDC, 2008).

The CDC (2008) estimates there are approximately 19 million new STD infections each year, with almost half occurring in people from 15 to 24 years of age. Many cases go undiagnosed, so the true burden is not fully known. In 2008, more than 1.5 million cases of chlamydia and gonorrhea occurred, making them the two most reported infectious diseases. Females are at greater risk for STDs as a result of biological differences and other factors. Syphilis, once close to elimination, has reemerged, primarily related to men who have sex with men (MSM), but not in all cases (CDC, 2008).

The CDC HIV/AIDS Facts (updated August 2009) indicate that at the end of 2006, in the United States, approximately 1.1 million people were diagnosed or undiagnosed with HIV infection (CDC, 2007). In 2007, the 42,655 new cases of HIV/AIDS diagnoses among adolescents and adults were male, with 53% of that number attributed to MSM. African Americans accounted for 51% of the HIV/AIDS cases, followed by whites (29%) and Hispanic/Latinos (18%). The rate of HIV transmission has decreased and the number of people living with HIV/AIDS has increased. Prevention efforts are proving effective (CDC, 2007).

The *Healthy People 2020* goal is to promote responsible sexual behaviors, strengthen community capacity, and increase access to quality services to prevent STDs and their complications (USDHHS, 2010). HIV-infected persons report reduced risk behaviors because they know they are infected (Hall et al, 2008).

Nurses serve as advocates by focusing on the high-risk behaviors of men and women, as well as on the factors in their communities that lead to STDs. High-risk populations should be considered when assessing for client's risk for STDs, including pregnant women, adolescents, MSM, women who have sex with women (WSW), and older clients (Wasik and Kachlic, 2009). Interventions to improve education, employment opportunities, and adequate housing—as well as those to decrease drug use, isolation, and poverty—can have a critical impact on this epidemic. The CDC/HRSA Advisory Committee on HIV/AIDS and STD Prevention (CHAC) recommend the following: (a) early detection and treatment of curable STDs should become a major, explicit component of comprehensive HIV prevention programs at national, state, and local levels, (b) in areas where STDs that facilitate HIV transmission are prevalent, screening and treatment programs should be expanded, (c) HIV testing should always be recommended for individuals who are diagnosed with or suspected to have an STD, and (d) HIV and STD prevention programs in the United States, together with private and public sectors partners, should take joint responsibility for implementing these strategies. A comprehensive HIV prevention program needs to include social, behavioral, and biomedical interventions (CDC, 2007).

HOW TO Prevent Sexually Transmitted Diseases (STDs)

Nurses play a vital role in preventing STDs. Five key concepts provide the foundation for the prevention and control of STDs: (1) education and counseling of persons at risk on ways to adopt safer sexual behavior, (2) identification of asymptomatically infected persons and of symptomatic persons unlikely to seek diagnostic and treatment services, (3) effective diagnosis and treatment of infected persons, (4) evaluation, treatment, and counseling of sex partners of persons who are infected with an STD, and (5) pre-exposure vaccination of persons at risk for vaccine-preventable STDs (Centers for Disease Control and Prevention: CDC fact sheet: the role of STD prevention and treatment in HIV prevention, 2007. Available at http://www.cdc.gov/std/hiv/stds-and-hiv-fact-sheet-press.pdf. Accessed February 23, 2011.

Weight Control

Americans spend a great deal of time, energy, and money in the never-ending pursuit of the beautiful body. One study indicated that spending on overweight and obesity could be as much as 10%, or $147 billion, of U.S. health care costs (Finkelstein et al, 2009). In 1998 the National Institutes of Health (NIH) began using the calculation of **body mass index** (BMI) to define overweight and obesity in individuals. BMI is the relationship

---

TABLE 30-2	**BMI DETERMINATION AND INTERPRETATION**
BMI*	**CATEGORY**
≤18.5-24.9	Normal weight
25.0-29.9	Overweight
30.0-39.9	Obesity
≥40	Extreme obesity

From National Institutes of Health: Do you know the health risks of being overweight? Rockville, MD, 2004, USDHHS.
*Body mass index is a method used to determine optimal weight for height and is an indicator for obesity or malnutrition. Two formulas may be used for its calculation:
BMI = Weight (in kilograms) / Height (in meters squared)
BMI = Weight (in pounds) / Height (in inches squared) × 703

---

of body weight and height. A BMI of 25 to 29.9 is defined as overweight, whereas a BMI of 30 and above is considered obese (WIN, 2008) (Table 30-2).

Overweight and obesity are topics addressed numerous times in *Healthy People 2020*. According to the AHA (2009), 145 million Americans age 20 and older are over weight or obese (BMI ≥25.0 kg/m²). This number is composed of 76.9 million men and 68.1 million women. Of the total 145 million, 74.1 million are obese (BMI ≥30.0).

Obesity has many effects on health and is linked to a number of major health problems. Nurses can provide education regarding obesity's risks to health. The educational offerings can be fashioned after a community health model using the levels of prevention to establish effective interventions for adults at risk for **weight control** issues. For example, only about one third of all adults meet the 2008 Physical Activity Guidelines (CDC, 2008). Therefore, a community prevention project aimed at increasing activity levels would help in prevention of obesity and subsequent illnesses of diabetes and heart disease.

In addition to obesity, other eating disorders have increased among U.S. women. Common eating disorders seen in women include anorexia nervosa and bulimia. **Anorexia** is defined as a fear of gaining weight coupled with disturbances in perceptions of the body. Excessive weight loss is the most noticeable clue. Individuals with anorexia rarely complain of weight loss because they view themselves as normal or overweight. Many of these women also struggle with psychological problems, including depression, obsessive symptoms, and social phobias. **Bulimia** is characterized by a persistent concern with the shape of the body along with body weight, recurrent episodes of binge eating, a loss of control during these binges, and use of extreme methods to prevent weight gain, such as purging, strict dieting, fasting, use of laxatives or diuretics, or vigorous exercise (NIMH, 2009).

Through comprehensive physical and psychosocial assessments, as well as histories of dietary practice, nurses identify women with eating disorders and provide appropriate referrals. Weight control strategies include promoting healthy eating habits and regular physical activity. At a population level, nurses advocate against advertising that promotes exceptionally thin bodies for women. They also promote community-wide exercise and healthy eating programs.

WOMEN'S HEALTH CONCERNS

It is preferable to emphasize prevention in adult health care. Screening, immunizations, and a healthy lifestyle are important for women of all ages. The Office of Women's Health (USDHHS) has compiled guidelines titled, "General Screenings and Immunizations for Women."

> **DID YOU KNOW?** *The Agency for Research and Health Quality (ARHQ) was mandated by Congress to provide annual reports on health care quality and disparities. Women are one of the populations addressed in this report.*

Reproductive Health

Women often use health care services for reproductive health concerns. A number of *Healthy People 2020* objectives address areas related to women's reproductive health (see the Maternal Infant and Child Health section of the *Healthy People 2020* table on p 679 (2010).

Nurses are in a unique position to advocate for policies that increase women's access to services for reproductive health. In addition, many nurses discuss contraception with women of child-bearing age. Contraceptive counseling requires accurate knowledge of current contraceptive choices and a nonjudgmental approach. The goal of contraceptive counseling is to ensure that women have appropriate instruction to make informed choices about reproduction. The choice of contraceptive method depends on many factors, including the woman's health, frequency of sexual activity, number of partners, and plans to have future children. Except for abstinence, no method provides a 100% guarantee against unintended pregnancy or disease (USDHHS, 2010).

Preconceptual counseling addresses risks before conception and includes education, assessment, diagnosis, and intervention. The purpose is to reduce and/or eliminate health risks for women and infants. One major health problem that could be significantly impacted by preconceptual counseling is the problem of neural tube defects. Approximately 1 in every 1000 pregnancies is affected. The CDC notes that two of the most common neural tube defects in 2005, spina bifida and anencephaly, had a combined incidence of 29 per 100,000 live births (Matthews, 2007). Research has shown that intake of folic acid can significantly reduce the occurrence of these very serious and often fatal neural tube defects by 50% to 70%. A recommendation was made that women capable of or planning a pregnancy take 0.4 to 0.8 mg of folic acid daily (USPSTF, 2009).

The goal of one *Healthy People 2020* objective is to increase the proportion of pregnancies begun with the recommended folic acid level. The CDC conducted a multimedia campaign regarding folic acid supplementation. In 2005, approximately 30% of women surveyed reported daily use of a supplement containing folic acid; in 2007 this had risen to 40% (MMWR, 2008).

Another concern critical to preconception awareness is exposure to substances such as alcohol. A major preventable cause of birth defects, mental retardation, and neurodevelopmental disorders is fetal exposure to alcohol during pregnancy. Although fetal alcohol syndrome (FAS) is declining in the United States, it still remains a preventable public health problem. According to the Substance Abuse and Mental Health Services Administration (SAMSHA), FAS affects between 5 and 20 per 10,000 live births. The rate is higher (15-25 per 10,000) among some Native American tribes (SAMSHA, 2009). The CDC and the American Academy of Pediatrics recommend no alcohol during pregnancy. One study showed that female children of women who drank less than one drink per week were more likely to have emotional and behavioral problems at 4 and 8 years of age, respectively (Sayal et al, 2007). Community interventions have been shown to help decrease the consumption of alcohol during pregnancy. A pilot study was conducted in six community settings in three large cities. One-hundred ninety women received four manual-guided motivational counseling sessions delivered by mental health clinicians and one contraceptive counseling session delivered by a family planning clinician. At the end of 6 months, 68.5% of the women were judged no longer at risk for having an alcohol-exposed pregnancy (AAP, 2003).

Nurses will want to be involved in community-based interventions for women. They can conduct motivational classes and participate in campaigns that print and broadcast advertisements informing women of child-bearing age that drinking during pregnancy can cause birth defects. Nurses can serve as advocates not only to encourage their clients to use prenatal care services, but also to work toward the establishment of services that are accessible, affordable, and available to all pregnant women.

Gestational Diabetes

Gestational diabetes mellitus (GDM) is a condition characterized by carbohydrate intolerance that is first identified or develops during pregnancy. The incidence of gestational diabetes is increasing in the United States. Gestational diabetes has a higher incidence among minorities—African Americans, American Indians, and Hispanic/Latino Americans. After the pregnancy ends, 5% to 10% of women will continue with diabetes, and they have a 40% to 60% chance of developing diabetes within the next 5 to 10 years. Because of this, Buchanan et al (2007) suggested that this is a step in the evolving process of diabetes and an opportunity to intervene to prevent the progression to Type 2 diabetes.

Menopause

During menopause the levels of the hormones estrogen and progesterone change in a woman's body. This change leads to the cessation of menstruation. Decline in these hormone levels can affect the vaginal and urinary tract, cardiovascular system, bone density, libido, sleep patterns, memory, and emotions (NIA, 2008).

Women's attitudes toward menopause vary greatly and are influenced by culture, age, support, and the recounted experiences of other women. For decades, however, the prevailing medical view of menopause was a state of deficiency that required hormone replacement to reduce heart disease and osteoporosis. A more positive outlook of menopause encourages women to view it as a transitional and natural stage in the life of a woman.

For decades, many U.S. women used hormone replacement therapy (HRT), although HRT remained untested by rigorous scientific study. A clinical trial launched in 1991, the Women's Health Initiative, set out to test specific effects HRT had on women's health, especially its effect on heart disease and osteoporosis. Researchers concluded that HRT did not prevent heart disease and that to prevent heart disease women should avoid smoking, reduce fat and cholesterol intake, limit salt and alcohol intake, maintain a healthy weight, and be physically active. Scientists also concluded that HRT should be used to prevent osteoporosis only among women who are unable to take nonestrogen medications (NOF, 2010).

Complementary and Alternative Therapies

The change in the recommendations regarding HRT led many women to seek alternative approaches for the management of menopausal symptoms. Women experiencing menopause frequently report symptoms including hot flashes, vaginal dryness, and irregular menses. Examples of alternative therapies are those actions that are taken by women instead of HRT. Complementary therapies are those taken to augment (or as a complement to) HRT. The listing of alternative/complementary therapies for menopausal symptoms can be an endless task, but Box 30-1 provides common examples. The National Center for Complementary and Alternative Medicine at the National Institutes of Health (2009) notes that alternative therapies may or may not be helpful in reducing menopausal symptoms and that more research should be done to determine the scientific benefits and risks of these therapies.

Breast Cancer

In 2009 an estimated 192,370 women were diagnosed with breast cancer. Of that number, an estimated 40,170 women would die. Although the incidence of breast cancer is higher in white women than in African-American women, the death rate for African-American women is higher. Secondary prevention that includes screening activities, such as mammography, clinical breast examination, and self-breast examination, makes a difference in death rates. Early detection can promote a cure whereas late detection typically ensures a poor prognosis. The Surveillance Epidemiology and End Results Study from the National Cancer Institute (NCI) using data from 2002 to 2006 showed that the age-adjusted incidence rate for breast cancer was 123.8 per 100,000 women per year. The age-adjusted death rate was 24.5 per 100,000 women, and the median age at death was 68 years (NCI, 2010).

DID YOU KNOW? *In November of 2009 the USPSTF, based on analysis of evidence, recommended biennial screening mammography for women aged 50 to 74 years of age. Screening mammography was not recommended for other age groups. In response to the reaction of others, in December of 2009, they updated the recommendation for women in the 40- to 50 age group to say, "The decision to start regular, biennial screening mammography before the age of 50 years should be an individual one and take client context into account, including the client's values regarding specific benefits and harms."*

USPSTF: Screening for Breast Cancer, 2009. Available at http://www.uspreventiveservicestaskforce.org/uspstf/uspsbrca.htm. Accessed February 22, 2011

Osteoporosis

Osteoporosis, "or *porous bone*", is a disease characterized by low bone mass and structural deterioration of bone tissue, leading to bone fragility and an increased risk of fractures of the hip, spine, and wrist" (NIAMSD, 2009). This disease affects 44 million people in the United States, and 68% of these individuals are women. Among women more than 50 years of age, approximately one out of every two women will have an osteoporosis-related fracture. Expenditures for osteoporosis-related fractures total $14 billion per year in the United States (NIAMSD, 2009).

Prevention includes diets rich in calcium and vitamin D and avoiding medications that cause bone loss. Always check with the pharmacist and medication labels to determine which medications to avoid. Exercise also improves bone density, especially weight-bearing activities such as walking, running, stair climbing, and weight lifting. Limiting alcohol consumption and avoiding smoking are also important. Finally, several medications are approved for the prevention of osteoporosis in the United States (NIAMSD, 2009).

MEN'S HEALTH CONCERNS

Men and women have a number of shared health concerns, as described previously. It is important to realize that the health status of one gender impacts the health status of the other, the children, and ultimately society. For example, when a male is ill and cannot work, the family and society is impacted economically and work productivity is reduced (Bonhomme, 2007). The family can suffer from lack of income. If the male dies, the widow generally experiences the loss of companionship and assumes the responsibilities of the lost spouse. Resources

---

BOX 30-1	**EXAMPLES OF ALTERNATIVE/ COMPLEMENTARY THERAPIES FOR MENOPAUSAL SYMPTOMS**

- Acupuncture
- Acupressure
- Massage therapy
- Healing touch
- Aromatherapy
- Guided imagery
- Chiropractic healing
- St. John's wort
- Black cohosh
- Soy and isoflavones
- Ginseng
- Kava
- Red clover
- Dong quai

to promote and sustain health outcomes of both genders must be balanced for the overall health of the community. However, although a vital aspect of community health, **men's health** is often overlooked and barriers exist that prevent men from reaching their full health potential (Bonhomme, 2007). Gender characteristics and society interact to influence who is healthy by determining health behaviors, treatment availability, and research funding (WHO, 2007).

Although health policies, campaigns, and community health organizations offer services for men, there is a bias where women's health is emphasized and other barriers that negatively impact men's health (Broom and Tovey, 2009). Treadwell and Marguerite (2008) noted that virtually no health services were offered to men, especially to men at the lowest socioeconomic levels or to those unable to work. They report that while working in communities and visiting clinics to address health needs, few men were in the waiting rooms where primary health care and prevention services were offered. Men often put work ahead of their own health needs (Mahalik, Burns, and Syzdek, 2007).

Several barriers to men reaching their full health potential have been identified. Men do not participate in health care to the same level as women, apparently because of the traditional masculine gender role learned through socialization (Bonhomme, 2007). Only 57% of U.S. men see a doctor, nurse practitioner, or physician assistant compared with 74% of women (AHRQ, 2010). Even fewer Hispanic (35.5%) and African-American (43.5%) men compared with white (63%) men made appointments for routine medical care. Men are socialized to ignore pain, be self-reliant, and be achievement oriented. Large numbers of men do not receive the **health screenings** intended to prevent and identify disease. Men are more often employed in dangerous jobs and incur more work-related injuries than women (Berdahl and Zodet, 2010). Not only do these behaviors limit the opportunity to prevent disease through screening, health education, and counseling, but also once they are diagnosed, management and treatment will be more difficult.

Barriers such as these provide opportunities and challenges for the nurse. By being aware of that bias and barriers in the health care system and recognizing that something should be done, nurses can help reduce the bias and remove barriers to health for both genders. The nurse will want to develop strategies to get men involved in lifestyle changes that prevent illness. All health care providers can do a better job at reaching out to men and offer the guidance and knowledge to improve men's health. The nurse can take an active role in public policy development and implementation. The role also includes encouraging men to identify primary care providers and obtain a physical examination and the recommended screening tests appropriate to that individual.

Men who can establish a working relationship with their health care provider and participate in the recommended screening tests may live healthier, happier, and longer lives. Refer to Box 30-2 for a variety of screening tests with suggested frequencies. Health screenings as well as other prevention strategies for adults are regularly updated by AHRQ.

Some health screenings are clearly beneficial while health care providers and researchers debate the benefit of other screening procedures. As a health care professional, it is important to keep up to date on current research and literature to identify the appropriate screenings for the specific population served.

The nurse can assume many roles to fulfill responsibilities to improve the health of men in the community. As an educator, the nurse provides the knowledge and skill for replacing unhealthy behaviors with a healthy lifestyle. As a client advocate, the nurse supports and interacts with those agencies to obtain the needed resources. The nurse acts as a change agent to assess needs and system influences, identify and set priorities, plan and implement programs for men, and evaluate results. Working within groups and communities, nurses can identify needs and priorities and develop interventions to reduce health risks and improve the health status not only of men, but also of their wives, mothers, daughters, and sisters and the communities in which they live.

BOX 30-2 PREVENTION STRATEGIES FOR ADULTS

Dental Health
- Regular dental examinations
- Floss; brush with fluoride toothpaste

Health Screening
- Blood pressure
- Height and weight
- Nutritional screening (obesity)
- Lipid disorders (men 35 and older; women 45 and older)
- Papanicolaou (Pap) test (all women sexually active with a cervix)
- Colorectal cancer (adults 50 and older)
- Mammogram (women 40 and older)
- Osteoporosis (postmenopausal women 60 and older)
- Problem drinking
- Depression screening
- Tobacco use/tobacco-causing diseases
- Rubella serology or vaccination (women of child-bearing age)
- Chlamydia (sexually active women age 25 and younger; women older than 25 with new/multiple sexual partners)
- Testicular cancer (symptomatic males)
- Coronary heart disease screening (EEG; exercise treadmill)
- Syphilis screening (for at-risk population only)
- Diabetes mellitus (adults with hypertension or hyperlipidemia)

Chemoprophylaxis
- Multivitamin/folic acid (women planning or capable of pregnancy)
- Aspirin prevention (CAD at-risk adults)

Immunizations
- Tetanus-diphtheria (TD) boosters
- Rubella (women of child-bearing age)
- Pneumococcal vaccine (adults 65 and older)
- Influenza vaccine (adults 65 and older/at risk/annually)

From Agency for Healthcare Research and Quality, U.S. Preventive Services Task Force: *The guide to clinical preventive services*, 2009. Available at http://www.ahrq.gov/clinic/pocketgd09/pocketgd09.pdf.

Cancers Unique to Men

Prostate Cancer

An estimated 217,730 men were expected to be diagnosed with prostate cancer in 2010. It is the most common non-skin cancer and the second leading cause of cancer deaths in the United States (NCI, 2010). The NCI estimated that 2,276,112 men will be alive with a history of prostate cancer and approximately one in six men will be diagnosed with prostate cancer in their lifetime. African-American men have higher rates of prostate cancer than other racial/ethnic groups (234.6 vs. 156.9 cases per 100,000 men). Prostate cancer is linked to changes in the DNA of a prostate cancer cell and high levels of male hormones (ACS, 2010). More research is needed to determine the cause.

The ACS recommends men be informed about risks and possible benefits of prostate cancer screening. The information should be provided at age 50 for men of average risk for prostate cancer and age 45 for men at high risk, such as African-American men and men who have had a father, brother, or son diagnosed with prostate cancer before age 65. If the men have had several of these family members diagnosed with prostate cancer at an early age, these men should be informed about prostate screening at age 40 (ACS, 2010).

Two screening tests include the prostate-specific antigen (PSA) and the digital rectal examination (DRE). The PSA test is not accurate in terms of sensitivity or specificity. This blood test produces many false-positive results because many factors can elevate the PSA, such as infections, ejaculation, exercise such as bike riding, and benign prostatic hyperplasia (BPH). The DRE is a procedure where the physician inserts a well-lubricated, gloved index finger into the rectum to palpate the prostate gland and examine the rectum for masses. The examiner is unable to palpate the anterior aspects of the prostate, reducing the accuracy of this examination. Men find this examination unpleasant and another reason for avoiding health care (ACS, 2010).

Testicular Cancer

Testicular cancer is the most common solid tumor diagnosed in males between the ages of 15 and 40 years, with the peak incidence between the ages of 18 and 40 years. The ACS predicted 8480 new cases of testicular cancer and 350 deaths in 2010 (ACS, 2010). Age-adjusted incidence showed 6.4 of 100,000 white men and 1.2 of 100,000 African-American men were diagnosed with testicular cancer, with a mortality rate of 0.3 of 100,000 and 0.2 of 100,000, respectively. Unfortunately, the cause of testicular cancer is unknown. The only established relationship to testicular cancer is cryptorchidism. The good news is that testicular cancer is rare, and the 5-year survival rate by race was reported as 95.7% for white men and 88.4% for African-American men.

Because painless testicular enlargement is commonly the first sign of testicular cancer, the testicular self-examination has traditionally been recommended for men. However, in 2004 the U.S. Preventive Services Task Force (USPSTF) updated previously published guidelines that significantly altered that tradition for asymptomatic adolescent and adult males (USPSTF, 2004). The new guidelines state:

The USPSTF found no new evidence that screening with clinical examination or testicular self-examination was effective in reducing mortality from testicular cancer. Even in the absence of screening, the current treatment interventions provided very favorable health outcomes. Given the low prevalence of testicular cancer, limited accuracy of screening tests, and no evidence for the incremental benefits of screening, the USPSTF concluded that the harms of screening exceeded any potential benefits.

Depression

More women than men are classified as having depression (6.6% and 4.4%, respectively) for all ages (Pratt and Brody, 2010). Wilhelm (2009) reported that the rates of depression vary between genders based on the type of depression. Of particular concern for men is that higher rates of depression can be found in the unemployed, socially disadvantaged, those who abuse substances, and those with more than one medical condition. There are reasons to believe that men with depression often go unrecognized and underreported. Men tend to be stoic and do not verbalize how they feel and are reluctant to talk about health issues, and men often do not have positive relationships with their health care provider (Bonhomme, 2007).

The suicide rate is four times greater for men, although women are diagnosed twice as often with major depression. Referring again to men being socialized into gender roles, Bonhomme (2007) states that "men are typically socialized to avoid introspection and awareness of helpless feelings, which lead men to not recognize that they may have a mental health problem requiring intervention" (p 126). Much of how gender is manifested in individuals is learned from socialization. How men manifest signs and symptoms of depression may result in low numbers of men diagnosed with depression because men are socialized to hide their feelings. Ultimately, men are seen with more incidences of avoidance behavior, anger, violence, and finally suicide (Branney and White, 2008). Further research is needed to explore how men manifest depression.

Erectile Dysfunction

Erectile dysfunction (ED), also known as impotence, is the consistent inability to achieve or maintain an erection sufficient for satisfactory sexual performance. Up to 40% of men between the ages of 40 and 70 are affected by ED, and the chances increase with aging. It can occur in association with cardiovascular disease, diabetes, hypertension, hypercholesterolemia, smoking, spinal cord injury, prostate cancer, genitourinary surgery, psychiatric disorders, and the use of alcohol and drugs (Douglass and Lin, 2010).

Although ED may be discussed more openly with health care providers since the increased publicity generated from the marketing of the medications for ED, many men will still be embarrassed and reluctant to discuss the subject. Men who respond positively to treatment for ED report significantly better quality of life (Latini and Penson, 2003). With this evidence of positive response, health care providers should be proactive in discussing ED with men.

In summary, regardless of the prevalence differences in the health problems described in this section between men and women, appropriate health care services must be provided and men and women need to be encouraged equally to take advantage of these services.

HEALTH DISPARITIES AMONG SPECIAL GROUPS OF ADULTS

Health disparities present political implications and influence government actions, including the commitment of resources to address them (Braveman, 2006). In the United States, the government describes health disparities as a continuing and persistent gap in health status between genders, ethnicities, economic status, and those who represent the majority populations (NPA, 2010). The causes are complex, but there are two major factors including inadequate access to care and substandard quality of care (NPA, 2010).

Certain groups have been recognized as experiencing health disparities and have become a priority for policy efforts. Many factors contribute to disparities in health and health care for special groups of adult men and women, including education, insurance status, segregation, immigration status, health behaviors and lifestyle choices, health care provider behavior, employment, and the nature and operation of the health system in communities (Kosoko-Lasaki, Cook, and O'Brien, 2009). In particular, poverty is a strong and underlying current throughout all of the special groups.

Adults of Color

In 2000, about 33% of the U.S. population identified themselves as members of racial or ethnic minority groups. By 2050, these groups are projected to account for almost half of the U.S. population (NHDR, 2008). Adults of color experience many of the same health problems as their white counterparts. Improvements in preventive care, chronic care, and access to care have led to improvements to the health of some populations in areas such as mammograms and smoking cessation counseling. However, the complete picture of disparities is different for each population. For African Americans, large disparities remain in new AIDS cases despite significant decreases in other groups. The proportion of new AIDS cases was 9.4 times as high for African Americans as for whites. Hospital admissions for lower extremity amputations in clients with diabetes and lack of prenatal care for pregnant women in the first trimester are the largest disparities for African Americans (NHDR, 2008).

Although addressing these disparities appears daunting, the intent is to close the gap with regard to the health disparities in adults of color while at the same time preserving and respecting the richness and unique influences of various cultures. Population-focused nurses are positioned to advocate for culturally sensitive and gender-sensitive programs necessary in communities where adults of color may reside.

NURSING TIP *Because of the known health disparities experienced by adults of color, it is essential that preventive services target diversity and cultural awareness throughout the entire program planning process.*

Incarcerated Adults

The U.S. prison population grew at the slowest rate (0.8%) since 2000, reaching 1,610,446 sentenced prisoners in 2008 (U.S. Department of Justice, Bureau of Justice Statistics, 2009). However, while this appears to be positive, it does create a challenge to nurses who will be caring for this special population in other community settings. An increase in the number of prison releases has led to offenders being released to the community without supervision. African-American males were incarcerated at a rate six and one half times higher than white males. The proportion of prisoners under state or federal jurisdiction was 93% men and 7% women (Sabol, West, and Cooper, 2009). Women are more likely to be serving time for property and drug offenses rather than violent crimes.

Over the past 40 years, legal, social, and political factors have led to the current epidemic of psychiatric disorders in the U.S. prison system. Incarcerated populations with major psychiatric disorders (major depressive disorder, bipolar disorders, schizophrenia, and non-schizophrenic psychotic disorders) have a substantially increased risk of multiple incarcerations. The greatest increase may be among inmates with bipolar disorders (Baillargeon et al, 2009). Nurses can support and deliver beneficial continuity of care reentry programs to help those who are mentally ill connect with community-based mental health programs at the time of release from prison to decrease recidivism rates (Baillargeon et al, 2009).

Welcome Home Ministries was an innovative program developed in southern California by a nurse/minister to ease the transition for women from jail to life on the "outside" (Box 30-3) (Parsons and Warner-Robbins, 2002).

Lesbian/Gay Adults

Lesbians/gay adults represent a sometimes hidden special population, in part because of the social stigma associated with homosexuality coupled with the fear of discrimination. Although it is

---

BOX 30-3 POPULATION-LEVEL INTERVENTION

Welcome Home Ministries is an innovative program developed in southern California by a nurse/minister to ease the transition for women from jail (population) to life on the "outside." In the program, a registered nurse and formerly incarcerated women help others recently released make this adjustment. The program is based on research in which women reported histories of poverty, physical and emotional abuse, addiction (usually to methamphetamine), and repeated incarceration. Many also reported grief over their lives and especially over their children. The program includes a protocol of jail visitations to women prisoners by formerly incarcerated women and transportation of newly released women to new homes. All women are encouraged to participate in gatherings where they support and encourage one another. Struggles of transitions and successes are shared, and goals are set to help women remain healthy and drug free.

From Parsons ML, Warner-Robbins C: Holistic nursing on the front lines, *Am J Nurs* 102:73-77, 2002; Parsons ML, Warner-Robbins C: Factors that support women's successful transition to the community following jail/prison, *Health Care Women Int* 23:6-18, 2002; Parsons ML, Warner-Robbins C: Formerly incarcerated women create healthy lives through participatory action research, *Holistic Nurs Pract* 16: 40-49, 2002.

well known that men who have sex with men are at a higher risk of contracting HIV and other sexually transmitted diseases, there is accumulating evidence that sexual orientation may also be an unrecognized risk factor for psychiatric morbidity, alcohol use, illicit drug use, cigarette smoking, and challenges with health care. Lesbian and gay adults report higher levels of psychological distress, which has been associated with more frequent reporting of some chronic conditions, health limitations, and poorer physical health status. This may be particularly true for minority groups (Cochran and Mays, 2007).

To improve the health of lesbian/gay adults, services that address their unique needs are warranted. Safe places where this special population can voice their concerns and receive effective health promotion, disease prevention, and treatment are critical. Clarification of ways in which sexual orientation is associated with health outcomes will be critical to developing appropriate health interventions (Bostwick et al, 2010).

Adults with Physical and Mental Disabilities

Many issues confront adults with disabilities. Concerns associated with health, aging, civil rights, abuse, and independent living are but a few examples of the types of problems facing this population. In 2007, 69 million adults 18 years of age and over had either basic actions difficulty (including movement or emotional difficulty or trouble seeing or hearing) or complex activity limitation (such as work or self-care limitations). This was an increase by 8 million in the past 10 years. One-quarter of adults 18 to 64 years of age had at least one basic actions difficulty or complex activity limitation in 2007, compared with 62% of adults 65 years of age and over (NCHS, 2009).

Those in poor physical and mental health face additional challenges in accessing care in the community setting, and these additional barriers may further worsen health outcomes. These problems are even more pronounced among those adults with disabilities. One study found that women with disabilities placed a high value on preventive health screenings, but they often did not participate in them because of the difficulties associated with living with a disability (Mele, Archer, and Pusch, 2005). This most likely is also true for men with disabilities, although this has not been studied. Women are more likely to seek treatment for most diseases, especially potentially stigmatized diseases such as those related to mental health. These differences appear to begin in the teen years (Chandra and Minkovitz, 2006).

Often adults with disabilities demonstrate multiple comorbidities. For instance, adults with developmental disabilities may be at a high risk for obesity and its sequelae (Bazzano et al, 2009). This may be due to individual and community factors including physical challenges, cognitive limitations, medications, lack of accessible adaptive fitness facilities, and a segregation from the community in general. A community-based health intervention program called "The Healthy Lifestyle Change Program" targeted adults with developmental disabilities. This program used a twice-weekly education and exercise program to increase knowledge, skills, and self-efficacy regarding health, nutrition, and fitness with peer mentors serving as participatory leaders and motivators. Outcomes were improved lifestyles, weight loss success, and increased life satisfaction (Bazzano et al, 2009).

Nurses can develop an awareness of the many health-related issues facing adults with disabilities. In particular, care should be taken to recognize the physical barriers that prevent disabled adults from accessing health care, such as structures that are not accessible despite the ADA recommendations. Developing health promotion programs targeted at this vulnerable, high-risk group can assist in overall well-being.

Impoverished and Uninsured Adults

In 2008, the nation's official poverty rate was 13.2%, up from 12.5% in 2007. Poverty affects acute and chronic conditions, accumulates over the life course, and is transmitted across generations. It limits education and employment opportunities, leaving individuals susceptible to weaker social integration, low control, depressive symptoms, and often a fatalistic outlook (Sanders, Lim, and Sohn, 2008). Often the stress of poverty may lead to poor dietary habits, tobacco use, and inconsistent personal hygiene. Health disparities, including chronic illness and health care services, are consistently associated with socioeconomic differences. The vulnerable homeless, impoverished rural, migrant, and public housing communities suffer from an increased burden of disease and greater morbidity and mortality than the general population (Custodio, Gard, and Graham, 2009).

The United States stands alone among industrialized nations in not providing health coverage to all its citizens (Wilper et al, 2009). The numbers of people without health insurance coverage rose from 45.7 million in 2007 to 46.3 million in 2008 (U.S. Census Bureau, 2009). Adults who are insured will access health care services more often, including obtaining recommended screening and care for chronic conditions, thus reducing the overall costs of potential catastrophic illness (Wilper et al, 2009). Although President Obama signed the Patient Protection and Affordable Care Act along with the Health Care and Education Reconciliation Act in March 2010, many changes such as health insurance mandates do not begin until 2014.

Nurses can be uniquely involved in community assessments to document pockets of poverty within their communities. For example, housing is a fundamental determinant of health and provides shelter and privacy. Exposure to cracks in ceilings and walls, inadequate heat, mold, poor ventilation, pesticide residue, excessive moisture, leaky pipes, and lead paint are all health hazards that can be addressed by nurses. Recent research has also found that health resilience to poverty was supported by protective factors in built and social environments. (See Chapter 29 for discussion of the built environment.) When poverty itself cannot be eliminated, improving the quality of the built and social environments can foster resilience to the harmful effects of poverty (Sanders et al, 2008).

Frail Elderly

In the past decade, the United States experienced a 15% increase in the population 65 years of age and older. By 2020, this group is expected to increase another 36% (A Profile of Older Americans, 2009). In addition, the population of those 85 years and older is projected to increase another 15% by 2020. Most older persons have at least one chronic condition and many have multiple conditions, putting them at risk of experiencing frailty while living in a community setting.

Frailty is a geriatric syndrome that places older adults at risk for adverse health outcomes, including falls, worsening disability, institutionalization, and death (Espinoza and Hazuda, 2008). It is a complex state of impairment that signifies loss in areas of physical functioning, physiological resiliency, metabolism, and immune response (Hackstaff, 2009).

The prevalence of frailty in the older population poses a major public health dilemma since the majority of this group will reside in a community setting, placing new demands on health care systems, family caregivers, and community resources. To improve the health of frail elderly, community-based nursing programs will need to address racial/ethnic and socioeconomic disparities.

The elder-friendly community model identifies four domains needed by the elderly including having basic needs met, social and civic engagement, physical and mental health and well-being, and independence for the frail and disabled (Feldman and Oberlink, 2003). This model identifies independence for the frail elderly as the ability to "age in place" with specific indicators that focus on activities of daily living, transportation, and caregivers' ability to complement formal services. Community-level characteristics, including security issues, accessible shopping, and adequate transportation services are important community resources (Weierbach and Glick, 2009). Nurses can use this model to incorporate both individual and community factors that are necessary for elderly to live and thrive in community settings.

Importance of Cultural Competence in Health Disparity

In the past two decades, more attention has been given to the importance of cultural competence in a nation that is increasingly multiethnic, multicultural, and increasingly diverse. Experts in the field have theorized that cultural competence may be viewed as a strategy to combat health disparities (Browne and Mokuau, 2008). The Office of Minority Health (OMH) provides the following definitions of cultural competence:

> Cultural and linguistic competence *is a set of congruent behaviors, attitudes, and policies that come together in a system, agency, or among professionals that enables effective work in cross-cultural situations. 'Culture' refers to integrated patterns of human behavior that include the language, thoughts, communications, actions, customs, beliefs, values, and institutions of racial, ethnic, religious, or social groups. 'Competence' implies having the capacity to function effectively as an individual and an organization within the context of the cultural beliefs, behaviors, and needs presented by consumers and their communities (NPA, 2010).*

Nurses who work with adults with health disparities will need knowledge, skills, and attitudes that honor diversity. This includes the need to continually engage in self-reflective activities that assess his or her world views and values regarding oppression, discrimination, and working with the diverse individuals (Browne and Mokuau, 2008).

COMMUNITY-BASED MODELS FOR CARE OF ADULTS

Nursing Roles

Communities are where people live, work, and socialize. Community health settings include public health departments, nurse-managed health centers, ambulatory care clinics, and home health agencies. Nurses are involved in direct care, providing self-care information, contributing to the supervision of paraprofessionals, or collaborating with other disciplines to provide the most appropriate, high-quality, cost-effective care at the most appropriate level and location.

Knowledge of community resources is a fundamental part of caring for the adult with special needs in any community. The nurse assesses the need for and helps develop the resources. Every community has an area agency on aging that coordinates planning and delivery of needed services, and it can be a good resource for the nurse. Most communities have information and referral systems as well as a public directory of services available.

The Doctor of Nursing Practice (DNP) role brings specific competencies and nursing backgrounds to the role of primary care provider. A recent community-based model to provide care for frail elders highlights three areas of expertise that advanced practice nurses in the DNP role can provide: management of complex chronic illness, illness and injury prevention, and promotion of quality of life (Auer and Nirenberg, 2008).

Community Care Settings

Senior Centers

Senior centers were developed in the early 1940s to provide social and recreational activities. Now many centers are multi-purpose, offering recreation, education, counseling, therapies, hot meals, and case management, as well as health screening and education. Some even offer primary care services. Nurses have a unique opportunity to provide services to a group of older persons who wish to remain independent in the community (Weierbach and Glick, 2009; Truncali et al, 2010).

Adult Day Health

Adult day health is for individuals whose mental or physical function requires them to obtain more health care and supervision. It serves as more of a medical model than the senior center, and often individuals return home to their caregivers at night. Some settings offer respite care for short-term overnight relief for caregivers. This provides caregivers the opportunity to work or have personal time during the day. Often, support groups for caregivers are offered by nurses (Jennings-Sanders, 2004).

Home Health and Hospice

Home health can be provided by multidisciplinary teams. Nurses provide individual and environmental assessments, direct skilled care and treatment, and short-term guidance and instruction. Nurses often function independently in the home and must rely on their own resources and knowledge to improvise and adapt care to meet the client's unique physical and social circumstances. They work closely with the family and other caregivers to provide necessary communication and continuity of care. (See Chapter 41 for more details.)

Hospice represents a philosophy of caring for and supporting life to its fullest until death occurs. The hospice team encourages the client and family to jointly make decisions to meet physical, emotional, spiritual, and comfort needs (see palliative care in the Content Resources section of the Evolve website).

Assisted Living

Assisted living covers a wide variety of choices, from a single shared room to opulent independent living accommodations in a full-service, life-care community. The differences are related to the type and extent of the amenities provided and the contract signed for them. The role of the nurse varies depending on the philosophy and leadership of the management of the facility. The nurse generally provides assessment and interventions, medication review, education, and advocacy (Counsell et al, 2006; Auer and Nirenberg, 2008).

Long-Term Care and Rehabilitation

Nursing homes, or long-term care facilities, house only about 5% of the older population at a given time; however, 25% of those adults older than 65 will spend some time in a nursing home. Nursing homes provide a safe environment, special diets and activities, routine personal care, and the treatment and management of health care needs for those needing rehabilitation,

as well as for those needing a permanent supportive residence. Rehabilitation is a combination of physical, occupational, psychological, and speech therapy to help debilitated persons maintain or recover their physical capacities. Rehabilitation is typically needed for older adults after a hip fracture, stroke, or prolonged illness that results in serious deconditioning (Olsson et al, 2009).

Like hospitals, nursing homes are paid using the prospective payment model based on the nursing assessment. A recent new model developed by nurse practitioners used collaborative practice techniques to change care management for frail and elderly nursing home residents, which reduced hospitalizations by 45%, reduced emergency room visits by 50%, and effectively reduced the incidence of acute episodes in the nursing home setting (Kappas-Larsen, 2008).

LINKING CONTENT TO PRACTICE

The information in this chapter focuses on the health issues of adult and older adult men and women from a population perspective as opposed to the individual or family. In practice, the knowledge, skills, and attitudes, such as those identified by the Quad Council for Public Health Nursing, transcend other public health disciplines. Therefore, nurses practicing in community health need to foster the ability to work effectively with interprofessional teams across a variety of organizations to accomplish goals to improve community health. Working in interprofessional teams is a core competency identified by the Institute of Medicine (IOM) and involves essential features such as "sections related to self, team, team communication and conflict resolution, effect of team on safety and quality, and the impact of systems on team functioning" (Cronenwett et al, 2007, p 123).

CHAPTER REVIEW

PRACTICE APPLICATION

During her community clinical time in nursing education, Laura had the opportunity to accompany Marie, her preceptor, on an initial home visit to a young woman named Josie. Josie was a 20-year-old single woman who had come to the public health center last week for a gynecological examination because she thought she might have some sort of infection. During the visit, Josie mentioned to the clinic nurse that she did not have any food in her house. After the examination the clinic nurse made a referral to the women's resource service center for a home visit and for inclusion of Josie into their case management program.

When Marie and Laura arrived at Josie's apartment, they immediately noted that the living areas were devoid of furniture; however, there was a soiled mattress on the floor of the living room. Dirty clothing was on the floor; empty take-out food sacks and trash littered the area. The kitchen area was also dirty, with evidence of cockroach infestation.

Marie and Laura noticed that Josie appeared to be uncomfortable and had difficulty interacting with either of them. Marie explained

that they were there because the nurse at the clinic had asked them to stop by and see if there was any way that they might help Josie with her health care needs and living situation. Immediately Josie began to cry. She had been with her abusive boyfriend until about 3 weeks ago when she asked him to leave. Marie and Laura learned that since that time, Josie had been prostituting as a way to survive. She was frightened and thought that her boyfriend was going to return and harm her. She also feared that she was pregnant.

Based on this situation, what would be potential actions that Laura and her preceptor Marie might take?

A. Make an appointment for Josie to return to the women's clinic for pregnancy testing.

B. Suggest to Josie that she focus on cleaning up her apartment, reminding her of the hazards of spoiled food.

C. Refer Josie to a safe-house shelter as a victim of domestic violence.

D. Make a referral for food delivery from a local church.
Answers are in the back of the book.

PRACTICE APPLICATION—cont'd

The nurse in a local public health department talks with the director of the department, who needs to determine what major public health issues exist in the community and prioritize them to better allocate resources. The director formed a committee to assist in this process. The director asks the nurse to participate on the committee because of the nurse's interest in men's health. The director asks the nurse to identify up to 10 major health issues in the community, prioritize them, and recommend strategies to improve men's health in the community. The director wants a report supporting conclusions and strategies that the department could implement.

Based on the above scenario, answer the following questions:

A. What information do you want to collect?

B. How would you identify priorities in your area?

C. What positive and negative factors may be influencing these issues?

D. How would you select strategies to improve health issues?
   1. What interventions, if any, are currently being used, and are they effective?
   2. Who are the key participants that would need to be involved in improving the issues?
   3. Have these issues been addressed effectively in other communities? If they have, what have they done?
   Answers can be found on the Evolve site.

KEY POINTS

- The health of adults is embedded in their communities.
- Societal factors influence the distribution of health and disease.
- Women's health advocates have widened the framework of women's health by focusing on social, psychological, cultural, political, and economic as well as biological factors.
- The complexities of women's lives—their educational levels, income, culture, ethnicity/race, and a host of other identities and experiences—shape their health.
- The Office on Women's Health (OWH) works to address inequities in research, health services, and education that have traditionally placed women at risk for health problems.
- The problem of unintended pregnancy exists among adolescents as well as adult women.
- Women's attitudes toward menopause vary greatly and are influenced by culture, age, support, and the shared experiences of other women.
- Cardiovascular disease (CVD) is the leading cause of death among U.S. adults.
- Diabetes has increased dramatically in the United States during the last decade.
- Women in the United States experience depression at higher rates than do men.
- Overall, white women have a higher incidence rate for all cancers while African-American women have higher mortality rates.
- Most U.S. women contract HIV/AIDS by heterosexual transmission.
- The Bureau of Justice reports a dramatic rise in the number of women in state and federal prisons.
- Research findings indicate that lesbians and bisexual women have higher prevalence rates of several risk factors than their heterosexual counterparts with regard to smoking, alcohol use, and lack of preventative cancer screening.

- Poverty among women heads-of-household reflects the disparities that exist in the United States among various ethnic/racial groups because female-headed African-American and Hispanic families suffer disproportionately higher rates of poverty than do other families.
- Research shows that older women, especially women of color from lower socioeconomic groups, experience higher rates of chronic illness and disability than their white and more affluent counterparts.
- One out of every two American women more than 50 years of age will experience an osteoporosis-related fracture in her lifetime.
- Men are reluctant to seek health care and are not well connected to the health care system.
- Large numbers of men do not receive the health screenings intended to prevent and identify disease.
- To improve health outcomes for men, chronic disease prevention and control programs should combine individual and population-based strategies developed in collaboration with community members and developing infrastructure to address environmental and policy change.
- Although adverse working conditions and numerous pathological conditions clearly are detrimental to men's health, there is a great need to focus on the mental health of men.
- The nurse acts as a change agent to assess needs and system influences, identify and set priorities, plan and implement programs, and evaluate results.

CLINICAL DECISION-MAKING ACTIVITIES

1. Interview three women, each from a different culture, about their experiences accessing health care. Are there differences in their stories about how they meet their health care needs? Do variances in ethnicity and culture present barriers to accessing health care?

2. Review current legislation that deals with women's health. Note patterns or trends in the issues that are being considered by the Senate or the House of Representatives. Are there obvious gaps in legislation that adversely affect women's health?

3. Considering breast cancer, apply the levels of prevention to women in underserved areas. Describe approaches to meeting their health care, social needs, and psychological needs. What barriers might prevent an effective program addressing breast cancer?

4. Contact your local public health office to determine what services are available for women. Identify community resources and agencies targeted for women. How do these organizations communicate their services to women in the community?

CLINICAL DECISION-MAKING ACTIVITIES—cont'd

5. Propose a community-based intervention for women with HIV. Describe various program components such as goals and objectives, evaluation methods, and program outcomes.

6. Identify a men's health issue in your community. Contact local health agencies in your area to determine what strategies are currently in place to address the issue.

7. Based on the issue identified in no. 6, search the Internet for evidence-based practices related to the issue.

8. Think about television, movie, or magazine portrayals of men and identify both positive and negative influences the media may have on men's health.

9. Locate several websites focusing on men's health topics. Using criteria for credible websites from Health on the Net Foundation (www.hon.ch), evaluate those sites for credible health information.

REFERENCES

Administration on Aging: *Long-term care ombudsman program complaint codes (n.d.).* Retrieved from http://webcache.googleusercontent.com/custom?q=cache:mLnql8x3maoJ:www.aoa.gov/AoARoot/AoA_Programs/Elder_Rights/Ombudsman/docs/Complaint_Code.doc+definitions&;cd=1&hl=en&ct=clnk&gl=us&client=google-coop-np.

Administration on Aging: *About AoA*, 2010. Available at http://www.aoa.gov/AoARoot/About/index.aspx. Accessed February 22, 2011.

Administration for Children and Families: *About ACF*, n.d. Available at http://www.acf.hhs.gov/acf_about.html. Accessed February 22, 2011.

Agency for Healthcare Research and Quality, U.S. Preventive Services Task Force: *The guide to clinical preventive services*, 2009. Available at http://www.ahrq.gov/clinic/pocketgd09/pocketgd09.pdf.

Agency for Healthcare Research and Quality: *Men shy away from routine medical appointments*, AHRQ News and Numbers, June 16, 2010. Available at http://www.ahrq.gov.

Alexander LL, LaRosa JH, Bader H, Garfield S: *New dimensions in women's health*, ed 4, Boston, 2007, Jones and Bartlett.

American Academy of Pediatrics: Fetal alcohol syndrome and alcohol-related neurodevelopmental disorders, *Pediatrics* 111(S1):1131–1135, 2003.

American Cancer Society: *Cancer facts and figures 2009*, Atlanta, 2009, ACS. Accessed at http://www.cancer.org.

American Cancer Society: *Prostate cancer overview*, 2010. Available at http://www.cancer.org/Cancer/ProstateCancer/OverviewGuide/prostate-cancer-overview-what-causes. Accessed February 22, 2011.

American Heart Association: *Overweight and obesity statistics*, 2009. Available at http://grfw.org/presenter.jhtml?identifier=3000947. Accessed February 23, 2011.

American Heart Association: *Women, heart disease, and stroke*, 2010. Available at www.americanheart.org. Accessed April 14, 2011.

Americans with Disabilities Act of 1990, as amended. Available at http://www.ada.gov/pubs/ada.htm. Accessed March 28, 2010.

Angel J, Angel R: Minority group status and healthful aging: social structure still matters, *Am J Public Health* 96(7):1152–1159, 2006.

Angell SY, Garg RK, Gwynn RC, et al: Relevance, awareness, treatment, and predictors of control of hypertension in New York City, *Circ Cardiovasc Qual Outcomes* 1(1):46–53, 2008.

Auer P, Nirenberg A: Nurse practitioner home-based primary care: a model for the care of frail elders, *Clin Schol Rev* 1(1):33–39, 2008.

Azad N, Nashtar S: A call for a gender specific approach to address the worldwide cardiovascular burden, *Prev Control* 1(3):223–227, 2005.

Baillargeon J, Binswanger I, Penn J, et al: Psychiatric disorders and repeat incarcerations: the revolving prison door, *Am J Psych* 166(1):103–109, 2009.

Bazzano A, Zeldin A, Diab I, et al: The Healthy Lifestyle Change Program: a pilot of a community-based health promotion intervention for adults with developmental disabilities, *Am J Prevent Med* 37(6S1):S201–S208, 2009.

Berdahl T, Zodet M: Medical care utilization for work-related injuries in the United States 2002-2006, *Med Care* 48(7):645–651, 2010.

Bonhomme J: Men's health: impact on women, children and society, *J Mens Health Gender* 4(2):124–130, 2007.

Bos A, Kanner D, Muris P, et al: Mental illness stigma and disclosure: consequences of coming out of the closet, *Issues Ment Health Nurs* 30:509–513, 2009.

Bostwick W, Boyd C, Hughes T, McCabe S: Dimensions of sexual orientation and the prevalence of mood and anxiety disorders in the United States, *Am J Public Health* 100(3):468–475, 2010.

Branney P, White A: Big boys don't cry: depression and men, *Adv Psychiatr Treat* 14:256–262, 2008.

Braveman P: Health disparities and health equity: concepts and measurement, *Annu Rev Public Health* 27:167–194, 2006.

Brittle C, Bird C: *Literature review on effectiveness of sex- and gender-based systems/model of care*, 2007. Available at http://www.womenshealth.gov/archive/owh/multidisciplinary/reports/GenderBasedMedicine/. Accessed February 22, 2011.

Broom A, Tovey P: *Men's health: body, identity and social context*, West Sussex, England, 2009, Wiley-Blackwell.

Browne C, Mokuau N: Preparing students for culturally competent practice among ethnic minority elders, *Educ Gerontol* 34:306–327, 2008.

Brownson R, Chriqui J, Stamatakis K: Policy, politics, and collective action, *Am J Public Health* 99(9):1576–1582, 2009.

Buchanan T, Xiang A, Kjos S, Watanabe R: What is gestational diabetes? *Diabetes Care* 30:S105–S111, 2007, doi:10.2337/dc07-s201.

Centers for Disease Control and Prevention: *National diabetes fact sheet: general information and national estimates on diabetes in the United States, 2007*, Atlanta, 2008, USDHHS, CDC. Available at http://www.cdc.gov/diabetes/pubs/factsheet07.htm. Accessed February 23, 2011.

Centers for Disease Control and Prevention (n.d.): Rates for new cancer cases and deaths by race/ethnicity and sex. Centers for Disease Control and Prevention. *The Futures Initiatives*, 2005. Retrieved from http://www.cdc.gov/futures/. Accessed February 22, 2011.

Centers for Disease Control and Prevention: *CDC fact sheet: the role of STD prevention and treatment in HIV prevention*, 2007. Available at http://www.cdc.gov/std/hiv/stds-and-hiv-fact-sheet-press.pdf. Accessed February 23, 2011.

Centers for Disease Control and Prevention: *Sexually transmitted disease in the United States*, 2008. Available at http://www.cdc.gov/std/stats08/trends.htm. Accessed February 23, 2011.

Chandra A, Minkovitz C: Stigma starts early: gender differences in teen willingness to use mental health services, *J Adolesc Health* 38(6):754–758, 2006.

Chang L, Toner B, Fukudo S, et al: Gender, age, society, culture, and the patient's perspective in the functional gastrointestinal disorders, *Gastroenterology* 130(5):1435–1446, 2006.

Clougherty JE: A growing role for gender analysis in air pollution epidemiology, *Environ Health Perspect* 118(2):167–175, 2010.

Cochran S, Mays V: Physical health complaints among lesbians, gay men, and bisexual and homosexually experienced heterosexual individuals: results from the California Quality of Life Survey, *Am J Public Health* 97(11):2048–2055, 2007.

Community Health Status Indicators Project Working Group: *Data sources, definitions, and notes for CHSI2008*, Washington, DC, 2008, USDHHS. Available at http://communityhealth.hhs.gov. Accessed February 23, 2011.

Counsell S, Callahan C, Buttar A, et al: Geriatric Resources for Assessment and Care of Elders (GRACE): a new model of primary care for low income senior, *J Am Geriatr Soc* 54(7):1136–1141, 2006.

Cronenwett L, Sherwood G, Barnsteiner J, et al: Quality and safety education for nurses, *Nurs Outlook* 55:122–131, 2007.

Custodio R, Gard A, Graham G: Health information technology: addressing health disparity by improving quality, increasing access, and developing workforce, *J Health Care Poor Underserved* 20:301–307, 2009.

Danielsson U, Bengs C, Lehti A, et al: Struck by lightning or slowly suffocating-gender trajectories into depression, *BMC Fam Pract* 10:56, 2009. doi:10.1186/1471-2296-10-56.

Douglass M, Lin J: Erectile dysfunction and premature ejaculation: underlying causes and available treatments, *Formulary J* 45:17–45, 2010.

Edwards BK, Ward E, Kohler BA, et al: Annual report to the nation on the status of cancer, 1975–2006, featuring colorectal cancer trends and impact of interventions (risk factors, screening, and treatment) to reduce stress, *Cancer* 16(3):544–573, 2009. Available at http://www3.interscience.wiley.com/cgi-bin/fulltext/123206036/HTMLSTART. Accessed February 22, 2011.

Emanuel L: Advanced directives, *Annu Rev* 59:187–198, 2008.

Espinoza S, Hazuda H: Frailty in older Mexican-American and European-American Adults: is there an ethnic disparity? *J Am Geriatr Soc* 56:1744–1749, 2008.

Feldman P, Oberlink M: The advantage initiative: developing community indicators to promote the health and well-being of older people, *Fam Community Health* 26:268–274, 2003.

Finkelstein EA, Trogdon JG, Cohen JW, Dietz W: Annual medical spending attributable to obesity: payer- and service-specific estimates, *Health Aff* 28(5):s822–s831, 2009.

Forchuk C, Jensen E, Csiernik R, et al: Exploring differences between community-based women and men with a history of mental illness, *Issues Ment Health Nurs* 30:495–502, 2009.

Glazier R, Kennie N, Bajcar J, Willson K: A systematic review of interventions to improve diabetes care in socially disadvantaged populations, *Diabetes Care* 29(7):1675–1688, 2006.

Hackstaff L: Factors associated with frailty in chronically ill older adults, *Soc Work Health Care* 48:798–811, 2009.

Hall H, An Q, Hutchinson A, Sansom S: Estimating the lifetime risk of a diagnosis of the HIV infection in 33 states, 2004-2005, *J Acq Immune Def Syndrome* 49(3):294–297, 2008.

Halphen JM, Sadowsky JM: Recognizing and reporting elder abuse and neglect. *Geriatrics* 64(7):13–18, 2009.

Heron MP, Hoyert DL, Murphy SL, et al: *Deaths: final data for 2006, national vital statistics reports,* vol 57(14), Hyattsville, MD, 2009, NCHS.

Holdcroft A: Gender bias in research: how does it affect evidence based medicine? *J Royal Soc Med* 100:2–3, 2007.

Jennings-Sanders A: Nurses in adult day care, *Geriatr Nurs* 25(4):227–232, 2004.

Jones DW, Peterson ED, Bonow RO, et al: Translating research into practice for healthcare providers: the American Heart Association's strategy for building healthier lives, free of cardiovascular disease and stroke, *Circulation* 118(6):687–696, 2008.

Kappas-Larson P: The evercare story: reshaping the health care model, revolutionizing long-term care, *J Nurse Pract* 4(2):132–136, 2008.

Kim J, Alley D, Seeman T, et al: Recent changes in cardiovascular risk factors among women and men, *J Womens Health* 15(6):737–746, 2006.

Kosoko-Lasaki S, Cook C, O'Brien R: *Cultural proficiency in addressing health disparities*, Sudbury, MA, 2009, Jones and Bartlett.

Latini D, Penson D: Longitudinal differences in disease specific quality of life in men with erectile dysfunction, *J Urol* 169:1437–1442, 2003.

Levin P, Cary A, Kulbok P, et al: Graduate education for advanced practice public health nursing: at the crossroads, *Public Health Nurs* 25(2):176–193, 2008.

Lloyd-Jones D, Adams RJ, Brown TM, et al: Heart disease and stroke statistics—2010 update: a report from the American Heart Association Statistics Committee and Stroke Statistics Subcommittee, *Circulation* 121:e1–e170, 2010.

Mahalik J, Burns S, Syzdek M: Masculinity and perceived normative health behaviors as predictors of men's health behaviors, *Soc Sci Med* 64:2201–2209, 2007.

Mathews TJ: *Trends in spina bifida and anencephalus in the United States, 1991-2005,* Hyattsville, MD, 2007, USDHHS, CDC, NCHS.

McWilliams JM, Meara E, Zaslavsky M, Ayanian JZ: Differences in control of cardiovascular disease and diabetes by race, ethnicity, and education: U.S. trends from 1999 to 2006 and effects of Medicare coverage, *Ann Int Med* 150(8):505–515, 2009.

Mele N, Archer J, Pusch B: Access to breast cancer screening services for women with disabilities, *JOGNN Clin Res* 34(4):453–464, 2005.

Messinger-Rapport B, Baum E, Smith M: Advance care planning: beyond the living will, *Cleve Clin J Med* 76(5):276–284, 2009.

Miller E, West D, Wasserman M: Health information websites: characteristics of US users by race and ethnicity, *J Telemed Telecare* 13(6):298–302, 2007.

Miniño AM, Xu J, Kochanek KD, Tejada-Vera B: *Death in the United States, 2007,* NCHS data brief, No 26, Hyattsville, MD, 2009, NCHS.

Model Elements: *Guide to implementing the chronic care model, annual clinic focus,* 2007. Available at www.aafp.org. Accessed February 11, 2011.

Morbidity and Mortality Weekly Report: *Center for Disease Control and Prevention. Life expectancy ranking at birth, by sex: selected countries and territories,* 2008. Available from http://www.cdc.gov/mmwr/. Accessed February 22, 2011.

Morbidity and Mortality Weekly Report: *Centers for Disease Control and Prevention: Prevalence of self-reported physically active adults—United States,* 2007, 57:1297-1300, 2008. Available from http://www.cdc.gov/mmwr/preview/mmwrhtml/mm5748a1.htm. Accessed February 22, 2011.

Mosca L, Mochari-Greenberger H, Dolor R, et al: Twelve-year follow-up of American women's awareness of cardiovascular disease risks and barriers to heart health, *Circ Cardiovasc Qual Outcomes* 3:120–127, 2010.

National Cancer Institute: *Surveillance epidemiology and end results (SEER): cancer stat fact sheets,* 2010. Available at http://www.seer.cancer.gov/statfacts/html/prost.html. Accessed February 22, 2011.

National Center on Elder Abuse: *Why should I care about elder abuse?* n.d. Available at http://www.ncea.aoa.gov/NCEAroot/Main_Site/Index.aspx. Accessed February 22, 2011.

National Center for Complementary and Alternative Medicine: *Alternative Therapies for managing menopausal symptoms,* 2009. Available at www.cccam.nih.gov. Accessed February 11, 2011.

National Center for Chronic Disease Prevention and Health Promotion (NCCDPHP): *Preventing chronic disease, public health research, practice and policies,* July 2007. Available at www.cdc.gov. Accessed February 22, 2011.

National Center for Health Statistics: *Health, United States, 2009: with special feature on medical technology,* Hyattsville, MD, 2009.

National Healthcare Disparities Report: *AHRQ Publication No. 09-0002,* 2008, USDHHS. Available at www.ahrq.gov/qual/qrdr08.htm. Accessed February 22, 2011.

National Institute of Arthritis and Musculoskeletal and Skin Diseases, *Osteoporosis Overview,* 2009. Available at www. osteo.org.

National Institute of Diabetes and Digestive and Kidney Diseases (NIDDK), National Diabetes Information Clearinghouse: *General information and national estimates on diabetes in the United States, 2006,* 2008. Available at www.diabetes.niddk.nih.gov.

National Osteoporosis Foundation: *Clinician's guide to prevention and treatment of osteoporosis,* 2010. Available at http://www.nof.org/professionals/pdfs/NOF_Clinician Guide2009_v7.pdf.

National Partnership for Action (NPA): Office of Minority Health, *Health disparities,* 2010. Available at http://minorityhealth.hhs.gov/. Accessed February 22, 2011.

Olsson L, Hansson E, Ekman I, Karlsson J: A cost-effective study of a patient-centered integrated care pathway, *J Adv Nurs* 65(8):1626–1635, 2009.

Parsons ML, Warner-Robbins C: Formerly incarcerated women create healthy lives through participatory action research, *Holist Nurse Practition* 16:40–49, 2002.

Pazoki R, Nabipour I, Seyednezami N, Seyed R: Effects of a community-based healthy heart program on increasing healthy women's physical activity: a randomized controlled trial guided by Community-Based Participatory Research (CBPR), *BMC Public Health* 7:216, 2007. doi:10.1186/1471-2458-7-216.

Pearlman R, Starks H, Cain K, et al: *Your life your choices: planning for future medical decisions: how to prepare a personalized living will,* n.d. Available at http://stevebuyer.house.gov.

A Profile of Older Americans: *Administration on Aging,* 2009, USDHHS. Available at http://www.aoa.gov/AoAroot/Aging_Statistics/Profile/2009/docs/2009profile_508.pdf. Accessed February 22, 2011.

Riska E: Men's mental health. In Broom A, Tovey P, editors: *Men's health: body, identity and social context,* West Sussex, UK, 2009, Wiley-Blackwell, pp 145–162.

Robine JM, Michel JP, Herrmann F: Who will care for the oldest people? *Br Med J* 334:570–571, 2007.

Rogers B, Franke J, Jeras J, et al: The Family and Medical Leave Act: implications for occupational and environmental nursing, *Am Assoc Occup Health Nurses J* 57(6):239–250, 2009.

Rose M, Arenson C, Harrod Salkey R, et al: Evaluation of the chronic disease self-management program with low-income, urban, African American older adults, *J Community Health Nurs* 25:193–202, 2008.

Rosland A, Piette J: Emerging models for mobilizing family support for chronic disease management: a structured review, *Chron Illness* 6(7), 2010. doi:10.1177/1742395309352254.

Roy K, Haddix A, Ikeda R, et al: Monitoring progress toward CDC's health protection goals: health outcome measures by life stage, *Public Health Rep* 124:304–316, 2009.

Sabol WJ, West HC, Cooper M: *Prisoners in 2008*. Bureau of Justice Statistics Bulletin, 2009, U.S. Department of Justice. Available at www.ojp.usdoj.gov/bjs/. Accessed February 22, 2011.

Sanders A, Lim S, Sohn W: Resilience to urban poverty: theoretical and empirical considerations for population health, *Am J Public Health* 98(6):1101–1106, 2008.

Sayal K, Heron J, Golding J, Ernond A: Prenatal alcohol exposure and gender differences in childhood mental health problems: a longitudinal population-based study, *Pediatrics* 119(2):e426–434, 2007.

Shin J, Martin R, Howren M: Influence of assessment methods n reports of gender differences in AMI symptoms, *Western J Nurs Res* 31(5):553–568, 2009.

Shuford JA: *What is the difference between sexually transmitted infection (STI) and sexually transmitted disease (STD)?* 2008. Available at http://www.medinstitute.org/public/132.cfm. Accessed February 22, 2011.

Smith-Campbell B: Politics and policy, In Larsen PD, Lubkin IM, editors: *Chronic illness Boston*, 2009, Jones and Bartlett, pp 555–575.

Stuenkel D, Wong V: Stigma. In Larsen PD, Lubkin IM, editors: *Chronic illness: impact and intervention*, Sudbury, MA, 2009, Jones and Bartlett.

Substance Abuse and Mental Health Services Administration: *Fetal alcohol syndrome thru the lifespan*, 2009. Available at www.samhsa.gov. Accessed February 11, 2011.

Travis MA: Lashing back at the ADA backlash: how the Americans with Disabilities Act benefits those without disabilities, *Tenn Law Rev* 76(2):311–378, 2009.

Treadwell M, Marguerite R: Poverty, race, and the invisible men. *Am J Public Health* 98(Suppl 1): S142–S144, 2008. (Original work published 2003.).

Truncali A, Dumanosvsky T, Stollman H, Angell S: Keep on Track: a volunteer-run community-based intervention to lower blood pressure in older adults, *J Am Geriatr Soc* 58(6):1177–1183, 2010.

U.S. Census Bureau: *Income, poverty, and health insurance coverage in the United States, 2008*, 2009. Available at http://www.census.gov/Press-Release/www/releases/archives/income_wealth/014227.html. Accessed April 16, 2011.

U.S. Department of Health and Human Services, National Women's Health Information Center: *Teen Talk II*, 2010. Available at http://www.womenshealth.gov/index.cfm. Accessed February 22, 2011.

U.S. Department of Health and Human Services: *Healthy People 2020*, 2010. Available at www.healthcare.gov.

U.S. Department of Justice, Bureau of Justice Studies: *Prisoners in 2008*, 2009. Available at http://bjs.ojp.usdoj.gov/index.cfm?ty=pbdetail&iiid=1763. Accessed February 22, 2011.

U.S. Preventive Services Task Force: Folic acid for the prevention of neural tube defects: U.S. Preventive Services Task Force recommendation statement. *Ann Intern Med* 150:626–631, 2009USPSTF.

U.S. Preventive Services Task Force: *Screening for testicular cancer: U.S. Preventive Services Task Force recommendation statement*, 2004. abaj, ab, e at www.guideline.gov. Accessed February 11, 2011.

Waski M, Kachlic M: A review of common sexually transmitted diseases, *Formulary* 44:78–85, 2009.

Weierbach F, Glick D: Community resources for older adults with chronic illness, *Holist Nurs Pract* 23(6):355–360, 2009.

Wilhelm K: Men and depression, *Austr Family Physician*, 38(3), 102–105, 2009.

Wilper AP, Woolhandler S, Lasser KE, et al: Health insurance and mortality in U.S. adults, *Am J Public Health* 99(12):2289–2295, 2009.

WIN, 2008. Available at http://win.niddk.nih.gov/Publications/tools.htm#bodymassindex. Accessed February 22, 2011.

World Health Organization: *Unequal, unfair, ineffective and inefficient gender inequality in health: why it exists and how we can manage it—final report to the WHO Commission on Social Determinants of Health*. Available at http://www.who.int/social_determinants/resources/csdh_media/wgekn_final_report_07.pdf. Accessed February 22, 2011.

World Health Organization: *Global health risks: mortality and burden of disease attributable to selected major risks*, 2009. Available at http://www.who.int/healthinfo/global_burden_disease/global_health_risks/en/index.html. Accessed February 22, 2011.

CHAPTER 31

Special Needs Populations

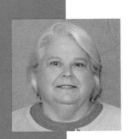

Lynn Wasserbauer, PhD, FNP, RN

Lynn Wasserbauer is a nurse practitioner at The University of Rochester Medical Center. Her current practice is in psychiatric nursing. Her bachelor's and master's degrees in nursing are from the University of Rochester. Her PhD in nursing and her post-master's certificate as a family nurse practitioner are from the University of Virginia.

ADDITIONAL RESOURCES

evolve WEBSITE

http://evolve.elsevier.com/Stanhope

- *Healthy People 2020*
- WebLinks
- Quiz
- Case Studies
- Glossary
- Answers to Practice Application
- Resource Tools
  - Resource Tool 5.A: Schedule of Clinical Preventive Services
  - Resource Tool 31.A: The Living Will Directive

- Resource Tool 31.B: Assessment Tools for Communities with Physically Compromised Members
- Resource Tool 31.C: Assessment Tools for Families with Physically Compromised Members
- Resource Tool 31.D: Assessment Tools for Physically Compromised Individuals

APPENDIX

- Appendix F.1: Instrumental Activities of Daily Living (IADLs) Scale

OBJECTIVES

After reading this chapter, the student should be able to do the following:

1. Define terms related to disability.
2. Discuss implications of developmental disability, physical disability, or chronic illness.
3. Identify the conditions that may contribute to disability.
4. Discuss the effects of being disabled on the individual, the family, and the community.

5. Describe the implications of being disabled for selected (low-income) populations.
6. Discuss selected issues for those who are disabled (abuse, health promotion).
7. Discuss the objectives of *Healthy People 2020* as they relate to disability.
8. Examine the nurse's role in caring for people who are disabled.

KEY TERMS

Americans with Disabilities Act, p. 698
burden of chronic disease, p. 701
Children with Special Health Care Needs (CSHCN), p. 700

chronic disease, p. 700
disability, p. 698
developmental disability, p. 700
dual diagnosis, p. 700
functional limitations, p. 700

Medical Model of Disability, p. 698
Social Model of Disability, p. 698
work disability, p. 699

Special thanks to Susan Kennel, PhD, RN, CPNP and Carol Lynn Maxwell-Thompson, MSN, RN, FNP-C, who authored this chapter in the seventh edition of the text.

Foundational to the American system of government is the belief that all citizens are entitled to protection of individual civil rights. Unfortunately, individuals with disabilities were among the last groups in the United States to receive civil rights protection. Until the late twentieth century, widespread discrimination against the disabled made it difficult for them to feel fully integrated into society. As a result of this discrimination, the disabled often were literally shut in and shut out of much of American society. The Americans with Disabilities Act (ADA) of 1990 was the first comprehensive civil rights legislation for individuals with disabilities. One effect of this legislation is a greater emphasis on community care for the disabled, rather than institutionalization, and there is a growing emphasis on providing that care in as "home-like" an environment as possible.

One of the many challenges for the disabled is access to appropriate health care. Although not all care can be delivered at home, public health nurses are uniquely positioned to serve as care providers and managers for community-dwelling disabled individuals. Having an understanding of disabilities, disability rights, and the legislation specifically enacted to decrease discrimination will assist nurses in intervening and advocating for the disabled.

This chapter provides an overview of disabilities, defines key terms, and reviews the effects of disabilities on individuals, families and communities. Also, relationships between disabling conditions and *Healthy People 2020* are discussed, as is the nurse's role in planning and providing or securing appropriate interventions for individuals, families, and communities to deal with or prevent these health problems.

UNDERSTANDING DISABILITIES

Models of Disability

There is no single accepted definition for disability. The definition of disability varies depending on common use of the word or the specific agency defining the term. With regard to

health care, the Medical Model of Disability is generally used to understand the disabled. In this model, disability is considered to be a function of physical characteristics or conditions that place an individual at a disadvantage compared with those lacking the characteristic or condition. This model places emphasis on the disabled person and the need to modify the course of illness, or as much as possible to give the disabled person a "normal" life. This model is used for determination of disability by the Social Security Administration. In the Social Model of Disability, emphasis is placed on systemic barriers as well as societal attitudes and stigmas that contribute to the perception that those with limitations or physical illnesses are disabled. In this model the focus is on the need to change society and not the individual with a disability. This model has led to a focus on civil rights for the disabled and the need for legislation addressing discrimination (Scullion, 2010).

Disability Defined

Disability is defined by Webster's as "the condition of being disabled; inability to pursue an occupation because of a physical or mental impairment; a program providing support to one affected by a disability; lack of legal qualification to do something or a disqualification, restriction, or disadvantage" (Merriam-Webster, 2010).

Census Determination of Disability

In the U.S. Census of 2000, the population was assessed to determine and define disability based on functional limitations. The census bureau collected data on the number of individuals with disabilities. Six specific subpopulations of disability were identified and include employment disability, sensory disability, mental disability, physical disability, self-care disability, and go-outside-the-home disability (U.S. Census Bureau, 2009b).

For the 2010 census the definition of disability was changed to improve the response rate and gather more reliable

LINKING CONTENT TO PRACTICE

This chapter focuses on the importance of understanding disabilities, the rights of the disabled, and nursing care for this population. Within public health nursing, there has been a commitment to caring for people in their communities and working to build the health of communities. The Council on Linkages (2009) has identified several core competencies for public health nursing.

The topics included in this chapter reinforce several of these core competencies. For example, being able to correctly define disability is important for the core competency of Analytical/Assessment Skills. Understanding disability policy meets the core competency of Policy Development/Program Planning Skills and to work effectively with individuals with disabilities requires Cultural Competence Skills. These are a few examples of the need for public health nurses to develop core competencies that can then be used in a variety of settings and with diverse populations.

BOX 31-1 RANKING OF CAUSES OF DISABILITIES AMONG CIVILIAN NON-INSTITUTIONALIZED PERSONS AGES 18 YEARS OR OLDER, UNITED STATES, 2005

1. Arthritis or rheumatism
2. Back or spine problems
3. Heart trouble
4. Mental or emotional problem
5. Lung or respiratory problem
6. Diabetes
7. Deafness or hearing problem
8. Stiffness or deformity of limbs/extremities
9. Blindness or vision problems
10. Stroke

From Centers for Disease Control and Prevention: Prevalence and most common causes of disabilities among adults—United States, 2005, *MMWR Morbid Mortal Wkly Report* 58:421-426, 2009.

---

information. The current definition of disability includes the following: no question is asked about employment disability, hearing difficulty/vision difficulty, cognitive difficulty, ambulatory difficulty, self-care difficulty, and independent living difficulty. These changes may appear subtle; however, they represent a conceptual change away from a strict medical model of disability (U.S. Census Bureau, 2009b). Box 31-1 lists the top ten causes of disability in the United States.

Work disability, as defined by the U.S. Census Bureau, refers to a person who meets one or more of the following conditions (U.S. Census Bureau, 2009a):

1. Has a health problem or disability that prevents the person from working or limits the kind or amount of work the person can do
2. Has a service-connected disability or retired or left a job for health reasons
3. Did not work because of a long-term physical or mental illness or disability that prevented the performance of any kind of work
4. Did not work at all in the past 12 months because of illness or disability

5. Is under 65 years of age and covered by Medicare
6. Is under 65 years of age and a recipient of Supplemental Security Income (SSI)
7. Received veterans' disability compensation

Social Security Disability

The Social Security Administration, who ultimately determines the individual's status for disability benefits, defines disability as "the inability to engage in any substantial gainful activity (SGA) by reason of any medically determinable physical or mental impairment(s), which can be expected to result in death or which has lasted or can be expected to last for a continuous period of not less than 12 months" (USSSA, 2008, p 1).

The Social Security Administration states that an impairment "results from anatomical, physiological, or psychological abnormalities which can be shown by medically acceptable clinical and laboratory diagnostic techniques" (USSSA, 2008, p 1). The Social Security Administration and Workman's Compensation Systems determine the patient's disability based on clinical evidence. The health care provider should consult the office of Disability Determination Services in the Social Security Administration or the Workman's Compensation Department for guidelines from individual states since requirements may vary.

NURSING TIP *Disability status is based on a person's ability to complete major life activities independently. Major life activities refer to self-care, receptive and expressive language, learning, mobility, self-direction, capacity for independent living and financial sufficiency.*

Americans with Disabilities Act

According to the ADA, the term *disability* means, with respect to an individual, (a) a physical or mental impairment that substantially limits one or more of the major life activities of such an individual, (b) a record of such an impairment, or (c) being regarded as having such an impairment (ADA, 1990, Section 3 [2]).

Thus, individuals who are clearly diagnosed with an illness that limits functioning in one or more major life activities are covered. According to ADA guidelines, hearing, seeing, speaking, walking, caring for oneself, or thinking are examples of major life activities. An individual must have significant difficulty independently performing one or more of these activities to meet the definition of disability.

Also covered by the ADA are individuals who have a history of an illness, those who have been considered (possibly erroneously) to have had an illness, or those who have been treated as if they had a disabling illness. The intent of the ADA is to reduce "discrimination based not only on simple prejudice, but also on stereotypical attitudes and ignorance about individuals with disabilities" (Jones, 1991, p 34). This means that individuals may have been misdiagnosed or inappropriately treated as if they had an illness or disability. Because of this, these individuals may not have had the same opportunities available to them as did non-disabled individuals. An example of this is intelligence testing or assessment of cognitive ability. If there was an underestimate of intelligence or functioning, an individual may not have been allowed full access in education. This then may have limited his or her ability to be prepared for higher education.

Functional Disability

The International Classification of Impairments, Disabilities and Handicaps from 1980 were most recently redefined by the World Health Organization (WHO) in 2001. This new classification, called the International Classification of Functioning, Disability and Health (ICF), provides standardized language for measuring, classifying, and defining disability. The new definition of disability considers not only medical problems, but also physical, social, attitudinal, and personal factors (WHO, 2010b). In the new classification, functioning and disability are determined by the complex interaction between the health condition of the individual and environmental and personal factors. It recognizes that external factors beyond body structures and functions contribute to the disability. The emphasis is on function rather than the condition or the disease. It is relevant across cultures, age groups, and genders and is a useful way to measure health outcomes (CDC, 2010b).

Functional limitations occur when individuals experience difficulty performing basic activities of daily living because of their disability. Examples of functional limitations include difficulty standing, walking, climbing, grasping, and reading. Emphasis is placed on the level of function rather than on the purpose of the activity, so that functional limitation can be associated with the disability. For example, impairment in the strength or range of motion of the arm could lead to functional limitations in grasping or reaching. Affected individuals may have difficulty performing basic self-care activities such as bathing and dressing.

Additional Definitions

In psychiatry the phrase dual diagnosis generally means a substance abuse disorder concurrent with a mental illness disorder (Horsfall et al, 2009). For children with developmental disabilities, dual diagnosis usually means that a mental illness disorder is present simultaneously with mental retardation. It is also possible for nurses to care for clients who have dual diagnoses involving physical limitations.

The term Children with Special Health Care Needs (CSHCN) is defined by the Maternal and Child Health Bureau of the USDHHS Administration as "those who have or are at increased risk for a chronic, physical, developmental, behavioral or emotional condition and who also require health and related service of a type or amount beyond that required by children generally" (Maternal and Child Health Bureau, 2008).

This definition is broad and includes children with many conditions and risk factors. The prevalence of special health care needs increases with age and varies with race and ethnicity. The children with the highest prevalence of special health care needs are Native American/Alaska Native children, multiracial children, and non-Hispanic white children. The lowest rates are in Hispanic children and non-Hispanic Asian children (Maternal and Child Health Bureau, 2008).

The term developmental disability, as defined by the National Center on Birth Defects and Developmental Disabilities of the Centers for Disease Control and Prevention (CDC), is a chronic impairment that occurs during development and up to age 22 and lasts throughout the person's lifetime. The disability limits the functioning of an individual in at least three of the following areas: self-help, language, learning, mobility, self-direction, independent living, and economic self-sufficiency (CDC, 2010c).

Chronic disease, or illness, refers to any long-lasting condition or illness. Disease processes (e.g., diabetes mellitus, cancer, heart disease) and congenital or acquired conditions (e.g., Down syndrome, severe burns, amputation of a limb) are examples of chronic diseases. Therefore, concepts related to disabilities and functional limitations may apply to individuals with a chronic disease or other conditions. For nurses working with these clients, the onset, course, outcome, and degree of limitation are important factors to consider when determining the meaning of the disease to individuals and the families.

Persons with disabilities have often been defined by their illness or disability. Defining someone by their disease or disability is devaluing and disrespectful. It can also place artificial limitations on an individual's potential and value. Language is powerful. The word *handicapped* symbolized the person with a disability begging with a "cap in his hand." The term *disabled* is often used to describe cars that are disabled, indicating they are broken, not functioning, or defective. Whereas we may refer to *things* that are broken or defective, people with disabilities are not broken. Rather than saying a baby has a birth defect, a better term would be to say a child has a congenital disability. The Person First Movement was initiated in an effort to promote acceptable language for people with disabilities. The Person First Movement advocates for political correctness in defining persons with disabilities. In other words, refer to a "woman who is blind" rather than a "blind woman" or a "person with diabetes" rather than a "diabetic" (Snow, 2010).

Definitions of disability need to take into account the degree of disability, the limitations it imposes, and the degree of dependence that occurs as a result of the disability. These definitions can range from minor to severe. Situational factors also affect the disability experience and influence the individual's ability to cope and function in society. Nurses and the interdisciplinary team need to be included, informed, and involved in the science of disability and rehabilitation to be influential in the decision making related to practice, policy, training, research, and funding.

SCOPE OF THE PROBLEM

Number of Disabled Americans

The American Community Survey (ACS) conducted by the U.S. Census Bureau is a yearly supplement to the Decennial Census. The ACS collects information on demographic, social, economic, and housing characteristics, as well as disability data. According to the most recent ACS data collected in 2008, approximately 12.1%, or 36 million, of non-institutionalized men, women, and children in the United States reported a disability. Prevalence rates by type of disability are as follows: vision 2.3%; hearing 3.5%; ambulating 6.9%; cognitive 4.8%; self-care 2.6%, and independent living 5.5% (Erickson, Lee, and von Schrader, 2010).

However, when the total U.S. population, including institutionalized individuals, is considered, the total number of individuals reporting a disability increases to 19%, or 54.4 million U.S. residents. That is, about one in five U.S. residents reports having a disability. Among those with a disability, approximately 12%, or 35 million residents, report having a serious disability. Approximately 28.9% of families, or about two in every seven families, reported a family member with a disability (U.S. Census Bureau, 2008).

> **DID YOU KNOW?** *Every hour, 3000 Americans become disabled. All these people will most likely require disability services.*

Number of Disabled Worldwide

According to the WHO, approximately 650 million people have some type of disability. This number is increasing annually in part because of the increase in chronic diseases, injuries, automobile crashes, violence, and an aging population. Of the disabled, 80% are poor and live in developing countries. Worldwide, most of the people with disabilities have limited access to basic public health services and rehabilitation (WHO, 2010a).

Data obtained from the Global Burden of Disease Study (WHO, 2008) indicated an increased prevalence of severe disability and dependency in Africa, the Middle East, Asia, and Latin America. Conversely, the former socialist economies of Europe have seen a decline in the numbers of disabled individuals who are dependent on others.

Burden of Chronic Disease

Another way to consider disability data is to look at the burden of chronic disease. Although not all individuals with chronic diseases are disabled, the following data from the CDC provide convincing evidence that chronic diseases contribute significantly to the development of disability. Chronic diseases such as heart disease, stroke, cancer, diabetes, and arthritis are some of the most common, costly, and preventable of all

health problems in the United States. Approximately 7 out of 10 deaths among Americans each year are from chronic diseases. Heart disease, cancer, and stroke account for more than 50% of all deaths each year. In 2005 nearly 50% of the adult population, or almost 133 million Americans, had at least one chronic illness (CDC, 2010a).

Disabilities among the chronically ill are common and the CDC reports that about one fourth of people with chronic conditions have one or more daily activity limitations. For example, arthritis is the most common cause of disability, with nearly 19 million Americans reporting activity limitations. Diabetes continues to be the leading cause of kidney failure, non-traumatic lower-extremity amputations, and blindness among adults ages 20 to 74 (CDC, 2009).

The WHO (2008) collected data on the Global Burden of Disease, and within this study, disability is defined as loss of health. They conceptualize heath as the ability or inability to function in areas such as hearing, vision, mobility, and cognition. The most recent data available are from 2004, and the three leading causes of disability worldwide are hearing loss, vision problems, and mental disorders.

Additional Causes of Disability

Several other conditions and inherited problems can cause disability (Figure 31-1). These include genetic disorders, acute and chronic illnesses, violence, tobacco use, lack of access to health care, as well as failure to eat correctly, exercise regularly, or manage stress effectively. In addition, substance abuse, environmental problems, and unsanitary living conditions can cause disability. The people reporting these causes identified difficulty with functional limitations, difficulty with activities of daily living (ADLs)/instrumental activities of daily living (IADLs), or inability to do housework, or to work at a job or business (CDC, 2009).

Older adults, especially the frail elderly, often develop disabilities resulting from illnesses or injuries. When these disabilities are associated with hospital admission, there is an increased fall risk (Sherrington et al, 2009). Falls in the elderly frequently result in injury which then leads to additional disability from loss of independence and mobility (Clough-Gorr et al, 2008). This loss of independence places additional burdens on family members and caregivers to provide assistance with ADLs and IADLs.

> **NURSING TIP** *A thorough nursing assessment can identify factors placing a community-dwelling elder at risk for falls. The assessment should include functional impairments, medications, and environmental factors that increase fall risk. Early assessment and intervention can prevent a fall and decrease development of additional medical problems and disability.*

Childhood Disability

An estimated 13.9% of children in the United States have special needs, which may be developmental, behavioral, or emotional in nature. Moreover, 21.8% of households with

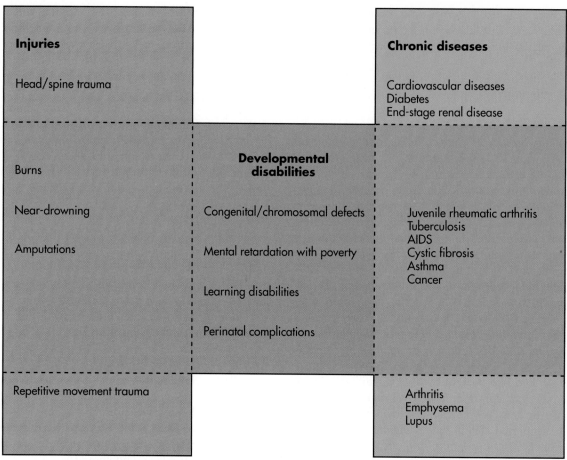

FIGURE 31-1 Examples of conditions related to being physically compromised.

children have at least one child with a special health need. Children with special health care needs require such things as prescription medication (86%), specialty medical care (52%), vision care (33%), mental health care (25%), specialized therapies (23%) and medical equipment (11%). Although most of the time these needs are met, it is estimated that 16% of children with special health needs report at least one unmet need (Maternal and Child Health Bureau, 2008; Newacheck and Kim, 2005).

Special health care needs increase with age; 8% of children under the age of 5 are considered to have special health care needs, 14.6% of children between the ages of 6 and 11 have special needs, and 15.8% of adolescents have special needs. In addition, special health care needs are more common in boys (15%) compared with girls (10.5%) (Maternal and Child Health Bureau, 2008).

Childhood disability may be developmental or acquired and may be a result of prenatal damage, perinatal factors, acquired neonatal factors, or early childhood factors. These may include genetic factors, prematurity, infections, traumatic or toxic exposure, or nutritional factors. In some cases, the etiology of many childhood disabilities remains unknown. Preventive screening for genetic disorders including developmental disabilities is critical for early detection and medical intervention. Newborn screening, immunization programs, and genetic counseling prevent disabilities.

Neonatal screening for phenylketonuria (PKU), hypothyroidism, thalassemias, and other disorders has greatly reduced childhood disabilities.

Mental Illness

An often overlooked source of disability is that related to mental disorders. According to the National Institute of Mental Health (2010), each year approximately 57.5 million Americans over the age of 18 (26.2%) have a diagnosable mental disorder. Major depressive disorder is the leading cause of disability in the United States for individuals ages 15 to 44. For individuals with one diagnosable mental illness, almost 45% meet criteria for a second or third mental illness. Multiple diagnoses, including individuals with a dual diagnosis, increase the severity of disability and functional impairment.

THE EFFECTS OF DISABILITIES

The costs of chronic disability to the injured persons, family, employers, and society are significant. In 2008 the ACS estimated that of the non-institutionalized population ages 21 to 64 who had any type of disability, only 39.5% were employed. Employment rates varied by type of disability, with hearing disability having the highest rate of employment (56%) and self-care disability having the lowest rate of employment (18.7%) (Erickson, Lee, and von Schrader, 2010).

Employment rates also vary based on educational level. In general, for individuals with any type of disability, the higher the educational level, the higher the rate of employment. Of disabled individuals with less than a high school education, only 25.3% were employed. Those with a high school education had an employment rate of 37.6% whereas 57.6% of those with a bachelor's degree or higher were employed (Erickson, Lee, and von Schrader, 2010).

Disability status also affects annual household income, as can be seen in a 2008 survey of the average annual household income among households with or without a disabled individual age 21 to 64. The annual household income for households with a disabled member was $39,600 whereas the income for households without a disabled member was $61,200. Of perhaps greater significance is the number of individuals living below the poverty line (25.3%) as opposed to non-disabled individuals living below the poverty line (11.2%) (Erickson, Lee, and von Schrader, 2010).

Nurses provide care for persons who are disabled, for their families, for the populations and subpopulations that they comprise, and for the communities in which they live. Remember that some clients prefer to be regarded as being physically or mentally challenged or compromised, whereas others may think such terms minimize the importance of the needs and problems of people who are disabled. The extent to which the disabled person may need extra support, care, and services from the family unit and the community is shown in Box 31-2. These relationships are best understood by looking at the stress placed on the individual.

Effects on the Individual

According to the USDHHS, disabilities are characteristics of the body, mind, or senses that affect a person's ability to engage independently in some or all aspects of day-to-day life. Many different types of disabilities exist, and they affect people in various ways. People may be born with a disability, develop a disability from being sick or injured, or acquire a disability with the aging process. Most men, women, and children of all ages, races, and ethnicities will experience disability at some time during their lives.

As the population ages, the likelihood of developing a disability increases. For example, 22.6% of individuals 45 to 54 years old have a disability, 44.9% of 65- to 69-year-olds have a disability, and 73.6% of those 80 years and older have a disability. Disability is not a sickness, and most people with disabilities are healthy without a documented chronic illness. However, persons with disabilities may be at greater risk for developing illnesses as a result of their condition. For example, someone with decreased mobility can suffer from the problems of immobility such as obesity, skin breakdown, osteoporosis, pneumonia, malnutrition, or loneliness. Most persons with disabilities can and do work, play, learn, and enjoy healthy lives (USDHHS, 2010b).

Many disabled people try to discourage the image that they are helpless and pitiful. For example, *Murderball* is a documentary film about several quadriplegic rugby players who play competitive rugby in wheelchairs. Their motto is "Smashing

---

BOX 31-2 POTENTIAL EFFECTS OF BEING PHYSICALLY COMPROMISED: INDIVIDUALS, FAMILIES, AND COMMUNITIES

Individuals
- Related health problems (e.g., nutrition, oral health, hygiene, limited activity/stamina)
- Self-concept/self-esteem
- Life expectancy and risk for infection and secondary injury
- Developmental tasks; change in role expectations

Families
- Stress on family unit
- Need for use of external resources to help family meet role expectations
- Options limited in use of any discretionary income
- Social stigma

Communities
- Need/demand to reallocate resources
- Discomfort or fear from lack of knowledge of disability
- Need to comply with legislation
- Services provided by health department, health care providers
- Need for other services beyond medical diagnosis (e.g., transportation)

---

stereotypes one hit at a time!" These individuals promote the idea of living and working independently (U.S. Quad Rugby Association, 2010).

Children: Infancy Through Adolescence

Children who live with a disability are affected in many ways. In an effort to decrease childhood obesity, greater emphasis has been placed on increasing children's physical activity. In spite of this goal, children with any type of disability continue to be less physically active and at greater risk of obesity than their healthy peers. This is in part due to the relative lack of available opportunities for disabled children to participate in organized and spontaneous play. Moreover, non-disabled children and parents have also had negative attitudes about interacting or playing with disabled children (Obrusnikova, Block, and Dillon, 2010; Reinehr et al, 2010).

Children and adolescents with special health care needs are also at higher risk to experience psychological maladjustment compared with their healthy peers. The risk of psychological problems such as depression and anxiety were correlated with the degree of physical impairment, not with the level of disease activity. For some, the inability to participate in certain physical activities affects their feelings of belonging and self-worth (Ding et al, 2008; Wilson and Clayton, 2010).

A particular problem for children with cognitive disabilities is difficulty with accurately interpreting social cues. These children are less likely to understand a social interaction that differs from usual and predictable interactions. As a result of misinterpreting social cues, children with cognitive disabilities are at a disadvantage in developing age-appropriate friendships. This can contribute to increased social isolation for many disabled children (Leffert, Siperstein, and Widaman, 2010).

For other children, managing the effects of their disability may cause embarrassment and they may choose to isolate themselves from others. For example, students who have spina bifida or renal disease might need to leave classrooms or other school settings quickly to use the bathroom. Having to explain this need to their classmates could call unwanted attention to these children and their diseases. However, disabled children can overcome some of these obstacles if they have families who are able to provide the support necessary for the development of more positive self-images and a feeling of inclusiveness. The use of assistive technology such as computers can enhance learning and decrease obstacles related to inadequate education (Kliebenstein and Brome, 2002; Heywood, 2010; Murchland and Parkyn, 2010).

The unique issues and challenges experienced by adolescents with disabilities have not been studied as well as those that affect younger children and adults. This population is often overlooked by advocacy groups for the disabled and by most of the new initiatives developed for disabled persons. However, the years between 10 and 18 are difficult ones for most adolescents, and the needs of those who are disabled are similar to those of their healthy peers (i.e., education, peer relationships, recreation, and planning for the future). In addition to the expected challenges experienced by adolescents, those who are disabled must also deal with prejudice, discrimination, and social isolation because of their disability (Groce, 2004; Redmon, 2010).

Disabled adolescents are often viewed as asexual by their healthy peers. However, they are as sexually active as healthy adolescents. They view themselves as "normal" even though they realize that others perceive them differently. Moreover, disabled adolescents are just as likely as their non-disabled peers to engage in risky sexual activity. This places them at risk for unplanned pregnancy and sexually transmitted diseases. Therefore, they should receive the same amount of sexual education as their unaffected peers (Skar, 2003; Maart and Jelsma, 2010).

EVIDENCE-BASED PRACTICE

This article describes the value of qualitatively driven research in understanding the experiences and health care needs of the chronically ill and presents literature-based recommendations to improve the management of chronic disease. Chronically ill persons encounter significant social and emotional challenges such as fatigue, pain, and stigmatization. They also face difficulties in navigating health care systems that have been designed to serve the acutely ill. The author suggests that an important factor in improving the health care and service delivery for the chronically ill is to move from a provider-dependent model to one of self-care management through increased and more effective patient–provider communication.

Nurse Use

Nurses should foster and facilitate open and consistent communications with the chronically ill. Effective patient–provider interactions promote health and improve care by encouraging individual patients to share their attitudes, beliefs, concerns, and questions.

From Thorne S: Patient-provider communication in chronic illness: a health promotion window of opportunity, *Fam Community Health* 29(1 Suppl):4S-11S, 2006.

Adults

According to The Center for an Accessible Society (2010), more than 3 million people in the United States require help from another person to live independently. Many adults receive some, but not enough, help to meet their needs. With inadequate community support, an individual may experience hunger, injuries, falls, or other problems that contribute to the development of secondary health problems, disabilities, and possibly early death. Becoming disabled increases the risk of placement in a nursing home or other long-term care facility, contributing to both decreased community participation and limited social integration for the disabled.

It is estimated that those persons who live by themselves receive only 56% of the help they need while those living with family members or friends receive 80% of what they need. Informal supports such as family members and friends frequently have multiple other work, family and community responsibilities. This makes it difficult for them to consistently meet the needs of the disabled. Those without informal supports must rely on formal supports, which are increasingly limited in difficult financial times (The Center for an Accessible Society, 2010).

In addition, millions of Americans depend on Medicaid to finance their long-term services (The Center for an Accessible Society, 2010). For example, 80% of all Medicaid long-term care funds go to nursing homes or other institutional service providers, even though many of these people could receive services in their own homes. A personal assistant could make it possible for a disabled person to live at home instead of in an institution. Many Americans think that nursing homes are the only alternative for long-term care. However, the elderly often prefer the freedom and control of living at home. Many states offer community-based services such as home health care services and senior services. In Home Supportive Services (IHSS) provide home health services to the aged, blind, or disabled. In addition, adult protective services exist to receive reports of abuse of elders or dependent adults.

According to The Center for an Accessible Society (2010), computer technology and the Internet can increase the independence of people with disabilities. Homebound persons can access a computer and order groceries, shop for needed items, research questions, participate in online discussions, and communicate with friends and family. With newer technologies, blind persons can access the computer as well as sighted persons. Even persons who cannot hold a pen or who lack fine-motor skills can use speech recognition and other technologies to write letters, pay bills, and perform other tasks using the computer and Internet.

However, only one fourth of persons with disabilities own computers, and only one tenth use the Internet. The elderly and African Americans with disabilities, especially low-income or low-education level elders, rarely take advantage of these new technologies. Fortunately, the cost of computers and associated equipment for the disabled has become less expensive. Moreover, there are organizations which

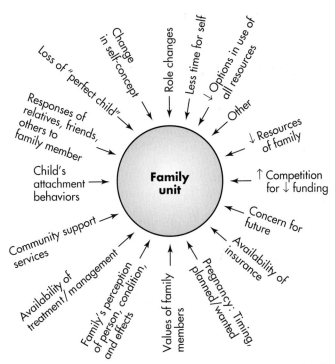

Change in self-concept
Role changes
Less time for self
↓ Options in use of all resources
Other
Loss of "perfect child"
Responses of relatives, friends, others to family member
Child's attachment behaviors
Community support services
Availability of treatment/management
Family's perception of person, condition, and effects
Values of family members
Pregnancy: Timing, planned/wanted
Availability of insurance
Concern for future
↑ Competition for ↓ funding
↓ Resources of family

Family unit

FIGURE 31-2 Factors influencing a family unit when a member is physically compromised.

provide low-cost or free computer equipment for qualified disabled individuals (The Center for an Accessible Society, 2010).

Effects on the Family

Most people who are physically disabled are cared for at home by one or more family members. Figure 31-2 lists some of the issues and concerns that occur when a family member is disabled and shows the effect of the disability on the family unit. As Figure 31-2 shows, the entire family system is affected when one of its members is disabled.

The WHO has also attempted to collect data to estimate the number of people worldwide requiring daily assistance from another person to carry out health, domestic, or personal tasks. The study concluded that many countries would be greatly affected by the increasing number of dependent people. Additional data are needed about these individuals, and the kinds of disabilities they have, to identify the human and financial resources that will be needed to support them (WHO, 2008).

Children: Infancy Through Adolescence

A child's disability may have long-term effects on the family, primary caregiver, and the marital relationship. Providing care for these children places additional demands on the family, particularly the mother. Mothers of children with special health care needs report higher levels of stress, anxiety, depression, and feelings of isolation compared with mothers of unaffected children. In addition, employment is difficult and sometimes impossible to secure for the parents of

children who require extensive care. This is especially true for mothers, single parents, and low-income families who may be unable to afford childcare for their disabled children. In addition to the day-to-day physical care these children require, the caregiver must also access and coordinate physical, occupational, and speech therapy as well as specialty care and additional educational services (Ha et al, 2008; Bilgin and Gozum, 2009).

The cost of caring for a child with a disability often affects the family's financial well-being. Children with special health care needs are more likely than the general population of children to have health insurance. However, one third of the children with disabilities who have insurance lack adequate coverage to meet their needs. This is due to high out-of-pocket expenses, the services required not being covered, or the child not having access to appropriate providers (Maternal and Child Health Care Bureau, 2008; Laskar et al, 2010).

Although children with special health care needs are more likely to have health insurance through Medicaid, children from low-income families who lack medical insurance are at a particular disadvantage because their families may be unable to afford the care they need. Siblings of children with special health care needs are at higher risk for developing emotional and psychological problems compared with their unaffected peers. For example, they tend to express more psychosomatic illnesses, anxiety disorders, and aggressive behaviors compared with siblings of non-disabled children (O'Brien, Duffy, and Nicholl, 2009; Dauz et al, 2010).

Conversely, these siblings are often found to be more mature, altruistic, responsible, and independent when compared with siblings of non-disabled children. Whether a child suffers or benefits from having a disabled brother or sister depends on the attitude of the parents toward the disability and their coping methods, the economic circumstances of the family, the communication among family members, and the degree of parental affection and attention received by the non-disabled child (Cate and Loots, 2000; Dyke, Mulroy, and Leonard, 2009).

Adults

Having a physically disabled adult in a family causes enormous stress on the rest of the members. There may be a significant loss of income when a parent is unable to work because of a disability. According to The Council for Disability Awareness (2009), 62% of the bankruptcies in the United States in 2007 were the result of the inability to pay medical expenses. Another effect on multi-generational families is caregiver burden. Well children in the family may have unmet needs due to the disability of a parent. Moreover, the children may have to assume the role of caregiver if other supports are not available. Adults who are responsible for caring for their own children as well as one or both of their parents have been termed the "sandwich generation." These adults often struggle with burnout as well as increased marital stress when faced with caring for an elderly parent with a disability (Pezzin, Pollak, and Schone, 2008; Roth et al, 2009).

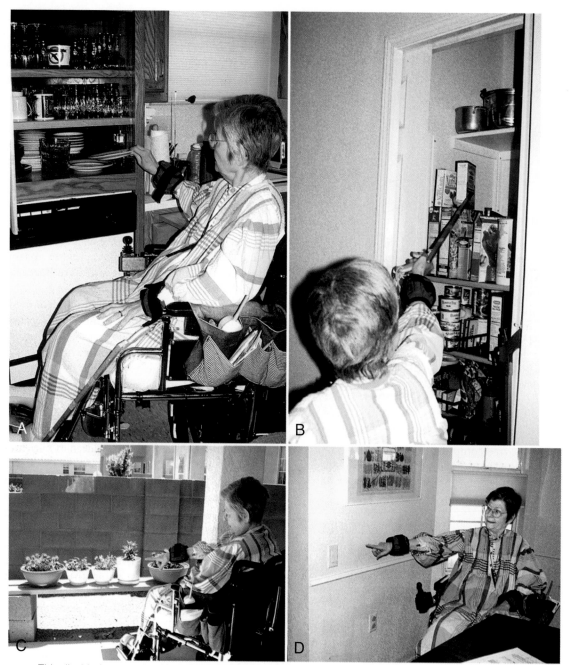

This disabled woman is able to live in and maintain her own home, including growing plants and flowers, with the help of easy-access devices and lower light fixtures and cabinets.

Effects on the Community

The presence of physically disabled people and their families in the community has far-reaching effects on all aspects of community life. The prevention of disability and providing community support for caretakers need to be priorities. The community may be called on to respond in new ways to these citizens as a result of federal laws affecting those who are disabled.

Children: Infancy Through Adolescence

Families of children with disabilities need the support of their communities as they care for their disabled children at home. Services that families find most helpful include respite care, family counseling, and genetic counseling. Low-income families and those without private insurance have more difficulty accessing these services compared with those from higher-income families (Johnson and Kastner, 2005).

Children who are chronically ill or disabled and who enter school for mainstream education require educational support from the public school system as mandated in the Individuals with Disabilities Education Act (IDEA). IDEA is outlined in Box 31-3. In addition, IDEA requires states to provide appropriate services to infants and children from birth to age 5 who have or are at risk for disability. Examples of such services include speech therapy, occupational therapy, physical therapy, play

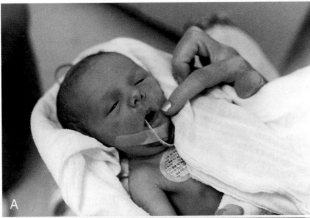

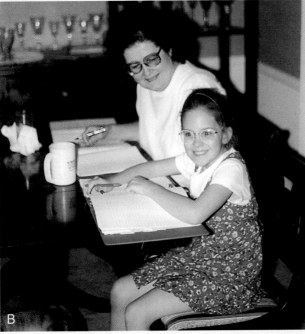

A, An at-risk infant girl who was 1 month premature and delivered by cesarean section because of abruption. This child's Apgar scores were 1 at 1 minute of age and 3 at 5 minutes of age.
B, The same child at 10 years of age. She is profoundly hearing impaired. Her parents' commitment has helped her to be mainstreamed successfully and she is able to do her own homework.

BOX 31-3   INDIVIDUALS WITH DISABILITIES EDUCATION ACT (IDEA)

The Individuals with Disabilities Education Act federal law was developed:
- To ensure that all children with disabilities have available to them a free, appropriate public education that emphasizes special education and related services designed to meet their unique needs and prepare them for employment and independent living
- To ensure that the rights of children with disabilities and their parents are protected
- To assist states, localities, educational service agencies, and federal agencies to provide for the education of all children with disabilities
- To assess and ensure the effectiveness of efforts to educate children with disabilities

From U.S. Department of Education: *Building the legacy: IDEA 2004*, 2010. Available at www.idea.ed.gov. Accessed March 2, 2011.

---

therapy, and behavioral therapy (U.S. Department of Education, 2010).

Although the provision of appropriate services for disabled infants and children is mandated by IDEA, states vary in the nature and quantity of services they provide for eligible children. In addition, public schools must evaluate their effectiveness with students who are disabled. This can add to the cost of educating children. Increased education for pediatricians and nurses can increase supportive and knowledgeable collaboration for the development of early intervention programs in the schools.

Adults

Former Surgeon General Richard H. Carmona sought to improve the health and wellness of persons with disabilities. To achieve this goal he encouraged (1) health care providers to see and treat the whole person, not just the disability, (2) educators to teach about disability, (3) the public to focus on a person's abilities, not just the disability, and (4) the community to ensure accessible health care and wellness services to persons with disabilities (Carmona, 2005).

To improve the health and wellness of persons with disabilities, Carmona advocated the following:
- People nationwide should understand that persons with disabilities can lead long, healthy, productive lives.
- Health care providers have the knowledge and tools to screen, diagnose, and treat with dignity the whole person with a disability.
- Persons with disabilities can promote their own good health by developing and maintaining healthy lifestyles.
- Accessible health care and support services promote independence for persons with disabilities (Carmona, 2005).

Persons with disabilities that affect mobility are at risk for health problems of the multiple body systems related to mobility/immobility. Persons with mobility associated problems can suffer damage to any system. Some of the problems that develop with the musculoskeletal system include foot drop, muscular atrophy, contractures, or fractures. Respiratory and circulatory function can be compromised by pneumonia or deep vein thrombosis. Renal problems such as infection, incontinence, or renal calculi are common problems related to immobility. Decubiti and skin breakdown and rashes can develop from immobility and/or incontinence of bowel and bladder. Malnutrition or obesity could also be related to effects of immobility.

SPECIAL POPULATIONS

Low-Income Populations

Physically compromised individuals often experience poverty, as do other special population groups including single parents and their children, the aged, the unemployed, and members of racial and ethnic minorities. Persons with low income have less access to health care throughout their lives and are less likely to participate in all levels of prevention. Therefore, they are at greater risk for the onset of disabling conditions and for more rapid progression of disease processes. Those in poverty could also be at greater risk for disabling conditions resulting from

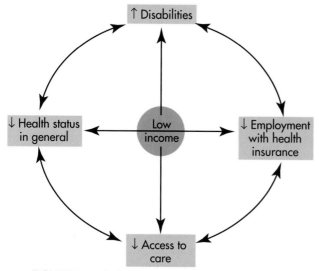

FIGURE 31-3 Relationships of poverty and disability.

lifestyle choices (e.g., injuries; tobacco, alcohol, or drug abuse; and inadequate nutrition).

People who are disabled and live in poverty are less likely to have the resources to provide for their own special needs. Those who are disabled are often unemployed, even though they may be able to work and are seeking jobs. Employers may be reluctant to hire people whose conditions may increase employer-provided health insurance costs. This is another barrier to adequate insurance and access to health care for the disabled. Other factors that affect low-income, physically compromised clients' access to needed services are inadequate transportation, lack of coordination of care, and limited locally available services for those who cannot pay for them. Figure 31-3 illustrates the relationship between poverty and disabilities.

SELECTED ISSUES

Abuse

Disabled persons are more likely to experience some form of abuse during their lifetime compared with individuals without disabilities. The most common type of abuse reported by disabled individuals is care related. Because many disabled individuals are dependent on others for basic care, they are at risk for experiencing negligent and sometimes cruel physical care from their care providers. Although abuse can occur at any age, it is more commonly found in children and the elderly (Govindshenoy and Spencer, 2007; Jaudes and Mackey-Bilaver, 2008).

Children with cognitive disabilities under the age of 6 and who are from low-income families are at the highest risk for abuse or neglect. Psychological and emotional problems, such as conduct disorders, appear to be associated with abuse. There is also an association between learning difficulties and abuse. However, children with developmental delay or mental retardation are not at increased risk. Several recent studies have shown that children with physical disabilities are also not at increased risk for abuse or neglect. Under IDEA a screening to detect mental or psychosocial health conditions is mandated as early as possible. Once identified, these children should be considered at risk for potential

abuse. Health care professionals and child protection agencies should be trained to recognize cognitive disabilities in children and to intervene quickly to decrease possible abuse (Govindshenoy and Spencer, 2007; Jaudes and Mackey-Bilaver, 2008).

Children with special health care needs are at higher risk for abuse for the following reasons (Figure 31-4): (1) because of the cost of their medical care, they place an additional strain on the family's financial status; (2) they may require concentrated parental supervision because of their disability, and this in turn places an additional emotional and physical stress on the caregivers; (3) respite care may be difficult for the parents to secure, which compounds an already stressful situation (Giardino, Hudson, and Marsh, 2003; Spencer et al, 2005).

Disabled women are more likely to suffer some form of abuse when compared with their non-affected peers. Women with physical disabilities have stated that abuse is their most critical health issue. In fact, 67% of disabled women report experiencing some type of abuse in their lifetime. The abuse may be related to dependence on others for basic physical care, or their disability may be the result of abuse at multiple points in a woman's life. In addition, many disabled women report feeling unattractive, undesirable, and socially unacceptable. Because of this negative self perception, they may enter into and remain in precarious intimate relationships that place them at high risk for abuse. Disabled women report that the abuse they experience negatively affects both their psychological and their physical health. For these reasons, disabled women who suffer abuse are less likely to live independently and seek employment outside the home (Hassouneh-Phillips, 2005).

Health Promotion

Health promotion usually focuses on the primary prevention of conditions that may lead to disability (e.g., smoking cessation to prevent lung cancer). Actually all three levels of prevention apply to physically compromised clients (see the Levels of Prevention box). They need information and counseling for health-promoting behaviors and for prevention of the progression of a condition or pathology.

Health promotion is a multidimensional concept that applies to all individuals regardless of disability. Strategies are needed to expand the knowledge base of health promotion for those who are disabled. Persons with chronic disabilities have frequently defined themselves in terms of their physical problems and sick role. However, they need all the prevention activities of the non-disabled. This includes immunizations, exercise, weight control, use of safety precautions, safe sex practices, stress reduction, as well as screening and treatment of disease not related to their disability.

In addition, health promotion and prevention programs for persons with disabilities should focus on preventing the complications from the effects of immobility and the disease process. The complications of immobility and the disease process need to be prevented to ensure optimal independent and healthy living, thus allowing the individual with disabilities the opportunity to have a productive and happy life.

Many health promotion and disease prevention needs are similar across the life span (e.g., exercise, diet, avoidance of

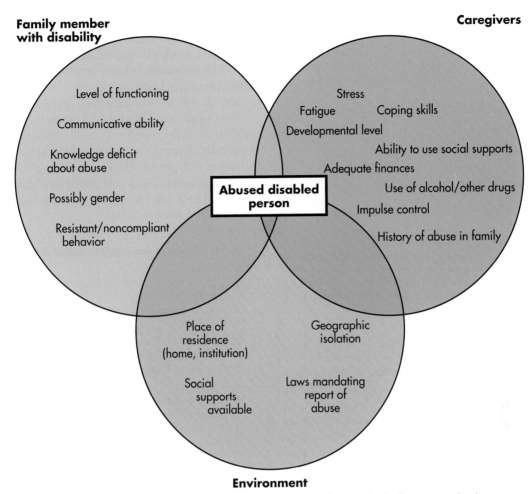

Family member with disability

- Level of functioning
- Communicative ability
- Knowledge deficit about abuse
- Possibly gender
- Resistant/noncompliant behavior

Caregivers

- Stress
- Fatigue
- Coping skills
- Developmental level
- Ability to use social supports
- Adequate finances
- Use of alcohol/other drugs
- Impulse control
- History of abuse in family

Abused disabled person

- Place of residence (home, institution)
- Social supports available
- Geographic isolation
- Laws mandating report of abuse

Environment

FIGURE 31-4 Factors influencing the abuse of those who are physically compromised.

excess substance use, and injury prevention). However, specific problems and interventions to deal with these needs vary according to age, specific disabling condition, and developmental status. For example, nutritional needs of premature infants are related to obtaining adequate energy, protein, fat, vitamins, and minerals. An older adult with type 2 diabetes mellitus may be concerned primarily with reducing the risk of experiencing a myocardial infarction.

Persons with disabilities need appropriate nutrition. Therefore, nurses may consult with dietitians or refer clients to them for assistance. Speech therapists may also be needed for persons with chewing or swallowing difficulties. Occupational health experts focus on the activities of daily living and often use adaptive equipment to promote success and independence with ADLs. Families and professionals can work together to meet the nutritional needs of persons with disabilities and chronic health care problems.

Health promotion and disease prevention for those who are physically compromised have not been emphasized in primary care or in rehabilitation. It is especially important to establish lifelong, health-promoting behaviors in children who are disabled. Unfortunately, parents may be so overwhelmed by caring for such children that this aspect of care is not considered.

LEVELS OF PREVENTION

Physically Compromised Clients

Primary Prevention
- Educate community residents about behaviors during pregnancy that will reduce the risk of having a baby with a disability.
- Push for a congressional mandate for addition of folic acid to cereals in the United States to reduce neural tube defect in infants.
- Promote exercise and physical fitness programs in schools to lessen obesity in that population and decrease incidence of dysmetabolic syndrome.

Secondary Prevention
- Initiate early detection actions to identify any chronic or disabling condition.
- Initiate blood pressure screening programs to identify those at risk for strokes or heart damage as soon as possible.
- Push programs for early detection of cancer (e.g., mammography, malignant melanoma), since co-occurring morbidities are more common with later detection of cancer.

Tertiary Prevention
- Take action to maintain or increase functional abilities for persons who have a physically compromising condition.
- Encourage exercise programs for sedentary clients with osteoporosis to reduce the likelihood of fractures.
- Initiate a diabetes type 1 education program for children and parents, with a focus on disease management and prevention of disease complications.

♥ HEALTHY PEOPLE 2020

Selected objectives are listed here that pertain to persons with disabilities.
- DH-5: Increase the proportion of youth with special health care needs whose health care provider has discussed transition planning from pediatric to adult health care.
- DH-7: Reduce the proportion of older adults with disabilities who use inappropriate medications.
- DH-8: Reduce the proportion of people with disabilities who report having physical or program barriers to local health and wellness programs.
- DH-9: Reduce the proportion of people with disabilities who encounter barriers to participating in home, school, work or community activities.
- DH-13: Increase the proportion of people with disabilities who participate in social, spiritual, recreational, community, and civic activities to the degree that they wish.
- DSC-14: Reduce the proportion of people with disabilities reporting delays in receiving primary and periodic preventive care due to specific barriers.

From U.S. Department of Health and Human Services: *Developing Healthy People 2020*. Available at www.healthypeople.gov. Accessed March 2, 2011.

HEALTHY PEOPLE 2020 OBJECTIVES

Selected objectives from *Healthy People 2020* for persons with disabilities are highlighted in the *Healthy People 2020* box. Many of the objectives address concerns discussed in this chapter regarding increasing health promotion and wellness activities for individuals with disabilities. In addition, there is greater emphasis on increasing access to services, which can increase independence and foster community living.

The *Healthy People 2020* objectives are a useful tool available to nurses to evaluate if individuals with disabilities are receiving adequate services. Moreover, these objectives can serve as national benchmarks for individuals with disabilities with regard to their health, use of community services, leisure activities, and overall quality of life.

THE CUTTING EDGE   *Nurses can use the Healthy People 2020 objectives to advocate for increased physical activity and wellness programs for the disabled. This can be done by working with community and disability organizations to ensure compliance with the ADA and by educating others about the Healthy People 2020 objectives.*

ROLE OF THE NURSE

Many factors influence the role of nurses who work with individuals with disabilities. These factors include the community's awareness of these persons and the commitment to their health needs. Also, the missions of the agencies where nurses work influence the type of services they provide to special groups. For example, the structure and priorities of a community-based agency determine whether a nurse will care for the general population or focus on service to a specific population. If funding sources are dedicated to particular programs (e.g., tuberculosis control, maternal-child health services), care for those who are disabled may be dispersed throughout several program areas and may be difficult to identify.

In dealing with those who are disabled, the nurses' roles may also change as the focus varies among the levels of individuals, families, groups, or entire communities. For example, at the level of the individual, nurses may provide nursing care for ventilated patients at home.

Nurses also serve as educators who provide clients at any level with sufficient knowledge to enable them to care for their own needs. At the community level, nurses may provide information about certain causes of disability and aim to reduce the behaviors that precede the development of disability, such as spinal cord injury. The closely related counseling role is of value because clients learn to improve their problem-solving skills with guidance from the nurse.

HOW TO   Promote Appropriate Use of Asthma Medications by Children

A. *Collaborate/coordinate efforts with health care provider managing child's asthma.*
   1. *Personnel in all areas in which child uses drugs need to be informed of regimen.*
   2. *Be aware of factors that could affect adherence to regimen:*
      a. *Prolonged therapy*
      b. *Medications used prophylactically*
      c. *Delayed consequences of non-adherence*
      d. *Drugs expensive, hard to use*
      e. *Family concerns about side effects*
      f. *Adherence less likely with mild or severe asthma; most likely with moderate asthma*
      g. *Child with cognitive or emotional problems*
      h. *Poorly functioning family*
      i. *Strong alternative health beliefs*
      j. *Multiple caregivers*
B. *Assess child's adherence to regimen.*
   1. *Count pills; use float test for remaining amount in inhalers (gross estimate).*
   2. *Ask child, "In an average week, how many puffs of your inhaler do you actually get?"*
   3. *Obtain refill history from pharmacist (information can be obtained from child's health care provider).*
C. *Interventions*
   1. *Educate child, parents, and other caregivers.*
   2. *Encourage adaptation of regimen to family's needs.*
      a. *Health care provider may need additional information about family situation.*
      b. *Signed, dated, written permission to exchange information with such a provider is needed.*
   3. *Encourage consideration of acceptability of medication to child, family.*
   4. *Be encouraging, caring, supportive, and willing to work with family.*
   5. *Follow up and monitor progress closely, including school attendance, when appropriate.*
   6. *Consider home visits (e.g., to assess/manage environmental triggers).*
   7. *Identify an "asthma partner" (i.e., another adult besides parents when they do not reliably monitor child).*
   8. *Use a contract for adherence.*
   9. *In extreme cases, especially with young and/or ill children, consider reporting family to child protective services for medical neglect.*

Nurses serve as advocates for individuals and families or groups. An advocate is a person who speaks on behalf of those who are unable to speak for themselves. One of the potential problems with this role is that nurses may unintentionally foster excessive dependence by individuals, families, or other groups. Nurses should focus on using advocacy to support those who need this service. At the same time, observing nurses' data-collecting and negotiating skills can serve as models for clients who are capable of using such knowledge. For example, nurses might advocate for a school environment that is adapted to the specific needs of children who require wheelchairs, but who do not necessarily have to be limited to their chairs, without explicitly telling the children when they should use their wheelchairs. Nurses may help family caregivers of disabled individuals by validating that the caregivers' own basic needs are being sacrificed and by identifying ways that this problem can be moderated.

As referral agents, nurses maintain current information about agencies whose services are of potential use to those who are disabled. Referral, one of the most important functions of nurses, is the process of directing clients to the resources that can meet their needs. For self-directed clients and families, information about an agency's services, phone number, and address may be adequate. For families with little understanding of how systems work, more specific guidance and case conferences may be necessary to coordinate clients' health-related and educational needs.

As health care providers with a goal of making basic care universally accessible, nurses are positioned well to ensure that the full range of prevention and information about health promotion are made available to individuals with disabilities. On a more individualized basis, the nurse in a case manager role works to meet the needs of clients by developing a plan of care for them to help them reach individual goals. Although nurses may direct others to carry out the plan, they are responsible for evaluating the plan's effectiveness. For example, clients who have been disabled because of complications from diabetes mellitus may have several immediate problems. They may need to adjust to the amputation of one or more limbs, as well as learn new skills to improve management of their diabetes in an effort to prevent additional complications. Nurses (as case managers) will develop plans with clients and families to meet these needs and establish time frames to evaluate specific outcomes.

THE CUTTING EDGE *The most up-to-date information on national and local resources for individuals with disabilities can be found on the Internet. Two excellent resources are Connecting the Disability Community to Information and Opportunities (www.disability.gov) and Disability Resource Directory (www.disability-resource.com).*

In the coordinator role, nurses are not responsible for developing overall plans of client care. Instead, responsibilities include assisting clients and families by organizing and integrating the resources of other agencies or care providers to meet clients' needs most efficiently. For example, with the family's agreement, a nurse may arrange for the family to see a social worker on the same day they bring their children to an appointment in a pediatric cardiology clinic.

Nurses are collaborators when they take part in joint decision making with clients, families, groups, and communities. Collaboration with other care providers is of particular importance in coordinating care and assisting a disabled person to understand the full range of services available to them. For example, nurses may work with agencies or groups who make decisions about community housing for those who are physically disabled.

In the nursing as case finder role, nurses identify individuals with disabilities who have unmet service needs. For example, nurses may arrange developmental, vision, and hearing screenings for young children. Although a nurse's efforts are for particular clients, the focus of case finding is on monitoring the health status of entire groups or communities. Nurses may also identify those who are members of vulnerable populations and who, although not presently affected by an illness, are at high risk for acquiring the disease. Such people may have limited or no access to health promotion or disease prevention services, or they may be unaware of those for which they are eligible.

Nurses may function as change agents at all levels, including the health care delivery system. A change agent is one who originates and creates change. This process includes identifying a need for change, enlightening and motivating others as to this need, as well as starting and directing the proposed change. Nurses may function in the role by helping to obtain more appropriate health care services for those who are disabled.

LEGISLATION

A nurse who works with physically disabled clients may have a caseload of clients of all ages, while another nurse, such as a school nurse, may see clients in a specific age group. Nurses need to be knowledgeable about the legislation that relates to populations for whom they provide nursing care. Box 31-4

BOX 31-4 CATEGORIES OF FEDERAL LEGISLATION FOR THOSE WITH DISABILITIES

Education
- Early childhood special education
- Elementary and Secondary Education Act and amendments
- Vocational education for those who are disabled

Rehabilitation
- Vocational
- Medical, including Medicare and Medicaid
- Rehabilitational

Services
- Economic assistance
- Facility construction and architectural design
- Deinstitutionalization and independent living
- Civil rights and advocacy

Based on data from National Information Center for Children and Youth with Disabilities. Available at www.icdri.org. Accessed July 12, 2010.

BOX 31-5 SUMMARY OF LEGISLATION

- Americans with Disabilities Act (ADA) of 1990
- Communications Act of 1934 and Telecommunications Act of 1996
- Rehabilitation Act of 1973
- The Fair Housing Act of 1988
- Civil Rights of Institutionalized Persons Act of 1980
- Voting Accessibility for the Elderly and the Handicapped Act of 1984
- National Voter Registration Act of 1993
- The Air Carrier Access Act of 1986
- Individuals with Disabilities Education Act of 1975
- No Child Left Behind Act of 2001
- Elementary and Secondary Education Act of 1965
- The Individuals with Disabilities Education Improvement Act of 2004
- The Developmental Disabilities Act and Bill of Rights Act of 2000

BOX 31-6 COMPONENTS OF THE AMERICANS WITH DISABILITIES ACT

The Americans with Disabilities Act (ADA) addresses four main areas:

Employment

- Employers may not discriminate against qualified persons with disabilities in hiring or promotion.
- Employers may ask about the person's ability to perform a job but may not subject a person to tests that are not job related.
- Employers must make reasonable accommodations that do not impose an undue hardship on business operations, such as job restructuring and modification of equipment.

Public Facilities

- Private businesses, such as restaurants, hotels, theaters, and stores, must not discriminate against persons with disabilities.
- Auxiliary aids and services must be provided for persons with visual or hearing impairments or other disabilities, unless it is with undue burden.
- Physical barriers in existing facilities must be removed if possible. If not, other methods must be provided so services may be offered.
- All new construction and alterations must be accessible.

Transportation

- New public buses and rail cars made after August 26, 1990, must be wheelchair accessible.
- New bus and train stations need to be accessible.
- Key stations in rapid, light, and commuter rail systems must be accessible by 1993 with extensions up to 20 years by commuter rail and 30 years for rapid and light rail.
- All Amtrak stations must be accessible by July 26, 2010.

Communication

- Telephone companies must offer telephone relay services to individuals who use telecommunication devices for the deaf (TDD).

From Americans with Disabilities Act, 2010. Available at www.ada.gov. Accessed July 10, 2010.

---

summarizes categories of historically significant federal legislation designed to benefit those who are disabled, and Box 31-5 summarizes key disability rights legislation.

The U.S. Department of Justice provides *A Guide to Disability Rights Law* (2006). This publication provides an overview of federal civil rights laws designed to ensure equal opportunity for people with disabilities. This guide is an excellent reference about legislation and disability rights information. The document is available in multiple formats including large print, Braille, audiotape, and CD from the ADA website (http://www.ada.gov).

Rehabilitation services were originally developed through legislation for veterans of World War I. In time, others who were physically disabled were regarded less as sources of embarrassment to their families and more as citizens who should participate as fully as possible in all aspects of society. This change in attitude was reflected in changing laws affecting the disabled.

The Rehabilitation Act of 1973 was the first legislation designed specifically to eliminate discrimination against the disabled. This act required all federal agencies and programs receiving federal funds to hire disabled workers. The Rehabilitation Act was an important piece of legislation that defined disability clearly and increased opportunities for some disabled Americans. However, additional legislation was needed to provide more inclusive protection for individuals with disabilities and to extend the benefits of the Rehabilitation Act to encompass more than federal programs. The ADA of 1990 was designed to decrease discrimination and increase opportunities for all disabled Americans by providing more comprehensive protection for them (Allarie, 2005; Lair and Kale, 2005).

The ADA was signed into law July 26, 1990. The act makes it illegal for state and local governments, private employers, employment agencies, labor organizations, and labor-management committees to discriminate against the disabled in employment, public accommodations, transportation, state and local government operations, and telecommunications (ADA, 1990). Cutting across the specific policy provisions of the ADA are four global goals that clarify the intent of the legislation. For persons with a disability, the ADA is designed to promote: (1) equality of opportunity, (2) full participation in society and social integration, (3) independent living, and (4) economic self-sufficiency (ADA, 1990). "The ADA provides comprehensive civil rights protection for qualified individuals with disabilities" (Walk et al, 1993, p 92). The ADA addresses four areas as shown in Box 31-6.

According to the ADA (1990), a qualified employee or applicant with a disability is a person who, with or without reasonable accommodation, can perform the essential functions of the job in question. Reasonable accommodations may include but are not limited to:

- Making existing facilities that are used by employees readily accessible to and usable by persons with disabilities
- Job restructuring, modifying work schedules, reassignment to a vacant position
- Acquiring or modifying equipment or devices; adjusting or modifying examinations, training materials, or policies; and providing qualified readers or interpreters

Employers may not ask qualified job applicants questions about the existence, nature, or severity of a disability. Qualified applicants may be asked about their ability to perform job functions. A job offer may be made conditional based on the results of a medical examination, but only if that examination is required for all applicants for the same job. In addition, the examination must be job related and consistent with the employer's business needs. Individuals who use illegal drugs or who are intoxicated at work are not covered under the ADA. Tests for illegal drugs are not subject to the ADA's restrictions on examinations. Employers may hold illegal drug users and alcoholics to the same performance standards as other employees.

Service animals are defined and protected under the ADA. Service animals are working animals that are individually trained to perform tasks for persons with disabilities. These tasks may include guiding someone who is blind, alerting persons who are deaf, pulling wheelchairs, and other special tasks. Under the ADA, businesses and other organizations who serve the public, including restaurants, hotels, taxis, stores, medical offices and hospitals, theaters, and parks, are required to allow service animals to accompany a disabled person into all areas open to the general public.

The Fair Housing Act of 1988 prohibits housing discrimination based on race, color, religion, sex, disability, familial status, and national origin. This includes private as well as public housing. The Act also requires new multifamily housing with four or more units to be accessible for persons with disabilities.

The Civil Rights of Institutionalized Persons Act of 1980 authorizes the attorney general to investigate conditions of confinement in state and local institutions such as prisons, detention centers, jails, nursing homes, and institutions for persons with psychiatric or developmental disabilities. Civil lawsuits may be initiated on the behalf of the person if harmful or neglectful conditions are found (Guiding Light Foundation, 2010).

According to the Department of Justice, the Voting Accessibility for the Elderly and the Handicapped Act of 1984 requires polling places across the United States to be accessible for persons with disabilities during federal elections. In addition, states are responsible for ensuring available registration and voting aids for disabled and elderly voters, including telecommunication devices for the deaf (Guiding Light Foundation, 2010).

The National Voter Registration Act of 1993, also known as the Motor Voter Act, makes it easier for all Americans to vote. Because of the low registration turnout of minorities and persons with disabilities, this act requires all offices of state-funded programs to provide program applicants with voter registration forms, to assist them in completing the forms, and to transmit the forms to the appropriate office (Guiding Light Foundation, 2010).

The Air Carrier Access Act of 1986 prohibits discrimination by airlines. Persons with disabilities do not have to give advance notice before they fly. Moreover, unless there is a safety concern, they cannot be discriminated against with regard to seat assignment (Guiding Light Foundation, 2010).

IDEA of 1975 is federal legislation that guarantees all children with disabilities ages 3 through 21 years the right to a free and appropriate public school education that will meet their individual needs. This law protects the rights of parents, guardians, and surrogate parents to fully participate in educational decisions. Special education including physical education is defined in this law, and special instruction is to be provided at no cost to parents. Special education was created to meet the special needs of children with disabilities.

According to IDEA, children with disabilities are those who have one or a combination of the following conditions and therefore would benefit from special education: autism, blindness, deafness, hearing impairment, mental retardation, multiple disabilities, orthopedic impairment, serious emotional disturbance, specific learning disabilities, traumatic brain injury, visual impairment, and other health impairments (USDE, 2010).

Basic Rights Under IDEA

Free and appropriate public education (FAPE)—The child's education must be designed to meet the child's special needs.

Appropriate evaluation/assessment—Each child with a disability must receive a complete educational assessment before being placed in a special education program.

Individualized education plan (IEP)—This plan must be focused and modified on a set of goals and objectives to meet the child's individual needs.

Education in the least restrictive environment (LRE)—Children with disabilities should be educated as much as possible with their peers who do not have disabilities.

Parent and student participation in decision making—Parent and student participation and communication are encouraged. Parents are members of the IEP team and are included in evaluation, eligibility, and placement.

Early intervention services for children and their families—Funds are allocated to infants who have disabling conditions and/or developmental delays. An individualized family service plan (IFSP) is developed that details the early intervention services to enhance the child's development and strengthen the family (Department of Developmental Services, 2005).

The No Child Left Behind Act of 2001 expands parental roles in their child's education. This law reauthorized the Elementary and Secondary Education Act of 1965, the principal federal law governing elementary and secondary education. According to the U.S. Department of Education, it is built on four concepts: accountability, doing what works according to the scientific research, expanding parental options, and expanding local control and flexibility. This bill:

- Supports learning in the early years, hopefully preventing learning disabilities
- Provides more information for parents about their child's programs
- Alerts parents to important information about their child's performance
- Gives more resources to schools
- Gives children and parents a lifeline
- Improves teaching and learning by providing better information to teachers
- Ensures that teacher quality is a high priority
- Allows more flexibility

The Individuals with Disabilities Education Improvement Act of 2004 is the nation's special education law and serves 6.8 million children and youth with disabilities (USDE, 2010).

The Developmental Disabilities Act and Bill of Rights Act of 2000 requires the Administration of Developmental Disabilities

---

BOX 31-7 FEDERAL AGENCIES WITH DEVELOPMENTAL DISABILITY ACTIVITIES

- Administration on Developmental Disabilities (ADD)
- Center for Medicaid and Medicare Services—Medicaid and the State Children's Health Insurance Program can help children and adults obtain health care coverage
- DisabilityInfo.gov—provides information about disability resources in the federal government
- Maternal and Child Health Bureau (MCHB)—promotes the health of mothers and children; provides newborn hearing screening, information on child health and safety and information on genetics
- Medline plus Health Information, National Library of Medicine—online resource for information
- National Council on Disability (NCD)—ensures that persons with disabilities have the same opportunities as others; promotes policies and programs that assist people with disabilities
- National Institutes of Health (NIH)—conducts and funds research on developmental disabilities

- National Institute on Disability and Rehabilitation Research (NIDRR)—promotes the participation of persons with disabilities in their communities
- Office of Disability Employment—focus is to increase job opportunities for people with disabilities; this office is within the U.S. Department of Labor
- Office of Special Education Programs (OSEP)—improves the lives of children and youth with disabilities from birth to adulthood through education and support services; this office is within the U.S. Department of Education
- Office on Disability—oversees the implementation of federal disability policies and programs; fosters interactions between the U.S. Department of Health and Human Services, other federal and state agencies, and private-sector groups
- Rehabilitative Services Administration (RSA)—helps persons with disabilities get jobs and live more independently; RSA is part of the U.S. Department of Education

From Centers for Disease Control and Prevention: *Federal agencies with developmental disability activities,* 2010. Available at www.cdc.gov. Accessed July 10, 2010.

(ADD) under the USDHHS to ensure that people with developmental disabilities and their families receive the services and support they need. The disabled and their families must also be given the opportunity to participate in the planning and implementation of these services. The ADD is a federal agency within the USDHHS and is responsible for implementation and administration of The Developmental Disabilities Act and Bill of Rights Act of 2000 and the disability provisions of the Help Americans Vote Act. There are eight areas of emphasis for ADD: employment, education, childcare, health, housing, transportation, recreation, and quality assurance. The ADD meets these requirements through four programs:

1. *State Councils on Developmental Disabilities (SCDD):* Each state has a council whose function is to increase the independence, productivity, inclusion, and community integration of persons with developmental disabilities.
2. *Protection and Advocacy Agencies (P&As):* Every state has a system to empower, protect, and advocate on the behalf of persons with developmental disabilities. The system investigates incidents of abuse, neglect, or discrimination based on disability.

3. *University Centers for Excellence in Developmental Disabilities—Education, Research, and Services (UCEDD):* This program provides support to a national network of university centers to carry out interdisciplinary training, services, technical assistance, and information dissemination activities. Its purpose is to increase independence, productivity, and integration into communities.
4. *Projects of National Significance:* The purpose of this program is to focus on emerging issues, provide technical assistance, conduct research regarding disability issues and develop state and federal policy (www.acf.hhs.gov). In addition, most states and many large cities and counties have their own laws prohibiting discrimination on the basis of disability. Such laws offer greater protection to employees by extending coverage to smaller employers, by using more expansive definitions of disability than those used under the ADA and by expanding the duty of employers to assist employees with disabilities to move to new positions for which they are qualified. Box 31-7 lists federal agencies with developmental disability activities.

CHAPTER REVIEW

PRACTICE APPLICATION

A referral was made to a public health department from a nearby regional level III neonatal intensive care unit (NICU) regarding discharge plans for a developmentally delayed infant. The infant, Joel, was born at 27 weeks' gestation and had remained in intensive care for 7 months. His hospital course was complicated by respiratory distress syndrome, bronchopulmonary dysplasia, and intraventricular hemorrhage. At the time of discharge, Joel was receiving neither supplemental oxygen nor medications and was taking all of his feedings orally. There were strong indications of spastic diplegia and he was diagnosed as having severe retinopathy of prematurity with the expectation of eventual blindness.

Family financial resources were extremely limited. Although Medicaid coverage was available for subsequent needs, the family owed more than $100,000 to the hospital. Joel's grandmother agreed to care for him while his 17-year-old mother Mary finished high school. Joel's father, who is also 17 years old and unemployed, had not been active with Mary and her mother in the hospital discharge-planning program. His involvement with Mary and Joel was expected to be minimal. The hospital was seeking a home evaluation before discharge.

What would you consider to be the first step in completing the home evaluation?

Answers can be found on the Evolve site.

KEY POINTS

- Nurses have many opportunities to influence the care of individuals with disabilities through health promotion activities. Health education is important for parents who might be at high risk for having a disabled child, for children at risk for accidents and injuries, and for adults with chronic illnesses who might prevent disability through careful health practices.
- Many of the *Healthy People 2020* objectives apply to physically compromised individuals, their families, and communities.
- Physically compromised individuals need to participate in health promotion to prevent the onset of a new health disruption, to strengthen their well-functioning aspects and to prevent further deterioration of their health.

- Nursing interventions for physically compromised clients require attention to their health as well as to the environment in which they live.
- Nurses influence policy decisions that affect the health and well-being of compromised individuals.
- Nurses must know both federal and state laws pertaining to disabilities to most effectively assist clients and their families.

CLINICAL DECISION-MAKING ACTIVITIES

1. Divide the class or the clinical group into two teams and debate the following: Children with developmental disabilities should or should not be mainstreamed into classrooms with non-disabled children.
2. During a home visit first to an adult and then to a child who have a chronic illness that leaves them physically compromised, answer the following questions:
   A. Could this disability have been prevented? If so, what steps could a nurse have taken to provide health promotion activities that would have prevented the occurrence of the disabling condition?
   B. What role, if any, does the environment play in the onset of this compromising health condition?
   C. What preventive activities are currently needed to ensure the highest possible quality of life for this person?

3. For the next week, look at each building you enter and consider the following:
   A. What accommodations have been made to allow physically compromised people to enter this building?
   B. What accommodations should still be made?
   C. Who should pay for these architectural accommodations?
4. Spend one day following your usual schedule using either crutches or a wheelchair, so that you can understand better what it means to be physically compromised and have special needs.
5. Using a telephone book, community resource directory, or the web pages for your town, identify all agencies whose scope of work is devoted to assisting special needs individuals and their families.

REFERENCES

Allarie SH: Employment and satisfaction outcomes from a job retention intervention delivered to persons with chronic diseases, *Rehabil Couns Bull* 48:100–109, 2005.

Americans with Disabilities Act of 1990, PL 101–336, 1990.

Americans with Disabilities Act: *Components of the act*, 2010. Available at www.ada.gov. Accessed July 10, 2010.

Bilgin S, Gozum S: Reducing burnout in mothers with an intellectually disabled child: an education programme, *J Adv Nurs* 65:2552–2561, 2009.

Carmona R: *The Surgeon General's call to action to improve the health and wellness of persons with disabilities*, 2005. Available at www.surgeongeneral.gov/library/calls. Accessed February 23, 2011.

Cate I, Loots G: Experiences of siblings of children with physical disabilities: an empirical investigation, *Disabil Rehabil* 22:399–408, 2000.

The Center for an Accessible Society, 2010. Available at www.accessiblesociety.org. Accessed July 8, 2010.

Centers for Disease Control and Prevention: Prevalence and most common causes of disabilities among adults—United States, 2005, *MMWR Morbid Mortal Weekly Report* 58:421–426, 2009.

Centers for Disease Control and Prevention: *Chronic diseases and health promotion*, 2010a. Available at www.cdc.gov/chronicdisease/overview/index.htm. Accessed February 23, 2011.

Centers for Disease Control and Prevention: *Classifications of diseases and functioning and disability*, 2010b. Available at www.cdc.gov. Accessed July 8, 2010.

Centers for Disease Control and Prevention: *Developmental disabilities*, 2010c. Available at www.cdc.gov. Accessed July 1, 2010.

Centers for Disease Control and Prevention: *Federal agencies with developmental disability activities*, 2010d. Available at www.cdc.gov. Accessed July 10, 2010.

Clough-Gorr KM, Erpen T, Gillmann G, et al: Preclinical disability as a risk factor for falls in community-dwelling older adults, *J Gerontol* 63A:314–320, 2008.

The Council for Disability Awareness: *Disability statistics*, 2009. Available at www.disabilitycanhappen.org. Accessed February 23, 2011.

Council on Linkages Between Academia and Public Health Practice: *Tier 1, tier 2 and tier 3 core competencies for public health professionals*, 2009. Available at www.phf.org. Accessed May 20, 2010.

Dauz WP, Piamjariyakul U, Graff JC, et al: Developmental disabilities: effects on well siblings, *Issues Compr Pediatr Nurs* 33:39–55, 2010.

Department of Developmental Services, 2005. *Parents' rights: an early start guide for families*, 2010. Available at www.matrixparents.org. Accessed July 10, 2010.

Ding T, Hall A, Jacobs K, David J: Psychological functioning of children and adolescents with juvenile idiopathic arthritis is related to physical disability but not to disease status, *Rheumatology* 47:660–664, 2008.

Dyke P, Mulroy S, Leonard H: Siblings of children with disabilities: challenges and opportunities, *Acta Pediatr* 98:23–24, 2009.

Erickson W, Lee C, von Schrader S: *Disability statistics from the 2008 American Community Survey (ACS)*, Ithaca, NY, 2010, Cornell University Rehabilitation Research and Training Center on Disability Demographics and Statistics. Available at www.ilr.cornell.edu/edi/disabilitystatistics. Accessed February 22, 2011.

Giardino A, Hudson K, Marsh J: Providing medical evaluations for possible child maltreatment to children with special health care needs, *Child Abuse Negl* 27:1179–1186, 2003.

Govindshenoy M, Spencer N: Abuse of the disabled child: a systematic review of population-based studies, *Child Care Health Dev* 33:552–558, 2007.

Groce N: Adolescents and youth with disability: issues and challenges, *Asia Pacific Disabil Rehabil J* 15:13–32, 2004.

Guiding Light Foundation: *Disability laws*, 2010. Available at www.guidinglightfoundation.com. Accessed July 10, 2010.

Ha JH, Hong J, Seltzer MM, Greenberg JS: Age and gender differences in the well-being of midlife and aging parents with children with mental health or developmental problems: report of a national study, *J Health Soc Beh* 49:301–316, 2008.

Hassouneh-Phillips D: Understanding abuse of women with physical disabilities: an overview of the abuse pathways model, *Adv Nurs Sci* 28:70–80, 2005.

Heywood J: Childhood disability: ordinary lives for extraordinary families, *Community Pract* 83:19–22, 2010.

Horsfall J, Cleary M, Hunt GE, Walter G: Psychosocial treatments for people with co-occurring severe mental illnesses and substance use disorders (dual diagnosis): a review of empirical evidence, *Harv Rev Psychiatry* 17:24–34, 2009.

Jaudes PK, Mackey-Bilaver L: Do chronic conditions increase young children's risk of being maltreated? *Child Abuse Negl* 32:672–681, 2008.

Johnson C, Kastner T: Helping families raise children with special health care needs at home, *Pediatrics* 115:507–511, 2005.

Jones NL: Essential requirements of the Act: a short history and overview, *Milbank Q* 69(Suppl 1-2):25–54, 1991.

Kliebenstein MA, Brome ME: School re-entry for the child with chronic illness: parent and school personnel perceptions, *Pediatr Nurs* 26:579–582, 2002.

Lair PL, Kale KD: Post-offer medical exam was premature, *HR Magazine* 50:163, 2005.

Laskar AR, Gupta VK, Kumar D, et al: Psychosocial effect and economic burden on parents of children with locomotor disability, *Indian J Pediatr*, April 17, 2010. [Epub ahead of print].

Leffert JS, Siperstein GN, Widaman KF: Social perceptions in children with intellectual disabilities: the interpretation of benign and hostile intentions, *J Intellect Disabil Res* 54:168–180, 2010.

Maart S, Jelsma J: The sexual behavior of physically disabled adolescents, *Disabil Rehabil* 32:438–443, 2010.

Maternal and Child Health Bureau: *The national survey of children with special health care needs chartbook 2005-2006*, 2008. Available at www.mchb.hrsa.gov. Accessed July 8, 2010.

Merriam-Webster On-Line Dictionary: *Disability*, 2010. Available at www.merriam-webster.com. Accessed April 30, 2010.

Murchland S, Parkyn H: Using assistive technology for schoolwork: the experience of children with physical disabilities, *Disabil Rehabil Assist Technol* May 7, 2010. [Epub ahead of print].

National Information Center for Children and Youth with Disabilities, 2010. Available at www.icdri.org. Accessed July 12, 2010.

National Institute of Mental Health: *The numbers count: mental disorders in America*, 2010. Available at www.nimh.gov/health/publications. Accessed May 6, 2010.

Newacheck P, Kim S: A national profile of health care utilization and expenditures for children with special health care needs, *Arch Pediatr Adolesc Med* 159:10–17, 2005.

O'Brien I, Duffy A, Nicholl H: Impact of childhood chronic illness on siblings: a literature review, *Br J Nurs* 18(1358):1360–1365, 2009.

Obrusnikova I, Block M, Dillon S: Children's beliefs toward cooperative playing with peers with disabilities in physical education, *Adapt Phys Act Q* 27:127–142, 2010.

Pezzin LE, Pollak RA, Schone BS: Parental marital disruption, family type, and transfers to disabled elderly parents, *J Gerontol B Psychol Sc* 63:S349–S358, 2008.

Redmon SJ: Healthcare transitions for adolescents and young adults with special healthcare needs and/or disabilities, *Prof Case Manag* 15:170, 2010.

Reinehr T, Dobe M, Winkel K, et al: Obesity in disabled children and adolescents: an overlooked group of patients, *Deutsch Arztebl Inter* 107:268–275, 2010.

Roth DL, Perkins M, Wadley VG, et al: Family caregiving and emotional strain: associations with quality of life in a large national sample of middle-aged and older adults, *Qual Life Res* 18:679–688, 2009.

Scullion PA: Models of disability: their influence in nursing and potential role in challenging discrimination, *J Adv Nurs* 66:697–707, 2010.

Sherrington C, Lord SR, Vogler CM, et al: Minimizing disability and falls in older people through a post-hospital exercise program: a protocol for a randomized controlled trial and economic evaluation, *BMC Geriatr* 9:1471–1489, 2009.

Skar L: Peer and adult relationships of adolescents with disabilities, *J Adolesc* 26:635–649, 2003.

Snow K: *People first language*, 2010, CDC. Available at www.disabilityisnatural.com. Accessed July 8, 2010.

Spencer N, Devereux E, Wallace A, et al: Disabling conditions and registration for child abuse and neglect: a population based study, *Pediatrics* 116:609–613, 2005.

Thorne S: Patient-provider communication in chronic illness: a health promotion window of opportunity, *Fam Community Health* 29(Suppl 1):S4–S11, 2006.

United States Quad Rugby Association, 2010. Available at www.murderball.quadrugby.com. Accessed July 12, 2010.

U.S. Census Bureau: *Press release*, 2008. Available at www.census.gov/Press-Release. Accessed May 6, 2010.

U.S. Census Bureau: *Methodology for identifying persons with a work disability in the current population survey*, 2009a. Available at www.census.gov/hhes/www/disability/acs.html. Accessed March 2, 2011.

U.S. Census Bureau: *Review of changes to the measurement of disability in the 2008 American Community Survey*, 2009b. Available at www.census.gov/hhes/www/disability/2008ACS_disability.pdf. Accessed February 22, 2011.

U.S. Department of Education: *Building the legacy: IDEA 2004*, 2010. Available at www.idea.ed.gov. Accessed March 2, 2011.

U.S. Department of Health and Human Services: *Developing Healthy People 2020*, 2010a. Available at www.healthypeople.gov. Accessed May 18, 2010.

U.S. Department of Health and Human Services: *Office on Disability*, 2010b. Available at www.hhs.gov/od. Accessed February 23, 2011.

U.S. Department of Justice: *A guide to disability rights laws*, 2006. Available at www.ada.gov/cguide.htm. Accessed February 23, 2011.

U.S. Social Security Administration: *Disability evaluation under social security*, 2008. Available at www.ssa.gov/disability/professionals/bluebook/general-info.htm. Accessed February 23, 2011.

Walk EE, Ahn HC, Lampkin PM, et al: Americans with Disabilities Act, *J Burn Care Rehabil* 14:92–98, 1993.

Wilson PE, Clayton GH: Sports and disability, *Phys Med Rehabil Clin North Am* 2:S46–S54, 2010.

World Health Organization: *Global burden of disease: 2004 update*, 2008. Available at www.who.int. Accessed May 6, 2010.

World Health Organization: *Disability: including prevention, management and rehabilitation*, 2010a. Available at www.who.int. Accessed July 10, 2010.

World Health Organization: *International classification of functioning, disability and health*, 2010b. Available at www.who.int/classification/icf/en. Accessed February 23, 2011.

PART 6

Vulnerability: Issues for the Twenty-First Century

As we proceed through the twenty-first century, the complexity of health and social problems is increasing. Solutions will require an integrated behavioral, social, and health care approach that begins with a commitment to primary health care. Primary health care involves a partnership between public health and primary care to address the problems of society as well as of individuals and families.

Communities increasingly experience significant problems as a result of conditions that are often expensive and hard to treat: violence against people and property, unresolved mental health illnesses, abuse of substances among people of all groups, teen pregnancy, and an increasing number of people who are disenfranchised from society. Some groups like those represented by people who are poor, homeless, or part of the growing migrant populations often have less access to health care and prevention services that would help maintain their health. Personal resources and access to health and social services are limited for these populations. Although there is hope that health care reform will ameliorate many of the concerns of people who have limited access to health care, at present there are still many uninsured and underinsured people in the United States. Some of the early implementation aspects of health care reform place nurses, including nurse practitioners, nurse midwives, home health care, and other public health nurses, at the forefront of helping to reduce health disparities and provide accessible care in communities.

The stage is set in this section of the text with a discussion of the concept of vulnerability and the implications for communities of the growing number of vulnerable people. Poverty and homelessness are two conditions that have profound effects on the health of individuals, families, and communities. The growing community health problems arising from increased rates of teen pregnancy and the implications of the growing migrant population in cities and rural areas across the country are highlighted. Problems that are escalating include mental health issues, substance abuse, interpersonal violence and abuse, and communicable diseases such as HIV, hepatitis, and sexually transmitted diseases. Over the last decade, many intentional and unintentional acts of violence, natural diseases and unintended human-made diseases have focused attention on the fragility of our ability to sustain health in the affected communities. These events have also demonstrated how essential public health nurses are and how often communities do not have access to essential public health services. The chapters in Part 6 discuss some of the most common problems seen in communities.

CHAPTER 32

Vulnerability and Vulnerable Populations: An Overview

Juliann G. Sebastian, PhD, RN, FAAN

Juliann G. Sebastian developed an interest in public health and community-based nursing while obtaining her BSN degree, when she provided care in rural Appalachia. Since then, she has cared for a range of vulnerable populations across the life span and in a variety of community settings, including adults who are homeless, low-income families, and frail elders in their home environments. Her doctoral preparation was in organization theory and health economics, and her research interests are in the area of community systems of care delivery for underserved populations. She was a member of the inaugural cohort of Robert Wood Johnson Nurse Executive Fellows (1998-2001), during which time she focused on development of models of academic clinical nursing practice. Her research and publications have focused on academic nurse-managed centers, community-based care, and primary care. She is a Fellow in the American Academy of Nursing and has held numerous leadership positions in professional nursing organizations. Dr. Sebastian serves as Dean of the College of Nursing at the University of Missouri–St. Louis.

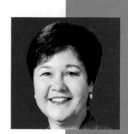

ADDITIONAL RESOURCES

Ⓔvolve WEBSITE
http://evolve.elsevier.com/Stanhope
- *Healthy People 2020*
- WebLinks
- Quiz
- Case Studies
- Glossary
- Answers to Practice Application

OBJECTIVES

After reading this chapter, the student should be able to do the following:

1. Define what is meant by vulnerable populations.
2. Analyze trends that have influenced the development of vulnerability among certain population groups and social attitudes toward vulnerability.
3. Analyze the effects of public policies on vulnerable populations and on reducing health disparities experienced by these populations.
4. Examine the multiple individual and social factors that contribute to vulnerability.
5. Evaluate strategies that can be used by nurses to improve the health status and eliminate health disparities of vulnerable populations, including governmental, community-based, and private programs.

KEY TERMS

This chapter introduces the concept of vulnerability and the nursing roles for meeting the health needs of vulnerable population groups. Selected population groups who have greater risk than others to poor health outcomes are described. Public policies that have influenced vulnerable groups and the effects of these policies are explored. The nature of vulnerability is analyzed, and factors that predispose people to vulnerability, outcomes of vulnerability, and the cycle of vulnerability are described. Nursing interventions are designed to help break the cycle of vulnerability and to eliminate health disparities. Numerous interventions are possible at the individual, family, group, community, and population levels. This chapter describes how nurses use the nursing process with vulnerable population groups and presents case examples throughout and at the end to clarify these ideas.

PERSPECTIVES ON VULNERABILITY

Definition and Health Risk

Shi and Stevens (2005a) describe vulnerable populations "as those at greater risk for poor health status and health care access" (p 148). In health care, **risk** is an epidemiological term meaning that some people have a higher probability of illness than others. In the familiar concept of the epidemiologic triangle, the agent, host, and environment interact to produce illness or poor health. The natural history of disease model explains how certain aspects of physiology and the environment, including personal habits, social environment, and physical environment, make it more likely that one will develop particular health problems (Friss, 2010). For example, a smoker is at risk for developing lung cancer because cellular changes occur with smoking. However, not everyone who is at risk develops health problems. Some individuals are more likely than others to develop the health problems for which they are at risk. These people are more *vulnerable* than others. The web of causation model better explains what happens in these situations. A **vulnerable**

population group is a subgroup of the population that is more likely to develop health problems as a result of exposure to risk or to have worse outcomes from these health problems than the rest of the population. Vulnerability is a global concern, with different populations being more vulnerable in different countries. Examples of vulnerable populations of concern to nurses are persons who are poor and homeless, pregnant adolescents, migrant workers and immigrants, individuals with mental health problems, people who abuse addictive substances, individuals who are abused or victims of violence, persons with communicable disease and those at risk, and persons who are HIV positive or have hepatitis B virus or a sexually transmitted disease (STD).

> **DID YOU KNOW?** *Vulnerable populations experience disparities in access to care and have poorer health status than the population as a whole. The proportion of vulnerable populations in the United States is increasing (Shi and Stevens, 2005b). This is occurring at a time when federal goals include eliminating health disparities (USDHHS, 2010).*

According to the web of causation model of health and illness (Friss, 2010), the interaction between numerous causal variables creates a more potent combination of factors predisposing an individual to illness (see Chapter 12 for more information on epidemiology). This means that the relative risk for illness or a poor health outcome is greater for vulnerable populations (Aday, 2001). Vulnerable population groups are those that are particularly sensitive to risk factors and who possess multiple, **cumulative risk factors.** This is referred to as the **differential vulnerability hypothesis** (Aday, 2001).

Vulnerable populations may be particularly sensitive to the effects of multiple risks. Risks may originate in environmental hazards (e.g., lead exposure from peeling, lead-based paint) or social hazards (e.g., crime and violence), in personal behavior (e.g., diet and exercise habits), or from biological or genetic makeup (e.g., congenital addiction or compromised immune status). Members of vulnerable populations often have comorbidities, or multiple illnesses, with each affecting the other. Risk factors may interact with each other, creating a more hazardous situation. For example, mothers who abuse substances are more likely to give birth to low-birth-weight infants, or to give birth prematurely, or to experience stillbirths or have infants treated for health complications following birth (Mayet et al, 2008). Another example of the interaction between social conditions and health is that perceptions of racial discrimination have been linked with poorer perceptions of health and less control over health outcomes (Pieterse and Carter, 2010). These elements of multiple risk factors, cumulative effects of risk factors, and low thresholds for risk must be addressed when assessing the needs of vulnerable populations and designing services for them.

Examples of Vulnerable Groups

There are many examples of vulnerable populations. Nurses may work with pregnant adolescents who are poor, have been abused, and are substance abusers. Nurses may also work with people who abuse substances, and with individuals who test positive for human immunodeficiency virus (HIV) and hepatitis B virus (HBV), as well as those with severe mental illnesses. Nurses work with individuals and families who are homeless and marginally housed. They also provide care for migrant workers and immigrants. Any of these groups may be victimized by abuse and violence. Each of these groups is discussed in detail in Chapters 33 through 38 and in Chapter 14.

Priority population groups differ in other countries. Priority population groups are groups targeted by national governments for special emphasis in health care goals because their health status is particularly poor. In Canada, Aboriginal Indians and people who live in remote rural areas of northern Canada need special attention to reduce health disparities. The infant mortality rate for Canada as a whole was 5.1 per 1000 live births in 2007. By comparison, the infant mortality rate for the Nunavut people who live in northern Canada was 15.1 per 1000 live births (Statistics Canada, 2010). This chapter highlights some of the problems that the vulnerable populations just described have with access to care, quality and appropriateness of care, and health outcomes.

Health Disparities

Nurses, other public health professionals, and policy makers target health care interventions toward vulnerable population groups because these groups suffer from disparities in access to care, uneven quality of care, and the poorest health outcomes. The Institute of Medicine (IOM, 2003) defined disparities in health care as "racial or ethnic differences in the quality of care that are not due to access-related factors or clinical needs, preferences, and appropriateness of intervention" (pp 3-4). Appropriate differences in care may result from client preferences or clinical needs. Disparities, on the other hand, refer to lower quality care or poorer outcomes. Disparities may result from client-level factors such as mistrust, provider-level factors such as conscious or unconscious stereotyping or prejudice,

or health systems factors such as lack of insurance coverage or fragmentation (IOM, 2003).

Healthy People 2020 (USDHHS, 2010) discusses vulnerable population groups and identifies illness prevention and health promotion objectives for them. One of the four goals of *Healthy People 2020* is elimination of health disparities. Thirty-eight topic areas in *Healthy People 2020* emphasize access, chronic health problems, injury and violence prevention, environmental health, food safety, education and community-based programs, health communication and health information technologies, immunization and infectious diseases, and public health infrastructure, among others.

Healthy People 2020 is an implementation guide for all federal and most state health initiatives, with a special emphasis on promoting systematic approaches to eliminating health disparities experienced by underserved and disadvantaged populations. Disadvantaged populations are those that have fewer resources for promoting health and treating illness than the average person in the United States. For example, a family or individual below the federal poverty line is considered disadvantaged in terms of access to economic resources.

Examples of areas that show health disparities across population groups are infant mortality, mortality among children under 5 years of age, and age-adjusted mortality rates. In 2006 African Americans had an infant mortality rate of 12.9 per 1000 live births, compared with 5.6 for whites (Mathews and MacDorman, 2010). Mortality rates in children under age 5 vary dramatically around the world, probably reflecting widely differing social, economic, and educational conditions for health (Hegevary, Berry, and Murua, 2008). Non-Hispanic African Americans in the United States had an age-adjusted death rate of 961.9 per 100,000 compared with a rate of 766.5 per 100,000 for non-Hispanic whites (Miniño et al, 2009).

Trends Related to Caring for Vulnerable Populations

Over the years there have been different focuses for care of vulnerable populations. An analysis of these trends can help nurses learn from lessons of the past and develop new approaches best

---

 HEALTHY PEOPLE 2020

Objectives for Vulnerable Populations

Following are examples of objectives that nurses who work with vulnerable populations might want to note:

- AHS-1: Increase the proportion of persons with health insurance.
- AHS-6: Reduce the proportion of individuals who are unable to obtain or delay in obtaining necessary medical care, dental care, or prescription medicines.
- HIV-2: Reduce new incident HIV infections and HIV diagnoses among adolescents and adults.
- HIV-4: Reduce the number of new HIV cases among adolescents and adults.
- EMC-2.5: Increase the proportion of parents with children under the age of 3 years whose doctors or other health care professionals talk with them about positive parenting practices.

From U.S. Department of Health and Human Services: *Healthy People 2020*, Washington, DC, 2010. Available at http://www.healthypeople.gov/2020/default.aspx. Accessed March 1, 2011.

BOX 32-1	TRENDS RELATED TO VULNERABLE POPULATIONS

- Growth in disparity between socioeconomically advantaged and disadvantaged populations around the world
- Increasing community-based care and community partnerships
- Increasing importance of academic nurse-managed centers and community health centers
- Outreach and case finding
- Comprehensive health care and social services in workplaces, schools, faith-based organizations
- Social justice activism and advocacy
- Culturally and linguistically appropriate care
- Partnerships between public and private payers

suited for the contemporary environment. Box 32-1 lists trends related to caring for vulnerable populations.

During colonial times, persons with chronic physical or mental conditions were cared for in their own communities. Later, the social reforms of the nineteenth century led to institutional care for many of these individuals. In the twenty-first century, there is a renewed emphasis on caring for vulnerable population groups in the community through partnerships between groups such as public health, managed care, and community groups (Aday, 2001).

Many of the vulnerable population groups described in this chapter and other chapters have less access to health services than other groups. The trend is toward more outreach and case finding to make access easier (IOM, 2000). **Outreach** is an approach to making health care more easily available to certain populations by implementing health education, counseling, or support services in places where people normally congregate, such as places of worship, schools, workplaces, and community centers. **Case finding** occurs when nurses design methods for finding populations and individuals especially in need of services. In some cases, lay health workers assist with outreach or case finding (Lewin et al, 2010). A related trend is to develop culturally and linguistically appropriate forms of outreach and care delivery to more effectively promote the health of these populations (USDHHS, 2001b). **Culturally and linguistically appropriate care** fits with the cultural expectations and norms of a particular group to the extent possible and that is provided in the language of that group. For example, in African-American communities in the United States, one of the most effective locations for outreach and community education is the neighborhood church or mosque. The American Cancer Society program Sister to Sister involves African-American women going door to door in African-American neighborhoods and providing individualized education about the importance of breast cancer screening.

> **NURSING TIP** *Nurses demonstrate respect to clients of different cultural backgrounds by learning about the cultural norms, values, and traditions of the groups within a particular community. Being fluent in a second language is especially important. Nurses who work in communities with a large Hispanic population find it useful to be fluent in Spanish. Similarly, nurses who work with people who are deaf should consider learning sign language.*

There is also a trend toward providing more comprehensive, family-centered services when treating vulnerable population groups. It is important to provide comprehensive, family-centered, "one-stop" services. Providing multiple services during a single clinic visit is an example of one-stop services. For example, providing all the immunizations a child needs during any clinic visit helps increase the extent to which children in a community are fully immunized (Larson, 2003). If social assistance and economic assistance are also provided and included in interprofessional treatment plans, services can be more responsive to the combined effects of social and economic stressors on the health of special population groups. This situation is sometimes referred to as providing **wraparound services,** in which comprehensive health services are available and social and economic services are "wrapped around" these services.

> **DID YOU KNOW?** *Vulnerable populations are often most effectively served by making a comprehensive set of services available in one place and at one time. If a mother brings a child to a community clinic for a simple acute problem, it may be a good time to check to see if the child has up-to-date immunizations. Any siblings who are present could also be evaluated for immunization status and each child provided with the necessary immunizations, assuming none are contraindicated.*

It is helpful to provide comprehensive services in locations where people live and work, including schools, churches, neighborhoods, and workplaces. **Comprehensive services** are health services that focus on more than one health problem or concern. For example, some nurses use mobile outreach clinics to provide a wide array of health promotion, illness prevention, and illness management services in migrant camps, schools, and local communities. A single client encounter might focus on an acute health problem such as influenza, but it may also include health education related to diet and exercise, counseling related to smoking cessation, and a follow-up appointment for immunizations once the influenza has resolved. Comprehensive services are provided in community health centers and nurse-managed clinics. These types of clinics are thought of as **safety net providers** because they increase access to health and social services for vulnerable populations with limited financial ability to pay for care (IOM, 2000; Hansen-Turton, 2005).

Nurses in the community focus on advocacy and issues of social justice. **Advocacy** refers to a set of actions one undertakes on behalf of another. Nurses may function as advocates for vulnerable populations by working for the passage and implementation of policies leading to improved public health services for these populations. For example, a nurse may serve on a local coalition for low-income mothers and children; another nurse may work to develop a plan where local health care organizations provide free or low-cost health care.

Social justice refers to providing equitable care and social supports for the most disadvantaged members of society (Boutain, 2008). Nurses can function as advocates for policy changes to improve social, economic, and environmental factors that predispose vulnerable populations to poor health. In one community, nurses worked with others to promote passage of a law banning smoking from restaurants and bars. This was done to protect customers and employees from the harmful effects of second-hand smoke.

Nurses also provide culturally and linguistically appropriate health care. Linguistically appropriate health care means communicating health-related assessment and information in the recipient's primary language when possible and always in a language the recipient can understand. National standards for culturally and linguistically appropriate care have been published (USDHHS, 2001b).

A major shift in providing care for certain vulnerable populations in the United States is the increasing reliance on private managed care by Medicaid and Medicare. Many states have waivers from the federal government that permit them to test innovative approaches to organizing care for Medicaid beneficiaries (Gilmer, Kronick, and Rice, 2005). A state is allowed to waive certain usual Medicaid requirements in order to test unique approaches to providing health care in specific local areas. These waivers have often been used to develop forms of managed care arrangements for all or part of the Medicaid beneficiaries in a state. An advantage of the waivers is that they allow states to develop strategies that work best in local communities, rather than mandating that all states use the same model.

Some vulnerable populations are such high financial risks and have such unique needs that their care is contracted to specialty groups. For example, mental health and substance abuse services are often contracted out to behavioral managed care firms. These contracts are referred to as carve outs because the care for a specific population has been carved out of an overall managed care plan for all other clinical populations. Other groups whose care may be carved out are older adults, people with disabilities, and children with special health care needs. Care may also be carved out as part of a block grant, in which funds are given in a block to a local region that focuses on a broad area, such as maternal and child health. Block grants are intended to enable local areas to have more control in deciding how to spend funds so that they can respond to local needs and conditions. In one city, funds from a block grant broadly focused on energy and home heating were used to help support a shelter for homeless adults.

The situation in Canada differs from the United States because control of local health care decisions rests largely at the provincial government level rather than at the federal level. This permits responsiveness to local conditions and needs. A major challenge in today's health care environment is developing flexible new care delivery strategies for high-risk populations that are responsive to local cultural mores and social context, and that result in improved clinical outcomes at an affordable cost. The Patient Protection and Affordable Care Act of 2010 provides new opportunities for innovative approaches to care for vulnerable populations through its provisions for funding for nurse-managed centers (Naylor and Kurtzman, 2010) and community health centers (Adashi, Geiger, and Fine, 2010).

BOX 32-2   LEGISLATION THAT HAS AFFECTED VULNERABLE POPULATION GROUPS IN THE UNITED STATES

Legislation That Provided Direct and Indirect Financial Subsidies to Certain Vulnerable Population Groups
- Social Security Act of 1935
- Medicare and Medicaid Social Security Act amendments of 1965
- State Child Health Insurance Program amendment, 1998
- Patient Protection and Affordable Care Act, 2010

Legislation That Provided Financial Support for Building Health Care Facilities
- Hill-Burton Act of 1946
- Community Mental Health Centers Act of 1963
- Stewart B. McKinney Homeless Assistance Act of 1988

Legislation That Affected How Health Care Resources Were Used
- National Health Planning and Resources Development Act of 1974
- Tax Equity and Fiscal Responsibility Act of 1982
- Federal Balanced Budget Act of 1997

Legislation Related to Health Information
- Health Insurance Portability and Accountability Act of 1996

PUBLIC POLICIES AFFECTING VULNERABLE POPULATIONS

Landmark Legislation

Public policy is shaped by legislation that specifies the general directions for government bodies to take. Even though laws may relate to only a certain proportion of the population, they tend to have a ripple effect and result in other groups following the general intent of the law. As seen in Box 32-2, various pieces of landmark legislation have affected vulnerable population groups throughout the twentieth century.

Three of these pieces of legislation provided direct and indirect financial subsidies to certain vulnerable groups. The Social Security Act created the largest federal support program for older adults and people living in poverty in history. This act sought direct payments to eligible individuals to ensure a minimal level of support for people at risk for problems resulting from inadequate financial resources. Later, the Medicare and Medicaid amendments to the Social Security Act of 1965 provided for the health care needs of older adult, poor, and disabled people who might be vulnerable to impoverishment because of high medical bills or because of poor health status from inadequate access to health care. These acts created third-party health care payers at the federal and state levels. Title XXI of the Social Security Act, enacted in 1998, provided for the State Child Health Insurance Program (CHIP) to provide funds to ensure currently uninsured children. The Patient Protection and Affordable Care Act of 2010 will increase the number of people eligible for Medicaid by expanding eligibility to those with incomes up to 133% of the federal poverty level beginning in 2014 (Newhouse, 2010).

Three of the other laws created financial support for building health facilities, thereby improving access to health services for vulnerable groups. The Hill-Burton Act of 1946 provided financial support to build hospitals that would provide care to indigent people. The Community Mental Health Centers Act of 1963 funded construction of community mental health centers and training of mental health professionals who provided community-based care for the severely mentally ill individuals who were discharged from state mental hospitals. Finally, the Stewart B. McKinney Homeless Assistance Act of 1988 resulted in money for clinics and a wide variety of educational and social services for homeless individuals and families.

Three additional pieces of legislation—the National Health Planning and Resource Development Act of 1974, the Tax Equity and Fiscal Responsibility Act of 1982, and the Balanced Budget Act of 1997—influenced the use of resources for providing health services. The National Health Planning and Resources Development Act was intended to provide local mechanisms for planning which types of health services and facilities were really needed so that duplication of expensive facilities and services would be avoided. Part of the planning process included community health needs assessment, with the goal of providing balanced services so all would have access to the care they needed.

The Tax Equity and Fiscal Responsibility Act (TEFRA) of 1982 focused on the cost of health services but did so in a very different way. This act was designed to limit the rapid increase in health care costs, but it did not focus on community planning. Instead, TEFRA mandated that payment for hospital services for Medicare recipients would be based on a list of common medical diagnoses (diagnosis-related groups [DRGs]) with predetermined rates of payment for these diagnoses. If hospitals provided services that cost more than the amount indicated on the list, those hospitals lost money. This led to an increased emphasis on shorter hospital stays, more emphasis on identifying cost-effective treatments, and more emphasis on community-based care and care in the home. This was difficult for certain vulnerable groups, such as the homeless, who did not have the same level of resources and support to continue with the care necessary after discharge.

A similar shift in payment occurred with the stipulations related to home health in the Balanced Budget Act of 1997. In an attempt to curb the rapid growth in spending on home health and financial fraud in that industry, the Health Care Financing Administration (now the Centers for Medicare and Medicaid Services [CMS]) instituted prospective payment for home health services. The goal was to ensure that care was needed, rather than to limit access. Nurses and other health care providers work closely with families to determine the kinds of services needed to foster self-care, and the optimal timing of these services. The Balanced Budget Act of 1997 also reduced payments for services for Medicare beneficiaries, with the result that some providers no longer treat Medicare beneficiaries. This means that those whose health needs may be high (some chronically ill and older adult persons) may have limited access to care. The Patient Protection and Affordable Care Act of 2010 also includes provisions for reductions in the growth of future Medicare expenditures (Newhouse, 2010).

> **WHAT DO YOU THINK?** *Who should assume responsibility for providing health services to vulnerable populations? Providers sometimes close their practices to people on Medicaid or Medicare because providers feel they cannot afford to give care to people whose insurers reimburse at levels below what it costs to provide care. What role do you think nurse-managed centers and community health centers should provide in caring for vulnerable populations?*

Finally, one law focuses on the privacy and security of personal health information. The Health Insurance Portability and Accountability Act of 1996 was intended to help people keep their health insurance when moving from one place to another. Ensuring the privacy and security of personal health information means that electronic and paper health records, case management, referrals, and physical space layouts (such as computer screen visibility and clinic registration sheets) must be managed to protect the client's privacy and safeguard the privacy of personal health information. In certain cases, health information for public health uses may be shared with appropriate public health agencies, such as in cases of suspected abuse or when investigating a communicable disease outbreak. As electronic health networks become more widely used, some provisions of this law may need to be updated (Greenberg, Ridgely, and Hillestad, 2009).

FACTORS CONTRIBUTING TO VULNERABILITY

Vulnerability is multidimensional; that is, several factors contribute to vulnerability. Flaskerud and Winslow's (1998, 2010) framework says that resource limitations, poor health, and health risks are related to vulnerability. It is important to emphasize, however, that vulnerability is not simply a state of deficiency. Social conditions contribute heavily to vulnerability, and changing conditions such as poverty or non-financial barriers to health care access can influence elimination of disparities (Shi and Stevens, 2005b). Social determinants of health are factors such as economic status, education, environmental factors, nutrition, stress, and prejudice that lead to resource constraints, poor health, and health risk (Wilensky and Satcher, 2009). Nursing interventions focus on helping vulnerable populations acquire the resources needed for better health and reduction of risk factors.

Social Determinants of Health

Lack of adequate social, educational, and economic resources predisposes people to vulnerability and disparities in health outcomes. Economic status is strongly related to health (Adler and Newman, 2002; Shi and Stevens, 2005a,b). Poverty, a primary cause of vulnerability, is a growing problem in the United States (Shi and Stevens, 2005a). Poverty is a relative state. The federal definition of poverty is used to develop eligibility criteria for programs such as Medicaid and welfare assistance. In 2011 the federal poverty guideline for a family of four was $22,350 for all states except Hawaii and Alaska (Federal Register, January 20, 2011). However, many people who earn just a little more than the federal poverty guideline are ineligible for assistance programs yet are unable to manage their living expenses. Poverty causes vulnerability by making it more difficult for people to function in society and by limiting people's access to the resources for living a healthy life.

Poverty is a global problem. The gap between rich and poor countries as well as between social strata within developing countries in particular has grown (Shi and Stevens, 2005a,b). This depletes human potential worldwide and creates economic, political, and cultural instability, all of which influence health.

Persons who do not have the financial resources to pay for medical care are considered medically indigent. They may be self-employed or they may work in small businesses and be unable to afford health insurance. A total of 46.3 million people (15.4% of the population) were uninsured in 2008 (DeNavas-Walt, Proctor, and Smith, 2009).

Some people have inadequate health insurance coverage. This may be because their deductibles and co-payments are so high they have to pay for most expenses out of pocket, or because few conditions or services are covered. In these situations, poverty in its relative sense causes vulnerability because uninsured and underinsured people are less likely to seek preventive health services because of the expense and are more likely to suffer the consequences of preventable illnesses. The Patient Protection and Affordable Care Act of 2010 will create new ways to insure more of these individuals (Newhouse, 2010).

People who are poor are more likely to live in hazardous environments that are overcrowded and have inadequate sanitation, work in high-risk jobs, have less nutritious diets, and have multiple stressors, because they do not have the extra resources to manage unexpected crises and may not even have adequate resources to manage daily life. Poverty often reduces an individual's access to health care. In the developed countries of the world, this is more likely to be a problem for those just above the poverty line who are not eligible for public support, whereas in developing countries, poverty is correlated with decreased access to health care.

Poverty seems to be a key contributor to health disparities across racial groups. Poverty levels have decreased among African Americans living in urban and suburban areas, but are still far higher than the rates for whites (Andrulis, Duchon, and Reid, 2003). According to the 2006-2008 American Community Survey, 31.0% of African Americans were below 125% of the poverty level compared with 28.8% of persons of Hispanic or Latino origin, and 14.2% of whites (ACS, 2010). Female-headed households, and in particular those of African-American and Hispanic descent, are more likely to live in poverty than others. It may also be that race and economic status interact in some situations, and that relationships between race and economic status vary by health problem (IOM, 2003). Health provider attitudes about race and poverty may contribute to disparities in health services (IOM, 2003; Ford and Airhihenbuwa, 2010).

Poverty is more likely to affect women and children than other groups (Shi and Stevens, 2005b). These populations are already vulnerable to poor health outcomes, and adding the stressors associated with poverty increases the effect of vulnerability. Adolescent pregnancy is a key contributing factor to familial cycles of poverty. Adolescents who choose to keep and raise their infants are more likely to remain poor themselves. This may result in interrupted education for one or both of the parents, limited job opportunities, expenses associated with child rearing, and a long-term cycle of economic problems that affect both the parents and their children (Koniak-Griffin and Turner-Pluta, 2001). If the teenage mother is a single parent, the economic stresses may be even greater.

Education plays an important role in health status. Although education is related to income (Shi and Stevens, 2005a,b), educational level seems to influence health separately. Higher levels of education may provide people with more information for making healthy lifestyle choices. More highly educated people are better able to make informed choices about health insurance and providers. Education may also influence perceptions of stressors and problem situations and give people more alternatives. Finally, education and language skills affect health literacy. "Health literacy is a measure of patients' ability to read, comprehend and act on medical instructions" (Schillinger et al, 2002, p 475). People with low levels of general literacy are not likely to have the health literacy needed to improve health and use health services (Nutbeam, 2009).

Access to health care may be more limited for low socioeconomic groups. Barriers to access are policies and financial, geographic, or cultural features of health care that make services difficult to obtain or so unappealing that people do not wish to seek care. Examples include offering services only on weekdays without providing evening or weekend hours for working adults, being uninsured or underinsured, not having reasonably convenient or economical transportation, or providing services only in English and not in the population's primary language. Removing these barriers by providing extended clinic hours, low-cost or free health services for people who are uninsured or underinsured, transportation, mobile vans, and professional interpreters helps improve access to care (Shi and Stevens, 2005b).

Subconscious discrimination can result in an inadequate number of providers who are willing to treat certain racial groups and people with certain diagnoses, such as HIV, as well as the health services clinicians offer to individual clients (IOM, 2003; Ford and Airhihenbuwa, 2010). Discrimination against certain diagnoses can influence which conditions insurers are willing to reimburse. Other non-financial barriers include having inadequate providers in rural areas and certain sections in urban areas, and cultural barriers.

The interactions among multiple socioeconomic stressors make people more susceptible to risks than others with more financial resources, who may cope more effectively. In the following example, Tammy's situation illustrates how living environment and practical problems such as transportation, cost, and access problems interact to make people who are poor particularly vulnerable to health problems.

Tammy is a 22-year-old single mother of three children whose primary source of income is Aid to Families with Dependent Children. She is worried about the future because she will no longer be eligible for welfare by the end of the year. She has been unable to find a job that will pay enough for her to afford childcare. Her friend, Stephanie, said that Tammy and her children could stay in Stephanie's trailer for a short time, but Tammy is afraid that her only choice after that will be a shelter.

Tammy recently took all three children with her to the health department because 15-month-old Jason needed immunizations. She was also concerned about 5-year-old Angie, whose temperature had been 100° to 101°F sporadically for the past month. Tammy and her friends in the trailer park think that some type of hazardous waste from the chemical plant next door to the park is making their children sick. Now that Angie was not feeling well, her mother was concerned. However, the health department nurse told her that no appointments were available that day and that she would need to bring Angie back to the clinic on the next day. She left, feeling discouraged because it was so difficult for her to get all three children ready and on the bus to go to the health department, not to mention the expense. She thought maybe Angie just had a cold and she would wait a little longer before returning to the clinic. However, she wanted to take care of Angie's problem before losing her medical card. Tammy is desperate to find a way to manage her money problems and take care of her children.

Extreme poverty, in the form of homelessness or marginal housing, is related to risk for physical, dental, and mental health problems; food insecurity; and limited access to health care (Baggett et al, 2010). Those who are homeless or marginally housed have even fewer resources than poor people who have adequate housing. Homeless and marginally housed people must struggle with heavy demands as they try to manage daily life. These individuals and families do not have the advantage of consistent housing and must cope with finding a place to sleep at night and to stay during the day, or moving frequently from one residence to another, as well as finding food, before even thinking about health care. Lack of access to nutritious

EVIDENCE-BASED PRACTICE

This study sought to determine the perspectives of young homeless adults about facilitators and barriers to health care, and their opinions about how to improve health care for this population. The investigators conducted focus groups with 24 young adults between the ages of 18 and 25 years who used services from a local drop-in center. Participants were asked about health problems, how they went about seeking services, what was important to them in terms of receiving services, barriers they experienced, ways to better communicate information about health, and their suggestions for improvement. They reported having a number of chronic and acute health problems for which they sought care, including problems with substance abuse, mental health issues, and chronic and acute physical problems. Barriers to care included access to care, perceptions of discrimination, lack of social support, restrictive eligibility policies, and limited hours for care.

Nurse Use

Young adults who are homeless need access to health and social services that are provided in a non-judgmental and supportive manner. They also need services that are integrated to make it easier and more likely to get the care needed. The authors of this study noted that outreach and drop-in centers may be particularly well equipped to provide integrated health and social services that study participants said would be helpful.

From Hudson AL, Nyamathi A, Greengold B, et al: Health-seeking challenges among homeless youth, *Nurs Res* 59:212-218, 2010.

food on a regular basis poses serious health problems for people (Borre, Ertle, and Graff, 2010). Health problems of those who are homeless include victimization from crime or abuse, communicable diseases, substance abuse, severe mental illness, and exacerbations of chronic illnesses (IOM, 2000).

Health Status

Changes in normal physiological status predispose individuals to vulnerability. This may result from disease processes, such as in someone with one or more chronic diseases. For example, HIV infection is a pathophysiological situation that increases vulnerability to opportunistic infections such as *Mycobacterium avium* complex because of immunodeficiency. Chapter 14 describes HIV, hepatitis, and STDs in detail. Physiological alterations may also result from accidents, injuries, or congenital problems leading to mental or physiological disability. Older adults may exhibit vulnerability because of both age-related physiological changes and multiple chronic illnesses, resulting in limitations in functional status and loss of independence. Chapter 30 discusses elder health. Special needs individuals are another example of a vulnerable group, as discussed in Chapter 31.

Vulnerable groups may share certain physiological and developmental characteristics that predispose them to unique risks. Among these, age is probably the most central variable. It has long been known that persons at the extreme ends of the age continuum are less able physiologically to adapt to stressors. For example, very-low-birth-weight infants are at risk for various physiological and developmental problems (Rautava et al, 2010). Older adults are more likely to develop active infections from communicable diseases such as tuberculosis (TB), and they generally have greater likelihood of mortality and more difficulty recovering from infectious processes than younger people because of their less effective immune systems (Salvadó et al, 2010). Chapter 37 discusses substance abuse, and Chapters 13 and 14 describe communicable and infectious disease risk and prevention.

Certain individuals are vulnerable at particular ages because of the interaction between crucial developmental characteristics and socioeconomic tensions. For example, adolescent girls are more likely to deliver low-birth-weight infants than women ages 20 to 40 (March of Dimes, 2010), probably because of physiological variables, although socioeconomic conditions may play an equally important role (Koniak-Griffin and Turner-Pluta, 2001). As discussed in Chapter 35, an inability to afford prenatal care, a lack of awareness of the existence of or importance of prenatal care, and a tendency to seek such care later in pregnancy than older mothers also contribute to poor pregnancy outcomes of adolescents.

OUTCOMES OF VULNERABILITY

Outcomes of vulnerability may be negative, such as lower health status than the rest of the population, or they may be positive with effective interventions. For example, culturally competent, family- and community-focused nursing interventions may improve vulnerable populations' health status and provide such groups with the tools and resources to promote their own health.

Poor Health Outcomes and Health Disparities

Vulnerable populations have worse health outcomes than more advantaged populations in terms of morbidity and mortality. This means that they experience health disparities. Health disparities occur in the areas of access to care, quality of care and cultural and linguistic appropriateness of care, and health outcomes (IOM, 2003; USDHHS, 2001a). These groups have a high prevalence of chronic illnesses, such as hypertension, and high levels of communicable diseases, such as TB, hepatitis B virus (HBV), STDs, and upper respiratory tract illnesses, including influenza. They have high mortality rates from crime and violence, including domestic violence. Other types of health outcomes that deserve further study in vulnerable populations include functional status, overall perception of physical and emotional well-being, quality of life, and satisfaction with health services. Apparently some vulnerable groups wait longer to obtain appointments to see a clinician, and they perceive the communications with their clinicians as less than desirable (AHRQ, 2002). Nursing interventions should target strategies aimed at increasing resources or reducing health risks in order to reduce health disparities between vulnerable populations and populations with more advantages (Flaskerud and Nyamathi, 2002; Flaskerud and Winslow, 2010).

Poor health creates *stress* as individuals and families try to manage health problems with inadequate resources. For example, if someone with AIDS develops one or more opportunistic infections and is either uninsured or underinsured, that person and the family and caregivers will have more difficulty managing than if the individual had adequate insurance. Vulnerable populations cope with multiple stressors, and doing so creates a sort of "cascade effect," with chronic stress likely to result.

The factors that predispose people to vulnerability and the outcomes of vulnerability create a cycle of vulnerability in which the outcomes reinforce the predisposing factors, leading to more negative outcomes. Nurses identify areas where they can work with vulnerable populations to break the cycle. The nursing process guides nurses in assessing vulnerable individuals, families, groups, and communities; developing nursing diagnoses of their strengths and needs; planning and implementing appropriate therapeutic nursing interventions in partnership with the vulnerable clients; and evaluating the effectiveness of interventions.

NURSING APPROACHES TO CARE IN THE COMMUNITY

Core Functions of Public Health

The core functions of public health are assessment, policy, and surveillance (U.S. Public Health Service, 1994, updated 2000). These functions refer to actions initiated on behalf of a group or population, rather than with individuals. However, these functions parallel the stages of the nursing process. Assessment of groups is similar to assessment of individuals. Policy development and implementation can occur within organizations or at local, state, or national levels. Policies are population-level interventions, much like interventions targeted toward individuals. A major difference is that policies create conditions that affect many people, such as healthy workplaces, health-promoting community resources (e.g., bike paths, safe places for walking), and laws related to seat belts. Policy interventions may be interpreted more broadly to include developing programs and initiatives for populations, such as nurse home visiting programs for underserved and first-time mothers (Temple, Lutenbacher, and Vitale, 2008), school-based smoking cessation programs (Jarrett, Horn, and Zhang, 2009), support groups for caregivers of people with Alzheimer disease, health literacy programs for newly settled immigrants, and health education programs for school children. Another example is developing health-related public service announcements or other ways of providing health messages to large groups. Surveillance refers to evaluation and monitoring to ensure that policies and programs are implemented as intended, that unplanned changes are managed effectively, and that goals and objectives are met. Each of these three core functions is similar to those in the nursing process, with the key distinction being their emphasis on assessing, planning, implementing, and evaluating health services for groups and populations. Many activities in which nurses engage with and on behalf of vulnerable populations are based on these core functions and represent forms of social advocacy and promotion of social justice for these groups.

As discussed in Chapter 1, 10 services are identified as essential public health services that ensure that the core functions of public health are being carried out (U.S. Public Health Service, 1994, updated 2000). These services include monitoring community health status, identifying community health hazards, providing people with the education and tools to promote health and prevent illness and injury, mobilizing community partnerships to solve community health problems, developing policies and plans to solve community health problems, and evaluating community health services and outcomes. Nurses

---

🌐 LINKING CONTENT TO PRACTICE

Generalist and staff public health nurses should have competencies in eight domains as defined by the Quad Council of Public Health Nursing Organizations (2003). Each of the eight competencies is important in working with vulnerable populations. Public health nurses working with vulnerable populations should be able to analyze data and determine when a problem exists with an individual and within a vulnerable population group. They should be able to identify options for programs or policies that could be helpful to these populations and communicate their ideas and recommendations clearly. Public health nurses should be able to provide culturally competent interventions for individuals or for vulnerable populations. As an example, a public health nurse should be able to collect and analyze data related to the prevalence of violence among women in the community, identify key stakeholders, evaluate the cultural preferences of the population, work with others to develop a program to meet a defined need within this population including preparation of a basic budget for the program, and ensure that the program is culturally appropriate for the population. The Council on Linkages Between Academia and Public Health Practice (2010) published a similar list for public health professionals including but not limited to public health nurses. This list includes an emphasis on evaluation and ongoing improvement of programs. In the current example, the public health nurse would evaluate the program developed for women who are victims of violence and work with others to develop and implement quality improvements on a regular basis.

BOX 32-3   GUIDELINES FOR ASSESSING MEMBERS OF VULNERABLE POPULATION GROUPS

Setting the Stage

- Create a comfortable, non-threatening environment.
- Learn as much as you can about the culture of the clients you work with so that you will understand cultural practices and values that may influence their health care practices.
- Provide culturally and linguistically competent assessment by understanding the meaning of language and non-verbal behavior in the client's culture.
- Be sensitive to the fact that the individual or family you are assessing may have other priorities that are more important to them. These might include financial, housing, or legal problems. You may need to give them some tangible help with their most pressing problem before you will be able to address issues that are more traditionally thought of as health concerns.
- Collaborate with others as appropriate; you should not provide financial or legal advice. However, you should make sure to connect your client with someone who can and will help them.

Nursing History of an Individual or Family

- You may have only one opportunity to work with a vulnerable person or family. Try to complete a history that will provide all the essential information you need to help the individual or family on that day. This means that you will have to organize in your mind exactly what you need to ask, and no more, and why the data are necessary.
- It will help to use a comprehensive assessment form that has been modified to focus on the special needs of the vulnerable population group with whom you work. However, be flexible. With some clients, it will be both impractical and unethical to cover all questions on a comprehensive form. If you know that you are likely to see the client again, ask the less pressing questions at the next visit.

- Be sure to include questions about social support, economic status, resources for health care, developmental issues, current health problems, medications, and how the person or family manages their health status. Your goal is to obtain information that will enable you to provide family-centered care.
- Does the individual have any condition that compromises his or her immune status, such as AIDS, or is the individual undergoing therapy that would result in immunodeficiency, such as cancer chemotherapy?

Physical Examination or Home Assessment

- Again, complete as thorough a physical examination (on an individual) or home assessment as you can. Keep in mind that you should collect only the data for which you have a use.
- Be alert for indications of physical abuse, substance use (e.g., needle marks, nasal abnormalities, presence of drug paraphernalia, or materials for producing methamphetamine), or neglect (e.g., being underweight or inadequately clothed).
- You can assess a family's living environment using good observational skills. Does the family live in an insect- or rat-infested environment? Do they have running water, functioning plumbing, electricity, adequate heat and air conditioning, and a telephone?
- Is perishable food (e.g., mayonnaise) left sitting out on tables and countertops? Are bed linens reasonably clean? Is paint peeling on the walls and ceilings? Is ventilation adequate? Is the temperature of the home adequate? Is the family exposed to raw sewage or animal waste? Is the home adjacent to a busy highway, possibly exposing the family to high noise levels and automobile exhaust?

design their population-level assessment, policy, and surveillance strategies to eliminate health disparities of vulnerable population groups in the 10 essential services of public health.

ASSESSMENT ISSUES

Box 32-3 lists guidelines for assessing members of vulnerable population groups, whether individuals, families, or larger groups. The following discussion expands on the points listed in that box.

Nursing Conceptual Approaches

Nursing assessment of vulnerable populations may be organized around any nursing conceptual framework that takes into account the multiple stressors experienced by these groups and the particular difficulties they have managing their health. The approaches of Neuman (Fawcett, 2001), Roy (Fawcett, 2002), and Orem (Denyes et al, 2001) are particularly appropriate to use with vulnerable populations. Neuman's focus on identifying stressors and lines of resistance is a useful framework for organizing a nursing assessment, because vulnerable populations experience multiple, overlapping stressors. Roy's emphasis on health-promoting modes of adaptation helps the nurse emphasize client strengths that are resources for coping with stressors. Orem's self-care approach directs the nurse to assess the client's self-care needs and abilities so that therapeutic nursing interventions can target self-care deficits.

Because members of vulnerable populations often experience multiple stressors, nursing assessment must balance the need to be comprehensive with the ability to focus only on information that the nurse requires and that the client is willing to provide. The discussion that follows focuses on assessment of individual clients and families and on assessment of entire vulnerable population groups. With individuals and families, assessment can be intrusive and tiring, so it is important that the nurse have a reason to obtain the data before asking the client. This means that assessing becomes an *iterative assessment process,* involving progressively more depth as the nurse refines hypotheses about the nursing diagnosis.

Socioeconomic Considerations

Assessment should include questions about the clients' perceptions of socioeconomic resources, including identifying people who can provide support and financial resources. Support from other people may include information, caregiving, emotional support, and help with activities of daily living, such as transportation, shopping, and babysitting. Financial resources may include the extent to which the client can pay for health services and medications, as well as questions about eligibility for third-party payment. Be sure to assess the extent to which individuals, families, groups, and populations can afford basic necessities such as food, safe housing, clean water, and reliable transportation. Ask the client about the perceived adequacy of both formal and informal support networks.

Physical Health Issues

Often, nurses see individual clients in a clinic. These clients may be concerned about specific problems, which should be the initial priority. However, because vulnerable populations often find it difficult to seek routine health promotion and illness prevention services, nurses should take the opportunity to explain to clients the value of preventive assessment. If clients agree, nursing assessment should include evaluation of clients' preventive health needs, including age-appropriate screening tests, such as immunization status, blood pressure, weight, serum cholesterol, Papanicolaou smears, breast examinations, mammograms, prostate examinations, glaucoma screening, and dental evaluations. It may be necessary to make referrals to have some of these tests done for clients. Assessment should also include preventive screening for physical health problems for which certain vulnerable groups are at a particularly high risk. For example, persons with AIDS should be evaluated regularly for presence of common opportunistic infections, including TB and pneumonia. Individuals who use illegal intravenous drugs should be evaluated for HBV, including liver palpation and serum antigen tests as necessary. Those with addictions to alcohol or hepatotoxic drugs should be asked about symptoms of liver disease and evaluated for jaundice and liver enlargement. Individuals with a severe mental health problem should be assessed for the presence of tardive dyskinesia, indicating possible toxicity from antipsychotic medications. General screening may be done as part of health fairs provided at places where people live (e.g., neighborhoods, community centers, shelters), work (occupational settings, including non-office settings such as farms, truck stops, and racetracks), pray (faith communities), or play (recreational settings).

Biological Issues

Vulnerable populations should be assessed for congenital and genetic predisposition to illness and either receive education and counseling as appropriate or be referred to other health professionals as necessary. For example, pregnant adolescents who are substance abusers should be referred to programs to help them quit using addictive substances during their pregnancies and ideally after delivery of their infants as well. Pregnant women older than age 35 should be informed about amniocentesis testing to determine if genetic abnormalities exist in the fetus. Specialized counseling about treatment and anticipatory guidance regarding the infant's needs can be provided by an advanced practice nurse or a physician.

Psychological Issues

Vulnerable family groups should be assessed for stress and the presence of healthy or dysfunctional family dynamics. Also evaluate them for effective communication patterns, caregiving capabilities, and the extent to which family developmental tasks are being met. Assess individuals for the presence of stressors, usual coping styles, levels of self-efficacy (or the belief that one is capable of meeting life's challenges), overall sense of well-being and level of self-esteem, and the presence of depression and anxiety (Shi and Stevens, 2005b). Assess vulnerable individuals and families for risks of or exposure to violence and abuse. Likewise, groups (such as a school population) should be evaluated for the presence of or potential for violence.

Lifestyle Issues

Nurses should assess lifestyle factors of vulnerable individuals, families, and groups that may predispose them to further health problems. Lifestyle factors include diet, exercise, rest, and the use of drugs, alcohol, and caffeine. For example, many homeless individuals eat their meals either at shelters or at fast-food restaurants. Because of the unpredictability of meals and food availability, it is often difficult for them to eat a diet that is low in fat, cholesterol, and sodium, and it is particularly difficult to eat the recommended five servings of fruits and vegetables per day. Assess these populations for food insecurity and the effects on health. Cultural preferences may also influence lifestyle and health risk behaviors.

Environmental Issues

Vulnerable groups are more likely to be exposed to environmental hazards such as pollutants or carcinogens than other groups. Nurses should assess the living environment and neighborhood surroundings of vulnerable families and groups for environmental hazards such as lead-based paint, asbestos, water and air quality, industrial wastes, and the incidence of crime. Nurses must often establish partnerships with vulnerable groups to put changes into place, such as persuading a local industry to reduce the levels of effluents from their plants or working with local government and law enforcement to develop crime prevention programs.

PLANNING AND IMPLEMENTING CARE FOR VULNERABLE POPULATIONS

In some situations, the nurse works with individual clients. In other cases, the nurse develops programs and policies for populations of vulnerable persons. In either case, planning and implementing care for members of vulnerable populations involve partnership between nurse and client. Nurses who direct and control the client's care cannot establish a trusting relationship and may inadvertently foster a cycle of dependency and lack of personal health control. In fact, the most important initial step is for nurses to establish that they are trustworthy and dependable. For example, nurses who work in a community clinic for people with substance use problems must overcome any suspicion that clients may have of them and eliminate any fears that they will manipulate them with "games."

Roles of the Nurse

Nurses working with vulnerable populations may fill numerous roles, including those listed in Box 32-4. These roles include the following:

- Identifying vulnerable individuals and families through outreach and case finding
- Encouraging vulnerable groups to obtain health services
- Developing programs that respond to their needs
- Teaching vulnerable individuals, families, and groups strategies to prevent illness and promote health

BOX 32-4 NURSING ROLES WHEN WORKING WITH VULNERABLE POPULATION GROUPS

- Case finder
- Health educator
- Counselor
- Direct care provider
- Population health advocate
- Community assessor and developer
- Monitor and evaluator of care
- Case manager
- Advocate
- Health program planner
- Participant in developing health policies

- Counseling clients about ways to increase their sense of personal power and help them identify strengths and resources
- Providing direct care to clients and families in a variety of settings, including storefront clinics, mobile clinics, shelters, homes, neighborhoods, worksites, churches, and schools

For example, a nurse in a mobile clinic for migrant farmworkers might administer a tetanus booster to a client who has been injured by a piece of farm machinery and may also check that client's blood pressure and cholesterol level during the same visit. A home-health nurse seeing a family referred by the courts for child abuse may weigh the child, conduct a nutritional assessment, and help the family learn how to manage anger and disciplinary problems. A nurse working in a school-based clinic may lead a support group for pregnant adolescents and conduct a birthing class. Nurses working with people being treated for TB monitor drug treatment compliance to ensure that they complete their full course of therapy. Nurses serve as population health advocates and work with local, state, or national groups to develop and implement healthy public policy. They also collaborate with other community members and serve as community assessors and developers, and they monitor and evaluate care and health programs. *Healthy People in Healthy*

LINKING CONTENT TO PRACTICE

This chapter focuses on vulnerability and vulnerable populations. Public health nurses have long been concerned with vulnerable populations, from the days of Lillian Wald to the present time. Nursing theories and social justice theories support the practice of public health nurses using the core functions and essential services of public health in designing programs and services for members of these populations. Public health nurses use their knowledge of epidemiology, risk factors, and the social determinants of health to understand which populations in their communities might be most vulnerable to poor health. They identify factors that predispose populations to vulnerability and develop interventions to reduce these factors. Public health nurses work closely with other members of interprofessional teams and community members in coalitions, neighborhoods, and interest groups to advocate for, and assist people who are vulnerable to poor health. The goal is to create environmental conditions that reduce the risks of vulnerability and to empower people through health education and sufficient resources to live healthy lifestyles.

Communities describes one approach for working collaboratively with communities to develop healthy communities and eliminate health disparities (USDHHS, 2001b). Nurses often function as case managers for vulnerable clients, making referrals and linking them with community services, and they serve as advocates. The nurse functions as an advocate when referring clients to other agencies, working with others to develop health programs, and influencing legislation and health policies that affect vulnerable populations.

THE CUTTING EDGE *Nurse-managed centers provide care for vulnerable populations. These centers often care for large numbers of uninsured and underinsured persons and focus on community health promotion. The Patient Protection and Affordable Care Act of 2010 included funding for nurse-managed centers because they provide innovative forms of care to meet the special needs of vulnerable populations.*

The nature of nurses' roles varies depending on whether the client is a single person, a family, or a group. For example, a nurse might teach an HIV-positive client about the need for prevention of opportunistic infections, or may help a family with a member who is HIV-positive to understand myths about transmission of HIV, or may work with a community group concerned about HIV transmission among students in the schools. In each case, the nurse teaches how to prevent infectious and communicable diseases, and the size of the group and the teaching method are different.

Client Empowerment and Health Education

Nurses should help all vulnerable groups achieve a greater sense of personal empowerment through effective health education and helping them access necessary resources. Nurses empower clients by helping them acquire the skills needed for healthy living and for being effective health care consumers. Health education is one key to working with vulnerable populations. As discussed in Chapter 16, nurses need to determine if the populations with whom they work have adequate health literacy to benefit from health education.

Foster empowerment by providing culturally and linguistically appropriate health-promoting strategies (IOM, 2002, 2003). The use of professional interpreters or clinicians who are fluent in the clients' language helps ensure language concordance with clients (IOM, 2003). This means that the language used by the person providing health information is the same as that of the client hearing the information.

Levels of Prevention

Healthy People 2020 (USDHHS, 2010) objectives emphasize health promotion and illness prevention. One way to do this is for vulnerable individuals to have a primary care provider who both coordinates health services for them and provides their preventive services. This primary care provider may be an advanced practice nurse or a primary care physician (e.g., a family practice physician). Another approach is for a nurse to serve as a case manager for vulnerable clients and, again, coordinate services and provide illness prevention and health promotion services.

One example of primary prevention is to give influenza vaccinations to vulnerable populations who are immunocompromised (unless contraindicated). Secondary prevention is seen in conducting screening clinics for vulnerable populations. For example, nurses who conduct blood pressure screening as part of health fairs are engaging in secondary prevention. Tertiary prevention is conducting a therapy group with the residents of a group home for people with severe mental illnesses. Nurses who work with abused women to help them enhance their levels of self-esteem are also providing tertiary preventive activities.

LEVELS OF PREVENTION

Vulnerable Populations

Primary Prevention
- Provide health teaching about balanced diet and exercise. Help clients identify how to maintain a healthy diet and exercise plan in low-cost ways.
- Give influenza shots to people who are immunocompromised or who live in high-risk environments, such as in shelters or in the streets. Follow annual CDC guidelines for the populations that should receive the vaccination.

Secondary Prevention
- Conduct screening clinics to assess for such problems as hypertension.
- Develop a portable immunization chart, such as a wallet card, that mobile population groups such as the homeless and migrant workers can carry with them.
- Develop healthy nutrition and exercise programs for those who are overweight.

Tertiary Prevention
- Work with a local coalition to reduce levels of drug abuse in the community.
- Participate with an interprofessional team providing health care in a geographic area affected by a disaster, such as a weather-related disaster.

Strategies for Promoting Healthy Lifestyles

Helping vulnerable persons develop healthy lifestyle behaviors requires great sensitivity by nurses. They should focus on identifying clients' priorities and helping them meet these priorities. For example, discussing exercise with a homeless person requires empathy and creativity. Often, vulnerable individuals and families are coping with crises, so the nurse must begin by using crisis intervention strategies. After the crisis has been managed, a trusting relationship is likely to exist between the nurse and client. This relationship forms the basis for health promotion interventions. Nurses must be sensitive to the lifestyles of their vulnerable clients and must develop methods of health promotion that recognize these lifestyle factors. *Healthy People 2020* objectives and *Healthy People in Healthy Communities* are useful guidelines.

Healthy People in Healthy Communities (USDHHS, 2001a) provides suggestions for community-wide strategies to develop and maintain healthier communities. These strategies use the MAP-IT approach, in which the focus is on building coalitions and improving community health through a wide range of community partnerships. Partnerships can include health professionals, business people, educators, politicians, and local

TABLE 32-1 TYPES OF CLINICS THAT SERVE VULNERABLE POPULATIONS AND FUNDING SOURCES

TYPES OF CLINIC	FUNDING SOURCES
Community health centers	Bureau of Primary Health Care
Migrant health clinics	Bureau of Primary Health Care
Health care for the homeless clinics	Bureau of Primary Health Care
Nurse-managed centers	Variety of types of funding, including grants, insurance, sliding scales
Mobile clinics	Variety of types of funding, including grants, insurance, sliding scales
Storefront clinics	Variety of types of funding, including grants, insurance, sliding scales
Neighborhood clinics	Variety of types of funding, including grants, insurance, sliding scales
School clinics	Bureau of Primary Health Care

community leaders, to name a few. MAP-IT is an acronym for *m*obilizing community resources, *a*ssessing, *p*lanning, *i*mplementing, and *t*racking results. Community partnerships can be helpful to nurses who wish to intervene at the population level to improve the socioeconomic environment in which vulnerable populations live (USDHHS, 2001a).

Comprehensive Services

In general, more agencies are needed that provide comprehensive services with non-restrictive eligibility requirements. For example, the Boston Health Care for the Homeless Program (O'Connell et al, 2010) found that it was effective to have an interprofessional team take care directly to people who are homeless in non-traditional settings. Communities often have many agencies that restrict eligibility for their services to people most likely to benefit from those services, or they limit eligibility to make it possible for more people to receive services. For example, shelters may prohibit people who have been drinking alcohol from staying overnight and sometimes limit the number of sequential nights a person can stay. Food banks may limit the number of times a person can receive free food. Agencies are frequently specialized as well. For vulnerable individuals and families, this means that they must go to many agencies to find services for which they qualify and that meet their needs. Examples of clinics that provide comprehensive services are community health centers, nurse-managed centers, school-based health centers, and migrant clinics. Other examples are listed in Table 32-1.

Resources for Vulnerable Populations

Nurses should know about community agencies that offer health and social services for vulnerable populations. They should also follow up with the client after the referral to ensure that the desired outcomes were achieved. Sometimes, excellent community resources are available but impractical for clients because of transportation or reimbursement problems. Nurses should identify those problems that will interfere with clients following through with referrals, and they should work with other team members to make referrals as convenient and realistic as possible. Although clients with social problems such as financial needs should be referred to social workers, nurses should understand the close connections between health and social problems and know how to work effectively with other professionals. A list of community resources can often be found in the telephone book, and many communities have publications that list them. Examples of agency resources found in most communities are as follows:

- Health departments
- Community mental health centers and community health centers
- American Red Cross and other voluntary organizations
- Food and clothing banks
- Missions and shelters
- Nurse-managed clinics
- Social service agencies such as Travelers' Aid and Salvation Army
- Church-sponsored health and social service assistance

Two other important categories of resources for vulnerable populations are their own personal coping skills and social supports (Aday, 2001). These groups must often be quite resourceful and creative to manage in the face of multiple stressors. Nurses should work with clients to help them identify their own personal strengths and draw on those strengths when managing their health needs.

Case Management

Case management involves linking clients with services and providing direct nursing services to clients, such as teaching, counseling, screening, and immunizing (Zander, 2002). Lillian Wald was the first nurse case manager. She linked vulnerable families with a variety of services to help them stay healthy (Buhler-Wilkerson, 1993). Linking, or brokering health services, is accomplished by making appropriate referrals and by following up with clients to ensure that the desired outcomes from the referral were achieved. Nurses are effective case managers in community nursing clinics, health departments, and case management programs where the focus includes both community and hospital care. Nurse case managers emphasize health promotion and illness prevention with vulnerable clients and focus on helping them avoid unnecessary hospitalization. Figure 32-1 illustrates the coordination and brokering aspect of the nurse's role as case manager for vulnerable populations.

HOW TO **Coordinate Health and Social Services for Members of Vulnerable Populations**

Nurses who work with vulnerable populations often need to coordinate services across multiple agencies for members of these groups. It is helpful to have a strong professional network of people who work in other agencies. Effective professional networks make it easier to coordinate care smoothly and in ways that do not add to clients' stress. Nurses can develop strong networks by participating in community coalitions and attending professional meetings. When making referrals to other agencies, a phone call can be a

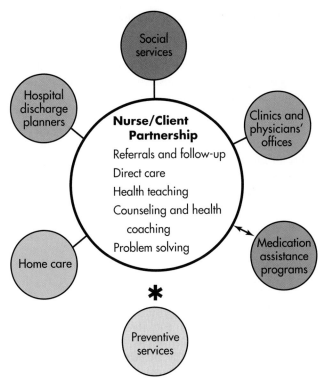

FIGURE 32-1 The nurse as case manager for vulnerable populations.

helpful way to obtain information that the client will need for the visit. When possible, have an interprofessional, interagency team plan care for clients at high risk for health problems. It is crucial to obtain the clients' written and informed consent before engaging in this kind of planning because of confidentiality issues. The following list of tips can be helpful:

- *Involve clients in making decisions about the kinds of services they will find useful.*
- *Work with community coalitions to develop plans for service coordination for targeted vulnerable populations.*
- *Collaborate with legal counsel from the agencies involved in the coalitions to ensure that legal and ethical issues related to care coordination have been properly addressed. You might include privacy and security of clinical data and ensuring compliance with the Health Insurance Portability and Accountability Act (HIPAA), contractual provisions for coordinating care across agencies, and consent for treatment from multiple agencies.*
- *Develop policies and protocols for making referrals, following up on referrals, and ensuring that clients receive coordinated care.*

EVALUATION OF NURSING INTERVENTIONS WITH VULNERABLE POPULATIONS

Evaluation of therapeutic nursing interventions begins with client goals and objectives and focuses on the extent to which client health outcomes are achieved, whether clients are individuals, families, groups, or populations. Nurses may evaluate individual client goal achievement, the extent to which a vulnerable family achieved goals developed in partnership with the nurse, or the extent to which a nursing program achieved its objectives for a particular population. Evaluation takes place while providing care and gives the nurse a basis for revising therapeutic interventions to make them more effective. Evaluation also takes place when a case is closed or when a program is completed, and then it gives nurses data to use in providing care to similar clients or programs in the future. The types of client outcomes that may be evaluated include improved quality of life, improved indicators of physical health status (e.g., blood pressure, skin integrity, mobility), reduced depression or anxiety, improved functional status, increased levels of knowledge about health behaviors, and satisfaction with care. Nurses use a variety of scales to evaluate these outcome indicators; they sometimes interview clients or administer short questionnaires; and they use laboratory reports and results of health assessments to help evaluate goal achievement with individuals and clients. Incidence and prevalence data, survey data, and service utilization data are used to evaluate health programs for vulnerable populations.

CHAPTER REVIEW

PRACTICE APPLICATION

Assume that you are a nurse working in a free health clinic for farmworkers from the local migrant community. Doris, a 46-year-old woman pregnant with her third child, comes to the clinic and requests treatment for swollen ankles. During your assessment, you learn that she was seen by the nurse practitioner (NP) at the local health department 2 months ago. The NP gave her some sample vitamins, but Doris lost them because she has moved twice since that time. She has not received regular prenatal care and has no plans to do so because she does not have a green card and is worried that she will be deported. Her previous pregnancies were essentially normal, although she said she was "toxic" with her second child. Doris is 5 feet 4 inches tall, weighs 190 pounds, and has a blood pressure of 160/90 mm Hg with pitting edema of the ankles and a mild headache. She shares with you that she used to have "spells" and occasionally took medication for her nerves.

You are aware that the client's situation, although acute, is not unusual in your community. The migrant farmworker population has grown in recent years and some of the families are beginning to accompany the primary wage earner in the household and settle in the community. Not all local residents are comfortable with this because they say that taxpayer money is being used to provide services for people who are not legal residents and who do not pay taxes. Complicating the debate is that some residents are legal immigrants and some are not. The situation is becoming tense and a few vocal community members have begun a drive to put forth a referendum addressing the issue. The nurses in your clinic have debated whether you should become involved in these local discussions and help raise community awareness of the health and social needs of the migrant farmworker population. Each of you understands that the immigration issues are complex and you respect local concerns, but you are also eager to be part of the solution.

Where should you and your colleagues begin to address the problems experienced by the migrant farmworker population (both legal immigrants and illegal aliens) and the local community's concerns?

A. Make a list of the issues and present it to the local city council.
B. Help develop the language for the referendum.
C. Mount vigorous opposition to the local group that is considering a referendum on the issues.
D. Gather data to describe the extent of the issues by meeting with local concerned citizens, migrant farmworkers, politicians and policy makers, and health care providers.

Answers can be found on the Evolve site.

KEY POINTS

- Vulnerable populations are more likely to develop health problems as a result of exposure to risk or to have worse outcomes from those health problems than the rest of the population. Vulnerable populations are more sensitive to risk factors than those who are more resilient and are more often exposed to cumulative risk factors. These populations include poor or homeless persons, pregnant adolescents, migrant workers, severely mentally ill individuals, substance abusers, abused individuals, persons with communicable diseases, and persons with sexually transmitted diseases, including HIV and HBV.
- All countries have special population groups that are more vulnerable to poor health than others. The identities of the groups vary across countries, depending on local political, economic, cultural, and demographic characteristics.
- Health care is increasingly moving into the community. This began with deinstitutionalization of the severely mentally ill population and is continuing today as hospitals reduce inpatient stays. Vulnerable populations need a wide variety of services, and because these are often provided by multiple community agencies, nurses coordinate and manage the service needs of vulnerable groups.
- Public policies sometimes provide financial assistance for vulnerable populations and sometimes provide money to build health facilities and train professionals to work with vulnerable groups. Unanticipated implementation problems often further disadvantage vulnerable populations. Health care reform in the United States is focusing heavily on community-based health promotion and illness prevention.
- Socioeconomic problems, including poverty and social isolation, physiological and developmental aspects of age, poor health status, and highly stressful life experiences, predispose people to vulnerability. Vulnerability can become a cycle, where the predisposing factors lead to poor health outcomes and chronic stress, and these outcomes in turn increase vulnerability.

KEY POINTS—cont'd

- Nurses assess vulnerable individuals, families, and groups to determine which socioeconomic, physical, biological, psychological, and environmental factors are problems for clients. They work as partners with vulnerable clients to identify client strengths and needs and develop intervention strategies designed to break the cycle of vulnerability.
- Nursing roles seen when working with vulnerable populations in the community include health teacher, counselor, direct care provider, case manager, advocate, health program planner, and participant in developing health policies. Nurses focus on empowering clients to prevent illness and promote health, and they work to achieve the *Healthy People 2020* national health objectives with vulnerable populations. Nurses link clients with resources in the community and monitor client outcomes to ensure that community referrals are effective.
- Evaluation of therapeutic nursing interventions with vulnerable populations occurs both during and after service delivery. Results of evaluations are used to make revisions in nursing care, with the ultimate goal of improving client outcomes.

CLINICAL DECISION-MAKING ACTIVITIES

1. Vulnerability implies that certain populations have both a higher relative risk for illness because of the presence of multiple risk factors and a greater sensitivity to the effects of individual risk factors. Identify populations in your community that you think are more vulnerable to poor health than others. List the risk factors members of these populations are more likely to have, and identify the prevalence of these risk factors in your community. Discuss with your classmates or a nurse in a clinical agency the effect you believe these risk factors are having on the health of vulnerable populations in your community. Analyze whether members of these populations seem to be more sensitive to the effect of the risk factors than the population as a whole. What are some of the complexities related to these issues?

2. Examine health statistics and demographic data in your geographic area to determine which vulnerable groups predominate in your area. Look through your phone book for examples of agencies that you think provide services to these vulnerable groups. Make appointments with key individuals in several of these agencies to discuss the nature of their target population, the types of services provided, and the reimbursement mechanisms for these services. Various class members should visit different agencies and then share their results during class. On the basis of your findings, identify gaps or overlaps in services provided to vulnerable groups in your community. Try to be specific and delineate the political and economic reasons for the gaps and overlaps. What might be some ways to manage these gaps and overlaps to help clients receive the services they need?

3. Debate with your class the nature and extent of services that you believe should be made available to the homeless. How do you think these services might be funded? What research evidence have you used in constructing your arguments?

4. To what extent do you think economic issues and social values play a role in the way that health services are offered to vulnerable population groups? Explain why you think the population as a whole should or should not pay for care for vulnerable groups. Base your argument on the concept of social justice. The book "Vulnerable Populations in the United States" by Shi and Stevens (2005b) will help you consider these issues in more depth.

5. Discuss the types of assistance you might provide to the following clients:
   A. A 33-year-old pregnant woman with developmental disabilities who is frequently homeless and her boyfriend who is currently unemployed
   B. A 14-year-old girl who has run away from her foster home and who is earning money through prostitution and has a drug habit
   C. A 22-year-old woman with four children who is receiving welfare and whose boyfriend uses methamphetamine
   D. A woman with AIDS who has three children, no other family, and few friends
   E. A 56-year-old male who is a migrant farmworker whose TB skin test just came back positive

What kinds of nursing needs do these clients have in common? What types of risks might you assess? In what ways would you choose to function as an advocate for the vulnerable populations represented by these individuals?

6. Examine the pros and cons of school-based reproductive care for adolescents. What does the research literature say about the optimal ways to provide such care? What are the ethical issues involved in providing reproductive information to adolescents, with or without parental consent? Check state and federal legal requirements related to privacy and confidentiality of personal health information in these situations. How would nurses be expected to balance confidentiality concerns of teens in school-based clinics, with parental interest in their children's health information?

7. Interview nurses at a health department to identify which personal care services they provide to vulnerable populations and which population-based services they provide. Discuss their opinions about whether personal care services should be provided only by private agencies. Analyze this issue from the perspectives of the core functions of public health, access to care for vulnerable populations, and cost-effectiveness of care provided by public health departments as compared with private agencies. Include research support for your arguments.

8. Read and analyze the Quad Council's Public Health Nursing Competencies (2003) and determine which of the Generalist/Staff PHN competencies you possess and which you wish to more fully develop. Design a learning plan for yourself that will help you gain the competencies with which you do not currently feel comfortable, and identify how you would use these in providing care to vulnerable populations.

REFERENCES

Adashi EY, Geiger HJ, Fine MD: Health care reform and primary care—the growing importance of the community health center, *N Engl J Med* 362:2047–2050, 2010: doi:10.1056/nejmp1003729.

Aday LA: *At risk in America: the health and health care needs of vulnerable populations in the United States*, ed 2, San Francisco, 2001, Jossey-Bass.

Adler NE, Newman K: Socioeconomic disparities in health: pathways and policies, *Health Aff* 21:60–76, 2002.

Agency for Healthcare Research and Quality: *Statistical brief #3: children's health care quality, fall 2000*, Rockville, MD, 2002. Available at http://www.meps.ahrq.gov/papers/st3/stat03.htm. Accessed November 10, 2005.

American Community Survey: *United States, selected characteristics of people at specified levels of poverty in the past 12 months, 2006-2008, American Community Survey 3-year estimates*, 2010. Available at http://factfinder.census.gov/servlet/STTable?_bm=y&-qr_name=ACS_2008_3YR_G00_S1703&-geo_id=01000US&-ds_name=ACS_2008_3YR_G00_&-lang=en&-format=&-CONTEXT=st. Accessed August 8, 2010.

Andrulis DP, Duchon LM, Reid HM: *Dynamics of race, culture and key indicators of health in the nation's 100 largest cities and their suburbs, The Social and Health Landscape of Urban and Suburban America Series*, Brooklyn, NY, 2003, SUNY Downstate Medical Center.

Baggett TP, O'Connell JJ, Singer DE, Rigotti NA: The unmet health care needs of homeless adults: a national study, *Am J Public Health* 100:1326–1333, 2010. doi:10.2105/AJPH.2009.180109.

Borre K, Ertle L, Graff M: Working to eat: vulnerability, food insecurity, and obesity among migrant and seasonal farmworker families, *Am J Ind Med* 53:443–462, 2010. doi:10.1002/ajim.20836.

Boutain DM: Social justice in nursing: a review of the literature. In de Chesnay M, Anderson A: *Caring for the vulnerable: perspectives in nursing theory, practice, and research*, ed 2, Sudbury, MA, 2008, Jones and Bartlett.

Buhler-Wilkerson K: Bringing care to the people: Lillian Wald's legacy to public health nursing, *Am J Public Health* 83:1778–1786, 1993.

Council on Linkages Between Academia and Public Health Practice: *Tier 1, tier 2, and tier 3 core competencies for public health professionals*, 2010. Available at http://www.phf.org/link/index.htm. Accessed May 3, 2010.

DeNavas-Walt C, Proctor BD, Smith JC: U.S. Census Bureau, Current Population Reports, P60-236, *Income, poverty, and health insurance coverage in the United States: 2008*, Washington, DC, 2009, U.S. Government Printing Office.

Denyes MJ, et al: Self-care: a foundational science, *Nurs Sci Quart* 14:48–54, 2001.

Fawcett J: The nurse theorists: 21st century updates—Betty Neuman, interview by Jacqueline Fawcett, *Nurs Sci Quart* 14:211–214, 2001.

Fawcett J: The nurse theorists: 21st century updates—Sister Callista Roy, interview by Jacqueline Fawcett, *Nurs Sci Quart* 15:308–310, 2002.

Federal Register: The 2011 HHS poverty guidelines, vol 76, No. 13:3637–3638, January 20, 2011.

Flaskerud JH, Winslow BW: Conceptualizing vulnerable populations health-related research, *Nurs Res* 47:69–78, 1998.

Flaskerud JH, Nyamathi AM: New paradigm for health disparities needed, *Nurs Res* 51:139, 2002.

Flaskerud JH, Winslow BW: Vulnerable populations and ultimate responsibility, *Issues Ment Health Nurs* 31:298–299, 2010. doi:10.3109/01612840903308556.

Ford CL, Airhihenbuwa CO: Critical race theory, race equity, and public health: toward antiracism praxis, *Am J Public Health* 100:S30–S35, 2010. doi:10.2105/AJPH.2009.171058.

Friss RH: *Epidemiology 101 (essential public health)*, Sudbury, MA, 2010, Jones and Bartlett.

Gilmer T, Kronick R, Rice T: Children welcome, adults need not apply: changes in public program enrollment across states and over time, *Med Care Res Rev* 62:56–78, 2005.

Greenberg MD, Ridgely MS, Hillestad RJ: Crossed wires: How yesterday's privacy rules might undercut tomorrow's nationwide health information network, *Health Aff* 28:450–452, 2009. doi:10.1377/hlthaff.28.2.450.

Hansen-Turton T: The nurse-managed health center safety net: a policy solution to reducing health disparities, *Nurs Clin North Am* 40:729–738, 2005.

Hegevary ST, Berry DM, Murua A: Clustering countries to evaluate health outcomes globally, *J Public Health Pol* 29:319–339, 2008. doi:10.1057/jphp.2008.13.

Hudson AL, Nyamathi A, Greengold B, et al: Health-seeking challenges among homeless youth, *Nurs Res* 59:212–218, 2010. doi:10.1097/NNR.0b013e3181d1a8a9.

Institute of Medicine (IOM): *America's healthcare safety net*, Washington, DC, 2000, National Academy Press.

Institute of Medicine (IOM): *Speaking of health: assessing health communication strategies for diverse populations*, Washington, DC, 2002, National Academy Press.

Institute of Medicine: *Unequal treatment: confronting racial and ethnic disparities in healthcare*, Washington, DC, 2003, National Academy Press.

Jarrett T, Horn K, Zhang J: Teen perceptions of facilitator characteristics in a school-based smoking cessation program, *J Sch Health* 297–303, 2009. doi:10.1097/GRF.0b013e31816f2952.

Koniak-Griffin D, Turner-Pluta C: Health risks and psychosocial outcomes of early childbearing: a review of the literature, *J Perinat Neonatal Nurs* 15:1–17, 2001.

Larson E: Racial and ethnic disparities in immunizations: recommendations for clinicians, *Fam Med* 35:655–690, 2003.

Lewin S, Munabi-Babigumira S, Glenton C, et al: Lay health workers in primary and community health care for maternal and child health and the management of infectious diseases, *Cochrane Database Syst Rev* 3:CD004015, 2010.

March of Dimes: *Peristats, from National Center for Health Statistics, Final Natality Data, 2004-06*, 2010. Available at http://www.marchofdimes.com/peristats/level1.aspx?dv=ls&reg=99&top=4&stop=44&lev=1&slev=1&obj=1. Accessed February 26, 2011.

Mathews TJ, MacDorman MF: Infant mortality statistics from the 2006 period linked birth/infant death data set, *National Vital Statistics Report*, vol 58, no 17, Hyattsville, MD, 2010, NCHS.

Mayet S, Groshkova T, Morgan L, et al: Drugs and pregnancy—outcomes of women engaged with a specialist perinatal outreach addictions service, *Drug Alcohol Rev* 27:497–503, 2008. doi:10.1080/09595230802245261.

Miniño AM, Xu J, Kochanek KD, Tejada-Vera B: *Death in the United States, 2007*, NCHS data brief, No 26, Hyattsville, MD, 2009, NCHS.

Naylor MD, Kurtzman ET: The role of nurse practitioners in reinventing primary care, *Health Aff* 29:893–899, 2010. doi:10.1377/hlthaff.2010.0440.

Newhouse JP: Assessing health reform's impact on four key groups of Americans, *Health Aff* 29:1–11, 2010. doi:10.1377/hlthaff.2010.0595.

Nutbeam D: Defining and measuring health literacy: what can we learn from literacy studies? *Int J Public Health* 54:303–305, 2009. doi:10.1007/s00038-009-0050-x.

O'Connell JJ, Oppenheimer SC, Judge CM, et al: The Boston Health Care for the Homeless Program: a public health framework, *Am J Public Health* 100:1400–1408, 2010. doi:10.2105/AJPH.2009.173609.

Pieterse AL, Carter RT: An exploratory investigation of the relationship between racism, racial identity, perceptions of health, and health locus of control among Black American women, *J Health Care Poor Underserv* 21:334–348, 2010. doi:10.1351/hpu.0.0244.

Quad Council of Public Health Nursing Organizations: *Core competencies for public health professionals: a project of the Council on Linkages between Academia and Public Health Practice funded by the Health Resources and Services Administration*, 2003. Available at http://www.sphtc.org/phn_competencies_final_comb.pdf. Accessed February 26, 2011.

Rautava L, Häkkinen U, Korvenranta E, et al for PERFECT Preterm Infant Study Group, Health and the use of health care services in 5-year-old very-low-birth-weight infants. *Acta Pædiatrica* 99:1073–1079, 2010. doi:10.1111/j.1651-2227.2010.01737.x.

Salvadó M, Garcia-Vidal C, Vázquez P, et al: Mortality of tuberculosis in very old people. *J Am Geriatr Soc* 58:18–22, 2010 doi:10.1111/j.1532-5415.2009.02619.x.

Schillinger D, Grumbach K, Piette J, et al: Association of health literacy with diabetes outcomes, *JAMA* 288:475–482, 2002.

Shi L, Stevens GD: Vulnerability and unmet health care needs: the influence of multiple risk factors, *J Gen Intern Med* 20:148–154, 2005a.

Shi L, Stevens GD: *Vulnerable populations in the United States*, San Francisco, Copyright 2005 by John Wiley and Sons, 2005b, Published by Jossey-Bass.

Statistics Canada: *Infant deaths and mortality rates, by age group, Canada, provinces and territories, annual*, CANSIM (database), 2010. Available at http://cansim2.statcan.gc.ca/cgi-win/cnsmcgi.exe?Lang=E&CNSM-Fi=CII/CII_1-eng.htm. Accessed August 8, 2010.

Temple P, Lutenbacher M, Vitale J: Limited access to care and home healthcare, *Clin Obstet Gynecol* 51:371–384, 2008. doi:10.1097/GRF.0b013e31816f2952.

U.S. Department of Health and Human Services: *Healthy people in healthy communities: a community planning guide using Healthy People 2010*, Washington, DC, 2001a, U.S. Government Printing Office.

U.S. Department of Health and Human Services: *National standards for culturally and linguistically appropriate services in health care*, Washington, DC, 2001b, IQ Solutions.

U.S. Department of Health and Human Services: *The HHS poverty guidelines for the remainder of 2010*, August 2010. Available at http://aspe.hhs.gov/10poverty.shtml. Accessed March 2, 2011.

U.S. Department of Health and Human Services: *Healthy People 2020*, Washington, DC, 2010. Available at http://www.healthypeople.gov/2020/ Default.aspx. Accessed March 1, 2011.

U.S. Public Health Service: *The core functions project*, Washington, DC, 1994, updated 2000, Office of Disease Prevention and Health Promotion.

Wilensky GR, Satcher D: Don't forget about the social determinants of health, *Health Aff* 28:w194–w198, 2009. doi:10.1377/hlthaff.28.2.w194.

Zander K: Nursing case management in the 21st century: intervening where margin meets mission, *Nurs Admin Quart* 26:58–67, 2002.

CHAPTER 33

Poverty and Homelessness

Jeanette Lancaster, PhD, RN, FAAN

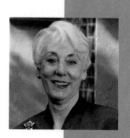

Dr. Jeanette Lancaster is the Medical Center Professor of Nursing at the University of Virginia. She has co-edited all prior editions of this text with Dr. Stanhope. She is grateful to Christine Di Martile Bolla, who authored this chapter in the last two editions. Dr. Bolla retired from Dominican University of California in 2009. Her thoughtful chapters added considerably to the sixth and seventh editions of the text.

ADDITIONAL RESOURCES

Evolve WEBSITE
http://evolve.elsevier.com/Stanhope
- *Healthy People 2020*
- WebLinks
- Quiz
- Case Studies
- Glossary
- Answers to Practice Application

OBJECTIVES

After reading this chapter, the student should be able to do the following:
1. Analyze the concept of poverty.
2. Discuss how nurses view and understand poverty, homelessness, and health.
3. Describe the social, political, cultural, and environmental factors that influence poverty and homelessness.
4. Discuss the effects of poverty on the health and well-being of individuals, families, and communities.
5. Analyze the concept of homelessness.
6. Discuss the effects of homelessness on the health and well-being of individuals, families, and communities.
7. Discuss nursing interventions for poor and homeless individuals.

KEY TERMS

consumer price index, p. 739
crisis poverty, p. 744
cultural attitudes, p. 738
deinstitutionalization, p. 746
Elizabethan poor laws, p. 738
emergency housing, p. 748
Federal Income Poverty Guidelines, p. 739
homelessness, p. 743
homeless persons, p. 743
Interagency Council on the Homeless, p. 748
low-income housing, p. 748
media discourses, p. 738
near poor, p. 739
neighborhood poverty, p. 739
persistent poverty, p. 739
personal beliefs, p. 737
poverty, p. 739
Poverty Threshold Guidelines, p. 739
Stewart B. McKinney Homeless Assistance Act of 1987, p. 743
supportive housing, p. 748
Temporary Assistance to Needy Families, p. 739
Women, Infants, and Children, p. 739
—*See Glossary for definitions*

American society values self-reliance, individual responsibility, and personal accountability. Although these cultural expectations are important, our beliefs about personal autonomy can work against the needs of persons who are unable to live independent, successful lives. Discussions about poor and homeless people arouse feelings in many Americans. Often we think that people should work hard, save some money, plan for the future, and be able to take care of themselves. The economic downturn that began in 2008 has altered these views. Many people who had always been able to take care of themselves and their families now needed help to provide such basic necessities as food and shelter. The weak job market had an especially negative effect on youth, recent college graduates, and older workers. Company lay-offs, plant closings, and businesses that were downsized, relocated, or closed affected workers and their income, health insurance, and retirement savings and plans.

Home foreclosures left many people homeless. These new homeless people had never imagined this would happen to them. Nurses encounter poor persons, families, and populations in a variety of settings, such as private homes, congregate living situations, schools, churches, clinics, and meal sites. To provide effective care and to advocate for individuals, families, and populations living in poverty, nurses need to understand poverty as a concept with historical, social, political, economic, biological, psychological, and spiritual dimensions. Understanding the concepts of poverty and homelessness begins with an examination of one's beliefs, values, and personal experience. It is also important to develop an appreciation for the history of public responses to poor and homeless persons, and the relationship of this history to contemporary public and personal debates. Nurses must be able to identify health care needs, barriers to care, and essential health care services for poor and homeless individuals, families, and aggregates. Providing effective nursing interventions requires an understanding of the epidemiology, health problems, and risk factors associated with poverty as well as sources of support and existing programs for these vulnerable populations.

This chapter describes the many ways that poverty and homelessness affect the health status of individuals, families, and communities, and it suggests effective nursing interventions for poor and homeless people. The concepts of poverty and homelessness are examined in historical, economic, political, and spiritual contexts.

CONCEPT OF POVERTY

Individual perceptions of poverty and poor persons are rooted in social, political, cultural, and environmental factors. Personal beliefs, social values, personal experience, cultural attitudes, media portrayals, and historical factors influence our understanding of poverty. It is important for each of us to be aware of our values and beliefs about poor and homeless persons.

To be effective, nurses must recognize and acknowledge the beliefs, values, and knowledge that form their worldviews and influence the way they practice. **Personal beliefs** are ideas about the world that a person believes to be true; these beliefs are rooted in societal values. Our attitudes toward poor persons are influenced by societal/cultural values of personal responsibility, individual autonomy, and personal accountability. Although these societal and cultural values have changed little throughout history, there is some evidence that they may be changing because of the magnitude of people affected by the current economic situation.

How Have People Historically Viewed Those Who Are Poor?

Public perceptions about poor persons and individual attitudes about what should be done for the poor go back to the Elizabethan poor laws. In seventeenth-century England, being poor was no disgrace because nearly everyone lived in poverty. Therefore, people often shared what they had with one another and frequently banded together to help those whose luck had taken a downturn. People become more mobile when the Industrial Revolution began. Increased migration from rural areas to urban industrial townships brought with it questions of whom among the downtrodden should be helped. In short, how could society distinguish poor persons deserving assistance from those who did not (Katz, 1989)? Elizabethan poor laws, established in the seventeenth century, said that persons who were born within the boundaries of the community should be given assistance by that community. Needy travelers from another community would not be helped and were sent back to their original community where they would be helped by their own folk.

Society changed to adapt to the Industrial Revolution. It became more difficult to differentiate between the deserving and the undeserving poor. Persons who were down-and-out were classified as deserving of assistance if their poverty was considered to be beyond their control. Widowed women, orphaned children, laborers who were injured on the job, and persons with chronic illness not caused by personal failure were considered deserving of public assistance. Alcoholics, prostitutes, mentally ill persons, and those considered to be lazy were the undeserving poor, and they were denied any type of aid (Katz, 1989).

Societal responses to poverty and homeless persons are deeply rooted in history. This history has helped to shape our cultural attitudes. Our cultural attitudes affect, and are affected by, the media. Therefore, it is important to consider the effects of cultural attitudes and the media on societal responses to poverty and homelessness. As will be seen in the next sections, there is no one definition of poverty. The definitions vary depending on the person or agency that is using the definition.

Cultural Attitudes and Media Discourses

Cultural attitudes are the beliefs and perspectives that a society values. Perspectives about individual responsibility for health and well-being are influenced by prevailing cultural attitudes. Media discourses, or views, are a way to communicate thoughts and attitudes through literature, film, art, television, newspapers, and the Internet. Media images of persons on welfare influence, and are influenced by, cultural attitudes and values. Poor persons may be cast as lazy, shiftless folk. These media images influence what we believe to be true about poor persons.

You can examine your own beliefs, values, and knowledge about vulnerable groups by thinking about the following clinical situations and questions:

- You are conducting health screening at a homeless shelter and one of the clients asks you for money for bus fare. Do you give it to her?
- You are in the home of an older person, and there are many roaches on the kitchen floor. What are your obligations in terms of the client's home environment? Where do you sit if he offers you a chair?
- What is your opinion of individual versus societal responsibility for health and well-being? In other words, who is responsible for helping poor and/or homeless persons? Is it society's responsibility? Is it up to poor or homeless persons to help themselves?
- What interventions would you initiate for a population of poor or homeless families in a local shelter? Would you begin with health screening or elsewhere?

- How could you effectively advocate for a group of medically indigent men?
- What do you think about your community conducting a town meeting to consider building a homeless shelter?

There are no easy answers to these questions. However, nurses' behaviors in these situations influence, and are influenced by, their relationships with clients who are poor. It is important to evaluate clients and populations in the context of the environment to develop effective nursing interventions. Treating medical problems alone is inadequate. Instead, care must be multidimensional and include biological, psychological, social, political, cultural, environmental, economic, and spiritual factors.

DEFINING AND UNDERSTANDING POVERTY

The official poverty measure in the United States is a specific dollar amount that varies by family size but is consistent across the country with the exception of Alaska and Hawaii. It does take into account the assets and debt a family has or other factors such as cost of living in different areas or urban versus rural differences. The 2011 poverty level was $22,350 for a family of four and $18,530 for a family of three in the 48 contiguous states and the District of Columbia. The levels are higher in both Alaska and Hawaii as shown in Table 33-1. These guidelines are used to determine if a family is eligible for public programs and in some instances, private programs (Federal Register, January 20, 2011). It is thought that across the nation, families actually need about twice the amount of the official poverty level to meet their basic needs. (See the National Center for Children in Poverty's [NCCP's] Basic Needs Budget calculator [http://www.nccp.org/tools/budget] for differentiation between basic needs for families of four living in urban [north vs. south], suburban, and rural towns).

In making their calculations, the NCCP assumes that the family comprises two parents and one child in school and a preschool child. The items that are included in the basic needs budgets are: rent and utilities, food, child care, health

TABLE 33-1	FEDERAL POVERTY GUIDELINES, 2011		
PERSONS IN FAMILY OR HOUSEHOLD	**48 CONTIGUOUS STATES AND DC**	**ALASKA**	**HAWAII**
1	$10,890	$13,600	$12,540
2	$14,710	$18,380	$16,930
3	$18,530	$23,160	$21,320
4	$22,350	$27,940	$25,710
5	$26,170	$32,720	$30,100
6	$29,990	$37,500	$34,490
7	$33,810	$42,280	$38,880
8	$37,630	$47,060	$43,270
For each additional person, add:	$3820	$4780	$4390

From Federal Register, Vol 76, No 13, January 20, 2011, pp 3637-3638.

insurance premiums, out-of-pocket medical costs, transportation, other necessities, payroll taxes, and income taxes. To compare the need versus the poverty level, in 2008, a family of four in Houston, Texas would need $50,624 compared with the same family in rural Decatur County, Iowa who would need $42,748 per year. The need in Houston is 239% greater than the federal poverty level, and the need is 202% greater in Decatur County.

In 2007, 37.3 million people had incomes below the federal poverty level; about 18% were younger than 18 years of age (U.S. Census Bureau, 2007). As mentioned, the number of people living in poverty increases during times of economic stress and when unemployment rates rise. Since people who live in poverty are not all alike, be sure to listen in order to individualize care and avoid making inappropriate assumptions about their needs. It is important to take the time to know clients by name and to listen to the stories of their lives. Getting to know your clients can begin to break down barriers caused by their fears and isolation as well as barriers caused by your fears as a nurse when those fears can lead to misunderstandings about people from different walks of life. It is also helpful to examine social and cultural definitions and considerations related to poverty.

Social and Cultural Definitions of Poverty

As mentioned, income level is used as the key criterion that determines whether someone is poor. Although income continues to be the measurement of choice, poverty is not adequately defined solely by income level. Understanding the social and cultural dimensions of poverty helps to broaden our view of the concept. Poverty refers to having insufficient financial resources to meet basic living expenses. These expenses include costs of food, shelter, clothing, transportation, and medical care. In addition to its economic outcomes, however, poverty has important physical, psychological, and spiritual consequences. People who are poor are more likely to live in dangerous environments, to work at high-risk jobs, to eat less nutritious foods, and to have multiple stressors, such as unemployment, inadequate housing, lack of affordable day care, and lack of access to regular health care.

Meanings and perceptions of poverty differ across cultures. Most Western cultures view poverty negatively, whereas other cultures often respect the poor. Religious and political differences affect the perceptions people hold of poor and underserved groups. Meanings of lower socioeconomic status can also vary among various groups within a culture.

Political Dimensions

It is important to examine poverty in terms of its political dimensions. Poverty involves a lack of control over critical resources needed to function effectively in society. The federal government uses two types of guidelines to define poverty. The Poverty Threshold Guidelines are issued by the U.S. Bureau of the Census and are used primarily for statistical purposes. The Federal Income Poverty Guidelines are issued by the U.S. Department of Health and Human Services (USDHHS) and are used to determine if a person or family is financially eligible for assistance or services from various federal programs. Eligibility for federal housing subsidies, Temporary Assistance to Needy Families (TANF, formerly called AFDC), Medicaid, food stamps, Women, Infants, and Children (WIC), and Head Start is based on the Federal Income Poverty Guidelines. Federal poverty guidelines are updated annually to be consistent with the consumer price index (CPI), also called the cost-of-living index. The CPI is a measure of the average change over time in the prices paid by households for a fixed market basket of consumer goods and services, including housing; electricity; food; clothing; fuels; doctor, dentist, and drug charges; transportation; and other goods and services that people buy for day-to-day living (United States Department of Labor. n.d.)

Many people who earn slightly more than the government-defined income levels (see Table 33-1) are unable to meet living expenses and are not eligible for government assistance programs. For example, in a family of four with an income of $22,000, the adult family members would not qualify for Medicaid in some states. Persons whose income is above the federal guidelines but whose income is inadequate are called the near poor.

The terms *persistent poverty* and *neighborhood poverty* are often used to describe social aspects of poverty. Persistent poverty refers to individuals and families who remain poor for long periods and whose poverty is multigenerational. Neighborhood poverty refers to geographically defined areas of high poverty, characterized by dilapidated housing and high levels of unemployment. Areas of neighborhood poverty also have higher rates of morbidity and mortality than nearby, more affluent, areas (Zenk et al, 2005). It is important for nurses who work with poor populations to know these definitions and to respect poor clients as human beings whose life situations influence their health and well-being.

Poverty in the United States was not recognized as a social problem before the Civil War (Katz, 1989). The prevalent attitude during that time was that poverty was an individual's problem, and poor individuals had only themselves to blame. Generally, society did not assume responsibility for alleviating the plight of the poor. However, during the post–Civil War industrialized era, this attitude changed significantly. Widespread unemployment, undesirable working conditions, insufficient wages, and substandard housing forced a rethinking of public responsibility for the poor (Wilson, 1990). Many laws concerning public health and housing were passed. The post–Civil War social reform movement led to an early interest in urban poverty research (Bremner, 1956; Miller, 1966). Despite influences of the Depression of the 1930s and national discussion of New Deal legislation, such as the Social Security Act of 1935, the public's interest in the plight of the poor declined (Wilson, 1990).

A resurgence of political activity on behalf of disadvantaged groups occurred during the late 1950s and early 1960s. In 1959 the Kerr-Mills Act increased funds for health care for aged persons (Fine, 1998). In 1961 President Kennedy approved a pilot food program in response to the hunger he observed on the campaign trail (Price, 1994); in 1963 he instructed his administration to develop a major policy effort to combat poverty.

After Kennedy's assassination, President Johnson sustained the interest in the antipoverty campaign. Johnson established the War on Poverty in 1964, which emphasized job-training programs and community organization and involvement (Pilisuk and Pilisuk, 1973; Wilson, 1990). In 1964 the Social Security Administration established the income level of the official poverty line. Individuals and families with incomes below the federal poverty line were considered to be living in poverty. In 1965 the Medicare amendments to the Social Security Act were passed. After 1965 considerable research focused on poverty as it related to education, health, housing, the law, and public welfare (Wilson, 1990).

Policy changes during the 1980s led to an emphasis on defense spending rather than on social programs. The visibility of the homeless and the media attention on an underclass of individuals seemed to blame the poor for being poor. However, being poor is often a result of the economic environment and is influenced by the degree that an area has a wide division in income levels and races (Zenk et al, 2005).

During the 1990s, record numbers of people received welfare benefits, and this stimulated enthusiasm for reform of health and the welfare systems (Zedlewski, 2002). In 1996 a bill creating the TANF program was enacted. This welfare reform legislation replaced the Aid to Families with Dependent Children (AFDC) program with a program of temporary welfare benefits. Under TANF, eligible persons are provided with benefits for a limited time, and are required to find jobs and/or to enroll in job-training programs. Low-income working families often do not bring home enough money to cover the costs of everyday living. Some do get help from government programs, notably tax credits, food stamps, WIC, and child care subsidies. However, often these supports are either too little or help too few families to fully meet the needs of the low-income working families (Zedlewski, Chaudry, and Simms, 2008). Low-income working families are at great risk during times of a weak economy. The loss of a job or a cut in hours of work can disrupt their precarious financial situation. Most of these persons cannot save for a time when times get rough since they barely earn enough to cover regular expenses. Also, many of these workers do not have employee-sponsored health insurance, and an illness can also be a devastating financial crisis.

WHAT DO YOU THINK? *Opinions and beliefs about welfare differ among recipients, taxpayers, politicians, economists, health care providers, and others. Some people believe that welfare benefits are inadequate, whereas others argue that welfare breeds dependency and illegitimacy. Families receiving welfare benefits also have differing views.*

There has been political debate about whether to abolish or to reform welfare. Aid to Families with Dependent Children (AFDC) was replaced with the Temporary Assistance to Needy Families (TANF) program. What is the relationship between welfare reform and health? What implications does welfare reform have on nurses working in the community? How would you have redesigned the welfare system? What issues will emerge in the twenty-first century?

Further Discussion

The causes of poverty are complex and interrelated. In recent decades the number of adult and older adult Americans living in poverty has decreased in part because of the support provided through Social Security and Medicare benefits, as discussed later. In contrast, the number of women and children living in poverty has increased. The following factors affect the growing number of poor persons in the United States:

- Decreased earnings
- Increased unemployment rates
- Changes in the labor force
- Increase in female-headed households
- Inadequate education and job skills
- Inadequate antipoverty programs
- Inadequate welfare benefits
- Weak enforcement of child support statutes
- Dwindling Social Security payments to children
- Increased numbers of children born to single women
- Trade deficits, debt, involvement in wars
- Outsourcing of American jobs

As most industrialized nations have moved from being industrial economies to service economies, job opportunities have increasingly excluded workers who do not have at least a high school education. Many manufacturing jobs do not pay sufficient salary to support a family, and many jobs at the lower end of the pay scale do not include health care benefits. Lack of access to health care benefits compounds the effects of poverty on health.

POVERTY AND HEALTH: EFFECTS ACROSS THE LIFE SPAN

Poverty directly affects health and well-being, leading to the following:

- Higher rates of chronic illness
- Higher infant morbidity and mortality
- Shorter life expectancy
- More complex health problems
- More significant complications and physical limitation from chronic diseases such as asthma, diabetes, and hypertension
- Hospitalization rates greater than those for persons with higher incomes

Poor health outcomes are related to decreased access to health care. Lack of access to health care can be related to inability to pay for health care, lack of insurance, geographic location, language, maldistribution of providers, transportation difficulties, immigration status, inconvenient clinic hours, and negative attitudes of health care providers toward poor clients. Access to health care is especially difficult for the working poor. Many employers, especially those paying low or minimum wage, do not provide health care insurance for their employees. These employees are often ineligible for public health insurance programs and unable to obtain affordable health care. The first topic area in *Healthy People 2020* deals with access to health services. This area and its objectives are relevant to meeting the needs of poor and homeless people. See the *Healthy People 2020* box for specific objectives.

❤ HEALTHY PEOPLE 2020

The following are a sampling of health access goals that affect poor and homeless people:

- AHS-1: Increase the proportion of persons with health insurance.
- AHS-2: Increase the proportion of insured persons with coverage for clinical preventive services.
- AHS-3: Increase the proportion of persons with a usual primary care provider.
- AHS-5: Increase the proportion of persons who have a specific source of ongoing care.
- AHS-6: Reduce the proportion of individuals that experience difficulties or delays in obtaining necessary medical care, dental care, or prescription medicines.

From U.S. Department of Health and Human Services: *Healthy People 2020*, Washington, DC, 2010, U.S. Government Printing Office.

TABLE 33-2 PERCENT OF CHILDREN IN LOW-INCOME FAMILIES BY RACE/ETHNICITY, 2007

ETHNIC GROUP	PERCENTAGE IN POVERTY (%)
African American	28
Latino	33
White	32
Asian	3
American Indian	1
Other	3

From National Center for Children in Poverty: Fass S, Dinan KA, and Aratani Y: *Child poverty and intergenerational mobility*, New York, December 2009, Columbia University. Available at www.nccp.org/publications/pub_911.html. Accessed February 26, 2011.

BOX 33-1 THE EFFECTS OF POVERTY ON THE HEALTH OF CHILDREN

- Higher rates of prematurity, low birth weight, and birth defects
- Higher infant mortality rates
- Increased incidence of:
  - Chronic disease
  - Traumatic death and injuries
  - Nutritional deficits
  - Growth retardation and developmental delays
  - Iron deficiency anemia
  - Elevated blood lead levels
  - Infections
- Increased risk for homelessness
- Decreased opportunities for education, income, and occupation

From Morrell-Bellai T, Goering PN, Boydell KM: Becoming and remaining homeless: a qualitative investigation, *Issues Ment Health Nurs* 21:581-604, 2000.

Poverty in Women of Child-Bearing Age

Poverty, which presents a significant obstacle to health across the life span, has an especially negative effect on women of child-bearing age. Women living in poverty have lower levels of physical functioning, as well as higher reported levels of body discomfort, than women in higher socioeconomic groups. Prevalence rates for ulcer disease, asthma, and anemia are significantly higher among women living in poverty. The reasons for these elevated rates are associated with the often poor living conditions and the limited resources to buy nutritious food. Also, poor women report significantly more risk behaviors for infection with human immunodeficiency virus (HIV) than more affluent women (Ellen et al, 2004).

Poverty has significant effects on adolescent women. Poor teens are four times more likely than their more affluent peers to have below-average academic skills. Regardless of their race, poor teens are nearly three times as likely to drop out of school as their non-poor counterparts. Teenage women who are poor and who have below-average skills are more likely to have children than non-poor teenage women. Poor pregnant women are more likely than other women to receive late or no prenatal care and to deliver low-birth-weight babies, premature babies, or babies with birth defects (Stein, Lu, and Gelberg, 2000).

Welfare reform affects the health and well-being of child-bearing women and their families. When changes in the benefit levels are made, women and their children are often affected. Also, the Personal Responsibility and Work Opportunity Reconciliation Act of 1996 requires that more families work to receive assistance. This may mean that funds are targeted to provide childcare subsidies so that women can work. If funds are limited, there may be less money available to assist other working poor women and their children when their need is not for childcare subsidies. More changes are expected as financial and health care reform in the United States continues and as state and federal budgets continued to be challenged to meet the many needs.

Children and Poverty

The poverty rate for children of 18% is higher than that for any other age group (U.S. Census Bureau, 2007). Moreover, poverty among young African-American and Hispanic children is more than three times that of white, non-Hispanic children (Table 33-2). Poverty among children (newborn to age 5 years) has increased in all racial and ethnic groups, as well as in all urban, suburban, and rural geographic areas.

Changes in welfare policy can affect family income, parenting behaviors, and children's access to services (NCCP, 2005). Decreases in family income can result in an increase in the number of children living in extreme poverty and can increase parental stress. Increased parental stress can have a negative effect on the well-being of children. Welfare changes that deny social and health services to the poor have negative effects on the health and well-being of poor children.

Young children (up to 5 years of age) are at highest risk for the most harmful effects of poverty, especially lack of adequate nutrition and brain development. Other risk factors include maternal substance abuse or depression, exposure to environmental toxins, trauma and abuse, and poor-quality daily care (Evans, Boxhill, and Pinkava, 2008). Some of the effects of poverty on children are listed in Box 33-1. Poverty increases the likelihood of chronic disease, injuries, traumatic death, developmental delays, poor nutrition, inadequate immunization levels, iron deficiency anemia, and elevated blood lead levels. Furthermore, children of poverty are more likely than non-poor children to be hungry and suffer from fatigue, dizziness, irritability, headaches, ear infections, frequent colds, weight loss, inability to concentrate, and increased school absenteeism (Emerson, 2004).

DID YOU KNOW?

- *Child poverty costs our society an estimated $500 billion a year in lost productivity and increased spending on health care and the criminal justice system.*
- *African-American children are more likely than white children to experience poverty.*
- *Among adults who experienced poverty as children, about 20% were poor in young adulthood and 13% to 14% were poor between the ages of 30 and 35.*

From Fass S, Dinan KA, Aratani Y: Child poverty and intergenerational mobility. *National Center for Children in Poverty, Mailman School of Public Health, Columbia University, NY, December 2009. Available at www.nccp.org/publications/pub-911. Accessed January 4, 2010.*

Deadbeat Parents

Under current federal law, non-custodial parents are required to provide financial support to their children. Current child support policies are designed to provide financial security to children, prevent single-parent families from entering the welfare system, help single-parent families get off welfare as quickly as possible, and decrease welfare expenditures (Kaplan et al, 2004). Individual states are responsible for locating non-supporting custodial parents, establishing paternity, and enforcing financial responsibility. In most states, government involvement in locating non-custodial parents begins when the custodial parent applies for TANF.

The current system is criticized because public expectations of financial responsibility for non-custodial parents are based on an assumption that the non-custodial parent is working full time. However, many low-income parents were never married, and many have intermittent work histories. Current policy requires the custodial parent to assign all financial support from the non-custodial parent to the state to equal the amount that the family receives from the welfare (TANF) system. In response to these regulations, many low-income parents often make private, informal arrangements for child support payments. Under these verbal arrangements, the non-custodial parent pays the custodial parent directly. The term "deadbeat" dad refers to fathers who do not contribute to the financial support of their children. As the number of custodial single fathers increases there may be greater attention to non-custodial mothers who do not contribute to the financial support of their children since non-custodial mothers are equally responsible under the law to provide for the economic well-being of their children. The term "deadbeat parent" is more gender-sensitive and appropriate.

Older Adults and Poverty

In 2007 an estimated 9.7% of older adults (65 years and older) lived in poverty (U.S. Census Bureau, 2007). This represents a decrease in the poverty rate for this age group, largely because of

improvements in Social Security and the Supplemental Security Income (SSI) program. SSI is a federal income supplement program funded by general tax revenues (not Social Security taxes). This program is designed to help older people, those who are blind or disabled, and those who have little or no income. SSI provides cash to meet basic needs for food, clothing, and shelter. The Social Security website (http://www.ssa.gov/pubs/index/html) has vast information about eligibility for SSI for children, survivors, retirees, and those with a disability. It also discusses the benefits available through Medicare and SSI via the Food Stamp and other nutrition programs. Despite the federal benefits available to older persons, certain groups of older adults remain vulnerable to the effects of poverty. Older African Americans, for example, are at significantly greater risk for chronic and nutrition-related diseases than older white persons (Kelley-Moore and Ferraro, 2004).

Older adults living in poverty are disproportionately more likely to have poor health outcomes than their more affluent counterparts (Liz et al, 2005). Prevalence rates for chronic illness and chronic illness complications, general morbidity, poor dental health, and overall mortality are significantly greater among poor older adults (Kelley-Moore and Ferraro, 2004). Moreover, poor older adults are more likely to seek acute crisis care rather than preventive health care. Older adults are particularly at risk because they may be alone and unable to manage their personal affairs. Many older adults are eligible for benefits but do not know how to access them.

NURSING TIP   *A client's advice to nurses caring for the poor:*

- *Treat the poor like everyone else.*
- *Do not be condescending.*
- *Do not make it obvious that someone is poor.*
- *Do not prejudge; ask if someone wants to pay his/her bill.*
- *Remember that people cannot always pay for their medicine.*
- *Suggest programs that might help, such as food banks, churches, and clothing centers.*
- *Poor people need a lot of support.*
- *Many poor people need help to learn how to promote their own health given limited resources.*

The Community and Poverty

Poverty can affect both urban and rural communities. Although there has been some decrease in disparities between poor neighborhoods and higher-income areas in terms of educational achievement, housing, and health status, poorer neighborhoods continue to have more minority residents, more single-parent families, higher rates of unemployment, lower wage rates, and higher rates of morbidity and mortality (Blank, 2001). Residents of poor neighborhoods are also more likely to be victims of crime, substance abuse, racial discrimination, and police brutality. Health care is often less available to residents of poor neighborhoods. Housing conditions in some areas are deplorable, with many families living in run-down shacks or condemned apartment buildings. Residents living in poverty are often exposed to environmental hazards, such as inadequate heating and cooling, exposure to rain and snow, inadequate water and plumbing, and the presence of pests and other vermin.

THE CUTTING EDGE *Poverty and homelessness are affected by the employment rate. When companies close or relocate, workers often go long periods of time without a steady income.*

Being poor affects the health and well-being of individuals, families, and communities. Nurses must examine individual and community strengths, resources, and sources of support in order to provide effective nursing interventions for persons living in poverty. Poverty and homelessness are linked in that poor people are often unable to pay for housing, food, childcare, health care, and education (National Coalition for the Homeless, 2009c). When people have limited resources, they must make difficult choices, one of which may be to give up housing. According to the National Coalition for the Homeless in the fact sheet, "Why are People Homeless," "If you are poor, you are essentially an illness, an accident, or a paycheck away from living on the streets" (National Coalition for the Homeless, 2009c, p 1). Similar to understanding poverty and its many implications, understanding the concept of homelessness requires reflection and analysis.

UNDERSTANDING THE CONCEPT OF HOMELESSNESS

Several variables, such as personal beliefs, personal/societal values, cultural norms, political debate, and personal knowledge/experience, influence nurses' perceptions of homelessness. Nurses who work with homeless persons need to understand homelessness from a conceptual perspective and be aware of the causes and effects of this public health problem. To implement effective nursing interventions for homeless clients, nurses need to be aware of their own beliefs and values about homelessness.

Personal Beliefs, Values, and Knowledge

Poverty can lead to homelessness. Homelessness, like poverty, is a complex concept. The term *homelessness* is defined in the following section on homelessness in the United States. Although people who have never been homeless cannot truly understand what it means to be homeless, nurses can increase their sensitivity about homeless persons and aggregates by examining their own personal beliefs, values, and knowledge of homelessness. The questions in the How To box can help nurses to constructively evaluate their own knowledge, beliefs, and values.

HOW TO Test Values and Beliefs About Poverty

Nurses should ask themselves the following questions about poverty and persons living in poverty:

1. *What do I believe to be true about being poor?*
2. *What do I personally know about poverty?*
3. *How have family and friends influenced my ideas about being poor?*
4. *Have I ever personally been poor?*
5. *How have media images of poor persons helped to shape our images of poverty and poor persons?*
6. *What do I feel when I see a hungry child? What do I feel when I see a hungry adult?*
7. *Do I believe that people are poor because they just do not want to work? Alternatively, do I believe that society has a significant influence on one's becoming poor?*
8. *What really causes poverty?*
9. *What do I really think can be done to prevent poverty and homelessness?*

Clients' Perceptions of Homelessness

People who live on the street are the poorest of the poor. They are often perceived by those more fortunate as faceless, nameless, invisible, inaudible entities. It is important for nurses to respect the individuality of all clients, including those who are homeless. People become homeless for many reasons and there is no one set of circumstances or patterns that lead to homelessness. The following sections provide an overview of what leads to homelessness and what some of the unique needs are of homeless persons and how nurses may meet those needs.

Homelessness in the United States

The **Stewart B. McKinney Homeless Assistance Act of 1987** (PL 100-77) defines homelessness as "lacking a fixed, regular, and adequate night-time residence and . . . has a primary nighttime residency that is: (a) a supervised publicly or privately operated shelter designed to provide temporary living accommodations; (b) an institution that provides a temporary residence for individuals intended to be institutionalized; or (c) a public or private place not designed for, or ordinarily used as, a regular sleeping accommodation for human beings" (cited in National Coalition for the Homeless, 2009b, p 1). This definition generally refers to persons who are homeless on the streets or who are in shelters, or who face eviction within 1 week.

There are two predominant ways to determine the number of people who are homeless: (1) point-in-time counts, counting the number of persons who are homeless on a given day or during a given week, or (2) period prevalence counts, which examines the number of people who are homeless over a given period of time (National Coalition for the Homeless, 2009a). It is hard to know exactly how many people are homeless for the following reasons:

- **Homeless persons** are often hard to find, since they may sleep in boxcars, on building roofs, in doorways, or under freeways or pedestrian overpasses. Others may stay temporarily with family or friends.
- Once located, many homeless persons refuse to be interviewed or they deliberately hide the fact that they are homeless.
- Some of them have only short or intermittent episodes of being without a home.
- It is hard to generalize from one location to another. For example, patterns of homelessness differ in large versus small cities and in rural areas.

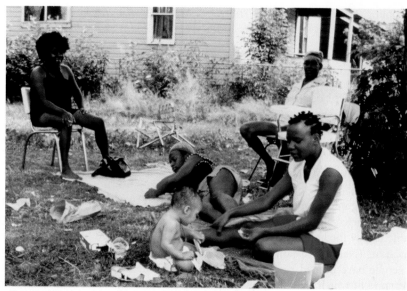

Many families find themselves living in poverty due to circumstances that they could not control. (Copyright © 1973, Picture History LLC. All rights reserved.)

The concept of homelessness encompasses two broad categories. The first category includes persons living in **crisis poverty**. These are people whose lives are generally marked by hardship and struggle. For them, homelessness is often transient or episodic. Persons living in crisis poverty may have brief stays in shelters or other temporary accommodations. Their homelessness may result from lack of employment opportunities, lack of education, obsolete job skills, divorce, or domestic violence. Such issues lead to persistent poverty and need to be addressed along with efforts to find stable housing.

Persons in the second category, persistent poverty, are chronically homeless men and women, many of whom have mental or physical disabilities. This is the group that is most frequently identified with homelessness in the United States. Physical and mental disabilities in this group often coexist with alcohol and other drug abuse, severe mental illness, other chronic health problems, and/or chronic family difficulties. These people lack money and family support, they often end up living on the streets, and their homelessness is often persistent. Members of this group need economic assistance, rehabilitation, and ongoing support.

Many homeless people previously had homes and managed to survive on limited incomes. Today's homeless include people of every age, sex, ethnic group, and family type. Surprisingly, the single homeless tend to be younger and better educated than stereotypes would suggest. Many are long-standing residents of their communities and have some history of job success (National Coalition for the Homeless, 2009a).

Homeless persons are found in both rural and urban areas. Many sleep at night in shelters that they must vacate during the day. This means that during the day, they sit or stand on the street; in parks, alleys, shopping centers, and libraries; and in places such as trash bins, cardboard boxes, or under loading docks at industrial sites. Homeless persons may seek shelter in public buildings, such as train and bus stations. Those who do not sleep in shelters may sleep in single-room-occupancy

(SRO) hotels, all-night movie theaters, abandoned buildings, and vehicles. Some people choose to be homeless rather than live with family, with friends, or in shelters.

Rural communities, despite their peaceful images, are not immune to homelessness. The extent of the problem is often somewhat more disguised in rural areas because rural people are often more likely to help one another. Therefore, family and friends often provide temporary housing to their neighbors who have no place to live. Homeless individuals and families living in rural areas suffer from the same types of health problems as their urban counterparts (Craft-Rosenberg, Powel, and Culp, 2000).

Who are most likely to be homeless? Single homeless adults are more likely to be male than female. The number of homeless families has increased significantly over the last decade. For many of these families, the length of time that they live in shelters is increasing, with studies showing stays of an average from 5.7 to 12 months (U.S. Conference of Mayors, 2007). Also, there is a higher percentage of African Americans in shelters (42%), compared with 38% white; 20% Hispanic; 4% Native American, and 2% Asian (U.S. Conference of Mayors, 2007). Victims of domestic violence and veterans within the armed forces also comprise sizable populations with the homeless cohort (National Coalition for the Homeless, 2009b).

Homeless children and youth fall into one of two groups: children and youth who are part of a homeless family and those who are unaccompanied youth. More than 1.5 million children live in families without a home, and about 42% are under the age of 6 (National Center for Children in Poverty, 2009a). Homeless families are often led by a single mother in her 20s with young children. It is estimated that between 1.6 and 1.7 million youth join the ranks of runaways and homeless people annually. There are more females than males in this category, and African-American and Native American youth are overrepresented in the category of runaway-homeless and independent youths (National Coalition for the Homeless, 2009b).

EVIDENCE-BASED PRACTICE

The effects of the duration of homelessness and gender on personal and social resources, cognitive and perceptual factors, and sexual health behaviors among homeless youth were examined. Data were gathered at a large drop-in center for runaway and homeless youth in central Texas. A sample of 805 youth between the ages of 16 and 23 years were recruited. Demographic data and the history of homelessness from surveys were collected. Valid scales were used to measure each of the conceptual variables that were assessed. Findings demonstrated that both the duration of homelessness and gender had direct and interaction effects on self-reports of personal and social resources, knowledge about AIDS, and sexual risk behaviors. Chronically homeless youth in the sample reported higher levels of sexual risk-taking behaviors. Young women, regardless of the length of time they were homeless, reported similar levels of being socially connected, whereas newly homeless young men had greater connectedness than those who were chronically homeless.

Nurse Use

Nurses working in the community may have opportunities to work directly with homeless youth and provide interventions to promote sexual health and decrease risk-taking behavior.

From Rew L, Grady M, Whittaker TA, et al: Interaction of duration of homelessness and gender on adolescent sexual health indicators, *J Nurs Schol* 4(2):109-115, 2008.

Factors that lead to homelessness among children and youth are similar to those affecting adults. See the Did You Know box for more details.

DID YOU KNOW? *Homelessness for children who live with their families most often results from lack of affordable housing, poverty, or domestic violence. Homelessness for unaccompanied youth is most often the result of mental illness, substance abuse, or lack of affordable housing.*

From The United States Conference of Mayors: Hunger and homeless survey: a status report on hunger and homelessness in America's cities, a 23-city survey, Washington, DC December 2007, The United States Conference of Mayors.

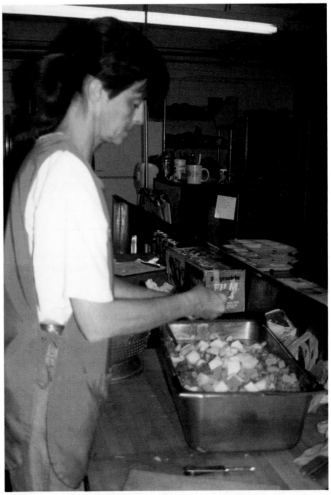

Women, many with children, are becoming part of the homeless population. This woman is a resident in a homeless shelter where residents help with the cooking, laundry, and other chores.

Why Are People Homeless?

Two trends are largely responsible for the growth in homelessness over the past 20 to 25 years. These trends are a growing shortage of affordable rental housing and a simultaneous increase in poverty. In recent times, foreclosures have increased the number of homeless people. Specifically between April 2008 and April 2009, there was a reported 32% increase in foreclosures caused by more than 6 million jobs that were lost, leading to a high unemployment rate (National Coalition for the Homeless, 2009c). As cities upgraded their housing stock, fewer low-cost housing options were available and former residents were unable to afford the new and improved housing. These residents were not able to move to new housing elsewhere. Specifically, in many older neighborhoods, people who are now homeless once lived in single-room-occupancy (SRO) buildings where they rented inexpensive rooms on a long-term basis. Urban renewal eliminated many of the SROs and in exchange

developed more attractive, better-maintained neighborhoods. It is often said that when neighborhoods were "gentrified" or upgraded, they reduced the ability of poor people to live in them because they became unaffordable for poorer former residents.

A worker in 2009 needed to earn $14.97 an hour to afford a one-bedroom apartment, and $17.48 an hour to afford a two-bedroom apartment. There was an increase of 41% from 2000 to 2009 in fair market rent for two bedroom units (National Low Income Housing Coalition, 2009). The lack of affordable housing has led to overcrowding, substandard housing, and increased homelessness. The wait to get into a shelter has grown since people are staying longer in shelters and new shelter beds are not opening quickly enough to meet the need.

There is an association between poverty and homelessness. As mentioned earlier, poor people are often unable to pay for housing, food, childcare, health care, and education. Not only have the number of available jobs decreased in recent years, but the availability of public assistance has simultaneously decreased as states and the federal government reduced their budgets and support for many programs. Programs such as TANF are unable to keep pace with inflation and the growing

---

BOX 33-2 WHO ARE AMERICA'S HOMELESS?

- Families
- Children
- Single women
- Female heads of household
- Adults who are unemployed, earn low wages, or are migrant workers
- People who abuse alcohol or other substances
- Abandoned children
- Adolescent runaways
- Older adults with no place to go and no one to care for them
- Persons who are mentally ill
- Veterans
- Immigrants and migrant workers

TABLE 33-3 COMMON HEALTH PROBLEMS OF HOMELESS PERSONS

PSYCHOSOCIAL	INFECTIOUS	OTHER
Depressive symptoms	HIV/AIDS	Trauma
Mental/psychiatric illness	TB/MDR TB	Preterm birth
Alcohol/substance abuse	Other infectious diseases	COPD
		Low birth weight
		Musculoskeletal problems
		Decreased access to care
		Foot problems
		Malnutrition
		Increased ED utilization rates

From Darmon N, Coupel J, Deheeger M, Briend A: Dietary inadequacies observed in homeless men visiting an emergency shelter in Paris, *Public Health Nutr* 4:155-161, 2001; Hwang SW: Homelessness and health, *CMAJ* 164(2):229-233, 2001; Kamieniecki GW: Prevalence of psychological distress and psychiatric disorders among homeless youth in Australia, *Austr N Z J Psych* 35:352-358, 2001; Stein JA, Lu MC, Gelberg L: Severity of homelessness and adverse birth outcomes, *Health Psychol* 19:524-534, 2000.
AIDS, Acquired immunodeficiency syndrome; *COPD*, chronic obstructive pulmonary disease; *ED*, emergency department; *HIV*, human immunodeficiency virus; *MDR TB*, multidrug-resistant tuberculosis; *TB*, tuberculosis.

---

numbers of people needing help. Box 33-2 summarizes the characteristics of America's homeless.

Deinstitutionalization of chronically mentally ill individuals from public psychiatric hospitals increased the number of homeless persons. The goal of deinstitutionalization was to replace large state psychiatric hospitals with community-based treatment centers. Clients were to have shorter stays in mental health facilities and to move into appropriately designed and readily available community-based care. Unfortunately, after the hospitals were downsized or closed, federal and state governments failed to allocate the needed funds to provide community-based services. Furthermore, few of the intended community mental health centers were ever built. Persons with severe mental illness account for about 26% of all homeless people in shelters (National Coalition for the Homeless, 2009b). Also, rates of alcohol and drug abuse are disproportionately high among homeless people (National Coalition for the Homeless, 2009b).

EFFECTS OF HOMELESSNESS ON HEALTH

Homelessness is correlated with poor health outcomes. The prevalence of illness in homeless people is estimated to be as high as 55%, and the average life expectancy in the U.S. population of a homeless person is 44 years compared with 78 years (Savage and Lee, 2010). Homeless individuals suffer significantly greater incidences of acute and chronic illness, acquired immunodeficiency syndrome (AIDS), and trauma (O'Connell et al, 2005). Even though they are at higher risk of physiological problems, homeless persons have greater difficulty accessing health care services. Health care is usually crisis oriented and sought in emergency departments, and those who access health care have a hard time following prescribed regimens.

Consider the case of an insulin-dependent diabetic man who lives on the street and sleeps in a shelter. His ability to get adequate rest and exercise, take insulin on a schedule, eat regular meals, or follow a prescribed diet is virtually impossible. Consider the following issues:

- How does a person buy an antibiotic without money?
- How is a child treated for scabies and lice when there are no bathing facilities?

- How does an older adult with peripheral vascular disease elevate his legs when he must be out of the shelter at 7 AM and is on the streets all day?

Just as people living in poverty have poor access to health care, so do homeless people. As discussed earlier, one of the topic areas in *Healthy People 2020* deals with access to health care. See the *Healthy People 2020* box for objectives that pertain to homeless persons.

In addition to facing challenges related to self-care, homeless people usually give lower priority to health promotion and health maintenance than to obtaining food and shelter. They spend most of their time trying to survive. Just getting money to buy food is a major chore. Although some homeless persons are eligible for entitlement programs, such as TANF, WIC, or Social Security, others must beg for money, sell plasma or blood products, steal, sell drugs, or engage in prostitution.

Some of the health problems accompanying homelessness include hypothermia, infestations, peripheral vascular disease, hypertension, respiratory tract infections, tuberculosis, AIDS, trauma, and mental illness (Roy et al, 2004). Table 33-3 lists significant health problems of homeless persons. Health problems caused by exposure include hypothermia in the winter and heat-related illnesses, such as heatstroke, and dehydration in the summer. Because they produce decreased sensitivity to hot and cold, the use of street drugs can lead to hyperthermia or hypothermia (Ford, Cantau, and Jeanmart, 2003).

The prevalence of diabetes, poor skin integrity, chronic disease, nutritional deficits, and trauma and the use and abuse of alcohol and illicit drugs compound the effects of exposure.

Cardiovascular and respiratory diseases in the homeless population include peripheral vascular disease, hypertension, tuberculosis, pneumonia, and chronic obstructive pulmonary disease. Homeless persons spend many hours on their feet and often sleep in positions that compromise their peripheral circulation. Hypertension among the homeless is often exacerbated by high rates of alcohol abuse and the high sodium content of foods served in fast-food restaurants, shelters, and other meal sites. Crowded living conditions place homeless persons at risk for exposure to viruses and bacteria that cause pneumonia and tuberculosis. High rates of tobacco, alcohol, and illicit drug use among homeless persons diminish immune responses and contribute to an increased prevalence of chronic obstructive pulmonary disease.

AIDS continues to be a concern among the homeless population. The sero-prevalence of HIV infection in the homeless is estimated to be at least double that found in the general population. The use of intravenous drugs and higher rates of sexual assault are other risk factors. Homeless persons with AIDS tend to develop more virulent forms of infectious diseases, to have longer hospitalizations, and to have less access to treatment (López-Zetina et al, 2001).

Trauma is a significant cause of death and disability in the homeless population. Major trauma includes gunshot wounds, stab wounds, head trauma, suicide attempts, and fractures. Minor trauma includes bruises, abrasions, concussions, sprains, puncture wounds, eye injuries, and cellulitis. Also, homeless people do not have regular access to dental care, places to bathe, and nutritious food, so be sure when assessing them to pay attention to their teeth, skin, and feet (Savage and Lee, 2010).

As mentioned, deinstitutionalization has contributed to the growing number of homeless persons who suffer from mental illnesses, including schizophrenia and affective disorders. The prevalence of alcohol and substance abuse compounds the effects of mental illness. Many homeless persons were mentally ill before becoming homeless, whereas others develop acute mental distress as a result of being homeless. Although treatment options may exist, homeless persons are often unable to gain access to mental health treatment facilities. Barriers to treatment include lack of awareness of treatment options, lack of available space in treatment facilities, inability to pay for treatment, lack of transportation, unsupportive attitudes of service providers, and lack of coordination of services (Dennis, Steadman, and Cocozza, 2000).

In addition to its effects on physical health, homelessness also affects psychological, social, and spiritual well-being. Becoming homeless means more than losing a home, or a regular place to sleep and eat; it also means losing friends, personal possessions, and familiar surroundings. Homeless persons live in chaos, confusion, and fear. Many describe experiencing loss of dignity, low self-esteem, lack of social support, and generalized despair.

Homelessness and At-Risk Populations

Being homeless affects health across the life span. Imagine the effect of homelessness on pregnancy, childhood, adolescence, or older adulthood; each group has different needs. Nurses need to recognize the unique needs of homeless clients at every age.

Homeless pregnant women are at high risk for complex health problems. Pregnancy outcomes for homeless pregnant women are significantly poorer than those for pregnant women in the general population. Pregnant homeless women present several challenges. They have higher rates of sexually transmitted diseases, higher incidences of addiction to drugs and alcohol, poorer nutritional status, and a higher incidence of poor birth outcomes (i.e., lower birth weight and lower Apgar scores). They are also often at risk for violence toward them. Although homeless women who are pregnant are at increased risk for pregnancy complications, they have less access to prenatal care. Being homeless has been shown to significantly predict lower birth weight and increase the incidence of preterm birth, even for homeless women receiving regular prenatal care (Stein, Lu, and Gelberg, 2000).

The health problems of homeless children, although similar to those of poor children, often have more serious consequences. Homeless children have poorer health than children in the general population, and they experience more symptoms of acute illness, such as fever, ear infection, diarrhea, and asthma, than their housed counterparts (Craft-Rosenberg et al, 2000). Homeless children living on the streets in urban areas are at greatest risk of poor health. Menke and Wagner (1998) compared mental health, physical health, and health care practices of homeless, previously homeless, and non-homeless school-age children; they found that homeless children demonstrated higher levels of anxiety, were significantly more depressed, and were at higher risk for physical and mental health problems than poor children who were not homeless. Homeless children are at greater risk for inadequate nutrition, which can lead to delayed growth and development, failure to thrive, or obesity. Homeless children also experience higher rates of school absenteeism, academic failure, and emotional and behavioral maladjustments. These children change schools frequently, which affects them and the school itself. When the children have inconsistent attendance or frequent school changes, they have a hard time keeping up with the work and progressing in a satisfactory way. The school also suffers when children drop in and out. This inconsistent attendance affects the teacher and classroom behavior, and it may affect school funding. That is, some schools are funded at the end of the year depending on how many students complete that year.

The stress of homelessness can be manifested in behaviors such as withdrawal, depression, anxiety, aggression, regression, and self-mutilation. Homeless children may have delayed communication, more mental health problems, and histories of abuse. As mentioned, they are less likely to have attended school than their housed counterparts (Craft-Rosenberg et al, 2000).

Statistics related to the number of homeless adolescents are often subsumed under the title *homeless children*. Homeless adolescents living on the streets have greater risk-taking behaviors, poorer health status, and decreased access to health care than teens in the general population. They are at high risk of contracting serious communicable diseases, such as AIDS and hepatitis B, and are more likely to use alcohol and illicit substances. Homeless teens often have histories of runaway behavior, physical abuse, and sexual abuse. Once on the streets, many homeless adolescents exchange sex for food, clothing, and shelter. In addition to the increased risk of sexually transmitted diseases and other serious communicable diseases, homeless adolescent girls who exchange sex for survival are at high risk for unintended pregnancy (Rew, 2002). Homeless youths often initiate sexual activity at an earlier age, are less likely to use contraception during the first sexual experience, are more likely to become pregnant, and are more likely to have multiple sex partners (Baer, Peterson, and Wells, 2004).

Homeless older adults are the most vulnerable of the impoverished older adult population. They have lived in long-standing poverty, have fewer supportive relationships, and are likely to have become homeless as a result of catastrophic events. Life expectancy for homeless older adults is significantly lower than for older, housed adults (Hwang, 2001). Permanent physical deformities, often resulting from poor or absent medical care, are common among homeless older adults. Homeless older adults suffer from untreated chronic conditions, including tuberculosis, hypertension, arthritis, cardiovascular disease, injuries, malnutrition, poor oral health, and hypothermia (Stergiopoulos and Herrmann, 2003). As with younger homeless persons, older adults who are homeless must focus their energy on survival, leaving little time for health promotion activities.

In sum, homelessness negatively affects the health of persons across the life span. Nurses must be able to identify the precursors to homelessness and anticipate the effects of homelessness on physical, emotional, and spiritual well-being in order to be able to advocate for effective prevention.

Federal Programs for the Homeless

The need for comprehensive, affordable, and accessible care for the nation's homeless population is huge. The federal government officially became involved with meeting the needs of the homeless in 1987 with the passage of the Stewart B. McKinney Homeless Assistance Act (PL 100-77). Title 11 of the McKinney Act provided funding for outpatient health services; however, the monies for these services were not large, and many needs go unmet. The McKinney Act grants homeless children the same access to education as permanently housed children. This act also created the Interagency Council on the Homeless (ICH) to coordinate and direct federal homeless activities. Housing assistance is available through the U.S. Department of Housing and Urban Development (HUD). HUD, along with many other federal agencies funds programs to help the homeless. In the section below on prevention, an illustration is given of how to access services in a state to assist homeless persons.

The ICH is made up of the heads of 16 federal agencies that have programs or activities for the homeless. The general goals of the ICH are to improve federal programs for the homeless through better coordination and linkages, decreasing the amount of documentation required to qualify for benefits. By targeting the most vulnerable segments of the homeless population, the ICH intends to influence the problem of homelessness. Children are a priority for the ICH.

Homeless families with children are eligible to receive shelter and nutrition assistance from the U.S. Department of Agriculture's WIC program. Persons receiving WIC benefits receive vouchers entitling them to free nutritious foods and infant formulas from local grocers. The TANF program can be a key source of income for homeless families.

Unfortunately, health care for homeless persons tends to be fragmented and limited in scope. Some of the most useful health care programs for the homeless begin with grants from private funding agencies, such as the Robert Wood Johnson Foundation and the Pew Charitable Trusts. Projects funded by these agencies have followed sound public health principles by encouraging community involvement, public/private partnerships, and commitment to outreach. Most of these projects rely heavily on nurse practitioners and physician assistants to deliver care in collaboration with physicians, nurses, and social workers. In recent years, many schools of nursing have received funding from the Division of Nursing in the USDHHS to establish nurse-managed centers for the homeless. Both faculty and students provide a range of services in these centers.

Levels of Prevention

Nurses need to understand how to apply the levels of prevention to homeless persons. When nurses advocate for preventive measures for people who are either poor or are homeless, they often invest time in activities outside the traditional areas of nursing practice. Nurses working in communities often need to advocate for affordable housing, community outreach services, preventive health services, and other assistance programs for poor and homeless persons.

DID YOU KNOW? *The website http://www.hud.gov has a wide range of services for homeless persons that are organized by state. Go to the website and choose, "Local homeless assistance," then select the state of interest followed by shelters that are organized by city or locality. Each state site offers extensive information for homeless persons beyond housing. Although each state has some unique offerings, they typically provide information about shelters, including special shelters for victims of domestic and sexual violence. The sites generally provide information about services for homeless veterans, persons with disabilities, transitional housing for offenders who are re-entering the community, and about meals, clothing, health care, skills training, counseling, and legal assistance. In each state, the agencies that provide the service are unique to the state. There are at least three common agencies in the states: the Salvation Army, United Way and Medicaid. (See http://www.hud.gov/homeless. Accessed July 19, 2010.)*

Preventive services related to homelessness include providing affordable, adequate housing. Aday (2001) identifies three major types of effective housing for prevention of homelessness and its complications: low-income, supportive, and emergency housing. Low-income housing refers to affordable housing that is available to all persons. Supportive housing refers to subsidized housing for vulnerable population groups, such as persons with physical and mental disabilities, women and children who are victims of abuse, and alcohol and drug users. Emergency housing refers to shelters for persons who are already homeless (Aday, 2001). Emergency housing is especially important for prevention of health problems for persons who are recently homeless.

It is difficult to separate services for homelessness into primary, secondary, and tertiary levels of prevention because interventions related to homelessness can be assigned to more than one level. Affordable housing, for example, may qualify as primary prevention, but it could also be an important secondary or tertiary preventive intervention.

Primary preventive services include affordable housing, housing subsidies, effective job-training programs, employer incentives, preventive health care services, multisystem case management, birth control services, safe sex education, needle exchange programs, and counseling programs. Nurses can form networks with other health professionals to educate policy makers and the public about the value of these preventive services. These programs could prevent homelessness from occurring at all, which would prevent many of its devastating sequelae.

Secondary preventive services target persons on the verge of homelessness as well as those who are newly homeless. Examples include supportive and emergency housing, targeted case management, housing subsidies, soup kitchens and meal sites, and comprehensive physical and mental health services. Nurses can work with homeless and near-homeless aggregates to provide education about existing services and strategies for influencing public policy that will provide more comprehensive services for homeless and near-homeless persons.

Tertiary prevention for homelessness includes comprehensive case management, physical and mental health services, emergency shelter housing, needle exchange programs, and drug and alcohol treatment. An important prerequisite for population-focused practice is a sound understanding of the sociopolitical milieu in which problems occur. Nurses can influence politicians and other policy makers at the federal, state, and local levels about the plight of vulnerable homeless populations in their community.

DID YOU KNOW? *Many states have programs that provide a broad spectrum of services that may interrupt the pattern of homelessness. Several follow the guidance of a program called HomeBase. The goal of HomeBase programs is to prevent and end homelessness. The HomeBase program in the Midlands of South Carolina was cited by the U.S. Department of Housing & Urban Development (HUD) as one of the 75 Best High Performance Projects that they sponsor. HomeBase in the Midlands of South Carolina is a project of MIRCI, which is a non-profit organization whose mission is to provide community-based services to persons recovering from mental illness or emotional disorders in their service area (Mental illness recovery center [MIRCI]. Available at http://www.mirci.org. Accessed April 17, 2011). HomeBase in New York City is a city-wide program that is part of the NYC Department of Homeless Services designed to help families and individuals overcome housing problems that could lead them to homelessness (New York City Department of Homeless Services. HomeBase. Available at http://www.nyc.gov.homebase. Accessed April 17, 2011). In Arizona, the HomeBase mission is to teach at-risk and homeless youth how to live healthy and independent lives (Homebase Youth Services, Phoenix, AZ. Available at http://www.hbys.org. Accessed April 17, 2011).*

LEVELS OF PREVENTION

Poverty and Homelessness

Primary Prevention
Provide health education in the local area for prevention of diseases related to multiuse of needles.

Secondary Prevention
Screen clients for early detection of drug use and the possibility of multiple users of needles; screen for diseases that may result from injection drug use: HIV, hepatitis, and other bloodborne diseases.

Tertiary Prevention
Implement more systematic programs for needle exchange; begin treatment for any diseases that are detected.

ROLE OF THE NURSE

Nurses play a critical role in the delivery of health care to poor and homeless people. To be effective, nurses need strong physical and psychosocial assessment skills, current knowledge of available resources, and an ability to convey respect, dignity, and value to each person. Nurses need to be able to work with poor and homeless clients to promote, maintain, and restore health. Nurses must be prepared to look at the whole picture: the person, the family, and the community interacting with the environment. The following strategies are important to consider when working with homeless individuals, families, and populations:

- *Create a trusting environment.* Trust is essential to the development of a therapeutic relationship with poor or homeless persons. Many clients and families have been disappointed by their interactions with health care and social systems; they become mistrustful and see little hope for change. By following through and doing what they say they will do, nurses can establish trusting relationships with clients. If the answer to a question is unknown, an appropriate response might be, "I don't know the answer, but I will try to find out. Let me make a few phone calls and I will let you know Friday." Reliability helps to build the foundation for a trusting relationship.
- *Show respect, compassion, and concern.* Poor and homeless clients are defeated so often by life's circumstances that they may feel they do not deserve attention. Listen carefully and empathize with clients so they know you believe they are worthy of care. Often, poor and homeless persons are not treated with respect and dignity by personnel in health care and social services. Because clients respond well to nursing interactions that demonstrate respect, it is helpful to use reflective statements that convey acceptance and understanding of their situation.
- *Do not make assumptions.* A comprehensive and holistic assessment is crucial to identifying underlying needs. Just because a young mother with three preschool children misses a clinic appointment does not mean that she does not care about the health of her children. She may not have transportation, one child may be sick, or she may be sick. Find out the reason for the absence and help solve the problem.

- *Coordinate a network of services and providers.* Working with poor and homeless people is challenging because of their multiple and complex needs. Many services exist, but often the people who could benefit are unaware of their existence. Developing a coordinated network of providers involves conducting a thorough assessment of the service area to identify federal, state, and local services available for poor and homeless clients. Where are the food banks? Where can you get clothing? What programs are available in the local churches and schools? How do people access these services? What are the eligibility requirements? How helpful are the people who work at the service agencies? What service is provided to eligible individuals and families? Nurses can identify these services and help link families with appropriate resources. In addition, a thorough assessment of available services for homeless persons in a nurse's service area can identify significant gaps in essential services. Once these gaps are identified, nurses can serve as case managers and work with other health care providers and with community members to advocate for necessary services for homeless clients.

- *Advocate for accessible health care services.* Poverty and homelessness create barriers that prevent access to health care services. Nurses can advocate for accessible and convenient locations of health care services. Neighborhood clinics, mobile vans, and home visits can bring health care to people unable to access care. Coordinating services at a central location often improves client compliance because it reduces the complexity and stress of getting to multiple places. Many homeless shelters and transitional housing units have clinics on site. These multiservice centers provide health care, social services, day care, drug and alcohol recovery programs, and comprehensive case management. Multiservice models are usually multidisciplinary. For example, midlevel practitioners (nurse practitioners and physician assistants), nurses, social workers, psychologists, child psychologists, and administrative personnel might provide a network of support for clients in shelters and low-income housing facilities.

- *Focus on prevention.* Nurses can use every opportunity to provide preventive care and health teaching. Important health promotion (primary prevention) topics include child and adult immunization, and education regarding sound nutrition, foot care, safe sex, contraception, and prevention of chronic illness. Screening for health problems such as tuberculosis, diabetes, hypertension, foot problems, and anemia is an important form of secondary prevention. Know what other screening and health promotion services are available in the target area, such as nutrition programs, job-training programs, educational programs, housing programs, and legal services. All these services may be included in a comprehensive plan of care.

| **HOW TO**   Evaluate the Concept of Homelessness |

- *What is it like to live on the streets?*
- *What issues might confront a young mother and her children inside a homeless shelter?*
- *How is it that people are so poor that they have no place to go?*

- *What really causes homelessness?*
- *How do you respond to the person on the street asking for money to buy a sandwich or catch a bus?*
- *How is your response different (or not) when a young mother with children asks you for money?*
- *How do you react to the smell of urine in a stairwell or elevator?*

- *Know when to walk beside the client and when to encourage the client to walk ahead.* This area is often difficult for the nurse to implement. Nursing interventions range from extensive care activities to minimal support. At times, nursing actions include providing encouragement and support, or providing information. At other times, nurses may actually call a pediatrician to set up an appointment for a sick child and may call again to see that the appointment was kept. Nurses assess for the presence of strengths, problem-solving ability, and coping ability of an individual or family while providing information on where and how to gain access to services. For example, a local hospital may provide free mammograms for uninsured women. Women who qualify for this free service may not take advantage of it because they are afraid that they may have breast cancer. Nurses can find out about this important service, inform the women of the service, teach them about the importance of preventive care, and assess and deal with fear and anxiety. The challenge for the nurse becomes choosing whether to schedule the appointments for the women or to simply provide them with a referral sheet, knowing that many will not follow through. The choice is not clear, but the goal is to make available a needed screening intervention without taking away the woman's right to decide what to do for herself.

- *Develop a network of support for yourself.* Caring for poor and homeless persons is challenging, rewarding, and at times exhausting. It is important to find a source of personal

---

🌐 LINKING CONTENT TO PRACTICE

When nurses provide care to people who are poor and/or homeless, they use the nursing process, which is a problem-solving process that is fully developed for public health nursing practice in the standards of practice (ANA, 2007). Specifically, nurses assess by "collecting comprehensive data pertinent to the health status of populations" (p 15); make a diagnosis and sets priorities; identify expected outcomes (standard 3) to develop a plan based on the population diagnosis and best practices (standard 4) for implementing and evaluating the chosen plan (standards 5 and 6).

Similarly, selected core competencies for public health professionals (Council on Linkages, 2009) can be clearly used in providing care to this vulnerable population. For example, two of the analytic and assessment skills call for assessing the health status of the population including related determinants of health and illness to describe the identified health problem. The competencies pertaining to cultural competency are important, such as "developing strategies for dealing with persons from diverse backgrounds" and considering the "role of cultural, social, and behavioral factors in the accessibility, availability, acceptability and delivery of public health services" (Public Health Foundation, 2009).

strength, renewal, and hope. The people you encounter are often looking to you to maintain hope and provide encouragement. Discover for yourself what restores and encourages you. For some nurses it is poetry, music, painting, or weaving. For others it is a walk in a peaceful place, a weekend retreat, a good run, a workout at the gym, or meeting with other nurses who are engaged in the same work. Be attentive to your own needs, and create the time and space to restore your spirit.

The Linking Content to Practice box describes how to apply selected core public health and public health nursing competencies to the care of poor and homeless people.

CHAPTER REVIEW

PRACTICE APPLICATION

Tonya Sims, a single mother with AIDS, lives in an apartment with seven other family members and her children, who are HIV positive. Ms. Sims does not often keep her children's numerous appointments at the immunology clinic. How do you respond?

A. Make an unsolicited telephone call or visit Ms. Sims and her family to let them know they are important and that you are thinking about them.

B. Call child protective services to report the failure of Ms. Sims to keep her children's appointments; she is non-compliant and neglectful of her children.

C. Do a more thorough assessment to determine why appointments are missed.

Answers can be found on the Evolve site.

KEY POINTS

- Poverty and homelessness affect the health status of people.
- To understand the concepts of poverty and homelessness, consider your personal beliefs and attitudes, your clients' perceptions of their condition, and the social, political, cultural, and environmental factors that influence poverty and homelessness.
- The definition of poverty varies depending on the source consulted. The federal government defines poverty on the basis of income, family size, age of the head of household, and number of children less than 18 years of age. Those who are poor insist that poverty has less to do with income and more to do with a lack of family, friends, love, and support.
- Factors leading to the growing number of poor persons in the United States include decreased earnings, unemployment, diminishing availability of low-cost housing, increased number of households headed by women (women's incomes are traditionally lower than men's), inadequate education, lack of marketable job skills, welfare reform, and reduced Social Security payments to children.
- Poverty has a direct effect on health and well-being across the life span. Poor persons have higher rates of chronic illness, higher infant morbidity and mortality, shorter life expectancy, and more complex health problems.
- Child poverty rates remain twice as high as those for adults. Children in single-parent homes are twice as likely to be poor as those who live in homes with two parents. Younger children (up to 5 years) are at highest risk for developmental delays and damage caused by inadequate nutrition or lack of health care.

- Poverty affects both urban and rural communities. The poorer the neighborhood, the greater the proportion of residents who are members of minority groups.
- At present, the following groups often constitute the homeless in both rural and urban areas: families, single mothers, single women, recently unemployed persons, substance abusers, adolescent runaways, mentally ill individuals, immigrants (legal and otherwise), migrant workers, and single men.
- Factors contributing to homelessness include an increase in the number of persons living in poverty, diminishing availability of low-cost housing, increased unemployment, substance abuse, lack of treatment facilities for mentally ill persons, domestic violence, and family situations causing children to run away.
- The complex health problems of homeless persons include inability to get adequate rest, exercise, and nutrition; exposure; infectious diseases; acute and chronic illnesses; infestations; trauma; and mental health problems.
- Nurses have a critical role in the delivery of care to persons who are poor and homeless. Nurses bring to each client encounter the ability to assess the client in context and to intervene in ways that restore, maintain, or promote health.
- In addition to interactions with individuals who are poor or homeless, nurses use the nursing process to assess and diagnose, and to plan, implement, and evaluate population-focused interventions.

CLINICAL DECISION-MAKING ACTIVITIES

1. Examine health statistics and demographic data to identify the rate of poverty and homelessness in your geographic area. What resources and agencies are available in your area to support homeless persons? What services are available from federal, state, and local sources? Identify a specific geographic region and assess this target area in terms of services for poor and homeless persons. Do a literature search to identify recommended state-of-the-art interventions for poor and homeless persons. Compare the recommended programs and interventions with those available in your target area. How does your area measure up? Give some specific recommendations about how you would fill the gaps.

2. Examine the specific programs identified in the preceding assessment. How do those who need services access them? Working with other students, make appointments with key persons in the agencies identified to find out what each agency offers, which particular aggregate is served, how clients access the services, who is eligible, how the agency receives funding, and what methods are used to evaluate the agency's ability to meet the needs of its targeted aggregates. Give some examples.

3. Identify nurses in your community who work with the homeless or with other vulnerable groups. Invite these nurses to come to a class meeting to share their experiences. What constitutes a typical workday? What are the rewards and challenges of working with vulnerable populations? How do they deal with the frustrations and challenges of their work? What advice might they offer to students working with vulnerable populations? What programs do they recommend? How would you advocate for vulnerable populations in your practice?

4. Imagine yourself as a nurse working in a homeless shelter or making a home visit to a family in an impoverished neighborhood. How have your life experiences and education prepared you (or not) for these situations?

5. Discuss welfare reform with other students. How does our welfare system work? Who receives welfare? Who is eligible for benefits? How do people apply for welfare? What are the strengths and weaknesses of welfare reform in the United States? What are the financial and personal costs of welfare reform? Identify federal and state senators and representatives in your districts. Where do they stand on the issue of welfare reform? Give details of your ideas for changing our welfare system.

REFERENCES

Aday LA: *At risk in America*, ed 2, San Francisco, 2001, Jossey-Bass.

American Nurses Association: *Scope & Standards of Practice: public health nursing*, Silver Springs, MD, 2007, ANA.

Baer JS, Peterson PL, Wells EA: Rationale and design of a brief substance use intervention for homeless adolescents, *Addiction Res Theory* 12:317–335, 2004.

Blank RM: An overview of trends in social and economic well-being, by race. In Smelsen NJ, Wilson WJ, Mitchell F, editors: *America becoming: racial trends and their consequences*, vol 1, Washington, DC, 2001, National Academies Press, pp 21–39.

Bremner RH: *From the depths: the discovery of poverty in the United States*, New York, 1956, University Press.

Craft-Rosenberg M, Powel SR, Culp K: Health status and resources of rural homeless women and children, *West J Nurs Res* 22:863–878, 2000.

Darmon N, Coupel J, Deheeger M, Briend A: Dietary inadequacies observed in homeless men visiting an emergency shelter in Paris, *Public Health Nutr* 4:155–161, 2001.

Dennis DL, Steadman HJ, Cocozza JJ: The impact of federal systems integration initiatives on services for mentally ill homeless persons, *Ment Health Serv Res* 2:165–174, 2000.

Ellen JM, Jennings JM, Meyers T, et al: Perceived social cohesion and prevalence of sexually transmitted diseases, *Sex Transm Dis* 31:117–123, 2004.

Emerson E: Poverty and children with intellectual disabilities in the world's richer countries, *J Intellect Dev Disabil* 20:319–339, 2004.

Evans GW, Boxhill L, Pinkava M: Poverty and maternal responsiveness: the role of maternal stress and social resources, *Internat J Behav Devel* 32(3):218–231, 2008.

Fass S, Dinan KA, Aratani Y: *Child poverty and intergenerational mobility*, NY, December 2009, National Center for Children in Poverty, Mailman School of Public Health, Columbia University. Available at http://www.nccp.org/publicatio ns/pub-911. Accessed January 4, 2010.

Federal Register: *The 2011 HHS Poverty guidelines*, Vol. 76, No. 13:3637–3638, January 20, 2011.

Fine S: The Kerr-Mills Act: medical care for the indigent in Michigan, 1960-1965, *J Med Allied Sci* 53:285–316, 1998.

Ford N, Cantau N, Jeanmart H: Homelessness and hardship in Moscow, *Lancet* 361:875, 2003.

Homebase Youth Services, Phoenix, AZ. Available at http://www.hbys. org. Accessed April 17, 2011.

Hwang SW: Homelessness and health, *CMAJ* 164(2):229–233, 2001.

Kamieniecki GW: Prevalence of psychological distress and psychiatric disorders among homeless youth in Australia, *Aust N Z J Psych* 35:352–358, 2001.

Kaplan GA, Siefert K, Ranjit N, et al: The black/white disability gap: persistent inequality in later life? *J Gerontol Ser B Psychol Sci Social Sci* 59B:S34–S44, 2004.

Katz MB: *The undeserving poor: from the war on poverty to the war on welfare*, New York, 1989, Pantheon Books.

Kelley-Moore J, Ferraro K: The black/white disability gap: persistent inequality in later life? *J Gerontol* 59:S34–S43, 2004.

Liz AK, Covinsky KE, Sands LP, et al: Reports of financial disability predict functional decline and death in older clients discharged from the hospital, *J Gen Intern Med* 20:168–175, 2005.

López-Zetina J, Kerndt P, Ford W, et al: Prevalence of HIV and hepatitis B and self-reported injection risk behavior during detention among street-recruited injection drug users in Los Angeles County, 1994-1996, *Addiction* 96:589–596, 2001.

Menke EM, Wagner JD: A comparative study of homeless, previously homeless, and never homeless school-aged children's health, *Issues Compr Pediatr Nurs* 20:153, 1998.

Mental Illness Recovery Center, Inc. [MIRCI]. Available at http://www. mirci.org. Accessed April 17, 2011.

Miller HP: *Poverty American style*, Belmont, CA, 1966, Dadsworth.

National Center for Children in Poverty: *Basic facts about low-income children in the United States*, 2005. Available at http://www.nccp.org.

National Coalition for the Homeless: *How many people experience homelessness?* July 2009a. Available at www.nationalhomeless.org. Accessed January 1, 2010.

National Coalition for the Homeless: *Who is homeless?* July 2009b. Available at www.nationalhomeless. org. Accessed January 1, 2010.

National Coalition for the Homeless: *Why are people homeless?* July 2009c. Available at www.national homeless.org. Accessed January 4, 2010.

National Low Income Housing Coalition: *Out of reach, 2007-2008*. Available from the National Low Income Housing Coalition, 1012 14th Street, Suite 610, Washington, DC. Available at http:www.nlihc.org/oor/oor2008. Accessed, April 17, 2011.

New York City Department of Homeless Services: *Homebase*. Available at http://www.nyc.gov.homebase. Accessed April 12, 2011.

O'Connell JJ, Mattison S, Judge CM, et al: A public health approach to reducing morbidity and mortality among homeless people in Boston, *J Public Health Manag Pract* 11:311–317, 2005.

Pilisuk M, Pilisuk P, eds: *How we lost the war on poverty*, New Brunswick, NJ, 1973, Transaction Publishers.

Price J: More mouths, more money, *Washington Times*:A6, April 19, 1994.

Public Health Foundation: *Council on Linkages: Core Competencies for Public Health Professionals* Washington DC, 2009, Author. www.phf.org/Link/competenciesinformation.htm. Retrieved 4/1/10.

Rew S: Relationships of sexual abuse, connectedness, and loneliness to perceived well-being in homeless youth, *J Specialists Pediatr Nurs* 7:51–74, 2002.

Roy E, Haley N, Leclerc P, et al: Mortality in a cohort of street youth in Montreal, *JAMA* 292:569–575, 2004.

Savage C, Lee RL: Caring for a homeless adult with a chronic disease. *Am Nurse Today* 5(3), March 2010. Available at www.AmericanNurse Today.com. Accessed March 2010.

Stein JA, Lu MC, Gelberg L: Severity of homelessness and adverse birth outcomes, *Health Psychol* 19:524–534, 2000.

Stergiopoulos V, Herrmann N: Old and homeless: a review and survey of older adults who use shelters in an urban setting, *Can J Psych* 48:374–380, 2003.

U.S. Census Bureau: *Current population survey*, Washington, DC, 2007, U.S. Government Printing Office.

U.S. Conference of Mayors: *Hunger and homeless survey: a status report on hunger and homelessness in America's cities, a 23-city survey*, Washington, DC, December 2007, The United States Conference of Mayors.

U.S. Department of Health and Human Services: *Healthy People 2020*, Washington, DC, 2010, U.S. Government Printing Office.

United States Department of Labor: Bureau of Labor Statistics. *Consumer Price Index*. Available at http://www.bls.gov/cpi. Accessed April 17, 2011.

Wilson WJ: *The truly disadvantaged: the inner city, the underclass, and public policy*, Chicago, 1990, University of Chicago Press.

Zedlewski SR: Family economic resources in the post-reform era, *Future Child* 12(1):120–145, 2002.

Zedlewski SR, Chaudry A, Simms M: *A new safety net for low-income families*, July 16, 2008, Urban Institute. Available at www.urban.org/url.cfm?ID=411738. Accessed February 26, 2011.

Zenk SN, Schulz AJ, Israel BA, et al: Neighborhood racial composition, neighborhood poverty, and the spatial accessibility of supermarkets in metropolitan Detroit, *Am J Public Health* 95(4):660–668, 2005.

CHAPTER 34

Migrant Health Issues

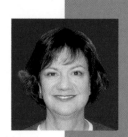

Marie Napolitano, PhD, RN, FNP

Dr. Marie Napolitano is an associate professor and the Director of the Doctor of Nursing Practice/Family Nurse Practitioner Program at the University of Portland. She has 22 years of clinical practice with migrant farmworkers and their families and has been a co-investigator on NIH pesticide exposure studies. Her areas of expertise include nurse practitioner education in the United States and internationally and the integration into practice of cultural considerations regarding immigrant and Latino populations. Her clinical interests include chronic illness self-care management for Latino individuals and families. She is Chair of the Migrant Clinician's Network Board and a member of the American Public Health Association's Caucus on Refugee and Immigrant Health.

ADDITIONAL RESOURCES

evolve WEBSITE
http://evolve.elsevier.com/Stanhope
- *Healthy People 2020*
- WebLinks
- Quiz

- Case Studies
- Glossary
- Answers to Practice Application
- Resource Tool 34.A: Resources for the Nurse Who is Working with Migrant Farm Workers

OBJECTIVES

After reading this chapter, the student should be able to do the following:
1. Define the term *migrant farmworker* and discuss the lifestyle and work environments that contribute to their health status.
2. Discuss the difficulties with obtaining epidemiological and health data on this population.
3. Describe occupational and common health problems of migrant farmworkers and their families and the barriers in securing health care.
4. Evaluate programs to determine effectiveness with encouraging health-seeking and health-promoting behaviors among migrant farmworkers and their families.
5. Analyze the role of the nurse in planning and providing culturally appropriate care to migrant farmworkers and their families.
6. Advocate for legislation and policy that would improve the lives and working conditions of migrant farmworkers and their access to health care services.

KEY TERMS

OUTLINE

Imagine yourself attempting to deliver treatment in a migrant camp to a toddler whose pertussis culture returned positive. The camp is located in an isolated rural community. The toddler lives in a trailer with her parents and siblings and extended family members (13 individuals). The family must also be treated as contacts. No one speaks English, so you have an interpreter with you. The family is just returning from picking strawberries all day in the fields, and they are tired and hungry. The family is willing to give medicine to the toddler because she is sick; however, they do not understand why they must take the medicine also, because they are not sick. The family tells you that they will not be able to take the noon dose because they have no water with them at work. Walking to the drinking barrel will take too long and they will lose income. As a nurse, what would you do? As a starting point, nurses need to be informed about the cultures, lifestyle, and health picture of the migrant and seasonal farmworkers and families that they serve.

Migrant and seasonal farmworkers (MSFWs) are essential to the agricultural industry in the United States. Although the availability and affordability of food in the United States depend on these individuals, their economic status and social acceptance have not reflected the importance of their work. Estimates of the numbers of MSFWs in the United States vary with the most commonly cited range between 3.0 and 4.5 million. Numbers vary because of differences in definition of migrants, divergent methodologies for estimating numbers, and difficulties in counting mobile populations. Standardized methodology for counting the farmworker population, developed by Dr. Alice Larson, has been used in 13 states with larger numbers of MSFWs. The majority of MSFWs are foreign born and predominantly Mexican (75%) (NCJN, 2009a). Traditionally, Mexican MSFWs have come from the west central states of Guanajuanto, Jalisco, and Michoacan; however, in 2009, 19 percent of MSFWs the non-traditional sending states of southern Mexico including Oaxaca, Guerrero, Chiapas, Puebla, Morelos and Veracruz (NCFH, 2009a "Migrant and seasonal farmworker demographics). Other workers include Central Americans, African Americans, Jamaicans, Haitians, Laotians, and Thais. The composition of the migrant and seasonal population can vary from region to region in the United States. Of the MSFWs, 47% are American citizens, legal permanent residents, or authorized to work in the United States (USDOL, 2005). Foreign-born farmworkers have spent an average of 10 years working in the United States. Approximately 29 percent have been in the United States for at least 14 years whereas 17 percent have been in the country for less than a year (NCFH, 2009a).

The definition of a migrant farmworker may vary depending on the level of government agency and by the type of service program. Federal statutes define a **migrant farmworker** as an individual whose principal employment within the past 24 months is in agriculture on a seasonal basis and who establishes for the purpose of such employment a temporary abode. **Seasonal farmworkers** work cyclically in agriculture but do not migrate. Although migrant and seasonal farmworkers comprise two distinct populations, they do share many demographic, cultural, and occupational characteristics. Much of the available information on agricultural farmworkers does not distinguish between migrant and seasonal farmworkers. Approximately 42% of hired farmworkers are migrants, but the numbers of migrants are decreasing as seasonal farmworker numbers are increasing (USDOL, 2005).

According to the National Agricultural Workers' Survey (NAWS) (USDOL, 2005), MSFWs are young with an average age of 33 years; 31% are less than 25 years of age. Interestingly, considering the nature of the work, 18% of MSFWs are older than 45 years of age. The majority of MSFWs are male (79%); they are married with an average of two children. Approximately two thirds of married migrant farmworkers based in the United States and 15% of those coming from another country are accompanied by family. The majority of MSFWs (81%) speak Spanish as their native language with nearly half unable to speak or read English. The average school grade completed is seventh grade, with 56% of U.S.-born farmworkers and 6% of foreign-born farmworkers completing the twelfth grade. In comparison, the recent Migrant and Seasonal Farmworker Descriptive Profiles Project (MCN, 2010) found more single men; fewer women and children (except on the West Coast); an increase in seasonal workers who no longer migrate; greater representation from Central America, the Caribbean, and Pacific; and shifting industry reducing traditional labor crops with less processing. Some regional results were that housing varied in terms of availability and quality, more indigenous individuals were found in the West with corresponding language challenges, and greater labor shortages exist in the West.

MIGRANT LIFESTYLE

Migrant farmworkers traditionally have followed one of three migratory streams: Eastern, originating in Florida; Midwestern, originating in Texas; and Western, originating in California. However, as workers increasingly travel throughout the country seeking employment, these streams are becoming less distinct. Migrant farmworkers are employed in fruit and nut (34%), vegetable (31%), horticultural (18%), field (14%), and miscellaneous (4%) agricultural venues (NCFH, 2009a). The cyclic nature of agricultural work along with its dependence on weather and economic conditions results in considerable uncertainty for migrant farmworkers. These individuals and families leave their homes with the expectation of work at certain sites. Word of mouth from friends or family, newspaper announcements, or previous employment help determine their destinations. However, upon arrival migrant farmworkers may find that other workers have arrived first or that the crops are late, leaving the farmworkers unemployed.

The way of life for a migrant farmworker is stressful. Some of the challenges of the **migrant lifestyle** are leaving one's home every year, traveling, and experiencing uncertainty regarding work and housing, isolation in new communities, and a lack of resources. The average farmworker spends approximately 6 months per year doing agricultural work, 8 weeks doing non-agricultural work, 8 weeks on the road, and 10 weeks of unemployment (NCFH, 2001). Farmworkers usually are paid an hourly rate (average $7.25) followed by piece rate pay. The specifics change depending on the location and type of work.

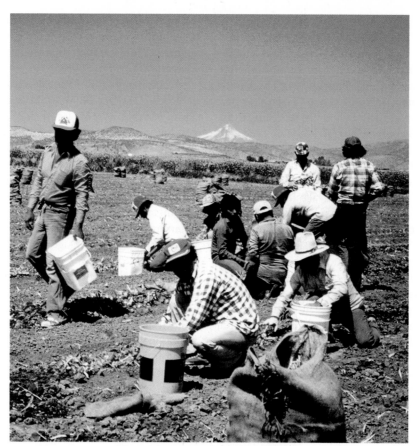

Migrant farmworkers working in fields.

Reports of average income for farmworkers have differed. The NAWS reported approximately 75% of MSFWs earn less than $10,000 per year and 60% of farmworker families have income totals below the federal poverty level.

Laws, such as the Fair Labor Standards Acts and the National Labor Relations Act, have been enacted to protect workers' rights (e.g., overtime pay, minimum age of employment). However, agricultural workers are exempt from these laws as well as from some Occupational Safety and Health Administration (OSHA) protective provisions. Where laws do exist to protect agricultural workers, they may be minimally enforced.

Migrant and seasonal agricultural workers are considered a unique vulnerable population because of their mobility, physical demands of work, social and often geographic isolation, language differences, and high rates of financial impoverishment (NCFH, 2009a). Although MSFW problems are numerous and creating solutions is difficult, some progress has been made in improving the condition of the farmworker population.

Housing

Migrant farmworkers often have trouble finding available, decent, and affordable housing. Housing conditions vary between states and localities, and housing arrangements and locations and types of housing differ for migrant and seasonal farmworkers. Housing for migrant farmworkers can be located in camps with cabins, trailers, or houses and be near farms. The author has seen migrant farmworker families living in cars and tents when housing was not available. The Housing Assistance Council (HAC), a non-profit organization whose mission is to improve affordable housing in rural areas, surveyed 4600 farmworker housing units across the country and found 52% of these units to be crowded by federal standards. More than half of the units lacked showers, a laundry machine, or both (Culp and Umbarger, 2004). This prevented farmworkers from removing pesticides from themselves and their clothing in a timely manner.

Because housing may be expensive, 50 men may live in one house or three families may share one trailer. Almost one third of migrant workers paid more than 30% of their total income for housing; those in the Western stream paid up to 43% of their total income. Many also support a home-base household. In addition to crowded conditions, housing may lack individual sanitation, bathing or laundry facilities, screens on windows, or fans or heaters. Housing may be located next to fields that have been sprayed with pesticides or where farming machinery poses a danger to children. Federal and state programs provide insufficient funds to meet the demand for farmworker housing.

HEALTH AND HEALTH CARE

The literature provides only a glimpse into the health status of migrant farmworkers. National data needed to present a clear picture of their health status are unavailable. Regional and local cross-sectional health status studies allow some insights. In the past, the most inclusive health data came from two reports from California: *Suffering in Silence: A Report on the Health of California's Agricultural Workers* (Villarejo et al, 2000) and the California Institute for Rural Studies (CIRS) Agricultural Workers' Health Study (Ayala et al, 2001). These reports showed a population at high risk for chronic disease, poor dental health, and mental health problems; higher rates of certain diseases such as tuberculosis (TB), anemia, diabetes, and hypertension; high levels of work injuries and chemical exposures; and detrimental physical and social environments for the children. Accurate morbidity and mortality data are difficult to obtain because of such factors as Mexican-born farmworkers returning to Mexico when no longer working, those farmworkers going back to Mexico to receive services, and easy-to-record infectious diseases decreasing (Villarejo, 2003).

Access to Health Care

The Migrant Health Act, signed in 1962, provides funds for primary and supplemental health services to migrant workers and their families. These funds are dispersed to 154 migrant health centers in 42 states that serve as models for delivery of services to a difficult-to-reach migrant population. Migrant health centers serve more than 760,000 individuals across the country (HRSA, 2008). However, estimates show that these clinics serve less than 20% of the entire migrant farmworker population (NCFH, 2005a). The others will seek medical care from an emergency department primarily or from a private physician, or they will not seek help at all.

Migrant farmworkers have limited access to health care. One survey indicated that one third of male farmworkers had never been to a physician or clinic and half had never been to a dentist (Ayala et al, 2001). Financial, cultural, transportation, mobility, language, and occupational factors are frequently cited as the major barriers that limit access to health care for farmworkers.

Factors that limit adequate provision of health care services include the following:

- *Lack of knowledge about services.* Because of their isolation, migrant farmworkers lack the usual sources for information regarding available services, especially if they are not receiving public benefits.
- *Inability to afford care.* The Medicaid program, which is intended to serve the poor, often is not available to migrant farmworkers. Workers may not remain in a geographic area long enough to be considered for benefits or they may lose benefits when they relocate to a state with different eligibility standards. Their salaries may fluctuate each month, making them ineligible during the times their salaries rise. Employers may not offer health insurance. Therefore, migrant farmworkers lack health insurance and state program assistance, which further hinders their access to care (Box 34-1).

BOX 34-1 WHAT MIGRANTS SAY ABOUT . . .

Health and Health Care

"What we have to do is reeducate our people and let them know that we have many rights to live and work and to educate and to have health care. And without health care, we cannot have the other three." Unidentified male farmworker, California

Work Conditions

"We're used to working. We don't want to be given things. We just want to be respected and to be paid the salaries." Teresa, California

"Right now, because I'm here today (testifying at hearing on work conditions), I may not have my job. Possibly I may not have my job tomorrow." Jose, California

"We have to get up at 4:00 in the morning so we can pick the strawberries until late—like 7 or 9—before they are too ripe." Unidentified male farmworker, Hillsboro, Oregon

Pesticide Exposure

"You go to the fields and you think that it's a foggy day because it's so pretty and it's white, but it's actually the chemicals that have been sprayed." Adelaide, California

"Pesticides presently occupy us tremendously during our work. We wear rubber gloves and that in itself creates a problem because it takes flesh, pieces of flesh from our hands." Guadalupe, California

"Pesticides only cause problems for people who are new to the work or have some physical problem or are weak." Unidentified male farmworker, Parksdale, Oregon

Housing

"My slogan is there must be a way to build houses. I believe we have the right to live in a decent way. We are the labor force. It's like we are foreigners—I am a U.S. citizen. Farmworkers come here with hope, but go home worse off than before." Unidentified male farmworker, Colorado

"We have no coolers in the summer and no heaters in the winter. Temperatures range up to 100 degrees in the summer and 30 degrees in the winter. We work out in the open for 12 or more hours and after working there for more than 12 hours, we have no place to rest. This creates a tremendous amount of frustration, not being able to provide the children with the minimum for comfort." Margarita, California

"The foremen even charged (the farmworkers) for sleeping under the trees." Teresa, California

Women

". . . Another thing I would like to mention is the way we are treated as women. As women we are discriminated with our co-workers because they see us as insignificant beings. The men think that they are superior." Maria, California

"I come with my uncle and cousin and I cook and clean for them—after I come home from the fields." Unidentified female farmworker, Cornelius, Oregon

Children and Youth

". . . (the children) go out to the fields. They lay under the trees and there is a residue falling on the children. They are picking grapes, what happens? The sprayers are there with the residue falling on the children." Irma, Oregon

"We have worked in the fields! Well, I'm not very young but I've left some of my youth in the work." Juliana, Washington

From Galarneau C, editor: *Under the weather: farm worker health,* Austin, TX, 1993, National Advisory Council on Migrant Health, Bureau of Primary Health Care, USDHHS.

- *Availability of services.* Immigrants are treated differently, depending on whether they were in the United States before the welfare reform legislation of 1996, and depending on the category of their immigration status. Each state determines whether to fill any or part of the services' gap to immigrants. As a result, many legal immigrants and unauthorized immigrants are ineligible for services such as Supplemental Security Income (SSI) and food stamps.
- *Transportation.* Health care services may be located a great distance from work or home, and transportation may not be available or may be too costly.
- *Hours of services.* Many health services are available only during work hours; therefore, seeking health care during work hours leads to loss of earnings.
- *Mobility and tracking.* While migrant families move from job to job, their health care records do not typically travel with them, leading to fragmented services in such areas as TB treatment, chronic illness management, and immunizations. For example, health departments are known to dispense TB medications on a monthly basis. Adequate treatment for TB requires 6 to 12 months of medication. The migrant farmworker who relocates must independently seek out new health services in order to continue medications. The Migrant Clinicians' Network (MCN) TB tracking program makes available to a farmworker's current provider any previous provider information that was entered into the tracking program. This tracking helps maintain continuity of TB care for a mobile population (MCN, 2005).
- *Discrimination.* Although migrant farmworkers and their families bring revenue into the community, they are often perceived as poor, uneducated, transient, and ethnically different. These perceptions foster attitudes and acts of discrimination against them.
- *Documentation.* Unauthorized individuals fear that securing services in a federally funded or state-funded clinic may lead to discovery and deportation.
- *Language.* The majority of migrant farmworkers speak another language as their first language, mostly Spanish, with a growing number speaking dialects. Although migrant health centers may hire bilingual staff, many emergency departments and private physicians' offices do not.
- *Cultural aspects of health care.* See the Cultural Considerations in Migrant Health Care section.

OCCUPATIONAL AND ENVIRONMENTAL HEALTH PROBLEMS

Agricultural work ranks as one of the most dangerous industries in the United States (Worker Health Chartbook, 2004). Agriculture has the highest fatality rate for foreign-born workers (AFL-CIO, 2005). Working conditions, such as standing on ladders, being exposed to chemicals, and using machinery, produce occupational health risks for the migrant farmworkers

who may be inadequately protected or educated. Lack of a comprehensive surveillance system makes it difficult to know the extent of all injuries within the migrant population. Injuries are unreported by farmworkers themselves for fear of loss of work and deportation. Injuries such as sprains and strains, fractures, and lacerations are the most common (Cooper et al, 2006). Other injuries include amputations; crush injuries from tractors, trucks, or other machinery; acute pesticide poisoning; electrical injuries; and drowning in ditches. Safety practices help prevent injuries; however, one study in North Carolina found that safety regulations are not consistently met especially during the middle of the season and that farmworkers tend not to practice safety behaviors, especially undocumented farmworkers (Whalley et al, 2009). This may be due to lack of knowledge, fear of losing time to work, or beliefs regarding who may be harmed.

The physical demands of harvesting crops 12 to 14 hours a day take their toll on the musculoskeletal system. Stooping to pick strawberries, reaching overhead while on a ladder to pick pears, or lifting heavy crates with straight legs all cause musculoskeletal pain. In one study, prevalence of chronic back pain among farmworkers and family members was 33% during the last migrant season (Shipp et al, 2009).

Naturally occurring plant substances or applied chemicals can cause irritation to the skin (contact dermatitis) or to the eyes (allergic or chemical conjunctivitis). The Bureau of Labor Statistics (2003) reported that farmworkers who work with crops have the highest incidence of skin disease of any industrial worker. Although skin diseases are common, farmworkers seldom seek care from health centers and mostly use self treatments (Feldman et al, 2009). Pesticides are found in both living quarters and the workplace of farmworkers. Pesticides include insecticides as well as pests such as insects, mice, and other animals and unwanted weeds, fungi, or microorganisms such as bacteria and viruses (Arcury and Quandt, 2009). Infectious diseases caused by poor sanitary conditions at work and home, poor quality drinking water, and contaminated foods take the form of acute gastroenteritis and parasites. Farmworkers have several risks for eye injuries because of the lack of eye protection devices, lack of knowledge about prevention of eye injuries, taking risks to save time (Verma, Schulz, Quandt et al, 2011) and exposure to chemicals, pollen, and dust. Heat-related deaths for crop workers exceed other types of workers (Luginbuhl et al, 2008). Cancer is another cited but not well-documented health problem for migrant farmworkers, mainly related to their exposure to chemicals. A high prevalence of breast cancer, brain tumors, non–Hodgkin's lymphoma, and leukemia has been found in agricultural communities (Larson, 2001; Ray and Richards, 2001). A registry-based case-control study of breast cancer in farm labor union members in California found that one crop (mushroom) and three chemicals (an organophosphate, malathion, and an organochlorine) were associated with breast cancer risk (Mills and Yang, 2005).

Pesticide Exposure

The vast majority of the North American food supply is treated with pesticides. Organophosphate pesticides make up the largest group of pesticides in current use. These pesticides are known to be potential hazards. Farmworkers are exposed not only to the immediate effects of working in fields that are foggy or wet with pesticides, but also to the unknown long-term effects of chronic exposure to pesticides. The location of the migrant farmworker's dwelling near fields or orchards can also be a major source of contamination for the worker and his or her family. The Environmental Protection Agency (EPA) and the Occupational Safety and Health Administration (OHSA) require that farmworkers be given information about pesticide exposure safety. However, migrant farmworkers may not receive this information, they may receive ineffectual training, or they may not understand the information (Napolitano, Philips, and Beltran, 2002; Whalley et al, 2009).

HOW TO Recognize the Signs and Symptoms of Pesticide Exposure

Signs and symptoms of pesticide exposure vary according to the amount and length of time of exposure. The majority of body systems can be affected by pesticide exposure.

- *Symptoms of acute poisoning include neuromuscular symptoms (headache, dizziness, confusion, irritability, twitching muscles, and muscle weakness), respiratory symptoms (shortness of breath, difficulty breathing, and nasal and pharyngeal irritation), and gastrointestinal symptoms (nausea, vomiting, diarrhea, and stomach cramps).*
- *Symptoms of chronic exposure will be related to such illnesses as cancer, Parkinson disease, infertility or sterility, liver damage, and polyneuropathy and neurobehavioral problems.*
- *Migrant workers may not understand exposure and may relate any symptom to pesticide exposure when the symptom cannot otherwise be explained.*
- *If symptoms of pesticide exposure are suspected, the nurse should develop a pesticide exposure history. A good example of an exposure form can be found at http://pesticide.umd.edu.*

Farmworkers may not have access to protective clothing or they may be unable to afford its purchase; alternatively, they may choose to disregard precautionary procedures and behaviors (such as wearing gloves) that affect their productivity (Arcury and Quandt, 2009; Napolitano, Philips, and Beltran, 2002). Some workers do not shower when they return from the fields because of their cultural beliefs about being exposed to cooler water while feeling hot from working. Although the worker protection standards are in effect to minimize pesticide risk, migrant farmworker families remain at high risk for exposure. Lack of resources for monitoring pesticide exposure, culturally inappropriate educational methods, migrants' fear of reporting violations and being fired, and language differences are just a few barriers that hinder a safer pesticide environment for migrant farmworkers.

Acute health effects of pesticide exposure include mild psychological and behavioral deficits such as memory loss, difficulty with concentration, mood changes, abdominal pain, nausea, vomiting, diarrhea, headache, malaise, skin rashes, and eye irritation. Not all health professionals are educated to recognize and treat pesticide illness and therefore might attribute the farmworkers' symptoms and physical findings to other causes. Death can result from acute severe pesticide poisoning (Moses, 1989; U.S. GAO, 2000). Also, chronic exposure may lead to cancer, blindness, Parkinson disease, infertility or sterility, liver damage, and polyneuropathy and neurobehavioral problems (U.S. GAO, 2000). Pesticides also lead to adverse reproductive and developmental outcomes (Arcury and Quandt, 2009). Goldman et al (2004) found pregnant women were not taking precautions against pesticide exposure; for example, they did not wash their hands before eating, wear protective clothing, or wash their clothes separately from other family members' clothing; they wore clothing and shoes from work into the home and ate fruits and vegetables directly from the fields.

COMMON HEALTH PROBLEMS

Migrant and seasonal farmworkers suffer from the same acute and chronic health problems as other populations in the United States. However, their lifestyle and racial or ethnic group membership place them at risk for health disparities compared with the general population. Migrants and their dependents have more frequent and more severe health problems than the general population in the United States (MCN, 2008). They experience many minor ailments. They also may not know that symptoms such as diarrhea or fever might indicate a more serious health problem, and they often do not seek early treatment. Migrants experience all of the health problems as does the general population. However, some health problems occur more frequently among migrant groups including diabetes, cardiovascular disease, asthma, tuberculosis and dental problems. In regard to dental problems an issue is that dental care is generally a low priority in migrant health seeking behavior (MCN, 2008). Lack of continuity of care and good record keeping often leads the children to being both over- and under-immunized. The most frequently seen minor pediatric problems are "rashes, strains, sprains, upper respiratory infections, otitis media, abdominal discomfort, diarrhea, urinary tract infections, anemia, lacerations, headaches, and dizziness" (MCN, 2008, p 2).

The financial status of 74.8% of farmworkers visiting federally funded health centers was at 100% below the federal poverty level (FPL). Over 54% were uninsured. Many employers do not offer health insurance, and migrant farmworkers may not be able to pay premiums or deductibles.

Because of the lack of access to health care and health care information, migrant women may not receive prenatal care. One study found that only 42% of farmworker women reported accessing prenatal services early in their pregnancy (first 3 months) compared with 76% nationally (Rosenbaum and Shin, 2005). The Pregnancy Nutrition Surveillance System found that more than 50% of migrant women had less than recommended weight gain throughout their pregnancies and almost 25% had undesirable birth outcomes, such as low-birth-weight, preterm births, and small-for-gestational-age babies (CDC, 1998). Pregnant women exposed to pesticides increases the newborn's risks for a variety of severe physical and neurological developmental abnormalities (Chelminski et al, 2004).

Food insecurity is a more prevalent problem in farmworkers than the general U.S. population (Cason, Snyder, and Jensen, 2004; Quandt et al, 2004). In Texas and New Mexico, 82% of farmworker families were found to have experienced food insecurity of which 49% experienced hunger (Weigel et al, 2007). Quandt et al (2004) found households with children have a higher prevalence of food hunger and used strategies such as borrowing money, reducing food variety, giving food to children first, and consuming less to cope with not having enough food.

Specific Health Problems

Among the Latino population in the United States, the prevalence of diabetes is estimated to be three to five times greater than that of the general population with higher rates of end-stage complications. In 2000, 2 million people, or 10% of Latinos (including farmworkers), were diagnosed with diabetes (Heuer, Hess, and Klug, 2004. The lifestyle of migrant farmworkers makes it difficult to obtain proper nutrition, adhere to weight control measures, and procure continuity of health care and medication administration necessary for good diabetes control. Migrant health centers participating in the Bureau of Primary Health Care's Diabetes Collaborative provide comprehensive and continuous diabetes care and monitoring for their clients. The MCN Diabetes Tracking Program allows providers to access information from any of the farmworkers' previous providers who participated in the tracking program, thereby allowing for better continuity of care (Box 34-2).

Dental disease is one of the most common health problems for farmworkers of all ages. According to the National Center for Farmworker Health (2005b), MSFWs have twice the rate of tooth decay and periodontal disease as the general population, and they experience more advanced periodontal disease. Migrant children also have significantly higher rates of tooth decay and lower rates of treatment (Quandt et al, 2007). Quandt et al (2007) found 80% of farmworkers in North Carolina had not received dental care in the last year and the few who had gotten care went to Mexico. Many of the people surveyed had inadequate knowledge of oral health and lack of access to care (and the resources to pay). Funding for increasing access to dental care has been insufficient to meet the needs of this

population. Without insurance or personal resources, private dentistry is usually not an option for the farmworker. Those migrant health centers with dental care have a high rate of use (HRSA, 2008).

Depression and stress are areas of concern among adult migrants, and this may be related to isolation, economic hardship, their legal status, poor living conditions and weather conditions that interrupt their work (MCN, 2008). Hiott et al (2008) found 38% of farmworkers report significant stress. MSFWs identify themselves as highly stressed even though they rate their physical health as good or excellent (Kim-Godwin and Bechtel, 2004). Magana and Hovey (2003) studied MSFWs' perceptions of stressors in their lifestyle in the Midwest. They identified 18 stressors, including being away from family, rigid work demands, low income, poor housing, exploitation by employers, limited access to medical care, and socialization of their children. High depression levels have been identified among migrant farmworkers and have been associated with such factors as high acculturative stress, low self-esteem, family dysfunction, ineffective social support, low religiosity, and lack of control and choice of lifestyle (Hovey and Magana, 2002).

Hovey and Magana (2002) found migrant women reported significantly more anxiety than migrant men and were at greater risk for anxiety from working all day, cooking, cleaning, taking care of children, experiencing sexual harassment, and seldom receiving maternity leave and prenatal care. Farmworkers, especially males, are reluctant to seek mental health care.

Drug and alcohol use in migrant communities has also been identified as a significant source of stress (Kim-Godwin and Bechtel, 2004). Drinking alcohol poses safety hazards for farmworkers, such as accidents while driving and workplace injuries. Alcohol can also contribute to health problems, violence in camps/home sites, and domestic violence.

Migrant farmworkers experience high rates of TB infection and positive TB tests (NCFH, 2005c) and significantly higher risk of dying from the disease. MSFWs are at greater risk for becoming infected with TB than the general population (Arcury and Quandt, 2007), at least six times more likely (Rhodes, 2009). One study in Connecticut suggested Latino migrant farmworkers may also have a high percentage of latent TB infection. MSFWs are at increased risk for TB because of higher rates in their countries of origin (Latin America, Haiti, and Southeast Asia), crowded housing, and malnutrition (NCFH, 2005c). Required long-term treatment is difficult to complete because of mobility, fear of deportation, language barriers, and lack of access to services. Incomplete treatment contributes to resistant TB. The MCN's TB tracking program fosters continuity and monitoring of TB treatment as migrant farmworkers move to different work and home sites.

It is difficult to obtain accurate HIV data for migrant farmworkers. Estimates are that HIV infection rates range from 2.6% of MSFWs with HIV to 13% (NCFH, 2005d, 2009b); however, the potential exists for already increasing rates to become epidemic (Sanchez et al, 2004). Risk factors for this population include lack of accurate knowledge, cultural, linguistic and geographic barriers to health care services, limited education, poverty, sharing needles for common medications such as

---

BOX 34-2   EXAMPLE OF ASSESSMENT WITH MIGRANT FARMWORKERS

The nurse, working with community partners and migrant camp gatekeepers, visits migrant camps to screen for diabetes (secondary prevention). If a high glucose level is obtained, the nurse refers the individual to a migrant health center or county health department clinic for a complete assessment. For those individuals in a given camp diagnosed with diabetes, the nurse plans and executes a culturally appropriate educational program on self care for diabetes (tertiary prevention).

vitamins and antibiotics, unprotected sexual activity, isolation and separation from families, available prostitution, and migration across borders that results in the spread of HIV (NCFH, 2005d, 2009b). Beliefs regarding AIDS/HIV also play a role in lack of preventive behaviors. Sanchez et al (2004) found that misconceptions existed, such as HIV no longer being a serious problem in the United States, that it only affects homosexuals, that one does not need be tested if the person looks healthy, and that HIV is curable. Farmworkers reported sexual issues are taboo and not discussed and that married men can have multiple partners (Washington Assoc of Community and Migrant Health Centers, 2003). Apostolopoulos et al (2006) stated that successful prevention efforts should include reducing migrants' social isolation and using their social networks while educating on condom use and increasing HIV awareness and testing.

Although a clear picture does not exist on the health status of the migrant farmworker population, available data indicate that this population suffers from challenging health problems and several health disparities that are difficult to address. Nurses can play a vital role in changing this situation.

CHILDREN AND YOUTH

Migrant farmworker parents want a better future for their children. In fact, this strong desire was the catalyst for many farmworkers to leave their country of origin. These children often appear to the outsider as happy, outgoing, and inquisitive. However, these children suffer from health problems including malnutrition (vitamin A and iron deficiencies), infectious diseases (upper respiratory tract infection, gastroenteritis), dental caries (from prolonged bottle-feeding, bottle-propping, and limited access to fluoride and dental care), inadequate immunization status, pesticide exposure, injuries, overcrowding and poor housing conditions, and disruption of their social and school life, which, not surprisingly, lead to anxiety-related problems. Only about 8 percent of farmworkers are covered by employer sponsored health insurance and 22 percent reported using needs-based services within the two years prior to the survey. The types of services were: Medicaid (15 percent); Women, Infants and Children (WIC) (11 percent); Food Stamps (8 percent) and Temporary Assistance for Needy Families (TANF) (1 percent) (NCFH, 2009c). Due to this limited health insurance it is no surprise that many farmworker children have unmet health needs, and those children who sought health care did not have a consistent provider and children were not on a well-child schedule (Gentry et al, 2007)

Some adolescents accompany their parents to work; however, other adolescents come alone or with others such as an uncle, cousin, or friend. Although the exact number of children who work in the fields is not known, farmworkers tend to be young. On average 33.5% are less than 31 years and 20% are between 20 and 24 years (NCFH 2009a). It is also estimated that about 6% of all farmworkers are between the ages of 14 to 17 years and that many of those children work "off the books" and cannot be documented as workers (NCFH, 2009c). Young workers experience greater health risks and loss of well-being. These youth are the most vulnerable to low wages, lack of education, social

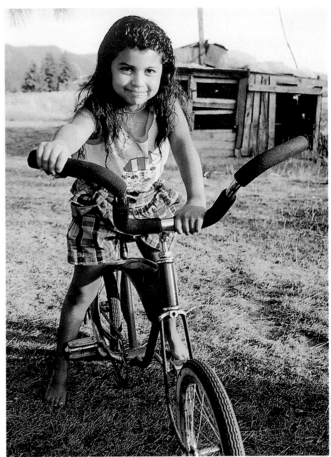

Children of migrant farmworkers experience many hardships. They may have to help with the agricultural work while trying to maintain their schoolwork and to fit into two different cultures. These can be difficult efforts, especially if the children have to move a lot or are frequently sick.

isolation, occupational hazards, and substance abuse and HIV exposure. Cooper et al (2005) found migrant youth were more likely to have been injured while working. Migrant adolescents have reported increasing substance use (Cooper et al, 2005). Salazar et al (2004) found that migrant adolescents believe that "weak" individuals were the most vulnerable to health problems and that being sick is an inevitable outcome of migrant lifestyle.

> **DID YOU KNOW?** *Farmworker children are excluded from the protection of the 1938 Child Labor Act. Children as young as 12 can work in the fields with parental permission. Children ages 16 and older may work in any farm job at any time, including performing hazardous work.*

Children of migrant farmworkers may need to work for the family's economic survival. The number of migrant farmworker children under age 14 is unknown. According to the Fair Labor Standards Act, the minimum age that a child can work in agriculture is 14 years, whereas the age is 16 in other industries. Children 12 to 13 years of age can work on a farm with the parents' consent or if the parent works on the same farm. Children younger than 12 years can work on a farm with fewer than seven full-time workers (Davis, 2001). Some additional protection is provided to children by the majority of states, such as limiting the number of hours per day and week a child can work.

Federal law does not protect children from overworking or from the time of day they work outside of school. Therefore, children may work until late in the evenings or very early in the mornings every day of the week if not protected by state law or if inadequately monitored. Personal communication with adolescent farmworkers in Oregon found that they were frequently too tired after working to do homework and to attend classes. In general, children of migrant farmworkers attend an average of 24 different schools by fifth grade (NCFH, 2005a). They leave school before the term ends to travel with their families and they arrive late to start school in the fall. Child farmworkers often attend three to five different schools each year as they migrate from one farm to another farm, and these frequent changes in schools and constant fatigue set these children up for failure. On average, farmworkers typically only complete the 7th grade. About 13% of child farmworkers complete 12 years of school (NCFH, 2001, 2009c).

Some children of migrant farmworkers stay home to care for younger children. Girls 8 to 10 years old remain at the camp site to care for their siblings and other children. The Migrant Head Start Program is a safe, healthy, and educative option for children 6 weeks to 5 years old (see Box 34-2). However, inadequate funding means there are not enough services for all migrant children. The Migrant Education Program is a state and nationally sponsored summer school program for farmworkers' children more than 5 years of age. However, this program is not available to all eligible migrant youth, especially those living in isolated rural areas.

Nurses can play an important role in the lives of migrant children, as portrayed by migrant children in southern Georgia. During focus groups, these children talked about the importance of nurses in their health and health care (Wilson, Pittman, and Wold, 2000). For example, one child said, "The nurses teach you how to stay healthy, like good things to eat, how to stay safe, and how to learn in school" (Wilson et al, 2000, p 143). Another child said, "The nurse also told us how to stay safe in our neighborhood, like staying away from people who drink and take drugs" (Wilson et al, 2000, p 143).

CULTURAL CONSIDERATIONS IN MIGRANT HEALTH CARE

To provide culturally effective care to migrant farmworkers, nurses need to become more knowledgeable about the cultural backgrounds of these individuals. Because the majority of migrant farmworkers are of Mexican descent, this section will focus on Mexican culture. Although certain health beliefs and practices have been identified with the Mexican culture, the nurse must remember that beliefs and practices differ between regions and localities of a country, and among individuals. Mexico is a multicultural country; therefore, the cultural backgrounds of Mexican immigrants vary depending on their place of origin. There are many indigenous groups in Mexico

that speak their own group dialect. Mexican immigrants may or may not understand or speak Spanish. Mexican immigrants who are less educated, have fewer economic resources, and are from rural areas tend to possess more traditional beliefs and practices.

Nurse–Client Relationship

The nurse is considered an authority figure who should respect (*respeto*) the individual, be able to relate to the individual (*personalismo*), and maintain the individual's dignity (*dignidad*). Mexican individuals prefer polite, non-confrontational relationships with others (*simpatia*). At times, because of simpatia, individuals and families may appear to understand what is being said to them (by nodding their heads) when in actuality they do not understand. The nurse should take measures to validate the understanding of these individuals. The Mexican individual expects to converse about personal matters (chit-chat) for the first few minutes of an encounter. They expect the nurse not to appear rushed and to be a good listener. Humor is appreciated and touching as a caring gesture is seen as a positive behavior.

Mexican clients may not seek care with health professionals first. Instead they may consult with knowledgeable individuals in their family or community (the popular arena of care) or with folk healers (the traditional arena of care). Examples of the members of the popular arena are the "senora," or wise, older woman living in the community; one's grandmother (*la abuela*); and the local parish priest.

> **NURSING TIP**   *If you work with Latino migrant workers, you may relate better with them if you learn some key Spanish words and phrases.*

Health Values

Family, in general, is a significant component of a Mexican individual's health care and social support system. The female in the household is considered to be the caretaker whereas the male is considered to be the major decision maker. However, Mexican females in certain families have significant influence over most matters including health decisions. Grandmothers and sisters are highly significant to the wife (female) in the immediate family. They provide advice, care, and support. Not all Mexican immigrants have extended families in the United States. If not present, communication may be maintained with family in Mexico, but a support system for these individuals may be lacking.

Love of their children, rather than concern for their own health, may encourage migrant parents to adopt healthier lifestyles. One example is when the parents of a child with asthma choose to stop smoking. In Oregon, when asked if they protected themselves from pesticide exposure, Mexican migrant parents responded negatively in general. However, they were willing to change their behaviors if, as a result, their children would be protected from pesticides (Napolitano et al, 2002).

The Mexican client may be more willing to follow the advice of another Mexican individual with a similar health problem rather than the advice of the health professional. The author found that Mexican women with type 2 diabetes were more willing to ask and adopt the practices of others with diabetes than follow the non-meaningful, redundant advice of physicians to take their meds, watch their diet, and exercise. One woman, who was unable to differentiate the symptoms of hyperglycemia and hypoglycemia, would drink a bottle of grape juice when she felt her "sugar high" as was recommended by her neighbor.

Although the majority of Mexican immigrants may identify themselves as Catholics, many Mexican individuals belong to other religious groups. The individual's religion may influence his or her health practices such as birth control; however, the nurse cannot assume that a Catholic, for example, will not use some method of birth control.

Health Beliefs and Practices

In the Mexican culture, health may be considered a gift from God. Another common perception of health is that a healthy person is one who can continue to work and maintain one's daily activities independent of symptoms or diagnosed diseases. The nurse should understand that a Mexican individual may not follow up with a clinic appointment because the client was capable of working that day. Mexican immigrants may believe that illness is a punishment from God and may cite this belief as a rationale for why therapies have not cured them. This more commonly occurs with chronic illnesses. There are four more common folk illnesses that a nurse may encounter with the Mexican client. These are *mal de ojo* (evil eye), *susto* (fright), *empacho* (indigestion), and *caida de mollera* (fallen fontanel). Symptoms and treatments may vary depending on the individual's or family's origin in Mexico. Other cultural beliefs related to hot-cold balance, pregnancy, and postpartum behaviors *(cuarentena)* have been documented. When experiencing a folk illness, the traditional Mexican individual would prefer to seek care with a folk healer. The more common healers are the *curanderos*, *herbalistas*, and *espiritualistas*. The most commonly used herbs are chamomile (manzanilla), peppermint (yerba buena), aloe vera, nopales (cactus), and epazote.

EVIDENCE-BASED PRACTICE

The High Plains Intermountain Center for Agricultural Health and Safety Risk Reduction Program uses long-term bilingual, intervention programs incorporating multiple integrative methods to improve farmworker safety. An evaluation study of this program showed that attitudes, beliefs, and knowledge of a farmworker influences his or her safety related behavior outcomes.

Nurse Use
Nurses can determine farmworker safety beliefs and practices on an individual level when assessing for health problems. In addition, nurses can develop focus groups of farmworkers to ask about work safety; they can plan and help deliver educational programs based on the results and evaluate effectiveness of these programs.

From Acosta MSD, Chapman P, Bigelow P, et al: Measuring success in a pesticide risk reduction program among migrant farmworkers in Colorado, *Am J Industr Med* 47:237-245, 2005.

HEALTH PROMOTION AND ILLNESS PREVENTION

The same principles of health promotion and illness prevention apply to migrant farmworkers as for the rest of the U.S. populations. However, health promotion and disease prevention may be difficult concepts for migrant workers to embrace because of their beliefs regarding disease causality, their irregular and episodic contact with the health care system, and their lower educational level.

Health promotion begins by asking farmworker families which health topics would be of interest to them and whether they are familiar with the available resources to improve their health. Several migrant health programs have recruited migrant workers to serve as outreach workers and lay camp aides to assist in outreach and health education of the workers. Nurses can be part of the planning and education of health workers for outreach educational programs. Evaluation to determine successful outreach educational methods can be undertaken by nurses. These activities demonstrate the core competencies related to the domain of community dimensions of practice skills for public health nursing (Quad Council, 2003). The skills include recognizing community relationships affecting health, collaborating with community partners to promote the health of the population, using group processes to advance community involvement, identifying community assets and resources, and promoting public health programs.

THE CUTTING EDGE *Nurses have the power to positively influence young persons to the profession by exposing them to our passions for practice, research, and education. One innovative program that provides Oregon nurses with an opportunity to influence high school students is the Apprenticeships in Science and Engineering (ASE) Program. This program was initiated in 1990 to address the growing concern over the quantity, quality, and cultural/gender diversity of the future workforce in the sciences, math, technology, and health arenas. Through the author, as an ASE mentor, several high school students have been exposed to migrant farmworker living situations and health needs in migrant camps in Washington County. They contributed to the evidence regarding the health needs of migrant farmworkers by completing a research project based on data obtained from a mobile van camp program.*

ROLE OF THE NURSE

As described below, nurses can use primary, secondary and tertiary prevention actions to help improve the health of migrant farmworkers. Primary prevention activities include education for the prevention of infectious diseases such as HIV, measures to reduce pesticide exposure, and immunizations in childhood and adulthood. Secondary prevention activities include screening for pesticide exposure, TB skin testing, diabetes screening and monitoring activities, and diagnostic testing done for prenatal care. Tertiary prevention includes rehabilitation for musculoskeletal injury, especially low back pain, and treatments for lead poisoning and anemia.

The health status of all people is a function of their ecology, or all that "touches" them. The nurse keeps a finger on the pulse

🔵 LINKING CONTENT TO PRACTICE

In this chapter, an overview of the lifestyle and health status of the migrant farmworker population has been presented. The public health nurse plays an important role in improving the health of this population. Core competencies within five of the Quad Council Domains of Public Health Nursing guide the nurse in working with migrant farmworkers. These domains are: (1) Analytic/Assessment Skills, which include identifying, describing and using data obtained from working with migrant individuals, families and groups; (2) Policy Development/Program Planning Skills, which are directed toward knowing and applying policies, laws, and regulations toward the delivery of health programs and the protection of the migrant population; (3) Communication Skills, which are used to identify health literacy of the migrant farmworker and to communicate in a linguistic and culturally appropriate style; (4) Cultural Competency Skills, which allow the nurse to function in a culturally appropriate manner and to assist the public health organization to become more culturally competent when serving migrant farmworker families; and, (5) Community Dimension of Practice Skills, which include use of community resources, establishing linkages between community partners to eliminate redundancy and better serve the migrant population, and maintaining partnerships with migrant leaders and agencies serving this population.

From Quad Council of Public Health Nursing Competencies, 2003. Available at http://www.sphtc.org/phn_competencies_final_comb.pdf. Accessed March 2010.

of the community by remaining active with political and social issues that involve the client. The nurse can be a catalyst for change to assess farmworker needs continually, to direct efforts to obtain needed health care services, and to evaluate the success of those efforts. Acting as a community educator, knowledgeable about how to obtain the latest information and resources, the nurse can work to assess the infrastructure and needs of the community. Follow-up on assessments by the nurse is critical. For example, the needs assessment might indicate inadequate child and adult immunizations in the migrant population, which may best be provided in the fields, camps, and schools. The nurse may instigate and lead in the creation of an immunization tracking system to share information with other counties and states as the farmworkers migrate.

Nurses can screen and monitor migrant farmworkers' health. Diseases such as TB, diabetes, and hypertension are often missed in a mobile population without regular access to care. Nurses can create screening programs in migrant camps and other farmworker housing. When problems are identified and treated, nurses can monitor the success of medication regimens, preventive measures, and follow-up with the health care system. The nurse can provide culturally specific health promotion and disease prevention programs and materials, as well as information about any further referral sources. The nurse can teach health promotion strategies to lay health promoters who then will educate the migrant community. Box 34-3 lists selected resources for the nurse working with migrant farmworkers. The Clinical Decision-Making Activities at the end of the chapter explore nurses' roles in various health care delivery settings.

The effectiveness of many existing programs dedicated to all levels of prevention and treatment for farmworkers have not

BOX 34-3 RESOURCES FOR THE NURSE WORKING WITH MIGRANT FARMWORKERS

Films and Videos
- Migrant Clinicians' Network (MCN) resource database: This comprehensive online database (http://www.migrantclinician.org/resources_intro.html) includes downloadable resources as well as links on a wide variety of primary care issues related to migrant farmworkers. Resources include links to other organizations, client education tools, clinical guidelines, MCN program materials, research guidelines, and others.
- *Un Lugar Seguro Para Sus Ninos:* Video developed as part of a research project with the Center for Research on Occupational and Environmental Health and Oregon Child Development Coalition (Oregon Migrant Head Start), 1999. (Contact the Oregon Child Development Coalition [phone: 503-570-1110] about availability.)

Written Materials
- National Center for Farmworker Health: *Monograph Series, Migrant Health Issues*
- National Center for Farmworker Health: *Factsheets on Migrant Farmworkers*

Organizations
Migrant Clinicians Network, Inc.
1515 Capital of Texas Highway South, Suite 220
Austin, TX 78746
(512) 328-7682
http://www.migrantclinician.org

National Center for Farmworker Health
1770 FM 967
Buda, TX 78610
http://www.ncfh.org

Farmworker Justice, Inc
1010 Vermont Ave NW, Suite 915
Washington, DC 20005
(202) 783-2628
http://www.fwjustice.org

📋 LEVELS OF PREVENTION

Migrant and Farmworker Health Issues

Primary Prevention
Teach migrant workers how to reduce exposure to pesticides.

Secondary Prevention
Conduct screening for diabetes in adult farmworkers and for anemia in children in camps.

Tertiary Prevention
Educate migrant families regarding appropriate nutrition for an adult with diabetes or a child with anemia.

been evaluated (Arcury and Quandt, 2007); therefore, opportunities exist for nurses to lead or participate in evaluation of these programs.

Nurses can be social and **political advocates** for the migrant population. Educating communities about these individuals, collecting necessary data on their lives and health, and communicating with legislators and other policy makers at local, state, and national levels are needed actions that nurses are prepared to undertake.

The health of the MSFW population warrants a variety of actions by nurses. Working with this population can be challenging. Insufficient resources, short-term stays in a community, barriers placed by growers, discrimination, and non-enforced legislation are just some of the obstacles that confront the nurse. However, nurses can make a difference in the health of migrant farmworkers and their families.

 HEALTHY PEOPLE 2020

Selected Objectives for Migrant Farmworker Populations

This box lists selected *Healthy People 2020* objectives that relate to health promotion and disease prevention in migrant farmworkers. They were selected on the basis of occupational, lifestyle, and socioeconomic factors that place migrant farmworkers and their families at unique risk for suboptimal health.

Environmental Health
- EH-10: Reduce pesticide exposures that result in visits to a health care facility.
- EH-19: Reduce the proportion of occupied housing units that have moderate or severe physical problems.

Immunization and Infectious Diseases
- IID-29: Reduce tuberculosis.
- IID-30: Increase treatment completion rate for all tuberculosis patients who are eligible to complete therapy.

Maternal, Infant, and Child Health
- MICH-10: Increase the proportion of pregnant women who receive early and adequate prenatal care.

Occupational Safety and Health
- OSH-2: Reduce nonfatal work-related injuries.
- OSH-8: Reduce occupational skin diseases or disorders among full-time workers.

From U.S. Department of Health and Human Services: *Healthy People 2020*, Washington, DC, 2010, Office of Disease Prevention and Health Promotion, U.S. Department of Health and Human Services.

CHAPTER REVIEW

PRACTICE APPLICATION

Maricela is 15 years old and has accompanied her uncle and male cousin to the camp to cook and clean the cabin for them. She also works in the fields picking crops in season. Maricela traveled the East Coast for 6 months with her uncle and cousin. Maricela is originally from Mexico and Florida is her homebase. One evening after finishing her work, Maricela asks to speak with Joan Lewis, the nurse practitioner whose medical van is parked outside the migrant camp where Maricela lives. She tells the nurse that her stomach has been hurting for awhile and asks Ms. Lewis for something to stop the pain. While assessing the complaint, Ms. Lewis asks Maricela what she believes has caused the pain. Maricela is very quiet and barely responds to the nurse. She does not make eye contact with Ms. Lewis. Maricela states that she probably ate something hot that upset her stomach. She seems to be in a great hurry and says she does not want her uncle to know she stopped by the van because he would be angry. Ms. Lewis, who speaks fluent Spanish, completes her history but Maricela does not permit the nurse to examine her abdomen. Maricela also would not talk about her last menstrual period. She asks for medicine again and gets up to leave.

A. What do you see as the important points regarding Maricela's situation?
B. What are cultural considerations that may impact the assessment of Maricela's complaint?
C. What could be the possible causes for Maricela's stomach pain? What is your rationale for each cause?

Answers can be found on the Evolve site.

KEY POINTS

- A migrant farmworker is a laborer whose principal employment involves moving from a homebase to another location to plant or harvest agricultural products and lives in temporary housing.
- An estimated 3 to 5 million migrant farmworkers are in the United States. These numbers are controversial because of the inconsistency in defining farmworkers and limitations in obtaining data.
- Migrant farmworkers are considered a vulnerable population because of their lifestyle and lack of resources.
- Health problems of migrant farmworkers are linked to their work and housing environments, limited access to health services and education, and lack of economic opportunities.
- Migrant farmworkers are faced with uncertainty regarding work and housing, inadequate wages, unsafe working conditions, and lack of enforcement regarding legislation for field sanitation and safety regulations.
- Farmworkers are exposed not only to the immediate effects in the fields (foggy or wet with pesticides), but also to unknown long-term effects of chronic exposure to pesticides.
- When harvesting is completed, the farmworker becomes simultaneously homeless and unemployed. Forced migration to find employment leaves little time or energy to seek out and improve living standards.
- Children of migrant farmworkers may need to work for the family's economic survival. They are most affected by the disruptive and challenging lifestyle.

CLINICAL DECISION-MAKING ACTIVITIES

1. Interview rural community leaders regarding migrant farmworkers in your area. What do business owners, teachers, clergy, politicians, and other health professionals say about this population? Can you identify misinformation or lack of information on their parts?
2. Outreach workers are personnel generally hired by an agency, such as a health department, to provide services such as education to migrant persons. Lay health promoters, often past migrants themselves, also provide community-based education. Find out if these roles exist in your community. Interview these individuals or accompany them in their work. Compare and contrast their roles. How are they complementary? How do they overlap? How can they work together to maximize health? How are their approaches to education different (e.g., does one use a protocol or template, whereas the other uses popular education techniques)? How does the outreach worker role and the lay health promoter role compare with the nursing role? How can the nurse work with the outreach worker and the lay health promoter?
3. Find an agency that visits migrant farmworkers in their housing. Ask to accompany them on subsequent visits. What is the condition of the housing? Are there deficits that could impact the health of the inhabitants?
4. Determine eligibility for Medicaid and Aid to Families with Dependent Children services in your state. You may consult the county health department and the state health department. Do migrant workers in your state qualify?
5. Design a temporary clinic to provide health care to migrant workers in your area during crop season. What services would you provide? What hours would you operate? How would you staff the clinic? Where would you get funds?
6. Below are a few settings and RN-delivered services for migrant clients. Can you propose others?

   Health department (generally state and county funded)—Nurses monitor communicable diseases and provide treatments for communicable outbreaks such as TB and pertussis.

   Migrant camps (generally funded through migrant clinics or health departments)—Nurses assess and triage, screen for disease, dispense medications under protocol, provide education, interview families, and coordinate care in conjunction with health department nurses.

   Migrant clinics (federally funded)—Nurses work with clinics' primary care providers, lead prenatal (both classes and home visits) and diabetes programs, educate regarding illnesses, and visit migrant camps to provide services or follow-up on clinic care.

REFERENCES

Acosta MSD, Chapman P, Bigelow P, et al: Measuring success in a pesticide risk reduction program among migrant farmworkers in Colorado, *Am J Ind Med* 47:237–245, 2005.

AFL-CIO: The urgent need for improved workplace safety and health policies and programs, *Immigrant Workers at Risk*, 2005. Report 1–22.

Apostolopoulos Y, Sonmez S, Kronefeld J, et al: STI/HIV risks for Mexican migrant laborers: exploratory ethnographies, *J Immigr Migratory Health* 8:291–302, 2006.

Arcury TA, Grzywacz JG, Talton JW, et al: Repeated pesticide exposure among North Carolina migrant and seasonal farmworkers, *Am J Ind Med* 53:802–813, 2010.

Arcury TA, Quandt SA: Delivery of health services to migrant and seasonal farmworkers, *Annu Rev Public Health* 28:345–363, 2007.

Arcury T, Quandt S, Cravey A, et al: Farmworker reports of pesticide safety and sanitation in the work environment, *Am J Ind Med* 39:487–498, 2001a.

Arcury TA, Quandt SA: Pesticide exposure among farmworkers and their families in the Eastern United States: matters of social and environmental justice. In Arcury TA, Quandt SA, editors: *Latino farmworkers in the Eastern United States: health safety and justice*, New York, 2009, Springer.

Ayala M, Clarke M, Kambara K, et al: *In their own words: farmworker access to health care in four California regions*, Davis, CA, 2001, California Institute for Rural Studies.

Bureau of Labor Statistics: *Incidence rates of nonfatal occupational illnesses, by industry and category of illness*, Washington, DC, 2003, U.S. Department of Labor. Available at www.bls.gov/iif/oschwc/osh/os/ostb1350.pdf. Accessed December 2009.

Cason K, Snyder A, Jensen L: *The health and nutrition of Hispanic migrant and seasonal farm workers*, Harrisburg, PA, 2004, The Center for Rural Pennsylvania.

Centers for Disease Control and Prevention: *Pregnancy-related behaviors among migrant farm workers—four states, 1989-1993*, 1998. Available at http://www.cdc.gov/mmwr/preview/mmwrhtml/00047114.htm. Accessed February 28, 2011.

Chelminski AN, Higgins S, Meyer R, et al: *Assessment of material occupational pesticide exposures during pregnancy and three children with birth defects: North Carolina*, 2004, North Carolina Health and Human Services Department.

Cooper SP, Burau K, Frankowski R, et al: A cohort study of injuries in migrant farm worker families in south Texas, *Ann Epidemiol* 16:313–320, 2006.

Cooper SP, Weller NF, Fox EE, et al: Comparative description of migrant farmworkers versus other students attending rural south Texas schools: substance use, work and injuries, *J Rural Health* 21:362–366, 2005.

Culp K, Umbarger M: Seasonal and migrant agricultural workers, *AAOHN J* 52:383–390, 2004.

Davis S: *Child labor. Migrant health issue—monograph series*, October 2001, National Center for Farmworker Health.

Feldman SR, Vallejos QM, Quandt SA, et al: Health care utilization among migrant Latino farmworkers: the case of skin disease, *J Rural Health* 25:98–103, 2009.

Gentry K, Quandt SA, Davis SW, et al: Child healthcare in two farmworker populations, *J Community Health* 32:419–431, 2007.

Health Resources and Services Administration: *Health Center: National Data*, 2008. Available at www.hrsa.gov/data-statistics/health-center-data/NationalData.html. Accessed February 2010.

Heuer L, Hess C, Klug M: Meeting the health care needs of a rural Hispanic migrant population with diabetes, *J Rural Health* 20:265–270, 2004.

Hiott AE, Grzywacz JG, Davis SW, et al: Migrant farmworker stress: mental health implications, *J Rural Health* 24:32–39, 2008.

Hovey J, Magana C: Cognitive, affective, and psychological expressions of anxiety symptomatology among Mexican migrant farmworkers: predictors and generational differences, *Community Ment Health J* 38:223–237, 2002.

Kim-Godwin Y, Bechtel G: Stress among migrant and seasonal farmworkers in rural southeast North Carolina, *J Rural Health* 20:271–278, 2004.

Larson A: *Environmental/occupational safety and health, migrant health issues—monograph series*, 2001, National Center for Farmworker Health. Available at http://www.ncfh.org. Accessed January 2006.

Luginbuhl RC, Jackson LL, Castillo DN, et al: Heat-related deaths among crop workers—United States, 1992-2006, Centers for Disease Control and Prevention, *Morbid Mort Wkly Rep* 57:649–653, 2008.

Magana C, Hovey J: Psychosocial stressors associated with Mexican migrant farmworkers in the midwest United States, *J Immigrant Health* 3:75–86, 2003.

Migrant Clinician's Network: *Migrant health issues*, 2008. Available at http://www.migrantclinician.org/migrant_info/health_problems.html. Accessed March 5, 2011.

Migrant Clinicians Network: *Tuberculosis*, 2005. Available at http://www.migrantclinician.org/excellence/tuberculosis. Accessed February 28, 2011.

Migrant Clinicians Network: *Migrant and seasonal farmworker descriptive profiles executive summary*, 2010. Available at http://www.migrantclinician.org/files/ExecSummFinal.pdf. Accessed February 28, 2011.

Mills P, Yang R: Breast cancer risk in Hispanic agricultural workers in California, *Int J Occup Health* 11:123–131, 2005.

Moses M: Pesticide-related health problems and farmworkers, *Am Assoc Occup Health Nurses J* 37:115–130, 1989.

Napolitano M, Philips J, Beltran M: Un lugar seguro para sus ninos: development and evaluation of a pesticide education video, *J Immigr Health* 4:35–45, 2002.

National Center for Farmworker Health: *Migrant and seasonal farmworker demographics*, 2009a, National Center for Farmworker Health. Available at http://www.ncfh.org. Accessed March 5, 2011.

National Center for Farmworker Health: *HIV/AIDS farmworker fact sheet*, 2009b, National Center for Farmworker Health. Available at http://www.ncfh.org. Accessed March 5, 2011.

National Center for Farmworker Health: *Child labor*, 2009c, National Center for Farmworker Health. Available at http://www.ncfh.org. Accessed March 5, 2011.

National Center for Farmworker Health: *Introduction. Migrant health issues—monograph series*, 2001, National Center for Farmworker Health. Available at http://www.ncfh.org. Accessed July 2005.

National Center for Farmworker Health: *Maternal and child health fact sheet*, 2005a, National Center for Farmworker Health. Available at http://www.ncfh.org/factsheets.php. Accessed December 2005.

National Center for Farmworker Health: *Oral health*, 2005b, National Center for Farmworker Health. Available at http://www.ncfh.org/factsheets.php. Accessed December 2005.

National Center for Farmworker Health: *Tuberculosis*, 2005c, National Center for Farmworker Health. Available at http://www.ncfh.org/factsheets.php. Accessed December 2005.

National Center for Farmworker Health: *HIV/AIDS farmworker fact sheet*, 2005d, National Center for Farmworker Health. Available at http://www.ncfh.org/factsheets.php. Accessed December 2005.

Quandt S, Arcury T, Early J, et al: Household food security among migrant and seasonal Latino farmworkers in North Carolina, *Public Health Rep* 119:568–576, 2004.

Quandt SA, Hiott AE, Grzywacz JG, et al: Oral health and quality of life of migrant and seasonal farmworkers in the US community/migrant health centers, *J Agricult Safety Health* 13:45–55, 2007.

Quad Council of Public Health Nursing Organizations: *Competencies for Public Health Nursing Practice*-Washington DC, 2003, ASTDN. Revised 2009.

Ray D, Richards P: The potential for toxic effects of chronic, low dose exposure to organophosphates, *Toxicol Lett* 120:343–351, 2001.

Rhodes SC: Tuberculosis, sexually transmitted diseases, HIV, and other infections among farmworkers in the Eastern United States. In Arcury TA, Quandt SA, editors: *Latino farmworkers in the Eastern United States: health safety and justice*, New York, 2009, Springer.

Rosenbaum S, Shin P: *Migrant and seasonal farmworkers: Health insurance coverage and access to care*, Washington, DC, 2005.

Salazar M, Napolitano M, Scherer J, et al: Hispanic adolescent farmworkers' perceptions associated with pesticide exposure, *West J Nurs Res* 26:146–166, 2004.

Sanchez M, Lemp G, Magis-Rodriguez C, et al: The epidemiology of HIV among Mexican migrants and recent immigrants in California and Mexico, *J Acquir Immune Defic Syndr* S37:S204–S214, 2004.

Shipp EM, Cooper SP, del Junco DJ, et al: Chronic back pain and associated work and non-work variables from farmworkers from Starr County, Texas, *J Agromed* 14:22–32, 2009.

U.S. Department of Labor: *A demographic and employment profile of the United States farm workers, findings from the National Agricultural Workers Survey (NAWS) 2001-2002*, Burlingame, CA, 2005, OSDOL, Office of the Assistant Secretary for Policy.

U.S. General Accounting Office: *Pesticides: improvements needed to ensure the safety of farmworkers and their children*, Washington, DC, 2000, GAO/RCED-00–40.

Verma A, Schulz MR, Quandt SA, et al: Eye health and safety among Latino farmworkers, *Agromedicine* 16(2):143–152, 2011.

Villarejo D: The health of U.S. hired farm workers, *Annu Rev Public Health* 24:175–193, 2003.

Villarejo D, Lighthall D, Williams D III, et al: *Suffering in silence: a report on the health of California's agricultural workers*, Davis, CA, 2000, California Institute for Rural Studies.

Washington Association of Community and Migrant Health Centers: *HIV/AIDS knowledge and prevention needs assessment of migrant seasonal farm workers*, 2003, p 11. Available at http:wacmhc.org.

Weigel MM, Armijos RX, Hall YP, et al: The household food insecurity and health outcomes of U.S.-Mexico border migrant and seasonal farmworkers, *J Immigr Minor Health* 9:157–169, 2007.

Whalley LE, Grzywacz JG, Quandt SA, et al: Migrant farmworker field and camp safety and sanitation in eastern North Carolina, *J Agromed* 14:421–436, 2009.

Wilson A, Pittman K, Wold J: Listening to the quiet voices of Hispanic migrant children about health, *J Pediatr Nurs* 15:137–147, 2000.

Worker Health Chartbook: *Chapter 3: Focus on Agriculture*, 2004. Available at http://www.cdc.gov/niosh/docs/2004-146/ch3/ch3-1.asp.htm. Accessed February 28, 2011.

CHAPTER 35

Teen Pregnancy

Dyan A. Aretakis, RN, FNP, MSN

Dyan A. Aretakis began her nursing practice in pediatrics at the University of Connecticut and at a regional residential facility for the mentally retarded. She went on to co-develop a model teen health center at the University of Virginia Health System in 1990 and currently practices in and directs its daily and long-term programs. This program is unique because it provides a range of adolescent primary health care services as well as community and professional outreach programs.

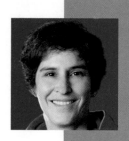

ADDITIONAL RESOURCES

evolve WEBSITE
http://evolve.elsevier.com/Stanhope
- *Healthy People 2020*
- WebLinks

- Quiz
- Case Studies
- Glossary
- Answers to Practice Application

OBJECTIVES

After reading this chapter, the student should be able to do the following:

1. Discuss approaches that could be used in working with the adolescent client.
2. Identify trends in adolescent pregnancy, births, abortions, and adoption in the United States.
3. Discuss reasons that may affect whether a teenager becomes pregnant.
4. Explain some of the deterrents to the establishment of paternity among young fathers.
5. Develop nursing interventions for the prevention of pregnancy problems that adolescents are at risk for experiencing.
6. Identify nursing activities that may contribute to the prevention of adolescent pregnancy.

KEY TERMS

abortion, p. 771
adoption, p. 773
birth control, p. 770
coercive sex, p. 773
gynecological age, p. 778
intimate partner violence, p. 777

long-acting contraceptive, p. 770
low birth weight, p. 779
non-genital sexual behavior, p. 771
paternity, p. 775
peer pressure, p. 773
prematurity, p. 779

prenatal care, p. 776
repeat pregnancy, p. 780
sexual debut, p. 772
sexual victimization, p. 773
statutory rape, p. 773
weight gain, p. 778
—*See Glossary for definitions*

OUTLINE

Teen pregnancy is an area of public concern because of its significant effect on communities. Resources to support the special needs of pregnant teenagers are decreasing, and the costs of sustaining young families are prohibitive. Many teenagers who become pregnant are caught in a cycle of poverty, school failure, and limited life options. Even under the ideal circumstances of adequate finances, loving and supportive families, and good birth outcomes, a teen mother must circumvent her own necessary developmental tasks to raise her child.

> **DID YOU KNOW?** *In 2004 the taxpayers' costs of teen childbearing in the United States were $9.1 billion. This includes costs of public health care, child welfare, incarceration, and lost tax revenue by the children born to teen mothers. In contrast, the decline by one third in the teen birth rate from 1991 to 2004 allowed a decrease in costs by $6.7 billion in 2004. Delaying a birth until the age of 18 saves over $2600 per individual per year (Hoffman, 2006).*

There is neither a uniform reason that teens become pregnant nor a universally acceptable solution. The causes of teen pregnancy are diverse and affected by changing moral attitudes, sexual codes, and economic circumstances. Teen pregnancy places an enormous strain on the health care and social service systems. Social concern is also raised about the lost potential for young parents when pregnancy occurs, and the academic and economic disadvantages that their children will experience. Nurses are in a key position to understand how teen pregnancy affects both the individual and the community. This chapter presents a variety of issues associated with teen pregnancy and proposes nursing interventions to promote healthy outcomes for individuals and communities.

ADOLESCENT HEALTH CARE IN THE UNITED STATES

Adolescents are generally healthy, and when they seek health care it is for reasons different from those of adults or young children. The main causes of teen mortality are high-risk behaviors: motor vehicle accidents (usually including alcohol), homicide, suicide, and accidental injuries (such as falls, fires, or drowning). Teens often engage in behaviors that put them at risk for life-threatening diseases. For example, each year, one fourth of both new human immunodeficiency virus (HIV) infections and newly identified sexually transmitted diseases (STDs) occur among adolescents. During the teen years, other behaviors are initiated (e.g., smoking, decreased activity, and poor nutrition) that can ultimately lead to poor health as well as influence behavior change that can significantly alter a young person's life.

National surveys highlight the health issues facing adolescents. There have been some improvements in risk behaviors as well as a worsening of others. Among ninth to twelfth graders participating in the 2007 Youth Risk Behavior Surveillance System, fewer teens reported riding in a car with a driver who had been drinking, currently smoking cigarettes or marijuana, trying methamphetamines, or attempting suicide. However, these and other significant risk behaviors continued at high rates. Of ninth to twelfth graders, 44.7% reported current alcohol use (26% reported episodic heavy drinking); 20% of teens were current cigarette smokers; and 38% had tried marijuana (19% were current users and 8% tried it before the age of 13). Mental health issues are also strongly associated with the adolescent years: 28.5% of students reported feeling sad or hopeless for more than 2 weeks; 35% of females and 21% of males reported these symptoms. Suicidal thoughts with a plan existed for 11.3% of students nationwide, and suicide was attempted by 9% of girls and 4% of boys (CDC, 2008).

Adolescents may not seek care for these problems for the following reasons: (1) access to health care may be hindered due to a limited number of professionals with expertise in dealing with teenagers, (2) costs of care or availability of insurance may limit services, (3) adolescents need to believe that their visits are confidential before they will honestly reveal information, and (4) health care professionals must be able to discuss sensitive topics in a non-judgmental and supportive manner and demonstrate a desire to work with youths. Nurses who want to promote the health of adolescents by providing anticipatory guidance about peer pressure, assertiveness, and future planning need to understand adolescent behaviors, health risks, and the social context in which they live. Involvement and education of the parents about youth culture and development can promote positive and supportive parenting of teens.

THE ADOLESCENT CLIENT

Adolescents have limited experience in independently seeking health care. When they do seek care, it is often to discuss concerns about a possible pregnancy or to find a **birth control** method. These teens may also need assistance negotiating complex health care systems. Special approaches in both client interview and subsequent client education are often warranted. The behavior of adolescents toward the nurse can range from mature and competent during one visit to hostile, rude, or distant at other times because behavior often reflects intense anxiety over what the teen is experiencing.

Because client interviews usually begin with evaluation of a chief complaint, teens need to know that their concerns are heard. Health care providers may have their own opinions about what teenagers need and may fail to take the chief complaint seriously. For example, when a teen expresses ambivalence about or a desire to become pregnant, this should be discussed in depth even though the nurse may feel uncomfortable when asked to provide information to a teen about how to conceive. During this interview, the nurse can provide preconception counseling and emphasize the need to achieve good health and to establish a health-promoting lifestyle before pregnancy. Health risks to the mother, as well as to fetal development, can be discussed. The nurse can encourage a young person to consider lifetime goals and discuss how parenthood might affect them. Not only does information presented this way demonstrate that the nurse has heard what the teen is saying, but it also allows the nurse to provide useful health information that may encourage the teen to examine her plans carefully, seriously, and maturely.

> **DID YOU KNOW?**   *One technique for contraceptive counseling is to have a young woman discuss her plans for childbearing. When the goal is to complete high school (or college) or reach a certain age/status prior to having children, that information can be a starting point in discussions about options for preventing pregnancy. A **long-acting contraceptive** (e.g., a 3- or 5-year method) can be an excellent option that would help her attain these goals.*

It is also important to pay attention to what the teen *fails* to verbalize. Knowledge of adolescent health care issues is valuable so that the nurse can anticipate other health concerns and provide an environment in which the adolescent feels safe about discussing other issues. By creating a caring and understanding atmosphere, the nurse can encourage the young person to discuss concerns about family violence, drugs, alcohol, or dating.

Discussing reproductive health care is a sensitive matter for both teens and many adults. Teens may have difficulty expressing themselves because of a limited sexual vocabulary or embarrassment resulting from their lack of knowledge. The

BOX 35-1	**SEXUALLY TRANSMITTED DISEASES AND TEEN PREGNANCY**

Sexually transmitted diseases (STDs) affect 25% of sexually experienced teenagers each year. STDs are more easily transmitted to women than men. STD infections among women can contribute to infertility, cancer, and ectopic pregnancy. When a young woman is pregnant, these infections can cause premature rupture of membranes, premature labor, and postpartum infection. Also, the baby can be affected by all STDs in several ways: prematurity and low birth weight, febrile infection after delivery, long-term infection, and even death (e.g., exposure to viral infections such as human papillomavirus and herpes simplex virus).

The pregnant adolescent is at high risk for acquiring an STD because she may not be using barrier protection (e.g., condoms). During the pregnancy, she will require periodic STD screening. STD education and counseling should accompany this screening. Information given should include ways to reduce risk, such as maintaining a mutually monogamous relationship and using latex condoms.

nurse must recognize this potential deficit and embarrassment and assist teens by anticipating concerns. It is also important to allow teens to express themselves in their own language, which may include crude or offensive words. Nurses must learn about common slang expressions and common misconceptions so they do not miss important concerns that a teenager might have. The nurse can offer more appropriate terms once trust is established.

Teens may have difficulty discussing topics that provoke a judgmental reaction, such as discussing STDs (Box 35-1). The nurse can choose neutral words to evaluate symptoms (e.g., "Has there been a change in your typical vaginal discharge?"). This approach also gives the nurse a chance to educate the young client about normal anatomy and physiology.

Considerable debate exists over whether adolescents should make reproductive health care decisions without their parents' knowledge. As seen in Box 35-2, the adolescent's right for access to contraceptive treatment is established by federal law. Obstacles to services do exist, however, and this may result in a teen not receiving contraceptive information and treatment. Obstacles can include lack of transportation to a health care facility, insufficient money to pay for services, or permission to leave school early to attend an appointment.

Although most minor teens can consent to birth control services in the United States, there is great variability in who may access and release their medical records. In recognition of the importance of confidentiality in reproductive health care, federal privacy rules were established in 2002 as follow up to the Health Insurance Portability and Accountability Act of 1996 (HIPAA). This rule, the HIPAA Privacy Rule (or more correctly, the Standards for Privacy of Individually Identifiable Health Information), established that if a minor consented to care, then only that individual could access and release those medical records. However, the Privacy Rule also deferred to existing state law. In many states the laws specify that parents can legally access all the medical records of their minor children (English, 2007; English and Kenney, 2010), which limits the

---

BOX 35-2 **REPRODUCTIVE HEALTH CARE AND ADOLESCENTS' RIGHTS**

No federal regulation requires a young person to have parents involved in decisions on contraception services provided by federal programs. States cannot prohibit an adolescent access to contraception. Several Supreme Court decisions protect this access:

- 1965: *Griswold v. Connecticut*—the right to prevent pregnancy through the use of contraceptives is protected by the right to privacy.
- 1972: *Eisenstad v. Baird*—the right to privacy in contraceptive use is extended to unmarried individuals.
- 1977: *Carey v. Population Services International*—the right to privacy is specifically extended to minors.

Modified from National Abortion and Reproductive Rights Action League Foundation: *Supreme Court decisions concerning reproductive rights, a chronology: 1965-2006,* Washington, DC, 2007, NARAL.

---

confidentiality assurances offered to a teen seeking reproductive health care. It is incumbent on nurses working with teens to be knowledgeable about state and federal laws so they can accurately inform teenagers of their rights and limitations in seeking reproductive health care.

> **THE CUTTING EDGE** *The nurse who is knowledgeable about **non-genital sexual behavior** among teens can incorporate appropriate safer-sex messages into educational programs.*

Abortion services for adolescents are not clearly defined. No federal protection is extended to adolescents requesting abortion services, and the adolescent's right to privacy and ability to give consent varies by state (Box 35-3). Confidential care to teenagers may mean the difference in preventing an unwanted pregnancy, an abortion, and a birth. This care can influence whether prenatal visits begin in the first trimester or in the second or third trimester. Teens have various reasons for pursuing confidential care, including seeking independence as well as serious and well-founded concerns about a parent's potential reaction (e.g., abuse of the teen). Once nurses recognize the reason for confidential care, they can work with teens to discuss reproductive health care needs with the family. To do so, first clarify family values about sexuality and family communication styles with the teen. In a non-healthy family, referral to community agencies (e.g., child protective services, Al-Anon) may be necessary. However, the nurse may need to honor the adolescent's need for confidentiality for an unknown period and proceed with the usual interventions, such as pregnancy testing, options counseling, and referral for clinical care.

TRENDS IN ADOLESCENT SEXUAL BEHAVIOR, PREGNANCY, AND CHILDBEARING

In 2009, there were 414,870 births to women under age 20. These numbers represent a 2-year increase in birth rates. The birth rate in the United States remains higher than in any other developed nation (Ikramullah, Barry, Manlove, and Moore, 2011). The

---

BOX 35-3 **ABORTION AND ADOLESCENT RIGHTS**

- *Parental consent laws:* One or both parents of a young woman who is under 18 years of age seeking an abortion must give permission to the abortion provider before the abortion is performed. There are 38 states with enforceable mandatory consent and notice laws. They are: Alaska, Alabama, Arkansas, Arizona, Colorado, Delaware, Florida, Georgia, Idaho, Indiana, Illinois, Kansas, Kentucky, Louisiana, Maine, Maryland, Massachusetts, Michigan, Mississippi, Minnesota, Missouri, Nebraska, North Carolina, North Dakota, Ohio, Oklahoma, Pennsylvania, Rhode Island, South Carolina, South Dakota, Tennessee, Texas, Utah, Virginia, West Virginia, Wisconsin, and Wyoming.
- *Parental notification laws:* One or both parents of a young woman seeking an abortion must be notified by the abortion provider before the abortion is performed. These laws are in 15 states: Colorado, Delaware, Florida, Georgia, Iowa, Illinois, Kansas, Maryland, Minnesota, Montana, Nebraska, Nevada, New Jersey, South Dakota, and West Virginia.
- *Parental notification and consent laws:* One or both parents of a young woman seeking an abortion must be notified and provide consent before the abortion is performed. These laws are enforced in 5 states: Oklahoma, Texas, Utah, Virginia, and Wyoming.
- *The following states (11) with parental notification or consent laws permit other trusted adults to stand in for a parent:* Arizona, Colorado, Delaware, Illinois, Idaho, Maine, North Carolina, Pennsylvania, South Carolina, Virginia, and Wisconsin.
- *The following states (6) have laws that have been found unconstitutional and unenforceable:* Arkansas, California, Montana, Nevada, New Jersey, and New Mexico.
- *Judicial bypass:* In a 1979 Supreme Court decision, it was ruled that any mandatory parental consent law must allow the young woman an opportunity to be granted an exception or waiver to the law. A young woman could appeal directly to a judge, who would decide either that she was mature enough to make this decision or that the abortion would be in her best interest.

Data from National Abortion and Reproductive Rights Action League Foundation: *Who decides? A state-by-state review of abortion and reproductive rights,* ed 19, Washington, DC, 2010, NARAL. Available at http://www.prochoiceamerica.org. Accessed March 9, 2011.

---

numbers of teens who become pregnant are generally identified in the following way: by age group (e.g., younger than 15, ages 15-17, ages 18-19, and under age 20); by states, by marital status; by rates (e.g., number of pregnancies, births, and abortions per 1000 young women); and by race/ethnicity (e.g., African American, white, Hispanic/Latino). Births to teenagers make up 11% of all births in the United States (Ikramullah et al, 2011). Teen birth rates increase by age, with the highest rates occurring among 19-year-olds. Pregnancy and birthrates increased steadily among teens of all ages from 1986 to 1991 and declined among teens of all ages and ethnicities from 1991 to 2005. Decreases from 25% to 19% were also noted in the teen repeat birth rate from 1991 to 2005 and increased in 2006 and 2007 (Ikramullah et al, 2009, 2011). Decreases in pregnancy among teens ages 15 to 17 have been attributed to reduced sexual activity (one fourth of the reduction) and the rest resulting from improved contraceptive use. For teens ages 18 to 19 the reduction is entirely attributed to increased contraceptive use (Kost, Henshaw, and Carlin, 2010).

NURSING TIP   *In providing care to teens, it is important to know some trends in teen pregnancies. Selected trends are:*

- *Hispanic teens have a higher birth rate than white or black teens.*
- *Hispanic teens and African-American teens have birth rates more than twice that of white teens.*
- *The states with the highest teen birth rates are mostly in the south.*
- *The states with the lowest teen birth rates are mostly in the north.*

In 2006 the teen birth rate began to rise for the first time since 1991. That year it rose by 5% and then another 1% in 2007. This increase was the greatest among white teens, followed by African-American teens. The Hispanic teen birth rate decreased between 2006 and 2007; however, the declines in the years previous were not as dramatic as with white and African-American teens. Even with these increases, the birth rate today is still less than half of the birth rate from 1960 for 15- to 17-year-olds and 18- to 19-year-olds. In addition, more than 86% of teens are unmarried at the time of their child's birth (Ikramullah et al, 2009).

The 2009 rate of 39.1 births per 1000 females age 15-19 was 6% lower than in 2008 (41.5) (Ikramullah et al, 2011).

In 2006, 27% of pregnancies of teenagers were ended by elective abortion, a decrease from 46% of teen pregnancies in 1986 (Guttmacher Institute, 2010). Elective abortion rates for teenagers increased from the time of legalization in 1973 until 1988 and then began to decline. This decrease was caused in part by decreases in the pregnancy rate, but may also have resulted from laws that required parental notification or consent for

♥ HEALTHY PEOPLE 2020

Selected Objectives Related to Adolescent Reproductive Health

Objectives Related to Adolescent Health
- HIV-13: Increase the percentage of adolescents who have been tested for HIV.

Objectives Related to Family Planning
- FP-1: Increase the proportion of pregnancies that are intended.
- FP-8: Reduce pregnancy rates among adolescent females.
- FP-9: Increase the proportion of adolescents aged 17 years and under who have never had sexual intercourse.
- FP-12: Increase the proportion of adolescents who received formal instruction on reproductive health topics before they are 18 years old.
- FP-13: Increase the proportion of adolescents who talked to a parent or guardian about reproductive health topics before they are 18 years old.

Objectives Related to Maternal, Infant, and Child Health
- MICH-10: Increase the proportion of pregnant women who receive early and adequate prenatal care.
- MICH-8.1: Reduce low birth weight (LBW) and very low birth weight (VLBW).
- MICH-12: Increase the proportion of pregnant women who attend a series of prepared childbirth classes.

From U.S. Department of Health and Human Services: *Healthy People 2020.* Available at http://www.healthypeople.gov/HP2020/. Accessed March 29, 2010.

minors requesting abortion services in some states. An adolescent might cite lack of maturity, an inability to afford a baby, and concerns about how a child would change his or her life as reasons for terminating a pregnancy by abortion (Guttmacher Institute, 2010).

BACKGROUND FACTORS

Many adults have difficulty understanding why young people would jeopardize their careers and personal potential by becoming pregnant during the teen years. Adolescents, however, do not view the world in the same way as adults. Teens often feel invincible and therefore do not recognize any risk related to their behaviors or anticipate the consequences. That is, they may not believe that sexual activity will lead to pregnancy. When teens become pregnant, they do not believe that the negative outcomes they are advised of could come true. Many teens believe that they are unique and different and that everything will work out fine. The developmental circumstances of adolescence, coupled with potential background disadvantages, can magnify the problems facing the pregnant and parenting teen. Pregnant teens often express the unrealistic attitude that they can do it all: school, work, parenting, and socializing.

Babies born to teenage mothers in the United States are at-risk for many of the same problems as their young mothers. These risks include school failure, poverty, and physical or mental illness (American Academy of Child & Adolecent Psychiatry, 2004).

Specifically, a disproportionate number of teens who give birth are poor (more than 75%), have limited educational achievements, and see few advantages in delaying pregnancy since they do not expect that their circumstances will improve at a later time (Kirby, 2002). Most teens report that their pregnancy was unplanned. They typically think that a pregnancy should be delayed until people are older, have completed their education, and are employed and married. Their behaviors, however, do not support the opinions they express. In fact, some teens actually seem ambitious about becoming pregnant. Several factors that often contribute to pregnancy are discussed next.

Sexual Activity and Use of Birth Control

The sexual debut, or first experience with intercourse, for a teen will have a significant impact on pregnancy risk. Although the percentage of sexually active teens today is much greater than it was in the 1970s, decreases between 1991 and 2007 have been noted. A reported 7.1% of students first had sex before the age of 13; in the ninth grade, approximately 33% of students are sexually active, 44% by tenth grade, 55% by the eleventh grade, and 65% by the twelfth grade. For each grade the percentage of males is greater than females in each racial group. Almost 15% of students have had sexual intercourse with four or more persons during their life. Male students and African-American students were more likely than white, Hispanic/Latino, or female students to initiate sexual activity before age 13. African-American students (67%) are more likely to report a history of sexual activity, followed by Hispanic/Latino (52%) and white students (44%) (CDC, 2008).

The *Healthy People 2020* goal is to increase the proportion of adolescents who have never engaged in sexual intercourse by age 17 (USDHHS, 2010).

> **DID YOU KNOW?** *In 1996 Congress passed the Personal Responsibility and Work Opportunity Reconciliation Act. This welfare reform package strives to discourage teen pregnancy and other non-marital births in a variety of ways. Emphasis is on the primary prevention of pregnancy through abstinence education and discouraging sex before marriage. Furthermore, benefits may be withdrawn if adolescent parents do not live in an adult-supervised home and attend school.*

Although more teens have begun using birth control in the past 10 years, there is still progress to be made. *Healthy People 2020* addresses this with goals to increase the proportion of 15- to 19-year-olds who use condoms and a hormonal contraceptive and increase the proportion of teens who receive reproductive health information through formal instruction as well as from their parents or guardians (USDHHS, 2010). Condoms are the most commonly used method of birth control, with 66% of adolescent females and 71% of adolescent males (Guttmacher, 2010) reporting their use at first voluntary coitus. Male teens use condoms with more frequency than female teens; ninth-grade males use condoms more than tenth-, eleventh-, or twelfth-grade males; and African-American males use condoms more often than any other group, male or female. Overall, 61% of teen couples reported that the male partner used condoms the last time they had intercourse, with the greatest use at last intercourse reported by African-American male teens (74%) and the lowest use reported by Hispanic/Latino female teens (52%) (CDC, 2008). Half of all first-time pregnancies occur within 6 months of initiating intercourse, and teens using a hormonal birth control method report sexual activity for up to 1 year before they see a health care provider to obtain a prescription (Klein and the Committee on Adolescence, 2005). Teens harbor many myths that contribute to poor use of birth control, such as believing women cannot get pregnant the first time, and some teens have erroneous knowledge about a woman's fertile time. Failure to use birth control can also reflect teens' embarrassment in discussing this practice with partners, friends, parents, and health care providers and the obstacles they encounter finding facilities that provide confidential and affordable birth control.

The earlier the sexual debut, the less likely a birth control method will be used, since younger teens have less knowledge and skill related to sexuality and birth control. School-based sex education can come too late or not at all. Birth control is usually discussed in the secondary-school curriculum, but this could be eighth grade in one school district and tenth in another; school curricula are not standardized. Younger teens may falsely believe that they are too young to purchase birth control methods such as condoms. Confidential reproductive health care services may be available for teens, but problems are still associated with transportation, school absences, and costs of care that ultimately restrict access to these services.

Inconsistent use of birth control can reflect teens' willingness to take risks, their dissatisfactions with available birth control methods, and their ambivalence about becoming pregnant. Real and perceived side effects of birth control methods can discourage use. Hormonal methods such as Mirena (an intrauterine device every 5 years), Implanon (a contraceptive implant every 3 years), Depo-Provera (an intramuscular injection every 3 months), NuvaRing (a monthly vaginal ring), and the Ortho Evra patch appeal to some women because the method is less directly tied to coitus. These methods may have nuisance-type effects (e.g., irregular bleeding or insertion into the vagina) that require the nurse to provide anticipatory guidance and management instructions to young women. Table 35-1 describes hormonal birth control methods that would be appropriate for the adolescent to consider.

As noted earlier, the use of alcohol and other substances is common among adolescents and can contribute to unplanned pregnancy. Mood-altering effects may reduce inhibitions about engaging in intercourse and interfere with the proper use of a chosen birth control method.

Peer Pressure and Partner Pressure

Peer pressure among teens is not a new phenomenon, but many of the influences have become more serious. Influence has expanded from fashion and language to cigarettes, substance abuse, sexuality, and pregnancy. Teens are more likely to be sexually active if their friends are sexually active (Hatcher et al, 2008). Peers reinforce teen parenting by exaggerating birth control risks, discouraging abortion and **adoption,** and glamorizing the impending birth of the child.

Both young men and young women may think that allowing a pregnancy to happen verifies one's love and commitment for the other. In addition, young men from socioeconomically disadvantaged backgrounds may be more likely to say that fathering a child would make them feel more manly, and they are less likely to use an effective contraceptive (Heavey et al, 2008).

Other Factors

Other factors influencing teen pregnancy are a history of **sexual victimization,** family structure, and parental influences. Pregnant teenagers have a greater likelihood of having been sexually abused during their lifetime, with rates recorded as high as 60% to 70% (Klein et al, 2005). Adolescent girls with a history of sexual abuse are at risk for earlier initiation of voluntary sexual intercourse, are less likely to use birth control, are more likely to use drugs and alcohol at first intercourse, and are more likely to have older sexual partners (Harner, 2005). The youngest women are more likely to experience **coercive sex** or **statutory rape** (65% of females who had intercourse before age 14 reported that it was involuntary) (Child Trends, 2005). Young women may also become pregnant as a result of forced sexual intercourse. A history of sexual victimization will influence a young woman's ability to exert control over future sexual experiences, which will affect the use of birth control and rejection of unwanted sexual experiences. All these factors contribute to an increased risk for becoming pregnant (Miller et al, 2010). In addition, young women who have experienced a lifetime of

METHOD	FAILURE RATE WITH TYPICAL USE (%/year)	PATTERN OF USE	NON-CONTRACEPTIVE BENEFITS
Mirena IUD	0.2	Placed in the uterus; effective continuously for 5 years	Less menstrual bleeding, often with amenorrhea after initial few months
Implanon	0.5	Placed subdermally in the upper arm; effective continuously for 3 years	Less menstrual bleeding
Depo Provera	3	IM injection into either the deltoid or the gluteal muscle every 3 months	Decreases sickle cell crisis Decreases the seizure threshold May become amenorrheic
NuvaRing	8	Vaginal ring inserted for 21 to 32 days; contains estrogen and progestin	For all estrogen/progestin combinations: • Risk of ovarian and endometrial cancer is reduced. • May use an extended regimen to reduce menses (except Ortho Evra patch) • May improve acne • Light regular menses (except POP)
Ortho Evra transdermal patch	8	A transdermal patch that is applied to specific skin sites weekly for 3 weeks, and removed for 7 days, containing estrogen and progestin	See above
Birth control pills	8	Take pill daily COC—estrogen and progestin POP—progestin only ("mini pill")	See above

TABLE 35-1   HORMONAL BIRTH CONTROL METHODS RECOMMENDED FOR TEENAGERS

Data from Hatcher RA, Trussell J, Stewart F, et al: *Contraceptive technology,* ed 19, New York, 2008, Ardent Media.

economic, social, and psychological deprivation may think that a baby will bring joy into an otherwise bleak existence. Some mistakenly believe that a baby can provide the love and attention that her family has not provided.

Family structure can influence adolescent sexual behavior and pregnancy. Adolescents raised in single-parent families are more likely to report having sexual experience as well as initiating sex at a younger age than those raised in two-parent families. This difference is striking: only 55% of youth living in one-parent families reported never having had intercourse compared with 70% of youth living in two-parent families. Other factors, such as parental higher education, family communication, and good family health practices, were also associated with decreased sexual risk behaviors (Oman, Vesely, and Aspy, 2005).

Parenting styles can influence a young woman's risk for early sexual experiences and pregnancy. Parents who are extremely demanding and controlling or neglectful and who have low expectations are least successful in instilling parental values in their children. Parents who have high demands for their children to act maturely and who offer warmth and understanding with parental rules have children more likely to exhibit appropriate social behavior and to delay early sexual experiences and pregnancy. Children of parents who are neglectful are the most sexually experienced, followed by children of parents who are very strict. Furthermore, parents who discuss birth control, sexuality, and pregnancy with their children can positively influence delay of sexual initiation and effective birth control use. Parents who do not communicate about sexuality with their teens may find them more at risk for sexual permissiveness and pregnancy (Bersamin et al, 2008).

WHAT DO YOU THINK?   *In response to federal welfare reform recommendations, there has been a recent trend toward the enforcement of statutory rape laws by individual states. These laws make it a crime to have sexual contact with a person before the age of consent is reached (which varies among states). Supporters of this action think that it will discourage adult men from relationships with minors and consequently reduce teen pregnancy. Opponents believe that this strategy does not take into account the complex issues involved in teen pregnancy (such as poverty and limited opportunities for young women) and think it may do more to distance a father from involvement in his child's life.*

YOUNG MEN AND PATERNITY

Although declines among pregnant female teenagers have been seen over the past 14 years, there are no published data showing the same decline among teen males. About 14% of sexually active teen males have gotten a partner pregnant and 4% have become teen fathers. These are conservative numbers since not all teen males are aware that a partner became pregnant nor are they always aware of the outcome of the pregnancy. Adolescent males who become fathers are often reported to be second-generation teen parents. Studies demonstrate that they came from poor families, did poorly in school, and engaged in many high-risk behaviors such as gang membership, drugs, and early sexual involvement. These young fathers face special challenges because of concomitant social problems and limited future plans or ability to provide support. There may also be an overlap between young fatherhood and delinquency. Adolescent males who demonstrate law-breaking behaviors, alcohol or substance use, school problems, and aggressive behaviors may have difficulty developing a positive fathering role, yet they are the highest-risk group to become young fathers (Marsiglio et al, 2006; Savio Beers and Hollo, 2009). Decreases have been reported about the numbers of adult men fathering teen pregnancies; however, the greatest risk for this exists with the youngest pregnant teens (Marsiglio et al, 2006).

Paternity, or fatherhood, is legally established at the time of the birth for a teen who is married. However, it is more difficult to establish paternity among non-married couples. Some of the difficulty lies in the complexity of the specific state system for young men to acknowledge paternity. In some states, a young man may have to work with the judicial system outside of the hospital after the birth; if he is under age 18, he may need to involve his parents.

Some young couples do not attempt to establish paternity and prefer a verbal promise of assistance for the teen mother and child. Although a verbal commitment may be acceptable when the child is born, the mother may become more inclined to pursue the establishment of paternity later when the relationship ends or for reasons related to financial, social, or emotional needs of the child. Young women who receive state or federal assistance (e.g., TANF, Medicaid) may be asked to name the child's father so the judicial process can be used to establish paternity.

Young men react differently when they learn that their partner is pregnant. The reaction often depends on the nature of the relationship before the pregnancy. Many young men will accompany the young woman to a health care center for pregnancy diagnosis and counseling. A large percentage of young men will continue to accompany the young woman to some prenatal visits and may even attend the delivery. These young men may also want to and need to be involved with their children regardless of changes in their relationships with the teen mother. It is not unusual for a young man to be excluded or even rejected by the young woman's family (usually her mother). He may then begin to act as though he is disinterested when he may really feel that he cannot provide resources for his child or know how to take care of him or her (Savio Beers and Hollo, 2009) (Figure 35-1).

Nurses can acknowledge and support the young man as he develops in the role of father. His involvement can positively affect his child's development and provide greater personal satisfaction for him and greater role satisfaction for the young mother. Young mothers who report less social support from their baby's father are more apt to be unhappy and distressed in the parenting role and consequently more at risk for abuse of their child (Savio Beers and Hollo, 2009). The immediate concerns revolve around his financial responsibility, living arrangements, relationship issues, school, and work. Establishing an opportunity to meet with the young man and both families is helpful to clarify these issues and identify roles and responsibilities.

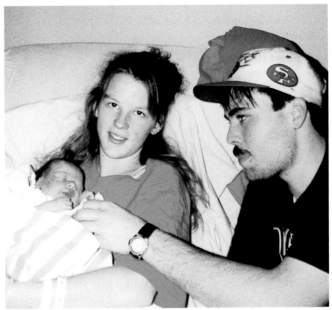

FIGURE 35-1 It is important to include both the teen mother and the father in teaching about child development.

Life experiences for a young man will influence behaviors that can lead to a teen pregnancy or prevent a teen pregnancy. Adverse childhood experiences including a history of abuse (especially physical and sexual abuse and domestic violence), mental illness and/or substance abuse in the childhood home, criminal behaviors in the home, and separated parents have been linked to negative behaviors such as early sexual intercourse, multiple partners, and substance use. These behaviors are possible antecedents to male involvement in teen pregnancy (Sipsma et al, 2010).

EARLY IDENTIFICATION OF THE PREGNANT TEEN

Some teens delay seeking pregnancy services because they fail to recognize signs such as breast tenderness and a late period, since they are experiencing a variety of other pubertal changes. Most young women, however, suspect pregnancy as soon as a period is late. These young women may still delay seeking care because they falsely hope that the pregnancy will just go away. A teen may also delay seeking care to keep the pregnancy a secret from family members, fearing either an angry or disappointed response or expecting to be forced into a decision that may not be hers.

Nurses must be sensitive to subtle cues that a teenager may offer about sexuality and pregnancy concerns. Such cues include questions about one's fertile period or requests for confirmation that one need not miss a period to be pregnant. Once the nurse identifies the specific concern, information can be provided about how and when to obtain pregnancy testing. The nurse should determine how a teenager would react to the possible pregnancy before completing the test. If the test is negative, the nurse should take the opportunity to assess whether the young woman would consider counseling to prevent pregnancy. A follow-up visit is important after a negative test to determine if retesting is necessary or if another problem exists.

LEVELS OF PREVENTION

Teen Pregnancy

Primary Prevention

Teach young people about sexual practices that will prevent untimely pregnancy.

Secondary Prevention

Provide services for early detection of teen pregnancy.

Tertiary Prevention

Counsel the young person or young couple about available options, including keeping the baby (and making appropriate plans to care for the child), abortion, and adoption.

BOX 35-4 GUIDELINES FOR ADOPTION COUNSELING

1. Assess your own thoughts and feelings on adoption. Do not impose your opinion on the decision-making process of teen mothers.
2. Know about state laws, local resources, and various types of adoption services.
3. Choose language sensitively. Examples follow:
   a. Avoid saying "giving away a child" or "putting up for adoption." It is more appropriate and positive to say "releasing a child for adoption," "placing for adoption," or "making an adoption plan."
   b. Avoid saying "unwanted child" or "unwanted pregnancy." A more appropriate term may be *unplanned pregnancy.*
   c. Avoid saying "natural parents" or "natural child," because the adopted parents would then seem to be "unnatural." The terms *biological parents* and *adoptive parents* are more appropriate.
4. Assess when a discussion of adoption is appropriate. It can be helpful to begin with information on adoption and then explore feelings and concerns over time. Individuals will vary in how much they may have already considered adoption, and this will influence the counseling session.
5. Assess the relationship between the pregnant teen and her partner and what role she expects him to play. Discuss the reality of this.
6. It may be helpful for a pregnant teen to talk with other teens who have been pregnant, are raising a child, have released a child for adoption, or have been adopted themselves.
7. A young woman can be encouraged to begin writing letters to her baby. These can be saved or given to the child when released to the adoptive family.

Modified from Brandsen CK: *A case for adoption,* Grand Rapids, MI, 1991, Bethany.

In looking at teen pregnancy from the perspective of levels of prevention, several steps could be taken. These are shown in the Levels of Prevention box.

A young woman with a positive pregnancy test requires a physical examination and pregnancy counseling. It is advantageous to offer these at the same time so that the counseling is consistent with the findings of the examination. The purpose of the examination is to assess the duration and well-being of the pregnancy, as well as to test for sexually transmitted infection. The pregnancy counseling should include the following: information on adoption, abortion, and child-rearing; an opportunity for assessment of support systems for the young woman; and identification of the immediate concerns she might have (Aruda et al, 2010).

The availability of affordable abortion services up to 13 weeks of gestation varies from community to community. Similarly, second-trimester services may be available locally or involve extensive travel and cost. The nurse should know about abortion services and provide information or refer the pregnant teenager to a pregnancy counseling service that can assist.

The pregnant teenager needs information about adoption, such as current policies among agencies that allow continued contact with the adopting family. Also, church organizations, private attorneys, and social service agencies provide a variety of adoption services with which the nurse should be familiar. Box 35-4 lists guidelines for adoption counseling.

> **NURSING TIP** *An important counseling opportunity presents itself when a teen has a negative pregnancy test. Use this time to clarify a desire or disinterest in pregnancy and help empower her to influence her reproductive future.*

Pregnancy counseling requires that the nurse and young woman explore strengths and weaknesses for personal care and responsibility during pregnancy and parenting. Young women vary in their interest in including the partner or their parents in this discussion. Issues to discuss include education and career plans, family finances and qualifications for outside assistance, and personal values about pregnancy and parenting at this time in their life. Often it is difficult to focus on counseling in any

depth at the time of the initial pregnancy testing results. A follow-up visit is usually more productive and should be arranged as soon as possible.

As decisions are made about the course of the pregnancy, the nurse can make referrals to appropriate programs such as WIC (a supplemental food program for women, infants, and children), Medicaid, and prenatal services. The young woman and her family also need to know about expected costs of care and, if there is a family insurance policy, whether it will cover the pregnancy-related expenses of a dependent child. For those without insurance, the family can apply for Medicaid or determine whether local facilities offer indigent care programs (e.g., Hill-Burton programs for assistance with hospital expenses). The nurse can also begin prenatal education and counseling on nutrition, substance abuse and use, exercise, and special medical concerns.

SPECIAL ISSUES IN CARING FOR THE PREGNANT TEEN

Pregnant teenagers are considered high-risk obstetric clients. Many of the complications of their pregnancy result from poverty, late entry into prenatal care, and limited knowledge about self-care during pregnancy. Nursing interventions through education and early identification of problems may dramatically alter the course of the pregnancy and the birth outcome.

Violence

Teens are more likely to experience violence during their pregnancies than adult women. Age may be a factor in their greater vulnerability to potential perpetrators that include partners, family members, and other acquaintances. Violence in pregnancy has been associated with an increased risk for substance abuse, poor compliance with prenatal care, and poor birth outcome. In the case of partner violence, young women may be protective of their partners because of fear or helplessness. Eliciting this history from an adolescent is not easy. Be sure to inquire about violence at every visit. Frequent routine assessments are more revealing than a single inquiry at the first prenatal visit. Research has demonstrated that 16% to 38% of pregnant adolescents reported violence during the pregnancy, a rate greater than that reported by adult women (Harner, 2004). Violence that began during the pregnancy may continue for several years after, with increasing severity. Variations by ethnicity have also been observed during this postpartum period; intimate partner violence may peak at 3 months postpartum among African-American and Hispanic/Latino new mothers and at 18 months for white mothers (Harrykissoon, Rickert, and Wiemann, 2002). The nurse must observe for physical signs of abuse, as well as for controlling or intrusive partner behavior (see the Evidence-Based Practice box).

> **WHAT DO YOU THINK?** *Public health nurses find their clients in unconventional settings. Approximately 24,000 pregnant teenagers are arrested annually and hundreds are incarcerated for various amounts of time in juvenile detention centers. The nurse can bring important interventions into this setting that include prenatal monitoring, reproductive health education, arrangements for infant care after delivery, attention to mental health issues, as well as guidance on parenting after the separation of incarceration (Hufft and Peternelj-Taylor, 2008).*

Initiation of Prenatal Care

Pregnant adolescents differ remarkably from pregnant adults in initiation and compliance with prenatal care. Inadequate prenatal care has been negatively associated with health risks to both the mother and the fetus. In 2003 6.4% of the pregnant 15- to 19-year-olds received late or no prenatal care (Neinstein, 2008). Teens report that the greatest barrier to care is real or perceived cost. Other barriers include denial of the pregnancy, fear of telling parents, transportation, dislike of providers' care, and offensive attitudes among clinic staff toward pregnant teens (Neinstein, 2008; Aruda et al, 2010).

Once a teen is enrolled in prenatal care, the nurse becomes an important liaison between personnel at the clinical site and the young woman. Confusion and misunderstandings occur easily when teens do not understand what a health care provider says to them. Often these misunderstandings are based on lack of knowledge about basic anatomy and physiology. For example, a teen may be told as she gets close to term that the head of the baby is down and it can be felt. This is an alarming piece of information for a young woman who imagines the entire baby could just pop out at any time!

EVIDENCE-BASED PRACTICE

As a group, adolescent mothers have lower rates of breastfeeding than adult mothers. Using data collected in Missouri among low-income adolescents, only 25% of these young mothers breastfed (for at least 1 week or longer). Continuing to increase the proportion of breastfeeding mothers is a goal of *Healthy People 2020*.

Nurses working with pregnant and parenting teens would benefit from a greater understanding of how teens make decisions to breastfeed and ways they can intervene to extend the duration of breastfeeding. Existing research has helped to articulate both the negative and positive aspects of breastfeeding that teen mothers have articulated.

In this study the authors gained qualitative information on this subject. They recruited teen mothers ages 14 to 18 at their 6-week postpartum visits from two university-based health care centers. Using either a focus group or individual interviews, they elicited information on how and when decisions to breastfeed occur throughout the pregnancy and when and why breastfeeding is terminated. By the time the 23rd participant was interviewed, the study ended because the information they were obtaining became repetitive. Clearly the themes had emerged.

Results were quite informative to nursing. For example, this study showed that the earlier in the pregnancy a teen makes the decision to breastfeed, the longer the duration of breastfeeding will be. However, many teens are still making the decision about breastfeeding late in their pregnancy and therefore are at risk for early weaning. An important source of support was the encouragement from friends and families. Information about the benefit to the infant was very persuasive in the decision-making process. When hospitalized, the responses from nursing staff (real or as perceived by the client) affected resolution of early breastfeeding problems (nipple pain, positioning issues) and affected decisions to provide supplemental formula, which subsequently can affect duration of breastfeeding. Repeatedly, teens reported the positive feelings of closeness to their babies from breastfeeding as well as the convenience.

Nurse Use

Nurses in public health can benefit tremendously from the information gleaned in this qualitative study design. Working closely with the pregnant teen and soon after delivery offers many opportunities to provide education and support that will endorse a positive breastfeeding experience.

From Wambach KA, Cohen SM: Breastfeeding experiences of urban adolescent mothers, *J Pediatr Nurs* 24(4):244-254, 2009.

Cooperation between the nurse and the clinical staff can also maximize the client's compliance with special health or nutritional needs. For example, a teen who has premature contractions may be restricted to bed rest and instructed to increase fluids. The nurse who makes home visits can provide additional assessment of the teen's condition and can solve problems about self-care, hygiene, meals, and schooling.

> **NURSING TIP** *Periodontal disease may appear between the ages of 12 and 17. Moderate to severe periodontal disease has been shown to be one of several risk factors for early pregnancy loss, preeclampsia, and premature and low-birth-weight babies. Nurses can promote awareness of oral hygiene and necessary interventions with pregnant teenagers and subsequently improve the health of their children (Murphy and Rew, 2009).*

Low-Birth-Weight Infants and Preterm Delivery

Teens are more likely than adult women to deliver infants weighing less than 5.5 lb or to deliver before 37 weeks of gestation. These low-birth-weight and premature infants are at

TABLE 35-2   ADOLESCENT NUTRITIONAL NEEDS DURING PREGNANCY

NUTRIENT	DAILY REQUIREMENT DURING PREGNANCY*	FOOD SOURCE
Calcium	1300 mg (decrease to 1000 mg for 19-year-olds)	Macaroni and cheese; pizza; puddings, milk, yogurt; also fortified juices, water, breakfast bars and fast foods, including Taco Bell's chili cheese burrito, McDonald's Big Mac
Iron	30 mg (recommendation is for 30 mg of elemental iron as daily supplement)	Meats; dried beans; peas; dark green, leafy vegetables; whole grains; fortified cereal; absorption of iron from plant foods improved by vitamin C sources taken simultaneously
Zinc	15 mg	Seafood, meats, eggs, legumes, whole grains
Folate (folic acid)	0.6 mg (prenatal vitamins contain 0.4-1.0 mg of folic acid)	Green, leafy vegetables; fruits
Vitamin A	800 μg	Dark yellow and green vegetables, fruits
Vitamin B$_6$	2.2 mg	Chicken, fish, liver, pork, eggs
Vitamin D	5 μg	Fortified milk products and cereals

*Higher ranges are especially important for the younger pregnant teen.

greater risk for death in the first year of life and are at increased risk for long-term physical, emotional, and cognitive problems (Neinstein, 2008). For example, low-birth-weight and premature infants can be more difficult to feed and soothe. This challenges the limited skills of the young mother and can further strain relations with other members of the household, who may not know how to offer support or assistance.

The risk for low-birth-weight infants and premature births can be averted by the teen's early initiation into prenatal care. Although such births still occur, it is important to work closely with the teen mother as soon as she is identified as pregnant to try to promote compliance with prenatal care visits and self-care during the pregnancy. After the pregnancy, these infants and their mothers will benefit from frequent nursing supervision to ensure that their care is appropriate and that everyone in the home is coping adequately with the strain of a small infant.

Nutrition

The nutritional needs of a pregnant teenager are especially important. First, the teen lifestyle does not lend itself to overall good nutrition. Fast foods, frequent snacking, and hectic social schedules limit nutritious food choices. Snacks, which account for approximately one third of a teen's daily caloric intake, tend to be high in fat, sugar, and sodium and limited in essential vitamins and minerals. Second, the nutritive needs of both pregnancy and the concurrent adolescent growth spurt require the adolescent to change her diet substantially. The growing teen must increase caloric nutrients to meet individual growth needs as well as to allow for adequate fetal growth. Third, poor eating patterns of the teen and her current growth requirement may leave her with limited reserves of essential vitamins and minerals when the pregnancy begins. The nurse can assess the pregnant teenager's current eating pattern and provide creative guidance. Identifying good choices that a teen can consume "on the run" might include snacks of drinkable yogurt, leftover pizza, string cheese, or energy/granola bars. The teen who often eats out can boost their protein intake at fast-food establishments by ordering milkshakes instead of soft drinks

and cheeseburgers or broiled chicken sandwiches instead of hamburgers (Stang and Story, 2005).

The recommended nutritional needs of the adolescent may depend on the **gynecological age** of the teen—that is, the number of years between her chronological age and her age at menarche, as well as her chronological age. Young women with a gynecological age of 2 or less years or under the age of 16 may have increased nutrient requirements because of their own growth. Furthermore, the younger and still-growing teen may compete nutritionally with the fetus. Fetuses may show evidence of slower growth in young women ages 10 to 16 years (Stang and Story, 2005). The nurse, in collaboration with the WIC nutritionist, can determine the nutritional needs of the pregnant teenager to tailor education appropriately. Table 35-2 describes adolescent nutritional needs in pregnancy.

Weight gain during pregnancy is one of the strongest predictors of infant birth weight. Although precise weight gain goals in adolescence are controversial, pregnant adolescents who gain 25 to 35 lb have the lowest incidence of low-birth-weight babies. Babies born to teenagers may be at risk for being small-for-gestational age despite adequate weight gain if there is very slow gain in the first 24 weeks. Teenagers who begin the pregnancy at a normal weight should be counseled to begin weight gain in the first trimester and to average gains of 1 lb per week for the second and third trimesters (Stang and Story, 2005). Younger teen mothers (ages 13-16), because of their own growth demands, may need to gain more weight than older teen mothers (ages 17 and older) to have the same-birth-weight baby. Table 35-3 shows the recommendations established by the Institute of Medicine for adolescent gestational weight gain by pre-pregnant weight categories.

It is important for the nurse to assess the attitudes of the pregnant teen about weight gain and to follow her progress, providing feedback on adequate weight gain and counseling if weight gain is excessive. Gaining weight beyond the recommendations raises the risk for infants to be hypoglycemic, to be large-for-gestational age, and to have a low Apgar score, seizures, and polycythemia (ADA Report, 2008). Family support

TABLE 35-3 GESTATIONAL WEIGHT GAIN RECOMMENDATIONS FOR ADOLESCENTS*

PRE-PREGNANT WEIGHT CATEGORIES†	RECOMMENDED TOTAL GAIN			
	KG	LB	TRIMESTER 1 (LB)	TRIMESTERS 2 AND 3 (LB/WK)
Underweight (BMI 19.8)	12.5-18	28-40	5	1.0
Normal weight (BMI 19.9-26)	11.5-16	25-35	3	1.0
Overweight (BMI 26-29)	7.0-11.5	15-25	2	0.66
Very overweight (BMI ≥29)	7.0-9.1	15-20	1.5	0.5

From Story M and Stang J, editors: *Nutrition and the pregnant adolescent: a practical reference guide,* Minneapolis, MN, 2000, University of Minnesota, Center for Leadership, Education, and Training in Maternal and Child Nutrition. Available at http://www.epi.umn.edu/let. Accessed March 28, 2010.
*Very young adolescents (14 years of age or younger, or less than 2 years post-menarche) should strive for gains at the upper end of the range.
†BMI (body mass index) is calculated as weight (in kilograms) divided by height (in meters squared).

of the pregnant teen can be a strong influence in adequate weight gain and good nutrition during the pregnancy. Nutrition education should emphasize what accounts for weight gain and how fetal growth will benefit.

Iron deficiency anemia is the most common nutritional problem among both pregnant and non-pregnant adolescent females (Stang and Story, 2005). Up to 11% of adolescents may begin a pregnancy with low or absent iron stores because of heavy menstrual periods, a previous pregnancy, growth demands, poor iron intake, or substance abuse. By the second trimester, at least 16% of pregnant adolescents will have iron deficiency anemia and even higher rates among lower income teenagers (ADA Report, 2008). The increased maternal plasma volume and increased fetal demands for iron (especially in the third trimester) can further compromise the adolescent. Iron deficiency in pregnancy may contribute to increased prematurity, low birth weight, maternal cardiovascular stress, increased risk of maternal urinary tract infection, decreased maternal well-being, postpartum hemorrhage, and slower wound healing (Stang and Story, 2005). The nurse can reinforce the need for the teen to take prenatal vitamins during pregnancy and after the baby's birth. Vitamins should contain 30 to 60 mg of elemental iron daily. The nurse should educate about iron-rich foods and foods that promote iron absorption, such as those containing vitamin C.

Infant Care

Many adolescents have cared for babies and small children and feel confident and competent. Few teens are ever prepared, however, for the reality of 24-hour care of an infant. The nurse can help prepare the teen for the transition to motherhood while she is still pregnant. The trend toward early discharge from the hospital has made prenatal preparation even more important. The nurse can enlist the support of the teen's parents in education about infant care and stimulation. Young fathers-to-be would benefit from this education as well. Family values, practices, and beliefs about childcare may be deeply embedded and require the nurse to work gently and persuasively to challenge any that may be detrimental to an infant (Savio Beers and Hollo, 2009). For example, a family may believe that corporal punishment is a necessary component of child-rearing.

Adolescents often lack the self-confidence and knowledge required to positively interact with their infants. They may also have unrealistic expectations about their children's development (Ryan-Krause et al, 2009). For example, they may expect their children to feed themselves at an early age or think that their children's behavior is more difficult than an adult mother might think. Teen parents often lack knowledge about infant growth and development, as seen in their limited verbal communication with their children, limited eye contact, and the tendency to display frustration and ambivalence as mothers. Over time, adolescents can improve their ability to foster their children's emotional and social growth. Children of adolescent mothers have also been found to be at risk for academic and behavior problems as they enter school (Terry-Humen, Manlove, and Moore, 2005). These risks can be reduced when the teen mother receives professional intervention and supervision in the area of infant social and cognitive development (Ryan-Krause et al, 2009).

Abusive parenting is more likely to occur when the parents have limited knowledge about normal child development. It may also be more likely to occur among parents who cannot adequately empathize with a child's needs. Younger teens are particularly at risk for being unable to understand what their infant or child needs. This frustration may be exhibited as abusive behavior toward the child. Nurses should continually assess for child abuse risk when dealing with teens who exhibit greater psychological distress or lack social supports (Lee, 2009).

After the birth of the baby, the nurse should observe how the mother responds to infant cues for basic needs and distress. Specific techniques that the new mother can be instructed to use in early childcare are listed in the How To box. Begin parenting education as early as possible. Adolescents who feel competent as parents have enhanced self-esteem, which in turn positively influences their relationship with their child. Recognizing these good parenting skills and providing positive feedback help a young mother gain confidence in her role (Ryan-Krause et al, 2009).

| HOW TO **Promote Interactions Between the Teen Mother and Her Baby**

The nurse can make the following suggestions to the teen mother:
1. *Make eye contact with your baby. Position your face 8 to 10 inches from your baby's face and smile.*
2. *Talk to your baby often. Use simple sentences, but try to avoid baby talk. Allow time for your baby to "answer." This will help your baby to acquire language and communication skills.*

3. *Babies often enjoy when you sing to them, and this may help soothe them during a difficult time or help them fall asleep. Experiment with different songs and melodies to see which your baby seems to like.*

4. *Babies at this age cannot be spoiled. Instead, when babies are held and cuddled, they feel secure and loved.*

5. *Babies cry for many reasons and for no reason at all. If your baby has a clean diaper, has recently been fed, and is safe and secure, he or she may just need to cry for a few minutes. What works to calm your baby may be different from other babies you have known. You can try rocking, gentle reassuring words, soft music, or remaining quiet.*

6. *Make feeding times pleasant for both of you. Do not prop the bottle in your baby's mouth. Instead, sit comfortably, hold your baby in your arms, and offer the bottle or breast.*

7. *When babies are awake, they love to play. They enjoy taking walks and looking at brightly colored objects or pictures and toys that make noises, such as rattles and musical toys.*

Repeat Pregnancy

Teen mothers who have a closely spaced second pregnancy, or a **repeat pregnancy,** have poorer birth, educational, and economic outcomes than teens who do not. In 2009, 19% of teen births were a repeat birth (Ikramullah et al, 2011). Some studies have shown that the younger the teen at first birth, the more likely she will have a second teen birth within 24 months (Savio Beers and Hollo, 2009). A *Healthy People 2020* objective is to reduce the proportion of pregnancies conceived within 18 months of a previous birth. Nurses should recognize which teens are at risk for a second teen pregnancy, such as lower educational and cognitive ability, mental health issues, physical trauma, losses (such as death of a loved one) and substance use. Also, some teens who report a planned first pregnancy are more likely to have an intentional second pregnancy within 24 months to complete their family (Savio Beer and Hollo, 2009; Patchen, Caruso, and Lanzi, 2009).

Discussions about family planning should begin during the third trimester of the current pregnancy. Nurses should review contraceptive options and help the young woman identify the methods she is most likely to use. It is helpful to determine at this time the methods she has used in the past, her satisfaction or dissatisfaction, and reasons for use or non-use. Many teens express unrealistic goals, such as "I am never going to have sex again" or "I need a break from guys," and they may erroneously believe that they are unable to conceive for some time after the delivery. After delivery, the nurse should follow up on the young woman's plan. Obstacles to obtaining contraceptives may exist, and the nurse can identify these and help problemsolve with the new mother.

Schooling and Educational Needs

Adolescents who become parents may have had limited school success before the pregnancy. However, coping with the demands of child-rearing coupled with the immaturity of the young mother may make school even less of a priority. As noted previously, the potential for a closely spaced second birth may be lessened by a return to school. Fifty-one percent of teen mothers earn a high school diploma compared with 89% of women who did not give birth during the teen years. Federal legislation passed in 1975 prohibits schools from excluding students because they are pregnant. Greater emphasis is placed on keeping the pregnant adolescent in school during the pregnancy and having her return as soon as possible after the birth. Several factors may positively influence a young woman's return to school. These include her parents' level of education and their marital stability, small family size, whether there were reading materials at home, whether her mother is employed, and whether the young woman is African American.

A practical challenge for young parents is locating and affording quality childcare; difficulties with this may prevent the highly motivated teenager from returning to high school. In the past 30 years, the percentage of parenting teens who return to high school and graduate has improved significantly. Attendance in college, now becoming the career requisite, is still less attainable for women who had children as teenagers than those who delayed childbearing, and less than 2% attain that college degree by the age of 30 (National Campaign to Prevent Teen Pregnancy, 2010).

Young women who have pregnancy complications may seek home instruction. This decision is made according to regulations issued by the state boards of education. Some young women have difficulty attending school because of the normal discomforts of pregnancy or because of social and emotional conflicts associated with the pregnancy. Teens who leave school without parental or medical excuses may face legal problems because of truancy. This increases the potential for them to become school dropouts. The nurse can determine if this has happened and try to coordinate with the school personnel (and school nurse, if one exists) to tailor efforts for a particular pregnant teen to keep her in school. Specific needs to be addressed include: (1) using the bathroom frequently, (2) carrying and consuming more fluids or snacks to relieve nausea, (3) climbing stairs and carrying heavy book bags, and (4) fitting comfortably behind stationary desks. Schools that are committed to keeping students enrolled are generally helpful and will assist in accommodating special needs.

TEEN PREGNANCY AND THE NURSE

Nurses can influence teen pregnancy through appropriate interventions at home and in the community.

Home-Based Interventions

Nurses can identify young women at risk for pregnancy in families currently receiving services. Younger sisters of pregnant teens are at a twofold increased risk for becoming pregnant themselves (Savio Beers and Hollo, 2009). Nurses can offer anticipatory guidance addressing sexuality issues to the parents of all preteens and teens during home visits to increase their knowledge and awareness.

Visiting the pregnant teen in her home allows the nurse to obtain an assessment of the facilities available at home for management of her pregnancy needs and the suitability of the environment for her child. Some specific areas to assess are

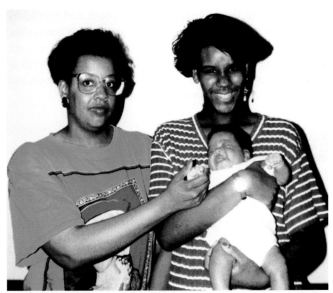

FIGURE 35-2 Both the teen mother and the teen's own mother can be included in health teaching.

adequacy of heating and cooling, a source of water, cleanliness of the home, cooking facilities, and food storage. The nurse may find it more convenient for parents and other family members to participate in education and counseling sessions in their own home. Also, the need for financial assistance and other social service support may be more easily identified. Home visiting by nurses during a young woman's pregnancy can be critical in achieving compliance with antepartum goals concerning weight gain, good nutrition, and prenatal medical concerns (Figure 35-2).

A teen pregnancy can shift the family dynamics. Families may go through stages of reactions. First, a crisis stage may occur, characterized by many emotions and conflict. By the third trimester, a honeymoon stage may occur, with greater acceptance and understanding of the teen and the impending birth. Finally, after the infant's birth, reorganization may occur, during which conflict may emerge again over issues of childcare and the young woman's role. The nurse can facilitate family coping and resolution of these stages by treating the family as client and assessing each person's role and strengths. Ultimately, family support for a teen parent can positively influence both mother and infant (Savio Beers and Hollo, 2009). A balance of moderate family guidance or supplementary care supports young mothers in their parenting role rather than replacing it.

> **DID YOU KNOW?** *Emergency contraception pills can reduce the risk for pregnancy up to 89% when used within 120 hours after unprotected intercourse. Although this is an effective and safe method, a long-acting birth control method provides greater protection.*

Community-Based Interventions

Many communities have broad-based coalitions and planning councils that facilitate a comprehensive approach to teen pregnancy. These groups usually include health care professionals,

social workers, clergy, school personnel, businessmen, legislators, and members of other youth-serving agencies. Nurses play a significant role on this team by participating in or organizing community assessments, public awareness campaigns, group education (for professionals, parents, and youths), and interprofessional programs for high-risk youths. Community acceptance is more likely when there is a broad base of support for activities directed at the reduction of teen pregnancy or reduction of consequences.

Research has evaluated years of pregnancy prevention programs. As less funding is available, programs must stand out to receive financial support. Research summaries that can be used by communities for strategic planning are available from the National Campaign to Prevent Teen Pregnancy (http://www.teenpregnancy.org), based in Washington, DC. Programs that have been evaluated fall into one of three categories: programs that focus on sexual factors (this includes educational programs addressing sexual behavior and STD/HIV); programs that focus on non-sexual behaviors (service learning that matches volunteerism with a didactic component); and programs that focus on both sexual and non-sexual factors (may bring other risk behaviors and/or protective factors into the curriculum). Since there is diversity available in the programs, communities can match their characteristics and needs with a program (Kirby, 2007).

The nurse can also be a valuable asset to schools. There are curriculum-based sex and STD/HIV education programs that have been evaluated and found to have positive effects on teens' sexual behavior (Kirby, 2007). Health teachers may ask nurses to provide educational materials or assistance with classroom instruction, especially in the areas of family planning, STDs, and pregnancy. Schools that do not have nurses may arrange to have a nurse from the health department available for health consultations with students during school hours. Schools may also request that nurses participate on their health advisory boards.

School-based health care clinics are operating in more than 1500 elementary, middle, and high schools in the United States. They are found primarily in urban areas (61%) but increasingly in rural (27%) and suburban (12%) regions. The services offered may include counseling, referrals, and primary care services. Some programs offer reproductive health counseling and services that can be vital in efforts to delay the onset of intercourse and increase the use of contraception. The nurse can assist school systems to design these programs as well as refer young women in need of reproductive health care services.

Nurses bring their knowledge about youth and reproductive behavior to any organization or group that has teens, their parents, or other professionals working with teens. Churches are becoming increasingly interested in addressing the needs of their youth, especially since teen sexual activity, pregnancy, and parenting are affecting more of their members.

CHAPTER REVIEW

■ PRACTICE APPLICATION

A local youth-serving agency requested the assistance of a nurse, Kristen Brown, in the implementation of a new high school–based program for pregnant and parenting teen girls. The primary goal of the program is to keep these teens in school through graduation. The secondary goal is to provide knowledge and skills about healthy pregnancy, labor and delivery, and parenting. After delivery, students enrolled in this program were paid for school attendance and this money could be used to defray the costs of childcare.

A nurse from the health department was the ideal choice to conduct the educational sessions. The group met weekly during the lunch hour. The curriculum that was developed had topics from early pregnancy through the toddler years. Occasionally, Ms. Brown recruited outside speakers such as a labor and delivery nurse or an early intervention specialist.

She also met individually with each enrolled student to provide case management services. Ideally, she would ensure that each student had a health care provider for prenatal care, that each was visited at home by a nurse, that each had enrolled in WIC and Medicaid if eligible, and that both the pregnant teen and her partner knew about other parenting and support groups.

One educational session that was particularly interesting was the discussion about the postpartum course—the 6 weeks after

delivery. There were many lively discussions about labor experiences as well as some emotional discussions about the reality of coming home with a baby and changes in the relationship with their male partner. Accurate contraception information was provided, which helped to clarify the many myths the girls had heard from friends and older women. Many girls benefited from understanding the normalcy of postpartum blues, but one young woman recognized that she had a more serious and persistent depression and privately approached the nurse for assistance.

At the end of the first school year, the dropout rate for pregnant and parenting teens had been reduced by half, and preterm labor rates had also declined. The local school board and a local youth-serving agency joined together to provide financial support to continue this program for an additional 2 years. Ms. Brown was asked to expand the educational programs and interventions she had developed.

What are some directions in which Ms. Brown might expand the program? List four.

Answers can be found on the Evolve site.

■ KEY POINTS

- The provision of reproductive health care services to adolescents requires sensitivity to the special needs of this age group. This includes knowing about state laws regarding confidentiality and services for birth control, pregnancy, abortion, and adoption.
- Pregnant teenagers have a substantial percentage of the first births in the United States. They are more likely to deliver prematurely and have a low-birth-weight baby. This risk can be reduced by early initiation of prenatal care and good nutrition.
- Factors that can influence whether a young woman becomes pregnant include a history of sexual victimization, family dysfunction, substance use, and failure to use birth control. Several factors may overlap.
- Nutritional needs during pregnancy can be challenged if the teenager has unhealthy eating habits and begins the pregnancy with limited reserves of vitamins and minerals. With education, the adolescent can make good food choices while still snacking or eating fast foods. Weight gain during pregnancy is a significant marker for a normal-weight baby.
- Young men need special attention and preparation as they become fathers. The interventions include information about pregnancy and delivery, declaration of paternity, care of infants and children, and psychosocial support in this role.

- The pregnant teen will need support during her pregnancy and in child-rearing. Families may provide most of this support. However, many communities have a variety of services available for adolescents. These services include financial assistance for medical care, nutritional programs, and school-based support groups.
- Adolescent parents often have unrealistic expectations about their children and may not know how to stimulate emotional, social, and cognitive development. The children born to adolescents are at risk for academic and behavioral problems as they become older. Teens who receive education on normal development and childcare are more likely to avert these problems with their children.
- During a pregnancy, teenagers are expected to attend school. Homebound instruction is reserved for those with medical complications. Teen mothers who return to school and complete their education after the birth of their child are less likely to have a repeat pregnancy. Problems finding childcare and the need to have an income can create an obstacle to school return.
- Community coalitions, which include nurses, can have a significant impact on teen pregnancy. These coalitions generally have diverse representation from the community, and therefore their activities meet with more community support.

CLINICAL DECISION-MAKING ACTIVITIES

1. Become familiar with statistics on teen pregnancy, births, miscarriages, and abortions in your area, and collect information on use of prenatal care, low-birth-weight and premature deliveries, high school completion, and repeat pregnancies. Compare the trends in statistics to the impact and costs to the individual, her family, and the community.

2. Call or visit local schools and interview the school nurse or guidance counselors about teen pregnancy. Determine what resources are available through the schools for pregnancy prevention. Assess the family life education curriculum, and identify a teaching project for nursing students. Can pregnancy prevention and parenting education be incorporated into the learning objectives in the existing school curriculum?

3. Design and offer a childbirth preparation class for pregnant teens and their support persons. Include a plan for identifying potential participants, select a site that is accessible, and develop an evaluation method. Develop teaching tools that acknowledge adolescent development.

4. Assess reproductive health care services for young men in your community. Design an awareness campaign targeting young men on paternity issues and the prevention of pregnancy. Be specific about ways to incorporate male role models and mentors.

REFERENCES

American Academy of Child & Adolescent Psychiatry: *Facts for families. When children have children,* No 31, July 2004. Available at http://www.aacap.org. Retrieved March 8, 2011.

American Dietetic Association Report: Position of the American Dietetic Association: nutrition and lifestyle for a healthy pregnancy outcome, *J Am Dietet Assoc* 108(3):553–561, 2008.

Aruda M, Wadicor K, Frese L, et al: Early pregnancy in adolescents: diagnosis, assessment, options counseling, and referral, *J Pediatr Health Care* 24(1):4–13, 2010.

Bersamin M, Todd M, Fisher DA, et al: Parenting practices and adolescent sexual behavior: a longitudinal study, *J Marriage Fam* 70(1):97–112, 2008.

Brandsen CK: *A case for adoption,* Grand Rapids, MI, 1991, Bethany.

Centers for Disease Control and Prevention: *Youth Risk Behavior Surveillance—United States,* 2007, Surveillance Summaries, *MMWR* 57(No SS-4), 2008.

Child Trends: *A demographic portrait of statutory rape,* Washington, DC, 2005, The Office of Population Affairs, USDHHS.

English A: Sexual and reproductive health care for adolescents: legal rights and policy challenges, *Adolesc Med State Art Rev* 18(3):571–581, 2007.

English A, Kenney KE: *State minor consent laws: a summary,* ed 3, Chapel Hill, NC, 2010, Center for Adolescent Health and the Law.

Guttmacher Institute: *Facts on American Teens' Sexual and Reproductive Health,* New York, 2010. Available at http://www.guttmacher.org/pubs/FB-ATSRH.html. Accessed March 29, 2010.

Harner H: Domestic violence and trauma care in teenage pregnancy: does paternal age make a difference? *J Obstet Gynecol Neonatal Nurs* 33:312–319, 2004.

Harner H: Childhood sexual abuse, teenage pregnancy, and partnering with adult men: exploring the relationship, *J Psychosoc Nurs Ment Health Serv* 43:20–28, 2005.

Harrykissoon SD, Rickert VI, Wiemann CW: Prevalence and patterns of intimate partner violence among adolescent mothers during the postpartum period, *Arch Pediatr Adolesc Med* 156:325–330, 2002.

Hatcher RA, Trussell J, Stewart F, et al: *Contraceptive technology,* ed 19, New York, 2008, Ardent Media.

Heavey EJ, Moysich KB, Hyland A, et al: Female adolescents' perceptions of male partners' pregnancy desire, *J Midwifery Womens Health* 53(4):338–344, 2008.

Hoffman S: *By the numbers: the public costs of teen childbearing,* Washington, DC, 2006, National Campaign to Prevent Teen Pregnancy.

Hufft AG, Peternelj-Taylor C: Ethical care of pregnant adolescents in correctional settings, *J Forensic Nurs* 4:94–96, 2008.

Ikramullah E, Cui C, Manlove J, Moore KA: *Facts at a glance.* Sponsored by the William and Flora Hewlett Foundation, Washington, DC, 2009, Child Trends. Available at http://childtrends.org. Accessed March 29, 2010.

Ikramullah E, Cui C, Manlove J, Moore KA: *Facts at a glance.* Sponsored by the William and Flora Hewlett Foundation, Washington, DC, Aprill 2011, Child Trends. Available at http://childtrends.org. Accessed June 1, 2011.

Kirby D: Antecedents of adolescent initiation of sex, contraceptive use and pregnancy, *Am J Health Behav* 26(6):473–485, 2002.

Kirby D: *Emerging Answers 2007: research findings on programs to reduce teen pregnancy and sexually transmitted diseases,* Washington, DC, 2007, National Campaign to Prevent Teen and Unplanned Pregnancy.

Klein JD and the Committee on Adolescence: Adolescent pregnancy: current trends and issues, *Pediatrics* 116:281, 2005.

Kost K, Henshaw S, Carlin L: *U.S. teenage pregnancies, births and abortions: national and state trends and trends by race and ethnicity,* 2010, The Alan Guttmacher Institute. Available at http://www.guttmacher.org/pubs/USTPtrends.pdf. Accessed March 29, 2010.

Lee Y: Early motherhood and harsh parenting: the role of human, social and cultural capital, *Child Abuse Neglect* 33:625–637, 2009.

Marsiglio W, Ries A, Sonenstein F, et al: *It's a guy thing: boys, young men, and teen pregnancy prevention,* Washington, DC, 2006, National Campaign to Prevent Teen Pregnancy.

Miller E, Decker MR, McCauley HL, et al: Pregnancy coercion, intimate partner violence and unintended pregnancy, *Contraception* 81:316–322, 2010.

Murphey C, Rew L: Three intervention models for exploring oral health in pregnant minority adolescents, *J Spec Pediatr Nurs* 14(2):132–141, 2009.

National Abortion and Reproductive Rights Action League Foundation: *Supreme Court decisions concerning reproductive rights, a chronology: 1965-2006,* Washington DC, 2007, NARAL.

National Abortion and Reproductive Rights Action League Foundation: *Who decides? A state-by-state review of abortion and reproductive rights,* ed 19, Washington, DC, 2010, NARAL.

National Campaign to Prevent Teen Pregnancy: *Why it matters: teen pregnancy and education,* Washington, DC, 2010. Available at www.teenpregnancy.org. Accessed April 1, 2010.

Neinstein LS, editor: *Adolescent health care,* ed 5, Philadelphia, 2008, Lippincott Williams and Wilkins.

Oman RF, Vesely SK, Aspy CB: Youth assets and sexual risk behavior: the importance of assets for youth residing in one-parent households, *Perspect Sex Reprod Health* 37:25, 2005.

Patchen L, Caruso D, Lanzi RG: Poor maternal mental health and trauma as risk factors for a short interpregnancy interval among adolescent mothers, *J Psychiatr Ment Hlt* 16:401–403, 2009.

Ryan-Krause P, Meadows-Oliver M, Sadler L, et al: Developmental status of children of teen mothers: contrasting objective assessments with maternal reports, *J Pediatr Health Care* 23(5):303–309, 2009.

Savio Beers LA, Hollo RE: Approaching the adolescent-headed family: a review of teen parenting, *Curr Probl Pediatr Adolesc Health Care* 39:216–233, 2009.

Sipsma H, Biello KB, Cole-Lewis H, et al: Like father, like son: the intergenerational cycle of adolescent fatherhood, *Am J Public Health* 100(3):517–524, 2010.

Stang J, Story M, editors: *Guidelines for adolescent nutrition services,* Minneapolis, MN, 2005, Center for Leadership, Education, and Training in Maternal and Child Nutrition, Division of Epidemiology and Community Health, School of Public Health, University of Minnesota. Accessed June 2, 2011.

Terry-Humen E, Manlove J, Moore KA: *Playing catch-up: how children born to teen mothers fare,* Washington, DC, 2005, National Campaign to Prevent Teen Pregnancy.

U.S. Department of Health and Human Services: *Healthy People 2020 Proposed Objectives.* Available at http://www.healthypeople.gov/HP2020/. Accessed March 29, 2010.

Wambach KA, Cohen SM: Breastfeeding experiences of urban adolescent mothers, *J Pediatr Nurs* 24(4):244–254, 2009.

CHAPTER 36

Mental Health Issues

Anita Thompson-Heisterman, MSN, PMHCNS-BC, PMHNP-BC

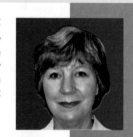

Anita Thompson-Heisterman began practicing community mental health nursing in 1983 as a psychiatric nurse in a community mental health center. Her community practice has included clinical and management activities in a psychiatric home care service, a nurse-managed primary care center in public housing, and an outreach program for rural older adults. Currently she is an assistant professor in the Division of Family, Community and Mental Health Systems at the University of Virginia School of Nursing, and her faculty practice is with the Memory and Aging Care Clinic at the University of Virginia Department of Neurology.

ADDITIONAL RESOURCES

evolve WEBSITE
http://evolve.elsevier.com/Stanhope
- *Healthy People 2020*
- WebLinks
- Quiz
- Case Studies
- Glossary
- Answers to Practice Application

OBJECTIVES

After reading this chapter, the student should be able to do the following:

1. Describe the history of community mental health and make predictions about the future.
2. Discuss the prevalence of mental illness in the United States and the world.
3. Describe essential mental health services and corresponding national objectives for improving mental health.
4. Discuss the health status of the population that has mental illness in the United States.
5. Evaluate standards, models, concepts, and research findings for use in community mental health nursing practice.
6. Describe the role of the community mental health nurse with individuals and with groups at risk for psychiatric mental health problems.
7. Apply the nursing process in community work with clients diagnosed with psychiatric disorders, families at risk for mental health problems, and vulnerable populations.
8. Examine strategies to improve the mental health of people who are at risk in a complex society.

KEY TERMS

Providing community services and nursing care to people suffering from mental illness or emotional distress is complex and influenced by many individual and community factors and requires a variety of approaches. Factors include: (1) the scope of emotional and mental disorders, (2) uncertainty about specific cause, cure, and treatment for most severe mental disorders, (3) severe chronic disabling nature of some mental disorders, and (4) complexity of the community mental health services sector. The scarcity of resources compounds the problems and presents challenges in community mental health work.

Cultural beliefs and economics influence the amount and types of services and treatment available in countries. However, two universal truths exist: services for people with mental disorders are inadequate in all countries, and mental illness has a significant effect on families, communities, and nations. Therefore, specialized knowledge and skills about severe mental illness and mental health problems are necessary for effective nursing practice in the community. It is helpful to understand both the organization of mental health services from a historical perspective and the trends in current health care demands and delivery. Knowledge about populations at risk for psychiatric mental health problems and understanding illness outcomes in terms of biopsychosocial consequences are even more important. Finally, it is necessary to refine and broaden nursing process skills in treatment planning to include the impact of mental illness on families and communities.

This chapter focuses on the scope of mental disorders, development of community mental health services, current health objectives for mental health and mental disorders, and the role of the nurse in community settings. Conceptual frameworks useful in community mental health nursing practice are also presented. Because other chapters in this book are devoted to high-risk groups such as the homeless population and those with substance abuse problems, this chapter's focus is on the variety of mental health problems encountered in communities, with an emphasis on populations who have long-term, severe mental disorders and groups who are most vulnerable to mental health problems.

SCOPE OF MENTAL ILLNESS IN THE UNITED STATES

Mental health is defined in *Healthy People 2020* (USDHHS, 2010) as encompassing the ability to engage in productive activities and fulfilling relationships with other people, to adapt to change, and to cope with adversity. The World Health Organization (WHO) expands the definition, describing mental health as a state of well-being in which a person can realize his or her potential and notes that mental health is essential if a person is to have health (WHO, 2008a). Mental health is an integral part of personal well-being, family and other interpersonal relationships, and contributions to community or society. Mental disorders are conditions that are characterized by alterations in thinking, mood, or behavior, which are associated with distress and/or impaired functioning. Mental illness refers collectively to all diagnosable mental disorders. Severe mental disorders are determined by diagnoses and criteria that include degree of functional disability (APA, 2000).

Mental disorders are indiscriminate. They occur across the life span and affect persons of all races, cultures, genders, and educational and socioeconomic groups. They are the leading cause of disability in North America (WHO, 2008b). In the United States, approximately 57.7 million adults (ages 18 and older), or 26.2% of the population, suffer from a mental disorder in a given year, and 6% of the population suffer from a serious mental illness such as schizophrenia. Nearly half of those with any mental disorder meet criteria for two disorders (Kessler et al, 2005; NIMH, 2010). At least 13% of children and adolescents between ages 8 and 15 years have a diagnosable mental disorder in a given year (Merikangas et al, 2009). Eight percent of youth between 12 and 17 suffer from a major depressive disorder, but only 39% receive treatment (SAMHSA, 2007). Nearly 17% of people over age 55 experience a mood or anxiety disorder (Byers et al, 2010), and these rates will rise as the number of older Americans increases over the next two decades. Alzheimer disease, the primary cause of dementia, affects about 5.3 million Americans each year and creates a significant mental health burden for individuals and families

(Alzheimer's Association, 2010). The number of cases in the population doubles every 5 years of age after age 60 and will become a public health crisis as the "baby boomer" generation ages. Affective disorders include major depression and manic-depressive or bipolar illness. Although bipolar illness may only affect a small proportion of the population, major depression is pervasive and is the leading cause of disability among adults ages 15 to 44. Anxiety disorders—including panic disorder, obsessive-compulsive disorder, posttraumatic stress disorder (PTSD), and phobias—are prevalent, affecting 18% of American adults each year. Mental disorders can also be a secondary problem among people with other disabilities. Depression and anxiety, for example, occur more frequently among people with disabilities (NIMH, 2010).

The impact of mental illness on overall health and productivity in the United States and throughout the world is often underrecognized. In the United States, mental illness causes about the same amount of disability as heart disease and cancer. Depression is the leading cause of years of productivity loss because of disability in the United States (WHO, 2008b). Despite the prevalence of mental illness, only 25% of persons with a mental disorder obtain help for their illness in any part of the health care system, and the majority of persons with mental disorders do not receive any specialty mental health care. Twenty-nine million persons 18 years and older received mental health care from a variety of providers in 2007. However, another 11 million who had a mental health need received no care (USDHHS, 2008). Of young people ages 4 to 17 years who have a mental disorder, 60% received help through private or community-based providers and 40% through schools (USDHHS, 2009). The WHO (2008b) reports the global burden of mental health, substance abuse, and neurological diseases at 14% and, in recognition of the lack of resources, launched a mental health global action program (mhGAP) to begin to address the needs (WHO, 2008a). Their poster "No Health Without Mental Health" effectively describes the need to integrate physical and mental health services. Given this information, it is critical that nurses recognize and provide health services for those with mental disorders in a variety of non-traditional community settings.

In addition to diagnosable mental conditions, there is growing awareness and concern about the public health burden of stress, especially following terrorist attacks around the world, natural disasters such as Hurricane Katrina in New Orleans and the earthquake in Haiti, and man-made disasters such as the 2010 oil spill in the Gulf of Mexico, the wars in Iraq and Afghanistan, and the effects of the economic crisis (NIMH, 2010). Strengthening the public health sector to respond to these events involves developing community mental health responses as well as addressing physical health concerns. Community mental health nurses (CMHNs) play an important role in identifying stressful events, assessing stress responses, educating communities, and intervening to prevent or alleviate disability and disease resulting from stress (Clark, 2010).

Although all of us are vulnerable to stressful life events and may develop mental health problems, persons with chronic and persistent mental illness have numerous problems. Mental illness is misunderstood, and those who suffer from it often experience stigma and lack of social support, which is so critical to health. Persons with mental illness are often identified by the illness as a schizophrenic instead of a person with the illness. The onset of the disruptive symptoms of schizophrenia often occurs just as young persons are attempting to finish schooling and develop a career, shattering lives and driving many into a lifetime of underemployment, poverty, and lack of access to adequate health services, housing, and social supports. Many accessible and coordinated services are needed to enable people with chronic mental illness to live in the community, yet these often are not available. Despite the inadequacy of resources, advances have been made in the treatment of mental illness. These advances have been influenced by two major movements: consumer advocacy, and better understanding of the neurobiology of mental illness (Tomes, 2006; Rick and Douglas, 2007; Weiss, 2007). Naturally the financing of mental health services impacts access to care and influences treatment. The system known as managed care had a significant impact on service delivery for the past 20 years, and passage of mental health parity and national health care reform will undoubtedly influence mental health care during the next decade.

Consumer Advocacy

Consumer advocacy movements for people with mental illness, like those for other illnesses, came about to fulfill unmet needs and to attempt to decrease the stigma associated with mental illness. Specifically, the National Alliance for the Mentally Ill (NAMI) was the first consumer group to advocate for better services. This consumer advocacy group worked to establish education and self-help services for individuals and families with mental illness. Efforts of the NAMI gained momentum in the early 1980s. Subsequently, political groups and legislative bodies responded with direct support. One example of direct support was funding for the Community Support Program (CSP) by the National Institute of Mental Health (NIMH). The CSP provided grant monies to states to develop comprehensive services for persons discharged from psychiatric institutions and invited consumers to participate (Tomes, 2006). These and similar efforts have helped bring consumers, families, and professionals together to work toward improvement in the treatment and care of persons with mental illness.

Neurobiology of Mental Illness

Mental illnesses are complex biopsychosocial disorders. Considerable emphasis in the past 20 years has focused on the biological basis of mental illness. The 1990s were declared the "decade of the brain" as great strides occurred through research in neurology, microbiology, and genetics that led to understanding the structural and chemical complexity of the brain. Consequently, more is now known about the functions of the brain than at any time in history. We have learned that the brain is not a static organ. The concept of brain plasticity demonstrates that new learning actually changes brain structure. For example, traumatic experiences change brain biochemistry, as do significant positive experiences (Rick and Douglas, 2007;

Weiss, 2007). This information supports the thought that both experience and psychosocial factors have effects on the etiology and on the treatment of mental illnesses. Both somatic and psychosocial interventions need to be used to treat mental illness. In addition to research, neuroradiological techniques aid diagnosis and treatment of people with psychiatric disorders. Angiography is used to screen for abnormalities of the vascular system, such as atherosclerosis and brain tumors, that can lead to behavior changes. The use of non-invasive scanning of the brain can help in making diagnoses. Computed axial tomography (CAT) scans provide a cross-sectional view of the brain, whereas nuclear magnetic resonance (NMR) imaging offers the advantage of imaging the brain from different planes. Still other techniques, such as positron-emission tomography (PET) and single photon emission computed tomography (SPECT), provide information about cerebral blood flow and brain metabolism. The information gained from these advanced technologies can lead to better understanding about mental illness and treatment.

> **THE CUTTING EDGE** *Using non-invasive imaging techniques, scientists soon will be able to study the effects of different forms of psychotherapeutic interventions on the brain.*

Discoveries in psychopharmacology have also revolutionized treatment of mental illness (Boyd, 2005). New atypical antipsychotic drugs used in the treatment of schizophrenia can improve the quality of life for many, primarily because of fewer side effects. However, new adverse effects, including weight gain, insulin resistance, and dangerously high blood glucose levels, known as metabolic syndrome, have created fresh concerns for consumers and providers (McElroy et al, 2005; Newcomer, 2005; Correll et al, 2006).

> **WHAT DO YOU THINK?** *Although psychopharmacology has dramatically improved the lives of people with severe mental illness, controversies exist about medication side effects and the costs of monitoring treatment. For example, side effects of antipsychotic drugs include central and peripheral nervous system manifestations. New or atypical antipsychotics have reduced some of these side effects but have caused weight gain, insulin resistance, and life-threatening hyperglycemia. Do the benefits offered by these medications justify their side effects and the additional costs of monitoring?*

Newer antidepressant medications known as selective serotonin reuptake inhibitors (SSRIs) are now considered the first choice in the treatment of depression as well as for many anxiety disorders because they lead to good responses with fewer side effects. They are now widely prescribed by primary care physicians as well as psychiatrists and are some of the most prescribed medications in the United States. Although considered safer than older agents, evidence suggests that the SSRIs accelerate bone loss and may lead to osteoporosis (Saag, 2007) and they may not be more effective than non-pharmacological interventions, such as exercise, in treating depression.

> **THE CUTTING EDGE** *The new science of pharmacogenetics will enable more individualized treatment of mental illness based on specific, genetically based responses to pharmaceuticals.*

SYSTEMS OF COMMUNITY MENTAL HEALTH CARE

Managed Care

Managed care is a system of managing health care to ensure access to appropriate and cost-effective services. Managed mental health care grew rapidly during the 1990s, and by 1999 nearly 80% of Americans were enrolled in a managed health care plan. Initially a method to control costs and access to mental health care in the private insurance sector, managed care became a significant factor in public mental health, and by the turn of the century more than half of all Medicaid recipients were enrolled in a managed mental health care plan. Consumer outcomes such as health status, quality of life, functioning, and satisfaction are considerations in deciding if services are effective. Since one purpose of managed care is to control costs, often by substituting less costly services for more costly ones, the findings about consumer outcomes are critical. For example, the provision of quality comprehensive services in the community is not inexpensive, but it is generally less costly than hospital care and frequent admissions. Services must fit the needs of the consumer, and outcomes research can help guide care and policy decisions.

> **DID YOU KNOW?** *Managed care programs tend to limit coverage to brief inpatient hospital stays for mental illness. However, community survival for people with serious mental illness requires a broad range of well-coordinated services, including mental and physical health, housing assistance, substance abuse treatment for some, and social and vocational rehabilitation.*

Changes continue to take place in mental health funding, and changes in one sector can have far-reaching consequences in many others. Although legislation was passed in 1996 ensuring parity for mental illness coverage in insurance plans, the implementation at the state level and the effects on insurance plans had been rather negligible for a variety of reasons, and further legislation passed in 2008 was needed to improve service access (Mental Health America, 2009). The seemingly constant changes in mental health funding present challenges for nurses, who need to make judgments about the positive and negative outcomes of these changes on the people they care for before research findings that can be generalized to the population are readily available.

Mental health problems and mental disorders are treated by a variety of caregivers who work in diverse and loosely connected facilities. The landmark surgeon general's report on mental health, in an attempt to delineate where Americans receive mental health services, defined four major ways through which people receive assistance: (1) the specialty mental health system, both public and private, (2) the general medical or primary care sector, (3) the human service sector, and (4) the voluntary support network, including advocacy groups (USDHHS, 1999). Nurses need to understand that delivery of mental health services may occur in any of these systems. In fact, most older adults receive mental health services through the primary care sector, whereas most children and adolescents are served through human services that include schools. Those with resources, less severe mental health problems, and access to primary care are more likely to have their mental health needs addressed within the context of a visit to their primary care provider. Because of the influence of managed care, access to a specialist, if indicated for psychiatric treatment, occurs via this route as well.

The community mental health model is the primary method of care for people with serious and persistent mental illness. Components of this model include team care, case management, outreach, and a variety of rehabilitative and recovery approaches to help prevent exacerbations of illness. In most states, services are provided through comprehensive community mental health centers (CMHCs). There is great variance in how each state and locality implements mental health service delivery and each version continues to evolve in this era of health care reform, as the CMHCs react to societal, political, and fiscal pressures. As resources diminish, the focus narrows and many CMHCs are unable to provide services to populations other than those with serious and persistent mental illness. It is unclear how the growing focus on integration of mental health into primary care, parity in insurance coverage, and the recent passage of national health care reform might impact the community mental health system of care (IOM, 2006; Manderscheid and Berry, 2006).

EVOLUTION OF COMMUNITY MENTAL HEALTH CARE

Historical Perspectives

The manner in which the community has perceived the etiology of mental and emotional illness across the ages has influenced the care and treatment of persons suffering from these disorders. These patterns were often cyclical. In ancient times, mental illness was viewed as resulting from supernatural forces and those afflicted were shunned. During the Greco-Roman era, mental and physical illnesses were seen as interrelated and resulting from physical conditions. Treatment was aimed at curing the disease by restoring balance. A return to a belief in supernatural etiologies occurred during the Middle Ages in Europe and continued in the colonies well into the eighteenth century. These beliefs led to poor treatment of the mentally ill, including incarceration, starvation, and torture. Near the end of the eighteenth century, the revolution in mental health care known as Humanitarian Reform took place. This reform movement, influenced by Philippe Pinel (1759-1820) in France and Benjamin Rush (1745-1813) in North America, led to hospital expansion, medical treatment, and the community mental health movements (Boyd, 2005).

Before the Humanitarian Reform, persons with mental illness were often housed in jails because health and social services had not been developed. Even later, after the development of hospitals as a site of treatment, persons with mental disorders were neglected and mistreated. Although the first psychiatric hospital in the United States was built in Williamsburg, Virginia, in 1773, approximately 50 years passed before widespread construction of facilities in other states took place. One person in particular, Dorothea Dix, led reform efforts to correct inhumane practices (Boyd, 2005).

Dorothea Lynde Dix (1802-1887) focused attention on criminals, those with mental disorders, and victims of the Civil War. She believed that people with mental disorders needed health and social services, and her efforts influenced the improved organization of mental health services. Her work led to the development of hospitals as the primary site of care, and she influenced standards for hospital administration and nursing care. Because of her lifetime efforts, often through political action, treatment for mentally infirm persons was altered in both North America and Europe (Boyd, 2005).

Hospital Expansion, Institutionalization, and the Mental Hygiene Movement

Psychiatric hospitals constructed during the expansion era were located in rural areas and were intended for small numbers of clients. However, they soon became overcrowded with people who had severe mental disorders, with older adults, and with immigrants who were poor and unable to speak English. Clients were essentially separated from the community and isolated from their families. Many were institutionalized for the rest of their lives, in response to both a continued fear of persons with mental disorders and a lack of community resources. Institutionalization of large numbers of people, combined with minimal information about cause, cure, and care, resulted in overcrowded conditions and exploitation of clients.

At the beginning of the twentieth century, institutional conditions were reported publicly in the United States by Clifford Beers, who had been hospitalized both in private and in public mental hospitals (Boyd, 2005). Beers urged reform and influenced the founding of the National Committee for Mental Hygiene. During the mental hygiene movement, attention shifted to ideas about prevention, early intervention, and the influence of social and environmental factors on mental illness. These ideas about treatment also influenced the development of multidisciplinary approaches to treatment. The mental hygiene and community mental health movements increased understanding about mental illness.

Further understanding about the scope of mental illness was gained during the conscription process for the armed services in World War II. Many of the persons screened for military service during World War II were found to have neurological and psychiatric mental health disorders. Even more military personnel required treatment for mental health problems associated with social and environmental stress during and after the war, not only in the United States but also in Europe, Russia, and Pacific Rim countries (Boyd, 2005). At the same time, the community mental health model continued to expand slowly while populations consisting of individuals with severe mental disorders and older adult persons with dementia grew larger in the state hospitals. Demands for mental health services in communities, combined with concerns about conditions of state psychiatric hospitals, prompted federal legislation that influenced development of the community mental health concept.

Federal Legislation for Mental Health Services

The first major piece of legislation to influence mental health services in the United States was the Social Security Act in 1935. This act, created in response to economic and social problems of the era, shifted the responsibility of care for ill people from the state to the federal government. The federal government's role expanded when the demand for mental health services increased during and after World War II. Key points of legislation that influenced the development of community mental health services are summarized in Table 36-1.

In 1946 the National Mental Health Act was passed and the National Institute of Mental Health (NIMH) administered its programs. Objectives included development of education and research programs for community mental health treatment approaches. The act also included financial incentives for training grants to increase the number of professional workers, including nurses, in mental health services. Education and research programs materialized readily, along with advances in science and technology and the development of psychotropic medications. In 1955 the Mental Health Study Act was passed and the Joint Commission on Mental Illness and Health was established by the NIMH. Members of the commission studied national mental health needs and submitted to Congress a report entitled *Action for Mental Health.* Recommendations of the report included continued development of research and education programs, early and intensive treatment for acute mental illness, and shifting the care of severely mentally ill persons away from the large hospitals to psychiatric wards in general hospitals

and to community mental health clinics. Along with prevention and intervention, community services were to include aftercare services following hospitalization for individuals with major mental illness (Boyd, 2005). The shift in the locus of care from state hospitals to community systems was begun.

The Community Mental Health Centers (CMHCs) Act was passed in 1963, and the CMHC concept was formalized. Federal funds were designated to match state funds to construct CMHCs and start programs. CMHCs were mandated to have five basic services: inpatient, outpatient, partial hospitalization, 24-hour emergency services, and consultation/education services for community agencies and professionals. In addition, regulations encouraged states to offer diagnostic and rehabilitative pre-care and aftercare services (Boyd, 2005). However, many CMHCs, especially those in poor and rural areas, were unable to generate adequate money for continuing their start-up programs. Funding did not follow the client to the community. The deinstitutionalization of persons with severe mental disorders was well underway before some of these shortcomings were recognized.

DEINSTITUTIONALIZATION

Deinstitutionalization involved transitioning large numbers of people from state psychiatric hospitals to communities. The cost of institutional care was perhaps the main reason for the movement; other influences included the discovery of psychotropic medications and civil rights activism (Boyd, 2005). The goal of deinstitutionalization was to improve the quality of life for people with mental disorders by providing services in the communities where they lived rather than in large institutions.

TABLE 36-1 LEGISLATION THAT INFLUENCED COMMUNITY MENTAL HEALTH SERVICES

YEAR	LEGISLATION	FOCUS
1946	National Mental Health Act	Education and research for mental health treatment approaches began (NIMH).
1955	Mental Health Study Act	Resulted in Joint Commission on Mental Illness and Health, which recommended transformation of state hospital systems and establishment of community mental health clinics.
1963	Community Mental Health Centers Act	Marked beginning of community mental health centers' concept and led to deinstitutionalization of large psychiatric hospitals.
1975	Developmental Disabilities Act	Addressed the rights and treatment of people with developmental disabilities and provided foundation for similar action for individuals with mental disorders.
1977	President's Commission on Mental Health	Reinforced importance of community-based services, protection of human rights, and national health insurance for mentally ill persons.
1978	Omnibus Reconciliation Act	Rescinded much of the 1977 commission's provisions and shifted funds for all health programs from federal to state resources.
1986	Protection and Advocacy for Mentally Ill Individuals Act	Legislated advocacy programs for mentally ill persons.
1990	Americans with Disabilities Act	Prohibited discrimination and promoted opportunities for persons with mental disorders.
1996	Mental Health Parity Act	Attempted to address discrepancy between mental health and medical–surgical benefits in employer-sponsored health plans.
2008	Mental Health and Addiction Equity Act	Prohibits discrepancy in coverage between mental health and physical health benefits in employer-sponsored and private insurance plans and added substance abuse as a covered mental health condition.
2010	Patient Protection and Affordable Health Care Act	Prohibits discrimination in coverage for preexisting conditions. Prohibits discontinuation of coverage because of illness.

To change the locus of care, large hospital wards were closed and persons with severe mental disorders were returned to the community to live. Many were discharged to the care of family members; others went to nursing homes. Still others were placed in apartments or other types of adult housing; some of these were supervised settings, and others were not.

Not surprisingly, as with any abrupt, dramatic change, problems related to unexpected service gaps between the hospitals and the CMHCs led to continuity-of-care problems. Although deinstitutionalization was a noble idea, there were not adequate resources to support the implementation. For example, families were not prepared for the treatment responsibilities they had to assume, and yet few mental health systems offered them education and support programs. Although many older adult clients were admitted to nursing homes and personal care settings, education programs were seldom available for staff members, who often lacked the skills necessary to treat persons with mental disorders. And finally, some clients found themselves in independent settings such as rooming houses and single-room occupancy hotels with little or no supervision and few skills to manage living in the community. Clients, families, communities, and the nation suffered as poor living and social conditions were associated with mental disorders. Homelessness and placement of the mentally ill in jails and prisons also occurred. These conditions may have increased the stigma associated with persons with mental illness. The placement of persons with mental illness in nursing homes, assisted living facilities, and jails was often referred to as "reinstitutionalization," since it only shifted people from one institution to another. These issues prompted additional legislation and advocacy efforts.

Civil Rights Legislation for Persons with Mental Disorders

The development of CMHCs was based partially on the principle that persons with mental disorders had a right to treatment in the least restrictive environment (Boyd, 2005). Although CMHCs were less restrictive than institutions, they lacked necessary services. For example, people with severe mental disorders require daily monitoring or hospitalization during acute episodes of illness. Even though hospital services were available, many individuals expressed their rights to refuse treatment and resisted admission. Also, transitional care following discharge for those persons who were admitted to hospitals was not available in most communities. In addition to the right to refuse treatment, advocates for mentally ill individuals focused on such civil rights issues as segregated services, inhumane practices in psychiatric hospitals, and failure to include clients in treatment planning. Activism for minorities and handicapped persons also influenced civil rights legislation for persons with mental disorders. In particular, during the 1970s institutional conditions of persons with developmental handicaps prompted the Developmental Disabilities Assistance Act and the Bill of Rights Act. Other legislation shifted funding from the federal to the state level. The Mental Health Systems Act was repealed in 1980. This action limited the federal leadership role, shifted more costs back to the states from the federal government, and

further impeded the implementation and provision of community mental health services.

State systems of mental health services developed in unique and diverse ways and were often inadequate. In general, individuals with severe mental disorders were vulnerable and neglected and either lacked or were unable to access health and social services. In an effort to offset these problems, in 1986 the federal Protection and Advocacy for Mentally Ill Individuals Act and the Mental Health Planning Act were passed. Advocacy programs for mentally ill persons became part of the same state advocacy systems developed earlier under the Developmental Disability Act, and consumer involvement in CMHCs was mandated (Boyd, 2005). In spite of advocacy efforts and legislation, the CMHCs were unable to meet the increased and diverse demands for mental health services in their communities. The lack of services, combined with concerns about discrimination against all people with disabilities, led to additional legislation.

The Americans with Disabilities Act (ADA) was passed in 1990. The ADA mandated that individuals with mental and physical disabilities must not be discriminated against and must be brought into the mainstream of American life through access to employment and public services (Boyd, 2005). History reveals that past legislation promoted the rights of persons with mental disorders, but litigation was also responsible for the lack of growth, if not the decline, in community mental health services. In 1996 the Mental Health Parity Act was passed to address discrimination in insurance coverage and in 2008 the Mental Health Parity and Addiction Equity Act (MHPAEA) was passed, prohibiting differential coverage for mental health disorders (Mental Health America, 2009). The community mental health nurse can advocate for clients to ensure equality in access to health services, housing, and employment.

Advocacy Efforts

Consumers or survivors, defined as persons who are current or former recipients of mental health services, along with their families have had a significant impact on mental health services. As in all areas of health care, the rights and wishes of consumers are important in planning and delivering services. However, consumers of mental health services have traditionally had difficulty advocating for themselves. In the past, treatment programs often fostered passivity in clients and excluded them from the treatment planning process. In addition, family members were responsible for care in the home, but they lacked resources and even information about treatment (Tomes, 2006). Like consumers, family members suffered from the stigma of mental illness and public attitudes that contributed to self-advocacy problems. In contrast, self-advocacy and involvement in treatment planning fosters self-confidence, promotes participation in services, and may have a significant influence on policy decisions (Tomes, 2006). Consumer and family groups fostered these objectives.

Family members led self-advocacy efforts in the 1970s, when small groups organized to challenge and change mental health services. These early efforts resulted in the formation of the National Alliance for the Mentally Ill (NAMI), which today has both state and local affiliates. Soon, consumer groups formed to advocate for better services, changes in mental health policy, self-help programs in treatment, and empowerment. Several advocacy groups that support these consumer efforts are summarized in Box 36-1. In their assessment of resources, nurses can identify community advocacy and support groups.

CONCEPTUAL FRAMEWORKS FOR COMMUNITY MENTAL HEALTH

The community mental health principles that are the underpinnings of practice include the right to mental health services delivered in the least restrictive environment, consumer involvement in treatment, advocacy, and rehabilitative and recovery services. Biopsychosocial theories are useful to understand the multidimensional aspects of community mental health nursing. These include theories and models that explain biological processes, systems, personality, lifespan development, family dynamics, and stress and coping. Focusing on wellness or recovery, relapse prevention, or relapse management and helping the client reach a maximal level of function are useful for nursing practice.

Another helpful framework for community mental health practice is systems theory, which emphasizes the relationship between the elements of a unit and the whole. An understanding of the whole occurs through the examination of interactions and relationships that exist between the parts. A holistic view of system and subsystems can be applied in a variety of ways in community mental health practice. One example of a subsystem in a community is its cultural groups. Subsystems of the cultural groups are families; subsystems of the

families are individuals. Using systems theory to explore the background, conditions, and context of situations will disclose information about the positive and negative forces that either promote or undermine the well-being of any unit in the system.

The diathesis-stress model is also useful in CMHN practice. This theory integrates the effects of biology and environment, or nature and nurture, on the development of mental illness. Certain genes or genetic combinations produce a predisposition to a disorder. When an individual with a predisposition to a disorder is challenged by an environmental stressor, the expression of the mental disorder may result (Boyd, 2005). The integration of psychosocial and neurobiological paradigms is critical to the practice of psychiatric nursing. Nurses must recognize the effects of environment and biology on people and actively work to mitigate psychosocial as well as biological stressors.

> **NURSING TIP** *Nurses need to teach individuals and groups strategies to promote mental health and reduce stress.*

Levels of Prevention

Health promotion and illness prevention are fundamental to community mental health practice as well as to national objectives for mental health (USDHHS, 2010). Therefore, the concepts of primary, secondary, and tertiary levels of prevention are useful in community mental health practice (see Levels of Prevention box).

Primary prevention refers to the reduction of health risks. It involves both health promotion and disease prevention. Health promotion strategies aim to enhance the well-being of healthy populations, whereas disease prevention strategies focus on the identification of populations at risk and conditions that may cause stress and illness. Providing education about stress reduction techniques to adults in the workplace is a form of mental

---

BOX 36-1 ADVOCACY AND SELF-HELP ORGANIZATIONS

- *Community Support Program (CSP):* A program of the U.S. Department of Health and Human Services (USDHHS), Substance Abuse and Mental Health Services Administration (SAMHSA), and the Center for Mental Health Services (CMHS), that developed plans for a model continuum of care, offers grants for demonstration programs including community rehabilitation projects, and provides money to states for development of consumer and family services and advocacy efforts
- *Consumer/Survivor Mental Health Research and Policy Work Group:* An endeavor sponsored by the Mental Health Statistics Improvement Program of the CMHS to initiate consumer representation in activities of the National Association of State Mental Health Program Directors (NASMHPD)
- *National Alliance for the Mentally Ill (NAMI):* A family organization that promotes family support groups, education programs, public campaigns to reduce stigma, and advocacy for mental health policy and services at local and national levels
- *NAMI Consumers' Council:* A consumer advocacy group that advocates for improved and effective psychiatric services and consumer empowerment
- *National Association of Psychiatric Survivors (NAPS):* A consumer organization that advocates for such things as involuntary treatment and some forms of treatment like electroconvulsive therapy
- *National Mental Health Association (NMHA):* An organization aimed at improving mental health in the population at large, emphasizing prevention
- *National Mental Health Consumers' Association (NMHCA):* A consumer organization that advocates for improvements in the mental health system

---

📋 LEVELS OF PREVENTION

In Community Mental Health

Primary Prevention
- Educate populations about mental health issues.
- Teach stress reduction techniques.
- Support and provide prenatal education.
- Provide parenting classes.
- Provide support to caregivers.
- Provide bereavement support.

Secondary Prevention
- Conduct screenings to detect mental health disorders.
- Provide mental health interventions after stressful events.

Tertiary Prevention
- Provide health promotion activities to persons with serious and persistent mental illness.
- Promote support group participation for those with mental health disabilities.
- Advocate for rehabilitation and recovery services.

health promotion. An example of disease prevention is to provide mental health information about depression and eating disorders to adolescents in schools.

Secondary prevention activities are aimed at reducing the prevalence or pathological nature of a condition. They involve early diagnosis, prompt treatment, and limitation of disability. Many functions of the practitioner role are aimed at secondary prevention for individuals. These include providing individual and group psychotherapy, case management, and referral. Screening members of a community for depression during National Depression Screening Day is an example of population-based secondary prevention. Counseling, referral, and treatment interventions after traumatic incidents, such as terrorist attacks or natural disasters, are other important community interventions.

Tertiary prevention efforts attempt to restore and enhance functioning. On a community level, tertiary prevention activities might include support of affordable housing, promotion of psychosocial rehabilitation and recovery programs, and involvement in advocacy and consumer groups for the mentally ill. Many nursing role activities in community mental health are aimed at tertiary prevention with individuals. They include working with individuals to monitor illness symptoms and treatment responses, coordinating transition from the hospital to the community, and identifying respite care options for caregivers.

Relapse management with a focus on recovery is central to many of the programs and activities that enhance coping skills and competence. The nurse may participate in assertive community treatment (ACT) programs, psychosocial rehabilitation (clubhouses), and intensive case management. ACT programs differ from intensive case management approaches in that they are based more on a medical model and team approach and provide crisis and case management services 24 hours a day, 7 days a week. They are sometimes referred to as hospitals without walls (Salyers and Tsemberis, 2008). Intensive case management models vary across programs but generally include contact with clients several times a week by an individual case manager. Nurses have critical roles in both treatment programs, as they have the knowledge and skills to provide comprehensive biopsychosocial care.

For example, the nurse visits the client at home, checks medication, assesses physical and emotional functioning, and may take the client shopping for nutritional food. The nurse may accompany the consumer to the physician's office and serve as an advocate for the client in this setting.

As case managers, nurses work with consumers, family members, and other caregivers to foster coping and competency aimed at managing illness symptoms. The goal of managing illness symptoms is to offset relapse and promote recovery. Relapse management and promotion of recovery are major goals of intervention in community mental health nursing. Assessment of the frequency, intensity, and duration of symptoms for the purpose of identifying biological, environmental, and behavioral triggers that may lead to illness relapse helps the consumer manage the illness and promotes recovery. Examples of triggers are poor nutrition, poor social skills, hopelessness, and poor

symptom management. Once triggers are identified, interventions aimed at fostering effective coping skills can be introduced to offset relapse of symptoms. For example, an intervention that may promote effective coping to offset social isolation is guiding the client to organized consumer group activities available in the community. Another is to promote consumer and family efforts at job training through community vocational agencies. Still another is to promote competency in family members by coordinating services that enhance their understanding of the illness, provide social support, and include respite care when needed. Finally, an alliance with the client to manage medication and side effects is an important component of relapse prevention and recovery promotion (Mynatt, 2005).

As previously discussed, scientific advances that led to the use of medications to treat mental illness revolutionized mental health care and services (Boyd, 2005). Atypical antipsychotics and new antidepressants with fewer side effects have further influenced mental health care in the community. Although these new drugs have dramatically improved the lives of many people with mental disorders, they are not without problems and are not a cure. The nurse has a critical role in monitoring side effects, detecting related health problems such as diabetes, and providing education and intervention. The most effective tertiary prevention is to combine medications with other relapse management approaches including culturally sensitive social, behavioral, and psychotherapeutic interventions (Kozuki and Schepp, 2005).

ROLE OF THE NURSE IN COMMUNITY MENTAL HEALTH

The role of the nurse in community mental health was shaped both by the evolution of services and by the work of nursing pioneers. Development of a knowledge base for the nursing discipline and the further expansion of mental health care services to non-traditional community sites called for more advanced community-based practitioners (ANA, 2007). Nursing practice standards reflect the values of the profession, describe the responsibilities of nurses, and provide direction for the delivery and evaluation of nursing care. These standards also describe the roles of nurses in both advanced and basic practice.

Advanced practice psychiatric nurses have graduate-level education. The psychiatric nurse practitioner title and role have been expanded to encompass primary care and specialty knowledge and skills. They provide primary, secondary, and tertiary care to individuals, groups, families, adults, children, and adolescents. Depending on state laws, some prescribe medications and have hospital admission privileges. For example, the advanced practice nurse may see clients individually to provide psychotherapy, may prescribe medications, and may conduct physical examinations or coordinate this care with other providers in primary care settings. The blended nurse practitioner role has been a response to a shift in the health care system away from specialization and toward comprehensive services that address both physical and mental health problems.

Nurses prepared at the undergraduate level provide basic primary, secondary, and tertiary services that are equally valuable. Specific roles and functions of nurses at the basic level (Box 36-2) are based on clinical nursing practice and standards (ANA, 2007). The functions suggest the overlapping roles of clinician, educator, and coordinator.

Clinician

Objectives of the practitioner role are to help the client maintain or regain coping abilities that promote functioning. This involves using the nursing process to guide the diagnosis and treatment of human responses to actual or potential mental health problems (ANA, 2007). Role functions at the basic practitioner level include case management, counseling, milieu therapy, and psychobiological interventions with individuals and with groups. Clinician skills are used with individual clients in a variety of settings, including the home, and often with large groups of people in specific neighborhoods, schools, and public health districts. For example, many clients who have schizophrenia live in personal care homes. These clients require biopsychosocial interventions related to medication management, milieu management for improved social interaction, and assistance with self-care activities for community living such as use of public transportation. Also, the practitioner increasingly coordinates these activities with both the consumer and with other staff members in community settings. Therefore, coordination of care is often the means for promoting recovery plan outcomes and enhancing quality of life for clients. These

---

BOX 36-2 ROLES AND FUNCTIONS IN PSYCHIATRIC/MENTAL HEALTH NURSING COMMUNITY PRACTICE

Roles
- Clinician
- Educator
- Coordinator

Functions
- Advocacy
- Case finding and referral
- Case management
- Community action and involvement
- Complementary interventions
- Counseling
- Crisis intervention
- Health maintenance
- Health promotion
- Health teaching
- Home visits
- Intake screening and evaluation
- Milieu therapy
- Promotion of self-care activities
- Psychiatric rehabilitation
- Psychobiological interventions

Modified from American Nurses Association, American Psychiatric Nurses Association, and International Society of Psychiatric Mental Health Nurses: *Scope and standards of psychiatric-mental health nursing*, Washington, DC, 2007, American Nurses Publishing.

---

activities can support positive outcomes for others in the community at large.

For example, family members are a primary support system for individuals with schizophrenia. Whether the client lives in a personal care home, a family residence, or another setting, counseling family members and the client about the illness may offset the stressors of caregiving. Moreover, educating the public may reduce the stigma and decrease social isolation for both clients and families, lead to public support for needed services, and decrease the costs of health care because of fewer hospitalizations. As suggested in these examples, clinician and educator roles overlap.

Educator

The educator role uses teaching/learning principles to increase understanding about mental illness and mental health. The educator role is foundational to health maintenance, health promotion, and community action. Teaching clients about illness symptoms and the benefits of medications promotes health maintenance and may reduce the risk for illness relapse. Research supports similar education programs for family members to increase their ability to monitor illness symptoms and to identify events that lead to relapse (Pickett-Schenk et al, 2006). The nurse may facilitate a combined support and education group for parents of children with schizophrenia or for consumers with major mental illness in weekly sessions at the community mental health center. The CMHN, both at the basic and at the advanced level, may participate in developing educational groups and programs for consumers, families, and other providers either alone or in collaboration with other organizations such as the Mental Health Association or the National Alliance for the Mentally Ill.

At the community level, both formal and informal teaching is important. One important objective for mental health promotion is to teach positive coping skills. Overmedicating is an example of an ineffective individual coping skill. Even when medications are properly used in treatment, the nurse requires specialized knowledge about drug interactions, pharmacokinetics, and pharmacodynamics. Factors that influence pharmacokinetics include anatomical and physiological changes that occur with aging or with co-existing mental and physical conditions. Use of non-prescription medications such as herbal remedies and over-the-counter drugs can influence pharmacokinetics. Because over one third of Americans use non-traditional remedies and many of these are specific for psychiatric conditions, nurses need to assess the use of these substances, be aware of interactions, and share this information with clients (Barnes, Bloom, and Nahin, 2009).

DID YOU KNOW? *Many people use herbal remedies such as ginkgo biloba for memory improvement, valerian root for sleep, and St. John's wort for depression to self-treat mental health symptoms.*

Coordinator

Coordination of care is a basic principle of the multidisciplinary team approach in community mental health services. Yet there is often a lack of coordination as well as limited services in many communities. Therefore, at a minimum, the role of coordinator must include case finding, referral, and follow-up to evaluate system breakdown and deficits. Because of current system deficits, nurses in community mental health function as coordinators who carry out intake screening, crisis intervention, and home visits. The nurse coordinator also tries to improve the client's health and well-being by promoting independence and self-care in the least restrictive environment. For example, the nurse may teach the client how to fill a medication box or how to use relaxation techniques to reduce stress. Health teaching related to nutrition, smoking cessation, and sleep promotion is essential for consumers with mental illness. These functions are consistent with descriptions of clinical case management that emphasize continuity of care for individuals who need complex services and with providing information for recovery (Caldwell, Sclafani, and Swarbrick, 2010).

To achieve these objectives and improve services, nurses work with a variety of professionals, including advanced practice nurses, social workers, physicians, psychologists, occupational and vocational therapists, and rehabilitation counselors. The nurse is often the advocate for the consumer who needs assistance making his or her needs clear and accessing both health and social services. Because non-licensed paraprofessionals are frequently involved in direct care activities, their services must be directed, coordinated, and evaluated within the context of treatment planning. Finally, coordination also involves work with individuals who may not have formal preparation but who are essential for positive treatment outcomes. These individuals include family members, shelter volunteers, consumer support groups, and community leaders who can influence development of services. For example, the nurse can teach others about mental illness and effective interventions for times when symptoms become apparent and behaviors become difficult to manage. In the coordinator role, nurses can identify and influence health system effectiveness and ineffectiveness.

> **NURSING TIP** *To assist your client in accessing community resources and services, it is as important to develop positive relationships with other community providers as it is with your clients.*

CURRENT AND FUTURE PERSPECTIVES IN MENTAL HEALTH CARE

Both nationally and internationally, too few mental health care services exist, and the available services are fragmented and often hard to access. In the United States, large segments of the population do not have basic health care services or insurance to cover both expected and unexpected illnesses. The Patient Protection and Affordable Health Care Act passed in 2010 hopes to close some of the gaps in coverage. Since health insurance coverage for most Americans is linked to employment, in an economic recession when jobs are lost, insurance is often lost as well, and people are no longer able to afford health care. Also, consumers, family members, and health care providers are concerned about issues of basic treatment, continuity of care,

housing, and costs for acute and long-term mental health services for persons with mental illness. As large numbers of baby boomers reach retirement age and Medicare eligibility, there is concern about whether Social Security and Medicare resources will continue to exist for older Americans. Declining state budgets and possible cuts in Medicaid funding may place community mental health services in peril. Therefore, implementation of health care reform continues to be a major political, social, and economic issue. Significant alterations in the current health care delivery system will occur slowly. In the meantime, nurses working in communities must understand the models of care, the scope of mental illness, and the national health objectives designed to promote the health and welfare of persons with mental health problems.

Managed care, as described previously, will continue to affect the delivery of mental health services. This will occur through a continued focus on providing services in primary care settings, through attempts to reduce inpatient stays, and through a more systematic evaluation of the outcomes of the care provided. The massive growth in managed care plans dramatically reduced hospital stays but also limited access to care. It is unclear how passage of national health care reform will affect the care of those with long-term care needs. Because the public mental health system is the only remaining state and federally supported treatment system for persons with serious and persistent mental disorders and Medicaid funds more than half of public mental health services, the high use of managed care approaches may not provide for adequate services. This could lead to gaps in service and large holes in the safety net for vulnerable consumers suffering from mental illness.

Nurses can be important providers in managed care models because of their emphasis on wellness and health promotion, skills at teaching and case management, and lower cost for service. In communities, nurses practice primary, secondary, and tertiary prevention activities by conducting comprehensive client histories to determine health problems and interventions that improve quality of care and cost-effectiveness. In home health settings, nurses screen for ineffective coping techniques such as use of alcohol or other substances to offset the stress of traumatic life events, thereby preventing further problems and costly care. They also screen for signs of psychiatric disorders in primary care and community health care settings. Community mental health services must include access to work and school settings for families and children. These types of nursing assessments and subsequent interventions may offset costly treatment in hospital settings.

Providing the range of community services necessary to handle persistent mental illness is difficult without sufficient funds for health and social services. It is important for nurses and others working in CMHCs to recognize the impact of changes in funding, target populations, restructuring, and disagreements between professions, agencies, and levels of government. Such information enables nurses to advocate for adequate services to meet the needs of individuals with severe and persistent mental illness. The nurse can build relationships with other providers, network with other agencies, and foster interagency collaboration to improve the quality of care for clients and their families.

NATIONAL OBJECTIVES FOR MENTAL HEALTH SERVICES

The goals of the community mental health movement are consistent with the health promotion and disease prevention objectives outlined in *Healthy People 2020* (USDHHS, 2010). The *Healthy People 2020* box illustrates the primary objectives of the national health agenda for mental health promotion and illness prevention. The objectives of *Healthy People 2020* address both settings where people receive care (e.g., primary care, juvenile justice systems) and populations at risk (e.g., children, adults with mental illness, and older adults). Increasing cultural competency and consumer satisfaction with mental health services are further objectives of the national agenda for mental health.

The new millennium brought recognition of the importance of addressing mental health and mental illness as part of disease prevention. Recognition of the burden of mental illness and the status of mental health in the United States was clarified by a landmark report from the surgeon general's office, *Mental Health: A Report of the Surgeon General* (USDHHS, 1999), followed by a report from the Surgeon General's Conference on Children's Mental Health in 2000. A national agenda for action described in *Healthy People 2010* and continued in *Healthy People 2020* (USDHHS, 2010) made mental health one of the 10 leading health indicators, which are chosen on the basis of relevance as a broad public health issue. The President's New Freedom Commission on Mental Health (2003) further highlighted the need to transform and heal system fragmentation to ensure access to quality mental health services. The goals of a transformed mental health system are found in Box 36-3.

Overall, the national goals of *Healthy People 2020* are to improve mental health and ensure access to quality and appropriate mental health services. Approaches emphasize prevention, maintenance, and restoration of mental health and independent functioning. The standards address mental health conditions of concern across the life span and with specific populations. Nurses can: (1) promote the standards in the agencies where they are employed, (2) use the standards in community assessment activities, and (3) introduce information about the standards to other groups and agencies, including local consumer and family organizations, to help prioritize mental health concerns.

BOX 36-3 NEW FREEDOM COMMISSION'S SIX GOALS OF A TRANSFORMED MENTAL HEALTH SYSTEM

1. Americans will understand that mental health is essential to overall health.
2. Mental health care will be consumer and family driven.
3. Disparities in mental health care will be eliminated.
4. Early mental health screening, assessment, and referral will be common practice.
5. Excellent mental health care will be delivered and research will be accelerated.
6. Technology will be used to access mental health care and information.

From President's New Freedom Commission on Mental Health: *Achieving the promise: transforming mental health care in America,* USDHHS Pub No SMA-03-3832, Rockville, MD, 2003, USDHHS.

 HEALTHY PEOPLE 2020

Examples of Targeted National Health Objectives for Mental Health and Mental Disorders

Goal: Improve mental health and ensure access to appropriate, quality mental health services.
- MHMD-1: Reduce the suicide rate.
- MHMD-4: Reduce the proportion of persons who experience major depressive episode (MDE).
- MHMD-6: Increase the proportion of children with mental health problems who receive treatment.
- MHMD-9: Increase the proportion of adults with mental disorders who receive treatment.
- MHMD-10: Increase the proportion of persons with co-occurring substance abuse and mental disorders who receive treatment for both disorders.

From U.S. Department of Health and Human Services: *Healthy People 2020 Objectives,* Office of Disease Prevention and Health Promotion, Washington, DC, 2010, USDHHS.

As indicated in the definitions at the beginning of this chapter, mental health is a dynamic process, influenced by both internal and external factors, that enables and promotes the individual's physical, cognitive, affective, and social functioning. In contrast, threats to mental health create stress that undermines relationships and diminishes the individual's ability to pursue and achieve life's goals. Values and beliefs influence the allocation of resources for neighborhoods and schools and can contribute to or undermine the mental health of people in communities.

Mental health problems are manifested in many ways. Untoward incidents or even anticipated life events can diminish physical, cognitive, affective, and social functioning. For example, in most situations, an anticipated or unexpected death of a family member results in grief that may temporarily interrupt the functioning of surviving family members and produce mental distress. Given adequate support and adaptation, most persons resume their lifestyles following the death of a loved one in spite of the sadness that they are likely to experience. When people do not have adequate resources, or when bereavement is complicated because of the conditions of the situation, there is an increased risk for threats to the mental health of surviving family members. Important interventions with individuals experiencing sorrow and grief are to encourage roles and activities that promote comfort and reduce isolation. Death of a family member can affect survivors of different ages in various ways. Infants and youths may be deprived of significant nurturing and care that will result in long-term emotional deficits, whereas adults are at increased risk for stress related to role changes, and older adults are vulnerable to social isolation as relatives and friends die. In any of these situations, individual or group therapy may be indicated not only for the immediate situation, but also for prevention of longer-term problems.

However, bereavement is not the only cause of diminished mental health. Other causes include, but are not limited to, physical health problems, disabilities resulting from trauma, exposure to violence in the neighborhood, job loss and unstable employment, and unanticipated environmental disasters that result in loss. Because multiple threats to mental health exist across the life span, it is useful to organize the study of problems according to life stages along life's continuum.

HOW TO Provide Interventions Following Community Disasters

Community mental health nurses can intervene immediately after a mass trauma by using interventions that promote:
- *A sense of safety*
- *Calming*
- *A sense of self and community efficacy*
- *Connectedness*
- *Hope*

From Hobfall SE, Watson P, Bell CC, et al: Five essential elements of immediate and mid-term mass trauma intervention: empirical evidence, Focus 70:221, 2009.

Children and Adolescents

Healthy People 2020 objectives aim to increase the number of children screened and treated for mental health problems. Children are at risk for disruption of normal development by biological, environmental, and psychosocial factors that impair their mental health, interfere with education and social interactions, and keep them from realizing their full potential as adults. For example, children may develop depression after a loss or behavior problems from abuse or neglect. Examples of environmental factors include crowded living conditions, violence, separation from parents, and lack of consistent caregivers. Exposure to community violence can be related to significant stress and depression in children (McClosky, Figuerdo, and Koss, 2008). Types of mental health problems typically diagnosed during childhood are depression, anxiety, and attention-deficit disorders. Examples of chronic disorders commonly seen are Down syndrome and autism. These problems affect growth and development and influence mental health during adolescence.

Suicide is the third leading killer of young persons between ages 15 and 24, and the second-leading cause of death in young adults, and in most cases there was a mental or substance abuse disorder (CDC, 2010). The second objective of *Healthy People 2020* is to reduce the rate of suicide attempts by adolescents. Some of the risk factors for both adolescents and adults include prior suicide attempts, stressful life events, and access to lethal methods. Increasing the number of adolescents screened for depression in primary health care settings is a new objective of *Healthy People 2020*. Early detection and treatment of depression can help prevent suicide. In addition to depression and substance abuse, adolescent problems include conduct disorders and eating disorders.

Another objective of *Healthy People 2020* is to reduce the proportion of adolescents with eating disorders. Many CMHNs do not directly work with persons with a primary eating disorder, but eating disturbances are frequently a symptom accompanying other conditions. Since most children are not seen in the mental health system, an important role of the CMHN is to educate other community providers, teachers, parents, and children. School nurses are in an ideal position to provide primary, secondary, and tertiary interventions for children with eating disorders. Nutrition education and early recognition, intervention, referral, and follow-up can help prevent eating disorders from becoming severe and can prevent relapses. Nurses can advocate in and beyond their communities for the provision of a nurse in all schools. This can increase the chances of early recognition of and treatment for persons with eating disorders.

Effective service expansion for children, particularly for those with serious emotional disturbances, depends on promoting collaboration across critical areas of support including schools, families, social services, health, mental health, and juvenile justice. Better services and collaboration for children with serious emotional disturbance and their families will result in greater school retention, decreased contact with the juvenile justice system, increased stability of living arrangements, and improved educational, emotional, and behavioral development. One of the objectives of *Healthy People 2020* is to ensure that children in the juvenile justice system receive access to mental health assessment and treatment (USDHHS, 2010). Children and adolescents require a variety of mental health services, including crisis intervention and both short- and long-term counseling. Nurses working in community settings, well-child clinics, and home health can help to offset this problem through prevention, education, and inclusion of parents in program planning. Because many children and adolescents lack services or access to services, community mental health assessment activities are essential. Assessment activities include identifying types of programs available or lacking in places where children and adolescents spend time. Assessments should be performed in schools and in the homes of clients served, and also in day care centers, churches, and organizations that plan and guide age-specific play and entertainment programs. Assessment data are essential for planning and developing programs that address mental health problems prevalent from the prenatal period through adolescence. Preventing problems during these developmental periods can reduce mental health problems in adulthood.

Adults

Adults suffer from varied sources of stress that contribute to their mental health status. Sources of stress include multiple role responsibilities, job insecurity, and unstable relationships. These and other conditions can undermine mental health and contribute to serious mental illness, depression, anxiety disorders, and substance abuse. *Healthy People 2020* objectives seek to help adults access treatment in order to decrease associated human and economic costs and to reduce suicide rates (USDHHS, 2010).

At some point, virtually all adults will experience a tragic or unexpected loss, a serious setback, or a time of profound sadness, grief, or distress. Major depressive disorder, however, differs both in intensity and in duration from normal sadness or grief. Depression disrupts relationships and the ability to function and can be fatal. Suicide was the eleventh leading cause of death in the United States in 2007 (NIMH, 2010), and the majority of those who kill themselves have a mental or substance abuse disorder. Other risk factors include prior suicide attempts, stressful life events, and access to lethal methods.

Women are twice as likely to experience depression, and women who are poor, unemployed, or victims of domestic violence are even more at risk. Available medications and psychological treatment can help 80% of those with depression, yet only a few seek help. Those with depression are more likely to visit a physician for some other reason, and the mental health condition may not be noted. Therefore, it is imperative that nurses in all settings recognize and screen for depression.

Anxiety disorders are common both in the United States and in other countries. An alarming 18% of the adult population will experience an anxiety disorder, many with overlapping substance abuse disorders (NIMH, 2010). Anxiety disorders may have an early onset and are characterized by recurrent episodes of illness and periods of disability. Panic disorder and agoraphobia along with depression are associated with increased risks of attempted and completed suicide.

The lifetime rates of co-occurrence of mental disorders and addictive disorders are strikingly high. About one in four persons in the United States experiences a mental disorder in the course of a year, and nearly one in three adults who have a mental disorder in their lifetime also experiences a co-occurring substance (alcohol or other drugs) abuse disorder (NIMH, 2010). Individuals with co-occurring disorders are more likely to experience a chronic course and to use services than are those with either type of disorder alone; however, the services are often fragmented and treatment occurs in different segments of the system.

How can nurses intervene? The general medical sector, including primary care clinics, hospitals, and nursing homes, is typically the initial point of contact for many adults with mental disorders; for some, these providers may be the only source of mental health services. Early detection and intervention for mental health problems can be increased if persons presenting in primary care are assessed for mental health problems. Nurses who work in the general medical sector and in other community settings are in an ideal position to assess and detect mental health problems. Nurses conduct comprehensive biopsychosocial assessments and are often the professional most trusted with sensitive information by clients in these settings. The use of screening tools for depression, anxiety, substance abuse, and cognitive impairment can assist the nurse in early detection and intervention for mental health problems. Suicide can be prevented in many cases by early recognition and treatment of mental disorders, and by preventive interventions that focus on risk factors. Thus, reduction in access to lethal methods and recognition and treatment of mental and substance abuse disorders are among the most promising approaches to suicide prevention. Nurses, long respected as important population-centered providers, can work with legislators for measures to limit access to weapons such as handguns.

Adults with Serious Mental Illness

Objectives of *Healthy People 2020* that address tertiary prevention and are targeted to persons with serious mental illness are to reduce the proportion of homeless adults who have serious mental illness, to increase their employment, and to decrease the number of adults with mental disorders who are incarcerated. Brief hospital stays and inadequate community resources have

LINKING CONTENT TO PRACTICE

This chapter describes the role of the nurse who works with seriously mentally ill persons in the community. The role is diverse and complex and relies on basic nursing knowledge as well as specific knowledge about mental illness. Applying this role in the community draws on many of the recommendations of nursing and public health groups. For example, the core competencies adopted by the Council on Linkages (2010) Between Academia and Public Health Practice include those related to assessment, policy development and program planning skills, communication and cultural competency skills, and involvement with the community in order to provide services effectively. The Quad Council of Public Nursing Organizations (2009) further develops these skills and makes clear application to nursing practice. Also, the American Nurses Association (2007) in its standards of practice documents identifies specific nursing competencies by specialty area.

resulted in an increased number of persons with serious mental illness living on the streets or in jail. It is estimated that 14% of males and one third of females in jail suffer from a mental illness (Steadman et al, 2009). Some people arrested for non-violent crimes could be better served if diverted from the jail system to a community-based mental health treatment program with linkage to mental health services. Approximately half of the homeless persons in the United States have a serious mental illness or a substance abuse problem and an astonishing 23% are veterans (National Association of State Mental Health Program Directors, 2007; National Coalition for Homeless Veterans, 2010). Most do not have any form of employment. Currently, many people with severe mental disorders live in poverty because they lack the ability to earn or maintain a suitable standard of living. Even people who live with family caregivers or in supervised housing are at risk for inadequate services since the long-term care they need often depletes human and fiscal resources. An effective approach for helping persons with serious mental illness is to partner with consumers to facilitate recovery through intensive case management. Persistent client outreach and engagement strategies are effective in helping persons with serious mental illness (Cook et al, 2009).

CMHNs are engaged in all forms of case management activities with persons with serious and persistent mental illness. They provide important case management services, coordinate resources for consumers, and function as important members of ACT programs, which provide continuous assistance to persons with mental illness. Nurses by philosophy and training promote independent living and provide support and encouragement for persons to achieve a maximal level of wellness and function. Nurses recognize the importance of the mental health benefits of meaningful work that improves self-esteem and independence. Nurses can support development of wellness recovery action plans both at the individual and agency level. Nursing health promotion interventions can be provided in shelters, soup kitchens, and other places where homeless persons receive food and protection.

Older Adults

In the United States, the population older than 65 years has steadily increased since the year 2000. As the life expectancy of individuals continues to grow, the number experiencing mental disorders of late life will increase. This trend will present society with unprecedented challenges in organizing, financing, and delivering effective preventive and treatment services for mental health in this population. Although many older people maintain highly functional lives, others have mental health deficits associated with normal sensory losses related to aging, failing physical health, difficulty performing activities of daily living, and social deprivation or isolation. Life changes related to work roles and retirement often result in reduced social contacts and support. Other previously described losses are associated with the death of a spouse, other family members, or friends. Reduced social networks and contacts triggered by these life events can influence mood and contribute to serious states of depression. However, depression is not a normal part of aging.

The depression rate among older adults is half that of younger people, but the presence of a physical or chronic illness increases rates of depression. Depression rates for older adults in nursing homes range from 15% to 25% (Blazer, 2009). In the United States men between the ages of 65 and 74 are in the highest risk category for suicide; men account for 80% of all suicides of those older than age 65 (NIMH, 2010). Alzheimer disease and vascular conditions can cause a severe loss of mental abilities with behavioral manifestations. Nearly half of those older than age 85 have symptoms of cognitive impairment severe enough to impair function. All these conditions affect the mental health status of individuals and their family caregivers.

Older adults, because they may be dependent on others for care, are at risk for abuse and neglect. Healthy aging activities such as physical activity and establishing social networks improve the mental health of older adults. Older adults underutilize the mental health system and are more likely to be seen in primary care or to be recipients of care in institutions. The nurse can reach them by organizing health promotion programs through senior centers or other community-based settings. Home health care nurses can assess and intervene to protect those at risk for abuse and neglect, and mental health nurses can provide stress management education for nursing home staff. Stress management for caregivers and respite day care programs for an older adult family member can increase coping and prevent abuse. Mental health outreach services for older adults have been very effective in reducing depressive symptoms (Van Citters and Bartels, 2004). Nurses can advocate with health authorities and localities to increase awareness of the importance of meeting the mental health needs of this growing population.

Most family caregivers are women who care for a spouse, an aging parent, or a child with a long-term disabling illness. These caregivers are also at risk for health disruption. The risk is particularly great for caregivers of persons with a chronic illness. Caregivers of persons with severely disabling mental disorders often have their mental health threatened by lack of social support, the stigma of the disease, and chronic strain. During stressful life events such as these, it is important for caregivers to know how to manage the many competing demands in their lives.

Activities to improve the mental health status of adults include public education programs, prevention approaches, and provision of mental health services in primary care. Specific approaches

to reduce stress include use of community support groups, education about lifestyle management, and worksite programs. Nevertheless, most programs currently available for adults, families, and caregivers with health problems primarily monitor or restore health rather than prevent problems. Therefore, the nurse can refer family caregivers and others to organizations such as the local Alliance for the Mentally Ill for group support services. In addition, many national organizations designed for groups with specific problems (Box 36-4) have local chapters or information that can be accessed on the Internet. Some state activities expand mental health services to older adults, and *Healthy People 2020* has objectives designed to increase services to older adults and cultural competence within the mental health system.

EVIDENCE-BASED PRACTICE

A systematic literature review of articles through May 2004 evaluated face-to-face psychiatric services provided to older adults (aged 65 and older) with mental illness residing in the community. Studies were included if they were randomized controlled trials, quasi-experimental outcome studies, uncontrolled cohort studies, or comparisons of two or more interventions. Articles that evaluated interventions provided in institutional settings or focused on persons with dementia or their caregivers were excluded. A total of 14 studies met all of the criteria. All of the randomized controlled trials reported improved depressive symptoms, and one reported improved overall psychiatric symptoms. The one study that employed nurse clinicians reported a decrease in overall symptom severity for individuals with a variety of psychiatric conditions. This evidence suggests home based mental health treatment, particularly that provided by nurses, is effective in improving psychiatric symptoms.

Nurse Use

Mental health outreach services for elders are critical since older adults do not use community mental health centers and depression is often undetected and undertreated in primary care settings. The nurse can help develop such programs and is the ideal clinician to provide comprehensive biopsychosocial assessment and intervention with older adults.

From Van Citters AD, Bartels SJ: A systematic review of the effectiveness of community-based mental health outreach services for older adults, *Psychiatr Serv* 55:1237, 2004.

Cultural Diversity

To work effectively, health care providers need to understand the differences in how various populations in the United States perceive mental health and mental illness and treatment services. These factors affect whether people seek mental health care, how they describe their symptoms, the duration of care, and the outcomes of the care received. Various populations use mental health services in different ways. People may not seek mental health services in the formal system, they may drop out of care, or they may seek care at much later stages of illness, which typically costs more. This pattern of use may be the result of a community-based mental health service system that is not culturally relevant, responsive, or accessible to select populations. Although all socioeconomic and cultural groups have mental health problems, low-income groups are at greater risk because they often lack minimal resources for meeting basic physical and mental health needs.

BOX 36-4   EXAMPLES OF SOURCES OF INFORMATION AND HELP FOR PEOPLE WITH MENTAL ILLNESS AND MENTAL HEALTH PROBLEMS

- Al-Anon
- Alcoholics Anonymous
- Alzheimer's Association
- American Anorexia/Bulimia Association
- American Association of Suicidology
- Anxiety Disorders Association of America
- Attention Deficit Information Network
- Children and Adults with Attention Deficit Disorder
- Depressive/Manic Depressive Association
- Gamblers Anonymous
- National Center for Post-Traumatic Stress Disorder
- National Center for Learning Disabilities
- Obsessive-Compulsive Foundation
- Overeaters Anonymous
- Schizophrenics Anonymous

See the Evolve website at http://evolve.elsevier.com/Stanhope for more information about these organizations.

In an effort to describe and remedy mental health disparities based on culture, a supplemental report was published in 2001 (USDHHS, 2001). Caution is needed, however, when discussing differences among racial and ethnic groups in the rates of mental illness. Studies of the number of cases of mental health problems among racial and ethnic populations, while increasing in number, remain limited and often inconclusive. Discussion of the rates of existing cases must consider differences in how persons of different cultures and racial and ethnic groups perceive mental illness. Behavioral problems, which Western medicine views as signs of mental illness, may be assessed differently by individuals in various racial and ethnic groups. With this caution in mind, along with the recognition that sample sizes for racial and ethnic groups may be limited, examination of existing large-scale studies for mental health trends among racial and ethnic groups remains important.

WHAT DO YOU THINK?   *Does the manner in which people of different cultures describe emotional distress affect the detection and treatment of mental illness?*

According to the surgeon general's report on culture, race, and ethnicity, the predominant minority populations in the United States are African Americans, Hispanics, Asian and Pacific Islander Americans, and Native Americans including Native Alaskans (USDHHS, 2001). A notable omission from this federal report is Middle Eastern Americans, and little information could be found either in the literature or through national websites, although there is a significant and growing population, particularly in the upper Midwest. Great diversity exists among people from the Middle East, although they may share some cultural traditions with Asians, Africans, or Europeans and in some cases have been included in those classifications. However, within each of the groups identified in the federal report, there is also much diversity, as each group consists of subgroups with unique cultural differences. Therefore, it is important to avoid simplification and overgeneralization in discussions about the characteristics and problems of minorities and to examine both individual and national bias. It is critical to conduct community assessments to determine unique characteristics and factors that contribute to mental health needs within specific aggregates of the population. The information presented here is intended to stimulate thinking and awareness for developing nursing activities in individual communities. Community assessments that include data about specific populations from organized agencies such as the Indian Health Service are important because assessment data guide role activities during all steps of the nursing process.

Nurses provide a variety of primary, secondary, and tertiary prevention interventions with populations at risk that help meet the objectives for improving mental health. Consumers have historically influenced mental health services, and the health care industry increasingly is using consumer opinion to gain information on service needs and changes. Objectives of *Healthy People 2020* are to increase state tracking of consumer satisfaction with mental health services and to increase the number of states who incorporate plans addressing cultural competence. Nurses working within broad-based coalitions of consumers, families, other providers, and community leaders can help to achieve the goals of accessible, culturally sensitive, quality mental health services for all people who are served.

African Americans

African Americans make up 12% of the population in the United States and are represented in all socioeconomic groups, yet 22% live in poverty (USDHHS, 2001). Ethnic and racial minorities in the United States may live in an environment of social and economic discrimination and inequality, which takes a toll on mental health and places them at risk for associated mental problems. African Americans are more likely to be exposed to, or to become victims of, violence, placing them at risk for the development of post-traumatic stress disorder (PTSD). They are overrepresented both in the homeless and in the correctional system populations, further increasing the risk of developing mental health problems. Although they were less likely to commit suicide, the suicide rate of young African-American men is now equal to that of whites (CDC, 2009). Despite these issues, African Americans are less likely to use mental health services and may have significant negative expectations about mental health services. Nurses can promote the mental health of African Americans by integrating mental health care into primary care settings, providing services in community centers, collaborating with African-American faith communities, providing education to decrease the stigma, working toward the provision of safer communities, and recruiting African Americans to work as community mental health providers.

Latino Americans

Latino Americans are the second largest minority group in America, and by 2050 they are projected to comprise 25% of the population (USDHHS, 2001). Although they live primarily in the Southwestern regions of the country, many have migrated to states in the Southeast and Midwest. Migrant farmworkers are also an important subpopulation among Latinos. As discussed in Chapter 34, migratory living patterns that are marked by low income, poor education, and lack of health services contribute to stressful living conditions. Nurses and nurse practitioners may be primary health care providers for migrant laborers and new immigrants. Their roles expand beyond traditional practice to encompass case management and interagency collaboration. Collaboration includes networking and referral to community mental health agencies and to advanced practice psychiatric nurses when either drug or alcohol abuse or mental illness is the primary health problem.

Latino Americans living in low-income urban areas are subject to many of the conditions described for low-income and disadvantaged African-American families. The surgeon general's report (USDHHS, 2001) indicates that recent Latino immigrants had lower rates of depression than those born in the United States, but evidence from the CDC (2009) found suicide to be the eighth-leading cause of death among Latino males and even higher rates of attempts among young Latina women. There are significant relationships between suicide and having a family history of suicide, physical or sexual abuse, and environmental stress. These findings suggest serious stressful living conditions for both individuals and families. Nurses working with Latino families need knowledge and skill in both the language and cross-cultural therapies, and they also need to include consumers in planning and evaluating mental health service delivery. Focus groups can be held to involve community members in the planning and implementation of culturally relevant mental health services.

Asian and Pacific Islander Americans

Asian and Pacific Islander Americans can be characterized by a diverse and rapidly increasing population (USDHHS, 2001). This group includes both settled citizens and new refugees. The largest segment of this population lives in California. Whereas Asian and Pacific Islander Americans, like other minority groups, are represented in all socioeconomic strata, the lower-income groups include refugees and recent immigrants who are dealing with the displacement issues of loss, adjustment, and adaptation. Losses often involve forfeiture of family, traditions, and lifestyles for cultures that may seem alien. Adjustments and adaptations include those basic to daily living: learning new languages, laws, and monetary systems and locating support systems. Finding support systems includes becoming acquainted with the health care delivery system. Our knowledge of the mental health needs of this population is limited, since they have the lowest utilization rates of mental health services of any cultural group (USDHHS, 2001). This avoidance of mental health care is associated with the stigma and shame related to having a mental disorder as well as to perceived discrimination by mental health providers (Spencer et al, 2009). Assessment, planning, and interventions with members of this diverse group must include information about their health beliefs, a key component in any program. This is the first step in providing culturally sensitive interventions.

EVIDENCE-BASED PRACTICE

The purpose of the qualitative study was to explore perceptions about barriers to mental health treatment for Korean-American women. Focus groups were conducted with 27 Korean-American participants, two groups of providers, and two groups of community women. Individual and contextual barriers to seeking mental health care were language, cultural differences, lack of time, financial limitations, lack of transportation, lack of knowledge, lack of funding for community agencies, lack of partnerships with churches, and perceived stigma.

Nurse Use

The following points should be kept in mind by population-focused nurses in the field of mental health:

- Nurses need to understand existing barriers that prevent people from seeking mental health services, and to design culturally sensitive approaches for vulnerable populations.
- Nurses can work to decrease the stigma of mental illness by educating minorities about the biological basis of many mental disorders.
- Designing services that integrate mental health services into primary care systems will help increase access and decrease barriers.
- Recruitment of a culturally diverse nursing workforce may increase use of mental health services.

From Wu MC, Kviz FJ, Miller AM: Identifying individual and contextual barriers to seeking mental health service among Korean American immigrant women, *Issues Ment Health Nurs* 30:78, 2009.

Native Americans

Native Americans represent 1.5% of the U.S. population. Although this is a small group, it is also diverse, with more than 551 tribes and more than 200 languages. Native Americans also appear to have significant rates of substance abuse, depression, and suicide (1.5 times the national rate), along with unintentional injury and homicide. They are exposed to violence at more than twice the national rate, which results in significant rates of PTSD (CDC, 2009). Use of mental health services has been difficult to determine, since only a small percentage of Native Americans use those provided by the Indian Health Service.

A promising intervention to address the needs of this diverse group is to build on the traditions of the specific tribe culture to foster identity and integration and enhance protective factors. A return to traditional values of community and group support has been shown to be effective in reducing rates of substance abuse (CDC, 2009). Nurses working with Native Americans, as with all population groups, need to learn the culture of the specific group and to mutually plan culturally sensitive mental health interventions at levels of primary, secondary, and tertiary prevention.

CHAPTER REVIEW

PRACTICE APPLICATION

Mr. B. is an 81-year-old white widowed man living in a rural area 20 miles from a small city. The nurse practitioner who had treated Mr. B. for sinusitis referred him to the outreach nurse for an evaluation. The nurse practitioner was concerned when she noted that Mr. B. had lost weight and had started to cry when talking about his wife who had died several years before. During the initial visit, the nurse noted that Mr. B. weighed only 110 lb, was not sleeping, had stopped going to church, and was quite anxious and sad about his finances, his limitations from arthritis, his relationship with his 27-year-old stepson, Bart, and the possibility of nursing home placement.

The nurse conducted a suicide assessment, knowing that Mr. B. was at high risk because of his age, his mood, and the presence of guns in the home. Mr. B. stated that he had considered shooting himself, but he was reluctant to have the rifles removed at the nurse's suggestion because Bart used the guns for hunting. Mr. B. agreed to a family meeting with his stepson, and Bart agreed to remove the guns from the house. Both Mr. B. and Bart needed significant education about the biological basis of depression and the efficacy of using a new antidepressant, along with support to treat his condition. Mr. B., like many older adults, did not wish to see a psychiatrist or use the community mental health system. He did agree to a trial of antidepressants, however.

The nurse, through the primary care nurse practitioner, arranged for a prescription of an antidepressant (a selective serotonin reuptake inhibitor) that is safe for use with older adults, and Mr. B. started the medication within 2 weeks of the initial visit. In addition to medication and counseling, Mr. B. needed help with nutrition. Because Bart was away 10 hours a day, at work in the city, Mr. B. was alone all day. Mr. B. was not able to prepare meals because of his arthritis. The nurse arranged with the local board for aging to provide home-delivered meals. This not only helped with nutrition, but also gave Mr. B. a visit from the volunteer twice a week.

Mr. B. and Bart needed help with financial planning, as they did not want to lose the farm should Mr. B. need more assistance or nursing home placement in the future. The nurse arranged for them to talk with a social worker regarding long-term care planning.

In addition to addressing the immediate concerns, the nurse continued to provide weekly visits to Mr. B. for support and counseling, medication monitoring, and case management activities. Family meetings with Bart and Mr. B. to discuss mutual concerns were arranged every 2 months and as needed. The significant improvement of depressive symptoms (that is, sleep, appetite, weight, and mood) in Mr. B. was monitored both clinically and through use of a depression rating scale.

Psychological, physical, and social problems of older adults are closely intertwined and are best evaluated and treated by a multidisciplinary team. Psychiatric illness often presents first with physical symptoms, and physical limitations create further psychological distress. Older adults often prefer not to use formal mental health services, so careful assessment in primary care settings is critical to detect their mental health problems.

A. In addition to his stepson and the nurse, who else might notice if Mr. B.'s condition began to deteriorate?

B. What nursing measures are important in monitoring Mr. B.'s response to the antidepressant?

C. What secondary prevention measures were used by the nurse?

D. What resources might be available for Bart should he need more information about depression?

Answers can be found on the Evolve site.

KEY POINTS

- Reform movements and subsequent federal legislation influenced the development of the current community mental health model that includes team care, case management, prevention, and rehabilitation and recovery components of service.
- During the past two decades, federal legislation in the United States focused on mainstreaming persons with mental disabilities into American life by legislating access to employment, services, and housing.
- Prevalence rates for mental health problems are very high, and people are at risk for threats to mental health at all ages across the life span. Low-income and minority groups are often at increased risk because they lack access to services and because programs may lack cultural sensitivity.
- National health objectives to promote health and services for persons who have mental health problems and severe mental disorders illustrate the scope of mental illness and provide direction for community mental health practice.
- Guidelines for attaining national health objectives were designed to help individuals at regional and local levels establish health priorities that include those for mental illness.
- The American Nurses Association standards provide a framework for the roles and functions of community mental health nurses.
- Frameworks that are useful in community mental health nursing include primary, secondary, and tertiary levels of prevention; biological theories including the effects of psychosocial factors on the brain, growth, and development; and rehabilitation and recovery models.

CLINICAL DECISION-MAKING ACTIVITIES

1. For 1 week, keep a list of incidents related to mental health problems that you learn about in the local media. Categorize the incidents according to age, sex, and socioeconomic, ethnic, or minority status. Which populations seem to have the most mental health problems?

2. Visit a local shelter or organization that offers temporary protection for persons with mental disorders. Determine services that are available or lacking for children, women, and men. Describe a nursing intervention that would improve services.

3. Visit with representatives of your local self-help organizations for consumers to determine their needs and the adequacy of resources for people with severe mental disorders and their caregivers; determine gaps in services. Develop a list of the agencies in your community that provide direct or indirect services for those with mental illness and their families.

4. Interview a school nurse, an occupational health nurse, an emergency department nurse, or a hospice nurse in your community to discuss types of mental health problems they see with clients in their practice settings. Determine resources that are available or lacking for primary, secondary, and tertiary prevention. Design a primary prevention intervention.

5. Interview a nurse working in a local community mental health agency to discuss roles, functions, programs, and resources available or lacking for primary, secondary, and tertiary prevention. Compare findings about prevention programs with information obtained from the preceding interview.

6. Visit a consumer-operated program or a psychosocial rehabilitation program. Interview members to learn how they view services and resources available or lacking in this setting. Describe how your attitudes about persons in recovery from mental illness changed after your visit.

7. Accompany a community mental health nurse on home visits to clients enrolled in an assertive community outreach program, and then accompany a psychiatric nurse in a home care agency. Compare and contrast how the services, funding, populations served, and philosophies of treatment differ.

8. As a class activity, arrange for a panel of speakers representing the minority populations described in this chapter. Discuss their views about the way culture shapes thinking about mental illness, and determine types of culturally sensitive services that are available or lacking in your community.

9. Review articles in at least four research journals to determine current research findings about mental disorders and mental health problems, and compare nursing care in the United States with that of other countries. Discuss the differences in mental health care between countries.

REFERENCES

Alzheimer's Association: Alzheimer's disease facts and figures 2010, Alzheimer's and dementia, *J Alzheim Assoc* 6:158, 2010.

American Nurses Association, American Psychiatric Nurses' Association, and International Society of Psychiatric Mental Health Nurses: *Scope and standards of psychiatric-mental health nursing*, Washington, DC, 2007, American Nurses Publishing.

American Psychiatric Association: *Diagnostic and statistical manual of mental disorders*, ed 4-TR, Washington, DC, 2000, APA.

Barnes PM, Bloom B, Nahin RL: *Complementary and alternative medicine use among adults and children, United States, 2007*, National Health Statistics Report, No 12, Hyattsville, MD, 2009, National Center for Health Statistics.

Blazer DG: Depression in late life: review and commentary, *Am Psychiat Assoc Focus* 7:118, 2009.

Boyd MA: Social change and mental health. In Boyd MA, editor: *Psychiatric nursing: contemporary practice*, ed 3, Philadelphia, 2005, Lippincott Williams & Wilkins.

Byers AL, Yaffe K, Covinsky KE, et al: High occurrence of mood and anxiety disorders among older adults, *Arch Gen Psychiatry* 67:489, 2010.

Caldwell BA, Sclafani M, Swarbrick M, et al: Psychiatric nursing practice and the recovery model of care, *J Psychosoc Nurs Ment Health Serv* 48(7):42–48, July 2010.

Center for Disease Control and Prevention, National Center for Injury Prevention and Control: *Suicide, facts at a glance*, Summer 2009. Available at http://www.cdc.gov. Accessed 2010.

Clark CC: Post traumatic stress disorder, *Nurs Spectrum* 26, March 8, 2010.

Cook JA, Copeland ME, Hamilton MM, et al: Initial outcomes of a mental illness self-management program based on wellness recovery action planning, *Psychiatr Serv* 60:246, 2009.

Correll CU, Frederickson AM, Kane JM, et al: Metabolic syndrome and the risk of coronary heart disease in 367 patients treated with second generation antipsychotic drugs, *J Clin Psychiatry* 67:575–583, 2006.

Council on Linkages Between Academic and Public Health Practice: *Core competencies for public health professionals*, Washington, DC, 2010, Public Health Foundation, Health Resources and Services Administration.

Hobfall SE, Watson P, Bell CC, et al: Five essential elements of immediate and mid-term mass trauma intervention: empirical evidence, *Focus* 70:221, 2009.

Indian Health Service: IHS Fact Sheet: *Indian health disparities*. Available at http://info.ihs.gov/disparities.asp. Accessed June, 2011.

Institute of Medicine: *Improving the quality of health care for mental and substance abuse conditions, Quality chasm series*, Washington, DC, 2006, IOM, National Academies of Science Press.

Kessler RC, Berglund PA, Demler O, et al: Lifetime prevalence and age of onset distributions of DSM-IV disorders in the National Comorbidity Survey Replication (NCS-R), *Arch Gen Psychiatry* 63(6), 2005.

Kozuki Y, Schepp KG: Adherence and non-adherence to antipsychotic medications, *Issues Ment Health Nurs* 26:379, 2005.

Manderscheid RW, Berry JT, editors: *Mental health, United States, 2004*, DHHS Pub No (SMA) 06-4195, Rockville, MD, 2006, Center for Mental Health Services, Substance Abuse and Mental Health Services Administration.

Merikangas KR, He JP, Brody D, et al: Prevalence and treatment of mental disorders among US children in the 2001-2004 NAHANES, *Pediatrics* 125(1):75–81, 2009.

McClosky LA, Figuerdo AJ, Koss MP: The effects of systemic family violence on children's mental health, *Child Devel* 66:1239, 2008.

McElroy JP, Meyer JM, Goff PC, et al: Presence of metabolic syndrome in patients with schizophrenia: baseline results from the clinical antipsychotic trials of intervention effectiveness (CATIE) and comparison with national estimates from NAHANES III Schizophrenia, *Research* 80:19, 2005.

Mental Health America: *Fact Sheet: Paul Wellstone and Peter Domenici Mental Health Parity and Addiction Equity Act of 2008*, Alexandria, VA, 2009, MHA.

Mynatt S: Patients with anxiety and depression wanted to know what to expect when they started their medication, *Evidence Based Nurs* 8:27, 2005.

National Association of State Mental Health Program Directors and Advocates for Human Potential, Inc: *Promoting independence and recovery through work: employment for people with psychiatric disabilities*, 2007, National Governors Association, Center for Best Practices.

National Coalition for Homeless Veterans: Available at http://www.nchv.org/background.cfm#facts. Accessed March 5, 2011.

National Institutes of Mental Health (NIMH), National Institutes of Health (NIH), U.S. Department of Health and Human Services: *The numbers count: mental disorders in America,* Washington, DC, 2010. Available at http://www.nimh.nih.gov/healthpublications. Accessed June 13, 2010.

Newcomer JW: Second generation (atypical) antipsychotics and metabolic effects: a comprehensive literature review, *CNS Drugs* 19:1, 2005.

Pickett-Schenk SA, Bennett C, Cook JA, et al: Changes in caregiving satisfaction and information needs among relatives of adults with mental illness: results of a randomized evaluation of a family led education intervention, *Am J Orthopsychiatry* 76:545–553, 2006.

President's New Freedom Commission on Mental Health: *Achieving the promise: transforming mental health care in America,* USDHHS Pub No SMA-03-3832, Rockville, MD, 2003, USDHHS.

Quad Council of Public Health Nursing Organizations: *Competencies for public health nursing Practice,* Washington, DC, 2003, ASTDN. revised 2009.

Rick S, Douglas DH: Neurobiological effects of childhood abuse, *J Psychosoc Nurs Ment Health Serv* 45:47–54, 2007.

Saag K: Mend the mind but mind the bones, *Arch Intern Med* 167:1231, 2007.

Salyers MP, Tsemberis S: Act and recovery: integrating evidence based practice and recovery orientation on assertive community treatment teams, *Community Ment Health J* 44:75, 2008.

Spencer MS, Chen J, Gee GG, et al: Discrimination and mental health related service use in a national study of Asian American, *Am J Public Health* 10:2105, 2009.

Steadman HJ, Osher FC, Robbins PC, et al: Prevalence of serious mental illness among jail inmates, *Psychiatr Serv* 60:761, 2009.

Substance Abuse and Mental Health Services Administration Office of Applied Studies: *The NSDUH report: major depressive episode among youth aged 12-17 in the US,* Rockville, MD, 2007, SAMHSA.

Tomes N: The patient as a policy factor: a historical case study of the consumer/survivor movement in mental health, *Health Aff* 25:721, 2006.

U.S. Department of Health and Human Services: *Mental health: a report of the surgeon general,* Rockville, MD, 1999, USDHHS.

U.S. Department of Health and Human Services: *Mental health: culture, race, and ethnicity—supplement to mental health: a report of the surgeon general,* Rockville, MD, 2001, USDHHS.

U.S. Department of Health and Human Services: Health Research Services Administration, Maternal and Child Health Bureau: *Woman's health USA, 2008,* Rockville, MD, 2008, USDHHS.

U.S. Department of Health and Human Services: *Health Research Services Administration, Maternal and Child Health Bureau: Child health USA 2008-2009,* Rockville, MD, 2009, USDHHS.

U.S. Department of Health and Human Services: *Healthy People 2020: mental health and mental disorders,* Washington, DC, 2010, Office of Disease Prevention and Health Promotion. Available at http://healthypeople.gov/hp2020/Objective/TopicArea. Accessed June 13, 2010.

Van Citters AD, Bartels SJ: A systematic review of the effectiveness of community-based mental health outreach services for older adults, *Psychiatr Serv* 55:1237, 2004.

Weiss SJ: Neurobiological alterations associated with traumatic stress, *Perspect Psychiatr Care* 43:114, 2007.

World Health Organization: *mhGP, mental health action programme: scaling up care for mental, neurological and substance abuse disorders,* Geneva, Switzerland, 2008a, WHO.

World Health Organization: *The global burden of disease: 2004 update. Table A2: burden of disease inDALYs by cause, sex and income group in WHO regions, estimated for 2004,* Geneva, Switzerland, 2008b, WHO.

Wu MC, Kviz FJ, Miller AM: Identifying individual and contextual barriers to seeking mental health service among Korean American immigrant women, *Issues Ment Health Nurs* 30:78, 2009.

CHAPTER 37

Alcohol, Tobacco, and Other Drug Problems

Mary Lynn Mathre, RN, MSN, CARN

Mary Lynn Mathre has 36 years of experience as an acute care nurse and has worked in the field of alcohol, tobacco, and other drugs for the past 25 years. From 1991 to 2003, she worked as the addictions consult nurse for the University of Virginia Health System. This role required much interaction with community resources to provide appropriate referrals and aftercare for the client population. From 2004 to 2007 she worked in an outpatient opioid treatment program as the executive director. Currently she works as an independent consultant on substance abuse prevention and brief interventions. She is an active member of the International Nurses Society on Addictions and serves on the editorial board for the *Journal of Addictions Nursing*.

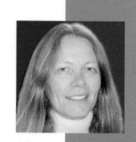

ADDITIONAL RESOURCES

evolve **WEBSITE**

http://evolve.elsevier.com/Stanhope

- *Healthy People 2020*
- Resource Tool 37.A: Smoking Cessation Resources
- Resource Tool 37.B: Useful Web Resources
- Resource Tool 37.C: Commonly Abused Drugs

- Quiz
- Case Studies
- Glossary
- Answers to Practice Application

OBJECTIVES

After reading this chapter, the student should be able to do the following:

1. Analyze personal attitudes toward alcohol, tobacco, and other drug problems.
2. Differentiate among these terms: substance use, abuse, dependence, and addiction.
3. Discuss the differences among the major psychoactive drug categories of depressants, stimulants, marijuana, hallucinogens, and inhalants.

4. Explain the role of the nurse in primary, secondary, and tertiary prevention of alcohol, tobacco, and other drug problems as it relates to individual clients, their families, and special populations.
5. Evaluate the role of the nurse in primary, secondary, and tertiary prevention of alcohol, tobacco, and other drug problems as it relates to the community and national policies on drug control.

KEY TERMS

addiction treatment, p. 820
Alcoholics Anonymous (AA), p. 822
alcoholism, p. 808
biopsychosocial model, p. 813
blood alcohol concentration, p. 809
brief interventions, p. 814
codependency, p. 819
cross-tolerance, p. 821
denial, p. 815
depressants, p. 808

detoxification, p. 819
drug addiction, p. 808
drug dependence, p. 807
enabling, p. 819
fetal alcohol syndrome, p. 809
hallucinogens, p. 808
harm reduction, p. 807
injection drug users, p. 817
mainstream smoke, p. 811
polysubstance use or abuse, p. 813
prohibition, p. 805

psychoactive drugs, p. 807
set, p. 812
setting, p. 812
sidestream smoke, p. 811
stimulants, p. 808
substance abuse, p. 805
tolerance, p. 811
withdrawal, p. 808
—*See Glossary for definitions*

OUTLINE

Substance abuse is the number one national health problem, causing more deaths, illnesses, and disabilities than any other health condition. The substance abuser is not only at risk for personal health problems, but may also be a threat to the health and safety of family members, co-workers, and other members of the community.

Substance abuse and addiction affect all ages, races, sexes, and segments of society. As seen in *Healthy People 2020* (USDHHS, 2010), tobacco use and substance abuse are two major topic areas, with many objectives and sub-objectives, as well as related objectives in other priority areas. The newer phrase of *alcohol, tobacco, and other drug (ATOD) problems* rather than *substance abuse* reminds us that alcohol and tobacco represent the major drugs of abuse when discussing substance abuse, drug addiction, or chemical dependency.

This chapter begins by providing a broad perspective of ATOD problems to clarify the relevant issues. A historical overview of ATOD problems and attitudes toward ATOD users and addicts is examined. Relevant terms are defined to decrease the confusion caused by frequent misuse of terms. The major drug categories are described, including information on commonly used substances and current ATOD use trends. The remainder of the chapter examines the role of the nurse in primary, secondary, and tertiary prevention and describes how the nurse can improve the outcomes for individuals, families, and various populations with ATOD problems when using a harm reduction model. The reader is encouraged to consider possible nursing strategies to apply the *Healthy People 2020* objectives for ATOD problems.

ALCOHOL, TOBACCO, AND OTHER DRUG PROBLEMS IN PERSPECTIVE

ATOD abuse and addiction can cause multiple health problems for individuals. Heavy ATOD use has been associated with many problems, including neonates with low birth weight and congenital abnormalities; accidents, homicides, and suicides; chronic diseases, such as cardiovascular diseases, cancer, lung disease, hepatitis, HIV/AIDS, and mental illness; violence; and family disruption. Factors that contribute to the substance abuse problem include lack of knowledge about the use of drugs; the war on drugs' emphasis on illicit drugs and law enforcement rather than the prevention and treatment of abuse and addiction of ATODs; lack of quality control of illegal drugs; and drug laws that label certain drug users as criminals, which encourages the negative attitudes and stigma toward these persons.

Historical Overview

Psychoactive drug use has been part of most cultures since the beginning of humanity. Often a culture encourages use of some drugs while discouraging the use of others. Caffeine, alcohol, and tobacco are socially acceptable drugs in the United States and Canada, whereas other cultures prohibit their use. Conversely, marijuana, cocaine, and opium use are not accepted in mainstream U.S. society, although these substances are considered sacred or beneficial and their use is accepted in various other cultures.

The United States' primary solution to various "drug problems" has been **prohibition.** During alcohol prohibition from 1920 to 1933, the United States experienced a sharp increase in violent crime and corruption among law officials as a result of the illicit marketing of alcohol. Distilled beverages were pushed because of the higher profit margin per bottle of liquor than for beer or wine. The high alcohol content in illicit moonshine caused severe health problems. The alcohol prohibition was eventually recognized as a failure and repealed (Rose, 1996).

Similar problems are occurring with the current war on drugs and the newer prohibition on marijuana, cocaine, and other drugs. An increase in both violent crime and reports of corruption among law officials as a result of the illicit market has become a major national problem (Common Sense for Drug Policy, 2007). Stronger drugs are pushed because of their greater profits. Some would say that drug prohibition laws have created mandatory sentences for drug offenders, violated civil liberties, and put more resources into law enforcement than into drug education and treatment (Common Sense for Drug Policy, 2007). As the drug war budget grows each year, most of that budget goes to law enforcement and punishment, leaving only a third for prevention and treatment. See Table 37-1 for a historical overview of the drug war budget.

A 3-year study by the National Center on Addiction and Substance Abuse (CASA) closely examined the 2005 federal, state, and local government budgets to measure the financial impact of ATOD problems on their health, social service, criminal justice, education, mental health, developmentally disabled, and other programs. The CASA study found that the government spent at least $467.7 billion ($238.2 billion, federal; $135.8 billion, state; and $93.8 billion, local) in 2005 on substance abuse and addiction, which amounted to 10.7% of the entire $4.4 trillion budgets. Of every dollar the federal and state governments spent on substance abuse and addiction, 95.6 cents was used to deal with the ATOD problems, while only 1.9 cents went to prevention and treatment, 0.4% to research, 1.4% to taxation or regulation, and 0.7% to interdiction. Almost half of this spending cannot be disaggregated by specific substance. However, of the $248 billion in ATOD-related spending, 92.3% was linked to alcohol and tobacco (National Center on Addiction and Substance Abuse, 2009).

Attitudes and Myths

Attitudes are developed through cultural learning and personal experiences. Attitudes toward ATOD problems are influenced by the way society inappropriately categorizes drugs as either "good" or "bad." In the United States, good drugs are typically over-the-counter (OTC) or those prescribed by a health care provider as *medicine,* yet this makes them no less problematic or addictive. Bad drugs are the illegal drugs, and persons who use these drugs are considered criminals regardless of whether the drug has caused any problems.

Americans rely heavily on prescription and OTC drugs to relieve (or mask) anxiety, tension, fatigue, and physical or emotional pain. Rather than learning non-medicinal methods of coping, many people rely on the "quick fix" and take pills to deal with their problems or negative feelings.

Addicts are often viewed as immoral, weak-willed, or irresponsible persons who should try harder to help themselves. Although alcoholism was recognized as a disease by the American Medical Association in 1954, and drug addiction was recognized as a disease some years later, much of the public and many health care professionals have failed to change their attitudes and accept alcoholics and addicts as ill persons in need of health care.

Nurses must examine their attitudes toward ATOD use, abuse, and addiction before working with this health problem. To be therapeutic, the nurse must develop a trusting, non-judgmental relationship with the client. Systematic assessment for ATOD problems is based on awareness that there may be problems with both legal and illegal drugs. If the nurse's attitude toward a client with a drug abuse problem is negative or punitive, the issue may never be directly addressed or the client may be avoided. If the client senses the negative attitude of the health care provider, either by words or from tone of voice, communication may cease and information may be withheld. To develop a therapeutic attitude, the nurse must realize that any drug can be abused, that anyone may develop drug dependence, and that drug addiction can be successfully treated.

TABLE 37-1   FEDERAL DRUG CONTROL SPENDING BY FUNCTION

Function	FY 2009 FINAL	FY 2010 ENACTED	FY 2011 REQUEST	2010-2011 CHANGE DOLLARS	PERCENT
Treatment	3561.9	3745.5	3882.5	136.9	3.7%
Percent	23.3	24.9	25.0		
Prevention	1854.7	1514.3	1717.7	203.3	13.4%
Percent	12.1	10.1	11.0		
Domestic Law Enforcement	3869.4	3843.5	3917.3	73.8	1.9%
Percent	25.3	25.6	25.2		
Interdiction	3910.2	3640.1	3727.0	86.9	2.4%
Percent	25.6	24.2	24.0		
International	2082.2	2288.0	2308.1	20.1	0.9%
Percent	13.6	15.2	14.8		
Total	**$15,278.40**	**$15,031.50**	**$15,552.50**	**$521.10**	**3.5%**
Supply/Demand Demand Reduction	5416.6	5259.9	5600.2	340.3	6.5%
Percent	35.5	35.0	36.0		
Supply Reduction	9861.8	9771.6	9952.4	180.8	1.9%
Percent	64.5	65.0	64.0		
Total	**$15,278.40**	**$15,031.50**	**$15,552.50**	**$521.10**	**3.5%**

WHAT DO YOU THINK? *Antiprohibitionists think that the pro-hibition of drugs causes greater societal problems than the use of those drugs and that the government has no right to forbid adults from what they choose to ingest. Although antiprohibitionists are often called "legalizers," this label is misleading because it implies that by "legalizing" a drug, the government is condoning its use. Do you understand the difference between the terms? Should some drugs be prohibited, and if so, who should decide which drugs to prohibit? Should persons be incarcerated because they have con-sumed a prohibited drug?*

Myths develop over years, and if myths are not questioned, many attitudes may be formed solely on the basis of fiction rather than fact. Some common myths are as follows:

- "An alcoholic is a skid row bum"—but less than 5% of persons with addictions fit this description.
- "If you teach people about drugs, they will abuse them"—although it is true that people may choose to use drugs if they have knowledge about them, it is more likely that people without knowledge about them will abuse them.
- "Addiction is a sin or moral failing"—addiction is recognized as a health problem involving biopsychosocial factors, and persons who use drugs do not do so with the intent to become addicted.

Paradigm Shift

We can hope to see a major shift in how the United States conceptualizes ATOD problems. The old criminal justice model is based on stereotypes, misinformation, and punishment, and it uses war tactics to fight the drug users, addicts, and suppliers. Campaigns have been launched using the slogans "zero tolerance" for drug users, "just say no" to drugs, and striving for a "drug-free America"—all of which vilify the drug user or drug addict. Gil Kerlikowske, the drug czar in the Obama administration, has said that he wants to move away from the "war on drugs" approach and that the Obama administration is likely to deal with drugs as a matter of public health rather than criminal justice alone, with the role of treatment growing relative to incarceration (Fields, 2009). Also, on the international level, experts are suggesting that national drug policies need to be more comprehensive rather than focusing on law enforcement strategies (Box 37-1).

The harm reduction model is a public health approach to ATOD problems initially used in Great Britain, The Netherlands, Germany, Switzerland, and Australia, and interest in it is spreading throughout Europe and in Canada. This new public health model recognizes the following:

- Addiction is a health problem.
- Any psychoactive drug can be abused.
- Accurate information can help people make responsible decisions about drug use.
- People who have ATOD problems can be helped.

This approach accepts the reality that psychoactive drug use is endemic, and it focuses on pragmatic interventions, especially education, to reduce the adverse consequences of drug abuse and get treatment for addicts. The United States has already taken a harm reduction approach with tobacco and alcohol.

Educational campaigns are used to inform the public about the health risks of tobacco use. Warnings have appeared on tobacco product labels since 1967 as a result of the surgeon general's 1966 report on the dangers of smoking. In 1971 a ban on television and radio cigarette advertising was imposed. Cigarette smoking has decreased since that time. Smoking is on the decline among eighth and twelfth graders. According to the 2007 report from *Monitoring the Future* drug survey data among secondary school students, 4% of eighth graders smoked in 2006, down from 5.5% in 2001. For twelfth graders in 2006, 12% smoked compared with 19% in 2001 (Johnston, O'Malley, and Bachman, 2007). Education is continuing to address the dangers of alcohol abuse and to establish guidelines for safe alcohol use.

Nurses need to seek the underlying roots of various health problems and plan action that is realistic, non-judgmental, holistic, and positive. A harm reduction model for ATOD problems facilitates such an approach.

Definitions

The terms *drug use* and *drug abuse* have virtually lost their usefulness because the public and government have narrowed the term *drug* to include only illegal drugs rather than including prescription, OTC, and legal recreational drugs. The current phrase *alcohol, tobacco, and other drugs* (ATODs) is a reminder that the leading drug problems involve alcohol and tobacco. The term *substance* broadens the scope to include alcohol, tobacco, legal drugs, and even foods. Substance abuse is the use of any substance that threatens a person's health or impairs social or economic functioning. This definition is more objective and universal than the government's definition of drug abuse, which is the use of a drug without a prescription or any use of an illegal drug. Although any drug or food can be abused, this chapter focuses on psychoactive drugs—drugs that affect mood, perception, and thought.

Drug dependence and drug addiction are often used interchangeably, but they are not synonymous. Drug dependence is

BOX 37-1 **HIGH-LEVEL PRINCIPLES FOR AN EFFECTIVE DRUG POLICY**
We propose that national drug strategies should always be based on five core principles: 1. Drug policies should be developed through a structured and objective assessment of priorities and evidence. 2. All activities should be undertaken in full compliance with international human rights law. 3. Drug policies should focus on reducing the harmful consequences rather than the scale of drug use and markets. 4. Policy and activities should seek to promote the social inclusion of marginalized groups. 5. Governments should build open and constructive relationships with civil society in the discussion and delivery of their strategies.

Adapted from the Suggested principles for an effective drug policy proposed by the International Drug Policy Consortium (IDPC), published in March 2010. Available at http://www.idpc.net/sites/default/files/library/IDPC%20Drug%20Policy%20Guide_Version%201.pdf. Each chapter of the guide fully integrates the above five core principles.

a state of neuroadaptation (a physiological change in the central nervous system [CNS]) caused by the chronic, regular administration of a drug; in drug dependence, continued use of the drug becomes necessary to prevent withdrawal symptoms. For example, when a person is given an opiate such as morphine on a regular basis for pain management, the morphine needs to be gradually tapered rather than abruptly stopped to prevent symptoms of withdrawal.

Drug addiction is a pattern of abuse characterized by an overwhelming preoccupation with the use (compulsive use) of a drug, securing its supply, and a high tendency to relapse if the drug is removed. Frequently, addicts are physically dependent on a drug, but there also appears to be an added psychological component that causes the intense cravings and subsequent relapse. In general, anyone can develop drug dependence as a result of regular administration of drugs that alter the CNS; however, only 7% to 15% of the drug-using population will develop a drug addiction. The process of becoming addicted is complex and related to several factors, including the addictive properties of the substance, family and peer influences, personality, age of first use, cultural and social factors, existing psychiatric disorders, and genetics.

Alcoholism is addiction to the drug called alcohol. Alcoholism and drug addiction are recognized as illnesses under a biopsychosocial model. Simply stated, the disease concept of addiction and alcoholism identifies them as chronic and progressive diseases in which a person's use of a drug or drugs continues despite problems it causes in any area of life—physical, emotional, social, economic, or spiritual.

PSYCHOACTIVE DRUGS

Although any drug can be abused, ATOD abuse and addiction problems generally involve the psychoactive drugs. These drugs, which can alter emotions, are used for enjoyment in social and recreational settings and for personal use to self-medicate physical or emotional discomfort. Psychoactive drugs are divided into categories according to their effect on the CNS and the general feelings or experiences the drugs may induce. The Internet or a pharmacology text can provide detailed information on these drug categories (e.g., depressants, stimulants [Box 37-2], hallucinogens, inhalants [Box 37-3] and marijuana), and a drug chart of commonly abused drugs is provided in the Evolve site for this book. This chapter focuses on alcohol, tobacco, and marijuana since alcohol and tobacco cause the greatest harm and marijuana is the most commonly used illicit drug. (Resource Tool 37.B on the Evolve website lists useful web resources with more information on handling substance abuse and addiction.)

BOX 37-2   COCAINE AND AMPHETAMINES: COMMON ILLICIT STIMULANTS

The most commonly used illicit stimulants include cocaine and amphetamines (not prescribed). Cocaine comes from the coca shrub cultivated by South American Indians in the Andes Mountains for thousands of years. Purified cocaine can be snorted, smoked, or injected. Crack is a cheap form of smokable cocaine that produces an intense high, but it lasts for a short period. Street cocaine ranges in purity from 50% to 60% and may be cut with other drugs, such as procaine or amphetamine, or any white powder, such as sugar or baby powder. High doses can cause extreme agitation, paranoid delusions, hyperthermia, hallucinations, cardiac dysrhythmias, pulmonary complications, convulsions, and possibly death (Cocaine, *MERCK MANUAL*, 2008).

Amphetamines are a class of stimulants similar to cocaine, but the effects last longer and the drugs are cheaper. Amphetamines have a chemical structure similar to adrenaline and noradrenaline and are generally used to decrease fatigue, increase mental alertness, suppress appetite, and create a sense of well-being. Historically, amphetamines have been issued to American soldiers and pilots to decrease fatigue and increase mental alertness. They are popular among people who need to stay awake for long hours to work or study. They can be taken as pills, injected, snorted, or smoked. "Ice," the smokable form of crystal methamphetamine, first appeared in Hawaii and the western states, but the market has moved across the United States. Methamphetamine is easy to manufacture on the illicit market and its effects can last up to 24 hours (Amphetamines, *MERCK MANUAL*, 2008).

Chronic administration of these stimulants can lead to a neurotransmitter depletion (especially of dopamine), which results in an extreme dysphoria characterized by apathy, sadness, and anhedonia (lack of joy). Thus, these users can get caught up in a dangerous cycle of gaining an extreme high followed by an extreme low. To avoid that low, the person consumes more of the stimulant. Addicts who use these drugs soon are overwhelmed by their cravings and may engage in criminal activities such as theft or prostitution to get drug money.

BOX 37-3   INHALANTS

Inhalants are often among the first drugs that young children use. The primary abusers of most inhalants are adolescents who are 12 to 17 years of age. The 2008 National Survey on Drug Use and Health found that 729,000 persons aged 12 or older had used inhalants for the first time within the past 12 months and 70% of them were under the age of 18 (SAMHSA, 2009a). Use often ends in late adolescence.

Inhalants are breathable chemicals, which include gases and solvents, and they do not fit neatly into other categories. The four categories of inhalants are volatile organic solvents, aerosols, volatile nitrites, and gases. These substances are inhaled ("huffed") from bottles, aerosol cans, or soaked cloth or put into bags or balloons to increase the concentration of the inhaled fumes and decrease the inhalation of other substances in the vapor (e.g., paint particles). (See www.inhalants.org for examples of products in these categories and specific drug information.) Inhalant users can get high several times in a short period since the inhalants are short acting and have a rapid onset. Users are predominately white. Experimental use is about equal for males and females, but males are more likely to engage in chronic use.

Depending on the dose, the user may feel a slight stimulation, less inhibition, or even lose consciousness. Other signs include paint or stains on clothes or the body; spots or sores around the mouth; red or runny eyes or nose; chemical breath odor; a drunk, dazed, or dizzy appearance; nausea and loss of appetite; and finally anxiety, excitability, and irritability. Chronic users may have poor school attendance or be delinquent and involved in theft and burglary (National Institute on Drug Abuse, 2009c). Users can die from "sudden sniffing death" syndrome, and this can occur from the first to the 100th time he or she uses the inhalant. This death appears to be related to acute cardiac dysrhythmia. Dangers with administration of gases increase when inhaling directly from pressurized tanks because the gas is very cold and can cause frostbite to the nose, lips, and vocal cords. Also, if a gas such as nitrous oxide is not mixed with oxygen, the user may die from asphyxiation (National Institute on Drug Abuse, 2009c).

Alcohol

Alcohol (ethyl alcohol or ethanol) is the oldest and most widely used psychoactive drug in the world. In 2006 a national survey found that young people between the ages of 12 and 20 are more likely to use alcohol than use tobacco or illicit drugs, including marijuana. Youth tend to drink less often than adults, but they consume more alcohol per occasion. On average, youth report consuming five drinks per occasion, and they increasingly binge drink. Alcohol abuse contributes to illness in each of the top three causes of death in the United States: heart disease, cancer, and stroke. In 2008, an estimated 22.2 million persons (8.9% of the population aged 12 or older) were classified with substance dependence or abuse in the past year based on criteria specified in the Diagnostic and Statistical Manual of Mental Disorders, 4th edition (DSM-IV). Of these, 3.1 million were classified with dependence on or abuse of both alcohol and illicit drugs, 3.9 million were dependent on or abused illicit drugs but not alcohol, and 15.2 million were dependent on or abused alcohol but not illicit drugs (SAMHSA, 2009a).

Alcohol abuse costs billions of dollars in lost productivity, property damage, medical expenses from alcohol-related illnesses and accidents, family disruptions, alcohol-related violence, and neglect and abuse of children.

> **DID YOU KNOW?** *Alcohol and cocaine use is independently associated with violence-related injuries, whereas opioid use is independently associated with non-violent injuries and burns.*
>
> *From Blondell RD, Dodds HN, Looney SW, et al: Toxicology screening results: injury associations among hospitalized trauma patients, J Trauma 58:561-570, 2005.*

Chronic alcohol abuse leads to profound metabolic and physiological effects on all organ systems. Gastrointestinal (GI) disturbances include inflammation of the GI tract, malabsorption, ulcers, liver problems, and cancers. Cardiovascular disturbances include cardiac dysrhythmias, cardiomyopathy, hypertension, atherosclerosis, and blood dyscrasias. CNS problems include depression, sleep disturbances, memory loss, organic brain syndrome, Wernicke-Korsakoff syndrome, and alcohol withdrawal syndrome. Neuromuscular problems include myopathy and peripheral neuropathy. Males may experience testicular atrophy, sterility, impotence, or gynecomastia, and females who consume alcohol during pregnancy may reproduce neonates with **fetal alcohol syndrome** (FAS) or fetal alcohol effects (FAE). Some of the metabolic disturbances include hypokalemia, hypomagnesemia, and ketoacidosis. Also, endocrine disturbances may result in pancreatitis or diabetes (Merck Manual, 2008).

The concentration of alcohol in the blood is determined by the concentration of alcohol in the drink, the rate of drinking, the rate of absorption (slower in the presence of food), the rate of metabolism, and a person's weight and sex. The amount of alcohol the liver can metabolize per hour is equal to about ¾ oz of whiskey, 4 oz of wine, or 12 oz of beer. Figure 37-1 shows the effects on the CNS as the **blood alcohol concentration** (BAC) increases. However, with chronic consumption, tolerance will develop, and a person can reach a high BAC with minimal CNS effects.

Alcohol use in moderation may provide health benefits by providing mild relaxation and lowering the serum cholesterol level. Controlled drinking organizations such as Moderation Management (http://www.moderation.org) provide guidelines for persons who want to have alcohol in their lives. See Box 37-4 for safe limits of alcohol consumption and Table 37-2 for standard drink equivalents.

Tobacco

Smoking is the foremost preventable cause of death and disease in the United States, with one in five deaths attributed to cigarettes. For every person who dies from tobacco use, another 20 will suffer from at least one serious tobacco-related illness (CDC, 2010). Table 37-3 highlights cigarette smoking–related mortality in the United States. The Centers for Disease Control and Prevention (CDC) estimates an average of 443,000 deaths per year are caused by complications of cigarette smoking (CDC, 2008a). In 2008, an estimated 70.9 million Americans aged 12 or older were current (past month) users of a tobacco product. This represents 28.4% of the population in that age range. In addition, 59.8

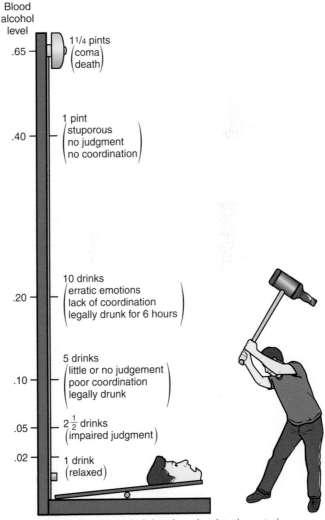

FIGURE 37-1 Blood alcohol level and related central nervous system effects of a normal drinker (160-lb man) according to the number of drinks consumed in 1 hour. (From Kinney J, Leaton G: *Loosening the grip,* ed 5, St Louis, 1995, Mosby.)

million persons (23% of the population) were current cigarette smokers; 13.1 million (5.3%) smoked cigars; 8.7 million (3.5%) used smokeless tobacco; and 1.9 million (0.8%) smoked tobacco in pipes (SAMHSA, 2009a). Young adults ages 18 to 25 reported the highest rate of current tobacco use at 44.8% (NIDA, 2009b).

BOX 37-4   WHAT ARE THE RECOMMENDED SAFE LIMITS FOR ALCOHOL CONSUMPTION?*

For healthy men up to age 65:
- No more than 4 drinks in a day AND
- No more than 14 drinks in a week

For healthy women (and healthy men over age 65):
- No more than 3 drinks in a day AND
- No more than 7 drinks in a week

From: National Institute on Alcohol Abuse and Alcoholism: *Helping patients who drink too much: a clinician's guide (update)*, NIH Pub No 07-3769, Rockville, MD, 2005, USDHHS.

*Depending on your health status, your doctor may advise you to drink less or abstain.

THE CUTTING EDGE   *Tobacco Control State Highlights 2010 is a call-to-action report that looked at six high-impact strategies to reduce tobacco use and provides key indicators for assessing progress in every state. The World Health Organization introduced a framework to describe these strategies using the acronym MPOWER. The strategies include: (1) Monitor tobacco use and prevention policies, (2) Protect people from tobacco smoke, (3) Offer help to quit tobacco use, (4) Warn about the dangers of tobacco use, (5) Enforce bans on tobacco advertising, promotion, and sponsorship, and (6) Raise taxes on tobacco (WHO, 2008).*

California has the longest running comprehensive tobacco control program, with adult smoking rates decreasing from 22.7% in 1988 to 13.3% in 2006. Compared with the rest of the states, heart disease deaths and lung cancer incidence in California have declined at accelerated rates. Research shows that the more states spend on evidence-based programs, the greater the reduction in smoking (CDC, 2010).

TABLE 37-2   WHAT IS A STANDARD DRINK?

A standard drink in the United States is any drink that contains about 14 g of pure alcohol (about 0.6 fluid oz or 1.2 tbsp). The U.S. standard drink equivalents shown here are approximate, since different brands and types of beverages vary in their actual alcohol content.

12 oz of beer or cooler	8-9 oz of malt liquor 8.5 oz shown in a 12-oz glass that, if full, would hold about 1.5 standard drinks of malt liquor	5 oz of table wine	3-4 oz of fortified wine (such as sherry or port) 3.5 oz shown	2-3 oz of cordial, liqueur, or aperitif 2.5 oz shown	1.5 oz of brandy (a single jigger)	1.5 oz of spirits (a single jigger of 80-proof gin, vodka, whiskey, etc.) Shown straight and in a highball glass with ice to show level before adding mixer*
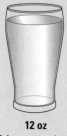	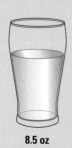	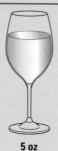	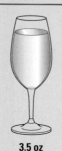	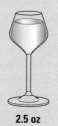	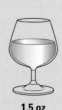	
12 oz	**8.5 oz**	**5 oz**	**3.5 oz**	**2.5 oz**	**1.5 oz**	**1.5 oz**

Many people do not know what counts as a standard drink and so they do not realize how many standard drinks are in the containers in which these drinks are often sold. Some examples:

- For **beer,** the approximate number of standard drinks in
  - 12 oz = 1
  - 16 oz = 1.3
  - 22 oz = 2
  - 40 oz = 3.3

- For **malt liquor,** the approximate number of standard drinks in
  - 12 oz = 1.5
  - 16 oz = 2
  - 22 oz = 2.5
  - 40 oz = 4.5

- For **table wine,** the approximate number of standard drinks in
  - a standard 750 mL (25 oz) bottle = 5

- For **80-proof spirits,** or "hard liquor," the approximate number of standard drinks in
  - a mixed drink = 1 or more*
  - a pint (16 oz) = 11
  - a fifth (25 oz) = 17
  - 1.75 L (59 oz) = 39

Note: It can be difficult to estimate the number of standard drinks in a single mixed drink made with hard liquor. Depending on factors such as the type of spirits and the recipe, a mixed drink can contain from one to three or more standard drinks.

The economic toll from tobacco use in the United States is enormous. Between 2000 and 2004, cigarette smoking was responsible for approximately $193 billion in annual health-related losses, with $96 billion in direct medical costs and $97 billion in lost productivity (CDC, 2008a).

Nicotine, the active ingredient in the tobacco plant, is a particularly toxic drug. To protect itself, the body quickly develops tolerance to the nicotine. If a person smokes regularly, tolerance to nicotine develops within hours, compared with days for heroin or months for alcohol. Pipes and cigars are less hazardous than cigarettes because the harsher smoke discourages deep inhalation. However, pipes and cigars increase the risk of cancer of the lips, mouth, and throat.

Smoke can be inhaled directly by the smoker (mainstream smoke), or it can enter the atmosphere from the lighted end of the cigarette and be inhaled by others in the vicinity (sidestream smoke). Sidestream or second-hand smoke contains higher concentrations of toxic and carcinogenic compounds than mainstream smoke. An estimated 3000 annual lung cancer deaths and over 1 million illnesses in children are attributed to sidestream smoke (Barry, 2007). Sidestream smoke is only about 20% less dangerous than actually smoking, and most of the toxic effects occur within the first 5 minutes of exposure (Barnoya and Glanz, 2005). Smoking bans are being adopted to reduce the discomfort and health hazards among non-smokers.

Nicotine is also used as chewing tobacco or snuff. Marketed as "smokeless tobacco," a wad is put in the mouth and the nicotine is absorbed sublingually. Higher doses of nicotine are delivered in the smokeless forms because the nicotine is not destroyed by heat. Nevertheless, this form is less addictive because nicotine enters the bloodstream less directly. Smokeless tobacco users are 20% more likely to die of heart disease than non-users (Henley et al, 2005), and they are at a higher risk for cancer of the mouth, pharynx, esophagus, stomach, and pancreas (Boffetta et al, 2005).

> **DID YOU KNOW?** *Snus is an old Scandinavian moist tobacco product that is packaged in a small "tea bag" and placed under the upper lip. It is not noticeable and eliminates the need for spitting that normally accompanies the use of oral snuff. It has recently come into the U.S. market by tobacco companies as a harm reduction alternative to smoking tobacco. It eliminates the hazards of smoking tobacco and is less carcinogenic than snuff. However, for some cigarette smokers, it offers them a method to continue their nicotine habit while in any smoke-free environment (Koch, 2007).*

> **DID YOU KNOW?** *Caffeine is one of the most widely used psychoactive drugs in the world, with a U.S. daily per capita consumption of 211 mg. Caffeine is found in coffee, tea, chocolate, soft drinks, and various medications (Table 37-4). Moderate doses of caffeine from 100 to 300 mg per day increase mental alertness and probably have little negative effect on health. Higher doses can lead to insomnia, irritability, tremulousness, anxiety, cardiac dysrhythmias, GI disturbances, and headaches. Regular use of high doses can lead to physical dependence, and the withdrawal symptoms may include headaches, slowness, and occasional depression (Mayo Clinic Staff, 2009). Treating afternoon headaches with analgesics containing caffeine may in reality be preventing a withdrawal symptom from heavy morning coffee consumption.*

TABLE 37-3 CIGARETTE SMOKING–RELATED MORTALITY

DISEASE	MEN	WOMEN	OVERALL
Cancers			
Lung	78,680	46,842	125,522
Other	25,792	9,534	35,326
Subtotal	104,472	56,376	160,848
Cardiovascular Diseases			
Heart disease	63,878	37,181	101,059
Stroke	7,896	8,026	15,922
Other	7,415	4,151	11,566
Subtotal	79,139	49,358	128,497
Respiratory Diseases			
Pneumonia/influenza	6,042	4,381	10,423
Bronchitis/ emphysema	7,536	6,391	13,927
Chronic airway obstruction	40,217	38,771	78,988
Subtotal	53,795	49,543	103,338
Total	**237,406**	**155,277**	**392,683**

Modified from Centers for Disease Control and Prevention: *Smoking-Attributable Mortality, Years of Potential Life Lost, and Productivity Losses—United States, 2000-2004.* Available at http://www.cdc.gov/tobacco/data_statistics/fact_sheets/health_effects/tobacco_related_mortality/index.htm. Accessed July 9, 2010.

TABLE 37-4 CAFFEINE CONTENT IN COMMONLY CONSUMED SUBSTANCES

DRINK/FOOD/ SUPPLEMENT	AMOUNT OF DRINK/FOOD	AMOUNT OF CAFFEINE
SoBe No Fear	8 oz	83 mg
Monster energy drink	16 oz	160 mg
Rockstar energy drink	8 oz	80 mg
Red Bull energy drink	8.3 oz	80 mg
Jolt cola	12 oz	72 mg
Mountain Dew	12 oz	55 mg
Coca-Cola	12 oz	34 mg
Diet Coke	12 oz	45 mg
Pepsi	12 oz	38 mg
7-Up	12 oz	0 mg
Brewed coffee (drip method)	5 oz	115 mg*
Iced tea	12 oz	70 mg*
Cocoa beverage	5 oz	4 mg*
Chocolate milk beverage	8 oz	5 mg*
Dark chocolate	1 oz	20 mg*
Milk chocolate	1 oz	6 mg*
Jolt gum	1 stick	33 mg
Cold relief medication	1 tablet	30 mg*
Vivarin	1 tablet	200 mg
Excedrin extra strength	2 tablets	130 mg

*Denotes average amount of caffeine.
Source: U.S. Food and Drug Administration, National Soft Drink Association, Center for Science in the Public Interest. Available at http://kidshealth.org/teen/drug_alcohol/drugs/caffeine.html#. Accessed July 10, 2010.

Marijuana

Marijuana (*Cannabis sativa,* or *C. indica*) is the most widely used illicit drug in the United States. Compared with the other psychoactive drugs, marijuana has little toxicity and is one of the safest therapeutic agents known (Marijuana, *Merck Manual,* 2008). Psychological dependence can occur with chronic use, but little is known about any potential physical dependence. However, because of its illegal status, there is no quality control, and a user may consume contaminated marijuana. Users enjoy a mild euphoria, a relaxed feeling, and an intensity of sensory perceptions. Some call the effect a dreamy state of consciousness in which ideas seem disconnected, unanticipated, and free flowing. Time, color, and spatial perceptions may be altered (Marijuana, *Merck Manual,* 2008). Side effects include dry and reddened eyes, increased appetite, dry mouth, drowsiness, and mild tachycardia. Adverse reactions include anxiety, disorientation, and paranoia.

The greatest physical concern for chronic users is possible damage to the respiratory tract from smoking the drug. For chronic users tolerance can develop, as well as physical dependence; however, the withdrawal symptoms are benign. Addiction can occur for some chronic users and is difficult to treat because the progression tends to be subtle.

Despite its therapeutic effects, especially in treating pain, the only legal access to marijuana was through the U.S. Food and Drug Administration's (FDA's) Compassionate Investigational New Drug Program. This program was closed in 1992. In response to this complete prohibition, some health care organizations support access to this medication through formal resolutions, including several state nurses' associations, the American Nurses Association, and the American Public Health Association. Fourteen states and Washington, DC have passed laws allowing clients to use marijuana as medicine under the recommendation of their physician, but the federal government continues its total prohibition efforts. See www.medicalcannabis.com for a full list of supporting organizations.

THE CUTTING EDGE *In 2002 a petition to remove cannabis from Schedule I of the Controlled Substances was submitted to the Drug Enforcement Administration. It went through an excessively long review, and the Department of Health and Human Services finally sent their recommendations back to the DEA in 2010. The DEA's final response is overdue, but it could end the prohibition of medical cannabis throughout the United States (http://www.drugscience.org).*

DID YOU KNOW? *Before marijuana prohibition, cannabis was a popular plant grown for its fiber (hemp), seed (popular birdseed), oil, and medicinal as well as psychoactive properties. During World War II, the hemp fiber was so valuable that farmers were required to grow marijuana to ensure a supply. Hemp fiber and seeds do not contain enough active tetrahydrocannabinol (THC) to produce any psychoactive effects. Hemp remains illegal to grow in the United States, but a growing number of hemp products are now available in the United States.*

PREDISPOSING/CONTRIBUTING FACTORS

In addition to the specific drug being used, two other major variables influence the particular drug experience: set and setting. To understand various patterns of drug use and abuse by individuals, all three factors (drug, set, and setting) should be considered.

Set

Set refers to the individual using the drug, as well as that person's expectations, including unconscious expectations, about the drug being used. A person's current health may alter a drug's effects from one day to the next. Some people are genetically predisposed to alcoholism or other drug addiction, and their chemical makeup is such that simply consuming the drug triggers the disease process. Persons with underlying mood disorders or other mental illness may try to self-medicate with psychoactive drugs. Sometimes the choice of drug exacerbates symptoms; for example, a depressed person might consume alcohol and become more depressed.

Setting

Setting is the influence of the physical, social, and cultural environment within which the use occurs. Social conditions influence the use of drugs. The fast pace of life, competition at school or in the workplace, and the pressure to accumulate material possessions are daily stressors. Pharmaceutical, alcohol, and tobacco companies are continuously bombarding the public with enticing advertisements pushing their products as a means of feeling better, sleeping better, having more energy, or just as a "treat." People grow up believing that most of life's problems can be solved quickly and easily through the use of a drug. For persons of a lower socioeconomic background and with minimal education or employment possibilities, many of life's opportunities may seem out of reach. Rather than seeking relief through medical care, the use of psychoactive drugs may offer a way to numb the pain or escape from a hopeless reality. They may also rely on alcohol or illicit drugs, which are more readily available. For some, dealing in illicit drugs may appear to be the only way to avoid a future of poverty and unemployment.

Biopsychosocial Model of Addiction

Many theories have been proposed to explain the etiological factors of addiction, and no consensus exists on specific causes. The underlying etiological factors include the belief that addiction is a disease, a moral failing, a psychological disturbance, a personality disorder, a social problem, a dysbehaviorism, or a maladaptive coping mechanism. Different people develop addiction in different ways. For example, some alcoholics say, "I knew I was an alcoholic from my first drink; I drank differently than others." Others have no family history of addiction, but when stressed (such as from chronic pain, significant losses, abusive relationships that lead to low self-esteem, or trauma resulting in posttraumatic stress disorder), they find that drugs may temporarily relieve their stress. Over time, heavy use of one or more drugs to cope with the stress may lead to addiction. Current research focuses on the neurochemistry of addiction, which shows actual brain chemistry changes among addicts. The **biopsychosocial model** provides a framework for understanding addiction as being the result of the interaction of multiple factors.

PRIMARY PREVENTION AND THE ROLE OF THE NURSE

The harm reduction approach to substance abuse focuses on health promotion and disease prevention. Primary prevention for ATOD problems includes: (1) the promotion of healthy lifestyles and resiliency factors, and (2) education about drugs and guidelines for their use. Nurses are ideally prepared to use health promotion strategies such as promoting and facilitating healthy alternatives to indiscriminate, careless, and often dangerous drug use practices and providing education about drugs to decrease harm from irresponsible or unsafe drug use practices.

> **NURSING TIP** *The Boston University School of Public Health offers a free online drug information service that provides news and funding coverage as well as resources and advocacy tools for ATOD policy, prevention, and treatment. The information provided by Join Together Online (JTO) may be reproduced and distributed freely. To sign up for this service, go to http://www.jointogether.org/jtodirect.*

Promotion of Healthy Lifestyles and Resiliency Factors

It is possible to teach clients to be assertive in their relationships with others and how to make more beneficial decisions by looking carefully at the pros and cons of each option and the related consequences. People may turn to medications, especially psychoactive drugs, when they have persistent health problems such as difficulty sleeping, muscle tension, lack of energy, chronic stress, and mood swings. Nurses can help clients understand that medications may mask problems rather than solve them. Stress reduction and relaxation techniques along with a balanced lifestyle may be more effective than medications. Lack of sleep, improper diet, and lack of exercise contribute to many health complaints. Assisting clients to balance their need for rest, nutrition, and exercise on a daily basis can reduce these complaints. Nurses can provide useful information to groups, assisting in the development of community recreational resources or facilitating stress reduction, relaxation, or exercise groups. Nurses can help people learn about drug-free community activities. The How To box lists community activities in which the nurse may become involved.

> **HOW TO Set Up Community-Based Activities Aimed at Substance Abuse Prevention**
> - *Increase involvement and pride in school activities.*
> - *Organize student assistant programs (students helping students).*
> - *Organize a Students Against Drunk Driving (SADD) chapter.*
> - *Mobilize parental awareness and action groups (e.g., Mothers Against Drunk Driving [MADD]).*
> - *Increase availability of recreational facilities.*
> - *Encourage parental commitment to non-drinking parties.*
> - *Encourage religious institutions to convey non-use messages, and provide activities associated with non-use.*
> - *Curtail media messages that glamorize drug and alcohol use.*
> - *Support and reinforce anti-drug use peer-pressure skills.*
> - *Provide general health screenings, including ATOD use.*
> - *Collaborate with community leaders to solve problems related to crime, housing, jobs, and access to health care.*

Lack of educational opportunities, job training, or both can contribute to socioeconomic stress and poor self-esteem, which can lead to drug use to escape the situation. Nurses can help clients identify community resources and solve problems to meet basic needs rather than avoid them.

In addition to decreasing risk factors associated with ATOD problems, it is important to increase protective or resiliency factors. Prevention guidelines to teach parents and teachers how to increase resiliency in youths include the following strategies:

- Help them develop an increased sense of responsibility for their own success.
- Help them identify their talents.
- Encourage them to dedicate their lives to helping society rather than believing that their only purpose in life is to be consumers.
- Provide realistic appraisals and feedback; stress multicultural competence; encourage and value education and skills training.
- Increase cooperative solutions to problems rather than competitive or aggressive solutions.

Drug Education

ATOD problems include more than abuse of psychoactive drugs. Today more than 450,000 different drugs and drug combinations are available, and prescription drugs are involved in almost 60% of all drug-related emergency room visits and 70% of all drug-related deaths. Nurses know about medication administration, the possible dangers of indiscriminant drug use, and the inability of drugs to cure all problems. Nurses can influence the health of clients by destroying the myth of good drugs versus bad drugs. This means (1) teaching clients that no drug is completely safe and that any drug can be abused, (2) helping persons learn how to make informed decisions about their drug use to minimize potential harm, and (3) teaching them to always tell their health care provider what supplements they are taking.

Drug technology is growing, yet the public receives little information about how to safely use this technology. Harm reduction as a goal recognizes that people consume drugs and that they need to know about the use of drugs and risks involved to make decisions about their drug use. Drug education should begin on an individual basis by reviewing the client's prescription medications. Because a physician or nurse practitioner has prescribed the medication, clients often presume little risk is involved.

Is the client aware of any untoward interactions this drug may have with other drugs being used or with food? A common occurrence with drug users is taking drugs from different categories together or at different times to regulate how they feel, known as **polysubstance use or abuse.** For example, a person may drink alcohol when snorting cocaine to "take the edge off"; or some intravenous drug users combine cocaine with heroin (speedball) for similar reasons. Polysubstance use can cause drug interactions that can have additive, synergistic, or antagonistic effects. Indiscriminant polysubstance abuse may lead to serious physiological consequences and can be complicated for the health care professional to assess and treat. It is important to encourage clients to ask questions about their drug use. The How To box lists seven key pieces of information that clients should obtain before taking a drug or medication to decrease the possible harm from unsafe medication consumption.

HOW TO **Determine the Relative Safety of a Drug for Personal or Client Use**

Before using a drug/medication, always determine the following:
- *The chemical being taken*
- *How and where the drug works in the body (main effects, side effects, and adverse reactions)*
- *The correct dosage and route of administration*
- *Whether there will be drug interactions, including interactions with herbal remedies or foods*
- *Awareness of the symptoms of a potential allergic reaction and know when to seek help*
- *If there will be drug tolerance*
- *If the drug will produce physical dependence**

From Mothers Against Misuse and Abuse: Drug consumer safety rules, Mosier, OR. Available at http://www.mamas.org/drugSafety.htm. Accessed July 9, 2010.

*Caution: Approximately 10% of the population may suffer from the disease of addiction. For them, responsible use of psychoactive drugs is limited because of their disease. They need to notify their physician of the addiction if use of psychoactive medicines is being considered as treatment.

Nurses can identify references and community resources available to provide the necessary information, and they can clarify the information. User-friendly reference texts and online resources are available that describe drug interactions among medications, other drugs (including alcohol, tobacco, marijuana, and cocaine), and other substances (food and beverages); they serve as excellent guides for nurses and their clients. (See http://www.drugdigest.org for more information.) Clients should learn about and ask questions about their prescription medications, self-administered over-the-counter drugs, including supplement and herbal remedies, and recreational drugs. This does not mean that nurses should encourage other drug use but, rather, that the potential harm from self-medication can be reduced if clients have the necessary information to make more informed decisions.

Parents should seek information about their use of medications so they can act as role models for their children. It can be confusing for children and adolescents to be told to "just say no" to drugs when they see their parents or drug advertisements try to "quick fix" every health complaint, feeling of stress, anxiety, or depression with a medication. The simple "just say no" approach does not help young people for several reasons. First, children are naturally curious, and drug experimentation is

often a part of normal development. Second, children from dysfunctional homes may use drugs to get attention or to escape an intolerable environment. And finally, the "just say no" approach does not address the powerful influence of peer pressure (Substance Use in Children and Adolescents, *Merck Manual,* 2008).

Drug education has moved into the school curriculum with Project DARE (Drug Abuse Resistance Education), the most widely used school-based drug-use prevention program in the United States. This program uses law enforcement officers to teach the material, but recent studies find that it is less effective than other interactive prevention programs and may even result in increased drug use (Kumpfer, 2008). Basic ATOD prevention programs for young people should combine efforts to increase resiliency factors with drug education. Nurses can serve as educators or as advisors to the school systems or community groups to ensure that all of these areas are addressed. Role playing is useful in teaching many of these skills.

SECONDARY PREVENTION AND THE ROLE OF THE NURSE

Screening for health problems has long been a basic tool used by public health nurses when working with various populations. There are numerous screening tools for ATOD problems that can be used independently or integrated with broader health screening tools. When drug abuse, dependence, or addiction is identified, nurses must assist clients to understand the connection between their drug use patterns and the negative consequences on their health, their families, and the community. Brief interventions include effective strategies nurses can initiate for early intervention before a person needs more extensive or specialized treatment.

THE CUTTING EDGE **Screening, Brief Intervention and Referral to Treatment (SBIRT)—What is SBIRT?**

SBIRT is a comprehensive, integrated, public health approach to the delivery of early intervention and treatment services for persons with substance use disorders, as well as those who are at risk of developing these disorders. Primary care centers, hospital emergency rooms, trauma centers, and other community settings provide opportunities for early intervention with at-risk substance users before more severe consequences occur.

- *Screening quickly assesses the severity of substance use and identifies the appropriate level of treatment.*
- *Brief intervention focuses on increasing insight and awareness regarding substance use and motivation toward behavioral change.*
- *Referral to treatment provides those identified as needing more extensive treatment with access to specialty care.*

A key aspect of SBIRT is the integration and coordination of screening and treatment components into a system of services. This system links a community's specialized treatment programs with a network of early intervention and referral activities that are conducted in medical and social service settings.

From Substance Abuse and Mental Health Services Administration: Screening, brief intervention and referral to treatment. Resource manual, n.d. Available at: http://sbirt.samhsa.gov/index.htm. Accessed March 10, 2011.

Assessing for Alcohol, Tobacco, and Other Drug Problems

The National Institute on Alcohol Abuse and Alcoholism (NIAAA) has published a clinician's guide for assessing problem drinking. This free booklet (NIAAA, 2005) is available in English and Spanish and provides a step-by-step guide for clinicians to use with their clients.

Self-assessment screening tools are available online at www. alcoholscreening.org and www.drugscreening.org. These screening tools are based on the Alcohol, Smoking, and Substance Involvement Screening Test (ASSIST) developed by the World Health Organization and allow for immediate feedback. People can participate in this screening anonymously.

DID YOU KNOW? *NIAAA also developed a nursing education model for the prevention and treatment of alcohol use disorders. This curriculum was designed for nurse educators to teach nurses about alcohol use disorders, but also serves as a self-teaching program for nurses who want to learn more.*

During health assessment, the nurse should assess for substance abuse problems including both self-medication practices and recreational drug use when taking a medication history. Thus, all relevant drug-use history is collected and aids in the assessment of drug-use patterns. Note any changes in drug-use patterns over time. After obtaining a medication history, follow-up questions can determine if problems exist. The following are examples:

- If using a prescription drug, is the client following the directions correctly?
- Has the client increased the dosage or frequency above the prescription level?
- Is the person using any prescribed psychoactive drugs?
- If so, for how long and what is the dosage?

The Levels of Prevention box shows the levels of prevention related to substance abuse.

NURSING TIP Use the 5 As when screening for ATOD problems:

- *Ask about use.*
- *Assess amount and pattern of use.*
- *Advise about safe use as appropriate.*
- *Assist with identifying help or resources.*
- *Arrange for follow-up as needed.*

LEVELS OF PREVENTION

Substance Abuse

Primary Prevention

Provide community education to teach healthy lifestyles; focus on how to resist getting involved in substance abuse.

Secondary Prevention

Institute early detection programs in schools, the workplace, and other areas in which people gather to determine the presence of substance abuse.

Tertiary Prevention

Develop programs to help people reduce or end substance abuse.

When assessing self-medication and recreational or social drug-use patterns, determine the reason the person uses the drug. Some underlying health problems (e.g., pain, stress, weight, insomnia) may be relieved by non-pharmaceutical interventions. The amount, frequency, and duration of use and the route of administration of each drug should be determined. To establish the presence of a substance abuse problem, it is necessary to determine if the drug use is causing any negative health consequences or problems with relationships, employment, finances, or the legal system. The How To box lists examples of questions to ask to determine the presence of socioeconomic problems that are often a result of substance abuse. If a pattern of chronic, regular, and frequent use of a drug exists, nurses should assess for a history of withdrawal symptoms to determine if there is physical dependence on the drug. A progression in drug-use patterns and related problems warns about the possibility of addiction. Denial is a primary symptom of addiction. Methods of denial include the following:

- Lying about use
- Minimizing use patterns
- Blaming or rationalizing
- Intellectualizing
- Changing the subject
- Using anger or humor
- "Going with the flow" (agreeing that a problem exists, stating the behavior will change, but not demonstrating any behavior changes)

A problem should be suspected if the client becomes defensive or exhibits other behavior indicating denial when asked about alcohol or other drug use.

HOW TO **Assess Socioeconomic Problems Resulting from Substance Abuse**

If the client admits to use of alcohol, tobacco, or other drugs, ask the following questions:

1. *Do your parents, spouse, or friends worry or complain about your drinking or using drugs?*
2. *Has a family member sought help about your drinking or using drugs?*
3. *Have you neglected family obligations as a result of drinking or using drugs?*
4. *Have you missed work because of your drinking or using drugs?*
5. *Does your boss complain about your drinking or using drugs?*
6. *Do you drink or use drugs before or during work?*
7. *Have you ever been fired or quit because of drinking or using drugs?*
8. *Have you ever been charged with driving under the influence (DUI) or being drunk in public (DIP)?*
9. *Have you ever had any other legal problems related to drinking and using drugs, such as assault and battery, breaking and entering, or theft?*
10. *Have you had any accidents while intoxicated, such as falls, burns, or motor vehicle accidents?*
11. *Have you spent your money on alcohol or other drugs instead of paying your bills (e.g., telephone, electricity, rent)?*

Drug Testing

During the 1980s, pre-employment or random drug testing in the workplace gained popularity. Drug testing can be done by examining a person's urine, blood, saliva, breath (for alcohol), or hair. Urine testing is the most common method of drug screening. Urine testing indicates only past use of certain drugs, not intoxication. Thus, persons can be identified as having used a certain drug in the recent past, but the degree of intoxication and extent of performance impairment cannot be determined with urine testing. Also, most drug-related problems in the workplace are related to alcohol, and alcohol is not always included in a urine drug screen. When is drug testing appropriate? Drug testing that follows documented impairment may help substantiate the cause of the impairment, and thus it serves as a backup rather than the primary screening method. It is also useful for recovering addicts. Part of their treatment is to abstain from psychoactive drug use; therefore, a urine test yielding positive results for a drug indicates a relapse.

Blood, breath, and saliva drug tests can indicate current use and amount. Any of these tests can help determine alcohol intoxication, and they are often used to substantiate suspected impairment. A serum drug screen can be useful when overdose is suspected to determine the specific drug ingested. The testing of hair is gaining attention because the results can provide a long history of drug-use patterns.

Alcohol and other drug testing should be used as a clinical and public health tool but not for harassment and punishment. For example, approximately 40% to 50% of people who are seen in trauma centers were drinking at the time of their injuries. Hence, it is recommended that breath alcohol testing should be routinely done for clients admitted to the emergency department for traumatic injuries (Physicians and Lawyers for National Drug Policy, 2008).

Employee assistance programs (EAPs) are a beneficial service in many work settings. Often a sizable number of EAP clients have substance use problems since most adults with these problems are employed. The 2008 national survey of drug use found that of the 20.3 million adults classified with dependence or abuse, 61.5% were employed full time (SAMHSA, 2009a). EAP programs can identify health problems among employees and offer counseling or referral to other health care providers as necessary. Such programs provide early identification of and intervention for substance abuse problems; they also offer services to employees to reduce stress and provide health care or counseling so that they may prevent substance abuse problems from developing. Nurses frequently develop and run these programs.

High-Risk Groups

Identifying high-risk groups helps nurses design programs to meet specific needs and to mobilize community resources.

Adolescents

The younger a person is when beginning intensive experimentation with drugs, the more likely dependence will develop. Underage drinking is seen as the most serious drug problem for youth in the United States. Almost one in five eighth graders and almost half of high school seniors report recent use of alcohol, compared with 21% of seniors reporting recent use of marijuana. In fact, the rate of illicit drug use has been declining, including drinking and the use of marijuana, cocaine, and heroin. Lifetime smoking trends for youths ages 12 to 17 years have also declined per a comparison of two national surveys. The Monitoring the Future survey results show a decrease from 33.3% of lifetime cigarette smoking for youths in 2002 to 22.9% in 2008. The National Survey on Drug Use and Health shows a decrease from 39.4% to 26.1% over the same years (SAMHSA, 2009a). There is more work to be done in the area of prevention since studies indicate that the younger the age at which youth begin substance abuse, the greater likelihood that the abuse will continue into adulthood.

THE CUTTING EDGE   *Prescription drug abuse is an emerging area of concern, especially among those ages 12 to 24. A 2010 high school survey of 16,460 students found that 20% of the students have taken a prescription medication that was not prescribed for them. The illicit use of prescription drugs was greatest among whites at 23%, followed by Hispanics at 17% and African-American students at 12% (HealthDay, 2010). Commonly abused classes of prescription drugs include opioids (prescribed to treat pain), CNS depressants (prescribed to treat anxiety and sleep disorders), and stimulants (prescribed to treat narcolepsy, attention-deficit/hyperactivity disorder [ADHD], and obesity). These drugs can be fairly safe when used as directed; however, some people with prescriptions begin using more than prescribed, mislead their primary care provider to get early refills, or do some "doctor shopping" to get more prescriptions. Many teens and college youth steal them from their family members, and others buy them off the Internet. The most commonly abused opioids among teens are hydrocodone (Vicodin) and oxycodone (OxyContin), and these are sometimes crushed and snorted or injected. Friends in school share their dextroamphetamine (Adderall) or methylphenidate (Ritalin), and often use them to help them study. Benzodiazepines such as diazepam (Valium) and alprazolam (Xanax) are the depressants of choice.*

A new trend called "pharming" is where young people bring prescription medications to a party to share with friends and they may take them alone, in combinations, or mix with alcohol. Students say that prescription drugs are often cheaper and easier to obtain, and some believe that they are "cleaner" or safer than illicit drugs such as marijuana or cocaine. They generally have no idea of the toxic effects when these drugs are taken in high doses or combined (NIDA, 2009a).

Heavy drug use during adolescence can interfere with normal development. Note that *Healthy People 2020* objectives SA-2 and TU-3 reduce the initiation of the use of tobacco, alcohol, and other drugs (see *Healthy People 2020* box). Family-related factors (genetics, family stress, parenting styles, child victimization) appear to be the greatest variable that influences substance abuse among adolescents. The co-occurrence with psychiatric disorders (especially mood disorders) and behavioral problems is also associated with substance abuse among adolescents, leaving peer pressure as a less-influential factor. Research suggests that successful social influence-based prevention programs may be driven by their ability to foster social norms that reduce an adolescent's social motivation to begin using ATODs. One particularly effective treatment approach for adolescents is the use of family-oriented therapy (SAMHSA, 2008).

HEALTHY PEOPLE 2020

Objectives Related to Substance Abuse
- SA-2: Increase the proportion of adolescents never using substances.
- SA-8: Increase the proportion of persons who need alcohol and/or illicit drug treatment and received specialty treatment for abuse or dependence in the past year.
- SA-17: Decrease the rate of alcohol-impaired driving (0.08+ blood alcohol content [BAC]) fatalities.

Objectives Related to Tobacco Use
- TU-3: Reduce initiation of tobacco use among children, adolescents, and young adults.
- TU-11: Reduce the proportion of non-smokers exposed to second-hand smoke.
- TU-14: Increase the proportion of smoke-free homes.
- TU-15: Increase tobacco-free environments in schools, including all school facilities, property, vehicles, and social events.
- TU-20: Increase the number of States and the District of Columbia, Territories, and Tribes with sustainable and comprehensive evidence-based tobacco control programs.

From U.S. Department of Health and Human Services: *Healthy People 2020: national health promotion and disease prevention objectives*, Washington, DC, 2010, U.S. Government Printing Office.

Older Adults

Older adults (65 years of age and older) represent 13% of the U.S. population and are the fastest growing segment of U.S. society, expected to represent 21% by the year 2030. Older adults are prescribed approximately one third of all medications in the United States (NIDA, 2005).

Alcohol and prescription drug misuse affects as many as 17% of adults age 60 and older. Problems with alcohol consumption, including interactions with prescribed and OTC drugs, far outnumber any other substance abuse problem among older adults (SAMHSA, 2009b). The free public education brochure, *As You Age... A Guide to Aging, Medicines and Alcohol* is available at http://www.asyouage.samhsa.gov/materials/.

The increased use of prescription drugs and alcohol by older adults may be related to coping problems. Problems of relocation, possible loss of independence, retirement, illness, death of friends, and lower levels of achievement contribute to feelings of sadness, boredom, anxiety, and loneliness. Factors such as slowed metabolic turnover of drugs, age-related organ changes, enhanced drug sensitivities, a tendency to use drugs over long periods, and a more frequent use of multiple drugs all contribute to greater negative consequences from drug use among older adults. Alcohol abuse may not be identified because its effects on cognitive abilities may mimic changes associated with normal aging or degenerative brain disease. Also, depression may simply be attributed to more frequent losses rather than the depressant effects of alcohol, and the older adult may subsequently receive medical treatment for depression rather than alcoholism.

Injection Drug Users

In addition to the problem of addiction, injection drug users (IDUs) (those who self-administer intravenously or subcutaneously) are at risk for other health complications. Intravenous (IV) administration of drugs always carries a greater risk of overdose because the drug goes directly into the bloodstream. With illicit drugs, the danger is increased because the exact dosage is unknown. In addition, the drug may be contaminated with other chemicals, such as sugar, starch, or quinine that can cause negative consequences. Often IDUs make their own solution for IV administration, and any particles present can result in complications from emboli.

Addicts often share needles. Human immunodeficiency virus (HIV), hepatitis C, and other bloodborne diseases can be transmitted through contaminated needles. Infections and abscesses may develop as a result of dirty needles or poor administration techniques. IDUs represent the most rapidly growing source of new cases of acquired immunodeficiency syndrome (AIDS), and they are at the greatest risk for the spread of the virus in the heterosexual community. The estimated number of diagnoses of HIV in injection drug users in 2009 was 2,449 men and 1,483 women (CDC, 2009). The number of diagnoses of HIV among adults and adolescents exposed through injection drug use decreased by 19% from 5,473 in 2005 to 4.4% in 2008 (CDC, 2009). In 2004, it was reported that 20% of all new HIV infection cases occurred among IDUs, with a disproportionate effect on those in minority groups (CDC, 2005a). Because of this trend, emphasis is being placed on reducing the transmission of this disease through contaminated needles. Abstinence is ideal but unrealistic for many addicts. Using the harm reduction model, the nurse should provide education on cleaning needles with bleach between uses and on needle exchange programs to decrease the spread of the virus. Studies indicate that needle exchange programs have not increased injection drug abuse but have, in fact, increased the number of people entering treatment programs (CDC, 2005b).

DID YOU KNOW? *In 2007, less than half of all substance abuse treatment facilities reported the availability of on-site infectious disease screening. However, in opioid treatment programs (OTPs) where many of the clients have been injection drug users, the incidence of screening was more likely: 93.3% screened for tuberculosis, 69.8% screened for HIV, 64.1% screened for hepatitis C, and 62.1% screened for hepatitis B (SAMHSA, 2010).*

Drug Use During Pregnancy

Most drugs can negatively affect a fetus. Thus, the use of any drug during pregnancy should be discouraged unless medically necessary. *Healthy People 2020* objectives address this issue under the Maternal, Infant and Child Health topic area with several objectives describe recommendations to improve the health of infants such as: reduce the occurence of fetal alcohol syndrome (FAS) (MICH-25), and increase abstinence from alcohol, cigarettes and illicit drugs among pregnant women (MICH-11). FAS is considered the leading preventable birth defect, causing mental and behavioral impairment. From 2003 to 2006 the percentage of pregnant women between the ages of 15 and 44 years who engaged in binge drinking in the first trimester dropped from 10.6% to 4.6%. This may be due to the extensive information available about the effects of alcohol on the fetus (SAMHSA, 2007). Estimates of illicit drug use during pregnancy range from 1.3% of women ages 26 to 44 years to 12.9% of adolescent girls ages 15 to 17 years. Tobacco remains the most-used addictive substance during pregnancy, with about 18% of pregnant women smoking (Jones, 2006).

> **WHAT DO YOU THINK?**   *In some states, pregnant women who are using illicit drugs are reported to child protective services because of the potential harm to the fetus. Will this practice do more harm than good? What about women who drink alcohol or smoke cigarettes?*

Despite the increased focus on drug abuse interventions, many pregnant women with drug problems do not receive the help they need. This may be a result of ignorance, poverty, lack of concern for the fetus, lack of available services,

and fear of the consequences of revealing drug use. The fear of criminal prosecution may push addicted women further away from the health care system, cause them to conceal their drug use from medical providers, and cause them to avoid the critical treatment and medical care that they need (Brady and Ashley, 2005).

Persons Who Use Illicit Drugs

The strategy of "just say no" to drugs is both simplistic and misleading. Indiscriminant use of "good" drugs has caused more health problems from adverse reactions, drug interactions, dependence, addiction, and overdoses than use of "bad" drugs. However, the war on drugs focuses on illicit drugs and punishes illicit drug users. The black market associated with illicit drug use puts otherwise law-abiding citizens in close contact with criminals, prevents any quality control of the drugs, increases the risk of AIDS and hepatitis as a result of needle sharing, and hinders health care professionals' accessibility to the abuser or addict. Lack of quality control (unknown strength and purity) can cause unexpected overdoses or secondary effects of the impurities; for example, a synthetic analog of fentanyl (3-methylfentanyl) marketed as "heroin" is 6000 times as potent as morphine. Unsafe administration (contaminated needles) leads to local and systemic infections. The high cost of drugs on the black market leads to crime to support the addiction. In 2006, approximately 20.4 million (or 8.3%) Americans ages 12 years and older had used illicit drugs in the past month. Illicit drugs include marijuana/hashish, cocaine (including crack), heroin, hallucinogens, inhalants, or prescription-type

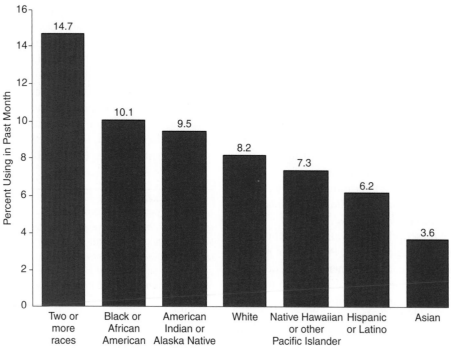

FIGURE 37-2 Past month illicit drug use among persons aged 12 or older, by race/ethnicity, 2008. (From Substance Abuse and Mental Health Services Administration: *Results from the 2008 National Survey on Drug Use and Health: National Findings,* Office of Applied Studies, NSDUH Series H-36, USDHHS Pub No SMA 09-4434, Rockville, MD, 2009.

psychotherapeutics that are used non-medically. Marijuana was the most frequently used illicit drug (SAMHSA, 2007). See Figure 37-2 for illicit drug use by race/ethnicity.

DID YOU KNOW? *The United States has approximately 5% of the world's population, yet Americans consume two thirds of all illicit drugs and incarcerate almost one quarter of the world's prisoners. Of the 2.3 million inmates in U.S. prisons, 65% meet the DSM-IV criteria for ATOD abuse and addiction and only 11% of those inmates receive any treatment during incarceration, few of which are evidence-based (NCASA, 2010).*

Codependency and Family Involvement

Drug addiction is often a family disease. One in four Americans experiences family problems related to alcohol abuse. People in a close relationship with the addict often develop unhealthy coping mechanisms to continue the relationship. This behavior is known as codependency—a stress-induced preoccupation with the addicted person's life, leading to extreme dependence and excessive concern with the addict.

Strict rules typically develop in a codependent family to maintain the relationships: don't talk, don't feel, don't trust, don't lose control, and don't seek help from outside the family. Codependents try to meet the addict's needs at the expense of their own. Codependency may underlie many of the medical complaints and emotional stress seen by health care providers, such as ulcers, skin disorders, migraine headaches, chronic colds, and backaches.

When the addicted person refuses to admit the problem, the family continues to adapt to emotionally survive the stress of the addict's irrational, inconsistent, and unpredictable behavior. Family members consequently develop various roles that tend to be gross exaggerations of normal family roles, and they cling irrationally to these roles, even when they are no longer functional.

One of the most significant roles a family member may assume is that of an enabler. Enabling is the act of shielding or preventing the addict from experiencing the consequences of the addiction. As a result, the addict does not always understand the cost of the addiction and thus is "enabled" to continue to use. Although codependency and enabling are closely related, a person does not have to be codependent to enable. Anyone can be an enabler: a police officer, a boss or co-worker, and even a drug treatment counselor. Health care professionals who do not address the negative health consequences of the drug use with the addicted person are enablers.

The nurse can help families recognize the problem of addiction and help them confront the addicted member in a caring manner. Whether or not the addicted family member is agreeable to treatment, the family members should be given some guidance about the literature and services that are available to help them cope more effectively. The nurse can help identify treatment options, counseling assistance, financial assistance, support services, and (if necessary) legal services for the family members. Children of ATOD abusers or addicts are themselves

at a greater risk for developing addiction and must be targeted for primary prevention.

WHAT DO YOU THINK? *Fatal heroin overdose has been a leading cause of death among injection drug users. In New York City, accidental overdoses kill more people than homicide or suicide. Partners of IDUs often delay or fail to get emergency care for an overdose because they fear arrest. Pilot programs that teach IDUs to perform CPR and administer naloxone have been successful in preventing deaths by overdose. These programs not only increased the awareness of the risk of overdose among IDUs, but also resulted in a decrease in heroin use among the participants (Seal et al, 2005). Programs to teach peer intervention to prevent fatal heroin overdoses appear to be another harm reduction strategy. Should these programs be expanded? Should naloxone be included in first aid kits? Should it be available over the counter for persons who are on prescribed opioids in case a child accidentally ingests the pills?*

TERTIARY PREVENTION AND THE ROLE OF THE NURSE

The nurse is in a key position to help the addict and the addict's family. The nurse's knowledge of community resources and how to mobilize them can significantly influence the quality of care clients receive.

Detoxification

Detoxification is the clearing of one or more drugs from the person's body and managing the withdrawal symptoms. Depending on the particular drug and the degree of dependence, the time required may range from a few days to several weeks. Because withdrawal symptoms vary (depending on the drug used) and range from uncomfortable to life threatening, the setting for and management of withdrawal depend on the drug used.

Drugs such as stimulants or opiates may produce withdrawal symptoms that are uncomfortable but not life threatening. Detoxification from these drugs does not require direct medical supervision, but medical management of the withdrawal symptoms increases the comfort level. On the other hand, drugs such as alcohol, benzodiazepines, and barbiturates can produce life-threatening withdrawal symptoms. These clients should be under close medical supervision during detoxification and should receive medical management of the withdrawal symptoms to ensure a safe withdrawal. Of those who develop delirium tremens from alcohol withdrawal, 15% may not survive despite medical management; therefore, close medical management is initiated as the blood alcohol level begins to fall.

A general rule in detoxification management is to wean the person off the drug by gradually reducing the dosage and frequency of administration. Thus, a person with chronic alcoholism could be safely detoxified by a gradual reduction in alcohol consumption. In practice, however, the switch to another drug, usually a benzodiazepine, often offers a safer withdrawal from alcohol as well as an abrupt end to the intoxication from the drug of choice. For example, chlordiazepoxide (Librium) is commonly used for alcohol detoxification.

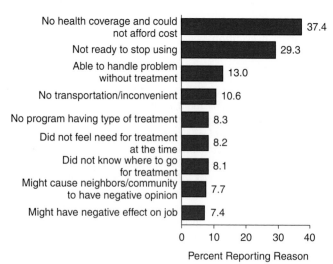

No health coverage and could not afford cost — 37.4
Not ready to stop using — 29.3
Able to handle problem without treatment — 13.0
No transportation/inconvenient — 10.6
No program having type of treatment — 8.3
Did not feel need for treatment at the time — 8.2
Did not know where to go for treatment — 8.1
Might cause neighbors/community to have negative opinion — 7.7
Might have negative effect on job — 7.4

Percent Reporting Reason

FIGURE 37-3 Reasons for not receiving substance use treatment among persons aged 12 or older who needed and made an effort to get treatment but did not receive treatment and felt they needed treatment, 2005-2008 combined. (From Substance Abuse and Mental Health Services Administration: *Results from the 2008 national survey on drug use and health: national findings,* Office of Applied Studies, NSDUH Series H-36, HHS Pub No SMA 09-4434, 2009, Rockville, MD.)

DID YOU KNOW? *Outpatient or home detoxification for persons requiring medical detoxification for alcohol withdrawal can be a cost-effective treatment. Nurses can monitor and evaluate the client's health status in the home environment to reduce the risk of medical complications related to alcohol withdrawal, and to provide encouragement and support for the client to complete the detoxification.*

Addiction Treatment

Addiction treatment differs from the management of negative health consequences of chronic drug abuse, overdose, and detoxification. Addiction treatment focuses on the addiction process. The goal is to help clients view addiction as a chronic disease and assist them to make lifestyle changes to halt the progression of the disease. According to the disease theory, addicts are not responsible for the symptoms of their disease; they are, however, responsible for treating their disease. In 2008, 23.1 million persons aged 12 or older needed treatment for an illicit drug or alcohol use problem (9.2% of the persons aged 12 or older). Of these, 2.3 million (0.9% of persons aged 12 or older and 9.9% of those who needed treatment) received treatment at a specialty facility. Thus, 20.8 million persons (8.3% of the population aged 12 or older) needed treatment for an illicit drug or alcohol use problem but did not receive treatment at a specialty substance abuse facility in the past year (SAMHSA, 2009b). Figure 37-3 shows the common reasons persons do not receive treatment. There are approximately 1.8 million annual admissions to treatment for abuse of alcohol and other drugs in facilities that report to state data systems. Of those, 62% of the admissions are to ambulatory outpatient programs, 18% to

residential programs, and 20% are admitted for detoxification (SAMHSA, 2009b).

Most treatment facilities are multidisciplinary because the intervention strategies require a wide range of approaches. Their programs involve interactions between the addict, family, culture, and community. Strategies include medical management, education, counseling, vocational rehabilitation, stress management, and support services. In addition, specific programs address the needs of various populations such as adolescents, pregnant women, specific ethnic groups, gays and lesbians, as well as health care professionals. The key to effective treatment is to match individual clients with the interventions most appropriate for them. Box 37-5 lists 13 fundamental principles for effective addiction treatment.

Total abstinence is the most recommended treatment goal for ATOD addiction. People who are addicted to a particular drug (e.g., cocaine) are advised to abstain from the use of all psychoactive substances. The use of another drug may simply reinforce the craving for the original drug and cause relapse. More commonly, the addiction merely transfers to the replacement substance.

Treatment may be on an inpatient or outpatient basis. In general, the more advanced the disease is, the greater the need for inpatient treatment. Inpatient treatment programs usually may range from less than 1 week to as long as 90 days. Once a person has completed detoxification (considered the first phase of the treatment process), the programs use counseling and group interaction to help the client stay clean long enough for the body chemistry to rebalance. This is often a difficult time for persons recovering from addictions because they may experience mood swings and difficulty sleeping and dealing with emotions.

The goal of the educational part of the programs is to provide information about the disease and how drugs affect a person physically and psychologically. Clients are informed of the various lifestyle changes that are recommended, and they learn about tools to assist them in making these changes. Discharge planning continues throughout treatment as clients build the support systems that they will need when they leave the controlled environment of a treatment center and face pressures and temptations (triggers) that may lead to relapse.

Long-term residential programs, also called halfway houses, have been developed to ease the person recovering from an addiction back into society. These facilities provide continued support and counseling in a structured environment for persons needing long-term assistance in adjusting to a drug-free lifestyle. The residents are expected to secure employment and take responsibility in managing their financial obligations.

Outpatient programs are similar in the education and counseling offered, but they allow the clients to live at home and continue to work while undergoing treatment. This method is effective for persons in the earlier stages of addiction who feel confident that they can abstain from drug use and have established a strong support network. The How To box provides resources to help locate treatment programs throughout the United States.

BOX 37-5   PRINCIPLES OF DRUG ADDICTION TREATMENT

More than three decades of scientific research have yielded 13 fundamental principles that characterize effective drug abuse treatment. These principles are detailed in *NIDA's Principles of Drug Addiction Treatment: A Research-Based Guide* (April, 2009).

1. No single treatment is appropriate for all individuals. Matching treatment settings, interventions, and services to each client's problems and needs is critical.
2. Treatment needs to be readily available. Treatment applicants can be lost if treatment is not immediately available or readily accessible.
3. Effective treatment attends to multiple needs of the individual, not just his or her drug use. Treatment must address the individual's drug use and associated medical, psychological, social, vocational, and legal problems.
4. At different times during treatment, a client may develop a need for medical services, family therapy, vocational rehabilitation, and social and legal services.
5. Remaining in treatment for an adequate period of time is critical for treatment effectiveness. The time depends on an individual's needs. For most clients, the threshold of significant improvement is reached at about 3 months in treatment. Additional treatment can produce further progress. Programs should include strategies to prevent clients from leaving treatment prematurely.
6. Individual and/or group counseling and other behavioral therapies are critical components of effective treatment for addiction. In therapy, clients address motivation, build skills to resist drug use, replace drug-using activities with constructive and rewarding non–drug-using activities, and improve problem-solving abilities. Behavioral therapy also facilitates interpersonal relationships.
7. Medications are an important element of treatment for many clients, especially when combined with counseling and other behavioral therapies. Buprenorphine, methadone, and levo-alpha-acetylmethodol (LAAM) help persons addicted to opiates stabilize their lives and reduce their drug use. Naltrexone is effective for some opiate addicts and some clients with co-occurring alcohol dependence. Nicotine patches or gum, or an oral medication, such as bupropion, can help persons addicted to nicotine.

8. Addicted or drug-abusing individuals with coexisting mental disorders should have both disorders treated in an integrated way.
9. Medical detoxification is only the first stage of addiction treatment and by itself does little to change long-term drug use. Medical detoxification manages the acute physical symptoms of withdrawal. For some individuals it is a precursor to effective drug addiction treatment.
10. Treatment does not need to be voluntary to be effective. Sanctions or enticements in the family, employment setting, or criminal justice system can significantly increase treatment entry, retention, and success.
11. Possible drug use during treatment must be monitored continuously. Monitoring a client's drug and alcohol use during treatment, such as through urinalysis, can help the client withstand urges to use drugs. Such monitoring can also provide early evidence of drug use so that treatment can be adjusted.
12. Treatment programs should provide assessment for HIV/AIDS, hepatitis B and C, tuberculosis and other infectious diseases, and counseling to help clients modify or change behaviors that place them or others at risk of infection. Counseling can help clients avoid high-risk behavior and help people who are already infected manage their illness.
13. Recovery from drug addiction can be a long-term process and frequently requires multiple episodes of treatment. As with other chronic illnesses, relapses to drug use can occur during or after successful treatment episodes. Participation in self-help support programs during and following treatment often helps maintain abstinence.

HOW TO   Find an Appropriate Treatment Program

1. *Look it up in the National Directory of Drug and Alcohol Abuse Treatment Programs (updated annually). This directory provides information on more than 11,000 alcohol and drug treatment programs in all 50 states, the District of Columbia, Puerto Rico, and 4 U.S. territories. Free copies are available by calling SAMHSA's Clearinghouse at 1-800-729-6686.*
2. *Look it up on the Substance Abuse and Mental Health Services Administration's (SAMHSA) website. Their Substance Abuse Treatment Facility Locator Internet-based service provides an easy-to-use directory to help you locate (including road maps to each facility) and contact public and private treatment programs (http://www.findtreatment.samhsa.gov).*

For those addicted individuals unwilling or unable to completely abstain from psychoactive drugs, other medications can assist them in abstaining from their drug of choice. Such is the case with methadone maintenance programs that treat heroin and other opioid addiction. Methadone, when administered in moderate or high daily doses, produces a **cross-tolerance** to other opioids, thereby blocking their effects and decreasing the craving for the drug of choice. The advantages of methadone are that it is long acting, does not produce a "high," and is inexpensive. The oral use of methadone eliminates the danger of the spread of AIDS and other bloodborne infections that

commonly occur among needle-sharing addicts. Although not recognized as a cure for heroin (or other opioid) addiction, methadone maintenance is a harm reduction intervention because it reduces deviant behavior and introduces addicted persons to the health care system.

Recovery from addiction involves a lifetime commitment and may include periods of relapse. The addicted person must realize that modern medicine has not found a cure for addiction; therefore, returning to drug use may ultimately reactivate the disease process.

Smoking Cessation Programs

Nearly 35 million Americans try to quit smoking each year. Fewer than 10% of those who try to quit on their own are able to stop for a year; those who use an intervention are more likely to be successful. Interventions that involve medications and behavioral treatments appear most promising (CDC, 2007; IOM, 2007). For example, nicotine replacement therapy can be used to help smokers withdraw from nicotine while focusing their efforts on breaking the psychological craving or habit. Four types of nicotine replacement products are available: nicotine gum and skin patches are available over the counter, and nicotine nasal spray and inhalers are available by prescription. These products are about equally effective and can almost double the chances of successfully quitting. Other treatments

EVIDENCE-BASED PRACTICE

The exploratory study of Courbasson et al (2007) examined the benefits of adding auricular acupuncture to a 21-day outpatient treatment program for women with concurrent substance abuse problems, anxiety, and depression. The structured treatment program was psychoeducational in nature and sought to determine if the acupuncture could be a viable alternative option to treatment as usual (TAU). The researchers also wanted to explore whether the addition of acupuncture would reduce the dropout rate of the treatment program.

The 185 women who received the acupuncture reported less physiological cravings for substances, felt significantly less depressed and anxious, and were better able to reflect on and resolve difficulties than the women in the control group. Because of these findings, the study concluded that auricular acupuncture showed promise as an adjunct therapy for addicted women in psychoeducational treatment programs.

Nurse Use

The use of auricular acupuncture seems to be an easily administered and cost-effective treatment alternative to medications for preventing substance abuse relapse and for improving overall health and well-being. The increased emergence of clinical studies recommending the use of acupuncture shows that such an alternative therapy could outweigh Western skepticism about such a practice. Further research is recommended in order to continue to explore the issue.

From Courbasson CMA, de Sorkin AA, Dullerud B: Acupuncture treatment for women with substance use and anxiety/depression: an effective alternative therapy? *Fam Community Health* 30:112-120, 2007.

LINKING CONTENT TO PRACTICE

Using the tools of primary, secondary, and tertiary prevention with individuals, families, and communities in whom alcohol and other drug use is an issue incorporates both public health and public health nursing guidelines and competencies. Specifically, the core competencies of the Council on Linkages Between Academia and Public Health Practice (2010) begin by identifying the analytic and assessment skills needed by public health professionals. The 12 skills in this competency category are used in providing services to the population described in this chapter. For example, you begin by assessing the "health status of populations and their related determinants of health and stress." You next move to skill #2, which is describing the "characteristics of a population-based health problem." These competencies are described through a set of eight domains. Each domain can be used with populations dealing with alcohol and other drug problems.

Similarly, the Intervention Wheel, which is the subject of Chapter 9, has many applications with this population. The Intervention Wheel specifies that "interventions are actions that PHNs take on behalf of individuals, families, and systems, and communities to improve or protect health status (Council on Linkages, 2010, p 1). This tool outlines 17 public health interventions. All 17 of these interventions have application with the populations described in this chapter. For example, case finding, referral and follow-up, health teaching, counseling, and policy development and enforcement are selected examples of ways in which public health nurses intervene in serving a vulnerable population with alcohol- and drug-related problems.

include smoking cessation clinics, hypnosis, and acupuncture. The most effective way to get people to stop smoking and prevent relapse involves multiple interventions and continuous reinforcement, and most smokers require several attempts at cessation before they are successful. Farrelly and colleagues (2008) evaluated whether state tobacco control programs were effective in decreasing the prevalence of adult smokers. They found that program expenditures more effectively influenced the habits of smokers 25 years of age and older versus those between ages 18 and 24. In the latter group the price of cigarettes had a greater effect on their smoking habits. Many resources are available on smoking cessation programs and support groups, including those listed in Box 37-6.

> **NURSING TIP** *There is a website developed specifically for nurses to help nurses quit smoking: http://www.tobaccofreenurses.org.*

Support Groups

The founding of Alcoholics Anonymous (AA) in 1935 began a strong movement of peer support to treat a chronic illness. AA groups have developed around the world. Their success has led to the development of other support groups such as the following:

- Narcotics Anonymous (NA) for persons with narcotic addiction
- Pills Anonymous for persons with polydrug addictions
- Overeaters Anonymous
- Gamblers Anonymous

AA and NA help addicted people develop a daily program of recovery and reinforce the recovery process. The fellowship, support, and encouragement among members provide a vital social network for the person recovering from an addiction.

Al-Anon and Alateen are similar self-help programs for spouses, parents, children, or others involved in a painful relationship with an alcoholic. Nar-Anon is a support group for those in relationships with persons with narcotic addictions. Al-Anon family groups are available to anyone who has been affected by their involvement with an alcoholic person. The purposes of Alateen include providing a forum for adolescents to discuss family stressors, learn coping skills from one another, and gain support and encouragement from knowledgeable peers. Adult Children of Alcoholics (ACOA) groups are also available in most areas to address the recovery of adults who grew up in alcoholic homes and are still carrying the scars and retaining dysfunctional behaviors.

For some persons, the AA program places too much emphasis on a higher power or focuses too much on the negative consequences of past drinking. Women for Sobriety focuses on rebuilding self-esteem, a core issue for many women with alcoholic problems. (See www.womenforsobriety.org for additional information.) Rational Recovery has a cognitive orientation and is based on the assumption that ATOD addiction is caused by irrational beliefs that can be understood and overcome. (See www.rational.org for additional information on this approach.)

Nurse's Role

Many people with alcoholism and drug addiction become lost in the health care system. If satisfactory care is not provided in one agency or the waiting list is months long, the person may give up rather than seek alternative sources of care. The nurse

BOX 37-6   SMOKING CESSATION RESOURCES

American Cancer Society
1-800-227-2345 (1-800-ACS-2345)
http://www.cancer.org, retrieved July 9, 2010
"Guide to Quitting Smoking" and more

American Heart Association
1-800-242-8721 (1-800-AHA-USA-1)
http://www.americanheart.org, retrieved July 9, 2010
"In Control: Freedom from Smoking" program

American Lung Association
1-800-548-8252
http://www.lungusa.org, retrieved July 9, 2010
"Freedom From Smoking Online" at www.ffsonline.org

Centers for Disease Control and Prevention
Office on Smoking and Health
1-800-232-4636 (1-800-CDC-INFO)
www.cdc.gov/tobacco
Free quit support line: 1-800-784-8669 (1-800-QUIT-NOW)

The Foundation for a Smoke-Free America
1-800-541-7741
http://www.tobaccofree.org, retrieved July 9, 2010
"Quitting Tips" and more

National Cancer Institute (NCI)
Toll-free tobacco number: 1-877-448-7848
http://www.cancer.gov, retrieved July 9, 2010
Tobacco quit line: 1-800-784-8669 (1-800-QUIT-NOW)
Quitting information, cessation guide, and counseling is offered, as well as information on state telephone-based quit programs

Smokefree.gov
Retrieved 7/9/10 from http://www.smokefree.gov
"Quit Smoking today! We can help"
Excellent source created by Tobacco Control Research Branch of NCI

Smokefree Women
Retrieved 7/9/10 from http://women.smokefree.gov
NCI collaborated with:
   Centers for Disease Control and Prevention - Office on Smoking and Health
   Centers for Disease Control and Prevention - Division of Reproductive Health
   Health Canada
   American Legacy Foundation
   The Robert Wood Johnson Foundation

SmokEnders
1-800-828-4357
http://www.smokenders.com, retrieved July 9, 2010
"The Quit Kit," an 11-week program

For more information, see the WebLinks on this book's Evolve website at http://evolve.elsevier.com/Stanhope.

EVIDENCE-BASED PRACTICE

Changes in Social Networks Contribute to Improved Drinking Outcomes

This project compared various strategies for helping alcohol dependent individuals change their social network from one that supports drinking to one that supports sobriety. Alcohol-dependent men and women were randomly assigned to one of three outpatient treatment conditions: Network Support (NS), Network Support + Contingency Management (NS+CM), or Case Management (CaseM, a control condition). Analysis of drinking rates indicated that the NS condition yielded up to 20% more days abstinent than the other conditions at 2 years posttreatment. NS treatment also resulted in greater increases at 15 months in social network support for abstinence, as well as AA attendance and AA involvement, than did the other conditions. The findings indicate that a network support treatment can effect long-term adaptive changes in drinkers' social networks, and that these changes contribute to improved drinking outcomes in the long term.

Nurse Use

This research supports the notion that AA and other sobriety support groups really can improve outcomes. It is important to have access to support group meetings in your local area.

From Litt MD, Kadden RM, Kabela-Cormier E, Petry NM: Changing network support for drinking: initial findings from the Network Support Project, *J Consult Clin Psychol* 754:542-555, 2007.

who knows the client's history, environment, support systems, and the local treatment programs can offer guidance to the most effective treatment modality (CSAT, 2006). Brief interventions by health care professionals who are not treatment experts can be effective in helping ATOD abusers and addicts change their risky behavior. Brief interventions may convince the ATOD abuser or addict to reduce substance consumption or follow through with a treatment referral (Moyer and Finney, 2005; NIAAA, 2005). Box 37-7 describes six elements commonly included in brief interventions, using the acronym FRAMES. Strategies used with clients can vary depending on their readiness for change. Understanding the stages of change listed in Box 37-8 and recognizing which stage a client is in are important factors for determining which interventions and programs may be most helpful to the client.

After the client has received treatment, the nurse can coordinate aftercare referrals and follow up on the client's progress. The nurse can provide additional support in the home as the client and family adjust to changing roles and the stress involved with such changes. The nurse can support addicted persons who have relapsed by reminding them that relapses may well occur, but that they and their families can continue to work toward recovery and an improved quality of life.

OUTCOMES

Health promotion and risk reduction are basic concepts in nursing. Promoting a healthy environment in the home and local community provides individuals and families a nurturing environment in which to achieve optimal health. Individuals with high self-esteem and access to health care and information about the health risks related to drug use can be responsible

---

BOX 37-7   BRIEF INTERVENTIONS USING THE FRAMES ACRONYM

- *Feedback.* Provide the client direct feedback about the potential or actual personal risk or impairment related to drug use.
- *Responsibility.* Emphasize personal responsibility for change.
- *Advice.* Provide clear advice to change risky behavior.
- *Menu.* Provide a menu of options or choices for changing behavior.
- *Empathy.* Provide a warm, reflective, empathetic, and understanding approach.
- *Self-efficacy.* Provide encouragement and belief in the client's ability to change.

From Center for Substance Abuse Treatment: *Brief interventions and brief therapies for substance abuse,* TIP 34, DHHS Pub No (SMA) 99-3353, Rockville, MD, 1999, USDHHS.

BOX 37-8   STAGES OF CHANGE

Pre-Contemplation

At this stage, the person does not intend to change in the foreseeable future. The person is often unaware of any problem. Resistance to recognizing or modifying a problem is the hallmark of pre-contemplation.

Contemplation

At this stage, the individual is aware that a problem exists and is seriously thinking about overcoming it but has not yet made a commitment to take action. The nurse can encourage the individual to weigh the pros and cons of both the problem and the solution to the problem.

Preparation

Preparation was originally referred to as *decision making.* At this stage, the individual is prepared for action and may reduce the problem behavior but has not yet taken effective action (e.g., reduces amount of smoking but does not abstain).

Action

At this stage, the individual modifies the behavior, experiences, or environment to overcome the problem. The action requires considerable time and energy. Modification of the target behavior to an acceptable criterion and significant overt efforts to change are the hallmarks of action.

Maintenance

In this stage, the individual works to prevent relapse and consolidate the gains attained during action. Stabilizing behavior change and avoiding relapse are the hallmarks of maintenance.

Modified from DiClemente CC , Schlundt D, Gemmell L: Readiness and stages of change in addiction treatment, *Am J Addict* 13(2):103-119, 2004.

---

for their personal health and make informed decisions about drug use. Nurses can assess the health of the community and its citizens, prioritize the needs, and identify local resources to collaborate with others to develop strategies that will improve the underlying health of the community.

Early identification and intervention for persons with ATOD problems can prevent many of the harmful physical, emotional, and social consequences that may occur if abuse continues and may also prevent abuse patterns from developing into addiction. The nurse needs to assess individual and community ATOD problems and target at-risk groups to develop strategies to increase assessment and provide appropriate interventions. Review the national health objectives (refer back to the *Healthy People 2020* box) for the tobacco and substance abuse areas and note how many can be achieved with secondary prevention strategies.

Besides saving taxpayers' money, treatment helps addicted individuals and their families recover from the devastating effects of addiction. Addicts and their families often become hopeless and helpless while actively addicted. The nurse can offer hope in affirming the addict's self-worth and can be the bridge to community resources to assist in treatment and recovery.

Many of these expected outcomes for ATOD problems have been lessened because a lack of funding has resulted from federal strategies that focus on law enforcement and punishment rather than on education and treatment. The greatest challenge for nurses is to influence policy makers to put the emphasis on health care for this major health problem.

CHAPTER REVIEW

▌ PRACTICE APPLICATION

Ms. Jane Doe, RN, is a home health case manager in a large, low-income housing area in her community. She designs care plans and coordinates health care services for clients who need health care at home. She makes the initial visits to determine the level and frequency of care needed and then acts as supervisor of the volunteers and nurses' aides who perform most of the day-to-day care. Single-parent families are the norm, and drug dealing is commonplace in this housing area.

Ms. Doe made a home visit to Ann Greene, a 26-year-old mother of three. She takes care of her 62-year-old maternal grandfather, Mr. Jones, who is recovering from cardiac bypass surgery. He has a smoking history of two packs per day for almost 40 years. Since

his surgery, he has reduced his smoking to one pack per day, but he refuses to quit. He has a history of alcohol dependence, reportedly consuming up to a fifth of liquor a day, and a history of withdrawal seizures. Four years ago he went through alcohol detoxification, but he refused to stay at the facility for continued treatment, stating he could stay sober on his own. Since that time he has had several binge episodes, but Ann says that he has not been drinking since the surgery. A widower for 5 years, Mr. Jones now lives with his granddaughter and her three children.

Ms. Greene is a widow and has two sons, ages 3 and 9, and a daughter, age 5. The oldest son's father is an alcoholic who is currently incarcerated for manslaughter while driving under the

PRACTICE APPLICATION—cont'd

influence of alcohol, and the father of her two youngest children was killed by a stray bullet in a cocaine bust 3 years ago. She and her husband had smoked crack cocaine for several months but both stopped when she became pregnant with their youngest child and remained cocaine free. She is angry at the system and frightened of police officers ever since the drug raid in which her husband was killed. Other residents were also hurt, and less than $500 worth of cocaine was found three apartments away from hers.

Ms. Greene does not consume alcohol, but she smokes one to two packs of cigarettes per day. She quit smoking during her pregnancies but restarted soon after each birth.

A. What type of interventions can the nurse provide for Mr. Jones regarding his smoking?
B. How can the nurse help Ms. Greene cope with the potential risk of Mr. Jones' drinking when he progresses to more independence?
C. How can the nurse help Ms. Greene with her cigarette smoking?
D. Knowing that there is a genetic link to alcoholism and being aware of the high rate of drug problems in the housing area, how can Nurse Doe help prevent this mother and her children from developing substance abuse problems?
E. What problems seem greater because of the drug laws, and what can Ms. Greene do to help make the environment safer and more nurturing?

Answers can be found on the Evolve site.

KEY POINTS

- Substance abuse is the number one national health problem, linked to numerous forms of morbidity and mortality.
- Harm reduction is an approach to ATOD problems that deals with substance abuse primarily as a health problem rather than as a criminal problem.
- All persons have ideas, opinions, and attitudes about the use of drugs that influence their actions.
- Social conditions such as a fast-paced life, excessive stress, and the availability of drugs influence the incidence of substance abuse.
- Important terms to understand when working with individuals, groups, or communities for whom substance abuse is prevalent are *drug dependence, drug addiction, alcoholism, psychoactive drugs, depressants, stimulants, marijuana, hallucinogens,* and *inhalants.*
- Primary prevention for substance abuse includes education about drugs and guidelines for use, as well as the promotion of healthy alternatives to drug use either for recreation or to relieve stress.

- Nurses can help develop community prevention programs.
- Secondary prevention depends heavily on careful assessment of the client's use of drugs. Such assessment should be part of all basic health assessments.
- High-risk groups include pregnant women, young people, older adults, intravenous drug users, and illicit drug users.
- Drug addiction is often a family, not merely an individual, problem.
- Codependency describes a companion illness to the addiction of one person in which the codependent member is addicted to the addicted person.
- Brief interventions by a nurse can be as effective as treatment.
- Nurses are in ideal roles to assist with tertiary prevention for both the addicted person and the family.

CLINICAL DECISION-MAKING ACTIVITIES

1. Read your local newspaper for 4 days and select stories that illustrate the effects of substance abuse on individuals, families, and the community. What interventions would you use? Who would you involve in your work? Are the interventions primary, secondary, or tertiary in nature? How would you evaluate your work?
2. For each of the stories in the newspaper related to substance abuse, describe preventive strategies that a nurse might have tried before the problem reached such a dire state.
3. Looking at your local community resources directory, the telephone book, or the Internet, identify agencies that might serve as referral sources for individuals or families for whom substance abuse is a problem.
4. Review popular magazine and television advertisements for alcohol, tobacco, and other medicines (e.g., sleep aids, analgesics, laxatives, stimulants). In small groups, discuss the messages conveyed in the advertisements, and discuss the implications of client education to reduce possible harm from misuse and abuse of these substances.

5. Attend an open AA or NA meeting and an Al-Anon meeting. Go alone if possible or with an alcoholic or a drug-addicted friend. As the members introduce themselves, give your first name and state, "I am a visitor." Plan to listen and do not attempt to take notes. Respect the anonymity of the persons present. Discuss your experiences later in a group.
6. In groups of four or five, review the national health objectives in *Healthy People 2020* (see www.healthypeople.gov) under Tobacco Use and under Substance Abuse. Pick an objective from each section, and brainstorm about possible community efforts a nurse could initiate to reach that objective.

REFERENCES

Amphetamines: *The Merck manual,* section 15, psychiatric disorders, chapter 198, drug use and dependence, 2008, Merck & Co, Inc. Available at http://www.merck.com/mmpe/sec15/ch198/ch198k.html. Accessed July 9, 2010.

Barnoya J, Glanz SA: Cardiovascular effects of secondhand smoke nearly as large as smoking, *Circulation* 111:2684–2698, 2005.

Barry M: *Health harms from secondhand smoke,* 2007, National Center for Tobacco-Free Kids. Available at http://tobaccofreekids.org/research/factsheets/pdf/0103.pdf. Accessed March 5, 2011.

Blondell RD, Dodds HN, Looney SW, et al: Toxicology screening results: injury associations among hospitalized trauma patients, *J Trauma* 58:561–570, 2005.

Boffetta P, Aagnes B, Weiderpass E, et al: Smokeless tobacco use and risk of cancer of the pancreas and other organs, *Int J Cancer* 114:992–995, 2005.

Brady TM, Ashley OS, editors: *Women in substance abuse treatment: results from the Alcohol and Drug Services Study (ADSS),* Office of Applied Studies, DHHS Pub No SMA 04-3968, Analytic Series A-26, Rockville, MD, 2005, SAMHSA.

Center for Substance Abuse Treatment: *Brief interventions and brief therapies for substance abuse,* TIP 34, DHHS Pub No (SMA) 99–3353, Rockville, MD, 1999, USDHHS.

Center for Substance Abuse Treatment: *Substance abuse: clinical issues in intensive outpatient treatment. Treatment Improvement Protocol (TIP) Series 47,* DHHS Pub No (SMA) 06–4182, Rockville, MD, 2006, Substance Abuse and Mental Health Services Administration.

Centers for Disease Control and Prevention: *Access to sterile syringes, fact sheet,* 2005a. Available at http://www.cdc.gov/idu/facts/AED_IDU_ACC.pdf. Accessed March 5, 2011.

Centers for Disease Control and Prevention: *Syringe exchange programs, fact sheet,* 2005b. Available at http://www.cdc.gov/idu/facts/AED_IDU_SYR.pdf. Accessed March 5, 2011.

Centers for Disease Control and Prevention: *Best Practices for Comprehensive Tobacco Control Programs—2007,* Atlanta, 2007, USDHHS, CDC, National Center for Chronic Disease Prevention and Health Promotion, Office on Smoking and Health.

Centers for Disease Control and Prevention: Smoking-attributable mortality, years of potential life lost, and productivity losses—United States, 2000-2004, *MMWR* 57(45):1226–1228, 2008a.

Centers for Disease Control and Prevention: *HIV surveillance in injection drug users (through 2008).* Available at http://www.cdc.gov/hiv/idu/resources/slides/index.htm. Accessed March 10, 2011.

Centers for Disease Control and Prevention: *Surveillance. Estimated numbers of diagnoses of HIV in injection drug users in 2009.* Atlanta, GA. Available at http://www.cdc.gov/hiv/topics/surveillance/basix.htm#hivaidsexposure. Accessed March 11, 2011.

Centers for Disease Control and Prevention: *Tobacco control state highlights 2010,* Atlanta, 2010, U.S. Department of Health and Human Services, Centers for Disease Control and Prevention, National Center for Chronic Disease Prevention and Health Promotion, Office on Smoking and Health.

Cocaine: *The Merck manual,* section 15, psychiatric disorders, chapter 198, drug use and dependence, 2008, Merck & Co, Inc. Available at http://www.merck.com/mmpe/sec15/ch198/ch198j.html. Accessed March 5, 2011.

Common Sense for Drug Policy: *Drug war facts,* ed 6, 2007. Available at http://www.drugwarfacts.org. Accessed July 10, 2010.

Courbasson CMA, de Sorkin AA, Dullerud B: Acupuncture treatment for women with substance use and anxiety/depression: an effective alternative therapy? *Fam Commun Health* 30:112–120, 2007.

Council on Linkages Between Academic and Public Health Practice: *Core competencies for public health professionals,* Washington DC, 2010, Public Health Foundation/Health Resources and Services Administration.

DiClemente CC, Schlundt D, Gemmell L: Readiness and stages of change in addiction treatment, *Am J Addict* 13(2):103–119, 2004.

Farrelly MC, Pechacek TF, Thomas KY, Nelson D: The impact of tobacco control programs on adult smoking, *Am J Public Health* 98(2):304–309, 2008.

Fields G: White house czar calls for end to "war on drugs," *Wall Street Journal* A3, May 14, 2009.

HealthDay: *20% of U.S. high schoolers abuse prescription drugs,* June 3, 2010. Available at www.nlm.nih.gov/medlineplus/print/news/fullstory_99556.html. Accessed July 9, 2010.

Henley J, Thun MJ, Connell C, et al: Two large prospective studies of mortalities among men who use snuff or chewing tobacco, *Cancer Causes Control* 16:347–358, 2005.

Institute of Medicine: *Ending the tobacco problem: a blueprint for the nation,* Washington, DC, 2007, The National Academies Press.

Johnston LD, O'Malley PM, Bachman JG: Monitoring the future national survey results on drug use, 1975-2006, NIH Pub No 07-6205, Bethesda, MD, 2007.

Jones HE: Drug addiction during pregnancy, *Cur Direct Psychol Sci* 15(3):126–130, 2006.

Kinney J, Leaton G: *Loosening the grip,* ed 5, St Louis, 1995, Mosby.

Koch W: As cigarette sales dip, new products raise concerns, *USA Today* 1A, August 7, 2007.

Kumpfer KL: Identification of drug abuse prevention programs: literature review. *NIDA Health Serv Res,* July 28, 2008. Available at http://www.drugabuse.gov/about/organization/despr/hsr/da-pre/KumpferLitReview.html. Accessed July 10, 2010.

Litt MD, Kadden RM, Kabela-Cormier E, Petry NM: Changing network support for drinking: Initial findings from the Network Support Project, *J Consult Clin Psychol* 77(2):229–242, 2007.

Marijuana: *The Merck manual,* section 15, psychiatric disorders, chapter 198, drug use and dependence, 2008, Merck & Co, Inc. Available at http://merck.com/mmpe/sec15/ch198/ch198i.html. Accessed July 10, 2010.

Mayo Clinic Staff: *Caffeine: how much is too much?* March 24, 2009. Available at http://www.mayoclinic.com/health/caffeine/NU00600/METHOD=print. Accessed July 10, 2010.

Merck manual: Alcohol: drug use and dependence, 2008, Merck & Co, Inc. Available at http://www.merck.com/mmpe/sec15/ch198/ch198g.html. Accessed July 10, 2010.

Mothers Against Misuse and Abuse: *Drug consumer safety rules,* Mosier, OR, 2010. Available at http://www.mamas.org/drugSafety.htm. Accessed July 9, 2010.

Moyer A, Finney JW: Brief interventions for alcohol problems: factors that facilitate implementation, *Alcohol Res Health* 28(1):44–50, 2004/2005.

National Center on Addiction and Substance Abuse: *Shoveling up II: the impact of substance abuse on federal, state and local budgets,* New York, 2009, Center on Addiction and Substance Abuse at Columbia University.

National Center on Addiction and Substance Abuse: *Behind bars II: substance abuse and America's prison population,* New York, 2010, Center on Addiction and Substance Abuse at Columbia University.

National Institute on Alcohol Abuse and Alcoholism: *Helping patients who drink too much: a clinician's guide (update),* NIH Pub No 07-3769, Rockville, MD, 2005, USDHHS. Available at http://pubs.niaaa.nih.gov/publications/Practitioner/CliniciansGuide2005/guide.pdf. Accessed March 5, 2011.

National Institute on Drug Abuse: *Research report series: prescription drugs—abuse and addiction,* NIH Pub No 05-4881, Rockville, MD, revised 2005, USDHHS. Available at http://www.nida.nih.gov/PDF/RRPrescription.pdf. Accessed March 5, 2011.

National Institute on Drug Abuse: *NIDA InfoFacts: Prescription and over-the-counter medications,* June 2009a. Available at http://www.drugabuse.gov/PDF/Infofacts/PainMed09.pdf. Accessed March 5, 2011.

National Institute on Drug Abuse: *NIDA InfoFacts: Cigarettes and other tobacco products,* June 2009b. Available at http://www.drugabuse.gov/infofacts/tobacco.html. Accessed July 10, 2010.

National Institute on Drug Abuse: *Research report series: inhalant abuse,* NIH Pub No 09-3818, Rockville, MD, 2009c, National Clearinghouse on Alcohol and Drug Information. Available at http://www.nida.nih.gov/PDF/RRinhalants.pdf. Accessed March 5, 2011.

National Institute on Drug Abuse: *Principles of drug addiction treatment: a research based guide,* ed 2, NIH Pub No 09-4180, Revised April 2009, 2009d. Available at http://www.nida.nih.gov/PODAT/. Accessed March 5, 2011.

Physicians and Lawyers for National Drug Policy: *Policy priorities: summary,* 2008. Available at http://www.plndp.org. Accessed July 9, 2010.

Rose KD: *American women and the repeal of prohibition,* New York, 1996, New York University Press.

Seal KH, Thawley R, Gee L, et al: Naloxone distribution and cardiopulmonary resuscitation training for injection drug users to prevent heroin overdose death: a pilot intervention study, *J Urban Health* 82:303, 2005.

Substance Abuse and Mental Health Services Administration: *Results from the 2006 national survey on drug use and health: national findings,* Rockville, MD, 2007, SAMHSA.

Substance Abuse and Mental Health Services Administration: *TIP 32: Treatment of adolescents with substance use disorders,* 2008, SAMHSA. Available at http://www.ncbi.nlm.nih.gov/bookshelf/br.fcgi?book=hssamhsatip&part=A56538. Accessed July 9, 2010.

Substance Abuse and Mental Health Services Administration: *Results from the 2008 National survey on drug use and health: national findings*, Office of Applied Studies, NSDUH Series H-36, HHS Pub No SMA 09-4434, Rockville, MD, 2009a.

Substance Abuse and Mental Health Services Administration, Office of Applied Studies: *Treatment Episode Data Set (TEDS). Highlights—2007, National Admissions to Substance Abuse Treatment Services*, DASIS Series: S-45, DHHS Pub No (SMA) 09–4360, Rockville, MD, 2009b.

Substance Abuse and Mental Health Services Administration, Office of Applied Studies: *The N-SSATS report: infectious disease screening*, Rockville, MD, February 25, 2010, SAMHSA.

Substance Use in Children and Adolescents: *The Merck manual,* section 15, psychiatric disorders, chapter 198, drug use and dependence, 2008, Merck & Co, Inc. Available at http://www.merck.com/mmpe/sec15/ch198/ch198qhtml. Accessed July 9, 2010.

U.S. Department of Health and Human Services: *Healthy People 2020: national health promotion and disease prevention objectives*, Washington, DC, 2010, U.S. Government Printing Office. Available at http://www.healthypeople.gov/HP2020/. Accessed July 9, 2010.

World Health Organization: *WHO Report on the Global Tobacco Epidemic, 2008: The MPOWER Package*, Geneva, 2008, WHO.

CHAPTER 38

Violence and Human Abuse

Kären M. Landenburger, RN, PhD

Kären M. Landenburger is a professor of nursing at the University of Washington, Tacoma. She received her PhD in nursing and her postdoctoral training in women's health from the University of Washington. Her area of expertise in community/public health nursing is the health and functioning of communities and populations, with an emphasis on community assessment, program planning and evaluation, and community partnerships. She is involved in community action research with communities focusing on public health issues and working on identifying field methods to use in collecting data on communities and populations. Her current research and practice focus on violence against women. She is involved on community and state levels in the education of health professionals about domestic violence as a social issue and about the needs of women who seek care.

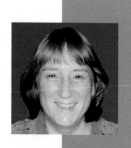

Jacquelyn C. Campbell, PhD, RN, FAAN

Jacquelyn C. Campbell is the Anna D. Wolf Chair and Professor in the Johns Hopkins University School of Nursing with a joint appointment in the Bloomberg School of Public Health. She is also the National Program Director of the Robert Wood Johnson Nurse Faculty Scholars Program. Her BSN, MSN, and PhD are from Duke University, Wright State University, and the University of Rochester schools of nursing. She has been conducting advocacy policy work and research in the area of domestic violence since 1980. Dr. Campbell has been the principle investigator on ten major National Institutes of Health, National Institute of Justice, and Centers for Disease Control and Prevention research grants and has published more than 220 articles and seven books on this subject. She is an elected member of the Institute of Medicine and the American Academy of Nursing, is Chair of the Board of Directors Family Violence Defense Fund, and was a member of the congressionally appointed U.S. Department of Defense Task Force on Domestic Violence, as well as a member of the board of directors and the House of Ruth Battered Women's Shelter.

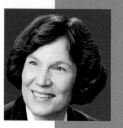

ADDITIONAL RESOURCES

@volve WEBSITE
http://evolve.elsevier.com/Stanhope
- *Healthy People 2020*
- WebLinks
- Quiz
- Case Studies
- Glossary
- Answers to Practice Application

OBJECTIVES

After reading this chapter, the student should be able to do the following:

1. Discuss the scope of the problem of violence in American communities.
2. Examine at least three factors existing in most communities that influence violence and human abuse.
3. Identify at least three types of community facilities that can help prevent violence.
4. Identify indicators of potential child abuse.
5. Define the four general types of child abuse: neglect, physical, emotional, and sexual.
6. Discuss abuse of older adults as a crucial community health problem.
7. Evaluate the roles that nurses can assume with rape victims.
8. Analyze primary preventive nursing interventions for community violence.
9. Evaluate the different responses that a nurse would expect to see in a battered woman from the beginning of the abuse until after the relationship has ended.
10. Discuss the principles of nursing intervention with violent families.
11. Describe specific nursing interventions with battered women.

KEY TERMS

OUTLINE

The word *violence* comes from the Latin *violare,* meaning to violate, injure, or rape. Indeed, violence is a violation, with both emotional and physical effects. Violent crime rates in the United States, including rape, robbery, homicide and assault, have declined by 41% since 1998. Although females were more likely to be victims of sexual assault, men experienced higher levels of stranger victimization in all other violent crimes. Women remain at greater risk in the home with 33% of female homicide victims killed by an intimate partner (USDOJ, 2007, 2009a,b). While rates may be decreasing in adult intimate partner violence (IPV) relationships, the incidence of violence among youth, especially adolescents, is increasing. For example, forms of aggression are becoming more commonplace in adolescent relationships, resulting in increased health risk for youth (CDC, 2006a, 2009). Teen dating violence is correlated with increased rates of suicide, alcohol use, and sexual activity (Kaminski and Fang, 2009). Male and female adolescents who are sexually harassed have increased rates of substance abuse and suicide. In young girls, particularly, sexual harassment is associated with eating disorders and self harm (Chiodo et al, 2009).

Although some violence may have decreased, the aftermath of the violence in our streets, in our schools and in our homes threatens the health and well-being of our entire population.

It is not clear from research if violence stems from an innate aggressive drive or is a primarily learned behavior. Clearly, all human beings have the capability for violence, yet what constitutes violence continues to be a subject for debate. Therefore, it is important to understand the theoretical and situational context in which violence is discussed (Malley-Morrison and Hines, 2004).

Violence is a public health nursing concern. Significant mortality and morbidity result from violence. Communities across the United States are concerned about crime and violence rates. Medical, nursing, psychology, and social service professionals have been slow to develop a response to violence that is part of their daily professional lives. As a result, the estimated 3.5 million victims of violence annually may not receive the best care possible. In addition, the extent of their pain that could have been avoided by community health prevention efforts is unknown. Nurses can take a more active role in the development of community responses to violence, public policy, and needed resources.

Violence is generally defined as those non-accidental acts, interpersonal or intrapersonal, that result in physical or psychological injury to one or more persons. Violent behavior is predictable and thus preventable, especially with community action. The Centers for Disease Control and Prevention's (CDC's) Initiative, "Choose Respect," was launched in 2006. The program has been adopted in multiple communities across the United States. The purpose of the program is to teach parents and adolescents about healthy relationships and to give them tools to deal with unhealthy relationships such as teen dating violence (CDC, 2006b). The Migrant Clinicians Network, an organization to help migrant and other poor transient workers, has developed a natural helper model for migrant workers, to work within their own community to identify and teach about IPV (Kugel et al, 2009). Based on models developed in the 1980s, communities are developing a coordinated response in which multiple agencies work together to assist with preventing IPV. In addition to the criminal justice system, advocates for women, health care providers, and employers are encouraged to learn about and assist their employees with issues of IPV (Pennington-Zoellner, 2009). The Wraparound Project (Dickers et al, 2009) is another program that focuses on prevention of interpersonal violence. Similar to models developed to assist clients recovering from myocardial infarctions, the project identified "teachable moments" to assist clients admitted to a hospital emergency room to receive culturally specific resources to prevent reoccurrence of interpersonal violence. All of these community programs have the same goal: to decrease the incidence and prevalence of violence in our communities. In order to guide prevention of violence, a section of the *Healthy People 2020* objectives is devoted to violence.

This chapter examines violence as a public health problem and discusses how nurses can help individuals, families, groups, and communities cope with and reduce violence and abuse. Nurses work with clients in a wide variety of settings, including the home. Since nurses are in key positions to detect and intervene in community and family violence, they need to understand how community-level influences can affect all types of violence.

 HEALTHY PEOPLE 2020

Objectives for Reducing Violence

- IVP-29: Reduce homicides.
- IVP-35: Reduce bullying among adolescents.
- IVP-37: Reduce child maltreatment deaths.
- IVP-39: Reduce violence by current or former intimate partners.
- IVP-40: Reduce sexual violence.

From U.S. Department of Health and Human Services: *Healthy People 2020 Objectives,* Washington, DC, 2010c, Office of Disease Prevention and Health Promotion, USDHHS.

SOCIAL AND COMMUNITY FACTORS INFLUENCING VIOLENCE

Many factors in a community can support or minimize violence. Changing social conditions, multiple demands on people, economic conditions, and social institutions influence the level of violence and human abuse. The following discussion of selected current social conditions helps to explain factors that influence violent behavior.

 LINKING CONTENT TO PRACTICE

According to the Quad Council Domains of Public Health Nursing Practice (Association of State and Territorial Directors of Nursing, 2003) and the American Public Health Association (2010), public health nurses must collaborate in partnership with communities to assess and identify community needs; plan, implement, and evaluate community-based programs; and assist in the setting of policy that will contribute to the needs of the community in relationship to all types of interpersonal violence. The Quad Council competencies in the analytic assessment domain direct nurses to conduct thorough health assessments of individuals, families, communities, and populations and to develop diagnoses for the population being assessed (Council on Linkages, 2010). Public health nurses can help the community in many ways as is described throughout this chapter.

Work

Productive and paid work is an expectation in mainstream American society. Work can be fulfilling and contribute to a sense of well-being; it can also be frustrating and unfulfilling, contributing to stress that may lead to aggression and violence. Unemployment and changing patterns of employment are also associated with violence both within and outside the home.

When jobs are repetitive, boring, and lacking in stimulation, frustration mounts. Some work environments discourage creativity and reward conformity and "following the rules." In many work settings, people try to get ahead regardless of the cost to others. Workers often go home feeling physically and psychologically drained. They may have worked at a back-breaking pace all day only to be yelled at by the boss for what seemed like a trivial oversight. It is hard to separate feelings generated at work from those at home. For example, a father arrives home feeling tired, angry, and generally inadequate because of a series of reprimands from his boss. Soon after he sits down, his 4-year-old son runs through the house pretending to fly a wooden airplane. After about three loud trips past his father, who keeps shouting for the child to be quiet and go outside, the airplane hits the father in the head. The father may hit the boy out of frustration and anger.

During economic downturns, people hesitate to give up jobs that are frustrating, boring, or stressful. Family needs may necessitate that they keep the hated job. Workers feel trapped and may resent those who depend on them. This frustration and resentment may lead to violence.

Unemployment may precipitate aggressive outbursts. The inability to secure or keep a job may lead to feelings of inadequacy, guilt, boredom, dissatisfaction, and frustration. Unemployment does not fit the image of the ideal man in American society, and these men are more likely to be violent both within and outside the family (Ellison et al, 2007; Peralta, Tuttle, and Steele, 2010). Women who experience IPV often lose their jobs because of constant harassment and stalking from the abuser and their subsequent absenteeism. Women who are stalked at work often find their jobs in jeopardy because of work interruption, continual stress, and decreased job performance. Slowly, employers are beginning to understand the implications of IPV. More women are finding support from employers when they disclose possible or actual abuse (Logan, Cole, and Capillo, 2007; Swanberg, Macke, and Logan, 2007).

Unemployment remains a risk factor associated with domestic violence (Ellison et al, 2007). Statistics from the U.S. Department of Labor (2010) showed that young, minority men have the highest rates of unemployment in the United States, ranging upward to 50% even in times of prosperity. This group also has the highest rate of violence. They live in a world of oppression, with lack of opportunity and enormous anger. They believe they are pushed out of mainstream society and are on the receiving end of the fallout of policies that ignore their dilemmas and give them no stake in mainstream America. Most analyses conclude that the differential rates of violence between African Americans and whites in the United States have more to do with economic realities, such as poverty, unemployment, and overcrowding, than with race (Ellison et al, 2007).

Education

In recent years, schools have assumed many responsibilities traditionally assigned to the family. Schools teach sexual development, discipline children, and often serve as a safe haven where children are fed and given the developmental support needed. Large classes often mean that teachers spend more time and energy monitoring and disciplining children than challenging and stimulating them to learn. As more and more social problems arise, it is often the expectation that the school system will teach children about these issues. One such issue is bullying. Bullying has become a major problem in U.S. schools. Bullying can be physical and/or psychological abuse, intimidation, or verbal abuse; the exclusion of some children in group activities is another form of bullying. Bullying takes place across ethnic groups and developmental age and is identified as an antecedent for perpetration of domestic violence (Corvo and deLara, 2010; Vervoort, Scholte, and Overbeek, 2010). Bullying can have devastating effects on health and can lead to self harm (Salmivalli, 2010). Cyberbullying, a form of hostile and intentional electronic communication, takes place constantly. It often leads to depression, isolation, and absenteeism. Many schools and parent groups are targeting bullying behavior on a larger scale by focusing on peer groups and population-based interventions (Berlan et al, 2010; Kiriakidis and Kavoura, 2010).

In large classes, children who do not conform to norms of expected behavior are often isolated. The non-conforming child is simply removed from the classroom because time is not available to help the child learn alternative forms of behavior. Often an end result is that there are two victims: children who are bullied and those who are the aggressor.

At times parents punish children for hitting or biting other children by spanking them. Also, spanking may be used in some schools. Such punishment only reinforces the child's tendency to strike out at others. Schools are often places where the stressors and frustrations that can contribute to violence are rampant, and violence is learned rather than discouraged; yet school can be a powerful contributor to non-violence. Classes can help adolescents learn peaceful conflict resolution and help young children deal with the threat of sexual abuse and the issues of date rape (Regan, 2010). Parents can be advised of the availability of such programs, and school boards should be urged to adopt them into the curriculum.

Media

The media can be instrumental in campaigns against violence. Recent television programs, both documentaries and dramatizations, and print articles have heightened public awareness about family violence. Programs that raise the social awareness of IPV may play a role in reducing violence in interpersonal relationships (Regan, 2010). Social marketing techniques and public service announcements serve as mechanisms to inform the public of community resources supporting victims of interpersonal violence and serve as mechanisms to prevent intimate violence (Grier and Kumanyika, 2010). Abused women and rape victims have especially benefited from media attention, which tends to lessen the stigma of such victimization. The media are also useful in publicizing services.

Television, movies, newspapers, and magazines show happy, fun-loving people. Television depicts all the wonders money can provide; yet for many Americans, the hope of buying many of the products being advertised is unrealistic. Such polarization between what is available and what is possible provides fertile ground for the development of abusive patterns. Frustration, unfulfilled dreams, and unmet wishes are often handled through hurting someone who cannot fight back. On the other hand recent research shows little direct correlation between television viewing and interpersonal violence (Ferguson and Kilburn, 2009; Ferguson, San Miguel, and Hartley, 2009).

The media cater to children by advertising products to buy and things to do. Parents may get angry when their children request the foods, toys, and clothes they see on television, in magazines, or in newspapers or hear advertised on the radio. In addition, many toys and video games encourage violence through play.

Too often, the media portray the world as a violent place. When people think that violence is rampant, there are two possible results. People may become blasé about violence and no longer feel outraged and galvanized to action when terrible things happen in their community. On the other hand, some people might become frightened of their neighbors, isolate themselves, and refuse to become involved when someone needs help. Neither response is useful in any community action program.

Organized Religion

Historically, a seemingly contradictory relationship exists between abuse and religion. For example, many religious groups uphold the philosophy of "spare the rod, spoil the child." Also, although divorce is socially accepted, some faiths uphold the victimization of people with their disapproval of divorce. Family members may stay together, although they are at emotional or physical war with one another, because of religious commitments. Although women have claimed that their spirituality has helped them in times of despair and victimization, they maintain that religious doctrine and some clergy become barriers to women seeking help or from leaving an abusive relationship (Beaulaurier et al, 2007; Potter, 2007).

Although churches have been slow to recognize domestic violence, some changes are taking place. Issues of male domination over women have become a major topic of discussion in some church groups, whereas in other groups women continue to be blamed for abuse that they sustain (Levitt and Ware, 2006). Religious affiliation and religious conservatism have been identified as risk factors for family violence, particularly child abuse (Hines and Malley-Morrison, 2005). Clergy need to be taught about the nature and dynamics of violence in the family, about religious messages and the potential for support, and about the need for collaboration between the church and advocates for the prevention of domestic violence. In religious groups where there is collaboration with advocates against abuse to children, women, and elders, there is a greater recognition of the harm of abuse and the clarity of the role of the clergy in dealing with abuse (Rodriguez and Henderson, 2010).

Population

A community's population can influence the potential for violence. Density, poverty, and diversity, particularly racial tension and overt racism, contribute to violence. In addition, one's perceptions of the safety in a community can be influenced by racism and perceptions of criminality (Lin, Thompson, and Kaslow, 2009; Howard, Budge, and McKay, 2010).

High-population-density communities can positively or negatively influence violence. Those with a sense of cohesiveness may have a lower crime rate than areas of similar size that lack social and cultural groups to support unity among members. Bonds formed among church groups, clubs, and professional organizations may promote harmony among members. Such groups provide members an opportunity to talk about stressors rather than to respond through violence. For example, residents of public housing often form neighborhood associations to deal with situations common to many or all residents. Tension can often be released in a productive way through projects carried out by the association.

Some high-population areas experience a community feeling of powerlessness and helplessness rather than one of cohesiveness. Lack of jobs and low-paying jobs may lead to feelings of inadequacy, despair, and social alienation. Social alienation and exclusion from opportunities can lead to decreased social cohesion and increased violence (Lee and Ousey, 2005; Rahn et al, 2009). Fear and apathy may cause community residents to withdraw from social contact. Withdrawal can foster crime because many residents assume someone else will report suspicious behavior, or they fear reprisals for such reports (Gracia and Herrero, 2007).

Youths often attempt to deal with feelings of powerlessness by forming gangs. Poverty and lack of education appear to be the overriding risk factors. A number of these young adults have attempted to deal with their feelings by turning to crime against people and property to release frustration. In many cities, these gangs have been highly destructive. Through community mobilization efforts, primary prevention programs have been developed to deal with the disenfranchisement of youth and gang violence (Pitts, 2009).

Other high-population areas may be characterized by a sense of confusion, resulting in disintegration and disorganization. These areas may have transient populations with limited physical or emotional investment in the community. Lack of community concern allows crime and violence to go unchecked and may become a norm for the area. Also, as crime increases, residents who are able to move leave the area. This increases community disintegration because the residents who leave are often the most capable members of the population.

The potential for violence also tends to increase among highly diverse populations. Differences in age, socioeconomic status, ethnicity, religion, or other cultural characteristics may disrupt community stability. Highly divergent groups may not communicate effectively and neither accept nor understand one another. Many such groups become hostile and antagonistic toward one another. Each group may see the other as different and not belonging. The alienated group may become the focal point for the others' frustrations, anger, and fears. Racism, classism, and heterosexism are examples of major causes of community disintegration resulting in a vicious cycle of dishonesty, distrust, and hate.

Community Facilities

Communities differ in the resources and facilities they provide to residents. Some are more desirable places to live, work, and raise families and have facilities that can reduce the potential for crime and violence. Recreational facilities such as playgrounds, parks, swimming pools, movie theaters, and tennis courts provide socially acceptable outlets for a variety of feelings, including aggression.

Spectator sports, such as football or hockey, also allow members of the community to express feelings of anger and frustration. However, viewing sports can encourage a sense of violence as participants hit or shove one another.

Although the absence of such facilities can increase the likelihood of violence, their presence alone does not prevent violence or crime. These facilities are adjuncts and resources that residents can use for pleasure, personal enrichment, and group development.

Familiarity with factors contributing to a community's violence or potential for violence enables nurses to recognize them and intervene accordingly. It is the nurse's responsibility to work with the citizens and agencies of the community to correct or improve deficits.

VIOLENCE AGAINST INDIVIDUALS OR ONESELF

The potential for violence against individuals (e.g., murder, robbery, rape, and assault) or oneself (e.g., suicide) is directly related to the level of violence in the community. Persons living in areas with high rates of crime and violence are more likely to become victims than those in more peaceful areas. The major categories of violence addressed in this chapter are described in terms of the scope of the problem in the United States and underlying dynamics.

Homicide

Homicide is the leading cause of death for children and youth between the ages of 1 and 9 years and the second leading cause of death for young African-American women ages 15 to 34; for young Native-American women ages 20 to 34; and the fourth-, third-, and fifth-leading causes of death for white women 15 to 19, 20 to 24, and 25 to 34, respectively (CDC, 2009). However, the African-American homicide rate has decreased significantly since 1970, whereas the white homicide rate has increased slightly (USDOJ, 2009b). Although the data are not adequate, it also appears that Hispanic-American men have a much higher rate of homicide than non–Hispanic-American whites. Homicide rates are highest among young adults followed by young adolescents (14 to 17 years old), but homicide occurs at an alarming rate even among very young children in the United States. Rates of homicide for children under the age of 1 year were highest in American Indian/Alaska Native and African-American infants (CDC, 2007). The majority of homicides of children are perpetrated by parents. Only 15% of male and 9%

of female homicides in the United States are caused by strangers (USDOJ, 2009b). When strangers are involved, many of these homicides are related to the illegal substance abuse network. The vast majority of homicides, however, are perpetrated by a friend, acquaintance, or family member. Therefore, prevention of homicide is at least as much an issue for the public health system as for the criminal justice system.

At least 16% of male homicides and 64% of female homicides in the United States occur within families, and half of these occur between spouses. These numbers, however, do not include unmarried couples who are living together or those who are either divorced or estranged, a group at higher risk. In total, approximately 14% of all homicides were committed by an intimate partner. Spouses or ex-spouses comprised about 24% of the perpetrators in female spousal homicides. Twenty-one percent of boyfriends or girlfriends and 19% of family members were responsible for female intimate partner homicides. Female homicides primarily are perpetrated by someone known to the victim. Only 10% of all female homicides were perpetrated by a stranger (Catalano et al, 2009).

An alarming aspect of family homicide is that small children often witness the murder or find the body of a family member (Lewandowski et al, 2004). No automatic follow-up or counseling of these children occurs through the criminal justice or mental health system in most communities. These children are at great risk for emotional turmoil and for becoming involved in violence themselves (Steeves and Parker, 2007).

The underlying dynamics of homicide within families vary greatly from those of other murders. Homicide within families is most often preceded by abuse of a family member, and homicides of intimate partners (male or female) are preceded by abuse of the female partner in 70% to 75% of cases (Campbell, Sharps, and Glass, 2000; Campbell et al, 2003). Thus, prevention of family homicide involves working with abusive families. Homicide is the leading cause of death for pregnant and postpartum women (Nannini et al, 2008). In fact, in a study of intimate partner homicide of women, 75% of the women who were killed by their husband, boyfriend, or ex-partner had been seen in a health care setting within the year prior to their homicide (Woods et al, 2008). Nurses have a duty to warn family members of the possibility of homicide when severe abuse is present, just as they warn of the hazards of smoking. Other nursing care issues are further discussed under Family Violence and Abuse in this chapter.

Assault

The death toll from violence is staggering, yet the physical injuries and emotional costs of assault are equally important issues in terms of the acute health care system. Twenty-two percent of females compared with 7.4% of males reported injury related to physical assault. Women are three times more likely than men to be killed by an intimate partner. Forty percent of women with disabilities claimed to have experienced IPV (VAWR, 2009). Age is the greatest risk factor for an individual's victimization through violence, and youths are at significantly higher risk. Although more males than females are victims of homicide and assault, women are more likely to be victimized

by a relative, especially a male partner (Catalano et al, 2009). Sometimes the difference between a homicide and an assault is only the response time and the quality of emergency transport and treatment facilities. The same community measures used to address homicide are useful to combat assault. Also, nurses often see assaulted persons in home health care with long-term health problems such as head injuries, spinal cord injuries, and stomas from abdominal gunshot wounds. In addition to physical care, nurses must also address the emotional trauma resulting from a violent attack by helping victims talk through their traumatic experience to try to make some sense of the violence, and by referring them for further counseling if anxiety, sleeping problems, or depression persists after the assault.

Rape

Currently, rape is one of the most underreported forms of human abuse in the United States with only about half (47%) of rapes in the National Crime Victimization Survey (NCVS) reported to police (Catalano et al, 2009), although reporting rates have improved over the past 15 years. According to the NCVS (Rand, 2009) sexual assault rates fell by 52% from 1999 to 2008. The rates of completed and attempted rape are almost equivalent. The incidence of rape exceeds the prevalence of rape victims because some victims experience more than one rape in a 12-month period. In 2008, according to the NCVS, there were an estimated 182,000 rapes or sexual assaults against females 12 or older, whereas males experienced 40,000 rapes or sexual assaults. This is a rate per 1000 of approximately 1.4 and 0.3, respectively. African-American females experienced higher rates of rape or sexual assault than white females and other women of color. Hispanic and non-Hispanic white females experienced comparable rates of sexual assault (Catalano et al, 2009). Over half the rapes or sexual assaults against females were committed by an offender whom they knew and one in five committed by an intimate partner. Strangers only committed about one third (31%) of all rape/sexual assaults. Nearly half (47%) of the rape and sexual assaults against females in 2009 were reported to the police. The rate of rape or sexual assault against females declined by 70% from 1993 to 2008 and by 36% during that period for males (Catalano et al, 2009). Since the majority of violence against women is IPV and women are raped more often by someone they know than by strangers, be alert for date and marital rape. In the National Violence Against Women Survey (Tjaden and Thoennes, 2000), 64% of rapes, physical assaults, and stalkings were committed against women by either current or former intimate partners. Official recognition of rape regardless of a victim's relationship to the perpetrator has led to an increased number of women reporting rape. Rape also happens to men, especially boys and young men, but the statistics on the incidence of male rape vary. In a survey of Air Force women, over 50% had reported being a victim of rape at some time in their lifetime. While the majority of rapes occurred prior to enlistment, 14% of women were raped for the first time in the military and 26% of women were victims of rape prior to and within the military (Bostock and Daley, 2007). It appears that the emotional trauma for a male rape victim is at least as serious as that for a woman.

For reported rapes, cities constitute higher risk areas than do rural areas, and the hours between 8 PM and 2 AM, weekends, and the summer months are the most critical times. In about half of rapes among strangers, the victim and the offender meet on the street, whereas in other cases the rapist either enters the victim's home or somehow entices or forces the victim to accompany him or her.

Prevention of rape, like that of other forms of human abuse, requires a broad-based community focus for educating both the community as a whole and key groups such as police, health providers, educators, and social workers. Rape rates and community-level variables such as community approval and legitimization of violence (e.g., violent network television viewing and permitting corporal punishment in schools) appear related and underscore the need for community-level intervention (Casey and Lindhorst, 2009).

> **DID YOU KNOW?** *Between 40% and 45% of physically abused women are also being forced into sex. This has implications for the prevention of unintended and adolescent pregnancies, human immunodeficiency virus (HIV), acquired immunodeficiency syndrome (AIDS), and sexually transmitted diseases (STDs), as well as for women's healthy sexuality and self-esteem.*

Attitudes

The first priority is to change attitudes about rape and about victims or survivors. Rape is a crime of violence, not a crime of passion. The underlying issues are hostility, power, and control rather than sexual desire. The defining issue is lack of consent of the victim. When a woman or man refuses any sexual activity, that refusal means "no." People have the right to change their mind, even when they seemed initially agreeable. Pressure from physical contact, threats, or deliberate inducement of drug or alcohol intoxication is a violation of the law. The myths that women say "no" to sex when they really mean "yes" and that the victims of rape are culpable because of the way they dress or act must end. On college campuses, negative attitudes toward acquaintance or date rape are slow to change. Women on college campuses underreport allegations of rape because of issues of confidentiality and fear of being discredited (Bachar and Koss, 2001). Another form of rape is forced sexual initiations, with as many as 21% of young women in the United States whose first sexual experience is below the age of 14 reporting that this initiation was physically forced, usually by a date or boyfriend (Stockman, Campbell, and Celentano, 2010). These early sexual experiences are associated with unplanned, adolescent pregnancies as well as HIV/STD risk behaviors.

Pornography

Although there is evidence of a relationship between the viewing of pornographic material showing violence against women and aggressive sexual behavior, it is not clear if the relationship is causal. In other words, our current research does not yet show that viewing pornography occurs before sexual aggressiveness or that young men who are sexually violent tend to watch pornography. The current research tends to minimize the relationship between sexual assault and pornography (Ferguson and Hartely, 2009). However, there is some evidence that claims that early exposure to pornography as a child may be related to sexual offense in the future (Seto and Lalumière, 2010). Prevention programs, or more accurately labeled risk reduction or avoidance programs, also involve providing information to women about self-protection, including using self-defense procedures, avoiding high-risk locations, and safeguarding one's home against unwanted entry. Most rape prevention programs have been oriented toward women. Men are beginning to take some steps toward prevention toward women via anti-rape websites (Masters, 2010). Many of these websites are community-based programs that promote education about violence against women and promote a positive male role model of gender equity.

Victim or Survivor?

During the act of rape, survivors are often hit, kicked, stabbed, and severely beaten. It is this violence that is most traumatic because of the survivors' fear for their lives, helplessness, lack of control, and vulnerability.

People react to rape differently, depending on their personality, past experiences, background, and support received after the trauma. Some cry, shout, or discuss the experience. Others withdraw and fear discussing the attack. During the immediate as well as the follow-up stages, victims tend to blame themselves for what happened. When working with rape victims, help them identify the issues behind self-blame. While not placing fault on survivors, teach them to take control, learn assertiveness, and therefore believe that they can take certain actions to prevent future rapes. Survivors need to talk about what happened and to express their feelings and fears in a non-judgmental atmosphere. Non-judgmental listening is important (Ullman, 2010).

In any psychological trauma, victims should be given privacy, respect, and assurance of confidentiality. They should also be told about health care procedures conducted immediately after the rape and should be linked with proper resources for ease of reporting the crime. Nurses often provide continuous care once the victim enters the health care system. Because many victims deny the event once the initial crisis is past, a single-session debriefing should be completed during the initial examination. The physical assessment, examination, and debriefing should be carried out by specially trained providers.

As discussed in Chapter 44, in most states, nurses trained as sexual assault nurse examiner (SANE), a subspecialty of forensic nursing, perform the physical examination in the emergency department to gather evidence (e.g., hair samples, skin fragments beneath the victim's fingernails, evidence from pelvic examinations using colposcopy) for criminal prosecution of sexual assault (Sheridan, 2004). This is an important nursing intervention because physicians may not be able to take the time required for this procedure; nurses can take advantage of this opportunity to provide therapeutic communication and support. Nurses can be trained to conduct the examination either in SANE trainings or in Forensic Nursing programs in many schools of nursing, and their evidence is credible and effective in resultant court proceedings (Houmes, Fagan, and Quintana,

2003; Campbell et al, 2006; Campbell et al, 2007). Nurses can lobby for changes in hospital policies and state laws to make this strategy a reality in all states.

Rape is a situational crisis for which advance preparation is rarely possible. Therefore, nursing efforts are directed toward helping victims cope with the stress and disruption of their lives caused by the attack. Counseling focuses on the crisis and the concomitant fears, feelings, and issues involved. Nurses can help survivors learn how to regroup personal strengths. If **posttraumatic stress disorder** (PTSD) occurs, professional psychological or psychiatric treatment is indicated.

Many rape victims need follow-up mental health services to help them cope with the short- and long-term effects of the crisis. The time after a rape is one of disequilibrium, psychological breakdown, and reorganization of attitudes about the safety of the world. Common, everyday tasks often tax a person's resources, and they may forget or fail to keep appointments. Nurses can make referrals and obtain the victim's permission to remain in telephone contact in order to assess support, provide encouragement, and offer resources.

Suicide

Suicide, according to the National Violent Death Reporting System (NVDRS), accounted for the highest rate of violent death in 2007, taking the lives of 9245 people. Firearms accounted for 50.7%, hanging/strangulation/suffocation for 23.1%, and poisoning for 18.8% of suicides. Firearms (56%) or hanging/strangulation/suffocation (24.4%) were the most common form of suicide for men. Women used poisoning (40.8%) most frequently, followed by firearms (30.9%). Precipitating factors for suicide were mental health (45%), IPV (30%) and physical health problems (21.4%) (CDC, 2010b). The risk for death by suicide is greater than for death by homicide. Rates of completed suicide are higher for men, especially older adults, non-Hispanic whites, and Native Alaskans/American Indians (NA/AI) (Karch, Dahlberg, and Patel, 2010). Affluent and educated people often have higher rates of suicide than do the economically and educationally disadvantaged except for NA/AI populations who are often poor and yet commit suicide in alarming numbers. The presence of a gun in the home is an important risk factor for both suicide and homicide (Campbell, 2007).

Suicide is the third-leading cause of death among young people ages 15 to 24. In 2007, for every 100,000 young people in each age group the following number died by suicide: Between the ages of 15 and 19, 6.9 per 100,000 and from 20 to 24, 12.7 per 100,000 (NIMH, 2010). Boys and young men between the ages of 15 and 19 were five times more likely to commit suicide than females and four times more likely if between the ages of 20 and 24 (Karch, Dahlberg, and Patel, 2010). Suicide was the cause of death for 12% for youth between the ages of 10 through 24 years. Attempted suicide was more prevalent for white, African-American, and Hispanic females than for these same males. Leading risk factors for adolescent suicide are mental health, unintended pregnancy, and sexually transmitted disease (STD), especially HIV (Eaton et al, 2010). An important risk factor for actual and attempted suicide in adult women is IPV.

Nurses need to be involved in the reduction of suicide and the care for victims because suicide affects the community, the family, and individuals. On a community level, nurses can be involved in a coordinated response to the prevention of suicide and the care of attempted suicides. Through their roles in public health and school nursing, they can help develop policies and protocols for suicide across the life span. Nursing care may focus on family members and friends of suicide victims. Survivors, while angry at the dead person, may turn the anger inward. They may question their own liability for the death and have difficulty dealing with their feelings toward the dead person; survivors may limit their social activities because it is difficult for them and their friends to talk about the suicide. Nurses can help survivors cope with the trauma of the loss and make referrals to a counselor or support groups.

FAMILY VIOLENCE AND ABUSE

Family violence, including sexual, emotional, and physical abuse, causes significant injury and death. These three forms of abuse tend to occur together as part of a system of coercive control. Generally, IPV is perpetrated by the most powerful against the least powerful. IPV is directed primarily toward women in heterosexual relationships (although they may physically fight back). According to the Bureau of Justice Statistics, 99% of IPV against females was perpetrated by males (Catalano et al, 2009). Although the rate of IPV has decreased for both females and males over the last 15 years, the rate of homicides perpetrated by a known other has remained the same (Catalano et al, 2009). IPV in same-sex relationships follows the same patterns of behavior as in heterosexual relationships. Similar to heterosexual relationships, males perpetrate the majority of IPV (Tjaden and Thoennes, 2000). Dynamics of power and control caused by race, gender expression, ability, immigration status, age, and class are methods of control in same-sex IPV (National Coalition of Anti-Violence Programs, 2010). Approximately 23% of gay males have been physically or sexually assaulted or stalked.

Recognizing the battered child or woman in the emergency department is relatively simple after the fact. It is unfortunate that, by the time medical care is sought, serious physical and emotional damage may have been done. Nurses are in a key position to predict and deal with abusive tendencies. By understanding factors contributing to the development of abusive behaviors, nurses can identify incidents of IPV.

Development of Abusive Patterns

Perpetrators of IPV often believe that violence within an interpersonal relationship is a normal behavior pattern (Stover et al, 2010). Factors that characterize people who become involved in IPV include upbringing, living conditions, and increased stress. Understanding how these factors influence the development of abusive behavior can help the nurse manage abusive families.

Upbringing

Of all the factors that characterize the background of abusers, the most predictable one is previous exposure to some form of violence (Whiting et al, 2009). As children, abusers were often beaten or witnessed the beating of siblings or a parent. These children learn that violence is a suitable way to manage conflict.

For both men and women, witnessing abuse as children was associated with abuse of their children. Factors of financial solvency and support tended to decease the incidence of child abuse (Dixon, Browne, and Hamilton-Giachritsis, 2009; Whiting et al, 2009). Childhood physical punishment teaches children to use violent conflict resolution as an adult. A child may learn to associate love with violence because a parent is usually the first person to hit a child. Children may think that those who love them are also those who hit them. The moral rightness of hitting other family members thus may be established when physical punishment is used to train children, especially when it is used more than occasionally. These experiences predispose children ultimately to use violence with their own children.

As well as having a history of child abuse themselves, people who become abusers tend to have hostile personality styles and be verbally aggressive. They have often learned these characteristics from their own childhood experiences. Their parents may have set unrealistic goals, and when the children failed to perform accordingly, they were criticized, demeaned, punished, and denied affection. These children may have been told how to act, what to do, and how to feel, thereby discouraging the development of normal attachment, autonomy, problem-solving skills, and creativity (Dixon, Hamilton-Giachritis and Brown, 2005). Children raised in this way grow up feeling unloved and worthless. They may want a child of their own so that they will feel assured of someone's love.

Because of their experiences of trauma and to protect themselves from feelings of worthlessness and fear of rejection, abused children form a protective shell and grow increasingly hostile and distrustful of others. The behavior of potential abusers reflects a low tolerance for frustration, emotional instability, and the onset of aggressive feelings with minimal provocation. Because of their emotional insecurity, perpetrators of abuse often depend on a child or spouse to meet their needs of feeling valued and secure. When their needs are not met by others, they become overly critical. Critical, resentful behavior and unrealistic expectations of others lead to a vicious cycle. The more critical these people become, the more they are rejected and alienated from others. Abusive individuals tend to perceive that the target of their hostility is "out to get" them. These distorted perceptions can be detected when parents talk about an infant crying or keeping them up at night "on purpose" (Dixon et al, 2005).

Increased Stress

A perceived or actual crisis may precede an abusive incident. Because a crisis reinforces feelings of inadequacy and low self-esteem, a number of events often occur in a short time to precipitate abusive patterns. Unemployment, strains in the marriage, or an unplanned pregnancy may set off violence, especially in people with other risk factors such as a history of trauma themselves.

The daily hassles of raising young children, especially in an economically strained household, intensify an already stressed atmosphere for which an unexpected and difficult event may provoke violence. Stressful life events, poverty, and cultural values and social isolation are often associated with family violence. Crowded living conditions may also precipitate abuse. The presence of several people in a small space heightens tensions and reduces privacy; tempers flare because of the constant stimulation from others.

Social isolation is associated with abuse in families (Hines and Malley-Morrison, 2005). Such isolation reduces social support, decreasing a family's ability to deal with stressors. The problem may be intensified if a violent family member tries to keep the family isolated to escape detection. Therefore, when a family misses clinic or home visit appointments, nurses need to keep in mind that abuse may be present. Nurses can encourage involvement in community activities and can help neighbors reach out to neighbors to help prevent abuse.

Frequent moves disrupt social support systems, are associated with an overall increased stress level, and tend to isolate people, at least briefly. Mobility can have a serious negative effect on the abuse-prone family. These families do not readily initiate new relationships; they rely on the family for support. Resources may be unfamiliar or inaccessible to them. Because frequent moving may be both a risk factor for abuse and a sign of an abusive family trying to avoid detection, nurses should assess such families carefully for abuse.

Types of Family Violence

Because various forms of family violence and violence outside the home often occur together, nurses who detect child abuse should also suspect other forms of family violence. When older adult parents report that their (now adult) child was abused or has a history of violence toward others, the nurse should recognize the potential for elder abuse. Physical abuse of women is frequently accompanied by sexual abuse both inside and outside the marital relationship. Severe wife abusers may have a history of other acts of violence. Families who are verbally aggressive in conflict resolution (e.g., using name calling, belittling, screaming, and yelling) are more likely to be physically abusive. Although the various forms of family violence are discussed separately, they should not be thought of as totally separate phenomena.

No member of the family is guaranteed immunity from abuse and neglect. Spouse abuse, child abuse, abuse of older adults, serious violence among siblings, and mutual abuse by members all occur. Although these examples are not inclusive, they demonstrate the scope of family violence.

Child Abuse

A national survey estimated that in 2009, 702,000 unique reports of children and adolescents who were subjected to neglect, medical neglect, physical and sexual abuse, and emotional maltreatment (USDHHS ACF, 2010a). Of these children, 78% were victims of neglect; 18% were victims of physical abuse, 10% were sexually abused, and 8% were psychologically maltreated. The remaining 2% were medically neglected. This is probably a conservative figure, since only the most severe cases are reported. Except for sexual abuse, which is four times as

BOX 38-1 DETERMINING RISK FACTORS FOR CHILD ABUSE

Ask the following questions or observe the following behaviors to determine if risk factors are present.

1. Are the parents unemployed?
2. Do the parents have the financial resources to care for a child?
3. Is there a support network that is willing to offer assistance?
4. Do one or both parents have a history of child abuse?
5. Is a parent a victim or perpetrator of intimate partner violence?
6. Do the parents have knowledge about child development?
7. Do one or both parents have problems with substance abuse?
8. Are the parents overly critical of the child?
9. Are the parents communicative with each other and the nurse?
10. Does the mother of the child seem frightened of her partner?
11. Does the child suffer from recurrent injuries or unexplained illnesses?

Data from Rodriguez CM: Personal contextual characteristics and cognitions: predicting child abuse potential and disciplinary style, *J Interpers Violence* 25(2):315-335, 2010; U.S. Department of Health and Human Services, Administration for Children and Families, Administration on Children, Youth and Families, Children's Bureau: *Child maltreatment, 2008,* 2010a. Available at http://www.acf.hhs.gov/programs/cb/stats_research/index.htm#can. Accessed August 20, 2010; Zimmerman F, Mercy JA: A better start: child maltreatment prevention as a public health priority, *Zero to Three* 30(5):4-10, 2010.

high for girls as for boys, victims are equally distributed among sexually abused male and female children (USDHHS, 2010a).

Children also witness domestic violence (Berman et al, 2010). When children witness domestic violence, they may experience many psychological and physical problems. Children living in homes with parental violence are more likely to feel guilt over the abuse and suffer from post-traumatic stress syndrome more than children who are not exposed to violence (Scott, 2007; Kletter, Weems, and Carrion, 2009). Children who experience abuse need to understand that the abuse experience is not their fault. From a practical sense, children need to understand safety issues and what they need to do when abuse occurs (Ernst et al, 2008). Risk factors for abused children include factors such as strain on the economic resources of the family, lack of social support, abuse between parents, and problems with substance abuse. Some of the risk factors are identified in Box 38-1 (USDHHS, 2010a; Zimmerman and Mercy, 2010). Children who witness abuse react differently according to their age, level of development, and sex; their reactions are influenced by the severity and frequency of the abuse witnessed (Kelly, Gonzalez-Guarda, and Taylor, 2010).

Children are often abused because they are small and relatively powerless. In many families only one child may be abused. Parents may identify with this child and be especially critical of the child's behavior. Also, this child may have certain qualities, such as looking like a relative, being handicapped, or being particularly bright and capable, that provoke the parent.

Child abuse signifies ineffective family functioning. Abusive parents who recognize their problem are often reluctant to seek assistance because of the stigma attached to being considered a child abuser and the legal ramifications of abuse. Parents with a history of abuse as a child or who have minimum education, a lack of social support, a tendency toward

depression, and multiple stress factors may be at risk for abusing their children (Whiting et al, 2009). Children are often used as leverage between parents when there is a history of abuse between the parents. The abusive parent is often coercive and manipulative toward the child as a mechanism to control the non-abusive parent. Abusive parents often have unrealistic expectations of a child's developmental abilities. They often use avoidance strategies to deal with behavioral issues and overreact with abusive discipline in times of stress (Rodriguez, 2010). Abusive parents use physical discipline more frequently, often in the form of physical punishment and verbal abuse. Spanking, although quite prevalent in the United States, can also be considered a form of child abuse (Hines and Malley-Morrison, 2005; Straus, 2005). The nurse must not only teach normal parental behavior, but also address the underlying emotional needs of the parents. These parents often experience pain and poor emotional stability and need intervention as much as their children. Following are some of the behavioral indicators of potentially abusive parents (Zimmerman and Mercy, 2010).

HOW TO Identify Potentially Abusive Parents

The following characteristics in couples expecting a child constitute warning signs of actual or potential abuse:

- *Denial of the reality of the pregnancy, as seen in a refusal to talk about the impending birth or to think of a name for the child*
- *An obvious concern or fear that the baby will not meet some predetermined standard: sex, hair color, temperament, or resemblance to family members*
- *Failure to follow through on the desire for an abortion*
- *An initial decision to place the child for adoption and a change of mind*
- *Rejection of the mother by the father of the baby*
- *Family experiencing stress and numerous crises so that the birth of a child may be the last straw*
- *Initial and unresolved negative feelings about having a child*
- *Lack of support for the new parents*
- *Isolation from friends, neighbors, or family*
- *Parental evidence of poor impulse control or fear of losing control*
- *Contradictory history*
- *Appearance of detachment*
- *Appearance of misusing drugs or alcohol*
- *Shopping for hospitals or health care providers*
- *Unrealistic expectations of the child*
- *Verbal, physical, or sexual abuse of mother by father, especially during pregnancy*
- *Child is not biological offspring of male stepfather or mother's current boyfriend*
- *Excessive talk of needing to "discipline" children and plans to use harsh physical punishment to enforce discipline*

Foster Care. When child abuse is discovered, the child is often placed in a foster home. It is the legal responsibility of the nurse to report all cases of child abuse. Ideally, the initial report begins a process in which both the child and the family can receive the care needed. Although the focus of care should be on the best interests of the child and the parents, the primary attention should be on the safety of the child. While in foster care the abused child should receive continuous nursing care. The nurse is often the one consistent person abused children can relate to as they are transferred from their home to foster care and hopefully back to their home. Abused children generally want to return to their parents, and the goal of most agencies is to help natural families stay together as long as it is safe for the child. However, a family preservation approach may not always keep children safe (O'Reilly et al, 2010). Often the nurse's role is to help monitor a family in which a formerly abused child is returned from foster care. Keen judgment and close collaboration with social services are necessary in these situations. The nurse must ensure the safety of the child while working with the parents in an empathetic way. The nurse's goal is to enhance parenting skills through education on child care and development, communication, and principles of social learning theory. Parents must also be given positive support and reassurance about their ability to provide proper care to their child.

One of the most distressing outcomes of child abuse is depression and other mental health problems, especially suicide. Adolescents who have been placed in the social service system many times or who move from one foster home to another are at risk for delinquency, severe depression, alcohol and substance abuse, and suicide. Nurses need to understand the dynamics of adolescent suicide and substance abuse (Fletcher, 2010; Ford et al, 2010).

Indicators of Child Abuse. It is essential that nurses recognize the physical and behavioral indicators of abuse and neglect. Child abuse ranges from violent physical attacks to passive neglect. Violence such as beating, burning, kicking, or shaking may lead to severe physical injury. Passive neglect may result in insidious malnutrition or other problems. Abuse is not limited to physical maltreatment but includes emotional abuse such as yelling at or continually demeaning and criticizing the child. Children who come from a family where IPV occurs are at greater risk for physical and psychological abuse and child neglect (Hines and Malley-Morrsion, 2005; Whiting et al, 2009; Fletcher, 2010).

HOW TO Recognize Actual or Potential Child Abuse

Be alert to the following:
- *An unexplained injury*
- *Skin: burns, old or recent scars, ecchymosis, soft tissue swelling, human bites*
- *Fractures: recent, or older ones that have healed*
- *Subdural hematomas*
- *Trauma to genitalia*
- *Whiplash (caused by shaking small children)*
- *Dehydration or malnourishment without obvious cause*
- *Provision of inappropriate food or drugs (alcohol, tobacco, medication prescribed for someone else, foods not appropriate for the child's age)*
- *Evidence of general poor care: poor hygiene, dirty clothes, unkempt hair, dirty nails*
- *Unusual fear of nurse and others*
- *Considered to be a "bad" child*
- *Inappropriate dress for the season or weather conditions*
- *Reports or shows evidence of sexual abuse*

- *Injuries not mentioned in history*
- *Seems to need to take care of the parent and speak for the parent*
- *Maternal depression*
- *Maladjustment of older siblings*
- *Current or history of IPV in the home*

Emotional abuse involves extreme debasement of feelings and may lead the child to feel inadequate, inept, uncared for, and worthless. These children learn to hide their feelings to avoid more scorn. They may act out by performing poorly in school, becoming truant, and being hostile and aggressive. Children who are abused or who witness domestic violence can suffer developmentally (Kletter, Weems, and Carrion, 2009; Rodriguez, 2010). Major responses of adolescents to physical and sexual abuse are substance abuse, severe depression, and running away from home (Fletcher, 2010; Ford et al, 2010).

Physical symptoms of physical, sexual, or emotional stress may include hyperactivity, withdrawal, overeating, dermatological problems, vague physical complaints, stuttering, enuresis (bladder incontinence), and encopresis (bowel incontinence). Ironically, bedwetting is often a trigger for further abuse, thereby creating a vicious cycle. When a child displays physical symptoms without clear physiological origin, the nursing assessment should rule out the possibility of abuse.

Child Neglect. The four categories of child neglect include physical, emotional, medical, and educational neglect. Physical neglect is failure to provide adequate food, proper clothing, shelter, hygiene, or necessary medical care and is most often associated with extreme poverty. In contrast, emotional neglect is the lack of the basic nurturing, acceptance, and caring essential for healthy personal development. These children are largely ignored or treated as non-persons, which affects the development of self-esteem. A neglected child has difficulty feeling self-worth because the parents have not shown that they value the child. Medical and educational neglect consist of the failure to provide for a child's basic medical and educational needs. Children with disabilities may be neglected because of inadequate resources. Medical neglect may be due to an inability to buy basic drugs needed for common diseases. All forms of neglect may be involved when a parent fails to teach children about risky behaviors such as smoking and substance abuse (Hines and Malley-Morrison, 2005). Astute observations of children, their homes, and the family can assist in a proper assessment of neglect and possible recommendations for care.

Sexual Abuse. Child abuse also includes sexual abuse. Approximately 1 of 4 female children and 1 of 10 males in the United States experiences some form of sexual abuse by the time he or she reaches 18 years of age. It is hard to determine the exact prevalence because not all children have the cognitive ability to describe these experiences. Rates based on reports to child protective services are that approximately 50 in every 1000 children suffer from child abuse and/or neglect (USDHHS, 2010a). This abuse ranges from unwanted sexual touching to intercourse. Most childhood sexual abuse is perpetrated by someone the child knows and trusts. Between one third and one half of all sexual abuse involves a family member (Hines and Malley-Morrison, 2005, USDHHS, 2010b). A child's risk for abuse is highest with parents, immediate family members, and non-related caregivers, although coaches, scout leaders, and even priests and other church workers have been reported sexual abusers. The long-term effects of sexual abuse are depression, sexual disturbances, suicide, and substance abuse. Individuals with a history of both physical and sexual abuse tend to experience more severe symptoms than children who experience one form of abuse (Fletcher, 2010; Stevenson, 2009). Many of the characteristics of physically abusive and sexually abusive parents, such as unhappiness, loneliness, and rigidity, are shared by both groups. However, sexually abused children have more gastrointestinal symptoms and post-traumatic stress disorders than physically abused children (Ross, 2005).

Father–daughter incest is the type of incest most often reported; however, mothers do engage in child sexual abuse. In recent years more males have discussed their experiences of child sexual abuse. It is estimated that one in five children is a victim of child sexual abuse. Cases of father–daughter, father–son, mother–daughter, and mother–son incest have been reported (Hines and Malley-Morrison, 2005). Many cases of parental sexual abuse go unreported because victims fear punishment, abandonment, rejection, or family disruption if the problem is acknowledged. Although stepfathers are considered the most common perpetrator of father–daughter incest, we know little about female perpetrators. Incest occurs in all races, religious groups, and socioeconomic classes. Incest is receiving greater attention because of mandatory reporting laws, yet all too often its incidence remains a family secret.

Nurses must be aware of the incidence, signs and symptoms, and psychological and physical trauma of incest. Symptoms include low self-esteem, depression, anxiety, and somatic symptoms of headaches, eating and sleeping disorders, menstrual problems, and gastrointestinal distress (Ross, 2005). Sexually abused children often exhibit premature sexual behavior, such as masturbation. Children often try to avoid or escape the abusive behavior. Avoidance can be through either behavioral or mental reactions, such as dressing to cover one's body or pretending that the abuse is not taking place. The child can escape either physically by running away or emotionally by withdrawing into other activities and thereby placing the sexual abuse in the background (Stevenson, 2009).

Adolescents may display inappropriate sexual activity or truancy or may run away from home. Running away is usually considered a sign of delinquency; however, an adolescent who runs away may be using a healthy response to a violent family situation. Therefore, the assessment should ask about sexual and physical abuse at home and plan appropriate intervention.

The effects of childhood sexual abuse can be mitigated by continual professional support. At different developmental stages, children may need assistance to overcome negative feelings about their own sexuality (Stevenson, 2009). Adult survivors of sexual abuse often are socially isolated and have significant health problems that need to be addressed in terms of the ongoing effects of their childhood and adult experiences (Mapp, 2006).

Abuse of Female Partners

Although women do abuse men, by far the greater proportion of what is often discussed as spouse abuse or domestic violence is actually wife abuse. Of the approximately 3.5 million reports of family violence between 1998 and 2002, 73% of the victims were female. The majority of perpetrators (75%) were men (USDOJ, 2005). Neither the term *wife abuse* nor the term *spouse abuse* takes into account violence in dating or cohabitating relationships or violence in same-sex relationships. IPV, a more inclusive term, refers to all kinds of violence between partners. All adults should be assessed for violence in their primary intimate relationship. The incidence of violence in same-sex relationships is considered to be the same as that in heterosexual relationships, but there is relatively little research on the topic (Glass et al, 2008). The abuse of female partners has the most serious community health ramifications because of the greater prevalence and greater potential for homicide (Campbell, 2007), the effects on the children in the household, and the more serious long-term emotional and physical consequences.

Victims of child abuse are 12 times more likely to abuse their children than individuals with no history of child abuse. Bower-Russa (2005) found that attitudes about discipline and severity of abuse as a child were factors that contributed to perpetration of child abuse. Community support and intervention programs that focus on positive child-rearing practices, especially discipline and positive recognition, assist parents in a positive developmentally appropriate approach to child reading (Daro and Dodge, 2009).

Signs of Abuse. Battered women often have bruises and lacerations of the face, head, and trunk of the body. Attacks are often carefully inflicted on parts of the body that are disguised by clothing. This pattern of proximal location of injuries (e.g., breasts, abdomen, upper thighs, and back) rather than distal and patterned injuries (in various stages of healing, in particular configurations matching the body part or object used as a weapon) is characteristic of abuse (Campbell and Sheridan, 2004; Sheridan and Nash, 2009). When a woman has a black eye or bruises about the mouth, the nurse should ask, "Who hit you?" rather than, "What happened to you?" The latter implies that the nurse is neither knowledgeable nor comfortable with violence, and this may prompt the woman to fabricate a more acceptable cause of her injury.

NURSING TIP *It is not difficult to assess for intimate partner violence. You might use the following questions:*

- *Is somebody hurting you?*
- *You seem frightened by your partner. Has he hurt you?*
- *Did someone you know do this to you?*

Once abused, women tend to exhibit low self-esteem and depression (Humphreys and Campbell, 2010). They have more physical health problems than other women, such as chronic pain (back, head, abdominal), neurological problems, problems sleeping, gynecological symptoms, urinary tract infections, and chronic gastrointestinal problems (Campbell, 2002). In addition, these women are more at risk for chronic diseases such as cardiovascular disease, atherosclerosis, and autonomic nervous system disorders (Symes et al, 2010). Although the focus tends to be on the victim of the abuse, it is important to note that there are health consequences to the perpetrator and children witnessing the abuse as well. These physical and mental health consequences incur health care costs that are preventable (Rivara et al, 2007).

Abuse as a Process. Nursing research by Ford-Gilboe et al (2010) suggests that there is a process of response to battering over time wherein the woman's emotional and behavioral reactions change. At first there is a great need to minimize the seriousness of the situation. The violence usually starts with a slight shove in the middle of a heated argument. All couples fight, and if there is any physical aggression, both the man and the woman tend to blame the incident on something external such as a particularly stressful day at work or drinking too much. The male partner usually apologizes for the incident, and as with any problem in a relationship, the couple tries to improve the situation. Although marital counseling may be useful at this early stage, it is generally contraindicated at all other stages because of the risk to the woman's safety. Unfortunately, abuse tends to escalate in frequency and severity over time, and the man's remorse tends to lessen. The risk is such that women who try to leave an abusive relationship are at significant risk for homicide (Campbell, 2007).

Because women have often been taught to take responsibility for the success of a relationship, they usually go through a period in which they try to change their behavior to end the violence. They may even blame themselves for infuriating their spouse. Women who blame themselves for provoking the abuse are more likely to have low self-esteem and be depressed than those who do not blame themselves. Some women experience a moral conflict between their need to leave an abusive relationship and their sense that it is their responsibility to maintain a relationship (Flinck, Paavilainen, and Åstedt-Kurki, 2005). Women find that no matter what they do, the violence continues. During this period, the woman tries to hide the violence because of the stigma attached. She tries to placate her spouse and feels she is losing her sense of self. She is also typically concerned about her children whether she leaves or stays. Children may create barriers to a woman's ability to leave or to remain out of the relationship. Feelings of guilt and social and financial responsibility often influences a woman's decision about how she responds to the abuse (Rhodes et al, 2010).

Some abuse escalates to the point of severe physical injuries and/or death (Piquero et al, 2006). A woman is constantly subjected to emotional degradation, absolute financial dependency, sadistic physical and sexual violence, and control of all her activities. She may fear for her life and the lives of her children. She is in terror that her partner will try to kill her, her children, or both if she attempts to leave. This fear is, in fact, often justified. Clinically, she may experience learned helplessness, traumatic stress syndrome, or both, and she will need intensive therapy. She may kill herself or her abuser to escape because she sees no other way out (Campbell, 2007). Because of the severity of the abuse, a woman may flee to a shelter to obtain physical safety for herself and her children (Harding and Helweg-Larsen,

2009). The frequency of abuse, presence of children, and severity of tactics of power and control used by the perpetrator influences a woman's decision to return to or leave the relationship (Sonis and Langer, 2008; Rhodes et al, 2010). The risk of homicide increases if the woman tries to leave, creating a catch-22 situation. The woman feels she will die if she stays or leaves. The safety of the woman and her children is a nursing priority. The woman will need the following: (1) an order of protection (a legal document to keep the abuser away from her), (2) help in getting to a safe place, such as a wife abuse shelter in an anonymous location, and (3) a carefully calculated plan for escape and arrangements for a neighbor or an adolescent child to call the police when there is another violent episode.

Battered women often try several times to leave. Each attempt is a gathering of resources, a trial of her children's ability to survive without a father, and a testing of her partner's promises to reform. When and if it becomes clear that he is not going to change and she has the emotional support and the financial resources to do so, she will end the relationship. Often, this will involve using a shelter for abused women or individual advocacy and support groups and/or the criminal justice system (Harding and Helweg-Larsen, 2009). Violence may continue after she leaves the relationship. Regardless of the risk, women have hope for ending the abuse and have the requisite strength to leave abusive relationships (Sonis and Langer, 2008; Rhodes et al, 2010).

The male partner may attend a program for batters as an alternative to ending the relationship. These programs are most effective if they are court-mandated. Effectiveness depends upon a discussion of values about women and the perpetrator's minimization of the abuse (Tilley and Brackley, 2005). Abused women need affirmation, support, reassurances of the normalcy of their responses, accurate information about shelters and legal resources, and brainstorming about possible solutions. Other women in similar situations and professionals such as nurses can meet these needs. Cultural factors that influence responses to IPV are important factors in the development of interventions (Ward and Wood, 2009; Belknap and VandeVusse, 2010). Avoid pushing women into actions they are not ready to take.

Once the abuse ends, a period of recovery ensues. Recovery includes a normal grief response for the relationship that has ended and a search for meaning in the experience. The formerly battered woman will typically feel depressed and lonely after the relationship has ended.

Intimate Partner Sexual Abuse. Battered women are often forced into sexual encounters. This sexual abuse is usually but not always accompanied by physical abuse. Women who are sexually abused are at risk for STDs (Coker et al, 2009). Sexual abuse increases the risk for mental health problems for all women who are involved in physically abusive relationships. Women who experience child abuse are at an even greater risk for depression than those not exposed to abuse as a child (Fogarty et al, 2009).

The belief that men have a right to force their wives to have sex comes from traditional English law that said a woman gave irrevocable and perpetual consent to her husband on marriage to have sex whenever and however he wanted.

EVIDENCE-BASED PRACTICE

Belknap and VandeVusse (2010) conducted a community-based research project to assess the needs of Latinas and their families who had experienced intimate partner violence (IPV). The research partners included individuals from a College of Nursing, a local Latina Resource Center, and Latinas in the local community. Qualitative data from listening sessions as well as quantitative data consisting of demographic data, resource usage, and experiences in relation to and/or knowledge about IPV were collected. Sixty-three women participated in seven facilitator-led listening groups that encouraged participant involvement and discussion about experiences, achievements and needs in their lives. The sessions were conducted in Spanish. Analysis of the data resulted in six themes consisting of unmet needs, responsibilities, goals, achievements, help seeking, and IPV. The experiences of women grounded in the context of their daily lives assisted in gaining knowledge about factors that may reduce the incidence of IPV in the community as well as culturally specific resources needed for the planning of services. Listening groups were found to be a good mechanism where women could share resources and assist each other with problems in their daily lives.

Nurse Use

Nurses need to be able to work with IPV on various levels of intervention. Community-based partnerships are essential collaborative actions that will assist in the reduction of IPV. In order to do so, nurses must understand cultural differences among women who experience IPV. Public health nurses can take an active role in leading groups and planning, implementing, and evaluating programmatic change.

Data from Belknap RA, VandeVusse L: Listening sessions with Latinas: documenting life contexts and creating connections, *Public Health Nurs* 27(4):337-346, 2010.

Marital rape was not considered a crime in the United States until 1993 (Yllo, 1999). Marital rape leads to serious physical and emotional damage. Women who suffer from IPV may not consider forced sex a form of abuse. It is essential when women come to the emergency room with injuries that they are assessed for the presence of both physical and sexual abuse (Catallo, 2006).

There is also an alarming incidence of date rape, the dynamics of which may parallel marital rape. Females are more likely than males to be victims of date rape (USDOJ, 2010b). Young women who have been victims of dating violence experience low self-esteem, depression, anger, and irritability as well as increased physical health problems (Fredland and Burton, 2010). To assess for sexual assault, the following question should be used in all nursing assessments to determine if marital rape, date rape, or rape of a male has occurred: "Have you ever been forced into sex you did not wish to participate in?"

Abuse During Pregnancy. Battering during pregnancy has serious implications for the health of both women and their children. As a conservative estimate, 3% to 8% of pregnant women in the United States are physically battered during pregnancy, with a larger proportion of women abused during the year before pregnancy. Even more (up to 20%) adolescents are abused during pregnancy than adult women (Bloom et al, 2010). Although abuse during pregnancy occurs across ethnic groups, Puerto Rican, white, and African-American women experience a significantly higher severity of abuse than Hispanic women from Mexico and Central America (Bloom et al, 2010).

Women abused during pregnancy are at risk for spontaneous abortion, premature delivery, low-birth-weight infants, substance abuse during pregnancy, and depression (McFarlane and Parker, 2005). A man's control of contraception, a form of abusive controlling, may lead to unintended pregnancy and subsequent abuse. In addition, a man's refusal to use a condom places a woman at an increased risk of STDs, including infection with human immunodeficiency virus (HIV) (Campbell et al, 2008).

Generally, the same dynamics of coercive control operate when a woman is battered during pregnancy. IPV is a common event during pregnancy. Pregnant adolescents may be at greater risk than young adults and older women (Chambliss, 2008). Women who are abused during pregnancy are more likely to experience health problems and are at risk for alcohol and drug abuse (Blake et al, 2007). This group of infants could be anticipated to be at particularly high risk of child abuse after they are born. Clearly, all pregnant women should be assessed for abuse at each prenatal care visit, and postpartum home visits should include assessment for child abuse and partner abuse. There is a significant overlap in wife abuse and child abuse, and in more than half of families where there is severe wife abuse, there is also child abuse (Humphreys and Campbell, 2010).

Elder Abuse

Elder abuse is becoming an apparent form of family violence. Like spouse and child abuse, most cases of older adult abuse go unreported. As assessment of this population increases, a better understanding of the incidence and scope of elder abuse should follow. Perpetrators of the abuse are usually family members and/or caregivers.

Types of Elder Abuse. The elderly experience some of the same abuse as children. Abuse includes physical, emotional, sexual, and financial abuse, as well as violation of rights and abandonment and neglect. Older adults are neglected when others fail to provide adequate food, clothing, shelter, and physical care or to meet physiological, emotional, and safety needs. Older adult neglect either through lack of care or through improper care can be considered criminal neglect. In addition, violation of an older adult's rights, medical abuse, abandonment, and forms of physical violence are forms of elder abuse (Post et al, 2010). Older adults are also at risk for financial abuse through fraud, coercion to relinquish property rights, and money mismanagement (CDC, 2010a). Nurses and other health professionals tend to underestimate the incidence of abuse, resulting in substandard care and placing the elderly at risk for further trauma (Cooper, Selwood, and Livingston, 2009; Daly and Coffey, 2010).

Roughness in handling older adults can lead to bruises and bleeding into body tissues because of the fragility of their skin and vascular systems. It is often difficult to determine if the injuries of older adults result from abuse, falls, or other natural causes. Careful assessment through both observation and discussion can help in determining the cause of injuries. Other physical abuse occurs when caregivers impose unrealistic toileting demands, and when the special needs and previous living patterns of the person are ignored.

Older adults can also be abused with regard to nutrition. They may be given food that they cannot chew or swallow or that is contraindicated because of dietary restrictions. Caregivers may overlook food preferences or social or cultural beliefs and patterns about food. Older adults may become undernourished if they can neither prepare their own food nor eat the food that is prepared for them.

Caregivers may give older adults medication to induce confusion or drowsiness so that they will be less troublesome and need less care, or will allow others to control their financial and personal resources. Once medicated, older adults have few ways to act on their own behalf.

The most common form of psychological abuse is rejection or simply ignoring older adults. This kind of treatment conveys that they are worthless and useless to others. Older adults may subsequently regress and become increasingly dependent on others, who tend to resent the imposition and demands on their time and lifestyles. The pattern becomes cyclical: the more regressed the person becomes, the greater the dependence. Further, older adults' past accomplishments and present abilities are not consistently acknowledged, causing them to feel even less capable. Indicators of actual or potential older adult abuse follow.

HOW TO   Identify Potential or Actual Elder Abuse

- *Financial mismanagement*
- *Withdrawal and passivity*
- *Depression*
- *Fear of relative or caregiver*
- *Unexplained or repeated physical injuries*
- *Untreated health problems such as decubitus ulcers*
- *Poor nutrition*
- *Unexplained genital infections*
- *Physical neglect and unmet basic needs*
- *Social isolation*
- *Rejection of assistance by caregiver*
- *Lack of compliance to health regimens*

Data from Centers for Disease Control and Prevention. Elderly maltreatment: definitions, 2010. Available at http://www.cdc.gov/ViolencePrevention/eldermaltreatment/definitions.html. Accessed August 10, 2010; Cooper C, Selwood A, Livingston G: Knowledge, detection, and reporting of abuse by health and social care professionals: a systematic review, Am J Geriatr Psychiatry 17(10):826-838, 2009; Post LA, Page C, Conner T, et al: Elder abuse in long-term care: types, patterns, and risk factors, Res Aging 32(3):323-348, 2010.

Precipitating Factors for Elder Abuse. Caregivers abuse older adults for a variety of reasons. Older family members may be a physical, emotional, or financial burden for the caregiver, leading to frustration and resentment. In many case of abuse, the perpetrator is dependent upon the elderly person. The abuser may be an acquaintance, intimate or extended family member, or a stranger (Krienert, Walsh, and Turner, 2009).

Often the abuse takes place in the home with some form of weapon and is classified as simple assault. Elder abuse in the family setting can be recent or long term. Many abused older female adults are battered women who have become old. In addition, children who have lived in abusive households learn

that behavior. Thus, although it is important to assess for elder abuse when older adults are in need of care from family members, all older adults should be assessed for abuse (Krienert, Walsh, and Turner, 2009).

Confused and frail older adults are a high-risk group for abuse. Large numbers of frail older adults, many with serious physical or mental impairments, live in the community and are cared for by their families. Also, those with cognitive impairments such as Alzheimer disease and other dementias have a greater risk for physical abuse than older adults with other illnesses. These illnesses place a high burden on the caregiver, with subsequent caregiver depression (Anetzberger, 2005). Living with and providing care to a confused older adult is difficult. The round-the-clock tasks often exhaust family members. In addition, clients with Alzheimer's may become verbally and even physically aggressive as part of their illness, which may trigger retaliatory violence. Family stress increases as members work harder to fulfill their other responsibilities in addition to the needs of the older adults.

Also, when families are planning to take care of an older family member at home, nurses must help them fully evaluate that decision and prepare for the stressors that will be involved. It will be essential to have a plan for regular respite care. Strategies for the primary and secondary prevention of abuse of older adults include victim support groups, senior advocacy volunteer programs, and training for providers working with older adults.

Elderly people need to retain as much autonomy and decision-making ability as possible. Nurses have many ways to detect elder abuse, and they have the skills and responsibility for discovering it, giving treatment, and making referrals. Many families who care for older adult members exhaust their resources and coping ability. Nurses can help them find new sources of support and aid.

NURSING INTERVENTIONS

Primary Prevention

A community approach is essential to prevent violence and human abuse. Public health nurses can help the community in the following areas.

First, the community can take a stand against violence and make sure their elected officials and the local media consider non-violence a priority. Public education programs can educate communities about different forms of violence and ways to get help and intervene (Campbell and Manganello, 2006; Post LA et al, 2010). Nurses as community advocates can help with this process. In the legislative arena, laws are needed to outlaw physical punishment in schools and marital rape. Nurses can become involved with faith-based communities and schools to set up prevention programs aimed at decreasing violence. Policies for different kinds of abuse should become standardized (Miller, 2005).

Strong community sanctions against violence in the home can reduce abuse levels (Sullivan et al, 2005). Neighbors can watch what is happening and work together to address problems in other families; this is not an invasion of privacy but a sign of community cohesiveness. Nurses can work with advocate groups to make sure police deal with assault within marriage as swiftly, surely, and severely as assault between strangers (Stover et al, 2010). Nurses can encourage others to interfere when they see children beaten in a grocery store, notice that an older adult is not being properly cared for, see a neighborhood bully beat up their classmates, or hear a neighbor hitting his wife.

Second, people can take measures to reduce their vulnerability to violence by improving the physical security of their homes and learning personal defense measures. Nurses can encourage people to keep windows and doors locked, trim shrubs around their homes, and keep lights on during high-crime periods. Many neighborhoods organize crime watch programs and post signs to that effect. One sign, often posted in a window, shows a hand and indicates that people in this home will assist children who need help. Also, many neighbors informally agree to monitor one another's property and safety, and many law enforcement agencies evaluate homes for security and teach individual or neighborhood safety programs. Individuals install home security systems, participate in personal defense programs such as judo or karate, and purchase firearms for their protection.

Unfortunately, handguns are far more likely to kill family members than intruders (Hahn et al, 2005). Firearm accidents are a leading cause of death for young children, and handguns kept in the home are easy to use when people are either depressed or very angry. A handgun is used in the majority of homicides between family members and in most suicides. Nursing assessments should include a question about guns kept in the home. The family should be made aware of the risk that a handgun holds for family members. If the family thinks that keeping a gun is necessary, safety measures should be taught, such as keeping the gun unloaded and in a locked compartment, keeping the ammunition separate from the gun and also locked away, and teaching children about the dangers of firearms. Lobbying for handgun-control laws is a primary prevention effort that can significantly decrease the rate of death and serious injury caused by handguns in the United States.

Assessment for Risk Factors

Identification of risk factors is an important part of primary prevention. Although abuse cannot be predicted with certainty, several factors influence the onset and support the continuation of abusive patterns. Nurses can identify potential victims of abuse because they see clients in a variety of settings. Factors to include in an assessment for individual or family violence, or for potential family violence, are identified in Figure 38-1. Both individual and familial factors must be assessed within the context of the larger community (Straus et al, 2009). Factors that must be included are found in Box 38-2.

WHAT DO YOU THINK? *Most experts on violence agree that all women entering the health care system should be asked about domestic violence and sexual assault experience; yet men are also victimized by violence, even though little is known about their responses to such experiences. Some experts think that health care professionals should ask men if they are perpetrators of violence as a secondary prevention activity, reasoning that if identified early, such behavior may be more amenable to interventions. Others are concerned that since it is not certain what health care*

system interventions are most effective for male perpetrators or victims of violence, it is premature to do routine screening. There is also some concern that perpetrators of domestic violence or child abuse may become angry if asked about their violent behavior and retaliate against the family member.

Individual and Family Strategies for Primary Prevention

Primary prevention of violence can take place through community, family, and individual interventions (Box 38-3). Nurses, in their work in schools, community groups, employee groups, day care centers, and other community institutions, can foster healthy developmental patterns and identify signs of potential abuse. For example, nurses may take part in media campaigns that identify risk factors for abuse. Nurses can lead in developing after-school programs and late-night programs that support young people to work toward positive goals and to develop a constructive support network. Nurses can identify community needs and resources by capacity mapping. The identification of strengths and weaknesses can assist in determining future goals and needed interventions for the good of the community.

Primary prevention of abuse includes strengthening individuals and families so they can cope more effectively with multiple life stressors and demands, and reducing the destructive elements in the community that support and encourage violence.

BOX 38-2 ASSESSING FOR VIOLENCE IN A COMMUNITY CONTEXT

Individual Factors
- Signs of physical abuse (e.g., abrasions, contusions, burns)
- Physical symptoms related to emotional distress
- Developmental and behavioral difficulties
- Presence of physical disability
- Social isolation
- Decreased role performance within the family, and in job- or school-related activities
- Mental health problems such as depression, low self-esteem, and anxiety
- Fear of intimate others
- Substance abuse

Familial Factors
- Economic stressors
- Presence of some form of family violence
- Poor communication
- Problems with child rearing
- Lack of family cohesion
- Recurrent familial conflict
- Lack of social support networks
- Poor social integration into the community
- Multiple changes of residence
- Access to guns
- Homelessness

Community Characteristics
- High crime rate
- High levels of unemployment
- Lack of neighborhood resources and support systems
- Lack of community cohesiveness

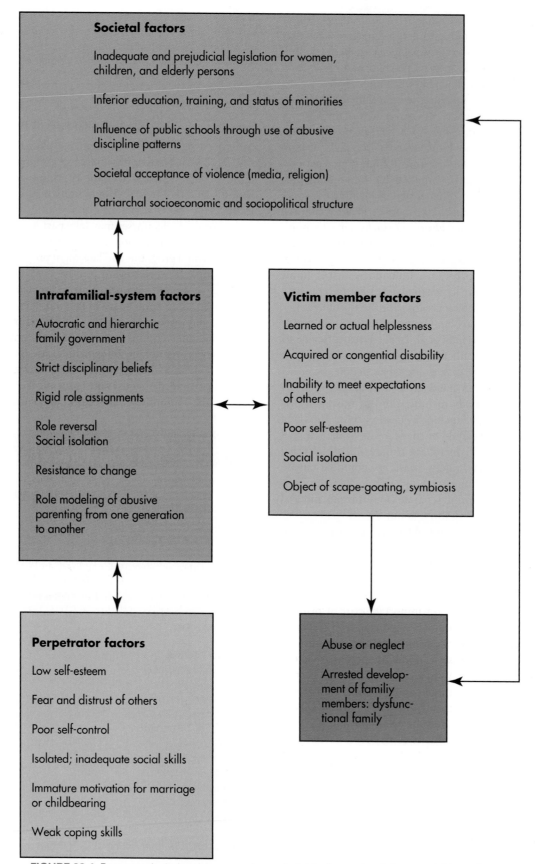

FIGURE 38-1 Factors to include when assessing an individual's or a family's potential for violence.

Providing support and psychological enrichment to at-risk individuals and families often prevents the onset of health disruption. For example, nurses can strengthen and teach parenting abilities. A class, clinic, or home visit can include basic skills such as diapering, feeding, quieting, and even holding and rocking. Parents also need to learn acceptable and effective ways to discipline children so that limits are maintained without causing the child emotional or physical harm. The Nurse Family Partnership model of professional nurse home visitation for at-risk pregnant women has been shown to significantly reduce the risk of child abuse and is being adapted to work toward primary and secondary prevention of IPV (Niolon et al, 2009).

Mutual support groups are valuable for new parents, families with special children, or abused people themselves. Such groups have variable formats and can provide information, support, and encouragement. Nurses can help establish such groups or can actually serve as group leaders. Chapter 16 describes the role of the nurse in working with community groups.

LEVELS OF PREVENTION

Violence

Primary Prevention
Strengthen individual and family by teaching parenting skills.

Secondary Prevention
Reduce or end abuse by early screening; teach families how to deal with stress and how to have fun and enjoy recreation.

Tertiary Prevention
When signs of abuse are evident, refer client to appropriate community organizations.

Secondary Prevention

When abuse occurs, nurses can initiate measures to reduce or terminate further abuse. Both developmental and situational crises present opportunities for abusive situations to develop. On a community level, nurses must form collaborative relationships to provide health services for battered women (McFarlane et al, 2005). Researchers must work effectively with community agencies to use current research to screen for domestic violence and to use model treatments that have a positive effect on decreasing domestic violence (Humphreys and Campbell, 2010).

Nurses can be primary leaders in the development of screening practices in the health care arena (Higgins and Hawkins, 2005). The development of training programs for health care providers can be an effective step in identifying and treating victims of violence. Nurses can work closely with shelters in identifying the needs of individuals who seek sanctuary from abusive situations.

On a family level, nursing intervention can help family members discuss problems and seek ways to deal with the tension that led to the abusive situations. Injured persons must be temporarily or permanently placed in a safe location. Secondary preventive measures are most useful when potential abusers recognize their tendency to be abusive and seek help. For children, there is often a need for 24-hour child protection services

BOX 38-3   PREVENTION STRATEGIES FOR VIOLENCE

Individual and Family Levels
- Provide education on developmental stages and needs of children (primary).
- Teach parenting techniques (primary).
- Teach stress-reduction techniques (primary).
- Provide assessment during routine examination (secondary).
- Assess for marital discord (secondary).
- Provide counseling for at-risk parents (secondary).
- Encourage assistance with controlling anger (secondary).
- Provide treatment for substance abuse (tertiary).

Community Level
- Develop policy.
- Conduct community resource mapping.
- Collaborate with community to develop systemic response to violence.
- Develop media campaign.
- Develop resources such as transition housing and shelters.

or caregivers who can take care of the child until the acute family or individual crisis is resolved. Respite care is extremely important in families with frail older adult family members. Telephone crisis lines can be used to provide immediate emergency assistance to families.

Effective communication with abusive families is important. Typically, these families do not want to discuss their problems and many are embarrassed to be involved in an abusive situation. Often a lot of guilt is involved. Effective communication must be preceded by an attitude of acceptance. It is often difficult for nurses to value the worth of an individual who willfully abuses another. The behavior, not the person, must be condemned.

In addition, families do not always know how to have fun. Nurses can assess how much recreation is integrated into the family's lifestyle. Through community assessment, nurses know what resources and facilities are available and how much they cost. Families may need counseling about the value of recreation and play in reducing tension and appropriately channeling aggressive impulses.

Tertiary Prevention: Therapeutic Intervention with Abusive Families

Although it may be hard for abusive families to form a trusting relationship with the nurse, nurses can act as a case manager, coordinating the other agencies and activities involved. Principles of giving care to families who are experiencing violence include the following:
- Intolerance for violence
- Respect and caring for all family members
- Safety as the first priority
- Absolute honesty
- Empowerment

Nurses must clearly indicate that any further violence, degradation, and exploitation of family members will not be tolerated, and that all family members are respected, valued human beings. However, everyone must understand that the safety of every family member is the first priority.

Abusers often fear they will be condemned for their actions, so it is often difficult to make and maintain contact with abusive families. Although nurses convey an attitude of caring and concern for them, families may doubt the sincerity of this concern. They may avoid being home at the scheduled visit time out of fear of the consequences of the visit or an inability to believe that anyone really wants to help them. If the victim is a child, parents may fear that the nurse will try to remove the child.

Nurses are mandatory reporters of child abuse, even when only suspected, in all states. They are also mandatory reporters of elder abuse and abuse of other physically and cognitively dependent adults as well as of felony assaults on anyone in most states. The mandatory reporting laws also protect reporters from legal action on cases that are never substantiated. Even so, physicians and nurses are sometimes reluctant to report abuse. They may be more willing to report abuse in a poor family than in a middle-class one, or they may think that an older adult or child is better off at home than in a nursing home or foster home. Referral to protective service agencies should be viewed as enlisting another source of help, rather than an automatic step toward removal of the victim or criminal justice action. This same attitude can be communicated to families, so that reporting is done with families rather than without their knowledge and prior input. Absolute honesty about what will be reported to officials, what the family can expect, what the nurse is entering into records, and what the nurse is feeling is essential.

To further empower the family, the nurse needs to recognize and capitalize on the violent family's strengths, as well as to assess and deal with its problems. The nurse must use a nurse–family partnership rather than a paternalistic or authoritarian approach. Families can often generate many of their own solutions, which tend to be more culturally appropriate and individualized than those the nurse generates. Victims of direct attack need information about their options and resources, and they need reassurance that abuse is unfortunately rather common and that they are not alone in their dilemma. They also need reassurance that their responses are normal and that they do not deserve to be abused. Continued support for their decisions must be coupled with nursing actions to ensure their safety.

Nursing Actions

The nurse can meet the family's therapeutic needs in a variety of ways. Besides referral to appropriate community agencies, nurses can act as role models for the family. During clinic and home visits, nurses can demonstrate constructive adult–child interactions. Nurses often teach mothers childcare skills such as proper feeding, calming a fretful child, effective discipline, and constructive communication.

Nurses can demonstrate good communication skills and discipline by teaching both parents and children in a calm, respectful, and informative manner. Caregivers, especially those caring for children, people with special needs, or older adults, may need to learn age-appropriate expectations. It is unreasonable to expect a 14-month-old infant to differentiate between right and wrong. Children at this age do not deliberately annoy caregivers by breaking delicate pieces of china. Likewise, a person with poor sphincter control does not willingly soil clothes or bedding.

BOX 38-4   COMMON COMMUNITY SERVICES

- Child protective services
- Child abuse prevention programs
- Adult protective services
- Parents Anonymous
- Domestic violence shelters
- Programs for children of battered women
- Community support groups
- 24-hour hotline
- Legal advocacy or information
- State/County coalition against domestic violence
- Batterer treatment
- Victim assistance programs
- Sexual assault programs
- Transition housing

Role modeling can be used with abuse victims of all ages. When providing nursing care to abused spouses or to older adults, nurses can demonstrate communication skills, conflict resolution, and skill training. For example, adult children often become abusive toward their older parents when they become frustrated in trying to care for them. During home visits, nurses can show how to physically and psychologically care for the relative. The nurse can work with caregivers to help them develop approaches that are acceptable to the individual older adult. Assessment, creativity, and critical thinking help the nurse, family, and client learn how to meet client and family needs without causing undue stress and frustration.

Considerable emotional investment and sheer drain of energy is used in working effectively with abusers and victims of abuse. Abusers present difficult clinical challenges since they are often reluctant to seek help or to remain actively involved in the helping process.

Referral is an important part of tertiary prevention. Nurses should know about available community resources for abuse victims and perpetrators. Some of these resources are listed in Box 38-4. If community attitudes and resources are inadequate, it is often helpful to work with local radio and television stations and newspapers to provide information about the nature and extent of human abuse as a community health problem. This also helps to acquaint people with available services and resources. Frequently, people do not seek services early in an abusive situation because they simply do not know what is available to them. Ideally, a program or plan for abused people begins with a needs assessment to identify potential clients and to determine how to effectively serve this group. Nurses can help to get programs started and provide public education.

Nursing Interventions Specific to Female Partner Abuse

Women in abusive relationships seek care for injuries in an emergency setting, a physician's office, or a prenatal clinic. These women may be seeking assistance for injuries sustained during physically abusive episodes (McFarlane et al, 2005), but even more often they are in the health care system for other health problems. Despite the overall incidence of battering and its resultant physical and emotional health problems for women, health professionals—even those in emergency departments—often fail to identify abused women and are often seen as paternalistic, judgmental, insensitive, and less effective and helpful than they could be.

Because of the stigma involved, women and health care providers may hesitate to initiate discussion about abuse. However, the majority of battered women claim they would have liked to talk about the issue with a health care professional if they were asked (Higgins and Hawkins, 2005). Because abuse develops slowly, starting with minor psychological abuse and building to more severe physical incidents, victims and health care providers alike may not recognize the abuse until a severe episode occurs.

The quality of health care that a battered woman receives often determines whether she follows through with referrals to legal, social service, and health care agencies. The emergency department is the point of entry for many women in abusive relationships. Care in the emergency department is often fragmented and necessarily oriented toward life-and-death situations. Therefore, women may not be adequately assessed and often receive little or no specific emotional support or intervention. A cycle persists in which women seek care and receive either no interventions or ineffective interventions. This cycle perpetuates feelings of anger and inadequacy in health care providers, resulting in blame placed on women for their lack of compliance to remedies offered.

Managed care and clinic settings may be the best places to routinely screen for domestic violence. Ideally a clinical nurse specialist who is an expert in screening for IPV should be available to coordinate efforts in the different health care settings. If battered women can be identified, perhaps effective interventions can be provided that will prevent the kind of serious injury that later results in emergency department visits or even a homicide.

However, some battered women hesitate to identify themselves as victims of domestic violence for several reasons. They may fear that revelation will further jeopardize their safety by increasing the violence, and they may also think that it will increase their sense of shame and humiliation. This hesitation to speak out often makes it difficult for health care professionals to identify the battered woman. In addition, the nature of the systems in which victims of violence introduce themselves can be barriers. Emergency departments, clinics, managed care settings, and health departments are busy places. Staff members work hard to maintain the functioning of these facilities. Sometimes it is difficult in such chaotic settings for staff members to realize their importance as the first or only health provider to recognize violence in their clients' lives, and that women need them to take the time to deal with this issue (Straus et al, 2009).

Studies have found that only a small percentage of battered women in emergency departments and other health care settings were identified as such and treated for the abuse, despite the significant prevalence (Furniss et al, 2007). Battered women present for treatment in a number of ways, including physical complaints (such as inability to sleep or chronic pain) related to the chronic stress of living in an abusive situation or to old injuries. They may be unaware of the relationship of their symptoms to the violence in their lives. Therefore, professional nursing organizations (American Nurses Association, Emergency Nurses Association, Association of Women's Health, Obstetric and Neonatal Nurses, American College of Nurse-Midwives) recommend that all women be routinely screened for domestic violence each time they come to a health care setting. For the battered woman and the staff to begin to make the connection between her life situation and the presenting complaints, the nurse needs to ask direct questions in a supportive, open, and concerned manner (Straus et al, 2009). Computerized inquiry is also effective in identifying abused women in health care settings (Trautman et al, 2007).

Assessment. Assessment for all forms of violence against women should therefore take place for all women entering the health care system. The assessment should be ongoing and confidential. A thorough assessment gathers information on physical, emotional, and sexual trauma from violence, risk for future abuse, cultural background and beliefs, perceptions of the woman's relationships with others, and stated needs. Conduct the assessment in private and direct other adults who are present to the waiting area and tell them that it is policy that initially women are seen alone. Women should be asked directly if they were in an abusive relationship as a child or are currently in an abusive relationship as an adult. They should also be asked if they have ever been forced into sex. Shame and fear often make disclosure difficult. Verbal acknowledgment of the situation and emotional and physical support assist women in talking about past or current circumstances (Humphreys and Campbell, 2010).

Women can be categorized into three groups: no, low, or moderate-to-high risk. Women with no signs of current or past abuse are considered at no risk. However, future visits should include questioning a woman about whether there have been any changes in her life or whether she has additional information or questions about topics discussed at previous visits. If there is a new intimate partner in her life, she should again be screened for abuse. The Abuse Assessment Screen (AAS) is a four-question screen that has been successfully used in almost every kind of health care setting and can be downloaded from the Nursing Network on Violence Against Women International (NNVAWI) website (http://www.nnvawi.org).

Women at low risk show no evidence of recent or current abuse. Education that helps a woman gain perspective on her situation and her needs should be discussed. Resource materials including group and individual formats can be suggested. The risk level should be recorded and preventive measures and teaching should be documented.

Assessment of moderate to high risk includes evaluation of a woman's fear for both psychological and physical abuse. Lethality potential should be assessed (Campbell, Webster, and Glass, 2009) and can be done with the Danger Assessment, also available at the NNVAWI website. Risk factors for lethality include behaviors such as stalking or frequent harassment, threats or an escalation of threats, use of weapons or threats with weapons, excessive control and jealousy, and forced sex. Statements from an abuser such as "If I can't have you, no one can" should be taken seriously. In all cases, a history of abuse and alcohol and drug use should be collected and carefully documented. The determined risk level should also be documented along with any past or present physical evidence of abuse from prior or current assault; this evidence should be photographed, shown on a body map, or described narratively. It is important that the assailant be identified in the record; this can take the form of either quotes from the woman or subjective information. These records can be very important for women in future assault or child custody cases, even if the woman is not ready to make a police report at the present time.

Immediate care for a woman in a potentially harmful or present abusive situation involves the development of a safety plan. A woman can be assisted to look at the options available to her (Dienemann, Neese, and Lowry, 2009). Discuss shelter information, access to counseling, and legal resources. If a woman wants to return to her partner, she can be helped in the development of plans that can be carried out if the abuse continues or becomes more serious. *The Domestic Violence Abuse Survivor Assessment* is an assessment tool that can help providers assist women in decision making and the identification of services to meet needs. The assessment covers discussion about the relationship and assessment of psychosocial needs, safety and danger issues, speaking with children, and issues of substance abuse. The assessment can be found on the Nursing Network on Violence Against Women, International website.

Whenever there is evidence of sexual assault within the prior 24 to 48 hours, a rape kit examination should be performed. Lists of resources such as rape crisis clinics and support groups for survivors of physical and emotional abuse should be made available.

Prevention. Prevention, public policy, and social attitudes are intertwined. Our society has taken a major step toward the secondary prevention of abuse through the establishment of programs that encourage women and children to speak about their experiences. Nurses need to support these programs further by believing the experiences they are told. In the development of laws that punish perpetrators of child and woman abuse, society has given some support to the victims of abuse. Often, however, the victims are again victimized by disbelief of their experiences, a devaluing of the effects of these assaults, and a focus on assisting the perpetrators of the crimes. Primary prevention includes a social attitudinal change. Both girls and boys need to be taught human values of interdependence, respect for human life, and a commitment to empathy and strength in the development of the human species regardless of sex, race, or socioeconomic status. We must urge continued progress toward eliminating the feminization of poverty and ensuring gender parity in economic resources. In addition, local communities must make it clear that violence against women is not tolerated by eliminating pornography, mandating arrests of abusers, and creating a general climate of non-violence.

Abused women need assistance in making decisions and taking control of their lives. Population-centered nurses, prenatal nurses, Planned Parenthood, primary care, and emergency department nurses are involved with women Iwhen they can be screened for the presence or absence of abuse. There are

mechanisms for routinely asking women who are either abused or at risk for abuse (Higgins and Hawkins, 2005; Dienemann, Neese, and Lowry, 2009). To intervene effectively, nurses must understand abuse as a cumulative process that must be examined as a continuum within the context of a relationship. During this process, the abuse, the relationship, and a woman's view of changes within herself require time-specific interventions. Women are often blamed and held responsible for the abuse inflicted on them by their male partners (Weaver et al, 2007; Copel, 2008; Saito et al, 2009; Ting and Panchanadeswaran, 2009). When this happens, either they are assisted in a way that discounts their feelings and further devalues them, or the abuse is ignored.

THE CUTTING EDGE *Capacity mapping can be both an approach and a tool for community assessment. It is an approach to planning based on building on community strengths rather than responding to deficits. As a tool, it is a method for identifying talents, skills, and resources within a community.*

Strategies for Addressing Education for Health Professionals. A variety of strategies have been reported that address the knowledge deficit of health practitioners on abuse issues. The National March of Dimes Birth Defects Foundation has sponsored a variety of training sessions for health professionals and produced an excellent training manual that addresses violence against women and battering during pregnancy (McFarlane and Parker, 2005). The program covers the assessment and planning of interventions to assist pregnant women in abusive relationships.

More and more nursing programs are implementing courses on how to intervene with IPV. Wallace (2009) developed and implemented a two-credit elective course focusing on attitudes, knowledge, and interventions in a structured learning environment to help nursing students acquire the expertise needed to work with women in abusive relationships. An educational program for nurses was developed in order to initiate systemwide routine inquiry in an urban health care system (Schoening et al, 2004). The program consisted of a mandatory 1-hour program for all nurses with an optional 3-hour program for nurses working in obstetrics. The program focused on the dynamics of abuse, screening procedures, and nursing interventions. The program showed an increase in positive responses to battered women for nurses involved in the 3-hour program and for nurses in the 1-hour program only if they had previous education on abuse. Short programs with skills' education as well as discussion can be a benefit to both nurses and the clients they serve.

Nurses are also joining in community-based efforts to prevent and intervene with IPV and child abuse. Nurses work in public health collaborating with shelters for women, community mental health centers, criminal justice and advocacy institutions, and community-based health care. Bloom et al (2009) developed a program to assist Latinas experiencing IPV. The program was developed specific to the cultural and linguistic needs of the population. Emphasis was placed on assisting the

Hispanic community in developing the knowledge and background to deal with the issue. At the same time, community efforts focused on expanding the knowledge base of the community at large about IPV.

VIOLENCE AND THE PRISON POPULATION

Many women currently in prison in the United States have experienced IPV. Similar to the general population of women who have experienced IPV, they are at risk for depression, posttraumatic stress disorder, anxiety, substance abuse, and suicide (Zust, 2009). Sexual assault or abuse, commonplace in U.S. prisons, increases these risks. Few studies have investigated the prevalence of sexual assault in the female population. The incidence of rape is higher in the female population than in the male prison population; the incidence of assault is higher for males than for women in the prison population; and the incidence of both rape and assault were higher for both men and women in prison than for the general population (Wolff, Blitz, and Shi, 2007; Wolff, Shi, and Bachman, 2008). The majority of women who have experienced abuse in prison have a history of experiencing multiple types of abuse as a child and as an adult (Zust, 2009). Currently, a significant number of women are imprisoned for killing their male partners. Before committing homicide, many of these women tried to use the social resources available to them. For many of these women, the homicide of their partners was an act of desperation that resulted from a system that failed to support them in remaining safe in their own homes. Nurses working in prisons must be aware of the complex histories of the prison population. It is essential to develop resources that can respond to the multiple social needs of prisoners. When women leave prison they need discharge planning and help to identify transition behaviors and resources that will decrease the likelihood of violence.

CHAPTER REVIEW

PRACTICE APPLICATION

Mrs. Smith, a 75-year-old bedridden woman, consistently became rude and combative when her daughter Mary attempted to bathe her and change her clothes each morning. During a home visit, Mary told the nurse, Mrs. Jones, that she had become so frustrated with her mother on the previous morning that she had hit her. Mary felt terrible about her behavior. She stressed that her mother's incontinence made it essential that she be kept clean; her clothes had to be changed every day for her own safety and physical well-being.

A. How should Mrs. Jones respond to this disclosure?
B. What specific nursing actions should be taken?
C. What ongoing services does the nurse need to provide?
   Answers can be found on the Evolve site.

KEY POINTS

- Violence and human abuse are not new phenomena, but they have increasingly become community health concerns.
- Communities throughout the United States are angry and frustrated about increasing levels of violence.
- Nurses can evaluate and intervene in incidents of community and family violence; to intervene effectively, the nurse must understand the dynamics of violence and human abuse.
- Factors influencing social and community violence include changing social conditions, economic conditions, population density, community facilities, and institutions within a community, such as organized religion, education, the mass communication media, and work.
- The potential for violence against individuals or against oneself is directly related to the level of violence in the community. Identification and correction of factors affecting the level of violence in the community constitute one way of reducing violence against family members and other individuals.
- Violence and abuse of family members can happen to any family member: spouse, older adult, child, or developmentally disabled person.

- People who abuse family members were often themselves abused and react poorly to real or perceived crises. Other factors that characterize the abuser are the way the person was raised and the unique character of that person.
- Child abuse can be physical, emotional, or sexual. Incest is a common and particularly destructive form of child abuse.
- Spouse abuse is usually wife abuse. It involves physical, emotional, and, frequently, sexual abuse within a context of coercive control. It usually increases in severity and frequency and can escalate to homicide of either partner.
- Nurses are in an excellent position to identify potential victims of family abuse because they see clients in a variety of settings, such as schools, businesses, homes, and clinics. Treatment of family abuse includes primary, secondary, and tertiary prevention and therapeutic intervention.

CLINICAL DECISION-MAKING ACTIVITIES

1. For 1 week, keep a log or diary related to violence.
   A. Make a note of each time you feel as though you are losing your temper. Consider what it might take to cause you to react in a violent way.
   B. Think back. When was the last time you had a violent outburst? What precipitated it? What were your thoughts? What were your feelings? How might you have handled the situation or those feelings without reacting in a violent way?
   C. During this same week, make note of the episodes of violent behaviors you observe. For example, do parents hit children in the supermarket? What seems to precipitate such outbursts? What alternatives might exist for reacting in a less violent way?

2. If you learned, after a careful assessment of your community, that family violence is a significant community health problem, what plan of action might you take to intervene? Remember that the goal is to promote health. Outline a plan of action with objectives, timetables, implementation strategies, and evaluation plans for intervening in family violence in your community.

3. Complete a partial community assessment to determine the actual incidence and types of violence in your community.

4. What resources are available in your community for victims of violence? Interview a person who works in an agency that seeks to aid victims of violence. What is the role of the agency? Do its services seem adequate? Who is eligible? Is there a waiting list? What is the fee scale?

5. Cut out all stories about violence that you find in your local newspaper every day for 2 weeks. Note the patterns. Is the majority of the violence perpetrated by strangers or family members? How are the victims portrayed? What kinds of families are involved? What kinds of stories and families get front-page treatment rather than a few lines in the back of the paper?

REFERENCES

Anetzberger GJ: The reality of elder abuse, *Clin Gerontol* 28:1–25, 2005.

American Public Health Association: *10 Essential public health services*, 2010. Available at http://www.apha.org/programs/standards/performancestandardsprogram/resexxentialservices.htm. Accessed August 20, 2010.

Association of State and Territorial Directors of Nursing: *Quad Council PHN Competencies*, 2003. Available at http://www.astdn.org/publication_quad_council_phn_competencies.htm. Accessed August 20, 2010.

Bachar K, Koss MP: From prevalence to prevention: closing the gap between what we know about rape and what we do. In Renzetti CM, Edleson JL, Bergen RK, editors: *Sourcebook on violence against women*, Thousand Oaks, CA, 2001, Sage Publications, pp 117–142.

Beaulaurier RL, Seff LR, Newman FL, Dunlop B: External barriers to help seeking for older women who experience intimate partner violence, *J Fam Violence* 22:747–755, 2007.

Belknap RA, VandeVusse L: Listening sessions with Latinas: documenting life contexts and creating connections, *Public Health Nurs* 27(4):337–346, 2010.

Berlan ED, Corliss HL, Field AE, et al: Sexual orientation and bullying among adolescents in the growing up today study, *J Adolesc Health* 46:366–371, 2010.

Berman H, Hardesty H, O'Connor A, Humphreys J: Children of abused women. In Humphreys J, Campbell JC, editors: *Family violence and nursing practice*, ed 2, New York, 2010, Springer, pp 154–185.

Blake SM, Kiely M, Gard CC, et al: Pregnancy intentions and happiness among pregnant black women at high risk for adverse infant health outcomes, *Perspect Sex Reprod Health* 39(4):194–205, 2007.

Bloom T, Bullock L, Sharps PW, et al: Intimate partner violence during pregnancy. In Humphreys J, Campbell JC, editors: *Family violence and nursing practice*, ed 2, New York, 2010, Springer, pp 279–398.

Bloom T, Wagman J, Hernandez R, et al: Partnering with community-based organizations to reduce intimate partner violence, *Hisp J Behav Sci* 31(2): 244–257, 2009.

Bostock DJ, Daley JG: Lifetime and current sexual assault and harassment victimization rates of active-duty United States Air Force women, *Violence against Women* 13:927–944, 2007.

Bower-Russa M: Attitudes mediate the association between childhood disciplinary history and disciplinary responses, *Child Maltreat* 10:272–282, 2005.

Campbell JC: Health consequences of intimate partner violence, *Lancet* 359:1331–1336, 2002.

Campbell JC: *Assessing dangerousness: violence by batterers and child abusers*, ed 2, New York, 2007, Springer.

Campbell JC, Baty ML, Ghandour RM, et al: The intersection of violence against women and HIV/AIDS: A review, *Int J Injury Control Safety Promotion* 15:221–231, 2008.

Campbell JC, Manganello J: Changing public attitudes as a prevention strategy to reduce intimate partner violence, *J Aggress Maltreat Trauma* 13(3-4):13–39, 2006.

Campbell JC, Sharps PW, Glass NE: Risk assessment for intimate partner homicide. In Pinard GF, Pagani L, editors: *Clinical assessment of dangerousness: empirical contributions*, New York, 2000, Cambridge University Press, pp 136–157.

Campbell JC, Sheridan DJ: Assessment of intimate partner violence and elder abuse. In Jarvis C, editor: *Physical assessment for clinical practice*, Philadelphia, 2004, Elsevier Science, pp 74–82.

Campbell JC, Webster DW, Glass NE: The Danger Assessment: Validation of a lethality risk assessment instrument for intimate partner femicide, *J Interper Viol* 24:653–674, 2009.

Campbell JC, Webster D, Koziol-McLain J, et al: Risk factors for femicide in abusive relationships: results from a multi-site case control study, *Am J Public Health* 93:1089–1097, 2003.

Campbell R, Long SM, Townsend SM, et al: Sexual assault nurse examiners' experiences providing expert witness court testimony, *J Forensic Nurs* 3:7–14, 2007.

Campbell R, Patterson D, Adams AE, et al: A participatory evaluation project to measure SANE nursing practice and adult sexual assault patients' psychological well-being, *J Forensic Nurs* 4(1):19–28, 2008.

Campbell R, Townsend SM, Long SM, et al: Responding to sexual assault victims' medical and emotional needs: a national study of the services provided by SANE programs, *Res Nurs Health* 29:384–398, 2006.

Casey EA, Lindhorst TP: Toward a multi-level, ecological approach to the primary prevention of sexual assault: prevention in peer and community contexts, *Trauma Violence Abuse* 10:91–114, 2009.

Catalano S, Smith E, Snyder H, Rand M: *Female victims of violence*, Washington, DC, 2009, Bureau of Justice Statistics Selected Findings. Available at http://bjs.ojp.usdoj.gov/content/pub/pdf/fvv.pdf. Accessed March 7, 2011.

Catallo C: Review: meta-analysis of qualitative studies generated recommendations for healthcare professionals meeting with women who had experienced intimate partner violence, *Evid Based Nurs* 9(4):125–134, 2006.

Centers for Disease Control and Prevention: Physical dating violence among high school students—United States, 2003, *MMWR Weekly* 55(19):532–535, 2006a.

Centers for Disease Control and Prevention: *Choose Respect: Annual Report 2005-2006*, 2006b. Available at http://www.cdc.gov/choose-respect/. Accessed March 10, 2011.

Centers for Disease Control and Prevention: Fatal injuries among children by race and ethnicity—United States, 1999–2002, *MMWR* 56(5):1–20, 2007.

Centers for Disease Control and Prevention: Data updates, *Injury Center Connection* 2(3):2, 2009.

Centers for Disease Control and Prevention: *Elderly maltreatment: definitions*, 2010a. Available at http://www.cdc.gov/ViolencePrevention/eldermaltreatment/definitions.html. Accessed August 20, 2010.

Centers for Disease Control and Prevention: *National suicide statistics at a glance*, 2010b. Available at http://www.cdc.gov/violenceprevention/suicide/statistics/index.html. Accessed August 20, 2010.

Chambliss LR: Intimate partner violence and its implication for pregnancy, *Clin Obstet Gynecol* 51(2):385–397, 2008.

Chiodo D, Wolfe DA, Crooks C, et al: Impact of sexual harassment victimization by peers on subsequent adolescent victimization and adjustment: a longitudinal study, *J Adolesc Health* 45:246–252, 2009.

Coker AL, Hopenhayn C, DeSimone CP, et al: Violence against women raises risk of cervical cancer, *J Womens Health* 18(8):1179–1185, 2009.

Cooper C, Selwood A, Livingston G: Knowledge, detection, and reporting of abuse by health and social care professionals: a systematic review, *Am J Geriatr Psychiatry* 17(10):826–838, 2009.

Copel LC: The lived experience of women in abusive relationships who sought spiritual guidance, *Issues Ment Health Nurs* 29(2):115–130, 2008.

Corvo K, deLara E: Towards an integrated theory of relational violence: is bullying a risk factor for domestic violence? *Aggress Violent Behav* 15(3):181–190, 2010.

Council on Linkages Between Academia and Public Health Practice: *Core competencies for public health professionals*, Washington, DC, 2010, Public Health Foundation/Health Resources and Service Administration.

Daly J, Coffey A: Staff perceptions of elder abuse, *Nurs Older People* 22(4):33–37, 2010.

Daro D, Dodge KA: Creating community responsibility for child protection: possibilities and challenges, *Future Children* 19(2):67–93, 2009.

Dickers RA, Jaeger S, Knudson MM, et al: Where do we go from here? Interim analysis to forge ahead in violence prevention, *J Trauma* 67:1169–1175, 2009.

Dienemann J, Neese J, Lowry S: Psychometric properties of the Domestic Violence Survivor Assessment, *Arch Psychiatr Nurs* 23(2):111–118, 2009.

Dixon L, Browne K, Hamilton-Giachritsis C: Patterns of risk and protective factors in the intergenerational cycle of maltreatment, *J Fam Viol* 24:111–122, 2009.

Dixon L, Hamilton-Giachritsis C, Browne K: Risk factors of parents abused as children: a mediational analysis of the intergenerational continuity of child maltreatment, *J Child Psychol Psychiatry* 46:59–68, 2005.

Eaton DK, Kann L, Kinchen S, et al: Youth risk behavior surveillance— United States, 2009, *MMWR* 59(SS-5):1–42, 2010.

Ellison CG, Trinitapoli JA, Anderson KL, Johnson BR: Race/ethnicity, religious involvement, and domestic violence, *Violence against Women* 13:1094–1112, 2007.

Ernst AA, Weiss SJ, Enright-Smith S, Hansen JP: Positive outcomes from an immediate and ongoing intervention for child witnesses of intimate partner violence, *Am J Emerg Med* 26(4):389–394, 2008.

Ferguson CJ, Hartley RD: The pleasure is momentary. the expense damnable? The influence of pornography on rape and sexual assault, *Aggress Violent Behav* 14:323–329, 2009.

Ferguson CJ, Kilburn J: The public health risks of media violence: a meta-analytic review, *J Pediatr* 154:759–763, 2009.

Ferguson CJ, San Miguel C, Hartley RD: A multivariate analysis of youth violence and aggression: the influence of family, peers, depression, and media violence, *J Pediatr* 155:904–908, 2009.

Fletcher J: The effects of intimate partner violence on health in young adulthood in the United States, *Soc Sci Med* 70(1):130–135, 2010.

Flinck A, Paavilainen E, Åstedt-Kurki P: Survival of intimate partner violence as experienced by women, *J Clin Nurs* 14(3):383–393, 2005.

Fogarty CT, Fredman L, Heeren TC, Liebschutz J: Synergistic effects of child abuse and intimate partner violence on depressive symptoms in women, *Prev Med* 46(5):463–469, 2009.

Ford JD, Elhai JD, Connor DF, Frueh BC: Poly-victimization and risk of posttraumatic, depressive, and substance use disorders and involvement in delinquency in a national sample of adolescents, *J Adolesc Health* 46(6):545–552, 2010.

Ford-Gilboe M, Varcoe C, Wuest J, Merritt-Gray M: Intimate partner violence and nursing practice, In Humphreys J, Campbell JC, editors: *Intimate partner violence and nursing practice*, ed 2, New York, 2011, Springer, pp 115–153.

Fredland NM, Burton C: Nursing care and teen dating violence: promoting healthy relationship development. In Humphreys J, Campbell J, editors: *Intimate partner violence and nursing practice*, ed 2, New York, 2011, Springer, pp 225–252.

Furniss K, McCaffrey M, Parnell V, Rovi S: Nurses and barriers to screening for intimate partner violence, *Am J Maternal Child Nurs* 32(4):238–243, 2007.

Glass N, Perrin N, Hanson G, et al: Risk for reassault in abusive female same-sex relationships, *Am J Public Health* 98:1021–1027, 2008.

Gracia E, Herrero J: Perceived neighborhood social disorder and attitudes toward reporting domestic violence against women, *J Interpers Violence* 22:737–752, 2007.

Grier SA, Kumanyika S: Targeted marketing and public health, *Annu Rev Public Health* 31:349–369, 2010.

Hahn RA, Bilukha O, Crosby A, et al: Firearms laws and the reduction of violence: a systematic review, *Am J Prev Med* 28(suppl 1):40–71, 2005.

Harding H, Helweg-Larsen M: Perceived risk for future intimate partner violence among women in a domestic violence shelter, *J Fam Violence* 24(2):75–85, 2009.

Higgins LP, Hawkins JW: Screening for abuse during pregnancy: implementing a multisite program, *MCN Am J Matern Child Nurs* 30:109–114, 2005.

Hines DA, Malley-Morrison K: *Family violence in the United States*, Thousand Oaks, CA, 2005, Sage.

Houmes BV, Fagan MM, Quintana NM: Violence: recognition, management and prevention: establishing a sexual assault nurse examiner (SANE) program in the emergency department, *J Emerg Med* 25:111–121, 2003.

Howard KAS, Budge SL, McKay KM: Youth exposed to violence: the role of protective factors, *J Community Psychol* 38:63–79, 2010.

Humphreys JC, Campbell JC: *Family violence and nursing practice*, New York, 2010, Springer.

Kaminski JW, Fang X: Victimization by peers and adolescent suicide in three US samples, *J Pediatr* 155(5):683–688, 2009.

Karch DL, Dahlberg LL, Patel N: Surveillance for Violent Deaths— National Violent Death Reporting System, 16 States, 2007, *MMWR* 59(SS04):1–50, 2010.

Kelly UA, Gonzalez-Guarda RM, Taylor J: Theories of intimate partner violence. In Humphreys J, Campbell JC, editors: *Intimate partner violence and nursing practice*, ed 2, New York, 2010, Springer, pp 253–278.

Kiriakidis SP, Kavoura A: Cyberbullying: a review of the literature on harassment through the internet and other electronic means, *Fam Community Health* 33:82–93, 2010.

Kletter H, Weems CF, Carrion VG: Guilt and posttraumatic stress symptoms in child victims of interpersonal violence, *Clin Child Psychol Psychiatry* 14(1):71–83, 2009.

Krienert JL, Walsh JA, Turner M: Elderly in America: a descriptive study of elder abuse examining National Incident-Based Reporting System (NIBRS) data, 2000-2005, *J Elder Abuse Negl* 21(4):325–345, 2009.

Kugel C, Retzlaff C, Hopfer S, et al: Familias con Voz: community survey results from an Intimate Partner Violence (IPV) Prevention Project with Migrant Workers, *J Fam Viol* 24:649–660, 2009.

Lee MR, Ousey GC: Institutional access, residential segregation, and urban Black homicide, *Sociol Inq* 75:31–54, 2005.

Levitt HM, Ware K: "Anything with two heads is a monster": religious leaders' perspectives on marital equality and domestic violence, *Violence against Women* 12:1169–1190, 2006.

Lewandowski L, McFarlane J, Campbell JC, et al: "He killed my mommy!" Murder or attempted murder of a child's mother, *J Fam Violence* 19:211–220, 2004.

Lin J, Thompson MP, Kaslow NJ: The mediating role of social support in the community environment - psychological distress link among low-income African American women, *J Community Psychol* 37:459–470, 2009.

Logan TK, Cole J, Capillo A: Sexual Assault Nurse Examiner program characteristics, barriers, and lessons learned, *J Forensic Nurs* 3(1):24–33, 2007.

Malley-Morrison K, Hines DA: *Family violence in a cultural perspective: defining, understanding, and combating abuse*, Thousand Oaks, CA, 2004, Sage.

Mapp SC: The effects of sexual abuse as a child on the risk of mothers physically abusing their children: a path analysis using systems theory, *Child Abuse Negl* 30:1293–1310, 2006.

Masters NT: "My strength is not for hurting": men's anti-rape websites and their construction of masculinity and male sexuality, *Sexualities* 13:33–46, 2010.

McFarlane J, Parker B: *Abuse during pregnancy: a protocol for prevention and intervention*, White Plains, NY, 2005, March of Dimes Birth Defects Foundation.

McFarlane JM, Groff JY, O'Brien JA, et al: Prevalence of partner violence against 7,443 African American, white, and Hispanic women receiving care at urban public primary care clinics, *Public Health Nurs* 22:98–107, 2005.

Miller C: Elder abuse: the nurse's perspective, *Clin Gerontol* 28:105–133, 2005.

Nannini A, Lazar J, Berg C, et al: Physical injuries reported on hospital visits for assault during the pregnancy-associated period, *Nurs Res* 57(3):144–149, 2008.

National Coalition of Anti-Violence Programs: *Lesbian, gay, bisexual and transgender domestic violence in the United States in 2007.* Available at http://www.ncavp.org/common/document_files/Reports/2007%20NCAVP%20DV%20REPORT.pdf. Accessed August 20, 2010.

NIMH: *suicide in the U.S.: Statistics and Prevention. NIH Pub No. 06-4594.* Available at http://www.nimh.nih.gov/health/publications/suicide-in-the-us-statistics-and-prevention/index.shtml. 2010. Accessed June 9, 2011.

Niolon PH, Whitaker DJ, Feder L, et al: A multicomponent intervention to prevent partner violence within an existing service intervention, *Prof Psychology Res Pract* 3:264–271, 2009.

O'Reilly R, Wilkes L, Luck L, Jackson D: The efficacy of family support and family preservation services on reducing child abuse and neglect: what the literature reveals, *J Child Health Care* 14(1):82–94, 2010.

Pennington-Zoellner K: Expanding "community" in the community response to intimate partner violence, *J Fam Viol* 24:539–545, 2009.

Peralta RA, Tuttle LA, Steele JL: At the intersection of interpersonal violence, masculinity, and alcohol use: the experiences of heterosexual male perpetrators of intimate partner violence, *Violence against Women* 16:387–409, 2010.

Piquero AR, Brame R, Fagan J, Moffitt TE: Assessing the offending activity of criminal domestic violence suspects: offense specialization, escalation and de-escalation evidence from the Spouse Assault Replication Program, *Public Health Rep* 121(4):409–418, 2006.

Pitts J: Youth gangs, ethnicity and the politics of estrangement, *Youth Policy* 102:101–113, 2009.

Post L, Page C, Conner T, et al: Elder abuse in long-term care: types, patterns, and risk factors, *Res Aging* 32(3):323–348, 2010.

Post LA, Klevens J, Maxwell CD, et al: An examination of whether coordinated community responses affect intimate partner violence, *J Interpers Violence* 25(1):75–93, 2010.

Potter H: Battered black women's use of religious services and spirituality for assistance in leaving abusive relationships, *Violence against Women* 13:262–284, 2007.

Rahn WM, Yoon KS, Garet M, et al: Geographies of trust, *Am Behav Sci* 52:1646–1663, 2009.

Rand MR: National Crime Victimization Survey: criminal victimization, 2008, *Bureau of Justice Statistics Bulletin*, 2009. Available at http://bjs.ojp.usdoj.gov/content/pub/pdf/cv08.pdf. Accessed August 19, 2010.

Regan ME: Implementation and evaluation of a youth violence prevention program for adolescents, *J Sch Nurs* 25:27–33, 2010.

Rhodes K, Cerulli C, Dichter M, et al: "I didn't want to put them through that": the influence of children on victim decision-making in intimate partner violence cases, *J Fam Violence* 25(5):485–493, 2010.

Rivara FP, Anderson ML, Fishman P, et al: Intimate partner violence and health care costs and utilization for children living in the home, *Pediatrics* 120(6):1270–1277, 2007.

Rodriguez CM: Personal contextual characteristics and cognitions: predicting child abuse potential and disciplinary style, *J Interpers Viol* 25(2):315–335, 2010.

Rodriguez CM, Henderson RC: Who spares the rod? Religious orientation, social conformity, and child abuse potential, *Child Abuse Negl* 34:84–94, 2010.

Ross CA: Childhood sexual abuse and psychosomatic symptoms in irritable bowel syndrome, *J Child Sex Abus* 14:27–38, 2005.

Saito AS, Cooke M, Creedy DK, Chaboyer W: Thai women's experience of intimate partner violence during the perinatal period: a case study analysis, *Nurs Health Sci* 11(4):382–387, 2009.

Salmivalli C: Bullying and the peer group: a review, *Aggression Violent Behav* 15:112–120, 2010.

Schoening AM, Greenwood JL, McNichols JA, et al: Effect of an intimate partner violence educational program on the attitudes of nurses, *J Obstet Gynecol Neonatal Nurs* 33:572–579, 2004.

Scott ST: Multiple traumatic experiences and the development of posttraumatic stress disorder, *J Interpers Viol* 22(7):932–938, 2007.

Seto MC, Lalumière ML: What is so sexual about male adolescent sexual offending? A review and test of explanations through meta-analysis, *Psychol Bull* 136:526–575, 2010.

Sheridan D: Legal and forensic nursing responses to family violence. In Humphreys J, Campbell JC, editors: *Family violence and nursing practice*, Philadelphia, 2004, Lippincott, Williams & Wilkins, pp 385–406.

Sheridan DJ, Nash KR: Acute injury patterns of intimate partner violence victims, *Trauma Violence Abuse* 8(3):281–289, 2009.

Sonis J, Langer M: Risk and protective factors for recurrent intimate partner violence in a cohort of low-income inner-city women, *J Fam Violence* 23(7):529–538, 2008.

Steeves RH, Parker B: Adult perspectives on growing up following uxoricide, *J Interpers Violence* 22:1270–1284, 2007.

Stevenson M: Perceptions of juvenile offenders who were abused as children, *J Aggression Maltreat Trauma* 18(4):331–349, 2009.

Stockman J, Campbell J, Celentano D: Sexual violence and HIV risk behaviors among a nationally representative sample of heterosexual American women: the importance of sexual coercion, *J Acquir Immune Defic Syndr* 53:136–143, 2010.

Stover CM, Berkman M, Desai R, Marans S: The efficacy of a police-advocacy intervention for victims of domestic violence: 12 month follow-up data, *Violence against Women* 16:410–425, 2010.

Straus M: Children should never, ever, be spanked no matter what the circumstances. In Loseke DR, Gelles R, Cavanaugh M, editors: *Current controversies on family violence*, Thousand Oaks, CA, 2005, Sage, pp 137–157.

Straus H, Cerulli C, McNutt LA, et al: Intimate partner violence and functional health status: associations with severity, danger, and self-advocacy behaviors, *J Womens Health* 18(5):625–631, 2009.

Sullivan M, Bhuyan R, Senturia K, et al: Participatory action research in practice: a case study in addressing domestic violence in nine cultural communities, *J Interpers Violence* 20:977–995, 2005.

Swanberg J, Macke C, Logan TK: Working women making it work intimate partner violence, employment, and workplace support, *J Interpers Violence* 22:292–311, 2007.

Symes L, McFarlane J, Frazier L, et al: Exploring violence against women and adverse health outcomes in middle age to promote women's health, *Crit Care Nurs Q* 33(3):233–243, 2010.

Tilley DS, Brackley M: Men who batter intimate partners: a grounded theory study of the development of male violence in intimate partner relationships, *Issues Ment Health Nurs* 26:281–297, 2005.

Ting L, Panchanadeswaran S: Barriers to help-seeking among immigrant African women survivors of partner abuse: listening to women's own voices, *J Aggress Maltreat Trauma* 18(8):817–838, 2009.

Tjaden P, Thoennes N: *Full report of the prevalence, incidence, and consequences of violence against women: findings from the National Violence Against Women Survey*, National Institutes of Justice, CDC, Washington, DC, 2000, U.S. Department of Justice.

Trautman D, McCarthy ML, Miller N, et al: Intimate partner violence and Emergency Department screening: Computerized screening versus usual care, *Ann Emerg Med* 49:526–534, 2007.

Ullman SE: The social context of talking about sexual assault, *Talking about sexual assault: Society's response to survivors*, Washington, DC, 2010, American Psychological Association, pp 13–27.

U.S. Department of Health and Human Services, Administration for Children and Families, Administration on Children, Youth and Families, Children's Bureau: *Child maltreatment 2008*, 2010a. Available at http://www.acf.hhs.gov/programs/cb/stats_research/index.htm#can. Accessed August 20, 2010a.

U.S. Department of Health and Human Services, Administration for Children and Families: *Defining child abuse and neglect*, 2010b. Available at http://www.childwelfare.gov/can/defining/. Accessed August 20, 2010.

U.S. Department of Health and Human Services: *Healthy People 2020 Objectives*, Washington, DC, 2010c, Office of Disease Prevention and Health Promotion, USDHHS.

U.S. Department of Health and Human Services: Administration for Children and Families: *Child maltreatment reports*, 2009. Available at http://www.acf.hhs.gov/program/cb/pubs/cm09/index.htm.

U.S. Department of Justice, Office of Justice Programs, Bureau of Justice, Statistics: *Family violence statistics: including statistics on strangers and acquaintances*, 2005. (NCJ 207846). Available at http://bjs.ojp.usdoj.gov/index.cfm?ty=pbdetail&iid=828. Accessed August 20, 2010.

U.S. Department of Justice, Office of Justice Programs, Bureau of Justice Statistics: *Homicide trends in the U.S*, 2007. Available at http://bjs.ojp.usdoj.gov/index.cfm?ty=pbdetail&iid=966. Accessed August 20, 2010.

U.S. Department of Justice, Office of Justice Programs, Bureau of Justice Statistics Bulletin: *National Crime Victimization Survey: Criminal Victimization, 2008* (NCJ 227777), 2009a. Available at http://bjs.ojp.usdoj.gov/content/pub/pdf/cv08.pdf. Accessed August 20, 2010.

U.S. Department of Justice, Office of Justice Programs, Bureau of Justice Statistics Selected Findings: *Female victims of violence* (NCJ 228356), 2009b. Available at http://bjs.ojp.usdoj.gov/content/pub/pdf/fvv.pdf. Accessed August 20, 2010.

U.S. Department of Justice, Office on Violence against Women: *Violence Against Women Act: 15 years working together to end violence*, 2010b. Available at http://www.ovw.usdoj.gov/docs/qa-factsheet.pdf. Accessed August 20, 2010.

U.S. Department of Labor, Bureau of Labor Statistics: *Demographics*, 2010. Available at http://www.bls.gov/cps/demographics.htm#race. Accessed August 20, 2010.

VAWR (Violence Against Women online Resources): *The facts about domestic violence*, 2009. Available at http://vaw.umn.edu/documents/inbriefs/domesticviolence/domesticviolence-color.pdf. Accessed August 20, 2010.

Vervoort MHN, Scholte RHJ, Overbeek G: Bullying and victimization among adolescents: the role of ethnicity and ethnic composition of school class, *J Youth Adolescence* 39:1–11, 2010.

Wallace CM: Measuring changes in attitude, skill and knowledge of undergraduate nursing students after receiving an educational intervention in intimate partner violence, doctoral dissertation, *College of Saint Mary*, 2009. ISBN: 978-110-924-5967967, 2009.

Ward C, Wood A: Intimate partner violence: NP role in assessment, *Am J Nurs Practitioners* 13(10):9–15, 2009.

Weaver TL, Turner PK, Schwarze N, et al: An exploratory examination of the meanings of residential injuries from intimate partner violence, *Women Health* 45(3):85–102, 200, 2007.

Whiting JB, Simmons LA, Havens JR, et al: Intergenerational transmission of violence: the influence of self-appraisals, mental disorders and substance abuse, *J Fam Viol* 24:639–6482009.

Wolff N, Blitz CL, Shi J: Rates of sexual victimization in prison for inmates with and without mental disorders, *Psychiatric Serv* 58(8):1087–1094, 2007.

Wolff N, Shi J, Bachman R: Measuring victimization inside prisons: questioning the questions. (includes abstract), *J Interpers Violence* 23(10):1343–1362, 2008.

Woods SJ, Hall RJ, Campbell JC, Angott DM: *J Midwifery Womens Health* 53(6):538–546, 2008.

Yllo K: Wife rape, *Violence Against Women* 5:1059–1063, 1999.

Zimmerman F, Mercy JA: A better start: child maltreatment prevention as a public health priority, *Zero to Three* 30(5):4–10, 2010.

Zust BL: Partner violence, depression, and recidivism: the case of incarcerated women and why we need programs designed for them, *Issues Ment Health Nurs* 30(4):246–251, 2009.

PART 7

Nurse Roles and Functions in the Community

At one time, the role of the public health nurse was primarily visiting clients at home and identifying cases of communicable disease. Over the decades, the role has become complex and now involves population-centered practice. The role of the nurse focuses on improving the health of individuals and families through the delivery of personal health services, with an emphasis on primary prevention, health promotion, and health protection. Population-centered nursing practice emphasizes the delivery of services and interventions aimed at protecting entire populations from illness, disease, and injury. As the health care system has changed, the need for a comprehensive, population-focused public health system has become more evident. Nurses are able to provide care to individuals, families, and populations including aggregates and communities in a variety of settings and roles.

With increasing emphasis being placed on the community as the client, nurses recognize that to address community health issues, they must be able to meet the needs of the individuals, families, and groups that are the nucleus of the community. In recent decades, the primary practice setting for the nurse was the hospital, but now nurses are caring for clients in many settings. Regardless of the type of client, practice setting, specialty area of practice, or the functional role of the nurse, nurses act as advocates for clients in meeting their needs through the health care system.

This section discusses the roles of manager, consultant, clinical nurse specialist, and nurse practitioner, with particular emphasis on the development of the advocacy role in population-centered practice. Throughout the text, content is applicable to a variety of practice settings, including the more traditional public health practice areas such as the health department. A few other practice settings with close association to population-centered nursing have been highlighted, such as school health, occupational health, home health/hospice, and congregational settings. In the community setting, the field of forensics is receiving increasing attention as an area of practice for public health nurses. This area of practice is a highlight of this text.

CHAPTER 39

The Advanced Practice Nurse in the Community

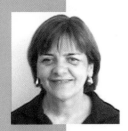

Molly A. Rose, RN, PhD

Molly A. Rose is a professor at Thomas Jefferson University in Philadelphia, Pennsylvania, and previous coordinator of the graduate community health/public health nursing program entitled Community Systems Administration. She is Co-Director of the Jefferson InterProfessional Education Center. She is a clinical nurse specialist in community health nursing and a family nurse practitioner. She has completed research in the areas of HIV and women, caregivers of children with HIV, HIV and the older adult, and interprofessional education and health promotion and the older adult. Dr. Rose's roles in community/public health nursing have included the areas of home health, camp, and parish nursing; she was president of the board of directors of a free clinic for older adults; she was a VISTA (Volunteers in Service to America) nurse in the rural South; and she has been involved in homeless shelters, program planning and evaluation, school health, clinics for the underserved, and academia.

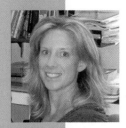

Kellie A. Smith, RN, MSN

Kellie A. Smith is an instructor at Thomas Jefferson University in Philadelphia, Pennsylvania, and is the coordinator of the graduate community health/public health nursing program entitled Community Systems Administration. She is a clinical nurse specialist in community health nursing. She has been involved in NIH/NIDDK (National Institute of Health/National Institute of Diabetes and Digestive and Kidney Diseases) research for type 2 diabetes prevention, the Diabetes Prevention Program. Ms. Smith was also involved with the trial's translational campaign, "Small Steps. Big Rewards," directed by The National Diabetes Education Program (NDEP). Ms. Smith has participated in health care professions' interprofessional education initiatives, including a chronic disease health mentor program. She has assisted students in community activism and philanthropy as the nursing student government faculty advisor.

ADDITIONAL RESOURCES

evolve WEBSITE
http://evolve.elsevier.com/Stanhope
- *Healthy People 2020*
- WebLinks

- Quiz
- Case Studies
- Glossary
- Answers to Practice Application

OBJECTIVES

After reading this chapter, the student should be able to do the following:
1. Briefly discuss the historical development of the roles of the advanced public health nurse and the nurse practitioner.
2. Describe the educational requirements for population-focused advanced practice nurses.
3. Discuss credentialing mechanisms in nursing as they relate to the role of the advanced practice nurse.
4. Compare and contrast the various role functions of population-focused advanced practice nurses.
5. Identify potential arenas of practice.
6. Explore current issues and concerns related to practice.
7. Identify five stressors that may affect nurses in expanded roles.

KEY TERMS

administrator, p. 861
advanced public health nurse, p. 856
certification, p. 858
clinical nurse leader, p. 857
clinical nurse specialist, p. 856
clinician, p. 859
competencies, p. 857
consultant, p. 861
educator, p. 860

faith community nursing, p. 863
Healthy People 2020, p. 864
independent practice, p. 862
institutional privileges, p. 866
interprofessional collaborative practice, p. 867
liability, p. 866
nurse practitioner, p. 856
nursing centers, p. 863

parish nursing, p. 863
portfolios, p. 866
prescriptive authority, p. 865
primary health care, p. 857
professional isolation, p. 866
protocols, p. 860
researcher, p. 862
third-party reimbursement, p. 862
—*See Glossary for definitions*

This chapter explores the roles of the advanced practice nurse in the community. Why, one might ask, is this chapter in the text? For a few good reasons, since it is the intent to provide the BSN student with an understanding of the career opportunities that may be chosen for continuing one's education to the graduate level. For the nurse in a graduate program, the chapter will provide an in-depth understanding of the role in the specialty area that has been chosen. The advanced practice nurse roles described in this chapter offer excellent choices for exciting careers, which will assure satisfaction that a major contribution can be made to making a difference in health outcomes and improved health status of clients at all levels.

The advanced practice nurse is a licensed professional nurse prepared at the master's level or doctoral level to take leadership roles in applying the nursing process and public health sciences to achieve specific health outcomes for the community; this nurse is often referred to as an advanced public health nurse (APHN) or public health clinical nurse specialist (CNS). Since both the American Nurses Association (2007) and the Association of Community Health Nursing Educators (ACHNE, 2007) refer to this specialized role as APHN, this is the title that will be used in this chapter. On the other hand, the advanced practice nurse in the community may be a nurse practitioner (NP). A nurse practitioner is generally a master's-prepared nurse who applies advanced practice nursing knowledge with physical, psychosocial, and environmental assessment skills to respond to common health and illness problems. Since about 2006, NPs were beginning to be prepared at the doctoral level through Doctorate of Nursing Practice Programs (AACN, 2006; NONPF, 2006). The APHN and NP often work in similar settings. However, their client focuses differ. The NP's client is an individual or family, usually in a fixed setting, who has the opportunity to identify individual trends in their practices. The APHN's clients may be individuals, families, groups at risk, or communities, but the ultimate goal is the health of the community as a whole (ANA/Quad Council, 2007; ACHNE, 2007). The APHN always has a population focus and obtains knowledge from nursing, social, and public health sciences to

achieve goals of promoting and protecting the health of populations by creating conditions in which people can optimize their health (ACHNE, 2007; ANA, 2007). Table 39-1 compares the functions taught to the APHN and the NP in their educational programs.

> **NURSING TIP**   *Advanced public health nurses generally view the community as their client even when caring for individuals, families, and groups.*

This chapter provides a history of the educational preparation of the advanced practice nurse. Functions in advanced practice and arenas for practice are discussed. Issues and concerns, role negotiation, and areas of role stress relative to the APHN and the NP in the community are also discussed.

HISTORICAL PERSPECTIVE

Changes in the health care system and nursing have occurred in the past few decades because of a shift in societal demands and needs. Trends that have influenced the roles of the APHN and NP include a shift from institution-based health care to population-focused health care, improvements in technology, self-care, cost-containment measures, accountability to the client, third-party reimbursement, and demands for making technology-related care more responsive to the client.

The CNS role began in the early 1960s and grew out of a need to improve client care. CNSs educate clients, communities, populations, families, and individuals; provide social and psychological support to clients; serve as role models to other nursing staff; consult with communities, nurses, and staff in other disciplines; and conduct clinical nursing research (Robertson and Baldwin, 2007).

In the United States during the 1960s, a shortage of physicians occurred, and there was an increasing tendency among physicians to specialize. The number of physicians who might have provided medical care to communities and families across

TABLE 39-1 HOW TO DISTINGUISH THE SIMILARITIES AND DIFFERENCES IN FUNCTIONS OF ADVANCED PUBLIC HEALTH NURSES (APHNs) AND NURSE PRACTITIONERS (NPs)

FUNCTION	NP PROGRAM	APHN PROGRAM
Comprehensive assessment	Always	Often
Physiology and pharmacology	Almost always	Often
Diagnosis and management	Always	Often
Systems	Individual/family focus	More systems focused
Leadership	Usually	Almost always
Program planning and evaluation	Less often	Always in community and public health
Research	Generally	Generally

the nation was reduced. As this trend continued, a serious gap in primary health care services developed. Primary health care includes both public health and primary care services.

The NP movement began in 1965 at the University of Colorado by Dr. Loretta Ford and Dr. Henry Silver. They determined that the morbidity among medically deprived children could be decreased by educating nurses to provide well-child care to children of all ages. Nursing practice for these pediatric nurse practitioners included the identification, assessment, and management of common acute and chronic health problems, with appropriate referral of more complex problems to physicians (Silver, Ford, and Stearly, 1967). The priorities of the nursing profession have traditionally been to care for and support the well, the worried well, and the ill, offering physical care services previously provided only by physicians. Preparing nurses as primary health care providers was not only consistent with traditional nursing, but also was responsive to society's critical need for primary health care services, including health promotion and illness prevention (Hooker and McCaig, 2001).

In 1965, the physician assistant (PA) role was initiated at Duke University. This program was intended to attract former military corpsmen for training as medical extenders (Hooker and Berlin, 2002). Nurse practitioners are often combined into a single category with other non-physician providers and are mistakenly portrayed as physician extenders. This misinterpretation of the intended role is addressed by one of the founders, Dr. Loretta Ford:

> As conceptualized, the nurse practitioner was always intended to be a nursing model focused on the promotion of health in daily living, on growth and development of children in families, and on the prevention of disease and disability. Nursing as a discipline and a profession evolved not because there was a shortage of physicians but because of societal needs. The early plans did not include preparing nurses to assume medical functions. The interests were in health promotion and disease prevention for aggregate populations in community settings, including underserved groups. These were the hallmarks of community-oriented nursing (Ford, 1986).

A report issued by the U.S. Department of Health, Education, and Welfare (now USDHHS), *Extending the Scope of Nursing Practice* (1971), helped convince Congress of the value of NPs as primary health care providers. The Nurse Training Act of 1971 (PL 92-150) and the comprehensive Health Manpower Act of 1971 (PL 92-157) provided education monies for many NP and PA programs through the 1970s and into the 1980s. Similarly, in the 1970s the concept of an expanded practice role for nurses was garnering interest in Canada. Canadian nurses saw the NP role as an opportunity to expand their scope of practice and perform the role in various settings largely outside tertiary care (Bajnok and Wright, 1993). The United Kingdom has increased their advanced practice nurse programs to educate and monitor the role that has been in place for about 20 years. They continue to define the role (RCN, 2010).

Graduate education for nursing is changing. AACN (2007) called for the creation of a new nursing role, clinical nurse leader (CNL). The clinical nurse leader is defined as a nurse who is a master's prepared generalist who functions at the micro-system level and assumes accountability for health care outcomes for a specific group of clients within a unit or area (AACN, 2007). In 2010, there were approximately 100 CNL programs in the U.S. (AACN, 2010). In addition, the AACN has determined that the degree for nurses seeking advanced practice should be the Doctor of Nursing Practice (DNP) (AACN, 2006). (See the Cutting Edge box.)

THE CUTTING EDGE *The AACN has determined that the preferred preparation for specialty advanced practice nursing should be the Doctor of Nursing Practice (DNP), which is defined by specialty nursing practices that focus on either advanced practice nursing (nurse practitioner) or on aggregates, systems, or organizations (APHN) (ACHNE, 2007; AACN, 2006). The latter designation includes Advanced Public Health Nursing (ACHNE, 2007). In 2010 over 100 DNP programs were accepting students (AACN, 2010).*

COMPETENCIES

The Quad Council of Public Health Nursing Organizations, in 2003, developed a set of national public health competencies specific for public health nursing practice that are based on the *Core Competencies for Public Health Professionals* authored by the Council on Linkages Between Academia and Public Health Practice (2001). The core competencies were designed to serve as a starting point for academic and practice organizations to understand, assess, and meet training and workforce needs for health professionals practicing in public health; they were updated in 2009 (Council on Linkages, 2009). The Quad Council competencies are more specific to public health nursing and were developed to assist agencies that employ public health nurses, as well as academic settings that prepare public health nurses, to facilitate education, orientation, training, and lifelong learning (Quad Council, 2003). The competencies are categorized into eight domains and are applied to two levels of public health nursing practice: the staff nurse/generalist role and the manager/consultant/CNS. The domains, which were updated, include core areas of analytic assessment, policy development/program planning, communication, cultural competency, community dimensions of practice, basic public health science, financial planning and management, and leadership and systems thinking skills (Quad Council, 2009). (See the Linking Content to Practice box.) The American Nurses Association (ANA, 2007) published *Scope and Standards for Public Health Nursing Practice*, which includes population-focused standards of care in the following areas: assessment, diagnosis, outcome identification, planning, assurance, evaluations and standards for professional performance in quality of care, performance appraisal, education, collegiality, ethics, collaboration, research, and resource utilization. This document is a collaboration between the ANA and the American Public Health Association-Public Health Nursing section's definition and role of Public Health Nursing Practice (1996).

LINKING CONTENT TO PRACTICE

In this chapter, emphasis is placed on the role of the advanced public health nurse in the community. The Quad Council's Domains of Public Health Nursing Practice (2009) are categorized into two levels of public health nursing practice: the generalist/staff role and the manager/CNS/consultant/executive role. The latter role includes a higher level mastery of skills and competencies. Their fifth domain, Community Dimensions of Practice Skills, lists the competencies as: establishes and maintains linkages with key stakeholders; utilizes leadership, team building, negotiation, and conflict resolution skills to build community partnerships; collaborates with community partners to promote the health of the population; identifies how public and private organizations operate within a community; accomplishes effective community engagements; identifies community assets and available resources; develops, implements, and evaluates a community public health assessment; and describes the role of government in the delivery of community health services. These skills are clearly consistent with the APHN role and are at an advanced mastery level. This is in contrast with the generalist/staff public health nurse where the expected level of performance mastery for this domain is at the knowledge level. Thus, if an agency planned to conduct health education programs within a community, the APHN would take leadership roles in developing, implementing, and evaluating a needs assessment and interacting with community stakeholders to assist with conducting the health education programs that would be most relevant and accessible to the community.

EDUCATIONAL PREPARATION

Educational preparation for the APHN includes a minimum of a master's degree and is based on a synthesis of current knowledge and research in nursing, public health, and other scientific disciplines. In addition to performing the functions of the generalist in population-focused nursing, the specialist possesses clinical experience in interprofessional planning, organizing, community empowerment, delivering and evaluating service, political and legislative activities, and assuming a leadership role in interventions that have a positive effect on the health of the community. ACHNE recommendations for graduate nursing education for the public health nurse specialty are guided by the IOM's 2003 report *Who Will Keep the Public Healthy?* (2003), ANA's *Public Health Nursing Scope and Standards of Practice* (2007), and AACN's *DNP Essentials* (2006). They identified five role characteristics of APHNs: (1) population-level health care focus, (2) ecological view, (3) responsibility for health outcomes for populations, (4) partnership/collaboration using an interprofessional approach, and (5) leadership in practice. The curriculum areas for the APHN that were identified are population-centered nursing theory and practice, interprofessional practice, leadership, systems thinking, biostatistics, epidemiology, environmental health sciences, health policy and management, social and behavioral sciences, public health informatics, genomics, health communication, cultural competence, community-based participatory research, global health, policy and law and public health ethics (ACHNE, 2007). In addition to didactic content, graduate education for the APHN must include practicum experience that takes place at the population level, be grounded in the ecological perspective, and include the measurement of outcomes (ACHNE, 2007).

In contrast to the APHN, educational preparation of the NP has not always been at the graduate level. Early NP programs were continuing education certificate programs, and the baccalaureate degree was not always a requirement. At present, however, NPs are required to hold master's degrees and encouraged to obtain a practice doctorate (AACN, 2006). The curriculum prepares NPs to perform a wide range of professional nursing functions including assessing and diagnosing, conducting physical examinations, ordering laboratory and other diagnostic tests, developing and implementing treatment plans for some acute and chronic illnesses, prescribing medications, monitoring client status, educating and counseling clients, and consulting and collaborating with and referring to other providers (AACN, 1996). Many institutions are offering combined CNS/NP programs. A 2006 AACN position statement calls for DNP education for advanced practice nurses and nurses seeking top systems/organizational roles. The eight foundational essentials for DNP programs are knowledge with a scientific underpinning; organizational and systems leadership; clinical scholarship; information systems; policy; collaboration; prevention and population health; and advanced nursing practice (AACN, 2006).

CREDENTIALING

Certification examinations for advanced practice nurses are offered by the American Nurses Credentialing Center (ANCC). The purpose of professional certification is to confirm knowledge and expertise and provide recognition of professional achievement in a defined area of nursing. Certification is a means of assuring the public that nurses who claim to be competent at an advanced level have had their credentials verified through examination (ANCC, 2009). Although certification itself is not mandatory, many state boards of nursing require that nurses in advanced practice, particularly those in an NP role, be nationally certified to practice.

The American Nurses Association (ANA) began its certification program in 1973 and has offered NP certification examinations since 1976. The American Nurses Credentialing Center was opened in 1991 and offers certification in NP, Advanced Practice, and CNS specialty areas. Until 2009 a nurse could also be certified as a generalist or as a BSN-prepared specialist in community health. Since 1985, the basic qualifications for certification as an NP have been a baccalaureate degree in nursing and successful completion of a formal NP program. As of 1992, a master's or higher degree in nursing is required for NP certification through the ANCC.

Examination topics for the NP certification examination include clinical management, professional role and policy, NP and client relationship, assessment, research, and health promotion and disease prevention (ANCC, 2010). The American Academy of Nurse Practitioners also has national competency-based certification examinations in three areas: family, adult, and gerontological nurse practitioners (AANP, 2010).

The certification examination for CNS in public/community health nursing was first offered in October 1990. Qualifications for this examination include a master's or higher degree in nursing with a specialization in community/public health nursing practice. Effective in 1998, eligibility requirements included holding a master's or higher degree in nursing with a specialization in community/public health nursing or holding a baccalaureate or higher degree in nursing and a master's degree in public health with a specialization in community/public health nursing. In 2009, the ANCC Commission renamed the certification exam from Clinical Nurse Specialist in Public/Community Health to Advanced Public Health Nursing. Along with the name change, the eligibility criteria were expanded to accept a variety of graduate education preparation in public/community health. (See the Did You Know? box.) Those who complete a master's degree in nursing in community/public health (which includes a minimum of 500 practicum hours), or a master's in public health degree and successfully pass the certification examination will be eligible to use the credential of Advanced Public Health Nurse–Board Certified (APHN-BC) (ANCC, 2010). Nurses who complete a master's degree in nursing in community/public health with additional courses in advanced pathophysiology, advanced pharmacology, and advanced health assessment, complete a minimum of 500 practicum hours and pass the examination, will be eligible to use the credential of Public Health Clinical Nurse Specialist–Board Certified (PHCNS-BC) (ANCC, 2010). Up until 2015, nurses who have a graduate degree in an area other than community/public health nursing and complete 2000 clinical hours of advanced practice public/community health nursing within the last 3 years are also eligible to sit for this examination and use the credential of APHN-BC. Examination topics for both distinctions include foundations of advanced public/community health; application of developmental theories; epidemiology; biostatistics; research evaluation; methods and utilization; public, community, and

environmental health assessment; strategies to improve public/community health; health promotion; disease prevention; risk reduction; theories and concepts of health behaviors; health screening and counseling; populations and communities education; health systems; organization and networks; and leadership concepts and professionalism (ANCC, 2010).

Certification for the APHN and NP is for 5 years. To maintain certification, the nurse must submit documentation of current RN licensure and meet a practice and continuing education requirement within the specialty area.

> **DID YOU KNOW?**   *There are two distinctions for APHN certification. The first is for those who complete a master's degree in nursing in community/public health, which includes a minimum of 500 practicum hours, or a master's degree in public health, and successfully pass the certification examination. They will be eligible to use the credential of Advanced Public Health Nurse–Board Certified (APHN-BC). The second is for those nurses who complete a master's degree in nursing in community/public health with additional courses in advanced pathophysiology, advanced pharmacology, and advanced health assessment, to complete a minimum of 500 practicum hours and pass the examination. They will be eligible to use the credential of Public Health Clinical Nurse Specialist–Board Certified (PHCNS-BC) (ANCC, 2010).*

ADVANCED PRACTICE ROLES

APNs holding a master's degree in nursing and specializing in public health nursing, in community health nursing, or as a nurse practitioner have many roles, some of which will be described here. It should be noted that the "nursing role in the APHN is not distinguished by the sites in which the nurses practice, but rather by the perspective, knowledge base, and principles that focus on care of populations" (ACHNE, 2007, p 16). The APHN's role characteristics include a focus on population health such as population and community assessment; advocacy and policy-setting at the organizational, community, and state levels; ecological view for large-scale program planning, project management; and leadership and partnership building. APHNs deliver population-focused services, programs, and research (ACHNE, 2007; Robertson and Baldwin, 2007).

Clinician

Most of the differences between the roles of the APHN and the NP are seen in clinical practice. Although the APHN's practice includes nursing directed at individuals, families, and groups, the primary responsibility is to take a leadership role in the overall assessment, planning, development, coordination, and evaluation of innovative programs to meet identified community health needs. The APHN provides the direction for population-focused health care by identifying and documenting health needs and resources in a particular community and in collaborating with population-focused nurse generalists, other health professionals, and consumers (ACHNE, 2007). Practicing within the role of clinician, the APHN is involved in conducting community assessments; identifying needs of populations at

BOX 39-1   EXAMPLE OF A *HEALTHY PEOPLE 2020* OBJECTIVE AND SELECTED ADVANCED PRACTICE NURSING ACTIVITIES

Objective

Under Mental Health (objective MHMD-1): Reduce suicide rate to no more than 10.2 suicide deaths per 100,000 people.

Activities

- Review recent literature and epidemiology of suicide.
- Provide in-service education programs to groups of health professionals related to groups at risk for suicide and related assessment and screening tools for early detection and treatment of depression.
- Become active in legislation activities related to firearm access.
- Assess individual clients for depression and suicide risk.

risk; and planning, implementing, and evaluating population-focused programs to achieve health goals, including health promotion and disease prevention activities. The APHN ultimately works toward the goals of promoting and protecting the health of populations by creating conditions in which people can optimize their health (ANA, 2007).

The NP applies advanced practice nursing knowledge and physical, psychosocial, and environmental assessment skills to manage common health and illness problems of clients of all ages and both sexes. The NP's primary client is the individual and family. In the direct role of clinician, the NP assesses health risks and health and illness status, as well as the response to illness of individuals and families. The NP also diagnoses actual or potential health problems; decides on treatment plans jointly with clients; intervenes to promote health, to protect against disease, to treat illness, to manage chronic disease, and to limit disability; and evaluates with the client and other primary care team members about how effective and comprehensive the nursing intervention may be in providing continuity of care (AACN, 1996; NONPF, 2006). Despite the setting of the practice nurse practitioner, the practice can be population focused. These interventions often include community assessment and analysis, case finding, an emphasis on prevention, and participation in public policy. An advanced practice nurse in the community may work in an agency or setting where the caseload consists of individuals who present themselves for services. The APHN goal would be to identify others in the community who may be at risk and in need of the services. Outreach activities can accomplish this while also trying to accomplish the goals and objectives of *Healthy People 2020* (Box 39-1).

The ability of NPs to diagnose and treat has increased the provision of health care, teaching, and client compliance with treatment plans. The amount of physician involvement in the NP's practice is generally directed through state legislation (Phillips, 2010). Frequently, the NP will use protocols or algorithms that have been previously agreed on by the physician and the NP. These documents, required by some states, serve as standing orders for the management of certain illnesses. As of 2010, all states have passed legislation, either partial or full, granting NP's supervisory, collaborative, or independent authority to practice.

Each state has differing regulatory and legislative mandates in regards to NP areas of practice authority, reimbursement, and prescriptive authority. Work is progressing on a Consensus Model for APRN Regulation that includes standardized regulatory language intended to improve access to client care by eliminating practice barriers across states (Phillips, 2010).

An important area for both APHNs and NPs to include in their advanced practice is health promotion/disease prevention. Within the past several decades, there has been a growing belief that the most effective way of dealing with major health problems is through prevention. This requires refocusing the health care system, identifying aggregates (populations) at risk, introducing risk reduction interventions, teaching people that they control their own health, and encouraging health promotion and disease prevention behaviors. It has been predicted that there will be an even greater emphasis on population-focused care and that nursing will increasingly be viewed as the way to address many of the health care problems that plague society in this new millennium (ACHNE, 2007; ANA, 2007). The U.S. Department of Health and Human Services (USDHHS, 2010) develops national objectives for promoting health and preventing disease. Since 1997, this initiative, called *Healthy People,* has set and monitored national health objectives to meet a broad range of health needs, encourage collaboration across sectors, guide individuals toward making informed health decisions as well as measure the impact of prevention activities. This campaign is essential for APHNs and NPs working toward the goal of a healthier nation. Nurses and advanced practice nurses may also use *The Guide to Clinical Preventative Services* to address health promotion and disease prevention (USDHHS/AHRQ/USPSTF, 2009). NPs and APHNs are especially involved in helping to meet the proposed objectives in the access to health services, educational and community-based programs, and public health infrastructure domains.

Population-Focused Intervention

The following example illustrates a population-focused intervention. An APHN was recently hired at a community hospital in the hospital's community health department. Traditionally, this department provided excellent health education and screening programs to individuals in the surrounding communities. However, outreach activities did not occur. After reviewing the data on attendance at community health events, the APHN developed and implemented a needs assessment in three neighboring communities not attending the events. In one neighborhood, consisting of 1800 apartments, 85% of the population was middle-income African Americans of all ages. The needs assessment revealed a strong interest in health promotion and disease prevention but nevertheless a lack of participation. The APHN developed a collaborative relationship with churches and community groups in the neighborhood. Health fairs and events were initiated. (See the Levels of Prevention box.)

Educator

Nurses in advanced practice function in several indirect nursing care roles. The educator role of the APHN and NP includes health education within a nursing framework (as opposed to health educators who may not have a nursing background) and professional nurse educator (faculty) roles.

The APHN identifies groups at risk within a community and implements, for example, health education interventions. The APHN and NP increase wellness and contribute to maintaining and promoting health by teaching the importance of good nutrition, physical exercise, stress management, and a healthy lifestyle. They provide education about disease processes and the importance of following treatment regimens. In addition, they provide anticipatory guidance and educate clients on the use of medications, diet, birth control methods, and other therapeutic procedures (Logan, 2005; NONPF, 2006; ACHNE, 2007). They also counsel clients, families, groups, and the community on the importance of assuming responsibility for their own health. This education may occur on an individual, family, or group level, in an institutional, ambulatory, or home setting, or it may occur in the community with vulnerable at-risk populations.

As professional nurse educators, the APHN and NP provide formal and informal teaching of staff nurses and undergraduate and graduate students in nursing and other disciplines (Figure 39-1). They also serve as role models by instructing (or being a preceptor to) students in advanced practice in the clinical setting.

Administrator

The APHN and NP may function in administrative roles. As a health **administrator,** they may be responsible for all administrative matters within an agency setting. They may be responsible for and have direct or indirect authority and supervision over the organization's staff and client care. In this capacity, nurses in advanced practice serve as decision makers and problem solvers. They may also be involved in other business and management aspects such as supporting and managing personnel; budgeting; establishing quality control mechanisms; and program planning and influencing policies, public relations, and marketing (Logan, 2005; ACHNE, 2007).

Consultant

Consultation is an important part of practice for APHNs and NPs. Consultation involves problem solving with an individual, family, or community to improve health care delivery. Steps of the consultation process include assessing the problem, determining the availability and feasibility of resources, proposing solutions, and assisting with implementing a solution, if appropriate (AACN, 1996; NONPF, 2006). The APHN and NP may serve as a formal or informal **consultant** to other nurses, providing them with information on improving client care. They may also consult with physicians and other health care providers or with organizations or schools to improve the health care

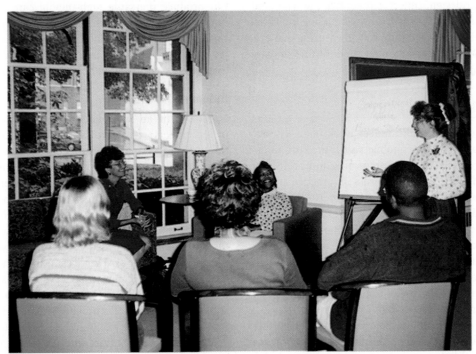

FIGURE 39-1 An advanced practice public health nurse leads a training session for a group of congregational nurses.

of clients. For example, nurse consultants are often used at the district or state level of public health departments. APHNs and NPs work closely with nurse supervisors, other nurse practitioners, and staff public health nurses to develop programs and improve the services provided to clients at clinics and in the home. Nurse consultants in the public health arena may work with all other public health nurses or may work in departments as members of an interprofessional team such as maternal–child health, chronic diseases, or family planning.

Researcher

Improvement in nursing practice depends on the commitment of nurses to developing and refining knowledge through research. Practicing APHNs and NPs are in ideal positions to identify researchable nursing problems related to the communities they serve. They can apply their research findings to the community health practice setting.

All APHNs and most NPs are trained in the research process and, as researchers, can conduct their own investigations and collaborate with doctorate-prepared nurses, answering questions related to nursing practice and primary health care. The acts of identifying, defining, and investigating clinical nursing problems and reporting findings encourages peer relationships with other professions and contributes to health care policy and decision making (Logan, 2005; Harne-Britner and Schafer, 2009). For example, APHNs in administrative, consultant, or practitioner roles encounter situations daily that need further investigating (e.g., non-compliance with certain public health regimens or immunization schedules). They may, anecdotally or through needs assessments, identify a trend that, if examined, could be dealt with through population-based strategies. (See the Evidence-Based Practice box.) APHNs and NPs may collaborate with population-focused nurses at all levels to develop the research design, collect and analyze the data, and determine the implications for further use of nursing interventions identified. APHNs play a critical role in ensuring that evidence-based research is shared and integrated into health care practice (Harne-Britner and Schafer, 2009).

ARENAS FOR PRACTICE

Regardless of where public health nurses work (e.g., schools, homes, clinics, jails, shelters, or mobile vans), the core interventions to accomplish the goals of promoting and protecting the health of populations is similar across all practice arenas. An Intervention Wheel model was developed to define the scope of public health nursing practice by type of intervention and level of practice (see Chapter 9). Interventions are actions that the public health nurse takes on behalf of individuals, families, systems, and communities (Minnesota Department of Health, 2001). Positions for NPs and APHNs vary greatly in terms of scope of practice, degree of responsibility, power and authority, working conditions, creativity, and reward structure (Logan, 2005; Robertson and Baldwin, 2007). These factors and the effects on practice are influenced by nurse practice acts and other legislation (e.g., reimbursement and prescriptive privileges) that govern the legal practice in each state (Phillips,

EVIDENCE-BASED PRACTICE

Based on results of a needs assessment survey of 10 questions that addressed the background and needs of ninth- and tenth-grade students at a local high school, a youth violence prevention program was implemented and evaluated by an advanced public health nurse. Results of the needs assessment showed that 88% (*n* = 53) of the students personally had been exposed to some form of violence, such as gun violence, hitting, and stabbings and 72% (*n* = 43) reported committing acts of violence. In addition, 68% (*n* = 41) of the students reported associating with individuals who commit various acts of violence, and 63% (*n* = 50) reported seeing a gun, while four students (7%) reported using a gun. Thirty-six students (60%) reported that they never had a class on violence-related topics. Content of the program developed and implemented by the APHN included material on gun and gang violence, dating violence, and anger management/conflict resolution. Teaching strategies were role-playing, group activities, and a field trip to a trauma program for youths at a local hospital. A pre-test was conducted prior to the program and again in one month at the end of the program. A one-way *t*-test identified an increase in knowledge and skills in several areas after program implementation. Skills acquired included therapeutically resolving violent disputes and methods to prevent different types of dating violence. This program provides a blueprint of an adolescent violence prevention program that could be replicated in other communities/settings.

From Regan ME: Implementation and evaluation of a youth violence prevention program for adolescents, *J School Nurs* 25(1):27-33, 2009.

2010). The following areas include traditional as well as alternative practice settings for APHNs and NPs.

Primary Care

Research indicates that the opportunities for APNs in primary care settings increased throughout the past decades, and this trend is expected to continue (Laurant et al, 2009). Evidence has supported that appropriately trained nurses in primary care can produce the same high-quality care and achieve equally positive health outcomes for clients as physicians. In general, preliminary research found no appreciable differences between physicians and nurses in health outcomes for clients, process of care, resource utilization, or cost (Laurant et al, 2009).

Independent Practice

Nurses form an independent practice for several reasons, including personal or professional desire to break new ground for nursing and to meet health care needs within a community. It is important to investigate the state's nurse practice act to determine the limitations and the laws related to this arrangement. For example, NPs may provide a more comprehensive array of health services in states where they have legislative authority to prescribe drugs. Nurses in many states have successfully lobbied for third-party reimbursement for all RNs who provide direct care services to individual clients (Phillips, 2010). The independent practice option is more likely to be chosen by NPs and APHNs in states that have established legislation to provide for this nursing practice.

Another option for NPs and APHNs interested in independent practice is to contract with physicians or organizations to provide certain services for their clients or staff. Nurses need to define a service package and market it attractively. An example is providing a home visit to new parents after 2 weeks to assess the newborn, respond to parental concerns, and provide counseling and anticipatory guidance about nutrition, development, and immunization needs. This service may be marketed to pediatricians and family practice physicians who would offer or recommend the service to their clients as an option. An NP may negotiate with a local school board to provide preschool children with health examinations or physical assessments before the children participate in sports. Under a contract, APHNs may develop and implement health and safety programs on accident prevention and health promotion activities for small companies.

Nursing Centers

Nursing centers or clinics, a type of joint practice developed by advanced practice nurses, provide opportunities for collaborative relationships for APHNs, NPs, baccalaureate-prepared nurses, other health care professionals, and community members (Anderko, Lundeen, and Bartz, 2006; Paterson, Duffett-Leger, and Cruttenden, 2009). Primary health services may be provided by NPs, depending on state legislation. Community APHNs, along with nurses and nursing students, may identify aggregates at risk and work in partnership with the community to implement risk-reduction activities (Anderko, Lundeen, and Bartz, 2006). A central mission of nurse-managed clinics is community development such as heath care accessibility and resources; public involvement; interprofessional practice; and health promotion and disease prevention supported by the principles of primary health care (Paterson, Duffett-Leger, and Cruttenden, 2009). Nursing center models are discussed in more detail in Chapter 21.

Faith Community Nursing/Parish Nursing

Faith community nursing, also known as parish nursing, is a concept that began in the late 1960s in the United States when increasing numbers of churches employed registered nurses to provide holistic, preventive health care to congregation members. Faith community nursing is a model of care that uses nurses based within faith communities such as churches and synagogues to provide health services to the members of those communities. The faith community/parish nurse functions as health educator, counselor, group facilitator, client advocate, and liaison to community resources (Health Ministries Association, 2005; McGinnis and Zoske, 2008).

Because these activities are complementary to the population-focused practice of APHNs, faith community nurses either have a strong public health background or work directly with both baccalaureate-prepared nurses and APHNs. Faith community nurses positively affect client outcomes by providing health services in health promotion and disease prevention, chronic disease management, and culturally sensitive services (McGinnis and Zoske, 2008). See Chapter 45 for further discussion about faith community/parish nursing.

> **NURSING TIP**　*The faith community nurse role, also known as parish nursing, has been integrated into some nurses' volunteer activities.*

Institutional Settings

Ambulatory/Outpatient Clinics

NPs and APHNs may be employed in the primary care unit of an institution (e.g., the ambulatory center or outpatient clinic). These centers/clinics generally provide hospital referral, hospital follow-up care, and health maintenance and management for non-emergent problems. The population served is usually more culturally and economically diverse and represents a larger geographic area than that served by private practices. In these outpatient settings, NPs typically practice jointly with physicians to provide acute and chronic primary care. Hospital acute care outpatient services may include clinics for general medicine or family practice, or specialty-oriented clinics, such as pediatric, obstetric-gynecologic, and ear-nose-and-throat clinics. Outpatient clinics organized for chronic care may be problem-oriented (e.g., hypertension, diabetes, or acquired immunodeficiency syndrome [AIDS] clinics).

Emergency Departments

Persons without access to health care, such as the medically uninsured and the homeless, often do not seek health care services until they become ill. Hospital emergency departments (EDs) are increasingly used for non-emergent primary care. Although this is an inappropriate use of expensive health services, it is a result of the current system, which limits access to routine and preventive health care. Emergency department care is one of the most expensive services offered in health care today (Wood et al, 2010).

Emergency services often require long waits for persons who have non-emergency problems. Fast-track/non-emergency sections of ERs have become commonplace to accommodate these situations. NPs in these settings see clients with non-emergent problems and provide the necessary treatment and appropriate counseling (Campo et al, 2008). APHNs may also help educate clients on the importance of health care and how to gain access to the preventive health care system. APHNs, with their knowledge of community health resources, can help ensure that psychosocial needs are assessed and met. APHNs can act as liaisons or go-betweens for community programs that serve the needs of special populations (Hooker et al, 2008).

Long-Term Care Facilities

The elderly age group represents the fastest growing population (especially those over 85 years of age) in the United States (Administration on Aging, 2009). The data reveal a long anticipated trend that we are living longer, resulting in higher percentages of elderly Americans. By 2030, it is projected that one in five people will be aged 65 or older (or 70 million people). Statistics reveal a shortage of advanced practice nurses specializing in gerontological nursing to care for the growing older adult population (Thornlow, Auerhahn, and Stanley, 2006).

Gerontology is an increasingly important field of study, and many courses are available on health needs of older adults. NPs and APHNs with an interest in geriatrics need to continue their education in this area to increase their knowledge and skills specific to this at-risk aggregate (Thornlow, Auerhahn, and Stanley,

2006). Many NPs and APHNs view long-term care facilities as exciting areas for practice and a way of increasing quality of care while containing costs for older adults and the disabled. U.S. federal legislation provides reimbursement for NPs and APHNs to provide care to clients in Medicare-certified nursing homes and to recertify eligible clients for continued Medicare coverage. In long-term care facilities where clients are not ambulatory, NPs and APHNs may make regular nursing home rounds, assess the health status of clients, and provide care and counseling as appropriate. In long-term care facilities in which the residents are more ambulatory, NPs and APHNs may also provide health maintenance and other primary health care services to the nursing home clients.

Industry/Occupational Health

The *Healthy People 2020* (USDHHS, 2010) objectives include a section on occupational health and safety with goals to reduce work-related injuries and deaths. Thousands of new cases of disease and death occur each year from occupational exposures.

APHNs and NPs are increasingly useful in occupational health programs as business and industry seek ways to control their health care costs and to provide preventive and primary on-site care services. These services help reduce absences from work and increase productivity of workers. The APHN in an industrial/occupational setting assesses the health needs of the organization on the basis of claims data, cost–benefit health research, results of employee health screening, and the perceived needs of employee groups (Mellor and St. John, 2007). With their advanced administrative and clinical skills, APHNs plan, implement, and evaluate company-wide health programs.

NPs in occupational settings generally practice independently, with physician consultation as needed. The health and welfare of the worker is the major concern. Responsibilities for maintaining employee health include direct nursing care for on-the-job injuries. Often clinical responsibility extends to monitoring work-related illnesses such as diabetes and hypertension. Employees may elect to see the NP for common problems and see a physician for more complicated problems. The role of the occupational health nurse is discussed in Chapter 43.

Government

U.S. Public Health Service

The U.S. Public Health Service operates the National Health Service Corps, which places health providers in federally designated areas with shortages of health workers, and the Indian Health Service, which provides health services to Native Americans.

During the 1970s, both the Corps and the Indian Health Service offered to pay to educate RNs to become nurse practitioners if they would promise to work for a designated period of time with the Public Health Service. These programs were discontinued during the 1980s when more emphasis was placed on physician recruitment. In 1988, Congress reauthorized two loan repayment programs for NPs' education—one with the Corps and one with the Indian Health Service. More recently in 2009, the American Recovery and Reinvestment Act invested an additional $300 million into the Health Corps hoping to double its

field strength by providing more scholarships and loan repayment options for health care providers. Depending on the needs of the area, an NP employed by the Public Health Service may be the only health care provider in the setting or may practice with a group of providers to serve a rural, an urban underserved, or a Native American population (USDHHS, 2010).

Armed Services

The increased availability of physicians reduced the active recruitment of nurses to advanced degree programs by the armed forces during the 1980s. NPs are used in ambulatory clinics serving active duty and retired personnel and their dependents. APHNs use their skills with needs assessment and program planning/evaluation to develop programs aimed at improving the health of the aggregate military population (U.S. Department of Defense/Today's Military, 2010).

Public Health Departments

Public health departments are increasingly employing advanced practice nurses with master's degrees. These APHNs and NPs have administrative and clinical skills to work collaboratively with physicians and to manage and implement clinical services provided by the health departments. Home care and hospice services are nursing sections in many public health departments and require the services of population-oriented nurse clinical specialists.

Health departments also provide primary care services in well-child clinics, family planning clinics, and general adult primary health care clinics. A public health department may use NPs and APHNs, depending on the size of the department, the department's health priorities in the community, and financial constraints.

APHNs should possess basic competencies for responding to disasters whether the health threats are natural, intentional, or technological (mass casuality incidents, unfolding infectious disease outbreaks, bioterrorism, or evolving environmental disasters). APHNs are well positioned to collaborate with leaders of the community to develop and implement systems level preparedness and response plans for popsulations before, during, and after an event (ACHNE, 2008; Jakeway et al, 2008; Kuntz et al, 2008).

Schools

School health nursing, discussed in Chapter 42, involves comprehensive assessment and management of care, with particular emphasis on health education, to promote healthy behaviors in children and their families. Innovative practice occurs in school nursing (Nelson, 2009). APHNs and NPs may be employed as school health nurses by school boards or county health departments to provide specific services to schools, such as confirming that immunization status is current; performing hearing and vision screenings; and providing many organizational, community assessment, and political functions. School-based health services may be staffed by APHNs and/or nurses prepared as school, pediatric, or family nurse practitioners. Services provided by these advanced nurse practitioners include not only basic health screening, but also monitoring of children with chronic health problems and finding health care for children with limited access to medical care. These nurses work collaboratively with parents, community leaders, educators, and physicians to ensure that each child within the school community receives needed services. APHNs and NPs may be well suited to manage school health services if they meet specific criteria developed by individual states.

Other Arenas

Home Health Agencies

Major legislative changes in Medicare and third-party reimbursement for hospital services resulted in unprecedented growth in the home health care industry through the 1990s. Home health care is less expensive than extended hospital care and thus is an attractive option for third-party payers (Madigan and Vanderboom, 2005; Schober, 2007). In addition, equipment and drug companies are developing products for home use, physicians and hospitals are exploring the development of home services, and consumers are demanding more services. Advanced practice nurses have traditionally been involved in home care in many capacities. Because of their knowledge and skills in the following areas, NPs and APHNs are well-qualified to provide home health care that yields positive outcomes for clients and their families. Home health APNs engage in holistic health assessments and coordinate services with an interprofessional team for clients with complex health needs; are involved in coaching, consultation, evaluating, and using research findings; provide leadership in both the clinical and professional arenas; and collaborate interprofessionally to accomplish client goals and outcomes (Barrett, Latham, and Levermore, 2007).

Many APNs today are practicing in telehealth environments. (See the What Do You Think? box.) Telehealth is the practice of health care delivery, diagnosis, consultation, treatment, and transfer of medical data and education using interactive video, visual, audio, and data telecommunication (Varghese and Phillips, 2009).

WHAT DO YOU THINK? *As telehealth moves into the mainstream of our present health care system, nurses must provide innovative ways to convey caring in their practices. What do you think are some solutions of incorporating the core nursing concept of caring while using telehealth technologies?*

Correctional Institutions

Residents of prisons and jails are a population with health needs that can be met by APHNs and NPs. APHNs are an asset within prison systems, planning and implementing coordinated health programs that include health education as well as health services. Where personnel resources are limited, APHNs provide health education and counseling for inmates and/or their families to prepare prison clients for going back into the community upon their release. NPs often practice in on-site health clinics at correctional institutions, providing both primary care services and health education programs (Walsh and Freshwater, 2006; Ferszt and Erickson-Owens, 2008).

ISSUES AND CONCERNS

Legal Status

The legal authority of nurses in advanced practice is determined by each state's nurse practice act and, in some states, by additional rules and regulations for practice (Phillips, 2010). In the 1970s, regulations for the direct care role performed by NPs, including diagnosis and treatment, were less defined in state nursing laws than they are today, and the legal statutes of NPs were being questioned. Since 1971, when Idaho revised its nurse practice act to include the practice of NPs, other states have amended their nurse practice acts or revised their definitions of nursing to reflect the new nursing roles. NPs are regulated by their state boards of nursing through specific regulations (Phillips, 2010). Legislative authority to prescribe has changed dramatically in the last several years. By 2002, NPs in all states (including the District of Columbia) had **prescriptive authority,** some with independent authority to prescribe and some dependent on physician collaboration (Phillips, 2010). Although legal problems and unresolved disputes still exist in a few states, tremendous gains have been made because of nurses' active involvement in the political and policy-making arenas (Phillips, 2010).

Reimbursement

The third-party reimbursement system in the United States, both public and private, is complicated. To practice independently or work collaboratively with physicians, NPs need to be reimbursed adequately. Because states regulate the insurance industry, available third-party private reimbursement depends in large part on state statute. Advanced practice nurses want direct access to third-party payers. The most common mechanism by which NPs get access to direct payment is through benefits-required laws. Laws also include the right to practice without being discriminated against by another provider or a health care agency (Phillips, 2010).

The Rural Health Clinic Services Act of 1977 (PL 95-210) was the first breakthrough in third-party reimbursement for nurses in primary care roles (Box 39-2). The law authorized Medicare and Medicaid reimbursement to qualified rural clinics for services provided by NPs and PAs, regardless of the presence of a physician (Wasem, 1990). The intent of the act was to improve access to health care in some of the nation's underserved rural areas; however, its use from state to state has varied dramatically. Recent legislative changes to include the coverage of services by certified nurse midwives, clinical psychologists, and social workers have improved the effectiveness of the Rural Health Clinic Services Act for reimbursement options.

In 1989, Congress mandated reimbursement for services furnished to needy Medicaid clients by a certified family nurse practitioner or certified pediatric nurse practitioner whether or not under the supervision of a physician. With the 1997 passing of the national reconciliation spending bill, NPs could be directly reimbursed, regardless of geographic setting, at 85% of what a physician would have been paid (if the service is covered under Medicare part B) (Pearson, 1998). Since January 1, 2003, individuals applying for Medicare provider numbers as

BOX 39-2 **LANDMARK U.S. LEGISLATION FOR ADVANCED PRACTICE NURSES**

- 1977: Rural Health Clinic Services Act authorized NP and PA services to be directly reimbursed when provided in a rural area.
- 1989: As part of the Omnibus Budget Reconciliation Act (OBRA), Congress recognized NPs as direct providers of services to residents of nursing homes.
- 1990: Congress established a new Medicare benefit through the Federally Qualified Health Centers where services of NPs are directly reimbursed when provided in these centers.
- 1997: Passage of the national reconciliation spending bill. NPs can now be directly reimbursed, regardless of geographic setting, at 85% of what the physician would have been paid (if the service is covered under Medicare part B).
- 2003: Individuals applying for Medicare provider numbers, such as NPs, must possess a master's degree from an NP program, as well as national certification and state licensure.

NPs must possess a master's degree from an NP program, as well as national certification and state licensure. Once an NP has a provider number, he or she submits bills using the standard government form to the local Medicare insurance carrier agency for each visit or procedure.

Institutional Privileges

Because of their direct care role, NPs in the community are more concerned than APHNs about institutional privileges. Traditionally it has been difficult for NPs to obtain hospital privileges within institutions where their clients are admitted. However, with the broadening scope of practice and professional responsibilities, more nurse practitioners are obtaining hospital privileges (often referred to as credentialing). An application process is generally required and reviewed by a group of physicians in the department of medicine. The criteria for nurse practitioners wishing to obtain hospital privileges vary by hospital and state; however, most hospitals require that nurse practitioners have national certification.

Employment and Role Negotiation

For NPs and APHNs to collaboratively provide comprehensive primary health care, they must understand and develop negotiating skills. Positive working relationships with health professionals, organizations, and clients require role negotiation, particularly when few guidelines exist for a role or a role is new and undeveloped. NPs and APHNs need to assess the internal politics of the organization as part of their role negotiation. Networking is another necessary skill. Forums, joint conferences, collaborative practice, and research provide opportunities to expand their functions.

Because NPs and APHNs in some locations often seek employment, as opposed to being sought by employers, assertiveness is needed. Increased financial constraints have reduced the number of job opportunities. This many change with the Obama health care reform initiatives. NPs and APHNs should feel comfortable about marketing their skills. Marketing strategies should

be designed to project an image that shows a nurse's individual achievement. In assessing and analyzing the needs of target markets, nurses must consider professional, institutional, and the target client groups' goals.

Methods of obtaining positions and negotiating future roles include providing portfolios of credentialed documents and samples of professional accomplishments such as audiovisual materials, program plans and evaluations conducted, client education packets, and history and physical assessment tools developed. Portfolios are folders that contain all of these documents to showcase the nurse's abilities. NPs and APHNs should keep current portfolios containing examples of their professional activities. Names, addresses, and telephone numbers of professional and personal references should be furnished in the portfolios (but only after the referring persons have granted permission). A new application that can assist in keeping current portfolios is an electronic portfolio or e-portfolio where information is housed on the Internet that can be easily updated and shared/transmitted to employers and others. Many websites provide e-portfolio management and services, such as Decision Critical (http://www.decisioncritical.com/Critical_Portfolio.asp).

ROLE STRESS

Factors causing stress for advanced practice nurses include legal issues (as discussed previously), professional isolation, liability, collaborative practice, conflicting expectations, and professional responsibilities. NPs and APHNs will want to identify self-care strategies to cope with predictable stressors, some of which are discussed here.

Professional Isolation

Professional isolation is a source of conflict for NPs and APHNs. Because they practice across all age groups, NPs and APHNs are likely to be hired in remote practice employment sites. Rural communities unable to support a physician, for example, may find the NP an affordable and logical alternative for primary care services. The autonomy of practice in these sites attracts many NPs and APHNs, who may fail to consider the disadvantages of isolated practice. Long drives, long hours, lack of social and cultural activities, and lack of opportunity for professional development are often experienced by these rural practitioners. These sources of stress, which could lead to job dissatisfaction, can be reduced or eliminated by negotiating the employment contract to include educational and personal leaves.

Liability

All nurses are liable for their actions. Because more legal action is appearing in the judicial system, specifically concerning NPs, the importance of liability and/or malpractice insurance cannot be overemphasized (ACNP, 2010). Although malpractice insurance may not be required to function as an NP or an APHN, most nurses carry their own liability insurance. It is in the best interest of NPs and APHNs to thoroughly investigate the coverage offered by different companies rather than to assume that the coverage is adequate. Practitioners who function without a physician on site are particularly vulnerable. The scope of the NP's and APHN's authority determines the liability standards applied. The limits of each practitioner's authority are legislated by individual states (Phillips, 2010).

Interprofessional Collaborative Practice

The future of NPs and APHNs depends on whether they make a recognized difference in the health of families and communities, and on their ability to practice collaboratively with physicians. Interprofessional collaborative practice defines a peer relationship with mutual trust and respect. Working out a collaborative practice takes a considerable amount of time and energy. Until such practice relationships evolve within joint practice situations, the quality health care that nursing and medicine can collaboratively provide will not be achieved. The arrangement demands the professional maturity to work together without territorial disputes, and the structure and philosophy of the organization must support joint practice as a mechanism for health care delivery. The growing pains of establishing such a practice produce stress for all involved; however, the results and benefits to clients and professionals are worth the effort.

Interprofessional collaborative practice for APHNs and NPs involves more disciplines than just medicine. Advanced practice nurses work with baccalaureate-prepared nurses and other nurses, social workers, public health professionals, nutritionists, occupational and physical therapists, and community leaders and members to meet their goals for the health of individuals, families, groups, and communities. To work toward the *Healthy People 2020* objectives, collaboration of multidisciplinary groups is essential. APHNs, NPs, and baccalaureate-prepared nurses can provide leadership in attaining this collaborative effort.

Conflicting Expectations

Services provided by NPs and APHNs in health promotion and maintenance are often more time consuming and complex than just the management of clients' health problems. NPs and APHNs frequently experience conflict between their practice goals in health promotion and the need to see the number of clients required to maintain the clinic's financial goals. The problem becomes worse when the clinic administrator or physician views NPs and APHNs only as medical extenders and limits reimbursement to the nurse. A practice model that can assist nurses in including health promotion and maintenance activities as well as medical case management into each client visit uses (1) flexible scheduling, (2) health maintenance flow sheets, and (3) problem-oriented recording with nursing goals and plans prominently displayed in the health record. For APHNs, program planning and evaluation based on systematic needs assessments conducted with communities are methods

to show the needs and benefits of health promotion/disease prevention. Being an educator and role model in carrying out *Healthy People 2020* objectives emphasizes the importance of health promotion and disease prevention in the health care system.

Professional Responsibilities

Professional responsibilities contribute to role stress. Most states require NPs and APHNs in expanded roles to be nationally certified and to maintain certification. Recertification requires documentation of continuing education hours. Because there may not be many nurse practitioners in an area, continuing education may not be locally available and may require travel and lodging expenses in addition to time away from the practice site. Anticipating professional responsibilities and travel expenses in financial planning decreases these concerns. Negotiating with the employer for educational leave and expenses should be part of any contract.

Quality of client care, however, cannot be measured or ensured by continuing education or the nurse's credentials. Professional responsibility includes monitoring one's own practice according to standards established by the profession and protocols, if used, and a personal feeling of responsibility to the community. Continuous quality improvement is another professional responsibility for NPs and APHNs. This process should evaluate need, cost, and effectiveness of care in relation to client outcomes (Austin, Luker, and Martin, 2006).

TRENDS IN ADVANCED PRACTICE NURSING

On the basis of data provided by state board of nursing authorities in 2009, there were 131,285 NPs; 12,227 CNSs; 7257 certified nurse midwives; and 37,550 certified registered nurse anesthetists in the United States (Phillips, 2010). These data show a continued increase in NPs and a decrease in CNSs. The loss of CNS positions in hospitals has occurred in financially stressed health care systems. Quality and cost of care have been adversely affected. Academics tended to emphasize NP programs as a result of the change. However, the need for NPs and APHNs is increasing, especially in light of health care reform, social changes, and complex specialized health problems of the twenty-first century (ANA, 2007).

APHNs and NPs in collaboration with nurses, community agencies and members, and other disciplines have the potential to make an impact on health promotion and disease prevention at the individual, family, group, and community levels. Population-focused APHNs and NPs are in excellent positions to use the *Healthy People 2020* National Health Promotion and Disease Prevention objectives and the Healthy People in Healthy Communities model in planning their advanced practice nursing interventions.

CHAPTER REVIEW

PRACTICE APPLICATION

CASE 1: APHN

Martha Corley is an APHN who coordinates the after-care services for a community hospital's early discharge clients. Martha has worked with the nursing staff to develop a nursing history form to identify family and social supports available to clients who are likely to need nursing or supportive care for a limited time after discharge. With this and additional information from head nurses, Martha visits selected clients to begin discharge planning. She consults with each client and family to validate assessed needs. The physician is also consulted about medical therapies to be continued at home. Martha has access to nurses and other resources throughout the community that accept cases on contract. She outlines the initial care plan with nurse case managers assigned to the client and receives regular progress reports. An essential aspect of her practice is to evaluate outcomes of her interventions.

Which of the following is the best example of evaluation of Martha's nursing care?
A. Assessment of client and family satisfaction of her services
B. Reported medical complications of her caseload
C. Review of related literature about home care programs
D. Collected data on hospital readmissions of her clients

CASE 2: FAMILY NURSE PRACTITIONER

Julie Andrews is an NP who practices with two board-certified family practice physicians in an urban office. Julie has her own appointment schedule and sees 12 to 20 adults and children on an average day. Although she sees some acutely ill clients, most of her appointments are for routine health maintenance visits. The two physicians also refer clients to Julie for management of stable chronic health problems such as hypertension and diabetes. She has received a number of referrals from Martha Corley (see case 1) of clients with hypertension and diabetes. Assignment of these clients to Julie by the physicians did not begin until Julie had been with the practice for about a year. During the first months of practice, Julie assessed the numbers and types of client problems seen in a typical week. She found that hypertension was the most frequent chronic problem. Julie reviewed a sample of records of clients with hypertension and found that many had recorded blood pressures indicating uncontrolled hypertension.

On the basis of this information, what advanced practice nursing intervention could Julie provide?
A. Continue to see the clients referred to her through the physicians and Martha.
B. Conduct an in-service education program on hypertension for the staff in the office.
C. Provide nurse practitioner visits for hypertensive clients and compare the outcomes to hypertension clients seen by the physicians in the office.
D. Provide care for all hypertensive clients in the office.
Answers can be found on the Evolve site.

KEY POINTS

- Changes in the health care system and nursing have occurred in the past few decades because of a shift in society's demands and needs.
- Trends such as a shift of health care from institution-based sites to the community, an increase in technology, self-care, cost-containment measures, accountability, third-party reimbursement, and demands for humanizing technical care have influenced the new roles of the APHN and NP.
- Educational preparation of the APHN has always been at the graduate level, whereas this has not been true of the NP; however, there are implications that both the NP and APHN educational preparation may be at the doctorate of nursing practice level.
- Specialty certification began through the ANA in 1976 for NPs, and through the ANCC in 1990 for APHNs.
- The major role functions of the NP and APHN in community health are clinician, consultant, administrator, researcher, and educator; typically, the NP spends a greater amount of time in direct care clinical activities and less time in indirect activities than the APHN.
- Major arenas for practice for NPs and APHNs in community health include primary care practice, institutional settings, industry, government, public health agencies, schools, home health, correctional health, nursing centers, and health ministry settings.
- Legal status, reimbursement, institutional privileges, and role negotiation are important issues and concerns to nurses who practice in an advanced role in public health nursing.
- Major stressors for NPs and APHNs include professional isolation, liability, collaborative practice, conflicting expectations, and professional responsibilities.
- The use of *Healthy People 2020* objectives is important in emphasizing health promotion and disease prevention in advanced practice nursing and in improving the health of the nation.

CLINICAL DECISION-MAKING ACTIVITIES

1. Explore the development of the NP and APHN in the community. Give details about the differences in the roles.
2. Investigate graduate programs in public health in the state or region to determine the requirements for admission, the type of degree awarded, and whether or not NP and/or APHN preparation is available. Do the similarities and differences make sense to you? Why?
3. Review your state's nurse practice act and any rules and regulations governing advanced practice roles. Are rules different for NPs and APHNs? Give examples.

4. Negotiate a clinical observation experience with an NP and an APHN in community and public health, and compare and contrast their roles. Discuss the roles as you see them with the NP and APHN. When you consider your thoughts about the roles, have you considered what the APHN and NP have told you about their roles? How has their input changed your views?

REFERENCES

Administration on Aging: *A profile of older Americans*, 2009. Available at http://www.aoa.gov/aoaroot/aging_statistics/Profile/index.aspx. Accessed March 7, 2011.

American Academy of Nurse Practitioners: *National competency-based certification examinations for adult and family nurse practitioner*, Austin, TX, 2010, AANP.

American Association of Colleges of Nursing: *The essentials of master's education for advanced practice nursing*, Washington, DC, 1996, AACN.

American Association of Colleges of Nursing: *The essentials of doctoral education for advanced practice nursing*, Washington, DC, 2006, AACN.

American Association of Colleges of Nursing: *White paper on the education and role of the clinical nurse leader*, Washington, DC, 2007, AACN.

American Association of Colleges of Nursing: *CNL and DNP program UPDATES*. Available at aacn.cche.edu. Accessed April 18, 2011.

American College of Nurse Practitioners: *Malpractice/liability*. Available at http://www.acnpweb.org/i4a/pages/index.cfm?pageid=3401. Accessed March 7, 2011.

American Nurses Association: *Scope and standards for public health nursing*, Silver Spring, MD, 2007, ANA.

American Nurses Credentialing Center: *Advanced practice certification information*, Washington, DC, 2009, ANA.

American Nurses Credentialing Center: *Advanced practice certification catalog*, Washington, DC, 2010, ANA.

American Public Health Association: *The definition and role of public health nursing practice in the delivery of health care*, Washington, DC, 1996, APHA, Public Health Nursing Section.

Anderko L, Lundeen S, Bartz C: The Midwest nursing centers consortium research network: translating research into practice, *Pol Poli Nurs Pract* 7(2):101–109, 2006.

Anderson C: Champions of advanced nursing practice, *Prof Nurs* 19:20–21, 2004.

Association of Community Health Nursing Educators: *Graduate education for advanced practice in community/public health nursing: at the crossroads*, Latham, NY, 2007, ACHNE.

Association of Community Health Nursing Educators: *Disaster preparedness white paper for community/public health nursing educators*, Latham, NY, 2008, ACHNE.

Austin L, Luker K, Martin R: Clinical nurse specialists and the practice of community nurses, *J Adv Nurs* 54(5):542–550, 2006.

Bajnok I, Wright J: Revisiting the role of the nurse practitioner in the 1990s: a Canadian perspective, *AACN Clin Issues Crit Care Nurs* 4(4):609, 1993.

Barrett A, Latham D, Levermore J: Defining the role of the specialist district nurse practitioner, *Brit J Comm Health* 12(11):522–526, 2007.

Campo T, McNulty R, Sabatini M, Fitzpatrick J: Nurse practitioners performing procedures with confidence and independence in the emergency care setting, *Adv Emer Nurs J* 30(2):153–170, 2008.

Council on Linkages Between Academia and Public Health Practice: *Core competencies for public health professionals*, Washington, DC, 2001. Available at http://www.phf.org/. Accessed April 18, 2011.

Council on Linkages Between Academia and Public Health Practice: *Core competencies for public health professionals*, Washington, DC, 2009. Available at http://www.phf.org/link/corecompetencies.htm. Accessed April 18, 2011.

Ferszt GG, Erickson-Owens DA: Development of an educational support groups for pregnant women in prison, *J Forens Nurs* 42(2):55–60, 2008.

Ford LC: Nurses, nurse practitioners: the evolution of primary care [book review], *Image J Nurs Scholar* 18:177, 1986.

Harne-Britner S, Schafer D: Clinical nurse specialists driving research and practice through research roundtables, *Clin Nurse Spec* 23(6):305–308, 2009.

Health Ministries Association: *American Nurses Association: Scope and standards for faith and community nursing*, Silver Spring, MD, 2005, Health Ministries Association and ANA.

Hooker RS, Berlin LE: Trends in the supply of physician assistants and nurse practitioners in the US, *Health Affairs* 21:174–181, 2002.

Hooker RS, Cipher DJ, Cawley JF, et al: Emergency medicine services: interprofessional care trends, *J Interprof Care* 22(2):167–178, 2008.

Hooker RS, McCaig LF: Use of physician assistants and nurse practitioners in primary care, 1995-1999, *Health Aff* 20(4):231–238, 2001.

Institute of Medicine: *Who will keep the public health?* Washington, DC, 2003, The National Academies Press.

Jakeway CC, LaRosa G, Cary A, Schoenfisch S: The role of public health nurses in emergency preparedness and response: A position paper of the Association of State and Territorial Directors of Nursing, *Public Health Nurs* 25(4):353–361, 2008.

Kuntz SW, Frable P: Quereshik, Strong LL: Association of Community Health Nursing Educators: Disaster preparedness white paper for community/public health nursing educators, *Public Health Nurs* 25(4):362–369, 2008.

Laurant M, Reeves D, Hermens R, et al: Substitution of doctors by nurses in primary care (review). *The Cochrane Collaboration* (Issue 4), 2009, John Wiley and Sons.

Logan L: The practice of certified community health CNSs, *Clin Nurse Spec* 19(1):43–48, 2005.

Madigan MA, Vanderboom C: Home health care nursing research priorities, *Appl Nurs Res* 18:221–225, 2005.

McGinnis SL, Zoske FM: The emerging role of faith community nurses in prevention and management of chronic disease, *Pol Polit Nurse Pract* 9(3):173–180, 2008.

Mellor G, St. John W: Occupational health nurses' perceptions of their current and future roles, *J Adv Nurs* 58(6):585–593, 2007.

Minnesota Department of Health: *Public health interventions: applications for public health nursing practice*, 2001, Saint Paul Minnesota Department of Health.

National Organization of Nurses Practitioner Faculties: *Domains and core competencies of nurse practitioner practice*, 2006. Available at http://www.nonpf.com/associations/10789/files/DomainsandCoreComps2006.pdf. Accessed March 7, 2011.

Nelson R: School nurses are needed more than ever, *Am J Nurs* 109(12):25–27, 2009.

Paterson B, Duffett-Leger L, Crutteden K: Contextual factors influencing the evolution of nurses' roles in a primary health care clinic, *Public Health Nurs* 26(5):421–429, 2009.

Pearson LJ: Annual updates of how each state stands on legislative issues affecting advanced practice nursing, *Nurs Pract* 23(1):14, 1998.

Phillips S: 22nd Annual legislative update: regulatory and legislative successes for APNs, *Nurs Pract* 35(1):24–47, 2010.

Quad Council of Public Health Nursing Organizations: *Quad Council Public Health Competencies*, 2003 with update in 2009. Available at http://www.cdphe.state.co.us/opp/phn/PHNcompetencies.pdf.

Regan ME: Implementation and evaluation of a youth violence prevention program for adolescents, *J School Nurs* 25(1):27–33, 2009.

Robertson JF, Baldwin KB: Advanced practice role characteristics of the community/public health nurse specialist, *Clin Nurs Spec* 21(5):250–254, 2007.

Royal College of Nursing Advanced Nurse Practitioners: An RCN guide to ANP role, competencies and programme accreditation.

Schober M: The global emergence of advanced practice nurses in providing home and community health care services, *Home Health Care Manag Pract* 20(1):34–40, 2007.

Silver HK, Ford LC, Stearly SA: A program to increase health care for children: the pediatric nurse practitioner program, *Pediatrics* 39:756, 1967.

Thornlow DK, Auerhahn C, Stanley J: A necessity not a luxury: Preparing advanced practice nurses to care for older adults, *J Prof Nurs* 22(2):116–122, 2006.

U.S. Department of Defense/Today's Military: *Health care practitioners*, 2010. Available at http://todaysmilitary.com/careers/career-fields/officer/health-care-practitioners. Accessed March 7, 2011.

U.S. Department of Health and Human Services: *Healthy people 2020*, Washington, DC, 2010, U.S. Government Printing Office. Available at www.health.gov/healthypeople/document. Accessed March 7, 2011.

U.S. Department of Health, Education, and Welfare: *Extending the scope of nursing practice*, Washington, DC, 1971, U.S. Government Printing Office.

U.S. Department of Health and Human Services: *National Health Service Corps*, 2010. Available at http://nhsc.hrsa.gov/about/. Accessed March 7, 2011.

U.S. Department of Health and Human Services: *Agency for Healthcare Research and Quality, U.S. Preventive Services Task Force*, Rockville, MD, 2009, The guide to clinical preventative services. Available at http://www.ahrq.gov/clinic/pocketgd09/pocketgd09.pdf. Accessed April 18, 2011.

Varghese SB, Phillips CA: Caring in telehealth, *Tele e-Health* 15(10):1005–1009, 2009.

Walsh L, Freshwater D: Managing practice innovations in prison health services, *Nurs Times* 102(7):32–34, 2006.

Wasem C: The Rural Health Clinic Services Act: a sleeping giant of reimbursement, *J Am Acad Nurs Pract* 2(2):85, 1990.

Wood C, Wettlaufer J, Shaha SH, Lillis K: Nurse practitioner roles in pediatric emergency departments: a national survey, *Pediatr Emerg Care* 26(6):406–407, 2010.

CHAPTER 40

The Nurse Leader in the Community

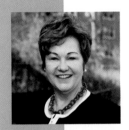

Juliann G. Sebastian, PhD, RN, FAAN

Juliann G. Sebastian developed an interest in public health and community-based nursing while obtaining her BSN degree, when she provided care in rural Appalachia. Since then, she has cared for a range of vulnerable populations across the life span and in a variety of community settings, including adults who are homeless, low-income families, and frail elders in their home environments. Her doctoral preparation was in organization theory and health economics, and her research interests are in the area of community systems of care delivery for underserved populations. She was a member of the inaugural cohort of Robert Wood Johnson Nurse Executive Fellows (1998-2001), during which time she focused on development of models of academic clinical nursing practice. Her research and publications have focused on academic nurse-managed centers, community-based care, and primary care. She is a Fellow in the American Academy of Nursing and has held numerous leadership positions in professional nursing organizations. Dr. Sebastian serves as Dean of the College of Nursing at the University of Missouri–St. Louis.

ADDITIONAL RESOURCES

OBJECTIVES

After reading this chapter, the student should be able to do the following:

1. Explain why nurses need effective leadership, management, and consultation skills in today's public health care environment.
2. Explore what is meant by partnership and interprofessional practice and describe how these concepts are related to nursing leadership, management, and consultation.
3. Analyze what is meant by systems thinking in community-based and public health settings.
4. Describe the major competencies required to be effective as a nurse leader, manager, and consultant in community-based and public health settings.
5. Examine nursing leadership strategies to enhance client safety and reduce health care errors in community settings.
6. Explain how nurses provide leadership in care coordination in the community.

KEY TERMS

Population-focused nurses have a responsibility to provide leadership in creating a new future for healthier communities. Members of the public ask whether better approaches to health care delivery might be developed that will ensure that all people around the world live in health-promoting communities and have access to quality health care as well as to health promotion and illness prevention services. Population-focused nurses practice in a variety of settings, including public health departments, community-based clinics, occupational health settings, schools, and managed care organizations. Leadership, management, and consulting skills are important to the success of client outcomes that depend heavily on cost-effective, efficient delivery of care. Care coordination and managing care transitions throughout the community, including acute and long-term care settings, is important to promoting a healthy community. Nurses need effective skills in communication, negotiation, and interprofessional practice and good leadership, management, and consultation skills, even if they do not have formal positions as managers or consultants.

Nurses must focus attention not only on the populations that are served by their organizations, but also on those that are not. Because they concern themselves with the total public, their focus is always on the future and on the interacting factors that influence the health of the public. Nurses work with partnerships of community members and community organizations. Partnerships can be complex and require time and thoughtful attention. This chapter examines the roles and functions of nurse leaders, managers, and consultants in the twenty-first century. It emphasizes nursing leadership in public health and community-based nursing practice, personnel management, and consultation with groups and individuals.

MAJOR TRENDS AND ISSUES

Ensuring client safety and quality of care, performing evidence-based practice, eliminating disparities in health care access and outcomes, and focusing on consumer participation in and satisfaction with care are key trends in health care.

The Institute of Medicine report titled *To Err Is Human* (Kohn, Corrigan, and Donaldson, 2000) focused attention on the incidence of health care errors. This is a concern in the community just as in hospitals and long-term care agencies. For example, studies in the United States (Metlay et al, 2005), Europe (Fialova et al, 2005), and Australia (Johnson et al, 2005) show that older adults living in the community are at high risk for medication errors. Sometimes this is because they are taking high-risk medications (Fialova et al, 2005), or because they cannot read instructions for medications (Georges, Bolton, and Bennett, 2004), or because they are not being taught how to take medications that have been prescribed for them (Metlay et al, 2005).

Evidence-based practice is another trend important for public health nurses. Basing clinical practice patterns and community programs on research and other forms of evidence such as best practice data is a key strategy for ensuring high-quality care. One example of evidence-based practice in a community setting is a smoking cessation relapse prevention program for new mothers (Groner et al, 2005) implemented by home health nurses. In this program, nurses used smoking cessation guidelines from the Agency for Health Care Policy and Research (now known as the Agency for Healthcare Research and Quality) to provide a cognitive-behavioral intervention for new mothers before hospital discharge, once in the home, and by telephone.

The health system in some local areas has been reorganized to provide a full continuum of services in a seamless system of care. Large, vertically integrated systems are able to do this. Vertical integration means that the system owns all of the services that clients might need (e.g., clinics, hospitals, and home health agencies). In other cases, free-standing agencies collaborate and contract with one another to achieve seamlessness. The goal is to reduce fragmentation, which should be helpful for vulnerable populations. Nurses coordinate clients' care across agencies, but this new trend in the health care system places added emphasis on relationships, such as alliances, agency partnerships, joint programs, and participation in service delivery networks (Provan and Milward, 2006). Nurses actively participate in these groups and need good negotiating and political skills to be effective.

Another important trend is related to the movement toward more community partnerships (El Ansari and Weiss, 2006).

The public has an increasing interest in becoming involved in planning for health services and in being active partners in their own care. Nurses need to be able to listen well and collaborate with lay community members, whose goals and ideas may differ from those of health care professionals. For example, people who were HIV positive who sought care in an infectious disease clinic were consulted about the implementation of an HIV prevention program within the clinic. The resulting input led to greater buy-in of key stakeholders and successful implementation of the prevention program.

> **DID YOU KNOW?** *Partnerships with community members and community agencies are essential to effective public and community health practice. Partnerships succeed when strong communication mechanisms are in place to ensure definition of needs and problems, timely problem resolution, and ongoing development of shared visions. In public and community health the development of shared visions and goals and the operational mechanisms to make those goals a reality is the key to success. Communication, the primary way to make this happen, can include regular advisory or coalition meetings, telephone calls, and clearly written policies and procedures.*

The public is increasingly using the Internet, a wide variety of publications, and lay support groups to obtain health information. People need help deciding which information is good and how to best work with their health care providers to adapt information to their own health profiles. Those with low health literacy (see Chapter 31) need special help obtaining the health information necessary to be effective partners in health care (Committee on Communication for Behavior Change in the 21st Century, 2002; Ryan, 2009).

To know whether an agency is performing as expected, nurses must be familiar with their professional standards of care, the standards held by accrediting bodies, such as The Joint Commission, and guidelines for practice, such as those published by the federal Agency for Healthcare Research and Quality, the U.S. Clinical Preventive Services Task Force (2009), and the Task Force on Community Preventive Services (Zaza, Briss, and Harris, 2005). Nurse leaders also need to know how to use electronic health records and management information systems to link client outcomes with clinical and administrative processes. Registries are examples of clinical databases dedicated to certain population groups, such as people with cancer, diabetes, injuries, or population groups such as women. Nurses should know how to work with the taxonomies for nursing diagnoses, interventions, and outcomes of nursing actions (Bulechek, Butcher, and Dochterman, 2007) because these are being included in electronic health records and will help nurses identify changing health needs (von Krogh, Dale, and Naden, 2005).

One trend that combines the idea of partnerships with a structured method for rapid performance improvement is the use of collaboratives. A **collaborative** is a group of similar organizations that agree to use common processes for providing clinical care and share certain types of data so all may learn. A well-known example is the Health Care Disparities Collaboratives

method used by the Federal Bureau of Primary Health Care (Martin et al, 2007). Community health centers may apply to participate in collaboratives that target certain chronic health problems, such as diabetes or cardiovascular disease.

A major trend in public health is a stronger focus on implementing the core functions of public health and providing the essential services of public health (PHF, 2010). Competencies have been identified for generalist public/community health nurses that build on the core function and essential services (Education Committee of the Association of Community Health Nurse Educators, 2010).

EVIDENCE-BASED PRACTICE

This paper describes the long-term results of a randomized trial of a nurse-led home visiting program for a group of women during and after pregnancy. Participants had low incomes, received health care in a large urban area, and were predominately African American. Follow-up occurred 12 years after the birth of their first child. Findings indicated that mothers who received the home visits had stayed with their partners longer, reported fewer problems from drug and alcohol use, and felt more capable than mothers who did not receive the nurse home visits. Governmental spending for families who had received the home visits was less than for those who did not receive the visits, suggesting long-term cost benefits of this model in addition to the improved health benefits for the mothers.

Nurse Use

This long-term research program and other papers published by researchers investigating this model suggest that nurse home-visiting programs for pregnant mothers and their infants lead to improved health and economic outcomes.

From Olds DL, Kitzman HJ, Cole RE, et al: Enduring effects of prenatal and infancy home visiting by nurses on maternal life course and government spending: follow-up of a randomized trial among children at age 12 years, *Arch Pediatr Adolesc Med* 164: 419-424, 2010.

DEFINITIONS

Nursing leadership refers to the influence that nurses exert on improving client health, whether clients are individuals, families, groups, or entire communities. Nursing management, on the other hand, refers to the ways nurses organize and use resources when providing clinical services. These resources might be people, as when a nurse coordinates an interprofessional team, or financial resources. An example of managing financial resources is when a nurse monitors the budget for an immunization program to make sure that personnel time, supplies, and equipment are being used efficiently. Nurses also manage time. For example, home health nurses must manage their time in order to provide clients with direct and indirect nursing services, such as health education and making referrals, respectively. Leadership sets the direction, and management ensures that goals will be achieved. Nurses must possess strong clinical leadership and management skills to be effective, whether or not they hold management positions.

Consultation has been described as a process in which the helper provides a set of activities that help the client perceive, understand, and act on events occurring in the client's environment. Clinical consultation increasingly focuses on ways to better coordinate the care delivery process across sites of care.

Population-focused nurses have a breadth of knowledge that makes them desirable consultants for colleagues both inside and outside the organizations in which they work. For example, a nurse working in a home health agency might be called on by a school nurse to give suggestions about the most effective way to intervene for a child using a respirator. Another example that occurs frequently is the informal consultation provided by nurses in the community, who help nurses working in hospitals make effective community referrals. At the population level, nurses who consult with a local health department about developing a program for obesity prevention in school-age children are focusing their efforts on a particular target population. An example would be the nurse leader of a community-based diabetes program who works with clinical colleagues in a hospital to improve the self-management education for people with diabetes.

Consultation is closely linked with the ideas of empowerment and self-management. When consultants help clients identify and work through problems and learn new skills that clients see as most important, they are enabling clients to solve more of their own problems. This is very similar to the traditional nursing philosophy of helping people to solve their own problems, whether they are individuals, families, groups, or communities. Empowerment is consistent with Dorothea Orem's nursing theory of self-care (Orem, 1991), in which she states that the nurse's role is to promote clients' self-care abilities.

| **THE CUTTING EDGE** *Agencies, localities, and professional organizations increasingly recognize the need for effective leadership in public health and community life. Nurses should watch for opportunities to participate in leadership development institutes or consider ongoing formal education through advanced public health nursing degree programs. Leadership development programs are available at various levels and are provided by civic and professional organizations. Civic programs introduce participants to the full range of leadership and quality-of-life issues in a community, including health, education, politics, the arts, and business. This breadth of concerns is consistent with nurses' understanding that health results from the interaction of many facets of social and economic influences. Other leadership development opportunities are provided by professional organizations (e.g., The International Honor Society for Nursing, the American Public Health Association), continuing education, and local groups. Local and statewide public health groups provide leadership institutes focused on developing leadership for solving public health problems (Wright et al, 2000; Porter et al, 2002; Wright, 2009). Finally, doctoral degree programs in public health nursing provide systematic academic development of public and leadership competencies and prepare nurses to sit for advanced nursing certification as public/community health nursing clinical specialists through the American Nurses Credentialing Center. Nurses should take advantage of opportunities such as these for lifelong learning and strengthening leadership skills.*

From Porter J, Johnson J, Upshaw VM, et al: The Management Academy for Public Health: a new paradigm for public health management development, J Public Health Manag Pract 8:66-78, 2002; Wright K, Rowitz L, Merkle A, et al: Competency development in public health leadership, Am J Public Health 90:1202-1207, 2000; Wright K: Environmental public health leadership development, J Environ Health 71: 24-25, 2009.

LEADERSHIP AND MANAGEMENT APPLIED TO POPULATION-FOCUSED NURSING

Goals

The goals of nursing leadership are as follows:
1. To work with others to ensure a healthy community
2. To serve as an advocate for vulnerable and high-risk populations and to work toward eliminating disparities in health care access, quality, and outcomes
3. To participate in establishing public and organizational policies and programs that promote a healthy living and working environment
4. To work with interprofessional teams to design ways to coordinate care across sites and over time, and to evaluate and continually improve health care outcomes

One way nurses achieve leadership goals is by participating in a *Healthy Communities* (CDC, 2010) initiative at the local level. Working with others to develop policies for smoke-free public spaces is an example of promoting healthy living and working environments. Another example is collaborating with consumers and professionals from other disciplines to evaluate root causes of medication errors in home-bound elders and design a process improvement strategy to reduce errors.

The goals of nursing management are as follows:
1. To achieve agency and professional goals for client services and clinical outcomes using a systems perspective
2. To help personnel perform their responsibilities effectively and efficiently
3. To mentor other staff members and foster lifelong learning
4. To develop new services that will enable the agency to respond to emerging community health needs
5. To monitor health outcomes for particular population groups and identify changes or variances suggesting new problems

An example of how nurses achieve management goals occurs when they develop plans for broad-based immunization clinics, such as smallpox vaccination clinics. Doing this in advance of confirmed bioterrorism is a way of preparing to meet an emerging community health need that achieves goals of protecting the public's health and helping personnel work effectively and efficiently. Table 40-1 shows examples of ways population-focused nurse leaders and managers facilitate primary, secondary, and tertiary preventive services.

Theories of Leadership and Management

Leadership and management theories help explain individual and group behavior as well as organizational and system dynamics. Theories that help explain and predict individual behavior often focus on employee motivation and job satisfaction. Some theories address interpersonal issues such as leadership, communication, conflict resolution, and group dynamics. Working with consumers, staff members, and other health professionals in an adult day-care facility to design a memory improvement program for participants exemplifies the use of these theories. This type of project requires knowledge of motivation and leadership, team work, change theory, and project planning, management, and evaluation.

TABLE 40-1 EXAMPLES OF LEVELS OF PREVENTION AND POPULATION-FOCUSED NURSING LEADERSHIP AND MANAGEMENT

LEVELS OF PREVENTION	NURSING LEADERSHIP (SETS GOALS)	NURSING MANAGEMENT (DIRECTS USE OF RESOURCES)
Primary (prevention of illnesses or problems before they begin)	Works with a community coalition to design a broad-based strategy for ensuring health and social needs of uninsured and underinsured populations are met. Works with nurses and interprofessional colleagues to develop goals related to preventing health care errors and ensuring client safety.	Develops policies and procedures for a referral program for low-income mothers and children to obtain nutrition services. Ensures that individuals and families understand care routines to promote adherence and reduce chances of health care error.
Secondary (screening for illness and treatment of health problems before they worsen)	Works with local government and health department to design lead screening and abatement programs in high-risk census tracks. Monitors data about a caseload of clients to determine if patterns are developing that might indicate a health problem or issue needs to be resolved.	Designs protocols for lead screening program and hires staff to implement program. Works with other members of care team to design protocols to improve specific health outcomes.
Tertiary (treatment of health problems to foster stabilization or delay exacerbation)	Participates on a planning commission with local health department, hospitals, police, and political leaders to update a community-wide disaster response plan that accounts for bioterrorism. Collaborates with interprofessional teams to set goals for performance improvement and rapid changes in quality of care problems.	Serves as chair of a committee that organizes, staffs, and monitors budget for a smallpox vaccination program. Monitors implementation of performance improvement activities to ensure timely and appropriate completion or revision as necessary.

Organizational and systems theories explain issues at a broader agency or community level. These theories focus on the best ways to organize work, on how to obtain the resources necessary to accomplish agency goals, on organizational level change, on power dynamics, and understanding systems. Systems theories help explain the dynamics of rapid, interconnected change and the emergence of patterns of activity (Holden, 2005).

WHAT DO YOU THINK? *Consider the management dilemma that Elizabeth Schaeffer faces in the following case:*

Elizabeth Schaeffer, RN, is the nurse manager of a mobile health clinic for migrant farmworkers. The clinic is owned by the local health department and is housed in a van that travels to migrant camps in a 10-county area, providing outreach, case finding, and primary care services. The clinic employs two nurses, one social worker, one physical therapist, and two lay community health workers. The health department commissioner wants to increase efficiency by instituting cross-training, meaning that the workers can do each other's jobs. The commissioner asked Elizabeth whether it would be possible to train the nurses in the van to do certain physical therapy procedures, and to train the community health workers to do phlebotomy and run electrocardiograms. Elizabeth is concerned about whether these actions would be outside the nurses' scopes of practice. She also wonders if there will be problems with quality of care and lower employee morale if this type of cross-training is implemented. Elizabeth questions whether asking lay community health workers to assume these additional responsibilities would violate the nurse practice act in the state. She begins her analysis by reading the Public Health Nursing: Scope and Standards of Practice (ANA, 2007a) and the standards for physical therapy services. What do you think Elizabeth should do next?

Good leadership skills are essential for nurse leaders and are among the key competencies for generalist public/community health nurses recommended by the Quad Council of Public Health Nursing Organizations (2009) and for "entry level public health professionals" by the Council on Linkages Between Academia and Public Health Nursing Practice (2010, p 1).

The transformational leader is able to transform, or change, the situation to one that differs from the status quo (Bass and Bass, 2008). Transformational leaders are sometimes found in learning organizations, or agencies that create cultures that support ongoing learning, experimentation, and creation of new knowledge (Roussel, Swansburg, and Swansburg, 2006). Transformational leadership is essential to promoting a culture of safety and positive work environments for others (Committee on the Work Environment for Nurses and Patient Safety, 2004).

Systems theories and systems thinking emphasize the interdependence of multiple parties. Nurses often recognize interdependence of units within an agency but may be less aware of agency interdependence. Economists analyze how distribution of resources affects policies, which players in a system will be influenced by policies, and how they will be influenced. These are called distribution effects. For example, if the federal government reduces money for health and social services, the clients of those services may be negatively affected. Employees of service agencies are also affected because agencies are likely to downsize to manage the reduced funding. Consequently, employees may either lose their jobs or experience wage cuts. Others likely to be affected include voluntary agencies and religious groups who might be expected to provide more services.

Roy's adaptation model of nursing has been extended to include nursing management (Roy, 2002). Roy argues that agencies are composed of interdependent systems. The role of nurse managers is to help the agency adapt to changing circumstances in the most effective way possible. Roy's model is particularly helpful for explaining and predicting how nurse managers and consultants can help agencies adapt to change. Nurse leaders should analyze how well interdependent units function to achieve agency goals. Furthermore, nurse leaders function as change agents because they foster agency adaptation. Complex adaptive systems theory accounts for the unpredictability of the behavior of people and organizations (Holden, 2005). The combination of unpredictability and interdependence leads to disequilibrium and potentially to adaptation and growth. Communities exemplify complex adaptive systems. Understanding the importance of relationships and tension in the midst of change led one group to design a primary care team-based approach to reflection as a way to improve care (Stroebel et al, 2005). Nurse leaders must understand the analytical, political, and communication skills needed to work effectively in these systems.

Clinical microsystems are the systems, people, information, and behaviors that take place at the point of client care (Nelson et al, 2008). Evidence-based clinical improvements can be implemented quickly in a clinical microsystem that has sufficient data about the practice, information systems that support clinical decision making, and a well-functioning team. For example, nurses working in a mobile health unit are part of a clinical microsystem. The team can make rapid changes in responses to quality problems if team members work well together and the mobile health clinic has an information system that makes it possible to track population health outcomes and clinical practice patterns.

> **HOW TO** Evaluate Risks to Client Safety
>
> *Population-focused nurse leaders should assess the systems within which they work to evaluate risks to client safety. In the community these risks might be related to communication problems, inadequate follow-up, or lack of continuity of care. Nurses should maintain accountability for the outcomes of individuals, families, and groups and should do their best to ensure that complete care is provided across the continuum and that clients feel empowered to manage their own care.*

Nurse Leader and Manager Roles

First-line nurse managers may be team leaders or program directors (e.g., director of a satellite occupational health clinic or director of a small migrant health clinic), whereas mid- or executive-level nurse managers may be division directors (including multiple programs or departments), local or state commissioners of health, or directors of large home health agencies with multiple offices. They function as coaches, facilitators, role models, evaluators, advocates, visionaries, community health program planners, teachers, and supervisors. Population-focused nurse leaders have ongoing responsibilities for the health of clients, groups, and communities, as well as for personnel and fiscal resources under their supervision. Nurse leaders may have positions as managers or they may be excellent clinicians and change agents who are seen as opinion leaders.

CONSULTATION

Goal

The goal of consultation is to help others empower themselves to take more responsibility, feel more secure, deal with their feelings and with others in interactions, and use flexible and creative problem-solving skills (Sabatino, 2009). The functions of a consultant differ from those of a manager because consultation is typically a temporary and voluntary relationship between a professional helper and a client. The similarities between consultants and leaders are in their emphases on empowerment and helping others develop. Consulting relationships are based on cooperation and respect between consultants and clients, who share equally in problem solving (Argyris, 1997).

The nurse's job responsibilities may include internal and external consultation. Internal consultants are members of the organization who work in a temporary capacity to help the client create or sustain change (Lacey and Tompkins, 2007). For example, a nurse may be employed to consult with other nurses in the agency about client care problems or, as an employee of the health department, may serve as a consultant to a local community retirement center about the public health care needs of its residents. If the nurse is an internal consultant, the nurse is employed on a full-time salaried basis by a community agency in which the consultation takes place. If the nurse is an external consultant, the nurse is employed temporarily on a contractual basis by the client. The client of the external nurse consultant may be a colleague, another health provider, or a community group or agency. Consulting may occur informally when a staff nurse asks a colleague for advice or help in solving a problem. The nature of the consultation relationship, whether it is internal or external, should not change the goal of consultation.

Theories of Consultation

Several models of consultation have been developed. Although nurses often consult with individuals about their own health care, or with another nurse or health professional about the needs of an individual client, this section emphasizes population-based consultation. At this level, the nurse focuses on the needs of a group, organization, or community. The client in this case is an organization or group. Content models emphasize the role of consultant as the expert who provides specific answers to problems or issues identified by the client. This approach has the advantage of being relatively quick and often responsive to client requests, but it does not help engage the client in problem solving and learning how to address similar issues in the future (Schein, 2009). This chapter focuses on Edgar Schein's model of process consultation because it is consistent with the nursing process and with nursing values of empowering clients and collaboratively working as partners with clients. The process model consultation focuses on the process of problem solving and collaboration between consultant and the client. The major goal of the process model is to help the client assess both the problem and the kind of help needed to solve it (Schein, 2009). Process consultation includes assessing the underlying agency culture that influences the problem and its solution (Schein, 2010). Both consultant and client participate in the problem-solving steps that lead to changes or to actions for problem solution.

Although consultants should emphasize process consultation, they should be willing to share their expert knowledge when appropriate. Because process consultation is collaborative, Schein (2009) recommends that consultants be willing to offer opinions and advice at all stages of the consultation process. Thus, although the major emphasis should be on process consultation, consultants may find it effective to integrate both context and process.

In the process model, the consultant is a resource person whose primary goal is to provide the client with choices for decision making. Process consultation includes the same steps as the nursing process: establishing a nurse–client relationship based on trust to assess the problem, planning and implementing actions, and evaluating the outcomes of nursing interventions. Nursing interventions may be described as direct client care or as consultation activities, depending on the goal of the intervention.

Consultation may occur before a problem occurs or after a problem exists. For example, a parent–teacher council developing a school-based family center contacts the nurse to assist with options for future nursing and health care for the students and their families. The board wishes to be proactive and plan for the needs of high-risk students and families. The administrator of a minimum-security prison has found that inmates are missing work for minor health problems and that health costs are skyrocketing. The nurse is asked to help explore solutions to the problem. Prison administration is reacting to an existing problem requiring immediate intervention.

The client is identified by determining who in the situation has the problem and needs to change. The following vignette illustrates this point:

> Barry Henderson, RN, has been asked by the pastor of his congregation to consult with the parish council regarding the potential establishment of a health ministry. Barry decides that the consultation contract needs to include representatives of the parish council and parishioners themselves to find effective answers to the question. He realizes that time would be wasted and resistance to change would still be present if the focus were on only one group at a time. If he met separately with the parish council, they may decide such a program should include only one set of services. The parishioners either may want a different set of services or may desire to have services and programming organized in a very different manner. For example, the parish council may be especially interested in blood pressure screening, whereas the parishioners may be interested in wellness classes to keep the congregation healthy and in home visiting for those who are ill. After spending much energy meeting with both groups separately, Barry believes that by being a messenger between the two groups rather than a facilitator for problem solving, the consultant role has been diluted. On the other hand, by meeting with both groups together, Barry could serve as a resource, helping them explore all viewpoints and alternatives for developing the new program. In this case, both the parish council and the parishioners are Barry's clients.

Consultation Contract

The consultation relationship is based on expectations. The consultant has expectations concerning time, money, resources, and the participation of the client in the process. Clients have expectations about what they will gain from the consultation relationship. Discussing the terms of a consultation contract makes expectations explicit, lessens the likelihood of violations of contract terms, and reduces the risk of additional demands being made on either party. Areas to include in the written consultation contract are as follows:

1. Client and consultant goals
2. The identified problem
3. The time commitment
4. Limitations of the contract
5. Cost
6. Conditions under which the contract may be broken or renegotiated
7. Intervention strategies suggested
8. Expected benefits for the client
9. Methods of data collection to be used
10. Potential interventions
11. Evaluation methods to be used
12. Confidentiality

Writing a contract for consultation relationships has a number of advantages. The contract terms assist the consultant in determining the number of hours that must be devoted to the interaction and in identifying needed resources and out-of-pocket expenses required to complete the interaction. Negotiation of the contract assists the client in identifying realistic expectations of the consultant and firmly establishes what the consultant will and will not do. The client has the opportunity during the negotiation to place limits on what the consultant can do, and the contract allows for future renegotiation of terms. Pricing methods for consultation services vary with the nature of the services. Consultants may price their services on the basis of the actual number of billable hours required to perform the service, or they may set a flat fee during the contract negotiation phase. Flat fees are more attractive to clients because they reduce uncertainty over the total cost of the consultation. They create an incentive for consultants to be efficient and to use an accurate method of estimating their services before the contract negotiation meeting.

The initial contact is made when the client or someone in a family, group, agency, or community communicates with the nurse about a potential problem that requires intervention. The communication may be a person-to-person contact during a home visit, may be written, or may occur by telephone. On initial contact, the client and the nurse have an exploratory meeting to define the problem, assess the nurse's interest and ability to help, and formulate future actions. If the nurse has little experience with the type of problem presented, the client may wish to seek assistance elsewhere. The nurse may also conclude that the situation is not within the nurse's expertise and will want to recommend someone else to work with the client.

Next, the terms of the relationship are discussed. The nurse consultant finds out what the client expects to gain from the relationship and develops terms for the interaction. Finally, in the initial exploratory meeting, the setting for the consultation is decided, the time schedule is set, the goals of the interaction are established, and the mode of intervention is chosen.

When the terms of the contract are agreed on, the data-gathering methods will be part of the agreement. Data-gathering methods used by consultants include direct observation, individual and group interviews, use of questionnaires or surveys, and tape recordings. While data are being gathered and after the diagnosis has been finalized, the nurse implements the intervention. After fulfilling the terms of the contract, the nurse must disengage or reduce the amount of involvement with the client. Decreased contacts allow each side to evaluate the effectiveness of the intervention. During disengagement, the nurse reassures the client that future interactions are possible at the client's discretion. When the agreed-on period of disengagement has passed, the relationship is terminated. The nurse typically provides the client with a written summary of the findings and recommendations resulting from the interactions during the disengagement and termination phases (Zuzelo, 2010).

An example of an internal consultative intervention follows:

> The director of nursing in a local health department telephoned the state public health nursing consultant for alcohol and other substance abuse prevention and requested a meeting at the local health department. The purpose of the meeting was to help staff analyze the evidence base and develop the protocols for a community-wide substance abuse prevention program they wished to provide. Several departments within the health department had been providing different aspects of substance abuse prevention but a coordinated effort was not in place. The nurse consultant, Paula, met with the client, Maggie, and reviewed her findings, sharing her analysis of the current situation and contributing factors. The central issue was defined as an organizational culture that did not promote interprofessional teamwork. This resulted in difficulties providing comprehensive and coordinated substance abuse prevention initiatives. Maggie then spoke with the other department directors to identify barriers and facilitators to interprofessional teamwork. Each director agreed to speak with staff in their departments to obtain their input on barriers and facilitators. One suggestion made by staff members was to hold an off-site retreat for team-based planning related to transitional care programs such as this one. Paula worked with Maggie to help develop suggestions for the agenda and logistics that Maggie shared with the other directors. The directors asked Paula to facilitate the retreat. Following revision of the program plan during the retreat, Paula met with Maggie and the other directors to help them develop additional strategies to foster an organizational culture that promoted interprofessional teamwork. She maintained contact with Maggie until the updated evidence base and program plan had been approved by the health department board and termination of the consultation occurred.

NURSING TIP *Two of the most important decisions a nurse makes before accepting or writing a consultation contract are to identify the real client in the situation and the nature of the problem. It is not a good idea to prematurely accept the problem as presented by the person seeking the consultation. Sometimes the person is not the actual client but defines only the problem as he or she views it. Using the process model of consultation, the consultant can help define the real client and the real problem in order to develop workable solutions.*

Nurse Consultant Role

An agency whose delivery of care is similar to that of an official public health service will most likely employ a nurse who provides traditional or nursing consultation for a broad range of community health activities (e.g., a community or public health nurse clinical specialist). A community health agency that provides a program approach to the delivery of community health services, such as family planning, maternity, child health, handicapped children's services, school health, or home health, will tend to employ specialist consultants. These consultants may have skills and training in specific clinical areas (e.g., a nurse with expertise in maternal and child health). Agencies providing primary health care require a consultant with both general knowledge of public health practice and specialized knowledge in a primary care clinical area. This is also a requirement in agencies involved in long-term and home health care.

The nurse consultant employed in an official public health agency functions as an internal consultant to the employing agency. As a representative of the agency, the nurse provides nursing and consultation to colleagues, other disciplines, agency administration, and other health and human service agencies and/or community groups. Two primary roles of the internal consultant are resource person and facilitator.

With knowledge of available resources, the nurse consultant can identify gaps in service, identify the critical services provided by the health care delivery system, and promote services for meeting health or social needs of the population. The consultant facilitates staff nurse problem solving about individual client and family needs, health needs of a group of clients, or professional concerns and attitudes. The consultant may assist managers and administrators in solving problems about personnel, program needs, organizational goals, community relationships, and client population needs. The consultant may also facilitate communication across agencies by working with interagency coalitions or alliances.

Consultants from federal agencies are often used as external nurse consultants. The nurse consultant from the federal agency may come to the local or state agency to serve on request as facilitator or resource person helping with program planning, development, and implementation. The primary role function of this consultant is to serve as a resource person, although the consultant may facilitate movement toward identifying actual program objectives.

An example of a vital role nurse consultants can play is in helping a community agency or a coalition conduct community needs assessments and develop strategic plans and associated action plans for achieving *Healthy People 2020* goals (see the *Healthy People 2020* box) (USDHHS, 2010).

COMPETENCIES FOR NURSE LEADERS

Leadership Competencies

Nurses need effective leadership, interpersonal, political, organizational, fiscal, analytical, and information competencies. Some competencies are similar to those required for leadership in other clinical areas, such as good communication skills and

HEALTHY PEOPLE 2020

Objectives Related to the Four Overarching Goals

The following are examples of some of the proposed objectives related to leadership, management, and consultation by public health nurses:

- AHS-2: (Developmental) Increase the proportion of persons with coverage of appropriate evidence-based clinical preventive services.
- HC/HIT-11: (Developmental) Increase the proportion of meaningful users of health information technology.
- PHI-1: Increase the proportion of federal, tribal, state, and local public health agencies that incorporate core competencies for public health professionals into job descriptions and performance evaluations.
- PHI-14: Increase the proportion of national and local public health jurisdictions that conduct a public health system assessment based on national performance standards.

From U.S. Department of Health and Human Services: *Healthy People 2020*, Washington, DC, 2010. Available at http://www.healthypeople.gov/HP2020/Objectives/TopicAreas.aspx. Accessed September 2, 2010.

 LINKING CONTENT TO PRACTICE

This chapter emphasizes the use of leadership, management, and consultative skills and knowledge in public health nursing practice, whether one has an official leadership or consulting role or not. Use of the theories and principles of leadership, management, and consultation with public health and nursing science is key to promoting healthy communities and achieving the goals of *Healthy People 2020* (USDHHS, 2010). Entry-level public health nurses are expected to possess competencies in these areas, including communication, collaboration, team building, analysis, program planning and management, managing budgets, and understanding and implementing policies (Quad Council of Public Health Nursing Organizations, 2009; Council on Linkages Between Academia and Public Health Practice, 2010). Public health nurses focus on working with communities in addition to other staff members and colleagues, and work with broad problems and issues that require systems thinking, leadership, and building coalitions (Koh and Jacobson, 2009). When a public health nurse thinks about empowerment, for example, he or she considers how to provide information and foster skill development for empowerment of other staff members and of community members. Thinking about working in partnership with community groups and policy makers influences a public health nurse's use of theories and principles of leadership, management, and consultation.

---

the ability to delegate effectively. Working in the community means being able to work with populations and groups, to build coalitions and work with partnerships. Leadership essential to these roles involves identifying a shared vision and influencing others to achieve the vision, emphasizing that client needs are the basis for health services, empowering others, delegating tasks and managing time appropriately, and making decisions effectively.

Nurse managers should be involved in developing agency-level vision, mission, and goal statements. The American Nurses Association (ANA), the American Public Health Association, Public Health Nursing Section, and the International Honor Society for Nursing offer guidance in these areas through conferences and various publications, as do other professional organizations.

Empowerment

Leaders help others empower themselves to make organizations more responsive to client needs. This means removing barriers to decision making and allowing staff nurses the authority to make client decisions in "real time," as needs demand, rather than requiring nurses to obtain numerous approvals. Empowerment is more than simply increasing nurses' authority—it includes ensuring that they have the necessary knowledge, skills, and resources to effectively make the decisions for which they are held accountable. For example, nurse managers who are responsible for preparing their own department or program budgets and for approving program spending must be given the opportunity to learn budgetary concepts. Nurses are likely to feel more empowered to do their work in a less bureaucratic environment that supports clinical autonomy and collaborative professional relationships (Spence Laschinger et al, 2010).

The concept of empowerment underpins the consulting process. Consultants assist others in identifying solutions to problems and, more importantly, in developing the ability to manage problems independently in the future.

Delegation

Effective delegation is a key competency of public health nurses. The Education Committee of the Association of Community Health Nurse Educators (2010) listed delegation among the competencies for community/public health nurses. This group noted that delegation is part of ensuring that care is appropriately coordinated within an interprofessional health care team. It has become increasingly necessary due to the complexity of care in public health and community settings (Resha, 2010).

Agency efficiency increases when tasks are assigned to the first level in the hierarchy where employees possess the necessary skills and knowledge to complete the task and where the task is related to the goals of those positions. Delegation develops others' talents and can contribute to job satisfaction. Asking a nurse in a nursing clinic for homeless families to develop a booklet describing community resources for this population helps the staff nurse learn more about community resources, the gaps that exist in local resources, and where opportunities exist for interagency collaboration. The nurse is also likely to learn about visual presentation, layout and brochure design issues, and how to present material at the appropriate reading level. Finally, delegation is an important tool in time management. A school nurse may delegate locating resources for a screening clinic to the parent–teacher association, and the time saved can be spent on developing a teaching plan for volunteers who will help with the actual screening. Strategies for effective time management and delegation are listed in Boxes 40-1 and 40-2. Figure 40-1 provides a sample timetable for conducting a health fair, showing how the nurse might decide which activities need to be completed and suggesting those that might be delegated.

Delegation has become an increasingly important skill for nurses, whether they have official roles as managers or not. As more agencies increase their use of unlicensed assistive personnel and lay community workers, nurses are increasingly delegating selected aspects of practice to others and supervising the completion of those tasks. Two types of delegation occur in clinical practice. Direct delegation involves speaking to an individual personally and transferring responsibility for a task to that person (ANA, 2007a). Indirect delegation results when an agency has policies and procedures in place that allow tasks to be

performed by someone other than the person who is accountable (ANA, 2007a). Sometimes nurses mistakenly think that they are not accountable for tasks that are indirectly delegated through agency policies (e.g., policies for cross-training). However, if nursing care has been delegated, then nurses and their organizations are accountable for the safe and effective completion of that care (NCSBN, 2005). Organizations are responsible for ensuring that staffing is sufficient to allow for safe and appropriate delegation of care (NCSBN, 2005; Block, 2009).

The first source of guidance for delegating tasks to unlicensed individuals is the state nurse practice act (NCSBN, 2005). The next source of assistance comes from specialty professional organizations. For example, the National Association of School Nurses and the ANA included care coordination, and working with parents, teachers, community members, and "adjunct personnel" (ANA, 2005, p 39) in the standards of professional performance for school nurses. Related responsibilities include ensuring optimal outcomes and quality of care.

In order to delegate effectively, public health nurses must understand the differences between responsibility, accountability, and authority (Weydt, 2010). The nurse may have the authority to delegate certain tasks to another individual or group. That individual or group accepts the responsibility to complete the task, but the nurse retains accountability to ensure the safety and quality of the outcome.

For example, a school nurse has the responsibility to assess a child with physical disabilities and develop a plan of care for that child. Selected aspects of that plan of care, such as assisting with feeding or emptying a catheter bag and recording output, could be delegated to an assistant, provided that person had received appropriate training and was competent to perform the task. This means that it is not adequate that the nurse know the individual has been certified as a nursing assistant; the nurse also needs to know that the individual is competent to safely perform the delegated task. It is important to ensure that those to whom certain tasks have been delegated have been

---

BOX 40-1   TIME MANAGEMENT TIPS

- List goals for 5 years, 1 year, and daily.
- Prioritize the goals.
- Identify the tasks that must be performed to accomplish the goals.
- Identify the tasks that can be delegated.
- Group the tasks in a meaningful way (e.g., geographically).
- Plan strategies to minimize time-wasters. For example, plan office hours when people can find you in your office available to respond to questions.
- Plan to work on tasks at times when you are at peak level of efficiency (e.g., plan tasks requiring mental alertness in the morning if you are more alert at that time).
- Plan plenty of time to accomplish tasks with adequate transitional time between tasks.
- Say no to tasks that are not essential to your position or your goals.
- Take adequate breaks from work, including breaks during the day and vacations.
- Maintain personal energy level through good health habits, including proper nutrition, adequate exercise, sleep, and stress management.

BOX 40-2   DELEGATING RESPONSIBILITY

Nurse managers share responsibility for any tasks they delegate to others. The nurse manager delegates responsibility for a task but retains final accountability for the safe, effective outcome of the task (ANA, 2010). It is critical, then, that nurse managers know that the individuals to whom they are delegating responsibility are both prepared and capable of effectively performing the tasks. Nurse managers should provide clear guidelines and plan specific times to obtain progress reports on task completion. This will allow the opportunity to manage problems as they arise and to provide staff with helpful feedback or instruction if needed.

Activity	Month 1	Month 2	Month 3	Month 4
Identify planning group	●——→			
Decide which displays to include		●——→		
Reserve location		●——→		
Invite exhibitors		●——→		
Develop referral policies for follow-up of screening tests		●————————→		
Arrange for publicity		●————————————→		
Conduct the health fair				●→

FIGURE 40-1 Sample timetable for conducting a health fair.

trained to accept the responsibility and carry it out effectively. Public health nurses must also provide adequate time to plan the delegation process and to communicate with the person or group to whom a task is being delegated (NCSBN, 2005). Communication should occur throughout the process to allow for feedback and clarifications when needed. The nurse retains the legal accountability for safe client care. This responsibility may be shared with the person to whom one is delegating, but accountability is never transferred (ANA, 2010).

Critical Thinking

Public health nursing leaders and consultants must be adept at critical thinking. Critical thinking includes analyzing and synthesizing data, using knowledge and values in making judgments, and using creative approaches in decision making and problem solving (Bittner and Gravlin, 2009). It includes reflection about the connections between sociocultural and biophysiological aspects of health status and services. Critical thinking may be fostered through the use of guided group discussions, in which group members are assisted to think about the connections just described and about the distribution effects that decisions may have on others. It is also fostered through activities to stimulate creativity, such as brainstorming. In the example of the occupational wellness program, the nurse manager would need to critically think about ways to increase program quality.

Decision Making

Finally, a core leadership skill is the ability to make decisions effectively. Decision making and problem solving are critical aspects of nursing practice in complex clinical environments (Bittner and Gravlin, 2009). This is a two-stage process in which the nurse first must decide how much input to seek from others and second must generate alternatives for the decision and choose among the alternatives. Including others in the decision-making process is beneficial in part because others may have information and ideas that would lead to a better decision, and also because others may support the decision more if they are involved in making it. This also fosters team building and collaboration, which are two competencies for public health nurses (Quad Council of Public Health Nursing Organizations, 2009; Council on Linkages Between Academia and Public Health Practice, 2010).

A decision tree can be used for selecting a leadership style that varies from a unilateral, independent decision process, to progressively more participative styles, with the most participative style involving delegating authority to a group that will be responsible for making the decision. Although many assume that autocratic decision making is not effective, in fact it may be both effective and efficient under certain circumstances, such as emergencies. In other situations, it is better to seek input from others, individually or as a group, to seek suggestions for solutions from the group, or to simply turn a problem over to a group to solve on their own.

The next stage of the decision-making process is to generate alternative solutions and to choose among those solutions. Both risk and cost are important dimensions in most situations. The goal involves low cost and low risk to clients and staff. Other dimensions might be unique to the situation. For example, if the nurse is trying to decide whether to develop an in-house wellness program for an occupational setting or to contract with a consulting group for that service, the nurse could compare the risks and benefits of both alternatives. The occupational health nurse might decide that the advantages of an in-house wellness program are that (1) it allows for staff participation in identifying key dimensions and goals and brainstorming creative solutions, (2) participants' values are built into the dimensions and goals, and (3) it allows for both creative and logical thinking processes.

Interpersonal Competencies

Nurse leaders, managers, and consultants need effective interpersonal skills in communicating, motivating, appraisal and coaching, contracting, supervising, team building, and promoting diversity.

Communication

Good communication skills, including skills in the use of assertiveness techniques and conflict resolution (Kritek, cited in IOM, 2010) as well as communicating through the media and professional and scientific literature, are essential to being effective in leadership roles. Nurses have a particular challenge in communicating because many of those with whom they work may be in a different health profession or in a different field altogether. Nurses often communicate with lay workers or with the public through media outlets such as newspaper columns, television and radio interviews, blogs, and public service announcements. It is especially critical to listen carefully, to make underlying assumptions clear, and to speak in the other's language. This may mean avoiding the use of professional jargon and speaking in more commonly shared language or speaking in the listener's primary language. It is increasingly important for nurses to be bilingual or multilingual, depending on the ethnic composition of the community.

Communication must be culturally competent to be effective. Because communication involves words, tone of voice, posture, eye contact, and spatial relationships, cultural norms often influence the meanings given to different aspects of body language. For example, whereas most advise direct eye contact when communicating, in some cultures this may be viewed as aggressive, especially when the eye contact is prolonged. Some cultures prefer the closer-space relationships that may make others feel they are being crowded. Other aspects of communication are important as well, such as the appropriate place for reprimands. It is never appropriate to reprimand or criticize in public, although public praise is usually an excellent idea. Nurse managers and consultants should be sensitive to the power of written communication and be aware that, although putting a message in writing is a good way to avoid confusion, it also may be seen as aggressive, distrustful, or a bid for power. The key is to make certain that the message that is communicated is the message that was intended. Effective communication skills are listed in Box 40-3.

BOX 40-3   EFFECTIVE COMMUNICATION SKILLS

- Listen actively.
- Restate the main points.
- Speak in the listener's language.
- Maintain culturally appropriate eye contact and body language.
- Provide an appropriate environment.
- Be aware of the power of written communication.
- Use simple, direct words.
- Use "I" statements and say how you feel.
- Provide frequent feedback.
- Reflect on the meaning of the message.

BOX 40-4   CREATING A MOTIVATING WORKPLACE

- Identify employees' needs and goals.
- Identify employees' beliefs about their abilities to meet their goals.
- Discuss with employees their strengths and areas for future development.
- Discuss how the employees' goals and the organization's goals can be aligned.
- Jointly develop job-related goals with employees, including timetables with checkpoints.
- Provide frequent, regular feedback to employees.
- Provide frequent thanks for a job well done and for progress toward goals.
- Facilitate the development of mentor–protégé relationships and role modeling.
- Provide opportunities for employees to learn new goal-related skills.
- Provide tangible signs of recognition, such as merit pay, employee of the month, and special bonuses for achievements.

Creating a Motivating Workplace

One of the more difficult skills to master is motivating other people; in fact, one cannot ever really motivate others, because motivation is internal. However, the skillful leader can create a motivating environment, working to make certain that both individual and agency goals are met to the extent possible. Sometimes individual motivation may be low because employees do not believe they have the skills necessary to achieve their goals, or they believe that the system will not allow them to do so. The effective nurse leader identifies which perceptions are inaccurate and helps individuals develop plans for improving their personal capacities for achieving goals. Although adequate salaries are important, compensation is not the only way to create a motivating environment for professionals. One home health aide supervisor is known for the high level of morale among her staff and the unusually low level of turnover. She makes a point of being available for discussion before the aides leave the agency in the morning and on their return in the afternoon. She always gives each person a birthday card, and thanks them for a job well done. For the long-term good, leaders should work with others in the community to increase salaries if they are not competitive. Other keys to creating a motivating workplace are listed in Box 40-4.

Appraisal and Coaching

Employee appraisal and coaching are closely related to motivation and individual development (Spence and Wood, 2007). The purpose of performance evaluation is to assist employees to more effectively meet the objectives of their roles and to help them develop their potential in ways that facilitate achieving agency goals. Performance evaluation should not take place just before an annual appraisal interview is scheduled. It should be a regular part of the job, with the manager providing regular feedback on employee progress toward goals. Performance appraisal is particularly challenging for nurse managers because so many community health workers practice independently in the field. For example, nurse managers in home health must plan either to make visits with the nursing staff on a regular basis or to obtain other forms of input on employee performance, such as planning telephone or office conferences with staff.

Coaching involves working one-on-one with others to improve clinical care delivery (Ervin, 2005). With coaching,

managers retain responsibility for decisions but request input and explain decisions. They support progress by helping the employee break the tasks into manageable parts, providing resources for accomplishing tasks and for acquiring the necessary skills, and praising task accomplishment. Coaching is most useful with people who may not yet be skillful in a particular area and who are not confident about their skills.

Contracting involves identifying expectations and responsibilities by both parties. Some contracts are informal, verbal agreements between individuals, whereas others (such as the consulting contract) are formal, written agreements.

Supervision

Nurse managers who delegate tasks to others must supervise the completion of those tasks and build in mechanisms to make certain that the tasks are completed safely and effectively (ANA, 2010; NCSBN, 2005). Supervision means decision making and implementation of activities in an ongoing relationship. It may occur either on site when the nurse manager is present and while the activity is being performed, or off site when the nurse is providing care in a community setting. It is important for nurse managers to build effective means of providing off-site supervision because so many community health activities do not take place within a single agency (e.g., home health care occurs in individual homes, and school health services are provided in individual schools).

Handling criticism is a difficult skill that involves both the giving and the taking of criticism related to job performance. Nurse managers should provide constructive critique as close as possible to the time they observe a problem with an employee's job performance. Constructive criticism focuses on the behaviors necessary to meet the job expectations and helps identify sources of problems, resources for managing problem behavior, and feedback. For example, if an employee is chronically tardy, the nurse manager should speak privately with the employee about the job expectation for promptness, identify why the employee is frequently tardy, establish a behavioral goal with time frames and consequences of achieving or not achieving the goal, and assist the employee to develop a plan for achieving the goal. The employee may be unaware of the importance of being punctual and can easily change the behavior. On the other hand, a behavior modification plan may be useful to help change the behavior. Behavioral consequences may include both positive reinforcers, such as praise, and disciplinary measures, such as oral and written warnings, limited raises, suspension, and termination. Suspension and termination are normally used only with problems related to safety, inability to perform job duties, breach of confidentiality, and illegal acts; they are detailed in agency policies and procedures.

Team Building

Finally, team building and managing diversity are group-level skills needed by nurse leaders, managers, and consultants (Phillips, 2009). Interprofessional teams increasingly are used to assess clients, plan client care or services, and manage quality improvement activities. Teams may include members of multiple health disciplines as, for example, with community health coalitions. They also may include people from other backgrounds, including lay community health workers. Nurse managers and consultants can facilitate team building by assisting the team to develop goals and ground rules, identifying who will fill various roles and determining how to share leadership, developing strategies for ongoing cooperation and recognition of contributions of each member, and resolving conflict.

Promoting Diversity

A key challenge to nurse managers is promoting and managing diversity in positive ways that value different perspectives and provide insights into culturally competent strategies to eliminate disparities. By the middle of the twenty-first century, today's minority groups will make up a majority of the U.S. population (The Sullivan Commission, 2004). Nurse leaders must work with others to create workplaces that build on the strengths of a diverse workforce to provide excellent health care and eliminate disparities in outcomes. Nurses should partner with schools, faith communities, health care agencies, and universities to encourage minority group members who are interested in nursing careers. This will help build a community nursing workforce that better reflects the population as a whole (The Sullivan Commission, 2004). Nurse managers must understand cultural values and norms to communicate effectively and interpret behavior accurately. They must know how to prevent any form of racial, sexual, or ethnic harassment and ensure a positive and welcoming environment in the workplace.

DID YOU KNOW? *When working with people from cultures different from their own, population-focused nurse leaders, managers, and consultants are more likely to be effective if they take the time to learn as much as possible about the culture. This helps clarify underlying beliefs, values, and assumptions that may influence managerial or consultative issues and improves communication effectiveness and the effectiveness of change processes. Differing cultural perspectives may be present across populations and across interprofessional groups (Reich and Reich, 2006).*

Power Dynamics and Conflict Resolution

Power imbalances can occur within groups, community organizations, and policy-making bodies, and affect health care professionals and community members. Managing power dynamics effectively requires that public health nurses understand community systems, collaboration, and strategies for providing information to empower others to work on their own behalf. Public health nurses work closely with community groups to build capacity for assessing strengths and needs, developing solutions to community health problems and promoting health and wellness, and managing long-term approaches for healthier communities. This is particularly important when working with vulnerable populations (Erwin, 2008).

Effective conflict resolution requires negotiation skills as well as skills in recognizing and managing power dynamics. Principled negotiation (Marriner-Tomey, 2008) emphasizes collaborative problem solving and development of mutually agreeable ways of achieving goals. Conflict resolution strategies can result in win-win, win-lose, or lose-lose outcomes. Strategies most likely to create win-win situations include collaborating, confronting problems directly, building consensus, and ensuring that all parties have an adequate opportunity for input (Marriner-Tomey, 2008).

Population-focused nurse leaders must understand power dynamics. Because nurses possess altruistic values, they may believe that being powerful is not necessary. However, it is impossible to create health-promoting public health services without some legitimacy in decision-making arenas. Membership on community agency boards and advisory committees puts nurse managers in the position to influence service delivery.

Consultants' advice may be followed because the client feels that the consultant possesses superior knowledge or skills and is trustworthy and credible. Internal nurse consultants may have power resulting from their roles in the organization. The client may not feel obligated to implement the recommendations of external consultants. On the other hand, external consultants may be viewed as influential because of an affiliation with other well-known consultants or a national organization. The consultant's ability to persuade clients by offering reasons, new techniques, or methods of problem solving may motivate clients to follow the consultant's advice.

Organizational Competencies

Nurses use organizational skills, such as planning, organizing, implementing, and coordinating as well as monitoring, evaluating, and improving quality. Nurses use these skills when managing programs and projects and when coordinating care for individuals, families, and groups.

Planning

Planning includes prioritizing daily activities to achieve goals. It also includes long-range planning, such as working with nurses in a department to plan a new program. Planning is a collaborative activity that can involve interprofessional teams, community groups, and policy makers. Developing a shared vision, goals, and measurable objectives provides the foundation for a plan. Nurses must be able to anticipate the cost of providing nursing services to a certain population over a period of time and to develop a proposal (or a business plan) for a contract to provide the services. Because planning is primarily a cognitive activity, nurse managers and consultants may tend to lessen its importance and allow little time for adequate planning. However, planning is the basis for direct nursing services and it is an essential competency for population-focused nurse care (ANA, 2007b; Quad Council of Public Health Nursing Organizations, 2009), so it is important to make adequate time for planning.

Several documents are available to help nurse managers and consultants plan nursing services. *Healthy People 2020* (USDHHS, 2010) defines the national health goals for the United States by the year 2020 and should be the basis for program planning. The *Healthy Communities Program* (CDC, 2010) describes strategies for working with community groups to achieve *Healthy People* goals at a local level. The Task Force on Community Preventive Services wrote *The Guide To Community Preventive Services* (Zaza, Briss, and Harris, 2005) to provide evidence-based strategies for community health planning.

Organizing

Organizing involves determining appropriate sequencing and timelines for the activities necessary to achieve goals and arranging for the appropriate people to carry out the plan. Flow sheets and timetables are helpful tools that allow nurse managers and consultants to visualize how tasks are organized and to identify gaps in the planning. Figure 40-1, as shown earlier, illustrates a timetable for conducting a health fair.

Implementing and Coordinating

Implementing and coordinating a plan includes not only following the timelines, but also making certain that the relevant regulations and policies are adhered to, that activities are appropriately documented, and that the work of all team members is coordinated. One strategy that helps ensure coordination is use of an action plan (Yoo et al, 2004). This is a table that includes the program goals and objectives, activities to meet the objectives, identification of those responsible for each activity, the timeframe for completing the activities, and the plan for evaluating achievement of the objectives. Team members should review the action plan at regular meetings and make changes as necessary. Action plans are also used to coordinate care for people with chronic illnesses such as asthma (see, for example, Borgmeyer et al, 2005). Nurse managers and consultants should give sufficient attention to the change process by helping those involved identify the need for change, keeping them informed, soliciting their input, and making modifications in the plan as necessary.

Monitoring, Evaluating, and Improving

Monitoring, evaluating, and making improvements are critical to nursing services. Nurses should monitor nursing services on a regular basis and make improvements as soon as the need for improvements becomes apparent. Professional standards and the standards of various accrediting bodies guide the focus of monitoring and evaluating. The Joint Commission standards for home health and ambulatory care clinics (http://www.jointcommission.org/) provide detailed and explicit minimum standards that all such agencies should be expected to meet.

In addition to professional standards of practice available from the ANA and specialty nursing organizations, the Agency for Healthcare Research and Quality has published clinical guidelines for prevention and treatment of selected health problems, such as wound care, pain, and tobacco cessation. Using evidence-based clinical guidelines is a key way to improve the quality of care. Finally, nurses should evaluate and monitor changes in client health outcomes. Effective outcomes management programs using information systems can be used for ongoing planning and program improvements for target populations such as women and children (Monsen et al, 2010).

Fiscal Competencies

Forecasting Costs

Nurse leaders must be skilled in the area of fiscal management. Nurse managers and consultants must be able to project the cost of public health nursing services. This is especially important in today's tight economic environment because the forecast should include an assessment of the risk rating of the likely health and illness experiences of a target population. Combining community health assessment skills, epidemiological projections, and consultation are key steps in this process and make it possible to design health programs to reduce health risks among various populations. After developing a profile of the anticipated health and illness experiences of a target population, the next step is anticipating the amount and kind of nursing resources needed by the population. These skills are basic to the development of proposals for new nursing services and contracts with external groups.

Develop and Monitor Budgets

Nurse managers have taken on more responsibility for developing and monitoring their own department budgets as agencies have decentralized. They must be able to develop a justifiable budget and monitor how actual spending compares with planned spending. Expenses commonly included in an operating budget are salaries and benefits, equipment, supplies, travel, and overhead. It is helpful to obtain staff input when developing a budget in order to make financial projections as realistic as possible. Nurse managers should review program action plans with staff to determine the resources necessary to implement the program. Combining anticipated volume, revenues, and expenses allows the nurse manager to anticipate a breakeven point for new services (i.e., determining when a new program can be expected to be financially self-sufficient).

Variance analysis means identifying the difference between actual and planned results, determining the cause of the variation, and correcting problems when they exist. Spending more than anticipated is not always negative; it may simply indicate that client or service volume was higher than anticipated. This could, however, be of concern in an agency that is fully capitated and receives a set amount of money to see a client for usually a year, regardless of the cost of the services the client needs. Additional services do not bring in additional revenues. Nurses in fully capitated environments have more opportunity than ever before to focus on health promotion and illness prevention services.

Higher expenses than planned are not always under the control of the nurse manager. For example, if the prevailing wage increases because of changes in the labor market, an agency may spend more than expected on salaries. On the other hand, spending less than predicted does not always indicate that a program is running efficiently; client volume may be down, or staff may not be providing adequate services. The most important thing for a public health nurse to do initially is to monitor expenses carefully and analyze why expenses might differ from the original plan.

For example, if a nurse manager observes that more has been spent on salaries and supplies than originally budgeted, and less on travel, should he or she think this is desirable or undesirable? To analyze the variance, the nurse should ask if the prices for labor and supplies were higher than expected or if the agency has used more nursing time or supplies than planned (Finkler, Kovner, and Jones, 2007). The answers to these questions will help determine whether the variance resulted from factors under the manager's control, such as inefficiency, or from factors outside of the manager's control, such as higher wages or higher prices than expected. The answers will also help determine whether the variance resulted from an increase in client volume or an alteration in case mix, with the agency serving sicker clients.

Conduct Cost–Effectiveness Analysis

Regardless of the type of reimbursement system in place, nurses should be able to conduct a simple cost-effectiveness analysis of their interventions. Such analyses are not measurements of the efficiency of a program (see Chapter 25 for a discussion of this distinction) but are comparisons of the money spent for the outcomes across two or more interventions. Cost-effectiveness analyses compare alternative approaches for achieving the same goals. The nurse should measure the full costs and benefits (or savings) of each alternative intervention and construct ratios to compare the alternatives. The final result might be stated as the number of people who were able to achieve a desired health outcome (e.g., losing weight or adhering to an exercise program) for each additional dollar spent. The results of cost-effectiveness analyses sometimes raise new questions that must be analyzed. For example, in a study of the cost-effectiveness of varying levels of worksite wellness programs in rural employment sites (Saleh et al, 2010), investigators found that the lower intensity interventions of screening and general awareness were more cost-effective than higher intensity interventions. However, the higher intensity interventions yielded better health outcomes in many areas. What would you recommend to management in an occupational setting based on these results?

Analytical and Information Competencies

It is increasingly important for nurses to have excellent analytical competencies and competencies in the use of information. For example, access to useful and needed data helps nurses and other health professionals monitor clinical outcomes, identify systems issues that can result in health care errors, and plan to better meet the health needs of their populations. Population-focused nurses need a good understanding of descriptive and clinical epidemiology as well as the ability to analyze graphical data displays such as histograms, flow charts, and line graphs. Use of aids such as checklists, reminders, and clinical decision support are all good ways to improve the quality of care and prevent errors (Nelson et al, 2008). Because nurses are interested in identifying patterns of health problems, care delivery, and outcomes in community settings, more nurses are including nursing taxonomies (or languages) in electronic client records. Nursing leaders who participate in incorporating electronic records and information systems should have a conceptual framework to guide the project (von Krogh, Dale, and Nåden, 2005).

CHAPTER REVIEW

PRACTICE APPLICATION

The nurse manager of a nursing clinic in a residential facility for frail older adults approached the local college of nursing for assistance with health promotion and health monitoring activities for the residents. The facility was undergoing renovation and was expected to more than triple its capacity by the time the renovation was completed. The nurse manager thought the health promotion activities that were already in place would be inadequate to serve the growing needs. Most of the residents were more than 70 years of age and had several chronic illnesses. The residential complex was 10 to 15 miles away from health care facilities.

Shirley, the nurse manager, supervised a staff of three nurses and one homemaker aide. She contracted with a local physical therapy firm for services as needed for the residents. Shirley had asked the staff if they thought they could realistically expand their services, and they suggested consultation. The staff commented that residents needed nurses who could provide health monitoring and skilled nursing services in their apartments, because so many were increasingly homebound. Staff members were hesitant about expanding into home care themselves because they feared it would mean a cutback in the health promotion activities they currently offered. They thought the needs, and the resources that would be required to meet the needs, should be evaluated before making any final decision.

What should the staff do to complete the evaluation of the problem?

A. Call a meeting of persons affected by the problem and decide on using an internal or external consultant to help evaluate the problem.

B. Write a contract and indicate how they want the evaluation to be done.

C. Develop a plan to implement home health services because the plan would include an analysis of needs and resources.

D. Continue with their health promotion activities and decide about home health services when more resources could be identified. Answers can be found on the Evolve site.

KEY POINTS

- Nurse leaders may function in formal roles as managers or consultants, or they may use managerial and consulting skills in their everyday clinical practice.
- Nurse leaders, managers, and consultants should work with organizations, coalitions, and community groups to design local strategies that will help achieve the *Healthy People 2020* goals.
- The goals of nursing leadership and management are (1) to achieve organization and professional goals for client services and clinical outcomes, (2) to empower personnel to perform their responsibilities effectively and efficiently, (3) to develop new services that will enable the organization to respond to emerging community health needs, and (4) to work with others for a healthy community.
- Systems thinking promotes sensitivity to the interdependence of parts of a system and the potential causes and consequences of organizational actions.
- Nurse managers may be team leaders or program directors, directors of home health agencies or community-based clinics, or commissioners of health. They function as visionaries, coaches, facilitators, role models, evaluators, advocates, community health and program planners, and teachers. They have ongoing responsibilities for clients, groups, and community health and for personnel and fiscal resources under their direction.
- The goal of consultation is to stimulate clients to take responsibility, feel more secure, deal constructively with their feelings and with others in interaction, and internalize skills of a flexible and creative nature.
- Consultation models can be categorized as content or process models. Process model consultation helps the client assess both the problem and the kind of help needed to solve the problem.

- Consultation involves seven basic phases: initial contact, definition of the relationship, selection of setting and approach, data collection and problem diagnosis, intervention, reduction of involvement and evaluation, and termination.
- Nurse consultants may function as internal consultants within an organization or external consultants outside the client organization.
- Nurse managers and consultants need a wide variety of competencies, including leadership, interpersonal, organizational, and political skills. Leadership skills include abilities to influence others to work toward achieving a vision, empower others, delegate tasks, manage time, and make decisions effectively.
- Interpersonal skills include communication, motivation, appraisal and coaching, contracting, team building, and diversity management skills.
- Organizational skills include planning, organizing, and implementing community nursing services; monitoring and evaluating services; quality improvement; and managing fiscal resources.
- Political skills are those used in negotiation and conflict management and managing power dynamics among health care teams and within the community.
- Population-focused nurses need analytical and informatics skills to be able to identify and monitor trends, improve health care safety, and evaluate outcomes.
- Generally, both nurse managers and consultants must hold a minimum of a baccalaureate degree in nursing. Organizations employing nurses without this credential should help them obtain additional education in the areas of community or nursing, management theories and principles, and theories and principles of consultation.

CLINICAL DECISION-MAKING ACTIVITIES

1. Discuss with your class members the implications that managed care and discounted fee-for-service preferred provider organizations have for nurse managers and consultants in community-based organizations and in the public health departments. What other implications can you think of in addition to those described in the text?

2. Draft a vision and mission statement for a nursing clinic with your classmates. Develop goals and objectives that follow the vision and mission you selected. What type of employees would you need to hire? List some of the policies and procedures you would need to have in such a clinic on the basis of your vision, mission goals, and objectives.

3. Have several class members obtain the vision, mission, and philosophy statements from agencies in which students have community health clinical experiences. Compare these statements in terms of the agencies' target populations, basic values, and essential functions.

4. Interview one or more practicing staff nurses working with populations. Ask them to describe the activities of their jobs that could be categorized as consultation. During the interview, attempt to determine the following:
   A. How they define consultation
   B. The goals they are attempting to achieve with their consulting activities
   C. The model they seem to be applying in their consulting activities
   D. The intervention strategies they use
   E. Whether their activities are of a generalist or a specialist nature and of an internal or external consultative nature
   F. The strengths and limitations they perceive in themselves regarding their consultative functions (e.g., education, experiential, organizational, relational, economic)

5. Interview one or more nurse consultants. During the interview, attempt to determine the answers to the preceding questions. Compare the responses of the two groups (public health nurse consultants and population-focused staff nurses). Analyze the factors you think account for the similarities and differences.

6. Visit a nurse-managed clinic for underserved populations. Talk with nurses and other staff members about how they work together as a team and what they do to promote client involvement in determining needed clinic services. Develop a case analysis of the microsystem within the clinic and how clinical care delivery is continuously monitored, evaluated, and improved within the system. What recommendations might you have for strengthening the clinical information system in the clinic?

REFERENCES

American Nurses Association: *Scope and standards of professional school nursing practice*, Washington, D.C., American Nurses Association and the National Association of School Nurses.

American Nurses Association: *Scope and standards for nurse administrators*, ed 2, Silver Spring, MD, 2010, ANA.

American Nurses Association: *Public health nursing: scope and standards of practice*, Silver Spring, MD, 2007a, Nursesbooks.org.

American Nurses Association: *Registered professional nurses and unlicensed assistive personnel*, Silver Springs, MD, 2007b, ANA.

Argyris C: Field theory as a basis for scholarly consulting, *J Soc Issues* 3:811, 1997.

Bass B, Bass R: *The Bass handbook of leadership: theory, research, and managerial applications*, New York, 2008, Free Press.

Bittner NP, Gravlin G: Critical thinking, delegation, and missed care in nursing practice, *J Nurs Adm* 39:142–146, 2009. doi:10.1097/NNA.0b013e31819894b7.

Block D: Reflections on school nursing and delegation, *PHN* 26:112–113, 2009. doi:10.1111/j.1525-1446.2009.00761.x.

Borgmeyer A, Jamerson P, Gyr P, et al: The school nurse role in asthma management: can the action plan help? *J Sch Nurs* 21:23–30, 2005.

Bulechek GM, Butcher K, Dochterman JM: *Nursing interventions classification*, ed 5, St Louis, 2007, Mosby.

Centers for Disease Control and Prevention: *Healthy communities program*, Atlanta, 2010, CDC.

Committee on Communication for Behavior Change in the 21st Century: *Improving the Health of Diverse Populations*, Washington, DC, 2002, Institute Of Medicine, National Academies Press.

Committee on the Work Environment for Nurses and Patient Safety: Board on Health Care Services: *Keeping Patient Safe: Transforming the Work Environment of Nurses*, Washington, DC, 2004, Institute of Medicine, National Academies Press.

Council on Linkages Between Academia and Public Health Practice: *Tier 1, tier 2, and tier 3 core competencies for public health professionals*, 2010. Available at http://www.phf.org/link/index.htm. Accessed May 3, 2010.

Education Committee of the Association of Community Health Nurse Educators: Essentials of baccalaureate nursing education for entry-level community/public health nursing. *PHN* 27:371–382, 2010. doi:10.1111/j.1525-1446.2010.00867.x.

El Ansari WE, Weiss ES: Quality of research on community partnerships: developing the evidence base, *Health Educ Res* 21:175–180, 2006. doi:10.1093/her/cyh/051.

Ervin NE: Clinical coaching: a strategy for enhancing evidence-based nursing practice, *Clin Nurse Spec* 19:296–301, 2005.

Erwin PC: Poverty in America: how public health practice can make a difference, *Am J Public Health* 98:1570–1572, 2008. doi:10.2105/AJPH.2007.127787.

Fialova D, Topinkova E, Gambassi G, et al: AdHOC Project Research Group: Potentially inappropriate medication use among elderly home care patients in Europe, *JAMA* 293:1348–1358, 2005.

Finkler SA, Kovner CT, Jones C: *Financial management for nurse managers and executives*, ed 3, St Louis, 2007, Saunders.

Georges CA, Bolton LB, Bennett C: Functional health literacy: an issue in African-American and other ethnic and racial communities, *J Natl Black Nurses Assoc* 15:1–4, 2004.

Groner J, French G, Ahijevych K, Wewers ME: Process evaluation of a nurse-delivered smoking relapse prevention program for new mothers, *J Community Health Nurs* 22:157–167, 2005.

Holden LN: Complex adaptive systems: concept analysis, *J Adv Nurs* 52:651–657, 2005.

Institute of Medicine: *A summary of the February 2010 Forum on the Future of Nursing: Education*, Washington, DC, 2010, The National Academies Press.

Johnson M, Griffiths R, Piper M, Langdon R: Risk factors for an untoward medication event among elders in community-based nursing caseloads in Australia, *Public Health Nurs* 22:36–44, 2005.

Koh HK, Jacobson M: Fostering public health leadership, *J Public Health* 31:199–201, 2009. doi:10.1093/pubmed/fdp032.

Kohn L, Corrigan J, Donaldson M, editors: *To err is human: building a safer health system*, Washington, DC, 2000, National Academies Press.

Lacey MY, Tompkins TC: Analysis of best practices of internal consulting, *Organizational Develop J* 25:123–131, 2007.

Marriner-Tomey A: *Guide to nursing management and leadership*, ed 8, St Louis, 2008, Mosby.

Martin M, Larsen BA, Shea L, et al: State diabetes prevention and control program participation in the Health Disparities Collaborative: evaluating the first five years, *Prev Chronic Dis (serial online)* 4:1–10, January 2007. (date cited 8/28/10). Available from http://www.cdc.gov/pcd/issues/2007/jan/06_0027.htm. Accessed March 8, 2011.

Metlay JP, Cohen A, Polsky D, et al: Medication safety in older adults: home-based practice patterns, *J Am Geriatr Soc* 53:976–982, 2005.

Monsen KA, Fulkerson JA, Lytton AB, et al: Comparing maternal child health problems and outcomes across public health nursing agencies. *Matern Child Health J* 14:412–421, 2010. doi:10.1007/s10995-009-0479-9.

National Council of State Boards of Nursing: *Working with others, a position paper*, 2005. Available at https://www.ncsbn.org/1625.htm. Accessed March 9, 2011.

Nelson EC, Godfrey MM, Batalden PB, et al: Clinical Microsystems, part 1: the building blocks of health systems, *Joint Comm J Qual Patient Saf* 34:367–378, 2008.

Olds DL, Kitzman HJ, Cole RE, et al: Enduring effects of prenatal and infancy home visiting by nurses on maternal life course and government spending: follow-up of a randomized trial among children at age 12 years, *Arch Pediatr Adolesc Med* 164:419–424, 2010.

Orem DE: *Nursing: concepts of practice*, ed 4, St Louis, 1991, Mosby-Year Book.

Phillips A: Realistic team building in a nurse-managed clinic setting, *Internet J Adv Nurs Pract* 10:1–14, 2009.

Porter J, Johnson J, Upshaw VM, et al: The Management Academy for Public Health: a new paradigm for public health management development, *J Public Health Manag Pract* 8:66–78, 2002.

Provan KG, Milward HB: Health services delivery networks: what do we know and where should we be headed? *HealthcarePapers* 7(2):32–36, 2006.

Public Health Foundation: *Workforce competencies*, Council on Linkages, Washington, DC, 2010, PHF.

Quad Council of Public Health Nursing Organizations: *Core competencies for public health nurses*, Clifton Park, NY, 2009, ASTDN.

Reich SM, Reich JA: Cultural competence in interdisciplinary collaborations: a method for respecting diversity in research partnerships. *Am J Community Psychol* 38:51–62, 2006. doi: 10.1007/s10464-006-9064-1.

Resha C: Delegation in the school setting: is it a safe practice? *Online J Issues Nurs* 15(2), 2010. doi:10.3912/OJIN.Vol15No-02Man05.

Roussel L, Swansburg RC, Swansburg RJ: *Management and leadership for nurse administrators*, ed 4, Sudbury, MA, 2006, Jones and Bartlett.

Roy SC: The nurse theorists: 21st century updates—Callista Roy, interview by Jacqueline Fawcett, *Nurs Sci Q* 15:308–310, 2002.

Ryan P: Integrated theory of health behavior change: background and intervention development, clinical nurse specialist, *J Adv Nurs Pract* 23(3):161–170, 2009.

Sabatino CA: School social work consultation models and response to intervention: a perfect match, *Children Schools* 31:197–206, 2009.

Saleh SS, Alameddine MS, Hill D, et al: The effectiveness and cost-effectiveness of a rural employer-based wellness program. *J Rural Health* 26:259–265, 2010. doi:10.1111/j.1748-0361.2010.00287.x.

Schein E: *Helping: how to offer, give, and receive help*, San Francisco, 2009, Berrett-Koehler.

Schein E: *Organizational culture and leadership*, San Francisco, 2010, John Wiley.

Spence Laschinger HKD, Gilbert S, Smith LM, Leslie K: Toward a comprehensive theory of nurse/patient empowerment: applying Kanter's empowerment theory to patient care, *J Nurs Manag* 18:4–13, 2010. doi:10.1111/j.1365-2834.2009.01046.x.

Spence D, Wood EE: Registered nurse participation in performance appraisal interviews. *J Prof Nurs* 23:55–59, 2007. doi:10.1016.j.profnurs.2005.11.003.

Stroebel CK, McDaniel RR Jr, Crabtree BF, et al: How complexity science can inform a reflective process for improvement in primary care practices, *Jt Comm J Qual Patient Saf* 31:438–446, 2005.

The Sullivan Commission: *Missing persons: minorities in the health professions: a report of The Sullivan Commission on diversity in the healthcare workforce*, Washington, DC, 2004, The Commission.

U.S. Clinical Preventive Services Task Force: *Guide to clinical preventive services, 2009: recommendations of the U.S. Preventive Services Task Force, AHRQ Pub No 09-IP006*, Rockville, MD, September 2009, Agency for Healthcare Research and Quality. Available at http://www.ahrq.gov/clinic/pocketgd.htm. Accessed March 9, 2011.

U.S. Department of Health and Human Services: *Healthy People 2020: proposed objectives and comments*, Washington, DC, 2010, USDHHS. Available at http://www.healthypeople.gov/HP2020/Objectives/TopicAreas.aspx. Accessed August 9, 2010.

von Krogh G, Dale C, Nåden D: A framework for integrating NANDA, NIC, and NOC terminology in electronic patient records, *J Nurs Scholar* 37:275–281, 2005.

Weydt A: Developing delegation skills, *Online J Issues Nurs* 15(2):1, 2010, doi:10.3912/OJIN.Vol15No-02Man01.

Wright K, Rowitz L, Merkle A, et al: Competency development in public health leadership, *Am J Public Health* 90:1202–1207, 2000.

Wright K: Environmental public health leadership development, *J Environ Health* 71:24–25, 2009.

Yoo S, Weed NE, Lempa ML, et al: Collaborative community empowerment: an illustration of a six-step process, *Health Promot Pract* 5:256–265, 2004.

Zaza S, Briss PA, Harris KW, editors: *The guide to community preventive services: what works to promote health?* 2005, CDC, Atlanta, GA.

Zuzelo P: *The clinical nurse specialist handbook*, Sudbury, MA, 2010, Jones and Bartlett.

CHAPTER 41

The Nurse in Home Health and Hospice

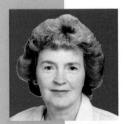

Karen S. Martin, RN, MSN, FAAN

Karen S. Martin is a health care consultant who has been in private practice since 1993. She works with service and educational settings nationally and internationally as they evaluate and improve their practice, documentation, and information management systems to meet quality and data exchange, as well as interoperability standards, for electronic health records. She is also a consultant to software developers. Karen has been employed as a staff nurse, director of a combined home care/public health agency, and, from 1978 to 1993, the Director of Research of the Visiting Nurse Association of Omaha, Nebraska, where she was the principal investigator of Omaha System research.

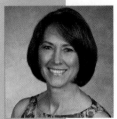

Kathryn H. Bowles, RN, PhD, FAAN

Kathryn H. Bowles is an Associate Professor at the University of Pennsylvania School of Nursing and the New Courtland Center for Transitions and Health. For several years, Dr. Bowles was the Director of Nursing Research at the Visiting Nurse Association of Greater Philadelphia and is currently the Beatrice Renfield Visiting Scholar at the Visiting Nurse Service of New York, with a focus on bringing evidence-based practice to home care. Her program of research focuses on improving care of the elderly using information technology such as decision support for hospital discharge planning and referral decision making, as well as testing telehealth technologies in community-based settings.

ADDITIONAL RESOURCES

evolve WEBSITE
http://evolve.elsevier.com/Stanhope
- *Healthy People 2020*
- WebLinks
- Quiz
- Case Studies
- Glossary

- Answers to Practice Application
- Resource Tools
  - Resource Tool 31.A: The Living Will Directive
  - Resource Tool 41.A: OASIS-C: Start of Care Assessment

OBJECTIVES

After reading this chapter, the student should be able to do the following:
1. Compare different practice models for home-based services.
2. Summarize the basic roles and responsibilities of home health and hospice nurses.
3. Explain the professional standards and educational requirements for nurses in home health and hospice.
4. Describe the three components of the Omaha System.
5. Analyze how nurses in home health and hospice use best practices, evidence-based practice, and quality improvement strategies to improve the care they provide.
6. Cite examples of trends and opportunities in home health and hospice involving technology, informatics, and telehealth.

KEY TERMS

accreditation, p. 904
benchmarking, p. 904
client outcomes, p. 898
documentation, p. 897
electronic health records, p. 896
evidence-based practice, p. 892
family caregiving, p. 891
home health care, p. 890
home health nursing, p. 890

hospice and palliative care,
   p. 890
hospice care, p. 892
information management,
   p. 897
interoperability, p. 908
interprofessional collaboration,
   p. 890
meaningful use, p. 908

medical home, p. 894
Medicare-certified, p. 894
nursing practice, p. 897
nursing process, p. 896
Omaha System, p. 896
Omaha System Intervention
   Scheme, p. 897
Omaha System Problem
   Classification Scheme, p. 897

Home health and hospice nurses are rapidly expanding practice specialties. For the purposes of this chapter, home health and hospice refer to a wide variety of holistic services provided to clients of all ages in their residences and other non-institutional settings. Assessment, planning, intervention, and evaluation are the focus of the services. Note that hospice care can be provided in acute care facilities, and many home health agencies offer these services in addition to home visits. Numerous references in this chapter describe home health research, economics, and client personal preference, suggesting that the home is the optimal location for diverse health and nursing services (Olds et al, 1997; Kitzman et al, 2000; Schumacher et al, 2006; Buhler-Wilkerson, 2007; Mader et al, 2008; NAHC, 2008; Beales and Edes, 2009; Homer et al, 2008; HAA, 2009; Ferrante et al, 2010; Naylor and Van Cleave, 2010). Client residences include houses, apartments, trailers, boarding and care homes, hospice houses, assisted living facilities, shelters, and cars. Home health and hospice services are provided by formal caregivers who include nurses, social workers, physical and occupational therapists, home health aides, chaplains, physicians, and others. Because of the nature of home health and hospice practice, a team approach and **interprofessional collaboration** are required. The specific disciplines who are involved vary with the program, the intensity of the client and family's needs, and the location of the program and home.

Access to other health care professionals, resources, and equipment is very different when home and institutional care settings are compared. Many nurses find home health and hospice practice very rewarding because they observe the impact of their services and practice with a high degree of autonomy. Nurses who make home visits need to have good organizational, communication, and documentation skills. Competence, integrity, adaptability, and creativity are essential characteristics. Nurses need to anticipate danger from people and circumstances in the physical environment to be savvy about their own safety as well as the safety of their clients (Humphrey and Milone-Nuzzo, 2010).

Home health care is a broad concept and approach to services. It includes a focus on primary, secondary, and tertiary prevention; the primary focus can involve aggregates, similar to other population-focused nurses. (See the Levels of Prevention box.) **Home health nursing** is "a specialized area of nursing practice, rooted in community health nursing, that delivers care in the residence of the client" (ANA, 2007, p 54). Home health nurses include generalist nurses, public health nurses, clinical nurse specialists, and nurse practitioners. They and their interprofessional team members provide diverse services to target populations such as new parents, frail elders, and clients who have injuries, surgery, disabilities, and acute or chronic health problems.

Hospice and palliative care are equally broad concepts and approaches to care. Hospice and palliative nursing are specialized areas of practice designed to "provide evidence-based physical, emotional, psychosocial, and spiritual or existential care to

LEVELS OF PREVENTION

Home Health

Primary Prevention

The nurse (a) administers seasonal and H1N1 flu vaccine, or (b) provides case management interventions so clients obtain the vaccines at convenient locations.

Secondary Prevention

The nurse monitors clients in their homes for early signs of new health problems in order to initiate prompt treatment. When the nurse works collaboratively with the physician and/or nurse practitioner, effective interventions can be provided. An example is monitoring clients for medication side effects.

Tertiary Prevention

The nurse provides instruction about dietary modifications and insulin injections to newly diagnosed diabetic clients. The purpose of these interventions is to prevent development of complications from diabetes. Diabetic clients and their families implement the therapeutic plan with the goal of maintaining the highest possible level of health.

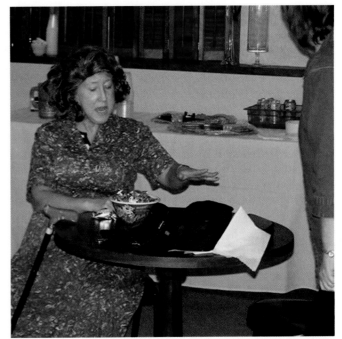

FIGURE 41-1 Nurses are guests in clients' homes. (From www. omahasystem.org/photogallery.html. Used with permission from Karen Martin, RN, MSN, FAAN.)

individuals and families experiencing life-limiting, progressive illness" (HPNA & ANA, 2007, p 1). Palliative services can be initiated whether or not cure is possible and can be considered a continuum of care. In contrast, hospice involves supportive services when a life-limiting illness does not respond to curative treatment, is the end-of-life portion of the continuum, and is regulated as a 6-month time period by Medicare (Viola et al, 2009; Perry and Parente, 2010). Advanced practice hospice and palliative nursing are emerging roles. Nurses work closely with members of other disciplines to provide comprehensive interprofessional care; volunteers are important team members.

WHAT DO YOU THINK? *Despite the current nursing shortage, increased client load, complex technological needs of clients in the home, and reimbursement regulations that focus on secondary and tertiary care, it remains an ethical responsibility of the home health or hospice nurse to promote health and prevent illness in the home and community.*

When entering a client's home, the nurse is a guest and needs to earn the trust of the family and establish a partnership with the client and family (Figure 41-1). It is essential that clients and families are involved in making decisions for home-based services to be efficient and effective. Family is defined by the individual client and includes any caregiver or significant other who assists the client with care at home. Family caregiving involves transportation, helping clients meet their basic needs, and providing care such as personal hygiene, meal preparation, medication administration, and simple as well as complex treatments. Today's clients and family caregivers provide many aspects of care in the home that were previously provided in hospitals or in home by professional care givers. Care can be confusing, challenging, stressful, and frightening for family caregivers (Schumacher et al, 2006; Buhler-Wilkerson, 2007; Altilio et al, 2008; Honea et al, 2008; Gorski, 2010). Clients need

to be monitored regularly, and some require 24-hour care. It is likely that family members are grieving when clients receive end-of-life care. Nurses need to identify support services that enable family caregivers to provide care while maintaining their own physical and emotional health status.

EVOLUTION OF HOME HEALTH AND HOSPICE

Home health care provided by formal caregivers in the United States originated in the nineteenth century, and was based on the district nursing model developed by William Rathbone in England. In many communities, the initial programs evolved into visiting nurse associations. The movement expanded rapidly in the United States, resulting in the formation of 71 agencies prior to 1900, and 600 organizations by 1909. Additional historical details are described in Chapter 2 and other publications (Buhler-Wilkerson, 2002; Donahue, 2011).

In 1893, Lillian Wald and Mary Brewster established the Henry Street Settlement House in New York City and developed a comprehensive program to address health and illness, poverty, education, shelter, and other basic needs. Nurses such as Lillian Wald, Mary Brewster, and Lavinia Dock were social activists who organized health care services, convinced community leaders to support their programs, provided national leadership, and published extensively. One of Lillian Wald's most impressive innovations was to convince the Metropolitan Life Insurance Company to include home visits as a benefit in the early 1900s and to examine the cost effectiveness of care. That partnership continued until 1952 (Buhler-Wilkerson, 2002; Donahue, 2011).

After World War I, the problems related to immigration and infectious diseases decreased. Simultaneously, the heightened public and professional interest in maternal-child health led to an increase in the number of public health departments and the nurses they employed (Buhler-Wilkerson, 2002; Donahue, 2011).

Home health services were included as a major benefit when Medicare legislation was passed in 1965, and resulted in significant changes nationally. The benefit was designed to provide intermittent, shorter visits with temporary lengths of stay to persons age 65 and older; health promotion and long-term care were not reimbursed. When a client was admitted to service, the home health agency was required to develop a plan of care and obtain the signature of a physician. During the next 30 years, the number of Medicare-certified agencies grew rapidly as a result of the aging population and prospective payment legislation that decreased the length of hospital stays. This trend changed when the Balanced Budget Act of 1997 was enacted; the legislation was designed to reduce federal home health reimbursement by initiating a per-beneficiary (or client) visit limit. The Act prompted the closure of more than 30% of the country's Medicare-certified home health agencies and a dramatic decline in the number of clients served (Schlenker et al, 2005; NAHC, 2008).

Hospice care was introduced in the United States in the 1970s by Florence Wald, often referred to as the mother of the hospice movement. She began her career as a staff nurse at the Visiting Nurse Service of New York and became Dean of the Yale University School of Nursing. Before establishing Connecticut Hospice in 1974, Dr. Wald collaborated with Dame Cicely Saunders, a British nurse, physician, and social worker who founded St. Christopher's Hospice in England in 1967 (Zerwekh, 2006; Gazelle, 2007). During the same era, Dr. Elisabeth Kübler-Ross, a physician, published *On Death and Dying* (1969), a book that was widely read by the public and health care professionals. Dr. Ross described the inhumanity of a death-denying society such as the United States, and the need to provide sensitive end-of-life care and involve clients in choices. The concept of hospice grew from a commitment to provide compassionate and dignified care to people in the comfort of their homes, and an emphasis on the quality of life (Zerwekh, 2006; Gazelle, 2007; Malloy et al, 2008; Perry and Parente, 2010; Sanders et al, 2010).

In 1987, the first comprehensive, integrated palliative care program was established at the Cleveland Clinic; it expanded from an inpatient unit to a comprehensive program that included a hospice affiliation. In 1999, the Robert Wood Johnson Foundation funded the Center to Advance Palliative Care to stimulate the development of high-quality palliative care programs in hospitals and other health care settings. Both home-based and inpatient hospice and palliative care models share a focus on comfort, pain relief, and mitigation of other distressing symptoms (Altilio et al, 2008; Viola et al, 2009; Perry and Parente, 2010; Sanders et al, 2010).

Medicaid reimbursement for hospice care began in 1980 and Medicare in 1983; reimbursement determines many aspects of the programs. Physicians need to indicate that clients have 6 months or less to live, and clients acknowledge that they have a terminal prognosis and select care that is comfortable, not life-extending. Because the time of death is difficult to predict and many people in this country are reluctant to acknowledge a terminal prognosis, hospice care often begins late in the disease process (Zerwekh, 2006; HAA, 2009; Viola et al, 2009; Perry and Parente, 2010).

EVIDENCE-BASED PRACTICE

Finding ways to help clinicians adopt and consistently use evidence-based practice illustrates the translation of research into practice. Murtaugh and colleagues (2005) tested two interventions designed to help home health nurses use evidence-based practice for clients with heart failure. Study participants were 354 nurses employed by a large non-profit agency in an urban area. Nurses were randomly assigned to the control group or one of two intervention groups. Nurses in the control group provided usual care. Nurses in one intervention group received basic e-mail reminders to follow the agreed-upon evidence-based practices when the clients were admitted for care. The other intervention group of nurses received the e-mail reminders, client education materials for use with their clients, and information regarding outreach and consultation with a clinical nurse specialist. Data were collected from clients' records. Although both intervention groups significantly increased their adherence to heart failure evidence-based practice guidelines, the group that also received client education materials and clinical nurse specialist consultation had the best outcomes.

Nurse Use

This study illustrates the importance of facilitating evidence-based practice and the effectiveness of simple reminder and support strategies.

From Murtaugh CM, Pezzin LE, McDonald MV: Just-in-time evidence-based email "reminders" in home health care: impact on nurse practices, *Health Serv Res* 40:849-864, 2005.

DESCRIPTION OF PRACTICE MODELS

Population-focused home care, transitional care, home-based primary care, home health, and hospice are models in current use. All involve interprofessional collaboration as well as interest in best practices and evidence-based practice. Best practices suggest using the best possible evidence from a variety of sources including research, experience, and expert practitioners; evidence-based practice suggests increased emphasis on programs of research that demonstrated consistently good outcomes. The models vary regarding the size and extent of participation, focus of the services, target population, research, political involvement, and funding. With each model, nurses have essential roles in the provision of care, documentation of services, program development and management, outcome and effectiveness analysis, and public education.

Population-Focused Home Care

Using an evidence-based and data-driven approach to population-focused home care, certain models of care delivery have produced superior outcomes. These models usually include structured approaches to regular visits with assessment protocols, focused health education, counseling, and health-related support and coaching. Examples of population-focused home care are described in the following paragraphs.

A group of researchers conducted studies involving clients who had psychiatric illnesses and lived in various community settings. During one interprofessional study, psychiatric nurses made home visits to elders who lived in public housing, had psychiatric symptoms, and were referred by building personnel (Rabins et al, 2000). The nurses conducted comprehensive psychiatric assessments; provided counseling, coaching, medication monitoring, and referrals; and coordinated care with social workers and physicians. Clients' psychiatric symptoms were reduced. The findings of another study indicated that clients who had dementia benefited when hospice care was provided, as did their family caregivers (Bekelman et al, 2005).

In Australia, a nurse and a pharmacist made home visits to older adults with diagnoses of atrial fibrillation and heart failure (Inglis et al, 2004). They conducted comprehensive health and medication assessments, provided health education, and made follow-up referrals. The nurse maintained telephone contact with clients for 6 months and provided care coordination. Clients in the experimental home visiting group had fewer hospital readmissions and shorter hospitalizations than those in a control group.

In Taiwan, public health and home health nurses participated in an extensive, interprofessional community-oriented program of research using home and clinic visits and telephone calls. Huang et al (2004) reported on the effectiveness of a 6-week home nursing program with elderly Chinese diabetic clients who lived alone. After weekly visits including structured education and monitoring, elders improved their levels of fasting blood glucose, post-meal blood glucose, and hemoglobin A1c. The researchers (Huang, 2005; Hsueh et al, 2010) also demonstrated successful outcomes when nurses have provided smoking cessation education and encouragement to long-term smokers. The Nurse-Family Partnership was initiated in 1977 by a researcher, David Olds, and a nurse, Harriet Kitzman; it is probably the best known and well-funded nurse home visit program in the United States (Olds et al, 1997; Kitzman et al, 2000). The Partnership involves nurses who provide structured education and case management during regularly scheduled home visits to pregnant women; visits continue until the children's second birthday. Recipients of care have been ethnically diverse, low-income, first-time mothers and their families who lived in New York, Tennessee, and Colorado. Longitudinal, randomized controlled trials documented numerous lifelong improvements in health outcomes that were statistically significant and economically sound. Mothers had fewer children, were more likely to become employed, and were less likely to enter the criminal justice system; children were less likely to be abused; and both mothers and children demonstrated improved health and development. The researchers estimate that nurses visit more than 30,000 families in nearly 40 states; federal and private funding continues to increase as the program maintains successful outcomes and grows (Olds et al, 1997; Kitzman et al, 2000; Donelan-McCall et al, 2009).

The Program of All-Inclusive Care for the Elderly (PACE) began in 1972, and is a managed care model of integrated health and personal care services for non-institutionalized individuals aged 55 and older who meet frailty criteria (Dobell and Newcomer, 2008). Interprofessional care is provided in adult day-care centers with home-based assessments and supportive services also provided as needed. Home health care and hospice can be services offered through this model. Because of the model's success, it is now included in Medicare and Medicaid capitation plans. As of 2009, 72 PACE programs operated in 30 states (National PACE Association, 2010).

Transitional Care

As a result of a fragmented health care system, increasing complexity of client care, and rising costs, transitional care has gained much needed attention. Transitional care is defined as "a set of actions designed to ensure the coordination and continuity of health care as clients transfer between different locations and different levels of care in the same location" (Coleman and Berenson, 2004, p 1). Challenges to quality care originate from a lack of depth, accuracy, and timeliness of information received from the referring site; the need for complex medication reconciliation; and difficulties with communication and coordination among community-based providers.

Transitional care programs that involve home health have emerged as low- and high-intensity interventions that include, but vary from, traditional home care interventions. Low-intensity interventions include coaching, telephone follow-up, and specific disease management programs (Boling, 2009). For example, a program by Coleman and colleagues (2006) proposes an intervention that emphasizes medication self management, use of a client-centered health record, arranged physician follow-up, and client education about warning signs, symptoms, and how to respond to them. The intervention includes a home visit and at least three telephone calls made by a nurse or trained provider after a transition.

High-intensity transitional care programs are designed for populations who have complex or high-risk health problems. An example is the Transitional Care Model where advanced practice nurses perform transitional care from hospital to home providing in-hospital visits and discharge planning followed with home visits, primary care office visits, and telephone follow-up for 1 to 3 months after discharge (Brooten et al, 2001; Naylor, 2004; Naylor and Van Cleave, 2010). Examples of high-risk groups for whom the Transitional Care Model has been tested in numerous studies include women with high-risk pregnancies, adults with cognitive impairments, older adults with common medical and surgical conditions, and older adults with heart failure (Brooten et al, 2001; Naylor, 2004; Naylor and Van Cleave, 2010). The research model is currently implemented in practice settings in collaboration with major insurance companies and home care agencies (Naylor and Van Cleave, 2010).

Outcomes achieved with the Transitional Care Model consistently show cost savings and improvements in clinical and quality outcomes for clients receiving the intervention compared with usual care. The most common outcome across all populations is a consistent reduction in readmissions to a hospital. The Transitional Care Model strategies emphasize screening in acute care for high-risk clients; engaging the elder/caregiver in designing personalized goals and the plan of care; managing symptoms; educating and promoting self-management; and collaborating with the multidisciplinary team members to assure continuity and collaboration.

NURSING TIP *Home health nurses can facilitate smooth transitions during and after hospitalization by working closely with the interprofessional team to educate them about the benefits of home health, and how to identify clients for referral (Bowles et al, 2009). Once the referral is made, the home health nurse should request specific information about the hospitalization to help establish a baseline and develop a care plan (Bowles et al, 2010b). Because clients and caregivers often find it difficult to learn during hospitalization, home health nurses should ask staff what clients were taught about their conditions, medications, self-care, and symptoms. The nurse can reinforce information, evaluate the client's ability to adhere to the treatment plan, and prevent unnecessary re-hospitalization. Nurses should also determine if clients have a follow-up appointment scheduled with their primary care provider and, if not, facilitate the appointment.*

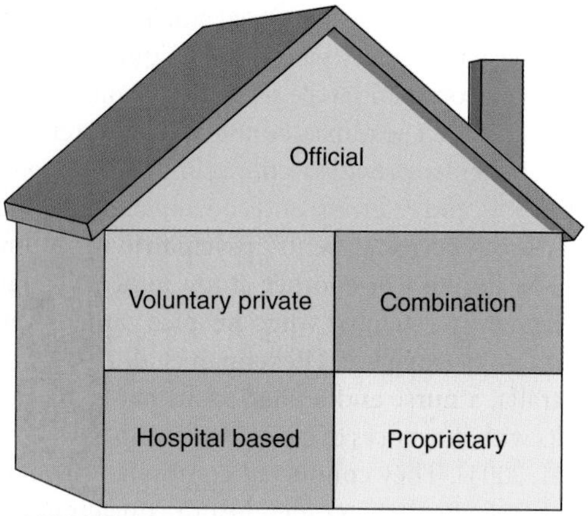

FIGURE 41-2 Types of home health agencies.

Home-Based Primary Care

The goal of home-based primary care is to offer clients an alternative to receiving services in a primary care clinic, community center, or physician's office. These clients have functional or other health problems that make the trip from their homes to other care sites very difficult.

The Veterans Affairs Administration Hospital-Based Home Care Program targets individuals who have complex chronic disabling diseases with the goal of maximizing the independence of the client and reducing preventable emergency room visits and hospitalizations (Beales and Edes, 2009). An interprofessional team provides comprehensive longitudinal primary care that incorporates telehealth and electronic health records (EHRs). Nurses serve as case managers, continually evaluate clients' needs, and deliver care. Approximately three fourths of Veterans Affairs facilities offer the home care program. The program has produced positive outcomes (Mader et al, 2008; Beales and Edes, 2009; Chang et al, 2009).

In 1967, the American Academy of Pediatrics originated the concept of medical home in an attempt to establish centralized, accessible health care records for medically complex, chronically ill children (Friedberg et al, 2009; Homer et al, 2008). Although there are distinct variations of medical home, the models typically include superb access to care; client engagement in care; EHRs that may be client controlled; care coordination; integrated, comprehensive care; ongoing, routine client feedback; and publicly available information about practices (Davis and Stremikis, 2010; Ferrante et al, 2010). More recently, the Centers for Medicare and Medicaid Services (CMS) and politicians supported medical home as a model to decrease costs and incorporated the concept into health care reform. Nurse practitioners are especially interested in policy implications and participating as leaders in this movement (Graham, 2010).

Home Health

Staff members of home health agencies provide care at home and help clients and their families achieve improved health and independence in a safe environment. According to CMS (2008) and NAHC (2008), approximately 7.6 million clients received Medicare-certified home health services in 2007. Persons who were 65 years and older accounted for more than 85% of all home health clients. Recipients of home health services had diverse needs, but circulatory disease was the most common diagnosis, followed by neoplasms and endocrine diseases, especially diabetes. It was estimated that 9284 Medicare-certified home health agencies employed up to 17,000 staff members. The size of individual agencies varied from those that employ a few nurses to the Visiting Nurse Service of New York with its 2500 nurses and more than 12,000 staff members (VNSNY, 2010). Annual national expenditures for home health care in 2007 and 2008 were approximately $57 to $64 billion. As the largest payer, Medicare accounted for 37% of total home health reimbursement. Home health payments represented 3.3% of the total Medicare reimbursement while hospitals represented approximately 35%. In addition to Medicare, state and local governments accounted for 19.9% of home health reimbursement, Medicaid for 19%, private insurance for 12%, out-of-pocket or private pay 10%, and other sources 3% (CMS, 2008; NAHC, 2008).

Home health agencies can be divided into five general categories with a description of each to follow:

- Official/public: approximately 13% of total home health agencies
- Private and voluntary: approximately 12% of total home health agencies
- Combination: approximately 0.5% of total home health agencies
- Hospital based: approximately 19% of total home health agencies
- Proprietary: approximately 56% of total home health agencies (Figure 41-2)

Official or public agencies receive tax revenue and are operated by state, county, city, or other local government units, such as health departments. Typically, official agencies also offer well-child clinics, immunizations, health education programs, and home visits for preventive health care.

Voluntary and private agencies are non-profit home health agencies and usually receive some funds from United Way, donations, and endowments. Currently, there are about the same number of voluntary and private agencies.

Combination agencies have characteristics of both governmental and voluntary agencies. The number of combination agencies continues to decrease although some are large agencies.

Hospital-based agencies grew rapidly during the 1970s and 1980s when the advent of diagnostic-related groups led to earlier hospital discharges. Some hospitals and their home health agencies are separating because of recent changes in Medicare reimbursement.

Proprietary agencies are free-standing, for-profit agencies that are required to pay taxes. Many are part of large chains. Proprietary agencies now dominate the industry.

In addition to Medicare-certified home health agencies, there are other agencies that are not certified. These are often private agencies, governed by individual owners or corporations that offer private duty, home health aide, and homemaker services.

Although the size, administrative, organizational, and board structures of Medicare-certified agencies differ, they must meet ever-changing licensure, certification, and accreditation regulations established by national and state groups (Buhler-Wilkerson, 2007; NAHC, 2008; Fazzi et al, 2010). The primary source of those regulations is CMS (2009). Because the conditions are lengthy and complex, many agencies employ a nurse to become an expert and ensure that the agency is in compliance. To be Medicare-certified, key criteria identified in the Conditions of Participation are: (a) the client must be home-bound, (b) services must be intermittent and include a skilled service provided by a nurse, physical therapist, or speech and language pathologist, (c) a plan of care must be initiated and followed, and (d) Medicare forms, physician orders, and client records must be completed on a timely basis. Skilled nursing services is the Medicare term that describes the duties of the registered nurse, and refers to the requirement of nursing judgment. Those services involve assessment, teaching, and selected procedures; using Omaha System terms, they may also be categorized as Teaching, Guidance, and Counseling; Treatments and Procedures; Case Management; and Surveillance (Martin, 2005).

Hospice

Slightly more than 1 million clients received Medicare-certified hospice services in 2007 with an average stay of 71 days. The average length of stay is rising as home health nurses and others provide information about end-of-life hospice care to clients and families, and hospice becomes more widely accepted by the public. Initially, cancer was the primary diagnosis of most clients; currently, cancer is the diagnosis of about one third of hospice clients and various neurological, cardiac, and other end-stage diseases comprise two thirds of the diagnoses (Zerwekh, 2006; NAHC, 2008; HAA, 2009; Perry and Parente, 2010).

Medicare, Medicaid, managed care, private insurance, and private donations fund most hospice services. The number of Medicare-certified hospices grew from 31 in 1984 to more than 3000 in 2009. Hospice services account for approximately 2.5% of the total Medicare budget, just less than home health services. Services are provided based on Medicare criteria. After the client acknowledges a terminal prognosis and selects comforting care rather than life-extending care, hospice organizations coordinate services in partnership with the client and family

and provide financial case management. The four types of care and the percentage documented in 2005 were: (1) routine home care with intermittent visits, 96.5%, (2) continuous home care when condition is acute and death is near, 1.1%, (3) general inpatient/hospital care for symptom relief, 2.2%, and (4) respite care in a nursing home of no more than 5 days at a time to relieve family members: 0.2% (NAHC, 2008; HAA, 2009).

Medicare-certified hospice providers can be divided into the following four general categories:

- Home health agencies: approximately 18% of total hospice providers
- Hospital-based facilities: approximately 16% of total hospice providers
- Skilled nursing facilities: approximately 0.6% of total hospice providers
- Free-standing facilities: approximately 65% of total hospice providers

Hospice programs are usually operated and staffed as independent entities or corporations even when they are part of a larger organization because of the specialized nature of the practice and complex regulations. The focus of hospice care is comfort, peace, and a sense of dignity at a very difficult time. Comprehensive services emphasize continuity of care. According to Zerwekh (2006), hospice addresses four foci: (1) attention to the body, mind, and spirit, (2) death is not a taboo topic, (3) health care technology should be used with discretion, and (4) clients have a right to truthful discussion and participation in treatment decisions.

The client's family and friends are essential hospice team members who are involved in symptom and medication management, personal care, and the use of supplies. Death produces intense emotions even when family members have prepared for it. Bereavement services involve attending the funeral or other services for the deceased client, and contact at anniversaries of death, holidays, and the client's birthday for 13 months after the client's death. Hospice organizations usually offer support group opportunities for families or refer them to support groups in the area (Altilio et al, 2008; Baker et al, 2008; Malloy et al, 2008).

The interprofessional hospice team includes nurses, physicians, social workers, therapists, chaplains, counselors, aides, pharmacists, and volunteers. In 2008, there were approximately 95,000 employees and 50,000 volunteers; nurses, aides, and social workers were the largest groups of employees (NAHC, 2008). There were more than 10,000 hospice-credentialed nurses and 271 certified advanced practice nurses in palliative care; the latter group included clinical specialists and nurse practitioners (HPNA/ANA, 2007). Working with clients who are dying involves unique emotional stress; hospice programs address the team's well-being as well as that of the clients and families (Hinds et al, 2005; Zerwekh, 2006; HPNA/ANA, 2007; Baker et al, 2008; HAA, 2009; Viola et al, 2009).

Home Care of Dying Children

"The death of a child alters the life and health of others immediately and for the rest of their lives" (Hinds et al, 2005, p S70). The needs of dying children and their families are unique because of the degree of emotional impact, and because the young are not expected to die or precede the death of their parents. It is essential that nurses understand the child's physical, cognitive, psychosocial, and spiritual development and family dynamics, cultural heritage, and spiritual beliefs in order to provide appropriate pain management, assist the child and family to communicate with each other, advocate for their needs in the community, and provide case management and continuity of care (Baker et al, 2008; Hinds et al, 2005).

Bereavement programs as described for hospice programs are especially important for families who have lost a child. Parents, grandparents, and siblings can participate in a variety of support groups offered by the hospice program or other bereavement organizations.

HOW TO Use a Hospice Approach to Care in Any Setting

The hospice philosophy of care means providing comfort measures to individuals before death and support for their families before and after death. Individuals may be any age. Death may occur in the individual's home, a hospital setting, or an uncontrolled setting such as the community. How does one adapt nursing care in any situation? What basic skills can professional caregivers use that can be applied in any situation or setting? How do caregivers adapt to the death of a hospice client, inpatient death, or a sudden, unexpected death where, for example, many people have died as a result of a natural disaster or a terrorist act?

- *Be prepared. Consider your own philosophy of death so that you can assist others without distraction when that time comes.*
- *Cultures vary in their beliefs about and responses to death. Know the differences in cultural responses so that you can effectively help people in their time of need.*
- *Death events cannot be totally controlled even in a hospice environment where the eventual death has been illustrated to family and friends and the dying individual before the death. Expect the unexpected and take cues from the client and the loved ones regarding their needs.*
- *Shock, disbelief, and crisis reactions occur even with prepared, hospice deaths. Ask family and caregivers what they need; provide them with the basics such as food or blankets; provide comfort; if it is not contraindicated, provide the family/friends with personal effects or mementos of the individual; give sensitive, caring support. Sit with them and listen.*
- *In a disaster, the philosophy of care is to provide the greatest good to the greatest number of people. Using triage, the needs of those with less severe injuries have priority over the needs of those who are closer to death. Responsibilities of caregivers and health professionals will be stretched to the maximum. A leader for a group of clients needs to be identified and must delegate responsibility to a caregiver who can assist the dying and their loved ones.*

From Mistovich JJ, Karren KJ: Prehospital emergency care, ed 9, Upper Saddle River, NJ, 2010, Pearson Education.

SCOPE AND STANDARDS OF PRACTICE

Nursing is a theory and practice-based profession that incorporates art and science. Examples of nursing, family, and systems theories are mentioned and summarized in other chapters of this book. Chapter 15 addresses evidence-based practice; the concept is addressed frequently in this chapter and two examples are included. Several chapters of this book describe the Quad Council's (2003) eight domains of practice; those domains are linked to information in this chapter in the Linking Content to Practice box.

⊕ **LINKING CONTENT TO PRACTICE**

The Nurse in Home Health and Hospice

The individuals, families, and communities served by home health and hospice nurses are described throughout this chapter as are the knowledge, skills, and attitudes of nurses who function well in those settings. The descriptions are evident in the text, clinical examples, boxes/figures/tables, references, and other parts of the chapter. The competencies in this chapter are congruent with the following core competencies of the Quad Council's Domains of Public Health Nursing: (1) Analytic/assessment skills, (2) Policy development/program planning skills, (3) Communication skills, (4) Cultural competency skills, (5) Community dimensions of practice skills, (6) Basic public health sciences skills, (7) Financial planning and management skills, and (8) Leadership and systems thinking skills. Students and new graduates cannot be expected to have developed all of these skills when they begin home health or hospice practice. However, as nurses proceed in their career development and gain valuable work experience, they will progress along the novice to expert continuum.

The **nursing process** is the theoretical framework used by the ANA, which notes that the nursing process is the essential methodology by which client goals are identified and achieved. Their scope and standards publications, including those for Home Health Nursing and Hospice and Palliative Nursing, are organized according to the nursing process and contain two sections: the Standards of Care and the Standards of Professional Performance (ANA, 2007; HPNA/ANA, 2007). Both include the six steps of the nursing process: assessment, diagnosis, outcomes identification, planning, implementation, and evaluation; the steps are linked to standards and more specific measurement criteria that are stated in behavioral objectives. The standards address quality of care, performance appraisal, education, collegiality, ethics, collaboration, research, and resource use.

OMAHA SYSTEM

According to Clark and Lang (1992), "If we cannot name it, we cannot control it, finance it, teach it, research it or put it into public policy" (p 27). The **Omaha System** was initially developed to operationalize the nursing process and provide a practical, easily understood, computer-compatible guide for daily use in community settings. It is the only ANA-recognized terminology developed inductively by and for nurses who practice in the community. From the initial home health and hospice focus, adoption has expanded so that current users and user sites represent the continuum of care. Approximately 9000 multi-professional practitioners, educators, and researchers use Omaha System point-of-care **electronic health records** (EHRs) in the United States and other countries, and 2000 more use

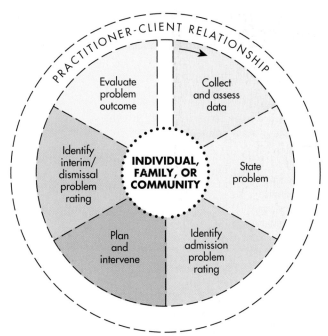

FIGURE 41-3 Omaha System model of the problem-solving process. (From Martin KS: *The Omaha System: a key to practice, documentation, and information management*, reprinted ed 2, Omaha, NE, 2005, Health Connections Press.)

paper-and-pen records. EHRs are longitudinal collections of clinical and demographic client-specific data that are stored in a computer-readable format. Details about Omaha System application, users, case studies, inclusion in reference terminologies, research, best practices/evidence-based practice, and listserv are described in publications and on the website (Martin, 2005; Omaha System, 2010, Martin et al, 2011).

Description of the Omaha System

As early as 1970, the nurses, other staff, and administrators of the Visiting Nurse Association (VNA) of Omaha, Nebraska, began addressing nursing practice, documentation, and information management concerns. At that time, practitioners were not using computers, and there was no systematic nomenclature or classification of client problems and concerns, interventions, or client outcomes to quantify clinical data and integrate with a problem-oriented record system. These realities provided the incentive for initiating research and involving community test sites throughout the country. Between 1975 and 1993, the VNA of Omaha staff conducted four extensive, federally funded development and refinement research studies that established reliability, validity, and usability of the Omaha System. Avedis Donabedian, the developer of the structure, process, and outcome approach to evaluation, was a valuable consultant (Donabedian, 1966; Martin, 2005). The result of the research was the Problem Classification Scheme, the Intervention Scheme, and the Problem Rating Scale for Outcomes. These three components of the Omaha System were designed to be used together, be comprehensive, relatively simple, hierarchical, multi-dimensional, and computer compatible. The Omaha System has existed in the public domain since the initial

research in 1975, and therefore is not held under copyright (Martin, 2005; Omaha System, 2010; Martin et al, 2011).

As depicted in Figure 41-3, the Omaha System conceptual model is based on the dynamic, interactive nature of the nursing or problem-solving process, the practitioner–client relationship, and concepts of diagnostic reasoning, clinical judgment, and quality improvement. The client as an individual, a family, or a community appears at the center of the model; this location suggests the many ways the Omaha System can be used and the essential partnership between clients and practitioners.

The Omaha System was intended for use by nurses and all the members of health care delivery teams. The goals of the research were to (1) develop a structured and comprehensive system that could be both understood and used by members of various disciplines, and (2) foster collaborative practice. Therefore, the Omaha System was designed to guide practice decisions, sort and document pertinent client data uniformly, and provide a framework for an agency-wide, multidisciplinary clinical information management system capable of meeting the daily needs of practitioners, managers, and administrators (Monsen and Martin, 2002b; Martin, 2005; Garvin et al, 2008; Correll and Martin, 2009; Westra et al, 2010; Martin et al, 2011).

THE CUTTING EDGE *More provider agencies are using portable computing devices and clinical information software so nurses can document their care and client outcomes wherever they are in the community. In Minnesota, 85% of all counties now have one or more public health or home care agencies or schools/colleges of nursing using Omaha System software.*

Problem Classification Scheme

The Omaha System Problem Classification Scheme is a comprehensive, orderly, non-exhaustive, mutually exclusive taxonomy designed to identify diverse clients' health-related concerns. Its simple and concrete terms are used to organize a comprehensive assessment, an important standard of nursing practice. The Problem Classification Scheme consists of four levels. Four domains appear at the first level and represent priority areas. Forty-two terms, referred to as client problems or areas of client needs and strengths, appear at the second level. The third level consists of two sets of problem modifiers: health promotion, potential, and actual, as well as individual, family, and community. Clusters of signs and symptoms describe actual problems at the fourth level. The content and relationship of the domain and problem levels depicted in Box 41-1 are further illustrated by the case example in this chapter. Understanding the meaning of and relationships among the terms is a prerequisite to using the scheme accurately and consistently to collect, sort, document, analyze, quantify, and communicate client needs and strengths.

Intervention Scheme

The Omaha System Intervention Scheme is an important standard of nursing practice in providing interventions. Four broad categories of interventions appear at the first level of the

BOX 41-1   DOMAINS AND PROBLEMS OF THE OMAHA SYSTEM PROBLEM CLASSIFICATION SCHEME

ENVIRONMENTAL DOMAIN

Material resources and physical surroundings both inside and outside the living area, neighborhood, and broader community:

  Income
  Sanitation
  Residence
  Neighborhood/workplace safety

PSYCHOSOCIAL DOMAIN

Patterns of behavior, emotion, communication, relationships, and development:

  Communication with community resources
  Social contact
  Role change
  Interpersonal relationship
  Spirituality
  Grief
  Mental health
  Sexuality
  Caretaking/parenting
  Neglect
  Abuse
  Growth and development

PHYSIOLOGICAL DOMAIN

Functions and processes that maintain life:

  Hearing
  Vision
  Speech and language

  Oral health
  Cognition
  Pain
  Consciousness
  Skin
  Neuro-musculo-skeletal function
  Respiration
  Circulation
  Digestion-hydration
  Bowel function
  Urinary function
  Reproductive function
  Pregnancy
  Postpartum
  Communicable/infectious condition

HEALTH-RELATED BEHAVIORS DOMAIN

Patterns of activity that maintain or promote wellness, promote recovery, and decrease the risk of disease:

  Nutrition
  Sleep and rest patterns
  Physical activity
  Personal care
  Substance use
  Family planning
  Health care supervision
  Medication regimen

From Martin KS: *The Omaha System: a key to practice, documentation, and information management,* reprinted ed 2, Omaha, NE, 2005, Health Connections Press.

BOX 41-2   CATEGORIES OF THE OMAHA SYSTEM INTERVENTION SCHEME

TEACHING, GUIDANCE, AND COUNSELING

Activities designed to provide information and materials, encourage action and responsibility for self-care and coping, and assist the individual, family, or community to make decisions and solve problems.

TREATMENTS AND PROCEDURES

Technical activities such as wound care, specimen collection, resistive exercises, and medication prescriptions that are designed to prevent, decrease, or alleviate signs and symptoms for the individual, family, or community.

CASE MANAGEMENT

Activities such as coordination, advocacy, and referral that facilitate service delivery; promote assertiveness; guide the individual, family, or community toward use of appropriate community resources; and improve communication among health and human service providers.

SURVEILLANCE

Activities such as detection, measurement, critical analysis, and monitoring intended to identify the individual, family, or community's status in relation to a given condition or phenomenon.

From Martin KS: *The Omaha System: a key to practice, documentation, and information management,* reprinted ed 2, Omaha, NE, 2005, Health Connections Press.

Intervention Scheme. An alphabetical list of 75 targets or objects of action and 1 "other" appear at the second level. Client-specific information generated by practitioners is at the third level. The contents of the category and target levels are depicted in Boxes 41-2 and 41-3, respectively. The Intervention Scheme enables practitioners to describe, quantify, and communicate their practice, including improving or restoring health, describing deterioration, or preventing illness.

Problem Rating Scale for Outcomes

The Omaha System Problem Rating Scale for Outcomes consists of three five-point, Likert-type scales for measuring the entire range of severity for the concepts of Knowledge, Behavior, and Status. Each of the subscales is a continuum providing a framework for measuring and comparing problem-specific client outcomes at regular or predictable times, because evaluation is an important standard of nursing practice. Suggested

BOX 41-3 TARGETS OF THE OMAHA SYSTEM INTERVENTION SCHEME

- Anatomy/physiology
- Anger management
- Behavior modification
- Bladder care
- Bonding/attachment
- Bowel care
- Cardiac care
- Caretaking/parenting skills
- Cast care
- Communication
- Community outreach worker services
- Continuity of care
- Coping skills
- Day care/respite
- Dietary management
- Discipline
- Dressing change/wound care
- Durable medical equipment
- Education

- Employment
- End-of-life care
- Environment
- Exercises
- Family planning care
- Feeding procedures
- Finances
- Gait training
- Genetics
- Growth/development care
- Home
- Homemaking/housekeeping
- Infection precautions
- Interaction
- Interpreter/translator services
- Laboratory findings
- Legal system
- Medical/dental care
- Medication action/side effects
- Medication administration

- Medication coordination/ordering
- Medication prescription
- Medication set-up
- Mobility/transfers
- Nursing care
- Nutritionist care
- Occupational therapy care
- Ostomy care
- Other community resources
- Paraprofessional/aide care
- Personal hygiene
- Physical therapy care
- Positioning
- Recreational therapy care
- Relaxation/breathing techniques
- Respiratory care
- Respiratory therapy care
- Rest/sleep
- Safety
- Screening procedures

- Sickness/injury care
- Signs/symptoms-mental/emotional
- Signs/symptoms-physical
- Skin care
- Social work/counseling care
- Specimen collection
- Speech and language pathology care
- Spiritual care
- Stimulation/nurturance
- Stress management
- Substance use cessation
- Supplies
- Support group
- Support system
- Transportation
- Wellness
- Other

From Martin KS: *The Omaha System: a key to practice, documentation, and information management*, reprinted ed 2, Omaha, NE, 2005, Health Connections Press.

TABLE 41-1 OMAHA SYSTEM PROBLEM RATING SCALE FOR OUTCOMES

CONCEPT	1	2	3	4	5
Knowledge: Ability of client to remember and interpret information	No knowledge	Minimal knowledge	Basic knowledge	Adequate knowledge	Superior knowledge
Behavior: Observable responses, actions, or activities of client fitting occasion or purpose	Not appropriate behavior	Rarely appropriate behavior	Inconsistently appropriate behavior	Usually appropriate behavior	Consistently appropriate behavior
Status: Condition of client in relation to objective and subjective defining characteristics	Extreme signs/symptoms	Severe signs/symptoms	Moderate signs/symptoms	Minimal signs/symptoms	No signs/symptoms

From Martin KS: *The Omaha System: a key to practice, documentation, and information management*, reprinted ed 2, Omaha, NE, 2005, Health Connections Press.

times include admission, specific interim points, and discharge. The ratings are a guide for the practitioner as client care is planned and provided; the ratings offer a method to monitor and quantify client progress throughout the period of service. The content and relationships of the scale are depicted in Table 41-1. Using the Problem Rating Scale for Outcomes with the Problem Classification Scheme and the Intervention Scheme creates a comprehensive problem-solving model for practice, education, and research.

PRACTICE GUIDELINES

Nursing practice is based on education, experience, and evidence. Because home health and hospice nurses usually work with clients and their families in their homes, they must develop skills to conduct home visits efficiently, effectively, and safely (Box 41-4). Accompanying skilled home health and hospice

nurses when they make home visits as well as having expert mentors are excellent strategies. However, novice home health and hospice nurses also need a commitment to life-long learning, practice, and self-evaluation (Zerwekh, 2006; Motyka and Nies, 2007; Humphrey and Milone-Nuzzo, 2010). The following is a brief summary of steps included in a home visit; these steps can be modified slightly for other non-institutional settings:

- Review client data, including the referral from the intake department, hospital discharge summary, orders, and plan of care to become familiar with the client's history, purpose of the visit, and expectations.
- Contact the client or family by calling the telephone number listed on the referral information to obtain agreement for the visit, schedule the day and time, and discuss the address.
- Gather agency and Medicare forms, a nursing bag, cellular phone or pager, portable computing device, teaching

BOX 41-4   GUIDELINES FOR HOME HEALTH AND HOSPICE

- You are a guest in your client's home and neighborhood. Your behavior and your manners must convey that you recognize this role.
- Respect the client's cultural, religious, and ethnic heritage. Hesitate before contradicting that heritage. Clients are more likely to follow their heritage than your advice.

The client may not respect your cultural, religious, and ethnic heritage. If you are a male nurse, the client may expect, and even request, a female nurse. Develop interpersonal skills—and a tough skin.

- Almost every home health client has family members or significant others who offer advice and can serve as either your advocate or your foe. Try to enlist them as your advocate.
- The client "owns" the health-related problem that initiated your services. That problem is just one portion of the client's past, present, and future. Thus it is the client who experiences, learns to understand, and ultimately solves the problem. It is your goal to help clients and their families become independent as quickly as possible. Talk to your peers and supervisors if you sense that you may be losing that perspective.
- Enjoy the unique autonomy and challenges of providing highly complex care in the home and community setting. Home health practice requires integration of high-technology skills, teaching, case management, and monitoring. Remember the need for communication with other members of the health care team. The nurse is usually responsible for judging whether or not the client can safely remain at home, and other team members need to share the information the nurse has through oral and written means.

From Black JM, Hawks JH: *Medical-surgical nursing,* ed 8, St Louis, 2009, Saunders, p 94.

materials, and supplies; understand the client's location; follow the agency policy when checking-out for the visit.

- Observe the neighborhood for resources and safety when approaching the client's home.
- Greet the client/family to begin developing a positive, appropriate professional relationship; involve them as much as possible during the visit and post-visit activities.
- Obtain signatures and complete needed forms.
- Provide care by completing a comprehensive assessment, identifying client problems, providing interventions, and evaluating client outcomes. Interventions may include teaching, guidance, and counseling; treatments and procedures; case management; and surveillance (Martin, 2005).
- Discuss the plan of care with the client and family and modify as needed.
- Document some or all of the visit details in the home, preferably while using a portable computing device and an EHR.
- Discuss the next visit as well as follow-up activities and referrals.
- Proceed to the next scheduled visit after checking in, according to the agency policy.
- Complete remaining visit documentation, submit forms, coordinate referrals to other community resources, and communicate with agency colleagues, the referral source, physicians, and others as appropriate. Obtain revised orders if needed.
- Revisit to re-assess the client and provide care.

NURSING TIP   *Convene a family-provider conference to discuss issues with a client and family, develop a consistent team approach, and clarify roles and responsibilities.*

CLINICAL EXAMPLES FROM PRACTICE

Three clinical examples from practice are presented in the following section; they illustrate the guidelines described in the previous section and Omaha System application. Those guidelines emphasize culturally sensitive, high-quality practice and demonstrate the assessment, intervention, and outcomes steps of the problem-solving process. Note that the first example is an individual who lives alone, the second is an individual whose family includes an involved spouse, and the third client is the community. Ideally, the student who visits Martha P. and the home health nurse who visits Mr. and Mrs. Jones use portable computing devices and EHRs in the home. The child care health consultants use a single electronic documentation system, can communicate easily about practice, and are creating a state-wide data base.

Martha P. is an older woman who lives in a deteriorating home. She is a relatively typical client for a student or home health nurse to visit. Box 41-5 consists of a story and answers designed to promote independent learning and group discussion. Note that the story and answers should be congruent: all pertinent data in the story should be reflected in the answers and all answers should match pertinent details in the story.

Mr. Jones, the second clinical example, is also a relatively typical client. After reading the example, identify the Omaha System problems, interventions, and ratings that are illustrated in the story. Discuss key characteristics of practice during this visit and an appropriate care plan for the next visit.

Mr. Jones, 70 years old, was discharged from the hospital yesterday after heart surgery for coronary artery disease and was referred to the local home health agency. Today, the home health nurse admitted him for **skilled nursing care** services. The nurse assessed Mr. Jones' cardiovascular status, the healing of his incisions, adjustment to his post-surgical status, and level of self-care. The nurse talked to Mr. and Mrs. Jones about exercise, nutrition, the signs and symptoms of possible post-operative cardiac problems, and their coping. Together, they looked at his medications. Mrs. Jones indicated that they were getting along well, but were concerned about the high cost of his new medications. They reviewed Mr. Jones' discharge packet. The nurse emphasized the need to maintain close communication with his physician and nurse practitioner, and the need to participate in the local exercise and nutrition rehabilitation program that they had prescribed. Mr. and Mrs. Jones indicated that they would do so. Before the visit ended, the nurse completed the necessary forms, documented the visit, and offered to call a local social service agency about financial assistance for medications. They made an appointment for the nurse's return visit.

The third clinical example describes the Arizona child care health consultant program. In 1987, two public health departments in Arizona began to offer child care health consultation

BOX 41-5   MARTHA P.: OLDER WOMAN LIVING IN A DETERIORATING HOME

Joan B. Castleman, RN, MS, Clinical Associate Professor
College of Nursing, University of Florida
Gainesville, Florida

INFORMATION OBTAINED DURING THE FIRST VISIT/ENCOUNTER

Martha P. was a 93-year-old woman who lived by herself in a deteriorating house. She had kyphosis and arthritis that contributed to her unsteady gait. Martha rarely used her cane in her house, but steadied herself by holding onto furniture.

When a student nurse arrived, Martha was shivering under a thin blanket. Boxes filled with old papers were stacked along the walls. The student nurse asked Martha if she had wood for the stove that heated the house. She replied that she ran out of wood yesterday and said, "I don't know what I'm going to do, but I'm not leaving this house." She reported that people from a church had brought the last load of wood. The student asked permission to contact Concerned Neighbors, a volunteer organization that could provide firewood. Martha was pleased. The student expressed concern that the boxes of paper, especially those near the stove, were a fire hazard. "Those boxes have been there for years, and I use them to light the stove," Martha said. When the student asked if she could help Martha move the four boxes near the stove to the other wall, she grudgingly agreed.

The student nurse noted that Martha was wearing a "Lifeline necklace," a fall alert system, and asked about her history of falls. Martha described how she moved around her home and fell in the bathroom last week when she was trying to take a sponge bath. She pushed the button, and "two nice gentlemen from the fire department came to pick me up." The student and Martha walked around her house. They talked about where she fell in the past, how fortunate she was not to have injuries, and ways to decrease her risk of falling in the future. Martha was willing to have a personal care assistant visit weekly to help her with a bath and shampoo as long there was no charge. Before leaving, the student took Martha's vital signs and blood pressure and noted that they were within normal limits. The student called Concerned Neighbors and arranged for firewood to be delivered that day; the student also telephoned a local health assistance organization to schedule a home health aide to provide personal care for the next week. Although Martha sounded grumpy, she asked the student to return.

APPLICATION OF THE OMAHA SYSTEM

Domain: Environmental
Problem: Residence (High Priority)

Problem Classification Scheme

Modifiers: Individual and Actual
Signs/symptoms of Actual:
   Inadequate heating/cooling
   Cluttered living space
   Unsafe storage of dangerous objects/substances

Intervention Scheme

Category: Teaching, Guidance, and Counseling
Targets and Client-specific Information:
   Safety (moved boxes away from stove; Martha unwilling to dispose of papers)
Category: Case Management
Targets and Client-specific Information:
   Other community resources (referred to Concerned Neighbors; arranged delivery of firewood)
Category: Surveillance
Targets and Client-specific Information:
   Home (needed wood)

Problem Rating Scale for Outcomes

Knowledge: 2—minimal knowledge (not aware/unwilling to recognize fire hazards)
Behavior: 2—rarely appropriate behavior (unable/unwilling to make changes)
Status: 2—severe signs/symptoms (residence was livable but needed changes)
Domain: Physiological

PROBLEM: NEURO-MUSCULO-SKELETAL FUNCTION (HIGH PRIORITY)

Problem Classification Scheme

Modifiers: Individual and Actual
Signs/symptoms of Actual:
   Limited range of motion
   Decreased balance
   Gait/ambulation disturbance

Intervention Scheme

Category: Teaching, Guidance, and Counseling
Targets and Client-specific Information:
   Mobility/transfers (ways to decrease risk of falling, absence of injuries, continue wearing "Lifeline necklace")
Category: Surveillance
Targets and Client-specific Information:
   mobility/transfers (how, when falls occurred)
   signs/symptoms—physical (falls/injuries; vital signs, blood pressure)

Problem Rating Scale for Outcomes

Knowledge: 2—minimal knowledge (knew few options to decrease falls)
Behavior: 2—rarely appropriate behavior (had not used cane in house; did wear and use "Lifeline necklace")
Status: 3—moderate signs/symptoms (activities restricted, fell last week)
Domain: Health-Related Behaviors

PROBLEM: PERSONAL CARE (HIGH PRIORITY)

Problem Classification Scheme

Modifiers: Individual and Actual
Signs/symptoms of Actual:
   Difficulty with bathing
   Difficulty shampooing/combing hair

Intervention Scheme

Category: Teaching, Guidance, and Counseling
Targets and Client-specific Information:
   Personal hygiene (needed help with bathing, shampoo)
Category: Case Management
Targets and Client-specific Information:
   Paraprofessional/aide care (referred to health assistance organization for home health aide)

Problem Rating Scale for Outcomes

Knowledge: 3—basic knowledge (knew she needed to bathe, but not aware of assistance)
Behavior: 3—inconsistently appropriate behavior (tried to take a sponge bath)
Status: 3—moderate signs/symptoms (cannot bathe safely without help)

This case illustrates use of the Omaha System with a client in the home. Talk with your classmates and other colleagues about how use of the Omaha System can guide your practice and documentation and can generate aggregate data to promote high-quality home health service. Identify Martha P.'s strengths and how to maximize those when providing care.

From Martin KS: *The Omaha System: a key to practice, documentation, and information management*, Omaha, NE, 2005, Health Connections Press.

services to child care programs. They recognized that if the health and safety of young children in child care environments was not addressed, related efforts to advance quality standards for children could not succeed (Ford and Linker, 2002). The nurses from Pima and Maricopa counties scheduled regular visits to child care centers, family child care homes, and Head Start centers. They worked collaboratively with providers to impact issues such as communicable disease, playground safety, safe infant sleep, medication management, and the inclusion of children with special health needs in the group setting. The nurses kept anecdotal notes and frequency counts for the number of consultation visits they made and how many staff members attended their educational programs. In time, they and their health departments realized that they had an information overload: their data were inconsistent and difficult to access, and were not organized in a way to produce meaningful reports.

In 2005, Kathi Ford and the Pima County Health Department participated in a pilot child care quality improvement project that involved child care health consultants. Such a consultant is a "health professional who has an interest in and experience with children, has knowledge of resources and regulations, and is comfortable linking health resources with facilities that provide primarily education and social services" (AAP/APHA, 2002, p 3). The Omaha System and an automated clinical information system were used to capture their data. Although their nursing practice did not change, the data collection, analysis, and reporting changed dramatically. Using community as the modifier, it was possible to describe and quantify common problems, interventions, and changes in Knowledge, Behavior, and Status. The clearly documented outcomes captured the interest of First Things First, a state agency whose mission is to ensure that children entering school are healthy and ready to succeed (First Things First, 2010). In 2009, funding increased to support approximately 47 child care health consultants in Arizona and created a quality improvement and rating system. Early in 2010, all First Things First–supported consultants began using the Omaha System to document their services in a single web-accessed charting system. Nationally, child care health consultants have documented reduction of communicable diseases, fewer injury incidents, increased access to health care for children and staff, and appropriate care for children with special health care needs (Ramler et al, 2006). Arizona consultants are developing a state-wide data base and plan to generate powerful outcome data and information in their reports.

PRACTICE LINKAGES

There are no limits to the diversity of clients who live in the community, their problems, and their strengths; the interventions that nurses provide; and the client outcome data that are generated. Although the three examples are diverse, they represent a small fraction of the actual roles and responsibilities of home health and hospice nurses. The examples illustrate fundamental principles of professional practice that are illustrated in Figure 41-3: (1) a holistic approach to the steps of the nursing or problem-solving process, (2) partnership with clients as

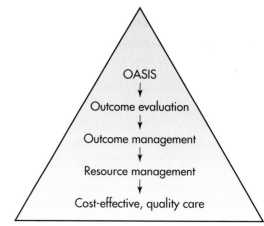

FIGURE 41-4 The outcome paradigm. (From Centers for Medicare and Medicaid Services: *Outcome-based quality improvement [OBQI] implementation manual,* August 2010, p 2.9.)

unique individuals, families, and communities, and (3) a focus on outcomes.

The following sections of the chapter are designed to increase the reader's understanding about the links between systematic best practices, evidence-based practice, and other aspects of the home health and hospice milieu. The typical nurse will not be involved with the theme of each section daily, but will over a period of months.

Setting short- and long-term goals provides criteria for evaluation, and increases continuity of care and the potential for improved outcomes. Research has shown that goals set with the client rather than for the client are more successful regarding self-motivation, adherence, and attainment (Naylor and Van Cleave, 2010).

Outcome and Assessment Information

The Centers for Medicare and Medicaid Services (CMS) mandated the Outcome and Assessment Information Set (OASIS) as part of the Conditions of Participation for Medicare-certified home health agencies in 1999 (CMS, 2009). Completion of OASIS provides a systematic comparative measurement of client outcomes at two points in time. It was designed to (1) provide a group of data elements representing core items that are part of a comprehensive assessment for an adult, non-maternity home health client, and (2) form the basis for measuring client outcomes for outcome-based quality improvement. The goal of OASIS is to demonstrate improved, cost-effective client outcomes as a result of home health services for agency reports and for public reporting (Figure 41-4).

OASIS has had several major revisions to improve its comprehensiveness, ease of use, reliability, and validity. Based on feedback from users, another revision began in 2008 and was implemented January 1, 2010. The newest revision, OASIS-C, consists of 116 data elements or structure/process/outcome items, each followed by a list of choices or fill-in-the-blanks. In contrast to previous versions, OASIS-C requires data about the plan of care and interventions. The process items represent "evidence-informed" practice. OASIS-C is approximately

40 pages long (CMS, 2009). (See Resource Tool 41.A on the Evolve website for one part of this assessment.)

Registered nurses or physical, occupational, or speech and language pathology therapists complete OASIS-C at the start of care, after hospitalization, at the 60-day recertification date following admission, at discharge, and at other points in time. Practitioners need to complete the initial OASIS-C accurately and consistently to reflect a client's actual status, and integrate OASIS-C with the rest of the agency's comprehensive assessment. They or their colleagues compare initial data to future versions as do Medicare surveyors and reimbursement reviewers. Many home health agencies use a computerized clinical information system so that the practitioner completes OASIS-C electronically; regardless, final data from OASIS-C must be submitted to the CMS electronically.

Target areas for emphasis on OASIS-C mirror challenges identified by nurses and home health agencies. Included are diabetic foot care, fall prevention, depression intervention, pain, pressure ulcers, safety, medication management, and infection control. Although all are important, the latter two are of special concern to many nurses employed in hospice as well as diverse public health and other health care settings; they are summarized below.

Medication Management

Medication management is an important component of home health practice. The goal is to assist clients and caregivers to become independent and reliable in managing medication administration. However, home health clients experience many challenges including the complexity of chronic conditions, coordination of their medical care, drug-drug interactions and side effects of medications, and cost. As experienced in an evidence-based practice improvement project at a large home care agency in the northeastern United States, other factors such as dementia and medication non-adherence present additional challenges. Home care nurses searched and critically evaluated the literature to find and use evidence-based screening tools to identify clients with cognitive impairment and medication adherence issues and created plans of care based on the latest published evidence to address these issues (Bowles et al, 2010a) (Figure 41-5).

Infection Prevention

In home health and hospice practice, infection prevention usually focuses on wound care, and invasive devices such as urinary and intravenous catheters as well as chest, tracheostomy, gastrostomy, and other tubes. Prevention of infection by promoting appropriate vaccinations such as flu and pneumonia is also a priority. Most importantly, nurses need to assume that every client is potentially infected or colonized with an organism that can be transmitted, and recognize that all blood and body secretions may contain transmissible agents. They need to be familiar with the infectious process, research evidence and best practices, bag technique, personal protective equipment, cleaning equipment, medical waste management, and infection control programs. Nurses need to practice sound technique during each and every client encounter (see How

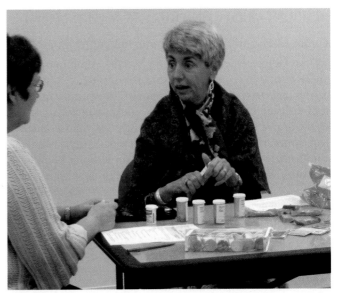

FIGURE 41-5 Medication management. (From www.omaha system.org/photogallery.html. Used with permission from Karen Martin, RN, MSN, FAAN.)

To box). Rhinehart and McGoldrick (2006) published a book that addresses the previous home health and hospice infection prevention and control topics as well as nosocomial and health-care acquired infections. Internet resources are available including guidelines from the Centers for Disease Control and Prevention (Siegel et al, 2006, 2007).

HOW TO   **Promote Infection Prevention Standards**

The practice of standard precautions means that all blood and body fluids must be treated as potentially infectious. Standard precautions are implemented to prevent exposure and infection of family caregivers and health care providers.

- *Use extreme care to prevent injuries when handling needles, scalpels, and razors. Do not recap, bend, break, or remove needles from syringes before disposal. Discard needles and syringes in puncture-resistant containers made of plastic or metal and dispose of them as directed by agency policy or community guidelines.*
- *Wear barrier precautions such as gloves, masks, eye covering, and gowns when contact with blood and body fluids is expected. Use masks in combination with eye protection to eliminate contact with respiratory secretions or sprays of blood or body fluids during invasive respiratory procedures or wound irrigations.*
- *Use aseptic technique with all sterile injection equipment.*
- *Double bag and discard soiled dressings or other materials contaminated with body fluids in polyethylene garbage bags.*
- *Clean kitchen counters, dishes, and laundry with warm water and detergent after use. Clean bathrooms with a household disinfectant.*
- *Hand hygiene is the single most important practice in preventing infections. Hand hygiene should be performed before and after providing client care and before and after preparing food, eating, feeding, or using the bathroom.*
- *For clients with multi-drug resistant organisms, limit the amount of non-disposable equipment brought into the home; use disposable stethoscopes, etc. when possible.*

ACCOUNTABILITY AND QUALITY MANAGEMENT

Evidence-Based Quality/Performance Improvement

All providers, whether they are within community-based settings, hospitals, long-term care, or private practices, are accountable to their clients, reimbursement sources, and professional standards. Accountability is directly linked to quality or the degree to which health services for individuals, families, and communities increase the likelihood of desired health outcomes, and are consistent with current professional knowledge. Florence Nightingale is often credited with establishing standards of care, demonstrating the value of evidence-based practice, and analyzing health-related outcome data successfully.

Most home health and hospice agencies have a long history of evaluating the quality of care they provided to their clients. Often, agencies use a systematic, triangulated approach in their pursuit of excellence that includes hiring qualified personnel, new employee orientation, mentoring programs, case conferences, supervisory shared visits, record audits, utilization reviews, quality studies, client satisfaction surveys, in-service education, recognition for outstanding performance, and annual evaluations. Some agencies became accredited as a way to distinguish themselves from other providers.

The sophistication of quality and performance improvement strategies used in home health and hospice has dramatically improved in recent years. Changes were prompted by the interest in research-based practice that has evolved into programs of research and evidence-based practice, use of computers and the Internet, guidelines developed by the National Quality Forum (2010), and the mandate from Medicare to use OASIS and Outcome-Based Quality Improvement. Nurses should have access to current research literature, critique that research, and apply it to their practice (Melnyk and Fineout-Overholt, 2005). Several frameworks have been described to guide evidence-based practice projects (Melnyk and Fineout-Overholt, 2005; Levin et al, 2010).

Evaluating the quality of care professionally and legally should be done in many ways, but documentation is of special significance. The steps of the nursing process must be documented and include communication with team members, physicians, and community resources. It is through the clinical record that nurses demonstrate that they are delivering quality care and identifying strategies to improve the quality of care.

Outcome-Based Quality Improvement

Outcome measurement and cost control are the focus of the CMS Outcome-Based Quality Improvement (OBQI) program. Their definition of outcomes is: (1) health status changes between two or more time points, where the term "health status" encompasses physiological, functional, cognitive, emotional, and behavioral health, (2) changes that are intrinsic to the client, (3) positive, negative, or neutral changes in health status, and (4) changes that result from care provided, or natural progression of disease and disability, or both (CMS, 2009).

Data from OASIS-C are part of the two-stage CMS OBQI framework to produce various reports (Figure 41-6). The first stage, outcome analysis, enables an agency to compare its

performance to a national sample, note factors that may affect outcomes, and identify final outcomes that show improvement in or stabilization of a client's condition. Comparing agency data and trends to a national sample is also known as benchmarking, an analysis process that has been used by many businesses but is relatively new to health care. The second stage, known as outcome enhancement, enables the agency to select specific client outcomes and determine strategies to improve care. Reports include agency-client–related characteristics (case mix), potentially avoidable events (adverse event outcomes), and end-result and utilization outcomes. The reports are for a 12-month period, the agency's previous 12-month period, and national reference or comparative data. Comparisons are risk adjusted for client differences, both over time for the agency and between the agency and the reference group. Similarly to OASIS, a detailed manual describes the OBQI program (CMS, 2009).

Accreditation

Home health and hospice providers participate in several different continuous quality improvement options. They may elect to meet the accreditation standards of the Joint Commission or the Community Health Accreditation Program of the National League for Nursing and complete their Medicare survey in that way. If they do not seek accreditation, Medicare surveyors will conduct regular reviews. In 2007, the Public Health Accreditation Board was established to offer national public health accreditation. Because some home health and hospice programs are integrated with health departments, they will participate in public health accreditation.

After an agency applies for accreditation, a lengthy self-study must be completed that addresses all aspects of the agency's operation, and an accreditation team schedules a site visit. Both accrediting organizations review agencies' organizational structure, compliance with Medicare Conditions of Participation, care provided during home visits and documentation of those visits, and the outcomes of client care with a focus on improved health status. Site visitors accompany nurses and other practitioners on home visits to observe the steps of the problem-solving process in action. To maintain accreditation, agencies must follow guidelines and undergo periodic reviews. In the

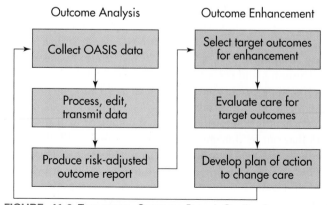

FIGURE 41-6 Two-stage Outcome-Based Quality Improvement framework. (From Centers for Medicare and Medicaid Services: *OASIS-C guidance manual*, September 2009, p F.3.)

future, accreditation may become a requirement for licensure of all home health agencies.

PROFESSIONAL DEVELOPMENT AND COLLABORATION

Education, Certification, and Roles

Nurses are employed in home health and hospice from a variety of educational and practice backgrounds. They should be educated to function at a high level of competency so that they can be relied on not only by their professional colleagues, but also by the community. They have diverse roles and responsibilities in their practice settings; autonomy is a fundamental characteristic that was described earlier in this chapter. Nurses are responsible for basing their practice on research evidence. A growing number of community research studies add to the body of knowledge for evidence-based practice. The application of existing evidence and generation of new research must be priorities to increase the quality and cost-effectiveness of care (Schumacher and Marren, 2004).

The educational preparation of nurses employed in home health agencies varies greatly. According to the ANA (2007), a baccalaureate degree in nursing should be the minimum requirement for entry into professional practice. Roles for nurses include care management and coordination of care, education, advocacy, administration, supervision, and quality improvement. The nurse with a baccalaureate degree functions in the role of a generalist, providing skilled nursing and coordinating care for a variety of clients. Nurses with a master's degree are prepared for roles as clinical specialists, nurse practitioners, researchers, administrators, or educators. Educational programs are increasing to prepare nurses for advanced practice roles in home health. The American Nurses Credentialing Center stopped offering the basic and clinical nurse specialist home health examinations when the number of applicants fell below their minimum standard; those who are already credentialed can continue to renew. As home health continues to expand, the need for specialized nurse clinicians will also increase to meet the highly technological and complex care needs of individuals, families, and communities. In managed care, more clinical specialists will be needed to provide case management and to develop programs to meet the needs of the population served by the managed care network. Nurse practitioners can provide primary care to frail older adults and other homebound clients.

The Hospice and Palliative Nurses Association (HPNA) offers certification examinations and credentialing (HPNA/ANA, 2007). By 2007, there were more than 10,000 credentialed registered hospice and palliative nurses. Licensed registered nurses may qualify for two levels of specialty practice certification that are differentiated by education, complexity of practice, and performance of certain nursing functions. Generalists provide direct care, function as educators, case managers, nurse clinicians, administrators, and other roles. The advanced practice certification is for a nurse prepared at the master's level or higher as a clinical nurse specialist or nurse practitioner. Roles of the advanced practice nurse include expert clinician, leader and facilitator of interprofessional teams, educator,

researcher, consultant, collaborator, advocate, case manager, or administrator.

Interprofessional Collaboration

Typically, home health and hospice nurses are members of interprofessional teams. The primary goal of the team is to help clients achieve their maximum level of health, self-care, and independent functioning in a safe environment. Medicare regulations, professional organizations, and state licensing boards influence team composition and functions. Box 41-6 shows successful interprofessional collaboration depending on the knowledge, skills, and attitudes of each team member. When team members work collaboratively in partnership with clients, families, and volunteers, the plan of care can be implemented effectively and reinforced by all. Although each team member has a specific responsibility, any overlap in responsibilities can be beneficial for reinforcement. Team members communicate through e-mail, phone calls, and face-to-face case conferences to review the plan of care, client progress, and team effectiveness (Martin, 2005; Zerwekh, 2006; Baker et al, 2008; Humphrey and Milone-Nuzzo, 2010).

Details about the role of nurses have been described in other sections of this chapter. Nurses often serve as the team leader or care manager in part because nursing service may be the client's primary need. Larger agencies may expand their nursing services to include wound and ostomy, intravenous, psychiatric/mental health, nurse practitioner, and other nursing specialists.

Physicians are an integral part of interprofessional teams; they submit initial and interim orders and review and sign the initial and updated plan of care. Many agencies hire a physician on a part-time basis or have an agreement with a physician who

---

BOX 41-6 FACTORS FOR SUCCESSFUL INTERPROFESSIONAL COLLABORATION

Knowledge
1. Understand how the group process can be used to achieve group goals.
2. Understand problem solving.
3. Understand role theory.
4. Understand what other professionals do and how they view their roles.
5. Understand the differences between client levels of acuity across levels of care, including acute care, home care, ambulatory care, and long-term care.

Skills
1. Use principles of group process effectively.
2. Communicate clearly and accurately.
3. Communicate without using the profession's jargon.
4. Express self clearly and concisely in writing.

Attitudes
1. Feel confident in role as a professional.
2. Trust and respect other professionals.
3. Share tasks with other professionals.
4. Work effectively toward conflict resolution.
5. Be flexible.
6. Adopt an attitude of inquiry.
7. Be timely.

serves as a voluntary consultant. Because state laws are changing, nurse practitioners are increasingly involved. In addition, agencies may have specialized services such as podiatrists, pharmacists, registered dietitians, respiratory therapists, music therapists, psychologists, and chaplains.

The services of physical therapists, occupational therapists, speech and language pathologists, social workers, and home health aides are available in most agencies. They may be employed by the agency or hired through contractual agreements. Their roles are summarized below.

- Physical therapists: Provide maintenance, preventive, and restorative treatment that includes strengthening muscles, restoring mobility, controlling spasticity, gait training, and teaching active and passive resistive exercises.
- Occupational therapists: Focus on upper extremities to restore muscle strength and mobility for functional skills and performance of activities of daily living.
- Speech and language pathologists: Evaluate speech and language abilities, develop a plan of care, and teach clients to improve their communication involving speech, language, or hearing.
- Social workers: Help clients and families manage social, emotional, and environmental factors that affect their well-being through identification and referral to appropriate community resources.
- Home health aides: Provide personal care and assist with activities of daily living under the supervision of nurses or physical therapists. Home health aides or homemakers may also help with light housekeeping, laundry, meal preparation, and shopping. (Figure 41-7).

LEGAL, ETHICAL, AND FINANCIAL ISSUES

The potential for human error as well as illegal and unethical activity exists in every health care organization. Examples of Medicare fraud and abuse in home health and hospice include inappropriate use of services, excessive payments to administrative staff or owners, "kickbacks" for referrals, and billing for visits and/or medical supplies that are not authorized or not provided. In addition, the complex regulations of CMS are difficult to understand and have not been interpreted consistently by Medicare surveyors.

Nurses are confronted with legal and ethical issues regularly. They need to be familiar with the living will, power of attorney for health care, and do-not-resuscitate documents. In addition, they need to be informed about local, state, and federal regulations that govern their profession and nursing license; and those that govern their employers. They need to be alert for potential problems or violations and identify solutions in a pro-active manner. The privacy guidelines of the Health Insurance Portability and Accountability Act of 1996 (USDHHS, 2003) ensures protection of clients' personal health information and includes provisions about informed consent. The legislation also allows clients full access to their health care records (Smith, 2007; Marquis and Huston, 2009).

Nurses are expected to follow professional, legal, and ethical standards to deliver care to clients, develop trusting relationships, act as client advocates, and help clients and families increase their self-advocacy skills. Because these responsibilities can produce tension, nurses need to recognize their personal values and biases to make certain they do not interfere with those of clients and families. Nurses should continually reassess

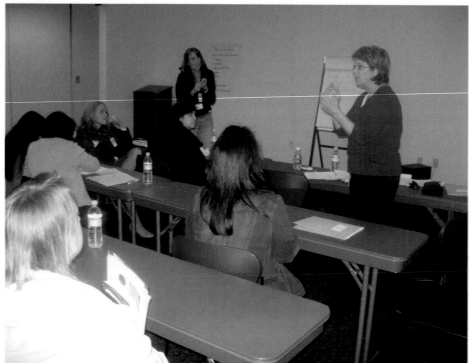

FIGURE 41-7 Interprofessional team. (From www.omahasystem.org/photogallery.html. Used with permission from Karen Martin, RN, MSN, FAAN.)

client and family needs to avoid inappropriate use and overuse of services. The safety of clients who live alone as well as family caregiver neglect and/or abuse are ethical concerns. If the clients' needs are greater than what reimbursement allows, nurses need to talk to the clients, their families, and agency personnel to consider alternatives. In addition, many agencies have established ethics committees to assist with ethical dilemmas.

Home health and hospice nurses are at risk for malpractice claims related to the complexity of care, failure to adhere to standards of practice, and other errors (Smith, 2007; Marquis and Huston, 2009). Nurses and their employers need to be proactive by taking responsibility for personal and agency actions. A focus on communication with clients, families, and the health care team; commitment to providing quality care; documentation refresher sessions; performance improvement programs; use of evidence-based practice guidelines; and appropriate use of information technology and telehealth are strategies that can help reduce risks.

Reimbursement for home health and hospice is complex; details about economics and reimbursement are included in Chapter 5. Medicare, state, and local governments; Medicaid; and managed care are the principal funding sources for home health and hospice (Buhler-Wilkerson, 2007; NAHC, 2008; HAA, 2009; Fazzi et al, 2010). If clients meet the eligibility criteria for the Conditions of Participation, Medicare is used as their primary payment source. When clients no longer meet those criteria and still require care, their services may be reimbursed by Medicaid, private insurance, donations, or the agency's United Way and other special needs funds.

Nurses who work in home health and hospice are involved with financial aspects of care to a greater extent than most other nurses. Nurses and their social work colleagues must be well informed about services that are covered by Medicare and other funding sources. Clients and families often ask for help to understand decisions about care and the numerous notices and bills that they receive. Nurses participate directly in decisions about the frequency, length, and type of client services, and their documentation needs to accurately support those decisions. Nurses must be knowledgeable about the reimbursement of medical supplies and should discuss problematic situations with clients, families, and agency personnel. Clients and families may be unhappy when their specific requests cannot be granted.

TRENDS AND OPPORTUNITIES

National Health Objectives

The overarching goals of the *Healthy People 2020* objectives (USDHHS, 2010a) are to:
- Attain high-quality, longer lives free of preventable disease, disability, injury, and premature death.
- Achieve health equity, eliminate disparities, and improve the health of all groups.
- Create social and physical environments that promote good health for all.
- Promote quality of life, healthy development, and healthy behaviors across all life stages.

Nurses who work with clients and families in the home and community have opportunities to promote achievement of key objectives. They can assess client status, identify available resources and gaps to meet client needs, encourage clients and families to use resources, and coordinate care with other providers and community agencies. They can participate in numerous population-level projects and campaigns.

The *Healthy People 2020* box highlights objectives relevant to home health and hospice nurses. Note that many objectives relate to lifestyle issues. With appropriate health education, referral to community resources, and follow-up, there is a potential to reduce morbidity and mortality and decrease chronic disabilities. Nurses can make important contributions on one-to-one and population-focused levels.

> ### ♥ HEALTHY PEOPLE 2020
>
> #### *Examples of National Health Objectives for the Year 2020*
>
> - AOCBC-11: Reduce hip fractures among older adults.
> - C-1: Reduce the overall cancer death rate.
> - C-13: Increase proportion of cancer survivors beyond 5 years.
> - CKD-9: Reduce kidney failure due to diabetes.
> - HD-3: Reduce stroke deaths.
> - HDS-1: (Developmental) Increase overall cardiovascular health in the U.S. population.
> - HDS-5: Reduce the proportion of persons in the population with hypertension.
> - IID-4: Reduce invasive pneumococcal infections.

From U.S. Department of Health and Human Services: *Healthy People 2020*, Washington, DC, 2010a, USDHHS.

Organizational and Professional Resources

It is increasingly important for nurses to be involved in political, economic, and regulatory issues at the local, state, and national levels before they affect practice and services to clients. Joining organizations, reviewing the Internet, networking with colleagues, and reading professional literature provide opportunities to become informed and influence decisions.

Nationally, several prominent home health organizations have extensive websites. The National Association for Home Care & Hospice (NAHC) is a trade organization formed in 1982. A few years later, the Hospice Association of America (HAA) and NAHC developed an organizational partnership. Many agencies join as members, but nurses can also participate in the nursing section after joining as individual members. Lobbying is NAHC's primary focus; it also schedules an annual meeting, publishes a journal (*CARING*), and offers educational opportunities. The Visiting Nurse Association of America, formed in 1983, has a similar focus, but membership is limited to community-based, non-profit home health and hospice providers. *Home Healthcare Nurse, Home Health Care Management and Practice, Family and Community Health, Journal of Community Health Nursing*, and *Home Health Care Services Quarterly* are additional journals for home health practitioners and managers.

Hospice organizations also have extensive websites. The National Hospice and Palliative Care Organization was formed in 1978 to stimulate public and professional interest. The

Hospice Foundation of America was founded in 1982; its initial mission was fundraising. The Hospice Nurses Association was formed in 1987; 10 years later, the organization expanded and became the HPNA. The organization schedules conferences, publishes the *Journal of Hospice and Palliative Nursing*, and offers certification and credentialing. The *American Journal of Hospice and Palliative Care*, *Journal of Pediatric Oncology Nursing*, *International Journal of Palliative Nursing*, and other related journals address nursing practice, pain control, oncology, and medical practice.

Technology, Informatics, and Telehealth

Technology

Advances in technology, informatics, and telehealth are pervasive in health care and nursing practice; they are a window to the future. Many home health and hospice nurses have developed specialized skills with the following: extensive dressing changes, parenteral nutrition, chemotherapy, intravenous therapy for hydration and antibiotics, intrathecal pain management, ventilators, and apnea monitors. As mentioned earlier in the chapter, clients and family caregivers must participate in certain procedures and equipment. It is the responsibility of the nurse and fellow team members to determine if such procedures and equipment can be used safely; when the answer is yes, team members must provide sufficient education, demonstrations, and monitoring so that care continues safely. Advances in technology, informatics, and telehealth should not be viewed as replacements for nurses and team members, but as tools to improve the quality of their practice.

Informatics

Informatics is one of the most important new trends and opportunities for nurses, including those employed in community settings (IOM, 2003; USDHHS, 2010b). Nurses face urgent information management challenges that include the need for timely, reliable, and valid quantified data and information about clients, the services they receive, and their outcomes of care. They also need verbal and automated methods to communicate with other nurses and health care providers (Monsen and Martin, 2002a, b; Martin, 2005; Lundberg et al, 2008; Correll and Martin, 2009; Fazzi et al, 2010; Westra et al, 2010; Martin et al, 2011) (Figure 41-8).

The American Nurses Association anticipated the impact of information technology on the profession, and took the first step early in the 1990s. They began to recognize standardized terminologies that could be used by nurses and other health care disciplines to describe, document, and quantify their daily practice accurately and consistently (ANA, 2006: Omaha System, 2010). The Omaha System and 11 more interface or point-of-care and reference terminologies have been recognized. The second step involves interoperability—the exchange of coded data and ability to use those data. SNOMED CT and Logical Observation Identifiers, Names, and Codes (LOINC) are examples of reference terminologies that facilitate interoperability by sharing data generated by the interface terminologies. The third step is meaningful use. This suggests that better health care does not come solely from the adoption of technology itself, but

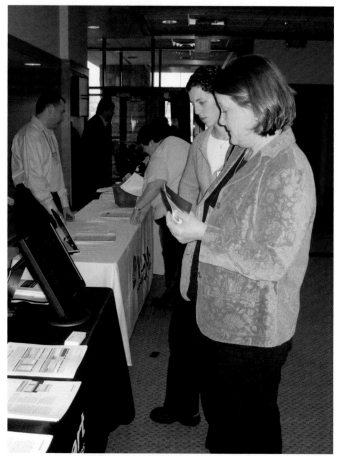

FIGURE 41-8 Use of information technology. (From www.omahasystem.org/photogallery.html. Used with permission from Karen Martin, RN, MSN, FAAN.)

through the exchange and use of electronic health information to best inform clinical decisions at the point-of-care (USDHHS, 2010; Martin et al, 2011). Meaningful use incorporates complex processes and workflow involving nurses and all health care practitioners, and it requires data integration and accessibility.

Health care providers throughout the United States have been given the mandate to convert to EHRs by 2014. As part of the American Recovery and Reinvestment Act of 2009, the CMS will provide reimbursement incentives for eligible professionals and hospitals to become "meaningful users" (Sensmeier, 2010). The privacy guidelines of HIPAA (USDHHS, 2003) ensure protection of clients' personal health information and include provisions about informed consent.

Telehealth

Telehealth supports long-distance clinical health care, client and professional health-related education, and public health and health administration using electronic information and telecommunications technologies (USDHHS, 2010c). The technology used varies to include videoconferencing, the Internet, store-and-forward imaging, streaming media, satellite, wireless communications, and plain old telephone systems. Telehealth equipment and program components include telephone triage and advice, and biometric telemonitoring equipment to measure vital signs, cardiac function, and point-of-care diagnostics.

The system may or may not include video technology for live-interaction (Finkelstein et al, 2006; Dansky et al, 2008). When conducted in the home, it is commonly referred to as *telehomecare.*

The increased availability of telehealth coincides with trends described in this and other chapters in this book: an aging population, increased chronic illness, a nursing shortage, and changes in health care reimbursement. Home health and hospice agencies face the challenge of managing increasingly complex clients in a highly constrained fiscal environment where patterns of care and reimbursement are based on client need and agency efficiency. Telehealth has been used successfully to improve health outcomes for clients who have diabetes (Chumbler et al, 2005), heart failure (Dansky et al, 2008; Dang et al, 2009), and chronic wounds (Kobza and Scheurich, 2000). Most often the clinical outcome achieved is a decrease in readmission to the hospital and emergency department use, especially for clients who are diagnosed with heart failure (Dang et al, 2009).

New trends promote new opportunities: innovations such as telehomecare can be used to monitor health status and symptom recognition, provide education, increase communication, and enable clients to become active partners in their own care offering more care at less cost than in-person visits only (Jovicic et al, 2006; Fazzi et al, 2010). Telehealth has emerged as a viable and acceptable way to supplement the delivery of health care.

Telemonitoring is increasingly being used with infants, women with high-risk pregnancies, and adults with various health problems. Smart homes are emerging to help the older adult to "age in place." Sensors can monitor activities and detect adverse events such as a fall or lack of movement and trigger a call for help. Medication management devices remind clients to take their medications, dispense medications, and send alerts to providers if devices are not accessed as expected. The next generation of devices is expected to focus on smart phone technology, making telemonitoring even more ubiquitous.

These are exciting times for home health and hospice. The need for nurses prepared to practice in these specialties is only expected to grow as the population ages, chronic illness rises, and more care is delivered in the community. Practice will increasingly require the use of sound judgment, interpersonal skills, and new technology. It is a good time to celebrate the past, embrace the present, and look forward to the future.

CHAPTER REVIEW

■ PRACTICE APPLICATION

The home visit is the hallmark of nursing in home health and hospice. Nurses are guests when they enter a client's home, and must recognize that their services can be accepted or rejected. The interpersonal relationship established during the first visit is critical, as is the initial assessment of the client, support system, and environment.

A. What strategies should the nurse use to develop a positive relationship during the first visit?

B. What are the most important elements to assess in the home environment?

C. What should the nurse do to establish a partnership with the client?

D. What is necessary for the nurse to include in the client contract?

E. How can the nurse determine the client's preferred learning style?

Answers can be found on the Evolve site.

■ KEY POINTS

- Home health, hospice, and palliative nursing practice provided in the client's home differ from care in institutional settings. The home setting affects practice in unique ways including establishing trust, developing care partnerships, selecting interventions, collecting outcomes and data, ensuring client safety, and promoting quality.
- Family members, including caregivers and significant persons who provide assistance and/or care, are essential members of the health care team.
- Home health has its roots in public health nursing, with an emphasis on health promotion, illness prevention, and caring for people in their communities.
- Home health and hospice practice and reimbursement changed when they became major Medicare benefits.
- Five models of care are described in this chapter: population-focused home care, transitional care, home-based primary care, home health, and hospice. Home health, hospice, and all other

nurses should become familiar with the models to inform clients and their families about options and educate providers who are potential referral sources.

- Medicare-certified home health and hospice agencies are divided into various types of the administrative and organizational structures. However, many aspects of nursing practice are the same in the various types.
- Standards of home nursing practice originate from the ANA and specialty organizations, and encourage adoption of evidence-based practice.
- Consistently demonstrating professional competency is essential for home health, hospice, and palliative care nurses.
- Home health nurses practice in accordance with the ANA (2007) *Home Health Nursing Scope and Standards of Practice.* Hospice and palliative nurses use the *Hospice and Palliative Nursing Scope and Standards of Practice* published by the Hospice and Palliative Nurses Association and the ANA (2007).

KEY POINTS—cont'd

- Interprofessional collaboration is inherent in home health and hospice.
- The Omaha System was developed and refined through a process of research. Reliability and validity were established for the entire system.
- The Omaha System is unique in that it is the only comprehensive vocabulary developed initially by and for nurses practicing in the community.
- The Omaha System consists of the Problem Classification Scheme (assessment), Intervention Scheme (care plans and services), and Problem Rating Scale for Outcomes (client change/evaluation).
- The Omaha System is designed to enhance practice, documentation, and information management. These areas are of concern to community health educators and students as well as practitioners and administrators.
- Interprofessional practitioners employed in Medicare-certified home health agencies use OASIS-C at designated intervals; it is the outcome measurement tool mandated by the Centers for Medicare and Medicaid Services' conditions of participation.
- Evidence-based quality/performance improvement is important in all home health and hospice agencies. Currently, Medicare's Outcome-Based Quality Improvement program is used for outcome measurement and cost control.
- Exciting trends and opportunities are pervasive in home health and hospice. Many nurses are developing skills using technology, informatics, and telehealth; a commitment to life-long learning is necessary.

CLINICAL DECISION-MAKING ACTIVITIES

1. Make a home visit with an experienced home health or hospice nurse and do the following:
   A. Evaluate the process and content of the nurse–client interaction to determine what aspects of the visit were based on evidence-based practice; describe the process of the visit.
   B. Compare actual roles and functions with the *Home Health Nursing Scope and Standards of Practice* (ANA, 2007), the *Hospice and Palliative Scope and Standards of Practice* (HPNA/ANA, 2007), or other specialty standards as appropriate for the client population.
   C. Observe and discuss whether that nurse uses a client problem/nursing diagnosis, intervention, or outcome measurement system or framework. Is it important to use a system or framework approach? Explain.
2. Work with a partner or in a small group. Select a client you have visited or invent a fictitious client, and list data for a typical referral and initial visit. Independently apply the three parts of the Omaha System to the client data. Compare each portion of your selections with that of your partner or group members.
3. Make a joint home visit with another health care professional and assess as in the preceding activity. Attend a client/family-provider conference and write a summary of the group process. Has your attitude changed after you listened to the opinions expressed by family members?

4. Review a client record. What client outcomes were met through home health care? What specific outcomes showed an improvement or a stabilizing condition?
5. Interview a home health or hospice nurse who uses electronic health records (EHRs). Ask about the advantages of EHRs and challenges associated with them. How can aggregate clinical data generated by EHRs help nurses better understand the needs of their clients? How might knowing the needs of their clinical population assist in reviewing the research literature and planning new interventions?
6. Review your state's laws governing advance directives. Consider the legal and ethical advantages and disadvantages of having such directives. How would you write an advance directive for yourself?
7. Participate in a telehomecare visit using video technology or observe the analysis of data from remote monitoring. Trace the nurse's decision making and changes in the plan of care based on the telemonitoring data. Determine what outcomes might be expected from this type of care.

REFERENCES

Altilio T, Otis-Green S, Dahlin CM: Applying the National Quality Forum Preferred Practices for Palliative and Hospice Care: a social work perspective, *J Soc Work End Life Palliat Care* 4:3–16, 2008.

American Academy of Pediatrics, American Public Health Association: *Caring for our children: national health and safety performance standards: guidelines for out-of-home child care*, ed 2, Elk Grove Village, IL, 2002, American Academy of Pediatrics.

American Nurses Association: *ANA recognized terminologies and data element sets*, 2006. Available at http://www.nursingworld.org/npii/terminologies.htm. Accessed March 12, 2011.

American Nurses Association: *Home health nursing scope and standards of practice*, Silver Spring, MD, 2007, Nursesbooks.org.

Baker JN, Hinds PS, Spunt SL, et al: Integration of palliative care practices into the ongoing care of children with cancer: individualized care planning and coordination, *Pediatr Clin North Am* 55:223–250, 2008. xii.

Beales JL, Edes T: Veteran's Affairs home based primary care, *Clin Geriatr Med* 25:149–154, 2009.

Bekelman DB, Black BS, Shore AD, et al: Hospice care in a cohort of elders with dementia and mild cognitive impairment, *J Pain Symptom Manage* 30:208–214, 2005.

Black JM, Hawks JH: *Medical-surgical nursing*, ed 8, St Louis, 2009, Saunders.

Boling PA: Care transitions in home health, *Clin Geriatr Med* 25:135–148, 2009.

Bowles KH, Holmes JH, Ratcliffe SJ, et al: Factors identified by experts to support discharge referral decision making, *Nurs Res* 58:115–122, 2009.

Bowles KH, Foust J, Lauder B: *Evidence-based medication management for cognitively impaired and non-adherent patients in home care. Symposium F4 evidence-based practice improvement: merging two paradigms*, Providence, RI, 2010a, Eastern Nursing Research Society. Available at http://www.proaccess.net/files/enrs-all-pres.pdf. Accessed March 12, 2011.

Bowles KH, Pham J, O'Connor M, Horowitz DA: Information deficits in home care: a barrier to evidence-based disease management, *Home Health Care Manag Pract* 22:278–285, 2010b.

Brooten D, Youngblut JM, Brown L, et al: A randomized trial of nurse specialist home care for women with high risk pregnancies: outcomes and costs, *Am J Manag Care* 7:793–803, 2001.

Buhler-Wilkerson K: No place like home: a history of nursing and home care in the U.S, *Home Healthc Nurse* 20:641–647, 2002.

Buhler-Wilkerson K: Care of the chronically ill at home: an unresolved dilemma in health policy for the United States, *Milbank Memorial Fund Q* 85:611–639, 2007.

Centers for Medicare and Medicaid Services: *National Health Expenditure Data*, 2008. Available at http://www.cms.gov/NationalHealthExpendData/downloads/highlights.pdf. Accessed March 12, 2011.

Centers for Medicare and Medicaid Services: *OASIS-C guidance manual*, 2009. Available at http://www.cms.gov/HomeHealthQualityInits/14_HHQIOASISUserManual.asp. Accessed March 12, 2011.

Chang C, et al: Impact of a home-based primary care program in an urban Veterans Affairs medical center, *J Am Med Directors Assoc* 10:133–137, 2009.

Chumbler NR, Neugaard B, Kobb R, et al: Evaluation of a care coordination home-telehealth program for veterans with diabetes, *Eval Health Prof* 28:464–478, 2005.

Clark J, Lang N: An international classification for nursing practice, *Int Nurs Rev 39* 27:109, 1992.

Coleman EA, Berenson RA: Lost in transition: challenges and opportunities for improving the quality of transitional care, *Ann Intern Med* 140:553–536, 2004.

Coleman EA, Parry C, Chalmers S, Min SJ: The care transitions intervention: results of a randomized control trial, *Arch Intern Med* 166:1822–1828, 2006.

Correll PJ, Martin KS: The Omaha System helps a public health organization find its voice, *CIN Comp Inform Nurs* 27:12–15, 2009.

Dang S, Dimmick S, Kelkar G: Evaluating the evidence base for the use of home telehealth remote monitoring in elderly with heart failure, *Telemed J E Health* 15:783–796, 2009.

Dansky KH, Vanskey J, Bowles K: Impact of telehealth on clinical outcomes in patients with heart failure, *Clin Nurs Res* 17:182–199, 2008.

Davis K, Stremikis K: Family medicine: preparing for a high-performance health care system, *J Am Board Fam Med* 23(Suppl 1):S11–S16, 2010.

Dobell LG, Newcomer RJ: Integrated care: incentives, approaches, and future considerations, *Social Work Public Health* 23:25–47, 2008.

Donabedian A: Evaluating the quality of medical care, *Milbank Memorial Fund Q* 44:166–206, 1966.

Donahue MP: *Nursing, the finest art*, ed 3, St Louis, 2011, Elsevier.

Donelan-McCall N, Eckenrode J, Olds DL: Home visiting for the prevention of child maltreatment: lessons learned during the past 20 years, *Pediatr Clin North Am* 56:389–403, 2009.

Fazzi R, Ashe T, Reissig M: The same but different: three insider's views of hospital-based, hospital affiliated, and freestanding agencies, *Caring* 29:32–36, 2010.

Ferrante JM, Balasubramanian BA, Hudson SV, et al: Principles of the patient-centered medical home and preventive services directory, *Ann Fam Med* 8:108–116, 2010.

Finkelstein SM, Speedie SM, Potthoff S: How telehealth improves clinical outcomes at lower cost for home health care, *Telemed J E Health* 12:128–136, 2006.

First Things First: 2010. Available at http://www.azftf.gov/. Accessed March 12, 2011.

Ford KM, Linker LA: Compliance of licensed child care centers with the American Academy of Pediatrics' recommendations for infant sleep positions, *J Community Health Nurs* 19:83–91, 2002.

Friedberg MW, Lai DJ, Hussey PS, Schneider EC: A guide to the medical home as a practice-level intervention, *Am J Manag Care* 15:S291–S299, 2009.

Garvin JH, Martin KS, Stassen DL, Bowles KH: The Omaha System: coded data that describe patient care, *J AHIMA* 79:44–49, 2008.

Gazelle G: Understanding hospice—an underutilized option for life's final chapter, *N Engl J Med* 357:321–324, 2007.

Gorski LA: Making a commitment to clinical data, *Home Health Care Manag Pract* 16:206–211, 2004.

Gorski LA: Central venous access device associated infections, *Home Healthc Nurse* 28:221–229, 2010.

Graham MC: Will we be included in medical home language? *Nurs Pract* 35:6, 2010.

Hinds PS, Schum L, Baker JN, Wolfe J: Key factors affecting dying children and their families, *J Palliat Med* 8(suppl 1):S70–S78, 2005.

Homer CJ, Klatka K, Romm D, et al: A review of the evidence for the medical home for children with special health care needs. *Pediatrics* 122:922–937, 2008.

Honea NJ, Brintnall R, Given B, et al: Putting evidence into practice: nursing assessment and interventions to reduce family caregiver strain and burden, *Clin J Oncol Nurs* 12:507–516, 2008.

Hospice Association of America (HAA): *Hospice facts and statistics*, Washington, DC, 2009, HAA. Available at http://www.nahc.org/facts/HospiceStats09.pdf. Accessed March 12, 2011.

Hospice and Palliative Nurses Association and American Nurses Association: *Hospice and palliative nursing scope and standards of practice*, Silver Spring, MD, 2007, Nursesbooks.org.

Hsueh KC, Chen CY, Yang YH, Huang CL: Smoking cessation program in outpatient clinics of Family Medicine Department in Taiwan: a longitudinal evaluation, *Eval Health Prof* 33:12–25, 2010.

Huang CL, Wu SC, Jeng CY, Lin LC: The efficacy of a home-based nursing program in diabetic control of elderly people with diabetes mellitus living alone, *Public Health Nurs* 21:49–56, 2004.

Huang CL: Evaluating the program of a smoking cessation support group for adult smokers: a longitudinal pilot study, *Nurs Res* 13:197–205, 2005.

Humphrey CJ, Milone-Nuzzo P: Transitioning nurses to home care. In Harris MD, editor: *Handbook of home health care administration*, ed 5, Sudbury, MA, 2010, Jones and Bartlett, pp 515–527.

Inglis S, McLennan S, Dawson A, et al: A new solution for an old problem? Effects of a nurse-led, multidisciplinary, home-based intervention on readmission and mortality in clients with chronic atrial fibrillation, *J Cardiovasc Nurs* 19:118–127, 2004.

Institute of Medicine (IOM): In Gebbie K, Rosenstock L, Hernandez LM, editors: *Who will keep the public healthy?* Washington, DC, 2003, National Academy Press. Available at http://www.nap.edu/openbook.php?record_id=10542&pageR1. Accessed March 12, 2011.

Jovicic A, et al: Effects of self-management intervention on health outcomes of patients with heart failure: a systematic review of randomized controlled trials, *BMC Cardiovasc Disord* 6:43–51, 2006.

Kitzman H, et al: Enduring effects of nurse home visitation on maternal life course: a 3-year follow-up of a randomized trial, *JAMA* 283:1983–1989, 2000.

Kobza L, Scheurich A: The impact of telemedicine on outcomes of chronic wounds in the home care setting, *Ostomy Wound Manag* 46:48–52, 2000.

Kübler-Ross E: *On death and dying*, New York, 1969, McMillan.

Levin R, Keefer JM, Marren J, et al: Evidence-based practice: merging two paradigms, *J Nurs Care Qual* 25:117–126, 2010.

Lundberg CB, Warren JJ, Brokel J, et al: Selecting a standardized language to increase collaboration between research and practice, *OJNI* 12:1–19, 2008. Available at http://ojni.org/12_2/lundberg.pdf. Accessed March 12, 2011.

Mader SL, Medcraft MC, Joseph C, et al: Program at home: a veterans affairs healthcare program to deliver hospital care at home, *J Am Geriatr Soc* 56:2317–2322, 2008.

Malloy P, Paice J, Virani R, et al: End-of-life nursing education consortium: 5 years of educating graduate nursing faculty in excellent palliative care, *J Prof Nurs* 24:352–357, 2008.

Marquis BL, Huston CJ: *Leadership roles and management functions in nursing: theory and application*, ed 6, Philadelphia, 2009, Lippincott, Williams & Wilkins.

Martin KS: *The Omaha System: a key to practice, documentation, and information management*, reprinted, ed 2, Omaha, NE, 2005, Health Connections Press.

Martin KS, Monsen KA, Bowles KH: The Omaha System and meaningful use: applications for practice, education, and research, *Comput Inform Nurs* 29:52–58, 2011.

Melnyk BM, Fineout-Overholt E: *Evidence-based practice in nursing and healthcare: a guide to best practice*, Philadelphia, 2005, Lippincott, Williams & Wilkins.

Mistovich JJ, Karren KJ: *Prehospital emergency care*, ed 9, Upper Saddle River, NJ, 2010, Pearson Education.

Monsen KA, Martin KS: Developing an outcomes management program in a public health department, *Outcomes Manag* 6:62–66, 2002a.

Monsen KA, Martin KS: Using an outcomes management program in a public health department, *Outcomes Manag* 6:120–124, 2002b.

Motyka CL, Nies MA: Home health and hospice. In Nies MA, McEwen M, editors: *Community/public health nursing: promoting the health of populations*, ed 4, St Louis, 2011, Elsevier, pp 671–693.

Murtaugh CM, Pezzin LE, McDonald MV, et al: Just-in-time evidence-based e-mail "reminders" in home health care: impact on nurse practices, *Health Serv Res* 40:849–864, 2005.

National Association for Home Care & Hospice (NAHC): *Basic statistics about home care*, Washington, DC, 2008, NAHC. Available at http://www.nahc.org/facts/08HC_Stats.pdf. Accessed March 12, 2011.

National PACE Association: *What is PACE?*. Available at http://www.npaonline.org/website/article.asp?id=12. Accessed March 12, 2011.

National Quality Forum: 2010. Available at http://www.qualityforum.org. Accessed March 12, 2011.

Naylor MD: Transitional care for older adults: a cost-effective model, *LDI Issue Brief* 9:1–4, 2004.

Naylor MD, Van Cleave J: The Transitional Care Model for Older Adults, In Meleis AI, editor: *Transitions Theory: middle range and situational specific theories in research and practice*, New York, 2010, Springer Publishing, pp 459–464.

Olds DL, Eckenrode J, Henderson CR Jr, et al: Long-term effects of home visitation on maternal life course and child abuse and neglect: fifteen year follow-up of randomized trial, *JAMA* 278:637–643, 1997.

Omaha System: 2010. Available at http://www.omahasystem.org. Accessed March 12, 2011.

Perry KM, Parente CA: Integrating palliative care into home care practice. In Harris MD, editor: *Handbook of home health care administration*, ed 5, Sudbury, MA, 2010, Jones and Bartlett, pp 863–875.

Quad Council: *Quad Council PHN Competencies*, 2003. Available at http://www.astdn.org/publication_quad_council_phn_competencies.htm. Accessed March 12. 2011.

Rabins PV, Black BS, Roca R, et al: Effectiveness of a nurse-based outreach program for identifying and treating psychiatric illness in the elderly, *JAMA* 283:2802–2809, 2000.

Ramler M, Nakatsukasa-Ono W, Loe C, Harris K: *The influence of child care health consultants in promoting children's health and well-being: a report on selected resources*, Newton, MA, 2006, Healthy Child Care Consultant Network Support Center. Available at http://hcccnsc.jsi.com/resources/publications/CC_lit_review_Screen_All.pdf. Accessed March 12, 2011.

Rhinehart E, McGoldrick M: *Infection control in home care and hospice*, ed 2, Boston, 2006, Jones & Bartlett.

Sanders S, Mackin ML, Reyes J, et al: Implementing evidence-based practices: considerations for the hospice setting, *Am J Hosp Palliat Care* 27:369–376, 2010.

Schlenker RE, Powell MC, Goodrich GK: Initial home health outcomes under prospective payment, *Health Serv Res* 40:177–193, 2005.

Schumacher KL, Beck CA, Marren JM: Family caregivers: caring for older adults, working with their families, *AJN* 106:40–48, 2006.

Schumacher KL, Marren J: Home care nursing of older adults, *Nurs Clin North Am* 39:443–471, 2004.

Sensmeier J: Alliance for Nursing Informatics statement to the Robert Wood Johnson Foundation Initiative on the future of nursing: acute care focusing on the area of technology, *Comput Inform Nurs* 28:63–67, 2010.

Siegel JD, Rhinehart E, Jackson M, Chiarello L: *Management of multi-drug resistant organisms in healthcare settings*, 2006. Available at http://www.cdc.gov/ncidod/dhap/pdf/ar/mdroGuideline2006.pdf. Accessed March 12, 2011.

Siegel JD, Siegel JD, Rhinehart E, Jackson M, Chiarello L: *Guideline for isolation precautions: preventing transmission of infectious agents in healthcare settings*, 2007. Available at http://www.cdc.gov/ncidod/dhap/pdf/guidelines/Isolation2007.pdf. Accessed March 12, 2011.

Smith MH: *Legal basics for professional nursing practice*, 2007. Available at http://www.nursingworld.org/mods/archive/mod995/canlegalnursfull.htm. Accessed March 12, 2011.

U.S. Department of Health and Human Services: *Understanding health information privacy: HIPAA-national standards for transactions, security and privacy*, 2003. Available at http://www.hhs.gov/ocr/privacy/hipaa/understanding/index.html. Accessed March 12, 2011.

U.S. Department of Health and Human Services: *Healthy People 2020: national health promotion and disease prevention objectives*, 2010a. Available at http://www.healthypeople.gov/hp2020/Objectives/TopicAreas.aspx. Accesssed March 12, 2011.

U.S. Department of Health and Human Services: *Health information technology*, 2010b. Available at http://www.healthit.hhs.gov/portal/server.pt. Accessed March 12, 2011.

U.S. Department of Health and Human Services—HRSA: *Telehealth*, 2010c. Available at http://hrsa.gov/telehealth/default.htm. Accessed March 12, 2011.

Viola D, Leven DC, LePere JC: End-of-life care: an interdisciplinary perspective, *Am J Hosp Palliat Care* 26:75–78, 2009.

Visiting Nurse Service of New York: 2010. Available at http://www.vnsny.org. Accessed March 12, 2011.

Westra BL, Oancea C, Savik K, Marek KD: The feasibility of integrating the Omaha System data across home care agencies and vendors, *Comput Inform Nurs* 28:162–171, 2010.

Zerwekh JV: *Nursing care at the end of life: palliative care for patients and families*, Philadelphia, 2006, FA Davis.

CHAPTER 42

The Nurse in the Schools

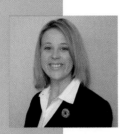

Lisa Pedersen Turner, RN, MSN, PCHCNS-BC

Lisa Pedersen Turner is the clinic coordinator of the Good Samaritan Nursing Center as well as a clinical instructor for public health nursing at the University of Kentucky. Her work at the Good Samaritan Nursing Center has focused on providing school health services to underserved populations as well as developing a K-12 school health curriculum for a county in rural Kentucky. She has lectured and supervised students studying public health nursing in a myriad of community settings, including school clinics, homeless shelters, and free clinics for adults and children. She has contributed to several projects to evaluate school health services and has presented at national and international symposia on nursing clinics in the community.

ADDITIONAL RESOURCES

ⓔvolve WEBSITE
http://evolve.elsevier.com/Stanhope
- *Healthy People 2020*
- WebLinks

- Quiz
- Case Studies
- Glossary
- Answers to Practice Application

OBJECTIVES

After reading this chapter, the student should be able to do the following:
1. Discuss professional standards expected of school nurses.
2. Differentiate between the many roles and functions of school nurses.
3. Describe the different variations of school health services and coordinated school health programs.
4. Analyze the nursing care given in schools in terms of the primary, secondary, and tertiary levels of prevention.
5. Anticipate future trends in school nursing.

KEY TERMS

advanced practice nurse, p. 916
American Academy of Pediatrics (AAP), p. 916
Americans with Disabilities Act, p. 915
case manager, p. 917
Centers for Disease Control and Prevention, p. 918
Child Nutrition and WIC Reauthorization Act of 2004, p. 915
community outreach, p. 918
consultant, p. 917
counselor, p. 917
crisis teams, p. 926
direct caregiver, p. 917
do-not-resuscitate orders, p. 930
emergency plan, p. 923
health educator, p. 917

Health Insurance Portability and Accountability Act of 1996 (HIPAA), p. 922
individualized education plans (IEPs), p. 915
individualized health plans (IHPs), p. 915
National Association of School Nurses, p. 915
No Child Left Behind Act of 2001, p. 915
PL 93-112 Section 504 of the Rehabilitation Act of 1973, p. 915
PL 94-142 Education for All Handicapped Children Act, p. 915

PL 105-17 Individuals with Disabilities Education Act (IDEA), p. 915
primary prevention, p. 920
researcher, p. 918
Safe Kids Campaign, p. 921
school-based health centers, p. 919
School Health Policies and Programs Study 2006, p. 917
school-linked program, p. 920
secondary prevention, p. 920
standard precautions, p. 924
tertiary prevention, p. 920
—*See Glossary for definitions*

In 2010 over 49.4 million children attended one of 132,700 schools every day (U.S. Department of Education, National Center for Education Statistics, 2010). These children need health care during their school day, and this is the job of the school nurse. There are approximately 45,000 school nurses in the public schools alone (American Federation of Teachers, 2008). Even parents expect a school nurse to be available for their children at school (Read et al, 2009).

It is commonly thought that school nurses only put bandages on cuts and soothe children with stomachaches. However, that is not their major role. School nurses give comprehensive nursing care to the children and the staff at the school. At the same time, they coordinate the health education program of the school and consult with school officials to help identify and care for other persons in the school community.

The school nurse provides care to the children not only in the school building itself, but also in other settings where children are found—for example, in juvenile detention centers, in preschools and daycare centers, during field trips, at sporting events, and in the children's homes (Nic Philibin et al, 2010).

The school nurse, therefore, must be flexible in giving nursing care, education, and help to those who need it. This chapter discusses the history of nursing in the schools and the functions of school nurses today. In addition, the standards of practice for school nurses are discussed, as the nurse takes on a variety of roles. Different types of school health services are reviewed, including government-financed programs.

The primary, secondary, and tertiary levels of nursing care that nurses give to children in the schools are presented. The most common health problems that the school nurse finds in children are also discussed under their appropriate prevention levels. The chapter ends with a discussion of the ethical dilemmas that may arise for school nurses. The future of nursing in the schools is predicted for ever-changing communities.

HISTORY OF SCHOOL NURSING

The history of school nursing began with the earliest efforts of nurses to care for people in the community. In the late 1800s in England, the Metropolitan Association of Nursing provided medical examinations for children in the schools of London.

By 1892 nurses in London were responsible for checking the nutrition of the children in the schools (Anonymous, 2008). These ideas spread to the United States where, in 1897, nurses in New York City schools began to identify ill children. They then excluded these children from classes so that other children would not be infected (Vessey and McGowan, 2006). Health education was also important during this time. Many states had laws in the late 1800s mandating that nurses teach within the schools about the abuse of alcohol and narcotics (Fee and Liping, 2007).

In the early 1900s in the United States, the main health problem in the community was the spread of infectious diseases. On October 2, 1902, in New York City, Lillian Wald's Henry Street Settlement nurses began going into homes and schools to assess children. These public health nurses were at first in only four schools caring for about 10,000 children. They made plans to identify children with lice and other infestations and those with infected wounds, tuberculosis (TB), and other infectious diseases (Vessey and McGowan, 2006; Judd, Sitzman, and Davis, 2009).

The need for school nurses was immediately recognized by the health care community. By 1910, Teachers College in New York City added a course on school nursing to their curriculum for nurses. In 1916 a school superintendent requested that a public health nurse be sent to the schools to care for children of immigrants (Judd, Sitzman, and Davis, 2009). By the 1920s school nurse teachers were employed by most municipal health departments. As the years went by and communities struggled with serious economic issues and hardships during the Depression, school nurses continued to provide health care to children in the schools through the federal Works Progress Administration program (WPA) (Judd, Sitzman, and Davis, 2009).

In the 1940s the nurses were mostly employed by the school districts directly. The nurses also provided home nursing and health education for the children and their parents (Vessey and McGowan, 2006). In addition, school nurses became concerned with the condition of school buildings (Judd, Sitzman, and Davis, 2009).

After World War II and into the 1950s, as a result of the increased use of immunizations and antibiotics, the number of children with communicable disease in the schools fell. School nurses then turned their attention to screening children for common health problems and for vision and hearing. School nurses were less likely to teach health concepts in the children's classrooms and more likely to consult with teachers about health education (Vessey and McGowan, 2006). However, there was an increased emphasis on employee health, and school nurses began screening teachers and other school staff for health problems (Fee and Liping, 2007).

The 1960s saw an upsurge in the call for higher levels of education for school nurses. A position paper delivered at the 1960 American Nurses Association (ANA) convention called for the Bachelor of Science in nursing degree as the minimum educational preparation for school nurses. By 1970 the first school nurse practitioner program was started at the University of Colorado. There, school nurses learned advanced concepts of school nursing practice to provide primary health care to children (Vessey and McGowan, 2006).

Federal Legislation in the 1970s, 1980s, 1990s, and 2000s

Community involvement in health in schools was a major thrust in the 1970s and 1980s. Counseling and mental health services were added to the responsibilities of school nurses, who began to directly teach children concepts of health. Children were no longer just being screened for illnesses (Vessey and McGowan, 2006). Because of federal laws that required schools to make accommodations for handicapped children, medically fragile children were attending schools, often for the first time. One of these laws, PL 93-112 Section 504 of the Rehabilitation Act of 1973, was an important step in helping all children enjoy a normal educational experience (Robert Wood Johnson Foundation, 2010). This law was followed by PL 94-142 Education for All Handicapped Children Act, which required that children with disabilities have services provided for them in the schools.

Following the passage of the Americans with Disabilities Act in 1992, PL 105-17 Individuals with Disabilities Education Act (IDEA) passed in 1997. Both of these laws required that more children be allowed to attend schools. Schools had to make allowances for their special needs, which included ensuring that their school experience was in balance with their health care needs by developing individualized education plans (IEPs) and individualized health plans (IHPs). That meant that more children with human immunodeficiency virus (HIV), acquired immunodeficiency syndrome (AIDS), chronic illnesses, or mental health problems were in the classrooms and needed more attention from the school nurse (Robert Wood Johnson Foundation, 2010). The No Child Left Behind Act of 2001 requires a healthy environment in the schools, which also affects children who have health problems (Adler, 2009). Table 42-1 summarizes the effects of these laws on school nurses and schoolchildren.

Also during the 1990s, the responsibilities of the school nurse were extended to include the development of complete clinics and health care agency centers within or attached to the schools (Vessey and McGowan, 2006). These school-based clinics will be discussed later in this chapter. By 2002, some school nurses were responsible for several schools, and they provided care under a variety of nursing roles. To address obesity and to promote healthy eating and physical activity through changes in school environments, Congress passed the Child Nutrition and

TABLE 42-1	FEDERAL LEGISLATION AFFECTING SCHOOL NURSING
LAW	**EFFECT ON SCHOOL NURSES AND CHILDREN**
1973: PL 39-112, Section 504 of Rehabilitation Act	Children cannot be excluded from schools because of a handicap. The school must provide health services that each child needs.
1975: PL 94-142, Education for All Handicapped Children Act	All children should attend school in least restrictive environment. Requires school district's committee on handicapped to develop individualized education plans (IEPs) for children.
1992: Americans with Disabilities Act	Persons with disabilities cannot be excluded from activities.
1997: PL 105-17, Individuals with Disabilities Education Act (IDEA)	Educational services must be offered by schools for all disabled children from birth through age 22 years.
2001: No Child Left Behind Act of 2001	All children must receive standardized education in a healthy environment.
2004: Child Nutrition and WIC Reauthorization Act of 2004	Every local education agency (LEA) participating in federal school meal programs must establish a local school wellness policy.

Compiled from Betz CL: Use of 504 plans for children and youth with disabilities: nursing application, *Pediatr Nurs* 27:347-352, 2001; Whalen LG, Grunbaum JA, Kann L, et al: *Profiles 2002. School health profiles. Surveillance for characteristics of health programs among secondary schools*, Washington, DC, 2004, Centers for Disease Control and Prevention, USDHHS.

WIC Reauthorization Act of 2004 (PL 108.265 Section 204). This act designated that each local education agency (LEA) participating in federal school meal programs, such as the National School Lunch or Breakfast Program, must establish a local school wellness policy. Table 42-2 gives the highlights of school nursing history over the last century.

STANDARDS OF PRACTICE FOR SCHOOL NURSES

The professional body for school nurses is the National Association of School Nurses (NASN), headquartered in Washington, DC. This association provides the general guidelines and support for all school nurses. It revised the standards of professional practice for school nurses in 2001. These standards require that all school nurses use the nursing process throughout their practice: assessment, analysis, planning, implementation, and evaluation.

In addition, the professional standards rely on nurses to give care based on 11 criteria (NASN, 2001). These criteria include the ability to do the following:

- Develop school health policies and procedures.
- Evaluate their own nursing practice.
- Keep up with nursing knowledge.

TABLE 42-2   HIGH POINTS IN SCHOOL NURSING HISTORY

DECADE	MAJOR EVENTS IN SCHOOL NURSING
1890s	English and American nurses are used in schools to examine children for infectious diseases and to teach about alcohol abuse.
1900s	Henry Street Settlement in New York City sends nurses into schools and homes to investigate children's overall health.
1910s	School nursing course added to Teachers College nursing program.
1920s and 1930s	School nurses are employed by community health departments.
1940s	School districts employ school nurses.
1950s	Children are screened in schools for common health problems.
1960s	Educational preparation for school nurses is debated.
1970s	School nurse practitioner programs begun. Increased emphasis put on mental health counseling in schools.
1980s	Children with long-term illness or disabilities attend schools.
1990s	School-based and school-linked clinics are started. Total family and community health care is offered.
2000s	School nurses give comprehensive primary, secondary, and tertiary levels of nursing care.

From Schlachta-Fairchild L, Varghese SB, Deickman A, Castelli D: Telehealth and telenursing are live: APN policy and practice implications, *J Nurse Pract* 6:98-106, 2010.

- Interact with the interprofessional health care team.
- Ensure confidentiality in providing health care.
- Consult with others to give complete care.
- Use research findings in practice.
- Ensure the safety of children, including when delegating care to other school personnel.
- Have good communication skills.
- Manage a school health program effectively.
- Teach others about wellness.

In general, the NASN standards (Box 42-1) compare very well with those developed by the American Academy of Pediatrics (AAP) regarding giving health care to students in the schools. The AAP (2008a) developed their own ideas about how nurses function in schools based on their assessment of schoolchildren's health needs. These guidelines are similar to those written by the NASN. The AAP stated that school nurses should ensure the following:

- That children get the health care they need, including emergency care in the school
- That the nurse keeps track of the state-required vaccinations that children have received
- That the nurse carries out the required screening of the children based on state law
- That children with health problems are able to learn in the classroom

BOX 42-1   SUMMARY OF MAJOR CONCEPTS OF NASN STANDARDS

- Give and evaluate appropriate up-to-date nursing care.
- Collaborate well with other health providers and school staff.
- Maintain school health office policies, including privacy and safety of health records.
- Teach health promotion and maintenance to children, families, and communities.

Modified from National Association of School Nurses: *Scope and standards of professional school nursing practice*, Washington, DC, 2001, American Nurses Association.

The AAP recommends that the nurse be the head of a health team that includes a physician (preferably a pediatrician), school counselors, the school psychologist, members of the school staff including the administrator, and teachers. The goal is for children to get complete health care in the schools.

EDUCATIONAL CREDENTIALS OF SCHOOL NURSES

The NASN recommends that school nurses be registered nurses who also have bachelor's degrees in nursing and a special certification in school nursing (NASN, 2001). The AAP has the same recommendations (AAP, 2008a). However, not all nurses have been educated this way. There are no general laws regarding the educational background of school nurses. School nurses in some states are required to be registered nurses, but licensed practical nurses are also seen in some schools. Box 42-2 lists the states that have laws regarding the education of school nurses. Only about half of all U.S. states require some form of additional study for school nurse specialty certification (CDC, 2006).

DID YOU KNOW? *The educational preparation for school nurses in the United States ranges from an associate's degree to a master's degree with certification credentials.*

School nurses in some schools may be advanced practice nurses who specialize in caring for children. They may be nurse practitioners that have specialized in child health nursing (pediatrics), in family nursing, or in the school nurse practitioner role. Clinical nurse specialists who are school nurses may also be found in child health nursing or community or public health nursing. The higher the educational level of the school nurse, the better that nurse is able to give complete care to children and their families. These advanced practice nurses may be certified by professional organizations such as the ANA or their own professional organization. Most hold master's degrees in nursing.

School nurses do not start their nursing careers in the schools. All have prior experience in nursing—most from working either in hospitals or with communities. In addition, most have spent years working with children, so they are aware of their special health needs.

ROLES AND FUNCTIONS OF SCHOOL NURSES

School nurses give care to children as direct caregivers, educators, counselors, consultants, and case managers. They must coordinate the health care of many students in their schools with the health care that the children receive from their own health care providers.

In *Healthy People 2020 Proposed Objectives,* goal ECBP HP2020-4 states that there should be 1 nurse for every 750 children in each school (USDHHS, 2010). Most schools have not achieved this objective. By 2006 approximately 45% of the nation's schools met that standard (CDC, 2010a). A study by the Centers for Disease Control and Prevention (CDC) (2006), the **School Health Policies and Programs Study 2006** (SHPPS 2006), found that by 2006 several states (Alabama, Arizona, Louisiana, Pennsylvania, Tennessee, Vermont, West Virginia, and Wyoming) specified a maximum student-to-school nurse ratio. Three states (Delaware, District of Columbia, and New Jersey) required schools to have a full-time school nurse. Having fewer nurses in the schools means that the nurses are expected to perform many different functions. It is therefore possible that they are unable to give the amount of comprehensive care that the students need (Ficca and Welk, 2006).

In 2003 the National Association of School Nurses adopted a resolution recommending that there be a school nurse at all times in every school. The recommendation was based on requirements of the IDEA Act and CDC health recommendations (NASN, 2003).

> **DID YOU KNOW?**   *Many schools do not have a nurse in the building every day.*

School Nurse Roles
Direct Caregiver

The school nurse is expected to give immediate nursing care to the ill or injured child or school staff member. **Direct caregiver** is the traditional role of the school nurse.

Although most school nurses are in public or private schools and give care only during school hours, the nurse in a boarding school provides nursing care to children 24 hours a day and 7 days a week. In boarding schools, the children live at school and go home only for vacations. The nurse also lives at the school and may be on call all the time. The nurse in the boarding school is very important to the children because this nurse is the gatekeeper to their complete health care (Thackaberry, 2001). The nurse makes all of the health care decisions for the child and has a referral system to contact other health care providers, such as physicians and psychological counselors, if needed.

Health Educator

The school nurse in the **health educator** role may be asked to teach children both individually and in the classroom. The nurse uses different approaches to teach about health, such as teaching proper nutrition or safety information. Many school nurses teach the older elementary girls and boys about the coming changes in their bodies as puberty arrives. Other school nurses may teach the health education classes that are required by the states to be included in the programs.

Case Manager

The school nurse is expected to function as a **case manager,** helping to coordinate the health care for children with complex health problems. This may include the child who is disabled or chronically ill and who may be seen by a physical therapist, an occupational therapist, a speech therapist, or another health care provider during the school day. The nurse sets up the schedule for the child's visits so that those appointments do not unnecessarily impact negatively on the child's academic day.

Consultant

The school nurse is the person best able to provide health information to school administrators, teachers, and parent–teacher groups. As a **consultant,** the school nurse can provide professional information about proposed changes in the school environment and their impact on the health of the children. The nurse can also recommend changes in the school's policies or engage community organizations to help make the children's schools healthier places (Nic Philibin et al, 2010). This is a population-level role for the school nurse; the population consists of all children, families, staff, and the surrounding community.

Counselor

The school nurse may be the person whom children trust to tell important secrets about their health. It is important that, as a **counselor,** the school nurse have a reputation as being a trustworthy person to whom the children can go if they are in trouble or if they need to confide about a personal matter (Nic Philibin et al, 2010). Nurses in this situation should tell children that if anything they reveal points out that they are in danger, the parents and school officials must be told. However, privacy and confidentiality, as in all health care, are important.

In addition, the school nurse may be the person to help with grief counseling in the schools. (See later discussion on the school crisis team.)

Community Outreach

When participating in community outreach, nurses can be involved in community health fairs or festivals in the schools, using that opportunity to teach others. They can be part of an influenza immunization program for the school staff and can promote a health education fair and do blood pressure screenings. They can initiate a liaison, coordinating with local health charities to provide education to the schools (Hamner, Wilder, and Byrd, 2007).

EVIDENCE-BASED PRACTICE

Because of the obesity epidemic in the United States, interventions to increase physical activity and reduce sedentary behaviors have become a priority for public health practitioners. This evidence-based guideline provides school-based strategies and tools to increase the level of physical activity and to reduce sedentary behavior in the kindergarten through eighth-grade population. The complete guideline, which contains additional assessment instruments, forms, and curriculum information, is available from the Research Translation and Dissemination Core (RTDC) of the University of Iowa College of Nursing. This guideline focuses on three methods that have a strong research base, are easy and inexpensive to implement, and show the greatest effect on behavior changes according to current research: increasing time spent in moderate to vigorous physical activity (MVPA) during physical education class, increasing time spent in MVPA during recess (free play time), and teaching skills to reduce sedentary behaviors.

Nurse Use

School nurses can use the information in this guideline as a resource for research-based interventions and methods for evaluation of their effectiveness. Using this guideline, school nurses can work with administrators to provide low-cost strategies to increase physical activity by children in schools without loss of educational instruction time.

From Bagby MA, Adams S: Evidence-based practice guideline: increasing physical activity in schools—kindergarten through 8th grade, *J Sch Nurs* 23(3):137-145, 2007.

Researcher

Little research has been done on nurses caring for children in the schools. The school nurse is responsible for making sure that the nursing care given is based on solid, evidence-based practice. Outcomes regarding school nurse services need to be studied (Nic Philibin et al, 2010). Therefore, the school nurse, as an educator, is in the right position to do studies as a researcher that advances school nursing practice.

SCHOOL HEALTH SERVICES

School health services vary in their scope. However, there are common parts to the programs.

Federal School Health Programs

The federal government, through the coordination of the Centers for Disease Control and Prevention, has developed a plan that school health programs should follow (CDC, 2008) (Figure 42-1).

LINKING CONTENT TO PRACTICE

School nurses play a primary role in the implementation of the CDC School Health Program components. These components are described below and addressed throughout this chapter. The emphasis in this program design is working with the school as a population or community. This plan has eight parts:

- *Health education*—This section includes teaching children about how to stay healthy and how to prevent becoming ill or being injured. The health education is offered in a planned, sequential, K-12 curriculum that addresses all dimensions of health.
- *Physical education*—Taking part in physical activity during the school day is recommended for all children. This is to provide regular exercise as well as to provide sports programs outside the normal school day. This, it is hoped, may help reduce obesity, high blood pressure, and other diseases later in life (Cole et al, 2006).
- *Health services*—The purpose of this segment is to reduce illness in children. Specifically, the schools can help children with asthma cope with their disease. This is also the section of comprehensive school health that promotes the school nurse to student ratio of 1:750 as discussed earlier in this chapter (USDHHS, 2010).
- *Nutrition services*—Information on nutrition and diet should be taught to all children. In addition, the schools should provide healthy food choices for students in their meal programs (both breakfast and lunch). The Team Nutrition Program called *Making It Happen* is a federal program sponsored by the U.S. Department of Agriculture that encourages schools to have nutritious foods available for all students (Team Nutrition, 2010).
- *Counseling, psychological, and social services*—This section promotes the health of children who receive special education services (IDEA), as well as children who have mental health needs. Working with families at risk because of socioeconomic needs is also part of this area (Stevenson, 2010).
- *Healthy school environment*—The emphasis in this area is to reduce tobacco use in teenagers as well as reducing violence overall in the schools. Education regarding the prevention of HIV/AIDS is also a part of this section (Hayter et al, 2008).
- *Health promotion for staff*—Nurses can help provide health care for teachers and other staff members in the schools. Staff can ask nurses about their health and obtain health education at school during their workday (Ryan, 2008).
- *Family/community involvement*—The school health program should contact families and community leaders to find out what health services are needed the most and how they can work together to emphasize health education for all. This includes being involved as health educators when adolescents take part-time jobs. Health in the workplace setting is just as important for the students (AAOHN/NASN, 2004).

This plan was originally developed in 1987 after the CDC began funding schools for HIV-prevention education programs. By 1992 this educational system was so successful that it was expanded to include school health programs to teach children prevention of other chronic illnesses. These include diseases caused in part by risk factors such as poor diet, lack of exercise, and smoking.

Then, in 1998, the government expanded the program again to include a more complete school health education program that included the parents and the community in the children's care. By 2009, 22 states had been funded for their school health programs by the CDC (CDC, 2009b). The

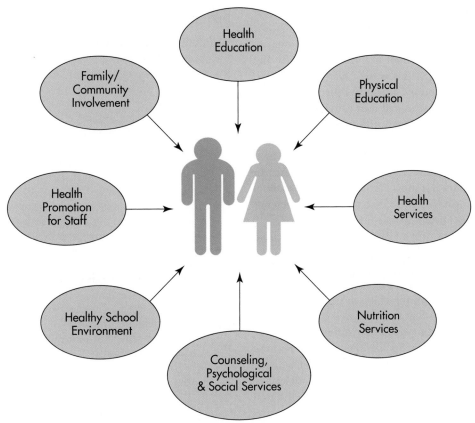

FIGURE 42-1 The eight components of a coordinated school health program. (From Centers for Disease Control and Prevention: *Healthy Youth! Coordinated school health program,* Washington, DC, 2008, CDC. Available at http://www.cdc.gov/HealthyYouth/CSHP/.)

funding has paid for the development of health education plans of study, or curricula, that include policies, guidelines, and training for these health programs. The states then use these courses to teach the children. The schools are actively involved in helping the children practice problem solving, communication, and other life skills so they can reduce their risk factors.

According to the CDC, two states in particular have been very successful with these programs. West Virginia has developed a program called the Instructional Goals and Objectives for Health Education and Physical Education, which increased the ability of the children to pass the President's Physical Fitness Test. In Michigan, the Governor's Council on Physical Fitness, Health, and Sports developed an Exemplary Physical Education Curriculum project that made up educational materials and plans for children to achieve high physical fitness scores. All of these programs were paid for by the federal school health program funding (CDC, 2009b).

School Health Policies and Program Study 2006

After the CDC began funding educational programs about prevention of HIV in the schools in 1987, there was clearly a need to expand these programs. By 1992 the CDC began giving money to fund other school health programs that taught students about heart disease, cancer, stroke, diabetes, and substance abuse prevention (Kann, Brener, and Wechsler, 2007). These programs have been evaluated by the School Health

Policies and Programs Study 2006 (CDC, 2006), which looked at all eight parts of the school health program in all 50 states and the District of Columbia. The study found that only half of the states had the recommended 1 school nurse for every 750 students that was discussed earlier in this chapter. It also found that most school health programs had access to mental health counselors, but that the food in the schools' cafeteria tended to be high in salt and fat. Most schools had rules forbidding weapons on the school grounds or use of tobacco. Parental involvement in the school health programs was only about 50% and, to make a difference in a child's health, parents are encouraged to be involved (Kann, Brener, and Wechsler, 2007).

School-Based Health Programs

Because many schoolchildren may not receive health care services other than screening and first aid care from the school nurse, the U.S. government began funding **school-based health centers** (SBHCs) during the 1990s. These are family-centered, community-based clinics run within the schools. These clinics give expanded health services, including mental health and dental care, as well as the more traditional health care services (Brown and Bolen, 2008). The SBHCs can range in size from small to large; some school clinics are open to the community only during the school year and others are open 24 hours a day all year round. An example of the more limited clinic is the SBHC in Worcester, MA, where six clinics are run in the schools (elementary through high school) by the Family Health Center of Worchester, Inc during the school year months of August through May (Family Health Center, 2010).

Another example of a clinic is the school-linked program, which is coordinated by the school but has community ties (Brown, 2008). An example of this is the *Collaborative Model for School Health* in Pitts County, North Carolina. The nurses employed by the local hospital in that area provide health care for children in kindergarten through fifth grade. There is collaboration between the county health department, the local university's nursing school, and other private health care providers to give primary, secondary, and tertiary nursing care. An evaluation of the program has shown that the children's school attendance and learning has increased as a result of the presence of more complete school health services (Trapp, 2010).

At a center in Texas, an urban SBHC is located in a school district where many of the children lack health insurance. The school nurses there are assisted by three part-time nurse practitioners and one public health nurse. The school nurse is responsible for the record keeping on the children's immunizations, does the screening, and gives first aid to injured children. Then the school nurse refers children who need additional health care to the SBHC in the school. Parents like the program because they trust the school nurse. They also like its location inside the school because everyone can receive health care without having to travel far to get to a clinic (Texas Association of School-Based Health Centers, 2010).

SCHOOL NURSES AND *HEALTHY PEOPLE 2020*

Many *Healthy People 2020* proposed objectives are directed toward the health of children. In addition, several point directly at the care that nurses give to children in the schools. The *Healthy People* box lists the objectives that involve school-age children. These objectives are concerned with the children with disabilities in the schools, the number of children with major health problems, and the ratio of nurses to children in the schools. Nurses can accomplish the goals using the three levels of prevention, as discussed next.

THE LEVELS OF PREVENTION IN SCHOOLS

The three levels of prevention—primary, secondary, and tertiary—have always been a part of health care in the schools (Selekman, 2006). Primary prevention provides health promotion and education to prevent health problems in children. Secondary prevention includes the screening of children for various illnesses, monitoring their growth and development, and caring for them when they are ill or injured. Tertiary prevention in the schools is the continued care of children who need long-term health care services, along with education within the community (Figure 42-2).

Primary Prevention in Schools

Children need continued health services in the schools. The school nurse sees them on an almost daily basis and is the person who is usually given the role of teaching them about and promoting their health.

♥ **HEALTHY PEOPLE 2020**

Objectives Related to School Health and School Nursing

- AH-5: Increase educational achievement of adolescents and young adults.
- AH-9: (Developmental) Increase the percentage of middle and high schools that prohibit harassment based on a student's sexual orientation or gender identity.
- ECBP-2: Increase the proportion of elementary, middle, and senior high schools that provide comprehensive school health education to prevent health problems in the following areas: unintentional injury; violence; suicide; tobacco use and addiction; alcohol or other drug use; unintended pregnancy, HIV/AIDS and STD infection; unhealthy dietary patterns; and inadequate physical activity.
- ECBP-5: Increase the proportion of the nation's elementary, middle, and senior high schools that have a nurse-to-student ratio of at least 1:750.
- IID-10: Maintain vaccination coverage levels for children in kindergarten.
- IID-11: Increase routine vaccination coverage levels for adolescents.
- IVP-27: Increase the proportion of public and private schools that require students to wear appropriate protective gear when engaged in school-sponsored physical activities.
- NW-2: Increase the percentage of schools that offer nutritious foods and beverages outside of school meals.
- RD-5: Reduce the number of school days or work days missed among persons with current asthma.
- TU-15: Increase tobacco-free environments in schools, including all school facilities, property, vehicles, and school events.

From U.S. Department of Health and Human Services: *Healthy People 2020*, 2010. Available at http://www.healthypeople.gov/hp2020/Objectives/TopicAreas.aspx. Accessed September 27, 2010.

The school nurse may have the opportunity to go into the classroom to teach health promotion concepts, such as handwashing or tooth-brushing skills. He or she may spend time with the teachers, giving them the latest information on healthy

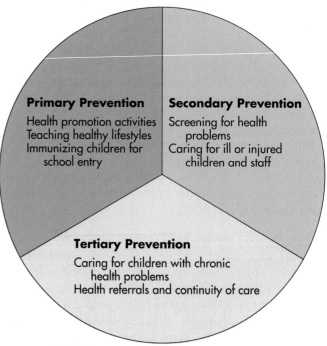

FIGURE 42-2 Levels of prevention in schools.

lifestyles for children or ways to spot a child who may be ill or in need of counseling.

HOW TO   Teach Young Children in School

When teaching children in preschools and elementary schools, keep the lesson to no more than 10 minutes. Use a lot of examples, pictures, and stuffed animals in the talk. Always remember the developmental stage of the children when teaching them.

In addition, nurses can teach healthy food choices and encourage school districts that allow vending machines to have nutritious foods instead of "junk food" available in the machines (Team Nutrition, 2010). The Food-Safe Schools (FSS) project sponsored by the American Nurses Foundation and the CDC Division of Adolescent School Health has educated many school nurses on how to promote proper food storage and preparation in the schools. The hope is to reduce the incidence of food-borne diseases in the schools (CDC, 2010b). These are examples of population-level health care for schools.

NURSING TIP   *To promote involvement of parents with the health of their children who are beginning school, some school nurses send out a questionnaire about the child's health to parents. The parents then meet with the nurse over coffee, return the questionnaire, and sign any needed health care consents. This also gives the nurse an opportunity to teach the parents about the child's health issues. This has greatly improved the communication between the nurse and the parents.*

From: Selekman J, editor: School nursing: a comprehensive text, Philadelphia, 2006, FA Davis.

School nurses use the nursing process while they care for children in the schools. In their primary prevention efforts, they assess children and families to determine their level of knowledge about health issues. Finding out whether children are at risk for preventable problems is also completed. The nurse then analyzes the assessment findings. Plans are made to develop teaching plans or health promotion activities. Once these activities are implemented, the nurse can evaluate and revise the plan.

The areas of primary prevention that the school nurse focuses on include preventing childhood injuries, preventing substance abuse behaviors, reducing the risk of the development of chronic diseases, and monitoring the immunization status of children. These primary prevention activities are completed for the population of children in the school. The activities for the population are determined by the analysis of the assessments completed on all of the children in the school to determine the most pressing priorities for the population.

Prevention of Childhood Injuries

Injuries to children and teenagers are the leading cause of death in this age group (Borse et al, 2008). The school nurse educates children, teachers, and parents about preventing injuries. Working with the national **Safe Kids Campaign,** the school nurse can

provide educational programs reminding children to use their seat belts or bicycle helmets to prevent injuries. Other classes can be on crossing the street, water safety, and fire safety. The school nurse, as the trusted person at school, is able to quickly give information to help prevent injuries from occurring, since most injuries are preventable (Hudson, 2008).

School nurses also provide health promotion to prevent playground injuries. These number over 100,000 injuries to children per year. School nurses assess school playgrounds for equipment safety on the basis of the U.S. Consumer Product Safety Commission guidelines (Hudson, 2008). School sports also have the potential to cause injuries to children, and the school nurse is usually involved in deciding with parents and coaches on how to best prevent injuries on the sports field (Kennedy, 2009).

School nurses also promote skateboard and scooter safety by providing health educational workshops to children and their families. Scooter and skateboard injuries are increasing (AAP, 2009).

The nurse on a community-wide scale can implement these programs. Research has shown that once behaviors of children related to safety are taught, their effects spread quickly throughout the community. This makes the entire community safer (Selekman, 2006).

Substance Abuse Prevention Education

Primary prevention interventions by the school nurse include educating children and adolescents about the effects of drugs and alcohol on their bodies. Preventing use of and "saying no" to drugs have been part of the school health program for many years. Teenagers are taught by the school nurse to stay away from drugs (such as marijuana, cocaine, crack, heroin) and alcohol.

There has been an increase in the use of "club drugs" such as lysergic acid (LSD), ketamine, gamma hydroxybutyrate (GHB), Rohypnol, and Ecstasy (MDMA). The school nurse can provide instruction about the serious side effects of Ecstasy, especially that it causes a very high body temperature that can lead to death. Teaching the teenagers about the dangers of all drugs is the responsibility of the school nurse. In addition, the school nurse can teach parents and other members of the community about the latest drug fads, increasing everyone's awareness of these dangerous trends (Buckley and White, 2007).

Disease Prevention Education

The nurse has the opportunity to teach children healthy lifestyles to reduce their risk of disease later in life. For example, children can be taught ways to reduce their risk from becoming obese by teaching and reinforcing healthy nutrition and exercise (Gorely et al, 2009). The school nurse can then reinforce the teachers' educational plans or develop the program further for other age groups to teach them how to take care of their heart.

Dissemination of health promotion information to the parents of the children is often a challenge for the school nurse. In Newark, Delaware, the school nurse at one of the elementary schools has a "School Nurse's Corner" webpage (Laudorn, 2010). On this page, the nurse shares important health information related to school-age children, such as immunization requirements and childhood obesity. In this way, the school nurse is able to promote the health of not only the schoolchildren, but also the community.

Vaccinations for Schoolchildren

All states have laws that require that children receive immunizations, or vaccinations, against communicable diseases before they attend school (CDC, 2010c). School nurses must be up to date on the latest laws on immunizations for children in their own state. For children entering kindergarten, these vaccinations include diphtheria, pertussis, and tetanus (the DTaP series); measles, mumps, and rubella (the MMR series); polio; and others. Table 42-3 lists the mandated immunizations for school entry for each state. Chapter 14 has a more complete discussion of communicable diseases and immunizations in children.

The school nurse must keep a complete file of all of the children's vaccination records in order to meet the state's laws. These files will contain the student's name, date of birth, address and telephone number, parents'/guardians' names, and contact information. It will also include the student's primary health care provider's name, telephone number, and address. Most important, the information should include all the vaccinations with the dates the child received booster shots. This makes it easy for the school nurse to find out which children still need immunizations or boosters.

The **Health Insurance Portability and Accountability Act of 1996 (HIPAA)** requires that all health information be private. However, there is conflicting information whether the immunization status of children is covered by the law. Whereas some believe that school clinics and school nurses are allowed to have that information without permission because they are considered to be public health officials, others state that this only applies to sharing medical information (EOHHS, 2010).

Because children are prevented from attending school if they have not had the required immunizations, the school nurse must make every effort to find missing data in the immunization record. The nurse will need to contact the parents to get the immunization history for the child. Written notes will need

---

TABLE 42-3 REQUIRED IMMUNIZATIONS FOR SCHOOL ENTRY: ELEMENTARY, JUNIOR, AND HIGH SCHOOLS COMBINED

IMMUNIZATION	STATES REQUIRING IMMUNIZATION	IMMUNIZATION	STATES REQUIRING IMMUNIZATION
Diphtheria	All 50 states	Hepatitis B—cont'd	District of Columbia
Tetanus	All states except New York		Florida
Polio	All 50 states		Georgia
Measles	All states except North Carolina		Hawaii
Chickenpox	Alabama		Idaho
	Alaska		Indiana
	Arkansas		Iowa
	California		Kentucky
	Colorado		Louisiana
	Connecticut		Maryland
	District of Columbia		Massachusetts
	Florida		Michigan
	Georgia		Minnesota
	Louisiana		Mississippi
	Maryland		Missouri
	Massachusetts		Nebraska
	Michigan		Nevada
	Mississippi		New Hampshire
	New York		New York
	North Carolina		North Dakota
	Oklahoma		Ohio
	Rhode Island		Oklahoma
	South Dakota		Pennsylvania
	Virginia		Rhode Island
Hepatitis B	Alaska		South Carolina
	Arizona		Texas
	Arkansas		Utah
	California		Virginia
	Colorado		Washington
	Connecticut		Wisconsin
	Delaware		Wyoming

From Centers for Disease Control and Prevention: *State level school health policies and practices: a state-by-state summary from the School Health Policies and Programs Study 2006,* Atlanta, 2006, CDC, USDHHS.

to be sent to each child's home at least one year before each new immunization is needed so that the parents have time to get the child to his or her health care provider for the shots. If the parents or guardians do not speak English, these notes will need to be translated into the family's language. If the parents have lost the information that gives the child's immunization history, they should be encouraged to contact their physician or nurse practitioner to get it.

Many problems with children not being immunized or having incomplete vaccination records may arise in families who have moved a great deal or who may not have a regular physician. The parents may have no idea whether the child has even received the shots. Families may also be without health care insurance to pay for the immunizations, or they may have insurance that does not pay for preventive care. In these cases, the parents have to pay for the immunizations, which can be expensive. Certain low-income families without health care insurance may qualify for federal programs that provide free immunizations to children. Each state has its own program, so school nurses will want to become familiar with what their state provides.

Some parents may request that their child be exempted from the required immunizations because of their belief that not all immunizations are good for their children, for medical reasons, or for religious or philosophical reasons. The school nurse will want to be aware of the laws in the state regarding acceptable reasons for immunization exemption. At the same time, the nurse has the opportunity to teach parents and the rest of the community about the overall benefits to society from the use of immunizations.

School nurses can also play an important role in immunizing children against seasonal flu. Up to 42% of school-age children have seasonal influenza each year (AAP, 2008b). Vaccination against influenza should begin as soon as that season's vaccine becomes available (Li and Freedman, 2009). During the 2009 H1N1 influenza outbreak, school nurses were at the front line of the epidemic. In fact, it was a school nurse in Queens, New York, who first notified the CDC that the influenza epidemic had reached U.S. soil (Robert Wood Johnson Foundation, 2010). School nurses were challenged to reduce the spread of the epidemic among school-age children.

Secondary Prevention in Schools

Because secondary prevention involves caring for children when they need health care, this is the largest responsibility for the school nurse. This includes caring for ill or injured students and school employees. It also involves screening and assessing children, and referral to appropriate health agencies or providers. The school nurse uses the nursing process during secondary prevention activities. When an ill or injured child comes to the school's health office, the nurse must immediately assess the child for the degree of illness or injury.

DID YOU KNOW?   *The health records of children in schools are to be kept private, just as they are in hospitals and other health agencies.*

Children seek out the school nurse for a variety of different needs:

- Headaches
- Stomachaches
- Diarrhea
- Anxiety over being separated from the parents
- Cuts, bruises, or other injuries

In addition, children may seek reassurance from the school nurse or even appear to hide in the nurse's office. This may be a result of harassment or bullying from other children in the school (Frisen and Bjarnelind, 2010).

Once the assessment data are gathered, the nurse determines the course of action and follows it through the implementation and evaluation phases. This occurs for direct child health care as well as for screening children for other health problems. If assessment data identify a child as having a health problem, the school nurse continues to follow the nursing process to further care for that child.

Nursing Care for Emergencies in the School

The school nurse cares for children who are injured or become ill in the schools. The school nurse must have an **emergency plan** in place so that a routine can be followed when emergencies occur. This plan includes making an assessment of the emergency and surveying the scene, treating the injured or ill children or teachers, and calling for back-up help from the community's emergency medical units if needed.

The AAP and the American Health Association (AHA) have recommended that plans be developed in the schools in case of an emergency when a child or staff member needs immediate care. The school nurse develops this plan so that a staff member in the school, such as the principal or an athletic coach, can follow it in case the nurse is not in the building at the time of the emergency. The following recommendations are based on both the AAP's and the AHA's guidelines (AAP, 2008c):

- The plan addresses when to call 911 for local emergency personnel. It includes how to make arrangements to transfer a child to the hospital via ambulance in case more care is needed. If the nurse is not in the school at all times, at least two different staff members are listed who are responsible for determining if emergency care is needed. These persons will be educated by the school nurse on proper first-aid techniques so that correct care is given until further help arrives.
- All staff in the schools must be taught standard precautions. These policies are written into the emergency plan. Members of the athletic staff such as coaches and physical education teachers need to be up to date on emergency health procedures. If they are not, the school nurse will teach them about the policies and provide a means to review first-aid procedures with them on a regular basis.
- Individualized emergency plans are made for all students who may have a health problem that could result in an emergency situation in the school. This plan could be for the child with food allergies (e.g., to peanuts), one who has sensitivity to insect bites that could result in

anaphylactic shock, or those with chronic illnesses such as asthma, diabetes, or hemophilia.

- The children in the schools can be taught by the nurse basic first-aid procedures, including standard precautions related to blood exposure. This lesson, depending on the age and grade level of the children, would allow the children to help in a playground accident while the adults are being summoned to the scene.

The nurse may not always be at the school and the emergency may have to be handled by a teacher, administrator, secretary, custodian, or coach. This issue is especially applicable to school nurses in rural settings, who may have several schools for which they are responsible when such schools may be far apart. Therefore, all emergency procedures are written and easily accessible to anyone in the school. Along with the procedures and an emergency manual written or obtained by the school nurse, an injury or illness log is available for personnel to fill out so that there is an accurate record of what happened. Along with this form, procedures for notifying the parents or legal guardians about the emergency are spelled out and include what was done for the child, and where the child was sent if transfer to a hospital or other medical agency was required.

Because the school nurse may have to give nursing care to a child or adult in respiratory or cardiac arrest, the nurse must have current certification in cardiopulmonary resuscitation (CPR) and the use of the automated external defibrillator (AED), which should be available to all school nurses per the American Hospital Association (AAP, 2008b). Other education in the area of emergency nursing would also be helpful to the school nurse, including pediatric advanced life support (PALS) or emergency nursing for pediatrics (ENPC) certification (USDE, 2010).

Emergency Equipment in the School Nurse's Office

The school nurse needs a great deal of equipment to deal with emergencies in the school. These needs are based on the guidelines of the AAP (AAP, 2008c). The health office will need to have basic emergency items on hand (Box 42-3). Necessary equipment includes full oxygen tanks with oxygen masks of different kinds (bag-valve masks, resuscitation masks), splints for sprained or broken limbs, cervical spine collars to keep a child's head in proper alignment, and sterile dressings. Various sizes of these items are needed since children may be of different ages

in the school. Another recommended item for the nurse's office includes an epinephrine auto injector kit (EpiPen auto injector) in case a child goes into anaphylactic shock after exposure to an allergen (AAP, 2008c). This should be locked in a medication cabinet because of the needle in the kit. The school nurse will need to teach other school personnel how to use the EpiPen auto injector in an emergency (Kruger et al, 2009).

Gloves to meet standard precautions guidelines and a telephone available for calling emergency personnel and parents are essential. Next to the telephone, paper and pen should be available so that instructions from the emergency personnel can be written down. The AED should be located in a central location at the school for easy access in an emergency. It should not be locked in the nurse's office but available for school staff to obtain in case the nurse is off site that day.

Giving Medication in School

The school nurse, as part of secondary prevention, may be responsible for giving medications to children during the school day (AAP, 2008a). These may include prescribed medications, medications that the parents have asked the school's nurse to give (such as cold remedies), or vitamins. In all instances, the nurse will want to develop a series of guidelines to help with the legal administration of medications in the school. The school nurse will inquire of parents if the child is taking any medications (AAP, 2008b). HIPAA requires that all of this information be confidential (Nic Philibin et al, 2010).

The prescribed drug must have the original prescription label on it and be in the original container so that there are no errors. In addition, the AAP (2008a) recommended that the physician inform the school nurse about possible side effects of the medication that may occur during the school day. If the physician does not contact the nurse first, the nurse will call the physician and ask. A current, signed parental consent form for giving the medication is essential for the student's file (AAP, 2008a).

A current drug reference in the nurse's office is necessary so that it can be consulted for information. The nurse is responsible for giving the medication and is expected by state law to know its action, side effects, and implications. The school nurse must have a means of contacting a pharmacist to ask questions regarding the medication if needed.

Assessing and Screening Children at School

The AAP's Committee on School Health (AAP, 2006) has developed guidelines for the school nurse to use when screening children in the schools. The plans are for the state-required screening of children as well as for more complete health examinations for children in the school.

Children should receive screening for vision, hearing, height and weight, oral health, tuberculosis, and scoliosis in the schools (CDC, 2006). For each of these areas, the school nurse will keep a confidential record of all of the screening results for the children in the school according to the HIPAA rules. In addition, each state has different laws regarding the screenings and the nurse will need to be aware of these laws.

In addition, some children may not have a regular physician or other primary health care provider such as a nurse

---

BOX 42-3   EMERGENCY ITEMS FOR THE SCHOOL NURSE

- Gloves
- Oxygen and oxygen masks
- Suction machine
- Sterile dressings
- Splints
- Bed or cot
- Locked medication cabinet
- Epinephrine auto injector kit
- Automated external defibrillator (AED) (placed in a central location away from the nurse's office)

practitioner to give them health care. For these children, the AAP (2006) has recommended that children have a physical and developmental examination in the school setting. This would include obtaining information on their language skills and their motor abilities. Their social abilities and their height and weight are also tested. As the children grow up, their level of physical growth can be noted as well as their sexual maturation. Dental assessments are also to be made. Some states are passing laws requiring these assessments and giving nurses the right to complete the assessment and refer to a dentist.

Physical examinations to participate in a school sport are also given in the school. The school nurse would arrange for the sports physicals and help to monitor the examinations being done by the school's physician or nurse practitioner.

Screening for tuberculosis (TB) in schoolchildren is also done in several states. This can be a problem since child has to have the Mantoux test or the TST test given to them first. Then they have to return to have the test site read by the nurse. If the site is positive, the child has been exposed to TB and needs further health screening. One study showed that it was more efficient to have the children screened for TB at a health clinic and then have the school nurse read the test and send that information to the health clinic for follow-up (Winje et al, 2008).

The school nurse can also screen children and adolescents for hypertension, or high blood pressure. One study found that 21.6% of students screened in grades K-12 in a rural area had an elevated blood pressure, with higher prevalence among the older students (King et al, 2006). These findings indicate the importance of the school nurse in providing effective prevention strategies related to screening, follow-up, and treatment.

Screening Children for Pediculosis (Lice)

School nurses must screen children for lice infestation. Prevalence of head lice in U.S. schools ranges from 10% to 40%, being found most commonly in school-aged children, typically in late summer and autumn (Wolfram, 2010). Lice are found most often in white middle-class children because of their oval hair shafts. Lice are more often seen in clean hair as well. Therefore, the suggestion that lice are associated with unclean homes in poverty areas is incorrect (Wolfram, 2010). The school nurse needs to check children for lice because in many areas, children with lice are excluded from school. During the "lice check," the nurse must check the children's hair for both lice and nits (HeadLice.org, 2010).

It is the responsibility of the school nurse to teach children, parents, and teachers how to prevent lice and treat cases of infestation. The nurse can do this by teaching children not to share combs and hats, and teaching parents to completely treat the child with anti-lice medications. Parents also need to be told to remove all nits from the head with a fine-toothed comb and to wash all bed linens and clothing (HeadLice.org, 2010).

Identification of Child Abuse or Neglect

The school nurse is mandated by state laws to report suspected cases of child abuse or neglect. These laws differ from state to state and the nurse must be aware of the particular requirements for reporting in his or her state.

When the nurse identifies a child who may be abused, or receives information from a teacher or other staff member that leads to the belief that a child has been abused, the nurse must contact the appropriate legal authorities as well as the school's principal. A confidential file should be made about the incident. However, the nurse contacts the government authorities, usually the state or county child protection department, who look into the suspected case. In all cases, the child must be protected from harm, and those who have no right to know that child abuse or neglect is suspected should not be given any information.

Communicating with Health Care Providers

The school nurse often makes an assessment of a child that requires referral to the child's family physician or other health care provider. The findings from these assessments must be communicated accurately to the child's parent and the provider. The nurse must be able to disseminate the information quickly and accurately to the child's parents. Again, HIPAA privacy rules must be followed (Nic Philibin et al, 2010).

HOW TO   Develop Good Relationships with Families

School nurses need to have good relationships with families. The nurse can make this possible by doing the following:

1. *Being visible at school events.*
2. *Sending home invitations for parents and guardians to call the nurse at any time.*
3. *Inviting parents to visit the school health office.*
4. *Calling parents or guardians to ask about ill children.*
5. *Offering to help families cope with children who have long-term illnesses.*
6. *Acting as a referral source for families with health care needs.*
7. *Including parents and members of the community in health education activities.*

One way to do this is to write a detailed report about the findings. This information can be given to the child to give to his or her parents. However, the child may lose the report on the way home. The information can be mailed to the parents, but this takes more time. Perhaps the best way is to telephone the parents, telling them that the child needs to see the physician or nurse practitioner and that the child will be bringing the information home that day. In this way, the parents can ask the child for the report and the child is aware that the parents expect it.

Efforts to Prevent Suicide and Other Mental Health Problems

Suicide is the third-leading cause of death in teenagers. Recommendations have been made about reducing the incidence of suicide in teenagers. A suicide prevention program developed in one school district (see later discussion) contains ideas for the school nurse to use. Suicide prevention must be addressed by school nurses. Nurses can lead educational programs within the schools to emphasize coping strategies and stress management techniques for children and adolescents who have problems, and to teach about the risk factors. The school nurse can teach faculty members to look for the risk factors. The school nurse can also help organize a peer assistance program to help teenagers cope with school stresses (Molock et al, 2007).

If a student threatens suicide at school, the school nurse can intervene by ensuring the safety of the student and by removing him or her from the school situation immediately. While parents are being notified, the nurse is able to assess the child's suicide risk and refer the child or teenager to crisis intervention or mental health services.

In the unfortunate instance in which a teenager who attended the school has committed suicide, the school nurse is called upon to help the school population, both students and teachers, cope with the death. Grief counseling is set up and coordinated by the school nurse. In addition, further assessments can be made regarding the suicide potential among the deceased teenager's friends, since suicide clusters have been noted.

Other mental health problems may affect students. Adolescents may have early signs of mental or emotional problems such as behavior problems in class or severe class or test anxiety. Families may be in crisis, and this translates into problems for the children.

Children who are homeless have special problems. Because these children do not have a stable address, this also means that they probably have frequently moved from school to school. Children whose parents are addicted to drugs or alcohol can also benefit from support from the school nurse. This lack of a stable environment may increase chances that they may develop a mental or emotional problem. The school nurse can be an advocate for these children and their families.

Violence at School

In 2009, in the previous 30 days prior to the survey, approximately 5.6% of high school students carried a weapon on school property and 5% of high school students missed at least one day of school because they felt unsafe (CDC, YRBS, 2010). Approximately 38% of public schools reported at least one incident of violence to police during the 2005-2006 school year (CDC, 2010d). In 2007, 23% of students reported gangs at their schools (CDC, 2010d). In 2006, there were 29 violent crimes (including rape, sexual and aggravated assault, and robbery) at school per 1000 students (CDC, 2010d). In 2007, about 32% of students reported being bullied during the school year and about 4% of students reported being cyber-bullied in 2007 (CDC, 2010d).

In the past several years, there have been school shootings by students or other attackers against other students and teachers. The school nurse may be able to help identify students who will act in this way. Furthermore, the nurse can provide health education classes to help children learn positive ways of dealing with conflict.

The mother of a murdered girl in Paducah, Kentucky, herself a registered nurse, stated that there are six characteristics that may help point out a student who may be thinking about such drastic violence (Steger, 2000):

- *Venting:* having mood swings
- *Vocalizing:* threatening others
- *Vandalizing:* damaging property
- *Victimizing:* seeing themself as a victim
- *Vying:* belonging to gangs
- *Viewing:* witnessing the abuse of others

By helping to identify the student who might be considering school violence or by teaching students and teachers about these warning signs in students, the school nurse may be able to help prevent violent actions through education and follow-up of children who need help. The U.S. federal government has many agencies that can be used as resources to help school nurses develop programs in their schools (CDC, 2010d).

School Crisis Teams: Responding to Disasters

Events that occur in or near schools may cause a crisis for children, teachers, and staff. Possible crises include the death of a student or teacher from accident, injury, homicide, or suicide; an accident or fire in the school or community; a terrorist attack; or a disaster in the community that affects many children's families, such as a tornado, hurricane, or earthquake (Lerner, Lindell, and Volpe, 2010).

The U.S. Department of Education recommends that all schools have crisis plans in place to help the children, teachers, parents, and community cope with the sudden event. **Crisis teams** are prepared to help everyone respond quickly to the crisis, to ensure the safety of the school, and to follow up on the effects of the crisis on the members of the school (Lerner, Lindell, and Volpe, 2010).

The crisis plan includes an administrative policy made either for the entire school district or, if the schools are large, for each individual school. The plan includes the names of the persons on the crisis team: the superintendent of the school district, the school nurse, the guidance counselor, the school psychologist or social worker, teachers, police or school security, clergy from the community, and parents. Plans to obtain and share information can be made quickly (Lerner, Lindell, and Volpe, 2010).

The school nurse as a first responder to the scene (NASN, 2005) is involved with triaging injured people, working with the emergency medical personnel as they care for the injured or ill, and assessing the degree of shock, stress, or grieving in the children, teachers, parents, and others in or near the school. The school nurse is also there to be a counselor to help everyone cope with the emotional aspects of this serious event (NASN, 2005) (Box 42-4).

The nurse can help the crisis team make a checklist for everyone to follow that explains what to do in every possible crisis situation. Then, at the end of the crisis, the crisis team will want to take time to counsel all of the people who helped in the crisis, including the teachers, emergency personnel, and parents, as well as the children. That way everyone can talk about the crisis. The crisis plan should be reviewed every year to see what parts of the plan need updating. Drills take place to act out the plan to see how it works and how it can be revised to make it more workable (Lerner, Lindell, and Volpe, 2010).

Tertiary Prevention in Schools

Using the nursing process, the school nurse gives nursing care related to tertiary prevention when working with children who have long-term or chronic illnesses or special needs. As

BOX 42-4   DEALING WITH A DISASTER: RESPONSIBILITIES OF THE SCHOOL NURSE

- Provide triage.
- Communicate with emergency medical personnel.
- Assess the school community for the presence of shock and stress.
- Recommend reduced television viewing of the disaster.
- Provide grief counseling.
- Communicate with the children, parents, and school personnel.
- Follow up with assessment of children for anxiety, depression, regression, and post-traumatic stress disorder.

Modified from Lerner MD, Lindell B, Volpe J: *A practical guide for crisis response in our schools*, 2010, American Academy of Experts in Traumatic Stress. Available at http://store.nc-cm.org/servlet/Detail ?no=1. Accessed March 19, 2011.

BOX 42-5   STATES THAT REQUIRE SCHOOL NURSES TO PARTICIPATE IN INDIVIDUALIZED EDUCATION PLANS FOR STUDENTS

• Alabama	• New Jersey
• Arizona	• New Mexico
• Colorado	• New York
• Delaware	• North Carolina
• District of Columbia	• Oklahoma
• Hawaii	• Rhode Island
• Illinois	• South Carolina
• Indiana	• Tennessee
• Iowa	• Texas
• Louisiana	• Utah
• Maryland	• Vermont
• Massachusetts	• Virginia
• Minnesota	• Washington
• Mississippi	• West Virginia
• Nevada	• Wisconsin

Compiled from Centers for Disease Control and Prevention: *State level school health policies and practices: a state-by-state summary from the School Health Policies and Programs Study 2006,* Atlanta, 2006, CDC, USDHHS.

prevalence for chronic conditions such as asthma and diabetes increases among children, today's school nurse faces a school population that is more medically diverse than ever seen in the past (Robert Wood Johnson Foundation, 2010). The nurse participates in developing an individual education plan (IEP) for students with long-term health needs (Box 42-5).

For example, nurses must have information about children's medications to be administered during school hours. They also need to know if the children need any therapy during the school day, such as physical or occupational therapy. If the child has a hearing or vision problem, the nurse may need to ask the teacher to seat the child in the best place in the classroom so the child can see or hear better. If a child is in a wheelchair or uses crutches, the school building itself may need to be altered so that the child can get around the school and use the restrooms. It is the responsibility of the nurse to tell the school's administrators about any needs such as these (AAP, 2008c).

DID YOU KNOW?   *Children with disabilities who live in residential care facilities because of their long-term health needs go to school every day.*

Children with Asthma

Asthma is the leading cause of children being absent from school because of a chronic illness (CDC, 2009a). Children may be hospitalized with an asthma attack or they may have just returned home from the hospital. Asthma can also be caused by allergic triggers that affect children in the school. Possible culprits are chalk dust from the blackboards, molds or mildew in the school, or dander from pets that live in some classrooms (CDC, 2009a).

There may also be concerns about the quality of the air in the school building because many doors are shut. Industrial arts' classes and other sources of air pollution can occur in the school (U.S. EPA, 2010). The school nurse can keep track of the indoor air quality of the school so that school administrators have data about what can affect the children. Figure 42-3 contains

the questions developed by the U.S. Environmental Protection Agency that the school nurse should answer regarding the air quality of the school.

The nurse uses tertiary prevention when helping children who have asthma. This includes administering, or helping them use, their inhalers or other asthma rescue medications (AAP, 2008c). It also includes instructing the teachers, children, and parents about asthma and ways to reduce allergens in the classroom (AAP, 2008c). Schools have management programs in place to help children with asthma (AAP, 2008c).

Children with Diabetes Mellitus

Diabetes is one of the most common chronic diseases in children and adolescents; about 151,000 people below the age of 20 years have diabetes (CDC, 2010e). Every year, more than 13,000 children and adolescents are diagnosed with type 1 diabetes (CDC, 2010e). In the last couple of decades, type 2 diabetes (formerly known as adult-onset diabetes) has been reported among U.S. children and adolescents with increasing frequency (CDC, 2010e). The school nurse must establish a plan of care for children with diabetes. This includes methods of monitoring blood glucose levels and administering insulin or other medications during the school day. Special nutritional needs also need to be discussed (NASN, 2006).

Children Who Are Autistic or Who Have Attention-Deficit/Hyperactivity Disorder

Because all children are expected to attend some school regardless of their illness, children with autism go to regular schools in most cases. Because a child with autism has severe communication problems, the school nurse provides help for the child, the teachers, and the parents so that the child's school day is pleasant. The nurse can give the child prescribed medications for

Health Officer/School Nurse

This checklist discusses three major topic areas:
Student Health Records Maintenance
Public Health and Personal Hygiene Education
Health Officer's Office

Instructions:
1. Read the IAQ *Backgrounder*.
2. Read each item on this Checklist.
3. Check the diamond(s) as appropriate or check the circle if you need additional help with an activity.
4. Return this checklist to the IAQ Coordinator and keep a copy for future reference.

Name: _____

Room or Area: _____

School: _____

Date Completed: _____

Signature: _____

MAINTAIN STUDENT HEALTH RECORDS

There is evidence to suggest that children, pregnant women, and senior citizens are more likely to develop health problems from poor air quality than most adults. Indoor Air Quality (IAQ) problems are most likely to affect those with preexisting health conditions and those who are exposed to tobacco smoke. Student health records should include information about known allergies and other medically documented conditions, such as asthma, as well as any reported sensitivity to chemicals. Privacy considerations may limit the student health information that can be disclosed, but to the extent possible, information about students' potential sensitivity to IAQ problems should be provided to teachers. This is especially true for classes involving potential irritants (e.g., gaseous or particle emissions from art, science, industrial/vocational education sources). Health records and records of health-related complaints by students and staff are useful for evaluating potential IAQ-related complaints.

Include information about sensitivities to IAQ problems in student health records
• Allergies, including reports of chemical sensitivities.
• Asthma.
◇ Completed health records exist for each student.
◇ Health records are being updated.
○ Need help obtaining information about student allergies and other health factors.

Track health-related complaints by students and staff
• Keep a log of health complaints that notes the symptoms, location and time of symptom onset, and exposure to pollutant sources.
• Watch for trends in health complaints, especially in timing or location of complaints.
◇ Have a comprehensive health complaint logging system.
◇ Developing a comprehensive health complaint logging system.
○ Need help developing a comprehensive health complaint logging system.

Recognize indicators that health problems may be IAQ
• Complaints are associated with particular times of the day or week.
• Other occupants in the same area experience similar problems.

• The problem abates or ceases, either immediately or gradually, when an occupant leaves the building and recurs when the occupant returns.
• The school has recently been renovated or refurnished.
• The occupant has recently started working with new or different materials or equipment.
• New cleaning or pesticide products or practices have been introduced into the school.
• Smoking is allowed in the school.
• A new warm-blooded animal has been introduced into the classroom.
◇ Understand indicators of IAQ-related problems.
○ Need help understanding indicators of IAQ-related problems.

HEALTH AND HYGIENE EDUCATION

Schools are unique buildings from a public health perspective because they accommodate more people within a smaller area than most buildings. This proximity increases the potential for airborne contaminants (germs, odors, and constituents of personal products) to pass between students. Raising awareness about the effects of personal habits on the well-being of others can help reduce IAQ-related problems.

Obtain *Indoor Air Quality: An Introduction for Health Professionals*
• Contact IAQ INFO, 800-438-4318.
◇ Already have this EPA guidance document.
◇ Guide is on order.
○ Cannot obtain this guide.

Inform students and staff about the importance of good hygiene in preventing the spread of airborne contagious diseases
• Provide written materials to students (local public health agencies may have information suitable for older students).
• Provide individual instruction/counseling where necessary.
◇ Written materials and counseling available.
◇ Compiling information for counseling and distribution.
○ Need help compiling information or implementing counseling program.

FIGURE 42-3 Indoor air quality checklist. (From U.S. Environmental Protection Agency: *School and child care-based asthma education programs,* 2010. Available from http://www.epa.gov/asthma/school-based.html.)

Provide information about IAQ and health
- Help teachers develop activities that reduce exposure to indoor air pollutants for students with IAQ sensitivities, such as those with asthma or allergies (contact the American Lung Association [ALA], the National Association of School Nurses [NASN], or the Asthma and Allergy Foundation of America [AAFA]). Contact information is also available in the IAQ Coordinator's Guide.
- Collaborate with parent-teacher groups to offer family IAQ education programs.
- Conduct a workshop for teachers on health issues that covers IAQ.
◇ Have provided information to parents and staff.
◇ Developing information and education programs for parents and staff.
○ Need help developing information and education program for parents and staff.

Establish an information and counseling program regarding smoking
- Provide free literature on smoking and secondhand smoke.
- Sponsor a quit-smoking program and similar counseling programs in collaboration with the ALA.
◇ "No Smoking" information and programs in place.
◇ "No Smoking" information and programs in planning.
○ Need help with a "No Smoking" program.

HEALTH OFFICER'S OFFICE

Since the health office may be frequented by sick students and staff, it is important to take steps that can help prevent transmission of airborne diseases to uninfected students and staff (see your IAQ Coordinator for help with the following activities).

Ensure that the ventilation system is properly operating
- Ventilation system is operated when the area(s) is occupied.
- Provide an adequate amount of outdoor air to the area(s). There should be at least 15 cubic feet of outdoor air supplied per occupant.
- Air filters are clean and properly installed.
- Air removed from the area(s) does not circulate through the ventilation system into other occupied areas.
◇ Ventilation system operating adequately.
○ Need help with ventilation-related activities.

☐ **No Problems to Report.** I have completed all the activities on this checklist, and I do not need help in any areas.

FIGURE 42-3, cont'd Indoor air quality checklist.

mood or prevention of seizures. The nurse is also responsible for preparing the teachers about the communication problems that the child may have. The nurse may recommend the use of sign language, picture boards, or other types of communication devices that are used by the child. In addition, the nurse can teach the parents about autism. The nurse can also help parents work with others in the health care system so that the child can have a positive learning experience at school (Bellando and Lopez, 2009).

WHAT DO YOU THINK? *Children with mental disabilities attend school. How would this affect other children in the classroom?*

Children with attention-deficit/hyperactivity disorder (ADHD) also attend school. As of 2006, 4.5 million children between 5 and 17 years of age have been diagnosed with ADHD (CDC, 2010f). The school nurse can help these children learn appropriate behaviors to reduce classroom disruptions (Dang et al, 2007).

Children with Special Needs in the Schools

Children who need urinary catheterization, dressing changes, peripheral or central line intravenous catheter maintenance, tracheotomy suctioning, gastrostomy or other tube feedings, or intravenous medication also attend schools. The nurse may supervise a health aide who is assigned to the child to care for complex nursing needs. In all these cases, the school nurse provides tertiary care to maintain the child's health. The nurse has the skills needed to assess the child's well-being. In addition, the nurse may have to teach another person in the school how to care for the child in case the nurse is not in the building when

the child needs help. It is the responsibility of the school nurse to keep up with the latest health care information through in-service programs (AAP, 2008c).

HOW TO **Help Injured Children Return to School After Long Absences**

This article discussed how a school nurse helped a sixth-grade boy who had received serious facial burns return to school. Enrique was afraid of how the children would respond to the pressure mask he wore to minimize future scarring. The nurse had a meeting with Enrique's mother and the school's principal and also contacted nurses from the hospital's burn unit. The school nurse developed the following plan:

1. *The school nurse taught the boy's classmates about burns and their treatment.*
2. *The boy came to class with the nurse and showed his classmates his face without this pressure mask. He then put the mask back on.*
3. *Both Enrique and the nurse answered the children's questions.*
4. *Changes were made in his schedule so he could be out of the sun during the school day and during gym time.*

The nurse found that Enrique's burns were soon forgotten and he was accepted by his friends.

From Kaffenberge CJ: School reentry for students with a chronic illness: a role for professional school counselors, Prof School Counsel 9(3):223-230, 2006.

Children with HIV or AIDS may also attend school. Because of privacy and confidentiality laws, the school nurse may not even know that the child attends the school. In these cases, the nurse may be aware of the child's HIV status either by direct notification from the parents or physician or just by knowing that certain drugs the child is prescribed during the school day are anti-HIV medications. In all cases, the nurse must maintain confidentiality. This means that information cannot be released to anyone, including teachers, other health professionals, other students, or staff as an example.

As part of regular health education in the school, the school nurse can provide education about HIV/AIDS prevention and risks to the children, school employees, and community. The school nurse should also be part of the school health advisory committee to develop an HIV/AIDS health curriculum that teaches not only about HIV/AIDS prevention, but also about the disease itself, so that children and families are not afraid to go to school with children who have the disease.

Children with DNR Orders and the School Nurse

As part of tertiary prevention, the school nurse also maintains the health of children with terminal diseases who go to school. These children have been largely mainstreamed into the regular school population. The PL 94-142 Education for All Handicapped Children Act stated in 1975 that all children should go to school in the "least restrictive environment" (AAP, 2010). Therefore, there may be children who have do-not-resuscitate orders (DNR orders) at school, and some may die at school. DNR orders are signed by the parents and the physician according to the state's law. Under law, the school nurse is bound to obey the DNR order; however, it is not clear how the schools view them.

The AAP's committees on school health and bioethics reaffirmed a set of guidelines to help school health providers and the schools decide what to do when a child with a DNR order attends the school (Hone-Warren, 2007; AAP, 2010). A formal request to the school and the school board from the physician is a must regarding the written DNR order. The school nurses should be involved in discussions regarding when to use the DNR order. The decision not to do anything for a dying child, and how to function if the child were to suddenly face death, is made in advance of discussions between the school nurse, the parents, the physician, and the school officials.

When a child dies in school, the nurse is responsible for helping the children who witnessed the death. The nurse becomes a grief counselor and helps the children and teachers cope with the death. Further education about death and dying given by the school nurse would also help the school community cope with death in the schools.

Homebound Children

Even though the laws regarding disabled persons state that all children should go to school, some children cannot. Instead, they may be taught in the home or in another institutional setting such as the hospital. In these situations, the school nurse can be a liaison between the child's teacher, physician, school administrators, and parents regarding the child's needs. The nurse helps these individuals develop the child's IEP so that it is appropriate for the child and does not remove necessary learning from the plan. The child should be allowed to go to school when he or she is able, at which point the school nurse

coordinates the child's health care needs and classes (Kaffenberge, 2006).

Pregnant Teenagers and Teenage Mothers at School

Many teenage girls who are pregnant attend school. Therefore, the school nurse may provide ongoing care to the mother (Norris et al, 2009). Although this may appear to be primary prevention, it is tertiary prevention because adolescent pregnancies are considered to be high risk. This is discussed in more detail in Chapters 29 and 35.

CONTROVERSIES IN SCHOOL NURSING

School nursing has evolved into a complex health care role, and some areas of the field still cause controversy, such as birth control education and giving out birth control to students in the schools. A study carried out in South Carolina regarding whether school-based health clinics should provide contraception services found that the community wanted gynecological health care available to the adolescents. However, it was not to be given at the school-based center. The community agreed that abstinence sex education could be provided in the schools, but they wanted all other services to be referred by the nurses to community agencies (Bleakley, Hennessy, and Fishbein, 2006).

Differences in opinion exist relating to sex education, reproductive services, and screening for sexually transmitted diseases in the schools (Bleakley, Hennessy, and Fishbein, 2006). The school nurse should make an effort to communicate with the community, school board, teachers, parents, and students about what they think about different types of services in the schools.

ETHICS IN SCHOOL NURSING

The school nurse may be faced with ethical issues in the schools. For example, a child may have a DNR order that the parents wish to be used if the child dies at school (see earlier text), but following the DNR order may be against the nurse's personal beliefs. Perhaps a girl asks the nurse where she can get an abortion and wishes to talk to the school nurse about how she feels, but the nurse is against abortions. Alternatively, a teenager asks for emergency contraception, which the nurse cannot condone. In these cases, the nurse must give nursing care to the student client and keep personal beliefs out of the discussion. However, if the nurse feels so strongly that he or she cannot work with the situation, another school nurse should be called for help, or the student should be referred to other health providers who can give the care the student needs. Care should never be denied or ignored; referral is a good option.

FUTURE TRENDS IN SCHOOL NURSING

The future of school nursing is strong. The amount of health care being given in the schools is increasing. In the future, school nursing will entail telehealth and telecounseling to teach health education (Schlachta-Fairchild et al, 2010). The Internet

TABLE 42-4	ONLINE RESOURCES FOR SCHOOL NURSES
ORGANIZATION	**INTERNET ADDRESS**
The American Academy of Child and Adolescent Psychiatry	http://www.aacap.org
American Academy of Pediatrics	http://www.aap.org
National Association of School Nurses	http://www.nasn.org
Center for Health and Health Care in the Schools	http://www.healthinschools.org
National Youth Violence Prevention Resource Center	http://www.safeyouth.org
U.S. Department of Education Emergency Preparedness	http://www2.ed.gov/admins/ lead/safety/emergencyplan/ index.html
Healthy Schools Network	http://www.healthyschools.org

will be used by school nurses to work with children and parents. Teleclinics operated out of the schools will be seen more frequently (Schlachta-Fairchild et al, 2010). Online resources are listed in Table 42-4. The school nurse is responsible for keeping up with the latest changes in health care and health practice so that the health of children in the schools can be enhanced by new trends in health care.

THE CUTTING EDGE *School nurses communicate with some families by using the Internet.*

CHAPTER REVIEW

PRACTICE APPLICATION

The elementary school principal has notified the school nurse that Melissa and John, 8-year-old twins who receive daily physical therapy for mild cerebral palsy, have transferred to the school. The nurse must comply with federal laws related to providing education and services to all children with disabilities.

A. What nursing responsibilities should the school nurse carry out?

B. What factors must be considered when the nurse coordinates the IEP and IHP plans?

C. How will this situation impact other children at school?

D. What is the central focus of Melissa's and John's education? Answers can be found on the Evolve site.

KEY POINTS

- School nurses provide health care for children and families.
- In the early 1900s, school nurses screened children for infectious diseases.
- By 2005, school nurses provided direct care, health education, counseling, case management, and community outreach.
- The National Association of School Nurses (NASN) is the professional organization for school nurses.
- School nurses have varying educational levels depending on state laws.
- The U.S. government supports school-based health centers, school-linked programs, and full-service school-based health centers.
- *Healthy People 2020* has objectives to enhance the health of children in schools.
- Primary prevention provides health promotion and education to prevent childhood injuries and substance abuse.
- The school nurse monitors the children for all of their state-mandated immunizations for school entry.
- HIPAA privacy rules regarding the health information of children apply in schools.

- Secondary prevention involves screening children for illnesses and providing direct nursing care.
- School nurses develop plans for emergency care in the schools.
- Giving medications to children in the school must be monitored carefully to prevent errors.
- School health nurses are mandated reporters to tell the authorities about suspected cases of child abuse and/or neglect.
- Disaster-preparedness plans should be set up for all schools with the school nurse as a member of the crisis response team.
- Tertiary prevention includes caring for children with long-term health needs, including asthma and disabling conditions.
- School nurses carry out catheterizations, suctioning, gastrostomy feedings, and other skills in the schools.
- Some ethical dilemmas in the schools are related to women's health care.
- Some school nurses use the Internet to help communicate with children and their families.

CLINICAL DECISION-MAKING ACTIVITIES

1. For the state where you live, make a list of the immunizations required for children attending schools. Then contrast this to the immunizations you received when in school. How has this changed over the years?

2. Contact the nurse in your former high school. Interview the nurse, focusing on the major focus of the role. Describe what the nurse likes best and least about the role. What changes can be made to make the responsibilities easier?

3. Arrange to visit an elementary school health office during screening activities. Observe the interaction between the nurse and the children. Describe how the nurse is using the nursing process during the screening process.

4. Organize a group of nursing students to volunteer at a school health fair. Develop a health education booth for the fair. Describe how the health information can be used by the children, families, and the community.

5. Attend the annual school board meeting that discusses the budget for the next year. Analyze the budget for health services. How will this be adequate to care for the children? What issues influence the budgetary process?

6. On the Internet, focus on your state's health department. What trends do you see relating to health in the schools?

7. Volunteer as a participant in your school district's emergency response drill. How did the school nurse's responsibilities work to help reduce confusion and increase the provision of emergency care?

REFERENCES

Adler JH: *Divided Sixth Circuit Court Dismisses No Child Left Behind Suit*, October 16, 2009. Available at http://the volokhconspiracy. Accessed March 19, 2011.

American Academy of Pediatrics, Council on Children with Disabilities: identifying infants and young children with developmental disorders in the medical home: an algorithm for developmental surveillance and screening, *Pediatrics* 118(1):405–420, 2006.

American Academy of Pediatrics, Council on School Health: The role of the school nurse in providing school health services, *Pediatrics* 121(5):1052–1056, 2008a.

American Academy of Pediatrics, Committee on Infectious Diseases: Prevention of influenza: recommendations for influenza immunization of children, 2007-2008, *Pediatrics* 121:e1016–e1031, 2008b.

American Academy of Pediatrics, Committee on School Health: Guidelines for emergency medical care in school, *Pediatrics* 122(4):887–894, 2008c. Available at http://aappolicy.aappublications. org/cgi/content/abstract/pediatr ics;122/4/887. Accessed March 19, 2011.

American Academy of Pediatrics, Committee on Injury and Poison Prevention: Skateboard and scooter injuries, *Pediatrics* 109:542–543, 2002. Reaffirmed 2009.

American Academy of Pediatrics, Council on School Health and Committee on Bioethics: Honoring do-not-attempt-resuscitation requests in schools, *Pediatrics* 125(5):1073–1077, 2010.

American Association of Occupational Health Nurses (AAOHN) and National Association of School Nurses (NASN): *Role of occupational and environmental health nurses and school nurses in promoting safe and healthful environments for working youths*, 2004. Available at https://www.aaohn.org/aaohn-in-action/quality-of-work-environments.html. Accessed March 19, 2011.

American Federation of Teachers: *Every child needs a school nurse: brochure*, 2008. Available at www. aft.org/pdfs/healthcare/br_school nursebrochure.pdf. Accessed March 19, 2011.

Anonymous: Role of the school nurse 100 years ago, *Br J Nurs* 17(21):1345, 2008.

Bagby MA, Adams S: Evidence-based practice guideline: increasing physical activity in schools—kindergarten through 8th grade, *J Sch Nurs* 23(3):137–145, 2007.

Bellando J, Lopez ML: The school nurse's role in treatment of the student with autism spectrum disorders, *J Spec Pediatr Nurs* 14(3):173–182, 2009.

Betz CL: Use of 504 plans for children and youth with disabilities: nursing application, *Pediatr Nurs* 27:347–352, 2001.

Bleakley A, Hennessy M, Fishbein M: Public opinion on sex education in US schools, *Arch Pediatr Adolesc Med* 160:1151–1156, 2006.

Borse NN, Gilchrist J, Dellinger AM, et al: *CDC Childhood Injury Report: patterns of unintentional injuries among 0-19 year olds in the United States, 2000-2006*, Atlanta, 2008, CDC, National Center for Injury Prevention and Control.

Brown MB, Bolen LM: The school-based health center as a resource for prevention and health promotion, *Psychol Schools* 45(1):28–38, 2008.

Buckley EJ, White DG: Systematic review of the role of external contributors in school substance use education, *Health Educ* 107(1): 42–62, 2007.

Centers for Disease Control and Prevention: *State level school health policies and practices: a state-by-state summary from the School Health Policies and Programs Study 2006*, Atlanta, 2006, CDC, USD-HHS. Available at http://www. cdc.gov/HealthyYouth/shpps/2006 /summaries/index.htm. Accessed March 19, 2011.

Centers for Disease Control and Prevention: *Healthy Youth! Coordinated school health program*, Washington, DC, 2008, CDC. Available at http://www.cdc.gov/Healthy Youth/CSHP/. Accessed March 19, 2011.

Centers for Disease Control and Prevention: *Asthma*, 2009a. Available at http://www.cdc.gov/ HealthyYouth/asthma/. Accessed March 19, 2011.

Centers for Disease Control and Prevention: *Healthy youth! funded partners: state, territorial, and local agencies and tribal governments coordinated school health programs (CSHPs)*, 2009b. Available at http://www.cdc.gov. Accessed March 19, 2011.

Centers for Disease Control and Prevention: *Data 2010, Objective 07-04*, 2010a. Available at http:// wonder.cdc.gov/.

Centers for Disease Control and Prevention: *Healthy youth! Food safety*, 2010b. Available at http:// www.cdc.gov/HealthyYouth/ foodsafety/index.htm. Accessed March 19, 2011.

Centers for Disease Control and Prevention: *State vaccination requirements*, 2010c. Available at http://www.cdc.gov/vaccines/vac-gen/laws/state-reqs.htm. Accessed March 19, 2011.

Centers for Disease Control and Prevention: *Understanding school violence-fact sheet*, 2010d. Available at www.cdc.gov/violenceprevention. Accessed March 19, 2011.

Centers for Disease Control and Prevention: *Children and diabetes—more information*, 2010e. Available from http://www.cdc.gov/ diabetes/projects/cda2.htm. Accessed March 19, 2011.

Centers for Disease Control and Prevention: *Attention-deficit/hyperactivity disorder (ADHD)*, 2010f. Available at http://www.cdc.gov/ncbddd/adhd/ data.html. Accessed March 29, 2011.

Centers for Disease Control and Prevention, Youth Risk Behavior Survey: *Behaviors that contribute to violence on school property*, 2010. Available at http://www.cdc. gov/HealthyYouth/yrbs/trends.htm. Accessed March 19, 2011.

Cole K, Waldrop J, D'Auria J, Garner H: An integrative research review: effective school-based childhood overweight interventions, *J Spec Pediatr Nurs: JSPN* 11(3):166–177, 2006.

Dang MT, Warrington D, Tung T, et al: A school-based approach to early identification and management of students with ADHD, *J Sch Nurs* 23(1):2–12, 2007.

Family Health Center: *Our programs and services*, 2010. Available at http://www.fhcw.org.

Fee E, Liping B: Models of public health education: choices for the future? *Bull World Health Org (BLT)* 85(12):901–980, 2007.

Ficca M, Welk D: Medication administration practices in Pennsylvania schools, *J Sch Nurs* 22(3):148–155, 2006.

Frisen A, Bjarnelind S: Health-related quality of life and bullying in adolescence, *Acta Paediatrica* 99(4):597–603, 2010.

Gorely T, Nevil ME, Morris JG, et al: Effect of a school-based intervention to promote healthy lifestyles in 7–11 year old children, *Int J Behav Nutr Phys Act* 6:5, 2009.

Hamner JB, Wilder B, Byrd L: Lessons learned: Integrating a service learning community-based partnership into the curriculum, *Nurs Outlook* 55(2):106–110, 2007.

Hayter M, Piercy H, Massey M, Gregory T: School nurses and sex education: surveillance and disciplinary practices in primary schools, *J Adv Nurs* 61(3):273–281, 2008.

HeadLice.Org: *10 Steps to staying ahead of lice*, 2010. Available at http://www.headlice.org/downloads/10steps.htm. Accessed March 19, 2011.

Hone-Warren M: Exploration of school administrator attitudes regarding do not resuscitate policies in the school setting, *J Sch Nurs* 23(2):98–103, 2007.

Hudson SD: An investigation of school playground safety practices as reported by school nurses, *J School Nurs* 24(3):138–144, 2008.

Judd D, Sitzman S, Davis M: *A history of American nursing: trends and eras*, Sudbury, MA, 2009, Jones & Bartlett.

Kaffenberge CJ: School reentry for students with a chronic illness: a role for professional school counselors, *Prof School Counsel* 9(3):223–230, 2006.

Kann L, Brener ND, Wechsler H: Overview and summary: School Health Policies and Programs Study 2006, *J Sch Health* 77:385–397, 2007.

Kennedy S: Can school nurses help prevent heat stroke fatalities in high school football? *Off the Charts AJN*, 2009. Available at http://ajnoffthecharts.com/2009/09/17/can-school-nurses-help-prevent-heat-stroke-fatalities-in-high-school-football/. Accessed March 19, 2011.

King CA, Meadows BB, Engelke MK, Swanson M: Prevalence of elevated body mass index and blood pressure in a rural school-aged population: implications for school nurses, *J Sch Health* 76(4):145–149, 2006.

Kruger BJ, Toker KH, Radjenovic D, et al: School nursing for children with special needs: does number of schools make a difference? *J Sch Health* 79(8):337–346, 2009.

Laudorn C: *School nurse's corner*, 2010. Available at http://www.christina.k12.de.us/downes/resources/nurse.html. Accessed March 19, 2011.

Lerner MD, Lindell B, Volpe J: *A practical guide for crisis response in our schools*, 2010, American Academy of Experts in Traumatic Stress. Available from http://store.nc-cm.org/servlet/Detail?no=1. Accessed March 19, 2011.

Li C, Freedman M: Seasonal influenza: an overview, *J School Nurs* 25(Suppl 1):4s–10s, 2009.

Molock SD, Barksdale C, Matlin S, et al: Qualitative study of suicidality and help-seeking behaviors in African American adolescents, *Am J Commun Psychol* 40(1):52–63, 2007.

National Association of School Nurses: *Scope and standards of professional school nursing practice*, Washington, DC, 2001, ANA.

National Association of School Nurses: *NASN resolution: access to a school nurse*, 2003. Available at http://www.nasn.org/Default.aspx?tabid=61. Accessed March 19, 2011.

National Association of School Nurses: *Protecting our children from bio-terrorism*, 2005. Available at http://www.nasn.org.

National Association of School Nurses: *School nurse role in care and management of the child with diabetes in the school setting*, 2006. Available at http://www.nasn.org/Default.aspx?tabid=216. Accessed March 19, 2011.

Nic Philibin CA, Griffiths C, Byrne G, et al: The role of the public health nurse in a changing society, *J Adv Nurs* 66(4):743–752, 2010.

Norris J, Howell E, Wydeven M, Kunes-Connell M: Working with teen moms and babies at risk: the power of partnering, *Am J Matern Child Nurs* 34(5):308–315, 2009.

Office of Health and Human Services (EOHHS): *Frequently asked questions on HIPAA and school health*, 2010. Available at http://www.mass.gov. Accessed March 19, 2011.

Read M, Small P, Donaher K, et al: Evaluating parent satisfaction of school nursing services, *J Sch Nurs* 25(3):205–213, 2009.

Robert Wood Johnson Foundation: Unlocking the potential of school nursing: keeping children healthy, in school, and ready to learn, *Charting Nurs Future* 14:2–5, 2010.

Ryan KM: Health promotion of faculty and staff: the school nurse's role, *J Sch Nurs* 24(4):183–189, 2008.

Schlachta-Fairchild L, Varghese SB, Deickman A, Castelli D: Telehealth and telenursing are live: APN policy and practice implications, *J Nurse Pract* 6:98–106, 2010.

Selekman J, editor: *School nursing: a comprehensive text*, Philadelphia, 2006, FA Davis.

Steger S: Killed at school, *RN* 63:36–38, 2000.

Stevenson BA: Evolving roles for school nurses: addressing mental health and psychiatric concerns of students, *NASN Sch Nurs* 25:30–33, 2010.

Team Nutrition, U.S. Department of Agriculture: *Making it happen! School nutrition success stories, About Team Nutrition, 2010*, 2010. Available at http://www.fns.usda.gov/TN/about.html. Accessed March 19, 2011.

Texas Association of School-based Health Centers: *89 Texas SBHCs*, 2010. Available at http://www.tasbhc.org/texas-school-based-health-centers/. Accessed March 19, 2011.

Thackaberry J: Who cares for the health of your school? *Independent School* 60:94–97, 2001.

Trapp D: *Medical homes for Medicaid: The North Carolina model*, 2010, Amednews.com. Available at http://www.ama-assn.org/amednews/2010/08/02/gvsa0802.htm. Accessed March 19, 2011.

U.S. Department of Education: *Emergency planning*, 2010. Available from http://www2.ed.gov/admins/lead/safety/emergencyplan/index.html. Accessed March 19, 2011.

U.S. Department of Education, National Center for Education Statistics: *Fast Facts*, 2010. Available at http://nces.ed.gov/fastfacts/display.asp?id=372. Accessed March 19, 2011.

U.S. Department of Health and Human Services: *Proposed Healthy People 2020 Objectives*, 2010. Available at http://www.healthypeople.gov/hp2020/Objectives/TopicAreas.aspx. Accessed March 19, 2011.

U.S. Environmental Protection Agency: *School and child care-based asthma education programs*, 2010. Available from http://www.epa.gov/asthma/school-based.html. Accessed March 19, 2011.

Vessey JA, McGowan KA: A successful public health experiment: school nursing, *Pediatr Nurs* 32(3):213, 255-256, 2006.

Whalen LG, Grunbaum JA, Kann L, et al: *Profiles 2002. School health profiles. Surveillance for characteristics of health programs among secondary schools*, Washington, DC, 2004, CDC, USDHHS.

Winje BA, Oftung F, Korsvold GE, et al: School based screening for tuberculosis infection in Norway: comparison of positive tuberculin skin test with interferon-gamma release assay, *BMC Infect Dis* 8:140, 2008.

Wolfram W: *Lice*, 2010. Available at http://emedicine.medscape.com/article/783877-overview. Accessed March 19, 2011.

CHAPTER 43

The Nurse in Occupational Health

Bonnie Rogers, DrPH, COHN-S, LNCC, FAAN

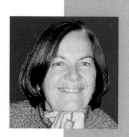

Bonnie Rogers is a Professor of Nursing and Public Health and is Director of the North Carolina Occupational Safety and Health Education and Research Center and the Occupational Health Nursing Program at the University of North Carolina School of Public Health, Chapel Hill, North Carolina. Dr. Rogers received her diploma in nursing from the Washington Hospital Center School of Nursing, Washington, DC; her baccalaureate in nursing from George Mason University, School of Nursing, Fairfax, Virginia; and her master of public health degree and doctorate in public health, the latter with a major in environmental health sciences and occupational health nursing from the Johns Hopkins University School of Hygiene and Public Health, Baltimore, Maryland. She holds a postgraduate certificate as an adult health clinical nurse specialist. She is a certified occupational health nurse and legal nurse consultant as well as a fellow in the American Academy of Nursing and the American Association of Occupational Health Nurses. In addition to managerial, consultant, and educator/researcher positions, Dr. Rogers has also practiced for many years as a public health nurse, occupational health nurse, and occupational health nurse practitioner. She has published more than 175 articles and book chapters and two books, including *Occupational Health Nursing: Concepts and Practice* and *Occupational Health Nursing Guidelines for Primary Clinical Conditions.* She is Associate Editor for the *Legal Nurse Consulting Principles and Practices* core book, and is Editor of the *Journal of Legal Nurse Consulting.* She is a member of several editorial panels and has given more than 450 presentations nationally and internationally on occupational health and safety issues. Dr. Rogers has had several funded research grants on clinical issues in occupational health, health promotion, research priorities, hazards to health care workers, and ethical issues in occupational health. She was invited to study ethics as a visiting scholar at the Hastings Center in New York and was granted a NIOSH career award to study ethical issues in occupational health. Dr. Rogers is a strong advocate of occupational health research and has served as Chairperson of the NIOSH National Occupational Research Agenda Liaison Committee for nearly 15 years. She has served on numerous Institute of Medicine committees including Vice Chairperson for the Protection for Healthcare Workers in the Workplace Against Novel H1N1 Influenza A. She is currently a member of the first IOM standing committee on Personal Protective Equipment for Workplace Safety and Health. Dr. Rogers is past president of the American Association of Occupational Health Nurses as well as the Association of Occupational and Environmental Clinics. She completed several terms as an appointed member of the National Advisory Committee on Occupational Safety and Health and was recently elected Vice President of the International Commission on Occupational Health. She is a consultant in occupational health and ethics.

ADDITIONAL RESOURCES

ⓔvolve WEBSITE
http://evolve.elsevier.com/Stanhope
- *Healthy People 2020*
- WebLinks—Of special note, see the link for this site:
  - OSHA
- Quiz
- Case Studies
- Glossary
- Answers to Practice Application

- Resource Tools
  - Resource Tool 43.A: Immunizing Agents and Immunization Schedules for Health Care Workers

APPENDIX
- Appendix F.3: Comprehensive Occupational and Environmental Health History

OBJECTIVES

After reading this chapter, the student should be able to do the following:
1. Describe the nursing role in occupational health.
2. Discuss current trends in the U.S. workforce.
3. Give examples of work-related illness and injuries.
4. Use the epidemiological model to explain work-health interactions.
5. Cite at least three host factors associated with increased risk from an adverse response to hazardous workplace exposure.

6. Explain one example each of biological, chemical, enviromechanical, physical, and psychosocial workplace hazards.
7. Complete an occupational health history.
8. Differentiate between the functions of OSHA and NIOSH.
9. Explain an effective disaster plan in occupational health.

KEY TERMS

OUTLINE

Nurses provide care to individuals to help them achieve optimal health; yet, at the same time in the course of their work, nurses face numerous hazardous substances such as blood, body fluids, or chemicals and often must lift heavy loads. Work can be both fulfilling and hazardous or risky. Many changes have occurred in the nature of work and workplace risks, the work environment, workforce composition and demographics, and health care delivery mechanisms. An analysis of the trends suggests that work-health interactions will continue to grow in importance, affecting how work is done, how hazards are controlled or minimized, and how health care is managed and integrated into workplace health delivery strategies. Although some workers may never face more than minor adverse health effects from exposures at work, such as occasional eyestrain resulting from poor office lighting, every industry has grappled with serious hazards (USDHHS, NIOSH, 2010).

In America, work is viewed as important to one's life experiences, and most adults spend about one third of their time at work (Rogers, 2011). Work—when fulfilling, fairly compensated, healthy, and safe—can help build long and contented lives and strengthen families and communities. No work is completely risk free, and all health care professionals should have some basic knowledge about workforce populations, work and related hazards, and methods to control hazards and improve health.

Important developments are occurring in occupational health and safety programs designed to prevent and control work-related illness and injury and to create **environments** that foster and support health-promoting activities. Occupational health nurses have performed critical roles in planning and delivering worksite health and safety services, which must continue to grow as comprehensive and cost-effective services. In addition, the continuing increase in health care costs and the concern about health care quality have prompted the inclusion of primary care and management of non–work-related health problems in the health services' programs. In some settings, family services are also provided.

Health at work is an important issue for most individuals for whom the nurse provides care. With many individuals spending so much time at work, the workplace has significant influence on health and can be a primary site for the delivery of health promotion and illness prevention. The home, the clinic, the nursing home, and other community sites such as the workplace will become the dominant areas where health and illness care will be sought (USDHHS/CDC/NIOSH, 2009).

This chapter describes the nurse's role in occupational health—working with employees and the workforce population. The focus is on the knowledge and skills needed to promote the health and safety of workers through occupational health programs, recognizing work-related health and safety and the principles for prevention and control of adverse **work-health interactions**. The prevalence and significance of the interactions between health and work underscore the importance of including principles of occupational health and safety in nursing practice. The types of interactions and the frequent use of the general health care system for identifying, treating, and preventing occupational illnesses and injuries require nurses to use this knowledge in all practice settings. The Epidemiologic Triangle is used as the model for understanding these interactions, as well as risk factors, and effective nursing care for promoting health and safety among employed populations.

DEFINITION AND SCOPE OF OCCUPATIONAL HEALTH NURSING

Adapted from the American Association of Occupational Health Nurses (AAOHN) (2004), occupational and environmental health nursing is the specialty practice that focuses on the promotion, prevention, and restoration of health within the context of a safe and healthy environment. It includes the prevention of adverse health effects from occupational and environmental hazards. It provides for and delivers occupational and environmental health and safety programs and services to clients. Occupational and environmental health nursing is an autonomous specialty, and nurses make independent nursing judgments in providing health care services.

The foundation for occupational and environmental health nursing is research based. Recognizing the legal context for occupational health and safety, this specialty practice derives its theoretical, conceptual, and factual framework from a multidisciplinary base including, but not limited to:

- Nursing science
- Medical science
- Public health sciences such as epidemiology and environmental health
- Occupational health sciences such as toxicology, safety, industrial hygiene, and ergonomics
- Social and behavioral sciences
- Management and administration principles

Guided by an ethical framework made explicit in the AAOHN Code of Ethics, occupational and environmental health nurses encourage and enable individuals to make informed decisions about health care concerns. Confidentiality of health information is integral and central to the practice. Occupational and environmental health nurses are advocates for client(s), fostering equitable and quality health care services and safe and healthy environments in which to work and live.

HISTORY AND EVOLUTION OF OCCUPATIONAL HEALTH NURSING

Nursing care for workers began in 1888 and was called industrial nursing. A group of coal miners hired Betty Moulder, a graduate of the Blockley Hospital School of Nursing in Philadelphia (now Philadelphia General Hospital), to take care of their ailing co-workers and families (AAOHN, 1976). Ada Mayo Stewart, hired in 1885 by the Vermont Marble Company in Rutland, Vermont, is often considered the first industrial nurse. Riding a bicycle, Miss Stewart visited sick employees in their homes, provided emergency care, taught mothers how to care for their children, and taught healthy living habits (Felton, 1985). In the early days of occupational health nursing, the nurse's work was family centered and holistic.

Employee health services grew rapidly during the early 1900s as companies recognized that the provision of worksite health services led to a more productive workforce. At that time, workplace accidents were seen as an inevitable part of having a job. However, the public did not support this attitude, and a system for workers' compensation arose that remains today (McGrath, 1945).

Industrial nursing grew rapidly during the first half of the twentieth century. Educational courses were established, as were professional societies. By World War II there were approximately 4000 industrial nurses (Brown, 1981). The American Association of Industrial Nursing (AAIN) (now called the American Association of Occupational Health Nurses) was established as the first national nursing organization in 1942. The aim of the AAIN was to improve industrial nursing education and practice and to promote interprofessional collaborative efforts (Rogers, 1988).

Passage of several laws in the 1960s and 1970s to protect workers' safety and health led to an increased need for occupational health nurses. In particular, the passing of the landmark Occupational Safety and Health Act in 1970, which created the Occupational Safety and Health Administration (OSHA) and the National Institute for Occupational Safety and Health (NIOSH), discussed later in this chapter, resulted in a great need for nurses at the worksite to meet the demands of the many standards being implemented. Under OSHA, the Act focuses primarily on protecting workers from work-related hazards. NIOSH focuses on education and research. In 1988 the first occupational health nurse was hired by OSHA to provide technical assistance in standards development, field consultation, and occupational health nursing expertise. In 1993 the Office of Occupational Health Nursing was established within the agency. In addition to direct health care delivery, nurses are more engaged than ever in policy making and management of occupational health services. In addition, in 1998, the AAOHN adopted the concept of environmental health as a significant component of the practice field. To this end, AAOHN has incorporated the term "environmental" as in occupational and environmental health nurse, in its documents and publications. In 1999, AAOHN published its first set of competencies in occupational health nursing, which have been updated, and established the AAOHN Foundation to support education, research, and leadership activities in occupational health nursing. Role expansion includes environmental health and forging sustainable relationships in the community to better improve worker health.

ROLES AND PROFESSIONALISM IN OCCUPATIONAL HEALTH NURSING

As U.S. industry has shifted from agrarian (agriculture) to industrial to highly technological processes, the role of the occupational health nurse has continued to change. The focus on work-related health problems now includes the spectrum of human responses to multiple, complex interactions of biopsychosocial factors that occur in community, home, and work environments. The customary role of the occupational health nurse has extended beyond emergency treatment and prevention of illness and injury to include the promotion and maintenance of health, overall risk management, care for the environment, and efforts to reduce health-related costs in businesses. The interprofessional nature of occupational health nursing has become more critical as occupational health and safety problems require more complex solutions. The occupational health nurse frequently collaborates closely with multiple disciplines and industry management, as well as with representatives of labor.

Occupational health nurses constitute the largest group of occupational health professionals. The most recent national survey of registered nurses indicates that there are approximately 22,000 licensed occupational health nurses (HRSA, 2006). Occupational health nurses hold positions as nurse practitioners, clinical nurse specialists, managers, supervisors, consultants, educators, and researchers. Data also show that approximately 60% of occupational health nurses report that they are employed in single-managed occupational health nurse units in a variety of businesses. The occupational health nursing role requires the nurse to adapt to an organization's needs as well as to the needs of specific groups of workers.

The professional organization for occupational health nurses is the American Association of Occupational Health Nurses. The AAOHN's mission is comprehensive. It supports the work of the occupational health nurse and advances the specialty. The AAOHN also does the following:

- Promotes the health and safety of workers
- Defines the scope of practice and sets the standards of occupational health nursing practice
- Develops the code of ethics for occupational health nurses with interpretive statements
- Promotes and provides continuing education in the specialty
- Advances the profession through supporting research
- Responds to and influences public policy issues related to occupational health and safety

The AAOHN provides the Standards of Occupational and Environmental Health Nursing Practice to define and advance practice and provide a framework for practice evaluation. The AAOHN Code of Ethics lists five code statements based on the goal of occupational and environmental health nurses to promote worker health and safety (AAOHN, 2004). Both documents can be obtained from the AAOHN at http://www.aaohn.org.

Occupational health nurses have many roles, such as clinician, case manager, coordinator, manager, nurse practitioner, corporate director, health promotion specialist, educator, consultant, and researcher (AAOHN, 2007). The majority of occupational health nurses work as solo clinicians, but increasingly additional roles are being included in the specialty practice. In many companies, the occupational health nurse has assumed expanded responsibilities in job analysis, safety, and benefits management. Many occupational health nurses also work as independent contractors or have their own businesses that provide occupational health and safety services to industry, as well as consultation.

Ethical conflict is nothing new in occupational and environmental health nursing practice. Traditional concerns about confidentiality of employee health records, hazardous workplace exposures, issues of informed consent, risks and benefits, and dual duty conflicts are now married with newer concerns of genetic screening, worker literacy and understanding, work organization issues, and untimely return to work (Rogers, 2011). With the current changes in health care delivery and the movement toward managed care, occupational health nurses will need increased skills in primary care, health promotion, and disease prevention. The aim of the occupational health nurse will be to devote much attention to keeping workers and, in some cases, their families healthy and free from illness and worksite injuries. Specializing in the field is often a requirement.

THE CUTTING EDGE *Occupational and environmental health nursing research priorities have been developed and published by The American Association of Occupational Health Nursing and are being updated.*

Academic education in occupational health and safety is generally at the graduate level. Training grants from NIOSH support Master's and doctoral education with emphases in occupational health nursing, industrial hygiene, occupational medicine, and safety. These programs, listed in Box 43-1, are offered through Occupational Safety and Health Education and Research Centers throughout the country. Certification in occupational health nursing is provided by the American Board for Occupational Health Nurses (ABOHN). ABOHN offers two basic certifications: the COHN (Certified Occupational Health Nurse) and COHN-S (Certified Occupational Health Nurse–Specialist). Eligibility for the COHN requires licensure as a registered nurse, whereas the COHN-S requires RN licensure plus a baccalaureate degree. In addition, certification is achieved through experience, continuing education, professional activities, and examination. Those interested in certification can view the requirements on the ABOHN website (www.abohn.org).

WORKERS AS A POPULATION AGGREGATE

The population of the United States was expected to increase from approximately 281.4 million people in 2000 to an estimated 335 million by the year 2025 (Hollmann, Mulder, and Kallan, 2000). In reality, the population had grown to 307 million plus by 2009 (U.S. Census Bureau, 2009). By 2010 the U.S. population had become older, with the greatest growth among those older than age 65, and a reduction in those younger than 25. Since 1995 there has been a dramatic increase in the number of workers older than 55 (Mosisa and Hipple, 2006). Between 1977 and 2007, employment of older workers over age 65 increased by 101% compared with 59% of the total employment (BLS, 2008c). BLS (2008a) data show total workforce projection to increase by 8.5% from 2006 to 2016 with workers aged 55 to 64 increasing by 36.5% and those over 65 years of age increasing by 80%. By 2016 workers older than 65 will comprise 6.1% of the labor force, up from 3.6% in 2006. The number of adults age 65 years and older is expected to more than double between now and the year 2050. By that year, one in five Americans will be an older adult.

In 2005 there were more than 131.6 million civilian wage and salary workers in the United States, employed in about 63,000 different worksites (BLS, 2007). More than 91% of those who are able to work outside of the home do so for some portion of their lives. Neither of these statistics indicates the full number of individuals who have potentially been exposed to work-related

BOX 43-1 DIRECTORS NIOSH EDUCATION AND RESEARCH CENTERS (ERCs)

Alabama Education and Research Center
University of Alabama at Birmingham
School of Public Health
1665 University Boulevard
Birmingham, AL 35294-0022
(205) 934-6208
Fax: (205) 975-5444
R. Kent Oestenstad, PhD, Director
E-mail: oestenk@uab.edu

California Education and Research Center—Northern
University of California, Berkeley
School of Public Health
140 Warren
Berkeley, CA 94720-7360
(510) 642-0761
Fax: (510) 642-5815
Robert C. Spear, PhD, Director
E-mail: spear@uclink4.berkeley.edu

California Education and Research Center—Southern
University of California
School of Public Health
650 Young Drive South
Los Angeles, CA 90095-1772
(310) 825-7152
Fax: (310) 206-9903
William C. Hinds, ScD, CIH, Director
E-mail: whinds@ucla.edu

Cincinnati Education and Research Center
University of Cincinnati
Department of Environmental Health
P.O. Box 670056
Cincinnati, OH 45267-0056
(513) 558-1749
Fax: (513) 558-2772 or 4397
C. Scott Clark, PhD, PE, CIH, Director
E-mail: clarkcs@uc.edu

University of Colorado at Denver and Health Sciences Center
4200 E. Ninth Avenue
Denver, CO 80262
(303) 315-0880
Fax: (303) 315-7642
Lee S. Newman, MD, MA, FCCP, FACOEM, Director
E-mail: lee.newman@uchsc.edu

Harvard Education and Research Center
Harvard School of Public Health
Department of Environmental Health
665 Huntington Avenue
Boston, MA 02115
(617) 432-3323
Fax: (617) 432-0219
David C. Christiani, MD, Director
E-mail: dchris@hohp.harvard.edu

Illinois Education and Research Center
University of Illinois at Chicago
School of Public Health
2121 West Taylor Street
Chicago, IL 60612-7260
(312) 996-7469
Fax: (312) 413-9898
Lorraine M. Conroy, ScD, CIH, Director
E-mail: lconroy@uic.edu

Iowa Education and Research Center
Heartland Center for Occupational Health and Safety
Department of Occupational and Environmental Health
100 Oakdale Campus—124 IREH
Iowa City, IA 52242-5000
(319) 335-4415
Fax: (319) 335-4225
Nancy L. Sprince, MD, MPH, Director
E-mail: nancy-sprince@uiowa.edu

Johns Hopkins Education and Research Center
Johns Hopkins University
School of Hygiene and Public Health
615 North Wolfe Street
Baltimore, MD 21205
(410) 955-4037
Fax: (410) 955-1811
Jacqueline Agnew, PhD, Director
E-mail: jagnew@jhsph.edu

Michigan Education and Research Center
University of Michigan
School of Public Health
1420 Washington Heights
Ann Arbor, MI 48109-2029
(734) 936-0758
Fax: (734) 763-8095
Thomas G. Robins, MD, Director
E-mail: trobins@umich.edu

Minnesota Education and Research Center
University of Minnesota
School of Public Health
Box 807 Mayo Memorial Building
Minneapolis, MN 55455
(612) 626-4855
Fax: (612) 626-0650
Ian A. Greaves, MD, Director
E-mail: igreaves@mail.eoh.emn.edu

health hazards. Although some individuals may currently be unemployed or retired, they continue to bear the health risks of past occupational exposures. The number of affected individuals may be even larger, as work-related illnesses are found among spouses, children, and neighbors of exposed workers.

Americans are employed in diverse industries that range in size from one to tens of thousands of employees. Types of industries include traditional manufacturing (e.g., automotive and appliances), service industries (e.g., banking, health care, and restaurants), agriculture, construction, and the newer high-technology firms, such as computer chip manufacturers. Approximately 95% of business organizations are considered small, employing fewer than 500 people (BLS, 2005a). Although some industries are noted for the high degree of hazards associated with their work (e.g., manufacturing, mines, construction, and agriculture), no worksite is free of occupational health and safety hazards. In addition, the larger the company, the more likely it is that there will be health and safety programs for employees. Smaller companies are more apt to rely on external community resources to meet their needs for health and safety services.

Characteristics of the Workforce

The U.S. workplace has been changing rapidly (BLS, 2005a). Jobs in the economy continue to shift from manufacturing to service. Longer hours, compressed workweeks, shift work, reduced job security, and part-time and temporary work are realities of the modern workplace. New chemicals, materials, processes, and equipment are developed and marketed at an ever-increasing pace.

The workforce is also changing. With the U.S. workforce expected to grow to approximately 166 million by the year 2018, it will become older and more racially diverse (BLS, 2008a). In 2005 there were 131.6 million employed workers (BLS, 2007). In 2008, the workforce was comprised of 48% women, 11% blacks, and 14% Hispanics (BLS, 2008b). These changes will continue to present new challenges to protecting worker safety and health.

The demographic trends in the U.S. workforce describe a changing population aggregate that has implications for the prevention services targeted to that group. Major changes in the working population are reflected in the increasing numbers of women, older individuals, and those with chronic illnesses who are part of the workforce. Because of changes in the economy, extension of life span, legislation, and society's acceptance of working women, the proportion of the employed population that these three groups represent will probably continue to grow.

For example, in the late 1990s while nearly 60% of all women were employed, women were predicted to account for 67% of the increase in the labor force in the twenty-first century (BLS, 2005b). These workers tended to be married, with children

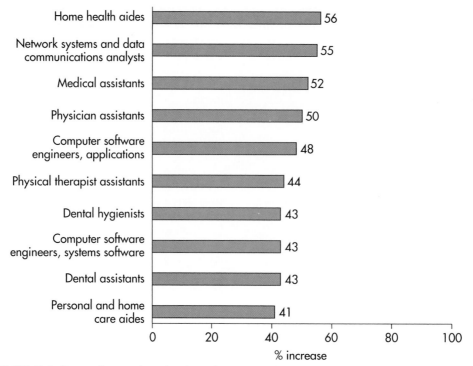

FIGURE 43-1 Occupations projected to have the most rapid growth during the period 2004 to 2014. (From Bureau of Labor Statistics, 2005a.)

and aging parents for whom they were responsible. This aggregate of workers presents new issues for individual and family health promotion, such as child care and elder care, that can be addressed in the work environment. In 1990 more than half of the female labor force was concentrated in three areas: administrative support/clerical (26%), service (14%), and professional specialty (14%). Twelve percent were employed in fields such as labor, transportation and moving, machine operation, precision products, crafts, farming, construction, forestry, and fishing. In the male labor force, nearly 20% worked in precision production, crafts, or repair occupations, 13% in executive positions, 11% in professional specialty occupations, and 10% in sales. Other trends shaping the profile of the workforce include more education and mobility. Increasing mismatches between skills of workers and types of employment were seen in the 1990s.

Future employment trends projected to 2014 are shown in Figure 43-1. Of the 20 fastest growing occupations in the economy, half are related to health care. Health care is experiencing rapid growth, due in large part to the aging of the baby-boom generation, which will require more medical care. In addition, some health care occupations will be in greater demand for other reasons. As health care costs continue to rise, work is increasingly being delegated to lower-paid workers in order to cut costs. For example, tasks that were previously performed by doctors, nurses, dentists, or other health care professionals increasingly are being performed by physician assistants, medical assistants, dental hygienists, and physical therapist aides. In addition, clients increasingly are seeking home care as an alternative to costly stays in hospitals or residential care facilities, causing a significant increase in demand for home health aides. Although not classified as health care workers, personal and

home care aides are being affected by this demand for home care as well (Bartsch, 2009).

Characteristics of Work

There has been a dramatic shift in the types of jobs held by workers. Following the evolution from an agrarian economy to a manufacturing society and then to a highly technological workplace, the greatest proportion of paid employment was in the occupations of trade, transportation, and utilities with 25 million workers (BLS, 2008b). During the 1996 to 2000 period, service-providing industries accounted for virtually all of the job growth. Only construction added jobs in the goods-producing business sector, offsetting declines in manufacturing and mining. According to the BLS (2008b), jobs in construction, transportation, wholesale and retail trade, health care, and service-producing industries are expected to increase by 2018. (Table 43-1 shows occupations with the fastest growth.)

The nature of work has been accompanied by many new occupational hazards, such as complex chemicals, nanotechnology, non-ergonomic workstation design (requiring the adaptation of the workplace or work equipment to meet the employee's health and safety needs), and many issues related to work organization such as job stress, burnout, and exhaustion. In addition, the emergence of a global economy with free trade and multinational corporations presents new challenges for health and safety programs that are culturally relevant.

Work-Health Interactions

The influence of work on health, or work-health interactions, is shown by statistics on illnesses, injuries, and deaths associated with employment. Employers reported 3.9 work injuries

TABLE 43-1   OCCUPATIONS WITH THE FASTEST GROWTH

OCCUPATIONS	PERCENT CHANGE	NUMBER OF NEW JOBS (IN THOUSANDS)	WAGES (MAY 2008 MEDIAN)	EDUCATION/TRAINING CATEGORY
Biomedical engineers	72	11.6	$ 77,400	Bachelor's degree
Network systems and data communications analysts	53	155.8	71,100	Bachelor's degree
Home health aides	50	460.9	20,460	Short-term on-the-job training
Personal and home care aides	46	375.8	19,180	Short-term on-the-job training
Financial examiners	41	11.1	70,930	Bachelor's degree
Medical scientists, except epidemiologists	40	44.2	72,590	Doctoral degree
Physician assistants	39	29.2	81,230	Master's degree
Skin care specialists	38	14.7	28,730	Post-secondary vocational award
Biochemists and biophysicists	37	8.7	82,840	Doctoral degree
Athletic trainers	37	6.0	39,640	Bachelor's degree
Physical therapist aides	36	16.7	23,760	Short-term on-the-job training
Dental hygienists	36	62.9	66,570	Associate's degree
Veterinary technologists and technicians	36	28.5	28,900	Associate's degree
Dental assistants	36	105.6	32,380	Moderate-term on-the-job training
Computer software engineers, applications	34	175.1	85,430	Bachelor's degree
Medical assistants	34	163.9	28,300	Moderate-term on-the-job training
Physical therapist assistants	33	21.2	46,140	Associate's degree
Veterinarians	33	19.7	79,050	First professional degree
Self-enrichment education teachers	32	81.3	35,720	Work experience in a related occupation
Compliance officers, except agriculture, construction, health and safety, and transportation	31	80.8	48,890	Long-term on-the-job training

From Bureau of Labor Statistics: Occupational Employment Statistics and Division of Occupational Outlook: Occupations with the fastest growth (2009), 2008. Available at www.bls.gov/emp/ep_table_103.htm.

and occupational illnesses per 100 workers in 2007 (BLS, 2009). That same year, occupational injuries alone cost over $100 billion in lost wages and lost productivity, administrative expenses, health care, and other costs (BLS, 2006) (Figure 43-2). This figure does not include the cost of occupational diseases. These figures are often described as the "tip of the iceberg," because many work-related health problems go unreported. However, even the recorded statistics are significant in describing the amount of human suffering, financial loss, and decreased productivity associated with workplace hazards. Health care, manufacturing, transportation, and service providing industries were among the top occupations representing days away from work in 2008 (BLS, 2009).

The high number of work injuries and illnesses can be drastically reduced. In fact, significant progress has been made in improving worker protection since Congress passed the 1970 Occupational Safety and Health Act. For example, vinyl chloride–induced liver cancers and brown lung disease (byssinosis) from cotton dust exposure have been almost eliminated. Reproductive disorders associated with certain glycol ethers have been recognized and controlled. Fatal work injuries have declined substantially through the years. Notably, from 1970 to 1995, fatal injury rates in coal miners were reduced by more than 75%, and the disease prevalence was reduced by 90% (USDHHS/NIOSH, 2004). However, since 1995 there has been a doubling of the disease incidence (NIOSH, 2008).

The U.S. workplace is rapidly changing and becoming more diverse. Major changes are also occurring in the way work is organized, with increased shift work, reduced job security, and part-time and temporary work as realities of the modern workplace. In addition, new chemicals, materials, processes, and equipment (such as nanotechnology, and fermentation processes in biotechnology) continue to be developed and marketed at an accelerating pace creating new work-related hazards. Figure 43-3 shows figures for employment and wages from 1986 to 2005.

APPLICATION OF THE EPIDEMIOLOGICAL MODEL

The epidemiological triad can be used to understand the relationship between work and health (Figure 43-4). With a focus on the health and safety of the employed population, the host is described as any susceptible human being. Because of the nature of work-related hazards, nurses must assume that all employed individuals and groups are at risk of being exposed

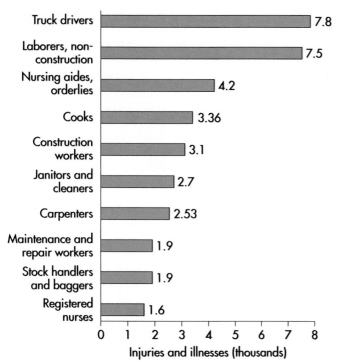

FIGURE 43-2 Ten occupations with the most injuries and illnesses involving days away from work, 2005. Total number of injuries and illnesses involving days away from work was 2.2 million. (From Bureau of Labor Statistics: Lost work time injuries and illnesses: characteristics and resulting time away from work, Washington, DC, 2006, U.S. Department of Labor.)

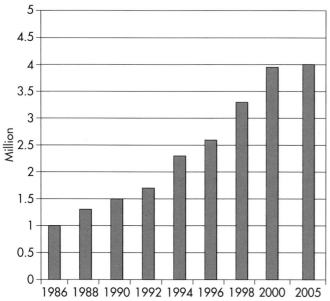

FIGURE 43-3 Employment and wages, 1986 to 2005 (wage and salary workers in millions). (From Bureau of Labor Statistics: *Career guide,* Washington, DC, 2005, U.S. Department of Labor.)

to occupational hazards. The **agents,** factors associated with illness and injury, are occupational exposures that are classified as biological, chemical, enviromechanical, physical, or psychosocial (Box 43-2). The third element, the environment, includes all external conditions that influence the interaction of the host and agents. These may be workplace conditions such

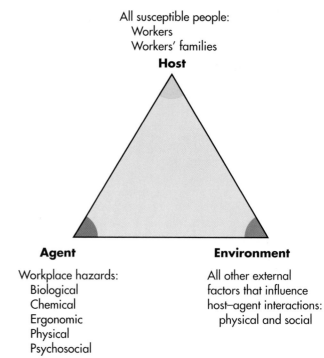

FIGURE 43-4 The epidemiological triad.

BOX 43-2 **CATEGORIES OF WORK-RELATED HAZARDS**

- Biological and infectious hazards—Infectious/biological agents, such as bacteria, viruses, fungi, or parasites, that may be transmitted via contact with infected clients or contaminated body secretions/fluids to other individuals
- Chemical hazards—Various forms of chemicals, including medications, solutions, gases, vapors, aerosols, and particulate matter, that are potentially toxic or irritating to the body system
- Enviromechanical hazards—Factors encountered in the work environment that cause or potentiate accidents, injuries, strain, or discomfort (e.g., unsafe/inadequate equipment or lifting devices, slippery floors, work station deficiencies)
- Physical hazards—Agents within the work environment, such as radiation, electricity, extreme temperatures, and noise, that can cause tissue trauma
- Psychosocial hazards—Factors and situations encountered or associated with one's job or work environment that create or potentiate stress, emotional strain, or interpersonal problems

From Rogers B: *Occupational health nursing: concepts and practice,* St Louis, 2011, Elsevier.

as temperature extremes, crowding, shift work, and inflexible management styles. The basic principle of epidemiology is that health status interventions for restoring and promoting health are the result of complex interactions among these three elements. To understand these interactions and to design effective nursing strategies for dealing with them in a proactive manner, nurses must look at how each element influences the others.

Host

Each worker represents a host within the worker population group. Certain host factors are associated with increased risk of adverse response to the hazards of the workplace. These include

TABLE 43-2   SELECTED JOB CATEGORIES, EXPOSURES, AND ASSOCIATED WORK-RELATED DISEASES AND CONDITIONS

JOB CATEGORIES	EXPOSURES	WORK-RELATED DISEASES AND CONDITIONS
All workers	Workplace stress	Hypertension, mood disorders, cardiovascular disease
Agricultural workers	Pesticides, infectious agents, gases, sunlight	Pesticide poisoning, "farmer's lung," skin cancer
Anesthetists	Anesthetic gases	Reproductive effects, cancer
Automobile workers	Asbestos, plastics, lead, solvents	Asbestosis, dermatitis
Butchers	Vinyl plastic fumes	"Meat wrappers' asthma"
Caisson workers	Pressurized work environments	Caisson disease ("the bends")
Carpenters	Wood dust, wood preservatives, adhesives	Nasopharyngeal cancer, dermatitis
Cement workers	Cement dust, metals	Dermatitis, bronchitis
Ceramic workers	Talc, clays	Pneumoconiosis
Demolition workers	Asbestos, wood dust	Asbestosis
Drug manufacturers	Hormones, nitroglycerin, etc.	Reproductive effects
Dry cleaners	Solvents	Liver disease, dermatitis
Dye workers	Dyestuffs, metals, solvents	Bladder cancer, dermatitis
Embalmers	Formaldehyde, infectious agents	Dermatitis
Felt makers	Mercury, polycyclic hydrocarbons	Mercurialism
Foundry workers	Silica, molten metals	Silicosis
Glass workers	Heat, solvents, metal powders	Cataracts
Hospital workers	Infectious agents, cleansers, radiation	Infections, latex allergies, unintentional injuries
Insulators	Asbestos, fibrous glass	Asbestosis, lung cancer, mesothelioma
Jack-hammer operators	Vibration	Raynaud's phenomenon
Lathe operators	Metal dusts, cutting oils	Lung disease, cancer
Office computer workers	Repetitive wrist motion on computers	Tendonitis, carpal tunnel syndrome, tenosynovitis, eye strain

age, sex, health status, work practices, ethnicity, and lifestyle factors (Rogers, 2011). For example, the population group at greatest risk for experiencing work-related accidents with subsequent injuries is new workers with less than 1 year of experience on the current job. Most non-fatal injuries and illnesses involving days away from work occur among new workers (the highest percentages were in mining [44%]; agriculture, forestry, and fishing [43%]; construction [41%]; and wholesale and retail trade [34%]). Nearly two thirds of injury and illness cases with days away from work occurred among workers with 5 or fewer years of service with their employer (BLS, 2007). The host factors of age, sex, and work experience combine to increase this group's risk of injury because of characteristics such as risk taking, lack of knowledge, and lack of familiarity with the new job.

Older workers may be at increased risk in the workplace because of diminished sensory abilities, the effects of chronic illnesses, and delayed reaction times. Another population group that may be very susceptible to workplace exposure is women in their child-bearing years. The hormonal changes during these years (along with the increased stress of new roles and additional responsibilities) and transplacental exposures are host factors that may influence this group's response to potential toxins.

In addition to these host factors, there may be other, less well-understood individual differences in response to occupational hazard exposures. Even if employers maintain exposure levels below the level recommended by occupational health and safety standards, 15% to 20% of the population may have health reactions to the "safe" low-level exposures (Levy and Wegman, 2006). This group has been termed *hypersusceptible*. A number of host factors appear to be associated with this

hypersusceptibility: light skin, malnutrition, compromised immune system, glucose-6-phosphate dehydrogenase deficiency, serum alpha$_1$-antitrypsin deficiency, chronic obstructive pulmonary disease, sickle cell trait, and hypertension. Individuals who have known hypersusceptibility to chemicals that are respiratory irritants, hemolytic chemicals, organic isocyanates, and carbon disulfide may also be hypersusceptible to other agents in the work environment (Levy and Wegman, 2006). Although this has prompted some industries to consider preplacement screening for such risk factors, the associations between these individual health markers and hypersusceptible response are speculative and require further research.

Agent

Work-related hazards, or agents (see Box 43-2), present potential and actual risks to the health and safety of workers in the millions of business establishments in the United States. Any worksite commonly presents multiple and interacting exposures from all five categories of agents. Table 43-2 lists some of the more common workplace exposures, their known health effects, and the types of jobs associated with these hazards.

Biological Agents

Biological agents are living organisms whose excretions or parts are capable of causing human disease, usually by an infectious process. Biological hazards are common in workplaces such as health care facilities and clinical laboratories where employees are potentially exposed to a variety of infectious agents, including viruses, fungi, and bacteria. Of particular concern in occupational health is infectious diseases transmitted by humans (e.g., from client to worker or from worker to worker) in a variety of work settings. Bloodborne and airborne pathogens represent a significant class of exposures for U.S. health care workers at risk. Occupational transmission of bloodborne pathogens (including the hepatitis B and C viruses and the human immunodeficiency virus [HIV]) occurs primarily by means of needlestick injuries as well as through exposures to the eyes or mucous membranes (Panlilio et al, 2005). The risk of hepatitis B virus infection following a single needlestick injury with a contaminated needle varies from 2% to greater than 40%, depending on the antigen status of the source person and the nature of the exposure. The risk of hepatitis C virus transmission depends on the same factors and ranges from 3.3% to 10%.

Transmission of tuberculosis (TB) within health care settings (especially multidrug-resistant TB) has reemerged as a major public health problem (USDHHS, CDC, NIOSH, 2009). Since 1989 outbreaks of this type of TB have been reported in hospitals, and some workers have developed active drug-resistant TB. In addition, among workers in health care, social service, and corrections' facilities who work with populations at increased risk of TB, hundreds have experienced tuberculin skin test conversions. Reliable data are lacking on the extent of possible work-related TB transmission among other groups of workers at risk for exposure. Many workers in these settings were employed as maintenance workers, security guards, aides, or cleaning people, who were not well protected from inadvertent exposure. Education should be provided to all health care workers, including those not having direct client care, in the proper handling and disposal of potentially contaminated linens, soiled equipment, and trash containing contaminated dressings or specimens (Jensen et al, 2005). (See Evidence-Based Practice box.)

Chemical Agents

More than 300 billion pounds of chemical agents are produced annually in the United States. Of the approximately 2 million known chemicals in existence, less than 0.1% have been adequately studied for their effects on humans. Of those chemicals that have been linked to carcinogens, approximately half test positive as animal carcinogens. Most chemicals have not been studied epidemiologically to determine the effects of exposure on humans (Levy and Wegman, 2006). As a consequence of general environmental contamination with chemicals from work, home, and community activities, a variety of chemicals have been found in the body tissues of the general population. These tissue loads may result in part from the accidental release of chemicals into the environment, such as that which occurred in Love Canal when chemicals leached out from buried industrial wastes.

In many workplaces, significant exposure to a daily, low-level dose of workplace chemicals may be below the exposure standards but may still carry a potentially chronic and perhaps cumulative assault on workers' health. Predicting human responses to such exposures are further complicated because multiple chemicals often combine and interact to create a new chemical agent. Human effects may be associated with the interaction of these agents rather than with a single chemical. Another concern about occupational exposure to chemicals is

EVIDENCE-BASED PRACTICE

The aim of this study was to evaluate self-reported compliance with personal protective equipment (PPE) use among surgical nurses and factors influencing compliance/non-compliance.

Health care workers still fail to adhere to standard precaution guidelines despite evidence that such a failure increases the risk of mucocutaneous blood and body fluid exposure resulting in bloodborne infection. The major infectious occupational hazards in the health care industry are hepatitis B and C viruses (HBV, HCV), and human immunodeficiency virus (HIV).

A total of 601 surgical nurses, from 18 randomly selected hospitals (7 urban and 11 rural) in the Pomeranian region of Poland, were surveyed using a confidential questionnaire. The survey indicated that compliance with PPE varied considerably. Compliance was high for glove use (83%), but much lower for protective eyewear (9%). Only 5% of respondents routinely used gloves, masks, protective eyewear, and gowns when in contact with potentially infective material. Adherence to PPE use was highest in the municipal hospitals and in the operating rooms. Nurses who had a high or moderate level of fear of acquiring HIV at work were more likely ($P < .005$ and $P < .04$, respectively) than staff with no fear to be compliant. Significantly higher compliance was found among nurses with previous training in infection control or experience of caring for an HIV client; the combined effect of training and experience exceeded that for either alone. The most commonly stated reasons for non-compliance were non-availability of PPE (37%), the conviction that the source client was not infected (33%), and staff concern that following locally recommended practices actually interfered with providing good client care (32%).

Nurse Use

Since both training programs and practical experience in working with HIV-positive clients positively influenced nurses' compliance to PPE use, and the combined effect was greater that either alone, it is important that surgical nurses receive effective teaching in infection control and safe work practice behavior. OHNs should work with infection control professionals to design programs to increase use of PPE to minimize work-related health hazard exposure.

From Ganczak M, Szych Z: Surgical nurses and compliance with personal protective equipment, *J Hosp Infect* 66:346-351, 2007.

reproductive health effects. Workplace reproductive hazards have become important legal and scientific issues. Toxicity to male and female reproductive systems has been demonstrated from exposure to common agents such as lead, mercury, cadmium, nickel, and zinc, as well as in antineoplastic drugs. Because data for predicting human responses to many chemical agents are inadequate, workers should be assessed for all potential exposures and cautioned to work preventively with these agents. High-risk or vulnerable workers, such as those with latex allergy—a widely recognized health hazard—should be carefully screened and monitored for optimal health protection (Petsonk and Levy, 2005; USDHHS, CDC, NIOSH, 2009). To accurately assess and evaluate the exposure and recommend changes for abatement, it is essential that the nurse have a good understanding of the basic principles of toxicology, including routes of exposure (i.e., inhalation, skin absorption, and ingestion), dose-response relationships, and differences in effects (i.e., acute versus chronic toxicity).

DID YOU KNOW?   *Only 0.1% of the nearly 2 million known chemicals produced have been tested for their effect on humans.*

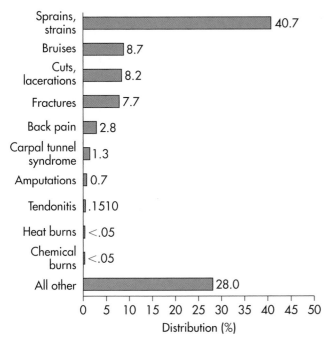

FIGURE 43-5 Distribution of injury and illness cases with days away from work in private industry, by nature of injury or illness, 2005. Total number of injury and illness cases with days away from work was 2.2 million. (From Bureau of Labor Statistics: *Lost work time injuries and illnesses: characteristics and resulting time away from work,* Washington, DC, 2006, U.S. Department of Labor.)

Enviromechanical Agents

Enviromechanical agents are those that can potentially cause injury or illness in the workplace. They are related to the work process or to working conditions, and they can cause postural or other strains that can produce adverse health effects when certain tasks are performed repeatedly. Examples are repetitive motions, poor or unsafe workstation-worker fit, slippery floors, cluttered work areas, and lifting heavy loads. In 2005 (BLS, 2006), sprains and strains were by far the most frequent disabling conditions, accounting for 503,530 of the cases (40.7%) of days away from work. Bruises accounted for 107,770 cases (8.7%), and cuts and lacerations accounted for another 101,660 cases (8.2%) (Figure 43-5). The back and shoulders were the body parts most often affected by disabling work incidents.

Severity of illness or injury can be estimated from the number of days away from work. Sprains and strains, bruises/contusions, cuts/lacerations, fractures, and multiple injuries accounted for more days away from work than for all types of injury and illness. Carpal tunnel syndrome (CTS), fractures, amputations, tendonitis, and multiple injuries had median days away from work greater than the 6-day median for all injuries and illnesses combined (Figure 43-6). The most frequently reported upper-extremity musculoskeletal disorders affect the hand/wrist region.

In 2003 CTS, the most widely recognized condition, occurred in 26,000 full-time workers. This syndrome required

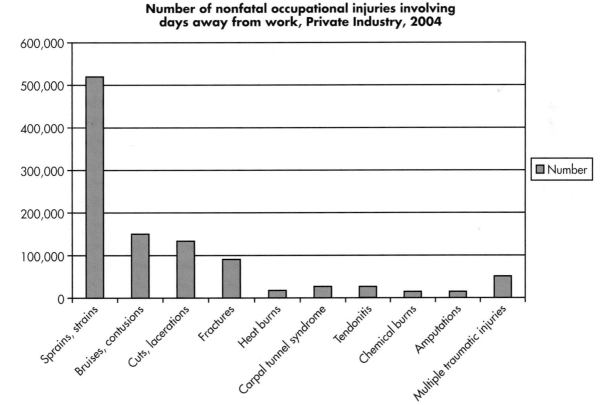

FIGURE 43-6 Number of non-fatal occupational injuries and illness involving days away from work, 2004. (From Bureau of Labor Statistics: *Lost work time injuries and illnesses: characteristics and resulting time away from work,* Washington, DC, 2006, U.S. Department of Labor.)

the longest recuperation period of all conditions resulting in lost work days, with a median 25 days away from work (USDHHS/NIOSH, 2004).

Back pain/injury is one of the most common and significant musculoskeletal problems in the world (USDHHS/NIOSH, 2004). In 2005 back injuries and disorders accounted for 37% of all non-fatal occupational injuries and illnesses involving days away from work in the United States. Although the exact cost of back disorders is unknown, the estimates are staggering and in the billions per year. Regardless of the estimate used, the problem is large both in health and in economic terms. Moreover, as many as 30% of U.S. workers are employed in jobs that routinely require them to perform activities that may increase the risk of developing lower back disorders. The research on these hazards, related human responses, and prevention is evolving. Injuries and illnesses related to this category of agents have been termed *cumulative trauma*—the largest category of work-related illness and disability claims in the United States. The most productive strategy in preventing these exposures appears to be redesigning the workplace and the work machinery or processes.

Physical Agents

Physical agents are those that produce adverse health effects through the transfer of physical energy. Commonly encountered physical agents in the workplace include temperature extremes, vibration, noise, laser, radiation, and electricity. For example, vibration, which accompanies the use of power tools and vehicles such as trucks, affects internal organs, supportive ligaments, the upper torso, and the shoulder-girdle structure. Localized effects are seen with handheld power tools; the most common is Raynaud's phenomenon. The control of worker exposure to these agents is usually accomplished through engineering strategies such as eliminating or containing the hazardous agent. In addition, workers must use preventive actions, such as practicing safe work habits and wearing personal protective equipment when needed. Examples of safe work habits include taking appropriate breaks from environments with temperature extremes and not eating or smoking in radiation-contaminated areas. Personal protective equipment includes hearing protection, eye guards, protective clothing, and devices for monitoring exposures to agents such as radiation.

Psychosocial Agents

Psychosocial agents are conditions that create a threat to the psychological and/or social well-being of individuals and groups (Rogers, 2011). A psychosocial response to the work environment occurs as an employee acts selectively toward the environment in an attempt to achieve a harmonious relationship. When such a human attempt at adaptation to the environment fails, an adverse psychosocial response may occur. Work-related stress or burnout has been defined as an important problem for many individuals (Rogers, 2011). Responses to negative interpersonal relationships, particularly those with authority figures in the workplace, are often the cause of vague health symptoms and increased absenteeism. Epidemiological work in mental health has pointed to environmental variables such as these in the incidence of mental illness and emotional disorder.

The psychosocial environment includes characteristics of the work itself, as well as the interpersonal relationships required in the work setting and shiftwork. About 10% of U.S. workers do some form of shiftwork that has the potential to lead to a variety of psychological and physical problems, including exhaustion, depression, anxiety, and gastrointestinal disturbance. Strategies to minimize the adverse effects of shiftwork, such as rotating shifts clockwise, are beneficial. Job characteristics such as low autonomy, poor job satisfaction, and limited control over the pace of work have been associated with an increased risk of heart disease among clerical and blue-collar workers.

Interpersonal relationships among employees and co-workers or bosses and managers are often sources of conflict and stress. Another aspect is organizational culture. This refers to the norms and patterns of behavior that are sanctioned within a particular organization. Such norms and patterns set guidelines for the types of work behaviors that will enable employees to succeed within a particular firm. Examples include following organizational norms for working overtime, expressing constructive dissatisfaction with management, and making work a top priority (USDHHS/NIOSH, 2002). These factors and the employee's response to them must be assessed if strategies for influencing the health and safety of workers are to be effective.

Non-fatal violence in the health care worker's workplace is a serious problem that is underreported. Much of the study of health care worker violence has been in psychiatric settings; however, reports in other areas such as the emergency department have been reported. Risk factors associated with this type of violence must be identified and strategies implemented to reduce the risk (Rogers, 2006).

Environment

Environmental factors influence the occurrence of host-agent interactions and may direct the course and outcome of those interactions. The physical environment involves the geological and atmospheric structure of an area and the source of such elements as water, temperature, and radiation, which may serve as positive or negative stressors. Although aspects of the physical environment (e.g., heat, odor, ventilation) may influence the host–agent interaction, the social and psychological environment can be equally important (Gordis, 2008).

New environmental problems continue to arise, such as an increase in industrial wastes and toxins and indoor and outdoor environmental pollution, which present opportunities for significant health threats to the working and general population. The social aspects of the environment encompass the economic and political forces affecting society and its health. This includes factors such as sanitation and hygiene practices, housing conditions, level and delivery of health care services, development and enforcement of health-related codes (e.g., occupational health and safety, pollution), employment conditions, population crowding, literacy, ethnic customs, extent of support for health-related research, and equal access to health care. In addition, addictive behaviors such as alcohol and substance abuse and various forms of psychosocial stress may be an outgrowth of negative social environments.

Consider an employee who is working with a potentially toxic liquid. Providing education about safe work practices and fitting the employee with protective clothing may not be adequate if the work must occur in a very hot and humid environment. As the worker becomes uncomfortable in the hot clothing, protection may be compromised by rolling up a sleeve, taking off a glove, or wiping the face with a contaminated piece of clothing. If the norms in the workplace condone such work practices (e.g., "Everyone does it when it's too hot"), the interventions that address only the host and agent will be ineffective; strategies to address the environment itself must be considered, such as cooling fans or minimization of exposure through job rotation. The epidemiological triad can be used as the basis for planning interventions to restore and promote the health of workers. These efforts are influenced by society and by organizational activities related to occupational health and safety (Rogers, 2011).

The occupational environment, within the context of the social environment, is represented by the workplace and work setting and the interactive effects of this environment on the worker. The nurse must consider the hazards and threats posed by this environment and the commitment of the employer to providing a safe and healthful workplace through use of preventive strategies and controls (e.g., engineering, substitution) (Rogers, 2011).

ORGANIZATIONAL AND PUBLIC EFFORTS TO PROMOTE WORKER HEALTH AND SAFETY

Promotion of worker health and safety is the goal of occupational health and safety programs. These programs are offered primarily by the employer at the workplace, but the range of services and the models for delivering them have been changing dramatically over the past few years. In addition to specific services, legislation at the federal and state levels has had a significant effect on efforts to provide a healthy and safe environment for all workers. Under the Occupational Safety and Health Act and because of increased public concern about worker health and safety, companies are cited for not meeting minimal occupational health and safety standards. Criminal charges have been filed against business owners when preventable work-related deaths occurred. These events have redirected an emphasis on preventive occupational health and safety programming.

Unless they have OSHA-regulated exposures, business firms are not required to provide occupational health and safety services that meet any specified standards. With few exceptions, there is no legal recourse for specific services or level of personnel provided by employers to protect worker health and safety. Therefore, the range of services offered and the qualifications of the providers of occupational health and safety vary widely across industries. An important stimulus for health and safety programs is avoiding cost that can be attributed to the effectiveness of prevention services, as well as the need to support occupational health and safety and health promotion at the worksite.

On-Site Occupational Health and Safety Programs

Optimally, on-site occupational health and safety services are provided by a team of occupational health and safety professionals. The core members of this team are the occupational health nurse, occupational physician, industrial hygienist, and safety professional. In addition, more and more ergonomists are playing an important role in the occupational health and safety team. The largest group of health care professionals in business settings is occupational health nurses; therefore, the most frequently seen model is that of the one-nurse unit. This nurse collaborates with a community physician or occupational medicine physician who provides consultation and accepts referrals when medical intervention is needed. The collaboration may occur primarily through telephone contact, or the physician may be under contract with the company to spend a certain amount of on-site time each week. As companies become larger, they are likely to hire additional nurses, safety professionals, industrial hygienists, and physicians, the latter usually on a part-time or consultant basis. An increasingly popular option is to contract some health, safety, and industrial hygiene work to external providers. The largest firms often have corporate occupational health and safety professionals who set policy and participate in company decision-making at the corporate level. These professionals work with the nurses employed at the individual sites within the company. Depending on the needs of the company and the workers, additional professionals may be on the occupational health and safety team, including employee assistance counselors, physical therapists, health educators, physical fitness specialists, and toxicologists.

The services provided by on-site occupational health programs range from those focused only on work-related health and safety problems to a wide scope of services that includes primary health care (Box 43-3). In industries that have exposures regulated by law, certain programs are required, such as

---

BOX 43-3   SCOPE OF SERVICES PROVIDED THROUGH AN OCCUPATIONAL HEALTH AND SAFETY PROGRAM

- Health/medical surveillance
- Workplace monitoring/surveillance
- Health assessments
- Preplacement
- Periodic, mandatory, voluntary assessments and services
- Transfer of clients/services
- Retirement/termination
- Executive
- Return to work
- Health promotion
- Health screening
- Employee assistance programs
- Case management
- Primary health care for workers and dependents
- Worker safety and health education related to occupational hazards
- Job task analysis and design
- Prenatal and postnatal care and support groups
- Safety audits and accident prevention
- Workers' compensation management
- Risk management, loss control
- Emergency preparedness
- Pre-retirement counseling
- Integrated health benefits programs

respiratory protection or hearing conservation. The ability of a company to offer additional programs depends on employee needs, management's attitudes and understanding about health and safety, acceptance by the workers, and the economic status of the company. A significant increase in the number of health promotion and employee assistance programs offered in industry has occurred over the past few years. Health promotion programs focus on lifestyle choices that cause risks to health (e.g., job stress, obesity, smoking, stress responses, or lack of exercise) (O'Donnell, 2009). Employee assistance programs are designed to address personal problems (e.g., marital/family issues, substance abuse, or financial difficulties) that affect the employee's productivity. Since such efforts are cost-effective for businesses, they should continue to increase.

Similar types of occupational health and safety programs are available on a contractual basis from community-based providers. These may be offered by free-standing occupational health clinics, health maintenance organizations, hospitals, emergency clinics, and other health care organizations. In addition, consultants in each discipline work in the private sector (self-employed, in group practice, or in insurance companies) and in the public sector (in local and state health departments or departments of labor and industry). These services may be provided on-site, delivered at a specific location in the community, or offered through a mobile van that visits companies. These multiple resources have increased the options for companies that need occupational health and safety services, and they have also broadened the employment opportunities for health and safety professionals.

NURSING CARE OF WORKING POPULATIONS

The nurse is often the first health care provider seen by an individual with a work-related health problem. Consequently, nurses are in key positions to intervene with working populations at all levels of prevention. Prevention may be accomplished in the pre-pathogenesis period by measures designed to promote general optimal health, by protection against specific disease agents, or by the establishment of barriers against agents in the environment. These procedures have been termed *primary prevention.*

As soon as the disease is detectable, early in pathogenesis, secondary prevention may be accomplished by early diagnosis and prompt and adequate treatment. When the process of pathogenesis has progressed and the disease had advanced beyond its early stages, secondary prevention may be accomplished by means of adequate treatment to prevent sequelae and limit disability. Later, when defect and disability have been resolved, tertiary prevention may be accomplished by rehabilitation.

The occupational health nurse practices all levels of prevention (Rogers, 2011). Delivery of primary prevention services to employees is directed toward promoting health and averting a problem. In the occupational health setting, the purpose of health promotion is to maintain or enhance the well-being of individuals or groups of employees, and the company in general. This may include programs designed to enhance coping skills or good nutrition and knowledge about potential health hazards both inside and outside of the workplace.

Health protection (i.e., taking primary prevention measures) is designed to eliminate or reduce the risk of disease in order to prevent the development of an illness or injury. Walk-throughs by the occupational health nurse and/or other team members to identify workplace hazards are aimed at health protection.

Specific protection programs or interventions often require active participation on the part of the employee. Participation in an immunization program, employment of personal protective equipment such as respirators or gloves, and cessation of smoking are examples of specific health protection measures.

Secondary prevention occurs after a disease process has already begun. It is aimed at early detection, prompt treatment, and prevention of further limitations. For employees, early detection involves health surveillance and periodic screening to identify an illness at the earliest possible moment in its course, and elimination or modification of the hazard-producing situation. Interventions aimed at disability limitation are intended to prevent further harm or deterioration, and they include referral for counseling and treatment of an employee with an emotional or mental health problem whose work performance has deteriorated, as well as removal of workers from heavy-metal exposure who manifest neurological symptoms.

Tertiary prevention is intended to restore health as fully as possible and assist individuals to achieve their maximum level of functioning. Rehabilitation strategies such as return-to-work programs after a heart attack or limited duty programs after a cumulative trauma injury are examples of tertiary prevention.

Worker Assessment

The initial step of assessment involves the traditional history and physical assessment, emphasizing exposure to occupational hazards and individual characteristics that may predispose the client to the increased health risk of certain jobs. The occupational health history is an indispensable component of the health assessment of individuals (Rogers, 2011). Because work is a part of life for most people, including an occupational health history into all routine nursing assessments is essential. Many workers in the United States do not have access to health care services in their workplaces, yet it is not unusual to find health care providers in the community who have little or no knowledge about workplaces or expertise in occupation-related illnesses and injuries. Because of the large number of small businesses that do not have the resources for maintaining on-site health care, injured and ill workers are first seen in the public and private health care sector (e.g., in clinics, emergency departments, physicians' offices, hospitals, health maintenance organizations, and ambulatory care centers). Nurses are often the first-line assessors of these individuals and perhaps the only contact for education about self-protection from workplace hazards.

Identifying workplace exposures as sources of health problems may influence the client's course of illness and rehabilitation and may also prevent similar illnesses among others with potential for exposure (Levy and Wegman, 2006). Including occupational health data into client assessments begins with recognizing the possible relationship between health and occupational factors. The next step is to integrate into the history-taking procedure some routine assessment questions that will provide the data necessary to confirm or rule out occupationally induced symptoms. Symptoms of hazardous workplace exposures may be indicated by vague complaints involving any body system. These complaints are often similar to common medical problems. Three points that occupational health histories should include are a list of current and past jobs the client has held; questions about exposures to specific agents and relationships between the symptoms and activities at work, job titles, or history of exposures; and other factors that may influence the client's susceptibility to occupational agents (e.g., lifestyle history such as smoking, underlying illness, previous injury, or disabling condition).

Questions about the employee's occupational history can be included in existing assessment tools. The more complete the data collected, the more likely the nurse is to notice the influence of work-health interactions. All employees should be questioned about their employment history. To describe only a current status of "retired" or "housewife" may lead to the omission of needed data. The nurse should be aware that not all workers are well informed about the materials with which they work or about potential hazards. For this reason, the nurse must develop basic knowledge about all of the types of jobs held by clients and the possible hazards associated with them. Because there is an increased likelihood of multiple exposures from other environments such as the home and the community that may interact with workplace exposures, the nurse should extend the questioning to include this information.

Identifying work-related health problems should be an integrated focus of any assessment effort. A systematic approach for evaluating the potential for workplace exposures is the most effective intervention for detecting and preventing occupational health risks. Figure 43-7 shows one short assessment tool that can be incorporated into routine history taking. Similar questions can be included in the assessment of workers' spouses and dependents, who may receive second-hand or indirect exposure to occupational hazards.

During these health assessments, the nurse has the opportunity to teach about workplace hazards and prevention measures the worker can use. At the same time, the nurse is obtaining information that will be valuable in optimizing the fit between the job and the worker. Such assessments can be done during pre-placement examinations before the client begins a job, on a periodic basis during employment, or when a work-related health problem or exposure becomes apparent. Work-related health assessments should also be conducted when an employee is being transferred to another job with different requirements and exposures. The goal of these assessments is to identify agent and host factors that could place the employee at risk and to determine prevention steps that can be taken to eliminate or minimize the exposure and potential health problem.

When the health data from such assessments are considered collectively, the nurse may determine some patterns in risk factors associated with the occurrence of work-related injuries and illnesses in a total population of workers. For example, a nurse practitioner in a clinic noted a dramatic increase in the number of dermatitis cases among her clients. When she looked at factors in common among these individuals, she determined that they all worked at a company with solvent exposure commonly associated with dermal irritations. She worked with the union and the company to assess the environment/agent exposure to the employees. This nursing intervention led to a safer work environment and a decrease in dermatitis in this population group. Such an approach can be used at the company, industry, and community levels. The initial collection of data and the questioning about workplace exposures are vital steps for any intervention.

WHAT DO YOU THINK? *There is an acceptable level of risk in any job.*

Workplace Assessment

The nurse may conduct a similar assessment of the workplace itself. The purpose of this assessment, known as a **worksite walk-through** or survey, is to become knowledgeable about the work processes and the materials, the requirements of various jobs, the presence of actual or potential hazards, and the work practices of employees (Rogers, 2011). Figure 43-8 shows a brief outline that can be used to guide a worksite assessment. More complex surveys are performed by industrial hygienists and safety professionals when the purpose of the walk-through is environmental monitoring using sampling techniques or a safety audit. However, most occupational health nurses have developed expertise in these areas and include such tasks as part of their functions. For all health care providers who assess workers, this information makes an important database. In addition, for the on-site health care provider, worksite walk-throughs assist the professional in developing rapport with and being seen as a credible worker among the employees.

A worksite survey begins with an understanding of the type of work that occurs in the workplace. All business organizations are classified within the North American Industry Classification System (NAICS) with a numerical code. This code, usually a two- to four-digit number, indicates a company's product and, therefore, the possible types of **occupational health hazards** that may be associated with the processes and materials used by its employees. NAICS codes are used to collect and report data on businesses. For example, illness and injury rates of one company are compared with the rates of other companies of similar size with the same code to determine whether the company is having an excess of illness or injury. In addition, by knowing the NAICS code of a company, a health care professional can access reference books that describe the usual processes, materials, and by-products of that kind of company.

The nurse will want to review the work processes and work areas by jobs or locations in the workplace. These preliminary data provide clues about what hazards may be present and an understanding of the types of jobs and health requirements that may be involved in a particular industry. A description of the work environment is next and provides an overall picture of general appearances, physical layout, and safety of the environment. Are safety signs posted and readable where needed? Is

I. Present Job

A. What is your job title? _____

B. What do you do for a living?_____

C. How long have you had this job? _____

D. Describe the specific tasks of this job: _____
_____

E. What product or service is produced by the company where you work? _____
_____

F. Are you exposed to any of the following on your present job?
Metals   Radiation   Stress
Vapors, gases   Vibration   Others: _____
Dusts   Loud noise
Solvents   Extreme heat or cold

G. Do you feel you have any health problems that may be associated with your work?
If yes, describe: _____
_____

H. How would you describe your satisfaction with your job? _____
_____

I. Have any of your co-workers complained of illness or injuries that they associate with their jobs?
If yes, describe: _____
_____

II. All Past Work

Starting with your first job, please provide the following information:

Job title	Years held	Description of work	Exposures	Injuries/Illnesses	Personal protection equipment used

III. Other Exposures

A. Do you have any hobbies that involve exposure to chemicals, metals, or any of the other agents mentioned before? If yes, describe: _____

B. Are any other members of your household exposed to any of the substances listed above? If yes, describe:
_____

C. Do you live near any factories, dump sites, or other sources of pollution? If yes, describe: _____
_____

FIGURE 43-7 Occupational health history form.

Name of company: _____   Date: _____
Address: _____
Telephone: _____
Parent company (if any): _____
Location of corporate offices: _____
SIC code: _____

The Work

Major products: _____
Major processes and operations, raw materials, by-products: _____
_____
Type of jobs: _____
_____
_____
Potential exposures: _____
_____

Work Environment
General conditions: _____
Safety signs: _____
Physical environment: _____

Worker Population
Employees
Total number: _____ Number in production: _____ Others: _____
% Full-time: _____ % Men: _____ % Women: _____
% First shift: _____ % Second shift: _____ % Third shift: _____
Age distribution: _____
% Unionized: _____ Names of unions: _____

Human Resources Management
Corporate commitment to health
Personnel
Policies/procedures
Input/surveys/committees
Record keeping

Health Data
Work-related illnesses, injuries, deaths per annum: _____
OSHA recordable: _____ Workers' compensation: _____
Other: _____ Most frequent complaints: _____
Average number of monthly calls to the health unit: _____
Absenteeism rate: _____

Occupation Health and Safety Services
Examinations
Employee assistance
Treatment of illness/injury
Health education
Physical fitness, health promotion activities
Mandatory programs
Safety audits
Environmental monitoring
Health risk appraisal
Screenings
Health promotion

Control Strategies
Engineering
Work practice
Administrative
Personal protective equipment

FIGURE 43-8 Worksite assessment guide.

there clutter or dampness on the floor that could cause slips or falls?

A description of the employee group is necessary information to understand the demographics and the work distribution in the company. Knowing about shiftwork and productivity can be helpful in pinpointing potential stressors. Human resources' management and corporate commitment to health and safety are needed to develop a supportive culture for effective and efficient programming. Reviewing the status of policies and procedures and assessing opportunities for input into improving service are important to establish the organization's strength in occupational health and safety management. Gathering data about the incidence and prevalence of work-related illnesses and injuries and the cost patterns for these conditions provides useful epidemiological trend data and helps to target high-cost areas. The types of occupational safety and health services and programs are important to know. This will show whether required programs are being offered and includes health promotion and disease prevention strategies.

HOW TO Assess a Worker and the Workplace

Assessing the worker for a work-related problem is a critical practice element. You need to do the following:
- *Complete general and occupational health history-taking with emphasis on workplace exposure assessment, job hazard analysis, and list of previous jobs.*
- *Conduct a health assessment to identify agent and host factors that interact to place workers at risk.*
- *Identify patterns of risk associated with illness/injury.*
- *Assessing the work environment is necessary to determine workplace exposures that create worker health risk. You need to do the following:*
  - *Understand the work being done.*
  - *Understand the work process.*
  - *Evaluate the work-related hazards.*
  - *Gather data about incidence/prevalence of work-related illness/injuries and related hazards.*
  - *Conduct a walk-though of the work environment.*
  - *Examine prevention and control strategies in place for eliminating exposures.*

Finally, examining control strategies that are effective in eliminating or reducing exposure is important in determining risk reduction. Control strategies follow a hierarchical approach. Engineering controls can reduce worker exposure by modifying the exposure source, such as putting needles in a puncture-proof container.

Work practice controls include good hygiene and proper waste disposal and housekeeping. Administrative controls reduce exposure through job rotation, workplace monitoring, and employee training and education. Finally, personal protective control is the last resort and requires the worker to actively engage in strategies for protection such as use of gloves, masks, and gowns to prevent exposures (Rogers, 2011).

The more information that can be collected before the walk-through, the more efficient the process of the survey will be. After the survey is conducted, the nurse can use the information with the aggregate health data to evaluate the effectiveness of the occupational health and safety program and to plan future programs.

NURSING TIP *Both corporate culture and cost-effective programs are key factors in influencing the development of occupational health services.*

HEALTHY PEOPLE DOCUMENTS RELATED TO OCCUPATIONAL HEALTH

In an attempt to meet the goal of increasing the span of healthy life for Americans, health promotion and protection strategies are proposed to address the needs of large population groups such as the American workforce. As part of the *Healthy People 2010* document (USDHHS, 2000), occupational safety and health objectives were identified to promote good health and well-being among workers, including the elimination and reduction of elements in occupational environments that cause death, injury, disease, or disability. In addition, this document promotes the minimizing of personal damage from existing occupationally related illness. The new or revised occupational health objectives are shown in the *Healthy People 2020* box.

♥ HEALTHY PEOPLE 2020

Objectives Related to Occupational Health

- OSH-1: Reduce deaths from work-related injuries.
- OSH-2: Reduce nonfatal work related injuries.
- OSH-3: Reduce the rate of injuries and illness cases.
- OSH-4: Reduce pneumoconiosis deaths.
- OSH-5: Reduce deaths from work-related homicides.
- OSH-6: Reduce work-related assault.
- OSH-7: Reduce the proportion of persons who have elevated blood lead concentrations from work exposures.
- OSH-8: Reduce occupational skin diseases or disorders among full-time workers.
- OSH-9: (Developmental) Increase the proportion of employees who have access to worksites that provide programs to prevent or reduce employee stress.
- OSH-10: Reduce new cases of work-related noise-induced hearing loss.

From U.S. Department of Health and Human Services: *Healthy People 2020*, Washington, DC, 2010, U.S. Government Printing Office.

LEGISLATION RELATED TO OCCUPATIONAL HEALTH

The occupational health and safety services provided by an employer are influenced by specific legislation at federal and state levels. Although the relationship between work and health has been known since the second century (Ramazzini, 1713), public policy that effectively controlled occupational hazards was not enacted until the 1960s. The Mine Safety and Health Act of 1968 was the first legislation that specifically required

BOX 43-4 **FUNCTIONS OF FEDERAL AGENCIES INVOLVED IN OCCUPATIONAL SAFETY AND HEALTH**

Occupational Safety and Health Administration (OSHA)

- Determines and sets standards and permissible exposure limits (PELs) for hazardous exposures in the workplace.
- Enforces the occupational health standards (including the right of entry for inspection).
- Educates employees and employers about occupational health and safety.
- Develops and maintains a database of work-related injuries, illnesses, and deaths.
- Monitors compliance with occupational health and safety standards.

National Institute For Occupational Safety and Health (NIOSH)

- Conducts research and reviews findings to recommend exposure limits for occupational hazards to OSHA.
- Identifies and researches occupational health and safety hazards.
- Educates occupational health and safety professionals.
- Distributes research findings relevant to occupational health and safety.

From Centers for Disease Control and Prevention, U.S. Department of Health and Human Services, National Institute for Occupational Safety and Health: *National occupational research agenda,* Pub No 99-108, Washington, DC, 2003, U.S. Government Printing Office.

BOX 43-5 **NATIONAL OCCUPATIONAL RESEARCH AGENDA (NORA) SECTORS**

- Agriculture, forestry, and fishing
- Construction
- Healthcare and social assistance
- Manufacturing
- Mining
- Services
- Transportation, warehousing, and utilities
- Wholesale and retail trade

certain prevention programs for workers. This was followed by the Occupational Safety and Health Act of 1970, which established two agencies, OSHA and NIOSH, each with discrete functions (Box 43-4) to carry out the act's purpose of ensuring "safe and healthful working conditions for working men and women" (PL 91-596, 1970).

In the context of the Occupational Safety and Health Act, OSHA, a federal agency within the U.S. Department of Labor, was created to develop and enforce workplace safety and health standards and regulations that regulate workers' exposure to potentially toxic substances, enforcing these at the federal and state levels. Specific standards and information about compliance can be obtained from federal, regional, and state OSHA offices, which can be found on the OSHA website. The National Institute for Occupational Safety and Health (NIOSH) was established by the Occupational Safety and Health Act of 1970 and is part of the Centers for Disease Control and Prevention (CDC). In 1996 NIOSH and its partners unveiled the National Occupational Research Agenda (NORA), a framework to guide occupational safety and health research into the following decade. The NIOSH agency identifies, monitors, and educates about the incidence, prevalence, and prevention of work-related illnesses and injuries and examines potential hazards of new work technologies and practices (USDHHS, NIOSH, 2010). NORA (Box 43-5) is focused on targeted sectors to reduce the still significant toll of workplace illness and injury.

Many standards have been established by OSHA and promulgated to protect worker health. One example is the Hazard Communication Standard. This standard is based on the premise that while working to reduce and eliminate potentially toxic agents in the work environment, an important line of defense is to provide the work community with information about hazardous chemicals in order to minimize exposures. The Hazard Communication Standard, which was first established in 1983, requires that all worksites with hazardous substances inventory their toxic agents, label them, and provide information sheets, called material safety data sheets (MSDSs), for each agent. In addition, the employer must have in place a hazard communication program that provides workers with education about these agents. This education must include agent identification, toxic effects, and protective measures. Numerous standards have been established by OSHA for specific chemicals and programs. A standard familiar to all health care professionals is the *Bloodborne Pathogens Standard.*

Workers' compensation acts are important state laws that govern financial compensation to employees who suffer work-related health problems. These acts vary by state, and each state sets rules for the reimbursement of employees with occupational health problems for medical expenses and lost work time associated with the illness or injury. Workers' compensation claims and the experience-based insurance premiums paid by industry have been important motivators for increasing the health and safety of the workplace.

NURSING TIP *NIOSH publications, many of which are free, are online at http://www.cdc.gov/niosh/homepage.html.*

DISASTER PLANNING AND MANAGEMENT

Although disaster planning and management have been functions of occupational health and safety programs, this is an area of legislation that affects businesses and health professionals. The legislation of the Superfund Amendment and Reauthorization Act (SARA) requires that written disaster plans be shared with key resources in the community, such as fire departments and emergency departments. Concern about disasters—such as the terrorist attacks on the World Trade Center and Pentagon on September 11, 2001; the methyl isocyanate leak in Bhopal, India; effects of hurricanes such as Katrina; or the community exposure to chemicals at Times Beach, Missouri, and exposure to radiation from crippled nuclear plants in Japan—has mandated more attention to disaster planning.

In occupational health, the goals of a disaster plan are to prevent or minimize injuries and deaths of workers and residents, minimize property damage, provide effective triage, and facilitate necessary business activities. A disaster plan requires the cooperation of different personnel within the company and community. The nurse is often a key person on the disaster planning team, along with safety professionals, physicians, industrial hygienists, the fire chief, and company management. The potential for disaster (e.g., explosions, floods, fires, leaks) must be identified, and this is best achieved by completing an exhaustive chemical and hazard inventory of the workplace. The material safety data sheet and plant blueprints are critical for correctly identifying substances and work areas that may be hazardous. Worksite surveys are the first step to completing this inventory.

Effective disaster plans are designed by those with knowledge of the work processes and materials, the workers and workplace, and the resources in the community. Specific steps must be detailed for actions to be put in place by specific individuals in the event of a disaster. The written plan must be shared with all who will be involved. Employees should be prepared in first aid, cardiopulmonary resuscitation, and fire brigade procedures. Plans must be clear, specific, and comprehensive (i.e., covering all shifts and all work areas) and must include activities to be conducted within the worksite and those that require community resources. Transportation plans, fire response, and emergency response services should be coordinated with the agencies that would be involved in an actual disaster. The disaster plan, emergency and safety equipment, and the first response team's abilities should be tested at least annually with a drill. Practice results should be carefully evaluated, with changes made as needed.

Hospitals and other emergency services, such as fire departments, should be involved in developing the disaster plan and should receive a copy of the plan and a current hazard inventory. It is imperative that the plan and hazard inventory be periodically updated. The occupational health nurse or another company representative should provide emergency health care providers with updated clinical information on exposures and appropriate treatment. It should never be presumed that local services will have current information on substances used in industry. Representatives of these agencies should visit the worksite and accompany the nurse on a worksite walk-through so that they are familiar with the operations.

In disaster planning, the nurse is often assigned or assumes the responsibility for coordinating the planning and implementing efforts, working with appropriate key people within the company and in the community to develop a workable, comprehensive plan. Other tasks include providing ongoing communication to keep the plan current; planning the drills; educating the employees, management, and community providers; and assessing the equipment and services that may be used in a disaster.

In the event of a disaster, the nurse should play a key role in coordinating the response. Principles of triage may be used as the response team determines the extent of the disaster and the ability of the company and community to respond. Post-disaster nursing interventions are also critical. Examples include identifying the ongoing disaster-related health needs of workers and community residents, collecting epidemiological data, and assessing the cause and the necessary steps to prevent a recurrence.

Occupational health nursing is a broad, dynamic specialty practice. The Public Health Foundation provides the basis for practice, supporting a health promotion and protection and prevention model. The occupational health nurse must have interprofessional skills and linkages to provide the most effective care and service. Occupational health nurses are involved in all levels of prevention in their practice (see the Levels of Prevention box).

LEVELS OF PREVENTION

Occupational Health

Primary Prevention
Nurse provides education on use of personal protective equipment in the workplace to prevent injury/exposure.

Secondary Prevention
Nurse screens for hearing loss resulting from noise levels in the plant.

Tertiary Prevention
Nurse works with chronic diabetic workers to ensure appropriate medication use and blood glucose screening to avoid lost work days.

CHAPTER REVIEW

PRACTICE APPLICATION

An insurance company recently renovated its claims processing office area and fitted the workstation with new computers. The company's occupational health nurse noticed an increase in visits to the health unit for complaints of headaches, stiff neck muscles, and visual disturbances consistent with computer usage.

To conduct a complete investigation of this problem, the nurse assessed the workers, the agent (computer), previously existing potential agents, and the work environment. Interventions focused on designing the health hazard out of the work process, if possible. In the present example, the first level of intervention was to refit the workstation for better worker use of the computer.

Minimizing the possible hazards of the agent involved recommendations for desks, chairs, and lighting designs that would accommodate the individual worker and allow shielding of the monitor. The nursing interventions included strengthening the resistance of the host by prescribing appropriate rest breaks, eye exercises, and relaxation strategies. Recognizing that previous cer-

vical neck injury or impaired vision may increase the risk of adverse effects from computer work, the nurse would include assessment for these factors in employees' preplacement and periodic health examinations.

For the environmental concerns, the nurse educated the manager about the health risks of paced, externally controlled work expectations and recommended alternatives.

This case is an example of which of the following?
A. The application of the occupational health history
B. A worksite assessment or walk-through
C. A work-health interaction
D. The use of the Epidemiologic Triangle in exploring occupational health problems

Answers can be found on the Evolve site.

KEY POINTS

- Occupational health nursing is an autonomous practice specialty.
- The scope of occupational health nursing practice is broad, including worker and workplace assessment and surveillance, case management, health promotion, primary care, management/administration, business and finance skills, and research.
- The workforce and workplace are changing dramatically, requiring new knowledge and new occupational health services.
- The type of work has shifted from primarily manufacturing to service and technological jobs.
- Workplace hazards include exposure to biological, chemical, enviromechanical, physical, and psychosocial agents.
- The Occupational Safety and Health Act of 1970 states that workers must have a safe and healthful work environment.
- The interprofessional occupational health team consists of the occupational health nurse, occupational medicine physician, industrial hygienist, and safety specialist.
- Work-related health problems must be investigated and control strategies implemented to reduce exposure.

- Control strategies include engineering, work practice, administration, and personal protective equipment.
- The Occupational Safety and Health Administration enforces workplace safety and health standards.
- The National Institute for Occupational Safety and Health is the education and research agency that provides grants to investigate the causes of workplace illness and injuries.
- Workers' compensation acts are important laws that govern financial compensation of employees who suffer work-related health problems.
- The occupational health nurse should play a key role in disaster planning and coordination.
- Academic education in occupational health nursing is generally at the graduate level.

CLINICAL DECISION-MAKING ACTIVITIES

1. Arrange to visit a local industry to observe work processes and discuss working conditions. See if you can identify the work-related hazards and make recommendations for eliminating them.
2. Interview the occupational health nurse in an industry setting and ask questions about scope of practice, job functions, and contributions to the business. Compare and contrast what you have learned about this nurse role to that of the school health nurse.

3. Contact the American Association of Occupational Health Nurses and ask what the most pressing trends are in the specialty. What are some of the complex issues related to these trends?
4. Obtain a proposed standard from the Occupational Safety and Health Administration, critique it, and submit your comments.
5. Attend a workers' compensation hearing, analyze the problem, and critique the outcome. How is your critique affected by what you thought the outcome should be?

REFERENCES

American Association of Occupational Health Nurses: *The nurse in industry*, New York, 1976, AAOHN.

American Association of Occupational Health Nurses: *Standards of occupational health nursing practice*, Atlanta, 2004, AAOHN.

American Association of Occupational Health Nurses: *Code of ethics*, Atlanta, 2004, AAOHN.

American Association of Occupational Health Nurses: *Foundation Blocks XII: Developing occupational health job description*, Pensacola, 2007, Florida.

Bartsch KJ: *The employment projections for 2008-18*. Available at www.bls.gov/opub/mlr/2009/11/art1exc.htm. Accessed March 19, 2011.

Brown M: *Occupational health nursing*, New York, 1981, MacMillan.

Bureau of Labor Statistics: A special issue: charting the projections—2004-2014, *Occupat Outlook Q* 43:2–38, 2005a.

Bureau of Labor Statistics: *Employment and wages*, Washington, DC, 2005b, U.S. Department of Labor.

Bureau of Labor Statistics: *Lost work time injuries and illnesses: characteristics and resulting time away from work*, Washington, DC, 2006, U.S. Department of Labor.

Bureau of Labor Statistics: *Handbook of labor statistics*, Washington, DC, 2007, U.S. Department of Labor.

Bureau of Labor Statistics: *Older workers*, 2008a. Available at www.bls.gov/spotlight/2008/older workers. Accessed August 5, 2010.

Bureau of Labor Statistics: *Overview of 2008-2018 population projection, Occupational outlook handbook*, 2008b. Available at www.bls.gov.

Bureau of Labor Statistics: *Occupations with the fastest growth (2009)*, 2008c. Available at www.bls.gov/emp/ep_table_103.htm. Accessed March 19, 2011.

Bureau of Labor Statistics: *Workplace injury and illness summary*, 2009. Available at www.bls.gov/news.release/osh.nr0.htm. Accessed March 19, 2011.

Bureau of Labor Statistics: *Handbook of labor statistics*, Washington, DC, 2007, U.S. Department of Labor.

Bureau of Labor Statistics: *Survey of occupational injuries and illnesses. Nonfatal (OSHA recordable) injuries and illnesses. Industry incidence rates and counts*, Washington, DC, 2009, U.S. Department of Labor.

USDHHS, CDC, NIOSH: *State of the Sector/Healthcare and Social Assistance*, Pub No. 2009-139, Washington, D.C, 2009, Author.

Felton J: The genesis of American occupational health nursing, part 1, *Occupat Health Nurs* 33:615, 1985.

Ganczak M, Szych Z: Surgical nurses and compliance with personal protective equipment, *J Hosp Infect* 66:346–351, 2007.

Gordis L: *Epidemiology*, ed 4, St Louis, 2008, Elsevier.

Health Resources and Services Administration, Bureau of Health Professions: *The National Sample Survey of Registered Nurses 2004, documentation for the general public use file*, 2006. Available at http://datawarehouse.hrsa.gov/nssrn.aspx. Accessed March 19, 2011.

Hollmann FW, Mulder TJ, Kallan JE: *Methodology and assumptions for population projections of the United States: 1999-2100*, Population division working paper no 38, Washington, DC, 2000, Bureau of Census, U.S. Department of Commerce.

Institute of Medicine: *Safe work in the 21st century*, Washington, DC, 2000, National Academy Press.

Jensen PA, Lambert LA, Iademarco MF, et al: Guidelines for preventing the transmission of mycobacterium tuberculosis in health care settings, *Morb Mortal Wkly Rep* 54(RR17), 2005.

Levy BS, Wegman DH: *Occupational health: recognizing and preventing occupational disease*, Philadelphia, 2006, Lippincott Williams & Wilkins.

McGrath B: Fifty years of industrial nursing, *Public Health Nurs* 37:119, 1945.

Mosisa A, Hipple S: Trends in labor force participation in the U.S, *Monthly Labor Review* 129:35–57, 2006. Available at www.bls.gov.

National Institute for Occupational Safety and Health: *Occupational respiratory disease surveillance*, 2008. Available at www.cdc/niosh.gov. Accessed March 19, 2011.

O'Donnell M: Definition of health promotion: Embracing passion, enhancing motivation, recognizing dynamic balance, and creating opportunities, *Am J Health Promot* 24(1):IV, 2009.

Panlilio A, Cardo DM, Grohskopf LA, et al: Updated U.S. Public Health Service guidelines for the management of occupational exposures to HIV and recommendations for post exposure prophylaxis, *Morbid Mortal Wkly Rep* 54(RR9), 2005.

Petsonk L, Levy B: Latex allergy. In Levy BS, Wagner GR, Rest KM, Weeks JL, editors: *Preventing occupational disease and injury*, Washington, DC, 2005, APHA, pp 298–301.

Public Law 91-596: *The Occupational Safety and Health Act*, Washington, DC, 1970, U.S. Department of Labor.

Ramazzini B: *De morbis artificum* [diseases of workers], 1713 (translated by Wright WC, Chicago, 1940, University of Chicago Press).

Rogers B: Perspectives on occupational health nursing, *AAOHN J* 36:100–105, 1988.

Rogers B: *Occupational health nursing: concepts and practice*, St Louis, 2011, Elsevier.

U.S. Census Bureau: *World and Population Clocks*, 2009. Available at www.census.gov. Accessed May 11, 2011.

U.S. Department of Health and Human Services, National Institute for Occupational Safety and Health: *National occupational research agenda*, Cincinnati, OH, 2010, USDHHS.

U.S. Department of Health and Human Services: *Healthy People 2010: understanding and improving health*, ed 2, Washington, DC, 2000, U.S. Government Printing Office.

U.S. Department of Health and Human Services, National Institute for Occupational Safety and Health: *The changing organization of work and the safety and health of working people*, Pub No 2002-116, Cincinnati, OH, 2002, USDHHS.

U.S. Department of Health and Human Services, National Institute for Occupational Safety and Health: *Workers health chartbook*, 2004, Pub No. 2004-16, Washington, DC, 2004, USDHHS/NIOSH.

CHAPTER 44

Forensic Nursing in the Community

Susan B. Patton, DNSc, PNP-BC

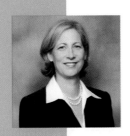

Dr. Susan Patton is a Board Certified Pediatric Nurse Practitioner and co-proprietor of East Arkansas Children's Clinic, in Forrest City, Arkansas, where she has lived for the past 25 years. She serves as Medical Consultant to Kids for the Future, a developmental preschool located in Forrest City. In addition, Dr. Patton works with victims of child abuse and sexual assault in her general pediatric practice. In her faculty position at the University of Tennessee College of Nursing, she is the Coordinator of the Doctor of Nursing Practice program focused on forensic nursing. Her major areas of research and practice are developmental pediatrics and injury/violence prevention. Dr. Patton has served on the Education Committee of the International Association of Forensic Nurses, President of the Forensic Nurse Certification Board, and Chair of the Ad Hoc Committee for Advanced Practice Portfolio Credentialing Committee. Dr. Patton has received a number of awards in her career including the Arkansas Advance Practice Nurse of the Year, a special recognition from the Arkansas General Assembly for her service to Arkansas, the Dr. John Runyan Award for Community Health Nursing, the UTHSC Excellence in Teaching award, the Arkansas Foundation for Medical Care Innovator's award, and the Arkansas Nurses Distinguished Service award.

ADDITIONAL RESOURCES

℮volve WEBSITE
http://evolve.elsevier.com/Stanhope
- *Healthy People 2020*
- Quiz

- Case Studies
- Glossary
- Answers to Practice Application

OBJECTIVES

After reading this chapter, the student will be able to do the following:

1. Describe the specialized competencies and skills of the forensic nurse within the nursing process.
2. Discuss the relationship of the forensic nurse with public health professionals in addressing injury as a public health concern.
3. List the health risks that result from incidents of injury.
4. Identify how forensic nurses deal with injuries in the three levels of prevention.
5. Discuss the health disparities that contribute to the occurrence and poor outcomes in marginalized groups who experience injury.
6. Explain the contribution of theoretical underpinnings to current models of forensic nursing practice.
7. Identify client populations and clinical arenas in the community where forensic nurses practice.
8. Define the key terms and concepts within forensic nursing theory.
9. Identify professionals who commonly work in collaboration with the forensic nurse in addressing injury care and prevention.

KEY TERMS

adjudication, p. 960
forensic, p. 958
forensic nurse examiner, p. 958
forensic nursing, p. 958

injury, p. 963
justice, p. 963
legal nurse consultants, p. 960
perceptivity, p. 963

sexual assault nurse examiner (SANE), p. 958
victimization, p. 963

Appreciation is given to Drs. Karen Landenburger and Jacquelyn Campbell for providing some content related to forensic nursing that was moved from Chapter 38, which discusses violence in the community.

PERSPECTIVES ON FORENSICS AND FORENSIC NURSING

Injuries resulting from crime and victimization cause pain and suffering and may cause disability, economic failure, and "distress of the human spirit" (Lynch, 2006, p 24). However, such injuries have often taken a back seat to treatment of disease and infection. Today forensic nurses expertly care for victims of injuries, largely as a community-based specialty, from a medical as well as a legal perspective. Whether the injury is caused by intentional violence or unintentional accident, forensic nurses are involved with not only the treatment but also the prevention of what is now the leading cause of death in the first four decades of life (CDC, 2009). The burden of injuries to individuals ranges from minimal and brief to debilitating or fatal. The economic burden worldwide is tremendous. In the United States, in 2000 alone, the 50 million injuries that required medical treatment were estimated to cost up to $406 billion. These total costs, for both fatal and non-fatal injuries, include estimates of $80.2 billion in medical care costs and $326 billion in productivity losses, which include lost wages and the accompanying fringe benefits, as well as the lost ability to perform normal household responsibilities (Finkelstein, Corso, and Miller, 2006). Because injuries result from a wide variety of physical, environmental, and behavioral causes, risk reduction comes from a variety of approaches. Forensic nurses have a unique set of skills for dealing with injury, and these skills will be discussed in this chapter.

Forensic means pertaining to the law. Forensic nursing synthesizes the biopsychosocial and spiritual aspects of nursing care with an expert understanding of forensic science and the criminal justice process. Forensic nursing is distinguished by its unique body of knowledge and skills as well as by the practice arenas and client population served. The skill set is defined by the scope and standards of practice, which includes skills such as collection, documentation, and preservation of evidence and other findings that may later have implications in the prosecution of a crime. Practice standards also reflect care given to both the living and the dead, victims of trauma and perpetrators of crime, as well as individuals and groups within a community. Forensic nurses often have experience in emergency and trauma services and can provide an expert analysis of wounding patterns and physiological response to injury. They are able to compassionately care for individuals and families who experience emotional reactions to trauma from a variety of causes. While the majority of forensic nurses in the United States are sexual assault nurse examiners (SANEs), other roles exist to care for survivors of other crimes, liability-related injury, and deaths. These include the clinical forensic nurse, forensic nurse examiner or investigator, forensic psychiatric nurse, forensic correctional nurse, legal nurse consultant, nurse attorney, and nurse coroner or death investigator. Arenas of care include but are not limited to emergency departments and community-based urgent care clinics, offices of the medical examiner and coroner, investigative units of law enforcement and criminal justice agencies, and governmental programs of safety prevention.

Forensic nursing care largely occurs in collaboration with professionals, both within and outside of nursing, including but not limited to public health professionals including epidemiologists, law enforcement and corrections officers, emergency department providers, and psychiatric practitioners. Forensic nurses also work collaboratively with public health nurses who bring a population focus to injury prevention programs. As part of a public health approach to crime, forensic nurses serve as content experts, clinician advisors, and/or the clinical managers of care facilities that may contribute to a community response to injury prevention.

INJURY PREVENTION

Not surprisingly, the health determinants of injury, identified in *Healthy People 2020*, mirror disease occurrence in a community. The rate of injury and crime is lower in communities that promote good health. Where inequities of resources and education exist, health disparity, violence, and other crimes rise and accidental injuries occur more often (Weissling, 2002). Trauma victims are overrepresented in minority, disenfranchised, and disadvantaged groups. Disparity can also be seen in the prosecution, conviction, and incarceration of individuals of minority groups in many countries. In the United States, one in three African-American males and one in six Latinos will be incarcerated sometime in their lives (Mauer, 2009). Populations that experience more disease also experience more violent as well as accidental injury, and more events that lead to prosecution. The measures that improve overall health, lower risk, and reduce disparity also reduce physical and emotional injury. Injury now joins certain categories of disease, disability, and premature death as a major preventable health state. Reducing injury reflects the goals of *Healthy People 2020* as well as goals of other organizations such as the U.S. Public Health Service, the Centers for Disease Control and Prevention (CDC), the World Health Organization (WHO), and the International Association of Forensic Nurses.

The National Center for Injury Prevention and Control, within the CDC, was established in 1997 to coordinate prevention of injuries, violence, and their consequences. The work of this center includes providing grants that fund prevention programs, dissemination of research findings, and maintenance of a website, blogs, podcasts, and electronic newsletters. This funding helps to inform the public of the epidemiology of injury and to provide other resources for professionals. The Center's website includes information about home and recreational safety, traumatic brain injury, injury data and statistics, injury response, motor vehicle safety, and violence prevention (CDC, 2009).

> **DID YOU KNOW?** *The International Association of Forensic Nurses (http://www.iafn.org) list 535 sexual assault centers in the United States. Forensic Nurse Death Investigators serve as trainers for the CDC's National Sudden Unexpected Infant Death Investigation program.*

HEALTHY PEOPLE 2020 GOALS, PREVENTION, AND FORENSIC NURSING

The *Healthy People 2020* goals that deal with reducing injury and violence in the United States reflect the breadth of concerns and problems that result in injury, both intentional and unintentional in communities. Objectives related to safety, violence, injury, and sexual assault are incorporated throughout the *Healthy People 2020* document. These objectives relate to injuries that are both intentional and unintentional.

♥ HEALTHY PEOPLE 2020

Objectives Pertaining to Injury

> The following proposed objectives are examples that pertain to injury and are relevant in forensic nursing:
> * IVP-29: Reduce homicides.
> * IVP-30: Reduce firearm-related deaths.
> * IVP-33: Reduce physical assaults.
> * IVP-34: Reduce physical fighting among adolescents.
> * IVP-36: Reduce weapon carrying by adolescents on school property.
> * IVP-40: Reduce sexual violence.

U.S Department of Health and Human Services: *Healthy People 2020.* Available at http://www.healthypeople.gov/2020/default.aspx. Accessed June 8, 2011.

Nurses who work in the area of forensics use all three levels of prevention. For example, forensic nurses (FNs) promote safety

in their involvement with projects that aim to prevent domestic violence, sexual assault, child abuse, and accidental injuries before they occur (primary prevention) in program development and management of care centers. Community awareness of violent crimes is achieved in concert with certain programs and the community-based professionals who work there. Secondary prevention is practiced following the occurrence of injuries and crime. Forensic nurses provide direct care to both victims and perpetrators. Their expertise serves the individual as well as the community in the collection of evidence for the legal justice system. Compassionate holistic care aims to minimize the spiritual, psychological, physical, and social trauma, as well as the financial burden. If disability, incarceration, or death occurs, FNs provide tertiary care in settings appropriate to address rehabilitation or identify factors that have put individuals at risk.

📋 LEVELS OF PREVENTION

Intentional injury

> **Primary Prevention**
> Develop programs that promote safety and avoidance of violence, including both intentional violence and unintentional accidents.
>
> **Secondary Prevention**
> Provide timely, sensitive, direct care to both victims of injury and perpetrators of crime and violent behavior.
>
> **Tertiary Prevention**
> When injury has occurred, refer clients to appropriate community services for appropriate follow-up care and rehabilitation of the effects of trauma.

> **NURSING TIP** *Evidence should be collected in such a way that the collection itself protects rather than destroys or alters the evidence.*

FORENSIC NURSING AS A SPECIALTY AREA THAT PROVIDES CARE IN THE COMMUNITY

Within communities, the growing prevalence of "criminal and negligence-based trauma" indicates a need for health professionals who can intercede with skills that address social justice as well as care for social offenders (Lynch, 2010, p 17). Thus, forensic nurses respond to sexual assault, drug- and alcohol-related crimes, incidents of human trafficking, elder mistreatment, child abuse, gang violence, as well as mass disaster, automobile accidents, and work-related injuries. In each situation, forensic nurses look for historical, behavioral, and physical indicators that a crime has been committed and intentional injury has occurred. For example, children who are abused may have cigarette burns, bite marks, pressure sores, and other physical signs that parents may claim to be the result of accidents. Münchausen syndrome by proxy is a form of child abuse in which the primary caregiver uses the child as a mechanism to gain attention. The caregiver often causes illnesses and subsequent symptoms in the child (Finn, 2010).

BOX 44-1   EMERGENCY RESPONSE TO ASSAULT VICTIMS

1. Use standardized medical treatment and forensic protocols.
2. Assess for sexual assault using "forced sex" terminology rather than "rape" or "sexual assault," and call a sexual assault nurse examiner if appropriate.
3. Support privacy of assault victim.
4. Explain procedures clearly to the assault victim.
5. Document location, date, and time of assault.
6. Collect evidence in a systematic format; take pictures if necessary.
7. Take care not to destroy evidence while giving care.
8. Maintain chain of evidence.
9. Maintain evidence integrity.
10. Document the following:
    a. Injuries
    b. Emotional state
    c. Medical history
    d. Victim's account of assault
11. Identify and refer to resources that can be used after the assault.

From U.S. Department of Justice, Office on Violence Against Women: *A national protocol for sexual assault medical forensic examinations adults/adolescents,* 2004. Available at http://www.ncjrs.gov/pdffiles1/ovw/206554.pdf. Accessed August 20, 2010.

abuse, and intimate partner violence. He states that documentation should include written documentation as well as forensic photography. Written forms of documentation should be as verbatim as possible, with the use of declarative statements and body maps. When possible, use a 35-mm or digital camera to take the necessary photographs. The photographs should be taken in context, with two or more photos focusing more clearly on the injury. Injuries should also be depicted on diagrams and recorded in the nurses' notes. The How To box describes how to label photographs taken after the injury.

HOW TO   Label photos

All photos should be clearly labeled with the following information:
- *Client's name*
- *Client's medical identification number*
- *Client's date of birth*
- *The data and time of the photograph*
- *The name of the photographer*
- *The body location of the injury*
- *The forensic case number*

From Sheridan DJ: *Legal and forensic nursing responses to family violence.* In Humphrey J, Campbell JC, editors: *Family violence and nursing practice,* Philadelphia, 2004, Lippincott Williams & Wilkins.

A client who is admitted to a hospital with traumatic injuries should be evaluated as to the potentially forensic nature of the injuries (Sheridan and Nash, 2009). The response to victims of assault includes a number of steps, as outlined in Box 44-1. The nurse most often comes in contact with police, victims, and perpetrators of violence or crime in the emergency department. The nurse provides a vital link between the investigative process, health care, and the court (Sachs, Weinberg, and Wheeler, 2008). Nurses should take specific actions when they come in contact with victims. It is important that evidence be carefully collected and that the person who is doing the collection be systematic in this process.

One example of appropriate forensic care is that when cutting a shirt off a victim who has been shot in the chest, avoid cutting through the bullet hole in the shirt. Rather, it should be cut to the side of the hole to protect the point of origin of the bullet for later criminal investigation. The collection of DNA provides a significant role in criminal investigations. It is essential that DNA be collected correctly and that elimination samples of DNA be collected from authorized people at the crime scene and from the victim (USDOJ/Office on Violence Against Women, 2004).

The most common types of trace evidence of victims of violence, including those who are raped, are clothing, bullets, bloodstains, hairs, fibers, and small pieces of material such as fragments of metal, glass, paint, and wood. In the investigation of sexual assault, an evidence kit should be used within 72 hours of the assault with specimens collected and preserved according to state crime lab procedures. Clothing should be handled only by the victim or nurse wearing protective gloves. Throughout the collection process, the nurse takes every opportunity to show compassion to the victim of the assault while maintaining objectivity in recording observations (Houmes, Fagan, and Quintana, 2003).

Sheridan (2004) provides a useful guide to assessment of all forms of violence, including child abuse and neglect, elderly

Forensic nurses may have alternative specialties that are combined for a special population. Advanced practice nurses (APNs) such as psychiatric, pediatric, geriatric and acute care nurse practitioners bring to forensic nursing skills that allow them to provide advanced assessment and prescription of medications and treatments needed by forensic clients. Notably, forensic psychiatric nurses treat both victims of post-traumatic stress disorder and seriously emotionally disturbed clients incarcerated for violent crimes. APNs in correctional facilities may identify themselves as forensic nurses when they manage acute and chronic illness, promote wellness, and work in these systems to develop policies around legal and ethical issues.

The specialty also incorporates three subspecialties of nursing practice that are located within the criminal justice system: forensic nurse, nurse attorney, and legal nurse consultant. Forensic nurses employed in the criminal justice arena generally provide care to individuals who are either victims of injury or perpetrators of a crime that is under investigation. **Legal nurse consultants** provide expert consultation regarding health care to attorneys in either civil or criminal court but do not render direct client care in that setting. Some of these situations might include medical malpractice, personal injury, workers' compensation, and probate. Nurse attorneys hold a license from a state bar association in addition to a nursing license and generally use their nursing knowledge for adjudication. **Adjudication** refers to a judicial decision or a sentence.

Finally, forensic nurses are advocates for programs that prevent injuries, which occur as a result of both intentional injury and health hazards related to environments that create injury. Relying on an understanding of epidemiology, these nurses have knowledge of occurrence as well as the mechanisms of injury in a community. Forensic nurses partner with public health professionals including nurses to design, implement, and evaluate projects and programs that have a forensic focus.

History of Forensic Nursing

Early writings about the evolution of modern nursing, particularly with regard to care given to victims of war, mental illness, and abuse, lays a foundation for the advent of forensic nurses in the twentieth century (Nutting and Dock, 1907). Chapter 1 discusses the history of public health nursing; this section emphasizes nursing history's linkages to forensic nursing. With public health nurses, forensic nurses celebrate the early pioneers working in communities that brought medical care to the most vulnerable and marginalized. They worked to develop national and international organizations such the National Organization for Public Health Nursing (1912), National Society of Nurses (later the American Nurses Association [ANA], 1912), the International Congress of Nursing (1912), and the WHO (1948). These organizations were designed to give structure and standards for care and education regarding issues of violence and neglect. These issues pertain to public health, mental health, and forensic nurses who are experts in dealing with the effects of trauma, and who advocate for care of the wounded, both physically and emotionally.

Contemporary practice of forensic nursing in the United States was largely propelled by early efforts to identify and prevent child abuse and neglect and sexual assault of women. In the 1940s through the 1960s, radiologists identified fractures that they linked to assault and pediatricians began describing indicators of "battered child syndrome" (Gurevich, 2010). Subsequently, nurses became aware of their role in identifying indicators of assault. In emergency departments, forensic nurses stepped forward to assist in "rape" kit collection, with compassion and competence in preserving crucial evidence and a strong understanding of the "rape trauma syndrome" first described by Burgess in 1973. Burgess and other advanced practice nurses initiated previously undescribed care with forensic clients. The first nurse-run sexual assault clinics opened in Memphis and Minneapolis in 1974 (Speck, n.d.) with subsequent development of the first protocols for sexual assault care (Ledray, 1998). In 1985 the U.S. Surgeon General identified violence as a health care issue, and health care providers such as nurses working with victims and perpetrators of crimes, as key agents in ameliorating the effects of violence in our communities (History of IAFN, 2010). In 1990, Virginia Lynch published her dissertation on the role description and integrated model of forensic nursing care of both living and deceased victims of trauma and perpetrators of crime (Lynch, 1990). By 1992, The Joint Commission began to require hospitals to develop protocols for the treatment of victims of sexual assault. At the present time most victims of sexual assault go to emergency departments. The lack of availability of trained providers spurred the development of SANE programs.

Today, the Integrated Model of Forensic Nursing is recognized internationally as the basis for practice as well as education of forensic nurses. Following efforts to describe the unique contribution of forensic nursing (Lynch, 1986), the specialty was recognized by the American Academy of Forensic Science in 1991. The following year SANEs from the United States and Canada established the International Association of Forensic Nurses (IAFN). Subsequently, the ANA designated forensic nursing as a specialty in 1995 and it is now recognized as one of the fastest growing specialties in nursing. IAFN boasts a membership of over 3000 nurses worldwide and has members in over 24 countries.

Educational Preparation

Historically, forensic nurses refined and developed their forensic skills through clinical practice and continuing education. Today, there are three primary routes for training in forensic nursing. First, nurses can gain additional skills and knowledge through continuing education courses or basic concepts introduced in generalist education. Second, certificate programs include specific content, entrance requirements, and often clinical opportunities. Third, graduate nursing academic programs are offering minors or concentrations in forensic nursing.

Formal graduate course work on forensic nursing was first introduced at the University of Texas, Arlington in 1986. To begin a specialty by starting with graduate preparation is both uncommon and courageous; more often content is introduced in the undergraduate studies, and graduate study assists in refining and developing the content until it is formalized in courses and majors. By 2000 there were 12 graduate programs preparing clinical nurse specialists and nurse practitioners with a focus on forensic nursing. The development of the scope and standards of practice and a core curriculum for graduate study in 2004 facilitated the development of new programs of study and formed the basis for advanced practice credentialing of students and practicing clinicians. A forensic focus in research became more prevalent in both master's and doctoral studies, which facilitated the opening of the first doctor of nursing practice (DNP) program focused on forensic nursing in 2002 at the University of Tennessee Health Science Center in Memphis. Now, new DNP programs are opening based on this model of advanced nursing practice.

The inclusion of forensic nursing content into undergraduate generalist education remains controversial. The American Association of Nurse Attorneys (TAANA) and the IAFN have recommended coursework regarding public and private legal proceedings. Students need to develop a working understanding of laws and procedures applicable to nursing practice and certain client situations, such as mandated reporting of child abuse (Morrison, 1999). In addition, nurses are prepared to care for families experiencing trauma. Many educators in the United States believe the complexity of forensic content has evolved so that the skills and competencies required to differentiate the specialty are not appropriate in a generalist educational curriculum. However, guidelines for the introduction of core concepts such as the physiological response to violence and risk factors for maltreatment are under development by educators in IAFN.

Theoretical Foundations of Forensic Nursing

Humans seek stability; they seek safety from physical trauma and emotional wounding from violent relationships; and they seek protection of their finances and freedom from fears that threaten their very understanding of human existence. Theories that contribute to our understanding of what constitutes safety and well-being have been extrapolated from a variety of sources outside of nursing. Maslow, an American psychologist, developed a hierarchy of needs and desires that are seen as influencing the development of an individual toward high levels of "self-actualization" and satisfaction (Maslow, 1943b). Nursing has embraced his conceptualization of the hierarchy of human need attainment. Specifically for this chapter, it is important to consider the need for safety and the desire for security that may be threatened by injury. In examining methods to identify the risk of injury, William Haddon, a physician and expert on automobile injury, developed a matrix that looks at factors related to personal attributes, vector or agent attributes, and environmental attributes before, during, and after an injury or death. He demonstrated that by using this framework, one can then evaluate the relative importance of different factors and design interventions (Haddon, 1972; O'Neill, 2002). Subsequently, community-based nurses such as those who work in public health and forensic nursing and increasingly hospital-based nurses have used the matrix to develop programs to prevent a wide variety of injuries including burns, falls, firearm injuries, and, most recently, critical incidents from medical error. More recently, forensic science has and continues to inform forensic nursing practice. This is particularly true in terms of the intricacies of evidence collection and the growing body of knowledge within criminalistics (James and Nordby, 2009). In addition, the influence of law, including structure of the court system, federal rules of evidence, principles of witness testimony, expert opinions, and rights of citizens, has shaped the unique body of knowledge that guides the specialty from outside of nursing.

> **DID YOU KNOW?** *Criminal justice principles and law inform practice and form the boundaries of many aspects of practice such as client consent, rules of evidence, and expert courtroom testimony.*

Professional organizations outside of nursing that address large scale health concerns such as the CDC and the WHO have contributed to nursing's understanding of injury. At the turn of the twenty-first century these organizations began a global campaign toward violence prevention that had a tremendous influence on developing a primary prevention approach within the forensic community (Krug, et al, 2002; Brown et al, 2007; Peden et al, 2009). For example, in 2002 the CDC initiated efforts to develop a national state-based surveillance system, National Violent Death Reporting System (NVDRS), that could identify the cause and manner of death leading to prevention efforts by pulling together data on violent deaths (including child maltreatment fatalities, intimate partner homicides, other homicides, suicides, and legal intervention deaths), unintentional firearm injury deaths, and deaths of undetermined intent (CDC, 2009). Subsequently, a task force was formed to uniformly prepare individuals to conduct Sudden Unexpected Infant Death Investigation. Forensic nurses practicing as death

investigators served in the development of training programs that are now used nationwide.

> **THE CUTTING EDGE** *Today, the NVDRS operates in 18 states pulling together data about violent deaths. This system says that to stop violent deaths, it is important to understand all the facts; this includes knowing the who, when, where, and how about the violent death (CDC, 2010).*

In nursing, the conceptualizations that have contributed the most to forensic nursing include holism through caring, ways of knowing including intuition and suspiciousness, human reaction to trauma including the Rape Trauma Syndrome, and models specific to forensic nursing. Hammer, Moynihan, and Pagliaro (2006) examined the connection between the construct of caring and the unique relationship between forensic nurses and their clients. Although caring was previously recognized as the "hallmark of professional nursing" (Hammer, Moynihan, and Pagliaro, 2006) by theorists in the 1980s, Hammer recognized that part of what makes forensic nursing a specialty is the manner in which caring is translated.

The caring component must address caring not only for clients, but also for one's self. A sense of self-worth must be cultivated and nurtured to the degree that caring is conscientious, objective, and demanding of the scientific truth. Caring must also be curious and questioning, it should also be directed toward colleagues, and finally, caring should be about firm and valued concepts that inform practice (Hammer, Moynihan, and Pagliaro, 2006).

In that regard, questioning and ways of knowing, particularly intuition, are viewed as vital for a successful practice. Winfrey and Smith (1999) have described the concept of knowing as, more accurately, being suspicious in forensic nursing. Questioning has also led to a greater understanding of what most would consider the unexplainable and the unimaginable: the manifestations of Rape Trauma Syndrome (Burgess and Holmstrom, 1974), behaviors of the seriously emotionally disturbed offender (Mason and Mercer, 1998), and widespread occurrence of intimate partner violence (Campbell and Humphreys, 2003). Lynch's Integrated Model of Forensic Nursing, as previously discussed, depicts the biopsychosocial and spiritual dimensions of nursing care with the legal expertise needed when trauma results in court-related issues. Lynch and Duval (2010) have credited several nursing theorists—including Paterson and Zderad; Conway and Hardy; Leininger, Giger, and Davidhizar; Chinn and Kramer; and Brenner—in the development of forensic nursing theory and practice. Subsequent to Lynch's efforts, Hufft (2006) described forensic nursing within the domains of nursing and delineated the theoretical foundations for advanced forensic practice. Together, these role descriptions have informed the scope and standards of practice as well as credentialing vehicles such as the Advanced Forensic Nursing Portfolio.

> **NURSING TIP** *Knowledge, observation, and intuition are aspects of forensic nursing.*

Key Concepts in Forensic Nursing

The core concepts or conceptual metaphors that underlie forensic and other nursing models are certainly not unique to nursing. Concepts when applied to the nursing process guide knowledge, skills, and attitudes found in practice. Concepts in forensic nursing theory include, but are not confined to, safety, injury, presence, perceptivity, victimization, truth, and justice.

Safety is among the five basic needs of humans, identified by Maslow, in his theory of self-actualization (Maslow, 1943a). Maslow describes the first basic need as meeting one's physiological needs. This need is followed by safety needs, which can be affected by levels of security. The need for safety can become acute during periods of emergent trauma or chronic during periods of collective violence or chronic abuse. Until an individual is safe and wounding has healed, he or she cannot move on to higher levels of understanding and satisfaction.

Injury involves trauma or damage that is physiological, emotional, financial, spiritual, intellectual, and societal. Injury may be intentional, often known as violence, or may be unintentional. The cause may be a single source or multifaceted; it may be of human etiology or of natural causes. Making the distinction between the causes of injury is key to forensic practice. Justice is the concept of moral rightness based on ethics, rationality, law, natural law, fairness, and equity. As such, justice is viewed in the context of bioethics of the health care professions and the prevailing law of a particular society and culture. Therefore, the fact that justice is an important goal in forensic nursing care must be viewed in the context of the environment in which the care is given.

Presence is used by nurses as a part of the humane, holistic approach to both victims of trauma and perpetrators of crime. Lynch (2010) has defined presence as "the invisible quality that commands and comforts while directing attention away from one's self and into the being of another, instilling confidence and respect in the self of that being" (p 12).

Perceptivity, as an element of intuitiveness, is one tool the forensic nurse uses to investigate injury. Perceptivity involves an increased awareness of human behavior and environment that is interpreted by knowledge and lived experience in making expert decisions.

Truth is conceptualized as an agreement with fact or reality but also reflects characteristics such as honesty and sincerity on the part of the truth teller. Conceptualization of truth is influenced by philosophies that view it as subjective, objective, relative, or absolute. Forensic nurses hold the ideal that the results of scientific inquiry form the basis for their interactions with clients, health care systems, and the judicial system, which interact with their care; they are not influenced by personal bias or outside influence.

Victimization occurs when individuals or groups are exploited or treated unfairly, generally when there is an imbalance of power. The harm may be systematic when groups are mistreated or witness violence or it may be the result of individual attacks. Psychological responses to victimization include heightened feelings of vulnerability, depression, and anger. Juxtaposed to victimization is client empowerment, often through advocacy.

Scope and Standards of Practice

The scope and standards of practice for forensic nursing were first published in 1995. Revisions based on the uniform template of the ANA with addition of advanced practice competencies were published in 2009. The standards are delineated in each of the recognized areas: Scientific Process, Quality of Practice, Education, Professional Practice, Evaluation, Collaboration, Ethics, Research, Resource Utilization, and Leadership. Although each of these parameters helps to differentiate forensic nursing from other specialties (ANA, 2004), competencies related to the scientific process, or nursing process, are perhaps the most indicative of the specialized nature of the specialty. For example:

- Assessment includes the collection of forensic data, which may involve interviewing the client for evidentiary purposes, reviewing medical legal documents, and collecting trace evidence to be used in a criminal investigation.
- Formulating a diagnosis or impression regarding the differentiation of intentional and unintentional injury is a skill that involves a unique understanding of mechanisms of injury and correlation of this with the history of the event. The impression of the forensic clinician has extraordinary legal implications beyond the realm of the health-related diagnosis.
- The identification of realistic outcomes of care are most commonly performed in collaboration with a team that frequently consists of professionals outside of nursing including law enforcement, criminal justice, community advocates, and social service agencies. Care may reflect a decision that is humane and ensures community safety, but not necessarily be reflective of the client's wishes.
- Formulation of the care plan involves collaboration with a team, and should support the integration of clinical, human, social, and financial resources with medical-legal parameters to complete the decision-making processes.
- Implementation of the plan involves skills and techniques that are derived from sound evidence related to the applied science of both nursing and forensics. Current knowledge of both is mandated.
- Coordination of care relevant to forensic outcomes often involves including education and other strategies to prevent injuries well after the occurrence, perhaps after the death of an individual who has been injured.
- Evaluation of outcomes, particularly when viewed in aggregate, may involve dissemination of the results to not only the client and others involved in the care or situation, but also to local, national, and international agencies as appropriate, for the development of laws and regulations to protect individuals in a community.

CURRENT PERSPECTIVES

Evidence-Based Practice and Research

Evaluation of competency is required of all professions. Evaluation of nurses begins in school and continues through testing for entry-level licensure, certification examination, peer review, and personal reflection. Reflection should be on practice as

LINKING CONTENT TO PRACTICE

This chapter discusses the role of forensic nurses in the prevention and treatment of victims of violence. In addition to using the ANA competencies for practice, the forensic nurse includes the public health competencies as described in the Council on Linkages Domains and Core Competencies. For example, the analytic/assessment skills that discuss assessment, data collection, and use of ethical principles are integral to this nursing role. In regard to applying ethical principles, the nurse would use them in the collection, maintenance, use, and dissemination of data and information. Clearly this skill is a part of forensic nursing.

From Public Health Foundation, Council on Linkages: *Core competencies for public health professionals,* Washington, DC, 2009, PHF.

well as during practice. As part of professional expectations and standards, forensic nurses are encouraged to participate in continuous quality improvement using the best evidence for practice or promising practice methods under evaluation (Nayduch and Fitzpatrick, 1999; Harkins, 2006). Scientific research in forensic nursing is in its infancy. Currently, research is largely a description of the forensic nursing role and client population (Evans, 2000; Lewis-O'Connor, 2009; Shelton, 2009). Recent descriptions of sexual assault teams promote practice observations that facilitate comparison and measurement of short-term outcomes such as client satisfaction and long-term outcomes such as prosecution rates (Campbell et al, 2005; Johnston, 2005; Speck, 2005; Campbell R et al, 2006; Bechtel, Ryan, and Gallagher, 2008; Campbell R et al, 2008). Studies in collaboration with other disciplines are currently underway to test the basis for distinctions among injuries such as bruising (Wiglesworth et al, 2009; Pierce et al, 2010). Forensic nurses are producing valuable information regarding DNA sampling (Maguire et al, 2008; Ledray, 2010). Scholarly contributions to forensic nursing practice have increased since professional journals such as the *Journal of Forensic Nursing* have increased publication of forensic specific content.

Certification

The scope and standards of forensic nursing practice have been used for the development of the certification examination and other credentials that are intended to demonstrate competence of the practitioner. Credentialing within forensic nursing, as with all new professional specialties, has become an increasingly important issue. Different types of credentials pertain to nursing—both within the discipline and without. While all nurses should have an understanding of credentialing and the implications and responsibilities that accompany such a designation, it is uniquely important for FNs who maintain close relationships to both the medical and the legal communities. FNs provide care when health and the law intersect and must therefore have credentials that speak to their unique qualifications to give that specialized care (Patton, 2010).

Certification examination for the pediatric, adolescent, and adult sexual assault nurse examiners (SANE A and SANE P) is available through the Forensic Nurse Certification Board. This certification along with the Legal Nurse Consultant, Corrections Nurse, Death Investigators, and Forensic Examiner are offered

EVIDENCE-BASED PRACTICE

The goal of this research study was to evaluate if the use of Sexual Assault Nurse Examiners (SANEs) in a pediatric emergency department improved the care of pediatric and adolescent sexual assault victims. The authors noted that sexual assault is a frequent violent crime in the United States and the victims with the highest level of incidence are women younger than 24 years. Their concern was that personnel in general (adult) emergency departments may not be adequately trained to evaluate and treat young sexual assault victims.

They reviewed the medical records of 114 victims who had received care at a pediatric emergency department with a history of sexual assault and who required a forensic evaluation (rape kit) over a 2-year period. They then evaluated the differences in selected documentation between the group for whom care was provided by a SANE and those who received care by a practitioner who was not a SANE. They found that many more clients when evaluated by a SANE after being sexually assaulted received sexually transmitted infection testing, pregnancy prophylaxis, and referrals to the Rape Crisis Center.

Nurse Use
SANEs play a key role in providing care for victims of sexual assault. The training to become a SANE is specialized and growing in importance and the recognition of its value to victims, their families, and the criminal justice system.

From Bechtel K, Ryan E, Gallagher D: Impact of sexual assault nurse examiners on the evaluation of sexual assault in a pediatric emergency department, *Pediatr Emerg Care* 24(7):442-447, 2008.

by other organizations to registered nurses meeting entry criteria but generally do not require a graduate degree. Recognition of the AFN by the American Nurses Credentialing Commission through a portfolio method of evaluation took place for the first time in 2009. Seen in light of the APRN Consensus Model for Regulation, forensic nursing is a specialty focus, beyond the role and population focus of the four categories of advanced practice (APRN Joint Dialogue Group, The APRN Consensus Work Group, & Committee, 2008). While the AFN credential represents a specialty focus for APNs, however, it is currently not an avenue for advanced practice certification or advanced practice licensure.

> **DID YOU KNOW?** *Forensic Nurse Examiners are most often referred to as Forensic Examiners, Medicolegal Death Investigators and Coroners, Sexual Assault Nurse Examiners, or Advanced Forensic Nurses.*

ETHICAL ISSUES

Ethical considerations in the practice of forensic nursing are unique because of the implications to not only a client's health, but in some cases, his freedom. Practice outcomes affect individuals and families, as well as society as a whole. Ethics and law are closely tied but are not equivalent. Ethical nursing practice involves adherence to law in most cases, but also to the ethics of nursing and the dictates of one's conscience (Walsh, 2005). Nurses maintain a different code of conduct than do certain colleagues. For example, law enforcement personnel answer singly to the law for its standard. Knowledge and understanding of these considerations is core to the specialty of forensic nursing (International Association of Forensic Nurses Ethics Committee, 2008).

WHAT DO YOU THINK? *Does the forensic nurse have a greater duty to the well-being of the victim, the accused, or to society under the ethics of the health care system? Who should be protected, and must the nurse make some ethical choice?*

Olsen (2006) organized ethical principles into five categories: respect for person, beneficence, distributive justice, respect for community, and contextual caring. Each of these categories reflects examples of the tension that may arise when the forensic nurse faces a dilemma imposed by conflicting interests. An overriding consideration is the need to respect each person and to develop contextual caring within the art of nursing. Respect for person means respect for autonomy while protecting vulnerable persons. The right of each human to self-determination is recognized within nursing but may not be respected by all societies. Therefore, respect for human rights may involve advocacy to some degree. Laws, cultural norms, and considerations of safety, which limit the liberty of an individual, may constrain the nurse's ability to fully exercise a therapeutic relationship. Questions raised pose dilemmas in a variety of medical and psychiatric settings.

Forensic environments include courtrooms, jails, prisons, and psychiatric facilities for the criminally insane. When criminal action or trauma to an individual requires care, the need for coercion is likely. Certain situations may make medical coercion necessary. These situations include incapacity (or inability) to make decisions and making decisions that could result in harm to self or harm to others in the absence of interventions. Paternalism has been defined as "the principle that allows one person to make decisions for another" (Williams, 2007, p 93). This may be necessary in the case of minors or older adults. Paternalistic intervention was viewed by the U.S. Supreme Court as lawful in the Case of *Washington v Harper* ("Washington versus Harper," 1990), when it ruled that mentally ill inmates could be compelled to take psychotropic medications against their will if the mental disorder is serious, the inmate is dangerous to himself, and the medication prescribed is in the inmate's best medical interest. Therefore, the ability of a psychiatric forensic nurse practicing in an advanced role to make a determination of rational autonomy is crucial in questions of coercion: to make judgments without being judgmental (Rose, 2005).

This same principle may be applied to clients who refuse treatment of infectious disease, whether or not they are incarcerated, in much the same manner public health law is used to guide treatment in community settings. Instructive guidelines on involuntary treatment are available from the American Correctional Association, the CDC, and the American Public Health Association (Finkelstein et al, 2006; Turner, 2006a).

Beneficence (care) and the complimentary principle of non-maleficence (without harm) go beyond autonomy in the responsibility of the nurse to not only support an individual's choices but to perform actions that enhance the health of others. Nurses provide care without prejudice of the circumstance or individual characteristics. They provide care to the injured, marginalized, and poor whether the individuals are victims or offenders. Nurses who care for pregnant teens in a youth facility or collect evidence from drug addicts each hold the same ethical responsibility as described previously (Muster, 1992; Hufft and Peternelj-Taylor, 2008). Questions may arise when the resources to achieve adequate health are not plentiful enough for all to receive adequate care. When economic restraints limit funds to process sexual assault evidentiary kits, treat victims of assault, and provide dental care to methamphetamine addicts in prison, where should the funds be applied? Principles of distributive justice address such questions in deciding what goods will be distributed to which persons in what proportions. Forensic nurses may find themselves in a policy-making position to answer such questions to ensure that their clients given similar circumstances are treated no better or worse than others in the application of protection and medical care. Also, when there are questions of retribution, whether withholding provisions or threatening harm, forensic nurses never participate in the punishment, however subtle, of another being.

Ethical decisions can be exceedingly difficult when the safety of a society is at risk. One approach to making decisions with respect for the community is utilitarianism, which appeals exclusively to outcomes or consequences in determining which choice to make. Williams (2009) explains:

Utilitarianism, with its mandate for the general good, rather than a specific interest, would place the safety of the community above the rights of any one individual. The forensic nurse expert, hired by the court to evaluate a client, as an example, testifies on behalf of society, not the individual. To that end, it may be argued that the nurse expert uses a utilitarian perspective that may not serve the interests of the client but instead, serves the interests of society. Traditional nursing mandates that the correct focus (and therefore the right moral choice) be placed on the individual. However, the burden of responsibility often shifts in forensic nursing from the individual to the community, a correct moral choice under utilitarianism (p 50).

WHAT DO YOU THINK? *During a forensic examination, the potential exists for withholding vital information in the investigation of wrongdoing. The temptation to "assist" the perceived victim's case may be justified by a desired outcome for that individual as well as the ultimate safety of a community. This dilemma of information can be carried to situations of privacy protection. The entitlement to privacy may be changed when someone's safety is at stake. If a specimen for DNA is collected during the investigation of a crime, should that information remain in the Combined DNA Index System (CODIS) for use in future crimes, regardless of the outcome of prosecution of that case and when there is the potential for repeat offense (Hackenschmidt, 2004)? Do hospitals have the right to videotape parents who are suspected of Münchausen syndrome, or is this a violation of fourth amendment rights (Morrison, 1999)? When victims give information to sexual assault examiners, are they informed that records may be released to law enforcement and attorney? Should they consent to the release of photographs that depict intimate areas of their body for anyone in law enforcement, attorneys and juries to see, even in the name of full disclosure (Ledray, 2008)?*

Finally, there are always questions regarding the relationship between forensic clients and nurses. Caring is the essence and core value of nursing (Watson, 2008). Olsen (2006) recognized that caring as well as ethics is influenced in the context of relationships and that nurses' "emotion is inextricably bound to moral good" (p 147). Contextual caring is not synonymous with beneficence but "entreats the forensic nurse to interact with each client, whether criminal or victim, as a person within an ethical relationship of caring concern grounded in the nurse's personal values" (Olsen, 2006, p 146). The care goes beyond the "obligatory dictates" of client rights. Unique problems are posed when the client is in denial about the role he or she plays in the problem or poses a safety risk to the nurse. In addition, forensic nurses must overcome the societal bias of establishing relationships with individuals believed to have injured another, perhaps intentionally. Finally, when personal bias or issues of conscience impair the ability to prescribe or participate in particular medical interventions, objections may be raised. Examples of situations at risk for bias in forensics include collection of trace evidence from individuals who have impaired consciousness or are coerced into consent, prescription of birth control following sexual assault, participation in capital punishment, and the use of unnecessary physical or medical restraint. Nurses and other health care professionals have well-established codes of ethics and other examined statements to guide practice and inform care (Walsh, 2005; Ferguson, 2006; Turner, 2006b; Committee on Bioethics, 2009; Lynch and Duval, 2010). It is imperative to view these statements that guide practice as a basis for conduct as well as for reflective dialogue in real client situations. The following two case studies demonstrate some of the aspects of forensic nursing care.

Case #1: Tamara Lynch is a 6-year-old child who lives in a busy household of four children, her grandmother, mother and stepfather. She is a client of the local pediatric clinic and has an appointment today for a school-related examination. She has been very interested in school in the past but recently her grades have declined and her mother describes her behavior as withdrawn. Shirley Meres is the pediatric nurse practitioner who has seen Tamara for her most recent health care. She too has noted the change in Tamara's affect. Based on the health history, Ms. Meres uses developmentally appropriate questions to ask Tamara about situations in which she may not feel safe or situations with adults that have made her feel uncomfortable about her body. Tamara describes repeated episodes with her stepfather during which she was inappropriately touched and fondled. The nurse meets with Tamara's mother and explains her role as a forensic nurse. She explains that Tamara will need a specialized physical examination with collection of evidence, including laboratory specimens and photographs. After obtaining permission from the mother, the evaluation is performed using enhanced lighting and visualization equipment to collect photographic evidence, and body fluids for diagnostic and forensic testing. The nurse tells Tamara and her mother that the examination is normal for her age; no indications of trauma are noted. All evidence is packed for preservation according to crime lab protocols. Following the interview and examination, Ms. Meres counsels the child and mother about predictable psychological reactions to child sexual assault and disclosure even though no evidence of abuse was found upon the

nurse's examination. The mother is given information on advocacy, the legal process that follows a report to law enforcement agencies, and mental health counseling that is available locally. Tamara is given an appointment at the clinic in 2 weeks. The nurse makes contact with law enforcement to report the child's disclosure and make arrangements for transfer of all evidence. Ms. Meres continues to follow the health care of the family in the months to follow for evaluation and prevention of common problems that present to families who experience child abuse.

Case #2: Mike Post is an 18-year-old male who is taken to the emergency department by ambulance for what appeared to be a motor vehicle collision. His condition is considered serious. Following resuscitative measures, he is pronounced dead. Staff members at the emergency department contact the medical examiner's office to report the death. Sean Miller is the forensic nurse investigator on duty who receives the call. When Mr. Miller arrives at the emergency department, he interviews paramedics and emergency department clinicians about the accident site and the appearance of the decedent on arrival. He photographs the body, clothing, and other sources of trace evidence, including items in the decedent's pockets. Mr. Miller performs a thorough examination of Mike Post and discovers a small bullet hole in the left postauricular tissue. All items are individually bagged, sealed, and labeled for further analysis by the crime laboratory. The nurse then meets with the family to explain the need for investigation of all sudden, unexpected deaths. He describes the process involved in the investigation and preparation of the body prior to transfer to a funeral home. Copies of the medical record and x-rays obtained at the facility are transported with the body for autopsy. Mr. Miller reports his findings to the forensic pathology team and law enforcement officers. The autopsy is performed and the ballistics analysis of the recovered bullet leads to the arrest of the alleged assailant. When the case goes to court, the nurse is subpoenaed to testify about the investigation and collection of evidence. The nurse maintains contact with the family to keep them informed of the progress of the case and the resources for legal and family grief counseling available in their community.

FUTURE PERSPECTIVES

Forensic nursing is predominantly a community-oriented specialty. Practice arenas are associated with health care facilities such as private clinics and emergency departments, criminal justice centers for victims of crime, medical examiner offices, police departments, correctional facilities, and mental health centers. What is consistent in each of these practice sites is the care of individuals who have experienced the effects of injury, either intentional or unintentional. Increasingly it is being recognized that hospitals need forensic nursing services. Clients routinely enter hospitals with conditions that have overlying legal implications (Markowitz, Steer, and Garland, 2005). In addition, injuries occur as a result of medical incidents and errors. Forensic nurses use their expert understanding of cause and effects of trauma and are in a position to investigate the circumstances in order to design a plan of care for individual as well as special groups of clients. They serve as a liaison between the hospital and the medical-legal community to reduce the effects of trauma.

CHAPTER REVIEW

PRACTICE APPLICATION

A 26-year-old woman arrived unaccompanied to the emergency department of an academic medical center with cuts on her face, hands, legs, and pelvic area. She was crying and said that she had been attacked and was afraid to have an examination or to provide the name of her attacker. What is the first action that the nurse should take:

1. Explain to her the importance of reporting this crime immediately.
2. Listen closely to her and reflect back to her the fear, anger, and other feelings you hear in her voice.
3. Immediately call law enforcement officials yourself.

Once you select the first action that you would take, explain your rationale and outline your exact actions.

Answers can be found on the Evolve site.

KEY POINTS

- Forensic nursing is a community-oriented specialty that addresses the prevention and treatment of accidental injury and violent crimes.
- The specialty reflects an integration of nursing, forensic science, and the law.
- Forensic nursing is needed whenever injury has legal implications.
- Forensic nurses need to maintain objectivity in rendering care to both victims of injury and perpetrators of crime.
- The scope and standards of forensic nursing practice guides forensic nurses with unique skills of the specialties such as expert courtroom testimony and documentation and security of evidence.
- Forensic nurses work in cooperation with public health professionals, including nurses, in developing programs of prevention such as automobile safety and intimate partner violence prevention.
- Educational programs for forensic nurses are offered through continuing education offerings and formal graduate degree programs.
- Credentialing for forensic nurses include Sexual Assault Nurse Examiners and Advanced Practice Forensic Nurses.

CLINICAL DECISION-MAKING ACTIVITIES

1. Think about injuries you have experienced and answer the following questions:
   A. How did the injury affect my ability to perform normal activities of my daily routine?
   B. What injury patterns did I have that would lead me to conclude it was violent or accidental?
   C. What could I have done to prevent the injury from occurring?
2. Discuss the effects of violence in your community with a fellow student. What situations exist that increase the risk that someone will be assaulted?
3. Write a list of the types of evidence that can be collected at a crime scene or in an emergency room based on a scenario of crime involving a young woman who is the victim of sexual assault.
4. In a short paragraph, explore how you might feel toward someone who commits a crime and needs nursing care. What ethical standards of nursing will influence your treatment of this individual?

REFERENCES

American Nurses Association: *Recognition of a specialty, approval of scope statements and acknowledgement of nursing practice standards*, Washington, DC, 2004, American Nurses Association.

APRN Joint Dialogue Group, The APRN Consensus Work Group, & Committee, NAA: *Consensus model for APRN regulation: licensure, accreditation, certification and education*, Washington, DC, 2008.

Bechtel K, Ryan E, Gallagher D: Impact of sexual assault nurse examiners on the evaluation of sexual assault in a pediatric emergency department, *Pediatr Emerg Care* 24(7):442–447, 2008.

Brown D, Butchart A, Harvey A, et al: *Third milestones of a global campaign for violence prevention report 2007: scaling up*, Geneva, 2007, WHO.

Burgess AW, Holmstrom LL: Rape Trauma Syndrome, *Am J Psychiatr* 131(9):981–986, 1974.

Campbell JC, Humphreys JC: *Family violence and nursing practice*, Baltimore, 2003, Lippincott, Williams & Wilkins.

Campbell R, Patterson D, Adams AE, et al: A participatory evaluation project to measure SANE nursing practice and adult sexual assault patients' psychological well-being, *J Forensic Nurs* 4(1):19–28, 2008.

Campbell R, Townsend SM, Long SM, Kinnison KE: Organizational characteristics of sexual assault nurse examiner programs: results from the National Survey Project, *J Forensic Nurs* 1(2):57–64, 88, 2005.

Campbell R, Townsend SM, Long SM, et al: Responding to sexual assault victim's medical and emotional needs: a national study of the services provided by SANE programs, *Res Nurs Health* 29:384–398, 2006.

Centers for Disease Control and Prevention: *Violence prevention: national violent death reporting system*, 2010. Available at http://www.cdc.gov/ViolencePrevention/NVDRS/index.html. Accessed November 7, 2010.

Centers for Disease Control and Prevention: *National Center for Injury Prevention and Control*, 2009. Available at http://www.cdc.gov/injury/. Accessed August 13, 2010.

Committee on Bioethics: Physician refusal to provide information or treatment on the basis of claims of conscience, *Pediatrics* 124(6):1689–1693, 2009.

Evans N: Special focus: mental health nursing: developing forensic nursing, *Nurs Manage* 6(10):14–17, 2000.

Ferguson C: Providing quality care to the sexual assault survivor: education and training for medical professionals, *J Midwifery Womens Health* 51(6):486–492, 2006.

Finkelstein EA, Corso PS, Miller TR: *The Incidence and economic burden of injury in the United States*, 2006. Available at http://www.us.oup.com/us/catalog/general/subject/Medicine/PublicHealth/?view=usa&ci=9780195179484. Accessed March 19, 2011.

Finn C: Child maltreatment: forensic biomarkers. In Lynch VA, Duvall JB, editors: *Forensic nursing science*, ed 2, St Louis, 2010, Elsevier.

Gurevich L: Parental child murder and child abuse in anglo-American legal system, *Trauma Viol Abuse* 11(1):18–26, 2010.

Hackenschmidt A: Advancing justice for sexual assault survivors and innocent inmates, or threat to privacy? a controversial DNA technology, *J Emerg Nurs* 30(6):575–577, 2004.

Haddon W: A logical framework for categorizing highway safety phenomena and activity, *J Trauma* 12:193–207, 1972.

Hammer RM, Moynihan B, Pagliaro E: *Forensic nursing: A handbook for practice*, Sudbury, MA, 2006, Jones and Bartlett.

Harkins T: Forensic nursing and quality assurance: a perfect match, *On the Edge* 12(3):5, 2006.

History of IAFN, 2010. IAFN Website. Accessed September, 2010.

Houmes BV, Fagan MM, Quintana NM: Violence: recognition, management, and prevention: establishing a sexual assault nurse examiner (SANE) program in the emergency department, *J Emerg Med* 25:111–121, 2003.

Hufft AG: Theoretical foundations for advanced practice nursing. In Hammer RH, Moynihan B, Pagliano EM, editors: *Forensic nursing: a handbook for practice*, Sudbury, MA, 2006, Jones and Barlett.

Hufft AG, Peternelj-Taylor C: Ethical care of pregnant adolescents in correctional settings, *J Forens Nurs* 4(2):94–96, 2008.

International Association of Forensic Nurses Ethics Committee: *The vision of ethical practice*, 2008. Available at http://www.iafn.org/displaycommon.cfm?an=1&subarticlenbr=56. Accessed March 19, 2011.

James SH, Nordby JJ, editors: *Forensic science: an introduction to scientific and investigative techniques*, ed 3, Boca Raton, 2009, CRC Press.

Johnston BJ: Outcome indicators for sexual assault victims, *J Forens Nurs* 1(3):118, 2005.

Krug EG, Dahlberg LL, Mercy JA, et al: *World report on violence and health*, Geneva, 2002, WHO.

Ledray L: *SANE development and operation guide*, Washington, DC, 1998, Sexual Assault Resource Service, U.S. Department of Justice, Office of Justice Programs, and Office of Victims of Crime.

Ledray LE: Consent to photograph: how far should disclosure go? *J Forensic Nurs* 4(4):188–189, 2008.

Ledray L: Expanding evidence, collection time: Is it time to move beyond the 72 hour rule? How do we decide? *J Forensic Nurs* 6(1):47–50, 2010.

Lewis-O'Connor A: The evolution of SANE/SART—are there differences? Sexual Assault Nurse Examiner/Sexual Assault Response Team, *J Forensic Nurs* 5(4):220–227, 2009.

Lynch VA: Forensic nursing: a new field for the profession. Paper presented at the 38th Annual Meeting of the American Academy of Forensic Science, 1986.

Lynch VA: *Clinical forensic nursing: a descriptive study in role development*, University of Texas, 1990, Arlington, TX.

Lynch VA: Concepts and theory of forensic nursing science. In Lynch VA, Duvall JB, editors: *Forensic nursing science*, ed 2, St Louis, 2010, Elsevier.

Lynch VA, Duval JB, editors: *Forensic nursing science*, ed 2, St Louis, 2010, Elsevier.

Maguire S, Ellaway B, Bowyer VL, et al: Retrieval of DNA from the faces of children aged 0–5 years: a technical note, *J Forensic Nurs* 4(1):40–44, 2008.

Markowitz JR, Steer S, Garland M: Hospital-based intervention for intimate partner violence victims: a forensic nursing model, *J Emerg Nurs* 31(2):166–170, 2005.

Maslow AH: A theory of human motivation, *Psychol Rev* 50(4):370–396, 1943a.

Maslow AH: A theory of human motivation, *Psychol Rev* 50:370–396, 1943b. Available at http://psychclassics.yorku.ca/Maslow/motivation.htm. Accessed March 19, 2011.

Mason T, Mercer D, editors: *Critical perspectives in forensic care: inside out*, Hampshire, London, 1997, Macmillan.

Mauer M: *Racial disparities in the criminal justice system*, Washington, DC, 2009, The Sentencing Project.

Morrison CA: Cameras in hospital rooms: the fourth amendment to the constitution and Munchausen syndrome by proxy, *Crit Care Nurs Q* 22(1):65–68, 1999.

Muster NJ: Treating the adolescent victim-turned-offender, *Adolescence* 27(106):441–441, 1992.

Nayduch DA, Fitzpatrick MK: The application of forensic findings to the trauma quality management process, *J Trauma Nurs* 6(4):98–102, 1999.

Nutting MA, Dock LL: *A history of nursing: the evolution of nursing systems from the earliest times to the foundation of the first English and American training schools for nurses*, vol 1, New York, 1907, G.P. Putnam's Sons.

O'Neill B: Accidents or crashes: highway safety and William Haddon Jr, *Contingencies* 24(1):30–32, 2002.

Olsen D: Ethical considerations in forensic nursing. In Hammer RH, Moynihan B, Pagliaro EM, editors: *Forensic nursing: a handbook for practice*, Sudbury, MA, 2006, Jones and Bartlett, pp 139–174.

Patton SB: Credential development for forensic nurses. In Lynch VA, Duvall JB, editors: *Forensic nursing science*, ed 2, St Louis, 2010, Elsevier Mosby.

Peden M, Oyegbite K, Ozanne-Smith J, et al: *World report on child injury prevention*, Geneva, 2009, WHO.

Pierce MC, Kaczor K, Aldridge S, et al: Bruising characteristics discriminating physical child abuse from accidental trauma, *Pediatrics* 125(1):67–74, 2010.

Rose DN: Respect for patient autonomy in forensic psychiatric nursing, *J Forensic Nurs* 1(1):23–27, 2005.

Sachs CJ, Weinberg E, Wheeler MW: Sexual assault nurse examiners' application of statutory rape reporting laws, *J Emerg Nurs* 34(5):410–413, 2008.

Shelton D: Forensic nursing in secure environments, *J Forensic Nurs* 5(3):131–142, 2009.

Sheridan DJ: Legal and forensic nursing responses to family violence, In Humphrey J, Campbell JC, editors: *Family violence and nursing practice*, Philadelphia, 2004, Lippincott Williams & Wilkins.

Sheridan DJ, Nash KR: Acute injury patterns of intimate partner violence victims, *Trauma Violence Abuse* 8:281–289, 2009.

Speck PM: *Program evaluation of current SANE services to victim populations in three cities*, Memphis, 2005, University of Tennessee Heath Science Center.

Speck PM: *The lived history of forensic nursing*, PowerPoint presentation, Memphis, n.d.

Turner M: Ethics and issues in prison, forensic, and other similar nursing settings, *Ethics and Human Rights Issues Update* 6(3), 2006a. Available at http://www.nursingworld.org/MainMenuCategories/EthicsStandards/Resources/IssuesUpdate/EthicsandIssuesinPrisonArticle.aspx. Accessed March 24, 2011.

Turner M: Ethics and issues in prison, forensic, and other similar nursing settings. Available at http://www.nursingworld.org/mainMenuCategories/EthicsStandards/Resources/IssuesUpdate/Ethicsandissuesinprisonarticle.aspx. Accessed June 8, 2011.

U.S. Department of Justice/Office on Violence Against Women: *A national protocol for sexual assault medical forensic examinations adult/adolescents, 2004*. Available at http://www.ncjrs.gov/pdffiles1/ovw/206554.pdf. Accessed June 8, 2011.

Walsh SJ: Legal perceptions of forensic DNA profiling: Part I: a review of the legal literature, *Forensic Sci Internat* 155(1):51–60, 2005.

Washington v Harper, 494 U.S., 1990.

Watson J: Social justice and human caring: a model of caring science as a hopeful paradigm for moral justice for humanity, *Creative Nurs* 14(2):54–61, 2008.

Weissling S: The case for forensic nursing, *Minority Nurse* (3), 2002. Available at http://minoritynurse.com/forensic-nursing/case-forensic-nursing. Accessed March 19, 2011.

Wiglesworth A, Austin R, Corona M, et al: Bruising as a marker of physical elder abuse, *J Am Geriatr Soc* 57(1):1191–1196, 2009.

Williams D: Forensic nursing and utilitarianism: the quest for being right, *J Forensic Nurs* 5(1):49–50, 2009.

Williams DL: Is there a case for paternalism in forensic nursing? *J Forensic Nurs* 3(2):93–94, 2007.

Winfrey ME, Smith AR: The suspiciousness factor: critical care nursing and forensics, *Crit Care Nurs Q* 22(1):1, 1999.

CHAPTER 45

The Nurse in the Faith Community

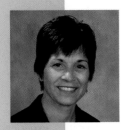

Jean C. Bokinskie, PhD, RN

Dr. Jean C. Bokinskie is an assistant professor at the Department of Nursing at Concordia College in Moorhead, Minnesota, and serves as the director of the Concordia College Parish Nurse Center. She teaches both didactic and clinical courses in adult health nursing in the undergraduate nursing program. She has also served as a parish nurse in her home congregation of Hope Lutheran Church since 1996. Dr. Bokinskie has been involved in the educational preparation of faith community nurses since 2000. In her role as Program Director, she provides consultative services to many faith communities for the initiation, development, and support of faith community nursing and health ministry programs. Dr. Bokinskie is active in updating the international curriculum for parish/faith community nurse preparation and in the current revision of the Scope and Standards document. She is an author and conference presenter for nurses and related health and healing professionals on faith community nursing/health ministries, both regionally and nationally. Her research interest areas include work place environments, perceptions of empowerment, outcome measures of faith community nursing actions, and resilience of individuals who have experienced spinal cord injury.

ADDITIONAL RESOURCES

⊝volve WEBSITE
http://evolve.elsevier.com/Stanhope
- *Healthy People 2020*
- WebLinks
- Quiz
- Case Studies

- Glossary
- Answers to Practice Application
- Resource Tools
  - Resource Tool 45.A: Resources for Faith Community Nursing

OBJECTIVES

After reading this chapter, the student should be able to do the following:
1. Describe the heritage of health and healing ministries in faith communities.
2. Relate models of faith community nursing to the current scope and standards of practice of faith community nursing.
3. Develop awareness of the nurse's role as a faith community or parish nurse within faith communities for spiritual care, health promotion, and disease prevention.

4. Use the nursing process in a faith community to assess, implement, and evaluate programs for healthy congregations using *Healthy People 2020* guidelines.
5. Examine the professional issues related to faith community nursing.

KEY TERMS

Faith community nursing or parish nursing is the dynamic process of working with faith communities to promote wholeness of body, mind, and spirit (Patterson, Wehling, and Mason, 2008). This specialty nursing practice has long-established roots in the healing and health professions. Throughout historical accounts of nursing, caring for members of communities has been important. The earliest accounts of caring and serving others stem from communities of faith. Religious texts abound with reference to the importance of caring for others as a foundational component of the faith tradition. Wholeness and being a in relationship with one's creator have sustained individuals and groups during times of illness, brokenness, and stress, and when cure was not possible (Hale and Koenig, 2003; Solari-Twadell and McDermott, 2006). In 1998 the American Nurses Association (ANA) accepted *parish nursing* as the most recognized term for the practice of nurses working with congregations or faith communities as published by the Health Ministries' Association (HMA) and the ANA in the *Scope and Standards of Parish Nursing Practice* (HMA/ANA, 1998). In the 2005 revision of the ANA's *Scope and Standards of Practice,* the term faith community nurse was adopted to be inclusive of the titles of parish nurse, congregational nurse, health ministry nurse, or health and wellness nurse (ANA/HMA, 2005). Currently the majority of faith community nurses serve in Judeo-Christian communities; however, the practice is expanding to other faith traditions as it attempts to respond to diverse faith perspectives and international needs (IPNRC, 2009a).

Faith community nurses work in close relationships with individuals, families, and faith communities to establish programs and services that significantly affect health, healing, and wholeness (Chase-Ziolek, 2005; Solari-Twadell and McDermott, 2006; Patterson, Wehling, and Mason, 2008). Faith community nurses balance knowledge and skill in their role in order to facilitate the faith community as it becomes a caring place—a place that is a source of health and healing for all members of the community. Nurses are drawn into faith community nursing because it encourages the expression of spirituality as a part of health and healing, whereas others become faith community nurses out of a sense of vocational calling (Mosack, Medvene, and Wescott, 2006).

Faith community nurses address health concerns of individuals, families, and groups of all ages. The members of faith communities, like other communities, experience birth, death, acute and chronic illness, stress, dependency concerns, challenges of life transitions, growth, and development; they also face decisions regarding healthy lifestyle choices. Serving as good stewards of resources, faith community nurses encourage partnering with other community health agencies, as well as lay and professional church leaders, to arrive at creative responses to health issues and to develop health promoting and spiritually healing activities. The nurse serves the faith community by focusing on the needs of the individual parishioner, the entire faith community, and the surrounding geographic area with attention to spiritual needs.

Faith community nursing continues to gain prominence as nurses reclaim their traditions of healing, acknowledge gaps in service delivery, and, along with the rise of nursing centers, affirm the independent functions of nursing (Nist, 2003; Solari-Twadell, 2006). The International Parish Nurse Resource Center (IPNRC) estimates that about 12,000 faith community nurses are practicing in all 50 states (IPNRC, 2009b). This estimation reflects a rather conservative estimate since it only includes the numbers reported by IPNRC-affiliated educating bodies and does not reflect the individuals who have completed non-affiliated IPNRC programs or who practice without additional education in the specialty area. Box 45-1 provides a demographic profile of a large sampling of parish nurses in the United States. In addition, the numbers of practicing faith community nurses continue to grow in other countries such as South Korea, Canada, New Zealand, Swaziland (Figure 45-1), Russia, and the United Kingdom (Daniels, 2009).

DEFINITIONS IN FAITH COMMUNITY NURSING

Faith communities are groups of people that gather in churches, homeless shelters, congregations, parishes, synagogues, temples, or mosques and acknowledge common values, beliefs, and practices within a single faith or multi-faith tradition(s) (ANA/HMA, 2005). It is a setting in which the members or guests are invited, but are not obligated, to participate in the rites and rituals of a faith tradition.

Parish nursing has been the most commonly used expression for the specialized practice of professional nursing in this context; however, the more inclusive term of *faith community nursing,* as

BOX 45-1   DEMOGRAPHIC PROFILE OF FAITH COMMUNITY NURSES

A large survey of faith community nurses (*n* = 1161) across the United States yielded the following description:

- Average age = 55 years
- 89% female
- 32% prepared at baccalaureate level in nursing, 24% prepared at the diploma level, 14% prepared at the associate's level, 12% hold a master's in nursing
- 68% serve as unpaid staff in towns (47%), cities (42%), and metro areas (11%)
- Majority are from Christian faith traditions with only 2% of the sample Jewish, 25% Lutheran, 23% Roman Catholic, 16% Methodist
- 17% have membership in the American Nurses Association

From Solari-Twadell PA: Uncovering the intricacies of the ministry of parish nursing practice through research. In Solari-Twadell PA, McDermott MA, editors: *Parish nursing: development, education, and administration*, St Louis, 2006, Mosby, pp 17–34

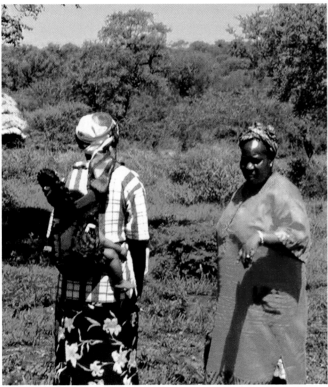

FIGURE 45-1 The parish nurse making a home visit in rural Swaziland, Africa.

throughout the life span. This includes active and less-active members, as well as those confined to home or those living in institutional settings. Often, the faith community's mission includes outreach to individuals and groups. These individuals or groups may be found in a geographic area near the traditional congregational setting, or in a common cultural community. These individuals or groups may not be designated members of the faith tradition. However, services may be extended to those beyond the congregational setting.

Health ministries are those activities and programs in faith communities organized around health and healing in order to promote wholeness in health across the life span (Chase-Ziolek, 2005). Health ministry services may be specifically planned or may be more informal. A professional or a layperson may provide them. These services include visiting the homebound, providing meals for families in crisis or when a family member returns home after hospitalization, participating in prayer circles, serving "healthy heart" meals, or holding regular grief support groups (Hale and Koenig, 2003). As a member of the health ministry team, the parish nurse emphasizes the nursing discipline's intentionality to include the spiritual dimension while incorporating physical, emotional, and social aspects of nursing with individuals, families, and faith communities.

EVIDENCE-BASED PRACTICE

The use of mind–body medicine and prayer was studied as part of a large exploratory, descriptive study of the use of complementary and alternative medicine in clients with hepatitis C (HVC) using services of a tertiary health care facility in the southeastern United States. The study's purpose was to identify the prevalence and reasons for the use of mind–body medicine by adult clients with HVC. The research was completed using an investigator-designed questionnaire and semi-structured interviews that explored the participants' use of CAM, including reasons and benefits from CAM use. Overall, 88% (*n* = 105) of the participants had used mind–body medicine in the past year. Clients with HVC most commonly used prayer for health reasons (91%, *n* = 95), prayed for their own health (88%, *n* = 92), and had others pray for their health (86%, *n* = 90). This was followed by participation group prayer (38%), deep breathing exercises (30%), and meditation (30%). Participants reported that prayer was used to give thanks for support of others and for themselves, whereas others reported that prayer allowed them to share their burden with a higher power. A few participants equated prayer with meditation, which evoked a calming state. Some participants did not equate prayer with being religious or with church attendance. This study affirms the use of prayer for health reasons, to facilitate relaxation, and to enhance emotional and physical well-being.

Nurse Use

Faith community nurses can be encouraged to continue to support members of faith communities through the use of individual and group prayer. It is important for the nurse to help members find the space and moments to pray during times of stress, illness, and grief; and encourage support groups to assist persons to enhance prayer and meditation practices. The faith community nurse may also integrate deep breathing exercises, meditation, and other complementary and alternative approaches to enhance the emotional and physical well-being of faith community members.

From Richmond JA, Bailey DE, McHutchison JG, Muir AJ: The use of mind-body medicine and prayer among adult patients with chronic hepatitis C, *Gastroenterol Nurs* 33:210-216, 2010.

adopted by the ANA and the HMA, better reflects the growing practice. The practice of faith community nursing is defined as the "practice of professional nursing that focuses on the intentional care of the spirit" in promoting "wholistic" health and prevention of illness (ANA/HMA, 2005, p 1). In addition, the practice is governed by each state's nurse practice act and standards of practice.

Faith community nurses respond to health and wellness needs within the context of populations of faith communities and are partners with the faith community in fulfilling the mission of health ministry in the intentional care for the spiritual needs of the population. The faith community includes persons

Faith community nurse models that have been widely implemented include congregation- and institution-based models. In the congregational model, the nurse is usually autonomous. The development of a faith community nurse/health ministry program arises from the individual community of faith. The nurse is accountable to the faith community and its governing body. The institutional model includes greater collaboration and partnership; the nurse may be in a contractual relationship with hospitals, medical centers, long-term care establishments, or educational institutions. In either model, nurses work closely with professional health care members, faith community pastoral staff, and lay volunteers. To promote healing, the nurse builds on strengths to encourage the connecting and integrating of inner spiritual knowing and healthy lifestyle choices to achieve optimal wellness in the many circumstances faced by individuals and families in life. Intentional and compassionate presence of a spiritually mature professional nurse in individual or group situations is vital. In this role, providing holistic care with congregation populations is important. Holistic care is concerned with the relationship between body, mind, and spirit in a constantly changing environment (Dossey, Keegan, and Guzzetta, 2005). The nurse and members of the congregation assess, plan, implement, and evaluate programs. The process of realizing holistic care is enhanced by an active wellness committee or health cabinet with members who are fully engaged in health ministry (Chase-Ziolek, 2005). These committees are most effective when members represent the broad spectrum of the life of the church. An active wellness committee provides leadership and influence throughout the faith community; ideas are not from one individual but generated out of a committee structure (McNamara, 2006). The faith community nurse uses all the knowledge and skills of this specialty to provide effective services. The outcome is a truly caring congregation that supports healthy, spiritually fulfilling lives. Resources for faith community nursing can be found on this book's Evolve website.

> **▌DID YOU KNOW?**   *As acute care registered nurses in the United States near retirement age, they will be searching for opportunities to serve in other capacities. One area of continued practice for these nurses may be in faith communities where they may have more scheduling flexibility and the opportunity to focus care on the spiritual needs of the congregants while using their expertise in providing health promotion services.*

HISTORICAL PERSPECTIVES

Faith Communities

In the roots of many faith traditions are concerns for justice, mercy, and the need for spiritual and physical healing. The appeal for caring, the healing of diseases, and acknowledging periods of illness and wellness is universal. Religion plays an important role in the lives of many individuals. In a 2005 poll, 64% of Americans described themselves as being religious and the same percentage indicated that they prayed daily (Adler, 2005). The relationship between spirituality, religion, and

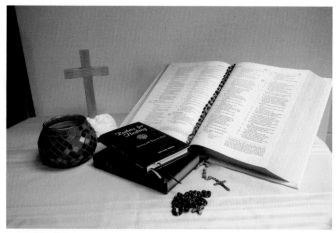

FIGURE 45-2 Religious symbols, images, rituals, and sacred places are a significant part of the ministry.

health is emerging as an important topic for nursing research. Schlundt and colleagues (2008) reported a positive association between religious involvement and perceptions of overall health, physical activity, healthy lifestyle behaviors, yet negative associations with eating patterns. An important aspect of living out one's spirituality and religion is being a part of a community of faith from birth to death, throughout wellness and illness (Figure 45-2). Whether participating as individuals or as families, all benefit from association with a supportive faith community or congregation through enhanced happiness, peace, hope and purpose (Koenig, 2009).

The biblical account of Phoebe (Romans 16:1-2) exemplifies the tradition of health and healing within a congregation. In addition, many Old Testament accounts and healing stories in the New Testament provide additional faith foundations (Psalms 106, 107, 113; Mark; Luke; Acts). The charge of the early Christian church was to preach, teach, and heal. The church provided access to services such as shelter and food; the church tended to wounds and offered comfort and safety. So, too, nuns, deacons, and deaconesses from the Christian tradition are all examples of the healing professions serving in communities as they encounter more caring congregations.

The origins of wholeness and salvation are derived from similar concepts of sodzo (Greek) and shalom, or wholeness. These terms and harmony in health are common to most faith communities. Writings in Christian and Jewish sources address the individual and community relationships with God as the source for a wise use of resources of self, environment, and one's community. Hygiene, health, and healing were a part of the Holiness Code of Leviticus. Throughout history, health existed at the center of the interaction between one's creator and humankind. The integration of faith and health within the caring community results in beneficial outcomes. Persons who encounter physical and emotional illness and who are able to call upon their faith beliefs and religious traditions are able to increase coping skills and realize spiritual growth. In a study of African-American men, prayer, spirituality, and trust in a higher power were important health maintenance strategies (Ravenell, Johnson, and Whitaker, 2006). In a study exploring perceived burden of caregivers, religious involvement in general, and church attendance in particular, seemed to provide both spiritual and social psychological benefits to dementia caregivers (Sun et al, 2009).

Using strengths from earliest memories of faith traditions and previous learning experiences, as well as the ability to accept support from family and friends, helps individuals and groups to interpret brokenness, disasters, joys, births, deaths, illness, and recovery. Encouraging growth in faith beliefs and honoring traditions and rituals of the faith community bring individuals, families, and congregations in closer connection with their creator. The consolation of sacred liturgies, religious rituals, sacred space, and communal events aids the grieving and the healing process; they also affirm transcendent life (O'Brien, 2003; Dossey, Keegan, and Guzzetta, 2005).

Some of the major Christian faith communities in the late nineteenth and early twentieth centuries used missionaries to develop multipurpose activities in communities, which included health activities and education along with religious messages. Hospitals were built in the United States and abroad, and underserved populations were targeted. As political and economic forces have changed through the years, health ministry strategies of faith communities have altered their approaches. Some faith groups have identified with community development efforts to help empower people to meet their needs for food, education, clean environments, social support, and primary health care. Congregations have also recognized the need to increase awareness in several areas including one's personal responsibility for healthy choices; the escalating cost of health care and the need for cost containment; the increasing numbers of the uninsured and underserved; the issues of domestic violence and substance abuse; and the ever-increasing dilemma of interpreting the complex changes within the health care delivery system.

The governing bodies of various faith communities have supported these efforts by endorsing statements related to health and wellness (ELCA, 2003; LCMS, 2003). The Presbyterian Church (USA) is cited as an example of a long-standing tradition of encouraging members to be good stewards or responsible managers of body, mind, the environment, and total resources. Studies in the late 1980s, the publication of essays titled "Health Care and Its Costs," and the meetings of the Task Force on Health Costs and Policies resulted in a 1988 policy statement, *Life Abundant: Values, Choices, and Health Care* (OGA, 1988). Congregations were asked to responsibly model holistic and compassionate concern for health and the provision of care. Furthermore, the policy statement endorsed employing parish nurses or other health professionals as agents of the congregation's mission to encourage the role of "communities of health and healing" (OGA, 1988, p 20). Similar efforts are present in the Episcopal Church USA, the United Church of Christ, the Catholic Church, and other national faith communities.

The revival of modern faith community nursing occurred in the 1940s when the Reverend Granger Westberg began to explore ways to address wholistic healing through the body-mind-spirit connection (1987). Believing that congregations should have a key role in wholistic health care, Westberg (1990) and his colleagues developed holistic health centers within faith community settings. He stated, "Care for all of the people of God is a part of the church's mission, of its understanding of the Christian gospel" (Westberg, 1990, p 9). The holistic health centers of the 1970s were a pivotal development that connected hospitals and faith communities and highlighted the role of the nurse in health and wellness promotion (Westberg, 1990). As Westberg noted, "It was clear that the nurses in each of these centers were the glue that bound these three professions together in a common appreciation of the healing talents of each" (1999, p 35). The centers emphasized a comprehensive team approach to total health care and holistic health care. The teams included physicians, nurses, and clergy working with families to encourage personal responsibility for health (Westberg, 1990).

The formulation of parish nursing in the early 1980s built on the strengths of these holistic health centers and focused on the nurse–clergy team working with individuals and their families. Nurses used their abilities to listen to the spoken and unspoken concerns of individuals and made assessments and judgments that were based on their knowledge of the health sciences and humanities. By the mid-1980s, Lutheran General Hospital and Reverend Westberg embarked on a pilot project with six Chicago congregations that included four Protestant and two Roman Catholic communities (Solari-Twadell and McDermott, 2006). Loyola University and Swedish Covenant Hospital were among the forerunners in revitalizing the nurse's role in the healing traditions; acknowledging the importance of body, mind, and spirit connections; incorporating education; and providing health promotion services within congregations.

Health Care Delivery

Early chapters in Parts 1 and 2 of this text familiarize the reader with the historical, economic, social, political, environmental, and ethical perspectives and influences on health care. The health care delivery system is challenged to work within parameters of tighter financial constraints while welcoming advanced technology and addressing new health concerns. Current health care reform reflects a shift in health care delivery to a more comprehensive wellness-focused program (ANA, 2010a). Faith community nurses are well positioned to provide holistic community-based care for vulnerable and underserved populations and to collaborate with care providers.

The following are examples of issues that are important to this chapter. After major hospitalizations, clients may return to their homes very sick with few, if any, care providers available. Caregivers are faced with the multiple tasks of managing finances, maintaining family responsibilities, and learning caregiving skills. Fragmented care and inadequate caregiver training and availability are problems for the disenfranchised, underserved, and uninsured, as well as for the economically well-situated and better-educated persons. Families are challenged to seek the best ways to meet the multiple demands of young children, teens, and aging parents whether in the metropolitan, micropolitan, or rural environment.

Consumer demand for involvement in health care decisions continues to increase, and society emphasizes individual responsibility for health. Simultaneously, consumers have increased interest in their own well-being and have expressed needs for health information to be available in a variety of formats (Loeb, O'Neill, and Gueldner, 2001; McGinnis and Zoske, 2008; Beacom and Newman, 2010). In addition to consumer interest and a heightened awareness of responsibility for one's own health, health care providers and managed care systems have found it financially advantageous for their participants to be healthy and remain out of the system. Thus, with rising costs of care, scarce resources for populations, and the complex system demands on individuals and families to seek health care, the challenge for the consumer now is how to cope with these forces.

The traditional health care delivery model will not meet the burgeoning needs of the future. The skills of professional nurses, such as faith community nurses, will become more important with the provision of health care services in non-traditional settings (McGinnis and Zoske, 2008). However, it is important to differentiate the unique practice of faith community nursing from other community-based specialty practices. Faith community nursing shares many similarities with home health, hospice, and public health nursing; but it is also shaped and guided by the worshipping community's traditions, rites, and rituals.

A primary focus of all nurses in the last few decades has been to coordinate care and to link health care providers, groups, and community resources as the client tries to understand diverse health plans. Negotiating with individuals, agencies, and community partnerships within the complex maze of the broader health care environment demands a knowledgeable and seasoned professional. Nurses are aware of the necessity of collaborative practices and the formation of partnerships to care for groups and individuals throughout the age span. These nurses recognize the need for diverse ways to address health promotion and disease prevention at all levels. They advocate for healthy lifestyle choices in exercise, nutrition, substance use, and stress management. They realize that information and guidance must be available via media, in schools, workplaces, faith communities, and residential neighborhoods. Faith community nurses need to partner with others as they serve populations through faith communities (Chase-Ziolek, 2005).

Holistic Health Care

Holistic health practices emphasize nurses' and clients' embrace of a commitment to optimal wellness. Such practices focus nurses and clients on seeking the meaning of wellness for the individual or situation, and on considering options from an array of therapies. Harmony between the physical, emotional, psychological, and spiritual self is sought. In addition to sharing backgrounds and functions similar to those of public health nursing, faith community nursing also parallels and benefits from commonalities and distinct practices of holistic nursing. Regardless of specialty or practice setting, nurses who practice in a holistic manner acknowledge wholeness as more than the sum of the individual parts (Dossey et al, 2005). The philosophy of holistic nursing practice (which is a subspecialty

in nursing) embraces concepts of the presence, healing, and holism. The interconnectedness of body, mind, and spirit is basic to holistic nursing and is embedded in the practice of faith community nurses. Like faith community nursing, holistic nursing emphasizes wholeness of persons across the life span.

The current standards of holistic nursing practice were approved by the *American Holistic Nurses Association (AHNA)* in 2000 (updated 2007) and contain five core values. These standards provide guidelines for practice, education, and research. The standards are a guide for all professional nurses, as are the five assumptions that underlie faith community nursing as found in *Faith Community Nursing: Scope and Standards of Practice* (ANA/HMA, 2005). Faith community nurses will find them helpful in embracing more holistic practices and interventions. Faith community nurses have already used some of the interventions commonly found in holistic nursing, and additional exploration by faith community nurses enhances practice possibilities to promote wellness and healing for practitioner and client (Denton, 2005). Both faith community nurses and holistic nurses share the skill of creating a healing environment (Dossey et al, 2005). Listening coupled with intentional compassion is basic to effective interventions. Selected interventions that are often used in both specialties of nursing are prayer, meditation, counseling, guided imagery, health promotion guidance, journaling, therapeutic touch, healing presence, and massage. Information about accessing AHNA can be found on this book's Evolve website.

FAITH COMMUNITY NURSING PRACTICE

Characteristics of the Practice

As in the early history of the development of public health nursing in this country, faith community nurses found that health promotion services were needed in underserved urban and rural areas (Baldwin et al, 2001; Wallace et al, 2002). Nurses identified gaps in the delivery of service. They found that congregants residing in communities that offered access to adequate health services also requested and benefited from health counseling and health promotion services at all levels of prevention.

The faith community nurse services emphasized health promotion and disease prevention and provided the benefits of holistic care through the supportive, caring faith community. Nurses acknowledged the inner strength and spirituality of persons and groups to increase healing. The nurses developed effective skills in negotiation, collaboration, and leadership. They also honed astute non-verbal and verbal communication skills. They embraced the vital role of families for healthy outcomes, and parish nurses knew that community support augmented the interventions chosen by individuals and families. Working with the congregation as the population group, parish nurses attempt to include in the wellness programs those persons who are less vocal or visible in the community of faith. The spiritual dimension of health was and is optimized by complementing the nursing role with pastoral care.

EVIDENCE-BASED PRACTICE

The study authors describe this collaborative program as a service focused on promoting health and preventing disease among vulnerable, underserved, low-income adults through a mobile health delivery project. In collaboration between a faith community nurse program, a religious order, and a university school of pharmacy, the project focused on the delivery of disease-screening services, counseling, health education, referrals, advocacy, and follow-up services through a mobile health van. Outcome measures indicated that low-income, medically underserved, older widowed women were most likely to use these services. The client population served was predominantly white. The most frequent health screening was blood pressure, followed by cholesterol, blood glucose, bone density, and body fat. Many of the women were being treated for hypertension, hyperlipidemia, and diabetes, but their measures were not in the appropriate ranges. The pharmacists and faith community nurses provided counseling and education on the importance of medication adherence as well as lifestyle modification, healthy food choices, and the need for exercise with each follow-up visit. Barriers to the project included client reluctance to access health screenings and lack of trust caused by past experiences with health care providers. These providers addressed these concerns by consistency in schedule at sites, using the same staff.

Nurse Use

Faith community nurses are encouraged to partner with other care providers to provide delivery of screening and follow-up services. This project fostered a positive, trusting client-provider relationship that formed the basis of the clients' motivation to make positive lifestyle changes. Assisting vulnerable individuals to decrease their health risks helps to empower people to care for themselves. As faith community nurses reach out to their surrounding community, they need to use creative strategies and collaborate with other care providers to positively impact health attitudes and behaviors.

From Mayernik D, Resick L, Skomo M, Mandock K: Parish nurse-initiated interdisciplinary mobile health care delivery project, *J Obstetr Gynecol Neonatal Nurs* 39:227-234, 2010.

TABLE 45-1 PHASES OF FAITH COMMUNITY NURSE PROGRAM DEVELOPMENT

PHASE	CHARACTERISTIC
Recognizing	Nurses describe a calling and desire to have a holistic practice
Preparing	Personal development: seek information and affirmation
	Professional development: educational preparation
	Coalition building: paving the way with the faith community
Planning	Assess community needs, market ideas, elicit volunteers, set goals
	Work with leaders, determine available resources, partnerships
Implementing	Team building, support and manage volunteers, self-development
Evaluating	Record keeping, outcome summaries

From Farrell SP, Rigney DB: From dream to reality: how a parish nurse program is born, *J Christian Nurs* 22:34-37, 2005.

spiritual care. Table 45-1 details the phases of faith community nurse program development.

NURSING TIP *Developing a keen sense of the mission of the faith community and appreciating its associations within the local and greater community are beneficial in the development of the health and healing activities by the faith community nurse.*

Faith communities and nurses have formed new and unique partnerships in response to societal and institutional needs (Hickman, 2006). Coalitions of networks were important as faith communities developed into centers of support and caring. Faith community nurses also began to affiliate with coalitions of inner city churches, networks of rural churches, individual hospitals, chaplaincy programs, and health departments. If the vision or mission of the congregation extended beyond its immediate membership, those outside of the immediate faith community who would benefit from the services are also potential recipients. Nurses then included arrangements with nearby community centers, visiting nurse associations, homeless shelters, community health centers, or forms of neighborhood nursing associations. Some nurses work with one or more faith communities and with one or more religious traditions.

Nurses in any of these arrangements consider the environment and population characteristics of congregations and the community. The strengths and assets of the congregation are the building blocks for services, and because faith communities traditionally value the talents and gifts of their members, efforts flourish within and beyond the faith community. Faith community nurses address the identified needs for health promotion and disease prevention, and they understand the importance of the body-mind-spirit connection with a primary focus on

To support the faith community nurse, the International Parish Nurse Resource Center (IPNRC) was established in 1986. The center's mission is the promotion and development of quality faith community nurse programs through research, education, and consultation (Patterson, 2003). Establishment of the philosophy, mission, assumptions, and strategic purpose of the specialty was conceived with the guidance of the IPNRC. In addition, core curricula as standard preparation for faith community nurses and coordinators were developed and continue to be revised (Patterson, 2003; Solari-Twadell and McDermott, 2006). Throughout the years, the IPNRC has been vigilant in addressing emerging issues such as documentation accountability, preparation for parish nurses, and accreditation concerns (related to The Joint Commission [TJC]) for parish nurses connected with institutional hospital systems. The IPNRC sponsors the annual Westberg Symposium for faith community nursing, which is an international forum to present the latest research and practice patterns in faith community nursing. Information about accessing the center can be found on this book's Evolve website.

The development of programs of study for the new specialty has evolved from the initial adoption of the HMA and ANA's *Scope and Standards of Practice of Parish Nursing Practice* (HMA/ANA, 1998) and the revised *Faith Community Nursing: Scope and Standards of Practice* (ANA/HMA, 2005). The document will be further revised in 2011. Faith community nurses active in the interfaith Health Ministries' Association (HMA) developed these documents. Professional and laypersons in both health and faith disciplines concerned about health ministries comprise the HMA, which also holds an annual symposium. Members of the faith community nurse section include professional nurse members committed to improving the practice and developing statements of agreement related to faith community nursing. Information about accessing the HMA can be found on this book's Evolve website.

As advanced practice nurse and faith community nurse practices increase in numbers and varieties of arrangements, evaluation of practice trends within the health care delivery system and the needs of society is necessary. Nursing must be accountable and responsive to those being served, as well as to those who provide opportunities to serve.

The goal of faith community nursing is to develop and sustain health ministries within faith communities. Faith community nursing is community-based and population-focused professional nursing practice with communities of faith to promote whole-person health. Faith community nurses must be fully aware of the beliefs, faith practices, and level of spiritual maturity of congregants served, and they link these with health and healing. Nurses work with a health cabinet or wellness committee to evaluate assets and areas of need in order to plan services that will attain outcomes congruent with goals established by the congregation and faith communities served (Patterson, 2003).

Many faith community nurses function in a part-time capacity and serve as salaried or unpaid staff. If salaried, the average faith community nurse earns around $17.00/hour (McCabe and Somers, 2009; Bokinskie, 2010). Some nurses are responsible for services for several faith communities, whereas others engage in faith community nursing as part of a full-time commitment in other capacities. For example, a nurse might be employed part time as a public health nurse and part time as a faith community nurse in the same community. Alternatively, a nurse employed full time in an acute care setting may spend time serving in an unpaid capacity working in a faith community with a group of other nurses. Depending on the practice model, the nurse has a narrowly defined or a wider realm of responsibility. Faith community nurse practices may be integrated into a health care system or into practices that collaborate with related professional practice areas such as health departments or colleges of nursing. Health care systems employ faith community nurse coordinators, who facilitate different arrangements with several faith communities of varying backgrounds (Hickman, 2006; Zurell and Solari-Twadell, 2006). Both rural and urban settings find these arrangements effective for facilitating health ministry programs (Solari-Twadell and McDermott, 2006). Practices in which several faith community nurses are supervised by a coordinator have built-in opportunities for networking, partnering, and mentoring.

At the first IPNRC-sponsored colloquium held in the early 1990s, five characteristics identified as central to the philosophy of parish nursing (faith community nursing) were conceived by nursing educators and practitioners (Solari-Twadell, 2006):

1. The spiritual dimension is central to the practice of parish nursing. Nursing embodies the physical, psychological, social, and spiritual dimensions of clients into professional practice. Although parish nursing includes all four, it focuses on intentional and compassionate care, which stems from the spiritual dimension of all humankind.

2. The roots of the role balance both knowledge and skills of nursing, using nursing sciences, the humanities, and theology. The nurse combines nursing functions with pastoral care functions. Visits in the office, home, hospital, or nursing home often involve prayer and may include a reference to scripture, symbols, sacraments, and liturgy of the faith community represented by the nurse. The values and beliefs of the faith community are integral to the supportive care given. Nurses also assist with worship services as appropriate within the faith community.

3. The focus of the specialty is the faith community and its ministry. The faith community is the source of health and healing partnerships, which result in creative responses to health and health-related concerns. Partnerships may be among individuals, groups, and health care professionals within the congregation. They may also be among various congregations or community agencies, institutions, or individuals. Partnerships also evolve as the congregation visualizes its health-related mission beyond the walls, stones, and steeples of its own place of worship.

4. Parish nurse services emphasize the strengths of individuals, families, and communities. Parish nurses endorse this fourth characteristic in their practice. As congregations realize the need for care and care for one another, their individual and corporate relationship with their Creator is often enhanced. This provides additional coping strength for future crisis situations within the family and community.

5. Health, spiritual health, and healing are considered an ongoing, dynamic process. Because spiritual health is central to well-being, influences are evident in the total individual and noted in a healthy congregation. Well-being and illness may occur simultaneously; spiritual healing or well-being can exist in the absence of cure.

The Third Invitational Parish Nurse Educational Colloquium sponsored by the IPNRC affirmed assumptions of the practice of faith community nursing, and these assumptions were confirmed in 2000 by the 600 participants of the Westberg Symposium (Solari-Twadell and McDermott, 2006; Solari-Twadell, McDermott, and Matheus, 2000). Box 45-2 details this vision. Those gathered affirmed that the client includes individuals, families, congregations, and communities across the life span. The practice includes the full cultural and geographic community regardless of ethnicity, lifestyle, sex, sexual orientation, or creed. The nurse in the practice incorporates faith and health, uses the nursing process in providing services to the faith community, and facilitates collaborative health ministries as an important component of the practice. In addition, the group affirmed that although the curricula stem from a Judeo-Christian theological framework, faith community nursing respects diverse traditions of faith communities and encourages adaptation of the programs to these faith traditions.

BOX 45-2 VISION OF PARISH NURSING

Root Assumptions

Parish nursing is rooted in the Judeo-Christian tradition, consistent with the basic assumption of all faiths that we care for self and others as an expression of God's love.

Mission

The mission of parish nursing is the intentional integration of the practice of faith with the practice of nursing so that people can achieve wholeness in, with, and through the community of faith in which parish nurses serve.

Purpose

- Challenge the nursing profession to reclaim the spiritual dimension of nursing care
- Challenge the health care system to provide whole person care
- Challenge the faith community to restore its healing mission

Strategic Vision

Access to a parish nurse ministry in every faith community

From the International Parish Nurse Resource Center, 2011. Available at http://www.parishnurses.org.

THE CUTTING EDGE *In response to the growing unmet needs for physical and mental health services for the homeless population, MeritCare Health System, Fargo, ND, is partnering with a local homeless shelter and a women's shelter to provide access to Shelter Faith Community Nurses (SFCN). An ultimate goal of shelter services is to assist the residents in achieving self-sufficiency; however, unmanaged health issues are a major barrier for the residents. The SFCN works collaboratively with the residents by empowering them to achieve optimal health and wellness by addressing the needs of mind, body, and spirit in a holistic manner with a focus on appropriate usage of health care services, access to care, and advocacy. Primary interventions of the SFCN are health assessment, health teaching/counseling, referral, and emotional support. Educational sessions include empowerment, problem-solving skills, self care, women and heart disease, and stress management. Preliminary findings from a research study on cost avoidance reflect health care cost savings through the implementation of the SFCN program.*

Scope and Standards of Faith Community Nursing Practice

Nursing: Scope and Standards of Practice (ANA, 2004) described what nursing is, what nurses do, and the responsibilities for which they are accountable. This document served as the template for the specialties within the profession, and therefore was the foundation for *Faith Community Nursing: Scope and Standards of Practice* (ANA/HMA, 2005). This revised scope and standards described the who, what, where, when, why, and how of the practice of faith community nursing. Nurses well versed in the parish nursing practice field compiled this revision of the 1998 *Scope and Standards of Parish Nursing Practice* by a thorough review of the practice, public comments, and dialogue of practicing parish nurses. Specialty areas within professional nursing achieve a major milestone when the standards and scope common to that practice are recognized.

The specialized practice of faith community nursing focuses on intentional *spiritual care* as an integral part of the process of promoting wholistic health and preventing or minimizing illness in the faith community (ANA/HMA, 2005). The scope and standards of care for the independent practice of the profession guide the nurse's practice and relate to the intentional care on spiritual health using the nursing interventions of "education, counseling, advocacy, referral, utilizing resources available to the faith community, and training and supervising volunteers from the faith community" (ANA/HMA, 2005, p 1). The faith community nurse's client focus includes the community as a whole; groups, families, and individuals from the designated membership; and groups, families, and individuals from the vicinity of the faith community or the greater community to which the congregation belongs. Nurses encourage individuals, families, and entire faith communities to promote health and healing within the context of the faith community to arrive at wellness outcomes. As in other arenas of nursing, the client level is multidimensional. Affliction of one member of the faith community can affect an entire community, and the response by the nurse needs to be complex. "Assessment focuses on identifying the educational and supportive needs of the whole faith community" (ANA/HMA, 2005, p 3). The faith community nurse uses professional skills that combine spiritual care and nursing care as well as services and resources from groups within and beyond the faith community to provide a holistic response (ANA/HMA, 2005).

The *Scope and Standards* delineate examples of the faith community nurse's independent functions. These functions are in compliance with and reflect the current boundaries of nursing practice, as well as specific legal standards to which nurses must adhere. Nurses function within the nurse practice act of their jurisdiction (i.e., their state). If advanced practice functions such as prescriptive authority and treatment are implemented, faith community nurses must be in compliance with the legal criteria of the jurisdiction's nurse practice act (ANA/HMA, 2005). For example, when influenza vaccine or immunization clinics are offered, appropriate arrangements are made to use nurses from a cooperating community agency (health department), or the faith community nurse must have a contractual policy agreement with the cooperating agency to provide the immunizations. In addition to a narrative description and glossary of terms, the document divides the standards the nurse must meet. It outlines standards of care and standards of professional performance. In keeping with wise use of persons and materials, standards of professional performance elaborate on coordination of care and consultation. Faith community nurses are "vital partners in advancing the nation's health initiatives" (ANA/HMA, 2005, p 9).

Educational Preparation for the Faith Community Nurse

Current educational preparation for the nurse includes the successful completion of extensive continuing education contact hours or designated coursework in faith community nurse preparation at the baccalaureate or graduate level, as well as a thorough grasp of the *Scope and Standards* of the practice (ANA/HMA, 2005; IPNRC, 2009c). Such preparation is held in colleges, universities, health care institutions, and faith community nurse networks across the United States and other countries as well as online and

BOX 45-3 RESOURCES FOR FAITH COMMUNITY NURSING

International Parish Nurse Resource Center
475 East Lockwood Avenue
St. Louis, MO 63119
http://www.parishnurses.org
(Publication: *Parish Nurse Perspectives*)

Health Ministries Association
1-800-280-9919
http://www.hmassoc.org
(Publication: *HMA Today*)

Interfaith Health Program of the Carter Center
1256 Briarcliff Road
Atlanta, GA 30306
http://www.cartercenter.org/health/index.html

Duke University Center for Spirituality, Theology and Health
Duke University Medical Center
Box 3825
Busse Building, Suite 0507
Durham, NC 27710
http://www.spiritualityandhealth.duke.edu

(Publication: *Crossroads*)
See the WebLinks on this book's Evolve website at http://evolve.elsevier.com/stanhope/foundations for further information about resources.

distance delivery (Gustafson, 2006). Many of these programs are in partnership with the IPNRC for ongoing support (IPNRC, 2009b). The philosophy of the IPNRC's curriculum embraces four major concepts: the spiritual dimension, professionalism, wholistic health, and community. With a primary focus on spiritual health and well-being, the faith community nurses promote wholistic health within a faith community practice (IPNRC, 2009b). These basic programs provide an orientation to the role and functions of the faith community nurse, as well as worship experiences for the process of ministry (McDermott and Solari-Twadell, 2006). Faith community nurses are then able to adapt this knowledge, combined with an in-depth understanding of the beliefs of their faith tradition, to meet the holistic health needs of their local community of faith. According to *Faith Community Nursing: Scope and Standards of Practice* (ANA/HMA, 2005), the preferred minimum preparation for the specialty is the following: educational preparation at the baccalaureate or higher level with content in community nursing, experience as a registered nurse, knowledge of the health care assets of a community, specialized knowledge of the spiritual practices of a given faith community, and specialized skills and knowledge to implement the *Scope and Standards*. Both the annual Westberg Symposium offered by the IPNRC and the annual meeting of the HMA offer comprehensive sessions for nurses to network, gain new knowledge, and stay abreast of current resources, trends, and issues in the practice (Box 45-3).

NURSING TIP *The faith community nurse benefits from several years of practice experience within acute and community based settings, following the basic undergraduate preparation, because the nature of the position demands a seasoned professional who practices independently.*

Advanced practice opportunities also enrich a specialty practice. Master's-prepared nurses (with specialization in congregational leadership, congregational health, public health nursing, or holistic nursing) and nurse practitioners have found niches in faith community nursing. Universities and seminaries have developed creative and unique partnerships to provide educational opportunities for faculty and students at the undergraduate and graduate levels.

HOW TO Work with Baccalaureate Nursing Students and Nursing Faculty

When exploring the possibility of using a faith community as a clinical site for nursing students, consider the following aspects:
- *Understanding: Explore with the nursing faculty member their knowledge of faith community nursing. What information about the specific faith community and the religious rites and rituals are needed prior to the start of the student experience?*
- *Curricular aspects: What is the focus of the course—community health, public health, maternal-child health, health promotion? What are the course objectives and the specific unit objectives? What is the academic level of the nursing student?*
- *Time/Students: Consider the number of hours available for this experience and the flexibility of the student's hours with those available to the faith community nurse. Can the setting accommodate multiple students or only one individual?*
- *Supervision: Who will provide the overall supervision of the student's activities? In what ways will the faith community nurse have input in the evaluation of the student's activities?*
- *Guidelines: Consider the guidelines needed for student safety, in-home or institutional visitation, confidentiality, and documentation.*
- *Activities: Formulate activities that include all aspects of the nursing process for the students to actively participate in. Identify areas from a variety of life stages and with different cultural backgrounds if possible.*

Formal educational preparation and continuing education options must continue to include the basics and enrichment courses in nursing practice, research, theology, and pastoral care. In addition, the nurse needs updates in areas of public health, medicine, sociology, cultural diversity, and human growth and development across the life span. Improving collaboration, negotiation, and coordination skills, as well as consultation, leadership, management, and research skills, is essential. Faith community nurses accept responsibility for ongoing professional education within nursing and ministry arenas (ANA/HMA, 2005; McDermott and Solari-Twadell, 2006).

The challenge for the practice is to document trends, maintain and enhance quality of preparation and services offered, engage in evidence-based practice, use increased numbers of advanced practice nurses, network within professional organizations, and become involved in outcomes-oriented research.

McDermott and Solari-Twadell (2006) described the history of the development of faith community education through the IPNRC and the current need to develop an evidence-based curriculum to adequately reflect current and anticipated parish nursing practice. The work of Solari-Twadell (2002) was used to define the differentiation of the ministry of faith community nursing using nursing standardized language of the Nursing Intervention Classification System (NIC). The results indicated that the basic preparation curriculum would need a major revision. This revision would prepare nurses for actual documented practice.

In a review of documentation of health records by faith community nurses, the standard language of NIC captured the spiritual dimension of care provided (Weis and Schank, 2000; Burkhart and Androwich, 2004). To remain at the cutting edge of the profession and recognize competency among practitioners, the specialty must pursue ongoing research in evidence-based practice for the continued documentation of actual interventions. This will enhance the development of the curricula needed for preparation and could lead to specialty certification.

A move to specialty certification has been pursued, but has been placed on hold due to lack of financial resources and minimal membership size (Patterson, 2009). There is also a question as to the need for this certification since faith community nurses work in "churches, synagogues, temples, mosques and other faith community settings and not in healthcare facilities, certification currently has little bearing on the decision of a committee or board in a community to engage the professional services of an FCN" (ANA/HMA, 2005, p 5).

Currently, faith community nurses may receive specialty certification in related areas such as community or public health nursing and holistic nursing or specific credentialed preparation from a religious body of the faith community served.

DID YOU KNOW? *Baccalaureate students can gain significant clinical practicum experience in population-focused care by working with faith community nurses. Nursing students assess community needs, plan, implement, and assist in the evaluation of programs to promote health and wellness within faith communities.*

Activities of the Faith Community Nurse

A description of the functions of parish nursing provides a framework for understanding the work of faith community nurses. These functions are derived from the primary roles of the parish nurse as envisioned by the founder of present-day parish nursing, Reverend Doctor Granger Westberg, and delineated by the IPNRC (Westberg, 1990; Patterson, 2003). The seven functions of the faith community nurse include personal health counseling, health education, referral or liaison activities, facilitating groups, integrating faith and health, health advocacy, and coordinating volunteer services. These functions and corresponding examples are displayed in Table 45-2. It is worthy to note that these functions often overlap into other categories. For example, the function of integrating faith and health can easily be found in the other functional areas and may be perceived more as a common theme of the other functions rather than a separate function to itself. Because of the uniqueness of the faith community as a practice setting, the nurse may have a broader practice than these seven functions; therefore, it is difficult to provide a comprehensive list of functions and actions for the faith community nurse.

Faith community nurses carry out their practice in groups or individually. They make visits to homes, to health care institutions, or at the faith community setting. Some nurses have designated office space, whereas others may use space that is most conducive to the particular need. Many parish nurses hold regular blood pressure screening events. These events not only screen for those who need medical follow-up, but also provide an opportunity for faith community members to approach the nurse about other personal health concerns in a non-threatening manner.

NURSING TIP *The faith community nurse can elevate the connection between faith and health using such strategies as meditation, song, and prayer to help control pain, or encouraging the ancient activity of walking a labyrinth as a way to calm anxiety.*

As one of the trusted members of the **pastoral care staff**, the faith community nurse will find it helpful to develop ease in inquiring about a few important areas of a persons' spiritual journey. Numerous instruments or tools are available for use in spiritual assessments (Carson and Koenig, 2002; Koenig, 2002; Dossey et al, 2005; Hodge and Limb, 2010). History of family relationships and past association with faith communities provide background information. Compassionate, careful listening involves being still, reflecting, and being intentionally in the present. Being sensitive to the differing needs of personal spirituality during various points along life's journey is important to consider while guiding persons through the spiritual assessment. The nurse then also helps individuals share necessary information about spirituality needs with other health care providers.

Ireland (2010) provides insight into how the nurse can use a culturally sensitive spiritual assessment tool to address spiritual needs. She describes how the client brought up spiritual issues with a joke or indirectly by addressing some of the difficulties in the client's life. Often these conversations occurred at night when the client's family was asleep. The nurse needs to be comfortable in the discussion with questions that lead clients to expand on their faith beliefs. This simple approach to spiritual assessment can be applied to many situations within all of professional nursing. Each nurse must guide the assessment to obtain the information needed to promote health and healing.

WHAT DO YOU THINK? *A young couple who has contributed their time, enthusiasm, and skills assisting as church youth group leaders are expecting their first child. The faith community nurse would contend this is a valuable learning experience for the teens. Having a couple experience healthy life events is indeed beneficial for youth. Upon birth, the infant is diagnosed with Down syndrome. Now there are not the normal celebrations and visions for the future. Instead of parties, what information is to be shared, and with whom, and when? How much privacy is granted? The manner in which the family, other youth leaders, and the nurse work with the team, use the strengths of the congregation, and reflect on the spiritual needs of all concerned is most important for healthy outcomes. The learning opportunities are valuable growth experiences for the couple, both as young teens and as new parents. Having opportunities to describe one's feelings and to deal with them in supportive groups is beneficial in the healing process.*

TABLE 45-2 FUNCTIONS AND RELATED ACTIVITIES OF THE FAITH COMMUNITY NURSE

FUNCTION	EXAMPLES OF RELATED ACTIVITIES
Personal health counseling	• Health risk appraisal/screenings including blood pressure, vision, depression, foot screenings • Perform spiritual assessments • Individual and group discussions on implementing healthy lifestyles through diet, exercise, and spiritual activities • Support and guidance related to acute and chronic actual and potential health problems
Health education	• Publish information in newsletter, website, or bulletin on physical, mental, and spiritual health issues • Distribute appropriate health-related pamphlets from local public health agency to teens, parents, elderly members • Hold classes to address identified educational needs • Coordinate a health fair to serve members across the life span • Provide one-on-one teaching related to defined health need • Provide education to create a fuller understanding of total physical, mental, and spiritual well-being
Resource referral/liaison activities	• Help clients know what resources are available in their community • Help individuals and families match the appropriate resource for their health situation • Link clients with appropriate resources within and outside of the faith community • Explain and assist members in considering choices when new care arrangements must be made for loved ones
Group facilitation	• Link individual's needs for the establishment of and referral to support groups • Facilitate or lead group activities • Facilitate change and enhance accessibility for physically or mentally challenged members
Coordination of volunteer services	• Work with volunteer coordinator or volunteers to ensure that persons acquire education to function as lay care providers to meet faith community needs • Provide supervision for respective volunteers
Integration of faith and health	• Lend support during times of joy by providing devotional materials for new parents • Use presence and skills to understand the individual's spiritual journey • Identify the individual's spiritual strengths that assist in healing and instill hope • Offer rites and rituals for the faith community • Participate in healing worship events • Offer prayer, hymns, scripture, pictures, and stories appropriate to the individual and for the faith tradition
Health advocacy	• Encourage faith community members to participate in political activities that impact the health and well-being of the faith community and surrounding area • Encourage individuals to implement healthy lifestyles • Offer services through the faith community including food pantries, day activities for children and seniors, congregant meals, tutoring, and latch-key activities • Provide outreach services for less-mobile members, non-members, vulnerable populations • Be present with members for questions that seem difficult to ask the health care provider • Provide service on a health care center's ethics committee

From Patterson DL: *The essential parish nurse,* Cleveland, 2003, The Pilgrim Press; Berry R: A parish nurse. In Office of Resourcing Committees on Preparation for Ministry: *A day in the life of . . . : a kaleidoscope of specialized ministries,* Louisville, KY, 1994, Presbyterian Church (USA), Distribution Management Service.

Faith community leaders are well aware that many of their members are part of the growing population of older adults in the country (Figure 45-3). They also witness increasing numbers of persons who are either uninsured or underinsured and see that many families have care needs for children and aging parents during working hours. They see a smaller pool of family members available for care-giving because of geographic distances or simply a lack of children (McGinnis and Zoske, 2008). They see a growing level of ethnic and cultural diversity within their neighborhoods and see the need to reach out.

Services offered to provide healthier living for these groups, day care for young children and elderly parents, language tutoring, and culturally appropriate outreach activities for vulnerable populations are examples of needed services (Bokinskie and Evanson, 2009) (Figure 45-4). Facilitating services for those in

and beyond the faith community benefit the recipients. Partnering with others provides opportunities for volunteers to serve and gain a feeling of worth. A growing model for this type of congregational care is being done through the work of "caring circles" or "care teams." This successful model surrounds a person in need with a group of trained volunteers ready to "share the care" in providing essential services for health support (Capossela and Warnock, 2004).

These service needs challenge the faith community nurse to be the catalyst for beneficial and healthy partnerships. Partnerships and facilitation of healthier living for older adults is the focus of community arrangements of the Elderberry Institute. For over 25 years, the community-owned block nursing programs (BNPs) and Living at Home (LAH) have assisted seniors to remain safe, independent, and socially active in their home

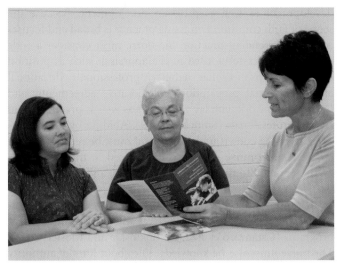

FIGURE 45-3 A visit with an older adult and family member provides referral information.

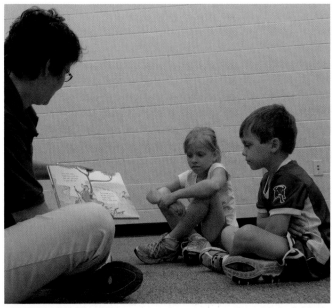

FIGURE 45-4 The faith community nurse works with individuals across the lifespan.

communities. Nurses in Minnesota, spearheaded by Martinson and Jamieson (1985) and following examples of public health nursing pioneer Lillian Wald, combined their professional nursing experience, their keen knowledge of the neighborhood, and the belief that communities could pool their own resources to meet the needs of its residents.

In the early St. Anthony BNP, residents received in-home support and health care with a mix of professionals and volunteers as caregivers (block companions). Residents from 6 to 85 years of age were served (Martinson and Jameison, 1985). One evaluation of the program indicated that 85% of the persons served were able to remain out of nursing homes. The Elderberry Institute provides technical assistance, training, and education for staff and volunteers and guides program operations for the new arrangements. Partnerships with hunger programs,

BOX 45-4	EVALUATING PROGRAM OUTCOMES IN FAITH COMMUNITIES

Faith community nurses provide health-promoting and disease-preventing activities within faith communities. These nurses need to provide these services with limited resources of money, time, and equipment. The following model for program development and evaluation can help in the creation of high-quality, effective programs:

Step 1: What is the problem or issue that the program is designed to address? Be specific about the problem as it guides the search for evidence-based information.

Step 2: Identify both short- and long-term goals. These help prioritize what you will need to monitor.

Step 3: Document the specific program outcomes. This may include numbers of attendees, participation rates, or desired changes in measurements.

Step 4: Develop and implement the interventions for the program, as determined by best practices, to achieve the goals identified in Step 2.

Step 5: Evaluate the short- and long-term goals and the specific program outcomes. Share the outcome results with individuals or in aggregate form to the faith community. Disseminate findings to other faith community nurses on the local and national levels.

Adapted from Timmons S: African American church health programs: What works? *J Christian Nurs* 2:100-106, 2010.

and other community resources such as faith community nursing services, keep these community groups viable. They strive to maintain a strong local citizen board. Faith community nurses in locations not served by Elderberry Institute programs are encouraged to become familiar with similar elder care resources and community groups in their locales. The strength of the foregoing program is in the demonstrated strong, collaborative, community partnerships. Additional resources for this topic can be found on this book's Evolve website.

Future Growth

Faith community nurses can develop comprehensive, population-focused practices. They may also implement programs at beginning levels of community-based practices to ensure comprehensive care for individuals and families. The continuing challenge for nurses, other health care providers, and the communities will be to garner government, foundation, and private funding and combine it with support from volunteer activities, family involvement, and community groups to create the unique mix needed for the distinctiveness of each community. Nurses are asked to partner with community members where they live, work, attend school, and gather for worship; to closely partner with these same members to advocate for those who are powerless; to keenly identify health and health-related needs; to detect and address those needs to prevent costly use of the health care system; and to be closely aligned with those who can implement visionary policy that improves health care for community members across the life span.

Uncovering and understanding the intricacies of the work of faith community nurses is a difficult task since very little research on the outcomes of faith community nursing interventions has been conducted. Box 45-4 provides a general guide to program evaluation for faith community nurses. Comprehending the distinctiveness of the role of faith community nursing is important to the maturation of the specialty because it allows for a clear recognition of the work done (Solari-Twadell, 2006). Ground-breaking research was conducted in 2002 by Solari-Twadell using the Nursing Intervention Classification (NIC) system (McCloskey, 2000). With data from more than 1000 parish nurses, essential or core nursing interventions were named that help to differentiate the practice of parish nursing. This research confirmed that spiritual care is the hallmark of the faith community nurse's practice as the top interventions used daily and weekly, including active listening, presence, spiritual support, emotional support, spiritual growth facilitation, humor, and hope instillation (Solari-Twadell, 2006).

ISSUES IN FAITH COMMUNITY NURSING PRACTICE

Every new discipline or care area must be alert to issues of accountability to populations served, as well as to those who entrust the nurse with the responsibility to serve a designated population. Because the role involves professional, legal, ethical, theological, and relational issues, the nurse will need to review, respect, and reflect on the parameters involved. Outcomes can be positive and the potential for conflicts reduced by the following:

- Discussions of health promotion activities must include the individual, the family, and the faith community leadership.
- Negotiations with the pastoral staff, congregations, institutions, and the wider community must be involved in job description preparation and program planning.
- Issues such as privacy, confidentiality, group concerns, access, and record management must be discussed with the pastoral staff or the contracting agency at the outset of any program agreement.

> **DID YOU KNOW?**   *Previous studies found that faith community nurses believe it is essential to work with health care providers, clergy, and congregational boards to effectively develop, facilitate, and implement health-promoting and spiritually focused activities for individuals and groups within faith communities (Blanchfield and McLaughlin, 2006; Bokinskie and Kloster, 2008).*

Professional Issues

A position description is a necessary tool for the development of the faith community nursing practice. The description should accurately reflect the functions, accountabilities, and responsibilities of the position (Hickman, 2006). Annual and periodic evaluations of faith community nurse practices, as well as assessments and evaluations of services needed, are certainly indicated. These evaluations will want to include self, peer, congregational, and/or institutional evaluations so that improvements can be made in practice if needed.

Professional appraisal, or a portfolio, is becoming a standard in nursing practice and therefore is needed within faith community nursing. The appraisals guide the nurse's professional

development as well as program development. Because the scope of faith community nursing practice is broad and focuses on the independent practice, the nurse must consider a wide variety of topics to be used in the appraisal, such as position description, professional liability, professional educational and experiential preparation, collaborative agreements, and the ability to work with lay volunteers as well as practicing and retired professionals (Smucker, 2009). Abiding by the professional nursing code is understood and must be reflected in the appraisal. The nurse must also be assessed in the application of skills related to the polity, expectations, and mission of the particular faith community.

It is important for the faith community nurse to serve in a collaborative relationship with the clergy to effectively implement programs (Catanzaro et al, 2006; Bokinskie and Kloster, 2008). The nurse must also be knowledgeable about lines of authority and channels of communication in the faith community as well as within collaborative institutions. Administrative personnel, such as clergy, or congregational committees provide guidance and contribute to the evaluation of faith community nurse programming. They also advocate for the nurse's services and raise awareness with the faith community's staff and membership.

Nurses advocate for well-being and thus are in unique positions to highlight justice issues in local and national legislation. As the faith community reflects on the implications of legislation on their congregation and the national faith community, the nurse contributes information to policy makers about the implications for health and well-being for the parish, for the local community, and for the global community. Active participation in political activities contributes to spiritual growth and healthy functioning.

> **WHAT DO YOU THINK?**   *Faith community nurses face much of the same ethical issues as other nurses in different practice settings. The nurse must respect the parishioner's wish for privacy and confidentiality, of veracity and truth telling, and of advocacy unless the client is in danger or laws mandate reporting of certain circumstances. However, the nurse must be keenly aware of the communal nature of the faith community—a setting where there is a commitment to pray for others, a setting where joys and struggles are shared (Hickman, 2006).*

Ethical Issues

Issues evolve from client, faith community, and professional arenas. The faith community nurse's interventions are guided by professional nursing responsibilities that will include the revised *Code for Nurses with Interpretive Statements* (ANA, 2008), *Nursing's Social Policy Statement* (ANA, 2010b), *Nursing: Scope and Standards of Practice* (ANA, 2010c), and *Faith Community Nursing: Scope and Standards of Practice* (ANA/HMA, 2005). In addition to these nursing responsibilities, the faith community nurse must be well versed on individual and group rights, statements of faith, polity, and doctrines of the faith community(ies) served.

Professional and therapeutic relationships are maintained at all times; consulting and counseling with minors and individual members of the opposite sex are conducted using professional ethical principles. Policies about these issues are established at the outset of the practice in conjunction with the pastoral team, the wellness committee, the faith community nurse, and the faith community's governing or judiciary body. As in other community health situations, the nurse, along with the client, identifies parameters of ethical concerns, plans ahead with clients to consider healthy options in making ethical decisions, and supports clients in their journey to choose alternatives that will strengthen coping skills and allow them to grow stronger in faith and health.

Communities of faith strive to be caring communities and value the fellowship among its members. However, confidentiality is of utmost importance in faith community nursing practice. The faith community nurse values client confidentiality but at the same time delicately assists the client and client's family at the appropriate time to "share" concerns with pastoral staff or fellow congregants. This sharing may gain valuable support to promote optimal healing. The nurse is often the staff member who helps the family to the stage of acceptance of a health concern. How much to share and when to share a concern are indeed a private affair and a part of the important journey of healing. A joyous event for one family may be a devastating event or even a depressing reminder of a past event for another family (like a birth for a new family and the loss of a child in another family).

Legal Issues

As an advocate of client and group rights, the nurse identifies and reports neglect, abuse, and illegal behaviors to the appropriate legal sources. The faith community nurse appropriately refers members to pastoral or community resources if the scope of the problem is not within the professional realm of the nurse. Referral is also indicated if conflict between nurse and client is such that no further progress is possible. The faith community nurse who has a positive relationship that values open dialogue with the pastoral team will be supported in efforts to select the most appropriate community resource for clients.

The nurse must personally and professionally abide by the parameters of the nurse practice act of the jurisdiction, maintain an active license of that state, and practice according to the Scope and Standards of Practice. Additional legal concerns are those of institutional contractual agreements, records' management, release of information, and volunteer liability. Resources to address legal issues of the practice related to the specific faith community include the faith community's legal consultant, the faith community's national position statements, and guidelines of any institutional partner, as well as resources from the HMA and IPNRC (Solari-Twadell and McDermott, 2006).

Financial Issues

Innovative arrangements for variations of the basic models mentioned previously call for sustained financial support. The nurse is called on to partner in finding funds and networking with potential supporters. The nurse is accountable for money spent and for fundraising, whether the position is salaried or volunteer. Educational and promotional materials, equipment,

---

BOX 45-5 RESOURCE ASSESSMENT FOR THE FAITH COMMUNITY NURSE

It is a challenge for the faith community nurse to assess what programs are really needed with limited resources available in faith communities. The following set of questions can help in coming to a clear understanding of what is possible and being aware in advance of the consequences of projects that are undertaken (Solari-Twadell and McDermott, 2006, p 104).

1. What resources are needed?
2. What resources are available?
3. Which of the available resources are accessible to the nurse for the accomplishment of a specific effort or project?
4. Can the work of the project or program be accomplished with what is available and accessible?

---

travel time, continuing education, and malpractice insurance are selected areas that need to be included in the budget of the parish nurse. If these materials are not budget items, services may be limited, and this needs to be interpreted to the faith community. Money, time, and people are never sufficient to meet the needs of the faith community nurse ministry, but it is up to the nurse to use a resource assessment in advance of a project in order to come to a clear understanding of what is possible given the specific faith community resources (Solari-Twadell and McDermott, 2006) (Box 45-5).

NATIONAL HEALTH OBJECTIVES AND FAITH COMMUNITIES

The *Healthy People 2020* indicators encourage communities to support individuals and families to attain high-quality lives free of preventable diseases across the life span, to reduce health disparities across groups, and to create environments that promote health. Faith communities have long held a position of esteem in communities. One of the oldest and strongest partnerships is that established between communities and religious or faith communities. The Carter Center in Atlanta and the Park Ridge Center for Health, Faith and Ethics in Chicago collaborated with health care professionals and leaders of faith traditions to identify roles of faith communities to address national health objectives and approaches to improving overall public health.

Because faith communities are rooted in healing traditions and hold issues of justice and mercy as a priority, the *Healthy People 2020* goals to attain high quality, longer lives free of preventable disease, disability, injury, and premature death, achieve health equity, eliminate disparities, and improve the health of all groups, create social and physical environments that promote good health for all, and promote quality of life, healthy development, and healthy behaviors across all life stages, can be readily addressed. Because values of health and faith institutions are closely aligned, evidence of partnering is becoming more prominent and necessary in the current socioeconomic environment. The National Heart, Lung and Blood Institute and the American Heart Association have long partnered with faith communities and offered resources for programs.

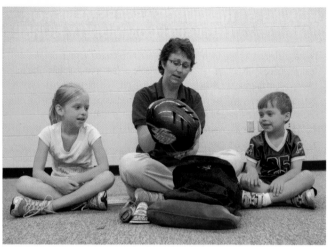

FIGURE 45-5 Health promotion activities are one aspect of the nurse's role.

Specific national objectives dealing with nutrition; physical activity; use of tobacco, alcohol, and other drugs; immunization status; environmental health; and injury and violence are within the realm of the health education role of the faith community nurse. Activities include age-appropriate discussions of preventive activities with various groups; classes on the use and misuse of alcohol, tobacco, and other drugs; and discussions regarding responsible sexual behavior in the context of faith values (Figure 45-5). As an outreach to the surrounding community, the nurse can create an environment within the faith community that promotes health and is a safe setting for activities.

Wellness committees and faith community nurses may regularly review the various health status objectives, make comparisons between national and specific state objectives, and then assess the extent to which the individual faith community member or group is in need of reducing risk.

- Regular blood pressure screening and monitoring activities focus on heart disease and stroke prevention and disability.
- Age-appropriate discussion of preventive activities can be held with various groups.
- Signs and symptoms of heart attack and stroke can be noted and described in newsletters and posted on bulletin boards throughout the facility.
- The nurse can coordinate healthy low-fat meals.
- The nurse can encourage youth groups to choose healthy fruit and vegetables as snacks after their activities.
- The nurse can coordinate a series of classes for families of adolescents on stress management and sessions on the use and misuse of alcohol, tobacco, and other drugs.
- The nurse can encourage or lead a faith-based exercise program for individuals as a part of ongoing faith community activity.

Examples of interventions related to selected portions of *Healthy People 2020* objectives that could be addressed by faith community nurses are listed in the *Healthy People 2020* box.

The faith community's wellness committee can also address other objectives to identify activities in which to engage the entire faith community or surrounding geographic area. Most advantageous for the faith community would be for the faith community nurse, wellness committees, and other interested persons to engage in partnership activities with community efforts such as health fairs. The teachers, principal, clergy, parent–teacher group, staff, students, wellness council, special education teachers, and recreation leaders are all potential participants (Figure 45-6). Health fairs are effective strategies for health promotion efforts guided by the *Healthy People 2020* framework. These and similar activities promote increased health of the entire community, and they include persons of all ages, encourage enthusiasm, offer fellowship and leisure, and reduce duplication of effort.

♥ HEALTHY PEOPLE 2020

Objectives Related to Nutrition and Weight and Physical Activity and Fitness for Youth in Faith Communities

Nutrition and Weight Status
- NWS-7: Increase the proportion of worksites that offer nutrition or weight management classes or counseling.
- NWS-10: Reduce the proportion of children and adolescents who are considered obese.
- NWS-11: (Developmental) Prevent inappropriate weight gain in youth and adults.
- NWS-14: Increase the contribution of fruits to the diets of the population aged 2 years and older.
- NWS-15: Increase the variety and contribution of vegetables to the diets of the population aged 2 years and older.
- NWS-16: Increase the contribution of whole grains to the diets of the population aged 2 years and older.
- NWS-17: Reduce consumption of calories from solid fats and added sugars in the population aged 2 years and older.

- NWS-18: Reduce consumption of saturated fat in the population aged 2 years and older.
- NWS-19: Reduce consumption of sodium in the population aged 2 years and older.
- NWS-20: Increase consumption of calcium in the population aged 2 years and older.

Physical Activity and Fitness
- PA-3: Increase the proportion of adolescents that meet current physical activity guidelines for aerobic physical activity and for muscle-strengthening activity.
- PA-8: Increase the proportion of children and adolescents who do not exceed recommended limits for screen time.
- PA-8.2: Increase the proportion of children and adolescents aged 2 years through 12th grade who view television, videos, or play video games for no more than 2 hours a day.

From U.S. Department of Health and Human Services: *Healthy People 2020: national health promotion and disease prevention objectives,* Washington, DC, 2010, USDHHS.

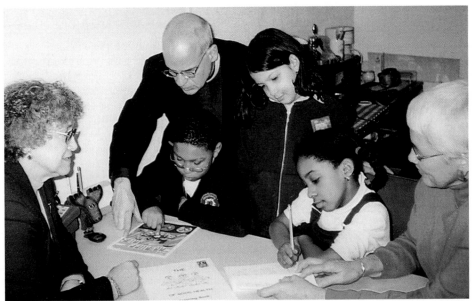

FIGURE 45-6 Planning a healthy lifestyle curriculum with principal, clergy, and pupils within a faith community school population.

LEVELS OF PREVENTION

Nutrition and Weight and Physical Activity and Fitness

Primary Prevention

- Hold classes for youth and parents on healthy eating appropriate for various age levels.
- Promote and encourage age-appropriate activities that include physical exercise in youth group meetings, retreats, summer camps, and nursery programs.
- Encourage a variety of activities and discourage extended inactivity (including television and video games).
- Encourage healthy snacks and meals for youth activities and parenting sessions.
- Write faith community newsletter articles informing parents of the need for adequate exercise and proper nutrition for healthy lifestyles in youth and teen years.
- Encourage parents to be proactive in school parenting councils as well as in neighborhood recreation leagues to ensure exercise programs and activities for youth.
- Encourage faith community leaders to sponsor a safe indoor/outdoor activity area for neighborhood or at-risk children.

Secondary Prevention

- Provide health assessment and counseling during home visits for health promotion initiated for other family members, such as visits after a hospitalization or a birth.
- Using an attitudinal/behavioral risk survey, identify factors for obesity in the faith community's youth.
- Be available for health counseling for youth and teens before and after activities.
- In schools associated with faith communities, assist with height and weight screening to identify youth and teens needing attention and referral.

Tertiary Prevention

- Collaborate closely with faith education teachers, youth ministers/counselors about sessions that deal with nutrition behavior change, exercise behavior modification with injury prevention guidelines, health problems of overweight young persons, and advantages of maintaining a healthy weight, and support, stress management, and improved quality-of-life sessions.
- Follow up and monitor health care provider's plan of care for young persons who have been identified as overweight; support and encourage them to withstand peer ridicule during behavior changes.
- Facilitate a faith-based activities program for overweight youth that includes age-appropriate exercises, health education, and spiritual development.
- Assist in making choices for behavior change (suggest avoiding calorie-rich or nutritionally lacking foods during school meal and snack times; suggest possible paths for walking and bicycling; suggest courts and gyms available for more strenuous exercise).
- Discuss in youth groups and parenting groups the need for loving, caring friends and the support needed for long-term behavior modification programs that are lifelong efforts.

From U.S. Department of Health and Human Services: *Healthy People 2020*, Washington, DC, 2010, USDHHS.

LINKING CONTENT TO PRACTICE

This chapter has stressed a population focus for faith community nursing. In Christian traditions, the scriptural story of the Good Shepherd who cares for the whole flock as well as for the lost, silent, or "out of bounds" individuals so that they may again become a part of the flock is an effective parallel with a population focus. The faith community nurse acts as a catalyst to facilitate efforts to address health indicators of the faith community and the related objectives for behavior change. The entire faith community is considered instrumental in this objective; those who find it difficult to voice their concern or those on the margins are intentionally sought to become part of the efforts to promote healthy behaviors and healthy environments.

Faith communities often work closely with other organizations closely aligned with their mission or outreach activities. These organizations may include an individual health care institution, a childcare or an adult day care center, an immigrant community, a homeless shelter, a crisis center, a preschool, or a local neighborhood, elementary, or high school. The example of the LAH/BNP programs or Care Team programs working with older, less mobile, or frail populations was cited earlier in this chapter. In all of these situations, faith community nurses use their best nursing skills to collaborate with all key individuals and groups involved.

Many faith communities may also administrate educational facilities from preschool level to high schools. If a faith community nurse is working in this type of setting, it is an example of another type of population-focused practice. The key players are gathered for discussions on assessment and programming for the health needs of this school population within the faith community setting. Assessing the school environment and population is advisable (see Chapter 42) prior to the implementation of programs. The group would consider the abilities of the faculty, staff, pupils, and parents. It would assess the physical environment for safe and healthy activities, and the program for enrichment opportunities in music, physical education, or dance. It would discuss health topics, curriculum appropriate for growth and development, healthy choice opportunities throughout the day's activities, and opportunities for parents and pupils to learn skills for lifelong learning, as well as other topics desired by the group. Suggestions can come from *Healthy People 2020,* state education requirements, and faith community school documents and guidelines. The agenda can be as comprehensive or as focused as the group wishes, but working within a timeline can be beneficial to see outcomes. The nurse would guide the group as it ascertains strengths and develops a plan for implementation of focused objectives and a plan for evaluating and reporting their efforts.

CHAPTER REVIEW

PRACTICE APPLICATION

The nursing process is a method that can be used to begin program planning and evaluation with faith communities. Such an approach can involve faith community members and faith community nurses in a dynamic endeavor to jointly learn about the members' individual health status, as well as that of the faith community and the local and broader geographic community. Faith community nurse programs are derived in various ways. Initially, the impetus for faith community nursing may stem from an unmet health need within the congregation or organization, from visions of lay or health professions members concerned about caring for vulnerable groups within the congregation, or from discussions of a committee dealing with health and wellness issues.

Which of the following activities is most likely to increase the interest and involvement of the faith community's members?
A. Writing a contract for the services of the faith community nurse
B. Surveying the faith community's environment
C. Gathering information on leaders and valued activities in the congregation through focus groups of pastoral staff
D. Assessing the needs of the congregational members through a survey
E. Holding a health fair
Answers can be found on the Evolve site.

KEY POINTS

- Faith community nurse services respond to health, healing, and wholeness within the context of the faith community. Although the emphasis is on health promotion and disease prevention throughout the life span, the spiritual dimension of nursing is central to the practice. The focus of the practice is on the "intentional care of the spirit" (ANA and HMA, 2005).
- Faith community nursing has evolved from roots of healing traditions in faith communities; early public health nursing efforts working with individuals, families, and populations in the community; and more recently the independent practice of nursing.
- The faith community nurse partners with the wellness committee and volunteers to plan programs that address the health-related concerns within faith communities.
- To promote a caring faith community, usual functions of the faith community nurse include health counseling and teaching for individuals and groups, facilitating linkages and referrals to

congregation and community resources, advocating and encouraging support resources, and providing spiritual care.
- Faith community nurses collaborate to plan, implement, and evaluate health promotion activities considering the faith community's beliefs, rituals, and polity. *Healthy People 2020* leading indicators and objectives are excellent and effective frameworks for health ministry efforts of wellness committees and basic to partnering for programs.
- Nurses in congregational or institutional models enhance the health ministry programs of the faith communities if carefully chosen partnerships are formed within the congregation, with other faith communities as well as with local health and social community organizations.
- Nurses working as faith community nurses must seek to attain adequate educational and skill preparation to be accountable to those served.

KEY POINTS—cont'd

- Nurses are encouraged to consider innovative approaches to creating caring communities. These may be in individual faith communities as nurses; among several faith communities in a single locale; or in partnership with other community institutions.

- To sustain oneself as a faith community nurse who provides spiritual care to support individuals, families, and communities in the healing and wholeness process, the nurse must be diligent to take time for self-nurture and renewal.

CLINICAL DECISION-MAKING ACTIVITIES

1. Contact the local organization of faith communities (such as the Council of Churches or health system) to see if there is faith community nursing in your area. If so, make contact and arrange to spend a day with a nurse.
   A. Interview the nurse about the faith community nurse role functions. Contrast the nurse's answers to what you learned in this chapter.
   B. Ask how the faith community nurse standards of practice are integrated into the practice. How can you verify the answer?
   C. If possible, have classmates spend time in different faith communities: in urban and rural settings, different faith traditions, non-traditional settings.
2. Discuss with classmates the similarities and differences between home health care nursing, school nursing, public health nursing, and faith community nursing. Compare your answers.
3. Choose a *Healthy People 2020* indicator to implement in a faith community setting. Discuss plans for implementing the objective and evaluating the outcomes with the faith community

nurse and wellness committee. What data did you use to develop a plan for implementation? How did you choose your population? How did you evaluate the outcomes of your goals and activities?
4. Interview a clergy member of a local church, temple, or mosque in your area (preferably with someone with a different background than your own). Ask the individual to elaborate on traditions of health and healing connections. Consider how you might be able to meet the unique needs of that faith community.
5. Visit a senior citizen daycare center and speak with participants about important events in their lives. Did they refer to rituals from faith traditions? Ask them about their associations with faith communities during their lives.
6. With classmates, interview a youth group leader and nurse in a local faith community about the concern of preventing risky behaviors among youths. What perspectives of this concern would the faith community staff need to consider?

REFERENCES

Adler NE: Special report: spirituality, *Newsweek*, August 20, 2005, pp 48–54.

American Holistic Nurses Association: *Holistic nursing: scope and standards of practice*, Washington, D.C, 2000, updated 2007, ANA.

American Nurses Association: *Nursing: scope and standards of practice*, Washington, D.C, 2004, ANA.

American Nurses Association: *Code for nurses with interpretive statements*, Washington, DC, 2008, ANA.

American Nurses Association: *Health care reform*, 2010a. Available at http://www.nursingworld.org/healthcarereform. Accessed July 1, 2010.

American Nurses Association: *Nursing's social policy statement*, ed 2, Washington, DC, 2010b, ANA. Available at http://www.nursesbooks.org.

American Nurses Association: *Nursing: scope and standards of practice* Silver Spring, MD, 2010c, ANA. Available at http://www.nursesbooks.org.

American Nurses Association and Health Ministries Association: *Faith community nursing: scope and standards of practice*, Silver Spring, MD, 2005, ANA. Available at http://www.nursesbooks.org.

Baldwin KA, Humbles PL, Armmer FA, Cramer M, et al: Perceived needs of urban African American church congregants, *Public Health Nurs* 18:295–303, 2001.

Beacom AM, Newman SJ: Communicating health information to disadvantaged populations, *Fam Community Health* 2:152–162, 2010.

Berry R: A parish nurse. In Office of Resourcing Committees on Preparation for Ministry: *A day in the life of… : a kaleidoscope of specialized ministries*, Louisville, KY, 1994, Presbyterian Church (USA), Distribution Management Service.

Blanchfield KC, McLaughlin E: Parish nursing: a collaborative ministry. In Solari-Twadell PA, McDermott MA, editors: *Parish nursing: development, education, and administration*, St Louis, 2006, Mosby, pp 65–81.

Bokinskie J: *Perceived levels of empowerment in parish nursing* (Doctoral dissertation), 2010. Available from ProQuest Information and Learning Company at disspub@proquest.com.

Bokinskie J, Evanson T: The stranger among us: ministering health to migrants, *J Christian Nurs* 26(4):202–211, 2009.

Bokinskie J, Kloster P: Effective parish nursing: Building success and overcoming barriers, *J Christian Nurs* 25(1):20–25, 2008.

Burkhart L, Androwich I: Measuring the domain completeness of the Nursing Interventions Classification System in parish nurse documentation, *Comput Inform Nurs* 22:72–82, 2004.

Capossela C, Warnock S: *Share the care*, ed 2, New York, 2004, Fireside of Simon & Schuster.

Carson VB, Koenig HG: *Parish nursing: stories of services and health care*, Philadelphia, 2002, Templeton Foundation Press.

Catanzaro A, Meador K, Koenig H, et al: Congregational health ministries: a national study of pastors' views, *Public Health Nurs* 24(1):6–17, 2006.

Chase-Ziolek M: *Health, healing and wholeness*, Cleveland, 2005, The Pilgrim Press.

Daniels M: News from the world forum for parish nursing, *Parish Nurse Perspect* 1:7, 2009.

Denton J, editor: *Good is the flesh: body, soul and Christian faith*, Harrisburg, PA, 2005, Morehouse Publishing.

Dossey BM, Keegan L, Guzzetta CE: *Holistic nursing: a handbook for practice*, ed 4, Sudbury, MA, 2005, Jones and Bartlett.

Evangelical Lutheran Church in America: *Caring for health: our shared endeavor*, 2003. Available at http://www.elca.org/What-We-Believe/Social-Issues/Social-Statements/Health-and-Healthcare.aspx. Accessed August 1, 2010.

Farrell SP, Rigney DB: From dream to reality: how a parish nurse program is born, *J Christian Nurs* 22:34–37, 2005.

Gustafson CZ: Distance delivery of parish nurse education. In Solari-Twadell PA, McDermott MA, editors: *Parish nursing: development, education, and administration*, St Louis, 2006, Mosby.

Hale WD, Koenig HG: *Healing bodies and souls: a practical guide for congregations*, Minneapolis, MN, 2003, Fortress Press.

Health Ministries' Association and American Nurses Association: *Scope and standards of parish nursing practice*, Washington, DC, 1998, ANA.

Hickman J: *Faith community nursing*, New York, 2006, Lippincott Williams & Wilkins.

Hodge DR, Limb GE: A Native American perspective on spiritual assessment: the strengths and limitations of a complementary set of assessment tools, *Health Social Work* 2:121–131, 2010.

International Parish Nurse Resource Center: *Parish nurse basic preparation curriculum*, St Louis, 2009a (revision), International Parish Nurse Resource Center.

International Parish Nurse Resource Center: *Parish nurse fact sheet*, 2009b. Available at http://parishnurses.org/Home_1.aspx. Accessed March 20, 2011.

International Parish Nurse Resource Center: *Ministry of parish nursing practice: job description for the ministry of parish nursing practice,* 2009c. Available at http://parishnurses.org/Home.aspx?ContentID+26. Accessed March 20, 2011.

Ireland J: Palliative care: a case study and reflections on some spiritual issues, *Br J Nurs* 4:237–240, 2010.

Koenig HG: *Spirituality and patient care,* Philadelphia, 2002, Templeton Foundation Press.

Koenig HG: *Religion and mental health: a review of previous research,* Durham, NC, August 2009, Paper presented at the Summer Research Workshop on Spirituality and Health.

Loeb SJ, O'Neill J, Gueldner SH: Health motivation: a determinant of older adults' attendance at health promotion programs, *J Community Health Nurs* 18:151–165, 2001.

Lutheran Church Missouri Synod: *Health ministries mission statement,* 2003. Available at http://www.lcms.org/pages/internal.asp?NavID=14348. Accessed March 20, 2011.

Martinson IM, Jamieson MK, O'Grady B, Sime M: The block nurse program, *J Community Health Nurs* 2:21, 1985.

Mayernik D, Resick L, Skomo M, Mandock K: Parish nurse-initiated interdisciplinary mobile health care delivery project, *J Obstetr Gynecol Neonatal Nurs* 39:227–234, 2010.

McCabe J, Somers S: Faith community nursing: meeting the needs of seniors, *J Christian Nurs* 2:104–109, 2009.

McCloskey JC, Bulechek GM: *Nursing Interventions Classification (NIC): Iowa intervention project,* St Louis, 2000, Mosby.

McDermott MA, Solari-Twadell PA: Parish nurse curricula. In Solari-Twadell PA, McDermott MA, editors: *Parish nursing: development, education, and administration,* St Louis, 2006, Mosby, pp 121–131.

McGinnis SL, Zoske FM: The emerging role of faith community nurses in prevention and management of chronic disease, *Pol Politics Nurs Pract* 9:173–180, 2008.

McNamara JW: *Health & wellness: what your faith community can do,* Cleveland, 2006, Pilgrim Press.

Mosack V, Medvene L, Wescott J: Differences between parish nurses and parish nurse associates: results of a statewide survey of an ecumenical network, *Public Health Nurs* 23(4):347–363, 2006.

Nist JA: Parish nursing programs: through them, faith communities are reclaiming a role in healing, *Health Progress* 84:50–54, 2003.

O'Brien ME: *Spirituality in nursing: standing on holy ground,* Sudbury, MA, 2003, Jones and Bartlett.

Office of the General Assembly: *Life abundant: values, choices, and health care,* Louisville, KY, 1988, Presbyterian Distribution Services.

Patterson DL: *The essential parish nurse,* Cleveland, 2003, The Pilgrim Press.

Patterson DL, editor: Update on specialty practice portfolio process a joint statement by the HMA and the IPNRC, *Parish Nurse Perspect* 4:8, 2009.

Patterson DL, Wehling G, Mason G: Parish nursing: reclaiming the spiritual dimensions of care, *Am Nurse Today* 10:38–39, 2008.

Ravenell JE, Johnson WE, Whitaker EE: African-American men's perceptions of health: a focus group study, *J Nat Med Assoc* 4:544–550, 2006.

Richmond JA, Bailey DE, McHutchison JG, Muir AJ: The use of mind-body medicine and prayer among adult patients with chronic hepatitis C, *Gastroenterol Nurs* 33:210–216, 2010.

Schlundt DG, Franklin MD, Patel K, et al: Religious affiliation, health behaviors and outcomes: Nashville REACH 2010, *Am J Health Behav* 32:714–724, 2008.

Smucker C: *Faith community nursing: developing a quality practice,* Silver Springs, MD, 2009, Nursesbooks.org.

Solari-Twadell PA: *The differentiation of the ministry of parish nursing practice within congregations,* 2002, Dissertation Abstracts International 63(06), 569A. UMI No. 3056442.

Solari-Twadell PA: Uncovering the intricacies of the ministry of parish nursing practice through research. In Solari-Twadell PA, McDermott MA, editors: *Parish nursing: development, education, and administration,* St Louis, 2006, Mosby, pp 17–34.

Solari-Twadell PA, McDermott MA, editors: *Parish nursing: development, education, and administration,* St Louis, 2006, Mosby.

Solari-Twadell PA, McDermott MA, Matheus R, editors: *Parish nursing education: preparation for parish nurse managers/coordinators: promoting congregational health, healing and wholeness for the twenty-first century,* Park Ridge, IL, 2000, IPNRC, Advocate Health Care.

Sun F, Kosberg JI, Leeper J, et al: Racial differences in perceived burden of rural dementia caregivers: the mediating effect of religiosity, *J Appl Gerontol* 3:290–307, 2009.

Timmons S: African American church health programs: What works? *J Christian Nurs* 2:100–106, 2010.

U.S. Department of Health and Human Services: *Healthy people 2020: the road ahead,* Rockville, MD, 2010, Office of Disease Prevention and Health Promotion. Available at http://www.healthypeople.gov/hp2020/default.asp, 2010. Accessed August 1, 2010.

Wallace DC, Tuck I, Boland CS, Witucki JM: Client perceptions of parish nursing, *Public Health Nurs* 19:128–135, 2002.

Weis D, Schank MJ: Use of a taxonomy to describe parish nurse practice with older adults, *Geriatr Nurs* 21:125–131, 2000.

Westberg GE: *The parish nurse: how to start a parish nurse program in your church,* Park Ridge, IL, 1987, Parish Nurse Resource Center.

Westberg GE: *The parish nurse,* Minneapolis, MN, 1990, Augsburg Fortress.

Westberg GE: A personal historical perspective of whole person health and the congregation. In Solari-Twadell P, McDermott M, editors: *Parish nursing: promoting whole person health within faith communities,* Thousand Oaks, CA, 1999, Sage.

Zurell LM, Solari-Twadell PA: Administration of parish nursing: describing roles, In Solari-Twadell PA, McDermott MA, editors: *Parish nursing: development, education, and administration,* St Louis, 2006, Mosby, pp 211–225.

CHAPTER 46

Public Health Nursing at Local, State, and National Levels

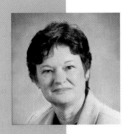

Diane V. Downing, RN, PhD

Diane V. Downing began practicing public health nursing in 1980 as a public health nurse with the Marion County Health Department in Indiana. She also worked at the local level as Assistant Commissioner for Nursing and Quality Assurance in the New York City Department of Health and Nurse Manager with Arlington Department of Human Services. She has worked at the state level in Indiana as the Sudden Infant Death Syndrome project coordinator, as division director for local health standards and evaluation, and as Division Director for the Maternal and Child Health Division. At the national level, she worked as the Director of the Policy and Research Division of the Public Health Foundation. She currently teaches public health nursing at Georgetown University School of Nursing and Health Studies in Washington, DC. She advocates for vulnerable populations and public health needs as a member of the Public Health Nursing Section Leadership, American Public Health Association. She represents Community-Campus Partnerships for Health on the Council of Linkages Between Academia and Public Health Practice. The Council on Linkages Between Academia and Public Health Practice, located in Washington, DC, and funded by the Centers for Disease Control and Prevention, is a coalition of representatives from 17 national public health organizations. The Council works to further academic/practice collaboration to ensure a well-trained, competent public health work force and a strong, evidence-based public health infrastructure.

ADDITIONAL RESOURCES

⊜volve WEBSITE
http://evolve.elsevier.com/Stanhope
- *Healthy People 2020*
- WebLinks—Of special note, see the links for these sites:
  - Council on Linkages Between Academia and Public Health Practice Core Public Health Competencies
  - Community-Campus Partnerships for Health Principles of Partnership
  - National Association of County and City Health Officials
  - Public Health Nursing Section of the American Public Health Association
  - Association of State and Territorial Health Officials
  - Nurse-Family Partnership Program

- Quiz
- Case Studies
- Glossary
- Answers to Practice Application
- Resource Tool 46.A: Core Competencies and Skill Levels for Public Health Nursing

APPENDIXES
- Appendix G.1: Examples of Public Health Nursing Roles and Implementing Public Health Functions
- Appendix G.2: American Public Health Association Definition of Public Health Nursing
- Appendix G.3: American Nurses Association Scope and Standards of Practice for Public Health Nursing

OBJECTIVES

After reading this chapter, the student should be able to do the following:
1. Define public health, public health system, public health nursing, and local, state, and national roles.
2. Identify trends in public health nursing.
3. Provide examples of public health nursing roles.
4. Differentiate the emerging public health issues that specifically affect public health nursing.
5. Describe collaborative partnerships.
6. Explain the principles of partnership.
7. Identify educational preparation of public health nurses and competencies necessary to practice.
8. Explore team concepts in public health settings.

KEY TERMS

federal public health agencies, p. 990
incident commander, p. 1001
local public health agencies, p. 991

partnerships, p. 990
public health, p. 990
public health nursing, p. 994
public health programs, p. 990

state public health agency, p. 991
—See Glossary for definitions

All of public health is built on partnerships. Public health programs are designed with the goal of improving a population's health status. They go beyond the administration of health care to individuals to a primary focus on the health of populations. Public health programs include community health assessment and interventions based on assessment results, analysis of health statistics, public education, outreach, case management, advocacy, professional education for providers, disease surveillance and investigation, emergency preparedness and response, compliance to regulations for some institutions/agencies and school systems, and follow-up of populations. Examples of follow-up care include communicating with persons with active, untreated tuberculosis, pregnant women who have not kept prenatal visits, and parents of under-immunized children. Public health programs are frequently implemented by the development of partnerships or coalitions with other providers, agencies, and groups in the location being served. Community-Campus Partnerships for Health (CCPH) defines partnerships as "a close mutual cooperation between parties having common interests, responsibilities, privileges and power" (CCPH, 2006). Partnerships are built on trust, mutual respect, and the sharing of power.

Box 46-1 presents principles of partnerships. Public health nurses are skilled at developing, sustaining, and evaluating community-wide partnerships. Public health nurses are involved in these activities in various ways depending on the public health agency (local, state, or federal) and the identified needs. Public health nurses may be the partnership facilitator or a member of the partnership representing their agency.

Public health is not a branch of medicine; it is an organized community approach designed to prevent disease, promote health, and protect populations. It works across many disciplines and is based on the scientific core of epidemiology (IOM, 1988, 2003a). Governmental agencies at the local, state, and federal levels are partners in the public health system that must work together to develop and implement solutions that will improve a community's health. Figure 46-1 represents the diverse and complex network of individuals and agencies making up the public health system (CDC, 2005a). Public health nurses partner with interprofessional teams of people within the public health areas (Figure 46-2), in other human services and public safety agencies, and in community-based organizations. The health of communities is a shared responsibility that requires a variety of diverse and often non-traditional partnerships. A critical partnership that shapes public health nursing practice in the United States is the interaction of local, state, and federal public health agencies.

ROLES OF LOCAL, STATE, AND FEDERAL PUBLIC HEALTH AGENCIES

In the United States, the local-state-federal partnership includes federal agencies, the state and territorial public health agencies, and the 3200 local public health agencies. The interaction of these agencies is critical to effectively leverage precious resources, both financial and personnel, and to protect and promote the health of populations. Public health nurses employed in all of these agencies work together to identify, develop, and implement interventions that will improve and maintain the nation's health.

Federal public health agencies develop regulations that implement policies formulated by Congress, provide a significant amount of funding to state and territorial health agencies for public health activities, survey the nation's health status and health needs, set practices and standards, provide expertise that facilitates evidence-based practice, coordinate public health activities that cross state lines, and support health services

---

BOX 46-1   PRINCIPLES OF PARTNERSHIP

Community-Campus Partnerships for Health (CCPH) involved its members and partners in developing the following "principles of good practice" for community partnerships:

- Partnerships form to serve a specific purpose and may take on new goals over time.
- Partners have agreed upon mission, values, goals, measurable outcomes, and accountability for the partnership.
- The relationship between partners is characterized by mutual trust, respect, genuineness, and commitment.
- The partnership builds upon identified strengths and assets, but also works to address needs and increase capacity of all partners.
- The partnership balances power among partners and enables resources among partners to be shared.
- Partners make clear and open communication an ongoing priority by striving to understand each other's needs and self-interests, and developing a common language.
- Principles and processes for the partnership are established with the input and agreement of all partners, especially for decision-making and conflict resolution.
- There is feedback among all stakeholders in the partnership, with the goal of continuously improving the partnership and its outcomes.
- Partners share the benefits of the partnership's accomplishments.
- Partnerships can dissolve and need to plan a process for closure.

From Community-Campus Partnerships for Health (CCPH): *Principles of good community-campus partnerships*, 2006. Available at http://www.ccph.info/.

research (IOM, 2003a). The U.S. Department of Health and Human Services (USDHHS) and the Environmental Protection Agency (EPA) are the federal agencies that most influence public health activities at the state and local levels (see Chapter 3). The USDHHS includes the Centers for Disease Control and Prevention (CDC), the Health Resources and Services Administration (HRSA), the Agency for Healthcare Research and Quality (AHRQ), and the Food and Drug Administration (FDA). The USDHHS is the agency that facilitates development of the nation's *Healthy People* objectives (USDHHS, 2010).

In the United States, states hold primary responsibility for protecting the public's health. Each of the states and territories has a single identified official state public health agency that is managed by a state health commissioner. The structure of state public health agencies varies. Some states require that the state health commissioner be a physician. A growing number of states do not limit the position to physicians but rather require specific public health experience. California, Maryland, Iowa, Oregon, Washington, and Michigan are examples of states that focus on public health experience as a requirement for the state health commissioner position. Public health nurses have been appointed to the state health commissioner positions in a number of states. For example, public health nurses have been appointed to health commissioner positions in the states of California, Oregon, Washington, and Michigan. The Association of State and Territorial Health Officials defines the **state public health agency** as the organizational unit of the state health officer, who works in partnership with other government agencies, private enterprises, and voluntary organizations to ensure that services essential to the public's health are provided for all populations. State public health agencies are responsible for monitoring health status and enforcing laws and regulations that protect and improve the public's health. In addition to state funds appropriated by state legislatures, these agencies receive funding from federal agencies for the implementation of public health interventions, such as communicable disease programs, maternal and child health programs, chronic disease prevention programs, and injury prevention programs. The agencies distribute federal and state funds to the **local public health agencies** to implement programs at the community level, and they provide oversight and consultation for local public health agencies. State health agencies also delegate some public health powers, such as the power to quarantine, to local health officers.

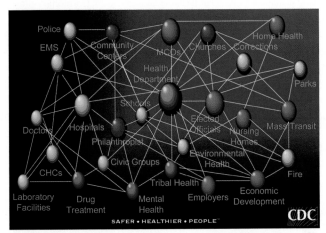

FIGURE 46-1 Adapted from The public health system. (From Centers for Disease Control and Prevention [CDC]: *The national public health performance standards, an overview, slide 9,* 2005. Available at http://www.cdc.gov/od/ocphp/nphpsp/Presentationlinks.htm.)

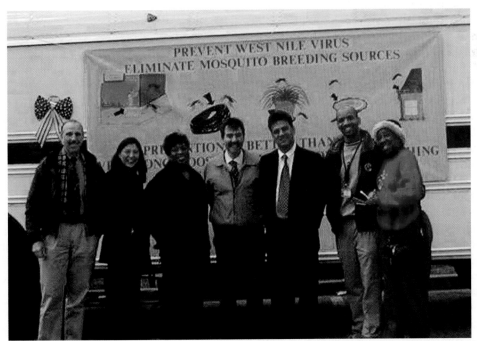

FIGURE 46-2 Public health nurses work on multidisciplinary teams that include environmental health specialists to increase public awareness about strategies to prevent transmission of West Nile virus. (Courtesy Arlington County Department of Human Services/Public Health Division, Arlington, VA.)

Local public health agencies have responsibilities that vary depending on the locality, but they are the agencies that are responsible for implementing and enforcing local, state, and federal public health codes and ordinances and providing essential public health programs to a community. The goal of the local public health department is to safeguard the public's health and to improve the community's health status. The health department's authority is delegated by the state for specific functions. The duties of local health departments vary depending on the state and local public health codes and ordinances and the responsibilities assigned by the state and local governments. Usually, the local public health department provides for the administration, regulatory oversight, public health, and environmental services for a geographical area. The National Association of County and City Health Officials' (NACCHO) operational definition of a local health department provides a description of the basic public health protections people in any community, regardless of size, can expect from their local health department. The definition provides standards within the 10 essential public health services (NACCHO, 2005). A sample of these standards can be found in Box 46-2. As with state health departments, some states require that local health directors be physicians, whereas other states focus on public health experience. For example, public health nurses in Maryland, Illinois, Washington, Wisconsin, and California hold local health director positions.

The majority of local, state, and federal public health agencies will be involved in the following:

- Collecting and analyzing vital statistics (Chapter 12)
- Providing health education and information to the population served (Chapter 16)
- Receiving reports about and investigating and controlling communicable diseases (Chapter 13)
- Planning for and responding to natural and man-made disasters and emergencies (Chapter 23)
- Protecting the environment to reduce the risk to health (Chapter 10)
- Providing some health services to particular populations at risk or with limited access to care (local public health agencies, guided by state and federal policies and goals and community needs) (Chapters 27 to 31, 38 to 46)
- Conducting community assessments to identify community assets and gaps (Chapter 18)
- Identifying public health problems for at-risk and high-risk populations (Chapter 18)
- Partnering with other organizations to develop and implement responses to identified public health concerns (Chapters 18 and 25)

Public health nurses practice in partnership with each other at the local, state, and federal levels and with other public health staff, other governmental agencies, and the community to safeguard the public's health and to improve the community's health status. Public health agency staffs include physicians, nutritionists, environmental health professionals, health educators, various laboratory workers, epidemiologists, health planners, and paraprofessional home visitors and outreach workers. Community-based organizations include the American Red Cross, free clinics, Head Start programs, daycare

---

BOX 46-2 LOCAL PUBLIC HEALTH AGENCY FUNCTIONS

The following are selected standards by selected essential public health service performed by local public health agencies:

Essential Public Health Service 1: Monitor Health Status to Identify Community Health Problems

- Obtain data that provide information on the community's health.
- Develop relationships with local providers and others in the community who have information on reportable diseases and other conditions of public health interest and facilitate information exchange.
- Conduct or contribute expertise to periodic community health assessments in order to develop a comprehensive picture of the public's health.
- Integrate data with other health assessment and data collection efforts conducted by the public health system.
- Analyze data to identify trends and population health risks.

Essential Public Health Service 4: Mobilize Community Partnerships to Identify and Solve Health Problems

- Engage the local public health system in an ongoing, strategic, community-driven, comprehensive planning process to identify, prioritize, and solve public health problems; establish public health goals; and evaluate success in meeting the goals.
- Promote the community's understanding of, and advocacy for, policies and activities that will improve the public's health.
- Develop partnerships to generate interest in and support for improved community health status, including new and emerging public health issues.

Essential Public Health Service 7: Link People to Needed Personal Health Services and Ensure the Provision of Health Care When Otherwise Unavailable

- Engage the community to identify gaps in culturally competent, appropriate, and equitable personal health services, including preventive and health promotion services, and develop strategies to close the gaps.
- Support and implement strategies to increase access to care and establish systems of personal health services, including preventive and health promotion services, in partnership with the community.
- Link individuals to available, accessible personal health care providers.

From National Association of County and City Health Officials: *Operational definition of a functional local health department*, November 2005. Available at http://www.naccho.org.

---

centers, community health centers, hospitals, senior centers, advocacy groups, churches, academic institutions, and businesses. Other governmental agencies include the fire/emergency services department, law enforcement agencies, schools, parks and recreation departments, and elected officials. Changes in local, state, and federal governments affect public health services, and public health nursing has to develop strategies for dealing with these changes. Public health nurses facilitate community assessments to identify emerging public health concerns within communities and, based on results of community assessments, help develop programs to provide needed services.

DID YOU KNOW? *States, not the federal government, hold primary responsibility for protecting the public's health. In an emergency the federal government expects the state to request assistance if needed. The federal agencies may contact the state to see if assistance is needed.*

HISTORY AND TRENDS IN PUBLIC HEALTH

A person born today can expect to live 30 years longer than a person born in 1900. Medical care accounts for 5 years of that increase. Public health practice, resulting in changes in social policies, community actions, and individual and group behavior, is responsible for the additional 25 years of that increase (USDHHS, 2009). Historically, public health nurses were valued by and important to society and functioned in an autonomous setting. They worked with populations and in settings that were not of interest to other health care disciplines or groups. Much public health service was delivered to the poor and to women and children, who did not have political power or voice. During the course of the twentieth century, public health responsibilities expanded beyond communicable disease prevention, occupational health, and environmental health programs to include reproductive health, chronic disease prevention, and injury prevention activities. As a result of Medicaid-managed care, many public health agencies were no longer providing personal health care services. Public health agencies began to shift emphasis from a focus on primary health care services to a focus on core public health activities such as the investigation and control of diseases and injuries, community health assessment, community health planning, and involvement in environmental health activities. As the twentieth century came to a close, developments in genetic engineering, the emergence of new communicable diseases, prevention of bioterrorism and violence, and the management and disposal of hazardous waste were emerging as additional public health issues (CDC, 1999). The Institute of Medicine (IOM, 2003a) identified the following seven priorities for public health in the twenty-first century:

- Understand and emphasize the broad determinants of health.
- Develop a policy focus on population health.
- Strengthen the public health infrastructure.
- Build partnerships.
- Develop systems of accountability.
- Emphasize evidence-based practice.
- Enhance communication.

Public health activities at the beginning of the twenty-first century were shaped by the September 11, 2001 terrorist attacks of the World Trade Center, the Pentagon, and a field in Pennsylvania, in which thousands were murdered. However, public health nursing activities at the federal, state, and local levels were even more dramatically affected by a series of anthrax exposures that occurred shortly after the terrorist attacks. In addition to anthrax exposures in Florida and New York, 1 month after the attacks of September 11, thousands of workers at the Brentwood Post Office and the Senate Building in Washington, DC, were exposed to an especially virulent strain of anthrax from a contaminated letter. These exposures required public health nurses to rapidly establish mass medication distribution clinics, while also responding to frightened calls from community members and requests for information from the media. The anthrax exposures alerted policy makers to the weakening public health infrastructure required to respond to bioterrorism events. As society grapples with the upheaval created by the reality of a bioterrorism event, public health nurses learn to leverage existing authority and expertise to ensure that all critical issues threatening the public's health are addressed. The shift of funding to support bioterrorism response efforts has the potential of weakening existing important public health programs. Nurses are well positioned to actively participate in policy decisions that will ensure that a public health infrastructure able to prevent and respond to bioterrorism will be strengthened and maintained within the context of general communicable disease surveillance and response. Public health nurses are facing issues such as unprecedented influenza, tetanus, and childhood vaccine shortages and emerging infections, such as SARS and the influenza A virus (H1N1) pandemic, that compete with bioterrorism activities for resources. One of these issues presented itself in the fall of 2009 and spring of 2010 when the world grappled with enough vaccine to prevent H1N1 as the virus was spread across the world. (See later discussion.)

During the twentieth century, public health nurses were a major force in the nation, achieving immunization rates that accounted for the dramatic decrease in measles. A policy brief issued by All Kids Count (2000, p 1) stated "in 1941, more than 894,000 cases of measles were reported in the U.S. In 1998, preliminary data indicated that just 100 cases were reported—a reduction of 99.9%." However, the general public was not informed about how this immunization activity was accomplished or about its effect on improving health and lowering health care costs. Public health nurses' difficulty explaining the value of ongoing prevention activities can result in a decrease in resources required to ensure adequate surveillance and containment of communicable disease outbreaks. For public health services to receive adequate funding, it is necessary for the public and the government to be aware of the benefits provided to a community by public health nurses. Public health nurses must be at the table, as advocates and experts, when issues are being discussed and decisions are being made to make certain that public health programs are provided for the populations at risk. For example, as the incidence of active tuberculosis (TB) cases decreases, officials will consider shifting funds for TB control to other efforts. Public health nurses at the national, state, and local levels work together to educate officials about the importance of continuing funding for surveillance and containment efforts if the lower TB incidence rates are to be maintained.

The twenty-first century public health nurse is working to develop a public health system able to monitor and detect suspicious trends and respond rapidly to prevent widespread exposure, whether the result of a deliberate or a natural epidemic. A prime example of emerging infectious diseases is severe acute respiratory syndrome (SARS), caused by a virus that brought illness and death to many in 2003. The disease spread quickly from China to other countries, being transported by airline passengers traveling internationally. The novel H1N1 influenza A virus pandemic provides another example of a natural epidemic that required a rapid, intensive, long-term response from public health nurses at the federal, state, and local levels. In 2009, the world was alerted to a new rapidly spreading influenza A virus (H1N1) when Mexico declared a state of emergency and closed schools and congregations in public settings in response to outbreaks of respiratory illness and increased reports of clients with influenza-like illness in several areas of the country (CDC, 2009). The first U.S. human cases of H1N1 were identified in April 2009 in California and Texas. On October 24, 2009, President Barack Obama declared H1N1 a national emergency in the United States. Public health nurses throughout the country shifted their activities to support the response to H1N1. Public health nurses who usually worked in areas such as family health services or school health services rapidly had to shift their focus to the H1N1 response. Family health service clinics and home visiting services were either cancelled or scaled back to free up public health nurse time to respond to the emerging pandemic.

WHAT DO YOU THINK? *Changes have occurred in public health nursing (Frank, 1959, p vii); they are occurring and will continue to occur in public health nursing. Public health nurses have to learn to function in an environment that must deal with many changes, since changes occur continually because of the many internal and external factors from people, programs, politics, and the unknown, as well as known local, state, and federal actions. Which skills help the public health nurse adapt to changes?*

SCOPE, STANDARDS, AND ROLES OF PUBLIC HEALTH NURSING

In 1920 C. E. A. Winslow defined public health as "the science and art of preventing disease, prolonging life and promoting health and efficiency through organized community effort" (Turnock, 2010, p 10). This definition is still used in public health textbooks because it focuses on the relationship between social conditions and health across all levels of society. The IOM defines public health practice as "what we as a society do collectively to assure the conditions in which people can be healthy" (IOM, 2003a, p 28). Reflecting these definitions, the Public Health Nursing Section of the American Public Health Association defined **public health nursing** as "the practice of promoting and protecting the health of populations using knowledge from nursing, social and public health sciences" (APHA, 1996, p 1). The American Nurses Association (ANA) adds that public health nursing is a population-focused practice that works to promote health and prevent disease for the entire population. Public health nursing is a specialty practice of nursing defined by scope of practice and not by practice setting (ANA, 2007).

Additional knowledge, skills, and aptitudes are necessary for a nurse to go beyond focusing on the health needs of the individual to focusing on the health needs of populations (see Chapters 1 and 18). This additional knowledge distinguishes the public health nurse from other nurses who are practicing in the community setting. Public health nursing practices arise from knowledge gained from the physical and social sciences, psychological and spiritual fields, environmental areas, political arena, epidemiology, economics, community organization, public health ethics, community-based participatory research, and global health. The Quad Council of Public Health Nursing Organizations identified eight principles (Box 46-3) that distinguish the public health nursing specialty from other nursing

---

BOX 46-3   TENETS OF PUBLIC HEALTH NURSING

The following eight tenets of public health nursing distinguish public health nursing from other nursing specialties, and are included in the *Scope and Standards of Public Health Nursing Practice* of the American Nurses Association (August 2007).

1. Population-based assessment, policy development, and assurance processes are systematic and comprehensive
2. All processes must include partnering with representatives of the people.
3. Primary prevention is given priority.
4. Intervention strategies are selected to create healthy environmental, social, and economic conditions in which people can thrive.
5. Public health nursing practice includes an obligation to reach out to all who might benefit from an intervention or service.
6. The dominant concern and obligation is for the greater good of all the people or the population as a whole.
7. Stewardship and allocation of available resources supports the maximum population health benefit gain.
8. The health of the people is most effectively promoted and protected through collaboration with members of other professions and organizations.

From American Nurses Association, *Public health nursing: scope and standards of practice*, 2007 Silver Springs, Md.

---

specialties. Although other nurses may practice some or all of these eight principles, they are not incorporated as a core foundation of the practice in other specialties. Public health nurses always adhere to all eight principles of public health nursing (ANA, 2007).

A variety of settings and a diversity of perspectives are available to nurses interested in developing a career in public health nursing. Public health nurses working at the federal, state, and local levels integrate community involvement and knowledge about the entire population with clinical understandings of the health and illness experiences of individuals and families in the population. They translate and articulate the health and illness needs of diverse, often vulnerable individuals and families in the population to planners and policy makers. As advocates, public health nurses help members of the community voice their problems and aspirations. Public health nurses are knowledgeable about multiple evidence-based strategies for intervention, from those applicable to the entire population, to those for the family and the individual. Public health nurses are directly engaged in the interprofessional activities of the core public health functions of assessment, assurance, and policy development. In any setting, the role of public health nurses focuses on the prevention of illness, injury, or disability, as well as the promotion and maintenance of the health of populations (ANA, 2007).

Public health nurses deliver services within the framework of ever-constricting resources coupled with emerging and complex public health issues. This requires the efficient, equitable, and evidence-based use of resources. The *Guide to Community Preventive Services* is a resource used by public health nurses to help determine which interventions to use (Task Force on Community Preventive Services, 2005). This guide provides recommendations about the effectiveness of selected health promotion/disease prevention guidelines. Box 46-4 presents

BOX 46-4 HOW TO USE EVIDENCE TO DETERMINE INTERVENTIONS

Selected Task Force on Community Preventive Services Recommendations: Vaccine-Preventable Diseases

RECOMMENDATION	INTERVENTIONS
Enhancing Access to Vaccination Services	
Recommended (strong evidence)	Expanding access in medical offices or public health clinics
Recommended (strong evidence)	Reducing out-of-pocket expenses
Recommended (sufficient evidence)	Vaccination programs in WIC settings
Recommended (sufficient evidence)	Home visits
Recommended (sufficient evidence)	Vaccination programs in schools
Insufficient evidence to determine effectiveness	Vaccination in childcare centers
Increasing Community Demand for Vaccines	
Recommended (strong evidence)	Client reminder/recall systems
Recommended (strong evidence)	Multicomponent interventions that include education
Recommended (sufficient evidence)	Vaccination requirements for childcare, school, and college attendance
Insufficient evidence to determine effectiveness	Clinic-based education only
Insufficient evidence to determine effectiveness	Client or family incentives
Insufficient evidence to determine effectiveness	Client-held medical records
Insufficient evidence to determine effectiveness	Community-wide education only

Task Force on Community Preventive Services: Centers for Disease Control and Prevention: *The guide to community preventive services,* 2005. Available at http://www.thecommunityguide.org/index.html. Accessed May 24, 2010.

selected Task Group recommendations. The *National Public Health Performance Standards Program* (CDC, 2004), a federal, state, and local partnership, has developed evaluation instruments that can be used to collect and analyze data on the programs provided through state and local public health systems. The instruments link with the 10 essential services of public health that define the core functions of public health (see Chapter 1) and help public health nurses at state and local health departments identify which essential services are met and which need additional resources.

Public health nurses make a significant difference in improving the health of a community by monitoring and assessing critical health status indicators such as immunization levels (Figure 46-3), infant mortality rates, and communicable diseases. On the basis of their assessment and in partnership with the community, public health nurses advocate for evidence-based interventions to respond to negative health status indicators. For example, a community assessment may indicate that a significant percentage of children have hemoglobin levels below 11 mg/dL. The public health nurse will know that additional information such as blood lead levels will be needed in order to implement an appropriate intervention.

Public health's shift from being the primary care provider of last resort to developing partnerships to meet the health promotion and disease prevention needs of populations has raised concerns about available health care for the uninsured and underinsured. The public health nurses' role in this ongoing shift in health care delivery is still being developed for many agencies. Public health nurses retain responsibility for assuring that all populations have access to affordable, quality health care services. They accomplish this by advocating for legislation that promotes universal health care, such as increased funding for community health centers and expansion of Medicaid

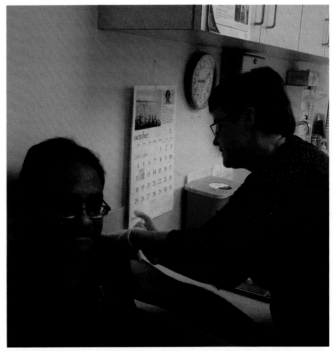

FIGURE 46-3 Public health nurses protect the population's health by providing immunizations. (Courtesy Arlington County Department of Human Services/Public Health Division, Arlington, VA.)

eligibility criteria; and by forming partnerships with hospitals, free clinics, and other organizations to guarantee health care for all populations in the community. Case management at the community level is a renewed effort in public health nursing. Through case management activities, public health nurses link populations with needed health care providers, as well as social services providers (see Chapter 22).

Uninsured individuals seek services on a sliding payment scale from such sources as university or public hospital clinics, neighborhood health centers, nurse-managed clinics, or community-based free clinics. Public health nurses serve as a bridge between these populations and the resource needs for this at-risk group by approaching health care providers on behalf of individuals seeking medical/health services and by keeping the needs of this population on the political agenda. Frequently, low-income populations or populations with multiple chronic illnesses lack the knowledge and skills to negotiate the complex health care system. This population needs education and training in identifying their problems, approaches to self-care, and illness prevention strategies and lifestyle choices that will have an effect on their health. The public health nurse understands barriers these populations confront, such as transportation issues, and difficulty understanding and following health care provider instructions.

Although vulnerable populations have always benefited from public health nursing services, the populations that are most acutely in need of public health nursing services have changed dramatically over the last couple of decades. Of particular concern are the number of young women and their partners who are substance abusers and have risky behaviors that put their pregnancy or children at high risk of injury or abuse. Public health nurses at the federal, state, and local levels have developed innovative, collaborative approaches to prepare staff to work effectively with this population.

EVIDENCE-BASED PRACTICE

The Nurse-Family Partnership home visitation program provides rigorously defined nurse home visits to first-time low-income mothers. It is an evidence-based public health program that has been rigorously evaluated in three randomized, controlled trials. Results demonstrated improvements in birth outcomes, prenatal health, child development, school readiness, and academic achievement, and reductions in child abuse and neglect and early childhood injuries. A recent study examined the effects of these nurse home visits on 594 urban mothers' birth spacing, partner relationships and government spending. The study design was a randomized controlled trial.

Results demonstrated that mothers receiving the nurse home visits, compared with the control group, experienced less role impairment from drug and alcohol use (0.0% vs 2.5%, $P = .04$) and longer partner relationships (59.58 vs 52.67 months, $P = .02$). It also demonstrated that over the 12-year study period, government spent less per year on Medicaid, food stamps, and Aid to Families with Dependent Children and Temporary Assistance for Needy Families for mothers receiving nurse home visits than the control group ($8772 vs. $9797, $P = .02$).

Nurse Use

On March 23, 2010, President Obama signed into law health care reform legislation that included $1.5 billion in funding for evidence-based home visitation to states over 5 years. Nurses can change outcomes for first-time low-income mothers by rigorously implementing the Nurse-Family Partnership model.

From Olds DL, Kitzman HJ, Cole RE, et al: Enduring effects of prenatal and infancy home visiting by nurses on maternal life course and government spending: follow-up of a randomized trial among children at age 12 years, *Arch Pediatr Adolesc Med* 164 (5):419-424, 2010.

ISSUES AND TRENDS IN PUBLIC HEALTH NURSING

The discovery and development of antibiotics in the 1940s, coupled with immunization programs and improvements in sanitation, contributed to the decrease in infectious disease related morbidity and mortality during the twentieth century (CDC, 1999). Twenty-first century issues facing public health nursing include increasing rates of drug resistance to community-acquired pathogens, societal issues such as health reform legislation, access to affordable housing, racial and ethnic disparities in health outcomes, behaviorally influenced issues (such as chronic diseases, violence in society, and substance abuse), emerging infections (such as SARS and H1N1 influenza), and unequal access to health care. Community assessments need to reflect the factors that affect the populations the public health nurse serves.

For example, a major twenty-first century public health challenge is emerging infections resulting from drug-resistant organisms. The widespread, often inappropriate, use of antimicrobial drugs has resulted in loss of effectiveness for some community-acquired infections such as gonorrhea, pneumococcal infections, and tuberculosis and in increasing rates of drug resistance in community-acquired pathogens such as *Streptococcus pneumoniae*, *Escherichia coli*, and *Salmonella* spp. The rise in antimicrobial resistance in community and health care settings is causing alarm among public health leaders, nurses, and infectious disease experts. "Staph" infections caused by methicillin-resistant *Staphylococcus aureus* (MRSA) have received increasing attention in recent years. MRSA is a type of staph bacteria that has developed resistance to certain antibiotics, including methicillin and other more common antibiotics such as oxacillin, penicillin, and amoxicillin (CDC, 2010a). Public health nurses are building partnerships, providing education, and making surveillance a top priority to prevent the spread of antimicrobial-resistant infections. Public health nurses can influence this trend by objecting to inappropriate use of antibiotics by providers and educating individuals, families, health care providers, elected officials, and the community about the dangers of misuse and overuse of antibiotics (CDC, 2010b).

Societal issues such as welfare and health insurance reform will influence a population's ability to obtain preventive health services either because of limited health care providers accepting government-sponsored health care coverage or because the low-wage jobs they take do not allow time off for health care. When childcare is an issue for the welfare mother returning to work, consideration must be given to effects on the individual, family, community, and population. Public health nurses assess the problem and determine what is wrong with a system that forces parents to go to work so they can be removed from welfare roles but that does not provide for childcare. The question to be answered by a nurse is "What will it take to change the system?"

Partnerships and collaboration among groups are much more powerful in making change than the individual client and public health nurse working alone. As another example, the depressed, non-functional mother in need of counseling is a significant public health concern because the mother's, children's, and family's needs are not being met. Frequently, the problem may not be obvious to the health professional who sees this woman for the first time. Public health nurses have special preparation to help them both identify the individual's problem and look at its effects on the broader community. In this example, the children may grow to be adults with mental health problems, and the community mental health services will need to be able to handle the increase in this population. Children may become violent adults, resulting in a need for more correctional facilities. Mothers may need additional mental health services. Children may be absent from school often and may not be able to contribute to society. They may be non-productive in the workplace because absence from school leads to lack of skills. One problem of the single individual can place great burdens on the community.

The IOM (2002) reported that disparities in health care treatment accounted for some of the gaps in health outcomes between racial and ethnic groups. This report found that minorities received lower-quality health care than white people, regardless of insurance status, income, and severity of the condition. Public health nurses work as case managers and at the policy level to promote equal access to health care, including health literature and spoken services that reflect the community in which the services are being delivered (see Chapter 8). The public health nurse working directly as a case manager or in a clinic setting or in the community can promote ethnicity-friendly services by partnering with other community agencies such as interpreter services. Identifying and alerting the community to gaps in available services can facilitate equal access to health care. For example, some communities may appear to have an adequate number of pediatricians to meet the community's needs. However, a community assessment may reveal that the community is home to a high number of children who rely on Medicaid as payment for services, or to families whose primary language is not English. Matching this information with the pediatrician population may reveal that none of the pediatricians accept Medicaid as payment for services, or they all deliver services in English only.

HOW TO Educate Nurses for Roles in Public Health: Curriculum Objectives for Public Health Nursing

The nurse should be able to do the following:

- *Articulate similarities and differences between individual-focused and population-focused nursing practice.*
- *Describe the history and current perspectives of public health nursing practice.*
- *Demonstrate skills used to apply key nursing contributions to public health practice (core functions and essential services) in a community.*
- *Apply principles and skills of population health to practice in the public health agency.*
- *Use current information and communication technology in all public health agencies.*
- *Communicate the benefits of public health and public health nursing practice.*

Population-focused public health nursing requires that public health nurses consider social determinants of health including social and environmental factors that influence the health of communities, families, and individuals. For example, a public health nurse providing communicable disease control services for the homeless population or the refugee population will also work for policies that ensure affordable housing. A public health nurse providing case management services for a new teen mother will include ensuring the mother returns to school; has safe, affordable housing; and has safe child care available while she attends school. The Nurse-Family Partnership Program (2010) is an example of a model program that considers the social determinants of health.

NURSING TIP *Many of the epidemics of the future will be defined by social problems such as lack of jobs, lack of affordable housing, substance abuse, and teen pregnancy, as well as newly identified communicable diseases such as SARS and novel H1N1 influenza.*

MODELS OF PUBLIC HEALTH NURSING PRACTICE

In response to the IOM (1988) report that described public health in a state of disarray and the need for all federal public health agencies to work to identify core public health functions, public health nurses have worked to develop models of practice that will operationalize the role of public health nursing. This section presents examples of models developed by local and state departments of health. These models also serve as examples of the important work that can be accomplished by local, state, and federal partnerships.

In Virginia, a statewide committee led an examination of the role of public health nursing in the context of increasing public expectation of accountability and the shift of public health nursing emphasis from clinical services to population-focused services. Their work resulted in a document that identifies public health nursing roles within the framework of the core public health functions (see Chapter 1). The work identifies the educational needs of staff that would prepare them to function effectively in the changing public health arena. Essential elements of the role were identified. These essential elements are being implemented through multiprofessional public health teams. The document includes a matrix that demonstrates the relationship of the public health functions defined by the essential elements to the public health nursing roles at the local level, as well as the role of the state in this responsibility (see Appendix G.1).

The Public Health Nursing Section of the Minnesota Department of Health (2001) developed a framework called the intervention model that defines public health nursing interventions by level of practice (see Chapter 9). Public health nurses deliver services within a framework of core interventions. The three levels of public health nursing practice are systems, community, and individual/family. The model identifies 17 population-based public health interventions delivered by public health nurses. It also identifies population-based interventions as those that do the following:

- Focus on entire populations possessing similar health concerns or characteristics.
- Are guided by an assessment of health status.
- Consider the broad determinants of health, such as housing, income, education, cultural values, and community capacity.
- Consider all levels of prevention, with primary prevention a priority.
- Consider all levels of practice (community, system, and individual/family) (see Appendix G.1).

The public health nursing practice model of Los Angeles County Department of Health describes public health nursing practice as population based. It synthesizes the 10 essential services of public health practice, principles identified by the Quad Council of Public Health Nursing Organizations and the Minnesota Department of Health, PHN Section and tenets of the ANA *Scope and Standards of Public Health Nursing Practice*. It includes the following criteria:

- Focuses on entire populations possessing similar health concerns or characteristics.
- Relies upon an assessment of population health status.
- Considers the broad determinants of health.
- Considers all levels of prevention, with a preference for primary prevention.
- Considers all levels of practice: Individual/Family Focused Practice, Community-Focused Practice, and Systems-Focused Practice
- Reaches out to all who might benefit, not focusing on just those who present themselves.
- Demonstrates a dominant concern for the greater good of all the people (the interest of the whole taking priority over the best interest of the individual or group).
- Creates healthy environmental, social, and economic conditions in which people can thrive. (Los Angeles County Department of Public Health/Public Health Nursing, 2007).

EDUCATION AND KNOWLEDGE REQUIREMENTS FOR PUBLIC HEALTH NURSES

The Council on Linkages Between Academia and Public Health Practice (2010) examined a decade of work to identify a list of core public health competencies that represent a set of skills, knowledge, and attitudes necessary for the broad practice of public health. Initially adopted in 2001 by the Council on Linkages Between Academia and Public Health Practice, the core competencies were revised and adopted unanimously by the Council in June 2009. The accomplishments of the Council on Linkages not only include developing the Core Competencies for Public Health Professionals to guide curriculum and workforce development, but also include promoting public health systems research to increase understanding of and improve public health infrastructure as well as focusing the field on evidence-based strategies to improve worker recruitment and retention and

combat emerging worker shortages. The Council is located in Washington, DC and is staffed by the Public Health Foundation. A list of member organizations is located at http://www.phf.org/link/membership.htm.

The competencies are built around the Essential Public Health Services. This is the only consensus set of core competencies in public health that apply to all practicing public health professionals. They capture the cross-cutting competencies necessary for all disciplines that work in public health, including public health nurses, physicians, environmental health specialists, health educators, and epidemiologists. The competencies are applied to three tiers. A detailed list of core competencies by job category and skill level is available. The core public health competencies have been applied to public health nursing (see the WebLinks on the Evolve website for both items).

🌐 **LINKING CONTENT TO PRACTICE**

In addition to having the core public health competencies, public health nurses have specialized competencies as described in the *Scope and Standards of Public Health Nursing Practice* (ANA, 2007). The core public health competencies are divided into the following eight domains. The content related to the domains can be found in the chapters noted.

1. Analytic assessment skills: Chapters 1, 9, 15, 17, 18, and 27 to 38
2. Basic public health sciences' skills: Chapters 3, 6, 8, 10, 12, 13, 14, 19, 23 to 26
3. Cultural competency skills: Chapters 4 and 7
4. Communication skills: Chapters 16 and 22
5. Community dimensions of practice skills: Chapters 18, 20, 21, and 41 to 45
6. Financial planning and management skills: Chapter 5
7. Leadership and systems' thinking skills: Chapter 40
8. Policy development/program planning skills: Chapters 8 and 25

In addition to being skilled in the areas of epidemiology, analytic assessment skills, environmental health, health services administration, cultural sensitivity, and social and behavioral science, the twenty-first century public health nurse must be competent in areas such as community mobilization, risk communication, genomics, informatics, community-based participatory research, policy and law, global health, and public health ethics (ANA, 2007).

THE CUTTING EDGE   *The Office of Public Health Genomics (OPHG) of the CDC promotes the integration of genomics and the education of public health providers in public health research, policy, and practice to learn more about how to prevent disease and improve the health of all people. The CDC says the study of genomics will help researchers and health practitioners, including public health nurses, understand why, in the same environment, some people get sick while others do not. This information could lead to new and better ways to improve health and prevent diseases in individuals and populations.*

Many of these core public health competencies are provided by public health nurses who have learned these skills in the workplace while gaining knowledge through years of practice. Rapid changes in public health are providing a challenge to public health nurses in that there is neither the time nor the staff to provide as much on-the-job training needed to learn and upgrade skills and knowledge of staff. Nurses with baccalaureate or master's preparation are needed to provide a strong public health system (see Chapter 1). In 2007 the ANA revised the 1999 *Scope and St andards of Public Health Nursing Practice* to reflect the increasing complexity and rapid changes faced by public health nurses. The revised standards include those that are expected of all baccalaureate degree nurses, the entry level into public health nursing practice, and the standards of the advanced practice public health nurse prepared at the master's level (ANA, 2007).

NATIONAL HEALTH OBJECTIVES

Since 1979 the U.S. Surgeon General has worked with local, state, and federal agencies; the private sector; and the U.S. population to develop objectives for preventing disease and promoting health for the nation. These objectives are revisited every 10 years. In 2009 proposed *Healthy People 2020* objectives were released for public comment (see the *Healthy People 2020* box).

 HEALTHY PEOPLE 2020

Selected National Health Objectives Related to the Public Health Infrastructure

- PHI-1: Increase the proportion of federal, tribal, state, and local public health agencies that incorporate core competencies for public health professionals into job descriptions and performance evaluations.
- PHI-4: Increase the proportion of 4-year colleges and universities that offer public health or related majors and/or minors.
- PHI-13: Increase the proportion of tribal, state, and local public health agencies that provide or assure comprehensive epidemiology services to support essential public health services.
- PHI-14: Increase the proportion of state and local public health jurisdictions that conduct performance assessment and improvement activities in the public health system using national standards.
- PHI-15: Increase the proportion of tribal, state, and local public health agencies that have implemented a health improvement plan and increase the proportion of local health jurisdictions that have implemented a health improvement plan linked with their State plan.

From the Office of Disease Prevention and Health Promotion, U.S. Department of Health and Human Services. Available at http://www. healthypeople.gov/hp2020/Objectives/TopicArea.aspx?id=40&Topic Area=Public+Health+Infrastructure. Accessed May 24, 2010.

Healthy People 2020 overarching goals are to:
- Attain high-quality, longer lives free of preventable disease, disability, injury, and premature death.
- Achieve health equity, eliminate disparities, and improve the health of all groups.
- Create social and physical environments that promote good health for all.
- Promote quality of life, healthy development and healthy behaviors across all life stages (Office of Disease Prevention

and Health Promotion, USDHHS, 2010). State health departments play a key role in implementing the *Healthy People* objectives. Examples of state *Healthy People 2020* goals can be located at http://www.healthypeople.gov.

State health departments help set local goals using the *Healthy People 2020* objectives as a framework. Knowing that public health departments do not have the resources to accomplish these goals independently, collaboration is essential to quality nursing practice and is encouraged at the local level with existing groups. New partnerships are developed related to specific goals. Communities develop coalitions to address selected objectives, based on community needs, to include all of the local community stakeholders such as social services, mental health, education, recreation, government, and businesses. Membership varies from community to community depending on that community's formal and informal structure. The groups join the coalition for a variety of reasons. For example, businesses see the value of developing a productive workforce that will be of importance to them and the community in the future.

Public health nurses help clients identify unhealthy behaviors and then help them develop strategies to improve their health. Some of the behaviors addressed by public health nurses are tobacco use, physical activity, and obesity, all of which affect quality and years of healthy life. Public health nurses also organize the community to conduct community health assessments to identify where health disparities exist and to target interventions to address those disparities. For example, community health assessments may disclose that certain populations are at higher risk for asthma, diabetes, low immunization rates, high cigarette smoking behavior, or exposure to environmental hazards.

Some *Healthy People 2020* communicable disease areas of focus are vaccine-preventable infectious diseases, emerging antimicrobial resistance, tuberculosis infection and disease, levels of human immunodeficiency virus (HIV), acquired immunodeficiency syndrome (AIDS), and sexually transmitted infections. To help clients reduce their risk of acquiring a communicable disease, public health nurses provide clients with instructions on the use of barrier methods of contraception and information on the hazards of multiple sexual partners and street drug use. Obtaining a complete sexual history on all clients coming to the health department for services takes special skills but is essential to determine the behaviors that have brought the client to the local health department. Education of young persons before they become sexually active has helped reduce the incidence of some sexually transmitted diseases in this population.

FUNCTIONS OF PUBLIC HEALTH NURSES

Public health nurses have many functions depending on the needs and resources of an area. Advocate is one of the many roles of the public health nurse. As an advocate, the public health nurse collects, monitors, and analyzes data and works with the client to identify and prioritize needed services, whether the client is an individual, a family, a community, or a population. The public health nurse and the client then develop the most effective plan and approach to take, and the nurse helps the client implement the plan so that the client can become more independent in making decisions and obtaining the services needed. At the community and population levels, public health nurses promote healthy behaviors, safe water and air, and sanitation. They advocate for healthy policies at the local, state, and federal levels that will develop healthy communities (see Chapter 18).

Legislation is a public health tool used to ensure the health of populations. Implemented with extreme concern for the balance between individual rights and community rights, public policy is a critical function for the public health nurse. Examples of legislation that has successfully improved the health of populations are required immunizations for school entry, seat belt use, smoke-free environments, and bicycle and motorcycle helmet use.

> **WHAT DO YOU THINK?** *Fewer than 40% of health care workers receive the flu vaccine, yet influenza is infectious in asymptomatic individuals. Unvaccinated health care providers place clients at risk of flu. Should health care providers be mandated to receive flu vaccinations?*

Case manager is a major role for public health nurses (see Chapter 22). The 2010 health reform legislation will increase the importance of the case management role as newly insured clients attempt to link with health care providers and the Nurse-Family Partnership program (2010) is expanded. Public health nurses use the nursing process of assessing, planning, implementing, and evaluating outcomes to meet clients' needs. Clear and complex communications are frequently an important component of case management. Other health and social agency providers may not be familiar with the home and community living conditions that are known to the public health nurse. It is the nurse who sees the living conditions and who can tell the story for the client or assist the individual, family, or community with the telling of their story. Case managers assist clients in identifying the services they need the most at the least cost. They also assist communities and populations in identifying and linking with services that will increase the overall population health status.

Public health nurses are a major referral resource. They maintain current information about health and social services available within the community. They know what resources will be acceptable to the client within the social and cultural norms for that group. The nurse educates clients to enable them to use the resources and to learn self-care. Nurses refer to other services in the area, and other services refer to the public health nurse for care or follow-up. For example, the mother and new baby may be referred to the public health nurse for postnatal care with postpartum home visit follow-up.

Assessment of literacy is a large part of public health nursing. Many individuals are limited in their ability to read, write, and communicate clearly. The public health nurse has to be culturally sensitive and aware of the specific areas of unique problems of clients, such as financial limitations that may in turn limit educational opportunities. Frequently, when a person goes to a physician's office, clinic, or hospital, they are clean and neatly dressed. The assumption is made that when they nod at the health care provider it means that they understand what has been said. This is frequently not the case, but the client is embarrassed to admit that he or she does not understand what has been said. Being illiterate does not mean a person is mentally slow. It is important for the public health nurse to follow up on the many contacts the individual or family has with medical, social, and legal services to clarify what is understood and to find an answer to the questions that have not been asked by the client or answered by the services.

The public health nurse is an educator, teaching to the level of the client so that information received is information that can be used. Patience and repetitions over time are necessary to develop the trust and to enable the client to use the relationship with the nurse for more information. As educator, the public health nurse identifies community needs (e.g., playground safety, hand hygiene, pedestrian safety, safe-sex practices) and develops and implements educational activities aimed at changing behaviors over time.

Public health nurses are direct primary caregivers in many situations, both in the clinic and in the community. Where the public health nurse provides primary care is determined by community assessment and is usually in response to an identified gap to which the private sector is unable to respond, coupled with an assessment of the impact of the gap in services on the health of the population. Examples include prenatal services for uninsured women, free or low-cost immunization services for targeted populations, directly observed therapy for clients with active tuberculosis, and treatment for sexually transmitted infections.

Public health nurses ensure that direct care services are available in the community for at-risk populations by working with the community to develop programs that will meet the needs of those populations. Currently, no system of outreach service in the medical models of care addresses the multiple needs of high-risk populations. High-risk populations frequently do not understand the medical, social, educational, or judicial system and the professional languages, codes of behavior, or expected outcomes of these services. Clients need a case manager, a health educator, an advocate, and a role model to enable them to benefit from these services and to teach them how to avoid complex and expensive problems in the future. The local public health nurse fills these roles and many more for this population. These are examples of the difficult clinical issues that public health nurses face in making ethical and professional decisions.

The public health nurse's role is unique and essential in many situations. Access to homes gives the nurse information that usually cannot be gathered in the hospital or clinic setting. The public health nurse learns to ask intimate questions creatively and to seek information that will facilitate case management and provide the clinical and social care needed, including other community resources. Careful attention must be paid to privacy and confidentiality in delivering public health nursing services. The credibility of the nurse and the agency depends on the professional handling of the public health information of each and every staff member.

> **DID YOU KNOW?** *It is important for public health nurses to practice confidentiality when they have knowledge about an individual, family, communicable disease outbreak, community-level problem, or any special knowledge obtained in the public health work setting.*

When a disaster (see Chapters 23 and 24) occurs, public health nurses at the local, state, and federal levels have multiple roles in assessing, planning, implementing, and evaluating needs and resources for the different populations being served. Whether the disaster is local or national, small or large, natural or man-made, public health nurses are skilled professionals essential to the team. As a health care facility, the local public health department has a disaster plan, as well as a role in the local, regional, and state disaster plans. Public health nurses' roles include providing education that will prepare communities to cope with disasters and professional triage for local shelters, conducting enhanced communicable disease surveillance, planning and implementing mass dispensing sites, working with environmental health specialists to ensure safe food and water for disaster victims and emergency workers, and serving on the local emergency planning committee. Their presence may be required in other regions of the state or country to provide official public health nursing duties in a time of crisis, such as a hurricane, that requires a lengthy period of recovery. Each governmental jurisdiction has an emergency plan. The public health agency is expected to provide planning and staffing during a disaster. These local emergency preparedness plans may be multigovernmental, which requires coordination between communities. Public health nurses have a critical role in ensuring that emergency preparedness plans address the special needs of vulnerable populations such as those with disabilities, or low-income populations who lack the resources to maintain the recommended 3- to 5-day supply of food and medication.

Essential and unique roles for public health nurses exist in the area of communicable disease control. Public health nursing skills are necessary for education, prevention, surveillance, and outbreak investigation. Public health nurses can find infected individuals; notify contacts; refer; administer treatments; educate the individual, family, community, professionals, and populations; act as advocates; and in general be state-of-the-art resources to reduce the rate of communicable disease in the community (see Chapters 13 and 14). The communicable disease role is one of the most important roles for public health nursing during disasters. During the terrorist attacks on September 11, 2001, the SARS outbreak, and the novel H1N1 pandemic, public health nurses at the federal, state, and local levels immediately implemented active enhanced surveillance activities and prepared for implementation of mass dispensing sites. Information about communicable diseases seen at the local level were passed on to the state public health agency and finally to the CDC. At each step, the data were analyzed for evidence of unusual disease trends.

> **DID YOU KNOW?** *HIPAA allows sharing of information for the purpose of treatment, payment, and operations without a signed consent.*

When October 2001 alerts from the CDC began presenting information about a photo editor in Florida who had been hospitalized with inhalation anthrax, public health nurses and hospital infection control practitioners throughout the nation increased activity. Public health response to disasters requires that resources be redirected temporarily from other programs while maintaining programs that will prevent additional outbreaks. Therefore, public health nurses not normally involved in communicable disease activities can be shifted to this function. The exposures resulting from the anthrax-tainted letters presented unprecedented public health challenges. The Washington, DC, anthrax exposures resulted in thousands of possible work-related exposures, five cases of inhalation anthrax in the region, and two deaths over a period of months. Public health at the federal, state, and local levels was looked to for coordinated leadership and answers to a situation in which experience was limited and answers were uncertain.

Although communicable disease control is a core public health service, the role of the public health nurse as **incident commander** in a widespread public health emergency is a new role (Figure 46-4). Issues such as how to conduct mass treatment in response to a bioterrorism event; which jurisdiction is in charge; how to communicate uncertain information to the public; and who should take antibiotics for how long had to be rapidly resolved across jurisdictional and agency lines. The anthrax exposures are typical of the nature of public health emergencies. They unfold as the communicable disease moves through communities.

Public health nurses are essential partners in disaster drills. In Virginia, an electrical company has a nuclear plant that requires annual multi-jurisdictional disaster drills. These disaster planning and practice sessions are an opportunity for local public health nurses to get to know other agencies' representatives and to let them know what public health nursing can offer. Because public health nurses are out in the communities and have assessment skills, they are essential in evaluating how the disaster was handled and making suggestions about how future events might be managed. To be most effective as disaster responders, public health nurses have to be a part of the team *before* an emergency. Knowing what type of disaster is likely to occur in a community is essential for planning. Types of disasters vary from place to place, but there is a history of past events and how they were handled, as well as resources and training from regional, state, and federal agencies. Public health nurses can help educate the public about the individual responsibilities and preparations that can be in place both for the person and for the community. The Levels of Prevention box presents additional examples of public health nurses' functions by level of prevention. Public health nurses at the local, state, and federal levels work in partnership to accomplish each function.

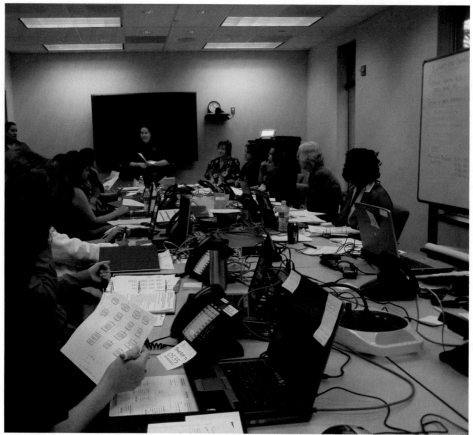

FIGURE 46-4 Public health nurses respond to community-wide disease outbreaks within the framework of the incident command structure. (Courtesy Arlington County Department of Human Services/Public Health Division, Arlington, VA).

📋 LEVELS OF PREVENTION

Public Health Nursing

Primary Prevention

- Partnering with the community to conduct a community health assessment to identify community assets and gaps
- Partnering with the community to develop primary prevention programs in response to identified gaps
- Providing information about safe-sex practices
- Providing individual and community-based education to increase knowledge and modify perceptions of risks
- Educating daycare centers and families about the dangers of lead-based paint
- Educating daycare centers, schools, and the general community about the importance of hand hygiene to prevent transmission of communicable diseases
- Inspecting daycare centers, nursing homes, and hospitals to ensure client safety and quality of care
- Providing immunizations
- Advocating for issues such as mandatory seat belt legislation, smoke-free environments, and universal access to health care

- Providing no-charge infant car seats accompanied by classes in use of safety seats
- Identifying environmental hazards such as housing quality, playground safety, pedestrian safety, and product safety hazards, and working with the community and policy makers to mitigate the identified hazards
- Developing social networking interventions to modify community norms related to sexual risk behaviors, condom use, and abstinence
- Larvaciding against mosquitoes in areas frequented by populations 55 years of age and over
- Working with communities to develop citizen emergency preparedness plans

Secondary Prevention

- Identifying and treating clients in a sexually transmitted disease clinic
- Identifying and treating clients with TB infection and disease in a TB clinic
- Providing directly observed therapy (DOT) for clients with active TB
- Conducting lead screening activities for children
- Conducting contacting/tracing for individuals exposed to a client with an active case of TB or a sexually transmitted disease

LEVELS OF PREVENTION—cont'd

Public Health Nursing

- Conducting ongoing disease surveillance for communicable diseases and implementing control measures when an outbreak is identified
- Implementing screening programs for genetic disorders/metabolic deficiencies in newborns; breast, cervical, and testicular cancer; diabetes; hypertension; and sensory impairments in children, and ensuring follow-up services for clients with positive results
- Conducting syndromic surveillance to ensure early identification of victims of an influenza epidemic or bioterrorism event
- Providing low-cost antibiotics for treatment of Lyme disease
- Conducting enhanced surveillance for novel influenza virus infection among travelers with severe unexplained respiratory illness returning from affected countries

- Establishing mass dispensing clinics for antibiotic distribution in response to a bioterrorism event or influenza pandemic

Tertiary Prevention
- Providing case management services that link clients with chronic illnesses to health care and community support services
- Providing case management services that link clients identified with serious mental illnesses to mental health and community support services
- Educating at rehabilitation centers to help clients with stroke optimize their functioning
- Establishing an alternative treatment site for victims of a smallpox epidemic

CHAPTER REVIEW

PRACTICE APPLICATION

A retirement community in a small town reported to the local health department 24 cases of severe gastrointestinal illness that had occurred among residents and staff of the facility during the past 24 to 36 hours. It was determined that the ill clients became sick within a short, well-defined period, and most recovered within 24 hours without treatment. The communicable disease outbreak team, composed of public health nurses, public health physicians, and an environmental health specialist, was called to respond to this possible epidemic.

How should they respond to this situation? (Refer to Chapter 12 for help in answering this question.)

A. Call the Centers for Disease Control and Prevention and ask for help with surveillance.
B. Send all the ill persons in the retirement community to the hospital.
C. Evaluate the agent, host, and environmental relationships to determine the cause of the problem.
D. Close the dining room and find another source to provide food to the residents.
Answers can be found on the Evolve site.

KEY POINTS

- Local public health departments are responsible for implementing and enforcing local, state, and federal public health codes and ordinances while providing essential public health services.
- The goal of the local health department is to safeguard the public's health and improve the community's health status.
- State health departments hold primary responsibility for promoting and protecting the public's health.
- Public health nursing is the practice of promoting and protecting the health of populations using knowledge from nursing and social and public health sciences.
- Public health is based on the scientific core of epidemiology.
- Marketing of public health nursing is essential to inform both professionals and the public about the opportunities and challenges of populations in public health care.

- A driving force behind public health nursing changes is globalization that allows rapid transmission of emerging infections and the expectation that public health nurses be active partners in emergency preparedness activities.
- Some of the roles public health nurses function in are advocate, case manager, referral source, counselor, educator, outreach worker, disease surveillance expert, community mobilizer, and disaster responder.
- Public health nurses have an important role in conducting community assessments including partnering with the community to collect and analyze data, developing community diagnosis, and implementing evidence-based interventions.
- Public health nurses base interventions on identified health status of populations and their related determinants of health.

CLINICAL DECISION-MAKING ACTIVITIES

1. What are some of the various roles of the public health nurse in the local, state, and federal public health systems? Contrast the roles. Explain why they may be different from one another.

2. How can public health nurses prepare themselves for change? Illustrate what you mean.

3. What can today's public health nurses learn from the past practice of public health nurses? How can you verify your answer?

4. Describe collaborative partnerships that public health nurses have developed. How do partnerships help solve public health problems?

5. What are some external factors that have an effect on public health nursing? How can you deal with the complexities of these factors?

6. What are core functions used by public health nurses as they plan interventions? Do these functions make sense to you? Explain.

7. If you were a public health nurse for a day, what would you like to accomplish? Why? Is your answer supported by evidence? Be specific.

8. How would you determine the most pressing public health issue in your community? Gather several points of view from key leaders in the community.

9. Give an example of a policy change or an effect from the work of public health nurses. How did this policy make a difference in client health outcomes?

REFERENCES

All Kids Count: *Policy brief: s. Sustaining financial support for immunization registries*, 2000. Decatur, GA.

American Nurses Association: *Public health nursing: scope and standards of practice*, 2007, Silver Springs, MD.

American Public Health Association: Definition and Background: A Statement of APHA Public Health Nursing Section (1996), Washington, D.C.

Centers for Disease Control and Prevention (CDC): 2002 Achievements in public health, 1900-1999: control of infectious diseases, *MMWR Morb Mortal Wkly Rep* 48:621–629, 1999.

Centers for Disease Control and Prevention: National public health performance standards program, users' guide, 2004, Atlanta, GA.

Centers for Disease Control and Prevention: *The national public health performance standards, an overview*, slide 9, 2005a. Available at http://www.cdc.gov. Accessed March 20, 2011.

Centers for Disease Control and Prevention: Outbreak of swine-origin influenza A (H1N1) virus infection—Mexico, March–April 2009. *Morb Mortal Wkly Rep* 58(17):467–470, 2009. Available at http://www.cdc.gov/mmwr/preview/mmwrhtml/mm5817a5.htm. Accessed March 20, 2011.

Centers for Disease Control and Prevention: *MRSA*, 2010a. Available at http://www.cdc.gov/mrsa/index.html. Accessed March 25, 2011.

Centers for Disease Control and Prevention: *Antibiotic/antimicrobial resistance campaign*, 2010b. Available at http://www.cdc.gov/drugresistance/campaigns.html. Accessed March 25, 2011.

Community-Campus Partnerships for Health (CCPH): *Principles of good community-campus partnerships*, 2006. Available at http://www.ccph.info/. Accessed May 24, 2010.

Council on Linkages Between Academia and Public Health Practice: *Core competencies for public health professionals,* Washington, DC, 2010, PHF. Available at http://www.phf.org/link/corecompetencies.htm. Accessed May 26, 2010.

Frank CM Sr: *Foundations of nursing*, ed 2, Philadelphia, 1959, Saunders.

Institute of Medicine: *The future of public health*, Washington, DC, 1988, National Academies Press.

Institute of Medicine: *Unequal treatment: confronting racial and ethnic disparities in health care*, Washington, DC, 2002, National Academies Press.

Institute of Medicine: *The future of public health in the 21st century*, Washington, DC, 2003a, National Academies Press.

Los Angeles County Department of Public Health-Public Health Nursing: *Public health nursing practice model*, 2007. Available at http://publichealth.lacounty.gov/phn/index.htm. Accessed March 20, 2011.

National Association of County and City Health Officials: *Operational definition of a functional local health department*, November 2005. Available at http://www.naccho.org. Accessed August 23, 2010.

Nurse-Family Partnership Program: 2010. Available at http://www.nursefamilypartnership.org/. Accessed June 3, 2010.

Office of Disease Prevention and Health Promotion, U.S. Department of Health and Human Services: *Healthy People 2020: the road ahead*, 2010. Available at http://www.healthypeople.gov/hp2020/default.asp. Accessed May 24, 2010.

Olds DL, Kitzman HJ, Cole RE, et al: Enduring effects of prenatal and infancy home visiting by nurses on maternal life course and government spending: follow-up of a randomized trial among children at age 12 years, *Arch Pediatr Adolesc Med* 164(5):419–424, 2010.

Public Health Nursing Section, Minnesota Department of Health: *Public health interventions—applications for public health nursing practice*, St Paul, MN, 2001, Department of Health, APHA.

Task Force on Community Preventive Services: Centers for Disease Control and Prevention, *The Guide to Community Preventive Services*, 2005. Available at http://www.thecommunityguide.org/index.html. Accessed May 24, 2010.

Turnock BJ: *Public health: what it is and how it works*, ed 3, Sudbury, MA, 2010, Jones and Bartlett.

USDHHS, *Healthy People 2020*: National health promotion and disease prevention objectives, 2009. Available at http://www.healthypeople.gov/hp2020/objectives/TopicAreas.aspx.

APPENDIX A

Resource Tools Available on the Evolve Website

CHAPTER 30

- Resource Tool 30.A: Lifestyle Assessment Questionnaire
- Resource Tool 30.B: A Health Risk Appraisal for Older Adults

CHAPTER 31

- Resource Tool 31.A: The Living Will Directive
- Resource Tool 31.B: Assessment Tools for Communities with Physically Compromised Members
- Resource Tool 31.C: Assessment Tools for Families with Physically Compromised Members
- Resource Tool 31.D: Assessment Tools for Physically Compromised Individuals

CHAPTER 34

- Resource Tool 34.A: Resources for the Nurse Working with Migrant Farmworkers

CHAPTER 37

- Resource Tool 37.A: Smoking Cessation Resources
- Resource Tool 37.B: Useful Web Resources
- Resource Tool 37.C: Commonly Abused Drugs

CHAPTER 41

- Resource Tool 41.A: OASIS-C: Start of Care Assessment

CHAPTER 43

- Resource Tool 43.A: Immunizing Agents and Immunization Schedules for Health Care Workers

CHAPTER 45

- Resource Tool 45.A: Resources for Faith Community Nursing

CHAPTER 46

- Resource Tool 46.A: Core Competencies and Skill Levels for Public Health Nursing

Program Planning and Design

Program planning is a process of outlining, designing, contemplating, and deliberating to develop actions to accomplish desirable goals and attain desirable outcomes.

PLANNING PROCESS

The successful program requires a lot of planning before implementation. The following need to be considered:

1. Who is in charge?
2. Who should be involved?
3. When is the best time to plan?
4. What data are needed?
5. Where should planning occur?
6. Will there be resistance?
7. Where will resistance come from?
8. Who will be early adopters?

Failing to plan can result in the inability to have a program that is viable and that will attain the goals and outcomes.

TIMETABLE

Timetables are very important to the success of planning. Two methods often used by planners are the following:
- Program Evaluation and Review Techniques (PERT)
- GANTT

PERT

The PERT method requires the planner to do the following:
- State the goal.
- List in sequence all the steps and activities for each step to accomplish the goal.
- Target dates for accomplishing each step are set.
- Diagram the process for easy use.

Student Activity

1. Go to literature and find a PERT application and diagram.
2. Draw a diagram of your program plan or a hypothetical one.
3. Be prepared to submit with end of module assignment.

GANTT

A GANTT chart is also a flow diagram that can be used to map out the activities needed to be accomplished so that one can maintain a timeline to achieve the goal. The GANTT chart looks much like a calendar.

Student Activity

1. Go to the literature and find a GANTT chart that has been applied to a project.

2. Complete a GANTT chart of the activities related to each objective in your project that are stated to meet the goal or do a hypothetical one.
3. Be prepared to submit at the end of the module.

People Planning

To have a successful plan one needs to involve the clients who are to be served by the program. Others to be involved are the following:
- Administrators
- Staff (providers)
- Other key stakeholders

Reasons

- Develop ownership
- Develop commitment
- Develop pride
- Develop understanding of problems
- Brainstorm
- Generate ideas

Data Planning

To have a successful program one must collect data on the following:
- Demographics of clients
- Disease statistics
- Vital statistics
- Existing similar programs
- Successes and barriers of similar programs
- Socioeconomic/environmental support
- Political issues

Student Activity

1. Find a source of data for one of the above categories.
2. Explain why it is a good data source for your program.

Performance Planning

Some programs, called projects, care planned for a one-time-only event. Most all programs are planned to be ongoing.

1. Question: Are problems that programs address usually solved?
   a. Explain your answer and give an example.
2. The following should be considered in planning for performance.
   a. Staff is the most expensive resource in planning.
   b. For efficiency, programs should be planned as ongoing activities.
   c. A 6-month start-up and a 5-year budget should be developed.

d. Long-term commitment of resources to a program is essential.

e. Planners must develop marketing tools, policies and procedures, and job descriptions before implementation.

f. Organizational structures including committees needs to be drafted.

g. Community partners and advisory board should be planned and contacted for agreement to serve.

Priority Planning

1. Plan programs for the greatest need and the best potential for making a difference.
2. Available resources to accomplish goal no. 1 must be sought. If resources are not available, the program plan is time wasted.
3. Be a comprehensive planner.
4. Complete ongoing needs assessments to determine community changes.
5. Prioritize the greatest needs.
6. Plan new programs or change existing ones for goal no. 5.

Plan for Measurable Outcomes

1. Collect baseline data on the problem and the target population.
2. Analyze needs assessment.
3. Look at incidence and prevalence of problems.
4. Look at available services currently addressing the problem.
5. Determine the impact of the current services, using SWOT.

Evaluation Planning

1. This must begin with the needs assessment.
2. Plan for process evaluation.
3. Plan for summative evaluation.
4. Develop a timeline for evaluation to occur.
5. Develop systems for records and data collection and choose evaluation instruments.

Questions To Be Answered

1. Do you have the right people doing the planning?
2. Do you have the essential data for planning?
3. Is this the right time to plan this program?'
4. Why should evaluation occur?
5. Who should do it?
6. What data should be gathered?
7. Should evaluation occur?

Planning Models

1. Choose a model for planning your program.
2. Two models developed for program planning by the Centers for Disease Control and Prevention are PATCH and APEX.

Student Activity

1. Read about these two models.
2. Briefly explain how these models can be applied to program planning.
3. Briefly explain the model you have chosen for planning. Include:
   a. Definition
   b. Goal

c. Model elements
d. Planning process

Mission

All programs will want to have a Mission Statement. Elements of a Mission Statement should include the following:
- Name of agency
- Name of program
- Who program serves
- Purpose of program
- Program goal
- Services offered

Student Activity

Write a Mission Statement for your program.

Vision

A Vision Statement is a brief one- or two-sentence statement that expresses the impact this program will have.

Student Activity

Write a Vision Statement for your program.

WORKSHEET FOR WRITING THE PHILOSOPHY

Questions for Discussion

What are our community's values and beliefs about health?

What is the purpose of our program?

What is our position on community involvement and responsibility for health?

What is our role in providing leadership?

WORKSHEET FOR FINDING AND OVERCOMING OBSTACLES

Goal:

Forces working against reaching goal (barriers/obstacles/challenges):

Forces working for reaching goal (existing resources/strengths):

Approaches to overcome obstacles:

WORKSHEET FOR WRITING OBJECTIVES

Health Issue:

Goal:

Objectives (write the most important objectives first)

1.

2.

3.

4.

CHECKLIST FOR PROGRAM PLANNING AND IMPLEMENTATION

1. Have you established a community advisory group with:
   ___ Representation of your targeted groups
   ___ The ability to provide valuable links with the community
   ___ Skills and resources that will be useful to the program
2. Have you identified community needs and concerns by way of:
   ___ Surveys/questionnaires
   ___ Focus groups
   ___ Public meetings or forums
   ___ Interested party analysis
3. Have you determined the community's priorities, taking into account:
   ___ Historical conditions
   ___ Traditional practices
   ___ Political and economic conditions
4. Have you developed program goals and objectives?
   ___ Yes
   ___ No
5. Have you decided on program strategies that:
   ___ Fit with the resources and needs of the community
   ___ Consider the beliefs, values, and practices of the community
   ___ Reflect field testing
   ___ Dispel health misconceptions
   ___ Change behavior
   ___ Change the environment
6. To implement your program, have you:
   ___ Prepared a timeline for program implementation
   ___ Listed people to be involved, and resources needed
   ___ Hired staff (preferably from the community)
   ___ Developed linkages with other community agencies, as appropriate
   ___ Planned to carry out an evaluation
7. Have you chosen appropriate methods and questions for:
   ___ Process evaluation
   ___ Outcome evaluation

REFERENCES

Green LW, Kreuter M: *Health promotion and planning: an education and ecological approach*, New York, 1999, McGraw-Hill.

Issel LM: *Health program planning and evaluation: a practical, systematic approach for community health*, Boston, 2004, Jones and Bartlett.

Posavac EJ, Carey RG: *Program evaluation: methods and case studies*, Englewood Cliffs, NJ, 2000, Prentice Hall.

Veney J, Kaluzny A: *Evaluation and decision making for health service programs*, Englewood Cliffs, NJ, 2005, Prentice Hall.

Herbs and Supplements Used for Children and Adolescents

HERB	ACTIONS	COMMON USES	SIDE EFFECTS/ TOXIC EFFECTS/ CONTRAINDICATIONS	CLINICAL RESEARCH
Aloe vera gel or liquid	Emollient Antiviral Anti-inflammatory Antifungal Antibacterial Laxative Immune modulator	*Topically:* Burns, skin irritation, diaper rash *Internally:* Digestive disorders, constipation, stomatitis	*Side effects:* Abdominal cramping, diarrhea	Accelerated healing in abrasions, burns, and psoriasis
Blue-green algae	Stimulant	ADHD Improves attention and hyperactivity	*Side effects:* Nausea, diarrhea, weakness, numbness *Cautions:* May be contaminated with microbes, heavy metals, and sewage	No clinical research
Calendula *Calendula officinalis* washes or ointments	Anti-inflammatory Antiseptic Spasmolytic	*Topically:* Skin rashes, irritation, cold sores, eczema, conjunctivitis	No known side effects	Accelerated wound healing and ulcers in adults
Chamomile *Anthemis nobilis* tea or tincture	Anti-inflammatory Spasmolytic Sedative	*Internally:* Anxiety, sleep problems, colic, irritability, teething *Topically:* Skin irritation, diaper rash	Considered very safe *Side effects:* Rare allergic reactions	Improved behavior in infants with colic
Echinacea *Echinacea angustifolia, E. pallida, E. purpurea* tinctures, capsules, tablets	Immune modulator Anti-inflammatory Antimicrobial	*Internally:* Upper respiratory tract infections, urinary tract infections, attention problems *Topically:* Eczema, ulcerations, burns	No reported side effects Considered very safe *Caution:* Not recommended for children under 2 years old	No controlled studies in children
Evening primrose oil *Oenothera biennis*	Anti-inflammatory Sedative Anticoagulant Astringent	Cough, asthma, allergies, eczema, acne, psoriasis, autoimmune diseases, PMS	*Side effects:* GI disturbances and headaches *Drug interactions:* Caution with seizure medications	Inconsistent results in clinical studies in children with attention problems No other pediatric studies
Feverfew *Tanacetum parthenium* fresh or dried leaves	Anti-inflammatory Spasmolytic Prostaglandin inhibitor	Rheumatoid arthritis, migraine prophylaxis, headaches, menstrual pain, insect repellent	*Side effects:* Allergic reactions, mouth ulcers, rebound headaches *Drug interaction:* May potentiate anticoagulants	No studies in children Efficacy in migraine prophylaxis in adults
Fish oil (omega-3 fatty acids)	Anti-inflammatory Lipid lowering	Hyperlipidemia, asthma, inflammatory bowel disease, ulcerative colitis, ADHD	*Side effects:* Flatus, halitosis, increased bleeding time *Caution:* May be contaminated with toxic chemicals	Improved visual processing and motor skills in children with dyslexia and dyspraxia Reduced risk of asthma

Continued

HERB	ACTIONS	COMMON USES	SIDE EFFECTS/ TOXIC EFFECTS/ CONTRAINDICATIONS	CLINICAL RESEARCH
Garlic *Allium sativum* capsules	Anti-inflammatory Antimicrobial Antioxidant Spasmolytic Lipid-lowering Hypotensive Expectorant Stimulant	Ear infections, upper respiratory tract infections, cough, atherosclerosis, hypertension, GI disorders, menstrual disorders, diabetes	*Side effects:* Flatus, heartburn, GI disturbances; may prolong bleeding time *Drug interactions:* Use caution with anticoagulants and anti-inflammatory agents	No change in cardiovascular risk factors in children with familial hyperlipidemia
Ginger *Zingiber officinale* capsules	Antiemetic Spasmolytic Immune modulator Antiviral	Nausea, vomiting, colic, upper respiratory infections, cough	*Side effects:* Heartburn *Drug interaction:* May potentiate anticoagulants	No studies in children Mixed results in studies for motion sickness and post-surgical vomiting
Ginkgo biloba	Vasoactive bronchodilator	ADHD, memory disorders, asthma	*Side effects:* Headache, dizziness, heart palpitations, GI disorders *Drug interaction:* May potentiate anticoagulants	No studies on efficacy in ADHD or asthma Positive results on memory in adults
Goldenseal *Hydrastis canadensis* tincture or fluid extract	Anti-inflammatory Antimicrobial Antiseptic Immune modulator	*Internally:* Colds, diarrhea, fever, sore throat *Topically:* Eczema, acne, conjunctivitis, cradle cap, hemorrhoids, fungal infections	*Side effects:* Hypotension, hypertension, local irritation, nausea, vomiting, diarrhea *Caution:* Not recommended for infants less than 1 month of age	Effective treatment for diarrhea associated with giardia in children No other clinical studies in children
Kava *Piper methysticum*	Sedative	Anxiety, depression, ADHD	*Side effects:* Weight loss *Drug interactions:* May potentiate sedatives, alcohol	No clinical studies in children Adult studies show effectiveness in management of anxiety and depression
Lemon balm *Melissa officinalis*	Spasmolytic Sedative Digestive aid Anti-inflammatory	Sleep disorders, anxiety, depression, ADHD Wounds and skin irritation	No known side effects *Drug interaction:* May inhibit thyroid hormones	No clinical studies in children, but in adults effective to improve sleep quality
Licorice *Glycyrrhiza glabra*	Anti-inflammatory Spasmolytic Antiviral Expectorant Antitussive Laxative	Asthma, sore throat, upper respiratory tract infection, colic, constipation, digestive disorder, arthritis, hypertonia	*Side effects:* Long-term use may have mineralocorticoid effect, hypertension, potassium loss, and arrhythmia *Drug interactions:* May potentiate digitalis and potassium loss in combination with steroids and diuretics *Contraindications:* Hypertension, diabetes, kidney disease, liver disease, hypokalemia	Effective in treating infant colic Effective with other Chinese herbs in treating severe eczema in adults No pediatric studies in other areas
Melatonin	Hormone produced by the pineal gland Antioxidant	Sleep disorders	*Side effects:* Reduced alertness, headache, dizziness, and irritability	Clinical trials show efficacy in sleep problems in children with ADHD

HERB	ACTIONS	COMMON USES	SIDE EFFECTS/ TOXIC EFFECTS/ CONTRAINDICATIONS	CLINICAL RESEARCH
Pycnogenol Grape seed or pine bark extracts	Antioxidant	ADHD	*Side effects:* Decreased platelet function *Caution:* There is no information related to safety in children	No clinical trials in children No studies on safety in combination with stimulant medications
St. John's wort *Hypericum perforatum*	Antidepressant Anti-inflammatory Astringent Sedative Immunomodulator	*Topically:* Wounds, burns, neuralgia *Internally:* Depression, anxiety	*Side effects:* GI symptoms, sedation, dizziness, confusion, rare photosensitivity *Drug interactions:* May potentiate antidepressants	Effective in treatment of depression in adults No clinical trials in children
Tea tree oil *Melaleuca alternifolia*	Antibacterial Antifungal	*Topically:* Skin infections, acne, vaginitis	*Side effects:* Contact dermatitis *Caution:* Not to be ingested	Positive results in acne management for adolescents
Valerian *Valeriana officinalis*	Hypnotic Sedative	Sleep disorders, restlessness, ADHD	*Side effects:* GI symptoms, headaches *Drug interactions:* May potentiate sedatives	No clinical trials in children or ADHD Improved quality of sleep in adults
Xylitol chewing gum, lozenges, or syrup	Bacteriostatic	Prevention of ear infections	*Side effects:* Diarrhea	Reduced the incidence of ear infections in preschool children

Modified from Blosser C: Complementary medicine. In Burns CG et al, editors: *Pediatric primary care,* ed 2, Philadelphia, 2000, Saunders; and Gardiner P, Kemper KJ: Herbs in pediatric and adolescent medicine, *Pediatr Rev* 21:44-57, 2000.
ADHD, Attention-deficit/hyperactivity disorder; *GI,* gastrointestinal; *PMS,* premenstrual syndrome.

Health Risk Appraisal

D.1: HEALTHIER PEOPLE HEALTH RISK APPRAISAL

Form C

The HEALTHIER PEOPLE NETWORK, Inc.

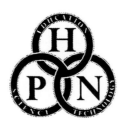

... linking science, technology, & education to serve the public interest ...

IDENTIFICATION NUMBER

The health risk appraisal is an educational tool, showing you choices you can make to keep good health and avoid the most common causes of death (for a person of your age and sex). This health risk appraisal is **not** a substitute for a check-up or physical exam that you get from a doctor or nurse; however, it does provide some ideas for lowering your risk of getting sick or injured in the future. It is NOT designed for people who already have HEART DISEASE, CANCER, KIDNEY DISEASE, OR OTHER SERIOUS CONDITIONS; if you have any of these problems, please ask your health care provider to interpret the report for you.

DIRECTIONS:
To get the most accurate results, **answer as many questions as you can.** If you do not know the answer leave it blank.

The following questions __must__ be completed or the computer program cannot process your questionnaire:

1. SEX   2. AGE   3. HEIGHT   4. WEIGHT   15. CIGARETTE SMOKING

Please write your answers in the boxes provided. ➡ (Examples: ⌧ or ☐ 98)	
1. **SEX**	1 ☐ Male 2 ☐ Female
2. **AGE**	☐ Years
3. **HEIGHT** (Without shoes) (No fractions)	☐ Feet ☐ Inches
4. **WEIGHT** (Without shoes) (No fractions)	☐ Pounds
5. Body frame size	1 ☐ Small 2 ☐ Medium 3 ☐ Large
6. Have you ever been told that you have diabetes (or sugar diabetes)?	1 ☐ Yes 2 ☐ No
7. Are you now taking medicine for high blood pressure?	1 ☐ Yes 2 ☐ No
8. What is your blood pressure now?	☐ / ☐ Systolic (High Number)/Diastolic (Low Number)
9. If you do **not** know the numbers, check the box that describes your blood pressure.	1 ☐ High 2 ☐ Normal or Low 3 ☐ Don't Know

Form   C

10.	What is your TOTAL cholesterol level (based on a blood test)?	[ ] mg/dl
11.	What is your HDL cholesterol (based on a blood test)?	[ ] mg/dl
12.	How many cigars do you usually smoke per day?	[ ] cigars per day
13.	How many pipes of tobacco do you usually smoke per day?	[ ] pipes per day
14.	How many times per day do you usually use smokeless tobacco? (Chewing tobacco, snuff, pouches, etc.)	[ ] times per day
15.	**CIGARETTE SMOKING** How would you describe your cigarette smoking habits?	1 ☐ Never smoked ☞ Go to 18 2 ☐ Used to smoke ☞ Go to 17 3 ☐ Still smoke ☞ Go to 16
16.	**STILL SMOKE** How many cigarettes a day do you smoke? ☞ **GO TO QUESTION 18**	[ ] cigarettes per day ☞ Go to 18
17.	**USED TO SMOKE** a. How many years has it been since you smoked cigarettes fairly regularly? b. What was the average number of cigarettes per day that you smoked in the 2 years before you quit?	[ ] years [ ] cigarettes per day
18.	In the next 12 months, how many thousands of miles will you probably travel by each of the following? (NOTE: U.S. average = 10,000 miles) a. Car, truck, or van: b. Motorcycle:	[ ] ,000 miles [ ] ,000 miles
19.	On a typical day, how do you USUALLY travel? (Check one only)	1 ☐ Walk 2 ☐ Bicycle 3 ☐ Motorcycle 4 ☐ Sub-compact or compact car 5 ☐ Mid-size or full-size car 6 ☐ Truck or van 7 ☐ Bus, subway, or train 8 ☐ Mostly stay home
20.	What percent of time do you usually buckle your safety belt when driving or riding?	[ ] %
21.	On the average, how close to the speed limit do you usually drive?	1 ☐ Within 5 mph of limit 2 ☐ 6-10 mph over limit 3 ☐ 11-15 mph over limit 4 ☐ More than 15 mph over limit
22.	How many times in the last month did you drive or ride when the driver had perhaps too much alcohol to drink?	[ ] times last month
23.	How many drinks of an alcoholic beverage do you have in a typical week? ☞ *MEN GO TO QUESTION 33*	(Write the number of each type of drink) [ ] Bottles or cans of beer [ ] Glasses of wine [ ] Wine coolers [ ] Mixed drinks or shots of liquor

Form C

WOMEN ONLY

24. At what age did you have your first menstrual period?	☐ years old
25. How old were you when your first child was born?	☐ years old (If no children, write 0)
26. How long has it been since your last breast x-ray (mammogram)?	1 ☐ Less than 1 year ago 2 ☐ 1 year ago 3 ☐ 2 years ago 4 ☐ 3 or more years ago 5 ☐ Never
27. How many women in your natural family (mother and sisters only) have had breast cancer?	☐ Women
28. Have you had a hysterectomy operation?	1 ☐ Yes 2 ☐ No 3 ☐ Not sure
29. How long has it been since you had a pap smear test?	1 ☐ Less than 1 year ago 2 ☐ 1 year ago 3 ☐ 2 years ago 4 ☐ 3 or more years ago 5 ☐ Never
★30. How often do you examine your breasts for lumps?	1 ☐ Monthly 2 ☐ Once every few months 3 ☐ Rarely or never
★31. About how long has it been since you had your breasts examined by a physician or nurse?	1 ☐ Less than 1 year ago 2 ☐ 1 year ago 3 ☐ 2 years ago 4 ☐ 3 or more years ago 5 ☐ Never
★32. About how long has it been since you had a rectal exam? ☛ **WOMEN GO TO QUESTION 34**	1 ☐ Less than 1 year ago 2 ☐ 1 year ago 3 ☐ 2 years ago 4 ☐ 3 or more years ago 5 ☐ Never

MEN ONLY

★33. About how long has it been since you had a rectal or prostate exam? ☛ **MEN CONTINUE ON QUES. 34**	1 ☐ Less than 1 year ago 2 ☐ 1 year ago 3 ☐ 2 years ago 4 ☐ 3 or more years ago 5 ☐ Never
★34. How many times in the last year did you witness or become involved in a violent fight or attack where there was a good chance of a serious injury to someone?	1 ☐ 4 or more times 2 ☐ 2 or 3 times 3 ☐ 1 time or never 4 ☐ Not sure
★35. Considering your age, how would you describe your overall physical health?	1 ☐ Excellent 2 ☐ Good 3 ☐ Fair 4 ☐ Poor

★ Questions with a star symbol are not used by the computer to calculate your risks; however, answering these questions may help you plan a more healthy lifestyle.

Form   C

★36. In an average week, how many times do you engage in physical activity (exercise or work which lasts at least 20 minutes without stopping and which is hard enough to make you breathe heavier and your heart beat faster)?	1 ☐ Less than 1 time per week 2 ☐ 1 or 2 times per week 3 ☐ At least 3 times per week
★37. If you ride a motorcycle or all-terrain vehicle (ATV), what percent of the time do you wear a helmet?	1 ☐ 75% to 100% 2 ☐ 25% to 74 % 3 ☐ Less than 25% 4 ☐ Does not apply to me
★38. Do you eat some food every day that is high in fiber, such as whole grain bread, cereal, fresh fruits or vegetables?	1 ☐ Yes 2 ☐ No
★39. Do you eat foods every day that are high in cholesterol or fat, such as fatty meat, cheese, fried foods, or eggs?	1 ☐ Yes 2 ☐ No
★40. In general, how satisfied are you with your life?	1 ☐ Mostly satisfied 2 ☐ Partly satisfied 3 ☐ Not satisfied
★41. Have you suffered a personal loss or misfortune in the past year that had a serious impact on your life? (For example, a job loss, disability, separation, jail term, or the death of someone close to you.)	1 ☐ Yes, 1 serious loss or misfortune 2 ☐ Yes, 2 or more 3 ☐ No
★42a. Race	1 ☐ Aleutian, Alaska native, Eskimo or American Indian 2 ☐ Asian 3 ☐ Black 4 ☐ Pacific Islander 5 ☐ White 6 ☐ Other 7 ☐ Don't know
★42b. Are you of Hispanic origin, such as Mexican-American, Puerto Rican, or Cuban?	1 ☐ Yes 2 ☐ No
★43. What is the highest grade you completed in school?	1 ☐ Grade school or less 2 ☐ Some high school 3 ☐ High school graduate 4 ☐ Some college 5 ☐ College graduate 6 ☐ Post graduate or professional degree

Name _____

Address_____

City _____State ___ ___   Zip ___ ___ ___ ___ ___

(Note: Name and address are optional, depending on how your report will be returned to you. If you wish to remain anonymous, copy your Identification Number onto a receipt form. You can then use this receipt to claim your computerized report.)

The
HEALTHIER PEOPLE NETWORK, Inc.

Participant's Guide to Interpreting the
HEALTH RISK APPRAISAL REPORT

Unhealthy habits lead to early death or chronic illness. Every year, 1.3 million people in the United States die prematurely from conditions which could be prevented or delayed. This Health Risk Appraisal may help you avoid becoming one of these statistics by giving you a picture of how your health risks relate to your particular characteristics and habits.

WHAT IS A HEALTH RISK APPRAISAL?

The Health Risk Appraisal is an estimation of your risk of dying in the next ten years from each of 42 causes of death. The twelve most important of these are printed individually on your report. The others are grouped together and printed as "All Other". These risks are calculated by a computer program which compares your characteristics to national mortality statistics using equations developed by epidemiologists. This Health Risk Appraisal does not tell you how long you will live, nor does it diagnose or treat disease.

RISK FACTORS

Most chronic diseases develop slowly in the presence of certain risk factors. Risk factors are either controllable or uncontrollable. Controllable risk factors include lifestyle habits that you can change such as smoking, exercise, diet, stress and weight. Uncontrollable risk factors include items such as your age and sex, and the health history of your family.

The Health Risk Appraisal uses both controllable and uncontrollable risk factors in calculating health risks. Your focus, however, should be on controllable risk factors.

To help you decide which controllable risk factors to concentrate on, the Health Risk Appraisal identifies your controllable risk factors for each cause of death. Your report gives you an idea of their relative importance by indicating the number of risk years you could gain by controlling these factors.

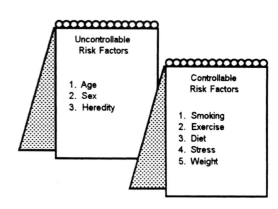

To identify your personal risks, to see what the numbers on your report mean, and to learn which risk factors you need to control, turn the page.

Participant's Guide to Interpreting the Health Risk Appraisal Report Form

An example using a 48 year old woman: 5'7", 250 mg/dl cholesterol, 160/95 BP, 30 cigarettes/day, 9 drinks/week, seat belt use 15%, drives 4,000 mi/yr, menarche 13 yrs, 1st child at 32

---

❶

YOUR RISK AGE	NOW 68.91	TARGET 60.82

◄—— Risks are elevated due to diabetes and family breast cancer

Mrs. Lopez **❻**
Female Age 48

THIS REPORT CONTAINS ESTIMATES DUE TO MISSING ITEMS, INCLUDING THE FOLLOWING **❼**
Cigars per day. Pipes smoked per day. Smokeless tobacco.

Many serious injuries and health problems can be prevented. Your Health Risk Appraisal lists factors you can change to lower your risk. For causes of death that are not directly computable, the report uses the average risk for a person of your age and sex.

MOST COMMON CAUSES OF DEATH	NUMBER OF DEATHS IN NEXT 10 YEARS FOR 1000 WOMEN AGE 48			MODIFIABLE RISK FACTORS
	❷ YOUR GROUP	**❸** TARGET	**❹** POPULATION AVERAGE	
Heart Attack	104	22	5	Avoid Tobacco Use, Blood Pressure, Cholesterol Level, **❽** HDL Level, Weight
Breast Cancer	42	42	5	A Low-Fat Diet and Regular Exercise Might Reduce Risk
Diabetes Mellitus	21	21	1	Control Your Weight and Follow Your Doctor's Advice
Stroke	19	5	2	Avoid Tobacco Use, Blood Pressure
Lung Cancer	13	7	5	Avoid Tobacco Use
Emphysema/Bronchitis	2	<1	1	Avoid Tobacco Use
Kidney Failure	2	2	<1	"
Colon Cancer	1*	1*	1	A High-Fiber and Low-Fat Diet Might Reduce Risk
Ovary Cancer	1*	1*	1	Get Regular Exams
Pancreas Cancer	1	1	1	Avoid Tobacco Use
Cirrhosis of Liver	1	1	1	Continue to Avoid Heavy Drinking
All Other	21	19	20	* = Average Value Used
TOTAL:	228	122	46	Deaths in Next 10 Years Per 1,000 Women, age 48

For Height 5'7" and Large Frame, 175 pounds is about 20% Overweight. Desirable Weight Range: 139-153 **❾**

GOOD HABITS **❺**	TO IMPROVE YOUR RISK PROFILE:	RISK YEARS GAINED **❿**
+ Regular pap tests + Safe driving speed	- Quit smoking <estimate>	3.57
	- Lower your blood pressure	1.88
	- Lower your cholesterol	1.56
	- Improve your HDL level	.92
	- Bring your weight to desirable range	.13
	- Always wear your seat belts	.03

Total Risk Years you could gain = 8.09 **⓫**

❶ Your **RISK AGE** compares your total risk from all causes of death to the total risk of those who are your age and sex. It gives you an idea of your risks compared with the population average in terms of an age. Your **TARGET** risk age indicates what your risk age would be if you made the changes recommended below.

❷ The numbers in the **YOUR GROUP** column refer to the number of predicted deaths for each cause of death in the next 10 years from among 1,000 people who have habits and characteristics just like you.

❸ The numbers in the **TARGET** column refer to those predicted to die in the next 10 years from among 1,000 people who have characteristics just like you, but who have adopted the habits recommended below in the **TO IMPROVE YOUR RISK PROFILE** box.

❹ The numbers in the **POPULATION AVERAGE** column refer to the national average of deaths in 10 years for people of your same sex and age.

❺ This box lists your **GOOD HABITS**. Congratulations!

❻ Your I.D., sex and actual age is here.

❼ If you did not answer items on the questionnaire which are used for calculations, these missing items will be listed here. The computer substitutes national average values for the items you left blank and calculates your risks with these numbers.

❽ Beside each cause of death are listed the modifiable risk factors which your questionnaire responses indicate you need to work on. The list is specific for you unless you have none of the risk factors or if there are no known risk factors for a cause of death. In this case, a short statement of general advice related to risk reduction is printed.

❾ Your **DESIRABLE WEIGHT RANGE** is based on your height and frame size.

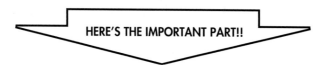

HERE'S THE IMPORTANT PART!!

❿ In this box is our prescription to lengthen your life and a prediction of how many **RISK YEARS** you can expect to gain by adopting these health habits.

⓫ The **TOTAL RISK YEARS** you could gain by making these habit changes are printed here. This is also the difference between your **Risk Age Now** and your **Target Age**. Also important are the recommendations on page 2.

Page 2 of your report lists some **ROUTINE PREVENTIVE SERVICES** that are specific for people of your age and sex. The report also lists some **GENERAL RECOMMENDATIONS FOR EVERYONE**. For the 48 year old woman used in this example, the following messages were printed:

ROUTINE PREVENTIVE SERVICES FOR WOMEN YOUR AGE	GENERAL RECOMMENDATIONS FOR EVERYONE
Blood Pressure and Cholesterol test	* Exercise briskly for 15-30 minutes at least three times a week.
Pap Smear test	* Use good eating habits by choosing a variety of foods that are low in fat and high in fiber.
Breast cancer screening (check with your doctor or clinic)	* Learn to recognize and handle stress - get help if you need it.
Rectal exam (or Sigmoidoscopy)	
Eye exam for glaucoma	
Dental Exam	
Tetanus-Diphtheria booster shot (every 10 years)	

The standard report can also print health education messages.

HEALTH RISK APPRAISAL LIMITS

Health Risk Appraisal is an educational tool. It does not take into consideration whether or not you already have a medical condition and it does not consider rare diseases and other health problems which are not fatal but can limit your enjoyment of life, such as arthritis.

Health Risk Appraisal does not predict when you will die or specifically what diseases you might get. It does tell you, however, your chances of getting a disease relative to a large group of people your age and sex, who answered the questionnaire just as you did.

Health Risk Appraisal does take into consideration lifestyle factors which account for a large number of premature deaths. When you become familiar with your particular risks, you can then do something about them!

CHOOSING A HABIT TO WORK ON

Health Risk Appraisal is intended to encourage you to work on habits you can change by showing you which behaviors should have top priority. If you can't change the behavior that is at the top of your list (the one that would give the largest number of **RISK YEARS GAINED**), try to concentrate on changing the next highest one. You don't have to change your entire lifestyle overnight. In fact, trying to change too many habits at once is probably the quickest way to become discouraged and fail.

MAKE A PLAN FOR CHANGING HABITS

Make a plan for changing the habit you choose as your first priority, write it down and keep it in sight. Be prepared for temptation! Observe the time, situation, or place that most often triggers your unhealthy habit and be ready to combat it when it appears. Let family and friends know of your goals and ask for their encouragement.

REWARD YOURSELF

Rewards are an important part of changing behavior. Give yourself a reasonable reward when you accomplish your goal. Don't eat half a gallon of ice cream after losing 10 pounds! Choose a healthy and enjoyable reward and you'll be on the road to good health!

2011 State and Local Youth Risk Behavior Survey

This survey is about health behavior. It has been developed so you can tell us what you do that may affect your health. The information you give will be used to improve health education for young people like yourself.

DO NOT write your name on this survey. The answers you give will be kept private. No one will know what you write. Answer the questions based on what you really do.

Completing the survey is voluntary. Whether or not you answer the questions will not affect your grade in this class. If you are not comfortable answering a question, just leave it blank.

The questions that ask about your background will be used only to describe the types of students completing this survey. The information will not be used to find out your name. No names will ever be reported.

Make sure to read every question. Fill in the ovals completely. When you are finished, follow the instructions of the person giving you the survey.

Thank you very much for your help.

DIRECTIONS

- **Use a #2 pencil only.**
- **Make dark marks.**
- **Fill in a response like this:** (A) (B) ● (D)
- **If you change your answer, erase your old answer completely.**

1. How old are you?
    - (A) 12 years old or younger
    - (B) 13 years old
    - (C) 14 years old
    - (D) 15 years old
    - (E) 16 years old
    - (F) 17 years old
    - (G) 18 years old or older
2. What is your sex?
    - (A) Female
    - (B) Male
3. In what grade are you?
    - (A) 9th grade
    - (B) 10th grade
    - (C) 11th grade
    - (D) 12th grade
    - (E) Ungraded or other grade
4. Are you Hispanic or Latino?
    - (A) Yes
    - (B) No
5. What is your race? (**Select one or more responses.**)
    - (A) American Indian or Alaska Native
    - (B) Asian
    - (C) Black or African American
    - (D) Native Hawaiian or Other Pacific Islander
    - (E) White

6. How tall are you without your shoes on?
   Directions: Write your height in the shaded blank boxes. Fill in the matching oval below each number.

Example

7. How much do you weigh without your shoes on?
   Directions: Write your weight in the shaded blank boxes. Fill in the matching oval below each number.

Example

The next 4 questions ask about safety.

8. **When you rode a bicycle** during the past 12 months, how often did you wear a helmet?
   - (A) I did not ride a bicycle during the past 12 months
   - (B) Never wore a helmet
   - (C) Rarely wore a helmet
   - (D) Sometimes wore a helmet
   - (E) Most of the time wore a helmet
   - (F) Always wore a helmet

9. How often do you wear a seat belt when **riding** in a car driven by someone else?
   - (A) Never
   - (B) Rarely
   - (C) Sometimes
   - (D) Most of the time
   - (E) Always

10. During the past 30 days, how many times did you **ride** in a car or other vehicle **driven by someone who had been drinking alcohol**?
    - (A) 0 times
    - (B) 1 time
    - (C) 2 or 3 times
    - (D) 4 or 5 times
    - (E) 6 or more times

11. During the past 30 days, how many times did you **drive** a car or other vehicle **when you had been drinking alcohol?**
    - (A) 0 times
    - (B) 1 time
    - (C) 2 or 3 times
    - (D) 4 or 5 times
    - (E) 6 or more times

The next 10 questions ask about violence-related behaviors.

12. During the past 30 days, on how many days did you carry **a weapon** such as a gun, knife, or club?
    - (A) 0 days
    - (B) 1 day
    - (C) 2 or 3 days
    - (D) 4 or 5 days
    - (E) 6 or more days

13. During the past 30 days, on how many days did you carry **a gun?**
    - (A) 0 days
    - (B) 1 day
    - (C) 2 or 3 days
    - (D) 4 or 5 days
    - (E) 6 or more days

14. During the past 30 days, on how many days did you carry a weapon such as a gun, knife, or club **on school property?**
    - (A) 0 days
    - (B) 1 day
    - (C) 2 or 3 days
    - (D) 4 or 5 days
    - (E) 6 or more days

15. During the past 30 days, on how many days did you **not** go to school because you felt you would be unsafe at school or on your way to or from school?
    - (A) 0 days
    - (B) 1 day
    - (C) 2 or 3 days
    - (D) 4 or 5 days
    - (E) 6 or more days

16. During the past 12 months, how many times has someone threatened or injured you with a weapon such as a gun, knife, or club **on school property?**
    - (A) 0 times
    - (B) 1 time
    - (C) 2 or 3 times
    - (D) 4 or 5 times
    - (E) 6 or 7 times
    - (F) 8 or 9 times
    - (G) 10 or 11 times
    - (H) 12 or more times

17. During the past 12 months, how many times were you in a physical fight?
    - (A) 0 times
    - (B) 1 time
    - (C) 2 or 3 times
    - (D) 4 or 5 times
    - (E) 6 or 7 times
    - (F) 8 or 9 times
    - (G) 10 or 11 times
    - (H) 12 or more times

18. During the past 12 months, how many times were you in a physical fight in which you were injured and had to be treated by a doctor or nurse?
    - (A) 0 times
    - (B) 1 time
    - (C) 2 or 3 times
    - (D) 4 or 5 times
    - (E) 6 or more times

19. During the past 12 months, how many times were you in a physical fight **on school property?**
    - (A) 0 times
    - (B) 1 time
    - (C) 2 or 3 times
    - (D) 4 or 5 times
    - (E) 6 or 7 times
    - (F) 8 or 9 times
    - (G) 10 or 11 times
    - (H) 12 or more times

20. During the past 12 months, did your boyfriend or girlfriend ever hit, slap, or physically hurt you on purpose?
    - (A) Yes
    - (B) No

21. Have you ever been physically forced to have sexual intercourse when you did not want to?
    - (A) Yes
    - (B) No

Continued

The 2 next questions ask about bullying. Bullying is when 1 or more students tease, threaten, spread rumors about, hit, shove, or hurt another student over and over again. It is not bullying when 2 students of about the same strength or power argue or fight or tease each other in a friendly way.

22. During the past 12 months, have you ever been bullied **on school property**?
    - (A) Yes
    - (B) No

23. During the past 12 months, have you ever been **electronically** bullied? (Include being bullied through e-mail, chat rooms, instant messaging, Websites, or texting.)
    - (A) Yes
    - (B) No

The next 5 questions ask about sad feelings and attempted suicide. Sometimes people feel so depressed about the future that they may consider attempting suicide, that is, taking some action to end their own life.

24. During the past 12 months, did you ever feel so sad or hopeless almost every day for **two weeks or more in a row** that you stopped doing some usual activities?
    - (A) Yes
    - (B) No

25. During the past 12 months, did you ever **seriously** consider attempting suicide?
    - (A) Yes
    - (B) No

26. During the past 12 months, did you make a plan about how you would attempt suicide?
    - (A) Yes
    - (B) No

27. During the past 12 months, how many times did you actually attempt suicide?
    - (A) 0 times
    - (B) 1 time
    - (C) 2 or 3 times
    - (D) 4 or 5 times
    - (E) 6 or more times

28. **If you attempted suicide** during the past 12 months, did any attempt result in an injury, poisoning, or overdose that had to be treated by a doctor or nurse?
    - (A) **I did not attempt suicide** during the past 12 months
    - (B) Yes
    - (C) No

The next 11 questions ask about tobacco use.

29. Have you ever tried cigarette smoking, even one or two puffs?
    - (A) Yes
    - (B) No

30. How old were you when you smoked a whole cigarette for the first time?
    - (A) I have never smoked a whole cigarette
    - (B) 8 years old or younger
    - (C) 9 or 10 years old
    - (D) 11 or 12 years old
    - (E) 13 or 14 years old
    - (F) 15 or 16 years old
    - (G) 17 years old or older

31. During the past 30 days, on how many days did you smoke cigarettes?
    - (A) 0 days
    - (B) 1 or 2 days
    - (C) 3 to 5 days
    - (D) 6 to 9 days
    - (E) 10 to 19 days
    - (F) 20 to 29 days
    - (G) All 30 days

32. During the past 30 days, on the days you smoked, how many cigarettes did you smoke **per day**?
    - (A) I did not smoke cigarettes during the past 30 days
    - (B) Less than 1 cigarette per day
    - (C) 1 cigarette per day
    - (D) 2 to 5 cigarettes per day
    - (E) 6 to 10 cigarettes per day
    - (F) 11 to 20 cigarettes per day
    - (G) More than 20 cigarettes per day

33. During the past 30 days, how did you **usually** get your own cigarettes? (Select only **one** response.)
    - (A) I did not smoke cigarettes during the past 30 days
    - (B) I bought them in a store such as a convenience store, supermarket, discount store, or gas station
    - (C) I bought them from a vending machine
    - (D) I gave someone else money to buy them for me
    - (E) I borrowed (or bummed) them from someone else
    - (F) A person 18 years old or older gave them to me
    - (G) I took them from a store or family member
    - (H) I got them some other way

34. During the past 30 days, on how many days did you smoke cigarettes **on school property**?
    - (A) 0 days
    - (B) 1 or 2 days
    - (C) 3 to 5 days
    - (D) 6 to 9 days
    - (E) 10 to 19 days
    - (F) 20 to 29 days
    - (G) All 30 days

35. Have you ever smoked cigarettes daily, that is, at least one cigarette every day for 30 days?
    - (A) Yes
    - (B) No

36. During the past 12 months, did you ever try **to quit** smoking cigarettes?
    - (A) I did not smoke during the past 12 months
    - (B) Yes
    - (C) No

37. During the past 30 days, on how many days did you use **chewing tobacco, snuff, or dip**, such as Redman, Levi Garrett, Beechnut, Skoal, Skoal Bandits, or Copenhagen?
   (A) 0 days
   (B) 1 or 2 days
   (C) 3 to 5 days
   (D) 6 to 9 days
   (E) 10 to 19 days
   (F) 20 to 29 days
   (G) All 30 days

38. During the past 30 days, on how many days did you use **chewing tobacco, snuff, or dip on school property?**
   (A) 0 days
   (B) 1 or 2 days
   (C) 3 to 5 days
   (D) 6 to 9 days
   (E) 10 to 19 days
   (F) 20 to 29 days
   (G) All 30 days

39. During the past 30 days, on how many days did you smoke **cigars, cigarillos, or little cigars?**
   (A) 0 days
   (B) 1 or 2 days
   (C) 3 to 5 days
   (D) 6 to 9 days
   (E) 10 to 19 days
   (F) 20 to 29 days
   (G) All 30 days

The next 6 questions ask about drinking alcohol. This includes drinking beer, wine, wine coolers, and liquor such as rum, gin, vodka, or whiskey. For these questions, drinking alcohol does not include drinking a few sips of wine for religious purposes.

40. During your life, on how many days have you had at least one drink of alcohol?
   (A) 0 days
   (B) 1 or 2 days
   (C) 3 to 9 days
   (D) 10 to 19 days
   (E) 20 to 39 days
   (F) 40 to 99 days
   (G) 100 or more days

41. How old were you when you had your first drink of alcohol other than a few sips?
   (A) I have never had a drink of alcohol other than a few sips
   (B) 8 years old or younger
   (C) 9 or 10 years old
   (D) 11 or 12 years old
   (E) 13 or 14 years old
   (F) 15 or 16 years old
   (G) 17 years old or older

42. During the past 30 days, on how many days did you have at least one drink of alcohol?
   (A) 0 days
   (B) 1 or 2 days
   (C) 3 to 5 days
   (D) 6 to 9 days
   (E) 10 to 19 days
   (F) 20 to 29 days
   (G) All 30 days

43. During the past 30 days, on how many days did you have 5 or more drinks of alcohol in a row, that is, within a couple of hours?
   (A) 0 days
   (B) 1 day
   (C) 2 days
   (D) 3 to 5 days
   (E) 6 to 9 days
   (F) 10 to 19 days
   (G) 20 or more days

44. During the past 30 days, how did you **usually** get the alcohol you drank?
   (A) I did not drink alcohol during the past 30 days
   (B) I bought it in a store such as a liquor store, convenience store, supermarket, discount store, or gas station
   (C) I bought it at a restaurant, bar, or club
   (D) I bought it at a public event such as a concert or sporting event
   (E) I gave someone else money to buy it for me
   (F) Someone gave it to me
   (G) I took it from a store or family member
   (H) I got it some other way

45. During the past 30 days, on how many days did you have at least one drink of alcohol **on school property?**
   (A) 0 days
   (B) 1 or 2 days
   (C) 3 to 5 days
   (D) 6 to 9 days
   (E) 10 to 19 days
   (F) 20 to 29 days
   (G) All 30 days

The next 4 questions ask about marijuana use. Marijuana also is called grass or pot.
46. During your life, how many times have you used marijuana?
   (A) 0 times
   (B) 1 or 2 times
   (C) 3 to 9 times
   (D) 10 to 19 times
   (E) 20 to 39 times
   (F) 40 to 99 times
   (G) 100 or more times

47. How old were you when you tried marijuana for the first time?
- (A) I have never tried marijuana
- (B) 8 years old or younger
- (C) 9 or 10 years old
- (D) 11 or 12 years old
- (E) 13 or 14 years old
- (F) 15 or 16 years old
- (G) 17 years old or older

48. During the past 30 days, how many times did you use marijuana?
- (A) 0 times
- (B) 1 or 2 times
- (C) 3 to 9 times
- (D) 10 to 19 times
- (E) 20 to 39 times
- (F) 40 or more times

49. During the past 30 days, how many times did you use marijuana **on school property**?
- (A) 0 times
- (B) 1 or 2 times
- (C) 3 to 9 times
- (D) 10 to 19 times
- (E) 20 to 39 times
- (F) 40 or more times

The next 10 questions ask about other drugs.

50. During your life, how many times have you used **any** form of cocaine, including powder, crack, or freebase?
- (A) 0 times
- (B) 1 or 2 times
- (C) 3 to 9 times
- (D) 10 to 19 times
- (E) 20 to 39 times
- (F) 40 or more times

51. During the past 30 days, how many times did you use **any** form of cocaine, including powder, crack, or freebase?
- (A) 0 times
- (B) 1 or 2 times
- (C) 3 to 9 times
- (D) 10 to 19 times
- (E) 20 to 39 times
- (F) 40 or more times

52. During your life, how many times have you sniffed glue, breathed the contents of aerosol spray cans, or inhaled any paints or sprays to get high?
- (A) 0 times
- (B) 1 or 2 times
- (C) 3 to 9 times
- (D) 10 to 19 times
- (E) 20 to 39 times
- (F) 40 or more times

53. During your life, how many times have you used **heroin** (also called smack, junk, or China White)?
- (A) 0 times
- (B) 1 or 2 times
- (C) 3 to 9 times
- (D) 10 to 19 times
- (E) 20 to 39 times
- (F) 40 or more times

54. During your life, how many times have you used **methamphetamines** (also called speed, crystal, crank, or ice)?
- (A) 0 times
- (B) 1 or 2 times
- (C) 3 to 9 times
- (D) 10 to 19 times
- (E) 20 to 39 times
- (F) 40 or more times

55. During your life, how many times have you used **ecstasy** (also called MDMA)?
- (A) 0 times
- (B) 1 or 2 times
- (C) 3 to 9 times
- (D) 10 to 19 times
- (E) 20 to 39 times
- (F) 40 or more times

56. During your life, how many times have you taken **steroid pills or shots** without a doctor's prescription?
- (A) 0 times
- (B) 1 or 2 times
- (C) 3 to 9 times
- (D) 10 to 19 times
- (E) 20 to 39 times
- (F) 40 or more times

57. During your life, how many times have you taken a **prescription drug** (such as OxyContin, Percocet, Vicodin, codeine, Adderall, Ritalin, or Xanax) without a doctor's prescription?
- (A) 0 times
- (B) 1 or 2 times
- (C) 3 to 9 times
- (D) 10 to 19 times
- (E) 20 to 39 times
- (F) 40 or more times

58. During your life, how many times have you used a needle to inject any **illegal** drug into your body?
- (A) 0 times
- (B) 1 time
- (C) 2 or more times

59. During the past 12 months, has anyone offered, sold, or given you an illegal drug **on school property**?
- (A) Yes
- (B) No

The next 7 questions ask about sexual behavior.

60. Have you ever had sexual intercourse?
    (A) Yes
    (B) No

61. How old were you when you had sexual intercourse for the first time?
    (A) I have never had sexual intercourse
    (B) 11 years old or younger
    (C) 12 years old
    (D) 13 years old
    (E) 14 years old
    (F) 15 years old
    (G) 16 years old
    (H) 17 years old or older

62. During your life, with how many people have you had sexual intercourse?
    (A) I have never had sexual intercourse
    (B) 1 person
    (C) 2 people
    (D) 3 people
    (E) 4 people
    (F) 5 people
    (G) 6 or more people

63. During the past 3 months, with how many people did you have sexual intercourse?
    (A) I have never had sexual intercourse
    (B) I have had sexual intercourse, but not during the past 3 months
    (C) 1 person
    (D) 2 people
    (E) 3 people
    (F) 4 people
    (G) 5 people
    (H) 6 or more people

64. Did you drink alcohol or use drugs before you had sexual intercourse the **last time**?
    (A) I have never had sexual intercourse
    (B) Yes
    (C) No

65. The **last time** you had sexual intercourse, did you or your partner use a condom?
    (A) I have never had sexual intercourse
    (B) Yes
    (C) No

66. The **last time** you had sexual intercourse, what **one** method did you or your partner use to **prevent pregnancy**? (Select only **one** response.)
    (A) I have never had sexual intercourse
    (B) No method was used to prevent pregnancy
    (C) Birth control pills
    (D) Condoms
    (E) Depo-Provera (or any injectable birth control), Nuva Ring (or any birth control ring), Implanon (or any implant), or any IUD
    (F) Withdrawal
    (G) Some other method
    (H) Not sure

The next 5 questions ask about body weight.

67. How do **you** describe your weight?
    (A) Very underweight
    (B) Slightly underweight
    (C) About the right weight
    (D) Slightly overweight
    (E) Very overweight

68. Which of the following are you trying to do about your weight?
    (A) **Lose** weight
    (B) **Gain** weight
    (C) **Stay** the same weight
    (D) I am **not trying to do anything** about my weight

69. During the past 30 days, did you **go without eating for 24 hours or more** (also called fasting) to lose weight or to keep from gaining weight?
    (A) Yes
    (B) No

70. During the past 30 days, did you **take any diet pills, powders, or liquids** without a doctor's advice to lose weight or to keep from gaining weight? (Do **not** include meal replacement products such as Slim Fast.)
    (A) Yes
    (B) No

71. During the past 30 days, did you **vomit or take laxatives** to lose weight or to keep from gaining weight?
    (A) Yes
    (B) No

The next 7 questions ask about food you ate or drank during the past 7 days. Think about all the meals and snacks you had from the time you got up until you went to bed. Be sure to include food you ate at home, at school, at restaurants, or anywhere else.

72. During the past 7 days, how many times did you drink **100% fruit juices** such as orange juice, apple juice, or grape juice? (Do **not** count punch, Kool-Aid, sports drinks, or other fruit-flavored drinks.)
    (A) I did not drink 100% fruit juice during the past 7 days
    (B) 1 to 3 times during the past 7 days
    (C) 4 to 6 times during the past 7 days
    (D) 1 time per day
    (E) 2 times per day
    (F) 3 times per day
    (G) 4 or more times per day

73. During the past 7 days, how many times did you eat **fruit**? (Do **not** count fruit juice.)
    (A) I did not eat fruit during the past 7 days
    (B) 1 to 3 times during the past 7 days
    (C) 4 to 6 times during the past 7 days
    (D) 1 time per day
    (E) 2 times per day
    (F) 3 times per day
    (G) 4 or more times per day

74. During the past 7 days, how many times did you eat **green salad**?
    - (A) I did not eat green salad during the past 7 days
    - (B) 1 to 3 times during the past 7 days
    - (C) 4 to 6 times during the past 7 days
    - (D) 1 time per day
    - (E) 2 times per day
    - (F) 3 times per day
    - (G) 4 or more times per day

75. During the past 7 days, how many times did you eat **potatoes**? (Do **not** count french fries, fried potatoes, or potato chips.)
    - (A) I did not eat potatoes during the past 7 days
    - (B) 1 to 3 times during the past 7 days
    - (C) 4 to 6 times during the past 7 days
    - (D) 1 time per day
    - (E) 2 times per day
    - (F) 3 times per day
    - (G) 4 or more times per day

76. During the past 7 days, how many times did you eat **carrots**?
    - (A) I did not eat carrots during the past 7 days
    - (B) 1 to 3 times during the past 7 days
    - (C) 4 to 6 times during the past 7 days
    - (D) 1 time per day
    - (E) 2 times per day
    - (F) 3 times per day
    - (G) 4 or more times per day

77. During the past 7 days, how many times did you eat **other vegetables**? (Do **not** count green salad, potatoes, or carrots.)
    - (A) I did not eat other vegetables during the past 7 days
    - (B) 1 to 3 times during the past 7 days
    - (C) 4 to 6 times during the past 7 days
    - (D) 1 time per day
    - (E) 2 times per day
    - (F) 3 times per day
    - (G) 4 or more times per day

78. During the past 7 days, how many times did you drink a **can, bottle, or glass of soda or pop**, such as Coke, Pepsi, or Sprite? (Do **not** count diet soda or diet pop.)
    - (A) I did not drink soda or pop during the past 7 days
    - (B) 1 to 3 times during the past 7 days
    - (C) 4 to 6 times during the past 7 days
    - (D) 1 time per day
    - (E) 2 times per day
    - (F) 3 times per day
    - (G) 4 or more times per day

The next 5 questions ask about physical activity.

79. During the past 7 days, on how many days were you physically active for a total of **at least 60 minutes per day**? (Add up all the time you spent in any kind of physical activity that increased your heart rate and made you breathe hard some of the time.)
    - (A) 0 days
    - (B) 1 day
    - (C) 2 days
    - (D) 3 days
    - (E) 4 days
    - (F) 5 days
    - (G) 6 days
    - (H) 7 days

80. On an average school day, how many hours do you watch TV?
    - (A) I do not watch TV on an average school day
    - (B) Less than 1 hour per day
    - (C) 1 hour per day
    - (D) 2 hours per day
    - (E) 3 hours per day
    - (F) 4 hours per day
    - (G) 5 or more hours per day

81. On an average school day, how many hours do you play video or computer games or use a computer for something that is not school work? (Include activities such as Xbox, PlayStation, Nintendo DS, iPod touch, Facebook, and the Internet.)
    - (A) I do not play video or computer games or use a computer for something that is not school work
    - (B) Less than 1 hour per day
    - (C) 1 hour per day
    - (D) 2 hours per day
    - (E) 3 hours per day
    - (F) 4 hours per day
    - (G) 5 or more hours per day

82. In an average week when you are in school, on how many days do you go to physical education (PE) classes?
    - (A) 0 days
    - (B) 1 day
    - (C) 2 days
    - (D) 3 days
    - (E) 4 days
    - (F) 5 days

83. During the past 12 months, on how many sports teams did you play? (Count any teams run by your school or community groups.)
    - (A) 0 teams
    - (B) 1 team
    - (C) 2 teams
    - (D) 3 or more teams

The next 3 questions ask about other health-related topics.

84. Have you ever been taught about AIDS or HIV infection in school?
    - (A) Yes
    - (B) No
    - (C) Not sure

85. Has a doctor or nurse ever told you that you have asthma?
    - (A) Yes
    - (B) No
    - (C) Not sure

86. Do you still have asthma?
    - (A) I have never had asthma
    - (B) Yes
    - (C) No
    - (D) Not sure

This is the end of the survey.
Thank you very much for your help.

Flu Pandemics

A pandemic is a global disease outbreak. An influenza pandemic occurs when a new type of influenza virus emerges, for which there is little or no immunity in the human population, begins to cause serious illness and then spreads easily person-to-person worldwide. A pandemic is determined by spread of disease, not its ability to cause death.

NEW FLU VIRUSES

There are three types of flu viruses. Type A viruses are found in many kinds of animals, including ducks, chickens, pigs, and whales, as well as humans. The type B virus widely circulates in humans. Type C has been found in humans, pigs, and dogs and causes mild respiratory infections, but does not spark epidemics.

Influenza virus is one of the most changeable of viruses. Changes may be small and continuous or large and abrupt.

Small, continuous changes happen in type A and type B influenza as the virus makes copies of itself. The process is called *antigenic drift*. The drifting is frequent enough to make the new strain of virus often unrecognizable to the human immune system. For this reason, a new flu vaccine must be produced each year to combat that year's prevalent strains.

Type A influenza also undergoes infrequent and sudden changes, called *antigenic shift*. Antigenic shift occurs when two different flu strains infect the same cell and exchange genetic material. The novel assortment of HA or NA proteins in a shifted virus creates a new influenza A subtype. Because people have little or no immunity to such a new subtype, their appearance tends to coincide with a very severe flu epidemic or pandemic.

SEASONAL FLU VERSUS PANDEMIC FLU

SEASONAL FLU	PANDEMIC FLU
Outbreaks follow predictable seasonal patterns; occur annually, usually in winter, in temperate climates	Occurs rarely (three times in twentieth century)
Usually some immunity built up from previous exposure	No previous exposure; little or no pre-existing immunity
Healthy adults usually not at risk for serious complications; the very young, the elderly and those with certain underlying health conditions at increased risk for serious complications	Healthy people may be at increased risk for serious complications
Health systems can usually meet public and patient needs	Health systems may be overwhelmed

SEASONAL FLU	PANDEMIC FLU
Vaccine developed based on known flu strains and available for annual flu season	Vaccine probably would not be available in the early stages of a pandemic
Adequate supplies of antivirals are usually available	Effective antivirals may be in limited supply
Average U.S. deaths approximately 36,000/year	Number of deaths could be quite high (e.g., U.S. 1918 death toll approximately 675,000)
Symptoms: fever, cough, runny nose, muscle pain; deaths often caused by complications, such as pneumonia	Symptoms may be more severe and complications more frequent
Generally causes modest impact on society (e.g., some school closings, encouragement of people who are sick to stay home)	May cause major impact on society (e.g., widespread restrictions on travel, closings of schools and businesses, cancellation of large public gatherings)
Manageable impact on domestic and world economy	Potential for severe impact on domestic and world economy

CHARACTERISTICS AND CHALLENGES OF A FLU PANDEMIC

1. Rapid Worldwide Spread
   - When a pandemic influenza virus emerges, its global spread is considered inevitable.
   - Preparedness activities should assume that the entire world population would be susceptible.
   - Countries might, through measures such as border closures and travel restrictions, delay arrival of the virus, but cannot stop it.
2. Health Care Systems Overloaded
   - Most people have little or no immunity to a pandemic virus. Infection and illness rates soar. A substantial percentage of the world's population will require some form of medical care.
   - Nations unlikely to have the staff, facilities, equipment, and hospital beds needed to cope with large numbers of people who suddenly fall ill.
   - Death rates are high, largely determined by four factors: the number of people who become infected, the virulence of the virus, the underlying characteristics and vulnerability of affected populations, and the effectiveness of preventive measures.
   - Past pandemics have spread globally in two and sometimes three waves.

3. Medical Supplies Inadequate
   - The need for vaccine is likely to outstrip supply.
   - The need for antiviral drugs is also likely to be inadequate early in a pandemic.
   - A pandemic can create a shortage of hospital beds, ventilators, and other supplies. Surge capacity at non-traditional sites such as schools may be created to cope with demand.
   - Difficult decisions will need to be made regarding who gets antiviral drugs and vaccines.
4. Economic and Social Disruption
   - Travel bans, closings of schools and businesses, and cancellations of events could have major impact on communities and citizens.
   - Care for sick family members and fear of exposure can result in significant worker absenteeism.

COMMUNICATIONS AND INFORMATION ARE CRITICAL COMPONENTS OF PANDEMIC RESPONSE

Education and outreach are critical to preparing for a pandemic. Understanding what a pandemic is, what needs to be done at all levels to prepare for pandemic influenza, and what could happen during a pandemic helps us make informed decisions both as individuals and as a nation. Should a pandemic occur, the public must be able to depend on its government to provide scientifically sound public health information quickly, openly, and dependably.

Source: U.S. Department of Health and Human Services: Pandemic flu. Available at www.flu.gov/individualfamily/about/pandemic/index.html.

APPENDIX D.4

Commonly Abused Drugs

SUBSTANCES: CATEGORY AND NAME	EXAMPLES OF *COMMERCIAL* AND STREET NAMES	DEA SCHEDULE*/ HOW ADMINISTERED†	*INTOXICATION EFFECTS*/POTENTIAL HEALTH CONSEQUENCES
Cannabinoids			
Hashish	Boom, chronic, gangster, hash, hash oil, hemp	I/swallowed, smoked	*Euphoria, slowed thinking and reaction time, confusion, impaired balance and coordination*/Cough, frequent respiratory infections; impaired memory and learning; increased heart rate, anxiety; panic attacks; tolerance, addiction
Marijuana	Blunt, dope, ganja, grass, herb, joints, Mary Jane, pot, reefer, sinsemilla, skunk, weed	I/swallowed, smoked	See above
Depressants			
Barbiturates	*Amytal, Nembutal, Seconal, Phenobarbital:* barbs, reds, red birds, phennies, tooies, yellows, yellow jackets	II, III, V/injected, swallowed	*Reduced anxiety; feeling of well-being; lowered inhibitions; slowed pulse and breathing; lowered blood pressure; poor concentration*/Fatigue; confusion; impaired coordination, memory, judgment; addiction; respiratory depression and arrest; death *Also: Sedation, drowsiness*/Depression, unusual excitement, fever, irritability, poor judgment, slurred speech, dizziness, life-threatening withdrawal
Benzodiazepines (other than fluni-trazepam)	*Ativan, Halcion, Librium, Valium, Xanax:* candy, downers, sleeping pills, tranks	IV/swallowed, injected	See above *Also: Sedation, drowsiness*/Dizziness
Flunitrazepam‡	*Rohypnol:* forget-me pill, Mexican valium, R2, Roche, roofies, roofinol, rope, rophies	IV/swallowed, snorted	See above *Also:* Visual and gastrointestinal disturbances, urinary retention, memory loss for the time under the drug's effects
GHB‡	*Gamma-hydroxybutyrate:* G, Georgia home boy, grievous bodily harm, liquid ecstasy	I/swallowed	See above *Also:* Drowsiness, nausea/vomiting, headache, loss of consciousness, loss of reflexes, seizures, coma, death
Methaqualone	*Quaalude, Sopor, Parest:* ludes, mandrex, quad, quay	I/injected, swallowed	See above *Also: Euphoria*/Depression, poor reflexes, slurred speech, coma
Dissociative Anesthetics			
Ketamine	*Ketalar SV:* cat valiums, K, Special K, vitamin K	III/injected, snorted, smoked	*Increased heart rate and blood pressure, impaired motor function*/memory loss; numbness; nausea/vomiting *Also:* At high doses, delirium, depression, respiratory depression and arrest
PCP and analogs	*Phencyclidine;* angel dust, boat, hog, love boat, peace pill	I, II/injected, swallowed, smoked	See above *Also: Possible decrease in blood pressure and heart rate, panic, aggression, violence*/Loss of appetite, depression

SUBSTANCES: CATEGORY AND NAME	EXAMPLES OF *COMMERCIAL* AND STREET NAMES	DEA SCHEDULE*/ HOW ADMINISTERED†	*INTOXICATION EFFECTS*/POTENTIAL HEALTH CONSEQUENCES
Hallucinogens			
LSD	*Lysergic acid diethylamide:* acid, blotter, boomers, cubes, microdot, yellow sunshines	I/swallowed, absorbed through mouth tissues	*Altered states of perception and feeling; nausea*/Persisting perception disorder (flashbacks) *Also: Increased body temperature, heart rate, blood pressure; loss of appetite, sleeplessness, numbness, weakness, tremors; persistent mental disorders*
Mescaline	Buttons, cactus, mesc, peyote	I/swallowed, smoked	See above *Also: Increased body temperature, heart rate, blood pressure; loss of appetite, sleeplessness, numbness, weakness, tremors*
Psilocybin	Magic mushroom, purple passion, shrooms	I/swallowed	See above *Also: Nervousness, paranoia*
Opioids and Morphine Derivatives			
Codeine	*Empirin with Codeine, Fiorinal with Codeine, Robitussin A-C, Tylenol with Codeine:* Captain Cody, schoolboy; (with glutethimide) doors & fours, loads, pancakes and syrup	II, III, IV, V/injected, swallowed	*Pain relief, euphoria, drowsiness*/Nausea, constipation, confusion, sedation, respiratory depression and arrest, tolerance, addiction, unconsciousness, coma, death *Also: Less analgesia, sedation, and respiratory depression than morphine*
Fentanyl and fentanyl analogs	*Actiq, Duragesic, Sublimaze:* Apache, China girl, China white, dance fever, friend, goodfella, jackpot, murder 8, TNT, Tango and Cash	I, II/injected, smoked, snorted	See above
Heroin	*Diacetyl-morphine:* brown sugar, dope, H, horse, junk, skag, skunk, smack, white horse	I/injected, smoked, snorted	See above *Also: Staggering gait*
Morphine	*Roxanol, Duramorph:* M, Miss Emma, monkey, white stuff	II, III/injected, swallowed, smoked	See above
Opium	*Laudanum, paregoric:* big O, black stuff, block, gum, hop	II, III, V/swallowed, smoked	See above
Oxycodone HCL	*Oxycontin:* Oxy, O.C., killer	II/swallowed, snorted, injected	See above
Hydrocodone bitartrate, acetaminophen	*Vicodin:* vike, Watson-387	II/swallowed	See above
Stimulants			
Amphetamine	*Biphetamine, Dexedrine:* bennies, black beauties, crosses, hearts, LA turnaround, speed, truck drivers, uppers	II/injected, swallowed, smoked, snorted	*Increased heart rate, blood pressure, metabolism; feelings of exhilaration, energy, increased mental alertness*/Rapid or irregular heart beat; reduced appetite, weight loss, heart failure, nervousness, insomnia *Also: Rapid breathing*/Tremor, loss of coordination; irritability, anxiousness, restlessness, delirium, panic, paranoia, impulsive behavior, aggressiveness, tolerance, addiction, psychosis
Cocaine	*Cocaine hydrochloride:* blow, bump, C, candy, Charlie, coke, crack, flake, rock, snow, toot	II/injected, smoked, snorted	See above *Also: Increased temperature*/Chest pain, respiratory failure, nausea, abdominal pain, strokes, seizures, headaches, malnutrition, panic attacks

Continued

SUBSTANCES: CATEGORY AND NAME	EXAMPLES OF *COMMERCIAL* AND STREET NAMES	DEA SCHEDULE*/ HOW ADMINISTERED†	*INTOXICATION EFFECTS*/POTENTIAL HEALTH CONSEQUENCES
MDMA (methyl-enedioxy-meth-amphetamine)	Adam, clarity, ecstasy, Eve, lover's speed, peace, STP, X, XTC	I/swallowed	See above *Also: Mild hallucinogenic effects, increased tactile sensitivity, empathic feelings*/Impaired memory and learning, hyperthermia, cardiac toxicity, renal failure, liver toxicity
Methamphet-amine	*Desoxyn:* chalk, crank, crystal, fire, glass, go fast, ice, meth, speed	II/injected, swallowed, smoked, snorted	See above *Also: Aggression, violence, psychotic behavior*/Memory loss, cardiac and neurological damage; impaired memory and learning, tolerance, addiction
Methylphenidate (safe and effective for treatment of ADHD)	*Ritalin:* JIF, MPH, R-ball, Skippy, the smart drug, vitamin R	II/injected, swallowed, snorted	See above
Nicotine	Cigarettes, cigars, smokeless tobacco, snuff, spit tobacco, bidis, chew	Not scheduled/ smoked, snorted, taken in snuff and spit tobacco	See above *Also:* Additional effects attributable to tobacco exposure; adverse pregnancy outcomes; chronic lung disease, cardiovascular disease, stroke, cancer, tolerance, addiction
Other Compounds			
Anabolic steroids	*Anadrol, Oxandrin, Dura-bolin, Depo- Testosterone, Equipoise:* roids, juice	III/injected, swallowed, applied to skin	*No intoxication effects*/Hypertension, blood clotting and cholesterol changes, liver cysts and cancer, kidney cancer, hostility and aggression, acne; in adolescents, premature stoppage of growth; in males, prostate cancer, reduced sperm production, shrunken testicles, breast enlargement; in females, menstrual irregularities, development of beard and other masculine characteristics
Dextromethorphan (DXM)	Found in some cough and cold medications; Robotripping, Robo, Triple C	Not scheduled/ swallowed	*Dissociative effects, distorted visual perceptions to complete dissociative effects*/For effects at higher doses, see Dissociative Anesthetics
Inhalants	*Solvents (paint thinners, gasoline, glues), gases (butane, propane, aerosol propellants, nitrous oxide), nitrites (isoamyl, isobutyl, cyclohexyl):* laughing gas, poppers, snappers, whippets	Not scheduled/ inhaled through nose or mouth	*Stimulation, loss of inhibition; headache; nausea or vomiting; slurred speech, loss of motor coordination; wheezing*/Unconsciousness, cramps, weight loss, muscle weakness, depression, memory impairment, damage to cardiovascular and nervous systems, sudden death

Source: U.S. Department of Health and Human Services, National Institutes of Health, National Institute on Drug Abuse. Available at www.drugabuse.gov/DrugPages/DrugsofAbuse.html.

*Schedule I and II drugs have a high potential for abuse. They require greater storage security and have a quota on manufacturing, among other restrictions. Schedule I drugs are available for research only and have no approved medical use; Schedule II drugs are available only by prescription (unrefillable) and require a form for ordering. Schedule III and IV drugs are available by prescription, may have five refills in 6 months, and may be ordered orally. Some Schedule V drugs are available over the counter.

†Taking drugs by injection can increase the risk of infection through needle contamination with staphylococci, HIV, hepatitis, and other organisms.

‡Associated with sexual assaults.

Friedman Family Assessment Model (Short Form)

Before using the following guidelines in completing family assessments, two words of caution. First, not all areas included below will be germane for each of the families visited. The guidelines are comprehensive and allow depth when probing is necessary. The student should not feel that every sub-area needs to be covered when the broad area of inquiry poses no problems to the family or concern to the health worker. Second, by virtue of the interdependence of the family system, one will find unavoidable redundancy. For the sake of efficiency, the assessor should try not to repeat data, but to refer the reader back to sections where this information has already been described.

IDENTIFYING DATA

1. Family Name
2. Address and Phone
3. Family Composition (see table)
4. Type of Family Form
5. Cultural (Ethnic) Background
6. Religious Identification
7. Social Class Status
8. Family's Recreational or Leisure-Time Activities

DEVELOPMENTAL STAGE AND HISTORY OF FAMILY

9. Family's Present Developmental Stage
10. Extent of Developmental Tasks Fulfillment
11. Nuclear Family History
12. History of Family of Origin of Both Parents

ENVIRONMENTAL DATA

13. Characteristics of Home
14. Characteristics of Neighborhood and Larger Community
15. Family's Geographic Mobility
16. Family's Associations and Transactions with Community
17. Family's Social Support Network (Ecomap)

FAMILY STRUCTURE

18. Communication Patterns
    Extent of Functional and Dysfunctional Communication (Types of recurring patterns)
    Extent of Emotional (Affective) Messages and How Expressed
    Characteristics of Communication within Family Subsystems
    Extent of Congruent and Incongruent Messages

Types of Dysfunctional Communication Processes Seen in Family
Areas of Open and Closed Communication
Familial and External Variables Affecting Communication
19. Power Structure
    Power Outcomes
    Decision-Making Process
    Power Bases
    Variables Affecting Family Power
    Overall Family System and Subsystem Power
20. Role Structure
    Formal Role Structure
    Informal Role Structure
    Analysis of Role Models (Optional)
    Variables Affecting Role Structure
21. Family Values
    Compare the Family to American or Family's Reference Group Values and/or Identify Important Family Values and Their Importance (Priority) in Family
    Congruence Between the Family's Values and the Family's Reference Group or Wider Community
    Congruence Between the Family's Values and Family Member's Values
    Variables Influencing Family Values
    Values Consciously or Unconsciously Held
    Presence of Value Conflicts in Family
    Effect of the Above Values and Value Conflicts on Health Status of Family

FAMILY FUNCTIONS

22. Affective Function
    Family's Need-Response Patterns
    Mutual Nurturance, Closeness, and Identification
    Separateness and Connectedness
23. Socialization Function
    Family Child-Rearing Practices
    Adaptability of Child-Rearing Practices for Family Form and Family's Situation
    Who Is (Are) Socializing Agent(s) for Child(ren)?
    Value of Children in Family
    Cultural Beliefs That Influence Family's Child-Rearing Patterns
    Social Class Influence on Child-Rearing Patterns
    Estimation About Whether Family Is At Risk for Child-Rearing Problems and, if so, Indication of High-Risk Factors
    Adequacy of Home Environment for Children's Needs to Play

24. Health Care Function
    Family's Health Beliefs, Values, and Behavior
    Family's Definitions of Health-Illness and Their Level of Knowledge
    Family's Perceived Health Status and Illness Susceptibility
    Family's Dietary Practices
    Adequacy of Family Diet (Recommended 24-hour food history record)
    Function of Mealtimes and Attitudes Toward Food and Mealtimes
    Shopping (and its planning) Practices
    Person(s) Responsible for Planning, Shopping, and Preparation of Meals
    Sleep and Rest Habits
    Physical Activity and Recreation Practices (not covered earlier)
    Family's Drug Habits
    Family's Role in Self-Care Practices
    Medically Based Preventive Measures (Physicals, eye and hearing tests, and immunizations)

    Dental Health Practices
    Family Health History (Both general and specific diseases—environmentally and genetically related)
    Health Care Services Received
    Feelings and Perceptions Regarding Health Services
    Emergency Health Services
    Source of Payments for Health and Other Services
    Logistics of Receiving Care

FAMILY STRESS AND COPING

25. Short- and Long-Term Familial Stressors and Strengths
26. Extent of Family's Ability to Respond, Based on Objective Appraisal of Stress-Producing Situations
27. Coping Strategies Utilized (Present/past)
    Differences in Family Members' Ways of Coping
    Family's Inner Coping Strategies
    Family's External Coping Strategies
28. Dysfunctional Adaptive Strategies Utilized (Present/past; extent of usage)

FAMILY COMPOSITION FORM

Name (Last, First)	Gender	Relationship	Date and Place of Birth	Occupation	Education
1. (Father)					
2. (Mother)					
3. (Oldest child)					
4.					
5.					
6.					
7.					
8.					

From Friedman MM, Bowden VR, Jones, EG: *Family nursing: research, theory, and practice,* ed 5, Stamford, CT, 2003, Prentice Hall.

Individual Assessment Tools

F.1: INSTRUMENTAL ACTIVITIES OF DAILY LIVING (IADL) SCALE

Name _____ Rated by _____ Date _____

1. **Can you use the telephone**
   without help, 3
   with some help, or 2
   are you completely unable to use the telephone? 1

2. **Can you get to places beyond walking distance**
   without help, 3
   with some help, or 2
   are you completely unable to travel unless special arrangements are made? 1

3. **Can you go shopping for groceries**
   without help, 3
   with some help, or 2
   are you completely unable to do any shopping? 1

4. **Can you prepare your own meals**
   without help, 3
   with some help, or 2
   are you completely unable to prepare any meals? 1

5. **Can you do your own housework**
   without help, 3
   with some help, or 2
   are you completely unable to do any housework? 1

6. **Can you do your own handyman work**
   without help, 3
   with some help, or 2
   are you completely unable to do any handyman work? 1

7. **Can you do your own laundry**
   without help, 3
   with some help, or 2
   are you completely unable to do any laundry at all? 1

8a. **Do you take medicines or use any medications?**
   Yes (If yes, answer Question 8b.) 1
   No (If no, answer Question 8c.) 2

8b. **Do you take your own medicine**
   without help (in the right doses at the right time), 3
   with some help (if someone prepares it for you and/or reminds you to take it), or 2
   are you completely unable to take your own medicine? 1

8c. **If you had to take medicine, could you do it**
   without help (in the right doses at the right time), 3
   with some help (if someone prepared it for you and/or reminded you to take it), or 2
   would you be completely unable to take your own medicine? 1

9. **Can you manage your own money**
   without help, 3
   with some help, or 2
   are you completely unable to manage money? 1

From Philadelphia Geriatric Center, Philadelphia, PA. Used with permission.

F.2: COMPREHENSIVE OLDER PERSONS' EVALUATION

Name (print): _____ Date of visit: _____

Chief complaint: _____

Today, I will ask you about your overall health and function and will be using a questionnaire to help me obtain this information. The first few questions are to check your memory.

Preliminary Cognition Questionnaire: Record if answer is correct with (+); if answer is incorrect with (−).

1. What is the date today? _____
2. What day of the week is it? _____
3. What is the name of this place? _____
4. What is your telephone number or room number?
   Record answer: _____
   If subject does not have phone, ask:
   What is your street address? _____
5. How old are you? Record answer: _____   _____
6. When were you born? Record answer from records if patient cannot answer: _____   _____
7. Who is the president of the United States now? _____

8. Who was the president just before him? _____
9. What was your mother's maiden name? _____
10. Subtract 3 from 20 and keep subtracting from each new number until you get all the way down _____
    Total errors: _____

If more than 4 errors, ask 11. If more than 6 errors, complete questionnaire for informant.

11. Do you think you would benefit from a legal guardian, someone who would be responsible for your legal and financial matters? Do you have a living will? Would you like one?
    a. no
    b. has functioning legal guardian for sole purpose of managing money — describe:
    c. has legal guardian
    d. yes

From Pearlman R: Development of a functional assessment questionnaire for geriatric patients: the comprehensive older persons evaluation, *J Chronic Disease* 40(56): 85S-94S, 1987.

I.2   Comprehensive Older Persons' Evaluation—cont'd

Demographic Section:
1. Patient's race or ethnic background—record: _____
2. Patient's gender (circle)   male   female
3. How far did you go in school?
   a. post-graduate education
   b. four-year degree
   c. college or technical school
   d. high school complete
   e. high school incomplete
   f. 0-8 years

Social Support Section: Now there are a few questions about your family and friends.
4. Are you married, widowed, separated, divorced, or have you never been married?
   a. now married
   b. widowed
   c. separated
   d. divorced
   e. never married
5. Who lives with you? (circle all responses)
   a. spouse
   b. other relative or friend—specify: _____
   c. group living situation (non-health)
   d. lives alone
   e. nursing home, number of years: _____
6. Have you talked to any friends or relatives by phone during the last week?
   a. yes
   b. no
7. Are you satisfied by seeing your relatives and friends as often as you want to, or are you somewhat dissatisfied about how little you see them?
   a. satisfied—skip to #8
   b. dissatisfied—ask A
      A. Do you feel you would like to be involved in a Senior Citizens Center for social events, or perhaps meals?
         1. no
         2. is involved—describe: _____
         3. yes
8. Is there someone who would take care of you for as long as you needed if you were sick or disabled?
   a. yes—Skip to C
   b. no—Ask A
      A. Is there someone who would take care of you for a short time?
         1. yes—Skip to C
         2. no—Ask B
      B. Is there someone who could help you now and then?
         1. yes—Ask C
         2. no—Ask C
      C. Who would we call in case of an emergency? Record name and telephone: _____
      _____

Financial Section: The next few questions are about your finances and any problems you might have.
9. Do you own, or are you buying, your own home?
   a. yes—skip to #10
   b. no—ask A
      A. Do you feel you need assistance with housing?
         1. no
         2. has subsidized or other housing assistance
         3. yes—describe: _____
      B. What type of housing did you have prior to coming here?
10. Are you covered by private medical insurance, Medicare, Medicaid, or some disability plan? (Circle all that apply)
    a. private insurance—specify and skip to #11:
    _____
    b. Medicare
    c. Medicaid
    d. disability—specify and ask A:
    _____
    e. none
    f. other—specify: _____
       A. Do you feel you need additional assistance with your medical bills?
          1. no
          2. yes
11. Which of these statements best describes your financial situation?
    a. my bills are no problem to me—skip to #12
    b. my expenses make it difficult to meet my bills—ask A
    c. my expenses are so heavy that I cannot meet my bills—ask A
       A. Do you feel you need financial assistance such as: (circle all that apply)
          1. food stamps
          2. social security or disability payments
          3. assistance in paying your heating or electrical bills
          4. other financial assistance? describe: _____

Psychological Health Section: The next few questions are about how you feel about your life in general. There are no right or wrong answers, only what best applies to you. Please answer yes or no to each question.
12. Is your daily life full of things that keep you interested? _____
13. Have you, at times, very much wanted to leave home? _____
14. Does it seem that no one understands you? _____
15. Are you happy most of the time? _____
16. Do you feel weak all over much of the time? _____
17. Is your sleep fitful and disturbed? _____

Continued.

I.2 Comprehensive Older Persons' Evaluation—cont'd

18. Taking everything into consideration, how would you describe your satisfaction with your life in general at the present time?
    a. good
    b. fair
    c. poor

19. Do you feel you now need help with your mental health; for example, a counselor or psychiatrist?
    a. no
    b. has—specify: _____
    c. yes

Physical Health Section: The next few questions are about your health.

20. During the past month (30 days), how many days were you so sick that you couldn't do your usual activities, such as working around the house or visiting with friends? _____

21. Relative to other people your age, how would you rate your overall health at the present time?
    a. excellent—skip to #22
    b. very good—skip to #22
    c. good—ask A
    d. fair—ask A
    e. poor—ask A
       A. Do you feel you need additional medical services such as a doctor, nurse, visiting nurse or physical therapy?
          1. doctor
          2. nurse
          3. visiting nurse
          4. physical therapy
          5. none

22. Do you use an aid for walking, such as a wheelchair, walker, cane or anything else? (circle aid usually used)
    a. wheelchair
    b. other—specify: _____
    c. visiting nurse
    d. walker
    e. none

23. How much do your health troubles stand in the way of your doing things you want to do?
    a. not at all—skip to #24
    b. a little—ask A
    c. a great deal—ask A
       A. Do you think you need assistance to do your daily activities; for example, do you need a live-in aide or choreworker?
          1. live-in aide
          2. choreworker
          3. has aide, choreworker or other assistance—describe: _____
          4. none needed

24. Have you had, or do you currently have, any of the following health problems? (if yes, place an "X" in appropriate box and describe; medical record information may be used to help complete this section.)

	HX	Current	Describe
a. Arthritis or rheumatism?			
b. Lung or breathing problem?			
c. Hypertension?			
d. Heart trouble?			
e. Phlebitis or poor circulation problems in arms or legs?			
f. Diabetes or low blood sugar?			
g. Digestive ulcers?			
h. Other digestive problem?			
i. Cancer?			
j. Anemia?			
k. Effects of stroke?			
l. Other neurological problem? specify: _____			
m. Thyroid or other glandular problem? specify: _____			
n. Skin disorders such as pressure sores, leg ulcers, burns?			
o. Speech problem?			
p. Hearing problem?			
q. Vision or eye problem?			
r. Kidney or bladder problems, or incontinence?			
s. A problem of falls?			
t. Problem with eating or your weight? specify: _____			
u. Problem with depression? specify: _____			
v. Problem with your behavior? specify: _____			
w. Problem with your sexual activity?			
x. Problem with alcohol?			
y. Problem with pain?			
z. Other health problems? specify: _____			

I.2   Comprehensive Older Persons' Evaluation—cont'd

Immunizations: _____
_____
_____

25. What medications are you currently taking, or have been taking, in the last month? (May I see your medication bottles?) (If patient cannot list, ask categories a-r and note dosage and schedule, or obtain information from medical or pharmacy records and verify accuracy with the patient.)

Allergies: _____

		Rx (Dosage and Schedule)
a.	Arthritis medication	_____
b.	Pain medication	_____
c.	Blood pressure medication	_____
d.	Water pills or pills for fluid	_____
e.	Medication for your heart	_____
f.	Medication for your lungs	_____
g.	Blood thinners	_____
h.	Medication for your circulation	_____
i.	Insulin or diabetes medication	_____
j.	Seizure medication	_____
k.	Thyroid pills	_____
l.	Steroids	_____
m.	Hormones	_____
n.	Antibiotics	_____
o.	Medicine for nerves or depression	_____
p.	Prescription sleeping pills	_____
q.	Other prescription drugs	_____
r.	Other nonprescription drugs	_____

26. Many people have problems remembering to take their medications, especially ones they need to take on a regular basis. How often do you forget to take your medications? Would you say you forget often, sometimes, rarely, or never?
   a. never
   b. rarely
   c. sometimes
   d. often

Activities of Daily Living: The next set of questions asks whether you need help with any of the following activities of daily living.

27. I would like to know whether you can do these activities without any help at all, or if you need assistance to do them. Do you need help to: (If yes, describe, including patient needs.)

		Yes	No	Describe (include needs)
a.	Use the telephone?			
b.	Get to places out of walking distance? (using transportation)			
c.	Shop for clothes and food?			
d.	Do your housework?			
e.	Handle your money?			
f.	Feed yourself?			
g.	Dress and undress yourself?			
h.	Take care of your appearance?			
i.	Get in and out of bed?			
j.	Take a bath or shower?			
k.	Prepare your meals?			
l.	Do you have any problem getting to the bathroom on time?			

28. During the past six months, have you had any help with such things as shopping, housework, bathing, dressing and getting around?
   a. yes—specify: _____
   b. no

Signature of person completing the form:

_____

F.3: COMPREHENSIVE OCCUPATIONAL AND ENVIRONMENTAL HEALTH HISTORY

Work History

1. List your current and past longest held jobs, including the military:

Company	Dates Employed	Job Title	Known Exposures

2. Do you work full-time?   NO ___ YES ___   How many hours per week? ___

3. Do you work part-time?   NO ___ YES ___   How many hours per week? ___

4. Please describe any health problems or injuries that you have experienced in connection with your present or past jobs:

5. Have you ever had to change jobs because of health problems or injuries? YES ___ NO ___
   If yes, describe:

   Did any of your co-workers experience similar problems?

6. In what type of business do you currently work?

7. Describe your work (what you actually do):

8. Have you had any current or past exposure (through breathing or touching) to any of the following?

__acids	__alkalies	__coal dust	__mercury	__silica powder
__chlorinated naphthalenes	__chloroprene	__lead	__radiation	__welding fumes
	__isocyanates	__phenol	__vibration	__carbon tetrachloride
__halothane	__perchloroethylene	__trichloroethylene	__beryllium	__fiberglass
__PBBs	__TDI or MDI	__asbestos	__ethylene dibromide	__noise (loud)
__styrene	__ammonia	__cold (severe)	__methylene chloride	__solvents
__alcohols	__chromates	__manganese	__rock dust	__x-rays
__chloroform	__ketones	__phosgene	__vinyl chloride	
__heat (severe)	__pesticides	__trinitrotoluene	__cadmium	
__PCBs	__toluene	__benzene	__ethylene dichloride	
__talc	__arsenic	__dichlorobenzene	__nickel	

9. Did you receive any safety training about these agents?   YES ___   NO ___
   Explain:

10. Are you involved in any work processes such as grinding, welding, soldering, or polishing that create dust, mists, or fumes? YES ___   NO ___
    If yes, describe:

11. Did you use any of the following personal protective equipment when exposed?

__boots	__respirator	__welding mask
__gloves	__sleeves	__glasses/goggles
__shield	__earplugs/muffs	
__coveralls	__safety shoes	

12. Is your work environment generally clean?   YES ___   NO ___
    If no, describe:

13. What ventilation systems are used in your workplace?

14. Do they seem to work? Are you aware of any chemical odors in your environment (if so, explain)?

15. Where do you eat, smoke, and take your breaks when you are on the job?

16. Do you use a uniform or have clothing that you wear only to work?   YES ___   NO ___

17. How is your work clothing laundered (at home, by employer, etc.)?

18. How often do you wash your hands at work and how do you wash them (running water, special soaps, etc.)?

19. Do you shower before leaving the worksite?   YES ___   NO ___

20. Do you have any physical symptoms associated with work?   YES ___   NO ___
    If yes, describe:

21. Are other workers similarly affected?   YES ___   NO ___

Home Exposures

1. Which of the following do you have in your home?
   __air conditioner   __fireplace   __electric stove
   __central heating (gas or oil)   __air purifier   __woodstove

2. In approximately what year was your home built?

3. Have there been any recent renovations?   YES ___   NO ___
   If yes, describe:

4. Have you recently installed new carpet, purchased new furniture, or refinished existing furniture?   YES ___   NO ___
   If yes, explain:

5. Do you use pesticides around your home or garden?   YES ___   NO ___
   If yes, describe:

6. What household cleaners do you use? (List most common and any new products you use.)

7. List all hobbies done at your home:

8. Are any of the agents listed earlier for work exposures encountered in hobbies or recreational
   activities?   YES ___   NO ___

9. Is any special protective equipment or ventilation used during hobbies?   YES ___   NO ___
   Explain:

10. What are the occupations of other household members?

11. Do other household members have contact with any form of chemicals at work or during leisure activities?
    YES ___   NO ___
    If yes, explain:

12. Is anyone else in your home environment having symptoms similar to yours?   YES ___   NO ___
    If yes, explain briefly:

Community Exposures

1. Are any of the following located in your community?
   __industrial plant   __major source of air pollution   __waste site
   __landfill   __toxic spill   __other_____
2. What is your source of drinking water?
   __private well   __public water source   __other
3. Are neighbors experiencing any health problems similar to yours?   YES ___   NO ___
   If yes, explain:

Key Occupational and Environmental Health Questions To Be Asked With All Histories

1. What are your current and past longest held jobs?
2. Have you been exposed to any radiation or chemical liquids, dusts, mists, or fumes?   YES ___   NO ___
3. Is there any relationship between current symptoms and activities at work or at home?   YES ___   NO ___

From Pope AM, Snyder MA, Mood LH, editors: *Nursing, health, and environment: strengthening the relationship to improve the public's health,* Washington, DC, 1995, National Academy Press.

Motivational Interviewing

Motivational interviewing (MI) is a collaborative strategy to promote behavioral change in clients and families. Clients and families are encouraged to set goals for making health changes, and the process allows the nurse to address ambivalence toward change and strengthen the client or family's commitment to behavioral change.

The core tenets of MI recognize the client and family as the experts who have the ability to make a change based on personal choices. The nurse provides a **collaborative** environment that supports change and has the client or family **share** their perceptions and knowledge about the behavior under discussion. The nurse then affirms the client or family's **autonomy** to make choices for change about the behavior.

There are four principles central to the spirit of MI to guide the nurse:

- *Expressing empathy* to communicate an understanding of the client or family's perspective
- *Rolling with resistance* and avoiding arguing with the client or family when ambivalence or unwillingness to change occurs
- *Supporting self-efficacy,* which is supporting the client's or family's confidence that change can be made
- *Developing discrepancy* is guiding the client or family when inconsistencies occur between current behavior and desired behavioral goals

The key components to interactions with clients and families during MI are guided by the acronym OARS:

- *Open-ended questions:* these questions allow the client or family to express their thoughts and share their personal experiences. It allows the nurse to develop a fuller understanding of barriers to change and individual values.

- *Affirmations of what the client and/or family says:* the nurse affirms the client or family's ability to change and how the behavior change is congruent with their values and goals.
- *Reflective listening:* this is the hallmark of MI. The nurse restates what the client or family shares and allows for clarifying what the client or family means to say or feels. This is an opportunity to focus on moving the client or family closer to behavioral change.
- *Summaries of the conversation and decisions made:* the nurse summarizes the MI session and the goals set by the client or family and reinforces the plan for change.

"Change" in health behavior is the overall goal of MI, and using strategies that promote movement toward change is important within the context of MI. This includes supporting statements expressing a desire for change, addressing perceived barriers to change, and having the confidence to make behavioral changes. Focus on linking the desired behavioral change to the client's or family's personal values, abilities, and goals. Developing small, achievable goals may be more attainable and less overwhelming for some clients and families in the beginning. Nurses can then continue to use MI in future interactions to promote progression in healthy behaviors.

Adapted from: Levensky ER, Forcehimes A, O'Donohue WT, Beitz K: Motivational interviewing, *Am J Nurs* 107(10):50-58, 2007.
Motivational Interviewing: Resources for clinical, researchers, and trainers. Retrieved from http://www.motivationalinterview.org.
Suarez M, Mullins S: Motivational interviewing and pediatric health behavior interventions, *J Develop Behav Pediatr* 29:417-428, 2008.

Essential Elements of Public Health Nursing

EXAMPLES OF PUBLIC HEALTH NURSING ROLES AND IMPLEMENTING PUBLIC HEALTH FUNCTIONS

This document is intended to clearly present the role of public health nurses in Virginia as members of the multidisciplinary public health team in a changing health care environment. The following matrices present the role of public health nursing in Virginia. The following definitions were used to develop these matrices.

Essential Element is taken from the National Association of City and County Health Officials' (NACCHO's) document *Blueprint for a Healthy Community*. The following public health essential elements are used as a framework to present the role of public health nursing in Virginia:

- Conducting Community Assessments
- Preventing and Controlling Epidemics
- Providing a Safe and Healthy Environment
- Measuring Performance, Effectiveness, and Outcomes of Health Services
- Promoting Healthy Lifestyles
- Providing Targeted Outreach and Forming Partnerships
- Providing Personal Health Care Services
- Conducting Research and Innovation
- Mobilizing the Community for Action

Public Health Function is defined as a broad public health activity needed to ensure a strong, flexible, accountable public health structure. It may require a multidisciplinary team to carry out.

Public Health Nurse Role is the activity the public health nurse is responsible for, either alone or as a member of a team, to accomplish the stated public health function. This can be the public health nurse at the local level or at the state level.

State Role is what public health nurses need from the state level to do their jobs (e.g., policy, aggregate data, training). This refers to any Central Office program or staff, not just nurses.

A process was implemented that would involve all public health nurses in Virginia. Although this lengthened the timeline to completion, it will ensure that the final document represents a consensus developed through creative open dialogue.

From National Association of City and County Health Officials: *Blueprint for a healthy community: a guide for local health departments*, Washington, DC, 1994, The Association.

ESSENTIAL ELEMENT 1: Conduct Community Assessment: Systematically collecting, assembling, analyzing, and making available health-related data for the purpose of identifying and responding to community- and state-level public health concerns and conducting epidemiological and other population-based studies.

Public Health Function	PHN Roles	State Roles
Develop frameworks, methodologies, and tools for standardizing data collection and analysis and reporting across all jurisdictions and providers.	• Provide, review, and comment on proposed methodologies and tools for data collection. • Field-test tools and methods.	• Collaborate with professional organizations and academic and governmental institutions to develop and test tools and methods. • Provide educational opportunities in areas of and use of tools. • Work with local-level agencies to standardize definitions, data collected, etc. across jurisdictions and among all stakeholders (schools, community-based organizations, and private providers).
Collect and analyze data.	• Collaborate with the community to identify population-based needs and gaps in service. • Analyze data and needs, knowledge, attitudes, and practices of specific populations. • Identify patterns of diseases, illness, and injury and develop or stimulate development of programs to respond to identified trends.	• Provide aggregated data to the local level in a timely and accurate manner. • Provide census tract–level aggregated data to the local level. • Provide national and state comparisons to be used with local data to obtain trends and assist localities in documenting need, progress, etc. to attain standard outcomes.

ESSENTIAL ELEMENT 2: Preventing and Controlling Epidemics: Monitoring disease trends and investigating and containing diseases and injuries.

Public Health Function	PHN Roles	State Roles
Develop programs that prevent, contain, and control the transmission of diseases and danger of injuries (including violence).	• Provide community-wide preventive measures in the form of health education and mobilization of community resources. • Ensure isolation/containment measures when necessary. • Ensure adequate preventive immunizations. • Implement programs that control the transmission of diseases and danger of injuries during disasters.	• Work with local jurisdictions to develop tools such as videos, PSAs, and/or posters that local jurisdictions can use. • Work with local jurisdictions to develop disaster plans for the control of the transmission of diseases and danger of injuries during disasters. • Facilitate state-level partnerships that promote health, healthy lifestyles, and wellness (individual and family).
Develop regulatory guidelines for the prevention of targeted diseases.	• Implement regulatory measures. • Implement OSHA Guidelines for Blood Borne Pathogens and the Prevention of the Transmission of TB in Health Care Settings.	• In partnership with localities, develop regulatory guidelines. • Serve as clearinghouse or source of information.

ESSENTIAL ELEMENT 3: Providing a Safe and Healthy Environment: Maintaining clean and safe air, water, food, and facilities both in the community and in the home environment.

Public Health Function	PHN Roles	State Roles
Develop methods/tools for collection and analysis of health-related data (occurrence of mortality and morbidity relating to both communicable and chronic diseases, injury registries, sentinel event establishment, environmental quality, etc.).	• Provide reporting guidelines and consultation regarding disease prevention, diagnosis, treatment, and follow-up of cases/contacts to physicians and institutions (emergency department, university and secondary school student health, prisons, industries, etc.). • Conduct/participate in community needs assessments to determine customer/provider knowledge deficits and perceptions of need. • Provide education to individuals, providers, targeted populations, etc., in response to knowledge deficits, disease outbreaks, toxic waste emissions, etc. • Provide individual follow-up/case management of communicable diseases that are transmitted by air, water, food, and fomites (TB, hepatitis A, salmonella, staphylococcus, etc.).	• Develop standard methodology and tools for collection and analysis of health-related data. • Provide training in area of data collection and analysis. • Evaluate activities and outcomes of interactions. • Work in partnership with localities to develop program based on data analysis needs.
Develop programs that promote a safe environment in the home.	• Provide childhood lead poisoning screenings and follow-up. • Teach clients to inspect homes for safety violations and toxic substances and to practice safe behaviors; assist families to access/use available resources/safety devices. • Assess/teach regarding safe food selection, preparation, and storage. • Train/supervise volunteers/auxiliary personnel in performance of the above tasks. • Teach families that all men, women, and children have a right to a safe environment free of physical or mental abuse.	• Provide consultation and technical assistance to state/local organizations regarding laws and regulations that protect health and ensure safety. • In partnership with localities, develop and evaluate educational programs.

ESSENTIAL ELEMENT 3: Providing a Safe and Healthy Environment—cont'd

Public Health Function	PHN Roles	State Roles
Develop programs that promote a safe environment in the workplace.	• Provide consultation in implementation of OSHA regulations relating to occupational exposure to diseases. • Provide educational program related to healthy lifestyles (smoking cessation, back protection, etc.). • Ensure provision of screenings for individuals to determine baselines and occurrence of infectious diseases and preventable deterioration of health and function: hearing, back soundness, lung capacity, RMS indicators, PPDs, etc. • Assist in policy/practice development to address prevention of the above. • Provide immunizations.	• Monitor and assist localities to implement prevention activities. • Assist localities in developing and evaluating educational programs. • Monitor outcomes of screening activities and evaluate interventions.
Develop programs that promote a safe environment in the school setting.	• Provide consultation on implementation of OSHA regulations relating to occupational exposure to diseases. • Provide educational programs related to healthy lifestyles (smoking cessation, etc.). • Ensure provision of screenings for students to determine baselines and occurrence of infectious disease and preventable deterioration of health and function. • Assist in policy/practice development to address prevention of the above. • Provide immunizations.	• Develop guidelines that ensure accountability in meeting standards set forth. • Ensure that policy is developed to protect children in the school environment. • Monitor immunization status of children and provide immunizations during outbreaks and evaluate activities.
Develop programs that promote a safe environment in the community.	• Identify population clusters exhibiting an unhealthy environment; provide consultation/group education regarding preventive measures. • Participate in development of local disaster plans to ensure provision of safe water, food, air, and facilities. • Respond in time of natural disasters such as floods, tornadoes, and hurricanes. • Participate in developing plans for shelter management during disasters, especially "Special Needs" shelters that may require nursing staff.	• In times of disaster, facilitate availability of resources across jurisdictions. • Have a statewide plan. • Ensure that localities have developed plans to protect the public in time of national and/or other disasters. • Coordinate efforts statewide. • Assist localities in responding. • Evaluate efforts.
Develop and issue standards that guide regulations and mandate policy and program development. Develop protocols to ensure accountability of all health care providers, public and private. Provide inservice to all providers of health care services.	• Survey worksites, schools, institutions, etc. for compliance to regulations that protect health and ensure safety. • Provide technical assistance (i.e., interpretation, implementation, and evaluation processes). • Share and implement knowledge gained in inservices.	• Develop a systematic evaluation tool for collection of data to measure trends. • Assist localities in developing standards to mandate accountability. • Provide consultation/technical assistance to localities.

ESSENTIAL ELEMENT 4: Measuring Performance, Effectiveness, and Outcomes of Health Services:

Monitoring health care providers and the health care system to identify gaps in service, deteriorating health status indicators, effectiveness of interventions, and accessibility and quality of personal and population-wide health services.

Public Health Function	PHN Roles	State Roles
Promote competency in public health issues throughout the health delivery system.	• Provide educational and technical assistance in areas such as case management and appropriate treatment and control of communicable diseases to the community.	• Develop appropriate regulatory, educational, and technical assistance programs. • Provide technical assistance and training to local health department for local forecasting and interpretation of data.
Collect data.	• Participate in data collection with a target population. • Ensure that the data collection system supports the objectives of programs serving the community by participating in the design and operation of data collection systems. • Collect data via surveys, polls, interviews, focus groups that will enable assessment of the community's perception of health status and understanding how the system works and how to obtain service needs.	• Work with localities (health districts, private providers, other state and local agencies) to develop standard data elements and definitions across jurisdictions and among all stakeholders, especially for consistency in coding of population-based data. • Identify data collection and analytic issues related to monitoring the impact of health system changes such as costs and benefits of record linkage, strategies for ensuring confidentiality, and strategies for analyzing trends in health within a broader social and economic context. • Advocate for uniform data collection from all managed care plans so that outcomes and health trends can be analyzed and tracked and sentinel events reported.
Analyze data to ensure accurate diagnosis of health status, identification of threats to health, and assessment of health service needs.	• Participate in a systematic approach to convert data into information that will identify gaps in service at the local and state level and will lead to action. • Monitor health status indicators to identify emerging problems and facilitate community-wide response to identified problems. • Facilitate data analysis as part of a local collaborative effort.	• Develop a systematic, integrated statewide approach to converting data into information that directs action. • Ensure that resources, such as hardware and software, to analyze data are available at the local level. • Work with localities (health districts, private providers, other state and local agencies) to address issues related to variable access to technology, confidentiality issues. • Educate and train currently employed public health nurses in areas of epidemiology and population-based services.
Monitor health status indicators for the entire population and for specific population groups and/or geographic areas.	• Identify target populations that may be at risk for public health problems such as communicable diseases, unidentified and untreated chronic diseases. • Conduct surveys or observe targeted populations such as preschools, childcare centers, and high-risk census tracks to identify health status. • Monitor health care utilization of vulnerable populations at the local and regional level.	• Develop methodology for identification, measurement, and analysis of key indicators of health care utilization of vulnerable populations.

ESSENTIAL ELEMENT 4: Measuring Performance, Effectiveness, and Outcomes of Health Services—cont'd

Public Health Function	PHN Roles	State Roles
Monitor and assess availability, cost-effectiveness, and outcomes of personal and population-based health services.	• Identify gaps in services (e.g., a neighborhood with deteriorating immunization rates may indicate lack of available primary care services). • Ensure that all receive the same quality of care, including comprehensive preventive services. • Monitor the impact of health system reforms on vulnerable populations. • Evaluate the effectiveness and outcomes of care. • Plan interventions based on the health of the overall population, not just for those in the health care system. • Identify interventions that are effective and replicable.	• Develop analyses that demonstrate the cost-effectiveness of investment in public health services. • Develop protocols and technical assistance for ensuring accountability of Medicaid managed care plans and other government-funded plans for service delivery and overall health status of their covered populations. • Identify standard theoretical, methodological, and measurement issues that are specific to population subgroups for monitoring the impact of health system changes on vulnerable populations.
Disseminate information.	• Disseminate information to the public on community health status, including how to access and use services appropriately. • Disseminate information to other health care providers regarding gaps in services or deteriorating health status indicators.	• Ensure a mechanism for public accountability of performance and outcomes through public dissemination of information and in particular ensure that underservice, a risk inherent in capitated plans, is measurable through available data. • Ensure that information is provided to communities, local health departments, managed care plans, and other appropriate state agencies.

ESSENTIAL ELEMENT 5: Promoting Healthy Lifestyles: Providing health education to individuals, families, and communities.

Public Health Function	PHN Roles	State Roles
Promote informed decision making of residents about things that influence their health on a daily basis.	• Exert influence through contact with individuals and community groups. • Accept and issue challenge of healthy lifestyles to all contacts. • Reinforce and reward positive informed decisions made for healthy lifestyles.	• Develop and monitor standards for the changes to determine changes in behavior.
Promote effective use of media to encourage both personal and community responsibility for informed decision making.	• Be a resource for the community. • Gather data and address findings as appropriate. • Work with community groups to promote accurate information for healthy lifestyle through the media. • Use current information and other agency's resources to maximize information accessible to the public.	• Assist localities to provide current information to community organizations and other state organizations. • Serve as a resource for localities and work with media.
Develop a public awareness/marketing campaign to demonstrate the importance of public health to overall health improvement and its proper place in the health delivery system.	• Provide education to special groups (e.g., local politicians, school boards, PTAs, churches, civic groups, news media) regarding the benefits of preventive health.	• Develop training activities to assist localities in marketing

ESSENTIAL ELEMENT 5: Promoting Healthy Lifestyles—cont'd

Public Health Function	PHN Roles	State Roles
Develop public information and education systems/programs through partnerships.	• Provide educational sessions/programs to public regarding components of healthy lifestyles. • Access grants/other funding sources to promote healthy lifestyle decisions (e.g., cervical and breast cancer prevention, bike helmets, hypertension). • Provide/promote teaching for individuals and families at every opportunity (home, clinic, community settings).	• Assist localities in developing and evaluating educational programs. • Assist localities in funding. • Hold regional/state training sessions. • Evaluate outcomes and plan ongoing educational systems/programs.

ESSENTIAL ELEMENT 6: Providing Targeted Outreach and Forming Partnerships: Ensuring access to services, including those that lead to self-sufficiency, for all vulnerable populations and ensuring the development of culturally appropriate care.

Public Health Function	PHN Roles	State Roles
Ensure accessibility to health services that will improve morbidity, decrease mortality, and improve health status outcomes.	• Provide family-centered case management services for high-risk and hard-to-reach populations that focus on linking families with needed services. • Improve access to care by forming partnerships with appropriate community individuals and entities. • Increase influence of cultural diversity on system design and on access to care, as well as on individual services rendered. • Ensure that translation services are available for the non–English-speaking population. • Participate in ongoing community assessment to identify areas of concern and above needs for rules. • Provide outreach services that focus on preventing epidemics and the spread of disease, such as tuberculosis and sexually transmitted diseases.	• Provide funds in cooperation with locality. • Ensure policy development that includes case management and is culturally sensitive. • Provide adequate ongoing continuing education for staff (especially in areas common to all localities). • Participate in state-level contract development to ensure that contracts with health plans require and include incentives for health plans to offer and deliver preventive health services in the minimum benefits package. • Educate financing officials about the roles of public health both in performing core public health services and in ensuring access to personal health services.

ESSENTIAL ELEMENT 7: Providing Personal Health Care Services: Providing targeted direct services to high-risk populations.

Public Health Function	PHN Roles	State Roles

Provide direct services for specific diseases that threaten the health of the community and develop programs that prevent, contain, and control the transmission of infectious diseases.	• Plan, develop, implement, and evaluate:
	  • Sexually transmitted disease services
	  • Communicable disease services
	  • HIV/AIDS services
	  • Tuberculosis control services
	  • Develop and implement guidelines for the prevention of the above targeted diseases.
		• Establish standards/criteria for personal health care.
		• Work with local health departments to assist in developing infrastructure and management techniques to facilitate record-keeping and appropriate financial monitoring and tracking systems, which enable local health departments to enter into contractual arrangements for preventive health and primary care services.

ESSENTIAL ELEMENT 7: Providing Personal Health Care Services—cont'd

Public Health Function	PHN Roles	State Roles
Provide health services, including preventive health services, to high-risk and vulnerable populations (e.g., the uninsured working poor), and in geographic areas where primary health care services are not readily accessible or available in a privatized setting.	• Provide coordination, follow-up, referral, and case management as indicated. • Integrate supportive services (such as counseling, social work, nutrition) into primary care services. • Assess existing community medical capacity for referral and follow-up.	• Continue to work at the state and local level to build capacity of primary and preventive health services, particularly in traditionally underserved areas, to ensure availability to providers and primary care sites essential to primary care access.

ESSENTIAL ELEMENT 8: Conducting Research and Innovation: Discovering and applying improved health care delivery mechanisms and clinical interventions.

Public Health Function	PHN Roles	State Roles
Ensure ongoing prevention research relating to biomedical and behavioral aspects of health promotion and prevention of disease and injury.	• Develop outcome measures. • Identify research priorities for target communities and develop and conduct scientific and operations research for health promotion and disease/injury prevention.	• Provide training in area of measuring program effectiveness.
Implement pilot or demonstration projects.	• Develop and implement linkages with academic centers, ensuring that clients and populations who participate in research projects benefit as a result of the research.	• Support evaluations and research that demonstrate the benefits of public health, as well as the consequences of failure to support public health interventions.

ESSENTIAL ELEMENT 9: Mobilizing the Community for Action: Providing leadership and initiating collaboration.

Public Health Function	PHN Roles	State Roles
Provide leadership to stimulate development of networks or partnerships that will ensure the availability of comprehensive primary health care services to all, regardless of ability to pay. Initiate collaboration with other community organizations to ensure the leadership role in resolving a public health issue.	• Advocate for improved health. • Disseminate health information. • Build coalitions. • Make recommendations for policy implementation or revision. • Facilitate resources that manage environmental risk and maintain and improve community health. • Provide information for a community group working on impacting policy at the local, state, or federal level. • Use results of community health assessments to stimulate the community to develop a plan to respond to identified gaps in service.	• Facilitate the establishment and enhancement of statewide high-quality, needed health services. • Administer quality improvement programs. • Use information-gathering techniques of assessment to assist policy/legislature activities to develop needed health services and functions that require statewide action or standards. • Recommend programs to carry out policies.

American Public Health Association Definition of Public Health Nursing

Public health nursing is a systematic process by which the following occur:

1. The health and health care needs of a population are assessed to identify subpopulations, families, and individuals who would benefit from health promotion or who are at risk of illness, injury, disability, or premature death.
2. A plan for intervention is developed with the community to meet identified needs that takes into account available resources, the range of activities that contribute to health, and the prevention of illness, injury, disability, and premature death.
3. The plan is implemented effectively, efficiently, and equitably.
4. Evaluations are conducted to determine the extent to which the interventions have an impact on the health status of individuals and the population.
5. The results of the process are used to influence and direct the current delivery of care, the deployment of health resources, and the development of local, regional, state, and national health policy and research to promote health and prevent disease.

This systematic process for public health nursing practice is based on and is consistent with (1) community strengths, needs, and expectations; (2) current scientific knowledge; (3) available resources; (4) accepted criteria and standards of nursing practice; (5) agency purpose, philosophy, and objectives; and (6) the participation, cooperation, and understanding of the population. Other services and organizations in the community are considered and planning is coordinated to maximize the effective use of resources and enhance outcomes.

The title "public health nurse" designates a nursing professional with educational preparation in public health and nursing science with a primary focus on population-level outcomes.

EXAMPLES OF ACTIVITIES OF PUBLIC HEALTH NURSES

The activities of public health nurses include the following:

1. They provide essential input to interdisciplinary programs that monitor, anticipate, and respond to public health problems in population groups, regardless of which disease or public health threat is identified.
2. They evaluate health trends and risk factors of population groups and help determine priorities for targeted interventions.
3. They work with communities or specific population groups within the community to develop public policy and targeted health promotion and disease prevention activities.
4. They participate in assessing and evaluating health care services to ensure that people are informed of programs and services available and are assisted in the use of available services.
5. They provide health education, care management, and primary care to individuals and families who are members of vulnerable populations and high-risk groups.

From American Public Health Association: *The definition and role of public health nursing: a statement of APHA Public Health Nursing Section,* Washington, DC, 1996, APHA.

American Nurses Association Scope and Standards of Practice for Public Health Nursing

STANDARDS OF CARE

Standard 1. Assessment

The public health nurse collects comprehensive data pertinent to the health status of populations.

Standard 2. Population Diagnosis and Priorities

The public health nurse analyses the assessment data to determine the population diagnoses and priorities.

Standard 3. Outcomes Identification

The public health nurse identifies expected outcomes for a plan that is based on population diagnoses and priorities.

Standard 4. Planning

The public health nurse develops a plan that reflects best practices by identifying strategies, action plans, and alternatives to attain expected outcomes.

Standard 5. Implementation

The public health nurse implements the identified plan by partnering with others.

Standard 5A: Coordination of Services

The public health nurse coordinates programs, services, and other activities to implement the identified plan.

Standard 5B. Health Education and Health Promotion

The public health nurse employs multiple strategies to promote health, prevent disease, and ensure a safe environment for populations.

Standard 5C: Consultation

The public health nurse provides consultation to various community groups and officials to facilitate the implementation of programs and services.

Standard 5D. Regulatory Activities

The public health nurse identifies, interprets, and implements public health laws, regulations, and policies.

Standard 6. Evaluation

The public health nurse evaluates the health status of the population.

STANDARDS OF PROFESSIONAL PERFORMANCE

Standard 7. Quality of Practice

The public health nurse systematically enhances the quality and effectiveness of nursing practice.

Standard 8. Education

The public health nurse attains knowledge and competency that reflect current nursing and public health practice.

Standard 9. Professional Practice Evaluation

The public health nurse evaluates one's own nursing practice in relation to professional practice standards and guidelines, relevant statutes, rules, and regulations.

Standard 10. Collegiality and Professional Relationships

The public health nurse establishes collegial partnerships while interacting with representatives of the population, organizations, and health and human services professionals, and contributes to the professional development of peers, students, colleagues, and others.

Standard 11. Collaboration

The public health nurse collaborates with representatives of the population, organizations, and health and human service professionals in providing for and promoting the health of the population.

Standard 12. Ethics

The public health nurse integrates ethical provisions in all areas of practice.

Standard 13. Research

The public health nurse integrates research findings into practice.

Standard 14. Resource Utilization

The public health nurse considers factors related to safety, effectiveness, cost, and impact on practice and on the population in the planning and delivery of nursing and public health programs, policies, and services.

Standard 15. Leadership

The public health nurse provides leadership in nursing and public health.

Standard 16. Advocacy

The public health nurse advocates to protect the health, safety, and rights of the population.

From American Nurses Association: *Public health nursing: scope and standards of practice,* Washington, DC, 2007, American Nurses Publishing.

The Health Insurance Portability and Accountability Act (HIPAA): What Does It Mean for Public Health Nurses?

Public Health Nursing Practice—definition: the synthesis of nursing and public health theory applied to promoting and preserving the health of populations. Practice focuses on the community as a whole, and the effect of the community's health status (resources) on the health of individuals, families, and groups. The goal is to prevent disease and disability and promote and protect the health of the community as a whole.

EXPLANATION

- Federal privacy standards were created by the Department of Health and Human Services (USDHHS) to protect patients' medical records and other health information provided to health plans, doctors, hospitals, and other health care providers.
- These standards took effect on April 14, 2003.
- Standardization of electronic transactions, and the elimination of inefficient paper forms, will save the health care industry over $29 billion in the next 10 years.

PRIVACY RULE

- Protects the confidentiality of individually identifiable health information, whether it is on paper, in computers, or communicated orally.
- Protected health information (PHI) is the name for this individually identifiable health information.
- Limits the ways that health plans, pharmacies, hospitals, and other covered entities can use patients' personal medical information.

PATIENT PROTECTIONS

- Patients should be able to see, obtain copies, and make corrections to their medical records.
- Patients should receive a notice from health care providers regarding how their personal medical information may be used by them and their rights under the privacy regulation. Patients can restrict this use.
- Limits have been set on how health care providers can use individually identifiable health information. Doctors, nurses, and other providers can share information needed to treat a patient. For purposes other than medical care, personal health information generally may not be used.
- Pharmacies, health plans, and other covered entities must obtain an individual's authorization before disclosing patient information for marketing purposes.

PUBLIC HEALTH SERVICES AND PHI

Overview: Although protection of health information is important, PHI is used for the public good by health officials to identify, monitor, and respond to disease, death, and disability among populations. Examples of ways PHI is used include public health surveillance, program evaluation, terrorism preparedness, outbreak investigations, direct health services, and public health research. Public health authorities have taken precautions in the past to protect the privacy of individuals and will continue to do so under HIPAA. The privacy rule, however, still permits PHI to be shared for important public health purposes.

PERMITTED PHI DISCLOSURES TO A PUBLIC HEALTH AUTHORITY

Without Authorization

- Reporting of disease, injury, and vital events
- Conducting public health surveillance, investigations, and interventions
- Reporting child abuse or neglect to a public health or other government authority legally authorized to receive such reports
- To a person subject to jurisdiction of the Food and Drug Administration (FDA) concerning the quality, safety, or effectiveness of an FDA-related product or activity for which that person has responsibility
- To a person who may have been exposed to a communicable disease or may be at risk for contracting or spreading a disease or condition, when legally authorized to notify the person as necessary to conduct a public health intervention or investigation
- To an individual's employer, under certain circumstances and conditions, as needed for the employer to meet the requirements of the Occupational Safety and Health Administration, Mine Safety and Health Administration, or similar state law

HIPAA AND NURSING RESEARCH

Definitions:

Covered entity: a health plan, a health care clearinghouse, or a health care provider who transmits any health information in electronic form.

Individually Identifiable Health Information (IIHI): information about an individual regarding his or her physical or mental health; the provision of health care; or the payment for the provision of health care; and which identifies the individual.

It is the covered entity's obligation not to disclose the information improperly when a researcher seeks data that includes PHI.

A covered entity can disclose IIHI for research purposes under any of the following conditions:

1. The IIHI pertains only to deceased persons.
2. The IIHI can be examined for reviews preparatory to research if it is not removed from the covered entity.
3. Information that has been deidentified can be disclosed; this information is no longer considered IIHI and thus not covered by HIPAA.
4. Data must be disclosed as part of a limited data set if the researcher has a data use agreement with the covered entity.
5. The researcher has a valid authorization from the research subject to disclose IIHI.
6. An IRB or privacy board has waived the authorization requirement.

Creating Data

Researchers may also be creating IIHI. If the researcher is part of a covered entity, any PHI obtained by any means is covered by HIPAA, and the researcher and his or her institution are bound by HIPAA regulations. Most universities with nursing schools will be hybrid entities (i.e., some parts of the university are a covered entity and some are not). Researchers should check their institution's policies.

Disclosing Data

Nurse researchers should be aware that sharing data with colleagues and students may constitute disclosures of IIHI and they should conform to HIPAA regulations. In this case, the researcher is the holder of the IIHI and can disclose it only under appropriate conditions:

1. Patients agree to specific disclosures in the initial authorization.
2. Former patients sign an additional authorization.
3. An IRB or privacy board waives the need for authorization.
4. The holder allows the colleague to review the data to prepare a research protocol if the colleague takes no information away.
5. A holder enters the data in a limited data set and signs a data use agreement with the recipient.
6. A holder deidentifies the data and shares it freely.

From Olsen DP: HIPAA privacy regulations and nursing research, *Nurs Res* 52(5):344-348, 2003; United States Department of Health and Human Services: *Fact sheet*. Retrieved Jan 26, 2004, from www.hhs.gov/news/press/2002pres/hipaa.html; CDC: *HIPAA privacy rule and public health*. Retrieved Feb 12, 2004, from www.cdc.gov/mmwr/preview/mmwrhtml/su5201a1.htm.

Focus on Quality and Safety Education for Nurses

Quality and Safety Education for Nurses (QSEN) addresses the challenge of preparing future nurses with the knowledge, skills, and attitudes necessary to continuously improve the quality and safety of the healthcare systems in which they work. This appendix shows how Quality and Safety Education in Nursing can be applied within a community health framework.

CH 1: Population-Focused Practice: The Foundation of Specialization in Public Health Nursing

✓ FOCUS ON QUALITY AND SAFETY EDUCATION FOR NURSES

Quality and Safety Education for Nurses (QSEN) Competencies

QSEN COMPETENCY	COMPETENCY DEFINITION
Client-Centered Care	Recognize the client or designee as the source of control and full partner in providing compassionate and coordinated care based on respect for client preferences, values, and needs.
Teamwork and Collaboration	Function effectively within nursing and interprofessional teams, fostering open communication, mutual respect, and shared decision making to achieve quality care.
Evidence-Based Practice	Integrate best current evidence with clinical expertise and client/family preferences and values for delivery of optimal health care.
Quality Improvement	Use data to monitor the outcomes of care processes and use improvement methods to design and test changes to continuously improve the quality and safety of health care systems.
Safety	Minimizes risk for harm to clients and providers through both system effectiveness and individual performance.
Informatics	Use information and technology to communicate, manage knowledge, mitigate error, and support decision making.

Prepared by Gail Armstrong, DNP, ACNS-BC, CNE, Associate Professor, University of Colorado Denver College of Nursing.

CH 10: Environmental Health

✓ FOCUS ON QUALITY AND SAFETY EDUCATION FOR NURSES

Targeted Competency: Function effectively within nursing and interprofessional teams, fostering open communication, mutual respect, and shared decision making to achieve quality client care.

Important aspects of safety include:

- **Knowledge:** Describe scopes of practice and roles of health care team members
- **Skills:** Assume role of team member or leader based on the situation
- **Attitudes:** Value the perspectives and expertise of all health team members

Safety Question: One of the objectives in *Healthy People 2020* related to environmental health is: "Reduce pesticide exposures that result in visits to a health care facility" (ED: 8-10). The public health nurse, who is working on a project to help mothers develop parenting skills, visits a new mother who lives and works on a large farm. When the nurse drives into the farm on her way to the housing where workers live, she sees that the fields are being sprayed with pesticides from a truck and that two young children are riding in the back of the truck. What action should she take?

Answer: *At the individual level, she should talk with the owner or manager of the farm and remind him or her of the toxicity of pesticides and the danger to those who are in the vicinity of the spraying. She should recommend that he or she not allow anyone to ride in the open portion of the vehicle and that the driver should leave the window closed and wear a mask to protect his or her nose and mouth.*

Systems level: *She should identify areas where the workers on the area farms congregate, such as churches, social halls, and so forth. Then she should ask if she could provide an educational program on the dangers of coming into contact with pesticides. She could distribute pamphlets about this hazard in local venues where both farm managers and workers will be able to access them. What else might the nurse do?*

CH 2: History of Public Health and Public and Community Health Nursing

✓ FOCUS ON QUALITY AND SAFETY EDUCATION FOR NURSES

Although the scope and responsibilities of public health nurses have changed over time, the commitment to quality and safety has remained constant. Since the beginning of population-centered nursing in the United States, the nurses who worked in this specialty have been committed to preserving health and preventing disease. They have focused on environmental conditions such as sanitation and control of communicable diseases, education for health, prevention of disease and disability, and at times care of the sick and aged in their homes. This long-standing commitment to quality and safety is consistent with the work of *Quality and Safety Education for Nurses* (QSEN), a national initiative designed to transform nursing education by including in the curriculum content and experiences related to building knowledge, skills and attitudes for six quality and safety initiatives (Cronenwett, Sherwood, and Gelmon, 2009). The QSEN work, led by Drs. Linda Cronenwett and Gwen Sherwood at the University of North Carolina, has made great progress in bridging the gap between quality and safety work in both practice and academic settings (Brown, Feller, and Benedict, 2010). The six QSEN competencies for Nursing are:

1. **Patient-centered care:** Recognizes the client or designee as the source of control and as a full partner in providing compassionate and coordinated care that is based on the preferences, values, and needs of the client.
2. **Teamwork and collaboration:** Refers to the ability to function effectively with nursing and interprofessional teams and to foster open communication, mutual respect, and shared decision making to provide quality client care.
3. **Evidence-based practice:** Integrates the best current clinical evidence with client and family preferences and values to provide optimal client care.
4. **Quality improvement:** Uses data to monitor the outcomes of the care processes and uses improvement methods to design and test changes to continually improve quality and safety of health care systems.
5. **Safety:** Minimizes the risk for harm to clients and provides through both system effectiveness and individual performance.
6. **Informatics:** Use information and technology to communicate, manage knowledge, mitigate error, and support decision making (Brown et al, 2010, p 116).

Of the six QSEN competencies, all but safety were derived from the Institute of Medicine report, *Health Professions Education* (2003). The QSEN team added safety because this competency is central to the work of nurses. Articles have been published to teach educators about QSEN, and national forums have been held. Also the American Association of Colleges of Nursing (AACN) has held faculty development institutes for faculty and academic administrators using a train-the-trainer model, and safety and quality objectives have been built in the AACN essentials for nursing education. Similarly, the National League for Nursing has incorporated the "NLN Educational Competencies Model" into their educational summits. The six QSEN competencies will be integrated in the chapters throughout the text to emphasize the importance of quality and safety in public health nursing today. *Note:* The terms *patient* and *care* will be changed to *client* and *intervention* to reflect a public health nursing approach.

Specifically related to the history of nursing, the following targeted competency can be applied:

Targeted Competency: Safety—Minimizes risk for harm to clients and providers through both system effectiveness and individual performance. Important aspects of safety include:

- **Knowledge:** Discuss potential and actual impact of national client safety resources initiatives and regulations
- **Skills:** Participate in analyzing errors and designing system improvements
- **Attitudes:** Value vigilance and monitoring by clients, families, and other members of the health care team

Safety Question

Updated definitions around client safety include addressing safety at the individual level and at the systems level. The history of public health nursing demonstrates the myriad ways that public health nurses have addressed client safety in their evolving practice. Public health nurses support safety through caring for individuals and providing care for communities and groups. Historically, how have public health nurses addressed safety at the individual client level? How have public health nurses addressed client safety at the systems level? How have public health nurses been involved in system improvements?

Answer: *Individual level: A rich part of public health nursing's history has been the development of home visitation, in which clients are cared for in their own environment. Similarly, public health nurses have improved client outcomes by pioneering new models of interventions for maternal–child health and individuals in rural communities.*

Systems level: *Through their work with communities, public health nurses were an integral part of reducing the incidence of communicable diseases by the mid-twentieth century. More recently, public health nursing has contributed to health care system improvements through the development of the hospice movement, birthing centers, daycare for elderly and disabled persons, and drug-abuse and rehabilitation services. These initiatives have updated the health care system to provide targeted care for previously overlooked populations.*

Prepared by Gail Armstrong, DNP, ACNS-BC, CNE, Associate Professor, University of Colorado Denver College of Nursing.

CH 6: Application of Ethics in the Community

✓ FOCUS ON QUALITY AND SAFETY EDUCATION FOR NURSES

One of the six tenets of Quality and Safety Education for Nurses (QSEN) is client-centered intervention (Sherwood and Drenkard, 2007). This chapter discusses many ways in which an understanding of basic principles of ethics can guide safe and effective nursing practice. Some key aspects of client-centered interventions in public health nursing include being certain that the information provided to individuals, families, and communities is accurate and reflects the most current evidence and that it is presented in a timely fashion. Community health education should take into account the age, gender, and cultural and religious backgrounds of those who receive the information. Giving health information that does not meet these criteria can be unsafe and clearly does not reflect attention to quality nursing care. One of the QSEN competencies related to client-centered care states: Recognize the client or designee as the source of control and full partner in providing compassionate and coordinated care (intervention) based on respect for client preferences, values, and needs. Specific aspects of client centered-care related to communication are:

- **Knowledge:** Integrate understanding of multiple dimensions of client-centered intervention: information, communication and education.
- **Skills:** Communicate client values, preferences, and expressed needs to other members of the health care team.

- **Attitudes:** Respect and encourage individual expression of client values, preferences, and expressed needs.

A second set of knowledge, skills, and attitudes included in this competency helps us understand the public health dilemma of serving the good of the population versus the good of the individual.

Consider this:

- **Knowledge:** Explore ethical and legal implications of client-centered interventions.
- **Skills:** Recognize the boundaries of therapeutic relationships.
- **Attitudes:** Acknowledge the tension that may exist between client rights and the organizational responsibility for professional, ethical interventions (Cronenwett, Sherwood, Barnsteiner, et al, 2007).

Client-centered ethical activity: Public health is more concerned about the good of the collective group than of the individual. Debate with a classmate whether children should be required to have all of the Centers for Disease Control and Prevention vaccines before they can enter school or remain in school. Some parents are choosing not to give their children all the recommended immunizations because of fear of side effects of the vaccine. To support your argument, see http://www.cdc.gov/vaccines/schedules/index.html for what is required. See web articles, such as those at http://www.responsibility-project.libertymutual.com.

CH 7: Cultural Diversity in the Community

✓ FOCUS ON QUALITY AND SAFETY EDUCATION FOR NURSES

The six quality and safety competencies for nurses that were identified in the Quality and Safety Education for Nurses (QSEN) project are client-centered care, teamwork and collaboration, evidence-based practice, quality improvement, safety, and informatics. Although each of these is important and pertinent to the nursing actions taken with people from cultural groups other than that of the nurse, perhaps the most significant is client-centered care. The chapter presents many guidelines and principles for aiding nurses in providing culturally competent care. Client-centered care is often less than effective when the nurse and client do not communicate effectively with one another. The lack of communication may occur when they speak different languages, when they have different cultural practices and expectations that lead them to hear messages differently, or when clients simply do not understand what the nurse is saying and are reluctant to acknowledge it. Nurses must observe for both verbal and nonverbal cues that a message is either understood or not understood. When the latter occurs, the nurse should take action to clarify the message, and this may include asking someone from that cultural group to assist or to enlist the aid of an interpreter (Issel and Bekemeier, 2010).

The following applies the QSEN competency of client-centered interventions that reflect cultural competence.

Targeted Competency: Client-Centered Intervention—Recognize the client or designee as the source of control and full partner in providing compassionate and coordinated interventions based on respect for client's preferences, values, and needs.

Important aspects of client-centered intervention include:

Knowledge: Describe strategies to empower clients or families in all aspects of the health care process.

Skills: Communicate client values, preferences, and expressed needs to other members of health care team.

Attitudes: Willingly support client-centered care for individuals and groups whose values differ from own.

Client-Centered Care Question: Competence in providing client-centered interventions involves not only effective interviewing of individual clients, but developing an awareness of their context. As a community-based clinician, it is helpful to familiarize yourself with the cultural context of your clients. Learning about community resources can sometimes be helpful in learning about the cultural context. You have just been hired as a visiting nurse in a Hispanic community. What community resources could you explore to assist you in providing effective client-centered care?

Answer:

- *You might explore community centers. Where are they? How well frequented are the community centers. Which programs are most popular? Which community center programs are health oriented?*
- *Are community members very involved with one or more churches? You might familiarize yourself with elements of this faith tradition.*
- *Are there community elders who are publicly recognized as leaders in the community? Can you meet with them to understand how the community has changed and evolved over time?*

Prepared by Gail Armstrong, DNP, ACNS-BC, CNE, Associate Professor, University of Colorado Denver College of Nursing.

CH 12: Epidemiology

✓ FOCUS ON QUALITY AND SAFETY EDUCATION FOR NURSES

Targeted Competency: Informatics—Use information and technology to communicate, manage knowledge, mitigate error, and support decision making. Important aspects of informatics include:

- **Knowledge:** Identify essential information that must be available in a common database to support client care.
- **Skills:** Use information management tools to monitor outcomes of care processes.
- **Attitudes:** Value nurses' involvement in design, selection, implementation and evaluation of information technologies to support client care.

Informatics Question
Determine If a Health Problem Exists in the Community
Nurses are involved in the surveillance and monitoring of health phenomena. Planning for resources and personnel often requires quantifying the level of a problem in the community. For example, to know how different districts compare in the rates of infants with very low birth weight, you would calculate the prevalence of infants with very low birth weight in each district:

1. Determine the number of live births in each district from birth certificate data obtained from the vital records division of the health department.
2. Use the birth-weight information from the birth certificate data to determine the number of infants born weighing less than 1500 g in each district.
3. Calculate the prevalence of births of infants with very low birth weights by district as the number of infants weighing less than 1500 g at birth divided by the total number of live births.
4. If the number of births of infants with very low birth weights in each district is small, use several years of data to obtain a more stable estimate.

Prepared by Gail Armstrong, DNP, ACNS-BC, CNE, Associate Professor, University of Colorado Denver College of Nursing.

CH 15: Evidence-Based Practice

✓ FOCUS ON QUALITY AND SAFETY EDUCATION FOR NURSES

Targeted Competency: Evidence-Based Practice—Integrate best current evidence with clinical expertise and client and family preferences and values for delivery of optimal interventions.
Important aspects of EBP include:

- **Knowledge:** Describe EBP to include the components of research evidence, clinical expertise and client and family values
- **Skills:** Locate evidence reports related to clinical practice topics and guidelines
- **Attitudes:** Value the need for continuous improvement in clinical practice based on new knowledge

Evidence-Based Practice Question:

As a nurse in the community you are working within a Native American community that has a high prevalence of diabetes. As you visit with clients in their homes, you notice that many have a standardized "Diabetes Care" hand-out they received from the same primary care clinic. Your clients comment that the nutritional recommendations are unrealistic in the context of their regular diet. You decide to initiate a focus group with clients who attend the diabetes clinic at the health department to customize nutritional diabetic guidelines for this community.

1. Go to The National Guideline Clearinghouse website at http://www.guideline.gov. This website is an initiative of the Agency for Healthcare Research and Quality and is a reservoir for evidence-based clinical guidelines.
2. On the home page, type "diabetes" in the search box.
3. The second result is: Guideline Synthesis: Nutritional Management of Diabetes Mellitus.

4. Review the various areas of the guidelines: Medical Nutritional Therapy, Carbohydrates, Protein, Fiber, Sucralose, Alcohol Consumption, Dietary Fat and Cholesterol, Micronutrients, Nutritional Interventions for Preventing and Managing Complications, and Physical Activity and Weight Management.
5. What baseline data might you gather from your focus group participants to be best informed in how to tailor the evidence-based recommendation for this community?
6. What might be effective strategies in writing up the community-specific guidelines and distributing them that might enhance their adoption?

Answer:
- Understanding the common elements of this community's diet is a good place to start. What are common carbohydrates, proteins, sources of sugar, dietary fat, and cholesterol that are commonly consumed?
- How does the common diet compare to the National Clearinghouse Guidelines? Are there healthy sources of carbohydrates, healthy fats that are part of the diet that can be emphasized?
- What are common patterns in the community around alcohol consumption? Would educational efforts around the deleterious effects of alcohol on diabetes be helpful?
- Writing up community-based guidelines with assistance from leaders in the community would be a helpful strategy. You could include healthy recipes from community leaders in your guidelines.

Your community-based guidelines might be distributed at a community celebration or gathering by members of the community who helped develop them.

Prepared by Gail Armstrong, DNP, ACNS-BC, CNE, Associate Professor, University of Colorado Denver College of Nursing.

CH 16: Using Health Education and Groups to Promote Health

✓ FOCUS ON QUALITY AND SAFETY EDUCATION FOR NURSES

Targeted Competency: Client-Centered Care—Important aspects of client-centered care include the following:

- **Knowledge:** Integrate understanding of multiple dimensions of client-centered care: information, communication, and education
- **Skills:** Communicate client values, preferences, and expressed needs to other members of the health care team
- **Attitudes:** Respect and encourage individual expression of client values, preferences, and expressed needs

Client-centered care question:

Providing health information in a way that is not understandable or useful to the recipient is a poor form of client-centered communication. If you were teaching a group of four women about wound care after surgery, what steps would you take to ensure that the message the women received was the message that you intended to send?

Answer: Generally you would begin by providing the needed information by describing each step; you might include an easy-to-understand hand-out in the language the four women understand, or you might give them a CD to take home that has the information on it. Next, you would demonstrate how to clean the wound. Then you would ask each woman to repeat the cleaning process that you just demonstrated. Finally, you would ask each woman if she had the facilities and supplies to clean the wound at home; and then you would ask each woman if she had any questions or concerns that you might answer. What else would you do?

Data from Cronenwett L, Sherwood G, Barnsteiner J, et al: Quality and safety education for nurses, *Nurs Outlook* 55:122-131 2007.

CH 23: Public Health Nursing and the Disaster Management Cycle

✓ FOCUS ON QUALITY AND SAFETY EDUCATION FOR NURSES

Targeted Competency: Safety—Minimize risk for harm to clients and providers through both system effectiveness and individual performance. Selected knowledge, skills, and attitudes are cited here to develop a disaster safety plan:

- **Knowledge:** Examine human factors and other basic safety design principles, as well as commonly used unsafe practices (such as workarounds and dangerous abbreviations). Specific steps might be:
  1. Learn how you can get information during the disaster or emergency.
     - Determine what types of disasters are most likely to happen.
     - Learn about warning signals in your community.
     - Ask about postdisaster pet care (shelters usually will not accept pets).
     - Review the disaster plans at your workplace, school, and other places where your family spends time.
     - Determine how to help older adult or disabled family members or neighbors.
     - WHAT should you do?
- **Skills:** Demonstrate effective use of strategies to reduce risk for harm to self or others.
  1. Create a disaster plan:
     - Talk with your family and create two places to meet, including outside your home and outside your neighborhood. Give each member of the family a copy of the plan.
     - Discuss the types of disasters that are most likely to happen, and review what to do in each case and make a plan.
     - Choose an out-of-state friend to be your family contact; this person will verify the location of each family member. After a disaster, it may be easier to call long distance than to make local calls.
     - Review evacuation plans, including care of pets. Have alternative routes for evacuation.
  2. Complete this checklist:
     - Post emergency phone numbers next to telephones.
     - Teach everyone how and when to call 9-1-1.
     - Determine when and how to turn off water, gas, and electricity at the main switches.
     - Check adequacy of insurance coverage for yourself and your home.
     - Locate and review the use of fire extinguishers.
     - Install and maintain smoke detectors.
     - Conduct a home hazard hunt and fix potential hazards.
     - Stock emergency supplies and assemble a disaster supplies kit.
     - Acquire first aid and cardiopulmonary resuscitation (CPR) certification.
     - Locate all escape routes from your home. Find two ways out of each room.
     - Find safe spots in your home for each type of disaster.
  3. Practice and maintain your plan:
     - Review the plan every 6 months.
     - Conduct fire and emergency evacuation drills.
     - Replace stored water every 3 months and stored food every 6 months.
     - Test and recharge fire extinguishers according to manufacturer's instructions.
     - Test your smoke detectors monthly and change the batteries at least once a year.
  4. What more should you do?
     - Attitudes: Appreciate the cognitive and physical limits of human performance.
- Monitor your personal reactions to the disaster and seek assistance if the stress of the losses and the potential work to reestablish a new normal seem overwhelming. Monitor also the reactions of your colleagues and the clients you serve and provide or refer to others anyone who needs stress management intervention.

Safety Question: To prepare more effectively for the event of a future disaster, list the steps that you would take to ensure the safety of your family, including any pets you may have.

CH 22: Case Management

FOCUS ON QUALITY AND SAFETY EDUCATION FOR NURSES

Targeted Competency: Teamwork and Collaboration—Function effectively within nursing and interprofessional teams, fostering open communication, mutual respect, and shared decision making to achieve quality client interventions and outcomes.

Important aspects of teamwork and collaboration include:

* **Knowledge:** Describe scopes of practice and roles of health care team members
* **Skills:** Clarify roles and accountabilities under conditions of potential overlap in team member functioning
* **Attitudes:** Value the perspectives and expertise of all health team members

Teamwork and Collaboration Question:

Observe a typical workday of a nurse in community health or public health nurse, noting the types of activities that are done in coordination and case management and the amount of time spent in these areas. Interview several staff members to determine whether they perceive that the amount of their time spent in case management is changing. To what degree are the staff members involved in care management activities? Ask about common colleagues with whom case managers collaborate. Besides primary care physicians, which health care team members are often involved in managing clients' care across time and across settings? What skills are needed by the case management nurse to best facilitate these interdisciplinary teams?

Prepared by Gail Armstrong, DNP, ACNS-BC, CNE, Associate Professor, University of Colorado Denver College of Nursing.

CH 26: Quality Management

FOCUS ON QUALITY AND SAFETY EDUCATION FOR NURSES

Targeted Competency: Quality Improvement—Use data to monitor the outcomes of intervention processes, and use improvement methods to design and test changes to continuously improve the quality and safety of health care systems.

Important aspects of quality improvement include:

* **Knowledge:** Recognize that nursing and other health professions students are parts of systems and intervention processes that affect outcomes for clients and families
* **Skills:** Identify gaps between local practices and best practice
* **Attitudes:** Value own and others' contributions to outcomes in local community settings

Quality Improvement Question:

You are working as a home care nurse and are discovering a trend of frequent readmissions to the hospital of many of your clients with heart failure. Using the quality assurance approach, consider the following questions:

* What is being done now?
* Why is it being done?
* Is it being done well?
* Can it be done better?
* Should it be done at all?
* Are there improved ways to deliver service?
* How much is it costing?
* Should certain activities be abandoned or replaced?

To which aspects of your clients' quality of life and care transitions will you apply these questions?

Answer: It would be helpful to look at a group of clients discharged from the hospital. Are they receiving adequate education and preparation to return home? You could also gather data about how clients are being managed by the community. How often are they following up with their primary care clinician? Are clients adequately educated to monitor their own fluid status, weight, and dietary restrictions? Are there community-based cardiovascular care programs that can help clients maintain optimum health and avoid exacerbations?

Prepared by Gail Armstrong, DNP, ACNS-BC, CNE, Associate Professor, University of Colorado Denver College of Nursing.

Page numbers followed by *b*, indicate box; *f*, figure, *t*, table.

HEALTHY PEOPLE 2020

Vision
A society in which all people live long healthy lives

Overarching goals
Achieve health equity, eliminate disparities, and improve the health of all groups

Eliminate preventable disease, disability, injury, and premature death

Promote healthy development and healthy behaviors across every stage of life

Create social and physical environments that promote good health for all

Foundation measures
General health status:
- Life expectancy
- Healthy life expectancy
- Year of potential life lost
- Physically and mentally unhealthy days
- Self-assessed health status
- Limitation of activity
- Chronic disease prevalence

Health-related quality of life and well-being
- Physical, mental, and social health–related quality of life
- Well-being/satisfaction
- Participation in common activities

Determinants of health
- A range of personal, social, economic, and environmental factors that influence health status are known as the determinants of health. They include things such as biology, genetics, individual behavior, access to health services, and the environment in which people are born, live, learn, play, work, and age.

Disparities
- Race/ethnicity
- Gender
- Physical and mental ability
- Geography

Focus areas
Access to health services
Adolescent health
Arthritis, osteoporosis, and chronic back conditions
Blood disorders and blood safety
Cancer
Chronic kidney disease
Dementias, including Alzheimer's disease
Diabetes
Disability and health
Early and middle childhood
Educational and community-based programs
Environmental health
Family planning
Food safety
Genomics
Global health
Health communication and health information technology
Health-related quality of life and well-being
Hearing and other sensory or communication disorders
Heart disease and stroke
Human immunodeficiency virus
Immunization and infectious disease
Injury and violence prevention
Lesbian, gay, bisexual, and transgender health
Maternal, infant, and child health
Medical product safety
Mental health and mental disorders
Nutrition and weight status
Occupational safety and health
Older adults
Oral health
Physical activity
Preparedness
Public health infrastructure
Respiratory diseases
Sexually transmitted diseases
Sleep health
Social determinants of health
Substance abuse
Tobacco use
Vision

Guidance is also provided on how to implement *Healthy People 2020* in the community via MAP-IT, which refers to the steps of: mobilize, assess, plan, implement, and track. In the *MAP-IT Guide to Using Healthy People 2020 in Your Community,* instructions are provided for ways to implement each of the five steps. See http://www.healthypeople.gov/2020/default/aspx for details about *Healthy People 2020.*